Handbook of Nonprescription Drugs

EDITION

Notices

The inclusion in this book of any drug in respect to which patent or trademark rights may exist shall not be deemed, and is not intended as a grant of or authority to exercise, any right or privilege protected by such patent or trademark. All such rights or trademarks are vested in the patent or trademark owner, and no other person may exercise the same without express permission, authority, or license secured from such patent or trademark owner.

The listing of selected trade names is intended only for ease of reference. The listed trade names are a representative sampling of drug products, not a comprehensive listing. The inclusion of a trade name does not mean the editors or publisher has any particular knowledge that the brand listed has properties different from other brands of the same drug, nor should its inclusion be interpreted as an endorsement by the editors or publisher. Similarly, the fact that a particular brand has not been included does not indicate the product has been judged to be in any way unsatisfactory or unacceptable.

The convention followed in this book to identify trade names of drugs and other products is to use initial capital letters (when appropriate). Nonproprietary, generic, or common names of such products are cited without initial capitalization.

The nature of drug information is that it is constantly evolving because of ongoing research and clinical experience and is often subject to interpretation. Although great care has been taken to ensure the accuracy of the information presented herein, the reader is advised that the authors, editors, reviewers, contributors, and publisher cannot be held responsible for the continued currency of the information or for any errors or omissions in this book or for any consequences arising therefrom. Readers are advised that decisions regarding drug therapy must be based on the independent judgment of the clinician, changing information about a drug (e.g., as reflected in the literature and manufacturer's most current product information), and changing medical practices.

The editors, authors, and contributors have written this book in their private capacities. No official support or endorsement by any federal or state agency or pharmaceutical company is intended or inferred.

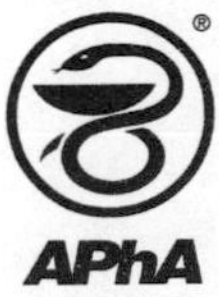

HANDBOOK OF NONPRESCRIPTION DRUGS

12th EDITION

Editors

Loyd V. Allen Jr., PhD
Editor-in-Chief, *International Journal of Pharmaceutical Compounding*
Edmond, Oklahoma

Rosemary R. Berardi, PharmD
Professor of Pharmacy, Department of Pharmacy Practice, College of Pharmacy,
The University of Michigan, Ann Arbor, Michigan

Edward M. DeSimone II, PhD
Professor of Pharmaceutical and Administrative Sciences, Department of Pharmaceutics,
School of Pharmacy and Allied Health Professions, Creighton University, Omaha, Nebraska

Janet P. Engle, PharmD
Associate Dean for Academic Affairs, Clinical Associate Professor, Department of Pharmacy Practice,
College of Pharmacy, University of Illinois at Chicago, Chicago, Illinois

Nicholas G. Popovich, PhD
Professor and Associate Head, Department of Pharmacy Practice, School of Pharmacy and Pharmacal Sciences,
Purdue University, West Lafayette, Indiana

Wendy Munroe Rosenthal, PharmD
President, MedOutcomes, Inc., Richmond, Virginia

Karen J. Tietze, PharmD
Professor of Clinical Pharmacy, Department of Pharmacy Practice, Philadelphia College of Pharmacy,
University of the Sciences in Philadelphia, Philadelphia, Pennsylvania

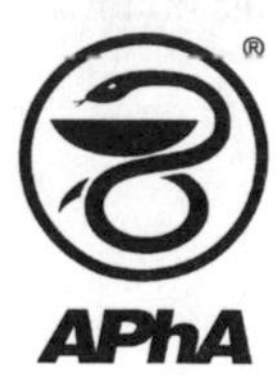

American Pharmaceutical Association
Washington, DC

Director, Books and Electronic Products Department
Julian I. Graubart

Development Editor/Managing Editor:
Linda L. Young

Editorial Assistant:
Kathy E. Anderson

Editorial Services:
Publications Professionals, Ltd.

Medical Research Services:
Robert Gutman

Composition Services:
Maryland Composition Company

Cover Design:
LaurelGraphx, Inc.

Anatomic Drawings:
Walter Hilmers, Jr., Judith M. Guenther, Alexa L. Chun, Marie A. Dauenheimer

Color Illustration Contributors:
Jean A. Borger, Richard C. Childers, Stanley Cullen, Alfred C. Griffin (deceased), Harold L. Hammond, R. Gary Sibbald

Printing:
Webcom Limited

Library of Congress Catalog Card Number: 86-71446
ISSN 0889-7816
ISBN 0-917330-97-8

How to Order This Book
By phone: 800-878-0729—VISA, MasterCard, and American Express cards accepted.

Table of Contents

Preface

The 12th edition of the *Handbook of Nonprescription Drugs* continues the APhA tradition of providing comprehensive and current information about self-care and nonprescription products. Since 1967, each new edition has broadened its scope to reflect the expanding role of pharmacists in self-care and the corresponding changes in pharmacy curricula. The major revision of the 12th edition involved the restructuring of chapters to provide an integrated therapeutic approach to patient care. This treatment model provides a basis for enhancing the level of pharmaceutical care provided to self-treating patients.

Elements that support the integrated therapeutic approach—discussions of the pathologic process and its manifestations, algorithms, dosage and administration tables, product tables, case studies, assessment question and answer sections, and patient education boxes—are standard features in chapters that discuss specific disorders. Students will learn from this model how to focus on patients instead of on nonprescription medications, a skill that will ease the transition to pharmacy practice and the important role of providing patient care. These features also make it easier for practitioners to access information and share it with patients.

Organization of the 12th Edition

As in the previous edition, chapters are grouped primarily according to body systems. The chapters are formally organized in the following sections:

- The Pharmacist's Role in Self-Care
- Pain and Fever Disorders
- Reproductive and Genital Disorders
- Respiratory Disorders
- Gastrointestinal Disorders
- Disorders Related to Nutrition
- Ophthalmic, Otic, and Oral Disorders
- Dermatologic Disorders
- Other Medical Disorders
- Home Medical Equipment
- Alternative Therapies

Chapter Format and Content

Chapter titles have changed to reflect the disorders that are discussed. This change completes the transition from a focus on products and the FDA review of ingredients to that of assessing patient complaints and recommending the appropriate treatment approaches.

The following primary headings are used (when applicable) in chapters that discuss disorders. To avoid duplicative discussion of anatomy and physiology, some chapters refer the reader to the leadoff chapter in a section for such discussion. Chapters that deal with prevention of disorders or supportive care for disorders or surgical procedures use some of these headings, along with others pertinent to the subject matter.

- Epidemiology
- Anatomy and Physiology
- Etiology
- Pathophysiology
- Signs and Symptoms
- Complications
- Treatment
- Patient Assessment
- Patient Counseling
- Evaluation of Patient Outcomes

Developing a format for chapters that discuss multiple disorders with similar manifestations was as challenging as it often is for a pharmacist to assess such complaints. Many of these chapters have tables that describe distinguishing characteristics of the conditions. A special treatment section titled "Treatment Overview" was developed for each disorder to identify specific treatment approaches, including specific pharmacologic agents. A detailed discussion of the pharmacologic agents follows the discussions of the conditions. Patient assessment, patient counseling, and evaluation of patient outcomes are also discussed collectively.

The treatment section underwent the most significant revision. The desired "Treatment Outcomes" are defined first, followed by a summary of the possible treatment approaches

("General Treatment Approach"). Patient or disease factors that preclude self-treatment are also explained in this treatment summary. These sections are followed by discussions of self-care options, both traditional and alternative. A renewed emphasis on nondrug measures and preventive measures reflects the philosophy of many self-treating individuals. The inclusion (when appropriate) of brief discussions of select herbal remedies and homeopathic products in chapters completes the discussion of self-care options. Some pharmacists may label discussions of alternative remedies slightly heretical, but patients voluntarily take these products, making it essential that pharmacists understand the philosophies of these remedies and the issues involved with the use of specific products.

Feedback from self-care instructors and previous contributors to the *Handbook* prompted the addition of more subheads and tables to make information more readily accessible. Authors added or updated tables that list drug interactions, and dosage and administration guidelines. Tables listing selected trade-name products and their primary ingredients were also incorporated in the chapters. Pharmacy students and practitioners can now quickly find all the information needed to make a treatment recommendation and to counsel patients.

Respondents to APhA surveys also requested easily accessible information on selecting the best product for a given patient's circumstances. To that end, authors provided therapeutic comparisons of agents based on available clinical studies of safety and effectiveness. They also addressed the issues related to use of a particular drug in high-risk patient populations, as well as provided product selection guidelines based on patient factors and preferences.

For many disorders, pertinent prescription therapies or diagnostic procedures are discussed in case a patient's medical or medication history precludes self-treatment. Some may view such discussion as a deviation from the scope of a book on self-care. Rather, this information provides balance and reflects the type of decisions that practitioners must make every day in the pharmacy setting.

New Topics

Since publication of the 11th edition, FDA reclassified three prescription drugs as nonprescription: ketoconazole, terbinafine, and nicotine transdermal system (patch). Discussions of these agents appear in the pertinent chapters. Discussions of new home testing/monitoring devices in Chapter 43 include tests for urinary tract infections, illicit drug use, acquired immunodeficiency syndrome (AIDS), and hepatitis C. This chapter also discusses a new method to detect ovulation by examining saliva patterns. FDA also issued a final monograph on sunscreen products; Chapter 33 discusses the details of this ruling.

This edition features one new chapter: "Homeopathic Remedies." This chapter explains the basics of homeopathy and also summarizes the results of numerous clinical studies on the use of homeopathic remedies in common disorders. The number of chapters increased because several chapters were divided into two or more chapters.

New Features

Most of the new features support the integrated therapeutic approach to self-care. Students and pharmacists can use these features to develop or hone problem-solving and critical-thinking skills.

Treatment Algorithms outline the major steps in selecting the appropriate treatment for a particular disorder. This feature provides a visual representation of the triage and treatment processes.

Patient Assessment Q&A sections teach the problem-solving skills required for the triage process. Rather than repeating text discussions, the "answers" explain the appropriate actions based on patient-specific factors. The referrals to preceding sections, which are set in italic, reinforce earlier explanations of facets of a disorder or its treatment, while underscoring the complex reasoning required to accurately assess a complaint and recommend appropriate treatment. Placement of the assessment section after the treatment section deviates from the patient–pharmacist consultation process outlined in Chapter 2. However, the pharmacy student is still amassing the drug knowledge already attained by the practitioner. To prepare the student for the triage process, contraindications to drug use and other facets of drug treatment need to be discussed first.

Patient Education boxes highlight the major points in self-treating a disorder. These boxes are a valuable tool for practitioners in counseling patients and for students in identifying which types of information the patient needs to properly self-treat a disorder.

"A Word about" boxes highlight facets of the integrated therapeutic discussion of the topic that do not fit within the framework of the chapter format. This feature allows an uninterrupted discussion of the disorder but also presents complementary clinical information.

Evaluation of Patient Outcomes sections reinforce follow-up of self-treating patients. This new section defines the parameters for confirming successful self-treatment and those that indicate medical referral is required.

Appendix I: FDA Pregnancy Risk Categories for Selected Nonprescription Medications provides critical information for pregnant patients. The table format allows quick access to the categories for the most common nonprescription medications.

Appendix II: Suggested Treatment Approaches for Case Studies is a new feature, although case studies are not new to the *Handbook*. The case studies present realistic pharmacist–patient encounters. The clinical considerations/strategies and patient education/counseling strategies guide the reader in how to apply the information provided in the scenarios. The reader can compare his or her treatment approach to that of the author by checking the pertinent case study in Appendix II.

Acknowledgments

The 12th Edition is based on the work of numerous authors, reviewers, and editors, who participated in this and/or past editions. Self-care encompasses a wide variety of disorders and treatments. To ensure that the discussions of chapter topics were the most authoritative and up-to-date, experts in these subjects were invited to write chapters, serve as peer reviewers, or serve as section editors.

Although the individuals who applied their demonstrated expertise to this edition are acknowledged in the list of contributors, the editors and the editorial staff express their deepest gratitude to the 59 authors and co-authors for their diligent efforts in updating and refocusing their chapters. The hours they spent preparing accurate, comprehensive, and practical discussions of their chapters' subjects are invaluable to the profession.

The peer reviewers were selected from many pharmacy practice settings and allied health professions, reflecting the interdisciplinary approach to patient care that is common in pharmacy and medical practice. These 107 health care professionals shared the perspectives of their particular practice settings or professions, ensuring that the chapters were thorough, balanced, and of the highest quality. Their contributions are also deeply appreciated.

The editors and editorial staff also thank Ruth Calloway, RPh, MS, for her research and review of the FDA pregnancy risk ratings for nonprescription medications. Her contribution will enhance the pharmaceutical care provided to patients who are or may become pregnant.

APhA editorial staff deserve special mention for their support and encouragement at every stage. Linda Young spent numerous hours preparing content guidelines, developing formats for chapters and supporting elements, and performing developmental editing of the chapters. Ms. Young also managed the design, editorial, and composition stages of the book, as well as the incorporation of product tables into the chapters. Kathy Anderson provided valuable support in document preparation and transmission of materials to contributors and editorial freelancers.

The combined efforts of all these individuals have maintained the *Handbook* as the worldwide standard and teaching resource on self-care and nonprescription products.

The Editors
June 2000

Contributors

Note: Numbers in parentheses denote chapter numbers.

Authors

Loyd V. Allen Jr., MS, PhD, APhA-APRS, FACA, FIACP (19)
Editor-in-Chief
International Journal of Pharmaceutical Compounding
Edmond, OK

Melvin F. Baron, PharmD, MPA (18)
Assistant Dean for Programmatic Advancement
Department of Clinical Pharmacy
College of Pharmacy
University of Southern California
Los Angeles, CA

Raymond L. Benza, MD (35)
Assistant Professor of Medicine
Department of Medicine, Division of Cardiovascular Diseases
University of Alabama Hospitals
Birmingham, AL

Rosemary R. Berardi, PharmD (14)
Professor of Pharmacy
Department of Pharmacy Practice
College of Pharmacy
The University of Michigan
Ann Arbor, MI

Joye Ann Billow, RPh, PhD (32)
Professor of Pharmaceutical Sciences
Department of Pharmaceutical Sciences
College of Pharmacy
South Dakota State University
Brookings, SD

John D. Bowman, BS, MSHP (34)
Assistant Professor
Department of Pharmacy Practice
McWhorter School of Pharmacy
Samford University
Birmingham, AL

Eddie L. Boyd, PharmD, MS (14)
Associate Professor of Pharmacy
Department of Pharmacy Practice
College of Pharmacy
The University of Michigan
Ann Arbor, MI

Geneva Clark Briggs, PharmD, BCPS (43)
MedOutcomes, Inc.
Richmond, VA

Kathryn K. Bucci, PharmD, BCPS (15)
Associate Professor of Family Medicine
Self Memorial Family Practice Residency Program
Montgomery Center for Family Medicine
Greenwood, SC

Demetris M. Butler, PharmD (12)
Director of Clinical Pharmacy Programs
Clinical Pharmacy Associates
Beltsville, MD

R. Keith Campbell, MBA (39)
Professor and Associate Dean
Department of Pharmacy Practice
College of Pharmacy
Washington State University
Pullman, WA

Edwina S. Chan, PharmD (35)
Associate Professor
McWhorter School of Pharmacy
Samford University
Birmingham, AL

Wendell L. Combest, PhD (45)
Associate Professor of Pharmacology
Department of Biopharmaceutical Sciences
School of Pharmacy
Shenandoah University
Winchester, VA

Timothy R. Covington, PharmD (1)
Bruno Professor of Pharmacy
Executive Director, Managed Care Institute
McWhorter School of Pharmacy
Samford University
Birmingham, AL

M. Lynn Crismon, PharmD, FCCP (40, 41)
Professor and Southwestern Drug Corporation Centennial Fellow in Pharmacy
Pharmacy Practice Division
College of Pharmacy
The University of Texas at Austin
Austin, TX

Clarence E. Curry Jr., PharmD (12)
Associate Professor of Pharmacy Practice
Department of Clinical and Administrative Pharmacy Sciences
College of Pharmacy, Nursing and Allied Health Sciences
Howard University
Washington, DC

Edward M. DeSimone II, MS, PhD (33)
Professor of Pharmaceutical and Administrative Sciences
Department of Pharmaceutics
School of Pharmacy and Allied Health Professions
Creighton University
Omaha, NE

Paul L. Doering, MS, FAPhA (21)
Distinguished Service Professor of Pharmacy Practice
Department of Pharmacy Practice
College of Pharmacy
University of Florida
Gainesville, FL

Judi Doerr, BS, RD/LD, CNSD (20)
Nutrition Consultant
Option Care of Oklahoma
Redmond, OK

Janet P. Engle, PharmD, RPh, FAPhA (23)
Associate Dean for Academic Affairs and Clinical Associate Professor
Department of Pharmacy Practice
College of Pharmacy
University of Illinois at Chicago
Chicago, IL

Jack E. Fincham, BS, PhD (42)
Dean and Professor
Department of Pharmacy Practice
School of Pharmacy
University of Kansas
Lawrence, KS

Andrew Glasnapp, RPh, FIACP (19)
Vice President and Director of Student Education and Projects
Professional Compounding Centers of America, Inc.
Houston, TX

Gary A. Goforth, MD, MTMH, FAAFP (15)
Medical Director, Faculty
Self Memorial Hospital Family Practice Residency Program
Montgomery Center for Family Medicine
Greenwood, SC

Kathryn L. Grant, PharmD, FASHP (46)
Assistant Professor of Pharmacy Practice and Science
College of Pharmacy
The University of Arizona
Tucson, AZ

Nina H. Han, PharmD (27, 28, 37, 38)
Manager, Dermatology Pharmacy
Department of Dermatology
Northwestern Medical Faculty Foundation
Chicago, IL

Robert P. Henderson, PharmD, FASHP, FCCP, BCPS (11)
Professor and Vice-Chair
Pharmacy Practice
McWhorter School of Pharmacy
Samford University
Birmingham, AL

Richard N. Herrier, PharmD (46)
Assistant Professor
Department of Pharmacy Practice
College of Pharmacy
The University of Arizona
Tucson, AZ

Martin D. Higbee, PharmD (44)
Associate Professor
Department of Pharmacy Practice and Science
College of Pharmacy
The University of Arizona
Tucson, AZ

Brian J. Isetts, RPh, PhD, BCPS (2)
Assistant Professor and Kellogg Fellow
Peters Institute of Pharmaceutical Care
College of Pharmacy
University of Minnesota
Minneapolis, MN

Arthur I. Jacknowitz, PharmD (5)
Professor and Chair
Department of Clinical Pharmacy
School of Pharmacy
West Virginia University
Morgantown, WV

Kenneth C. Jackson II, PharmD (3,4)
Clinical Assistant Professor
School of Pharmacy
University of Mississippi
Jackson, MS

Jenifer C. Jennings, PharmD, CDE (16, 17)
Pharmacy Consultant/Clinical Pharmacist
Kunkel Pharmaceuticals, Inc.
Loveland, OH

Donna M. Jermain, PharmD, BCPP (40, 41)
CNS Medical Service Liaison, Southwest Region
Pfizer Pharmaceuticals
Georgetown, TX

Claudia Kamper, PharmD (20)
Pharmaceutical Care Coordinator
Department of Pharmacy
Integris Health
Baptist Medical Center
Oklahoma City, OK

Kenneth R. Keefner, RPh, PhD (29)
Associate Professor and Director
Nontraditional Doctor of Pharmacy Program
School of Pharmacy and Allied Health Professions
Creighton University
Omaha, NE

Michael L. Kleinberg, PharmD, MS, FASHP (18)
Vice President
Professional Services
Immunex Corporation
Seattle, WA

Wendy Klein-Schwartz, PharmD, MPH (2)
Associate Professor
University of Maryland School of Pharmacy
Maryland Poison Center
Baltimore, MD

Linda Krypel, PharmD (24)
Assistant Professor
Department of Pharmacy Practice
College of Pharmacy and Health Sciences
Drake University
Des Moines, IA

Arthur G. Lipman, PharmD, FASHP (3, 4)
Professor of Clinical Pharmacy
College of Pharmacy and Pain Management Center
University Hospitals and Clinics
University of Utah Health Science Center
Salt Lake City, UT

R. Leon Longe, PharmD (13)
Professor
Clinical Pharmacy Program
College of Pharmacy
University of Georgia
Augusta, GA

David L. Lourwood, PharmD, BCPS (8)
Pharmacy Supervisor
Coram Health Care
Earth City, MO

Robert H. Moore III, PhD (34)
Professor
Department of Pharmaceutical Sciences
McWhorter School of Pharmacy
Samford University
Birmingham, AL

George Nemecz, PhD (45)
Assistant Professor
School of Pharmacy
Campbell University
Buies Creek, NC

Gail D. Newton, PhD, RPh (36)
Associate Professor
Department of Pharmacy Practice
School of Pharmacy and Pharmacal Sciences
Purdue University
West Lafayette, IN

Gary M. Oderda, PharmD, MPH (16, 17)
Professor and Chair
Department of Pharmacy Practice
University of Utah
Salt Lake City, UT

Victor A. Padrón, RPh, PhD (30)
Associate Professor of Pharmaceutical and Administrative Sciences
School of Pharmacy and Allied Health Professions
Creighton University
Omaha, NE

Louise Parent-Stevens, PharmD, BCPS (8)
Clinical Assistant Professor
Department of Pharmacy Practice
College of Pharmacy
University of Illinois at Chicago
Chicago, IL

Nicholas G. Popovich, PhD (36)
Professor and Associate Head
Department of Pharmacy Practice
School of Pharmacy and Pharmacal Sciences
Purdue University
West Lafayette, IN

Wendy Munroe Rosenthal, PharmD (43)
President
MedOutcomes, Inc.
Richmond, VA

Farid Sadik, PhD (31)
Dean and Professor
College of Pharmacy
University of South Carolina
Columbia, SC

Rosalie Sagraves, PharmD, FCCP (20)
Dean and Professor
College of Pharmacy
University of Illinois at Chicago
Chicago, IL

Timothy H. Self, PharmD (10)
Professor of Clinical Pharmacy
Department of Clinical Pharmacy
College of Pharmacy
University of Tennessee
Memphis, TN

Leslie A. Shimp, PharmD, MS (6, 7)
Associate Professor of Pharmacy
College of Pharmacy
The University of Michigan
Ann Arbor, MI

Condit F. Steil, PharmD, CDE (39)
Associate Professor of Pharmacy Practice
Director of the Center for Advancement of Pharmaceutical Care
Development in Community Practice
McWhorter School of Pharmacy
Samford University
Birmingham, AL

Mark W. Swanson, OD (22)
Assistant Professor
Department of Optometry
University of Alabama at Birmingham
Birmingham, AL

Karen J. Tietze, PharmD (9)
Professor of Clinical Pharmacy
Philadelphia College of Pharmacy
University of the Sciences in Philadelphia
Philadelphia, PA

Dennis P. West, PhD, FCCP (27, 28, 37, 38)
Professor of Dermatology
Department of Dermatology
Northwestern University Medical School
Chicago, IL

John R. White Jr., PharmD (39)
Associate Professor
Drug Studies Unit
Washington State University
Spokane, WA

Dennis M. Williams, PharmD, FASHP, FCCP (10)
Assistant Professor
Department of Pharmacy Practice
School of Pharmacy
University of North Carolina
Chapel Hill, NC

Reviewers

Ann B. Amerson, PharmD (3, 4)
Professor
Division of Pharmacy Practice and Science
College of Pharmacy
University of Kentucky
Lexington, KY

Robert J. Anderson, PharmD (1)
Professor
Department of Pharmacy Practice
Southern School of Pharmacy
Mercer University
Atlanta, GA

Kenneth A. Bachmann, PhD, FCP (40, 41)
Distinguished University Professor
Chair, Department of Pharmacology
College of Pharmacy
The University of Toledo
Toledo, OH

Danial E. Baker, PharmD, FASHP, FASCP (2, 39)
Director, Drug Information Center
Professor of Pharmacy Practice
College of Pharmacy
Washington State University
Spokane, WA

Chris Bapatla, PhD, MBA (22)
Director, Pharmaceutical Technical Affairs
Alcon Laboratories, Inc.
Fort Worth, TX

Connie Lee Barnes, PharmD (6, 7)
Associate Professor
Department of Pharmacy Practice
School of Pharmacy
Campbell University
Buies Creek, NC

Robert L. Beamer, PhD (21)
Distinguished Professor Emeritus
College of Pharmacy
University of South Carolina
Columbia, SC

R. Randolph Beckner, PharmD, MHS, BCPS (12)
Senior Regional Medical Associate
SmithKline Beecham Pharmaceuticals
Chesterfield, MO

J. Fred Bennes, BS Pharm (15, 27, 28, 37, 38)
Director of Quality and Resource Management
Promedicus Health Group
Appleton, NY

Darrell F. Bennett, BS (27, 28, 37, 38)
Pharmacist in Charge
California Polytechnic Student Health Center
California Polytechnic Health Center Pharmacy
California Polytechnic State University
San Luis Obispo, CA

Robert W. Bennett, MS (32, 34)
Associate Professor of Clinical Pharmacy
Department of Pharmacy Practice
School of Pharmacy and Pharmacal Sciences
Purdue University
West Lafayette, IN

Heather Boon, BScPhm, PhD (46)
Research Consultant
The Michener Institute for Applied Health Sciences
Toronto, Ontario, Canada

John A. Borneman III, BS, RPh (46)
President
Homeopathic Pharmacopoeia of the United States
Wayne, PA

Eddie L. Boyd, PharmD, MS (11)
Associate Professor of Pharmacy
Department of Pharmacy Practice
College of Pharmacy
The University of Michigan
Ann Arbor, MI

Donald J. Brideau Jr., MD (42)
Family Practitioner
Telegraph Corner Family Medicine
NOVA Medical Group
Alexandria, VA

Kim Broedel-Zaugg, RPh, MBA, PhD (43)
Associate Professor of Pharmacy Practice
Department of Pharmacy Practice
Raabe College of Pharmacy
Ohio Northern University
Ada, OH

Anthony T. Buatti, BA, BS Pharm, MBA (12)
Vice President
Pedinol Pharmacal, Inc.
Farmingdale, NY

Stephen M. Caiola, MS (11, 43)
Associate Professor and Director
Postgraduate Education Program
Department of Pharmacy Practice
School of Pharmacy
University of North Carolina
Chapel Hill, NC

Miriam P. Calhoun, BS (30, 34, 35, 44)
Consultant, Pharmaceutical Regulatory Affairs
Miriam P. Calhoun Associates
Potomac, MD

Bruce C. Carlstedt, PhD (9)
Professor of Clinical Pharmacy
Pharmacy Programs at Indianapolis
School of Pharmacy and Pharmacal Sciences
Purdue University
Indianapolis, IN

R. Frank Chandler, Bsc Pharm, MSc, PhD (45)
Professor Emeritus
Dalhousie University
President, Chandler Herbal Consulting
Halifax, Nova Scotia, Canada

Bruce D. Clayton, PharmD, RPh (11)
Professor of Pharmacy Practice
College of Pharmacy and Health Sciences
Butler University
Indianapolis, IN

Kim Coccodrilli Coley, PharmD (8)
Assistant Professor
Department of Pharmacy Practice
School of Pharmacy
University of Pittsburgh
Pittsburgh, PA

Thomas D. DeCillis, Captain USPHS Ret., BSc Pharmacy (14)
Panel Administrator
Food and Drug Administration
North Port, FL

Jeffrey C. Delafuente, MS, FCCP (9)
Professor and Director of Geriatrics
Department of Pharmacy
School of Pharmacy
Virginia Commonwealth University
Richmond, VA

Alexander F. Demetro, PharmD (22)
Pharmacist
Westwood Prescriptionists
San Jose, CA

Joseph T. DiPiro, PharmD (13)
Professor and Head
Department of Clinical and Administrative Sciences
College of Pharmacy
The University of Georgia
Augusta, GA

Paul L. Doering, MS (25, 26)
Distinguished Service Professor of Pharmacy Practice
Department of Pharmacy Practice
College of Pharmacy
University of Florida
Gainesville, FL

Herbert L. DuPont, MD (13)
Chief
Department of Internal Medicine
St. Luke's Episcopal Hospital
Houston, TX

Carl F. Emswiller Jr., BS Pharmacy, FACA (24)
Pharmacist
Emswiller Pharmacy
Leesburg, VA

Donald O. Fedder, DrPH, MPH (15, 36)
Professor of Social and Administrative Sciences
Department of Pharmacy Practice and Science and Epidemiology and Preventive Medicine
School of Pharmacy
University of Maryland
Baltimore, MD

Richard G. Fiscella, RPh, MPh (22)
Clinical Associate Professor
Department of Pharmacy Practice
College of Pharmacy
University of Illinois at Chicago
Chicago, IL

Rex W. Force, PharmD, BCPS (11)
Assistant Professor of Family Medicine and Pharmacy Practice
Department of Family Medicine
College of Pharmacy
Idaho State University
Pocatello, ID

Eric L. Foxman, RPh (46)
Secretary
American Association of Homeopathic Pharmacists
Clinton, WA

Janice A. Gaska, PharmD (12)
Associate Director, Medical Communications
Zeneca Pharmaceuticals
Wilmington, DE

William C. Gong, PharmD, FASHP (2)
Associate Professor of Clinical Pharmacy
School of Pharmacy
University of Southern California
Los Angeles, CA

Metta Lou Henderson, RPh, PhD (1)
Professor Emeritus of Pharmacy
Associate Dean Emeritus for Pharmacy Student Affairs
Raabe College of Pharmacy
Ohio Northern University
Portage, MI

Thomas J. Holmes Jr., PhD (36)
Associate Professor of Pharmaceutical Sciences
School of Pharmacy
Campbell University
Buies Creek, NC

Daniel A. Hussar, BS Pharmacy, MS, PhD (2)
Remington Professor of Pharmacy
Philadelphia College of Pharmacy
University of the Sciences in Philadelphia
Philadelphia, PA

Timothy J. Ives, PharmD, MPH, BCPS, FCCP (32)
Associate Professor of Pharmacy
School of Pharmacy
Clinical Associate Professor of Family Medicine
School of Medicine
University of North Carolina
Chapel Hill, NC

H. Won Jun, PhD (9)
Professor of Pharmaceutics
Department of Pharmaceutical and Biomedical Sciences
College of Pharmacy
The University of Georgia
Athens, GA

Jerry D. Karbeling, BS Pharmacy (29)
Vice President, Public Affairs
Iowa Pharmacy Association
Polk City, IA

H. William Kelly, PharmD, FCCP (10)
Professor of Pharmacy and Pediatrics
College of Pharmacy
University of New Mexico Health Sciences Center
Albuquerque, NM

Michael Kendrach, PharmD (29)
Assistant Professor
Director, Drug Information Services
McWhorter School of Pharmacy
Samford University
Birmingham, AL

William D. King, RPh, MPH, DrPH (16, 17)
Division Director and Professor of Pediatrics
Department of Pediatrics
The University of Alabama at Birmingham
Southeast Child Safety Institute
Birmingham, AL

Allen M. Kratz, PharmD (45)
Founder and CEO
HSV Laboratories, Inc.
Naples, FL

William Sanford Lackey, BS, FACA (21)
President
Wil-Sant, Inc.
Tucson, AZ

Lowell S. Lakritz, DDS (25, 26)
Private Practitioner
Drs. Lakritz & Salzman, SC
Madison, WI

Anthony J. LaMonica, BS Pharmacy, FACA, FAPhA, FNCPA, FMPhA, FBARD (27, 28, 37, 38)
President
Prescription Shoppe, Inc.
Everett, MA

E. Paul Larrat, BS, MBA, PhD (24)
Associate Professor of Pharmacoepidemiology
College of Pharmacy
University of Rhode Island
Kingston, RI

Alan H. Lau, PharmD, FCCP (16, 17)
Professor
Department of Pharmacy Practice
College of Pharmacy
University of Illinois at Chicago
Chicago, IL

Lisa A. Lawson, PharmD (5)
Associate Professor of Clinical Pharmacy
Philadelphia College of Pharmacy
University of the Sciences in Philadelphia
Philadelphia, PA

Timothy S. Lesar, PharmD (23)
Director of Pharmacy
Albany Medical Center
Pharmacy Department
Albany, NY

Nancy A. Letassy, PharmD, CDE (21)
Associate Professor of Pharmacy Practice
College of Pharmacy
University of Oklahoma
Edmond, OK

Michael S. Maddux, PharmD (24)
Professor and Assistant Dean
Department of Pharmacy Practice
College of Pharmacy
St. Louis College of Pharmacy
St. Louis, MO

Howard Maibach, MD (27, 28, 31, 37, 38)
Dermatology Department
University of California Hospital
San Francisco, CA

Carl J. Malanga, BS Pharmacy, PhD (19)
Professor and Associate Dean
School of Pharmacy
West Virginia University
Morgantown, WV

Robert A. Mangione, RPh, EdD (15)
Dean and Clinical Professor of Pharmacy
College of Pharmacy and Allied Health Professions
St. John's University
Jamaica, NY

Linda Gore (Sutherland) Martin, PharmD, MBA, BCPS (6, 7)
Coordinator, Drug Information Services
Drug Information Center
School of Pharmacy
University of Wyoming
Laramie, WY

James K. Marttila, PharmD, MBA, FASCP, FACA (3, 4)
Pharmaceutical and Special Projects Manager
Mayo Foundation for Medical Education and Research
Mayo Medical Ventures
Rochester, MN

Charles Y. McCall, PharmD, FASHP (39)
Associate Professor
Department of Clinical and Administrative Sciences
College of Pharmacy
The University of Georgia
Athens, GA

June H. McDermott, MS Pharmacy, MBA, FASHP (45)
Clinical Assistant Professor
School of Pharmacy
The University of North Carolina
Chapel Hill, NC

Susan M. Meyer, BS Pharmacy, MS, PhD (43)
Senior Vice President
American Association of Colleges of Pharmacy
Alexandria, VA

Timothy D. Moore, MS, RPh (8)
Administrative Director and Clinical Professor
The Ohio State University Medical Center
Columbus, OH

Merlin V. Nelson, PharmD, MD (19)
Neurologist
Affiliated Community Medical Center
Willmar, MN

Cheryl Nunn-Thompson, PharmD, MBA (42)
Clinical Assistant Professor
Department of Pharmacy Practice
College of Pharmacy
University of Illinois at Chicago
West Dundee, IL

Phillip Oppenheimer, PharmD (5)
Professor and Dean
School of Pharmacy
University of the Pacific
Stockton, CA

Victor A. Padrón, RPh, PhD (31)
Associate Professor
Department of Pharmacy Practice
School of Pharmacy and Allied Health Sciences
Creighton University
Omaha, NE

Somnath Pal, BS Pharmacy, MBA, PhD (30, 44)
Associate Professor
College of Pharmacy and Allied Health Professions
St John's University
Jamaica, NY

Henry A. Palmer, PhD (32)
Clinical Professor and Associate Dean for Professional Affairs
School of Pharmacy
University of Connecticut
Storrs, CT

Anthony Palmieri III, MS Pharmacology, PhD (14)
Manager, Technology Protection
Pharmacia and Upjohn
Kalamazoo, MI

Thomas F. Patton, PhD (23)
President
St. Louis College of Pharmacy
St. Louis, MO

John J. Piecoro Jr., MS, PharmD (13)
Professor
Division of Pharmacy Practice and Science
College of Pharmacy
University of Kentucky
Lexington, KY

Karen Plaisance, PharmD (35)
Associate Professor
Department of Pharmacy Practice and Science
School of Pharmacy
University of Maryland
Baltimore, MD

Charles D. Ponte, PharmD, CDE, BCPS, FASHP, FCCP, FAPhA (32)
Professor of Clinical Pharmacy and Family Medicine
Department of Clinical Pharmacy
Schools of Pharmacy and Medicine
Robert C. Byrd Health Sciences Center
West Virginia University
Morgantown, WV

Cathy Y. Poon, PharmD (20)
Associate Professor of Pharmacy
Department of Pharmacy Practice and Pharmacy Administration
Philadelphia College of Pharmacy
University of the Sciences in Philadelphia
Philadelphia, PA

June E. Riedlinger, RPh, PharmD (46)
Assistant Professor of Clinical Pharmacy, Department of Pharmacy Practice
Massachusetts College of Pharmacy and Allied Health Sciences
Boston, MA

Ronald J. Ruggiero, PharmD (8)
Clinical Professor and Pharmacist Specialist in Women's Health
Department of Clinical Pharmacy
Schools of Pharmacy and Medicine
University of California at San Francisco
San Francisco, CA

Katheryn W. Russi, BS Pharm, MPA (33, 34)
Associate Director, Clinical Services
Merck-Medco Managed Care, LLC
Livonia, MI

Robert B. Sause, PhD (29, 31)
Professor
Department of Pharmacy and Administrative Sciences
College of Pharmacy and Allied Health Professions
St. John's University
Jamaica, NY

David A. Sclar, B Pharm, PhD (39)
Professor of Health Policy and Administration
Boehringer Ingelheim Scholar in Pharmaceutical Economics
Director, Pharmacoeconomics and Pharmacoepidemiology Research Unit
College of Pharmacy
Washington State University
Pullman, WA

Steven A. Scott, PharmD (40, 41)
Associate Professor of Clinical Pharmacy
Department of Pharmacy Practice
School of Pharmacy and Pharmacal Sciences
Purdue University
West Lafayette, IN

Joan Lerner Selekof, BSN, CWOCN (18)
ET Nurse
University of Maryland Medical Center
Columbia, MD

Jeff Shapiro, RPh (42)
Manager, Retail Pharmacy
University Medical Center—Mesabi Retail Pharmacy
Hibbing, MN

Debra Sibbald, BSc Phm (30, 44)
Coordinator, Pharmaceutical Care I
Faculty of Pharmacy
University of Toronto
Mississauga, Ontario, Canada

Anthony J. Silvagni, PharmD, DO (16, 17)
Dean
College of Osteopathic Medicine
Nova Southeastern University
Ft. Lauderdale, FL

Kevin M. Sims, DMD, MS, BS Pharm (25, 26)
Private Practitioner
Birmingham, AL

Stewart B. Siskin, PharmD (33)
Director, Dermatology Clinical Research
Bristol-Myers Squibb
Buffalo, NY

Kenneth A. Skau, PhD (39)
Associate Professor of Pharmacology
Division of Pharmaceutical Sciences
College of Pharmacy
University of Cincinnati
Cincinnati, OH

Geralynn B. Smith, MS (6, 7)
Assistant Professor
Department of Pharmacy Practice
College of Pharmacy and Allied Health Professions
Wayne State University
Detroit, MI

John G. Sowell, BA, BSc Pharmacy, MS, PhD Pharmacology (35)
Professor
McWhorter College of Pharmacy
Samford University
Birmingham, AL

E. John Staba, PhD (45)
Professor Emeritus, Pharmacognosy
Department of Medicinal Chemistry
College of Pharmacy and Medicinal Chemistry
University of Minnesota
Minneapolis, MN

Mark Stiling, PharmD (10)
Medical Sciences Manager
Bristol-Myers Squibb
Louisville, KY

Carl Stone, DDS, MA, MBA (25, 26)
Associate Professor
Department of Restorative Dentistry
School of Dentistry
University of Detroit Mercy
Detroit, MI

Donald L. Sullivan, PhD (43)
Assistant Professor of Pharmacy Practice
Department of Pharmacy Practice
College of Pharmacy
Ohio Northern University
Ada, OH

Larry N. Swanson, PharmD (14, 21)
Professor and Chairman
Department of Pharmacy Practice
School of Pharmacy
Campbell University
Buies Creek, NC

Jeff G. Taylor, PhD (9)
Assistant Professor
College of Pharmacy and Nutrition
University of Saskatchewan
Saskatoon, SK

Michael S. Torre, MS, RPh, CDE (39)
Clinical Professor of Pharmacy
Department of Clinical Pharmacy Practice
College of Pharmacy and Allied Health Professions
St. John's University
Jamaica, NY

J. Edwin Underwood Jr., PharmD (3, 4)
Associate Professor
McWhorter School of Pharmacy
Samford University
Birmingham, AL

Paul C. Walker, PharmD (20, 30, 44)
Manager, DMC Clinical Pharmacy Services
Department of Pharmacy
Detroit Medical Center
Harper Hospital
Detroit, MI

J. Ken Walters, PharmD (19)
Director of Pharmacy Services
Department of Pharmacy Services
Sheppard Pratt Hospital
Baltimore, MD

C. Wayne Weart, PharmD (11)
Professor and Chairman of Pharmacy Practice
Associate Professor of Family Medicine
College of Pharmacy
Medical University of South Carolina
Charleston, SC

Dennis M. Williams, PharmD, FASHP, FCCP (1)
Assistant Professor
Department of Pharmacy Practice
School of Pharmacy
University of North Carolina
Chapel Hill, NC

Michael Z. Wincor, PharmD, BCPP (40, 41)
Associate Professor of Clinical Pharmacy, Psychiatry, and the Behavioral Sciences
Schools of Pharmacy and Medicine
University of Southern California
Los Angeles, CA

Eric T. Wittbrodt, PharmD, BCPS (10)
Assistant Professor of Clinical Pharmacy
Department of Pharmacy Practice
Philadelphia College of Pharmacy
University of the Sciences in Philadelphia
Philadelphia, PA

Letitia J. Wright, BS Pharmacy, PharmD (36)
Clinical Assistant Professor
Department of Pharmacy Practice, Wishard Health Services
School of Pharmacy and Pharmacal Sciences
Purdue University
Indianapolis, IN

John R. Yuen, PharmD (22, 23)
Pharmacist Specialist
Kaiser Permanente
Los Angeles Medical Center
South Pasadena, CA

Joel L. Zatz, PhD (29)
Professor of Pharmaceutics
College of Pharmacy
Rutgers University
The State University of New Jersey
Piscataway, NJ

SECTION I

THE PHARMACIST'S ROLE IN SELF-CARE

CHAPTER 1

Self-Care and Nonprescription Pharmacotherapy

Timothy R. Covington

Chapter 1 at a Glance

The place of nonprescription drug therapy should not be undervalued in a contemporary system of health care delivery and financing. The sales volume of nonprescription drugs currently exceeds $30 billion annually and should reach more than $36 billion by the year 2002. A host of professional, economic, and public interest issues and opportunities are converging to enhance the position of nonprescription drug therapy in the disease management process.

The domain of nonprescription drug therapy has often been neglected, undervalued, and/or underappreciated by many pharmacy practitioners and other health care professionals. This neglect has resulted in a substantial loss of market share by the pharmacy profession. Not too long ago, America's pharmacies sold approximately 70% of all nonprescription drugs. Today, America's 60,000-plus pharmacies sell less than 40% of nonprescription drugs, with the majority of sales occurring in the nation's other 1 million-plus retail outlets. This situation is less than optimal if the public interest is to be served, if therapeutic outcomes are to be maximized, and if therapeutic misadventures are to be minimized.

Nonprescription drugs are powerful chemical entities that should be viewed just like prescription drugs relative to their pharmacology, toxicology, contraindications (absolute and relative), precautions for use, adverse-effect profile, drug interaction potential, and special considerations in dosage and administration. Indeed, scores of nonprescription drugs were formerly prescription drugs. Moreover, all the expertise that is focused on the safe, appropriate, and effective use of prescription drugs should also be applied to nonprescription drug pharmacotherapy.

With numerous clinical and economic factors fostering growth of nonprescription drug therapy, the pharmacy profession needs to seriously rethink its professional and business role in this regard. The following market forces and factors should be considered if pharmacy's professional and economic opportunities with nonprescription drug therapy are to be expanded:

- The public's value system, attitudes, priorities, and level of sophistication are changing with regard to health matters. The public is becoming increasingly health conscious and wants a better understanding of disease and disease management. Individuals want more control over their personal health care and want to self-medicate when appropriate.
- The reclassification of prescription drugs to nonprescription status has accelerated markedly and is ex-

pected to continue at a significant pace. At any point in time, approximately 50 prescription drugs are in various stages of consideration for nonprescription status by the Food and Drug Administration (FDA).

- Cost containment initiatives for managed care continue to erode profit margins on legend drug dispensing. More frequently, profit margins on a $15 to $25 sale of nonprescription drugs exceed the profit margin on a $30 to $50 prescription dispensed at the average wholesale price minus a fixed percentage plus a dispensing fee. Further, nonprescription drug sales are typically cash and carry with no third-party constraints (e.g., claim submission, 3- to 6-week wait for payment).
- America is aging, and, significantly, the elderly consume a disproportionately large share of both prescription and nonprescription drugs. Although people aged 65 years and older in the United States make up approximately 14% of the total population, those 38 million Americans consume 25% of all prescription drugs and 33% of all nonprescription drugs sold.
- Approximately 60% of all dosage units consumed (prescription and nonprescription) are nonprescription drugs.
- Of approximately 3.5 billion health problems treated annually in the United States, some 2 billion (57%) are treated with a nonprescription drug.
- More than 400 medical disorders are treatable with one or more nonprescription drugs as the primary or major adjunctive therapy, and many of these disorders occur millions of times each year. Table 1–1 lists some of the most commonly self-treated disorders.
- The per capita expenditure for nonprescription drugs is approximately $90 per year and growing.
- The cost–benefit ratio of appropriately used nonprescription drugs is very high. Nonprescription drugs account for less than three cents of every dollar spent on health care in the United States, yet the benefit derived is vast.
- The pharmacist is the most accessible health professional, is the only health care professional who receives

Table 1–1

Selected Medical Disorders Amenable to Nonprescription Drug Therapy[a]

Abrasions	Colds (viral upper respiratory infection)	Flatulence	Ovulation prediction
Aches and pains (general, mild to moderate)	Congestion (chest, nasal)	Gastritis	Periodontal disease
Acne	Conjunctivitis	Gingivitis	Pharyngitis
Albumin testing	Constipation	Hair loss	Pinworm infestation
Allergic reactions	Contact lens care	Halitosis	Premenstrual syndrome
Allergic rhinitis	Contraception	Head lice	Pregnancy (diagnostic)
Anemia	Corns	Headache	Prickly heat
Arthralgia	Cough	Heartburn	Psoriasis
Asthma	Cuts (superficial)	Hemorrhoids	Ringworm
Athlete's foot	Dandruff	Impetigo	Seborrhea
Bacterial infection (topical, superficial, uncomplicated)	Deficiency disorders (mineral, vitamin, enteral food supplements)	Indigestion	Sinusitis
Blisters	Dental care	Ingrown toenails	Smoking cessation
Blood pressure monitoring	Dermatitis (contact)	Insect bites and stings	Sprains
Boils	Diabetes mellitus (insulin, monitoring equipment, supplies)	Insomnia	Strains
Bowel preparation (diagnostic)	Diaper rash	Jet lag	Stye (hordeolum)
Burns (minor, thermal)	Diarrhea	Jock itch	Sunburn
Calluses	Dry skin	Motion sickness	Teething
Candidal vaginitis	Dysmenorrhea	Myalgia	Thrush
Canker sores	Dyspepsia	Nausea	Toothache
Carbuncles	Feminine hygiene	Nutrition (infant)	Vomiting
Chapped skin	Fever	Obesity	Warts (common and plantar)
Cold sores		Occult blood in feces (detection)	Xerostomia
		Ostomy care	Wound care

[a] The pertinent nonprescription drugs or drugs for a particular disorder may serve as primary or major adjunctive therapy.

formal university-based education and training in nonprescription drug pharmacotherapy, and is perceived very favorably by the public. Thus, the pharmacist can and should differentiate himself or herself from other providers by offering value-added informational services. Several of these factors will be discussed in more detail later in this chapter.

The Self-Care Revolution

Many consumers desire, and are taking, a much more informed and active role in managing their own health care. Dr. Art Ulene coined the term "lifestyle medicine" to describe the partnership between informed health care consumers and health care providers. Documentation of the self-care revolution lies in the hundreds of self-help books, health-related newspaper features, television and radio programs, instructional audio and videotapes, articles that proliferate in various magazines for the mass market, and Internet Web sites and portals. A host of factors may influence individual attitudes, values, and practices relative to self-care. (See Table 1–2). Those attitudes, values, and practices vary from individual to individual. This stratification of the U.S. population should be taken into account by health care providers, and patients should be viewed as individuals with unique backgrounds and needs.

Surveys consistently demonstrate that consumers are increasingly self-medicating with nonprescription drugs. The following points reveal selected consumer attitudes about this practice:[1]

- Almost 7 of 10 consumers prefer to fight symptoms without taking medication, if possible.
- Approximately 9 of 10 consumers realize they should take medication only when absolutely necessary.
- Among consumers, 85% believe it is important to have access to nonprescription medications to help relieve minor medical problems.
- Of consumers who discontinued their nonprescription medication, 90% did so because their medical problem or symptoms were resolved.
- For problems treated with nonprescription medications, 94% of consumers report they would use the same product again for the same condition.
- Even though a medication may be available without a prescription, 94% of consumers agreed that care should be taken when using it.
- Nearly all (93%) consumers report that they read instructions before taking a nonprescription medication for the first time. Among consumers, 81% believe that the pharmacist is a good source of nonprescription drug information.
- Among consumers, 54% believe that the availability of products reclassified from prescription to nonprescription status has made it possible to save the time and expense of going to a physician for managing some conditions.
- Two of every three consumers favor the reclassification process.

Table 1–2

Selected Attitudes, Values, and Practices Likely to Influence Self-Care Behavior

Attitudes/Beliefs

- Appreciation of the value of wellness and prevention initiatives in managing illness
- Willingness to accept a significant degree of personal responsibility for one's own health
- Motivation and commitment to become a learner relative to the disease in question and its proper treatment
- Perception of the degree of seriousness of the medical condition one wishes to prevent or treat
- Acceptance of traditional health care providers
- Acceptance of the traditional process of health care delivery
- Willingness to communicate with legitimate, informed, mainstream health care providers
- Tendency to be influenced by friends, relatives, alternative health care providers, and printed "health information" that is not mainstream

Demographics

- Age
- Family size
- Gender differences
- Socioeconomic position

Economics

- Economic status (individual)
- Cost of care (products, services, or both)
- Convenience or access to health care products, services, or both
- Availability of health care products, services, or both

Education/Knowledge

- Educational level of individual (public education, college or university education)
- Baseline knowledge about the relevant medical condition(s)
- Baseline knowledge about the relevant treatment regimen
- Ability to comprehend or interpret consumer health information (verbal and written), package labeling, and package insert information
- Access to quality consumer health information through the lay press, electronic media, and so forth
- Access to mentors or learned intermediaries who can assist in interpreting consumer health information as well as offer additional advice and counsel
- Susceptibility to vague or misleading advertising or to claims regarding alternative health care (e.g., acupuncture, chelation therapy, herbalism, holism, megavitamin therapy, naturalism)

Over the past decade, the health problems most likely to be treated with a nonprescription drug have not changed substantially. Headache leads the list, followed by the common cold; muscle aches and pains (including sprains and strains); dermatologic conditions (e.g., acne, cold sores, dandruff, dry skin, athlete's foot, jock itch); minor wounds (e.g., cuts, scratches); premenstrual and menstrual symptoms; upset stomach; and sleeping problems.

Reports indicate that the average American experiences one potentially self-treatable health problem every 3 to 4 days and that approximately 90% of the U.S. population consider themselves "a bit under the weather" one or more times each month. Individuals are more likely to self-treat or to treat their children when they perceive their illness to be not serious enough to require medical intervention. In one survey, more than 50% of mothers had given their 3-year-olds one or more nonprescription medications within the previous 30 days.[2] An anecdotal report documented the fact that 16 nonprescription medications were on hand in the average home for treatment of a child's various conditions. From an economics perspective, a patient was overheard extolling the virtues of nonprescription drugs, "I can treat my headache for a dime. When I go to my doctor, my copayment for the office visit is $15, and my copayment on prescription drugs is $5 for generics and $15 for brand-name drugs. I try to take care of myself when I can."

Self-medication with nonprescription drugs is often the initial level of care in a tiered system of health care. To say that patients have choices in self-care therapy is an understatement. It is estimated that more than 300,000 nonprescription drug formulations are available to consumers. Many products are sold on a local or regional basis only. However, thousands of products have national distribution, and the many choices consumers have can be bewildering.

The self-care revolution involves and should encourage development of knowledge and skill in promoting wellness as well as in treating medical conditions. Informed, appropriate, and responsible use of nonprescription drugs is a large part of self-care. Data suggest that most patients respect these drugs, recognize their limitations, and read labeling information carefully. Yet other consumers are uninformed and misinformed. Casual and inappropriate use of nonprescription drugs can lead to serious adverse consequences of both a direct (e.g., adverse drug reaction, drug–drug interaction) and indirect (e.g., delays in seeking appropriate medical attention) nature. Such practices should be discouraged and addressed through (1) adequate package labeling, (2) direct-to-consumer advertising that has a strong educational emphasis about the medical condition(s) being treated and the proper use of the nonprescription drug to ensure an optimal health outcome, and (3) patient education and counseling by pharmacists and other qualified health care professionals regarding proper drug selection and use.

The Pharmacist's Responsibility in Pharmaceutical Care

In an era of health care reform and cost containment, numerous issues concerning the quality and cost of health care present practice opportunities to pharmacists. One significant practice opportunity is to serve and assist patients in using nonprescription drugs to manage numerous self-limiting conditions and some chronic conditions.

Self-care with nonprescription drugs should not be a random, uninformed process in which the patient acts alone by default. Many consumers want and need more information on the appropriate use of such drugs. In addition to highly readable, understandable, and usable package labeling, patients need access to a qualified, learned intermediary to assist in nonprescription drug selection, use, and monitoring. That person is most logically the community-based pharmacist.

The pharmacist is uniquely qualified to serve the public interest in nonprescription pharmacotherapy because he or she receives university-level education and training, which is undergirded by in-depth instruction in pathophysiology, pharmacology, medicinal chemistry, pharmaceutics, and pharmacokinetics. The pharmacist's knowledge and ability are often enhanced by electronic and print databases. Further, the pharmacist is accessible to the public and strategically positioned in the community to serve as a provider of not only the drug but also the information on how to maximize the value of drug therapy while minimizing any potential adverse consequences.

In the initial encounter with a patient seeking assistance with nonprescription drug use, the pharmacist should do the following:

- Assess, by interview and observation, the patient's physical complaint or symptoms and the medical condition.
- Differentiate self-treatable conditions from those requiring medical intervention.
- Advise and counsel the patient on the proper course of action (i.e., no treatment with drug therapy, self-treatment with nonprescription products, or referral to a physician or other health care provider).

If self-treatment with one or more nonprescription drugs is appropriate, the pharmacist is positioned and intellectually equipped to perform the following patient care services:

- Assist in product selection.
- Assess patient risk factors (e.g., contraindications, warnings, precautions, comorbidity, age, organ function).
- Counsel the patient regarding proper drug use (e.g., dosage, administration technique, monitoring parameters).

- Maintain a patient drug profile that includes nonprescription as well as prescription drugs.
- Monitor drug therapy for the following:
  —Drug allergies or hypersensitivities
  —Adverse drug reactions
  —Drug–drug interactions
  —An appropriate response to therapy
  —Signs and symptoms of drug overuse and/or dependency.
- Discourage the use of fraudulent and "quack" remedies.
- Assess the potential of nonprescription drugs to mask symptoms of a more serious condition.
- Prevent delays in seeking appropriate medical attention.

The public's ability to appropriately discern critical information about the condition being treated and about the clinical risk and benefit of the product is highly variable. The array of product choices, line extensions, and overstated or vague and misleading marketing messages create confusion at the very least. Package labeling is generally limited in the breadth and depth of the message it communicates; it can never address the informational needs of patients for all clinical circumstances, and it can be difficult to read. Moreover, comorbidity and polypharmacy create infinite special considerations in ensuring the safe, appropriate, and effective use of nonprescription drugs. Thus, the pharmacist–patient interaction is vital to optimal nonprescription pharmacotherapy. Further, the pharmacist and other health care providers should recognize the great difference between providing information to and educating patients. Validation of understanding is critical. Patients should be strongly encouraged to comment and ask questions.

FDA Regulation of Drugs

The first major federal legislation enacted to regulate drugs was the Pure Food and Drugs Act of 1906. "Unsafe" and "nonefficacious" drug products were not actually prohibited by the statute; drugs were required to meet only the standards of strength and purity claimed by manufacturers. Drug safety was not mandated by law until passage of the 1938 Federal Food, Drug, and Cosmetic Act (1938 Act). Legislation for that law had been under consideration since 1933, but final passage was compelled by the deaths of more than 100 individuals, many of them children, who used the newly marketed elixir of sulfanilamide, which contained the toxic solvent ethylene glycol (antifreeze) as the vehicle.

The 1962 amendments to the 1938 Act require that all new drugs be shown to be effective for their intended uses. This legislation thus required an FDA review of the effectiveness of 4500 new drug products, including 512 nonprescription drugs that had been approved for safety since 1938. In the mid-1960s, FDA contracted the National Academy of Sciences/National Research Council (NAS/NRC) to review these drugs. FDA took the information from NAS/NRC and, by a procedure called the Drug Efficacy Study Implementation (DESI), determined the effectiveness of all prescription drugs. As DESI was nearing completion, clearly it became time for an extensive examination of the nonprescription drug marketplace. In 1972, FDA initiated a massive scientific review of the active ingredients in nonprescription drug products to ensure that they were safe and effective and that they bore fully informative labeling. This review process is often referred to as the over-the-counter (OTC) drug review.

FDA is also responsible for reclassifying drugs from prescription to nonprescription status and for establishing regulations for package labels.

The Drug-Approval Process

The 1938 Act required that all new drugs—that is, new drug products introduced after 1938—be proven safe for human use before being marketed and be cleared in advance through a new drug application (NDA). Products marketed before 1938 were exempted from NDA provision under what is commonly referred to as the grandfather clause. Some currently marketed nonprescription drugs, such as aspirin, still fall under this clause. However, FDA's OTC drug review has evaluated all nonprescription drugs for safety, effectiveness, and labeling, regardless of the date of marketing entry.

Even today, the 1938 Act, as amended, defines a market divided into "new" drugs, which are defined by law as being recognized as safe and effective (RASE), and those that are generally recognized as safe and effective (GRASE). Although those latter drugs are referred to as "old" drugs, such a legal definition does not exist. A new chemical entity never before marketed in the United States would be classified as a new drug and, in most cases, initially approved for prescription use only.

Through NDA procedures, a prescription drug may be reclassified to nonprescription status but remain a new drug. An NDA for a nonprescription drug product can also be approved directly (without reclassification), such as occurred with ibuprofen 200 mg (a dose that was never available by prescription). When a new drug is used for many years by many patients (referred to in the law as "used for a material time and material extent"), it can be considered GRASE. Another mechanism to gain general recognition status for nonprescription drugs has been provided by FDA's OTC drug review.

New Drug Applications

An NDA is necessary for a drug that is defined by law as not being recognized as safe and effective (NRASE) until it has been precleared and approved by FDA. Under existing public procedures, some data related to the approval and contained in the NDA (e.g., a summary of the safety data and clinical studies) are publicly available. However, trade information (e.g., final formulation ingredients and quantities) is held confidential.

The approved NDA is manufacturer specific and allows only the sponsor to market the product. Any other manufacturer interested in marketing a similar product would first need to seek FDA approval through an appropriate NDA. In some cases, a full NDA is not necessary for the second manufacturer; an abbreviated application may be submitted instead, eliminating the need for duplicative testing.

All NDAs must contain complete (exact) labeling information, with final printed labeling being the usual last step before approval. (See the section Nonprescription Drug Labeling.) Most subsequent revisions in labeling require preapproval through a supplement to the application. Therefore, labeling is highly restricted and often takes considerable time to change. Similarly, except for some minor changes, the final product formulation cannot be changed without an approved supplement to the application. Finally, periodic submissions—for example, a brief summary of significant new information from the previous year that might affect the safety, effectiveness, or labeling, including any actions taken by the sponsor as a result of those findings—are required to report postmarketing information. Distribution data, minor labeling revisions, chemistry, and manufacturing and control changes must also be reported.

Monographs

An OTC monograph is developed for a drug that is defined by law as GRASE. A manufacturer desiring to market a monographed drug need not seek FDA's prior clearance. In this case, marketing is not exclusive; any manufacturer may market a similar product without specific approval. Under the monograph approach, all data and information supporting GRASE status are publicly available. The OTC drug review has established the monographs through a complex, public process. Each individual rulemaking has resulted in an administrative public record that is extensive.

For the final monograph, the manufacturer has considerable flexibility in labeling. All the required monograph labeling must be included; for example, antacids must include terms such as heartburn, acid indigestion, and sour stomach. In addition, language not included in the monograph may be used in the label without prior approval. For example, hospital-tested or pleasant-tasting antacid are terms considered outside the scope of the monograph but permissible in antacid labeling. However, even though these permissible terms are not precleared, they are subject to the general labeling provision of the 1938 Act and may not be false or misleading.

Monographs primarily address active ingredient(s) in the product, and, in most cases, final formulations are not subject to monograph specifications. Manufacturers are free to include any inactive ingredients that serve a pharmaceutical purpose, provided those ingredients are safe and do not interfere with either product effectiveness or any required final product testing. In a few instances, even though the product contains GRASE ingredients, it may need to meet a monograph testing procedure; for example, antacids must pass an acid-neutralizing test.

Because the drugs in the monograph system are GRASE, no requirement has yet been made to report adverse events. Historically, any changes in ingredient status and labeling have occurred as a result of adverse drug findings reported in the literature or through similar public mechanisms. With the ever-increasing use of nonprescription drugs, however, FDA believes it is important to develop a new and more effective formal mechanism to monitor and to screen reports of adverse drug effects and unexpected events associated with drug use.

Nonprescription Drug Labeling

Labels on nonprescription drug containers and packaging material should provide detailed information so that consumers can properly select and use the drugs. The message should not be constrained by the size of the container or package. Significant concerns about labeling comprehensibility, readability, and comprehensiveness continue to be expressed.

Comprehensibility

FDA regulations require that nonprescription drug labeling contain terms that are likely to be read and understood by the average consumer, including the person of low comprehension, under the customary conditions of purchase and use. This requirement is indeed challenging because, as manufacturers standardize labeling information for the average consumer, a significant percentage of people will always be "below average" in their ability to read, comprehend, discern, and act properly on label information. An estimated 20% of the U.S. adult population is functionally illiterate (e.g., reading below a fifth-grade level, plus experiencing difficulty in reading and accurately comprehending a food package label or a restaurant menu). In population subsets, the rate of functional illiteracy may exceed 40%. Approximately 35% of the U.S. population reads and comprehends at a sixth- to tenth-grade level.

Labeling information that exceeds an individual's ability to interpret, comprehend, and apply that information produces major obstacles to the safe, appropriate, and effective use of nonprescription drugs. An estimated one-half of all consumers of nonprescription drugs would benefit from counseling on how to interpret product labels properly.[3]

Readability

FDA and manufacturers of nonprescription drugs have been actively engaged in initiatives to increase drug label readability over the past several years. Label standardization that addresses text, format, and the provision of essential information in the same order and in the same area of every drug label is becoming a reality. The key goals have been uniformity in print size, pictograms, icons, color, color contrast, type face, type size, type spacing, columns, margins, paragraphs, uppercase versus lowercase lettering, bulleting, numbering, and language simplification. One option being evaluated is the use of a "drug facts" box similar to the "nutrition facts" box on food labeling.

Label format should continue to focus on special populations with impaired vision. For example, a 45-year-old needs 50% more light than a 20-year-old, and a 70-year-old needs approximately three times as much light as a 20-year-old to read well. Nonprescription drug manufacturers cannot control light, but they can compensate for low light and poor visual acuity by using larger print for the most critical messages. A threshold print size of 4.5 points, while not optimal, has been suggested as a minimum in nonprescription drug package labeling. Given that the U.S. population is aging rapidly and that most people over 40 cannot read 4.5-point print without reading glasses, many people consider a threshold print size of 6.0 points to be more appropriate.

Essential Information

Essential information that should be displayed prominently on all nonprescription drug labeling consists of the following elements.

Product Name/Ingredients

Large print on the package label should enable the reader to accurately identify the product trade name, generic name, classification, and strength of all therapeutic ingredients. Inactive ingredients (e.g., formulation factors, adjuvants) should also be listed by name and amount present.

Product Indications/Claims

Labels should include only FDA-approved indication (use) for the active ingredient(s). It would be useful if package labeling linked the ingredient with its specific indication (e.g., dextromethorphan for cough, pseudoephedrine for upper respiratory congestion).

Package Contents

In addition to strength, concentration, and net quantity, package labeling should include the dosage form used (e.g., tablet, chewable tablet, capsule, syrup, suspension, elixir, suppository, ophthalmic preparation); (2) the dosage units or volume contained in the package; (3) an indication that a tamper-resistant seal has been applied; and (4) the course of action to take if the seal or band is broken or missing.

Directions for Use

Labels must clearly instruct the patient on the proper way to take the product (e.g., orally, topically); the proper dosage and the frequency of administration (given the patient's age, pregnancy, and other special considerations); and, in some cases, the length of time to take the medication. Special storage procedures (e.g., refrigerate, avoid heat or cold extremes, avoid overexposure to sunlight) must be included.

Contraindications/Warnings/ Precautions/Adverse Effects

If a drug is contraindicated, all appropriate circumstances requiring the contraindication (e.g., pregnancy, glaucoma, hypersensitivity) should be included on the label. Label information should caution women who are pregnant or breast-feeding to check with a health care professional before taking the medication. Pediatric and geriatric populations may have special informational needs that should be on the label, particularly with regard to dosing and safety closures. Precautionary statements (e.g., time limits on use, removal from the reach of children, and action to take in case of an accidental overdose) should be on the label. Potential side effects (e.g., drowsiness, dizziness, nausea, diarrhea, blurred vision, elevation of blood pressure, tachycardia) that might debilitate or endanger the user to any degree should also be listed, as should drug–drug interactions of greatest potential clinical significance.

Indications for Seeking Medical Attention

Package labeling that recognizes the limitations of nonprescription drugs and advises consultation with a health care professional if symptoms persist or worsen over a relatively short period of time is strongly encouraged.

Manufacturer's Information

The manufacturer's and/or distributor's name, address, and toll-free telephone number are useful information in matters related to recalls, unexpected adverse effects, and other unanticipated issues.

Expiration Date and Batch Code

The expiration date is required and should remain distinguishable over time. The batch code is necessary for recall purposes.

Label Flags

Flags or side panels in prominent type should be readily apparent on package labels when significant changes are made in a product (e.g., its formulation) or its label information (e.g., indications, contraindications, warnings, precautions, adverse effects, drug interactions, and/or dosage or administration guidelines).

Limitations

Overreliance on package labeling as the primary patient education resource is fraught with potential patient risk. A package label can never address the infinite management issues associated with drug use, particularly in the presence of multiple disease states (comorbidity) and a complex regimen of prescription and/or nonprescription drugs (polypharmacy). Thus, package labeling should acknowledge and encourage a dialogue with the pharmacist as well as with the physician when patients have questions or concerns about nonprescription drug use.

Package Inserts

Finally, FDA, nonprescription pharmaceutical manufacturers, and manufacturer trade associations may ultimately acknowledge that the breadth and depth of patient information, which is needed to ensure the maximization of positive health outcomes and the minimization of adverse consequences from drug use, may not be achievable through total reliance on a package label or container. Accordingly, patient package inserts for nonprescription drugs may be necessary to communicate the complete information to patients in a readable and user-friendly format.

Drug Reclassification: Prescription to Nonprescription

FDA's OTC drug review is responsible for reclassifying many drugs from prescription to nonprescription status. In 1991, FDA announced the establishment of the Nonprescription Drug Advisory Committee to review and evaluate the safety and effectiveness of nonprescription drug products and to serve as a forum for exchanging views about the prescription and nonprescription status of various drugs. This process has produced more than 50 reclassifications from prescription-only to nonprescription status over the past 20 years.

Criteria for Reclassification

Until 1951, federal law did not contain criteria for determining whether a drug should be limited to prescription use. This decision was left to the manufacturer, and different manufacturers made different decisions about the same drug formulations, leading to confusion among manufacturers, regulators, health care professionals, and the general public. Questions arose about FDA's authority to permit refill authorizations or to limit drug prescribing to physicians. To end the confusion, in 1951, Congress enacted an amendment to the 1938 Act. It specified the following three classes of drugs that were limited to prescription use:

- Certain habit-forming drugs listed by name;
- Drugs not safe for use except when supervised by a licensed practitioner because of their toxicity or other potential for harmful effect, their method of use, or the collateral measures necessary for use;
- Drugs limited to prescription under an NDA.

These statutory definitions, along with the basic statutory language requiring adequate directions for use, are still the principal criteria for determining prescription versus nonprescription drug classification.

The second criterion is probably the most essential when FDA considers reclassification. The assessment of the overall margin of safety includes not only those considerations described in the statute (toxicity, potential for harmful effects, method of use, and collateral measures necessary to use) but also the potential for abuse and misuse and the benefit-to-risk ratio.

Drugs administered to treat serious disease conditions may cause adverse effects. Those drugs must be used carefully to achieve the appropriate level of effectiveness without endangering patient safety. Some drugs are, therefore, too toxic to be used for self-treatment and will continue to be classified as prescription drugs. However, because any drug can be misused with some toxic result, such a possibility is not the sole basis for prescription classification. Because all drugs have both benefits and risks—for example, most antihistamines may cause drowsiness—some degree of risk must be tolerated for patients to receive the benefits. However, product labels with adequate directions for use can inform patients about risks.

Exact standards or reclassification criteria are very difficult to set because so many factors must be carefully considered. The classification process is judgmental and is based on many factors related to an individual drug's use, risks, and benefits. The information that must be gathered from the expert opinions of advisors and consultants regarding a drug's nonprescription status includes, but is not limited to, the following:

- Is the condition self-diagnosable?
- Is the condition self-treatable?
- What is the product's toxicity?
- Does the product possess misuse and/or abuse potential?
- Is the product habit-forming?
- Do methods of use preclude nonprescription availability?
- Do the benefits of availability outweigh the risks?
- Can adequate directions for use be written?
- Can warnings against inappropriate and/or unsafe use be written?
- Can labeling be read and understood by the ordinary person?

Further scientific scrutiny typically addresses the following questions as well:

- Does the reclassification candidate have special or unique toxicity within its pharmacologic class?
- Does the reclassification candidate have an adequate margin of safety?
- Does the reclassification candidate's frequency of dosing affect its safe use?
- Has the reclassification candidate been used for a sufficiently long time (e.g., 3 to 5 years) on the prescription market to yield a full characterization of its safety profile?
- Has the reclassification candidate's safety profile been defined at high doses?

- Has a vigorous risk analysis been performed? If so, what are the results?
- Is there a full understanding of the pharmacodynamics of the reclassification candidate?
- Is the minimally effective dose of the proposed nonprescription indication known?
- Has the efficacy literature been reviewed in a way that supports the expected use and labeling of the reclassification candidate?
- Have potential drug interactions for the reclassification candidate been characterized?
- What is the worldwide clinical and marketing experience of the reclassification candidate?

Many FDA personnel and external experts are consulted in an effort to form a consensus on each reclassification candidate. The process is lengthy and thorough.

Mechanisms for Reclassification

Four basic mechanisms exist for reclassifying a prescription drug to nonprescription status.

Mechanism 1

A full NDA may be submitted for a currently marketed prescription drug. The application might contain new clinical studies to support a specific nonprescription indication using a lower prescription strength. In this case, because new studies have been conducted, the sponsor of the approved NDA will have marketing exclusivity for several years. Other manufacturers would need to duplicate the studies during that period.

Mechanism 2

The "switch regulation" provides that drugs limited to prescription use under an NDA can be exempted from that limitation if FDA determines that the prescription requirements are unnecessary for protecting the public health. The regulation allows a petition for such an exemption to be initiated by FDA or by any interested person.

Mechanism 3

A prescription drug that already has an approved NDA can be reclassified to nonprescription status through the filing and agency approval of a supplement to the NDA. FDA determines whether the drug, which was previously limited under the terms of its NDA, has now been shown to be safe for nonprescription use. In some cases, the same prescription dosage is considered for nonprescription status. Heavy reliance is placed on the extent of marketing experience and the degree of adverse findings. Under either the reclassification regulation or the supplement to the NDA, the reclassified drug product remains a "new drug" requiring premarket approval and periodic reports to FDA.

Mechanism 4

Finally, using a completely different process, nearly 40 ingredients have been reclassified through OTC drug review. Asked to make recommendations on any drugs that could be safely converted to nonprescription status, the advisory panels recommended changing many ingredients—including hydrocortisone, diphenhydramine, nystatin, and oxymetazoline—from prescription use to nonprescription drug availability. In some cases, the dosage was increased for marketed nonprescription ingredients (e.g., 2 mg of chlorpheniramine was elevated to 4 mg).

Table 1–3 shows a selected list of former prescription drugs that are now available over the counter.

A Third Class of Drugs?

It is becoming increasingly apparent that optimal drug therapy is the single most critical process in managing most medical conditions. Drug therapy represents 10% to 12% of the nation's total health care cost. By reliable estimates, it is solely or primarily responsible for managing 85% to 90% of all acute and chronic illness. Drug therapy (prescription and nonprescription) is the "best buy" in American health care; its return on investment is unrivaled in the health care process.

Drug therapy should not, however, be viewed as a benign panacea for managing acute and chronic illness. Rather, every drug should be viewed as a "two-edged sword" that has the potential to do great good but may do harm if not used properly. Package labeling addresses the potential risks associated with drug use under categories of information familiar to all pharmacists and physicians. Those categories include contraindications, warnings, precautions, adverse reactions, drug interactions, and administration and dosage guidelines.

The black-or-white, all-or-none classification system of prescription-only or nonprescription access leaves no room for shades of gray—drugs in a transitional category—and no consistent opportunity for a pharmacist to confer with a patient on nonprescription drug selection and use issues. In the nonprescription drug domain, no regulation or legislation exists that differentiates the pharmacist from any employee in any retail sales outlet that sells nonprescription drugs (e.g., department store, gas station, quick-shop, grocery store, hardware store). Drugs that were formerly in prescription-only status are even sold in vending machines as soon as they are reclassified. This practice raises serious public interest questions.

The National Consumer League notes that most developed and industrialized nations of the world have at least three classes of drugs. Many groups favor moving prescription drugs to nonprescription status when it is safe to do so, but most acknowledge that some drugs fall somewhere in between. Great Britain enjoys a three-class system (i.e., prescription only, general sales nonprescription, and restricted sales by pharmacists). This last category is often referred to as a "third class of drugs." In supporting a third class of drugs that fosters patient–pharmacist interaction, John Ferguson, secretary-registrar of the Royal Pharmaceutical Society of Great Britain, suggests that general availability of nonpre-

Table 1–3

Selected List of Reclassified Drugs

Ingredient	Use/Indication	Ingredient	Use/Indication
Acidulated phosphate fluoride	Dental rinse	Miconazole	Antifungal
Brompheniramine maleate	Antihistamine	Minoxidil	Baldness
Butoconazole	Antifungal	Naproxen	Analgesic
Chlorpheniramine maleate	Antihistamine	Nicotine	Smoking cessation
Cimetidine	Heartburn	Nicotine polacrilex	Smoking cessation
Clemastine fumarate	Antihistamine	Nizatidine	Heartburn
Clotrimazole	Antifungal	Oxymetazoline	Decongestant
Cromolyn sodium	Allergy prevention and treatment	Permethrin	Pediculicide
Dexbrompheniramine	Antihistamine	Phenylephrine	Decongestant
Diphenhydramine	Antihistamine	Phenylpropanolamine	Decongestant
Doxylamine	Sleep aid	Pseudoephedrine	Decongestant
Dyclonine	Oral anesthetic	Pyrantel pamoate	Pinworm treatment
Ephedrine sulfate	Bronchodilator, vasoconstrictor	Ranitidine	Heartburn
Famotidine	Heartburn	Sodium fluoride	Dental rinse
Haloprogin[a]	Antifungal	Stannous fluoride	Dental rinse or gel
Hydrocortisone	Antipruritic, anti-inflammatory	Terbinafine	Antifungal
Ibuprofen	Analgesic	Tioconazole	Antifungal
Ketoconazole	Antifungal (shampoo only)	Tolnaftate	Antifungal
Ketoprofen	Analgesic	Triprolidine	Antihistamine
Loperamide	Antidiarrheal	Xylometazoline	Decongestant

[a] Although FDA approved haloprogin for nonprescription use, no currently available nonprescription antifungals contain this agent.

scription drugs makes potent pharmaceuticals a mere commodity to be distributed like soap, cornflakes, and pantyhose; he notes that Great Britain's three-class system has withstood the test of time.

Since 1964, the American Pharmaceutical Association has supported a third class of drugs that would require pharmacist consultation before consumer purchase. Since 1987, it has specifically proposed that all drugs being considered for reclassification from prescription to nonprescription status be placed in a third class for a period of 2 or more years as a way to increase surveillance. Many available nonprescription drugs, as well as many prescription drugs being considered for reclassification, would qualify for transitional status because of their side-effect profile, drug interaction potential, and/or potential for misuse or abuse. For drugs in this transitional third class, the pharmacist could assist patients in selection and use, counsel patients, identify potential problems, resolve actual problems, and monitor the patient's progress. This active clinical involvement and surveillance, which is not possible in the approximately 1 million nonpharmacy retail outlets in the United States that now sell nonprescription drugs, could help to determine whether a drug is too toxic or is subject to misuse or abuse to the extent that it should not be moved from the transitional class to general use. Advocates of a third class of drugs have confidence in the pharmacist's specialized ability to operate in the best interest of the public relative to the use of a few drugs of particularly noteworthy risk.

In 1995, the General Accounting Office (GAO) of the U.S. Congress completed a 3-year study requested by Representative John Dingell (D–Mich.) to determine whether significant benefits or costs associated with a third class of drugs existed according to experience in 10 countries. The GAO report concluded that, at this time, no major improvements in nonprescription drug use are likely to result from restricting the sale of some nonprescription drugs to only pharmacies or only by pharmacists. This conclusion disappointed many consumer groups and the organized pharmacy group because it contradicts the marketplace reality as well as problems such as ephedrine misuse and abuse, laxative dependency, rebound congestion from overuse of topical nasal decongestants, and hypervitaminosis, to name a few. Some would argue that the GAO report did not research public interest issues in adequate depth. Arguments that a transitional third class of drugs is anticompetitive or anticonsumer and would create a pharmacist's monopoly, increase consumer costs, and restrain trade are arguably superficial, flawed, and diminished by public interest issues.

More groups are declaring that a third class of drugs is an idea whose time has come. The current environment for health care reform emphasizes disease management initiatives, optimal drug therapy outcomes, and quality health care at a reasonable cost. That emphasis creates a positive environment for further initiatives to create a real or de facto third class of drugs.

Marketing Issues

Product Line Extensions

The nonprescription drug manufacturers and FDA must more vigorously address the matter of line extensions (e.g., new doses, new formulations) although they are not a pure labeling issue. From a marketing perspective, it is understandable that a manufacturer would see a potential benefit in trading on the name recognition of a previously successful brand-name product. However, if product line extensions create redundancy, distortion, misinterpretation, consumer confusion, and inappropriate patient drug selection and use decisions, then marketing considerations must not override the safety and efficacy issues, which should be paramount.

Some companies capitalize on consumer recognition, trust, and loyalty to a brand name that originally applied to a single ingredient at a specific dose to treat a specific symptom (e.g., fever) or symptom complex (e.g., headache, fever, joint and muscle pain). When brand names are used as the prefix with numerous suffixes (e.g., PM, EX, DM, AF, Cold and Flu, Non-Drowsy, Extra, Allergy-Sinus-Headache, Advanced Formula, PH, Day/Night, and Plus), most consumers can and do become confused, if not bewildered.

Some product line extensions that carry the innovator brand name as the prefix retain the active ingredient of the innovator product, but strengths may vary. A few manufacturers with six or more product line extensions continue to use the innovator brand name as the prefix, but use none of the active ingredient of the innovator products and attach a vague suffix that provides little indication of any active therapeutic ingredients in the extension product. Such practices are contrary to the public health interest and fly in the face of labeling initiatives designed to assist patients' understanding.

Manufacturers of nonprescription drugs should be encouraged to consider the following guidelines in addressing the inherent problems of line extensions.[4]

- Product line extensions should be discouraged unless they meet a significant consumer need. In such cases, packaging and labeling should clearly distinguish the new product from existing products marketed under the same brand name.
- Brand names should be restricted to products that contain the same active ingredient(s). A change in the product ingredient profile should warrant a new brand name.
- Application of truly descriptive suffixes to existing brand-name products should be allowed only when one or more active ingredients have been added to an existing formulation (e.g., Robitussin DM).
- Standard nomenclature should be used for abbreviations for individual active ingredients commonly added to existing nonprescription formulations.
- A product reclassified from prescription-only to nonprescription status should be allowed to retain its brand name only if the nonprescription product contains the same active ingredient(s).

Nonprescription Drug Advertising

Although it can prohibit the sale of falsely advertised products, FDA does not regulate or have authority over nonprescription drug advertising. Such authority rests with the Federal Trade Commission. As defined in the Federal Trade Commission Act, advertisement shall mean the following:

> Any written or verbal statement, illustration, or depiction, other than a label or in the labeling, which is designed to promote the sale of a product, whether the same appears in television or radio broadcast, newspaper, magazine, leaflet, circular, book insert, catalog, sales promotional material, billboard, or in any display intended for use at the point of sale of the product.[5]

In the 1970s, the Federal Trade Commission Act was amended to prohibit advertisers, when describing the therapeutic benefits of nonprescription products, from using language not approved by FDA for labeling. In 1973, the National Association of Broadcasters and the Nonprescription Drug Manufacturers Association (now the Consumer Healthcare Products Association) developed a code of guidelines for manufacturers to follow in creating television advertisements for nonprescription drugs. According to those guidelines, which set standards for truthfulness and honesty, an advertisement should do the following:[6]

- Urge the consumer to read and follow label directions.
- Emphasize uses, results, and advantages of the product advertised.
- Present actual research performed, and interpret results honestly and accurately if that advertisement references scientific or consumer studies.
- Contain no claims of product effectiveness that are unsupported by clinical or other scientific evidence.
- Reference no doctors, hospitals, or nurses unless such representations can be supported by independently conducted research.
- Present no information in a manner that suggests the product prevents or cures a serious condition that must be treated by a licensed practitioner.
- Use no presentation to dramatize ingesting a medication unless it is informing the consumer of proper medication administration.

- Present no negative or unfair reflections about competing nonprescription products unless those reflections can be scientifically supported and presented in a manner so that consumers can perceive differences in the uses.

Print advertising should be held to the same integrity standards as the electronic media. Vigilance is warranted in monitoring advertising, however, to ensure that advertisements do not contain false or misleading claims.

Both consumers and health care professionals should become students of advertising messages. Our society should be more analytical as we receive marketing messages, particularly those that are subjective, superficial, vague, or potentially misleading. Health care professionals, particularly the pharmacist and physician, should assist patients in separating fact from ambiguity with regard to nonprescription drug use. Public health educators-at-large (e.g., the pharmacist and physician) are well qualified and positioned to protect and serve the public interest as an objective, informed source of nonprescription drug information. This counterbalance to marginal advertising is necessary and appropriate.

CONCLUSIONS

Self-care will play an increasingly important role in health care, and nonprescription pharmacotherapy represents a significant element in that self-care process. Consumers, manufacturers, governmental agencies, and professional groups—particularly pharmacists—should become even more intent on recognizing that each group fulfills essential functions in ensuring the safe, appropriate, effective, and economical use of nonprescription drugs.

References

1. *Self-Medication in the '90s: Practices and Perceptions.* Washington, DC: Nonprescription Drug Manufacturers Association; 1992:9–13.
2. Gadomski A. Rational use of over-the-counter medications in young children. *JAMA.* 1994;272:1063–4.
3. FDA office would be established under house FDA reform bill. *FDC Reports–The Tan Sheet.* April 1, 1996:3–4.
4. Hewitt NM, Lausier JM, Rosenbaum S. Labeling and advertising of TC medicines: special emphasis on Rx to OTC switch products. *Clin Res Reg Affairs.* 1994;11:207–23.
5. *Voluntary Codes and Guidelines for the OTC Medicines Industry.* Washington, DC: Nonprescription Drug Manufacturers Association; 1991.
6. Rupp MT, Parker JM. Drug names: when marketing and safety collide. *Am Pharm.* 1993;33:39–42.

CHAPTER 2

Patient Assessment and Consultation

Wendy Klein-Schwartz and Brian J. Isetts

Chapter 2 at a Glance

Assessment represents the first set of clinical judgments made by the pharmacist when caring for a patient. The purpose of assessment is for the pharmacist to determine, describe, and define the patient's drug-related needs including the goals of therapy and identification of the patient's drug therapy problems. Assessment provides the practitioner with a basis for consulting with a patient to decide what drug therapy problems the patient has that the pharmacist will take responsibility to resolve.

The purpose of this chapter is to describe the assessment process and to place it within the context of developing a consistent and systematic approach to caring for patients who have self-care needs. Special considerations for assessing pediatric, geriatric, pregnant, and breast-feeding patients are addressed in detail. Consumers expect pharmacists to assist them with an array of health care concerns and to help them interpret treatment options within the health care delivery system. The chapter is divided into six sections: (1) an evaluation of the demands for self-care; (2) an introduction to the consistent and systematic patient care process that pharmacists engage in when assuming responsibility for a patient's drug-related needs; (3) a description of the rational and ordered process for conducting an assessment and a follow-up evaluation of a patient's drug-related needs; (4) a discussion of the skills necessary to care for patients with self-care needs, including development of a care plan; (5) examples of providing this level of pharmaceutical care to selected high-risk and special patients (pediatric, geriatric, pregnant, and nursing patients); and (6) conclusions about how to implement and integrate those principles into pharmacy practice.

The Demand for Self-Care

The U.S. health care system is in a dynamic state of flux marked by rapid changes and confusing priorities. Access, cost, and quality of health care are extensively debated at a public policy level among a milieu of complex factors that affect the health care delivery system. Our complicated, diverse, and fractionated health care system can leave consumers bewildered and frustrated when confronted with personal health care concerns. Fortunately, patients have come to trust and depend on their pharmacist when faced with their own personal health care needs.[1]

Pharmacists, who are often on the front line of the health care delivery system, are called upon to help patients assess alternatives to meet their needs. In most cases, the pharmacist can help patients by making one of three basic recommendations: (1) recommend no treatment at all, (2) recommend self-care therapy, or (3) refer patients to other health care professionals. A new series of self-care protocols is available to assist pharmacists in making decisions about self-care, including appropriate medical care referral.[2]

Self-care, self-diagnosis, and self-medication are important components of the health care system in the United States. Instead of seeking the advice of a physician, many people self-diagnose and treat their symptoms with nonprescription drugs, herbal products, and home remedies. Several factors increase the extent of self-treatment: people who are older than 75 years, patients who are female, people of a certain socioeconomic status, and people with a number of distinct and separate symptoms.[3] Another factor is the trend of reclassifying certain prescription drugs to nonprescription status.

Nonprescription drugs allow individuals to manage their many medical problems rapidly, economically, and conveniently and may prevent unnecessary visits to a physician. In 1998, more than $19 billion was spent on nonprescription drugs. Of those purchases, 42.8% were made in pharmacies;[4] the rest were made in food stores and mass merchandising outlets. Similarly, the use of herbal products is growing, with U.S. sales estimated at $3.24 billion in 1996.[5]

The appropriate use of a nonprescription product, like that of any other drug, requires attention to the intended use, effectiveness, safety, and convenience of administration. Although warnings are required on the labels of such products, labeling alone may be inadequate, and the patient may need assistance in selecting and properly using nonprescription drugs. Inappropriate use and misuse of nonprescription drugs can increase the risk of "drug misadventures,"[6] resulting in increased health care costs and a more serious illness. Thus, the pharmacist's role is crucial in assessing a patient's need for nonprescription medications.

The magnitude of drug misadventures has been described in terms of drug-induced morbidity and mortality.[7] For every dollar spent on medications in the United States, at least an additional dollar is spent addressing the adverse consequences, or drug therapy problems, arising from their use. Drug therapy problems are defined as any aspect of a patient's drug therapy that interferes with a desired, positive therapeutic outcome.[8]

Many patients do not appreciate, or are not aware of, the need for professional assistance in selecting nonprescription drugs. This attitude has recently become more evident from the large number of nonprescription products purchased in nonpharmacy outlets, such as supermarkets and convenience stores, where a pharmacist is not generally available.[4] Figure 2–1 gives a general indication of the percentage of nonprescription products purchased in nonpharmacy outlets.

The presence of a pharmacist differentiates the nonprescription drug department in a pharmacy from a similar department in a food store. To serve patients better, pharmacists need to maximize the personal service they offer. Patient inquiries should always be referred to pharmacists, who must actively promote the value of their guidance in selecting and monitoring treatment with a nonprescription drug. It is essen-

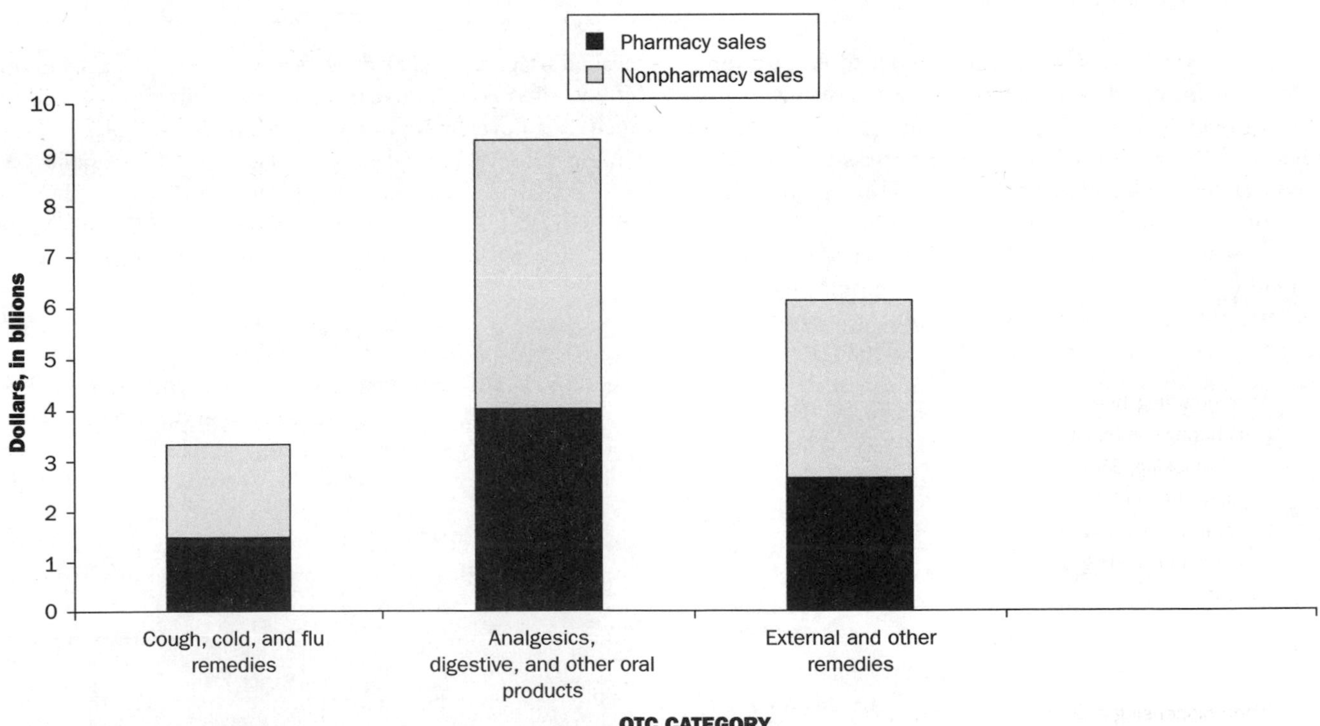

Figure 2–1 Expenditures for nonprescription drugs in 1998.

tial to increase a patient's awareness of the importance of consulting a pharmacist, not only when considering a drug for the first time, but also when making subsequent purchases.

Service, convenience, and price are important considerations in a patient's choice of pharmacy.[9] An analysis of patient use of nondispensing pharmacy services found that, although patients had not used most of the services available, most had obtained advice on nonprescription medications and minor health problems. Patients have ranked providing nonprescription drug information as a very important pharmacy service.[10] Most patients consider pharmacists to be competent and to have a professional relationship with their patients.[11]

Introduction to the Patient Access Process

Hepler and Strand describe the concept of assuming responsibility for achieving definitive drug therapy outcomes that will improve a patient's quality of life.[12] The definition of pharmaceutical care has been further refined as: "a practice in which the practitioner takes responsibility for all of a patient's drug-related needs and is held accountable for this commitment."[8] Three components make up a pharmaceutical care practice: the philosophy of practice, the patient care process, and the practice management system. All three components must be present for a true practice to exist. The reader is referred to *Pharmaceutical Care Practice*, by Cipolle, Strand, and Morley, for a detailed description of these practice components.[8]

The goal when assuming responsibility for all of a patient's drug-related needs is to help the patient achieve intended therapeutic goals and to ensure positive patient outcomes. Drug therapy problems that are identified must be addressed because they can impede progress toward achieving the intended therapeutic goals. A drug therapy problem is defined as any undesirable event that is experienced by the patient, that involves—or is suspected to involve—drug therapy, and that actually or potentially interferes with a desired patient outcome.[13] Drug therapy problems can adversely affect treatment goals and, therefore, must be identified and resolved before creating a plan for achieving those goals and for ensuring positive outcomes. Although each practitioner may execute the process differently, there is only one patient care process in pharmaceutical care.

A systematic, comprehensive, and efficient process must be present to meet this responsibility consistently and completely. The patient care process to meet this objective involves three major steps:[8]

1. Assessing or systematically reviewing the patient's drug-related needs, including identifying any and all drug therapy problems.
2. Creating a care plan or detailed schedule outlining the practitioner's and the patient's activities and responsibilities designed to

   —Resolve any drug therapy problems.
   —Achieve treatment goals.
   —Prevent any potential drug therapy problems.
3. At planned follow-up intervals, having the practitioner evaluate the patient's outcome and current status.

The care plan and evaluation provide the accountability and results or outcomes that are often lacking in the health care delivery system. Table 2–1 presents information to be documented in the assessment, care plan, and evaluation.[8] The following section will focus on conducting an assessment of a patient's drug-related needs, including examples of why an assessment is important.

Assessment of a Patient's Drug-Related Needs

Identifying drug therapy problems is a primary clinical decision-making process for the pharmacist. From a historical perspective, this responsibility represents a significant change in a societal demand that has occurred within a single generation of pharmacists. In the early 1960s, pharmacists were precluded by a code of ethics from providing any information to

Case Examples of Drug-Related Needs

Case Study 1

After browsing briefly in the vitamin aisle of a pharmacy in a neighboring community on Friday afternoon at about 5:00 pm, a healthy-looking, 35-year-old man asks the pharmacist, "What is the best vitamin?" What would happen if the pharmacist directed the man to take the best-selling generic multivitamin with minerals without finding out that he was a 3-day-per-week dialysis patient?

Case Study 2

When dispensing a prescription for erythromycin 333 mg taken 3 times a day for 10 days, a pharmacist instructs a patient to take 1 tablet 3 times daily with food, until the tablets are gone. What would happen if the pharmacist does not find out that the patient is taking an over-the-counter (OTC) terfenadine product that she stockpiled while visiting New Zealand?

Case Study 3

A patient, who is stabilized on warfarin 5 mg daily, walks into her local pharmacy looking for something to help improve her memory. As she presents a bottle for sustained-release Gingko 120 mg capsules to the clerk at the cash register, she mentions that she is glad there are herbal remedies available because most everything else interacts with her "blood thinner."

Table 2–1

Information Included in the Assessment, Care Plan, and Evaluation

Completeness of patient demographics in assessment	● Weight, height, and age (birth date) of patient must be documented to determine appropriateness of drug and dosage selections. ● Current phone number preferred by patient should be recorded to support follow-up contact. ● Current mailing address for each patient should be recorded to facilitate follow-up contact and to support billing systems. ● Insurance carrier should be recorded to support billing processes; if none, write "self," indicating self-pay. ● Allergies to medications or other substances along with any adverse reactions to past medications must be documented to ensure patient safety. ● Alerts describing patient-specific information required to ensure safe and effective drug therapy should be recorded, including alcohol, tobacco, and caffeine use. ● Medical devices needed by the patient, such as canes, wheelchairs, or contact lenses, should be recorded to support patient comfort and safety.
Appropriateness of care plan	● All medications the patient is taking must be documented, including prescription drugs, nonprescription drugs, samples, and others. ● An appropriate indication must be documented for each medication the patient is taking. ● For each medication, the dosage schedule must be documented. ● For each prescription medication, the prescriber should be recorded. ● For each care plan, all drug therapy problems must be documented. ● "None known at this time" is used to document the practitioner's determination that the patient does not have any drug therapy problems. ● For all drug therapy problems identified, when and how each problem was resolved should be documented. ● The specific services provided, including patient consultation and education, should be documented. ● For each patient, mutually agreed-upon directives including follow-up plans must be documented. ● Follow-up dates should be recorded to facilitate follow-up contact to monitor patient progress and outcomes. ● Follow-up dates for a patient's various care plans should be synchronized to ensure that the pharmacist can assess the patient's drug therapy in a comprehensive manner.
Clarity of follow-up evaluation	● For every episode in which pharmaceutical care services are provided, the pharmacist's evaluation of the status of each patient problem and the overall status of the patient must be documented. ● Each evaluation of patient status must be dated, and the initials of the pharmacist making the evaluation must be documented. ● If no comprehensive professional evaluation was made, but the patient's status demands a note in the pharmacy chart, a status "note" should be recorded. ● Written descriptions, explanations, and any other comments germane to the patient's condition or progress should be recorded in a progress note evaluation field.

Source: Page 305 of reference 8; used with permission.

the patient regarding the names or intended actions of prescription medications. The consumer movement of the 1970s and 1980s prompted pharmacists to inform patients of the name, action, and side effects of the medications being dispensed. Today, consumers seek the personal attention of a trusted professional to help them make sense of the deluge of available information in the medication-use process. The rational and ordered process for conducting an assessment helps the pharmacist maintain a disciplined approach when confronted with this rapidly changing societal demand.

The three cases presented in the box "Case Examples of Drug-Related Needs" demonstrate that a systematic assessment of a patient's drug-related needs would resolve or prevent likely drug misadventures and drug-therapy problems.

To identify drug therapy problems, help patients achieve therapeutic goals, and prevent potential drug therapy problems, the pharmacist must establish an efficient method of gathering pertinent information. In the three sample cases presented in the box, the pharmacist must find out, at a minimum, which medications the patients are taking and their intended uses. The pharmacist can then begin to assess (in this order) the indication, effectiveness, safety, and convenience of all medications used to treat each medical condition. This systematic and ordered process leads the pharmacist to determine potential drug therapy problems and to obtain information specific to the needs of each patient. Table 2–2 presents a general outline of the categories of drug therapy problems and their causes.[8]

Table 2–2

Causes of Drug Therapy Problems

Drug Therapy Problem	Possible Causes of Drug Therapy Problem
Indication	
Need for additional drug therapy	The patient has a new medical condition requiring initiation of new drug therapy.
	The patient has a chronic disorder requiring continuation of drug therapy.
	The patient has a medical condition that requires combination pharmacotherapy to attain synergism/potentiation of effects.
	The patient is at risk to develop a new medical condition preventable by using prophylactic drug therapy and/or premedication.
Unnecessary drug therapy	The patient is taking a medication for which there is no valid medical indication at this time.
	The patient accidentally or intentionally ingested a toxic amount of a drug or chemical, resulting in the present illness or condition.
	The patient's medical problem(s) are associated with drug abuse, alcohol use, or smoking.
	The patient's medical condition is better treated with nondrug therapy.
	The patient is taking multiple drugs for a condition for which only single-drug therapy is indicated.
	The patient is taking drug therapy to treat an avoidable adverse reaction associated with another medication.
Effectiveness	
More effective drug	The patient has a medical problem for which this drug is not effective.
	The patient is allergic to this medication.
	The patient is receiving a drug that is not the most effective for the indication being treated.
	The patient has risk factors that contraindicate using this drug.
	The patient is receiving a drug that is effective but not the least costly.
	The patient has an infection involving organisms that are resistant to this drug.
	The patient has become refractory to the present drug therapy.
	The patient is receiving an unnecessary combination product when a single drug would be appropriate.
Dosage too low	The dosage used is too low to produce the desired response for this patient.
	The patient's serum drug concentrations are below the desired therapeutic range.
	Timing of prophylaxis (presurgical antibiotic given too early) was inadequate for this patient.
	Drug, dose, route, or formulation conversions were inadequate for this patient.
	Dose and interval flexibility (insulin sliding scales, "as needed" analgesics) were inadequate for this patient.
	Drug therapy was altered before adequate therapeutic trial for this patient.
Safety	
Adverse drug reaction	The drug was administered too rapidly for this patient.
	The patient is having an allergic reaction to this medication.
	The patient is receiving a drug that is effective but not the safest available agent.
	The patient has identified risk factors that make this drug too dangerous to be used.
	The patient has experienced an idiosyncratic reaction to this drug.
	The bioavailability of the drug is altered because of an interaction with another drug or food the patient is taking.
	The effect of the drug has been altered because of enzyme inhibition/induction from another drug the patient is taking.
	The effect of the drug has been altered because of a substance in the food the patient has been eating.
	The effect of the drug has been altered because of displacement from binding sites by another drug the patient is taking.
	The patient's laboratory test result has been altered because of interference from a drug the patient is taking.

(continued)

Table 2–2

Causes of Drug Therapy Problems (continued)

Drug Therapy Problem	Possible Causes of Drug Therapy Problem
Dose too high	Dosage is too high for this patient.
	The patient's serum drug concentrations are above the desired therapeutic range.
	The patient's drug dose was escalated too rapidly.
	The patient has accumulated drug from chronic administration.
	Drug, dose, route, and formulation conversions were inappropriate for this patient.
	Dose and interval flexibility (insulin sliding scales, "as needed" analgesics) were inappropriate for this patient.
Convenience	
Adherence	The patient did not receive the appropriate drug regimen because a medication error (prescribing, dispensing, administration, monitoring) was made.
	The patient did not comply (adherence) with the recommended directions for using the medication.
	The patient did not take the drug as directed because of the high cost of the product.
	The patient did not take the drug(s) as directed because of a lack of understanding of the directions.
	The patient did not take the drug(s) as directed because it would not be consistent with the patient's health benefits.

Source: Pages 82 and 83 of reference 8; used with permission.

Skills Necessary to Care for Patients with Self-Care Needs

Advising patients on self-treatment is an important part of pharmacy practice and provides the pharmacist with an opportunity to act in the role of primary health care provider. Often the pharmacist is a patient's first contact with the health care system and can both assess the situation and recommend a course of action. This role may include recommending a nonprescription drug, dissuading patients from buying a medication when drug therapy is not indicated, recommending a nondrug treatment, or referring patients to another health care practitioner. If the pharmacist deters healthy people from using more costly health care services or products and refers more seriously ill patients to physicians, health care delivery in the United States can be improved and health care costs can be conserved.

Working with patients to identify their drug-related needs rests at the center of the pharmacist's communication process. A drug-related need is defined as a patient's health care needs that have some relationship to drug therapy and for which the pharmacist is able to offer professional assistance.[8] Patients will tell their story or present a picture (e.g., "when I urinate, I feel as though I am giving birth to a flaming lobster")[14] in a random fashion. It is the practitioner's job to interpret a patient's explicit and implicit needs. This skill is somewhat analogous to throwing a deck of cards into the air and being asked to reassemble the deck by suits.

The ordered process for "reassembling the deck" begins by assessing a patient's current medications, supplements and remedies for indication, effectiveness, safety, and convenience of use. Proceeding systematically in this order is critical so as not to miss an important piece of information or jump to an erroneous conclusion. Patients express their drug-related needs as understanding (or, more accurately, as a lack of understanding), expectations, concerns, and behavior (compliance or noncompliance). The pharmacist must translate a patient's expression of drug-related needs into an assessment of drug therapy problems. Table 2–3 provides a useful reference for translating those needs into drug-therapy problems.[8]

A final determination of drug therapy problems is conducted in consultation and agreement with a patient. Practitioners cannot force their will on patients. For instance, a 54-year-old female who smokes two cigarettes when her

Table 2–3

Translating Drug-Related Needs into Drug Therapy Problems

Patient's Expression	Drug-Related Needs	Drug Therapy Problems
Understanding	Indication	1. Additional drug therapy
		2. Unnecessary drug therapy
Expectations	Effectiveness	3. More effective drug
		4. Dosage too low
Concerns	Safety	5. Adverse drug reaction
		6. Dosage too high
Behavior	Convenience	7. Compliance (adherence)

Source: Page 77 of reference 8; used with permission.

husband conducts business out of town 1 day per month might not believe that she has a drug therapy problem. Classifying this as a drug therapy problem and pushing a smoking cessation intervention onto the patient may be detrimental to the therapeutic relationship.

Communication

Interventions by pharmacists through consultation and effective assessment strategies can enhance patient outcomes. Patients are the most important source of the information that pharmacists need to provide pharmaceutical care related to nonprescription drugs. Each step of the patient-care process involves communicating with patients, gathering information from them, and transmitting information to them. This process is particularly important during the assessment step because these data form the basis for the care plan and subsequent follow-up evaluation. Good communication between pharmacists and patients requires that pharmacists have effective communication skills.[15,16] Discussion of some of these communication skills follows.

Interaction between the pharmacist and patient establishes a therapeutic relationship, which is a partnership between the patient and the practitioner formed to identify the patient's drug-related needs. It is characterized by trust, empathy, respect, authenticity, and responsiveness.[8] This relationship allows the pharmacist to gather detailed, sometimes intimate, information from patients. In return, patients rely on the pharmacist to use knowledge, skills, and experience to ensure safe and effective drug therapy. Scheduled patient follow-up and reassessment are vital components of this therapeutic relationship and are used to determine actual patient outcome and progress towards meeting therapeutic objectives. These components allow a pharmacist to reassess whether a patient is experiencing drug therapy problems.

The patient–pharmacist relationship is dynamically affected by numerous variables. A positive interaction one day could be followed by a negative interaction a few days later for reasons unrelated to the pharmacist's care (e.g., loss of employment, marital turmoil, a cloudy day). The pharmacist must become adept at searching for and interpreting nonverbal cues (e.g., facial expression or body position), as well as at responding to voice tones, inflection, and mood. If a patient is experiencing a drug therapy problem but does not have the time or inclination to deal with it during the current encounter, the pharmacist must try to schedule an alternative time to gather additional information in order to assess the problem and determine an appropriate intervention. The potential severity of a drug therapy problem will dictate the timetable for this intervention.

General Principles of Communication

To establish an effective patient–pharmacist relationship, the pharmacist must be a capable and empathetic source of information. Because the pharmacist's underlying attitude toward the patient will influence the quality of communication, the effective pharmacist must eliminate barriers by avoiding biases toward a patient's level of education, socioeconomic or cultural background, interests, or attitude. In addition, the pharmacist must assure patients that any information they discuss will be strictly confidential.

A first step in a patient encounter is to assess what the patient already knows and to determine where gaps in knowledge exist. This step is important because patients may resent being told what they already know and, simultaneously, may be confused if the pharmacist wrongly assumes that patients understand more than they do. When interacting with patients, the pharmacist should use words that a layperson can understand.

Effective communication occurs when the receiver of a message hears and understands exactly what the sender wishes to communicate. One way to ensure understanding is through active listening, a process in which the receiver repeats the information back to the sender. As information is exchanged, the participants change roles as receivers and senders of information. The message received is influenced by its content and context, as well as by how it is sent. Pharmacists can improve communication by paying attention to the interaction between sender and receiver.

Effective Questioning Skillful questioning is the mark of a good communicator. Patients should feel that the pharmacist's questions convey a genuine interest in them and a desire to help. Because a patient may be uncooperative if the questions suggest only superficial curiosity, the pharmacist should explain the reason for asking personal questions (e.g., "I need additional information so I can select a product for your specific problem"). It is important to avoid cutting off the patient in the middle of a response, which can occur when a busy pharmacist is thinking ahead to the next question without adequately processing the current response.

The pharmacist should start the patient encounter by stating, "My name is ________, and I'm the pharmacist." The pharmacist should begin the exchange with an open-ended question such as, "How can I help you?" or "Would you please tell me more about the symptoms/problems you have?" Such valuable open-ended questions allow for increased flexibility and provide greater information than will questions that can be answered with only yes or no. Such open-ended questions enable a good practitioner to collect information faster and to establish better communication. If a patient's response wanders, however, the pharmacist must keep the interaction focused. To be sure that a patient understands dosage instructions, the pharmacist could ask, "So I know that I haven't forgotten to tell you anything, would you please tell me how you plan to take this medicine?"

Summarizing the important points or redirecting the interaction with a specific, closed-ended question can sometimes be useful. A question such as, "How long have you had this pain?" may help the pharmacist to gather specific information or to clarify information obtained through earlier open-ended questions. It is important to ask one question at a time; asking two questions in rapid succession or multiple-choice questions will cause confusion and restrict communication. It is also important to avoid leading questions or judgmental questions such as "Surely you've given up smoking, haven't you?"

Effective Listening Effective listening is a vital component of communication. When the pharmacist really listens, patients are free to state their problem completely and are assured of receiving the pharmacist's undivided attention. The pharmacist must focus on the patient and exclude distractions such as a telephone or a computer screen. The pharmacist may need to clarify the details of a patient's problem and should be receptive to a patient's response to questions. The pharmacist should respond with empathy, perhaps by paraphrasing a patient's words or by reflecting on what was said in terms of the patient's own experience. For instance, after listening to a complaint of pain, the pharmacist could say, "You have a sharp, stabbing pain in your wrist; is that right?" and end with a statement such as "That must be very uncomfortable." Interrupting or demonstrating disinterest or disapproval may inhibit a patient's discussion of problems and concerns. Encouraging a patient to talk, exploring a patient's comments, and expressing understanding will all facilitate communication. The pharmacist should reinforce correct decisions a patient has made while reserving judgment and should communicate warmth, understanding, and interest in the patient's concerns.

Nonverbal Communication

Nonverbal communication skills are important when conducting an assessment. A pharmacist's body language, such as posture and facial expression, communicates strong, direct messages. Pharmacists should be aware of their own nonverbal behavior as well as that of the patient. An open body posture—facing the patient with arms and legs uncrossed—indicates openness, honesty, and a willingness to communicate and listen. Maintaining an appropriate distance from a patient will facilitate confidential communication without making patients uncomfortable. If a patient backs away or moves closer, the pharmacist should maintain the new distance that the patient has established. Pharmacists should maintain eye contact with a patient and control their facial expressions to avoid showing negative emotions such as disapproval or shock.

The patient's nonverbal communication is equally important. If a patient has a closed body posture—arms crossed, legs crossed, body turned away from the pharmacist—the pharmacist may need to find out why the patient is uncomfortable and then try to allay any concerns. The pharmacist should watch a patient's facial expressions for signs of anxiety, nervousness, and physical symptoms such as pain.

Physical Barriers to Communication

High counters, glass separators, and elevated platforms inhibit communication and provide physical barriers. Pharmacists should try to be at eye level with their patients. A tall pharmacist may need to sit on a stool or lower his or her body position to avoid "hovering over" the patient. Discussions between patient and pharmacist should be as private and uninterrupted as possible. If the pharmacist expects or perceives that a patient is uncomfortable discussing the problem, a quiet or private consultation area should be sought and used. Ideally, a specific, private area of the pharmacy should be designated for patient consultations.

Communication Techniques for Special Populations

Special communication techniques may be required with some patients.[17,18] Writing or word processing the information to provide a quality copy may be necessary if the patient is deaf or hearing impaired. If a hearing-impaired patient reads lips, the pharmacist should be physically close to and directly in front of the patient, and should maintain eye contact while speaking. The pharmacist should speak slowly and distinctly in a low-pitched, moderately toned voice because yelling further distorts the sound and might embarrass the patient. A quiet, well-lit environment is essential because background noise and dimness can markedly diminish a hearing-impaired individual's ability to communicate. The pharmacist should use visual reinforcement, such as pointing to the part of the body that hurts or to the directions on a container. In planning for follow-up evaluation, the pharmacist should consider the fact that these patients will benefit from written or in-person follow-up rather than a telephone call.

When interacting with a patient who is blind or visually impaired, the pharmacist should first state, "I am the pharmacist." Because a patient who is blind cannot perceive most nonverbal communication, the pharmacist should depend on tone of voice and verbal feedback to convey empathy and interest in the patient's problem. If touching seems appropriate, the pharmacist should first ask the patient if it would be acceptable to do so.

Up to 20% of Americans are functionally illiterate.[19] For these patients, written information or directions on a label are barriers and cannot be relied on to reinforce information provided verbally by the pharmacist. Patients with reading impairments may be less inclined to ask questions or express their concerns. Therefore, the pharmacist must build a caring relationship to provide effective communication and consultation.[20] The pharmacist can facilitate communication by using simple language and pictorial labels.

Language and cultural barriers to communication may exist among some ethnic minorities.[21] For patients who are unable to communicate well in English, pharmacists may have to demonstrate proper medication use (e.g., eye drops, inhalers) and to develop visual aids (e.g., pictorial labels, illustrated pamphlets) or pamphlets in the patient's language. Pharmacists may ask questions related to cultural beliefs to assess how these beliefs may influence the patient's use of medications. Similarly, cultural behaviors may result in failure to make eye contact and should not be interpreted as lack of interest or understanding.

The Patient Consultation

Interacting with a patient about self-treatment is a primary care activity that carries with it a great professional responsibility. Patients with self-care needs present differently from patients who have been to a physician, where a treatment decision has already been made. In the past, when faced with a question such as "What product do you recommend for allergies?" the pharmacist may have considered the appropriate response as pointing out the best-selling allergy product. Today, pharmacists need to perform an assessment by eliciting information from the patient, integrating these data to determine if any drug therapy problems exist, and then developing a patient care plan.

The initial interaction can be initiated either by the patient or the pharmacist. (See Figure 2–2.) Although the patient often initiates the consultation, an increasing number of pharmacists greet patients entering the self-care section of the practice and initiate an assessment of the patient's self-care needs. The patient may approach the pharmacist with a symptom, often in the form of a question such as "What do you recommend for . . . ?" Or the patient may ask a product-related question such as "Which of these two products do you recommend?"

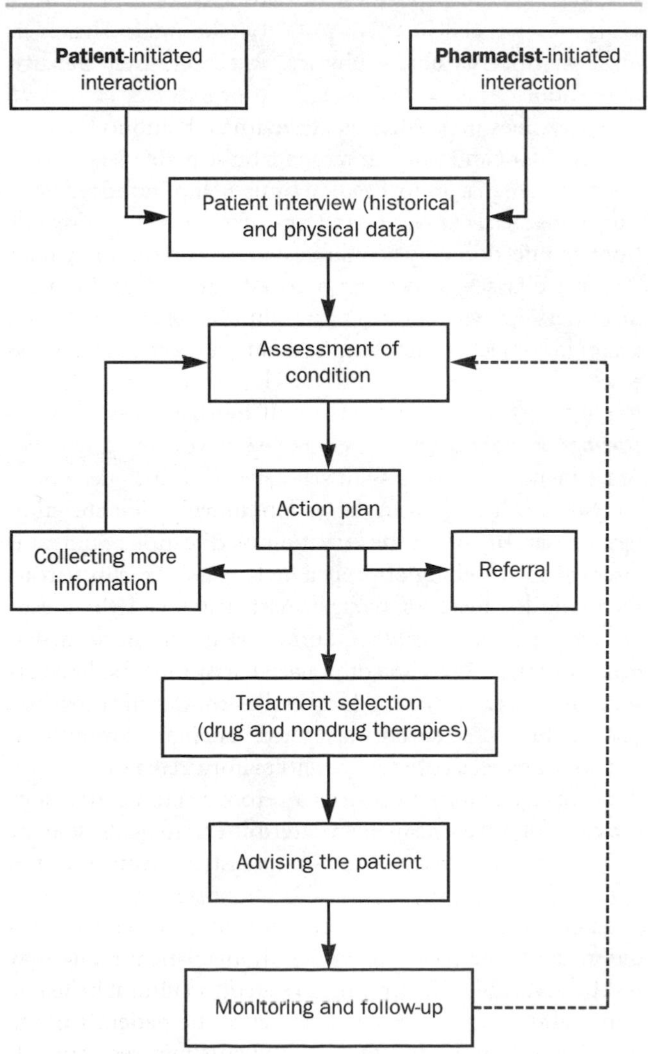

Figure 2–2 Patient–pharmacist consultation process.

Information Gathering Process

Before formulating a plan for self-treatment or physician referral, the pharmacist must obtain enough information to identify and assess the patient's medical and drug therapy problem. Important data include the patient's perceived needs and concerns, demographics (i.e., patient-related variables), diseases, medications, and a review of systems.[8] A verbal review of the patient's physiologic systems, from head to toe, can help the practitioner account for all of a patient's drug-related needs.

Other important information is an accurate accounting of each medication a patient is using to treat all medical conditions. This list includes prescription, nonprescription, and herbal products; vitamins; and dietary supplements. The pharmacist should have the patient's medication profile available at the start of the patient consultation.

The pharmacist can explain the need to review all medications by saying, "I would like to review each of the medications you are currently taking so that the medication we select (or is prescribed) for you fits with your current regimen. Here is a list of medications you have received at our pharmacy. Let's take a minute to see which ones you are currently taking, as well as what other medications you may be using." It may be helpful for the pharmacist to have a patient describe his or her daily activities and medication schedule.

When an accurate picture of the patient's active medication list has been attained, the pharmacist should tie all active medications to each of the patient's medical conditions. A patient's drug allergies and relative medical history may be taken at this point. The assessment process is dictated by the patient's knowledge level, as well as by the amount of time available to continue the interaction. Thus, to obtain the needed information quickly and efficiently, the pharmacist should approach the problem logically and should keep the questioning direct and to the point. With experience, the pharmacist will be able to gather the necessary information to assess a particular condition within a few minutes.

Fortunately, within the context of providing pharmaceutical care, the pharmacist need not try to obtain all relevant information in one encounter. The planned follow-up evaluation extends the initial assessment process and allows the pharmacist to obtain additional information. The weight of a 10-month-old child, the smoking history of a patient with emphysema, the allergy history of a patient with a sinus infection, and the calcium intake of a postmenopausal woman are examples of information that may be important during the patient encounter but that may be obtained during the follow-up evaluation. With continual practice, the pharmacist will learn to use every patient encounter to gather whatever additional information is needed. The pharmacist will develop a sense, based on the patient's expression of needs, for when to bring the initial assessment to a close and how to establish appropriate follow-up.

The Patient History

A broad overview of a patient's health enables the pharmacist to identify the condition that a patient seeks to treat and to make the most appropriate recommendation, which may or may not include a drug. Pharmacists should start out by determining a patient's needs with an open-ended question such as "How may I help you?" Patients may initially present incomplete and vague information. To determine what the specific symptoms are and whether they are amenable to self-treatment, the pharmacist can ask the following open-ended questions:

- Please describe your problem.
- When did the problem start?
- How long does it last? Does it come and go, or is it continuous?
- How does the problem limit your daily activities (sleeping, eating, working, walking, etc.)?
- Is this a new problem, or is it the recurrence or worsening of an old one? What other problems occur concurrently?
- What food, drug, and/or physical activity make the problem worse?
- Does anything you do relieve the problem? What has relieved it in the past?
- What has been done so far to treat the problem?

The next step is to gather patient-specific data, including demographic information and medical history. The pharmacist should selectively elicit the following information:

- Who is the patient? Is the patient the person in the pharmacy or someone else?
- How old is the patient?
- Is the patient male or female? If the patient is female, is she pregnant or breast-feeding?
- Does the patient have any other medical problems that may alter the expected effects of a nonprescription drug or may be aggravated by the drug's effects? Is the complaint related to a chronic illness?
- Does the patient have any allergies?
- Is the patient on a special diet? Does the patient have special nutritional requirements?
- Is the patient using any prescription, nonprescription, or social drugs (e.g., vitamins or food supplements, caffeine, nicotine, alcohol, or marijuana)? How long has the patient been taking those drugs?
- Has the patient experienced adverse drug reactions in the past?
- Who is responsible for administering medication (the patient or a caregiver)?

Throughout the encounter, the pharmacist is formulating a hypothesis based on identifying actual or potential drug-therapy problems. The pharmacist should determine whether the patient has misinterpreted the condition, done any harm by waiting to seek advice, or worsened the condition by previous attempts at self-treatment.

Observed Physical Data

Besides the historical data, physical data are helpful in assessing a medical problem. Physical data include pulse rate, heart sounds, respiration rate, age, and weight. Pharmacists routinely collect physical data, and some have acquired additional skills that have expanded their ability to assess and monitor patients' medical conditions. Depending on training and skills, the pharmacist can collect physical data by all or some of the following techniques: observation or inspection, palpation or manipulations, percussion, and auscultation. The importance of each technique in the process of data collection depends on the body system involved. For example, the skin is easily assessed by inspection and palpation, the lungs require percussion and auscultation, and all four skills are essential in examining the abdomen. However, most pharmacists obtain physical data exclusively through observation.

Many clues to a patient's general health and to the seriousness of a condition can come from simple observation. The degree of discomfort caused by pain may be judged from a patient's facial expressions or lack of use of a limb. Toxicity from an infection may be manifested by lethargy and pallor. The pharmacist would need to inspect the patient's skin before offering advice about a skin rash, which may result from a simple contact phenomenon or may suggest systemic disease.

Patient Assessment

Assessment of a patient with self-care needs includes evaluating data collected from the patient to determine the etiology and severity of the medical condition. This assessment is essential for reaching appropriate conclusions about treatment and the need for referral. Assessing severity will vary depending on the problem. Some conditions, such as diabetes with hyperglycemia or polyuria, may be considered severe only when they reach certain levels. Other conditions may be considered severe only when patients become symptomatic or when a patient's activity is impaired. For instance, the pharmacist may elect not to recommend a cough suppressant for a patient with an intermittent cough unless the cough is nonproductive and is keeping the patient awake at night.

Many times, however, the etiology and severity of a condition cannot be conclusively determined because data may not be accessible. Referral may be required when available information suggests that a certain etiology is responsible or that a condition may be particularly severe. For example, an acutely inflamed joint that is swollen, warm to the touch, tender, and painful may be caused by trauma, bacterial infection, gout, or rheumatoid arthritis. Because a final assessment may require examination of the joint fluid, such a patient should be referred to a physician. In general, the more severe the problem, the greater is the potential for referral.

Elderly patients, infants, children, patients with chronic diseases such as diabetes or renal or heart disease, patients with multiple medical conditions, those taking multiple medications, recently hospitalized patients, and patients who are receiving treatment from several physicians are at greater risk for complications and require more careful evaluation.

Care Plan Development

After collecting all available information and assessing the patient's condition, the pharmacist must formulate a care plan. A care plan is a detailed schedule that outlines the practitioner's and patient's activities and responsibilities.[8] Its structure is for two individuals, the patient and the practitioner, to work together to achieve common goals.

A care plan is constructed for three different purposes:

1. Resolve drug therapy problems identified during the assessment.
2. Meet the goals for each of the patient's medical conditions.
3. Prevent future drug therapy problems from developing.

Often, the pharmacist may create a care plan without having all desired information. Areas of uncertainty will most likely exist, but a well-considered plan can help ensure proper management of the patient. A sound care plan for a patient with self-care needs will most likely pay careful attention to the following five specific areas:

1. Collect additional information.
2. Select physician referral.
3. Select self-treatment.
4. Advise the patient about self-treatment.
5. Maintain follow-up contact.

Collecting Additional Information

The pharmacist may need more information to assess the patient's condition, which may require specific action such as either talking to a parent/caregiver or calling a physician. Communication between the pharmacist and the physician is often desirable to avoid conflict in managing the patient and to overcome problems of overlapping responsibilities. When such communication becomes necessary, the pharmacist must do the following:

- Obtain data on preexisting medical conditions to determine whether self-treatment is appropriate.
- Determine whether the physician wants to address the problem over the telephone with the patient.
- Determine whether the physician wants to see the patient, or whether the patient should be referred to an urgent care center or a hospital emergency department.
- Provide information on the reason for referral.

Selecting Physician Referral

When enough information is available to assess the condition, the pharmacist must decide whether to refer the patient to a physician or advise self-treatment. If the plan involves physician referral, the pharmacist must consider both the type of treatment center to which the patient will be referred (physician's office or emergency care facility) and the urgency for treatment. Some conditions do not require the immediate attention or extensive evaluation of emergency care treatment.

When advising a patient to see a physician, the pharmacist should discuss with the patient why the referral is being made. The pharmacist must use tact and firmness so that the patient is not unnecessarily frightened but is convinced of the need for concern. Referral to a physician is indicated in any of the following situations:

- The symptoms are too severe to be endured by the patient without definitive diagnosis and treatment.
- The symptoms are minor but have persisted and do not appear to be the result of some easily identifiable cause.
- The symptoms have repeatedly returned for no readily recognizable cause.
- The pharmacist is in doubt about the patient's medical condition.

Selecting Self-Treatment

Advising self-treatment requires the pharmacist to consider several factors. First, the pharmacist must identify a measurable and achievable therapeutic objective that is based on the condition and the patient. A therapeutic modality—either drug or nondrug—may then be recommended. For example, the objective in a patient who has a productive cough but is having difficulty producing sputum would be to increase sputum production. Thus, an expectorant would be the agent of choice. However, for a patient with a dry, nonproductive cough, the therapeutic objective may be to suppress the cough, in which case a cough suppressant would be selected. Choosing a specific treatment requires reviewing drug variables (e.g., dosage forms, ingredients, side effects, adverse reactions, relative effectiveness, price) and matching them with patient variables (e.g., age, sex, drug history, other physiologic problems, ability to pay).

Should self-treatment without drugs be indicated, selection of the nondrug modality would similarly be modified using patient variables. For example, the pharmacist may recommend that a patient with vomiting and diarrhea only drink fluids for a 24-hour period to provide bowel rest. However, if the patient has insulin-dependent diabetes, the pharmacist must modify this recommendation because patients with diabetes must maintain a specific caloric intake. Communicating with the physician about modifying the dose of insulin is necessary in this situation because of the change in caloric intake.

To measure the success of treatment, the pharmacist should set goals and measurement parameters that are based on the therapeutic objective, the toxic or adverse effects of treatment, the nature and severity of the condition, and the patient's ability to understand the condition and its treatment. The objectives in treating sinusitis with decongestants, for example, are to facilitate drainage and relieve symptoms such as headache. Achievement of the first objective can be determined by observing or asking about the nature of nasal discharge (e.g., quantity, color, viscosity); achievement of the second, by simply asking about the headache. Indices of toxicity are those symptoms associated with an excessive dose or an untoward reaction. The pharmacist should identify indices that suggest the problem may be worsening and may require special attention. Finally, indices relating to the patient's understanding the condition and its treatment can include determining the appropriateness of the patient's questions to the pharmacist as well as the patient's response to the pharmacist's queries.

Advising a Patient on Self-Treatment

The fourth area in the action plan is to advise the patient about self-treatment. The primary purposes are to educate the patient and obtain the consent necessary to enact the plan. Specifically, the pharmacist should give advice in the following areas:

- Reasons for self-treatment.
- Description of the drug and/or treatment.
- Administration of the drug and/or treatment.
- Side effects and precautions.
- General treatment guidelines.

Reference 2 is a tool to help pharmacists consult with patients regarding self-treatment decisions.[2] These drug treatment protocols can help pharmacists transition their practices toward pharmaceutical care and can serve as a guide for pharmacists to institute more sophisticated self-treatment counseling. The protocols help determine exclusions to self-care, identify patient-related variables that affect recommendations, suggest drug and nondrug therapies, provide recommendations, and suggest follow-up intervals. Self-care protocols are available for the common cold, constipation, cough, self-limited pain, and sun protection.

In advising the patient about a suggested treatment plan, the pharmacist should summarize the patient's condition, explain the significance of the symptoms, and outline the reasons for treatment. The pharmacist should clearly explain the therapeutic objectives and a realistic time frame for achieving the objectives. If the patient desires information on alternative treatments, the pharmacist should be prepared to present such information about their relative merits and drawbacks without biasing the information and jeopardizing the patient–physician relationship. The pharmacist should then discuss the nonprescription drugs selected, describing both the therapeutic action of the ingredients (e.g., decongestants, antihistamines, or laxatives) in lay terms and the effect the products will have on the patient's symptoms and condition. The pharmacist should inform the patient about the available dosage forms and the availability of any generic product.

The pharmacist should explain administration guidelines clearly and concisely. Because many patients may remember only part of the information, some thought should be given to deciding what is most important for the patient to remember. Covering a few of the most important points is better than overwhelming a patient with a lot of information. Additionally, patients will remember dosage instructions better if administration is linked to specific times of the day rather than just assigned "three times daily." Having a patient review normal daily activities will help establish the best times to take the medication. It is also important to include information about the duration of treatment.

The patient should be told about the most common side effects or adverse reactions associated with a drug and should be instructed on how to manage them. The pharmacist should discuss special warnings about activities, other drugs, foods, or beverages that should be avoided, as well as about the patient's medical conditions that may be complicated by use of the drug. Information should be written down if it is extensive or complex.

The pharmacist should offer to the patient some general treatment guidelines that may be helpful in managing the condition. These guidelines might include lifestyle changes, additional products or services, informational sources, and a list of signs and symptoms that indicate whether the drug is working, whether it is causing adverse effects, and when a physician's advice is needed. The patient should be told what the normal response time is to the treatment, what time is required for the condition to resolve, and what to do if response is delayed.

Evaluating the Progress

The final area in the patient care process is a follow-up evaluation. Evaluation is defined as the practitioner's determination—at planned intervals of follow-up—of the patient's outcome and current status.[8] The purpose of the evaluation is to determine whether previous drug therapy problems have been resolved, to evaluate the patient's progress toward therapeutic goals, and to assess whether new problems have developed from the drug therapy.

Documentation systems used by practitioners should include an evaluation of outcomes for each of the patient's medical conditions and a resolution status of drug therapy problems. Practitioners typically include progress notes in a patient's pharmaceutical care chart after each patient encounter. Evaluation notes help practitioners convey important aspects of the patient's care in a clear and concise manner to fellow practitioners.

Aspects of patient care that pharmaceutical care practitioners convey, in written format, may include the patient's expression of drug-related needs, goals of therapy, monitoring parameters, assessment of drug therapy problems, and a plan for resolving and preventing drug therapy problems and achieving treatment goals. An evaluation note can take on an appearance similar to the SOAP (*S*ubjective, *O*bjective, *A*ssessment, *P*lan) format used in medicine for the Problem-Oriented Medical Record system. Within pharmaceutical care, the practitioner assumes responsibility for all of a patient's drug-related needs within each of the patient's medical conditions.

Maintaining Follow-up Contact

Follow-up allows the pharmacist to determine whether self-treatment has resulted in an appropriate therapeutic response and whether the patient has used medications appropriately or experienced any drug therapy problems, including drug-related toxicity. On follow-up, the pharmacist may determine the need to reassess the patient's drug therapy and may either modify or develop a new patient care plan. The pharmacist should decide whether active monitoring and follow-up are necessary and, if they are, should arrange a follow-up plan. The pharmacist may either tell the patient to call after an appropriate time interval or inform the patient that the pharmacist will make a follow-up contact.

Some problems encountered by the pharmacist do not need follow-up. However, the patient should be encouraged to check back if the condition does not improve within a specific period of time or if problems with the medication develop. To this end, the pharmacist might state, "Please let me know whether you feel better in a couple of days," or, "If your cough is not better in a few days, you should see your physician. Be sure to tell your physician that you have been taking this medicine."

Follow-up provides feedback that allows pharmacists to assess whether their communication skills require modification and whether useful information has been provided. At the same time, the patient will sense that the pharmacist cares. The pharmacist's concern for the correct use of nonprescription drugs will also reinforce the notion that these products are drugs and must be used carefully.

Pharmaceutical Care for High-Risk and Special Groups

Four specific groups of patients—pediatric patients, elderly persons, pregnant patients, and nursing mothers—may experience a higher incidence of drug therapy problems than other patients. Because such problems could have dire consequences, these "high-risk" patients require special attention. Awareness of the physiologic state, possible pathologic conditions, and social context of these patients is necessary to properly assess their medical conditions and recommend treatment.

These special populations are addressed in some of the APhA drug treatment protocols.[2] One protocol, "Self-Care for Sun Protection," excludes infants younger than 6 months from self-treatment and has specific recommendations for children ages 6 months to 12 years. "Self-Care of Self-Limited Pain" provides preferred nonprescription analgesics and lists drugs that should be used with caution in pregnant patients or in children with influenza symptoms. "Self-Care of the Common Cold" indicates some nonpharmacologic measures to consider, especially for young children and pregnant women. "Self-Care of Cough" provides cautions on the use of oral codeine in young children with recommendations for the use of a medication-dispensing device for use in children younger than 6 years. Caution is advised, for example, in breast-feeding women and in patients ages 60 years or older who intend to use diphenhydramine.

In many respects, geriatric and pediatric patients require surprisingly similar considerations. Both groups share a need for drug dosages that are different from those for other age groups because of the following:

- They have altered pharmacokinetic parameters.
- Their ability to cope with illness or drug side effects is decreased because of physiologic changes associated with either normal aging or child development.
- Their patterns of judgment are impaired because of either altered sensory function or immaturity.
- They have different drug effects that are unique to their age groups.
- They have adverse drug effects that are unique to their age groups.
- They have a need for special consideration in administering medications.

Yet, because each of these four groups of patients is heterogeneous, it is important to consider these features for each individual patient.

Pediatric Patients

A study of the prevalence of nonprescription drug use in 3-year-old children found that 53.7% were given some nonprescription drugs within the past 3 months. The most commonly used medications were acetaminophen and cough or cold products.[22] In considering nonprescription drugs for the pediatric age group, the pharmacist should note that the pediatric population may vary substantially among age groups. It is appropriate to differentiate among relatively distinctive pediatric ages as follows:[23,24]

- *Premature*: gestational age of less than 36 weeks.
- *Neonate*: first postnatal month of life.
- *Infant (baby)*: ages 1 to 12 months.
- *Toddler*: ages 1 to 3 years.
- *Preschool or early childhood*: ages 3 to 6 years.
- *Middle childhood*: ages 6 to 12 years.
- *Adolescence*: ages 13 to 18 years.

Package labeling often discourages self-medication without medical evaluation in children younger than 1 or 2 years. For most products, the Food and Drug Administration (FDA) recommends against self-medication in children younger than 2 years. Some package labeling provides dosage guidelines by age group rather than by weight.

Physiologic Differences

Pediatric patients are at risk for drug therapy problems because their body and organ functions are in a continuous state of development. Whereas hepatic metabolism and renal elimination of drugs are usually slower in neonates and young infants, they improve rapidly over the first year of life. Additionally, children metabolize some drugs more rapidly than adults do. Illness in children is potentially more serious than in adults because their physiologic state is less tolerant of changes. Children are susceptible to fluid loss, so fever, vomiting, or diarrhea represent greater potential risks to them. Therefore, the pharmacist should consider physician referral after a shorter duration of a condition in a child than in an adult with the same condition.

Effects of Altered Drug Pharmacokinetics

The pharmacokinetic properties of drugs (e.g., absorption, distribution, metabolism, elimination) in pediatric patients may be quite different from those seen in adults, and those properties may vary significantly in pediatric age periods.

Absorption The gastrointestinal (GI) absorption of drugs is influenced by many factors, including gastric pH, gastric emptying time, motility of the GI tract, enzymatic activity, blood flow/perfusion of the GI mucosa, permeability and maturation of the mucosal membrane, and concurrent disease process.[25,26] Significant changes in these factors occur during the first few years of life.

The pH of the stomach changes significantly during the first few months of life. At birth, the pH is higher, ranging from 6 to 8.[24] It decreases rapidly to between 1 and 3 within a few days, then slowly increases during the next few weeks.[25] The gastric acidity then falls slowly until adult values are reached at about ages 2 or 3 years.[25,26] Changes in pH affect the absorption of drugs that are weak acids and weak bases. The higher gastric pH early in life increases absorption of some drugs such as penicillin and ampicillin but decreases absorption of acetaminophen, phenobarbital, and phenytoin.[25]

Gastric emptying in neonates and infants is prolonged and reaches adult values after 6 to 8 months.[25,27] Intestinal transit time is initially prolonged in neonates, but intestinal motility increases within several months, leading to variable and unpredictable drug absorption.

Bile acids and pancreatic enzymes are both reduced in newborns. The effect is most noticeable in the absorption of lipid-soluble drugs such as vitamins D and E.[28]

Disease states can have a pronounced effect on drug absorption. Pediatric patients with previous GI surgery may have a shortened intestinal length, which results in decreased bioavailability of a drug. Infantile diarrhea and gastroenteritis also decrease transit time, leading to lower absorption of drugs.[29]

Distribution The distribution of a drug in the body is most often expressed in terms of its volume of distribution (Vd). A higher Vd means that more drug is concentrated in other areas of the body (e.g., fat, muscle, body water) than in the blood.

Several differences in pediatric patients affect the distribution of drugs when compared with that in adults.[30] One major factor in determining the distribution of water-soluble drugs is total body water (TBW), which represents the relationship of body water to total body weight. In adults, water makes up about 55% of total body weight. However, neonates have a much higher Vd because their TBW is about 75%, which decreases rapidly in the first year of life. Adult values are reached by about age 12 years.[31] Water-soluble drugs such as aspirin, phenobarbital, and theophylline have lower serum concentrations for a given milligram-per-kilogram dose in a neonate or infant than for the same milligram-per-kilogram dose in an adult.[24,26]

The changes in body fat with age are just the opposite. A full-term infant will have an average of 12% body fat. This percentage increases with age to about 21% and 33%, respectively, in adult males and females.[30]

Plasma protein binding is another important parameter in the Vd of a drug. The higher the amount of drug bound to plasma proteins, the lower the amount of "free" drug is available to exert a pharmacologic action. Drugs such as aspirin, phenobarbital, phenytoin, and theophylline have lower protein binding in neonates and infants than in adults; adult values occur at about age 1 year.[32] Lowered protein binding is a result of decreased serum proteins and of a decreased drug affinity for binding to proteins.[25] Drugs that have a high degree of protein binding exert a greater effect in younger age groups because of the relatively low quantities of binding proteins.

Metabolism The metabolism of drugs is primarily the responsibility of the liver. The liver handles drugs in one of two ways: (1) by changing the structure of the drug through oxidation, reduction, demethylation, or hydrolysis or (2) by conjugating the drug molecule to make it more water-soluble. Nonconjugating reactions are primarily the function of mixed-function oxidase systems (cytochrome P-450). The activity of these enzymatic systems remains low in neonates, and each hepatic metabolic process matures at a different rate. This delayed maturation of metabolic processes makes it difficult to characterize the elimination of drugs undergoing biotransformations, but the metabolic processes begin in neonates at 20% of the adult activity level.[25] Conjugating reactions are even more variable and probably slower to mature in developing neonates and infants. Glucuronidation does not approach adult values until about ages 1.5 to 2.0 years.[25] Examples of drugs with reduced metabolism in newborns include acetaminophen, diazepam, phenobarbital, phenytoin, and salicylates.[32]

Once the metabolic function of the liver matures, it may actually exceed the adult capacity to metabolize drugs on a milligram-per-kilogram-per-day basis. This increased capacity probably occurs because the liver weighs proportionately more in children than it does in adults, which creates a higher relative metabolic surface area.[33] Theophylline doses are higher in children because of an increased rate of metabolism.

Excretion/Elimination Excretion or elimination is primarily the function of the kidneys; this process also undergoes significant age-related changes. At birth, the glomerular filtration rate (GFR) is approximately 30% that of adults.[26] Lower doses are required for drugs with reduced renal elimination, such as acetaminophen and salicylates, as well as for antibiotics, such as aminoglycosides and penicillins.[32] In contrast, newborns require higher doses of thiazide diuretics because of low GFR and tubular function.[32] GFR increases significantly in the first 2 weeks of life and reaches adult values by ages 6 to 12 months.[26] Therefore, drugs eliminated primarily by glomerular filtration require special dosage considerations during this period. Renal tubular secretion and reabsorption also mature with age but at a rate slightly slower than GFR.[27]

Other Potential Drug Therapy Problems

The pharmacist should be sensitive to the potential for drug therapy problems among children. In some illnesses such as diarrhea, nondrug therapy is often more appropriate than therapy with nonprescription antidiarrheal drugs. In some situations, specific drugs are contraindicated; for example, aspirin should not be administered to young children with certain viral illnesses because of its association with Reye's syndrome. (See Chapter 4, "Fever.") A 1994 survey[22] found that aspirin was still being used in this population despite publicity and warnings. Pharmacists should counsel parents of children and adolescents with febrile viral illnesses against using aspirin. For younger children, solid dosage forms are inappropriate, and the pharmacist will need to guide parents to liquid medications or chewable tablets.

Inaccurate Dosing Inaccurate dosing is another potential problem. Labeling on nonprescription drugs generally uses age-based guidelines for determining dosages; however, many products do not provide dosage information for children younger than 6 years. Following the nonprescription drug's label instructions for dosing a child older than 6 years can result in too high a dose and potential toxicity for the younger child. Inaccurate dosing by parents can result from determining an incorrect dose from the label instructions, by measuring out an incorrect amount, or both. A study of 100 caregivers found that only 40% were able to select the correct acetaminophen dose, and only 43% measured out a correct amount for their child.[34] Both a correct dose and an accurately measured dose were demonstrated by only 30% of caregivers. Pharmacists must better educate parents about dosing and administering nonprescription drugs by helping parents interpret labels and by demonstrating the appropriate use of measuring devices.

Children require a larger milligram-per-kilogram dose for some drugs than adults do because they metabolize the drugs more rapidly. Body surface area may be the best measure because it correlates well with all the body parameters, but body surface area is not easily determined. Because nonprescription medications have a wide therapeutic index (the ratio of the toxic dose to the therapeutic dose), safe doses may generally be determined by weight. Average weight at different ages appears in Table 2–4.[35]

Improper Administration Selecting the proper drug and dosage is of no benefit unless the medication is administered. Proper administration of medications to pediatric patients requires an appreciation of dosage forms, delivery methodology, routes of administration, palatability, and other factors. The discussion that follows focuses on oral medications.

Liquids are relatively easy to administer, and the dose can be titrated to the patient's weight; therefore, liquid medications are often used in pediatric populations. Because elixirs and syrups can have a high alcohol and sugar content, respectively, these liquid forms may be less desirable than suspensions and solutions. A suspension may also mask the disagreeable taste of a drug.

Problems with drug administration can result in the child's receiving the wrong dose. In a mock dosing scenario in which caregivers had the choice of teaspoons, tablespoons, syringes, droppers, measuring cups, and measuring tubes,

Table 2–4

Average Pediatric Weight by Age Groupings

	Average Weight	
Age	**Pounds**	**Kilograms**[a]
Birth	7.3	3.3
6 months	17.0	7.7
1 year	21.6	9.8
15 months	23.0	10.5
2 years	27.0	12.3
3 years	32.0	14.5
4 years	36.4	16.5
5 years	41.0	18.6
6 years	46.0	20.9
7 years	52.0	23.6
8 years	57.2	26.0
9 years	62.0	28.2
10 years	68.0	30.9

[a] 1 kg equals 2.2 lb.

Source: Reference 35.

only 67% of caregivers accurately measured the dose they intended to measure.[34] The volume delivered by household teaspoons ranges from 2.5 to 7.8 mL and may also vary greatly when the same spoon is used by different individuals. The American Academy of Pediatrics Committee on Drugs highly recommends the use of appropriate devices for liquid administration, such as a medication cup, cylindrical dosing spoon, oral dropper, and oral syringe. Ease of administration and accuracy should be considered when choosing a dosing device. Plastic medication cups are fairly accurate for volumes of exact multiples of 5 mL (i.e., 5 mL, 10 mL, 15 mL). An oral syringe is preferable to the other oral dosing devices for higher-viscosity liquids because the syringe completely expels the total measured dose. Potent liquid medications should be administered with an oral syringe to ensure that the correct dose is given; the pharmacist should briefly explain to caregivers how to use and read an oral syringe. However, drawing up the dose in the syringe requires dexterity.

The use of precision devices for oral dosing helps to ensure adequate therapeutic response by reducing the incidence of underdoses and by eliminating adverse drug effects from potential overdoses. These devices may also enhance acceptance of medication by infants and children. Parents or caregivers may need instructions on using these devices to measure doses accurately, as well as advice on giving medications to reluctant or struggling children. The pharmacist may need to demonstrate to parents and older children how to take the medication.

Tablets or capsules can usually be swallowed by a child older than 4 years. Tablets that are not sustained-release or enteric-coated formulations may be crushed. Most capsules may be opened and the contents sprinkled on small amounts of food (applesauce, jelly, or pudding) to ensure that all the drug is taken. If the child does not eat the full portion, underdosing can occur. If multiple drugs are prescribed, the child may be more cooperative if allowed to choose what flavored drink to use and which medication to take first. Table 2–5 presents selected guidelines for administering oral medications to pediatric patients.

Table 2–5

Selected Medication Administration Guidelines for Oral Medications

Infants

- Use a calibrated dropper or oral syringe.
- Support the infant's head while holding the infant in the lap.
- Give small amounts of medication to prevent choking.
- If desired, crush nonenteric-coated or slow-release tablets to a powder and sprinkle them on small amounts of food.
- Provide physical comforting while administering medications to help calm the infant.

Toddlers

- Allow the toddler to choose a position in which to take the medication.
- If necessary, disguise the taste of the medication with a small volume of flavored drink or small amounts of food. A rinse with a flavored drink or water will help remove an unpleasant aftertaste.
- Use simple commands in the toddler's jargon to obtain cooperation.
- Allow the toddler to choose which medications (if multiple) to take first.
- Provide verbal and tactile responses to promote cooperative taking of medication.
- Allow the toddler to become familiar with the oral dosing device.

Preschool children

- If possible, place a tablet or capsule near the back of the tongue; then provide water or a flavored liquid to aid the swallowing of the medication.
- If the child's teeth are loose, do not use chewable tablets.
- Use a straw to administer medications that could stain teeth.
- Use a follow-up rinse with a flavored drink to help minimize any unpleasant medication aftertaste.
- Allow the child to help make decisions about dosage formulation, place of administration, medication to take first, and type of flavored drink to use.

Adverse Drug Effects

Adverse reactions are another potential drug therapy problem in children. Side effects in children may be different from those in adults. For example, as in the elderly population, antihistamines and central nervous system (CNS) depressants may cause excitation in children. Thus, FDA recommends not administering antihistamines to children younger than 6 years.[36] In contrast, sympathomimetics such as ephedrine or pseudoephedrine may cause drowsiness in children. Administration of repeated above-therapeutic doses of acetaminophen over a period of 2 to 4 days can result in hepatotoxicity in children.[37,38]

Nonadherence

Nonadherence may occur when children refuse to take medication or when caregivers give up before the child receives the entire dose. Adherence may be improved by recommending a sweetly flavored product because children may be more willing to take a medication if they like the flavor, consistency, or texture.[39] Nonadherence can also occur when caregivers do not understand instructions or do not pass them on to daycare providers, teachers, or school nurses. Separate written instructions for drug administration may be necessary for these individuals.[40]

Assessment and Consultation

Assessment and consultation for pediatric patients usually involve the parents or caregivers. For younger children, the pharmacist works with parents to recommend treatment and to assess drug therapy problems. For older children, the pharmacist can also involve the child to enhance the effectiveness of the consultation.[40] Some tips for pediatric consultation include explaining what the medication is; using the word *medicine,* not *drug;* discussing different dosage forms and the importance of medication timing; preparing special vials for school; preparing the child for the medicine's taste; and demonstrating how to take the medicine.

Geriatric Patients

Social, economic, physiologic, and age-related health factors place elderly patients at high risk for medical problems and prompt them to be large consumers of nonprescription drugs. Indeed, the elderly as a group consume more drugs than any other age segment of our society. A 10-year study of more than 4509 elderly individuals found that nonprescription drug use in this population increased significantly from 1978 through 1988.[41] Close to two-thirds of ambulatory elderly patients use nonprescription drugs.[42] The response to drug therapy by elderly patients is more scattered and unpredictable than that of other populations. Pharmacokinetic, pharmacodynamic, and various nonpharmacologic factors predispose the elderly to potential problems with nonprescription drugs.[42] To deliver comprehensive pharmaceutical care to ambulatory elderly patients, pharmacists must recognize the special needs and risks of this group. Preexisting medical conditions in the elderly may preclude or require caution with the use of some nonprescription drugs.[42] For example, antihistamines should be avoided in patients with emphysema, bronchitis, glaucoma, and urinary retention from prostatic hypertrophy. Nasal and oral decongestants should be used with caution in patients with heart disease, hypertension, thyroid disease, and diabetes.

Effects of Physiologic Aging

Normal aging is associated with physiologic changes that predispose patients to disease. The elderly often suffer from impaired vision (e.g., difficulty reading and differentiating colors) and hearing loss. The pharmacist should be aware of patient behaviors that indicate visual or hearing loss and should take these impairments into consideration when communicating with elderly patients.[43] Additional instructions for nonprescription drugs may need to be provided in larger, high-contrast, dark print. Asking the patient to repeat counseling instructions can ensure that the elderly person heard correctly and understood the directions.

Subtle changes in mental status, such as confusion, may be anticipated in elderly patients who are anxious about their state of health. Elderly patients with cognitive impairments may have difficulty comprehending directions. Patients may not remember the names of all their medications or may not be able to remember instructions. Because of memory lapses, some elderly patients may require special drug delivery systems (e.g., transdermal patches or sustained-release preparations) to help them adhere to their dosage regimen. Elderly patients with cognitive impairments are less likely to read and interpret labels correctly,[44] which further emphasizes their need for special-dosage-form considerations.

Elderly patients are believed to confuse at least one-third of their problems with age-associated problems and therefore to misreport their symptoms.[45] Accurate perception and reporting of symptoms is vital to the successful use of any drug. In addition, elderly patients are often reluctant to share health information with others.

Aging alters the absorption, distribution, metabolism, and elimination of certain drugs, which increase the susceptibility of elderly patients to drug therapy problems. (See Table 2–2.) Such pharmacokinetic changes can result in an unexpected accumulation of these drugs to toxic levels.[43,46]

The aging process, as well as many chronic diseases, can alter a patient's nutritional status. Elderly patients who are most at risk for undernourishment or malnutrition are homebound patients and nursing home residents. Poverty, multiple chronic diseases, multiple drug therapy, or a combination of these factors may cause malnutrition in these patients. The patient's nutritional status and weight are important because they can alter the pharmacokinetics and pharmacodynamics of drugs.

Effects of Altered Drug Pharmacokinetics

Absorption Pharmacokinetic changes, which have been well described in literature, are caused not only by advancing age but also by the effects of disease states and often by multiple drug use. Antacids can alter absorption either by chelation or by pH changes of drugs such as chlordiazepoxide, digoxin, and tetracycline as well as of some vitamins and trace elements.[47] A decrease in GI fluid volume may result in slower absorption of some poorly soluble drugs such as ampicillin and digoxin. An age-related decrease in the acidity of gastric fluids can result in decreased absorption of calcium from calcium carbonate.[48]

Distribution Similarly, drug distribution is age and disease dependent, and changes can lead to altered drug action. As the ratio of lean body weight to lipid tissue changes with age—lean body weight decreases whereas lipid tissue increases—the Vd of water-soluble drugs decreases, possibly promoting more intense action of those drugs. Extracellular and other body fluids also decrease with age, thereby decreasing the Vd of water-soluble drugs. a_1-Acid glycoprotein, a plasma protein, increases with age in healthy elderly patients, whereas albumin levels decrease by 4% per decade of life.[49,50] The effect is greater in patients ages 70 years and older, and a high prevalence of abnormally low serum albumin exists in the very old. Therefore, drugs that are highly protein bound, such as warfarin and phenytoin, should show altered distribution patterns in elderly patients.

Metabolism It is generally agreed that elderly patients have diminished capacity to metabolize drugs because the oxidative drug-metabolizing mechanism changes with age. Theoretically, elderly patients should have reduced rates of hepatic drug metabolism because of their age-related changes. The weight of the liver is correlated with body weight; both decrease beginning in the fifth or sixth decade of life. Both hepatic function and blood flow decrease with age. Anatomic and physiologic changes are also effected by other factors, such as smoking and alcohol intake. Chronic use of alcohol or enzyme inducers such as phenobarbital can increase the risk of hepatotoxicity with long-term use of acetaminophen.

Excretion/Elimination Renal function declines with age but to a variable degree and at a variable rate; thus, age-related changes in renal function and drug elimination must be considered.[51,52] GFR declines with age, even in the absence of cardiovascular, renal, or acute illnesses. The decline is more rapid in men than in women. Altered physiologic processes, such as reduced cardiac output, cardiac contractility, total vascular resistance, and hypotension, may reduce GFR. Furthermore, renal function in geriatric patients is more vulnerable to insults imposed by drug therapy and to overall stress. Examples of drugs that may accumulate because of decreased renal clearance include digoxin, some antibiotics (aminoglycosides and penicillins), phenobarbital, and salicylates.

Effects of Altered Drug Pharmacodynamics

Pharmacodynamics (e.g., the hypoglycemic effect, the extent and duration of pain relief, and the effect of a drug on heart rate) represent the physiologic and psychologic responses to a drug or a combination of drugs and are integral to the pharmacologic management of chronic diseases of the elderly. Pharmacodynamics change with age and disease, but are difficult to differentiate between normal aging effects and pathophysiologic effects on the one hand and their influence on pharmacodynamics on the other. Advancing age heightens the interplay between the aging processes and chronic diseases, which has made it difficult to clearly identify those pharmacodynamic changes that are associated with age only.

Few studies have simultaneously investigated both pharmacokinetics and pharmacodynamics in geriatric patients. In general, drug action altered with age has been ascribed to the elderly's reduced reserve capacity and changes in the CNS, autonomic nervous system, cardiovascular system, endocrine system, and drug receptors.

Reduced Physiologic Reserve Elderly patients are more susceptible to decompensation under stress because of the loss of physiologic reserve. For example, perfusion of vital organs is often diminished in elderly patients, and small changes in blood flow, perhaps induced by drugs, can endanger organ function because functional reserve capacity is reduced. Geriatric patients are less able to regulate blood glucose levels, blood pH, pulse rate, blood pressure, and oxygen consumption; therefore, it is not unreasonable to assume that drugs can bring about unanticipated, although not unpredictable, adverse effects on functional reserve in elderly patients.

Altered Hemostatic and Thermoregulatory Mechanisms There is evidence that the efficiency of postural stability is reduced with advancing age.[53] Any drugs that affect this homeostatic mechanism (e.g., antihistamines that affect the CNS) can decrease the body's ability to maintain balance, possibly leading to a greater incidence of falls and fractures.

The efficiency of the thermoregulatory mechanism, which controls body temperature, decreases with advancing age.[54] Impaired shivering, defective vasoconstriction, and poor perception and recognition of cold weather effects are more prevalent in the elderly.

Altered Drug-Receptor Interactions A drug has affinity and intrinsic activity in relation to each of its receptors. Affinity is the efficiency with which a drug binds to its receptors; intrinsic activity is the drug's power to generate a stimulus. Drugs with both affinity and intrinsic activity are defined as agonists. Drugs that have affinity but lack intrinsic activity are defined as antagonists.

Most drugs bind to receptors and, thus, initiate their action. Age-related altered drug action may be related to altered drug-receptor interactions. It has been postulated that a given receptor site or drug concentration produces a greater pharmacodynamic effect in the elderly than in younger patients. However, generalizations cannot be drawn because the number of receptors is not fixed but is regulated by other factors, including diseases (e.g., ischemia, hypertension, heart failure, cardiac hypertrophy); drugs (e.g., glucocorticoids, hormones, adrenergic agonists, and antagonists); and the aging process itself. There may be age-associated receptor changes in some parts of the body but not in others. The CNS cholinergic receptors decline in the basal ganglia but probably not in other brain regions.

In adapting to drug therapy, receptors may become supersensitive or desensitized. For example, alterations in insulin receptors account for some forms of insulin resistance. Age-related changes have been documented for benzodiazepine receptors in the brain and for several hormone receptors.[55,56] Most studies, however, have concentrated on the cholinergic, the dopaminergic, and the β-adrenergic receptors. Recent studies[57] have shown that normal aging is associated with loss of serotonergic function and that elderly persons with late life depression and Alzheimer's disease are more markedly affected. There is also evidence of interplay between disturbances in cholinergic and serotonergic function in the elderly. These findings have an impact on drug therapy, especially with regard to management of neuropsychiatric disorders.

Drug-receptor response, which is defined as the pharmacologic response after a drug–end organ interaction, may be increased or decreased in geriatric patients. It has been suggested for some time that the elderly appear to have more sensitivity to some drugs. Drugs whose pharmacodynamic effects in the elderly have been most intensively studied include the barbiturates, the benzodiazepines, warfarin, heparin, and morphine.[47,52]

Altered Neurologic Functions In people between ages 20 and 80 years, brain weight is reduced by 20%, and up to a 25% loss of neurons may occur in some areas of the brain.[58] Neuronal loss in the superior frontal and temporal regions and in the striatum has been reported.[59] An age-related decline in dopamine receptors also occurs.[60]

Evidence indicates that with advanced age comes increased conduction time, decreased cerebral blood flow, and possibly increased permeability of the blood–brain barrier.[47] Both subjective and objective evidence indicates that geriatric patients have an enhanced CNS sensitivity to drugs, especially CNS depressants such as sedatives and antidepressants. Enhanced sensitivity may prompt a reduced dose requirement; decreasing the dose by as much as 50% has been recommended for some drugs such as fentanyl.[61]

Increased brain sensitivity and other changes (e.g., decreased coordination, prolongation of reaction time, and impairment of short-term memory) manifest as increased frequency of confusion, frequency of urinary incontinence, and increased number of falls, especially among elderly women. Drug therapy may exaggerate all these changes, particularly if drugs are used in the "usual" dose or if multiple drugs are used.

The most clear-cut evidence of enhanced brain sensitivity to the action of some drugs and thus of altered and age-associated pharmacodynamic drug actions exists for the benzodiazepines.[62] Confusion, ataxia, immobility, and incontinence have been demonstrated when some of those drugs are given in the normal adult dose to geriatric patients.[63] Impairment of neurologic function in geriatric patients who have been prescribed these drugs appears to be the rule rather than the exception.

Control of bowel and bladder function is lessened with advancing age. A further decrease in efficiency is likely with laxative use. Anticholinergic drugs and CNS drugs may lessen neurologic control. Antihistamines have sedative properties that may reduce bladder control in the elderly.[64] Adverse effects of nonprescription drugs are often increased when such drugs are added to an existing medication regimen.

Altered Cardiovascular Functions The action of cardiac drugs in geriatric patients is assumed to differ from that in younger people because measurements start from a different point. For example, the cardiac index changes with age; older people have a higher peripheral resistance and intrinsic heart rate plus a lower vagal restraint. Sinus node and atrioventricular node dysfunction increase with age; maximum heart rate decreases. Peak cardiac output at exercise also declines.

The maximal response of the myocardium to catecholamines is reduced with aging.[65] The heart manifests an increased sensitivity to the toxic effects of some drugs (e.g., digoxin), which is heightened in the presence of hypokalemia but manifests as a lesser increase in contractility to cardiac glycosides.[65]

Changes in the cardiovascular system also involve changes in blood vessels. Between ages 20 and 80 years, vessel elasticity and distensibility (i.e., ability to stretch and enlarge) are reduced by 90%, which leads to increased arterial blood pressure.[66] An increase in peripheral resistance is mainly responsible for essential hypertension. In both normotensive and hypertensive geriatric patients, plasma renin and aldosterone concentrations decline. Increases in plasma renin activity in response to sodium depletion or diuretics may also be reduced. Geriatric patients generally present with a relatively reduced fluid volume; extracellular volume is decreased to the greatest degree. Therefore, these hemodynamic and fluid volume changes are expected to change the drug response in geriatric patients.

Additionally, the elderly are more likely than younger people to become symptomatically orthostatic, even without drugs. The sensitivity and responsiveness of the baroreceptor reflex decreases with age, which does not allow an older patient to efficiently compensate for either elevated or reduced blood pressure.[52] Therefore, all drugs that could cause orthostatic hypotension, particularly if used in combination, should be used with caution in the elderly. The risk of orthostatic hypotension is further increased in geriatric patients either with volume depletion caused by salt or water depletion or both, or with circulatory changes caused by infections or fever.

Altered Endocrine Functions Age-related changes in the endocrine system have been documented. The reduced availability of hormones results in diminished endocrine regulatory mechanisms with age, as well as with deficiencies in hormonal feedback mechanisms.

Alterations in pancreatic and adrenal hormone levels result in decreased glucose tolerance with age and in an increased susceptibility to drug-induced hypoglycemia. Some geriatric patients suffer from a decreased release of insulin, whereas others have a decreased number of insulin receptors, postreceptor abnormalities, or both.[67] Production of sex hormones also decreases with age.[47] In women, reduced estrogen levels have been correlated with a greater incidence of osteoporosis. Because of hormonal changes, women are more susceptible to orthostatic hypotension. Decreased thyroid hormone levels make elderly patients more sensitive to the action of digitalis and increase the risk of drug-induced hypothermia.[68]

Altered Immunologic Functions Some, but not all, immunologic functions show a gradual decline with age. The thymus probably has less power than the central immunologic organs and the bone marrow to maintain functional levels of peripheral T-lymphoid cells.

The immune function is under complex regulatory control, and immunologic changes are probably caused by disturbances in that regulatory process. Indeed, age-related changes in immune function reflect several different alterations. Overall, T cells are diminished in function. The deficiency includes most T-cell effector and regulatory functions, with the possible exception of T-cell suppression. All these factors combine to decrease cellular immune response.[69,70] Infections are more prevalent in geriatric patients; however, infections that are common in older people (e.g., influenza, pneumococcal pneumonia) are not usually associated with immune deficiency as are infections caused by opportunistic organisms.

Altered Gastrointestinal Functions Aging is associated with secretory and morphologic changes in the stomach. Muscular atrophy, thinning of gastric mucosa, and infiltration of the submucosa with elastic fibers are evident in the stomach.[71,72] Intestinal blood flow may be reduced by as much as 50% by age 65 years and is further diminished by stress, congestive heart failure, hypoxia, and hypovolemia. Tension, depressive illness, anxiety, worry, and fear of disease and death influence the stomach's motility and secretory function. Chronic gastritis, irritable colon, heartburn, ulcer-like distress, and nausea can result.

Gastric secretion declines with age, gastric cell function decreases, and gastric pH is generally elevated. Furthermore, gastric secretion is diminished in patients with diabetes.

Gastric emptying is about 2.5 times faster in younger people than in older people because it is under the control of the CNS, which may lose efficiency with advancing age. Slowing of gastric emptying follows a reduction in gastric acid secretion. Gastric emptying is also negatively affected by stress, lack of ambulation, gastric ulcer, intestinal obstruction, myocardial infarct, and diabetes mellitus. Some drugs (e.g., antacids, anticholinergics, isoniazid, lithium, narcotic analgesics) delay gastric emptying. Fatty meals delay gastric emptying more in the elderly than in younger people. A delay in gastric emptying gives gastrotoxic agents a longer residence time, and, therefore, more opportunity to exert their toxic effect.

Nonsteroidal Anti-Inflammatory Drug–Induced Adverse Effects Nonsteroidal anti-inflammatory drugs (NSAIDs) are widely used, especially by patients with osteoarthritis and rheumatoid arthritis. GI complications from NSAIDs are responsible for approximately 107,000 hospital admissions and at least 16,500 deaths annually among patients with arthritis.[73] One of the risk factors for GI complications is increasing age. Some data suggest that age is not an independent risk factor. However, the absolute number of events of NSAID-related toxicity is greater for geriatric patients because of their frequent use of NSAIDs and the increased prevalence of comorbid conditions and concomitant drug therapies.[74] As people age, their use of NSAIDs increases, and the adverse effects of these drugs increase disproportionately. The potential GI toxicity of NSAIDs may be enhanced by their simultaneous administration with other GI toxic drugs, coffee, or alcohol. Through inhibition of the protective effects of GI prostaglandins and through local noxious effects, salicylates and other NSAIDs can cause superficial gastric and duodenal erosions and ulcer formation, which could then result in GI bleeding and perforations. Decreased platelet aggregation can enhance the potential for bleeding. All NSAIDs can interfere with platelet function and can prolong bleeding time. Mucosal lesions of the stomach and duodenum are often reported in patients who take NSAIDs. Geriatric patients may be especially susceptible to NSAID-associated peptic ulcer disease.

With advancing age, renal blood and plasma flow decrease, while the kidney's ability to concentrate urine decreases, as does its maximum diluting ability and its ability to compensate for abnormalities of the acid–base balance and electrolytes. Geriatric patients do not conserve sodium efficiently. Therefore, the two broad excretory functions of the kidneys—preservation of body fluid volume and maintenance of their composition—are adversely affected by aging. NSAIDs can exacerbate the severity of renal disease by blocking inter-renal cyclo-oxygenase (reduction of renal prostaglandin secretion). This risk is increased in volume-depleted geriatric patients.

Other Potential Drug Therapy Problems

Duplicate Therapy Geriatric patients can receive unnecessary drug therapy when drugs are added to their therapeutic regimen without a reevaluation of the entire regimen to determine whether certain drugs should be deleted. Duplicate therapy may occur because elderly patients may be seeing multiple health care providers for their various medical problems. Use of a single pharmacy can significantly lower the risk of inappropriate drug combinations.[75] Nonprescription drugs commonly involved in drug interactions in the elderly include aspirin, other NSAIDs, antacids, cimetidine, and antihistamines.[76] Many geriatric patients have serious and multiple diseases such as coronary artery disease, chronic renal failure, or congestive heart failure, which can be aggravated by concurrent therapy for other acute problems. Concomitant illnesses or certain drugs may contraindicate the use of other drugs. It is important to consider whether a geriatric patient is requesting a nonprescription drug to treat an adverse reaction from another medication.

Appropriate Dosing/Dosage Forms Normal drug doses may be too high for geriatric patients because of their impaired hepatic and renal function. This condition would necessitate either lowering the dose or increasing the dosing interval. Furthermore, geriatric patients may experience difficulty with some dosage forms (e.g., swallowing large tablets, using inhalers) because of physical impairments. Geriatric patients may have difficulty opening and closing containers because of arthritis or tremors. Child-resistant containers may be especially difficult for geriatric patients to open if they have deficits in physical dexterity. A pharmacist should direct geriatric patients to products without child-resistant containers, but should warn them of the potential poisoning hazard for their visiting grandchildren.

Poor Adherence The prevalence of nonadherence with medications is high in the geriatric population and is often the result of inadequate understanding of their medication regimen.[77] Poor adherence may result from difficulty swallowing or administering the drug. It may also result from an inability to afford the drug because of a limited or fixed income. Geriatric patients may lack a social support network to supply the aid required by an illness. Pharmacists may need to involve caregivers in medication administration. Pharmacists can also discourage geriatric patients from sharing medications with others.

Pregnant Patients

Drug therapy during pregnancy may be necessary to treat medical conditions or to manage common complaints of pregnancy such as vomiting or constipation. However, because most drugs cross the placenta to some extent, a mother who takes a drug might expose her fetus to it. Thus, the desire to ease the mother's discomfort must be balanced with concern for the developing fetus.

A study among 4186 women during the first trimester found that 66% used at least 1 drug; the mean number of drugs for all subjects and for drug users was 1.3 and 2.9, respectively.[78] Nonprescription drugs accounted for 68% of the drugs used; the drugs used most often were oral analgesics (acetaminophen and aspirin), antacids, and cold and allergy products.

Potential Drug Therapy Problems

Pregnant women should never presume that a nonprescription medication is safe to use during pregnancy. They should first consult with a pharmacist or physician to determine whether a medication is teratogenic (causes abnormal embryo development). Nausea and vomiting can cause another medication-related problem: difficulty in taking oral medications.

Teratogenic Effects Several factors are important in determining whether a drug taken by a pregnant woman will adversely affect the fetus. Two such factors are the stage of pregnancy and the ability of the drug to pass from maternal circulation to fetal circulation through the placenta. The first trimester, when organogenesis occurs, is the period of greatest teratogenic susceptibility for the embryo and is the critical period for inducing major anatomic malformations. However, exposure at other periods of gestation may be no less important because the exact critical period depends on the specific drug in question.

Drug therapy problems are also important considerations for the pregnant patient. Although dosage guidelines for some prescription drugs are different in the pregnant patient from those in other patients, no information on dosage adjustments exists for nonprescription drugs. Unnecessary drug therapy should be avoided. Nondrug therapy is often more appropriate than drug therapy for pregnant women. Use of cigarettes and alcohol should be avoided or limited because they have been associated with increased risk to the fetus.[79–83] Consumption of moderate doses of caffeine appears to be safe.[84]

In the pregnant patient, the primary concern is related to drug safety. All pharmacists should be familiar with the A-B-C-D-X system for evaluating the safety of drugs in pregnancy.[84] (See Appendix 1 in the back of the book.) Often the issue is not whether a more effective drug is available but whether a safer drug is available. For example, evidence exists that aspirin is associated with congenital defects, incidence of stillbirths, neonatal deaths, and reduced birth weight.[78,84] Use of aspirin late in pregnancy has been associated with increases in length of gestation and duration of labor. These effects are related to aspirin's inhibition of prostaglandin synthesis. In addition, because aspirin affects platelet function, perinatal aspirin ingestion has been found to increase the incidence of hemorrhage in both the pregnant woman and the newborn during and following delivery. Therefore, a women should avoid using aspirin during pregnancy, especially during the last trimester. Instead, because acetaminophen is generally considered safe for use during pregnancy, it is the nonprescription drug of choice for antipyresis and analgesia when taken in standard therapeutic doses.[78] NSAIDs such as ibuprofen and naproxen can be taken early in pregnancy.[84] However, they should not be used late in pregnancy because they are potent prostaglandin synthetase inhibitors. Not only can they cause problems in the newborn but also they can affect the duration of gestation and labor. Vitamins may pose a risk for congenital anomalies and adverse effects in the neonate when taken in doses above the recommended daily allowance.[85] Chronic use of large doses of antitussives that contain codeine may cause withdrawal in the newborn after delivery.[86]

Nonadherence Nausea and vomiting associated with the pregnancy may make it difficult for the pregnant woman to comply with taking oral medications. Pharmacists can recommend eating small meals, frequent snacks, and crackers to alleviate or minimize nausea and vomiting.

Management of the Pregnant Patient

The pharmacist can aid the self-treating pregnant woman in deciding which drug or nondrug treatments she should consider and when self-treatment may be harmful to her or her unborn child. The decision to suggest a drug must be based on both an up-to-date knowledge of the literature and a critical risk:benefit evaluation of the mother and the fetus. The pharmacist should choose drugs for which large studies or meta-analyses of several studies demonstrate that they can be safely used during pregnancy. When the pharmacist chooses between two drugs, the drug of choice will be the one that has been in use for a long time rather than a newer drug.[87] Ascertaining the trimester of pregnancy is important because it is a factor in determining whether some nonprescription drugs can be used safely. The pharmacist should discourage pregnant women from self-medicating with nonprescription drugs without receiving counseling from a physician or pharmacist. The assessment and management of the pregnant patient require observation of the following principles.

First, the pharmacist must be alert to the possibility of pregnancy in any woman of childbearing age who has certain key symptoms of early pregnancy, such as nausea, vomiting, and frequent urination. Any woman who fits this description should be warned not to take a drug that might be of questionable safety if she is pregnant.

Second, the pharmacist should advise the pregnant patient to avoid using drugs, in general, at any stage of pregnancy unless such use is deemed essential by the patient's physician. Also, the safety and effectiveness of homeopathic and herbal remedies in pregnancy have not been established, and their use should be discouraged.

Third, the pharmacist should advise the pregnant patient to increase her reliance on nondrug modalities as treatment alternatives. For example, the first approach to nausea and vomiting should be eating small, frequent meals and avoiding foods, smells, or situations that cause vomiting. Next, taking an effervescent glucose or buffered carbohydrate solution may be effective. Only if those measures are ineffective should she consider an antihistamine or antiemetic. Physician consultation may be indicated at this point.

Fourth, the pharmacist should refer the patient to a physician for certain problems that carry increased risk of poor outcomes in pregnancy (e.g., high blood pressure, vaginal bleeding, urinary tract infections, rapid weight gain, or edema).

The Nursing Mother

Drug use while breast-feeding can cause an adverse effect in the infant. The concentration of a drug in the mother's milk depends on a number of factors, including the drug's concentration in the mother's blood; the drug's molecular weight, lipid solubility, degree of ionization, and degree of binding to plasma and milk proteins; and the drug's active secretion into the milk. Other important considerations include the relationship between the time of taking a drug and the time of a breast-feeding, as well as the drug's potential for causing toxicity in infants. Also, some drugs (e.g., decongestants) may decrease milk supply.

When advising a nursing mother on self-treatment, the pharmacist should decide if a drug is really necessary, should recommend the safest drug (e.g., acetaminophen instead of aspirin) if one is necessary, and should then advise the mother to take the medication just after breast-feeding or just before the infant's lengthy sleep periods.[88,89] It is preferable to select a drug that has been in use for a long time that has shown no apparent harm to nursing infants. If appropriate, topical or local therapy may be preferred to oral systemic therapy.[88]

When taken in therapeutic dosages, most drugs are not present in breast milk in sufficient amounts to cause significant harm to the infant. However, several drugs are contraindicated for use while breast-feeding, and others should be used with caution by nursing mothers. The amount of caffeine in caffeine-containing beverages is not harmful, but higher doses (i.e., more than 1 g daily) have been reported to cause irritability and poor sleep patterns in infants.[89] Many nonprescription drugs exist for which there are no data on their transfer into breast milk and their possible clinical effects.

In a statement on drugs in human milk published by the American Academy of Pediatrics Committee on Drugs,[88] aspirin and other salicylates are the only nonprescription drugs that were considered to have had significant effects on some nursing infants and that nursing mothers should therefore take with caution. Nonprescription drugs that are usually considered compatible with breast-feeding include[84,87,90]

- Analgesics: acetaminophen, ibuprofen, flurbiprofen, naproxen, and ketoprofen.
- Antacids.
- Antidiarrheals: kaolin–pectin, attapulgite, and loperamide.
- Antihistamines: brompheniramine, chlorpheniramine, diphenhydramine, and triprolidine.
- Antisecretory agents: cimetidine, famotidine, ranitidine, and nizatidine.
- Cough preparations: dextromethorphan.
- Decongestants: phenylephrine, phenylpropanolamine, and pseudoephedrine.
- Fluoride.
- Laxatives: bran type, bulk-forming type, docusate, glycerin suppositories, magnesium hydroxide, and senna.
- Vitamins.

CONCLUSIONS

Pharmacy practitioners can begin to efficiently introduce the principles discussed in this chapter by viewing the initial patient consultation as a three-phase process: (1) development of the therapeutic relationship (encouraging patients to tell their stories), (2) assessment of drug-related needs, and (3) review of systems (or a verbal accounting of all patient systems from head to toe). The pharmacist should devote attention to assessing drug-related needs in which the identification of drug therapy problems and establishment of treatment goals takes place. Care planning involves doing what is necessary to meet and fulfill the patient's drug-related needs; then follow-up evaluation documents the patient's actual results or outcomes. Recognizing the special needs of pediatric, geriatric, pregnant, and breast-feeding patients is essential in avoiding or minimizing drug therapy problems in these high-risk groups.

The use of nonprescription drugs represents an important component of the health care system. Many people diagnose their own symptoms, select a nonprescription drug product, and monitor their own therapeutic response. If properly used, nonprescription drugs can relieve patients' minor physical complaints and can permit physicians to concentrate on more serious illnesses. If used improperly, however, nonprescription products can create a multitude of problems.

To be of greatest service to patients, pharmacists must continually update their therapeutic knowledge and must improve their interpersonal communication skills. As pharmacists continue to expand their patient-care services, people will learn of those services and will seek their pharmacist's assistance whenever they are in doubt about self-treatment. The result will be better-informed patients who will not only use the professional services of pharmacists but also recognize the pharmacists' contributions to health care.

References

1. Nurses Displace Pharmacists at Top of Expanded Honesty and Ethics Poll. Available at: http://www.gallup.com/poll/releases/pr9911116.asp. Accessed April 13, 2000.
2. Albrant, DH, ed. *The American Pharmaceutical Association Drug Treatment Protocols.* Washington, DC: American Pharmaceutical Association; 1999:367–411.
3. Montagne M, Bleidt B. How to help the elderly self-medicate. *US Pharm.* 1989;14:53–60.
4. Smith EA. OTC pharmacy trends. *Drug Topics.* 1998;142(suppl):4S–7S.
5. Johnston B. One-third of this nation's adults use herbal remedies with an herbal market estimated at $3.24 billion. *HerbalGram.* 1997;40:49.
6. Manasse HR Jr. Medication use in an imperfect world: drug misadventuring as an issue of public policy: Parts 1 and 2. *Am J Hosp Pharm.* 1989;46:929–44, 1141–52.
7. Johnson JA, Bootman JL. Drug-related morbidity and mortality: a cost of illness model. *Arch Intern Med.* 1995;155:949–56.
8. Cipolle RJ, Strand LM, Morley PC. *Pharmaceutical Care Practice.* New York: McGraw Hill; 1998.
9. Meade V. Patients satisfied with pharmacy services, survey shows. *Am Pharm.* 1994;34:26–8.
10. Hirsch JD, Gagnon JP, Camp R. Value of pharmacy services: perceptions of consumers, physicians, and third-party prescription plan administrators. *Am Pharm.* 1990;30:20–5.
11. Monsanto HA, Mason HL. Consumer use of nondispensing professional pharmacy services. *Drug Intell Clin Pharm.* 1989;23:218–23.
12. Hepler CD, Strand LM. Opportunities and responsibilities in pharmaceutical care. *Am J Hosp Pharm.* 1990;47:533–43.
13. Strand LM, Morley PC, Cipolle RJ, et al. Drug-related problems: their structure and function. *Ann Pharmacother.* 1990;240:1093–7.
14. Wagner A. Listen to the picture. *JAMA.* 1988;259:420.
15. Fisher RC. Patient education and compliance: a pharmacist's perspective. *Patient Educ Counselor.* 1992;19:261–71.
16. McNally DL, Wertheimer D. Strategies to reduce the high cost of patient noncompliance. *Md Med J.* 1992;41:223–5.
17. Chermak G, Jinks M. Counseling the hearing-impaired older adult. *Drug Intell Clin Pharm.* 1981;15:377–82.
18. Smith DL. The patient and his medications. In: *Medication Guide for Patient Counseling.* 2nd ed. Philadelphia: Lea and Febiger; 1981:3–46.
19. Epstein D. More counseling called for in medicating the illiterate. *Drug Topics.* 1988;132:15.
20. Olson RM, Blank D, Cardinal E, et al. Understanding medication-related needs of low literacy patients. *J Am Pharm Assoc.* 1996;36:425–9.
21. Siganga WW, Huynh TC. Barriers to the use of pharmacy services: the case of ethnic populations. *J Am Pharm Assoc.* 1997;37:335–40.
22. Kogan MD, Pappas G, Yu SM, et al. Over-the-counter medication use among U.S. preschool-age children. *JAMA.* 1994;272:1025–30.
23. Wong DL. Developmental influences on child health promotion. In: Wong DL, ed. *Essentials of Pediatric Nursing.* 5th ed. St. Louis: CV Mosby Co; 1997:83–103.
24. Skaer TL. Dosing considerations in the pediatric patient. *Clin Ther.* 1991;13:526–44.
25. Morselli PL. Clinical pharmacology of the perinatal period and early infancy. *Clin Pharmacokinet.* 1989;17(suppl 1):13–28.
26. Stewart CF, Hampton EM. Effect of maturation on drug disposition in pediatric patients. *Clin Pharm.* 1987;6:548–64.
27. Kearns GL, Reed MD. Clinical pharmacokinetics in infants and children: a reappraisal. *Clin Pharmacokinet.* 1989;17(suppl 1):26–67.
28. Matthews LW, Drotar D. Cystic fibrosis—a challenging long-term chronic disease. *Pediatr Clin N Am.* 1984;31:133–52.
29. Greene HL, McCabe DR, Merenstein GB. Protracted diarrhea and malnutrition in infancy: changes in intestinal morphology and disaccharidase activities during treatment with total intravenous nutrition or oral elemental diets. *J Pediatr.* 1975;87:695–704.
30. Friss-Hansen B. Body composition during growth: in vivo measurements and biochemical data correlated to differential anatomical growth. *Pediatrics.* 1971;47:264–74.
31. Friss-Hansen B. Body water compartments in children: changes during growth and related changes in body composition *Pediatrics.* 1961;28:69–81.
32. Morselli PL. Clinical pharmacokinetics in neonates. *Clin Pharmacokinet.* 1976;1:81–98.
33. Haley TJ. Metabolism and pharmacokinetics of theophylline in human neonates, children, and adults. *Drug Metab Rev.* 1983;14:295–335.
34. Simon HK, Weinkle DA. Over-the counter medications: do parents give what they intend to give? *Arch Pediatr Adolesc Med.* 1997;151:654–6.
35. Nykamp D. Nonprescription medications in the pediatric population. *Am Pharm.* 1995;35:10–29.
36. Pray WS. The pharmacist as self-care advisor. *J Am Pharm Assoc.* 1996;36:329–41.
37. Henretig FM, Selbst SM, Forrest C, et al. Repeated acetaminophen overdosing causing hepatotoxicity in children. 1989;28:525–8.
38. Heubi JE, Barbacci MB, Zimmerman HJ. Therapeutic misdaventures with acetaminophen: hepatotoxicity after multiple doses in children. *J Pediatr.* 1998;132:22–7.
39. Compounding for the pediatric patient. *Pharma Compounding.* 1997;1:84–6.
40. Martin S. Catering to pediatric patients. *Am Pharm.* 1992;32:47–50.
41. Stewart RB, Moore MT, May FE, et al. Changing patterns of therapeutic agents in the elderly: a ten-year overview. *Age Ageing.* 1991;20:182–8.
42. Lamy PP. Nonprescription drugs and the elderly. *Am Fam Physician.* 1989;39:175–9.
43. Mallet L. Counseling in special populations: the elderly patient. *Am Pharm.* 1992;32:71–81.
44. Meyer ME, Schuna HH. Assessment of geriatric patients' functional ability to take medication. *Drug Intell Clin Pharm.* 1989;23:171–4.
45. Levkoff SE, Cleary PD, Wetle T, et al. Illness behavior in the aged: implications for clinicians. *J Am Geriatr Soc.* 1988;36:622–9.
46. Montamat SC, Cusack BJ, Vestal RE. Management of drug therapy in the elderly. *N Engl J Med.* 1989;321:303–9.
47. Lamy PP. *Prescribing for the Elderly.* Littleton, Mass: PSG Publishing; 1980.
48. Wood RJ, Serfaty-Lacrosniere C. Gastric acidity, atrophic gastritis, and calcium absorption. *Nutr Rev.* 1992;50:33–40.
49. Cooper J, Gardner C. Effect of aging on serum albumin. *J Am Geriatr Soc.* 1988;36:660.
50. Brown EM, Winograd CH. Prevalence and impact of malnutrition on morbidity and mortality in the oldest old. *J Am Geriatr Soc.* 1988;36:653.
51. Muhlberg W, Platt D. Age-dependent changes of the kidneys: pharmacological implications. *Gerontology.* 1999;45:243–53.
52. Hammerlein A, Hartmut D, Lowenthal DT. Pharmacokinetic and pharmacodynamic changes in the elderly: clinical implications. *Clin Pharmacokinet.* 1998;35:49–64.
53. Swift CG. Prescribing in old age. *Br Med J.* 1988;296:913–5.
54. Collins KJ, Dore C, Exton-Smith AN, et al. Accidental hypothermia and impaired temperature homoeostasis in the elderly. *Br Med J.* 1977;1:353–6.
55. Severson JA. Neurotransmitter receptors and aging. *J Am Geriatr Soc.* 1984;32:24–7.
56. Bar RS, Roth J. Insulin receptor status in disease states of man. *Arch Intern Med.* 1977;137:474–81.
57. Meltzer CC, Smith G, Dekosky ST, et al. Serotonin in aging, late-life depression, and Alzheimer's disease: the emerging role of functional imaging. *Neuropsychopharmacology.* 1998;18(6):407–30.
58. Anderson JM, Hubbard BM, Coghill GR, et al. The effect of advanced old age on the neurone content of the cerebral cortex: observations with an automatic image analyser point counting method. *J Neurol Sci.* 1983;58:235–46.
59. Ball MJ. Neuronal loss, neurofibrillary tangles and granulovacuolar de-

generation in the hippocampus with ageing and dementia. *Acta Neuropathologia.* 1977;37:111–8.
60. Wagner HN, Burns HD, Dannals RF, et al. Imaging dopamine receptors in the human brain by positron tomography. *Science.* 1983;221:1264–6.
61. Scott JC, Stanski DR. Decreased fentanyl and alfentanil dose requirements with age: a simultaneous pharmacokinetic and pharmacodynamic evaluation. *J Pharmacol Exper Ther.* 1987;240:159–66.
62. Schmucker DL. Aging and drug disposition: an update. *Pharmacol Rev.* 1985;37:133–48.
63. Evans JG, Jarvis EH. Nitrazepam and the elderly. *Br Med J.* 1972;4:487.
64. Willington FL. Urinary incontinence: a practical approach. *Geriatrics.* 1980;35:41–8.
65. Lakatta EG, Gerstenblith G, Angell CS, et al. Diminished inotropic response of aged myocardium to catecholamines. *Circ Res.* 1975;36: 262–9.
66. Fleisch JH. Age-related changes in the sensitivity of blood vessels to drugs. *Pharmacol Ther.* 1980;8:477–87.
67. Davidson MB. The effect of aging on carbohydrate metabolism: a review of the English literature and a practical approach to the diagnosis of diabetes mellitus in the elderly. *Metabolism.* 1979;28:688–705.
68. Orlander P, Johnson DG. Endocrinologic problems in the aged. *Otolaryngol Clin North Am.* 1982;15:439–49.
69. Makinodan T, Kay MMB. Age influence on the immune system. *Adv Immunol.* 1980;29:287–330.
70. Price GB, Makinodan T. Immunologic deficiencies in senescence I. Characterization of intrinsic deficiencies. *J Immunol.* 1972;108:403–12.
71. Lamy PP. A consideration of NSAID use in the elderly. *Geriatr Med Today.* 1988;7:30–48.
72. Lamy PP. Non-steroidal anti-inflammatories in the elderly. In: Rainsford KD, Velo GP, eds. *Side Effects of Anti-inflammatory Drugs.* Lancaster, England: MTP Press; 1987:151–72.
73. Singh G. Recent considerations in nonsteroidal anti-inflammatory drug gastropathy. *Am J Med.* 1998;105:31S–38S.
74. Solomon DH, Gurwitz JH. Toxicity of nonsteroidal anti-inflammatory drugs in the elderly: is advanced age a risk factor? *Am J Med.* 1997;102: 208–15.
75. Tamblyn RM, McLeod PJ, Abrahamowicz M, et al. Do too many cooks spoil the broth? Multiple physician involvement in medical management of elderly patients and potentially inappropriate drug combinations. *Can Med Assoc J.* 1996;54:1174–84.
76. Seymour RM, Routledge PA. Important drug–drug interactions in the elderly. *Drugs and Aging.* 1998;12:485–94.
77. Tamblyn R. Medication use in seniors: challenge and solutions. *Therapie.* 1996;51:269–82.
78. Buitendijk S, Bracken MB. Medication in early pregnancy: prevalence of use and relationship to maternal characteristics. *Am J Obstet Gynecol.* 1991;165:33–40.
79. American Academy of Pediatrics Committee on Environmental Hazards. Effects of cigarette smoking on the fetus and child. *Pediatrics.* 1976;57:411–3.
80. Fielding JE. Smoking and pregnancy. *N Engl J Med.* 1978;298:337–9.
81. Clarren SK, Smith DW. The fetal alcohol syndrome. *N Engl J Med.* 1978;298:1063–7.
82. Shaywitz SE, Cohen DJ, Shaywitz BA. Behavior and learning difficulties in children of normal intelligence born to alcoholic mothers. *J Pediatr.* 1980;96:978–82.
83. Wagner CL, Katikaneni LD, Cox TH, et al. The impact of prenatal drug exposure on the neonate. *Obstet Gynecol Clin North Am.* 1998;25: 169–94.
84. Briggs GG, Freeman RK, Yaffe SJ. *Drugs in Pregnancy and Lactation: A Reference Guide to Fetal and Neonatal Risk.* 5th ed. Baltimore: Williams & Wilkins; 1998:73a–81a, 125c–31c, 524i–6i, 757n–8n.
85. Kacew S. Fetal consequences and risks attributed to the use of prescribed and over-the-counter (OTC) preparations during pregnancy. *Int J Clin Phamacol Ther.* 1994;32:335–43.
86. Hill RM, Craig JP, Chaney MD, et al. Utilization of over-the-counter drugs during pregnancy. *Clin Obstet Gynecol.* 1977;20:381–94.
87. Koren G, Pastuszak A, Ito S. Drugs in Pregnancy. *N Engl J Med.* 1998;338:1128–37.
88. American Academy of Pediatrics Committee on Drugs. Transfer of drugs and other chemicals into human milk. *Pediatrics.* 1994;93: 137–50.
89. Dillon AE, Wagner CL, Wiest D, et al. Drug therapy in the nursing mother. *Obstet and Gynecol Clin North Am.* 1997;24:675–96.
90. Logsdon BA. Drug use during lactation. *J Am Pharm Assoc.* 1997;37: 407–18.

SECTION II

PAIN AND FEVER DISORDERS

CHAPTER 3

Headache and Muscle and Joint Pain

Arthur G. Lipman and Kenneth C. Jackson II

Chapter 3 at a Glance

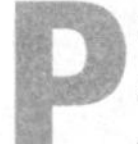ain is the most common ailment for which patients seek medical care. Patients also come to pharmacies to purchase systemic analgesics more often than they do for any other type of nonprescription medication. Yet pain is perhaps the most misunderstood of the common ailments, perhaps because of the limited coverage that pain management receives in most health professional curricula. Much of what we now know about the pathophysiology of pain and the appropriate use of analgesics has been discovered in the past two decades.

Editor's Note: This chapter is based, in part, on the 11th edition chapter "Internal Analgesic and Antipyretic Products," which was written by Arthur G. Lipman.

The International Association for the Study of Pain defines pain as an unpleasant sensory and emotional experience associated with actual or potential tissue damage or described in terms of such damage.[1] The definition recognizes that pain can have physical, affective, and learned components and is not necessarily a result of physical injury. This definition is in contrast to many traditional definitions of pain that discuss pain as solely a physical phenomenon.

The Integrated Approach to the Management of Pain,[2] a 1986 consensus document of the National Institutes of Health, concluded that pain should be considered as three distinct entities: acute pain, chronic pain associated with malignant disease, and chronic pain not associated with malignant disease.

Acute pain is an immediate reaction to noxious stimuli such as mechanical (e.g., fracture and muscle sprain) or thermal injuries. Effective analgesia prevents acute pain from progressing to more serious disorders.

Chronic pain associated with malignant disease includes the pain of any advanced, progressive disorder, not just cancer. Examples of such disorders are multiple sclerosis, amyotrophic lateral sclerosis (Lou Gehrig's disease), acquired immunodeficiency syndrome (AIDS), end-stage renal or hepatic failure with pain, congestive heart failure, dementia, and painful end-stage respiratory disease.

Chronic pain not associated with malignant disease is the most complex, most misunderstood, and least well managed of the three major categories of pain. This type of pain is related to a progressive, debilitating process. Arthritides may or may not be classified as chronic nonmalignant pain, depending on whether the disease is truly progressive or is manifested as periodic exacerbations and remissions.

Nonprescription analgesics may be useful in treating all three types of pain, but these drugs are only adjunctive for most chronic nonmalignant pain syndromes. Readers are referred to the listings under "Additional Information Sources" (see end of chapter) for information about management of chronic nonmalignant pain.

This chapter addresses treatment of minor pain with oral (systemic) analgesics. (See Chapter 5, "Musculoskeletal Injuries and Disorders," for a discussion of topical nonprescription analgesics.)

Nonprescription analgesic/antipyretic use has increased in the United States during the past decade as a result of reclassification of several nonsteroidal anti-inflammatory drugs (NSAIDs) to nonprescription status and the increased consumer demand for these products. As many as 47% of patients using nonprescription pain relievers do not read the labeling on the container, and 43% of people surveyed were unaware of the risks associated with taking these nonprescription agents along with prescription medications.[3] Providing accurate information on pain and its management is both a real need and an excellent opportunity for pharmaceutical care.

Physiology of Pain Perception

The sensory component of pain derives from transmission of peripheral nociceptive impulses to the central nervous system (CNS), specifically to the somatosensory cortex. By definition, these noxious impulses are not pain until they reach the cerebral cortex, where intellectual functions occur and recognize them as pain. Proximal to the cerebral cortex, these impulses are more correctly identified as nociceptive. Nociceptors are peripheral pain receptors that are activated by noxious stimuli in the periphery and that send the pain stimulus to the spinal cord by afferent, nociceptive nerve fibers. (See Figure 3–1.) The afferent nerve impulses pass through the dorsal root ganglion where neurotransmitters

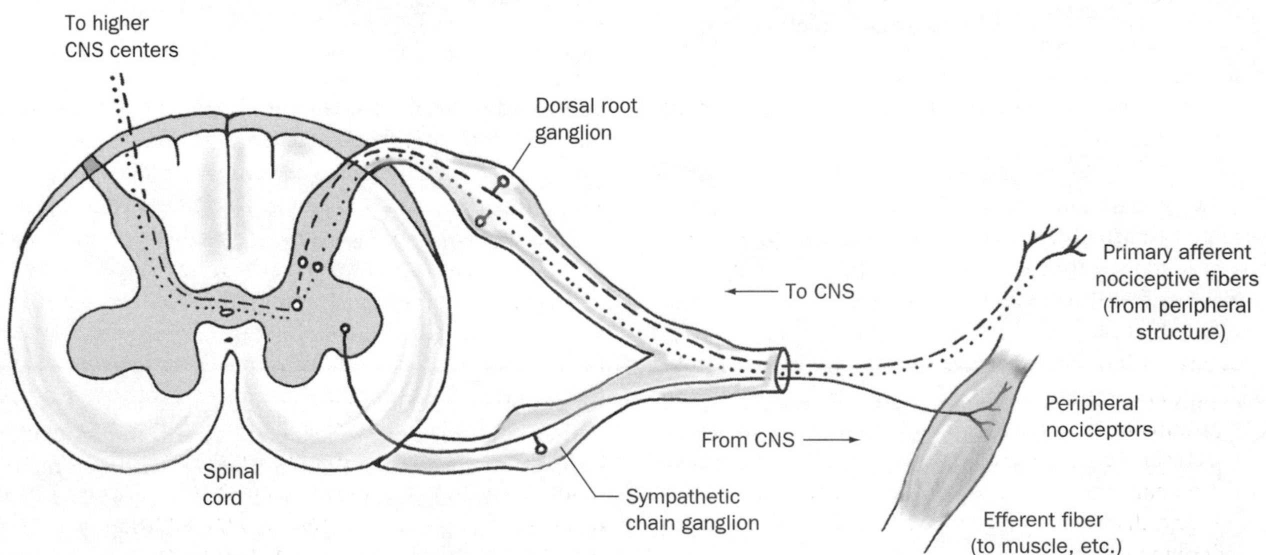

Figure 3–1 Pain pathways from the periphery to the central nervous system.

are synthesized. From there, the impulses go into the dorsal horn of the spinal cord, where the dorsal root ganglia synapse both with ascending fibers that send the pain message to the brain and with efferent fibers that return to the periphery to complete the nerve circuit. It is important to note that the efferent fibers pass through the sympathetic chain ganglia. This physiology helps to explain the chronic pain syndromes that are maintained by sympathetic nervous stimulation. Pain previously called sympathetically maintained pain is now referred to as a complex regional pain syndrome (CRPS). Generally, nonprescription medications are not useful for CRPS.

Numerous substances found in the dorsal horn of the spinal cord are involved in the transmission and modulation of pain. Current research has focused on the role of the amino acid glutamate, which activates *N*-methyl-D-aspartate (NMDA) receptors located on postsynaptic membranes.

The dorsal horn of the spinal cord contains large numbers of nociceptive nerve endings. High concentrations of opioid receptors, endorphins (endogenous opioid substances), α_2 sympathetic receptors, and serotonin-containing neurons are also found here. When activated by endorphins or opioid drugs, opioid receptors impede the release of excitatory neurotransmitters. α_2 Sympathetic receptors also decrease pain when activated by norepinephrine. Increased serotonin levels within the nerves may also have an antinociceptive effect. These drugs are assumed to increase levels of norepinephrine and serotonin in the nerves through inhibition of the reuptake of these neurotransmitters. The action of these drugs at sodium channels leading to nerve membrane stabilization appears to be the major mechanism. Nonprescription analgesics have minimal effect within the dorsal horn.

Headache

Headache is the most common pain complaint, and patients make 10 million visits annually to their primary care physician for this reason. Recurrent headaches afflict more than 40% of the U.S. population, and more than 50% of these sufferers do not consult a physician.[4]

Most of the 129 different types of headache are rare. In 1988, the International Headache Society classified headaches into two broad categories: primary and secondary. Primary headaches (approximately 90% of headaches) are recurrent and not associated with an underlying illness. Examples include episodic and chronic tension-type headaches, migraines with and without aura, cluster headaches, and rebound headaches. Secondary headaches are symptoms of an underlying disease. Head trauma, vascular defects (e.g., infarct, intracerebral hemorrhage, aneurysm), substance abuse or withdrawal, bacterial or viral diseases, and disorders of craniofacial structures are among the underlying causes.[5]

Many headaches, including some severe vascular headaches, respond well to nonprescription analgesics. This chapter focuses on the self-treatable headaches: tension-type headaches, diagnosed migraine (vascular) headache, muscular–vascular headaches (coexisting migraine and tension-type headaches), and sinus headache.

Tension-Type Headache

Tension-type headaches are also called muscle contraction headaches. Such headaches can be episodic or chronic.

Epidemiology/Etiology of Tension-Type Headache

More than 75% of the U.S. population will experience tension-type headaches at some time. These headaches are a type of myofascial pain that manifests in response to stress, anxiety, depression, emotional conflicts, fatigue, and repressed hostility. Tight muscles in the upper back, neck, or scalp or myofascial trigger points in the muscles of the cervical area, occiput, or scalp can cause headaches. Referred pain from remote trigger points can also initiate or exacerbate headaches.

Pathophysiology of Tension-Type Headache

The pathophysiology of tension-type headaches is still hypothetical and is likely to involve interaction among three factors: myofascial nociception, pericranial muscle strain, and descending (limbic) control of nociceptive brainstem neurons. The contribution of these factors is likely to vary from patient to patient and from episode to episode. Muscle strain might contribute to pain development in episodic tension-type headaches, but susceptibility would still depend on excitability of the nociceptive brainstem neurons. (See the section "Pathophysiology of Muscle Pain.") Thus, mental strain could predispose individuals to this type of headache by exciting the nociceptive neurons, and each repeated episode might lower the threshold for myofascial nociception and for successive episodes. Chronic tension-type headache is thought to result from establishment of these changes in the central limbic system.

Signs and Symptoms of Tension-Type Headache

Tension-type headaches commonly present as bilateral, diffuse pain, often over the top of the head and extending to the rear and base of the skull. The pain may radiate to other areas, such as the neck and shoulders. Patients often describe the pain as "tight" or "pressing," as if a band constricted the head. The pain is usually more gradual in onset than the pain of vascular headaches and produces more of an aching than a throbbing sensation. Shivering or cold temperatures may increase the pain. Episodic tension-type headaches may last for minutes to several days. Chronic tension-type headaches are distinguished from episodic tension-type headaches by having a frequency of at least 15 days per month for at least 6 months. Chronic tension-type headaches are often a manifestation of psychologic conflict, depression, or anxiety and may be associated with sleep disturbances, shortness of breath, constipation, weight loss, fatigue, decreased sexual drive, palpitations, and menstrual changes.

Treatment Overview of Tension-Type Headache

Episodic tension-type headaches often respond well to nonprescription analgesics. (See the section "Treatment of Headache.") However, chronic tension-type headaches usually require treatment by physical therapy and relaxation exercises. Generally, physical therapy emphasizing stretching and strengthening of the affected muscles is safer and more effective than prescription medications for tension-type headaches. Chronic tension-type headaches will probably require prescription medication. If nonprescription analgesics are used to treat chronic headache, use should be monitored (records kept) and episodic to prevent rebound headache. Caffeine-containing analgesics in particular should be avoided because of the risk of caffeine-withdrawal headaches.

Vascular Headache

Vascular headaches include migraine and cluster headaches, but migraine headaches account for most vascular headaches. Diagnosed migraine headache is self-treatable, whereas cluster headaches require medical referral.

Epidemiology of Vascular Headache

Of the U.S. population, 20% to 25% experience migraine headaches. This type of headache is uniformly distributed in that its prevalence in Third World countries is the same as in Western countries. Migraine without aura is almost twice as frequent as migraine with aura, and many individuals may have both types of headaches. Women have a five times higher incidence of migraine headaches than do men; women have a seven times higher incidence of migraine with aura and twice the incidence of migraine without aura. In children, boys and girls are affected equally, but attacks usually disappear in boys after puberty. Up to 70% of patients with migraine have family histories of migraine, suggesting that this disease is influenced by heredity.

Stress, fatigue, oversleeping, fasting or missing a meal, vasoactive substances in food, caffeine, alcohol, menses, and changes in barometric pressure and altitude may trigger migraine. Medications (reserpine, nitrates, indomethacin, oral contraceptives, and postmenopausal hormones) can trigger migraine. Although still debated, personality features of migraine sufferers include perfectionism, rigidity, and compulsiveness. Menstrual migraines appear at the menstrual stage of the ovarian cycle and occur in less than 10% of women.[6] Most affected women suffer attacks in the premenstrual period and, for some women, migraine headaches recur at specific times before, after, or during the menstrual cycle.

Cluster headache is rare (less than 0.1%) and occurs 10 times more frequently in males than in females. The disease can first appear at any age, but onset is usually between age 20 and 40 years. Unlike migraine headaches, heredity has much less influence on cluster headache: Only 7% of patients with cluster headache report a family history.

Alcohol, physical exertion (exercise), smoking or being in smoke-filled rooms, food that dilates the blood vessels (e.g., those containing nitrites), and rapid change of temperature can trigger cluster headaches. Emotional upset is not a trigger of this disease, in contrast to tension-type and migraine headaches.[7]

Etiology/Pathophysiology of Vascular Headache

Vascular headaches may be caused by distention or dilation of intracranial arteries or by traction or displacement of large intracranial veins or their meningeal covering.

Similar to tension-type headaches, the pathophysiology of migraine is still a patchwork of conjecture. The best evidence suggests that migraine occurs through a dysfunction of the trigeminovascular system. Stimulation (by an axon reflex) of trigeminal sensory fibers in the large cerebral and dural vessels causes neuropeptide release with concomitant neurogenic inflammation, vasodilatation, and platelet and mast cell activation. A reduction of blood flow has been reported only in migraine-with-aura patients. This reduction occurs initially in the cortical region identified as responsible for aura symptoms and later spreads anteriorly. Consistent cerebral blood flow changes have not been observed in patients with migraine only.[8] Another hypothesis is based on nuclear magnetic resonance studies that show reduced magnesium in brains of migraine-with-aura patients. Low magnesium could increase the excitability of NMDA receptors and could reduce the brain's ability to process energy demands.[9]

The pathophysiology of cluster headache is still unknown; current theories do not explain all features of this disorder. The rhythmical pattern of neuroendocrine data and of symptoms suggests a dysfunctioning "biological clock" in the hypothalamus.[6]

Signs and Symptoms of Vascular Headache

Migraine headaches are recurrent, hemicranial, and throbbing. They are classified as either migraine with or without aura. The aura associated with migraine manifests as a series of neurologic symptoms: shimmering or flashing areas or blind spots in the visual field, difficulty speaking, visual and auditory hallucinations, and (usually) one-sided muscle weakness. These symptoms may last for up to half an hour, and the throbbing headache pain that follows may last from several hours to 2 days. Migraines without aura begin immediately with the throbbing headache pain. Both forms of migraine are often associated with nausea, vomiting, photophobia, phonophobia, tinnitus, light-headedness, vertigo, and irritability and are aggravated by routine physical activity. A migraine attack may have a prodrome of a burst of energy or fatigue, extreme hunger, and nervousness.

Treatment Overview of Vascular Headache

Many patients use the term migraine to denote any bad headache. Therefore, a clinician's diagnosis is required to ensure that the headache is truly migraine before treatment is suggested. General treatment measures for migraine include

(1) maintaining a regular schedule for sleeping and eating meals to avoid fatigue, oversleeping or hunger and (2) practicing methods for coping with stress.

Nutritional strategies are intended to prevent migraine and are based on (1) dietary restriction of foods that contain triggers, (2) avoidance of hunger and low blood glucose (a trigger of migraine), and (3) magnesium supplementation. Those professionals who advocate nutritional therapy recommend foods without nitrites because nitrites dilate blood vessels. Other foods to be avoided contain substances that constrict blood vessels but cause rebound dilation. These substances are tyramine (found in red wine and aged cheese), phenylalanine (found in the artificial sweetener aspartame), monosodium glutamate (often found in Asian food), caffeine (in coffee, tea, cola beverages, chocolate), and theobromines (in chocolate). Any food allergen can also be a trigger.[10]

Another strategy is to elevate the low magnesium levels that are present in migraine sufferers. Magnesium supplements are safe and cheap, and many migraine patients might benefit from supplementation.[11]

Migraine patients have used cold packs for many years. Some migraine patients may benefit from the use of ice (ice bags or cold packs) combined with pressure to reduce the pain associated with acute migraine attacks.

For some patients, an NSAID or acetaminophen effectively controls migraine headache pain if dosed properly. Such nonprescription analgesics may actually abort a migraine headache if taken soon after onset. The NSAIDs can be used to prevent headache when the onset is predictable. For example, initiating NSAIDs 2 days before menses and continuing this medication through menstrual flow can prevent menstrual migraine. Recently, the Food and Drug Administration (FDA) approved the labeling of a nonprescription combination dosage form, Excedrin Migraine, for use in the temporary relief of mild-to-moderate pain associated with migraine headache. (See the section "Treatment of Headache.")

Coexisting Migraine and Tension-Type Headache

Mixed vascular–muscle contraction headaches (now identified as coexisting migraine and tension-type headaches) may occur. Patients with this disorder have daily muscle contraction headaches and occasional migraines. Most headache specialists view headaches across a spectrum, with tension-type on one end and vascular headaches on the other end. The current opinion is that either type of headache can precipitate the other. Treatment of the initiating headache type can abort the mixed headache problem. It is not always necessary to treat both types. Medications that may lead to dependency problems (e.g., caffeine-containing analgesics) should be strictly avoided in patients with coexisting migraine and tension-type headache.

Sinus Headache

Etiology/Signs and Symptoms of Sinus Headache

Sinus headache occurs when infection or blockage of the paranasal sinuses causes inflammation or distention of the sensitive sinus walls. (See Chapter 9, "Disorders Related to Cold and Allergy," for further discussion of the etiology and pathophysiology of sinus inflammation.)

Sinus headache is usually localized to the forehead or periorbital area. Pain tends to occur on awakening and may subside gradually after the patient has been upright for a while. Stooping or blowing the nose often intensifies the pain. Persistent sinus pain and/or discharge suggests possible bacterial infection and requires referral for medical evaluation.

Treatment Overview of Sinus Headache

Decongestants (e.g., pseudoephedrine) are often useful in facilitating drainage of the sinuses. (See Chapter 9, "Disorders Related to Cold and Allergy.") Concomitant use of decongestants and nonprescription analgesics can relieve the pain of sinus headache.

Other Headaches

Headaches can also be associated with fever, excessive alcohol or opioid consumption, fatigue, eye strain, or infection. Headache can also be a manifestation of anxiety or depression.

Headaches caused by fever or excessive alcohol consumption are amenable to nonprescription drug treatment. Hangovers from alcohol ingestion are caused by an accumulation of acetaldehyde, a toxic metabolite of ethyl alcohol. Hangover headaches often respond to acetaminophen or an NSAID. The metabolite is eliminated slowly, and the condition does not fully resolve for several hours until the acetaldehyde is eliminated from the body by normal metabolic and excretory processes.

Nonprescription stimulants, such as caffeine, may provide some relief from headaches related to fatigue, but making up any sleep deficit is important in reducing the incidence and severity of this type of headache. Nonprescription medications are usually not effective in treating anxiety or depression headaches.

Rebound headaches are another challenging area for clinicians. Overuse of abortive agents, such as NSAIDS and caffeine, can actually predispose patients to rebound headaches. Frequent and excessive use of analgesics (even nonopioid analgesics) or ergotamine formulations can exacerbate the following symptoms: asthenia; nausea and other gastrointestinal (GI) symptoms; restlessness, irritability, and anxiety; and depression, memory problems, and difficulty concentrating. When rebound headache is suspected, use of offending agent(s) should be tapered and subsequently eliminated.

Treatment of Headache

Treatment Outcomes

The primary goal of treating headaches is relieving or moderating pain. Analgesics are used to prevent, abort, or treat headaches, depending on when (just before, at onset, or during) therapy can be started.

General Treatment Approach

Nonprescription analgesics can usually relieve the pain of episodic tension-type headache and mild-to-moderate migraine. Patients with tension-type headaches should take an analgesic as soon as the headache starts. Migraine sufferers who can predict the occurrence of the headache (e.g., during menstruation) should take an NSAID (ibuprofen, ketoprofen, or naproxen) before the event known to trigger the headache as well as throughout the duration of the event. Taking an NSAID at the onset of symptoms can abort a migraine headache. Once a migraine has evolved, NSAIDs sometimes will relieve the pain. Excedrin Migraine, whose active ingredients are aspirin, acetaminophen, and caffeine, has been approved for use in the temporary relief of mild-to-moderate pain associated with migraine headache. Patients with coexisting tension and migraine headache should treat the initiating headache with the preferred analgesic for that type of headache. The algorithm in Figure 3–2 outlines the self-treatment of headaches.

Exclusions to self-treatment include (1) headaches that persist for 10 days with or without treatment, (2) a patient who is in the last trimester of pregnancy, (3) a patient who is 7 years of age or younger, (4) any patient with a high fever or signs of a serious infection, and (5) any headache associated with underlying pathology (secondary headache).

Nonpharmacologic Therapy

See the discussion of nondrug measures in the treatment overviews of the various types of headaches.

Pharmacologic Therapy

Nonprescription analgesics include an acetylated salicylate (aspirin), nonacetylated salicylates (magnesium salicylate, choline salicylate, and sodium salicylate), acetaminophen, and the three nonsalicylate NSAIDs (ibuprofen, ketoprofen, and naproxen). Because these agents can cause serious problems for certain disease states and can interact with several medications, selection of an analgesic should be based on a careful review of a patient's medical and medication histories. The dosages of nonprescription analgesics/antipyretics commonly used for minor pain such as headache are listed in Table 3–1. Dosages recommended by FDA are given in the following discussions of specific agents.[12]

Salicylates

Acetylated Salicylate (Aspirin) Aspirin is the only available acetylated salicylate. The active moiety of all salicylates is salicylic acid, but that compound is too irritating to be used systemically. Therefore, esters of salicylic acid and salicylate esters of organic acids that can be administered orally and rectally have been formulated. Table 3–2 lists adult dosages of commercially available nonprescription salicylates. FDA-recommended dosages are given in text discussions of the individual salicylates.

Mechanism of Action Salicylates inhibit prostaglandin synthesis from arachidonic acid by inhibiting both isoforms of the enzyme cyclooxygenase (COX-1 and COX-2). This enzyme is essential for prostaglandin synthesis. Prostaglandins sensitize nociceptors to the chemical or mechanical initiation of pain impulses. The resulting decrease in prostaglandins reduces the sensitivity of pain receptors to the initiation of pain impulses at inflammation and trauma sites. Although some evidence suggests that aspirin also produces analgesia through a central mechanism, its site of action is primarily peripheral.

Pharmacokinetics Salicylates are absorbed by passive diffusion of the non-ionized drug in the stomach and small intestine. Factors affecting absorption include dosage form, gastric pH, gastric emptying time, dissolution rate, and the presence of antacids or food. Because enteric-coated aspirin is absorbed only from the small intestine, its absorption is markedly slowed by food, which prolongs the gastric emptying time. Buffered-aspirin products are absorbed more rapidly than nonbuffered products, but this more rapid absorption has little therapeutic significance in terms of onset of drug effect. Rectal absorption of salicylate is slow and unreliable. By the rectal route, aspirin is only 60% to 75% bioavailable and produces peak salicylate levels of about half those achieved with an equivalent oral dose.[13]

Sustained-release aspirin is formulated to prolong the product's duration of action by slowing dissolution and absorption. Because of this delayed absorption, such products are not useful for rapid pain relief but may be useful as bedtime medication. A bioavailability comparison of a single 1.3 g dose of plain aspirin versus 1.3 g of a timed-release formulation (Measurin) revealed plasma salicylate concentrations to be higher for the first 4 hours following administration with the plain aspirin product and higher during the 4- to 8-hour interval with the timed-release product.[14] Although comparisons of three timed-release aspirin products (Measurin, Verin, and Zorprin) demonstrated all three to be equally bioavailable, they were not bioequivalent. Of the administered dose, 50% was recovered in the urine approximately 9 hours following administration of Measurin compared with 18 to 19 hours for both Verin and Zorprin.[15] These data suggest that the pharmacokinetic profiles are not identical for the various sustained-release aspirin products and that the duration of therapeutic efficacy, therefore, depends on the product.

Effervescent aspirin solutions (e.g., Alka-Seltzer) are rapidly absorbed because disintegration does not have to occur. However, there is no evidence that such products produce more rapid or effective analgesia than oral solid

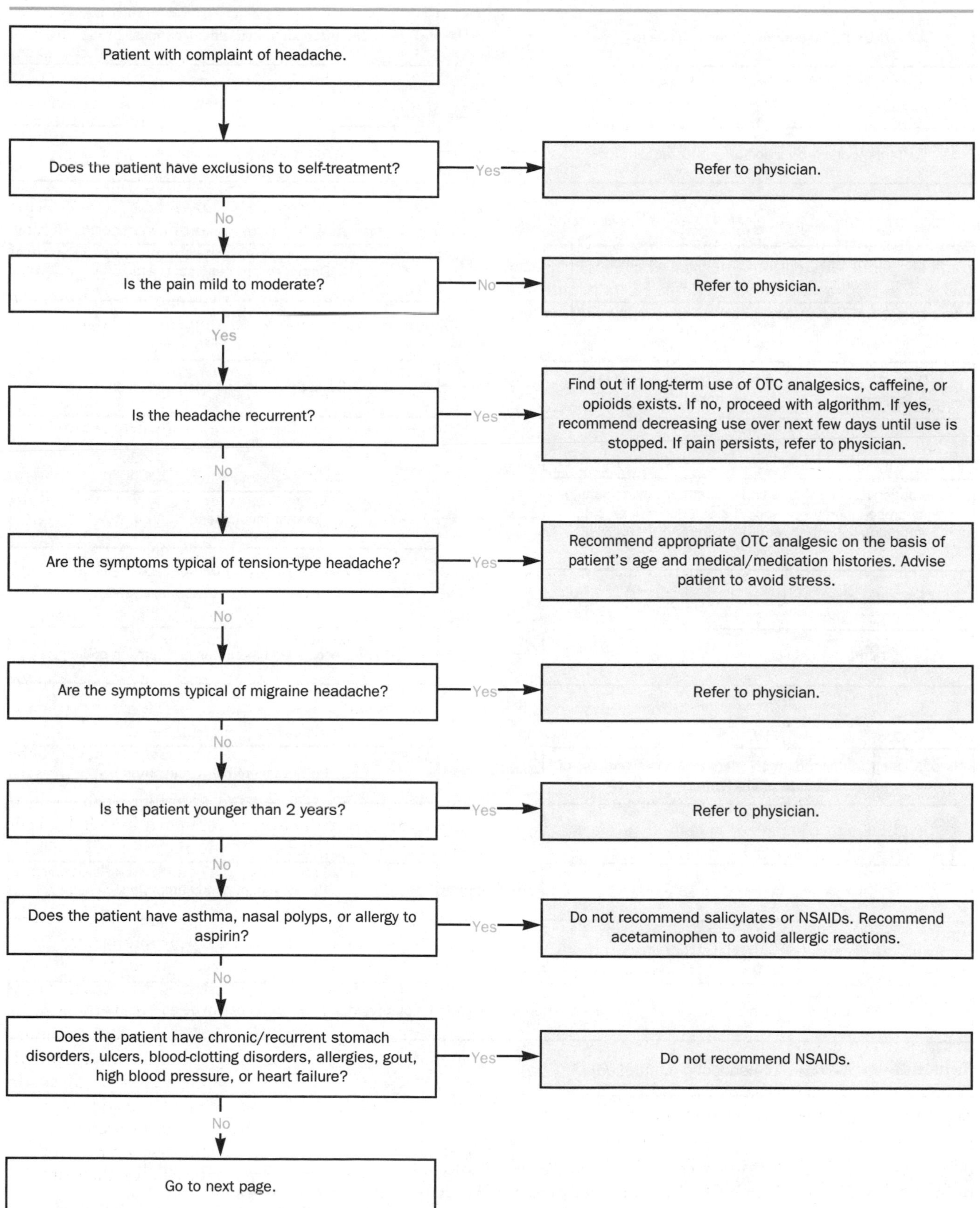

Figure 3–2 Self-care of headache.

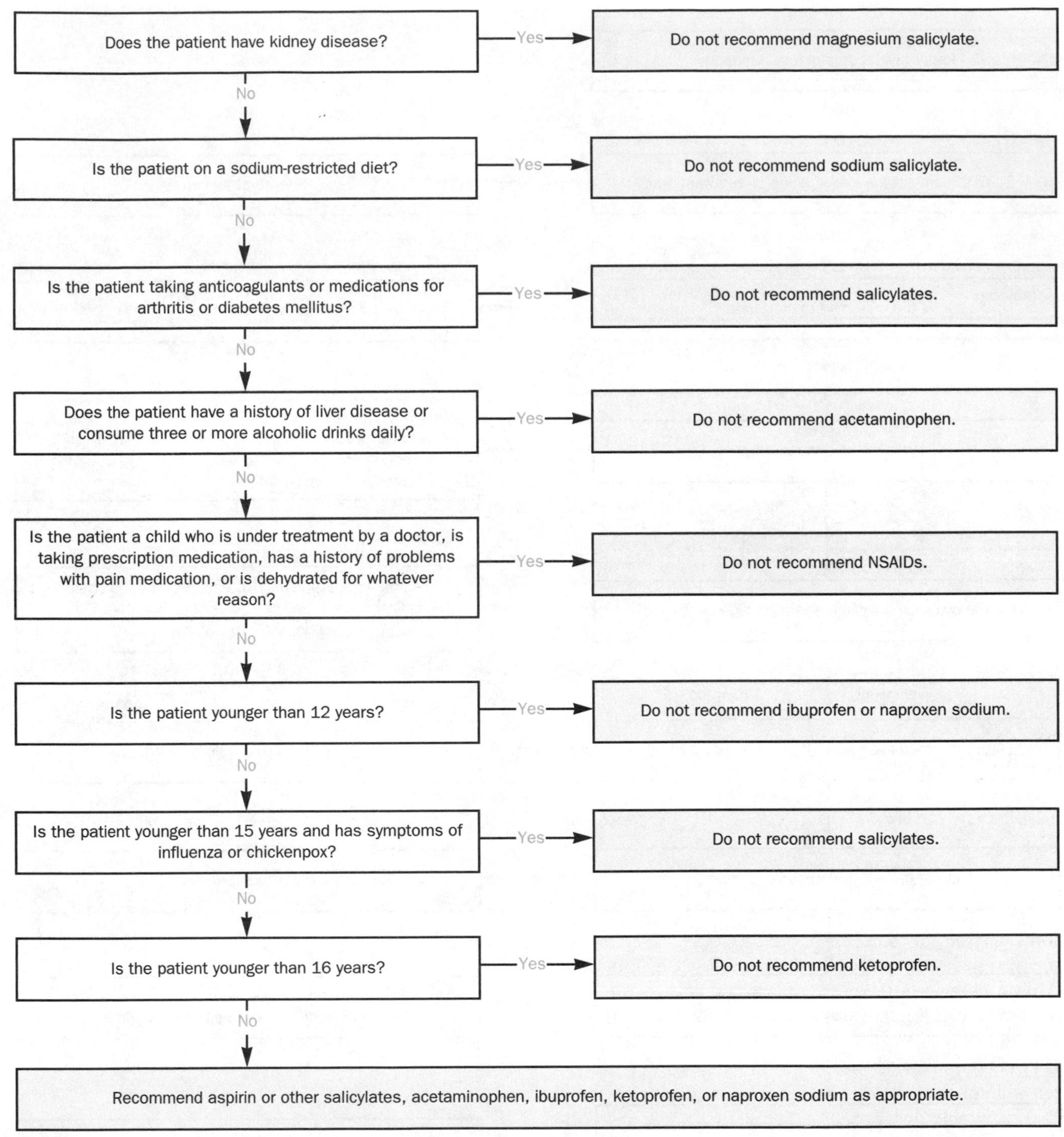

Figure 3–2 Self-care of headache (continued).

dosage forms of salicylates. Moreover, some effervescent aspirin solutions contain large amounts of sodium and must be avoided by patients requiring restricted sodium intake (e.g., patients with hypertension, heart failure, or renal failure).

Indications Salicylates are effective in treating mild-to-moderate pain and fever. These agents are most commonly used for musculoskeletal indications, but they are usually ineffective in pain of visceral origin.

Dosage/Administration Guidelines The adult oral aspirin dosage recommended by FDA for mild-to-moderate pain and fever is 325 to 650 mg every 4 hours, or 325 to 500 mg every 3 hours, or 65 to 1000 mg every 6 hours while symp-

Table 3–1

Dosages of Nonprescription Analgesic/Antipyretic Agents Commonly Used for Pain or Inflammation

Agent	Dosage (maximum)	
	Analgesic	**Anti-inflammatory**
Acetaminophen	650–1000 mg, 3–4 times/day (4000 mg/day)	—
Aspirin	650–1000 mg every 4 hours (4000 mg/day)	2400–3900 mg/day for 5–7 days
Ibuprofen	200–400 mg every 4–6 hours (1200 mg/day)	400–800 mg, 3–4 times/day[a] (3200 mg in 2 weeks)
Naproxen sodium	220 mg every 6–8 hours (660 mg/day)	275–550 mg, 2 times/day[a] (1650 mg/day for 2 weeks)
Ketoprofen	12.5–25 mg every 6–8 hours (75 mg/day)	50–75 mg, 3–4 times/day[a,b] (300 mg/day)

[a] Dosage exceeds that recommended in nonprescription product labeling.

[b] Dosage should be reduced in patients who are elderly and renally impaired.

Source: Extracted from: Whelton A. Renal effects of over-the-counter analgesics. *J Clin Pharmacol.* 1995;35:453–63.

Table 3–2

Recommended Adult Dosages of Nonprescription Salicylates

Agent	Dosage Forms	Usual Adult Dosage
Aspirin	Tablets, effervescent, enteric coated, buffered; suppositories; chewing gum	650–975 mg (three 325 mg doses) or 1000 mg (two 500 mg doses) every 4–6 hours, not to exceed 4000 mg/day
Choline salicylate	Oral solution (870 mg/5 mL)	870 mg every 3–4 hours not to exceed 6 daily doses
Magnesium salicylate	Tablets (325 and 500 mg)	650 mg every 4 hours or 1000 mg, 3 times/day
Sodium salicylate	Tablets, enteric coated (325 and 650 mg)	650 mg every 4 hours

Table 3–3

FDA-Recommended Pediatric Antipyretic Doses for Acetaminophen and Aspirin

Agent	Body Weight	Age (years)	Single Dose (mg)[a]
Acetaminophen	(10–15 mg/kg)	<2	Physician directed
		2–3	160
		4–5	240
		6–8	320
		9–10	400
		11–12	480
		Adult	650
Aspirin	(10–15 mg/kg)	<2	Physician directed
		2–3	162
		4–5	243
		6–8	324
		9–10	405
		11–12	486
		Adult	650

[a] Individual doses may be repeated every 4–6 hours as needed, up to four to five daily doses. Do not exceed five doses in 24 hours.

toms persist, not to exceed 4 g in 24 hours.[12] The recommended pediatric antipyretic doses are listed in Table 3–3. Aspirin dosages in the range of 4 to 6 g per day are often needed to produce anti-inflammatory effects. Because the maximum analgesic dosage for self-medication with aspirin is 4 g per day in divided doses, anti-inflammatory efficacy often will not occur unless the drug is used at the high end of the acceptable dosage range. Therefore, NSAIDs are the drugs of choice in inflammatory disorders such as rheumatoid arthritis.

Overdosage Mild salicylate intoxication (salicylism) occurs with chronic therapy that produces toxic salicylate plasma concentrations. Chronic intoxication in adults generally requires taking salicylate doses of approximately 90 to 100 mg/kg within 24 hours for at least 2 days. Symptoms include headache, dizziness, tinnitus, difficulty in hearing, dimness of vision, mental confusion, lassitude, drowsiness, sweating, thirst, hyperventilation, nausea, vomiting, and occasional diarrhea. These symptoms, which may mimic the signs and symptoms of the disease being treated, are all reversible on lowering the plasma concentration to a therapeutic range. Pharmacists should keep in mind that patients may not manifest all of the signs and symptoms of toxicity. Tinnitus should not be used as a sole indicator of salicylate toxicity.

Acute salicylate intoxication is categorized as mild (less than 150 mg/kg), moderate (150 to 300 mg/kg), or severe (greater than 300 mg/kg). Symptoms depend on serum salicylate levels and include lethargy, tinnitus, tachypnea and pulmonary edema, convulsions, coma, nausea, vomiting, hemorrhage, and dehydration. Acid–base disturbances are prominent and range from respiratory alkalosis to metabolic acidosis. Initially, salicylate affects the respiratory center in the medulla, producing hyperventilation and respiratory alkalosis. In severely intoxicated adults and in most salicylate-poisoned children younger than 5 years, respiratory alkalosis rapidly progresses to metabolic acidosis. Children are more prone to develop high fever in salicylate poisoning. Hypoglycemia resulting from increased tissue glucose use may be especially serious in children. Bleeding may occur from the GI tract or mucosal surfaces, and petechiae (minute hemorrhagic spots) are a prominent feature at autopsy.

Emergency management of acute salicylate intoxication is directed toward preventing the absorption of salicylate from the GI tract. Emergency medical personnel and poison control centers commonly advocate using ipecac syrup at home to empty the stomach for mild-to-moderate unintentional ingestions by children younger than 6 years. When the patient is to be seen in an emergency department, the emetic, gastric lavage, or activated charcoal may be used depending on the attending physician's preference and on the clinical situation. Ipecac syrup or activated charcoal should be used only if recommended by poison control or emergency department personnel. Vomiting should be induced even if the patient has vomited spontaneously. Adults and children older than 12 years should be given 30 mL of ipecac syrup followed by 8 ounces of water, clear liquids, or carbonated beverages and should be ambulated to stimulate emesis. If emesis does not occur in 20 to 30 minutes, the process should be repeated with the same ipecac dose.

For children ages 1 to 12 years, the recommended dose of ipecac syrup is 15 mL followed by 8 ounces of water, clear liquids, or carbonated beverages. The same 15 mL dose of ipecac syrup should be repeated if vomiting does not occur within 20 to 30 minutes. In children younger than age 1 year, vomiting should be induced only under medical supervision.

Administering ipecac syrup or other oral liquids to a person who is convulsing or not completely conscious is absolutely contraindicated because of the potential for aspiration. Further guidelines on the use of ipecac syrup or activated charcoal in preventing absorption of salicylate are included in Chapter 17 "Poisoning."

Adverse Effects Aspirin produces local GI damage by penetrating the protective mucous and bicarbonate layers of the gastric mucosa and by permitting the back diffusion of acid, thus causing cellular and vascular erosion. Two distinct mechanisms cause this problem: (1) a local irritant effect from the drug contacting the gastric mucosa and (2) a systemic effect from prostaglandin inhibition. Gastritis is a local effect that can occur without risk of ulceration. Conversely, ulceration is caused by systemic activity, and it can be asymptomatic until it is advanced. Contributing mechanisms include inhibition of mucosal prostaglandin synthesis, reduction and alteration of mucus secretion, and reduction of bicarbonate secretion.

Endoscopic evaluation of healthy volunteers showed that 650 mg of aspirin produced multiple gastric petechiae and erythema within 1 hour in all subjects. A second group taking 650 mg of aspirin every 6 hours for 24 hours showed multiple antral erosions in all subjects and duodenal erosions and petechiae in half the volunteers.[16] In a prospective endoscopic analysis of patients taking 2.5 g of aspirin per day for at least 3 months, 20% had gastric ulcers, 40% had gastric erosions, 75% had gastric erythema, and 4% had duodenal ulceration.

Endoscopic evaluation comparing the gastric damage produced by buffered and nonbuffered aspirin products suggests that either product can cause the same amount of gastric damage.[17] However, enteric coating eliminates the local gastric irritation produced by aspirin.[18,19] Equivalent doses of plain, buffered, or enteric-coated aspirin produce essentially the same plasma levels of salicylate; however, the time to peak is delayed with the enteric-coated product. Thus, for patients requiring rapid pain relief, enteric-coated aspirin is inappropriate because of the delay in absorption and the time to analgesic effect. However, for patients requiring prolonged aspirin therapy to manage rheumatoid arthritis, enteric-coated aspirin may be preferred because it produces less gastric mucosal injury than either plain or buffered aspirin.

GI blood loss with aspirin is dose dependent. Normal subjects with no aspirin exposure lose approximately 0.5 mL of blood per day in the stool. Moderate aspirin intake increases this amount to 2 to 6 mL per day, and up to 15% of patients will lose in excess of 10 mL per day. Chronic GI bleeding of this magnitude can deplete total body iron and can produce iron deficiency anemia. Patients experiencing aspirin-induced blood loss may or may not be positive for fecal occult blood, depending on the dose and duration of aspirin therapy. Aspirin use should be discontinued for at least 3 days before a test for fecal occult blood.

In a small percentage of patients, aspirin use can produce massive GI bleeding (acute hemorrhagic gastritis), resulting in hematemesis or melena. Recent aspirin ingestion has been associated with about half of all cases of acute hemorrhagic gastritis, and the incidence of hospital admissions for major upper GI bleeding attributable to regular aspirin use is estimated to be about 15 cases per 100,000 admissions per year.[20] Elderly patients, patients with a history of gastric ulceration or bleeding, and those with alcoholic liver disease are at increased risk for acute hemorrhagic gastritis with aspirin use and, therefore, should avoid aspirin. In addition, patients who take aspirin should be advised that ingesting aspirin with alcohol appears to increase the incidence of GI bleeding.

Many patients report that they are allergic to aspirin because they have experienced gastritis or heartburn following its use. These are common side effects, not allergy or hypersensitivity, and they are not contraindications to future trials of aspirin. True aspirin allergy is uncommon, occurring in less than 1% of patients. Manifestations of aspirin allergy include urticaria, edema, difficulty in breathing, bronchospasm, rhinitis, or shock. These adverse effects usually occur within 3 hours of aspirin ingestion. Aspirin allergy is usually to the moiety, not the salicylate. Therefore, many patients who are allergic to aspirin may use nonacetylated salicylates. Aspirin is the only acetylated salicylate available in the United States.

Aspirin allergy occurs most commonly in patients with urticaria, asthma, and nasal polyps. In patients with only one of these conditions, the incidence of aspirin allergy has been reported to range from 10% to 30%.[21] Patients with chronic urticaria often develop an urticarial reaction to aspirin, and those with asthma or nasal polyps more typically develop bronchospasm and/or rhinorrhea. However, the level of these adverse effects may not be clinically problematic.

Patients intolerant to aspirin may also cross-react to other chemicals or drugs. Up to 15% of patients who are allergic to aspirin may cross-react when exposed to tartrazine (Food Drug and Cosmetic yellow dye #5), which can be found in many drugs, in foods such as soft drinks and colored candy, and in colored desserts such as puddings and frostings. The cross-reaction rates for acetaminophen and ibuprofen in documented aspirin-intolerant patients are 6% and 97%, respectively. High cross-reaction rates in aspirin-intolerant patients are reported with some prescription NSAIDs. Thus, patients with a history of aspirin intolerance should be advised to avoid all aspirin- and NSAID-containing products and to use acetaminophen for analgesic self-medication.

Even though the cross-reaction rate for acetaminophen is low, aspirin-intolerant patients may exhibit urticarial or bronchospastic symptoms with this drug. Other nonprescription analgesics that have a low risk of cross-reactivity include sodium salicylate and choline salicylate. No symptoms of intolerance were observed in 182 documented aspirin-intolerant patients given either sodium or choline salicylate.[22]

Sustained-release aspirin products may produce less GI irritation than regular aspirin. However, aspirin-induced reversible deafness has been reported to occur to a much greater extent with high-dose sustained-release aspirin than with equivalent daily doses of plain aspirin.[23]

Drug–Drug Interactions Aspirin and the other nonprescription salicylates interact with several other important drugs and drug classes. Adverse effects of the drugs are additive with other agents or diseases that cause similar disorders. Patients at increased risk of toxicity from salicylates include those with (1) marked renal or hepatic impairment (uremia, cirrhosis, hepatitis); (2) metabolic disorders (hypoxia or hypothyroidism); (3) unstable disease (i.e., cardiac arrhythmias, intractable epilepsy, brittle diabetes); and (4) status asthmaticus. Elderly patients in general are at increased risk because of the increased incidence of multiple-system disorders. Table 3–4 lists clinically important drug interactions that have been reported with aspirin and other nonprescription analgesic/antipyretic drugs.

Analgesic doses of aspirin may increase the free fraction of valproic acid in plasma, thereby markedly causing enhanced neurologic toxicity such as drowsiness and behavioral disturbances. The mechanism appears to be a combination of protein-binding displacement and decreased clearance of valproic acid. Patients taking valproic acid should avoid salicylates; naproxen and acetaminophen are safe nonprescription analgesic alternatives.

Hypoglycemic effect of sulfonylurea oral antidiabetic agents may be enhanced by the concurrent administration of more than 2 g per day of any salicylate that increases insulin secretion. The decreased protein binding of the sulfonylurea may also play a role. Patients taking sulfonylurea oral hypoglycemic drugs to control diabetes should avoid all salicylate-containing products and consider acetaminophen as an appropriate alternative.

The uricosuric effect of both probenecid and sulfinpyrazone may be antagonized by the concurrent administration of salicylate, resulting in the worsening of hyperuricemia and the possible exacerbation of gout. The effect and magnitude of this interaction are salicylate-dose dependent. Aspirin doses of greater than 5 g per day are not only uricosuric but also toxic. An occasional dose of aspirin or other salicylate is unlikely to cause serious problems in patients taking uricosuric drugs, but all salicylates should be avoided in such patients to minimize risk. Acetaminophen is the best nonprescription alternative.

Ethyl alcohol can interact with acetaminophen, salicylates, and nonsalicylate NSAIDs, thereby increasing the risk of hepatic toxicity with acetaminophen and gastropathy with the salicylates and NSAIDs. Alcohol also increases fecal blood loss resulting from aspirin ingestion, possibly doubling daily GI blood loss when compared with that induced by aspirin alone. This effect results from both the GI erosive effects of alcohol and aspirin and from an extended bleeding time prolonged by alcohol's potentiation of the antiplatelet effect of aspirin. The ingestion of alcohol plus 1 g of aspirin 1 hour after a standard breakfast significantly elevated the blood alcohol concentration compared with that of subjects who did not receive aspirin. In such patients, alcohol bioavailability is increased because gastric alcohol dehydrogenase is inhibited, thus allowing greater GI absorption of alcohol.[24] Pharmacists should advise patients not to consume alcohol and aspirin together because of the potential for enhanced irritation or GI bleeding or because of enhanced neurologic impairment from the alcohol. If alcohol is to be consumed during analgesic use, acetaminophen should be recommended for self-medication as a "safer" alternative to salicylates or other NSAIDs.

Salicylates may increase the toxicity of methotrexate by displacing the drug from protein-binding sites and by decreasing its renal excretion. Serious sequelae, including pancytopenia, have been reported with this drug combination. Patients taking methotrexate must be warned against self-medication with any nonprescription analgesic containing any form of salicylate. Acetaminophen has been used concurrently with methotrexate without an increase in methotrexate toxicity.

Table 3–4

Clinically Important Drug Interactions with Nonprescription Analgesic/Antipyretic Agents

Analgesic/ Antipyretic	Drug	Potential Interaction	Management/Preventive Measures
Ibuprofen, high-dose salicylates	Phenytoin	Phenytoin displaced from serum protein–binding sites if phenytoin metabolism is saturated or if folate levels are low	Monitor unbound phenytoin levels; adjust dose, if indicated; ensure that patient has sufficient folate
Aspirin	Valproic acid	Oxidation of valproate inhibited; up to 30% reduction in clearance	Avoid concurrent use; use naproxen instead of aspirin (no interaction)
NSAIDs (several)	Digoxin	Renal clearance inhibited	Monitor digoxin levels; adjust doses as indicated
NSAIDs (several)	Aminoglycosides	Renal clearance inhibited	Monitor antibiotic levels; adjust doses as indicated
NSAIDS (several)	Antihypertensive agents; β-blockers, ACE inhibitors, vasodilators, diuretics	Antihypertensive effect antagonized; hyperkalemia may occur with potassium-sparing diuretics and ACE inhibitors	Monitor blood pressure and cardiac function; monitor potassium levels
NSAIDs	Oral anticoagulants	Risk of bleeding, especially GI bleeding, increased	Avoid concurrent use, if possible; risk is lowest with salsalate and choline magnesium trisalicylate
NSAIDs (some)	Lithium	Renal clearance inhibited	Monitor lithium levels; adjust doses as indicated; interaction less likely with aspirin than with ibuprofen or naproxen
NSAIDs	Alcohol	Increased risk of GI bleeding	Avoid concurrent use, if possible; minimize alcohol intake when using NSAIDs
NSAIDs (several)	Methotrexate	Methotrexate clearance decreased	Avoid NSAIDs with high-dose methotrexate therapy; monitor levels with concurrent treatment
Naproxen	Probenecid	Naproxen clearance inhibited	Monitor for adverse effects
Naproxen	Aluminum hydroxide	Naproxen absorption decreased	Increase naproxen dose as needed
Salicylates	Antacids in high doses	Salicylate levels possibly reduced 25%	Determine if salicylate doses should be increased
Salicylates (moderate to high doses)	Sulfonylureas	Hypoglycemic activity increased	Avoid concurrent use, if possible; monitor blood glucose levels when changing salicylate dose
Salicylates	Corticosteroids	Salicylate clearance possibly increased with long-term, high-dose salicylate therapy	Monitor salicylate levels when changing steroid dose; adjust salicylate dose, if indicated

Note: NSAIDs include the salicylates.

Aspirin in doses greater than 3 g per day can have a hypoprothrombinemic effect that can be additive to that produced by oral anticoagulants such as warfarin. In addition, the GI erosion and the inhibition of platelet aggregation produced by aspirin may further increase the bleeding risk—if aspirin is used concurrently with an oral anticoagulant. An increased incidence of GI bleeding has been reported in patients receiving warfarin and as little as 500 mg per day of aspirin. Thus, patients receiving oral anticoagulants should be cautioned to avoid all nonprescription analgesic products containing aspirin or other salicylates and to consider acetaminophen as an appropriate nonprescription analgesic alternative.

A large number of additional drug–drug interactions have been documented, many of which are not as clinically significant as those already mentioned. Pharmacists should review current drug interaction references for newly identified interactions when monitoring the therapy of patients taking high-dose salicylates.

Contraindications Aspirin is the prototype NSAID. Chemically, aspirin is acetylsalicylic acid. The acetyl moiety makes aspirin a more effective anti-inflammatory agent than other salicylates, and aspirin is the salicylate of choice for most patients. However, that moiety also acetylates platelets, causing irreversible inhibition of platelet aggregation. This effect provides a special advantage by preventing blood clots, but it can also be a disadvantage by increasing the risk of bleeding.

Platelet aggregation is an important, secondary hemostatic mechanism. Aspirin can potentiate bleeding from capillary sites such as those found in the GI tract (with ulcers), tonsillar beds (following tonsillectomy), and tooth sockets

A Word about Aspirin's Role in Preventing Cardiovascular/Cardiocerebral Events and Cancer

Cardiovascular/Cardiocerebral Disease

Aspirin inhibits prostaglandin synthesis within the platelet irreversibly and retards platelet aggregation for the life of the aspirin-exposed platelet. Because platelet aggregation has a role in thrombin clot formation, aspirin's antithrombotic activity has been used clinically under medical supervision to prevent transient ischemic attack, thrombotic stroke, myocardial infarction (MI) in unstable angina patients, and vascular reocclusion following both percutaneous transluminal coronary angioplasty and coronary artery bypass grafts. Aspirin has also been used clinically in post-MI patients to prevent the risk of future thromboembolic events.

Ongoing studies of new indications for aspirin have suggested new potential uses and the need for some caution in self-medication with these drugs. There is good evidence of the usefulness of aspirin in preventing and treating primary vascular events (i.e., for acute MIs and unstable angina).[25] Daily ingestion of low-dose aspirin provided significant protection against MI, stroke, and death among high-risk patients (i.e., those with unstable angina, suspected MI, or transient ischemic attacks). Low-dose aspirin taken daily or on alternate days may also be beneficial for other at-risk patients, including those with stable angina or peripheral vascular disease or those undergoing vascular procedures. The effectiveness of antiplatelet therapy in patients at low risk has not yet been demonstrated.

In 1998, FDA approved new labeling for all nonprescription drug products containing aspirin, buffered aspirin, and aspirin in combination with an antacid. FDA's ruling recognizes the role that aspirin plays in preventing future events for patients with cardiovascular and cerebrovascular disease.[26]

Cancer

Aspirin has been associated with decreased risk of colorectal cancer in men.[27] Epidemiologic evidence[28] has suggested that regular aspirin use may also reduce the risk of lung, colon, and breast cancers. These associations are not definitive and do not apply equally to both sexes and across all ages. A recent report[29] has cast some doubt on the ability of low-dose aspirin to prevent colorectal cancer. More studies will be needed to determine the utility of aspirin in reducing cancer risks.

(following dental extractions). A single 650 mg dose of aspirin can double the bleeding time. Aspirin therapy should be discontinued at least 48 hours before surgery and should not be used to relieve the pain following tonsillectomy, dental extraction, or other surgical procedures, except under the close supervision of a physician or dentist. Some surgeons and dentists routinely recommend cessation of aspirin a week before surgery. That recommendation probably is not necessary for patients with normal hematopoietic systems. These patients will produce sufficient new platelets within 48 hours to provide efficient platelet aggregation-induced blood clotting.

Because of this effect on hemostasis, aspirin is contraindicated in patients with hypoprothrombinemia, vitamin K deficiency, hemophilia, history of any bleeding disorder, or history of peptic ulcer disease. When peripheral anti-inflammatory activity is not needed and aspirin's effect on hemostasis is a concern, acetaminophen is an appropriate analgesic for self-medication. Most other NSAIDs impair platelet aggregation when the drugs are at analgesic serum levels, but these effects resolve as the drug is cleared from the serum. The prescription salicylate compounds salsalate and choline magnesium trisalicylate do not have appreciable effects on platelet aggregation and are reasonable alternatives when a peripheral anti-inflammatory agent is indicated. Sodium salicylate does not affect platelets, but it does increase prothrombin time.

Salicylates do not normally affect leukocyte, platelet, or erythrocyte counts; hematocrit; or hemoglobin. However, chronic blood loss from the GI tract, which results from continued use of aspirin-containing products, can cause iron-deficiency anemia and can alter hematologic indices.

Salicylates can affect uric acid secretion and reabsorption by the renal tubules. The resulting effect on plasma uric acid is dose related. Doses of 1 to 2 g per day inhibit tubular uric acid secretion without affecting reabsorption and may increase plasma uric acid levels, which can precipitate or worsen an attack of gout. Moderate doses of 2 to 3 g per day have little effect on uric acid secretion. High doses of more than 5 g per day may decrease plasma uric acid by increasing its renal excretion, but because these are toxic salicylate doses, they should not be used in the clinical management of gout or hyperuricemia. All salicylates should be avoided in patients with a history of gout or hyperuricemia.

Precautions/Warnings Chronic alcohol users should be warned that concurrent aspirin use may risk increased GI bleeding. Patients with preexisting coagulopathies should use caution because salicylate use can cause hemolysis in these patients. Patients with asthma or nasal polyps may experience bronchospasm when using salicylates. Patients with hemophilia or with renal or hepatic dysfunction should use salicylates with caution as should patients taking anticoagulants.

Special Population Considerations Aspirin consumption during pregnancy may produce adverse maternal effects, including anemia, antepartum or postpartum hemorrhage, and prolonged gestation and labor. The inhibition of prostaglandin synthesis will increase duration of gestation and labor. Aspirin ingestion on a regular basis during pregnancy may increase the risk for complicated deliveries, including cesarean sections as well as breech and forceps deliveries. However, controlled study data supporting this concern are lacking. In 1990, FDA required oral and rectal nonprescription drug products that contain aspirin to carry labels that warned against using the drugs during the last 3 months of pregnancy unless the patient is directed to do so by a physician.

Aspirin readily crosses the placenta and can be found in higher concentrations in the neonate than in the mother. Salicylate elimination is slow in the neonate because of the immature and underdeveloped capacity to form glycine and glucuronic acid conjugates in the liver and because of reduced urinary excretion resulting from low glomerular filtration rates.

Fetal effects of in utero aspirin exposure include intrauterine growth retardation, congenital salicylate intoxication, decreased albumin-binding capacity, and increased perinatal mortality. In utero mortality results, in part, from antepartum hemorrhage or premature closure of the ductus arteriosus. In utero aspirin exposure within 1 week of delivery can produce hemorrhagic episodes and/or pruritic rash in the neonate. Reported neonatal bleeding complications include petechiae, hematuria, cephalhematoma, subconjunctival hemorrhage, and bleeding following circumcision. An increased incidence of intracranial hemorrhage in premature or low-birth-weight infants has also been reported after maternal aspirin use near birth.[30] The relationship between maternal aspirin ingestion and congenital malformation is unresolved. An association between maternal aspirin ingestion, oral clefts, and congenital heart disease has been reported. However, other studies have failed to demonstrate any increased risk for fetal malformation resulting from maternal aspirin exposure.

Aspirin and other salicylates are excreted into breast milk in low concentrations. Following single-dose oral salicylate ingestion, peak milk levels occur at about 3 hours, producing a milk-to-maternal plasma ratio of 3:8. Although adverse effects on platelet function in the nursing infant exposed to aspirin through the mother's milk have not been reported, they still must be considered a potential risk.[31]

In summary, both increased maternal morbidity and fetal morbidity and mortality have been reported with perinatal aspirin exposure. The role of salicylates in producing fetal malformation during first-trimester exposure is unresolved. Women should be advised to avoid aspirin during pregnancy, especially during the last trimester, and when breast-feeding. During pregnancy, acetaminophen is the preferred analgesic for self-medication. Acetaminophen is also the preferred agent for nursing mothers; however, ibuprofen can be used.

Reye's syndrome is an acute, potentially fatal illness occurring almost exclusively in children younger than 15 years. The syndrome produces fatty liver with encephalopathy. It is characterized by vomiting, progressive CNS damage, signs of hepatic injury, and hypoglycemia. The onset usually follows a viral infection with influenza (type A or B) or varicella-zoster (i.e., chickenpox). Within 1 to 7 days, persistent vomiting generally occurs along with stupor, possibly progressing to generalized convulsions and coma. Other neurologic symptoms include listlessness, lethargy, disorientation, hostility, combativeness, inability to recognize family members, incessant moaning or screaming, twitching, and jerking. The mortality rate may be as high as 50%.

Although the cause of Reye's syndrome is unknown, viral and toxic agents, especially salicylates, have been associated with it. The Centers for Disease Control and Prevention (CDC) has been consistently monitoring for an association between Reye's syndrome and ibuprofen since 1977, and none has been identified.[32] The data suggest that nonsalicylate NSAIDs and this syndrome are not associated.

During the mid-1980s, the Reye's Syndrome Task Force of the Public Health Service (PHS) conducted an extensive study that found the risk of children's developing Reye's syndrome correlated with the salicylate dose, and children who received higher doses were at greater risk.[33] To address concerns for potential bias, an epidemiologic investigation confirmed the strong association between the use of salicylate during an antecedent viral infection and subsequent development of Reye's syndrome.[34]

After reviewing available data, the American Academy of Pediatrics, FDA, CDC, and PHS's Surgeon General issued a warning that aspirin and other salicylates should be avoided in children and young adults who have influenza or chickenpox. Since 1988, FDA has required that the following Reye's syndrome warning be added to all labels of nonprescription aspirin and aspirin-containing products:

> Children and teenagers should not use this medicine for chickenpox or flu symptoms before a doctor is consulted about Reye's syndrome, a rare but serious illness associated with aspirin use.

In 1993, FDA proposed that the warning be revised slightly and extended to all nonprescription products containing bismuth subsalicylate (which is not an analgesic/antipyretic, per se) except for those products marketed solely for diarrhea.[35] The Aspirin Foundation of America and manufacturers of nonaspirin salicylate drugs objected to the proposed change, and a final rule had not been published by early 2000.

It is imperative that pharmacists warn against giving products containing aspirin or nonaspirin salicylates to children and teenagers who have influenza or chickenpox. In such cases, acetaminophen is the preferred nonprescription analgesic/antipyretic. A simple viral upper respiratory infection (e.g., a common cold) is not a contraindication to aspirin use; however, symptoms of this type of infection may mimic some of those seen in influenza and chickenpox. Therefore, many clinicians recommend a conservative approach of avoiding aspirin when symptoms resembling influenza are present. The use of aspirin as a pediatric antipyretic has all but ceased in the United States, as have reports of Reye's syndrome.

Nonacetylated Salicylates Discussions of mechanism of action, indications, drug–drug interactions, precautions/warnings, and special population considerations for acetylated salicylates also apply to nonacetylated salicylates. (See the appropriate sections above.) Table 3–5 lists examples of commercially available acetylated and nonacetylated salicylates.

Choline Salicylate Choline salicylate (Arthropan) is an oral liquid salicylate preparation. Comparative analgesic/anti-inflammatory efficacy studies are not available for choline salicylate. The product was found to be less effective than either aspirin or acetaminophen as an antipyretic in children.[36]

Choline salicylate is more water soluble than aspirin and offers the advantage of being stable in an oral solution. It is absorbed from the stomach more rapidly than are aspirin tablets, but this rapidity may not be clinically important. A 5 mL dose of choline salicylate (174 mg/mL, or 870 mg) is equivalent to 650 mg of aspirin in salicylate content. FDA-recommended adult dosage is 435 to 870 mg every 4 hours, or 435 to 670 mg every 3 hours, or 87 to 1340 mg every 6 hours, not to exceed 5325 mg in 24 hours. For patients who find the fishy odor of the liquid product unacceptable, the oral solution of choline salicylate may be mixed with fruit juice, a carbonated beverage, or water just before administration. However, it should not be mixed with any alkaline solution, including antacids, because the liberation of choline exaggerates the fishy odor of the product.

Magnesium Salicylate Magnesium salicylate may be used by patients who are allergic to aspirin. Magnesium salicylate is available as the tetrahydrate salt (Arthriten, Backache). As a consequence, the salicylate content of 377 mg of magnesium salicylate tetrahydrate is equivalent to that of 325 mg of sodium salicylate. FDA-recommended adult dosage of magnesium salicylate for nonprescription use is 377 to 754 mg every 4 hours, or 377 to 580 mg every 3 hours, or 754 to 1160 mg every 6 hours, not to exceed 4640 mg in 24 hours.

The maximum 24-hour dose of magnesium salicylate contains 264 mg (11 mEq) of magnesium. Thus, patients with compromised renal function must avoid using magnesium salicylate because of the potential for decreased renal excretion of magnesium with its subsequent accumulation and the production of systemic magnesium toxicity.

Sodium Salicylate Patients who are allergic to aspirin may be able to tolerate sodium salicylate. Sodium salicylate is less effective than an equal dose of aspirin in reducing pain or fever. FDA-recommended adult dosage for nonprescription anti-inflammatory use of sodium salicylate is the same as that for aspirin (i.e., 325 to 650 mg every 4 hours, 325 to 500 mg every 3 hours, or 650 mg to 1 g every 6 hours, not to exceed 4 g in 24 hours).

The maximum 4 g dose of sodium salicylate contains 560 mg (25 mEq) of sodium. Consequently, patients on strict sodium restriction should avoid using sodium salicylate.

Table 3–5

Selected Single-Entity Salicylate Products

Trade Name	Primary Ingredients
Acetylated Salicylates (Aspirin)	
Anacin Caplets/Tablets	Aspirin 400 mg
Anacin Maximum Strength Tablets	Aspirin 500 mg
Ascriptin Arthritis Pain Caplets	Aspirin 325 mg
Ascriptin Enteric Adult Low Strength Tablets	Aspirin 81 mg
Bayer 8-Hour Aspirin Extended-Release Caplets[a]	Aspirin 650 mg
Bayer Aspirin Extra Strength Caplets/Tablets[a]	Aspirin 500 mg
Bayer Aspirin Regimen Regular Strength Caplets[a]	Aspirin 325 mg
Bayer Children's Aspirin Chewable Tablets[a,b]	Aspirin 81 mg
Bufferin Arthritis Strength Caplets/Tablets[a]	Aspirin 500 mg
Bufferin Low Dose Enteric Aspirin Caplets	Aspirin 81 mg
Bufferin Tablets[a]	Aspirin 325 mg
Ecotrin Adult Low Strength Tablets	Aspirin 81 mg
Ecotrin Maximum Strength Caplets/Tablets	Aspirin 500 mg
Ecotrin Regular Strength Tablets	Aspirin 325 mg
Nonacetylated Salicylates	
Alka-Seltzer Caplets	Acetaminophen 500 mg
Anacin Aspirin Free Maximum Strength Tablets	Acetaminophen 500 mg
Arthropan Liquid[a]	Choline salicylate 174 mg/mL
Backache Caplets[a]	Magnesium salicylate tetrahydrate 580 mg
Doan's Extra Strength Caplets[a]	Magnesium salicylate tetrahydrate 580 mg
Doan's Regular Strength Caplets	Magnesium salicylate tetrahydrate 377 mg
Mobigesic Tablets[a–c]	Magnesium salicylate 325 mg
Momentum Caplets[a]	Magnesium salicylate tetrahydrate 580 mg

[a] Sodium-free product.
[b] Sucrose-free product.
[c] Dye-free product.

Acetaminophen

Mechanism of Action Acetaminophen is an effective analgesic and antipyretic. Animal studies of acetaminophen at high doses have demonstrated weak anti-inflammatory activity that is not useful clinically. Unlike salicylates, acetaminophen produces analgesia through a central rather than a peripheral effect.

Pharmacokinetics Acetaminophen is rapidly absorbed from the GI tract and is extensively metabolized in the liver to inactive conjugates of glucuronic and sulfuric acids. In addition, acetaminophen is metabolized to a hepatotoxic intermediate metabolite by the cytochrome P450 enzyme system. This intermediate metabolite is detoxified by glutathione, but this system can become saturated in overdose situations. (See the section "Overdosage," which follows.)

Rectal bioavailability of acetaminophen is approximately 50% to 60% of that achieved with oral administration.

Indications Acetaminophen is effective in relieving mild-to-moderate pain of nonvisceral origin. Acetaminophen does not decrease peripheral inflammation, but it may help with pain caused by inflammation. Equal doses of acetaminophen and aspirin administered by the same route produce equivalent degrees of analgesia.

Dosage/Administration Guidelines FDA-recommended adult dosage of acetaminophen is 325 to 650 mg every 4 hours, 325 to 500 mg every 3 hours, or 650 to 1000 mg every 6 hours, not to exceed a total of 4 g in 24 hours. Table 3–3 lists recommended oral pediatric doses.

Acetaminophen is available for oral administration in various oral liquid and solid dosage forms. Additionally, acetaminophen is available in rectal suppositories. Acetaminophen oral capsules contain tasteless granules that can be emptied onto a spoon containing a small amount of drink or soft food. Patients and parents should not add the contents of the capsules to a glass of liquid because large numbers of granules may adhere to the side of the glass. Mixing with a hot beverage can result in a bitter taste. (See Table 3–6 for examples of commercially available products.)

Table 3–6

Selected Single-Entity Acetaminophen Products

Trade Name	Primary Ingredients
Liquiprin for Children Drops[a,b]	Acetaminophen 48 mg/mL
Tempra 1 Infant Drops[a–c]	Acetaminophen 80 mg/0.8 mL
Tempra 2 Toddler Syrup[a–c]	Acetaminophen 160 mg/5mL
Tempra Quicklets, Quick Dissolving Children's Strength Chewable Tablets[b,d]	Acetaminophen 80 mg
Tempra Quicklets, Quick Dissolving Junior Strength Chewable Tablets[b,d]	Acetaminophen 160 mg
Tylenol Extended Relief Timed-Release Caplets[d,e]	Acetaminophen 650 mg
Tylenol Extra Strength Tablets/Caplets/ Gelcaps/Geltabs[d]	Acetaminophen 500 mg
Tylenol Extra Strength Adult Liquid	Acetaminophen 166.7 mg/5 mL
Tylenol Junior Strength Swallowable Caplets[b,d,e]	Acetaminophen 160 mg
Tylenol Junior Strength Chewable Tablets[b]	Acetaminophen 160 mg
Tylenol Regular Strength Tablets/Caplets[d]	Acetaminophen 325 mg
Tylenol Children's Bubble Gum Flavor Chewable Tablets[b]	Acetaminophen 80 mg
Tylenol Children's Elixir/Suspension[a,b]	Acetaminophen 160 mg/5 mL
Tylenol Infants' Drops[a,b]	Acetaminophen 80 mg/0.8 mL

[a] Alcohol-free product.
[b] Pediatric formulation.
[c] Sulfite-free product.
[d] Sucrose-free product.
[e] Dye-free product.

Overdosage Symptoms are often absent for hours following an acute overdose of acetaminophen. During the first 2 days after an acute overdose, symptoms may not reflect the potential seriousness of the exposure. Early symptoms of acetaminophen intoxication include nausea, vomiting, drowsiness, confusion, and abdominal pain. Clinical manifestations of hepatotoxicity begin 2 to 4 days after the acute ingestion of acetaminophen and include increased plasma transaminases (both aspartate and alanine aminotransferase), increased plasma bilirubin with jaundice, and prolonged prothrombin time. In nonfatal cases, the hepatic damage is reversible over a period of weeks or months. The most serious adverse effect of acute acetaminophen overdose is dose dependent, potentially fatal hepatic necrosis. Renal tubular necrosis and hypoglycemic coma may also occur. In adults, hepatotoxicity may occur after ingestion of a single dose of 10 to 15 g (150 to 250 mg/kg) of acetaminophen; doses of 20 to 25 g or more are potentially fatal.

Because of the potential seriousness of acetaminophen overdose, all cases should be referred to a poison control center or other medical personnel experienced in managing such cases. Approximately 65% of acetaminophen overdoses in children are effectively managed in the home, compared with only about 18% of adult acetaminophen overdoses.[37] Immediate first-aid management of acute acetaminophen poisoning includes the induction of vomiting with ipecac syrup. Activated charcoal may also be effective in reducing the absorption of acetaminophen. However, it can adsorb the specific antidote for acetaminophen hepatotoxicity, *N*-acetylcysteine, and presumably reduce its efficacy. If activated charcoal is administered on an in-home, first-aid basis for acetaminophen overdose, this information must be made known to emergency medical personnel who administer *N*-acetylcysteine so that appropriate dose adjustments can be made. Dosing recommendations for both ipecac syrup and activated charcoal are included in Chapter 17, "Poisoning." Pharmacists and other caregivers are strongly encouraged to coordinate with a poison center any non–hospital-based management of poisoning or drug overdose.

Adverse Effects Acetaminophen has no effect on the urinary excretion of uric acid, on prothrombin synthesis, or on platelet aggregation and bleeding time. In addition, it produces less GI irritation, erosion, and bleeding than aspirin or other salicylates. Acetaminophen has a very low incidence of cross-reactivity in aspirin-intolerant patients. Thus, for patients who cannot take aspirin or another salicylate because of contraindications resulting from adverse effects on bleeding time, uric acid excretion, GI bleeding, aspirin intolerance, or concurrent drug therapy, acetaminophen is an appropriate nonprescription analgesic alternative.

Drug–Drug Interactions Clinically important drug interactions of acetaminophen are listed in Table 3–4. Acetaminophen doses in excess of 2275 mg per week have been associated with increases in the international normalized ratio (INR) of patients taking warfarin.[38] Periodic increases in acetaminophen usage should be discouraged in patients on anticoagulant regimens. Patients should continue to be counseled against using aspirin or NSAIDS while on warfarin therapy. However, patients should also be warned about the potential problem associated with continued acetaminophen use while on warfarin therapy. Patients who may require higher routine doses (e.g., osteoarthritis) should have their warfarin adjusted as the INR indicates.

Studies suggest that concurrent administration of short-term acetaminophen (less than 7 days) and zidovudine does not produce increased plasma levels of zidovudine and the subsequent increased risk of myelosuppression and neutropenia in AIDS patients.[39,40] Reportedly patients with AIDS and AIDS-related complex who were taking zidovudine experienced an increased incidence of bone marrow suppression if they concurrently used acetaminophen.[41] Chronic acetaminophen usage with zidovudine may produce increased levels of zidovudine, resulting in myelosuppression. For these patients, the short-term or intermittent use of acetaminophen is the recommended nonprescription analgesic for self-medication. Aspirin should probably be avoided by AIDS patients receiving zidovudine because the prolonged antiplatelet effect of aspirin could increase their bleeding risk.

Contraindications/Precautions/Warnings Use of this drug is contraindicated in patients who are hypersensitive to it. Acetaminophen is potentially hepatotoxic in doses exceeding 4 g per day. Chronic use may predispose patients to toxicity, and more conservative dosing may be warranted in such cases. Patients should use caution if they have liver disease and are taking other potentially hepatotoxic drugs, do not eat regularly, and ingest alcohol more than occasionally. These patients are at increased risk for acetaminophen-induced hepatotoxicity. Patients should be advised to avoid alcohol and fasting, if possible, when taking acetaminophen. Patients with G-6-PD deficiency should also use caution when medicating with acetaminophen.

Special Population Considerations Acetaminophen sometimes is underdosed, especially in young patients. This situation occurs when parents reuse the 0.8-mL dropper provided with infant drops (80 mg/0.8 mL) to measure a dose of an equivalent volume of acetaminophen elixir that contains 160 mg/5 mL, incorrectly assuming the same strength. In addition, rapidly growing infants quickly outgrow previous dose requirements. Therefore, recalculation of the pediatric dose according to present age and body weight is appropriate at the time of each treatment course.

Acetaminophen crosses the placenta but is considered safe for use during pregnancy. It appears in breast milk, producing a milk-to-maternal plasma ratio of 0.5 : 1.0. On the basis of a 1 g maternal dose, the estimated maximum infant dose is 1.85% of the maternal dose. The only adverse effect reported in nursing infants exposed to acetaminophen through breast milk is a rarely occurring maculopapular rash, which subsides when drug exposure is discontinued. The American Academy of Pediatrics considers acetaminophen use to be compatible with breast-feeding.[31]

Nonsalicylate NSAIDs

Ibuprofen, ketoprofen, and naproxen are alternative nonprescription NSAIDs to the salicylates.

Mechanism of Action The nonsalicylate NSAIDs apparently relieve pain by the peripheral inhibition of cyclo-oxygenase and subsequent inhibition of prostaglandin synthesis.

Pharmacokinetics All of the nonprescription NSAIDs are rapidly absorbed from the GI tract with consistently high bioavailability. The NSAIDs are extensively metabolized in the liver to inactive compounds, mainly by glucuronidation. Elimination occurs primarily through the kidneys. Naproxen sodium has a similar onset of activity, but its duration of action may be somewhat longer than the other nonprescription NSAIDs.

Indications NSAIDs have analgesic, antipyretic, and anti-inflammatory activity and are useful in managing mild-to-moderate pain of nonvisceral origin and dysmenorrhea. (See Chapter 7, "Disorders Related to Menstruation" for discussion of dysmenorrhea.) In 1994, naproxen sodium (Aleve) was approved for use as a nonprescription analgesic, anti-inflammatory agent, and antipyretic. The labeled indications for the nonprescription naproxen sodium include relieving minor pain associated with headache, the common cold, toothache, muscle ache, backache, arthritis, and muscle cramps as well as reducing fever. Like ibuprofen and naproxen sodium, ketoprofen is a propionic acid derivative

NSAID. Therefore, its indications (analgesia, anti-inflammatory activity, and antipyresis) and pharmacologic activity are the same as these two agents. Ketoprofen has been used effectively in juvenile rheumatoid arthritis in children ages 2 to 16 years. However, labeling of the nonprescription product recommends that the drug be used only in patients older than 16 years.

Dosage/Administration Guidelines Table 3–7 lists analgesic/antipyretic dosages for nonsalicylate NSAIDs, whereas Table 3–1 also lists the analgesic/anti-inflammatory dosages for NSAIDs and acetaminophen.

The analgesic dosage of nonprescription ibuprofen for patients older than 12 years is 200 to 400 mg every 4 to 6 hours, not to exceed 1200 mg in 24 hours. A dose–effect relationship has been demonstrated for ibuprofen analgesia in the range of l00 to 400 mg. On a milligram-to-milligram basis, ibuprofen is approximately 3.5 times more potent than aspirin as an analgesic, and the analgesic effect may last up to 6 hours.[42]

In 1995, FDA approved the oral pediatric suspension of ibuprofen as a nonprescription drug. This 100 mg/5 mL suspension (Children's Motrin) is indicated for children ages 2 to 11 years as an antipyretic and for relief of minor aches and pains caused by colds, influenza, sore throat, headaches, and toothaches. The duration of action may be as long as 8 hours. Besides the pediatric suspension, other nonprescription formulations of ibuprofen are now available. The products include an orange-flavored 50 mg chewable tablet (Children's Motrin Chewable Tablet), a berry-flavored dropper formulation (Children's Motrin Drops 50 mg per 1.25 mL), and 100 mg tablets and caplets (Junior Strength Motrin). The Junior Strength Motrin 100 mg tablets are orange flavored and can be chewed similar to the 50 mg product.

The maximum daily dosage of naproxen sodium according to the labeling for patients ages 12 to 15 years is three 220 mg tablets; doses should be taken 8 to 12 hours apart. Patients older than age 65 years should not take more than one tablet every 12 hours unless directed to do so by a physician. The labeling stipulates that children younger than 12 years should use the drug only under a physician's supervision.

In 1995, ketoprofen was approved for nonprescription use as an analgesic and antipyretic (Orudis KT, Actron). One 12.5 mg tablet of ketoprofen appears to be equivalent to one 200 mg tablet of ibuprofen. The recommended dose for patients older than 16 years is 12.5 mg every 6 to 8 hours, not to exceed 75 mg in 24 hours. If needed, a second dose may be taken after 1 hour.

In the event a patient misses a dose and it is almost time for the next regular dose, the patient should skip the missed dose and resume taking medication at the next scheduled time. The patient should not take two doses at the same time. These medicines may be taken with food, milk, or antacids if they upset the stomach. Tablets should be taken with a full glass of water, suspensions should be shaken thoroughly, and enteric-coated or sustained-release preparations should be neither crushed nor chewed. Table 3–8 lists examples of var-

Table 3–7

Recommended Analgesic/Antipyretic Dosages for Nonsalicylate Nonsteroidal Anti-Inflammatory Drugs

Agent	Age	Dosage (maximum)
Ibuprofen	6 months–12 years	7.5 mg/kg (30 mg/kg/day)
	>12 years	200–400 mg every 4–6 hours (1200 mg/day)
Naproxen sodium	<12 years	Not recommended
	12–65 years	220–440 mg every 8–12 hours (660 mg/day)
	>65 years	220 mg every 12 hours (440 mg/day)
Ketoprofen	<16 years	Not recommended
	>16 years	12.5 mg every 6–8 hours; may take second dose after 1 hour, if needed (75 mg/day)

Table 3–8

Selected Nonsalicylate Nonsteroidal Anti-Inflammatory Drugs

Trade Name	Primary Ingredients
Ibuprofen Products	
Advil Gel Caplets	Ibuprofen 200 mg
Advil Children's Suspension[a]	Ibuprofen 100 mg/5 mL
Advil Junior Strength Tablets	Ibuprofen 100 mg
Motrin IB Caplets/Tablets/Gelcaps	Ibuprofen 200 mg
Motrin Children's Chewable Tablets[a,b]	Ibuprofen 50 mg
Motrin Children's Drops[b,c]	Ibuprofen 50 mg/1.25 mL
Motrin Children's Suspension[b,c]	Ibuprofen 100 mg/5 mL
Motrin Junior Strength Chewable Tablets[a,b]	Ibuprofen 100 mg
Motrin Junior Strength Caplets[a,d]	Ibuprofen 100 mg
Nuprin Caplets/Tablets[e]	Ibuprofen 200 mg
PediaCare Fever Drops[a,c]	Ibuprofen 50 mg/1.25 mL
PediaCare Fever Suspension[a,c]	Ibuprofen 100 mg/5 mL
Ketoprofen Products	
Actron Caplets/Tablets	Ketoprofen 12.5 mg
Orudis KT Caplets/Tablets	Ketoprofen 12.5 mg
Naproxen Products	
Aleve Caplets/Tablets	Naproxen sodium 220 mg

[a] Pediatric formulation.
[b] Product containing phenylalanine.
[c] Alcohol-free product.
[d] Sucrose-free product.
[e] Sodium-free product.

ious dosage forms of commercially available nonsalicylate NSAIDs.

Overdosage Overdoses of nonsalicylate NSAIDs usually produce minimal symptoms of toxicity and are rarely fatal. In an analysis of more than 1500 reports of overdose with ibuprofen, only 0.4% of children and 1.6% of adults exhibited major or life-threatening effects. No fatalities were reported, and 86% of children and 41% of adults evidenced no symptoms from the drug exposure.[37] In a prospective study of 329 cases of ibuprofen overdose, it was found that GI and CNS symptoms (in 42% and 30% of patients, respectively) were most common and included nausea, vomiting, abdominal pain, lethargy, stupor, coma, nystagmus, dizziness, and lightheadedness. Hypotension, bradycardia, tachycardia, dyspnea, and painful breathing were also reported. In this study, 43% of ibuprofen-overdose patients were asymptomatic.[43] Unless contraindicated by convulsions or unconsciousness, appropriate first-aid treatment of ibuprofen overdose includes the induction of vomiting with ipecac syrup or the administration of activated charcoal. (See Chapter 17, "Poisoning.")

The occurrence of severe metabolic acidosis has been reported to follow naproxen sodium overdose.[44] Movement disorder has also been associated with naproxen sodium poisoning.

Adverse Effects The most frequent adverse effects of nonsalicylate NSAIDs involve the GI tract and include dyspepsia, heartburn, nausea, anorexia, and epigastric pain. These agents produce less GI upset and bleeding than does aspirin. In patients receiving one of these two medications for at least 1 year, aspirin produced a 15 mL blood loss over 4 days in contrast to only a 3 mL loss with ibuprofen.[45] Gastroscopic evaluation of patients on either ibuprofen or aspirin for 3 to 12 months revealed that 50% of the patients receiving aspirin evidenced gastric lesions compared with only 18% of those receiving ibuprofen.[46]

One case of naproxen photosensitivity was reported more than a decade ago.[47] The patient initially presented with an acute pruritic erythematous eruption on his face and neck before naproxen therapy. The lesion was treated with topical steroids and subsequently resolved. Approximately 6 weeks later, the patient received 250 mg of oral naproxen and the eruption reappeared within 7 hours. The eruption was again treated with a topical steroid, and the patient avoided NSAIDs without further incidence for 18 months. Photosensitivity may be an underreported problem with all NSAIDs.

When administered at doses higher than nonprescription doses, ketoprofen has produced headache in more than 3% of patients. Other dose-related side effects include visual disturbance in 1% to 3% of patients, peripheral edema in 2% of patients, and hepatic dysfunction in less than 1% of patients. At normal nonprescription doses, these effects are rare.

Drug–Drug Interactions Clinically important drug interactions of ibuprofen and other NSAIDs are listed in Table 3–4. A brief discussion of drug interactions with ibuprofen and ketoprofen follows.

Digoxin Ibuprofen has been reported to increase plasma digoxin concentrations in patients receiving digoxin. The clinical significance of this interaction is uncertain. Worsening heart failure with fluid overload and blunting of furosemide responsiveness may occur with the administration of ibuprofen to patients with congestive heart failure. Because of the uncertainty of a possible ibuprofen–digoxin interaction and the potential for ibuprofen-induced furosemide refractoriness with symptomatic deterioration, pharmacists should advise patients with a history of congestive heart failure to avoid self-medicating with any ibuprofen-containing products.[48]

Antihypertensive Drugs NSAIDs antagonize the blood pressure–lowering effects of certain antihypertensive drugs, including diuretics, angiotensin-converting enzyme inhibitors, β blockers, and centrally acting antihypertensives. Forty-five patients who had essential hypertension that was controlled with at least two antihypertensive drugs were given ibuprofen (400 mg every 8 hours), acetaminophen (1 g every 8 hours), or placebo (2 capsules every 8 hours) for 3 weeks. At the end of 3 weeks, the ibuprofen-treated group experienced a 5.8 mm Hg increase in sitting mean arterial pressure and a 6.6 mm Hg increase in supine mean arterial pressure, both of which were statistically significant when compared with placebo treatment. By contrast, the acetaminophen-treated group showed no change in blood pressure during the 3-week test interval.[49] Some studies suggest that naproxen may decrease the antihypertensive activity of some β blockers.[50] Other reports, however, suggest that this interaction may not be clinically important.[51] Thus, pharmacists should advise hypertensive patients who are selecting a nonprescription analgesic that NSAIDs may antagonize their blood pressure medication and that acetaminophen is a better choice.

Lithium The concurrent use of ibuprofen in lithium-stabilized patients is reported to produce increased plasma lithium levels and enhanced lithium toxicity. In a study of nine psychiatric patients on chronic lithium therapy (600 to 900 mg per day), the administration of ibuprofen (1800 mg per day for 6 days) decreased lithium clearance by 34% and increased serum lithium by 34% (range 12% to 66%). Three patients showed increased tremor, a dose-dependent adverse reaction to lithium.[52] Similar results have been obtained in healthy subjects concurrently given lithium (900 mg per day) and ibuprofen (1200 mg per day) for 7 days.[53] Limited controlled studies indicate that aspirin does not adversely affect lithium clearance.[54] Consequently, it is imperative that pharmacists advise patients taking lithium to avoid all ibuprofen containing nonprescription analgesics. Acetaminophen is considered the best alternative analgesic because it has little, if any, effect on renal prostaglandin synthesis. Lithium-treated patients may also safely self-medicate with aspirin.

Methotrexate A potentially serious interaction exists between methotrexate and NSAIDs. An anecdotal report of an 18-year-old male undergoing intravenous methotrexate therapy for osteogenic sarcoma supports the potential severity of the methotrexate–ibuprofen interaction. Unknown to the oncology team, this patient was self-medicating with ibuprofen (400 mg every 4 hours) for his leg pain. Twenty hours into his methotrexate infusion, his serum creatinine, which was 0.9 mg/dL before he began infusion, was found to be 2.3 mg/dL, and folinic acid rescue was begun immediately. It is postulated that ibuprofen competes with methotrexate for renal proximal tubular secretion, causing decreased renal clearance of methotrexate and resulting in nephrotoxicity.[55]

A life-threatening interaction of ketoprofen and methotrexate has been reported. Of four patients who experienced severe methotrexate toxicity resulting from concurrent ketoprofen administration, three ultimately died from methotrexate toxicity.[56]

According to limited reports, it is imperative that patients receiving methotrexate as outpatient therapy be warned not to self-medicate with nonprescription analgesics containing nonsalicylate NSAIDs or aspirin. For such patients, acetaminophen is the only nonprescription analgesic considered safe.

Contraindications Nonsalicylate NSAIDs are contraindicated in patients with a history of intolerance to aspirin or to any other NSAID. Cross-reactivity with ibuprofen is reported to be 97% in patients who are documented as aspirin intolerant. Patients with a history of asthma may experience a worsening of their bronchospastic symptoms with ibuprofen. According to FDA-class labeling requirements, all nonsalicylate NSAIDs carry the same warning about cross-reactivity. Nonacetylated salicylates are better tolerated than nonsalicylate NSAIDs in patients with a documented aspirin hypersensitivity.

Precautions/Warnings Patients should be cautioned that, in doses of 60 to 1800 mg per day, ibuprofen increased bleeding time by inhibiting platelet aggregation. However, ibuprofen's effect on platelet aggregation, unlike that of aspirin, is reversible within 24 hours after medication is discontinued.[57] In doses of 1200 to 2400 mg per day, ibuprofen does not appear to affect the hypoprothrombinemia produced by warfarin. However, ibuprofen should not be recommended for self-medication to patients who are concurrently taking anticoagulants because it can displace plasma protein-bound warfarin and because its antiplatelet activity could increase GI bleeding.

Alcohol ingestion has been shown to increase by 3.5-fold the prolongation of bleeding time produced by ibuprofen. Patients self-medicating with ibuprofen should be cautioned against the concurrent use of alcohol.[58]

Patients with preexisting renal impairment or congestive heart failure should also use nonsalicylate NSAIDs cautiously. These agents may decrease renal blood flow and glomerular filtration rate as a result of inhibition of renal prostaglandin synthesis. These effects may increase blood urea nitrogen and serum creatinine values, often with concomitant sodium and water retention. Advanced age, hypertension, use of diuretics, diabetes, and atherosclerotic cardiovascular disease appear to increase the risk of renal toxicity with ibuprofen. As a result, patients with a history of impaired renal function, congestive heart failure, or diseases that compromise renal hemodynamics should not self-medicate with ibuprofen.

Special Population Considerations No evidence exists that nonsalicylate NSAIDs are teratogenic in either humans or animals. However, use of these agents is contraindicated during the third trimester of pregnancy because all potent prostaglandin synthesis inhibitors can cause delayed parturition, prolonged labor, and increased postpartum bleeding. These agents can also have adverse fetal cardiovascular effects (e.g., delay closure of the ductus arteriosus). Lactating women taking up to 2.4 g of ibuprofen per day showed no measurable excretion of ibuprofen into breast milk. The American Academy of Pediatrics considers ibuprofen compatible with breast-feeding.[31]

The safety of ibuprofen use in children was demonstrated by a practitioner-based, randomized clinical trial of ibuprofen at doses of 5 mg/kg or 10 mg/kg and acetaminophen at a dose of 12 mg/kg. This study,[59] which involved a total of 84,192 children, demonstrated that the risk of hospitalization for GI bleeding, renal failure, or anaphylaxis was not increased following short-term use of ibuprofen as compared with acetaminophen in children.

The American Academy of Pediatrics also considers naproxen compatible with breast-feeding.[31] No evidence of teratogenicity or toxicity to embryos has been uncovered in studies of pregnant animals given high doses of ketoprofen. No evidence exists of adverse effects on fertility. The product labeling, however, recommends that nursing mothers not use this drug.

Prescription Therapies

Some NMDA antagonists may become useful drugs for the management of neuropathic pain in the future. However, currently available NMDA antagonists cause major adverse effects that are unacceptable to patients. It is doubtful whether clinically useful NMDA antagonists will be available without a prescription. Dextorphan, a metabolite of dextromethorphan an antitussive agent in many nonprescription cough formulations, has been studied as an NMDA antagonist.[60,61] Doses of several hundred milligrams per day are required for analgesia, and produce side effects. The doses needed for analgesia far exceed the recommended doses for antitussive activity. Dextromethorphan use in pain should be considered experimental at this time.

Recently, two new NSAIDs have been approved by the FDA for prescription use in both forms of arthritis. These drugs, celecoxib (Celebrex) and rofecoxib (Vioxx), differ from the traditional NSAIDs in their selectivity for the enzyme cyclooxygenase-2 (COX-2). This enzyme is present mainly in inflamed tissue. Conversely, cyclooxygenase-1 is found in most tissues and serves to protect the gastrointestinal mucosa and kidneys. The new COX-2 specific NSAIDs appear to have a decreased gastrointestinal toxicity profile, however they do not seem to afford protection to the kidneys. Therefore, it is important for patients to be well hydrated.

Therapeutic Comparisons

Aspirin versus Nonacetylated Salicylates When equivalent amounts of salicylates are given, it appears that aspirin and the nonacetylated salicylates are equally well absorbed and produce similar plasma salicylate levels. However, an oral solution of choline salicylate produces peak plasma salicylate levels sooner than the oral solid dosage forms.

Aspirin's irreversible effect on platelet aggregation with a prolongation of bleeding is caused by the acetyl moiety. Nonacetylated salicylates do not affect platelet aggregation or bleeding time significantly. With the exception of this difference, the nonacetylated salicylates have the same contraindications and interactions as aspirin because all other salicylate effects result from the production of salicylic acid. However, nonacetylated salicylates are weaker prostaglandin synthesis inhibitors than aspirin and, as such, appear to cause less GI erosion and bleeding, fewer renal complications, and a low level of cross-reactivity in aspirin-intolerant patients.[62,63]

A study[64] comparing the analgesic efficacy of 500 mg of aspirin taken four times daily with 500 mg of magnesium salicylate taken four times daily in patients with chronic degenerative arthritis found similar reductions in objective pain scores for the two drugs at the end of 12 weeks.

Aspirin versus Acetaminophen Numerous controlled studies have demonstrated the equivalent analgesic efficacy of aspirin and acetaminophen on a milligram-for-milligram basis in various pain models, including postoperative pain, cancer pain, episiotomy pain, and oral surgery pain. Aspirin and acetaminophen have similar dose–response and time–effect curves and are equipotent and equianalgesic for the relief of most pain. In a controlled study involving 269 patients, acetaminophen (1 g) and aspirin (650 mg) produced similar efficacy in the treatment of moderate-to-severe headache. The apparent superiority of aspirin on a milligram-for-milligram basis may be the result of an inflammatory component to the headache pain that would be unresponsive to acetaminophen. Acetaminophen (1 g) has been shown to be superior to aspirin (650 mg) in the control of pain secondary to dental surgery or episiotomy.[65] This difference is most probably a result of the dose differences, not superiority of acetaminophen as an analgesic.

Aspirin versus Ibuprofen Ibuprofen has been shown to be at least as effective as aspirin in treating various types of pain, including dental extraction pain, dysmenorrhea, and episiotomy pain. A double-blind, single-dose study of postepisiotomy pain found ibuprofen (400 mg) to be more effective than aspirin (600 mg).[66] Another double-blind, single-dose study that compared the efficacy of oral ibuprofen (100, 200, or 400 mg) with that of aspirin (650 mg) in treating moderate-to-severe pain after the extraction of impacted teeth estimated 100 mg of ibuprofen to be as effective as 650 mg of aspirin.[67] Single-dose analgesic studies often provide outcomes different from those of multiple dose studies, which characterize more accurately how the drugs are used clinically.

Controlled clinical trials have shown that ibuprofen is as effective as, but not superior to, aspirin in treating rheumatoid arthritis. A double-blind, crossover, randomized study with 18 rheumatoid arthritic patients compared aspirin (3.6 g per day), ibuprofen (1.2 g per day), and placebo. Both aspirin and ibuprofen were superior to placebo for symptomatic control but were not different from each other. Both drugs reduced morning stiffness and improved grip strength to an equivalent degree. However, aspirin appeared superior to ibuprofen in the reduction of joint size. It is noteworthy that the daily aspirin dose approached the maximum for safe use, whereas the ibuprofen dose was relatively low.

Ibuprofen versus Acetaminophen In postpartum patients with moderate-to-severe episiotomy pain, a single ibuprofen dose (400 mg) was found to be superior to acetaminophen (1 g) in producing analgesia. This superior analgesic effect was manifested by a more rapid onset and prolonged effect and by a greater area under the analgesic time–effect curve.[68] In reducing the severity and duration of migraine headache, ibuprofen 400 mg taken every 4 hours was significantly superior to acetaminophen 900 mg taken every 4 hours.[69] And in a multicenter study involving 706 patients, a single 400 mg oral dose of ibuprofen provided superior analgesia following oral surgery compared with 1 g of acetaminophen.[70] Numerous comparisons of oral ibuprofen and acetaminophen in various pain models suggest that 10 to 200 mg of ibuprofen is approximately equianalgesic to 650 mg of acetaminophen. Ibuprofen has a clear superiority, however, in pain conditions associated with inflammation.

A double-blind, randomized, parallel group study of 7.5 mg/kg ibuprofen syrup and 10 mg/kg acetaminophen syrup demonstrated no significant difference in temperature reduction over time among 154 children with infectious diseases that produced fever. However, the ibuprofen produced significantly greater temperature reductions during the first 4 hours of treatment.[71]

Naproxen versus Ibuprofen One 220 mg nonprescription naproxen sodium tablet appears to be very similar in indications and efficacy to one 200 mg ibuprofen tablet. The onset of activity is similar between the two NSAIDs. Naproxen sodium's duration of action is somewhat longer than that of ibuprofen, but the clinical significance of that difference is not clear. Naproxen sodium and ibuprofen are very similar pharmacologically and similar effects should be expected. Both are derived from propionic acid, and extensive clinical experience with these agents has demonstrated great similarity. Nonetheless, some patients with rheumatoid arthritis do report better response to one NSAID than to another for reasons that are unclear. It is less probable, but still possible, that such differences will occur at the maximum nonprescription doses of an NSAID; arthritic patients often require higher doses.

Combination Products

Many nonprescription analgesics are available as combination products containing aspirin, ibuprofen, or acetaminophen as primary ingredients plus caffeine or an antihistamine. Combination products containing two nonprescription analgesics are also available. (See Table 3–9 for examples of commercially available products.)

The adjuvant ingredients are claimed to enhance the analgesic efficacy of the product. Some evidence supports the enhanced efficacy of such combination products. Other studies have failed to demonstrate a benefit from the adjuvants.

Thirty clinical studies involving more than 10,000 patients have been analyzed to assess the value of caffeine as an analgesic adjuvant. These studies were based on various pain models, including postpartum uterine cramping, episiotomy pain, oral surgery pain, and headache. Caffeine was combined with aspirin or acetaminophen alone and with aspirin–acetaminophen combinations.

In 21 of 26 studies reviewed, the relative potency of the analgesic with caffeine was greater than that of the analgesic without caffeine. The pooled relative potency estimate for caffeine-containing analgesics is 1.41 (with a 95% confidence interval of 1.23 to 1.63), as compared with 1.0—the potency for the analgesic in the absence of caffeine. This analysis suggests that to obtain the same amount of response from an analgesic without caffeine would require a dose approximately 40% greater than that required in the presence of caffeine.[69]

Table 3–9

Selected Combination Analgesic Products

Trade Name	Primary Ingredients
Arthriten Tablets[a,b,c]	Acetaminophen 250 mg; magnesium salicylate tetrahydrate 377 mg
Excedrin Extra Strength Geltabs	Acetaminophen 250 mg; aspirin 250 mg; caffeine 65 mg
Excedrin Extra Strength Caplets/Tablets[a]	Acetaminophen 250 mg; aspirin 250 mg; caffeine 65 mg
Excedrin Extra Strength Aspirin Free Geltabs[b]	Acetaminophen 500 mg; caffeine 65 mg
Excedrin Extra Strength Aspirin Free Caplets/Geltabs	Acetaminophen 500 mg; caffeine 65 mg
Excedrin Migraine Caplets/Tablets[a]	Acetaminophen 250 mg; aspirin 250 mg; caffeine 65 mg

[a] Sodium-free product.

[b] Sucrose-free product.

[c] Dye-free product.

Excedrin Migraine was approved for the temporary relief of mild-to-moderate pain associated with migraine headache in 1998. This product is the same chemical formulation as Extra Strength Excedrin. Both products contain 250 mg each of acetaminophen and aspirin, and 65 mg of caffeine. Recent studies have shown that this product is superior to placebo in alleviating pain associated with migraine headaches.[72] Because this product contains caffeine, patients should be counseled about the possibility of rebound headaches. Patients who use this combination for more than three episodes weekly should be referred to a headache specialist for further evaluation.

The adjuvant effect of caffeine has also been reported for ibuprofen analgesia. In a double-blind study, a single oral dose of ibuprofen (100 or 200 mg) with and without caffeine (100 mg) was evaluated for pain relief in 298 patients with postoperative pain after the surgical removal of impacted third molars (wisdom teeth). Subjects self-rated their pain relief hourly for 8 hours. Relative potency estimates indicated that the caffeine–ibuprofen combination was 2.4 to 2.8 times as potent as ibuprofen alone. The combination also had a more rapid onset and a longer duration of analgesic action than ibuprofen alone.[73]

In addition, enhanced analgesia has been reported for various antihistamine–analgesic combinations, including orphenadrine–acetaminophen and phenyltoloxamine–acetaminophen. The adjuvant effect of phenyltoloxamine citrate (60 mg) in combination with acetaminophen (650 mg) was evaluated in 200 female inpatients experiencing episiotomy pain using a self-rating pain relief scale. Compared with acetaminophen alone, the phenyltoloxamine–acetaminophen combination produced significantly greater pain relief at all points from 30 minutes through 6 hours after administering acetaminophen alone.[74] An increasing amount of published date support the enhancement of analgesia by including either caffeine or an antihistamine with a nonprescription analgesic.

Combination dosage forms containing a decongestant and either acetaminophen or an NSAID are also available. Such combinations appear logical for use in sinus headaches or other indications in which both analgesia and decongestion are needed.

Product Selection Guidelines

Patient Factors Age is an important consideration when selecting an appropriate nonprescription medication. Parents of patients younger than 2 years should seek the advice of their pediatrician on what treatment option they should pursue. Children older than 2 years, but younger than 12 years, may use acetaminophen or ibuprofen. Naproxen sodium has been approved for use in patients at least 12 years of age, and ketoprofen is approved for individuals 16 years of age or older. Parents should not use aspirin or aspirin-containing products in children younger than 15 years unless directed to do so by a physician because of the risk for Reye's syndrome.

Salicylates and other NSAIDs should be avoided in the last trimester of pregnancy. Acetaminophen is a safe and effective alternative during this time. Acetaminophen, ibuprofen, and naproxen are compatible with breast-feeding, whereas current labeling advises against ketoprofen use in nursing mothers.

Patient Preferences Nonprescription analgesics and antipyretics are available in a number of dosage forms. During the patient assessment, pharmacists should determine which dosage form will provide the patient with an optimum outcome. In the majority of cases, patients will have a preference for route of administration and dosage form (e.g., oral or rectal, capsule or tablet).

One area in which the pharmacist can be instrumental in affecting outcomes is determining what dosing frequency will be needed for an individual patient. Naproxen sodium can be dosed two to three times daily and may improve patient compliance. Ketoprofen may be effective given three to four times daily. Conversely, acetaminophen, ibuprofen, and salicylates may require dosing as frequently as every 4 hours.

Pharmacoeconomics

Although individual agents may be warranted in certain circumstances (e.g., pregnancy, children, concurrent illness), no agent can claim superior efficacy at this time. All agents except naproxen sodium and ketoprofen are currently available as generic products. This difference may provide rationale for using less-expensive agents initially, unless patients prefer or require medications that can be dosed less frequently.

Patient Assessment of Headache

Before a nonprescription medication can be recommended, the pharmacist must find out about the patient's headache—the type, severity, location, frequency, intensity over time, age at onset, and medical and psychosocial history. The pharmacist should inventory all current medications and determine all past and present headache treatments and what treatments, if any, were successful or preferred.

As noted previously, secondary headaches other than minor sinus headache are excluded from self-treatment. A brief description of the signs and symptoms of some secondary headaches is presented here to aid in differentiating between primary and secondary headaches. Headache associated with seizures, confusion, drowsiness, or intellectual impairment may be a sign of brain tumor, subdural hematoma, or subarachnoid hemorrhage. Headache accompanied by nausea, vomiting, fever, and stiff neck may indicate brain abscess (arising from bacterial, fungal, or parasitic infection) or meningitis. The presence of headache with night sweats, aching joints, fever, weight loss, and visual symptoms (such as blurring) in patients with a history similar to rheumatoid arthritis may indicate cranial arteritis. Headache associated with localized facial pain, muscle tenderness, limited motion of the jaw may indicate temporomandibular joint disorder.[5]

Asking the patient the following questions will help elicit the information needed to accurately assess the type of headache and to recommend the appropriate treatment approach.

Assessment of Symptoms and Etiology

Q~ Describe the kind, intensity, and location of the pain? Are the headaches getting worse? Do you experience other effects just before the headaches start? Do you have muscular pain in the head, neck, or along the spine?

A~ *Identify the quality, location, and prodrome typical of primary headaches. (See the sections that describe signs and symptoms of the various headaches.)* Determine whether the patient's symptoms are typical of one of these headaches. If the pain extends to the neck or spine, determine whether the patient has had a recent facial, head, or spinal injury.

Q~ Are you under stress? Do you feel anxious, depressed, frustrated, or angry? Do you have insomnia?

A~ Suspect tension-type or migraine headaches in patients who are emotionally upset. Advise the patient that nonprescription medications are not effective in treating headaches related to anxiety or depression.

Q~ Do the headaches occur predictably? Do you know what triggers them? Do you have allergies, including those to medications?

A~ *Identify triggers for the primary headaches. (See the sections that discuss epidemiology of the various headaches.)* Determine whether triggers for the patient's headache are typical for one of these headaches. If the headaches are predictable, suspect cluster headache.

Q~ Do you take any medications for headache? If so, how long have you been taking them? Do you drink alcohol or caffeinated beverages, take opioids, or smoke?

A~ Suspect rebound headache in patients who consume a lot of caffeine or who have been on long-term analgesic therapy. If use of these agents is not excessive, suspect smoking as a potential cause.

Assessment of Medical and Medication Histories

Q~ What medications have or have not worked well for you in the past?

A~ If self-treatment is appropriate, base product recommendations on the patient's success or lack of success with previous self-treatments.

Q~ What medications have you already taken? How much and for how long? How effective were the medications?

A~ Be vigilant for polypharmacy in the self-treating patient. Determine whether attempts at self-management have placed the patient in a situation that requires a physician's intervention.

Q~ Do aspirin or other pain relievers upset your stomach? Have you ever had an ulcer or stomach problem?

A~ If yes, do not recommend aspirin or other NSAIDs. Advise patients with ulcers that these medications can predispose some patients to ulceration.

Q~ Have you ever had an allergic reaction to aspirin or any other medication for pain, swelling, or fever?

A~ If the patient is sensitive to aspirin, do not recommend analgesics containing aspirin or other NSAIDs. Medication allergy and intolerance should be one of the first questions asked by pharmacists of patients. This information is crucial in designing a therapeutic plan.

Q~ What allergies or reactions have you ever had to foods, dyes, or food additives?

A~ If needed, check labels of analgesics for problematic ingredients, especially tartrazine.

Q~ Do you now have or have you ever had asthma, allergies, nasal polyps, kidney disease, ulcers, gout, high blood pressure, heart failure, or a blood-clotting disorder?

A~ Do not recommend salicylates or other NSAIDs for patients with asthma and nasal polyps. These patients are at greater risk of allergy to NSAIDs. Do not recommend magnesium salicylate for patients with kidney disease. Do not recommend salicylates or other NSAIDs for patients with the remaining conditions.

Q~ Are you now taking medication for gout, arthritis, asthma, high blood pressure, or diabetes? Are you currently taking any drug that may thin your blood? Have you taken any such drug within the past week? What other prescription and nonprescription medications are you taking?

A~ *Identify possible drug interactions with internal analgesics. (See Table 3–4.)* On the basis of the patient's medication use, determine which internal analgesics are appropriate for self-treatment.

Q~ (If the patient is younger than 15 years) Has your child had recent symptoms of influenza or chickenpox?

A~ To avoid the risk of Reye's syndrome, do not recommend aspirin in such situations.

Q~ (If the patient is a woman of child-bearing age) Are you pregnant? Are you breast-feeding? If you are pregnant, do you plan to breast-feed?

A~ If yes to any of the questions, advise the patient not to use aspirin or other salicylates. Acetaminophen is the analgesic of choice for pregnant or breast-feeding women.

Patient Counseling for Headache

The pharmacist should stress that nonprescription analgesics are not appropriate long-term treatments for headache. Patients need to know that long-term use can actually cause rebound headache. The pharmacist should explain appropriate drug and nondrug measures for treating headaches. The use of nonprescription analgesics to preempt or abort migraine headaches should also be explained to migraine sufferers. The pharmacist should stress that nonprescription analgesics are potent medications and should make sure the patient understands possible adverse effects, interactions, and precautions/warnings for the selected agent. The box "Patient Education for Headache" lists specific information to provide patients.

Evaluation of Patient Outcomes for Headache

Pharmacists should communicate with patients in a timely manner to reinforce the need for appropriate medical attention for cases in which patients require therapy past the appropriate self-treatment time periods. The pharmacist should verify the patient's progress after 10 days of self-treatment. If a tension-type headache persists or has become worse, the patient should see a physician for evaluation.

Patients should know that continuing or escalating pain can be a sign of a more serious problem and that prompt medical attention is warranted. Patients should also know that continued use of analgesics can predispose them to toxicity because such medications affect multiple organ systems. The pharmacist should stress that chronic use of these medications, even for diagnosed migraine headaches, must be done under the supervision of a qualified physician.

Muscle Pain

This chapter discusses muscle pain in a broad context. Readers are referred to Chapter 5, "Musculoskeletal Injuries and Disorders," for further discussion of the epidemiology, etiology, pathophysiology, and signs and symptoms of particular types of muscle pain.

Epidemiology of Muscle Pain

Every adult has experienced skeletal muscle strain and pain. Usually, this pain is the result of minor trauma and is temporary. Most of these injuries are self-treated and go unreported. Hence, the incidence and prevalence of reported skeletal muscle injuries may well be underestimates. Because

Patient Education for Headache

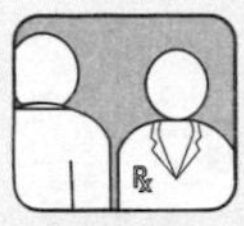

The objectives of self-treatment are (1) to relieve the pain of self-treatable headaches once they have set in, (2) to prevent or abort migraine headaches when possible, and (3) to prevent rebound headaches by avoiding chronic use of nonprescription analgesics. For most patients, carefully following product instructions and the self-care measures listed below will help ensure optimal therapeutic outcomes.

Tension-Type Headaches

- Nonprescription analgesics are usually effective for episodic tension-type headaches. However, consult a physician before using them for chronic tension-type headache.
- If these medications are used for chronic headaches, keep records of how often they are used and share this information with your physician.
- Do not use analgesics containing caffeine because of the risk of caffeine-withdrawal headaches.

Migraine Headache

- Avoid substances (food, caffeine, alcohol, medications) or situations (stress, fatigue, oversleeping, fasting, or missing meals) that you know can trigger a migraine.
- Use the following nutritional strategies to prevent migraine:
  —Avoid foods or food additives known to trigger migraines: red wine, aged cheese, aspartame, monosodium glutamate, coffee, tea, cola beverages, and chocolate.
  —Avoid foods to which you are allergic.
  —Eat regularly to avoid hunger and low blood glucose.
  —Take magnesium supplements.
- If onset of migraines is predictable (e.g., headache occurs during menstruation), take a nonsteroidal anti-inflammatory drug (NSAID) such as aspirin or other salicylates, ibuprofen, ketoprofen, or naproxen to prevent the headache. Start taking the analgesic 2 days before menstruation as well as during the menstrual cycle.
- Try to abort a migraine by taking acetaminophen or one of the NSAIDs mentioned previously at the onset of headache pain.
- Note that a nonprescription combination analgesic called Excedrin Migraine has been approved for use in the temporary relief of mild-to-moderate pain associated with migraine headache.
- If desired, use an ice bag or cold pack applied with pressure to reduce the pain associated with acute migraine attacks.
- If you have had cluster headaches, avoid substances (alcohol, cigarette smoke, or food such as nitrites that dilate blood vessels) or situations (exercise) known to trigger this type of headache. Consult a physician for medical treatment of these headaches.

Other Headaches

- If you have coexisting migraine and tension-type headaches, avoid caffeine-containing analgesics and other medications such as opioids that cause dependency. These substances can cause rebound headache.
- Consider concomitant use of decongestants and nonprescription analgesics to relieve the pain of sinus headache.
- Take acetaminophen or an NSAID for headaches related to excessive alcohol consumption (hangover) or fever.
- Note that nonprescription stimulants such as caffeine may provide some relief from headaches related to fatigue, but making up any sleep deficit is the best treatment.

Precautions for Nonprescription Analgesics

- If you are pregnant or breast-feeding, consult a physician before taking any nonprescription analgesics.
- Consult a pharmacist or a physician before taking any of these medications if you have a medical condition or are taking prescription medications. Nonprescription analgesics are known to interact with several medications. (See Table 3–4.)
- Do not take these medications for longer than 10 days unless a physician has recommended prolonged use.
- Do not exceed recommended dosages. (See Table 3–1.)

Nonsteroidal Anti-inflammatory Agents

- Note that aspirin, other salicylates (sodium salicylate, magnesium salicylate, and choline salicylate), ibuprofen, ketoprofen, and naproxen are nonsteroidal anti-inflammatory agents (NSAIDs).
- Do not take aspirin during the last 3 months of pregnancy unless a physician is supervising such use. Unsupervised use of this medication could harm the unborn child or cause complications during delivery.
- Do not give aspirin or other salicylates to children 15 years of age or younger who are recovering from chickenpox or the symptoms of influenza. To avoid the risk of Reye's syndrome, a rare but potentially fatal condition, give these patients acetaminophen for pain relief.
- Do not take NSAIDs if you drink a lot of alcohol. Concurrent use of these substances increases the risk of gastrointestinal bleeding.

(continued)

Patient Education for Headache (continued)

- Do not take aspirin or other NSAIDs if you are allergic to aspirin or have asthma or nasal polyps. Take acetaminophen instead.
- Do not take aspirin or other NSAIDs if you have stomach problems or ulcers, liver disease, kidney disease, or heart failure.
- Do not take aspirin if you are taking medication for bleeding problems (anticoagulants), gout, diabetes mellitus, or arthritis unless such use is supervised by a physician.
- Do not take other NSAIDs if you are taking anticoagulants.
- Do not take magnesium salicylate if you have kidney disease.
- Do not take sodium salicylate if you are on a sodium-restricted diet.
- Do not give ibuprofen to a child who is under treatment by a doctor, is taking prescription medication, has a history of problems with pain medication, or is dehydrated for whatever reason.
- Do not give ketoprofen to a child younger than 16 years.
- Do not give ibuprofen or naproxen to a child younger than 12 years.

⚠ Stop taking aspirin or other NSAIDs, and consult a physician if the following symptoms occur:

—Headache, dizziness, ringing in the ears, difficulty in hearing, dimness of vision, mental confusion, lassitude, drowsiness, sweating, thirst, hyperventilating, nausea, vomiting, and occasional diarrhea. These symptoms indicate mild salicylate toxicity.

—Dizziness, nausea and mild stomach pain, constipation, ringing in the ears, and swelling in the feet or legs. These symptoms are common side effects of NSAIDs.

—Rash or hives, or red, peeling skin; swelling in the face or around the eyes; wheezing or trouble breathing; bloody or black tarry stools; severe stomach pain or bloody vomit; bloody or cloudy urine; or unexplained bruising and bleeding. These symptoms require immediate medical attention.

Acetaminophen

- To avoid possible damage to the liver, do not take more than 4 g of acetaminophen a day.
- Avoid fasting, and do not drink alcohol while taking this medication.
- If you have had an adverse reaction to acetaminophen, have a history of liver disease, and consume the equivalent of three or more drinks of alcohol daily, do not take acetaminophen. These factors increase the risk of toxicity from acetaminophen.
- Do not give an acetaminophen product containing aspartame to a child with phenylketonuria.
- Follow dosage instructions for acetaminophen carefully if you have G-6-PD deficiency.

⚠ Stop taking acetaminophen and consult a physician if you experience the following symptoms: nausea, vomiting, drowsiness, confusion, and abdominal pain.

lower back pain is perhaps the most prevalent occupational hazard, more accurate estimates of its occurrence are available. At some time, more than 70% of the population has had lower back pain.[75]

Etiology of Muscle Pain

Ischemic muscle pain is caused by intramuscular pressure during activity that reduces blood supply to the muscle. Normally, this effect disappears within seconds of muscle relaxation. Ischemic muscle pain lasting for longer periods is probably the effect of histamine, acetylcholine, serotonin, and bradykinin. Potassium and adenosine may also contribute.

Overexertion or repeated unaccustomed eccentric muscle contraction is associated with delayed (8 hours) onset muscle pain, which can last for days. This pain reflects muscle damage that was presumably initiated by force generated in the muscle fibers. The mechanism by which delayed onset muscle pain is generated is unknown.

Myalgia can result from systemic infections (e.g., influenza, Coxsackie virus, measles, other illnesses) and from strenuous exertion. Prolonged tonic contraction produced by exercise, tension, or poor posture and by body mechanics can also produce muscle pain. Myalgia may be drug induced (e.g., by cancer chemotherapeutic agents such as doxorubicin). Abuse of alcohol may precipitate acute alcoholic myopathy. Bone and muscle pain (from osteomalacia) is associated with a diet deficient in vitamin D. Muscle pain is also frequently associated with insomnia.

Pain caused by noxious stimuli, such as mechanical or thermal insults, is immediate (acute). Numerous chemical substances, including prostaglandins, bradykinin, and histamine, normally mediate pain derived from ongoing tissue damage and many diseases. These pain-facilitating chemicals are present in normal tissue, but their production and release are enhanced by tissue damage. Pain itself enhances the production and release of these chemical mediators, a process that helps explain why untreated (or undertreated) acute pain may progress to a chronic pain syndrome. When acute pain is not adequately managed, the sympathetic "fight or flight" phenomenon may be maintained, causing ongoing adrenaline release. This ongoing release, in turn, results in increased, ongoing pain and anxiety. This situation helps to explain why anti-anxiety and centrally acting α_2-agonist medications sometimes are useful adjuncts in management of pain.

Pathophysiology of Muscle Pain

Somatic pain occurs when pain impulses are transmitted from peripheral nociceptors to the CNS by nociceptive nerve fibers. Common sites of origin of somatic pain are muscles, fascia, bones, and nerves. Somatic pain is most commonly myofascial (i.e., arising from muscles or the fascia that surround them) or musculoskeletal as in arthritis. Myofascial pain arises from localized tender areas in muscle or the surrounding fascia. These trigger points, which can occur following injury or immobility of the affected tissues, cause a reproducible, referred pain pattern when pressed.

Mechanoreceptors and chemoreceptors mediate muscle pain. These nerve endings are heterogeneous in that only a single chemical can stimulate some, whereas a variety of chemical, mechanical, and thermal triggers can stimulate others. Bradykinin, 5-hydroxytryptamine (serotonin), and histamine, as well as potassium and hydrogen ions are the primary chemical stimuli.

Erythema or redness, edema, and tenderness or hyperalgesia at the affected site characterize the inflammatory response, which develops through participation of multiple mediators, including histamine, bradykinin, 5-hydroxytryptamine, leukotrienes, and prostaglandins of the E series. Recently discovered opioid receptors found in peripheral tissues may play a role in the inflammatory response and may exert antihyperalgesic activity.[76] Because pain and inflammation increase prostaglandin production, drugs that inhibit peripheral prostaglandin production (e.g., NSAIDs) reduce the transmission of pain impulses from the periphery to the CNS.

[Note: Extemporaneously compounded topical agents containing nonsteroidal agents remain investigational at this time. Pharmacists compounding nonprescription analgesics into topical formulations for resale violate the Food, Drug, and Cosmetic Act and are advised to find other avenues to provide analgesia to their patients.]

Signs and Symptoms of Muscle Pain

Myalgia is a common diffuse muscle pain, which tends to be a dull, constant ache. Sharp pain is relatively rare. Muscle pain is usually exacerbated by contraction. Diffuse muscle soreness and aching may also be the initial symptom of rheumatoid arthritis, preceding joint involvement by weeks or months. Patients with myalgia complain of weakness, fatigue, and sometimes swelling, although swelling is rare.

Pain may be differentiated into nociceptive (visceral and somatic) pain and neuropathic pain. Patients describe somatic pain as aching, throbbing, or stabbing; visceral pain as dull or crampy; and neuropathic pain as burning, sharp, shocking, prickly, or numbing. Examples of nociceptive pain are cancer pain and arthritic pain, whereas neuropathic pain stems from nerve damage. The pain of neuroma is neuropathic.[77] Myofascial pain is characteristically referred from trigger points and is described by patients as debilitating, dull, aching, and deep and of varying intensity.[78]

Treatment of Muscle Pain

Acute pain is the body's alarm system; it signals injury by trauma, disease, muscle spasms, or inflammation. Chronic pain conversely may or may not be indicative and does require a physician's assessment.

Treatment Outcomes

The goals of treating muscle pain are to reduce the pain and discomfort and to prevent ongoing damage caused by inflammation. Assessing treatment effectiveness is not objective and relies on patients' perception of their pain.

General Treatment Approach

Nonprescription analgesics are often appropriate for managing acute pain such as muscle pain, if it is not too severe and if the complaints are not suggestive of a serious underlying disorder. Patients with muscle pain that has lasted longer than is normally expected from the underlying cause, or pain of more than 2 weeks' duration, should usually be referred for medical evaluation. Other exclusions to self-treatment include (1) pain that persists or worsens after 10 days of treatment, (2) a patient who is in the last trimester of pregnancy, (3) a patient who is 7 years of age or younger, and (4) any patient who has a high fever or signs of a serious infection.

Chronic nonmalignant pain management is often inappropriately treated with pharmacotherapeutic agents. Analgesic medications, as well as other CNS depressant drugs, are not effective as primary treatment modalities. These agents can produce adverse effects and may actually worsen pain. Patients with severe (chronic nonmalignant) pain often take excessive doses of acetaminophen and NSAIDs, which can lead to toxicities. The management of chronic nonmalignant pain often requires an interdisciplinary approach. Nonprescription analgesics may be useful adjuncts for some chronic nonmalignant pain, but these drugs are of limited value in most such syndromes. Not all pain and relatively few cases of chronic nonmalignant pain respond to analgesics alone. Physical therapy and behavioral therapies are the main treatment modalities for this type of pain.

Myofascial pain is amenable to treatment with nonprescription drugs, whereas neuropathic pain is usually treated with prescription drugs or other forms of treatment. Tricyclic antidepressants are often used as hypnotics in various types of chronic pain and are the agents of choice in managing neuropathic pain. The algorithm in Figure 3–3 outlines the self-treatment of muscle and joint pain.

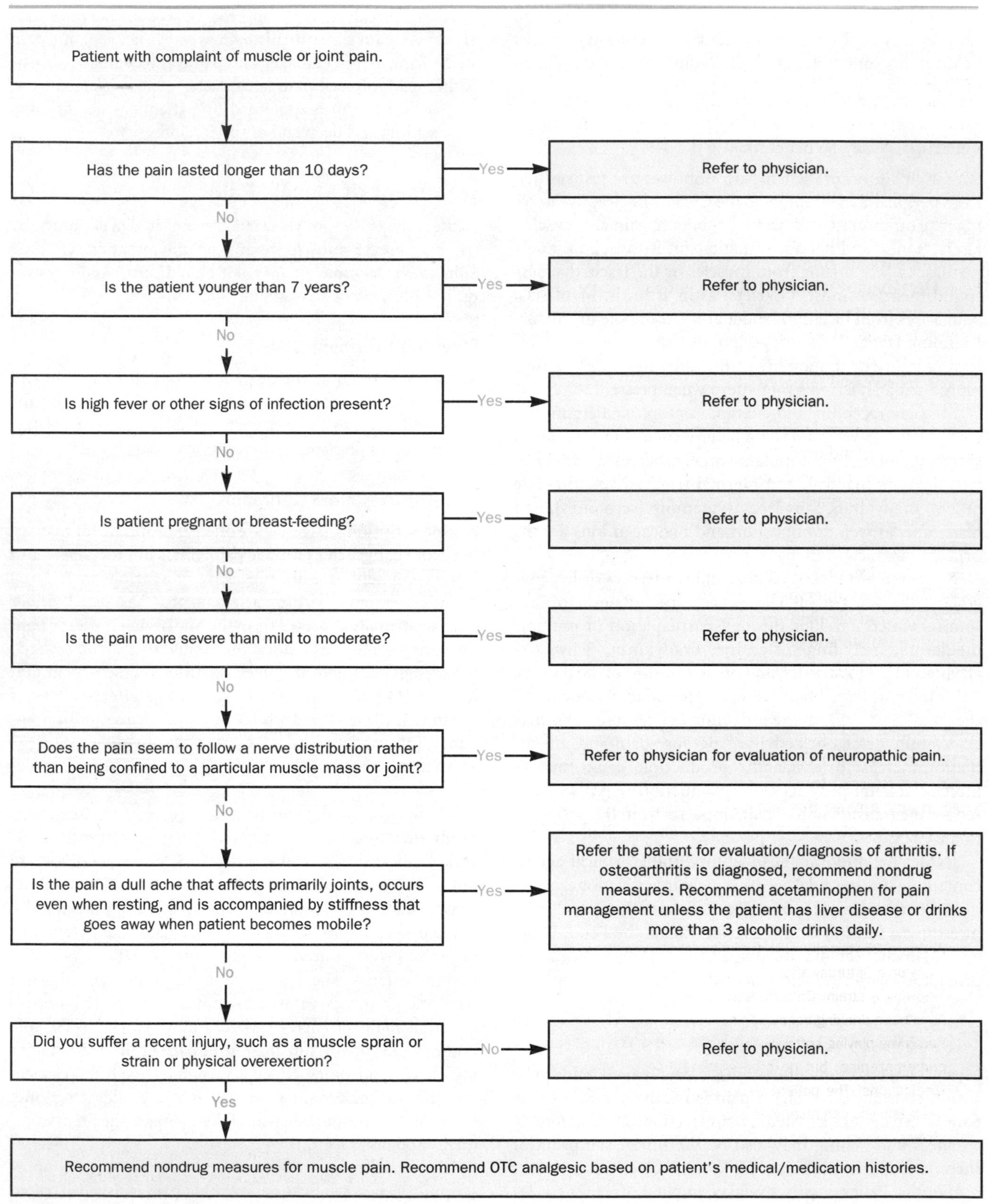

Figure 3–3 Self-care of muscle and joint pain.

Nonpharmacologic Therapy

RICE (rest, ice, compression, elevation) therapy promotes healing and helps reduce swelling and inflammation of muscle injuries. Table 5–1 in Chapter 5, "Musculoskeletal Injuries and Disorders," describes this therapy. For most injuries, rest may be beneficial for the first 48 to 72 hours. Mobilization of injured areas promotes healing and helps to maintain proper function. In most cases, physical activity should be encouraged after 48 to 72 hours. Consultation of a physical therapist may be beneficial for some patients.

Some patients find ice uncomfortable and may prefer heat. Heat therapy is usually recommended to begin 48 to 72 hours after injury and is applied for 15 to 20 minutes three to four times a day. Heat can promote healing and minimize muscle spasms. A heating device is never used on an area of skin with decreased sensation; this practice can lead to a skin burn.

For chronic muscle pain, a wide range of physical therapies is available and used, particularly for treatment of lower back pain and injuries from sports trauma and repetitive stress. These therapies aim to (1) stretch muscles that have been shortened by chronic pain and muscle spasm, (2) restore range of motion, and (3) strengthen the muscle. Massage (one of the therapies) may relieve pain by increasing blood flow to an otherwise ischemic area of the muscle.

Chronic muscle pain often requires structured physical therapy to isolate and stretch affected muscles. Although it may be appropriate to rest an injured muscle for a few days, failure to mobilize the area once the acute injury is healing will often result in the muscle becoming tight, weak, and overly contracted (guarded). Once guarding happens, patients can develop a tight band of muscle tissue. The tight bands are referred to as trigger points. Trigger points can arise in any muscle but are most commonly seen in large muscle groups. If muscle pain becomes chronic, the painful area may require application of ice or vapo-coolant sprays, or injections, typically using local anesthetics (trigger point injections, or TPIs) to facilitate remobilization. Analgesics and TPIs facilitate physical therapy for chronic muscle pain syndromes; however, the drugs are not curative. Pharmacists should keep in mind that physical therapy should occur within 2 hours of a TPI and should counsel patients appropriately.

Pharmacologic Therapy

Acute muscle pain usually responds well to nonprescription analgesics, especially when used in conjunction with heat and/or massage. Nonprescription analgesics should be started soon after the injury, taken on a regular schedule while the noxious stimulus is present, and taken in sufficient doses. (See the section "Treatment of Headache" for discussion of the dosages and properties of nonprescription systemic analgesics. Also see Chapter 5, "Musculoskeletal Injuries and Disorders," for discussion of nonprescription topical analgesics.)

Patient Assessment of Muscle Pain

Pharmacists can perform a brief assessment of pain with a few well-chosen questions. Assessment should include inquiry about the cause, duration, location, and severity of pain as well as factors that relieve and exacerbate it. The pharmacist should inventory all past and present medications, including pain medications, and should note the patient's satisfaction with or preference for past treatment medication. The pharmacist should inquire into the patient's medical history that bears directly either on the origin or treatment of pain.

Case Study 3–1

Patient Complaint/History

Andre, a 25-year-old male graduate student, stops by the pharmacy on a Saturday afternoon complaining of pain in his right leg following a strain. On further evaluation, the patient admits to have been drinking beer when he and his friends got a little carried away playing softball. Andre is currently taking lithium and carbamazepine, but no other prescription or nonprescription medications. The patient wants to know what nonprescription analgesic you can recommend to help him get on the road to recovery.

Clinical Considerations/Strategies

Readers can use the following considerations/strategies to determine whether treatment of this patient's disorder with nonprescription medications is warranted:

- Recommend appropriate nondrug measures for this patient's injury.
- Suggest an appropriate nonprescription analgesic on the basis of the patient's current medication use.
- Identify the precautions and adverse effects associated with the recommended regimen of using nonprescription medication.

Patient Education/Counseling

Readers can use the following strategies to develop a patient education/counseling plan that will help ensure optimal therapeutic outcomes:

- Explain the appropriate use of the recommended medication.
- Explain the signs and symptoms that indicate medical attention is needed.

Asking whether the pain is mild, moderate, or severe often leads to inconsistent reports. Simple, validated rating scales should be used. The two most common methods are the verbal numerical rating scale and the visual analog scale (VAS). If using the verbal scale, the pharmacist should ask patients to rank the present pain on a scale of zero to 10, with zero being no pain and 10 being pain as bad as the patient can imagine. The VAS allows patients to graphically quantify their pain by marking on a 10-cm line the distance along the line that indicates the level of the present pain. To quantify the pain, the pharmacist measures the line with a metric ruler and records the pain level, using a scale of 1 to 100. Using validated scales to quantify pain scores, such as the numerical rating scale (NRS), has proven to be a helpful tool for clinicians working with patients in pain. NRS scores greater than 3 indicate the need for an intervention, as do any scores that increase 2 or more points on the 10-point scale. Initially, pain scores establish a baseline for pain before treatment. In addition, a high pain score can be used to screen for patients who would be better served by seeking an appropriate medical evaluation. Pain scores also serve as a measuring stick for therapeutic outcomes. In general, nonprescription analgesics are appropriate for NRS scores of 1 to 3. These medications may be appropriate for scores of 4 or 5. Scores of 6 or higher indicate pain that requires medical referral.

Other scales are available for pain rating in children, adolescents, non-English speakers and other special populations.[79] It is important to use validated scales, not empirical ratings such as mild, moderate, or severe.

Asking the patient the following questions will help elicit the information needed to accurately assess the severity and cause of the pain. The questions about patients' medical and medication histories in the section "Patient Assessment of Headache" should also be asked. Responses to these questions will help to recommend the appropriate treatment approach.

Q~ Where is the pain? Is it in one place, such as a particular muscle or area of skin, or does it spread to other parts of the body?

A~ Suspect nociceptive pain if it is confined to a particular area (e.g., large muscle mass or joint). Suspect pain associated with nerve injury if the pain follows a nerve distribution and is described as burning, electrical, tingling, or paresthetic.

Q~ On a scale of zero to 10, with zero being no pain and 10 being pain as bad as you can imagine, what is your level of pain now? Have you ever had pain like this before? If so, what caused it and what helped it?

A~ Refer patients with chronic pain or pain rated 6 or higher which has existed for more than 10 days. Definitely consider use of nonprescription analgesics for acute pain rated 1 to 3. Consider past treatments when recommending an analgesic.

Q~ Is any part of your body red and swollen? Have you recently sustained a physical injury?

A~ Suspect inflammation if erythema and swelling are present. If a recent injury is ruled out, suspect arthritis. (See the section "Patient Assessment of Joint Pain.")

Q~ How long have you had this pain? Has it changed or remained constant in character and intensity?

A~ Chronic, consistent pain is rarely an emergency, but refer the patient to a physician for a careful medical examination. If the pain is increasing, advise the patient to see a physician as soon as possible.

Q~ What words best describe your pain (e.g., sharp, dull, aching, burning, electrical, stabbing)? Is it constant, or does it come and go? Did it develop suddenly or gradually?

A~ *Identify the signs and symptoms of visceral versus somatic pain and nociceptive versus neuropathic pain. (See the section "Signs and Symptoms of Muscle Pain.")* Try to determine the patient's type of pain by using the description of symptoms. Refer patients with suspected visceral and neuropathic pain to physician.

Q~ Does the pain occur with any particular event? What makes it worse or better?

A~ Using the patient's responses, try to determine whether the pain is associated with any particular activity, foods or beverages, or drug ingestion. Also, try to determine whether the pain is related to emotional, psychologic, or environmental factors.

Patient Counseling for Muscle Pain

The pharmacist should advise patients with chronic pain that nonprescription analgesics are ineffective for this disorder. Instead, the pharmacist should encourage patients to incorporate nondrug measures such as physical therapy into their prescription drug therapy. Patients with acute minor pain need to know what drug and nondrug measures will relieve their pain. The pharmacist should explain dosage guidelines for the various medications and should advise the patient of possible adverse effects, interactions, and precautions/warnings. Signs and symptoms that indicate medical attention is needed should also be explained. The box "Patient Education for Muscle Pain" lists specific information to provide patients.

Evaluation of Patient Outcomes for Muscle Pain

The pharmacist will have to assess treatment effectiveness according to the patients' perception of pain relief. If a patient reports the pain is still present or has worsened after 10 days of using nonprescription analgesics, the pharmacist should refer the patient to a physician.

Patient Education for Muscle Pain

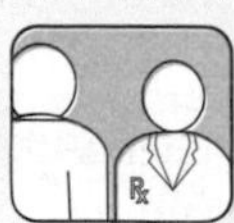

The objectives of self-treating acute pain are (1) to moderate or abolish pain and (2) to prevent chronic pain from developing by adequately treating acute pain. For most patients, carefully following product instructions and the self-care measures listed below will help ensure optimal therapeutic outcomes.

Nondrug Measures

- For a muscle strain, sprain, or other acute injury, rest the injured body part and try to keep it elevated for 48 to 72 hours.
- For further relief, apply a compression bandage such as Ace and either an ice bag or a cold wrap to the injured area three to four times a day. Apply cold therapy to the injured area for no more than 10 minutes at a time.
- If preferred to ice therapy, apply heat (heating pad or hot water bottle) to the injured area for 15 to 20 minutes three to four times a day. Do not apply heat to an area of skin with decreased sensation; this practice can lead to a skin burn.
- To keep the muscle functioning properly, resume normal daily physical activity after 48 to 72 hours.
- For chronic muscle pain such as lower back pain or repetitive strain injury, consult a physician or physical therapist.

Nonprescription Medications

- Ask your pharmacist to help you select the appropriate type of analgesic on the basis of your medical and medication history.
- For mild-to-moderate muscle pain, take a nonprescription analgesic for no longer than 10 days. (See Table 3–1 for dosages.)
- See the precautions for nonprescription analgesics listed in the box "Patient Education for Headache."

⚠ If the pain persists after 10 days of treatment with nonprescription analgesics, consult a physician and continue the medication only if guided by a physician.

Patients should know that continuing or escalating pain can be a sign of a more serious problem. The pharmacist should explain that a physician must supervise continued use of analgesics because these medications affect multiple organ systems, and chronic use can cause toxicity.

Joint Pain

Joints consist of cartilage covering the articulating surfaces of bones, the surrounding synovial membrane, and the periarticular supporting structures including ligaments and tendons. Bursae resemble synovial membranes and provide the surface and lubrication on which these supporting structures move.

Epidemiology of Joint Pain

The prevalence rate of arthritis and other rheumatic conditions in the United States is predicted to rise from 15.0% (37.9 million) in 1990 to 18.2% (59.4 million) in 2020. Correspondingly, the number of people who are severely disabled will rise from 2.8% (7.0 million) in 1990 to 3.6% (11.6 million) in 2020.[80]

The most prevalent form, osteoarthritis, affects 85% of people older than 70 years, and symptoms usually begin in the fifth or sixth decade of life. Pain is most commonly found in the back (23%), followed by the knee (19%) and shoulder (16%). The highest prevalence of disability occurs among the elderly who have multiple joint problems.[81] Up to 50 years of age, osteoarthritis is relatively infrequent and has a similar frequency in both men and women. But after the age of 50, women are markedly more susceptible. Also, geographic differences occur in the joints affected. For example, knee disease is common but hip disease is rare in Asia, whereas the reverse is true in the West.[82]

Rheumatoid arthritis affects roughly 1% of the population, commonly appears between the third and seventh decade of life, and occurs more often in women than in men. Although unexplained, the female excess suggests a hormonal basis. This hypothesis is supported by the noted protective effect of oral contraceptives and possibly by the massive increase in serum prolactin levels.[83] Genetic factors contribute to the cause in roughly 30% of cases, while the rest remain unexplained.[84]

Etiology of Joint Pain

Injury or inflammation of the tissues surrounding a joint (i.e., the joint capsule, tendons, ligaments, and bursae) can cause pain. Localized tenderness is often present, and the pain can be elicited by maneuvers that stress the structure but not the associated joint. Periarticular pain tends to be nocturnal and often involves the shoulder, elbow, or knee. It responds well to nonprescription analgesics and to limitation of motion in the affected joint.

By contrast, joint pain (arthralgia) often involves inflammation of the synovial membrane (synovitis) and cartilage loss. Synovitis-associated cartilage loss can be caused by mechanical stress and wear, such as in osteoarthritis (degenerative joint disease), or by erosive processes, such as in rheumatoid arthritis. (See Chapter 5, "Musculoskeletal Injuries and Disorders," for further discussion of causes of this disorder.)

Pathophysiology of Joint Pain

Ordinary joint pain is mechanical (caused by tension) or chemical (caused by exposure to irritants such as lactic acid, histamine, kinins, prostaglandins, and neuropeptides) in the joint. The noncorpuscular type IV nerve endings, which penetrate the synovium, capsule, and fat pads of the joint, are largely responsible for conduction of pain impulses.

In osteoarthritis, the main target is articular cartilage, which lacks nerve endings. This absence of nerve endings may explain why patients with mild disease often have no pain. As the disease progresses, the anatomy of the joint changes (capsule fibrosis occurs, marginal osteophytes proliferate, and the periosteum stretches). Pain from moving these physically misshapen joints is more likely to be mechanically stimulated. In addition, some inflammation occurs in osteoarthritis, initiating chemical pain stimuli.[82]

In rheumatoid arthritis, pain is more likely to be associated with inflammation and to progress to include mechanical, stress-associated pain derived from movement of malformed and eroded joints.[85]

Signs and Symptoms of Joint Pain

As opposed to rheumatoid arthritis, osteoarthritis is a local disease that occurs primarily in weight-bearing joints (e.g., knees, hips, and ankles). The primary complaint is joint stiffness and aching in the affected joint. The stiffness is temporary and lasts only a few minutes following initiation of joint motion. Degenerative changes of the upper extremities usually affect the joints of the fingers but rarely involve wrists, elbows, or shoulders. Osteoarthritis of the hip, knee, and spine does occur and can be disabling. Bursitis is common around osteoarthritis joints. Tendinitis may also be found, as well as tender spots. The latter may be either referred or caused by the underlying pathology. Dull, aching pain, which persists at rest, has been associated with venous stasis (congestion resulting from high pressure or blockage) or engorgement of the affected bones.

Rheumatoid arthritis is a systemic disease that may begin with a prodrome of fatigue, weakness, joint stiffness, arthralgia, and myalgia appearing several weeks before joint swelling. Multiple joints of the hands, wrists, and feet show symmetrical involvement. Involved joints become warm, red, and swollen, and range of motion is limited. Rheumatoid arthritis is a progressive disease that persists in affected joints and can produce joint deformity. Duration of morning stiffness can be used to assess severity and progression. Rheumatoid arthritis may have many extra-articular clinical features or complications, such as anemia, renal impairment, pleurisy, keratoconjunctivitis, Sjögren's syndrome, and potentially fatal septic arthritis.

Treatment of Joint Pain

Treatment Outcomes

The goals of treating joint pain are to reduce the pain and discomfort and prevent ongoing damage of joints resulting from inflammation.

General Treatment Approach

Nonprescription analgesics are approved for treating the aches and pains of minor arthritis. Such treatment should not be initiated, however, unless a physician has diagnosed the disorder.

Earlier stages of osteoarthritis respond well to nonprescription analgesics. Weight loss is also indicated to relieve stress on the affected joints of obese patients with osteoarthritis. Acetaminophen is the analgesic of choice for most osteoarthritic pain. For acute flares when inflammation exacerbates the problem, NSAIDs and local heat can be useful. Progressive disease, especially of weight-bearing joints, requires orthopedic management beyond the scope of nonprescription analgesics. (See Figure 3–3 for a summary of self-treatment of joint and muscle pain.)

Because the onset and progression of rheumatoid arthritis are slow and often subtle, many patients attempt self-medication in its initial stages. The therapeutic goal of managing rheumatoid arthritis—to control inflammation and induce remission—normally requires more than just nonprescription analgesics. NSAIDs have been the mainstay of therapy. Disease-modifying antirheumatic drugs (DMARDs), including the recently approved leflunomide and etanercept, are used earlier in disease progression than was common in the past. Education, exercise, and good nutrition are important in the control of rheumatoid arthritis. Many patients with rheumatoid arthritis have progressive, disabling disease that is best managed with a multimodal approach that includes education, physical therapy, nutritional counseling, and medications. Pharmacists should ensure that patients receive referral for appropriate care by clinicians with expertise in managing this disease.

Exclusions to self-treatment other than more severe arthritis pain include (1) a pain that does not respond to medication or worsens while taking medication for 10 days, (2) a patient who is in the last trimester of pregnancy, (3) a patient who is 7 years of age or younger, and (4) any patient who has a high fever or signs of a serious infection.

Nonpharmacologic Therapy

In addition to patient education, nutritional counseling, and physical therapy, nondrug measures discussed in the section "Treatment of Muscle Pain" apply to joint pain.

Pharmacologic Therapy

Acetaminophen is the preferred analgesic for minor pain of osteoarthritis unless inflammation is present. Nonprescription NSAIDs are appropriate for minor pain of rheumatoid arthritis. Dosages and properties of this agent are discussed in the section "Treatment of Headache."

Patient Assessment of Joint Pain

Differentiating joint pain from muscle pain can be difficult, especially in the early stages of arthritis. Once muscle pain has been eliminated, focusing on the characteristics of the pain and joint stiffness will help in determining whether arthritis is possibly causing the pain. The rating systems for pain measurement discussed in the section "Patient Assessment of Muscle Pain" also apply to joint pain. The presence of swelling is important in differentiating osteoarthritis from rheumatoid arthritis. If arthritis is suspected but undiagnosed, the pharmacist should advise the patient to see a physician for evaluation.

Asking the patient the questions in the section "Patient Assessment of Muscle Pain," as well as the following questions, will help elicit the information needed to determine the origin of the pain. The questions about patients' medical and medication histories in the section "Patient Assessment of Headache" should also be asked. Responses to these questions will help to recommend the appropriate treatment approach.

Q~ Is the pain a dull ache that persists even when you are resting?

A~ If yes, suspect joint pain rather than muscle pain.

Q~ Do some parts of your body feel stiff even when you are resting? Does the stiffness go away after you begin moving or change body position?

A~ Suspect arthritis if joint stiffness accompanies the pain.

Q~ Is the pain primarily in weight-bearing joints such as knees, hips, and ankles? Or are the hands, fingers, and feet primarily involved?

A~ Suspect osteoarthritis if the pain is limited to weight-bearing joints. Suspect rheumatoid arthritis if hands, fingers, and feet are the primary affected body parts. Advise the patient to see a physician for a definitive evaluation.

Q~ Are any of your joints swollen and red? Is the range of motion limited in these joints?

A~ If yes, suspect rheumatoid arthritis. Advise the patient to see a physician for a definitive evaluation.

Patient Counseling for Joint Pain

The pharmacist must stress that only minor pain of arthritis is amenable to treatment with nonprescription analgesics. If the patient's arthritis has been diagnosed and the pain meets this criterion, the pharmacist should recommend the appropriate analgesic for the patient's type of arthritis. The pharmacist should explain dosages as well as possible adverse effects, drug interactions, and precautions/warnings for the selected analgesic. Conditions that warrant medical attention should also be explained. The box "Patient Education for Joint Pain" lists specific information to provide patients.

Evaluation of Patient Outcomes for Joint Pain

Assessing the effectiveness of self-treating arthritis is not objective and relies on the patient's perception of the severity of the pain. If nonprescription analgesics are not relieving the pain, the patient should see a physician to determine whether prescription medications are in order. The pharmacist should explain that nonprescription agents are indicated for minor arthritis pain only and that they are effective only in the very early stages of rheumatoid arthritis.

CONCLUSIONS

Acute pain should be treated aggressively to prevent further damage and lessen the risk of chronic pain syndrome. Nonprescription analgesics are indicated only for mild-to-moderate pain and should not be used in excess of 14 consecutive days. Frequent use of nonprescription analgesics for headaches may lead to a rebound headache phenomenon. Physicians should evaluate pain that does not improve within 10 days or that worsens at any time.

Salicylates and other NSAIDs have clinically proven anti-inflammatory properties, acetaminophen does not. NSAIDs and salicylates should be used with caution in patients with hypertension, diabetes mellitus, kidney, liver, or heart disease and should be avoided in the last trimester of pregnancy. NSAIDs and salicylates should be avoided in patients with renal dysfunction, current or previous history of GI ulcers, and bleeding diathesis. Patients should be counseled to avoid combining different salicylates and other NSAIDs.

Acetaminophen is the drug of choice in treating osteoarthritis and should be used with extreme caution in patients who use alcohol or who have liver dysfunction. Acetaminophen and aspirin usage should not exceed 4 g per day.

In determining which medication to recommend, pharmacists should consider the condition being treated; the nature and origin of the complaint; the accompanying symptoms; and the concomitant history of asthma, urticaria, aspirin or NSAID intolerance, peptic ulcer disease, gout or hyperuricemia, clotting disorders, and concomitant hypertension or diabetes. It is also important to review concurrent prescription and nonprescription medications. In addition to efficacy, factors to be considered in recommending a medication will include formulation factors that may give the patient more prompt relief or fewer side effects as well as the potential for adverse effects and drug interactions. Because of decreased rectal bioavailability, acetaminophen or aspirin doses may need to be increased if administered rectally.

Patient Education for Joint Pain

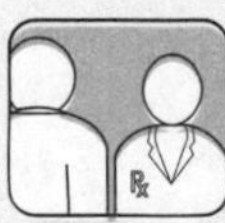

The objectives of self-treatment are (1) to reduce joint pain and discomfort and (2) to prevent ongoing damage of joints caused by inflammation. For patients with minor arthritis pain, carefully following product instructions and the self-care measures listed below will help ensure optimal therapeutic outcomes.

Osteoarthritis

- If you are overweight and have osteoarthritis, consider losing weight to relieve stress on your joints.
- Take acetaminophen to relieve minor pain of diagnosed arthritis. (See Table 3–1 for dosages.) If inflammation causes flare-up of joint pain, check with a physician about taking a nonsteroidal anti-inflammatory drug such as aspirin, ibuprofen, ketoprofen, or naproxen.
- See the precautions for nonprescription analgesics listed in the box "Patient Education for Headache."

Rheumatoid Arthritis

- Note that nonprescription analgesics may not effectively relieve the pain of rheumatoid arthritis.
- See a physician for a care plan that involves physical therapy, nutritional counseling, and, if needed, prescription medications.

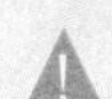

Consult a physician if the pain is not relieved or it worsens while taking nonprescription analgesics.

Under most circumstances, nonprescription NSAIDs and acetaminophen are equally effective and have similar times to onset of effect, similar times to peak antipyretic activity, and similar duration of action. When concurrent anti-inflammatory effects are desired, an NSAID should be used because acetaminophen lacks significant peripheral anti-inflammatory activity. All of these agents are effective analgesics and antipyretics, and they contribute to the relief of numerous discomforting symptoms (e.g., myalgia, arthralgia, headache) that often accompany fever.

Adverse reactions to nonprescription analgesics continue to be a concern.[86] NSAID-induced GI bleeding and nephropathy, as well as acetaminophen-induced hepatic damage, are real phenomena that mandate patients use these medications wisely. Pharmacists can markedly improve the outcomes of nonprescription analgesic/antipyretic use by discussing risk factors with patients and by recommending drugs with the best risk-to-benefit ratios for specific patients.

Nonprescription analgesic/antipyretic agents are effective medications that can greatly increase patient comfort when used correctly. Correct use of these drugs is more apt to occur if pharmacists (1) educate patients on how to manage pain, (2) counsel patients on drug selection and use when these symptoms occur, and (3) refer patients to physicians for more comprehensive evaluation and treatment when indicated. By monitoring patients who take these medications for therapeutic and toxic outcomes, pharmacists can make meaningful contributions to their patients' comfort and well-being and provide good pharmaceutical care.

References

1. Mersky H. Pain terms: a list with definitions and notes on usage. Recommended by the IASP Subcommittee on Taxonomy. *Pain.* 1979;6: 249–53.
2. National Institutes of Health Consensus Development Conference. The integrated approach to the management of pain. *J Pain Symptom Manage.* 1987;2:35–44.
3. *Am J Health Syst Pharm.* 1998;55:2597.
4. Mauskop A. Head pain. In: Ashburn MA, Rice LJ, eds. *The Management of Pain.* New York: Churchill Livingstone; 1998:249.
5. Classification and diagnostic criteria for headache disorders, cranial neuralgia, and facial pain. *Cephalagia.* 1988;8(suppl 7):1.
6. Schoenen J, de Noordhout AM. Headache. In: Wall PD, Melzack R, eds. *Textbook of Pain.* 3rd ed. Edinburgh, Scotland: Churchill Livingstone; 1994;498.
7. Saper JR, Magee KR. *Freedom from Headaches.* New York: Simon and Schuster; 1981:124–5.
8. Oleson J. Cerebral blood flow in migraine with aura. *Pathologie et Biologie.* 1992;40:318–24.
9. Ferbert A, Busse D, Thron A. Microinfarction in classic migraine? A study with magnetic resonance imaging findings. *Stroke.* 1991;22 : 1010–4.
10. Khalsa DH, Stauth C. *The Pain Cure.* New York: Warner Books; 1999: 236–41.
11. Mauskop A, Altura BM. Role of magnesium in the pathogenesis and treatment of migraines. *Clin Neurosc.* 1998;5:24–7.
12. *Federal Register.* 1988;53:46255–7.
13. Kanto J, Kiossner J, Mantyla R, et al. Bioavailability of rectal aspirin in neurosurgical patients. *Acta Anaesthesiol Scan.* 1981;25:25–6.
14. Hollister L. Measuring Measurin: problems of oral prolonged-action medications. *Clin Pharmacol Ther.* 1972;13:1–5.
15. Lobeck F, Spigiel R. Bioavailability of sustained-release aspirin preparations. *Clin Pharm.* 1986;5:236–8.
16. Ivey K. Mechanisms of nonsteroidal anti-inflammatory drug-induced gastric damage. *Am J Med.* 1988;84:41–8.
17. Lanza F. Endoscopic studies of gastric and duodenal injury after the use of ibuprofen, aspirin, and other nonsteroidal anti-inflammatory agents. *Am J Med.* 1984;77:19–24.
18. Hawthorne A, Mahida YR, Cole AT, et al. Aspirin-induced gastric mucosal damage: prevention by enteric-coating and relation to prostaglandin synthesis. *Br J Clin Pharmacol.* 1991;32:77–83.
19. Hoftiezer JW, Silvoso GR, Burks M, et al. Comparison of the effects of regular and enteric-coated aspirin on the gastroduodenal mucosa of man. *Lancet.* 1980;2(8195, pt 1):609–12.
20. Levy M. Aspirin use in patients with major upper gastrointestinal bleeding and peptic ulcer disease: a report from the Boston Collaborative Drug Surveillance Program, Boston University Medical Center. *N Engl J Med.* 1974;290:1158–62.

21. Lee T. Mechanism of aspirin sensitivity. *Am Rev Resp Dis.* 1992;1456(suppl):S34–6.
22. Samter M, Beers RJ. Intolerance to aspirin: clinical studies and consideration of its pathogenesis. *Ann Intern Med.* 1968;68:975–83.
23. Miller RR. Deafness due to plain and long-acting aspirin tablets. *J Clin Pharmacol.* 1978;18:468–71.
24. Roine R, Gentry RT, Hernandez-Munoz R, et al. Aspirin increases blood alcohol concentrations in humans after ingestion of ethanol. *JAMA.* 1990;264:2406–8.
25. Collaborative overview of randomised trials of antiplatelet therapy—I: Prevention of death, myocardial infarction, and stroke by prolonged antiplatelet therapy in various categories of patients. Antiplatelet Trialists Collaboration. *Br Med J.* 1994;308:81–106.
26. *Federal Register.* 1998;63:56802–19.
27. Giovannucci E, Rinun EB, Stampfer MJ, et al. Aspirin use and the risk of colorectal cancer and adenoma in male health professionals. *Ann Intern Med.* 1994;121:241–6.
28. Schreinemachers D, Everson R. Aspirin use and lung, colon, and breast cancer incidence in a prospective study. *Epidemiology.* 1994;5:138–46.
29. Sturmer T, Glynn R, Lee I, et al. Aspirin use and colorectal cancer: post-trial follow-up data from the Physicians' Health Study. *Ann Intern Med.* 1998;128:713–20.
30. Briggs G, Freeman R, Yaffe S. *Drugs in Pregnancy and Lactation.* 5th ed. Baltimore: Williams & Wilkins; 1998.
31. Committee on Drugs, American Academy of Pediatrics. The transfer of drugs and chemicals into human breast milk. *Pediatrics.* 1994;93: 137–50.
32. Rosefsky J. Ibuprofen safety. *Pediatrics.* 1992;89:166–7.
33. Hurwitz E, Barrett MJ, Bregman D, et al. Public Health Service study of Reye's syndrome and medications: report of the main study. *JAMA.* 1987;257:1905–11.
34. Forsyth B, Horwitz RI, Acampora D, et al. New epidemiologic evidence confirming that bias does not explain the aspirin/Reye's syndrome association. *JAMA.* 1989;261:2517–24.
35. *Federal Register.* 1993;58:14228.
36. Wilson J, Brown RD, Boccidni JA, et al. Efficacy, disposition and pharmacodynamics of aspirin, acetaminophen and choline salicylate in young febrile children. *Ther Drug Monit.* 1982;4:147–80.
37. Veltri J, Rollins D. A comparison of the frequency and severity of poisoning cases for ingestion of acetaminophen, aspirin, and ibuprofen. *Am J Emerg Med.* 1988;6:104–7.
38. Hylek E, Heiman H, Skates S, et al. Acetaminophen and other risk factors for excessive warfarin anticoagulation. *JAMA.* 1998;279:657–62.
39. Sattler F, Ko R, Antoniskis D, et al. Acetaminophen does not impair clearance of zidovudine. *Ann Intern Med.* 1991;114:937–40.
40. Steffe E, King JH, Inciardi JF, et al. The effect of acetaminophen on zidovudine metabolism in HIV-infected patients. *J Acquir Immune Defic Syndr Hum Retrovirol.* 1990;3:691–4.
41. Ricliman D, Fischl MA, Grieco MR, et al. The toxicity of azidothymidine (AZT) in the treatment of patients with AIDS and AIDS-related complex: a double-blind, placebo-controlled trial. *N Engl J Med.* 1987;317:192–7.
42. Miller R. Evaluation of the analgesic efficacy of ibuprofen. *Pharmacotherapy.* 1981;1:21–7.
43. McElwee N, Veltri JC, Bradford DC, et al. A prospective, population-based study of acute ibuprofen overdose: complications are rare and routine serum levels not warranted. *Ann Emerg Med.* 1990;19:657–62.
44. Martinez R, Smith D, Frankel L. Severe metabolic acidoses after acute naproxen sodium ingestion. *Ann Emerg Med.* 1989;18:129–31.
45. Schmid F, Culic D. Anti-inflammatory drugs and gastrointestinal bleeding: a comparison of aspirin and ibuprofen. *J Clin Pharmacol.* 1976;16:418–25.
46. Caruso I, Bianchi Porro G. Gastroscopic evaluation of anti-inflammatory agents. *Br Med J.* 1980;280:75–8.
47. Shelley W, Elpern D, Shelley E. Naproxen photosensitization demonstrated by challenge. *Cutis.* 1986;38:169–70.
48. Johnson AG, Siedemann P, Day RO. NSAID-related adverse drug interactions with clinical relevance: an update. *Int J Clin Pharmacol Ther.* 1994;32:509–32.
49. Radack K, Deck C, Bloomfield S. Ibuprofen interferes with the efficacy of antihypertensive drugs: a randomized, double-blind, placebo-controlled trial of ibuprofen compared with acetaminophen. *Ann Intern Med.* 1987;107:628–35.
50. Wong D, Spence JD, Lamid L, et al. Effect of nonsteroidal anti-inflammatory drugs on control of hypertension by beta-blockers and diuretics. *Lancet.* 1987;1:997.
51. Schuna AA, Vejraska BD, Hiatt JG, et al. Lack of interaction between sulindac or naproxen and propranolol in hypertensive patients. *J Clin Pharmacol.* 1989;29:524.
52. Ragheb M. Ibuprofen can increase serum lithium level in lithium-treated patients. *J Clin Psychiatry.* 1987;48:161–3.
53. Kristoff C, Hayes PE, Barr WH, et al. Effect of ibuprofen on lithium plasma and red blood cell concentrations. *Clin Pharm.* 1986;5:51–5.
54. Ragheb M. The clinical significance of lithium-nonsteroidal anti-inflammatory drug interactions. *J Clin Psychopharmacol.* 1990;10:350–4.
55. Cassano W. Serious methotrexate toxicity caused by interaction with ibuprofen. *Am J Pediatr Hematol Oncol.* 1989;11:481–2.
56. Thyss A, Milano G, Kubar J, et al. Clinical and pharmacokinetic evidence of a life-threatening interaction between methotrexate and ketoprofen. *Lancet.* 1986;1:256–8.
57. Royer G, Seekman C, Welshman I. Safety profile: fifteen years of clinical experience with ibuprofen. *Am J Med.* 1984;77:25–34.
58. Deykin D, Janson P, McMahon L. Ethanol potentiation of aspirin-induced prolongation of the bleeding time. *N Engl J Med.* 1982;306:852–4.
59. Lesko S, Mitchell A. An assessment of the safety of pediatric ibuprofen. *JAMA.* 1995;273:929–33.
60. Mercadante S, Casuccio A, Genovese G. Ineffectiveness of dextromethorphan in cancer pain. *J Pain Symptom Manage.* 1998;16:317
61. Kixinman E, Nygards E, Hansson P. Effects of dextromethorphan in clinical doses on capsaicin-induced ongoing pain and mechanical hypersensitivity. *J Pain Symptom Manage.* 1997;14:195–201.
62. Roth S. Salicylates revisited: are they still the hallmark of anti-inflammatory therapy? *Drugs.* 1988;36:1–6.
63. Savitsky M, Wiens J. Cross-reactivity in aspirin-sensitive patients. *Drug Intell Clin Pharm.* 1987;21:338–9.
64. Stern S. Clinical evaluation of the analgesic effect of magnesium salicylate. *Med Times.* 1967;95:1072–6.
65. Mehlisch D, Frakes L. A controlled comparative evaluation of acetaminophen and aspirin in the treatment of postoperative pain. *Clin Ther.* 1984;7:89–97.
66. Sunshine A, Olson NZ, Laska EM, et al. Ibuprofen, zomepirac, aspirin, and placebo in the relief of postepisiotomy pain. *Clin Pharmacol Ther.* 1983;34:254–8.
67. Jain A, Ryan JR, McMahon FG, et al. Analgesic efficacy of low-dose ibuprofen in dental extraction pain. *Pharmacotherapy.* 1986;6:318–22.
68. Schachtel B, Thoden W, Baybutt R. Ibuprofen and acetaminophen in the relief of postpartum episiotomy pain. *J Clin Pharmacol.* 1989;29:550–3.
69. Laska E, Sunshine A, Mueller F, et al. Caffeine as an analgesic adjuvant. *JAMA.* 1984;251:1711–8.
70. Mehlisch D, Sollecito WA, Helfrick JF, et al. Multicenter clinical trial of ibuprofen and acetaminophen in the treatment of postoperative dental pain. *J Am Dent Assoc.* 1990;121:257–63.
71. Autret L, Breart G, Jonville AP, et al. Comparative efficacy and tolerance of ibuprofen syrup and acetaminophen syrup in children with pyrexia associated with infectious diseases and treated with antibiotics. *Eur J Clin Pharmacol.* 1994;46:197–201.
72. Lipton R, Steward W, Saper J, et al. Efficacy and safety of acetaminophen, aspirin, and caffeine in alleviating migraine headache pain: three double-blind, randomized, placebo-controlled trials. *Arch Neurol.* 1998;55:210–7.
73. Forbes J, Beaver WT, Jones KF, et al. Effect of caffeine on ibuprofen analgesia in postoperative oral surgery pain. *Clin Pharmacol Ther.* 1991;49:674–84.
74. Sunshine A, Zighelboim I, De Castro A, et al. Augmentation of acetaminophen analgesia by the antihistamine phenyltoloxamine. *J Clin Pharmacol.* 1989;29:660–4.
75. Waddell G. A new clinical model for the treatment of low back pain. *Spine.* 1987;12:632.
76. Yaksh T. Pharmacology and mechanisms of opioid analgesic activity. *Acta Anaesthesiol Scand.* 1997;41:94–111.
77. Portenoy RK. Mechanisms of clinical pain. In: Portenoy RK, ed. *Neurologic Clinics.* Vol. 7. Philadelphia: WB Saunders; 1989:206–8.

78. Long SP, Kephart W. Myofascial pain syndrome. In: Ashburn MA, Rice LJ, eds. *The Management of Pain*. New York: Churchill Livingstone; 1998:306–7.
79. Acute Pain Management Guideline Panel. *Acute Pain Management: Operative or Medical Procedures and Trauma. Clinical Practice Guideline.* AHCPR Pub. No. 92–0032. Rockville, MD: Agency for Health Care Policy and Research, Public Health Service, US Department of Health and Human Services; 1992.
80. Helmick CO, Lawrence RC, Pollard RA, et al. Arthritis and other rheumatic conditions: who is affected now, who will be affected later? National Arthritis Data Workgroup. *Arthritis Care Res.* 1995;8:203–11.
81. Urwin M, Symmons D, Allison T, et al. Estimating the burden of musculoskeletal disorders in the community: the comparative prevalence of symptoms at different anatomical sites, and the relation to social deprivation. *Ann Rheum Dis.* 1998; 57:648–55.
82. McCarthy C, Cushnagan J, Dieppe P. Osteoarthritis. In: Wall PD, Melzack R, eds. *Textbook of Pain*. 3rd ed. Edinburgh, Scotland: Churchill Livingstone; 1994;387–9.
83. Silman AJ. Epidemiology of rheumatoid arthritis. *APMIS.* 1994;102: 721–8.
84. Alarcom GS. Epidemiology of rheumatoid arthritis. *Rheum Dis Clin North Am.* 1995;21:589–604.
85. Grennan DM, Jayson MIV. Rheumatoid arthritis. In: Wall PD, Melzack R, eds. *Textbook of Pain*. 3rd ed. Edinburgh, Scotland: Churchill Livingstone; 1994; 397–8.
86. Strom B. Adverse reactions to over-the-counter analgesics taken for therapeutic purposes. *JAMA.* 1994;272:1866–7.

Additional Information Sources

www.ahcpr.gov/clinic

National Cancer Institute Cancer Information Service ([800] 422-6237)

Jacox A, Carr DB, Payne R, et al. *Management of Cancer Pain. Clinical Practice Guideline.* No. 9. AHCPR Pub. No. 94–0592. Rockville, MD: Agency for Health Care Policy and Research, Public Health Service, US Department of Health and Human Services; 1994.

American Pain Society. *Principles of Analgesic Use in the Treatment of Acute Pain and Chronic Cancer Pain.* 4th ed. American Pain Society: Glenville, IL; 1999.

World Health Organization. Cancer pain relief and palliative care: report of a WHO Expert Committee. *Techanical Report Series 804.* Geneva: World Health Organization; 1990.

Portenoy R, Hagen N. Breakthrough pain: definition, prevalence and characteristics. *Pain.* 1990;41:273–81.

Russel S. Interdisciplinary versus multidisciplinary pain management. *J Pharm Care Pain Symptom Control.* 1993;1:89–94.

CHAPTER 4

Fever

Arthur G. Lipman and Kenneth C. Jackson II

Chapter 4 at a Glance

Most fevers are self-limited and nonthreatening; however, fever can cause a great deal of discomfort and, in some cases, may indicate serious underlying pathology (e.g., acute, infectious process) for which prompt medical evaluation is indicated. The principal reason for treating fever is to alleviate discomfort. Treatment should target the underlying cause whenever possible. Serious complications of fever are uncommon, and overly aggressive fever management may be more dangerous than the fever itself.

Epidemiology of Fever

Fever is one of the most common reasons that parents seek medications for their children. One of five emergency room visits for children is related to fever, and more than 10% of children between the ages of 1 month to 24 months who are seen in pediatricians' offices have fever.

Other epidemiologic variables correlate with the causes of fever discussed in the section "Etiology of Fever."

Editor's Note: This chapter is based, in part, on the 11th edition chapter titled "Internal Analgesic and Antipyretic Products," which was written by Arthur G. Lipman.

Physiology of Body Thermoregulation

Body temperature is regulated by the thermoregulatory center located in the anterior hypothalamus. Temperature-sensitive neurons in both the hypothalamus and the skin continuously transmit information about body temperature to the hypothalamic "thermostat." Physiologic and behavioral homeostatic mechanisms can then be invoked to maintain body temperature within the normal range. Examples of behavioral adaptations to temperature changes or extremes include putting on additional clothing, rubbing the hands together, adjusting air conditioning, and seeking shade for relief from the hot sun. Compensatory physiologic mechanisms include heat dissipation (e.g., sweating, vasodilation, hyperventilation) in response to heat, as well as heat production or conservation (e.g., shivering, vasoconstriction) in response to cold.

Compensatory effects are mediated by alterations in the secretory rates of thyroid-stimulating hormone and catecholamines. Normal thermoregulation prevents wide fluctuations in body temperature so that the average body temperature is usually maintained at 97.7°F to 99.5°F (36.5°C to 37.5°C).

Normal body temperature varies throughout the day, peaking daily between 5 pm and 7 pm and reaching its lowest point between 3 am and 5 am.[1–12] This consistent rhythm occurs at all ages older than 2 years and is more pronounced in children than in adults. Body temperature can vary by as much as 1.8°F (1°C) in adults and as much as 2.5°F (1.4°C) in children each day. Because circadian variation continues during febrile illness, patients may be incorrectly described as febrile when they have a relatively normal temperature in the early morning, and a moderately high evening temperature may be misinterpreted as fever.

Fever is defined as a body temperature that is higher than the normal core temperature of 98.6°F (37°C). Fever is a sign of an upward displacement of the body's thermoregulatory set point. A rectal temperature above 101.8°F (38.8°C), an oral temperature above 100°F (37.8°C), or an axillary (armpit) temperature above 99°F (37.2°C) is considered abnormal. Axillary temperatures range from 0.7°F (0.4°C) higher to 3.6°F (2°C) lower than rectal temperatures. This discrepancy is normal; it should not be ascribed to improper measurement technique. Axillary temperatures are considered indicative of fever when they exceed 100.4°F (38°C), whereas rectal temperatures will usually exceed 100.4°F. As noted previously, normal body temperature may range 1.8°F to 2.5°F (1°C to 1.5°C) from these norms, and diurnal rhythm causes variances in body temperature during the day. The average rectal temperature for an 18-month-old baby is 100°F (37.8°C); therefore, 50% of infants have normal rectal temperatures above 100°F. Rectal temperatures of healthy children may approach 101°F (38.3°C) in the late afternoon or after physical activity. Children commonly have elevated temperatures after vigorous play. For that matter, adults can experience elevations in temperature after exercise or other strenuous activities.

Pathophysiology of Fever

Pyrogens are fever-producing substances that activate the body's host defenses, resulting in an increase in the hypothalamic heat regulatory set point. Pyrogens can be exogenous (originating outside the body) or endogenous (originating within the body).

Prostaglandins of the E series are produced in response to circulating pyrogens and act on the anterior hypothalamus to elevate the thermoregulatory set point. In response to these prostaglandins and to changes in monoamine concentration, the hypothalamus appears to direct the reestablishment of body temperature to correspond to the elevated set point. Within hours, body temperature reaches this new set point and fever occurs. During the period of upward temperature readjustment, the patient experiences chills caused by peripheral vasoconstriction, and then skeletal muscle tone increases to maintain homeostasis. Because the new set point is regulated by negative feedback, body temperature rarely exceeds 106°F (41.1°C). Nonsteroidal anti-inflammatory drugs (NSAIDs) and acetaminophen, which inhibit the synthesis of E series prostaglandins in the central nervous system (CNS) in response to endogenous pyrogens, possess antipyretic activity.

Patients' ability to perceive fever varies. Some individuals quite accurately perceive elevations in their body temperature. Others (e.g., those with tuberculosis) are unaware of temperatures as high as 102.9°F (39.4°C). Furthermore, fever may be ignored because of more unpleasant concomitant symptoms.

Etiology of Fever

Fever is usually caused by a microbiologic agent, often a virus for which specific anti-infective therapy is not available. Fever may also be induced by certain drugs or physiologic processes or may be of unknown origin.

Microbe-Induced Fever

Most febrile episodes are caused by infection by exogenous pyrogens, including viruses, bacteria, fungi, yeasts, and protozoa. Persistent or increasing fever usually indicates an infectious process. Elevated temperatures associated with bacterial infections are generally higher than those associated with viral infections, but no absolute temperature exists at which these infections can be differentiated. Nor is there any basis for differentiating viral from bacterial infections according to the magnitude of temperature reduction from antipyretic drug therapy. Fever from exogenous pyrogens, such as infectious organisms, is often less marked in elderly patients than in younger individuals. Consequently, infection may not be easily recognized in geriatric patients if fever is the primary assessment criterion.

Pathology-Induced Fever

Noninfectious pathologic causes of fever include malignancies, tissue damage (e.g., myocardial infarct or surgery), antigen–antibody reactions, dehydration, and metabolic disorders such as hyperthyroidism or gout. Each of these etiologies can trigger the production and release of endogenous pyrogens from liver and spleen cells, monocytes, eosinophils, and neutrophils.

Signs and symptoms that help distinguish among fever-inducing disorders include headache, sweating, generalized malaise, tachycardia, arthralgia, myalgia, back pain, irritability, and anorexia. However, fever caused by the release of endogenous pyrogens from malignant cells is difficult to distinguish from fever caused by infections in cancer patients. High body temperature dulls intellectual function and causes disorientation and delirium, especially in individuals with preexisting dementia, cerebral arteriosclerosis, or alcoholism. Reducing high temperature may alleviate CNS symptoms in some individuals.

Drug-Induced Fever

Many drugs may induce fever. (See Table 4–1.) The incidence of drug-induced fever is unknown, but the condition may account for more than 3% of all adverse drug reactions.

Failure to discontinue the offending agent can result in substantial morbidity and even mortality. However, drug-induced fever often goes unrecognized because consistent signs and symptoms are lacking.[13]

Drug-induced fever probably is not related to atopy, sex, age, or systemic lupus erythematosus, as was previously believed. It is now believed to be a hypersensitivity reaction or idiosyncrasy in most cases. However, drugs may cause fever by interfering with peripheral heat dissipation, increasing basal metabolic rate, invoking cellular immune response, structurally mimicking endogenous pyrogens, or inflicting direct tissue damage.

Some drugs elevate body temperature by altering normal thermoregulatory mechanisms. Large doses of phenothiazines or anticholinergic agents decrease sweating and, thus, reduce heat dissipation. Thyroid hormones may increase the metabolic rate and, thus, increase heat generation. Other drugs may modify the behavioral response to the climatic temperature. For example, obtundation (dulling of body sensations) from sedatives may impair the normal behavioral withdrawal response from high environmental temperature.

Occasionally, fever may be a direct result of the pharmacologic effect of a drug. For example, the release of endotoxin from bacteria following the initiation of antibiotic therapy (e.g., penicillin for syphilis) can result in high fever, chills, hypotension, myalgia, and leukocytosis. This phenomenon (the Jarisch–Herxheimer reaction) may occur within hours after parenteral antibiotic therapy is begun. Fever may also result from the release of endogenous pyrogens associated with cellular injury or death following cancer chemotherapy. Similarly, the administration of drugs that possess oxidizing activity to individuals who have a glucose-6-phosphate dehydrogenase deficiency may cause fever as a result of the release of endogenous pyrogens from damaged erythrocytes.

Some drugs or their metabolites as well as some biologic preparations have antigenic properties that can produce a hypersensitivity reaction. Although drug fever usually develops after 7 to 10 days of treatment, fever and other symptoms may occur shortly after initiation of therapy when previous exposure and sensitization have occurred.[14] The onset of drug fever caused by antineoplastic agents often occurs within 7 days of initiation of therapy. Fever caused by cardiac drugs may not occur until more than 10 days have passed.[13]

Drug fever is distinguished by (1) fever occurring during or shortly after treatment with a drug previously reported to cause fever or other allergic symptoms, (2) fever accompanied by other manifestations of allergy, and (3) temperature elevation despite patient improvement. One study of drug-induced fever identified skin rash in only 18% of patients, and fewer than half of those individuals experienced urticaria (hives). Furthermore, a generally mild eosinophilia was present in only 22% of the patients. The presence of high fever and shaking chills may make it hard to differentiate drug fever from infection. Bradycardia is uncommon with drug fever.[14] Drug fever should not be excluded on the basis of a shift to the left in the white blood cell differential count because this shift occasionally accompanies drug-induced fever.[15] Diurnal temperature variation in drug fever is often minimal.

Fever in persons taking neuroleptic medications (e.g., phenothiazines, butyrophenones, thioxanthenes) could be caused by neuroleptic malignant syndrome, a potentially life-threatening condition.[16,17] The high fever of neurolep-

Table 4–1

Selected Agents That Induce Fever

Cardiovascular Agents	Methicillin	L-Asparaginase	**Anti-inflammatory Agents**
Hydralazine	Nitrofurantoin	6-Mercaptopurine	Aspirin
Methyldopa	Para-aminosalicylic acid	Procarbazine	Ibuprofen
Nifedipine	Penicillin G	Streptozocin	Tolmetin
Procainamide	Streptomycin[a]		
Quinidine	Sulfamethoxazole–trimethoprim	**CNS Agents**	**Other Agents**
	Sulfonamide	Amphetamine	Allopurinol
Antimicrobial Agents	Tetracycline	Benztropine[a]	Cimetidine
Ampicillin	Vancomycin	Carbamazepine	Clofibrate
Cefamandole		Chlorpromazine	Folate
Cephalothin	**Antineoplastic Agents**	Haloperidol	Interferon
Cephapirin	Bleomycin	Nomifensine	Iodide
Cloxacillin	Chlorambucil	Phenytoin	Levamisole
Colistin	Cytarabine	Thioridazine	Metoclopramide
Isoniazid	Daunorubicin	Triamterene	Propylthiouracil
Lincomycin	Hydroxyurea	Trifluoperazine[a]	Prostaglandin E_2
Mebendazole			Ritodrine

[a] Fever seen during drug overdose.

Source: Reference 13; adapted with permission.

tic malignant syndrome is often accompanied by muscle rigidity, abnormal body movements, sweating, tachycardia, high or low blood pressure, incontinence, and altered consciousness including delirium, stupor, or coma. Although neuroleptic malignant syndrome may occur in anyone taking these medications, it is most common in young males and possibly in people who are dehydrated. When this syndrome is suspected, the neuroleptic medication should be discontinued, and a physician should be contacted immediately.

The management of drug-induced fever involves discontinuing the suspected drug whenever possible. If feasible, all medications should be temporarily discontinued. If the fever is drug induced, the patient's temperature will generally decrease within 24 to 48 hours after the offending drug is withdrawn. After patient safety and the need to definitively identify the offending drug have been considered, each medication may be restarted, one at a time, while monitoring for fever recurrence. If an implicated drug cannot be discontinued, systemic corticosteroids may be given to suppress fever and to minimize other allergic symptoms. Dosage reduction of phenothiazines, anticholinergic agents, and thyroid hormone may decrease temperature and should be considered if these drugs are suspected of causing fever, particularly in elderly patients.

Complications of Fever

Serious complications of fever are rare. Harmful effects (e.g., dehydration, delirium, seizures, coma, irreversible neurologic or muscle damage) are most likely to occur at temperatures above 106°F (41.1°C). However, even lower body temperature elevations may be life-threatening in patients with heart disease because of an increased demand for oxygen in conjunction with increased cardiac output and heart rate. Increased risk and lower tolerance to elevated body temperature exist in infants and in patients with brain tumors or hemorrhage, CNS infections, preexisting neurologic damage, and decreased ability to dissipate heat.

Febrile seizures are seizures associated with fever in the absence of another cause, such as acute metabolic disorder or CNS inflammation. These seizures occur in about 2% to 4% of all children between the ages of 6 months and 5 years.[18] Simple febrile seizures generally last no longer than 15 minutes, have no features characteristic of focal origin, and do not recur during a single febrile episode. Significant neurologic sequelae (e.g., impaired intellectual development) are unlikely following a single pediatric febrile seizure that is not complicated by status epilepticus.[19] Status epilepticus, which is characterized by recurrent or repetitive seizures without intervening periods of normal consciousness, occurs in only about 1% to 2% of children who experience a febrile seizure. If not controlled, status epilepticus can result in permanent brain damage, renal failure, cardiorespiratory arrest, and death. Any person experiencing such seizures requires immediate medical attention.

Unlike simple febrile seizures, complex febrile seizures in children are repetitive during the course of a single febrile episode and generally last longer than 15 minutes. Such seizures exhibit signs characteristic of a focal origin. Complex seizures are believed to be precipitated by fever in children with preexisting or latent epilepsy.

Although both the magnitude and rate of temperature increase appear to be critical determinants in precipitating febrile seizures, the temperature at which a particular child will seize is unpredictable. Most initial febrile seizures occur in children younger than 3 years. Seizures occurring after

Case Study 4–1

Patient Complaint/History

The mother of a 4-year-old girl, Heather, calls the pharmacy to refill the child's phenytoin prescription. She asks the pharmacist what dose of acetaminophen she should give her daughter for fever. Heather has been seizure-free for about 6 months and is taking no other anticonvulsants. Her medication profile reveals only the use of fluoride and vitamin tablets, as well as a prescription for amoxicillin filled 9 days ago.

Clinical Considerations/Strategies

Readers can use the following considerations/strategies to determine whether treatment with nonprescription medications is warranted:

- Consider the appropriateness of a nonprescription antipyretic for this child's fever.
- Assess the complications that could result from fever in this child.
- Assess the possible causes of fever in this child.

Patient Education/Counseling

Readers can use the following strategies to develop a patient education/counseling plan that will ensure optimal therapeutic outcomes:

- Explain to the mother the possible complications of fever in a child with a history of seizures.
- Explain the possible relationship between the recent infection and the fever.
- Explain the need for medical supervision of this child's treatment for fever.

that age are usually unrelated to fever. The risk for a febrile seizure is increased in children (1) who have experienced a previous febrile seizure (especially if it occurred before age 1 year or was a complex febrile seizure), (2) who have a documented seizure or other CNS disorder, or (3) whose family history includes febrile seizures.[18,19] Prophylaxis against febrile seizures with antiepileptic drugs should be reserved for patients at high risk of subsequent epilepsy. Antipyretics rarely will prevent febrile seizures in children predisposed to them.

Detection of Fever

Subjective assessment of fever typically involves feeling a part of the body, such as the forehead. However, this method often does not detect a fever. If done properly, measuring body temperature with a thermometer is the most accurate method of detecting fever. However, normal body temperature varies according to the patient's age and level of physical and emotional stress, the environmental temperature, the time of day, and the anatomic site at which the temperature is measured.[13–17] These factors must be considered when evaluating temperature measurements.

Body temperature may be measured by using various types of thermometers. During the course of an illness, the same thermometer should be used because the readings from different thermometers may vary. Regardless of the site or method used, thorough hand washing should precede and follow all temperature measurements.

Types of Thermometers

Mercury-in-glass and electronic thermometers are commonly used for temperature measurement. Tympanic (ear canal) and skin thermometers are more recent innovations for measuring body temperature.

Glass Thermometers

Glass thermometers intended for oral use have a long, thin bulb designed to reach well under the tongue. In contrast, the bulb of the rectal thermometer is short and thick, permitting insertion in the rectum with little risk of breakage. Although a rectal thermometer can be used for oral temperature measurement, an oral thermometer should never be inserted into the rectum because oral thermometers are more fragile; they may break and injure rectal tissue. The same thermometer should never be used both rectally and orally because effective disinfection is difficult. To ensure reliable measurement, the patient should neither engage in vigorous physical activity nor heat or cool the oral cavity artificially by smoking or by drinking hot or cold beverages for at least 5 minutes (preferably 20 minutes) before temperature is measured.

The advantages of mercury-in-glass thermometers over electronic thermometers are (1) patient familiarity, (2) low cost, (3) light weight, and (4) compact size. Both are accurate when used appropriately. However, mercury-in-glass thermometers can break, rendering them useless and potentially dangerous. Although the elemental mercury contained in the thermometers manufactured today is nonabsorbable through the gastrointestinal tract and is nontoxic, many patients still fear mercury poisoning from a broken thermometer. The real danger is from glass fragments; patients should discard chipped thermometers. In addition, mercury-in-glass thermometers register slowly and must be disinfected before each use. Such thermometers should be stored in a cool location and out of direct sunlight because they may be damaged by excessive heat.

Electronic Thermometers

Electronic thermometers are available for oral, rectal, and axillary temperature measurement. These instruments may require about 30 seconds for equilibration. They register readings quickly and are not subject to glass breakage and the attendant risk of cuts. The use of disposable covers with these thermometers eliminates the need for disinfection following their use. In addition, the electronic digital temperature display makes these thermometers easier to read than the traditional glass thermometers.

Tympanic Thermometers

Body temperature can also be determined by measuring tympanic membrane blood temperatures with instruments developed for that use only. The tip of the instrument, which is placed in the ear canal, measures body temperature by sensing infrared radiation from the blood vessels in the eardrum. The tympanic membrane is close to the hypothalamus, and the blood supply to these two anatomic areas is at the same temperature. This measurement, therefore, provides an accurate reading of the body core temperature. The instructions that come with the instrument and that describe inserting the thermometer into the ear canal and properly positioning it should be followed carefully to ensure that the measured infrared radiation is from the tympanic membrane, not adjacent areas. The technique varies somewhat for young infants and older patients. The instrument provides an error message if the measurement is not performed correctly. The measurement takes only 1 second, is simple and accurate, and can be performed on a sleeping child. Inexpensive, disposable lens covers (sheaths) for the filter probe eliminate the need to disinfect the instrument between uses. The instruments are still relatively expensive, but the cost has decreased in recent years, and many families with young children now find the convenience of one of these thermometers sufficient to offset the cost.

Skin Thermometers

Skin thermometers, adhesive temperature strips that are applied to the skin and change color over a particular temperature range, are not sufficiently accurate or reliable. In one study, temperature strips failed to detect 66% of fevers of 100°F (37.8°C) or higher.[20] This method of temperature measurement is less reliable than either glass or electronic thermometers; however, these strips may be useful in noting temperature trends.[21]

Types of Temperature Measurement

Body temperature may be measured at rectal, axillary, oral, or ear canal sites. The rectal method is more consistently accurate than the oral or axillary readings. However, most patients, especially children, prefer the other, more comfortable methods of temperature measurement.

The difference between the Celsius and Fahrenheit scales often causes confusion about the presence of a fever. The normal variations in temperature among rectal, oral, and axillary sites of measurement can also confuse patients or caregivers. These differences should be emphasized when instructing individuals on the proper use of fever thermometers. Table 4–2 compares Fahrenheit and Celsius temperatures.

Oral Temperature Measurement

Oral temperature should not be taken when an individual is mouth breathing or hyperventilating; has recently had oral surgery; is not fully alert; or is uncooperative, lethargic, or confused. Oral thermometers are not appropriate for use in most children younger than 3 years because young children usually find it difficult to maintain a tight seal around the oral thermometer. Electronic thermometers can be used for children as young as 3 years because these instruments are not breakable if bitten and they pose no risk of accidental cuts.

Table 4–3 describes the proper methods for taking oral measurements with glass and electronic thermometers.[22]

Rectal Temperature Measurement

Risks associated with taking a rectal temperature include injury from broken glass, retention of the thermometer, rectal or intestinal perforation, and peritonitis (inflammation of the membrane lining the abdominal cavity). The patient should never be left unattended while the rectal thermometer remains in place because a positional change may cause the thermometer to be expelled or broken. Rectal temperature measurement is relatively contraindicated in patients who are neutropenic, who have had recent rectal surgery or injury, or who have rectal pathology (e.g., obstructive hemorrhoids). Use of rectal thermometers is also contraindicated in newborns, who are more susceptible to mucosal perforation. Further, many parents cannot use a rectal thermometer correctly or read it accurately.

Table 4–4 describes the proper methods of taking rectal temperatures in children and adults.

Table 4–2

Selected Temperatures in °Celsius and Equivalent °Fahrenheit

Celsius	Fahrenheit
36°	96.8°
37°	98.6°
38°	100.4°
39°	102.2°
40°	104.0°
41°	105.8°
42°	107.6°

Conversion formulas: Celsius = 5/9 (°F − 32); Fahrenheit = (9/5 × °C) + 32.

Table 4–3

Guidelines for Oral Temperature Measurements

Glass Thermometers

1. Inspect the thermometer for cracks or imperfections before taking a temperature.
2. Disinfect the thermometer by drawing it through a swab moistened with an antiseptic such as alcohol or povidone–iodine solution.
3. Rinse the thermometer with cool water. Never use hot water, which may break the thermometer. Rotate the thermometer at or slightly below eye level to confirm that the displayed temperature is below 96°F (35.6°C). If the reading is higher, shake the thermometer over a bed, carpet, or other soft surface, using a rapid, downward, snapping motion until the mercury column falls below the 96°F level.
4. Place the thermometer under the tongue, and position it slightly to one side of the mouth.
5. Keep the lips closed around the thermometer to hold it in place and to prevent air from flowing over the thermometer.
6. Leave the thermometer in place until the temperature reading is consistent. (Although the literature recommends insertion for 6 to 10 minutes, 3 to 4 minutes is usually sufficient.[22])
7. Remove saliva from the thermometer by wiping it from the stem toward the bulb.
8. After the recorded temperature is noted, shake the mercury down to less than the 96°F (35.6°C) level.
9. Disinfect the thermometer as described in step 2 for glass thermometers above.

Electronic Thermometers

1. Remove the probe from the thermometer base in which it is stored.
2. Verify the temperature set point as specified by the manufacturer.
3. Insert the thermometer probe into a probe sheath.
4. Insert the probe into the mouth as described in steps 5 and 6 above for glass thermometers.
5. After the electronic thermometer indicates the temperature has been measured, remove the probe from the mouth.
6. Discard the contaminated probe sheath.
7. Read the temperature display and record the measurement.
8. Reset the thermometer by returning the probe to the base.

Table 4–4

Guidelines for Rectal Temperature Measurements

1. Use a mercury-in-glass rectal, not an oral, thermometer to take rectal measurements.
2. Disinfect the thermometer by drawing it through a swab moistened with an antiseptic such as alcohol or povidone–iodine solution.
3. Rinse the thermometer with cool water. Never use hot water, which may break the thermometer. Rotate the thermometer at or slightly below eye level to confirm that the displayed temperature is below 96°F (35.6°C). If the reading is higher, shake the thermometer over a bed, carpet, or other soft surface, using a rapid, downward, snapping motion until the mercury column falls below the 96°F level.
4. Lubricate the bulb with a water-soluble lubricant to allow easy passage through the anal sphincter and to reduce the risk of trauma.
5. When taking rectal temperatures of infants and young children, place the child face down over your lap, separate the buttocks with the thumb and forefinger of one hand, and insert the thermometer gently and calmly in a direction pointing toward the child's umbilicus with the other hand. For infants, insert the thermometer to the length of the bulb. For young children, insert it about 1 inch into the rectum.
6. When taking an adult's rectal temperature, have the patient lie on one side with the legs flexed to about a 45° angle from the abdomen. Insert the bulb ½ to 2 inches into the rectum by holding the thermometer ½ to 2 inches from the bulb and inserting it until the finger touches the anus. To facilitate passage of the thermometer through the anal sphincter, have the patient take a deep breath. If the patient has hemorrhoids, gently insert the thermometer to avoid causing pain and injury.
7. Hold the thermometer in place (in a straight line along its angle of insertion) for at least 3 minutes.
8. Remove the thermometer and clean it by wiping from the stem toward the bulb.
9. Read the temperature at or slightly below eye level, and record the results.
10. Disinfect the thermometer as described in step 2.
11. Wipe any remaining lubricant from the anus.

Axillary Temperature Measurement

Axillary temperature measurement is recommended for adults who are not candidates for oral or rectal temperature measurement (e.g., somnolent individuals recovering from rectal surgery or severe diarrhea). Axillary temperature measurement may also be preferred in children 3 months to 5 years of age because intrusive rectal procedures can be very frightening to preschool children, to children with diarrhea, or to infants with severe diaper rash. However, because axillary temperature measurement is generally considered unreliable for detecting fever in infants and young children, rectal temperature measurement is preferred for infants 1 to 3 months of age.

Most oral thermometers can also be used to measure axillary temperature.

Table 4–5 describes the proper method for taking axillary temperature measurements.

Ear Canal Temperature Measurements

Tympanic thermometers provide digital readouts, and many can be set to provide either a rectal or an oral temperature equivalent. Table 4–6 describes the proper method for using this type of thermometer.

Treatment of Fever

The decision to treat fever is based on several considerations. Patient discomfort associated with fever is an indication for antipyretic therapy, but arguments against such treatment include (1) the generally benign and self-limited course of fever, (2) the possible elimination of a diagnostic or prognostic sign, (3) the attenuation of enhanced host defenses (i.e., possible therapeutic effect of fever), and (4) the untoward effects of antipyretic drugs.

No correlation exists between the magnitude or pattern of temperature elevation (i.e., persistent, intermittent, recurrent, or prolonged) and the underlying etiology or severity of the disease. Furthermore, when associated with an infectious

Table 4–5

Guidelines for Axillary Temperature Measurements

1. Use an oral mercury-in-glass thermometer to take axillary temperatures.
2. Inspect the thermometer for cracks or imperfections before taking a temperature.
3. Rotate the thermometer at or slightly below eye level to confirm that the displayed temperature is below 96°F (35.6°C). If the reading is higher, shake the thermometer over a bed, carpet, or other soft surface, using a rapid, downward, snapping motion until the mercury column falls below the 96°F level.
4. Place thermometer in the armpit.
5. Hold the arm pressed against the body for at least 10 minutes or as long as the thermometer instructions indicate.
6. Read and record the temperature.

Table 4–6

Guidelines for Ear Canal Temperature Measurements

1. Place a clean disposable lens cover over the insertion end of the instrument.
2. Do not insert the thermometer into the ear canal until the digital instruction panel indicates the thermometer is ready for use.
3. Aim the instrument tip into the canal by pointing the lens of the instrument toward the patient's eye.
4. Press the button for the length of time indicated in the instructions, typically 1 second.
5. Read the digital panel immediately, and record the temperature.
6. Discard the contaminated lens cover.

disease, effective antibiotic therapy is generally guided by microbiologic cultures and sensitivity, epidemiologic data, and other diagnostic data. In the febrile neutropenic patient with negative cultures, antipyretic therapy should be periodically interrupted to determine the need for continued anti-infective therapy. An agent lacking anti-inflammatory activity, such as acetaminophen, should be used when anti-inflammatory effects may mask the clinical signs of a particular disease (e.g., septic joint, rheumatic fever).

The argument is often overstated that fever is an adaptive response and that elevated body temperature may be beneficial. Although the growth of some pathogenic microorganisms is impaired by higher than normal temperatures, the benefits of fever appear to be limited to regional cutaneous infections. Fever itself is rarely beneficial to the host response to infection. Fever increases oxygen consumption, production of carbon dioxide, and cardiac output. The minimal benefits of low-grade fever on host defense mechanisms (e.g., antigen recognition, T helper lymphocyte function, leukocyte motility) do not appear to favorably alter the course of infectious diseases.[23]

Treatment Outcomes

The goal of self-treatment is to alleviate the discomfort of fever by reducing the body temperature to a normal level.

General Treatment Approach

Treatment of fever with oral antipyretic agents is indicated if the oral temperature exceeds 102°F (38.9°C). When a lower temperature and its associated discomfort are present, nonpharmacologic or pharmacologic intervention may be used. (See Figure 4–1.) All nonprescription antipyretic agents are also analgesics, and the discomfort associated with a fever of

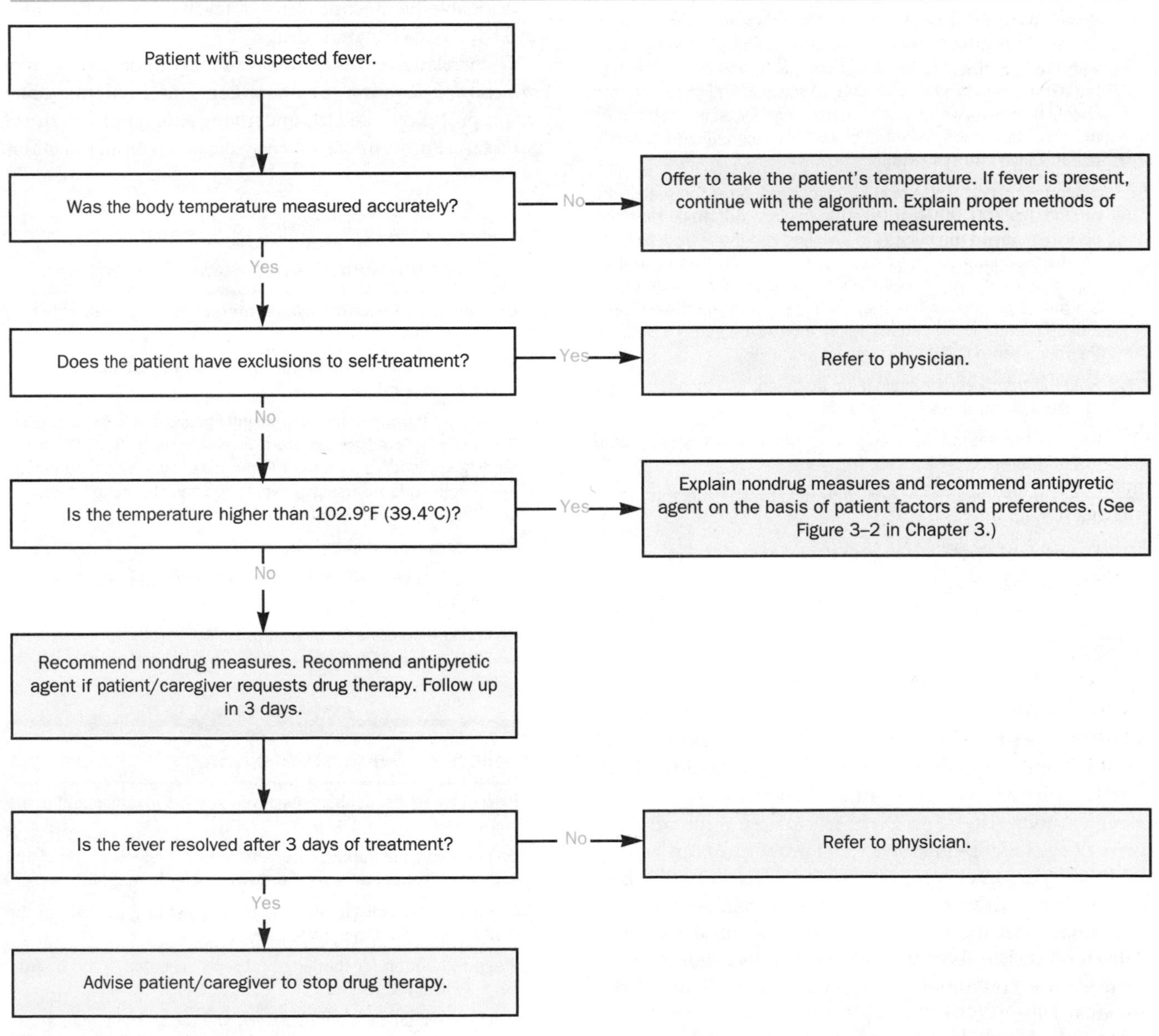

Figure 4–1 Self-care of fever.

less than 102°F may be the primary indication for any of the nonprescription analgesic/antipyretic medications.

A physician should be contacted at the first sign of fever in a child predisposed to seizures. In such individuals, antipyretic medication should be administered every 4 hours with one dose given during the night, and therapy should be continued for at least 24 hours. The physician should determine the need for additional therapy, such as anticonvulsant medication. If a fever-induced seizure occurs, sponging with lukewarm (not cold) water should be initiated and the physician should be notified immediately.

Because infants younger than 3 months are at greater risk of serious outcomes from fever than are older children, they should be evaluated by a physician when their temperature rises above 100°F. For infants older than 3 months, a rectal temperature reading above 104°F is cause for contacting a physician immediately and withholding antipyretic medication pending the physician's directive. Any patient exhibiting symptoms of an infection should also be referred to a physician. (See the section "Microbe-Induced Fever.")

Nonpharmacologic Therapy

When the body temperature exceeds 104°F (40°C), body sponging with tepid water can be started to facilitate heat dissipation. However, body sponging is not routinely recommended for children with a temperature below 104°F because this procedure is usually uncomfortable and often causes the child to shiver, which could raise the temperature even higher. Ideally, sponging should follow oral antipyretic therapy by 1 hour to permit the therapeutic reduction of the hypothalamic set point and thereby permit a more sustained temperature-lowering response. Unlike acetaminophen and NSAIDs, topical sponging does not reduce the hypothalamic set point. Sponging can be useful, however, because only a small temperature gradient between the body and the sponging medium is necessary to achieve an effective antipyretic response. Ice water baths or spongings with hydroalcoholic solutions (e.g., isopropyl or ethyl alcohol) are uncomfortable, unnecessary, and not recommended. Alcohol poisoning can result from cutaneous absorption or inhalation of topically applied alcohol solutions.

Nondrug measures for all degrees of fever consist of providing or wearing light clothing, removing blankets, maintaining room temperature at 78°F (25.6°C), and drinking or supplying sufficient fluid intake to replenish insensible losses. Fluid intake in febrile children should be increased by at least 1 ounce of fluids per hour (e.g., soft drinks, fruit juice, water, or other fluids), unless oral fluids are contraindicated.

Pharmacologic Therapy

Any of the nonprescription analgesic/antipyretic medications (i.e., acetaminophen, aspirin, ibuprofen, naproxen sodium, ketoprofen) are appropriate for treating fever. Chapter 3, "Headache and Muscle and Joint Pain," discusses these agents in detail. These medications should not be used longer than 3 days to treat fever. Patients with persistent fever should be referred to a physician.

Patient Assessment of Fever

The pharmacist must first determine whether a patient actually has a fever. Subjective or inaccurate methods of temperature measurement must be ruled out. If fever is present, a quick assessment of the severity is important, especially in patients at risk for seizures. For other patients, the seriousness of the underlying cause should also be evaluated.

Children who are capable of providing and understanding information should be included in any dialogue concerning their care. Asking patients or caregivers the following questions will help elicit the information needed to accurately assess the severity of the fever and to recommend the appropriate treatment approach.

Q~ How high is your (your child's) fever? How long has the fever been present?

A~ Consider the severity of the elevated temperature, as well as its duration, in determining the appropriate course of action. Refer patients with fever of greater than 48 hours to a physician.

Q~ How did you measure the temperature (i.e., by the oral, axillary, rectal, or ear canal method)?

A~ *Identify the range of "normal" temperatures for the different routes of measurement. (See the section "Physiology of Body Thermoregulation.")* Determine whether the measured temperature indicates a fever.

Q~ Describe how you measured the temperature.

A~ Determine whether the temperature was measured properly. If not, offer to take the patient's temperature.

Q~ What activities preceded this fever?

A~ Determine whether the activities were strenuous enough to cause a temporarily elevated temperature.

Q~ What other symptoms do you have?

A~ Refer to a physician any patients with symptoms related to infection.

Q~ Have you ever had a convulsion, seizure, or brain disorder?

A~ If yes, refer the patient immediately to a physician to avoid possible fever-induced seizures.

Q~ What medication or other treatment have you used to treat the fever?

A~ Consider previous treatment attempts to avoid duplicating therapy or recommending ineffective treatments.

Q~ Are you currently seeing or have you seen a health care professional for other medical conditions (e.g., recent surgery, cancer, gout, hyperthyroidism)?

A~ *Identify medical conditions that can cause fever. (See the section "Pathology-Induced Fever.")* Refer to a physician any patients with a serious underlying pathology.

Q~ Are you taking any nonprescription or prescription medications other than those for fever?

A~ *Identify medications known to induce fever. (See Table 4–1.)* If such a medication is being taken, refer the patient to a physician for possible temporary discontinuation of the medication, dosage reduction until the fever subsides, or use of corticosteroids to suppress the fever.

Patient Counseling for Fever

Although fever is a common symptom, it is often misunderstood and poorly treated. One study revealed that 20% of the population apparently does not know how to measure body temperature properly; many more people do not know how to interpret the results.[24] Pharmacists and other health professionals can improve patient outcomes by teaching patients self-assessment skills and the proper methods for measuring body temperature. Such instruction should include demonstration of measurement techniques. Pharmacists should also explain the appropriate nonpharmacologic and pharmacologic treatments for fever. The box "Patient Education for Fever" lists specific information to provide patients.

Evaluation of Patient Outcomes for Fever

Treatment of fever with antipyretic agents should not exceed 3 days. Timeliness of patient follow-up is important in reinforcing the need for appropriate medical attention if fever persists after 3 days of treatment or increases during the treatment period.

CONCLUSIONS

Fever is an elevation of body temperature above the body's normal thermoregulatory set point. An elevated body temperature is not a medical disorder in itself; rather, it is a symptom of underlying pathology. Fever can accompany a serious or a minor medical condition. It can also be induced by medications. Treatment should be directed at eliminating the underlying cause, as well as at alleviating the discomfort of fever.

Nonprescription analgesics/antipyretics resolve fever by lowering the elevated hypothalamic set point primarily through inhibition of prostaglandin synthesis and release at the thermoregulatory center. The duration of treatment with these agents should not exceed 3 days. Persistent fever or an increase in body temperature during treatment requires medical referral.

Patient Education for Fever

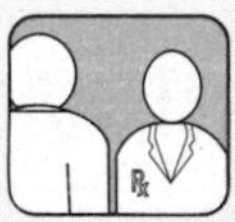

The objective of self-treatment is to relieve the discomfort of fever by returning the body temperature to the normal level. For most patients, carefully following product instructions and the self-care measures listed below will help ensure optimal therapeutic outcomes.

Measurement of Body Temperature

- For adults, use the oral method of temperature measurement. (See Table 4–3 for instructions.)
- For children 1 to 3 months of age, use the rectal method of temperature measurement. (See Table 4–4 for instructions.)
- For children 3 months to 5 years of age, the axillary method of temperature measurement can be used. (See Table 4–5 for instructions.)

Nondrug Measures

- When the body temperature exceeds 104°F (40°C), sponge the body with lukewarm (not cold) water. Wait 1 hour after a dose of an antipyretic before sponging the body.
- Do not use isopropyl or ethyl alcohol in body sponging. Alcohol poisoning can result from cutaneous absorption or inhalation of topically applied alcohol solutions.
- For all degrees of fever, wear light clothing, remove blankets, and maintain room temperature at 78°F (25.6°C).
- Unless advised otherwise, drink or give sufficient fluids to replenish body fluid losses. For children, increase fluids by at least 1 ounce per hour. Soft drinks, fruit juice, or water are acceptable.

Nonprescription Medications

- See the drug treatments listed in the box "Patient Education for Headache" in Chapter 3, "Headache and Muscle and Joint Pain."

 Seek medical attention if the fever persists after 3 days of drug treatment.

 Seek medical attention if the fever continues to increase during treatment.

Counseling of patients and caregivers should include proper instruction on taking body temperatures at the various body sites (oral, rectal, axillary, and ear canal) and with various types of thermometers (glass, electronic, tympanic, and skin). Patients should also be counseled on the proper use of antipyretic medications.

References

1. Jacox A, Carr DB, Payne R, et al. *Management of Cancer Pain. Clinical Practice Guideline No. 9.* AHCPR Publication No. 94–0592. Rockville, MD: Agency for Health Care Policy and Research, Public Health Service, US Department of Health and Human Services; March 1994.
2. Mercadante S, Casuccio A, Genovese G. Ineffectiveness of dextromethorphan in cancer pain. *J Pain Symptom Manage.* 1998;16: 317–22.
3. Kinnman E, Nygards E, Hansson P. Effects of dextromethorphan in clinical doses on capsaicin-induced ongoing pain and mechanical hypersensitivity. *J Pain Symptom Manage.* 1997;14:195–201.
4. Mersky H. Pain terms: a list with definitions and notes on usage, IASP Subcommittee on Taxonomy. *Pain.* 1979;6:249–53.
5. American Pain Society. *Principles of Analgesic Use in the Treatment of Acute Pain and Chronic Cancer Pain.* 4th ed. Glenville, IL: American Pain Society. 1999.
6. World Health Organization. *Cancer Pain Relief and Palliative Care: Report of a WHO Expert Committee.* Technical Report Series 804. Geneva: World Health Organization; 1990.
7. Yaksh T. Pharmacology and mechanisms of opioid analgesic activity. *Acta Anaesthesiol Scand.* 1997;41:94–111.
8. Chan W. Prostaglandins and nonsteroidal antiinflammatory drugs in dysmenorrhea. *Ann Rev Pharmacol Toxical.* 1983;23:131–49.
9. Portenoy R, Hagen N. Breakthrough pain: definition, prevalence and characteristics. *Pain.* 1990;41:273–81.
10. Russell S. Interdisciplinary versus multidisciplinary pain management. *J Pharm Care Pain Symptom Control.* 1993;1:89–94.
11. Mackowiak P. *Fever: Basic Mechanisms and Management.* New York: Raven Press; 1991.
12. Stephenson L, Kolka M. Effect of gender, circadian period, and sleep 1055 on thermal responses during exercise. In: Pandoff K, Sawka M, Gonzalez R, eds. *Human Performance Physiology and Environmental Medicine at Terrestrial Extremes.* Indianapolis: Benchmark Press; 1988: 267–304.
13. Mackowiak PA, LeMaistre CF. Drug fever: a critical appraisal of conventional concepts. *Ann Intern Med.* 1987;106:728–33.
14. Johnson D, Cunha B. Drug fever. *Infect Dis Clin North Am.* 1996;10: 85–91.
15. Lysy J, Oren R. Drug fever with a shift to the left. *DICP Ann Pharmacother.* 1990;24:782.
16. Chan T, Evans S, Clark R. Drug-induced hyperthermia. *Crit Care Clinic.* 1997;13:785–809.
17. Velammor V. Neuroleptic malignant syndrome: recognition, prevention, and management. *Drug Saf.* 1998;19:73–82.
18. Verity C, Butler N, Golding J. Febrile convulsions in a national cohort followed up from birth: I. Prevalence and recurrence in the first five years of life. *Br Med J.* 1985;290:1307–10.
19. Verity C, Butler N, Golding J. Febrile convulsions in a national cohort followed up from birth: II. Medical history and intellectual ability at 5 years of age. *Br Med J.* 1985;290:1311–15.
20. Lewit E, Marshall C, Salzer J. An evaluation of a plastic strip thermometer. *JAMA.* 1982;247:321–5.
21. Allen G, Horrow J, Rosenberg H. Does forehead liquid crystal temperature accurately reflect "core" temperature? *Can J Anaesth.* 1990;37: 659–62.
22. Baker N, Cerone SB, Gaze N, et al. The effect of type of thermometer and length of time inserted on oral temperature measurements of afebrile subjects. *Nurs Res.* 1984;33:109–11.
23. Roberts NJ. Impact of temperature elevation on immunologic defenses. *Rev Infect Dis.* 1991;13:462–71.
24. Eskerud J, Hoftvedt B, Laerum E. Fever: management and self-medication. Results from a Norwegian population study. *Fam Pract.* 1991;8: 148–53.

CHAPTER 5

Musculoskeletal Injuries and Disorders

Arthur I. Jacknowitz

Chapter 5 at a Glance

Skeletal muscles, ligaments, and tendons hold together the body's skeletal system and coordinate body movement. The muscle is much like a cable made up of an array of bundles—each bundle a collection of muscle fibers, nerves, blood vessels, and connective tissue. A muscle fiber is made up of muscle strands called myofibrils, which contain the contractile elements—actin and myosin. These structures move the muscle and are responsible for the muscle's resilience. With disuse, the muscle loses resilience. Similarly, with age, the resilient muscle fibers are replaced by less-resilient connective tissue, and consequently the muscle weakens, its contraction weakens, and the tissue becomes more susceptible to injury.[1]

Tendons attach muscles to bones, and ligaments attach

Editor's Note: This chapter is based, in part, on the 11th edition chapter titled "External Analgesic Products," which was written by Arthur I. Jacknowitz.

bones to other bones, thus holding joints together. Excessive use, sudden twisting, or stretching may damage muscle, tendon, or ligament. The extent of injury may vary from easily treated stiff muscles or tendinitis to much more serious problems such as joint dislocations that require a physician's attention. This chapter covers self-care of tendinitis and bursitis; strains, sprains, and cramps; repetitive strain injury; lower back pain; and arthritis. Pharmacologic therapy for these disorders is similar; therefore, nonprescription external analgesics are discussed in one section: "Treatment of Musculoskeletal Injuries and Disorders." Therapeutic or preventive measures specific to a disorder are included in the individual treatment overview of each disorder.

The pharmacist's greatest challenge in self-care of these disorders is determining which disorder is causing the symptoms. For that reason, patient assessment of self-treatable disorders is covered in one section: "Patient Assessment of Musculoskeletal Injuries and Disorders." Collective discussions of patient counseling and evaluation of patient outcomes for the various self-treatable disorders are also presented at the end of the chapter.

Physiology of Pain

Nociceptors are nerve endings that are sensitive to pain. The three types of nociceptors are distinguished by their sensitivity to either mechanical stress (such as a cut or a blow), heat, or certain chemicals. The skin, muscles, tendons, ligaments, and certain parts of the skull contain all three types of nociceptors.

Pain-producing substances, chemical mediators, are released or synthesized in response to tissue damage. When present in sufficient quantity, these mediators (called algogens) trigger nociceptor sites. Among the algogens is the breakdown product of arachidonic acid, prostaglandin E. Trauma also liberates inflammatory mediators (called leukotrienes) and blood platelet serotonin, which causes vasoconstriction. Mast cells that are recruited to the site of injury degranulate and release histamine, which causes local edema. Nociceptor stimuli originating in the damaged skin, blood vessels, muscle, ligaments, and joint capsules are conducted through peripheral nerves to the dorsal root ganglia of the spinal cord where they ascend to the substantia gelatinosum, cross to the opposite side of the spinal cord, and eventually signal the thalamus. A brief and perhaps oversimplified explanation of pain perception is that the cortex perceives pain as the interpretation of thalamic input.[2] If stimuli travel first to the reticular and limbic systems before entering the thalamus, then the cortex also perceives pain-related emotions.[2]

Stimuli entering the substantia gelatinosum may also return to the injured muscle through neurons exiting the anterior horn of the spinal cord and may cause the muscle to spasm. Thus, the muscle acting as both the initiator and recipient of nociception perpetuates a cycle of pain.

More than 30 years ago, Wall and Melzak proposed a gate-control theory, which postulated a neural gate mechanism to explain the modulation of pain.[3] According to this theory, pain signals are carried from specialized pain receptors to the spinal cord by two types of nerve fibers: (1) small, unmyelinated (type C) fibers and (2) large, myelinated (type A delta) fibers. (See Figure 5–1.) The small fibers conduct impulses slowly and are associated with dull, aching, and lingering pain. The large fibers are linked with immediate pain, which is characterized as sharp and precise with a pricking sensation.

A gating effect on the movement of impulses to the brain occurs when small and large nerve fiber impulses oppose each other. In fact, mild stimulation of large fibers can attenuate pain felt by the activation of small fibers, a finding that helps to explain the efficacy of topical counterirritants. An example is the effect of applying an external analgesic (stimulating large fibers) to diminish the pain caused by a sports-related knee injury (activating small fibers).

Pain perception is highly subjective. Pain may cause nausea, tears, and depression in some people but not in others. Psychologic state and circumstances seem to govern pain perception and responses. During extreme stress, individuals may experience stress-induced analgesia, which enables them to endure major trauma with little pain. This phenomenon has been described as an endogenous response involving induction of hormonal pain relievers and mood elevators. These substances—endorphins and enkephalins—are morphine-like but much more powerful.

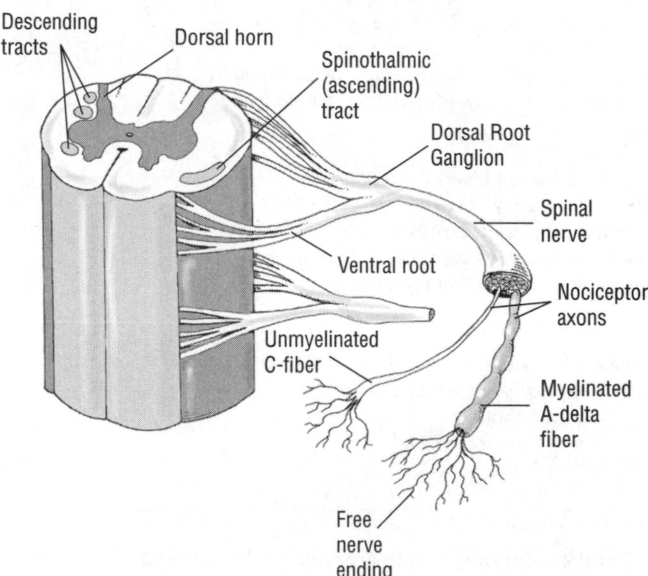

Figure 5–1 Afferent "pain" fiber input into the spinal cord. These specialized sets of afferent units carry pain signals to the spinal cord by either small, unmyelinated fibers (type C fibers) or large, myelin-containing nerve cells (type A delta fibers). Adapted from: *Hosp Formul.* September 1985;20:973; used with permission.

Tendinitis and Bursitis

Epidemiology of Tendinitis and Bursitis

Tendinitis and bursitis are two of the most common musculoskeletal injuries. The tendons of the heel, elbow, shoulder, knee, hand, and wrist are particularly vulnerable to injury. In young athletes, the most common injury is Achilles tendinitis.[4] (See Chapter 36, "Minor Foot Disorders.") Less-common injuries include tennis elbow, epicondylitis (inflammation of tissues adjoining the epicondyle of the humerus), or biceps tendinitis, which occurs in the throwing athlete such as a football quarterback or baseball pitcher; patellar tendinitis, which occurs in the volleyball and basketball player; and iliotibial-band tendinitis, which occurs in the runner.[5] In a prospective study of sports injuries in elderly athletes (those over 60 years of age),[6] the investigators found that shoulder, Achilles tendon, and calf complaints were significantly more common. In addition, although both young and old athletes sustained primarily knee-joint injuries, young athletes suffered this injury more often. Most (70%) of the injuries in the elderly were overuse injuries, but such injuries accounted for less than half (41%) of the injuries in young athletes.[6]

Notably, most cases of bursitis are due to overuse. This situation is particularly true in sports that involve repetitive, overhead throwing motions, such as baseball, swimming, gymnastics, skiing, and weight lifting. Runners commonly are afflicted with bursitis of the knees, hips, ankles, and feet.[7]

Pathophysiology of Tendinitis and Bursitis

Tendinitis, resulting from a strain or injury of tendons, is often seen at times of maximum physical effort, such as during athletic competition. (See Figure 5–2.) Three distinct pathologic phases follow injury.[8] An acute inflammatory response develops at first. As inflammation continues and remains untreated, excessive proliferation of connective tissue occurs. Microscopically, this second phase is characterized by the development of young, vascular elements with fibroblastic growth. In the third phase, persistent and chronic inflammation causes further overgrowth of connective tissue plus tendon degeneration, which may lead to rupture. The pathologic changes occurring in each phase appear to be related primarily to repetitive intrinsic tension overload in the muscle–tendon unit.

Bursae are sacs formed by two layers of synovial tissue that are located at sites of friction between tendon and bone or between skin and bone. The bursae enable the tendons and muscles to move over bony prominences. In bursitis, repetitive trauma from either friction of the overlying tendon or external pressure may cause the bursa to become inflamed, with resultant fluid buildup in the bursal wall. Bursal enlargement occurs by two mechanisms. The first involves an irritation of the endothelial cell lining of the bursal sac, which causes serous fluid to collect and press against the surrounding structures. The second and more probable mechanism, in the case of joint-enveloping bursae, involves irritation, fluid collection in the joint, and subsequent fluid movement into the adjacent bursa through a congenital or acquired vent in the joint.

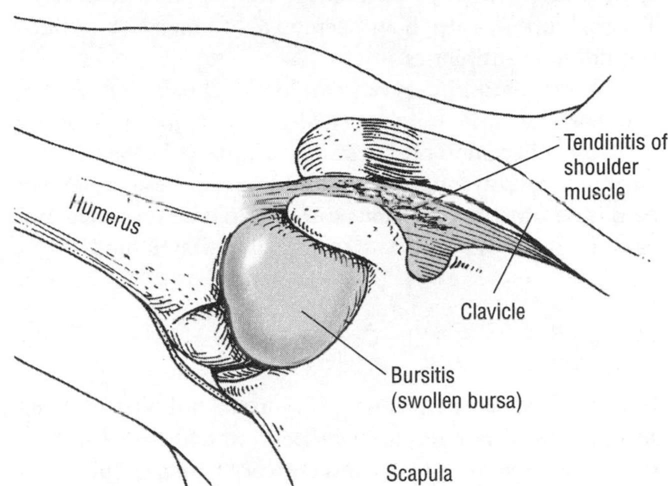

Figure 5–2 Bursitis and tendinitis. These two painful injuries, which often result from overuse of a joint or tendon, can cause inflammation, swelling, and tenderness in the injured area. Adapted from: *US Pharm.* January 1995;20(1); used with permission.

Etiology of Tendinitis and Bursitis

These injuries are caused by equal and opposite reactions, which result in either macrotrauma or microtrauma.[9] Macrotrauma, a sudden catastrophic injury, occurs when an equal and opposite force exceeds the inherent tensile strength of a body structure such as a bone, ligament, muscle, or tendon, thereby causing the structure to collapse. In contrast, microtrauma is a microscopic subclinical injury that results from repeated activity that, over time, overwhelms the tissue's ability to repair itself. By definition, this pain and dysfunction are described as overuse syndrome and are most often encountered in the form of tendinitis.[4] Repetitive microtrauma from exercise-related activities can also break down bursae, cartilage, bone, and nerve.

In industry, factors such as poorly designed equipment, awkward working positions, lack of job variation, long work hours, inadequate rest breaks, and bonuses for high work rates and overtime contribute to overuse injuries.[10] In athletics, contributing factors can include the athletes' age, poor technique and improper conditioning, exercise of prolonged intensity or duration, and poorly designed equipment for specific activities (e.g., poor cushioning of athletic shoes).[9] Tendon ruptures also have been linked to ingestion of fluoroquinolone antibiotics.

Bursitis is a common cause of localized pain, tenderness, and swelling, which is worsened by any movement of the structure adjacent to the bursa. (See Figure 5–2.) Pain caused by either macrotrauma or microtrauma may be acute. When pain is chronic, an infectious cause should be suspected and documented by appropriate studies of aspirated fluid.

Signs and Symptoms of Tendinitis and Bursitis

Inflammation is an indication of injury. Tendinitis and bursitis present with tenderness and pain, which may be accompanied by warmth, edema, and even erythema. Crepitus (an audible grating of the joint) may occur when the synovial sheath is inflamed.[11] The pain of bursitis and tendinitis can be distinguished in that the former appears to be constant while the latter tends to decrease with exercise. Symptoms of bursitis that mimic arthritic pain can be distinguished by a physical examination. For instance, direct pressure over the joint capsule of the shoulder does not cause pain in bursitis although it does in arthritis. (See Chapter 3, "Headache and Muscle and Joint Pain.") Septic bursitis (most frequently preceded by trauma and caused by *Staphylococcus aureus*) presents with fever and acute painful swelling, in much the same way as septic arthritis.

Treatment Overview of Tendinitis and Bursitis

Injury from playing sports or exercising is preventable by warming up and stretching muscles before exertion. Warming and stretching muscles are particularly important steps for preventing reinjury.

RICE (rest, ice, compression, and elevation) therapy applied to the affected area, and nonprescription internal and external analgesics are the recommended self-treatment of tendinitis and bursitis. (See the section "Treatment of Musculoskeletal Injuries and Disorders" for discussion of these therapies.) In addition, Achilles tendinitis can be treated with heel lifts and better-fitting shoes.

The use of fluoroquinolone antibiotics may be contraindicated for some patients. As of October 1994, the Food and Drug Administration (FDA) received reports of 25 fluoroquinolone antibiotic-associated tendon ruptures (22 of them occurring outside the United States).[12] The ruptures occurred 2 days to 6 weeks after the initiation of therapy. Of the 25 patients, 16 had relevant risk factors, including concomitant corticosteroid therapy, advanced age, and chronic renal dialysis. Although almost all fluoroquinolones have been reported to cause tendon rupture, pefloxacin appears to be the most common and ciprofloxacin the least common cause.[13,14] Acting on these reports, the FDA required the labels on all commercially available fluoroquinolones to warn of possible tendon rupture, and it advised that at the first sign of tendon pain or inflammation one should discontinue antibiotic treatment and should refrain from exercise until the diagnosis of tendinitis is excluded.[15]

Strains, Sprains, and Cramps

Sprain and strain are terms used to characterize injury to soft tissue. A sprain is a partial or complete rupture of a ligament, whereas a strain is a partial tear of muscles.[16] A cramp is a painful spasmodic contraction of a muscle.

Epidemiology of Strains, Sprains, and Cramps

Skeletal muscle pain is quite common, especially among persons who are not accustomed to strenuous exercise. Because active lifestyles and enthusiasm for sports and exercise by more Americans of all ages has in recent years produced the so-called "weekend warrior," an increasing number of muscle strains and back pains have been noted. A review indicated that approximately 50% of all sports participants will be injured at one point, and at least half of those injuries will be attributed to overuse.[17]

Strains, sprains, and cramps are very common among all age groups. One study of school-aged children indicated that strains and sprains were 27% of all sports injuries.[18] A prospective study of 766 emergency room subjects indicated that the incidence of ankle and foot sprains was highest among males before age 40 years and highest among females after age 40 years. Most sprains were sports-related, but other activities became the dominant cause in older subjects.[19] Strains and sprains were the most common of all lower-extremity injuries sustained by young men during their army training. Researchers identified older age, smoking, previous injury, and low levels of previous occupational and physical activity as risk factors.[20]

Nocturnal leg cramps occurred in 7.3% of 2527 children surveyed in a recent study. The incidence was noted in children older than 8 years and peaked in children ages 16 to 18 years.[21] In adults, rest cramps were more prevalent in older than in younger adults. The overall prevalence was 37% of the 218 subjects studied.[22]

Pathophysiology of Strains, Sprains, and Cramps

Tendons and ligaments are made up of mostly parallel collagen fibers. These fibers are disrupted by injury and develop adhesions to the surrounding tissues. The loose connective tissue around ligaments and tendons that normally would allow them to move freely then attaches and restricts ligament and tendon movement. If immobilized, certain ligaments lose their elastin and then weaken, thus predisposing them to reinjury.

Sprains are graded I, II, or III. A Grade I sprain is a microscopic injury that causes pain but joint stability remains normal. Grade II sprains are more serious and involve abnormal joint motion. Grade III sprains completely disrupt the ligament.

The tearing of collagen fibers within a muscle defines a strain. A scar forms in muscles (as well as in damaged ligaments and tendons) between the torn ends of the fibers, but this scar usually does not impair the restoration of function.

Etiology of Strains, Sprains, and Cramps

Sprains occur as a result of a joint being forced beyond its normal range of motion (e.g., a hyperextended knee) or forced in a plane through which little or no motion actually exists (e.g., a lateral ankle sprain). The abnormal forces producing the sprain can be rapid, as exemplified by a clipping injury in football, or slow, as observed with a slow, twisting fall in skiing. Although ligaments behave differently, depending on how quickly or slowly they are stretched, either mechanism can induce injury. Most strains, however, occur during forceful muscle action. The injury might occur soon after an activity has begun, such as coming out of the blocks when a race has just started, or with an interruption of some motion, such as momentarily losing one's footing on a slippery surface.[23] When these injuries occur, the muscles become sore and painful, and movement becomes difficult.

Muscle and tendon strain injuries occur in passively elongated or stretched muscle. Eccentric contraction of the muscle while the muscle is lengthening causes the injury.[24] To explain the etiology of the muscle damage and repair, researchers have hypothesized a number of mechanisms that involve disturbances of calcium homeostasis, inflammatory response, and synthesis of stress (heat shock) proteins.[25] No single hypothesis is favored or proven.

Similarly, at least five causes have been hypothesized to explain exercise-induced muscle cramps. Inherited abnormal substrate metabolism, abnormal fluid balance, abnormal serum electrolyte concentrations, extremes of heat or cold, and abnormal spinal reflex activity are among the causes suggested.[26]

Signs and Symptoms of Strains, Sprains, and Cramps

Because pain, swelling, bruising, loss of some function, and gradual stiffening are symptoms common to both of these injuries, strains and sprains may be difficult to distinguish. The extent of swelling may not indicate the extent of damage but rather the time between the injury and the application of ice.

Sprains and their symptoms occur at the joints and, thus, might be distinguished from a strain. In addition, a sprain may loosen a joint, giving it a greater range of motion when it is manipulated. If visibly deformed, a joint is probably ruptured or fractured, and it requires emergency help. Sprains and strains (unlike ruptures and fractures) are likely to allow limited use of the affected limbs.

Case Study 5–1

Patient Complaint/History

For 5 days before coming to the pharmacy, Sergei, an 18-year-old, male, high school athlete, complained of swelling and pain in his left ankle immediately following a track meet. The pain continued for several days.

The physician's examination of the ankle revealed tenderness and warmth over the ankle area; however, no indication of bone, joint, or ligament damage was noted on the x-rays or computerized axial tomography (CAT) scan. The physician instructed Sergei to wrap the injured ankle and to refrain from adding any stress to it.

Except for the ankle injury and a seasonal allergy for which he takes fexofenadine 60 mg bid, Sergei is in good general health.

Clinical Considerations/Strategies

Readers can use the following considerations/strategies to determine whether treatment of the patient's condition with nonprescription medications is warranted:

- Assess the need for nonpharmacologic therapy, including resting the ankle, applying ice, and elevating the ankle.
- Determine whether the patient has other allergies that would contraindicate the use of certain formulations of external analgesics.
- Select the most appropriate analgesic (i.e., external versus internal) and provide instructions for appropriate use.

Patient Education/Counseling

Readers can use the following strategies to develop a patient education/counseling plan that will help ensure optimal therapeutic outcomes:

- Explain the selection and proper use of external analgesics (e.g., indications, warnings/precautions, adverse effects, interaction potential, and administration and dosage guidelines).
- Discuss the concomitant use of bandages when applying external analgesics.
- Identify appropriate nonpharmacologic therapy for the management of sprains and strains.

Muscle cramps or spasms can occur in any skeletal muscle but are most frequently in calf and abdominal muscles. They occur after overexertion, when exercising soon after eating, and after jumping into cold water. Leg cramps frequently occur at night during sleep. Abdominal cramps may be a sign of gastrointestinal difficulties, including food poisoning. Cramps also could be (1) an adverse reaction to diuretic drugs and (2) a symptom of alcoholism, anemia, and arthritis. Also, increased frequency of cramps has been associated with cardiovascular problems.[27]

Treatment Overview of Strains, Sprains, and Cramps

A visibly deformed joint (Grade III sprain) indicates a possible ruptured or fractured joint and requires emergency treatment. Grade II sprains involve abnormal joint movement and should be treated by a physician. RICE therapy, internal analgesics, and external analgesics are self-treatments for Grade I strains and sprains. (See the section "Treatment of Musculoskeletal Injuries and Disorders" for discussion of these therapies.)

For muscle cramps, stretching and massaging the affected area immediately followed by rest or at least reduced activity will loosen the muscle. Stretching must be done cautiously to avoid muscle strain. For persistent cramps, heat should be applied to the area in the form of a warm wet compress, heating pad, or hot-water bottle. Warming up and stretching, drinking sufficient fluids, and not exercising to the point of exhaustion may prevent cramps. In addition, raising the foot of the bed may prevent nocturnal leg cramps.

Repetitive Strain Injury

Repetitive motion, stress, or stretching can lead to repetitive stain or to overuse injuries. Hence, repetitive strain injury is also called cumulative trauma disorder, regional pain syndrome, and overuse syndrome. Parts of the body that are forced to assume an awkward posture or to move in a repetitive manner (shoulder, hip, elbow, hand, and wrist) are particularly susceptible to such injuries.

Epidemiology of Repetitive Strain Injury

This type of injury occurs primarily in the workplace and has been described as the new industrial epidemic.[28] Although assembly line workers and typists are particularly prone, anyone who performs a repetitive physical task can develop this type of strain injury.[29] A recent warning indicated that filling 100 prescriptions a day qualifies as repetitive motion and that pharmacists and others who work at computer keyboards are at risk for developing muscle and tendon injuries.[30] However, a recent investigation has advocated that a thorough systematic search for concurrent medical diseases be performed before the injury is identified definitively as work related.[31] The diagnosis and treatment of underlying diseases, including diabetes, hypothyroidism, and inflammatory conditions, such as rheumatoid arthritis, can lead to improvement of symptoms in many instances.

Perhaps the most-common repetitive strain injury is called carpal tunnel syndrome. Repetitive motion disorders account for more than 50% of all work-related disorders, and 41% of work-related disorders are carpal tunnel syndrome. According to a 1998 British study,[32] between 7% and 16% of the population experience this problem and the incidence appears to be increasing. People ages 54 years and older are at higher risk than are younger adults. Even though the publicity about carpal tunnel syndrome has centered on people who use computer keyboards, an analysis of two national data sets of occupational illnesses identifies dentists, dental hygienists, butchers, and sewing machine operators as occupations with great risk for carpal tunnel syndrome.[33] Meat, poultry, and fish packers, assembly line workers, cake decorators, postal workers, and persons who assemble airplanes are also at high risk for carpal tunnel syndrome. In addition, leisure activities, such as computer games, sports, and card playing, may contribute to the risk.[34]

Pathophysiology of Repetitive Strain Injury

Repetitive stress injuries lead to inflammation that causes tissues to swell around nerves. Compression of nerves by swollen tissues (such as tendons and ligaments) slows the movement of signals through nerves, which then is perceived as pain, numbness, and tingling.

Etiology of Repetitive Strain Injury

The etiology of repetitive strain injury is often, but not always, related to work conditions. Other contributing factors include bone dislocations and fractures; certain medical conditions such as rheumatoid arthritis, diabetes, and hypothyroidism; long-term hemodialysis and diseases such as multiple myeloma (a tumor of bone marrow); Waldenström macroglobinemia (an increase in macroglobulins in the blood); and non-Hodgkin's lymphoma. These factors cause amyloid (a waxy starchlike protein) to build up in bone and joint tissues. Pregnancy (fluid retention) and menopause (hormonal changes) can cause swelling and thereby the symptoms of carpal tunnel syndrome.

It is of interest that in 1993, a British court ruled that repetitive strain injury does not exist as a separate medical condition. Rather than referring to this disorder as an injury, the court described it as a pain syndrome occurring in the workplace. However, the association of that pain with a specific type of work has yet to be clearly defined and has led to a strongly worded editorial advising employers and employees to pay attention to workplace factors (e.g., stress and appropriate work breaks) in order to reduce the incidence of this syndrome.[35] In the United States, although repetitive strain injury claims have been touted as the "asbestos of the

1990s," litigation against major corporations such as IBM has been stalled by a vigorous defense involving the work ethic of both employer and employee rather than the equipment.[36]

To help clarify this controversy, two British researchers[37] found that patients and office workers whose jobs involved intensive use of the computer keyboard sustained damage to sensory nerves supplying the hand. This study is the first to show a quantitative sensory deficit in patients with occupational repetition strain injuries. The authors express hope that the test used to monitor its development can lead to early detection of those at risk and can decrease the occurrence of this condition.

Signs and Symptoms of Repetitive Strain Injury

Repetitive strain injuries have all the features of sympathetically maintained pain: impairment of function, allodynia (pain induced by ordinarily nonpainful stimuli such as a cold breeze), paresthesia (an abnormal sensation such as tingling), numbness, and hyperesthesia (abnormal acuteness of sensitivity to touch or other sensory stimulus) throughout the entire extremity. Autonomic disturbances such as Raynaud's phenomenon may be present. (Raynaud's phenomenon is characterized by episodic aching or burning associated with artery constriction in the extremities and is related to nerve injury, occupational trauma, and other systemic and vascular diseases.) Symptoms usually progress over weeks and months and, in some cases, years. In addition to pain, numbness, or tingling, patients with carpal tunnel syndrome may experience a sense of heat or cold, a sense their hands are swollen when they are not, a weakness, and a tendency to drop things. Symptoms persist during sleep and even when the hand is not being used, which is a characteristic of this disorder that can be used to distinguish it from similar disorders.

Treatment Overview of Repetitive Strain Injury

Physicians recommend preventing repetitive strain by exercising the muscles vulnerable to injury. The other major preventive measure is to use ergonomic controls that reduce risk of predisposing factors. (Ergonomics is the control of posture, stresses, motions, and other physical factors that can injure the human body engaged in work or play.)

The mainstay of conservative treatment is RICE—with emphasis placed on resting the affected area. This treatment includes the use of splints or braces (if appropriate). Nonprescription nonsteroidal anti-inflammatory drugs (NSAIDs) and external analgesics may help reduce pain and swelling. (See the section "Treatment of Musculoskeletal Injuries and Disorders" for discussion of these therapies.) An exercise program administered by an occupational therapist can be helpful. However, if pain persists, a doctor may inject an anesthetic or corticosteroid (to shrink swollen tissues). A discussion of other alternative treatments is beyond the scope of this chapter, but invasive options are available.

Lower Back Pain

Just as the prehensile grasp has imposed a stress on the shoulder girdles of humans, so has erect posture predisposed the lower spine to the painful twinge of an aching back.

Epidemiology of Lower Back Pain

At least 70% of people experience lower back pain at some time in their lives. Lower back pain rivals the common cold as the leading cause of absenteeism from work,[38] and is the leading cause of disability among workers younger than 45 years.[39]

Pathophysiology of Lower Back Pain

The pathophysiology of lower back pain may be related to temporary impingement of nerve roots by swollen lower back muscles and ligaments. The impingement may sensitize nerves to transmit pain sensations.

Etiology of Lower Back Pain

Unlike the overuse injuries described previously, this regional musculoskeletal disorder is due primarily to a sedentary lifestyle (particularly one disrupted by bursts of activity), as well as to poor posture, improper shoes, excess body weight, poor mattresses and sleeping posture, and improper technique in lifting heavy objects. Thus, back pain is primarily a disease of living. Although most victims recover within a few days to a few weeks with conservative treatment, lower back pain is significantly likely to recur if the initial episode of pain is severe; advancing age increases the risk of recurrence.

Of all lower back pain causes, 30% to 90% is postural secondary to primary or secondary injury of supporting muscles and ligaments. Other causes include (1) congenital anomalies; (2) osteoarthritis; (3) spinal tuberculosis; and (4) referred pain from diseased kidneys, pancreas, liver, or prostate.

Emotional factors, including tension, anxiety, repressed anger, and other manifestations of "psychosocial prestress," have been postulated to correlate with the occurrence of lower back pain, but a comprehensive review of the literature could not confirm a relationship between lower back pain and temperament.[40]

Signs and Symptoms of Lower Back Pain

The principal symptom is pain (soreness) or tightness in the lower back. The pain impairs movement to the extent that the patient may not be able to bend, move, sit, or walk.

Treatment Overview of Lower Back Pain

Self-treatment is limited to acute lower back pain. Chronic pain (i.e., lasting more than 6 or 7 weeks) requires medical evaluation and treatment. The mainstay of treatment is RICE, nonprescription NSAIDs, and nonprescription external analgesics. (See the section "Treatment of Musculoskeletal Injuries and Disorders" for discussion of these therapies.) Other therapeutic interventions include alternating heat with cold; massage with traction (contraindicated for people with osteoporosis, tumor, pregnancy, or spine infection); and mobilization (a program of techniques and exercises to restore back mechanics and movement).

Arthritis

Rheumatoid arthritis, suppurative arthritis, gouty arthritis, Lyme arthritis, and osteoarthritis all cause arthritic pain, but only the pain of osteoarthritis may be self-treated after an initial diagnosis by a physician.

Epidemiology of Arthritis

Osteoarthritis is a "wear and tear" disease seen primarily in older individuals. By the year 2005, there will be 14 million more people between the ages of 40 and 54 years than there were in 1995. Indeed, in the next 5 years, an average of 12,000 people per day will reach the age of 50 years, and many will require external analgesics to alleviate the pain of arthritis.[41]

Approximately 40 million Americans currently suffer from all forms of arthritis, and the Centers for Disease Control and Prevention (CDC) expects that number to increase by 50% by the year 2020. In fact, 40% of adults ages 50 years and older regularly use external pain relievers, and arthritis patients account for more than 75% of total usage.

Most people ages 65 years and older have radiologically detectable osteoarthritis even if they are symptom free. The total number of people who have osteoarthritis is about 20 million and that number is increasing.[42]

Pathophysiology of Arthritis

Endogenous neuropeptides have been implicated in the pathogenesis of both rheumatoid arthritis and osteoarthritis.[43] Both substance P and interleukin-1 β (present in inflamed joints) enhance cartilage destruction by stimulating collagenase activity.[44] In experimental studies in animals, the degree of joint inflammation in rheumatoid arthritis correlates directly with release of the neurotransmitter substance P by specific joints. In addition, substance P activates rheumatoid synovial cells to produce prostaglandins and metalloproteinases.[45]

Etiology of Arthritis

Osteoarthritis is also known as degenerative joint disease because its main feature is deteriorating joint cartilage. In time, the cartilage loses proteoglycan and chondrocytes and becomes pitted. To compensate for this erosion, the underlying bone scleroses (hardens) and forms spurs. The disease is caused by genetic, metabolic, dietary, and hormonal factors. Physical activity, repetitive movement, and lifting heavy weights may aggravate this condition.

Signs and Symptoms of Arthritis

Osteoarthritis is marked by pain, swelling, occasional redness, warmth, tenderness, and stiffness in a joint not unlike the symptoms of a ligament or tendon injury. The symptoms are so much like those of the previously discussed injuries that a differential diagnosis to sort out other medical conditions is required before attempting self-treatment. Rheumatoid arthritis is a systemic disease that results in symmetrical joint inflammation along with constitutional symptoms such as depression and fatigue.

Acute, temporary stiffness and muscle pain can also result from cold, dampness, rapid temperature changes, and air currents. In some cases, visceral stimuli resulting from cardiovascular disease (e.g., angina pectoris) or gastrointestinal complaints (e.g., disorders of the gallbladder and esophagus) are felt as referred pain in the skeletal muscles of the shoulder. These episodes tend to be sudden in onset but are self-limiting (i.e., the condition will resolve with or without treatment in a short time). Elimination of the cause or symptomatic treatment generally provides relief.[2]

Treatment Overview of Arthritis

Although both types of rheumatic disorders are chronic systemic diseases, local treatment of painful joints coupled with rest may give temporary symptomatic relief. If the condition is minor, physician diagnosed, and uncomplicated by serious underlying problems, nonprescription internal or external analgesics may be appropriate. (See the section "Treatment of Musculoskeletal Injuries and Disorders" below.)

However, if the preparation does not relieve the symptoms within 7 days, or if the symptoms clear up and then return within a few days,[46] the medication should be discontinued and a physician should be consulted. Rheumatoid arthritis may require treatment with prescription antirheumatic drugs. Other modalities for long-term care include heat or cold application, splinting to provide support, and range-of-motion and strength maintenance exercises—but not during periods of inflammation.

Treatment of Musculoskeletal Injuries and Disorders

Treatment Outcomes

The goals of self-treating musculoskeletal injuries are to (1) relieve symptoms, especially pain and swelling, (2) restore function of the affected area, and (3) prevent further injury.

Additional treatment goals for arthritis are to maintain or increase joint motion and reduce stiffness.

General Treatment Approach

Patients with musculoskeletal injuries or disorders present with similar symptoms, especially pain and swelling of the affected area.

Tendon, muscle, and ligament injuries and bursitis are all treated in the same general fashion. Rehabilitation is divided into four overlapping phases.[47] In Phase I, patients use the RICE protocol and nonprescription internal or external analgesics to reduce inflammation, swelling, and pain. Ice is replaced by heat after 24 to 48 hours. For minor or moderate injuries, this phase lasts 1 to 2 weeks. In Phase II, patients work on restoring and maintaining normal range of motion. Superficial or deep heat is used to facilitate restoration of flexibility. In Phase III, patients do exercises to strengthen the affected area. To prevent reinjury, patients must gradually be reintroduced to the physical activity that caused the injury (Phase IV).

The algorithm in Figure 5–3 presents a stepwise approach to the management of pain associated with these complaints. Exclusions to self-care include nausea or severe vomiting; weakness in any limb; pain in a red, hot, or swollen joint (with or without fever); suspected fracture; any increase in pain intensity or character; and pain lasting longer than 2 weeks except in minor cases of diagnosed arthritis.

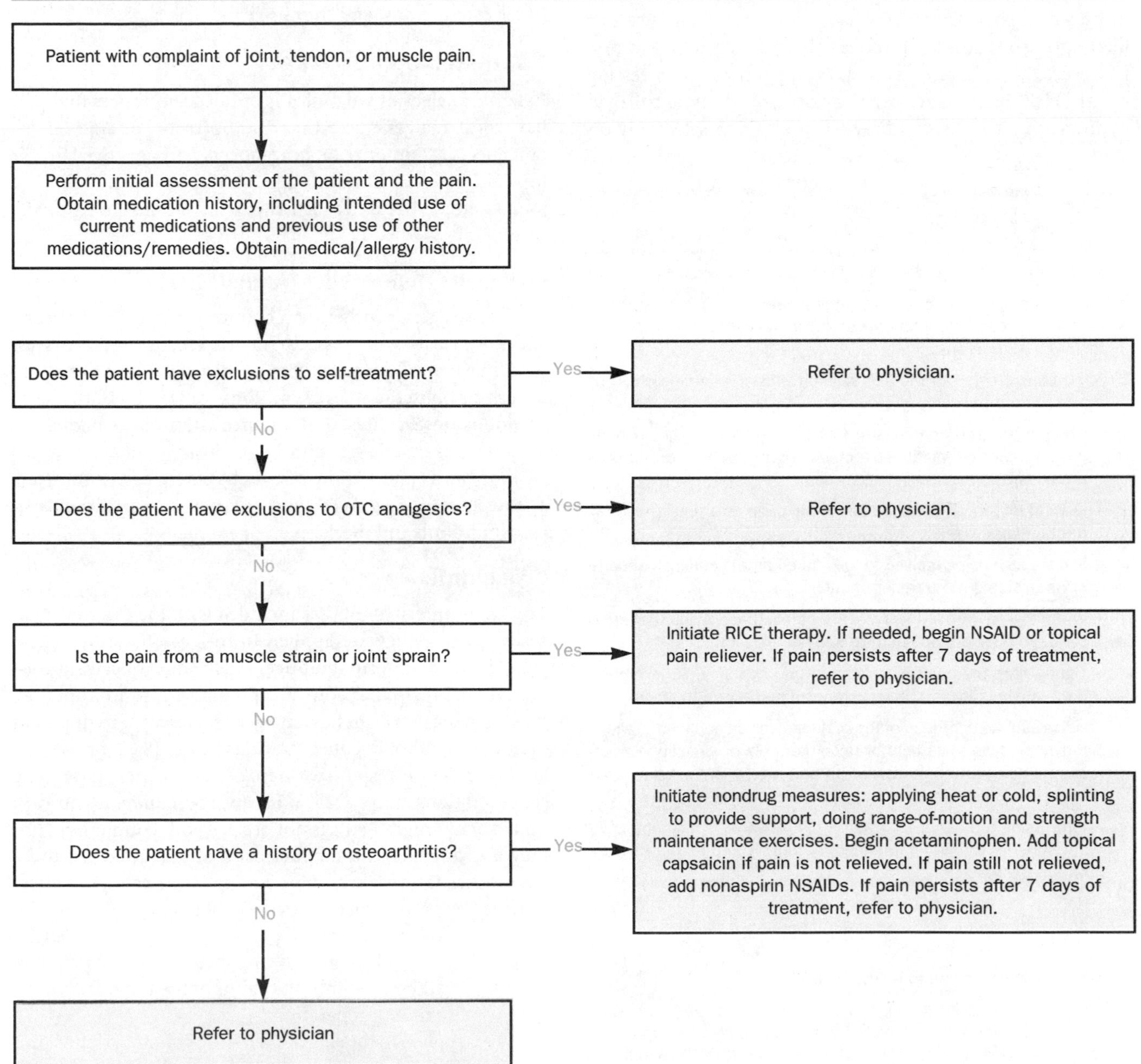

Figure 5-3 Self-care of musculoskeletal injuries and disorders.

Nonpharmacologic Therapy

The acronym RICE signifies the basic steps of nonpharmacologic therapy for strains, sprains, ruptures, repetitive stress, and other injuries. If the patient's pain is secondary to a muscle strain or joint sprain, RICE is the initial treatment of choice. Table 5–1 describes the steps in this therapy. As a general rule, heat treatment should not be used for at least 24 hours after an injury occurs. If swelling remains, heat is contraindicated in most cases because it may produce erythema by increasing blood flow to the area.

Although the nonprescription preparations described in this chapter have their own merit as therapeutic agents, simple physical methods of inducing counterirritation are available. Perhaps the most frequently used method is heat applied by means of a heat lamp, hot-water bottle, heating pad, or moist steam pack. Under normal conditions, collagen recoils like a spring once the load is released. After a stretching injury, however, the collagen tissue does not return to its resting length. Heat helps to restore the elastic property of collagen by increasing the viscous flow. Heat also acts selectively on free nerve endings in the tissue and on peripheral nerve fibers to increase the pain threshold. This action results in an analgesic effect.[48] However, heat should be applied with extreme caution, if at all, in conjunction with a counterirritant preparation. Severe burning or blistering of skin, muscle and skin necrosis, and interstitial nephritis have resulted from the simultaneous use of a counterirritant preparation and heat.[49]

Massaging the painful area is another method of producing counterirritation. The therapeutic benefits of massage have been known for centuries. The beneficial effects of some counterirritants used in treating musculoskeletal disorders may be largely the result of the massaging involved when applying the medication. Massage increases the flow of blood and lymph in the skin and underlying structures. Many clinicians have found that massage is therapeutically beneficial in select situations, and they use it extensively.

Table 5–1

Guidelines for RICE Therapy

- Rest the injured area, using slings or splints if necessary.
- Apply ice as soon as possible to the injured area in 20-minute increments, three to four times a day. Continue the ice-pack therapy for 24 to 48 hours.
- Apply compression to the injured area with an elastic support or an elasticized bandage as follows:
  - —Choose the appropriate size of bandage for the injured body part. If preferred, purchase a product designed for the appropriate body part.
  - —Unwind about 12 to 18 inches of bandage at a time and allow the bandage to relax.
  - —If ice is also being applied to the injured area, soak the bandage in water to aid the transfer of cold.
  - —Wrap the injured area by overlapping the previous layer of bandage by about one-third to one-half its width.
  - —Tightly wrap the point most distal from the injury. For example, if the ankle is injured, begin wrapping just above the toes.
  - —Decrease the tightness of the bandage as you continue to wrap. If the bandage feels tight or uncomfortable or circulation is impaired, remove the compression bandage and rewrap it. Cold toes or swollen fingers would indicate a bandage is too tight.
  - —After using the bandage, wash it in lukewarm, soapy water; do not scrub it. Rinse the bandage thoroughly and allow to air dry on a flat surface.
  - —Roll up the bandage to prevent wrinkles and store it in a cool, dry place. Do not iron the bandage to remove wrinkles.
- Elevate the injured area at or above the level of the heart to decrease swelling and to relieve pain.
- Do not apply heat to the injured area for at least 24 hours after the injury occurred. If swelling is not present, apply heat (warm wet compress, heating pad, or hot-water bottle) at 20- to 30-minute intervals every 2 to 4 hours.

Pharmacologic Therapy

External analgesics are topically applied substances that may have local analgesic, anesthetic, antipruritic, or counterirritant effects. Counterirritants are specifically approved for the topical treatment of minor aches and pains of muscles and joints (simple backache, arthritis pain, strains, bruises, and sprains).[50]

Analgesics/Anesthetics/Antipruritics

Topical analgesics (other than counterirritants), anesthetics, and antipruritics depress cutaneous sensory receptors for pain, burning, and itching; they act directly on the skin to diminish or obliterate these symptoms caused by burns, cuts, abrasions, insect bites, and cutaneous lesions. Chapter 31, "Insect Bites and Stings and Pediculosis," and Chapter 34, "Minor Burns and Sunburn," discuss these agents in detail. This section focuses on counterirritants because of their specific indication and mechanism of action.

Counterirritants

Topical counterirritants are included with the external analgesics because they are applied to the intact skin to relieve pain. Some counterirritant agents (in low concentrations) actually depress cutaneous receptor response in a manner similar to local anesthetics, analgesics, and antipruritics. For example, menthol in concentrations below 1% depresses cutaneous receptor response, whereas it stimulates response in concentrations above 1.25%. Because percutaneous absorption of active ingredients is not desired with counterirritants, they are considered a distinct class of analgesic products. Counterirritation is the paradoxical pain-relieving effect achieved by producing less-severe pain to counter a more intense one. To counter pain of pathologic origin, pain sufferers produce bearable pain by biting their lips, clenching their fists, digging their nails into the palms of their hands,[51] or using counterirritant preparations.

When applied to the skin at pain sites, counterirritants produce a mild, local, inflammatory reaction, which provides relief at another site that is usually adjacent to, or underlying, the skin surface being treated. Counterirritants relieve pain indirectly by stimulating rather than suppressing sensations of cold, warmth, and sometimes itching.[46] These induced sensations distract from the deep-seated pain in muscles, joints, and tendons. Pain is only as intense as it is perceived to be, and the perception of other sensations caused by the counterirritant or its application (e.g., massage, warmth, or redness) causes the sufferer to disregard the sensation of pain. The intensity of response depends on the irritant used, its concentration, the solvent in which it is dissolved, and the duration of its contact with the skin.[51] One theory of the mechanism of counterirritation proposes that stimulation of sensory nerve endings in the skin causes reflexive stimulation of vasomotor fibers to the viscera, thereby dilating the visceral vasculature and producing the sensation of warmth.[52]

A second theory proposes that stimulation of sensory nerve endings in the skin may have a reflex effect on axons, resulting in peripheral vasodilation. The vasodilation increases blood flow to the muscles by changing the thermal gradient that extends from the skin to the deeper structures.[53] A third theory proposes that summation of pain stimuli produces intense stimulation of the areas of pain interpretation of the brain, partly abating visceral pain stimuli. According to this theory, stimuli originating in the viscera or muscles are transmitted, along with sensations from the skin, over fibers in a common pathway and are referred to the same area of the spinal cord as the stimuli from the skin. (See Figure 5–1.) If the intensity of the stimulation from the skin is increased by a drug's irritant action, the character of the visceral or muscle pain is modified. With intense skin stimulation, the referred pain stimuli may be partly or completely obliterated insofar as the sensorium is concerned. The patient's attention is diverted from the muscular or visceral structure by the application of the counterirritant drug.[54]

Some counterirritants also cause vasodilation of cutaneous vasculature. These drugs, known as rubefacients, produce reactive hyperemia; it is hypothesized that this increase in blood pooling and/or flow is accompanied by an increase in localized skin temperature, which then may exercise a counterirritant effect. Thermography has documented this positive thermal response for some agents.[55] An increase in skin temperature and underlying muscle temperature has also been observed after topical applications of a commercially available preparation containing menthol and eucalyptus oil.[56] Table 5–2 groups counterirritants according to their specific mechanism of action.

Undoubtedly, the action of counterirritants in relieving pain has a psychologic component. Indeed, these agents may exert a placebo effect through pleasant odors or by the sensation of warmth or coolness they produce on the skin.

By whatever means it is produced, the degree of irritation must be controlled because strong irritation may cause allergic reactions (erythema and blistering). No evidence exists that the risk of adverse reactions to counterirritants increases when the application site is lightly bandaged. However, an increased risk of irritation, redness, or blistering does exist with tight bandaging or occlusive dressing.[46] Heating pads used in conjunction with counterirritants containing methyl salicylate have produced the elevated temperature, vasodilation, and occlusion necessary to greatly enhance percutaneous absorption of menthol and methyl salicylate, causing full-thickness skin and muscle necrosis as well as persistent interstitial nephritis.[49] In addition, heat exposure and exercise after applying methyl salicylate have shown a threefold increase in systematic availability of salicylate; this resultant increase in absorption of topically applied preparations could lead to adverse systemic reactions.[57] Therefore, patients should be told not to use heating pads or other heating devices

Table 5–2

Classification and Dosage Guidelines[a] for Nonprescription Counterirritant External Analgesics

Group	Mechanism of Action	Ingredients	Dosage/ Concentration (%)	Frequency/Duration of Use
A	Induce redness and irritation; are more potent than other commonly used counterirritants	Allyl isothiocyanate	0.5–5.0	For all counterirritants: Apply no more often than 3–4 times/day for up to 7 days
		Ammonia water	1.0–2.5	
		Methyl salicylate	10–60	
		Turpentine oil	6–50	
B	Produce cooling sensation; have strong organoleptic properties	Camphor	3–11	
		Menthol	1.25–16	
C	Cause vasodilation	Histamine dihydrochloride	0.025–0.1	
		Methyl nicotinate	0.25–1.0	
D	Incite irritation without rubefaction; are equal in potency to Group A ingredients	Capsicum	0.025–0.25	
		Capsicum oleoresin	0.025–0.25	
		Capsaicin	0.025–0.25	

[a] Dosages approved for adults and children ages 2 years and older.

Adapted from: *Federal Register*. 1979;44:69874.

in conjunction with any external analgesic and not to apply such products after strenuous exercise, especially during hot and humid weather. Rather, these products should be applied after the body has cooled down.

On the basis of topical effects, four types of counterirritants exist. (See Table 5–2.) Allyl isothiocyanate, ammonia water, methyl salicylate, and turpentine oil are rubefacients (cause redness). Camphor and menthol have a cooling effect. Histamine and methyl nicotinate cause vasodilation. Capsicum and capsaicin irritate without causing redness.[46] (See Table 5–3 for examples of commercially available products.)

These ingredients have been recognized as safe and effective (Category I) counterirritants for use in adults and in children ages 2 years or older by the FDA's Advisory Review Panel on Over-the-Counter (OTC) Topical Analgesic, Antirheumatic, Otic, Burn, and Sunburn Prevention and Treatment Drug

Table 5–3

Selected External Analgesic Products

Trade Name	Primary Ingredients
Menthol-Containing Products	
Absorbine Jr. Liquid	Menthol 1.27%
Absorbine Jr. Extra Strength Liquid/Absorbine Jr. Power Gel	Menthol 4%
BenGay Spa Cream	Menthol 10%
Flexall 454 Maximum Strength Gel	Menthol 16%
Therapeutic Mineral Ice Gel	Menthol 2%
Therapeutic Mineral Ice Exercise Formula Gel	Menthol 4%
Capsaicin-Containing Products	
Capzasin-HP Lotion/Cream	Capsaicin 0.075%
Capzasin-P Lotion/Cream	Capsaicin 0.025%
Icy Hot Arthritis Therapy Gel	Capsaicin 0.025%
Zostrix Cream	Capsaicin 0.025%
Zostrix Sports/Zostrix-HP Cream	Capsaicin 0.075%
Trolamine Salicylate–Containing Products	
Aspercreme Cream/Lotion	Trolamine salicylate 10%
Aspergel	Trolamine salicylate 10%
Myoflex Cream	Trolamine salicylate 10%
Sportscreme Cream/Lotion	Trolamine salicylate 10%
Combination Products	
Absorbine Arthritis Strength Liquid	Menthol 4%; capsaicin 0.025% (from capsicum oleoresin)
ArthriCare Pain Relieving Rub Cream	Menthol 1.25%; methyl nicotinate 0.25%; capsicum oleoresin 0.025%
ArthriCare Ultra Gel	Menthol 2%; capsaicin 0.075%
Arthritis Hot Cream	Methyl salicylate 15%; menthol 10%
BenGay Original Formula Pain Relieving Ointment	Methyl salicylate 18.3%; menthol 16%
BenGay Ultra Strength Pain Relieving Cream	Methyl salicylate 30%; menthol 10%; camphor 4%
Flexall Ultra Plus Gel	Menthol 16%; methyl salicylate 10%; camphor 3.1%
Icy Hot Chill Stick	Methyl salicylate 30%; menthol 10%
Menthacin Cream/Menthacin EZ Lotion	Menthol 4%; capsaicin 0.025%
Mentholatum Ointment	Camphor 9%; natural menthol 1.3%
Mentholatum Deep Heating Lotion	Methyl salicylate 20%; menthol 6%
Mentholatum Deep Heating Arthritis Formula Cream	Methyl salicylate 30%; menthol 8%
Minit-Rub Cream	Methyl salicylate 15%; menthol 3.5%; camphor 2.3%
Sloan's Liniment	Turpentine oil 47%; capsaicin 0.025% (from capsicum oleoresin)
Soltice Quick Rub Cream	Camphor 5.1%; menthol 5.1%
Vicks VapoRub Ointment	Camphor 4.8%; menthol 2.6%; eucalyptus oil 1.2%

Products. According to the FDA's proposed ruling on external analgesic products, issued in February 1983, "Although it is true that by 6 months of age a child's skin is similar to an adult's with regard to any absorption, there are enough other differences between adults and children under 2 years of age to require different standards of practice in the use of drugs."[46]

Allyl Isothiocyanate

Allyl isothiocyanate, also known as volatile oil of mustard and essence of mustard, is derived from powdered seeds of the black mustard plant and other species of mustard. It can also be prepared synthetically or by distillation after expression of the fixed oil. Depending on the variety of mustard, the yield of allyl isothiocyanate is approximately 1%.

Dosage/Administration Guidelines See Table 5–2 for dosing information.

Adverse Effects In high concentrations, allyl isothiocyanate is absorbed rapidly from intact skin as well as from all mucous membranes. Because penetration into the skin is rapid, ulceration may occur if the agent is not removed soon after application. A poultice, erroneously termed a *mustard plaster*, has often been used as a home remedy. It is prepared by mixing equal parts of powdered mustard and flour and moistening with water to form a paste. The paste is then spread on a towel or piece of material and placed on the affected area. The person who is preparing a mustard plaster should take care to avoid inhaling this powerful irritant; allyl isothiocyanate is one of the most toxic essential oils and should never be tasted or inhaled undiluted.[58] The continuous release of allyl isothiocyanate by the presence of water and body heat may cause the inflammatory action to go beyond redness to blistering; therefore, the poultice should not remain on the skin for more than a few minutes.

Contraindications/Precautions/Warnings The preceding drugs are not for internal use and are not to be applied to damaged or abraded skin or to eyes. Patients with sensitive skin should discontinue use if blistering occurs.

Ammonia Water (or Ammonia Liniment)

Ammonia solution is made by diluting strong ammonia solution with water (27% to 30% by weight of ammonia). This agent, also known as stronger ammonium hydroxide solution or Spirit of Hartshorn, is seldom found in nonprescription external analgesics.

Dosage/Administration Guidelines See Table 5–2 for dosing information.

Adverse Effects Because ammonia is caustic and the vapors are irritating, this product should be handled with care and the vapors should not be inhaled. Inhalation of ammonia vapor causes sneezing and coughing and, in high concentration, can cause pulmonary edema. Asphyxia has been reported following edema or spasm of the glottis. In addition, ammonia vapor is an eye irritant and can cause weeping, conjunctival swelling, and temporary blindness.[59]

Methyl Salicylate

Methyl salicylate occurs naturally as wintergreen oil or sweet birch oil; gaultheria oil and teaberry oil are other names for the natural compound. In some areas of the United States, it is still referred to as "mountain tea."[60] Synthetic methyl salicylate is prepared by the esterification of salicylic acid with methyl alcohol. In either form, methyl salicylate is the most widely used counterirritant.

Mechanism of Action The exact mechanism by which salicylates produce their analgesic effect is not known, but it is generally accepted that they act in part centrally and in part peripherally as anti-inflammatory agents that inhibit prostaglandins.

Pharmacokinetics Studies on the rate and extent of percutaneous absorption of various commercially available methyl salicylate preparations show direct tissue penetration rather than redistribution by the systemic blood supply.[61] One bioavailability study[62] showed that only about 12% to 20% of the amount of salicylate applied to the skin and covered with an occlusive bandage was absorbed systemically after 10 hours. Another more recent study[63] demonstrated an increase in the rate and extent of absorption after multiple applications. Bioavailability increased from 15% after the first two doses to 22% after 4 days of treatment. Furthermore, both the skin permeability coefficient for methyl salicylate and the percentage of salicylate absorbed decreased when the agents were applied to different areas of the body in this order: abdomen, forearm, instep, heel, and plantar.[62] The slower absorption from the foot regions was primarily attributed to fewer hair follicles and a thicker stratum corneum. The authors concluded that topical application of products containing methyl salicylate results in low plasma salicylate concentrations and that the usefulness of these preparations is limited to their local effects.

Dosage/Administration Guidelines See Table 5–2 for dosing information.

Overdosage At very low concentrations (0.04%), methyl salicylate is used in oral preparations for its pleasant flavor and aroma. Although the average lethal oral dose of methyl salicylate is estimated to be 10 mL for children and 30 mL for adults,[64] as little as 4 mL has caused death in infants and 5 mL has caused death in children.[65] Thus, although a survey by the FDA's advisory review panel considering methyl salicylate found that oral ingestion of this ingredient from products formulated as ointments caused no deaths and that few cases manifested severe symptoms,[50] regulations require the use of child-resistant containers for liquid preparations containing more than 5% methyl salicylate.[66] Severe, rapid onset of salicylate poisoning has been reported in a suicide attempt involving ingestion of Chinese herbal medicines.[67] (See the section "Alternative Remedies.")

Drug–Drug Interactions Concomitant use of salicylate-containing external analgesics and maintenance warfarin therapy has been implicated in prolonging prothrombin time.[68] Both methyl salicylate and trolamine salicylate were implicated. A later study showed that 11 patients had an abnormally elevated international normalized ratio after significant usage of topical methyl salicylate ointment.[69] Chapter 3, "Headache and Muscle and Joint Pain," describes other potential drug interactions for salicylates.

Contraindications/Precautions/Warnings Because percutaneous absorption can occur, this product should be used with caution in individuals who are sensitive to aspirin or who suffer from severe asthma or nasal polyps, conditions associated with aspirin sensitivity.

Turpentine Oil

Turpentine oil is commonly misnamed "turpentine." The oil used for medicinal purposes must be of higher quality than that used commercially. Medicinal turpentine oil, known as spirits of turpentine or rectified turpentine oil, is prepared by steam distillation of turpentine oleoresin collected from various species of pine trees.

Dosage/Administration Guidelines See Table 5–2 for dosing information.

Overdosage Several human fatalities from the ingestion of turpentine oil have been reported. An oral dose of 140 mL in adults (15 mL in children) may be fatal.

Adverse Effects Applying turpentine to skin may cause irritation, and large amounts of turpentine passing through the skin may cause excitement, coma, fever, tachycardia (rapid heart rate), liver damage, hematuria (presence of blood in the urine), and albuminuria (presence of serum albumin or globulin in the urine).

Turpentine oil is both a primary irritant and a sensitizer. As an irritant, it usually acts by defatting the skin, causing dryness and fissuring. It is often used as a cleanser for removing paints and waxes, and it can cause hand eczema by irritating sensitive skin. Application of turpentine liniments to the skin in greater amounts than recommended may cause local burning and irritation, gastrointestinal upset, and respiratory symptoms in susceptible individuals.[70] Cutaneous application of large enough amounts of turpentine has been associated with vesicular eruptions, urticaria, and vomiting. This remedy is used to relieve "seed ticks" among adults in rural Mississippi, and the CDC recommended that "health-care providers should be aware of potential drug interactions, toxicity, and adverse reactions as well as possible treatment benefits that may be associated with plant-derived therapies."[71]

Contraindications/Precautions/Warnings Use of turpentine is contraindicated in people with a known hypersensitivity to the agent.

Menthol

Menthol is either extracted from peppermint oil (which contains 30% to 50% concentration of menthol) or prepared synthetically. Menthol may be used safely in small quantities as a flavoring agent and has found wide acceptance in candy, chewing gum, cigarettes, cough drops, toothpaste, nasal sprays, and liqueurs. Menthol is usually combined with other ingredients with antipruritic or analgesic properties, such as camphor.[46] To facilitate applying the active agent, a soft, flexible pad containing a layer of menthol in a gel formulation was introduced in 1994.

Mechanism of Action When used in concentrations of 1.25% to 16%, menthol acts as a counterirritant: Applied to the skin, menthol stimulates the nerves that perceive cold while depressing the nerves that perceive pain. The initial feeling of coolness is soon followed by a sensation of warmth. An experimental study demonstrated that exposure to 2% menthol solution caused the threshold for warmth to rise significantly, whereas the threshold for heat pain remained unchanged.[72] Although masking sensations of warmth with menthol-induced sensations of cold may explain these results, the author considers that a direct inhibition or desensitization of the warmth receptors is more likely. Menthol may exert its action on the perception of cold and warmth by influencing calcium movement in thermoreceptors.[73] A published review summarizes the pharmacology, mechanism of action, therapeutic use, and toxicology of this naturally occurring substance.[74]

Dosage/Administration Guidelines See Table 5–2 for dosing information.

Overdosage The fatal dose of menthol in humans is approximately 2 g.[75] However, this amount may be an underestimate because, in acute studies, menthol appears to be a substance of very low toxicity.[74]

Adverse Effects A review of reactions to menthol has been published.[76] Menthol causes sensitization in certain individuals although the sensitization index is low.[77] Symptoms include urticaria, erythema, and other cutaneous lesions, such as contact dermatitis. Peppermint-flavored toothpaste has even been implicated in exacerbating wheezing and dyspnea (difficulty in breathing) in a young woman with a history of asthma.[78] Despite menthol's widespread record of safety, two patients were identified who experienced allergic contact dermatitis caused by the menthol content of peppermint oil: one experienced cheilitis (inflammation of the lips); the other, eczema affecting the upper lip. Of interest was the 18- to 24-month history of these conditions before their diagnosis.[79]

Contraindications/Precautions/Warnings Menthol is contraindicated in patients with hypersensitivity to the agent. Menthol treatment should be discontinued if the patient develops irritation, rash, burning, stinging, swelling, or infection.

Case Study 5–2

Patient Complaint/History

Maria, a 75-year-old female with a previous history of congestive heart failure, was admitted to the hospital with a chief complaint of difficulty in breathing. She was subsequently found to have an acute pulmonary embolism. While in the hospital, she developed atrial fibrillation and received anticoagulation therapy with heparin followed by warfarin. After a 10-day hospitalization, she was discharged with an international normalized ratio (INR) level of 2.4.

One month later, Maria presented to the hospital emergency room with vaginal bleeding, irregular heartbeat, and orthostatic hypotension. Ecchymoses were seen on the extremities; gross bleeding from the vagina was also evident. The hemoglobin level, which had been 110 g/L during her previous hospitalization, was now 80 g/L. Her INR level was 5.5, her platelet count was 2.85×10^9/L, and her blood salicylate levels were 0.80 mmol/L.

After fluid replacement, blood transfusions, and parenteral vitamin K were administered, the patient had an uncomplicated recovery. Her INR level returned to 2.6. Before her discharge from the hospital, Maria revealed that she had frequently applied large quantities of topical methyl salicylate and menthol to the skin over her foot, knee, elbow, shoulder, and finger joints to treat joint pain.

Clinical Considerations/Strategies

Readers can use the following considerations/strategies to determine whether treatment of the patient's condition with nonprescription medications is warranted:

- Describe the probable etiology of the bleeding.
- Determine which ingredients in external analgesic formulations should not be used by patients receiving warfarin therapy.
- Propose an alternative nonprescription external analgesic for this patient.

Patient Education/Counseling

Readers can use the following strategies to develop a patient education/counseling plan that will help ensure optimal therapeutic outcomes:

- Explain the risk of using nonprescription salicylates concurrently with warfarin.
- Explain the indications for which use of external analgesics is appropriate as well as what precautions should be observed during therapy.
- Discuss the overt signs and symptoms of complications related to excessive levels of unbound warfarin in the blood.

Camphor

Although camphor occurs naturally and is obtained from the camphor tree, approximately three-fourths of the camphor used is prepared synthetically. The natural product is dextrorotatory; the synthetic product is optically active.

Mechanism of Action In concentrations of 0.1% to 3%, camphor depresses cutaneous receptors and is used as a topical analgesic, anesthetic, and antipruritic. In concentrations exceeding 3%, particularly when combined with other counterirritant ingredients, camphor stimulates the nerve endings in the skin and induces relief of pain and discomfort by masking moderate to severe.[80] When applied vigorously, it produces a rubefacient reaction.

Dosages/Administration Guidelines See Table 5–2 for dosing information.

Higher concentrations than those recommended are not more effective and can cause more serious adverse reactions if accidentally ingested.[46] (The risk of toxicity relates to both the concentration of camphor in the ingested product and the rate of absorption of camphor into the body.) Accordingly, preparations with camphor concentrations exceeding 11%, such as camphorated oil (camphor liniment), which is a solution of 20% camphor in cottonseed oil, are not considered safe for nonprescription use and have been removed from the market.[81]

Overdosage In children, 5 mL of a 20% camphor liniment is a potentially lethal dose, and death resulting from respiratory depression or complications of status epilepticus can occur.[82]

Adverse Effects High doses of camphor can cause nausea, vomiting, colic, headache, dizziness, delirium, convulsion, and coma.

Contraindications/Precautions/Warnings Placing camphor into the nostrils of an infant may cause immediate collapse. In 1994, the American Academy of Pediatrics Committee on Drugs noted that, although nonprescription camphor-containing preparations cannot exceed 11%, camphor toxicity continues. The academy advised parents to be aware of this potential danger and recommended use of modalities that do not contain camphor.[83]

It is of interest that in 1980, the FDA's review panel recommended that camphor products for external use be limited to a concentration of 2.5% because of camphor toxicity concerns and the agent's low benefit-to-risk ratio.[84] However, the FDA has yet to take final action on the panel's recommendation.

Histamine Dihydrochloride

Although histamine dihydrochloride is an FDA-approved counterirritant, it is seldom found in nonprescription external analgesic products.

Mechanism of Action Applying products containing histamine dihydrochloride results in vasodilation and causes percutaneous absorption of histamine from an ointment vehicle containing other medicinal agents. Aqueous vehicles seem to be superior to ointments for percutaneous absorption.[50]

Dosage/Administration Guidelines See Table 5–2 for dosing information.

Methyl Nicotinate

Methyl nicotinate is a safe and effective counterirritant if used according to the FDA's guidelines.

Mechanism of Action Although nicotinic acid is inactive topically, this ester possesses a marked power of diffusion and readily penetrates the cutaneous barrier. Vasodilation and elevation of skin temperature result from very low concentrations. A recent comparative study on the release kinetics of methyl nicotinate from topical formulations found that the highest penetration rate occurred when methyl nicotinate was incorporated into hydrophilic gels.[85] Studies have shown that indomethacin, ibuprofen, and aspirin significantly depress the skin's vascular response to methyl nicotinate. Because these three drugs suppress prostaglandin biosynthesis, it was concluded that the vasodilator response to methyl nicotinate is mediated, at least in part, by prostaglandin biosynthesis.[86]

Dosage/Administration Guidelines See Table 5–2 for dosing information.

Adverse Effects Generalized vascular dilation can occur when methyl nicotinate passes through the skin into the circulation system.

Contraindications/Precautions/Warnings Susceptible persons who apply methyl nicotinate over large areas may experience a drop in blood pressure, pulse rate, and syncope caused by generalized vascular dilation.[50]

Special Population Considerations To address the potential for variability in response, a study was undertaken to explore the possibility of age and racial differences in methyl nicotinate–induced vasodilation of human skin.[87] The results indicated an equivalent response among young Caucasian and African American subjects (ages 26 to 30 years) and elderly Caucasian subjects (ages 63 to 80 years) when calculating the time-to-peak response, the area under the time–response curve, and the time for the response to decline to 75% of its maximum value. These results were unexpected because differences in percutaneous absorption between black and white human skin have been described in several studies.[88]

Capsicum Preparations

Capsicum preparations (capsaicin, capsicum, and capsicum oleoresin) are derived from the fruit of various species of plants of the nightshade family. Capsicum contains about 1.5% of an irritating oleoresin, the major component of which is capsaicin (0.02%). Capsaicin is the major pungent ingredient of hot (chile) pepper.

Mechanism of Action When applied to normal skin, capsaicin elicits a transient feeling of warmth. More concentrated solutions produce a sensation of burning pain. However, as a result of tachyphylaxis, this local effect diminishes with repeated applications. Capsicum preparations do not cause blistering or reddening of the skin, even in high concentrations, because they do not act on capillaries or other blood vessels.

To determine the reason for this feeling of warmth, investigators applied a solution of capsaicin to the skin, followed by an intradermal injection of histamine to test for chemical responsiveness.[89] Although the capsaicin-treated sites responded by developing a wheal and itch, the flare response did not occur. This latter response, also known as axon reflex vasodilation, is postulated to be under the control of substance P, a neurotransmitter that is thought to function in the passage of painful stimuli from the periphery to the spinal cord and higher structures.[90] (See Figure 5–4.) High concentrations of substance P are also present in sensory nerves supplying sites of chronic inflammation.[91]

Substance P is found in slow-conducting, unmyelinated type C neurons that innervate the dermis and epidermis. It is released in the skin in response to endogenous (stress) and exogenous (trauma or injury) factors. It appears that pruritic stimuli along with pain impulses are conveyed to central processing centers by type C fibers in the skin, for which capsaicin has selective activity. Local application of capsaicin to the peripheral axon appears to affect substance P primarily by depleting it from sensory neurons that have been implicated in mediating cutaneous pain. The depletion occurs both peripherally and centrally, presumably as the result of impulse initiation. When substance P is released, burning pain and redness occur initially but abate with repeated applications. The net effect may be analogous to cutting a nerve or ligating it, which also depletes the substance P content of the neuron.[92] No evidence exists to date, however, that topical application of low concentrations of capsaicin causes any permanent neurologic injury.[93]

Capsaicin has been shown to reduce the pain, but not the inflammation, of rheumatoid arthritis and the pain from osteoarthritis.[94,95] Altman et al. [96] have discussed the role of neuropeptides and capsaicin in the treatment of musculoskeletal pain related to osteoarthritis and rheumatoid arthritis.

On the basis of results from a recent in vitro study in which capsaicin enhanced the penetration of naproxen through human skin, it may be possible in the future, if or when topical NSAIDs become commercially available, to create a combination product that provides more effective topical analgesia than that produced by either agent alone.[97]

Capsaicin has assumed a role in treating certain cutaneous disorders (e.g., postherpetic neuralgia, psoriasis, postmastectomy pain, reflex sympathetic dystrophy, diabetic

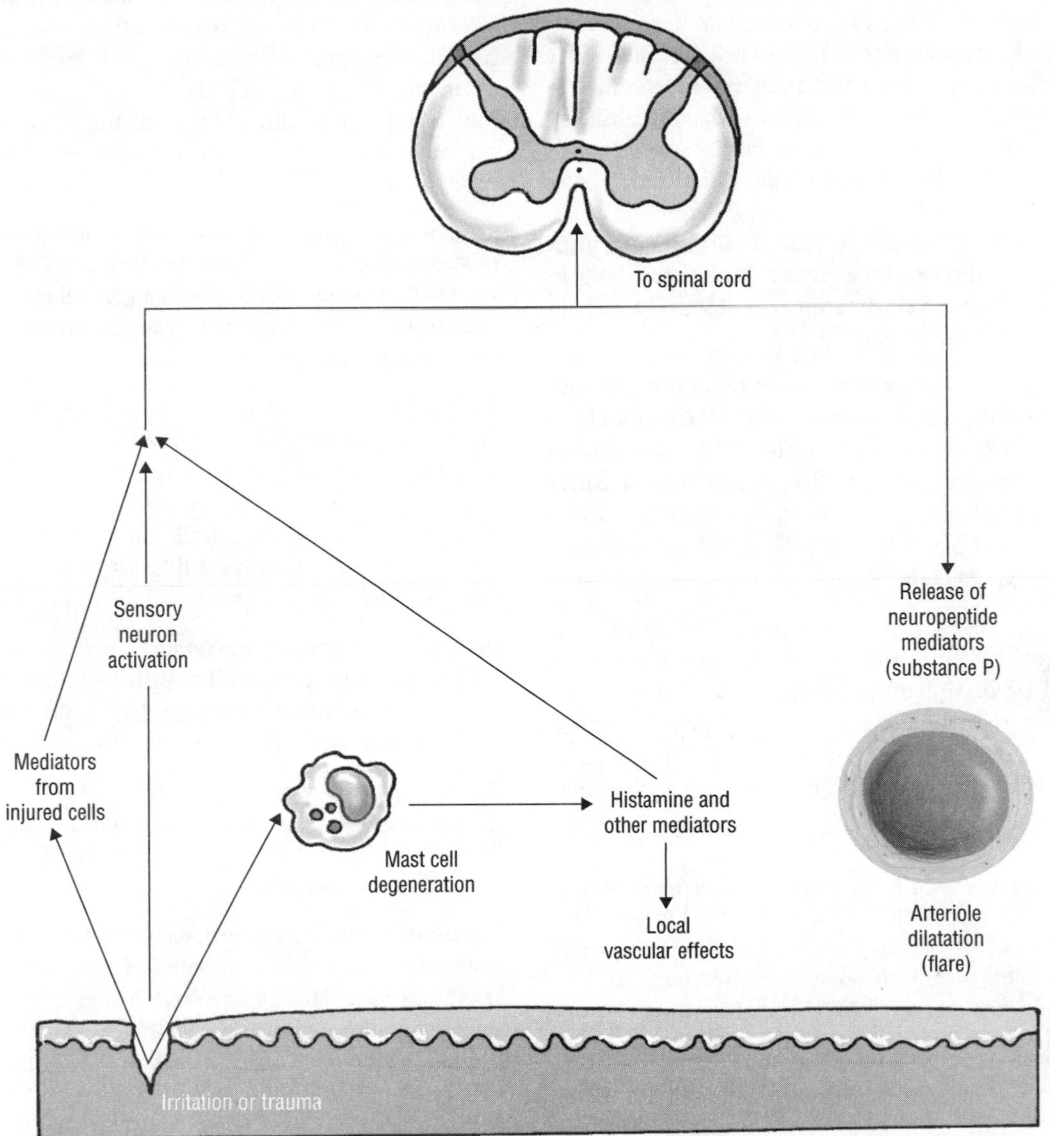

Figure 5–4 The axon reflex concept. Impulses created by the noxious stimulus of a peripheral branch of a sensory neuron are conducted not only in the usual direction to the spinal cord but also into neuron branches located near blood vessels. (Arrowheads show the direction of impulse propagation.) The axon flex enables the spread of vasodilation (flare) beyond the site of the original stimulus. Histamines and other mediators contribute to activation of axon reflexes and to local vascular effects. Adapted from: *Neuroscience.* 1988;24 : 748; used with permission.

neuropathy), posttraumatic amputation stump pain, itching associated with hemodialyis, notalgia paresthetica, erythromelalgia, idiopathic trigeminal neuralgia, fibromyalgia, foot pain accompanying Guillain-Barré syndrome, and, most recently, peripheral neuropathy associated with human immunodeficiency virus (HIV) infection. Further discussion of these disorders is outside the scope of this chapter. Readers are referred to the literature citations listed under "Additional Readings" for more information about capsaicin's effect on these disorders.

Dosage/Administration Guidelines Table 5–2 lists dosing information for capsaicin. The dose of this agent, however, may differ among patients. It appears that efficacy decreases and local discomfort increases when capsaicin is applied less often, because the drug's duration of action is 4 to 6 hours. Pain relief is usually noted within 14 days after therapy has begun but will occasionally be delayed by as much as 4 to 6 weeks. Notably, because capsicum lots vary, the concentration range for capsaicin cannot be expressed as a percentage and must be calculated for each lot.

Capsaicin must be used regularly every day as directed if it is to work effectively. Even then, it may not relieve pain immediately. The length of time it takes to work depends on the type of pain. In persons with arthritis, pain relief usually begins within 1 to 2 weeks. In most persons with pain caused by nerve damage, relief usually begins within 2 to 4 weeks, although, with head and neck nerve pain, relief may take as long as 4 to 6 weeks.

Once capsaicin has begun to relieve pain, its use must continue regularly three or four times a day to keep the pain from returning. If capsaicin treatment is stopped and pain returns, treatment can be resumed.

Adverse Effects Burning, stinging, and redness occur with the application of capsaicin in 40% to 70% of patients. However, this effect usually decreases within 72 hours with repeated use. If capsaicin gets into eyes or on other sensitive areas of the body, it will cause a burning sensation. Topical preparations greater than 1% have been associated with neurotoxicity and hyperalgesia.

Contraindications/Precautions/Warnings Use in patients with hypersensitivity to capsaicin is contraindicated. The agent should be discontinued temporarily if skin breaks down (weeping, red, small ulcers) and should not be applied to wounds or damaged skin. Pretreatment of skin subject to severe persistent reactions with topical lidocaine (5%) may be indicated.

Ingredients of Unproven Effectiveness and/or Safety

Eucalyptus oil, trolamine salicylate, and topical NSAIDs are currently classified as Category III ingredients (insufficient data are available to establish safety and effectiveness). Several commercial products are available containing trolamine salicylate as the primary ingredient. (See Table 5–3.)

Eucalyptus Oil Eucalyptus oil is a naturally occurring volatile oil with a characteristic, aromatic, camphoraceous odor. One of the chief constituents of eucalyptus oil is eucalyptol.

Mechanism of Action Eucalyptol and eucalyptus oil have been categorized as flavors and have mild irritant and rubefacient actions causing a sensation of warmth.

Dosage/Administration Guidelines The recommended topical dosage of eucalyptus oil for adults and for children ages 2 years and older is a 0.5% to 3% concentration applied to the affected area not more than three or four times a day.

Safety and Effectiveness A marketing experience of a topical analgesic product containing small amounts of eucalyptus oil revealed no evidence of toxicity. Nevertheless, a case report emphasized the profound depression that the central nervous system experienced after accidental ingestion.[98] In a status report of certain Category II and III active ingredients in external analgesic products, the FDA advised that eucalyptus oil "had not been shown to be generally recognized as safe and effective" for its intended use and that it should be eliminated from nonprescription counterirritant products.[99] However, a product has been recently introduced containing natural eucalyptus oil as an inactive ingredient in a "mucocutaneous adsorption gel" that when dry forms an invisible, moisture-resistant film that holds the active ingredients—capsaicin and menthol—in place to provide long-acting relief.[100]

Trolamine Salicylate After a comprehensive review of submitted documents, the FDA concluded in 1983 that the data were still insufficient to support a general recognition of the effectiveness of trolamine salicylate as a nonprescription external analgesic.[46]

Mechanism of Action Trolamine salicylate (formerly known as triethanolamine salicylate), although a salicylate salt, is not a counterirritant analgesic. Data exist to show that trolamine salicylate is absorbed from the skin;[101] 10 g of a 10% cream, if applied topically, may result in a concentration of salicylate in synovial fluid of approximately 60% of that obtained from a 500-mg oral dose of aspirin.

Dosage/Administration Guidelines The recommended topical dosage of trolamine salicylate for adults and for children ages 2 years and older is a 10% to 15% concentration applied to the affected area not more than three or four times a day.

Drug–Drug Interactions Trolamine salicylate has the same drug interactions as other salicylates. (See Chapter 3, "Headache and Muscle and Joint Pain," for discussion of these drug interactions.)

Contraindications/Precautions/Warnings Use is contraindicated in people with renal insufficiency or with hypersensitivity to trolamine or salicylates. People who have liver disease, hypoprothrombinemia (a deficiency of thrombin in the blood), vitamin K deficiency, or impending surgery or who are chronic alcohol users should not use this agent. During use, the agent should not contact the eyes or mucous membranes.

Safety and Effectiveness Although the FDA's review of data indicated that trolamine salicylate studies did not show any significant differences between active drug and placebo, several reports published after the review suggest that trolamine may be effective in alleviating neuralgia caused by unaccustomed strenuous exercise[102] and muscle soreness induced by a reproducible program of weight training.[103] A study documenting a specific use of trolamine was designed to evaluate the degree of pain relief and the increase in playing time among musicians with moderate or severe localized pain in the arms, wrists, hands, and fingers. After 750 mg of trolamine given over a 6-hour period was compared with placebo in a double-blind crossover trial, the investigators concluded that topical use of trolamine was associated with less pain and more playing time.[104] Additional studies should help clarify the use of this agent as an external analgesic.

In 1994, a major manufacturer of external analgesics containing trolamine salicylate asked the FDA to reopen the administrative record for this category of nonprescription drugs; the double-blind, placebo-controlled clinical trial indicated that trolamine salicylate provided significant improvement over placebo in arthritis relief.[105] The FDA has yet to act on this request.

A randomized, double-blind, placebo-controlled parallel study[106] conducted in 81 patients evaluated the effect of trolamine salicylate for the relief of pain and rigidity of osteoarthritis of the hands. The investigators found that trolamine was significantly superior to the placebo in improving pain and stiffness at 45 minutes after application. In addition, as noted in studies cited previously,[61,63] salicylic acid could not be detected or was substantially reduced in serum after trolamine application when compared with methyl salicylate. The FDA thus far has been unmoved by the evidence; it continues to rate the product as safe but not shown to be effective.

Topical Nonsteroidal Anti-Inflammatory Drugs

Current clinical investigations are ongoing with topical NSAIDs that have been marketed for a number of years in Europe.[107] The section "Safety and Effectiveness" below describes the results of these investigations.

Mechanism of Action Topical NSAIDs presumably act locally in a manner analogous to their systemic mechanism of action. Therefore, their application on acute soft tissue strains and sprains, where the target tissue is situated closer to the skin surface, may prove to be their optimal use as therapeutic agents.[108]

Adverse Effects A report suggests that even when applied topically, NSAIDs can cause renal disease and should be used with caution in those patients at risk.[109] Yet another case-control study of more than 1000 patients who were treated for upper gastrointestinal bleeding or perforation showed that topical NSAIDs are not significantly associated with these adverse reactions.[110]

Safety and Effectiveness A 1992 clinical study showed minimal systemic absorption of topical NSAIDs, consequent low plasma concentrations, and high tissue penetration, supporting their use as convenient and safe alternatives for treating painful and inflammatory musculoskeletal conditions.[111] A recent review[112] concluded that "evidence for a role for topical NSAIDs in acute and subacute soft tissue injuries is accumulating, but trials over longer periods will help to define the realistic extent of their value." In addition, according to the authors, "long-term data regarding adverse reactions are still awaited, but it appears likely that the lower plasma concentrations achieved with topical administration are likely to be associated with reductions in serious systemic adverse reactions." A second review published earlier that year reported that the results of a quantitative systematic review of randomized controlled clinical trials involving more than 10,000 patients indicated that "topical nonsteroidal anti-inflammatory drugs are effective in relieving pain in acute and chronic conditions."[113]

However, the recently published evidence-based guidelines[114] for NSAIDs in treating the pain of osteoarthritis sounded a cautionary note on the use of these agents. The investigators were unable to find any well-designed large-scale, randomized trials in which topical agents were compared with oral NSAIDs. They, therefore, could not recommend topical therapy as an evidence-based treatment.

More than a decade ago, the FDA's Arthritis Advisory Committee discussed problems associated with evaluating these products and offered recommendations for enhancing the ability to discriminate between the topical NSAID and the comparison topical placebo. No additional information has been forthcoming.[115]

Combination Products

General guidelines for nonprescription drug combination products state that Category I active ingredients from the same therapeutic category should not ordinarily be combined unless the combination is more effective, safer, and has enhanced patient acceptance or quality of formulation.[46] Four separate chemical and/or pharmacologic groups of counterirritants provide four qualitatively different types of irritation. Many marketed preparations aim for at least two such effects when greater potency is desired. Table 5–2 lists the individual ingredients and classifies them according to their relative potency and acceptable concentration ranges. Manufacturers may combine active ingredients from one group of counterirritants with one, two, or three other active ingredients, provided that each active ingredient is from a different group. Combination products currently available contain only camphor and menthol as active ingredients.[46]

It is irrational to combine counterirritants with local anesthetics, topical antipruritics, or topical analgesics. Because these agents depress sensory cutaneous receptors, their effects would oppose the counterirritant stimulation of cutaneous sensory receptors. It is also irrational to combine counterirritants with skin protectants because the protectants oppose and may nullify counterirritant effects.[50]

Dosage Forms of Counterirritants

Because percutaneous absorption of counterirritant drugs is generally undesirable, the finished product should consist of ingredients and vehicles that keep skin penetration to a minimum. The ideal topical drug vehicle should be (1) easy to apply and remove; (2) nontoxic, nonirritating, and nonallergenic; (3) cosmetically acceptable, nongreasy, and nondehydrating; (4) homogeneous; (5) bacteriostatic; (6) chemically stable; and (7) pharmacologically inert.[116]

Dosage forms referred to as "greaseless" are oil-in-water formulations, are "water washable," and are usually preferred for daytime use. In the past, many formulations contained lanolin or anhydrous lanolin as a vehicle. However, because both of these vehicles are obtained from wool fat (to which many people are allergic), these animal waxes are no longer used in contemporary formulations.

The longer any active ingredient remains in contact with the skin, the longer its duration of action. Little agreement exists on how long the preparations should be left in contact with the skin for optimal results; however, a practical guideline is that preparations should be used no more than three or four times a day. Although it is desirable to protect clothing from stains by covering the application site, the covering should not be tightly applied.

The FDA urged manufacturers to list all inactive ingredients voluntarily,[46] and this listing has been implemented for the most part. The nonprescription counterirritant preparations are usually available as liniments, gels, lotions, sprays, creams, and ointments.

Liniments Solutions or mixtures of various substances in oil, alcoholic solutions of soap, or emulsions are called liniments. They are intended for external application and should be so labeled. They are applied to the affected area of the skin with friction and rubbing; the oil or soap base facilitates application and massage. The vehicle selection for a liniment is based on the kind of action of the desired components.[117] Liniments with an alcoholic or hydroalcoholic vehicle are useful when rubefacient or counterirritant action is desired; oleaginous liniments are used primarily when massage is desired. By their nature, oleaginous liniments are less irritating to the skin than are alcoholic liniments.[117] Liniments should not be applied to skin that is broken or bruised.

Gels Gels used for the delivery of counterirritants are more appropriately classified as jellies because they are generally clear, are composed of water-soluble ingredients, and have a more uniform and semisolid consistency. A greater sensation of warmth is experienced with a gel than with equal quantities of the same product as a lotion or ointment. Products formulated as gels promote a more rapid and extensive penetration of the medication into the skin and hair follicles. Patients should be advised against using excessive amounts of gels or rubbing them vigorously into the skin because increased penetration may cause an unpleasant burning sensation.[117]

Lotions Lotions—suspensions of solids in an aqueous medium—are applied to the skin, usually without friction, for the protective or therapeutic value of their constituents. Depending on the ingredients, lotions may be alcoholic or aqueous and are often emulsions. Their fluidity allows for rapid and uniform application over a wide surface area and makes them especially suited for application to hairy body areas. Lotions are intended to dry on the skin soon after application, leaving a thin layer of their active ingredients on the skin's surface. In many instances, the cosmetic aspects of the lotion are of great significance. Because lotions tend to separate while standing, the label should include the instruction to shake the product before each use.[117]

Ointments Ointments are semisolid preparations that are applied to the skin to elicit one of three general effects: a surface activity, an effect within the stratum corneum, or a more deep-seated activity requiring penetration into the epidermis and dermis. These semisolid dosage forms are particularly desirable for counterirritation because the agents are applied with massage.[118]

Labeling of Counterirritants

The labels for these preparations list the indication as "the temporary relief of minor aches and sprains of muscles and joints." In addition, the labeling recommended by most of the FDA's review panel includes claims for "simple backache, arthritis pain, strains, bruises, and sprains."[50] Labeling approved by the FDA's advisory review panel on topical analgesics identifies the product as an "external analgesic" or as a "topical" or a "pain-relieving" cream, lotion, or ointment. However, these terms may not necessarily be similar to manufacturer's advertising claims.[50]

Preparation labels must list the active ingredients, including their concentrations, and must identify them by their officially recognized, established names. Recently, manufacturers have voluntarily listed inactive ingredients on the label. The manner of usage and the frequency of applications should also be indicated.[50]

It is acceptable to use terms describing certain physical or chemical qualities of the counterirritant preparations as long as the terms do not imply that any therapeutic effects occur. Terms such as *nongreasy, soothing, cooling action, penetrating relief, warming relief,* and *cool comforting relief* are considered acceptable in labeling.

As with all nonprescription drug products, external analgesics are intended to achieve a beneficial effect within a reasonable period of time. However, claims related to product performance are unacceptable unless they can be substantiated by scientific data. Claims such as fast, quick, prompt, swift, immediate, and remarkable are misleading and would not signal any property that is important to the safe and effective use of these products.[46]

Alternative Remedies

With the acceptance of capsaicin as an external analgesic agent, other components derived from natural sources have been incorporated into medications to relieve aches and pains.

These pain relievers contain ingredients such as arnica and calendula. External preparations derived from the flowering heads of arnica have been used for hundreds of years as topical counterirritants. Studies have shown that feelings of stiffness associated with strenuous physical exertion were improved following application of arnica. Indeed, the extract is found as an ingredient in a new, liquid gel, roll-on formulation (Absorbine Jr). However, numerous cases of arnica-associated contact dermatitis have been reported, and accidental ingestion can lead to significant toxicity.[119]

A second natural ingredient also found in the product discussed above is calendula. Although without clear evidence of a therapeutic effect, calendula has been used topically to promote wound healing and to reduce inflammation. However, unlike arnica, and despite its longstanding use, no serious adverse effects have been reported for calendula extract use.[120]

Liquid concentrated forms of methyl salicylate are found in some Chinese herbal medications. The concentrated form contains 5 cm^3 of 98% methyl salicylate, equivalent to 7000 mg of aspirin, and is highly lipid soluble. Its ingestion poses the threat of severe, rapid-onset salicylate poisoning.[67]

Although touted as treatment for osteoarthritis and other ailments involving injury to cartilage, glucosamine's efficacy is not recognized. The recommended dose of 500 mg is taken three times a day either orally, intramuscularly, intravenously, or intraarterially. Glucosamine serves as a preferred substrate for synthesis of proteoglycans, which are components of cartilage. Presumably, exogenous administration retards cartilage degradation. Interactions with other drugs have not been reported as yet. Adverse effects are minimal and include peripheral edema, tachycardia, gastrointestinal symptoms, drowsiness, headache, and skin rash. People who are hypersensitive to glucosamine should not be users, and users should be advised to continue conventional therapy.[1]

Chondroitin sulfate in combination with glucosamine has been a popular alternative therapy for osteoarthritis for several years. The recommended dose of 800 to 2400 mg per day is based on the patient's weight. The mechanism by which chondroitin exerts a beneficial effect is unclear. What is clear is that chondroitin binds to proteoglycans in cartilage. Advocates of this medication claim that chondroitin helps rebuild damaged cartilage. Neither efficacy nor harm has been shown. Chondroitin has been administered up to 6 years without any adverse effect. Nevertheless, patients should be warned of the possibility of chondroitin hypersensitivity or other allergic reactions and should be advised to stop medicating if these symptoms appear.[1]

S-adenosyl-L-methionine (also known as SAMe and ademetionine) is naturally occurring in all body tissues and fluids where it serves as a methyl group donor in transmethylation reactions and a sulfhydryl donor in transsulfuration reactions. *S*-adenosyl-L-methionine may be an innovative approach to the treatment of osteoarthritis and several other diseases. At present, it is not the indicated treatment for any disease. Its mechanism of action is undefined but believed to involve cartilage protection. The recommended dose for SAMe ranges from 400 to 1200 mg per day and is taken orally. The drug has rare gastrointestinal side effects (nausea, vomiting, and diarrhea), and only a single case of near-fatal allergic shock involving a high dose given intravenously has been reported.[121]

Patient Assessment of Musculoskeletal Injuries and Disorders

Before recommending treatment, the pharmacist will need to know the cause, location, type, intensity, duration, and other features of the symptoms. If the patient attributes the symptoms to arthritis, the pharmacist should find out whether a physician has diagnosed the disorder before recommending any treatment. Once the problem is identified, the pharmacist should ask whether it is a recurrent complaint, how the patient treated the symptoms in the past, and whether the therapy was effective. A thorough medical and drug history, especially the use of any pain medications, should also be taken. Asking the patient the following questions will help elicit the information needed to accurately assess the disorder and to recommend the appropriate treatment approach.

Q~ How long has the pain been apparent? How did it first appear? Is there any apparent cause for the pain? Can you relate the pain to a specific event, such as an accident, overwork, or a sports-related activity?

A~ If the pain is chronic, refer the patient to a physician. If it is acute, determine whether the injury is from sustained use of a body part or from a sudden eccentric movement of a poorly conditioned muscle, tendon, or ligament. If the latter, recommend the appropriate self-treatment unless the injury is a ruptured ligament or fracture. Refer the latter injuries for medical care.

Q~ What kind of pain is it? Is it sharp, dull, burning, shooting, aching, or stabbing?

A~ *Identify the type of pain associated with each musculoskeletal disorder or injury. (See the sections that discuss the signs and symptoms of the various disorders.)* On the basis of the patient's response, determine the cause of the pain and then recommend the appropriate treatment. Refer the patient to a physician if the origin of the pain is unclear.

Q~ Can you locate the pain? Does the pain move to other areas of the body?

A~ *Identify painful conditions that can be felt as referred pain in the back muscles or other muscles. (See the sections "Etiology of Lower Back Pain" and "Signs and Symptoms of Arthritis.")* If the location of the pain varies, refer the patient to a physician to determine whether visceral pain from an underlying pathology is present.

Q~ Has any specific treatment been helpful in alleviating the pain? What makes the pain better or worse?

A~ Determine what measures relieved the pain. If they are appropriate treatments, recommend the patient use them again with any needed modifications.

Q~ Using a scale of zero to 10, how bad is the pain? Is it debilitating? Is it recurrent?

A~ If the pain is debilitating or recurrent and the patient has no apparent physical injury, medical referral is appropriate. The patient could be suffering visceral pain from an underlying pathology.

Q~ Is the pain in a joint or muscle? If the pain is in a joint, is the joint red, swollen, warm, and tender to the touch?

A~ These signs and symptoms could indicate arthritis or a fractured, ruptured ligament or tendon. Refer the patient to a physician if these symptoms are present.

Q~ Is the pain secondary to a muscle strain or joint sprain?

A~ *Identify the appropriate self-treatment for these injuries. (See the section "Treatment of Strains, Sprains, and Cramps.")* If the patient has either injury, recommend the appropriate treatment.

Q~ Have you been diagnosed by a physician as having any type of arthritic condition?

A~ If yes, ask which type of arthritis the patient has and find out which nonprescription medications the physician recommended.

Q~ Are you taking any prescription or nonprescription medications or alternative remedies?

A~ Evaluate the patient's medication history for possible interactions with nonprescription counterirritants and external analgesics. Determine whether the patient has any drug allergies.

Patient Counseling for Musculoskeletal Injuries and Disorders

Counseling for musculoskeletal conditions begins with an explanation of the appropriate drug and nondrug measures for treating the patient's particular complaint. The patient should receive specific guidelines for usage of any recommended nonprescription external analgesics, including an explanation of possible adverse effects, drug interactions, and precautions and warnings. The pharmacist can minimize the risk of drug interactions with warfarin by (1) knowing all the drugs the patient is taking, (2) restricting drugs to those that are genuinely indicated, (3) keeping therapy as simple as possible, (4) educating the patient as to the importance of not changing or adding to a prescription or nonprescription medication without first consulting a physician or pharmacist, (5) avoiding occasional use of drugs (e.g., salicylates) known to cause clinically important interactions, and (6) keeping changes in drug therapy to a minimum and monitoring coagulation status closely for a number of weeks after any changes. Because external analgesic drug products temporarily relieve only minor pain, patients should understand the degree of relief that can reasonably be expected and the amount of time that it takes for relief to occur. The pharmacist should explain signs and symptoms that indicate the condition is worsening and requires medical attention. The box "Patient Education for Musculoskeletal Injuries and Disorders" lists specific information to provide patients.

Evaluation of Patient Outcomes for Musculoskeletal Injuries and Disorders

Patients with musculoskeletal injuries should return for evaluation after 7 days of self-treatment. If the symptoms are not relieved by the preparation within 7 days, or if the symptoms clear up and then return within a few days, the patient should discontinue the medication and see a physician for further evaluation. Patients with diagnosed arthritis should return after 7 days of self-treatment for a review of the condition to prevent prolonged ineffective self-treatment that might allow a more serious underlying disease to progress.

CONCLUSIONS

The increasing number of participants in strenuous exercise programs and various sporting events has led to the identification of the "weekend warrior." This phenomenon, coupled with the growing number of baby boomers who are entering their sixth decade of life and who also have active lifestyles, is providing increasing numbers of individuals seeking relief of aches and pains. This aging process is also giving rise to an expanding population of arthritis patients. In view of these cultural and demographic changes, external analgesics have assumed an important role in the nonprescription therapeutic armamentarium.

Counterirritant external analgesic agents contribute to decreasing the pain and discomfort associated with many minor aches and pains of muscles and joints. They can provide hours of relief from pulled muscles and painful joints. However, they must be used correctly to be safe and effective. It is important to note that self-treatment with nonprescription counterirritant preparations may result in harm if directions are not followed exactly.

Patients should be advised that the oral toxicity of counterirritant preparations is variable; some agents such as capsicum preparations have a low oral toxicity, whereas other agents, such as methyl salicylate and camphor, are highly toxic when ingested. Although some percutaneous absorption occurs when counterirritants are topically applied, the amount absorbed is insignificant if the ingredients do not exceed the maximum recommended effective concentrations and if the environmental conditions are normal (i.e., the counterirritant is not applied during or after strenuous exercise in high outdoor heat.)

Pharmacists can play an important role in educating patients about preventive and nondrug measures for musculoskeletal injuries and disorders. As drug information specialists, pharmacists are the best source of information

Patient Education for Musculoskeletal Injuries and Disorders

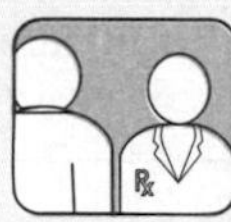

The objectives of self-treatment are to (1) reduce pain, (2) restore function of the affected area, and (3) prevent reinjury. Certain nondrug measures and nonprescription counterirritants can relieve the symptoms of pain from a sudden and recent muscle, tendon, or ligament injury; an overuse injury (tendinitis, bursitis, or repetitive stress injury); lower back pain; or arthritis. For most patients, carefully following product instructions and the self-care measures listed below will help ensure optimal therapeutic outcomes.

Nondrug Measures

- For pain related to a **muscle strain or joint sprain**, begin treatment with RICE therapy. (See Table 5–1.)
- For **periodic muscle cramps**, stretch and massage the affected area immediately; then rest or reduce activity of the muscle to allow it to loosen.
- For **persistent cramps**, apply heat to the affected area in the form of a warm wet compress, a heating pad, or a hot-water bottle.
- For **osteoarthritis**, try a combination of nondrug measures, including applying heat or cold to the affected area, supporting the area with splints, and doing range-of-motion and strength maintenance exercises.

Preventive Measures

- To prevent **cramps**, warm up and stretch muscles before physical activity, drink sufficient fluids, and do not exercise to the point of exhaustion. To help prevent nocturnal leg cramps, raise the foot of the bed. If you suffer from Achilles tendinitis, try wearing better-fitting shoes and heel lifts to reduce the symptoms.
- To prevent **strains and sprains**, do warm-up and stretching exercises before playing sports or exercising.
- To prevent **repetitive strain**, exercise the muscles vulnerable to injury and use ergonomic controls to adjust posture, stresses, motions, and other damaging physical factors.
- To prevent or reduce the occurrence of **lower back pain**, do exercises to strengthen the muscles of the lower back.

Nonprescription Medications

- See Table 5–2 for recommended dosages of counterirritants.
- Do not use counterirritants if your skin is abraded, sunburned, or otherwise damaged.
- When using counterirritants, wash your hands before touching your eyes or mucous membranes or before handling contact lenses.
- Do not put a tight bandage or dressing over an area treated with a counterirritant. Do not use warming devices with counterirritants.
- Do not treat a child younger than 2 years with counterirritants unless a physician supervises the use.
- If you suffer from arthritis, consult your doctor before attempting to treat your pain with counterirritants, or with topical or internal analgesics.
- If you have asthma and symptoms of wheezing and shortness of breath worsen while you are using a mentholated formulation, stop using it.
- Do not use any product containing salicylates (including aspirin, methyl salicylate, and trolamine salicylate) if you are receiving anticoagulation therapy (especially warfarin).

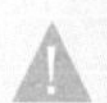

If a counterirritant causes excessive redness and blistering or hives and vomiting, stop using it.

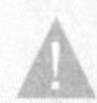

If you experience nausea, vomiting, colic, and other unusual symptoms while using a product containing camphor, seek medical care immediately.

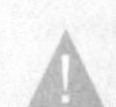

If the pain was present for more than 2 weeks before you sought treatment, consult a physician.

If the symptoms persist after more than 7 days of treatment or if the pain is constant and felt in any position, consult a physician.

about the usage and potential adverse effects or drug interactions of external analgesics.

References

1. Micromedex Healthcare Series, vol 102 [database online]. Englewood, CO: Micromedex, Inc.; 1999.
2. Reisner-Keller LA. Pain management. In: Herfindal ET, Gourley DR, eds. *Textbook of Therapeutics—Drug and Disease Management.* 6th ed. Baltimore: Williams & Wilkins; 1996:1047–51.
3. Melzack R, Wall PD. Pain mechanisms: a new theory. *Science.* 1965;150:971–79.
4. Herring SA, Nilson KC. Introduction to overuse injuries. *Clin Sports Med.* 1987;6:225–39.
5. Järuinen M. Epidemiology of tendon injuries in sports. *Clin Sports Med.* 1992;11:493–514.
6. Kannus P, Niittymäki S, Järuinen M, et al. Sports injuries in elderly athletes: a three year prospective controlled study. *Age Ageing.* 1989; 18:263–70.
7. McCarthy P. Managing bursitis in the athlete: an overview. *Physician Sports Med.* 1989;17(11):115–25.

8. Nirschi RP. Shoulder tendinitis. In: Petron PA, ed. *Symposium on Upper Extremity Injuries in Athletes.* St Louis: CV Mosby; 1986:322–36.
9. Puffer JC, Zachazewski MS. Management of overuse injuries. *Am Fam Physician.* 1988;38:225–32.
10. Evans G. Tenosynovitis in industry: menace or misnomer. *Br Med J.* 1987;294:1569–70.
11. Simon, H. Current topics in medicine: sports medicine. In: Rubenstein E, Federman DD, eds. *Medicine.* New York: Scientific American; 1987;I:1–23.
12. Szarfman A, Chin M, Blum MD. More on fluoroquinolone antibiotics and tendon rupture [letter]. *N Engl J Med.* 1995;332:193.
13. Carrasco JM, Garcia B, Andujar C, et al. Tendinitis associated with ciprofloxacin [letter]. *Ann Pharmacother.* 1997;31:120.
14. Cobeta JC, Juyol MC, Rodilla F. Ciprofloxacin—associated achilles tendinitis. *Eur Hosp Pharm.* 1997;3(5)178–9.
15. Nightingale SL. New fluoroquinolone warning label. *JAMA.* 1996; 276 :774.
16. Strains, sprains and bruises. *Drug Ther Bull.* 1976;14:66–7.
17. Barry NN, McGuire JL. Overuse syndromes in adult athletes. *Rheum Dis Clin North Am.* 1996;22:515–30.
18. Sorensen L, Larsen SE, Rock ND. The epidemiology of sports injuries in school-aged children. *Scand J Med Sci Sports.* 1996;6:281–6.
19. Holmer P, Sondergaard L, Konradsen L, et al. Epidemiology of sprains in the ankle and foot. *Foot Ankle Int.* 1994;15:72–4.
20. Jones BH, Cowan DN, Tomlinson JP, et al. Epidemiology of injuries associated with physical training among young men in the army. *Med Sci Sports Exerc.* 1993;25:197–203.
21. Leung AK, Wong BE, Chan PY, et al. Nocturnal leg cramps: incidence and clinical characteristics. *J Natl Med Assoc.* 1999;91:329–32.
22. Naylor JR, Young JB. A general population survey of rest cramps. *Age Ageing.* 1994;23:418–20.
23. Garrick JG, Webb DR. Sprains. In: *Sports Injuries: Diagnosis and Management.* Philadelphia: WB Saunders Co; 1990:14–22.
24. Zarins B, Ciullo JV. Acute muscle and tendon injuries in athletes. *Clin Sports Med.* 1983;2:167–82.
25. Clarkson PM, Sayers SP. Etiology of exercise-induced muscle damage. *Can J Appl Physiol.* 1999;24:234–8.
26. Schwellnus MP, Derman EW, Noakes TD. Aetiology of skeletal muscle 'cramps' during exercise: a novel hypothesis. *J Sports Sci.* 1997;15: 277–85.
27. Mayell M. *The Natural Health First-Aid Guide.* New York: Pocket Books (Simon and Shuster); 1994.
28. Ferguson D. The "new" industrial epidemic. *Med J Aust.* 1984;140: 318–9.
29. Brown CD, Nolan BM, Faithful DK. Occupational repetition strain injuries: guidelines for diagnosis and management. *Med J Aust.* 1984; 140 :329–32.
30. Pharmacy Newswire—Don't hurt yourself. *NARD J.* 1993;115(4):11.
31. Atcheson SG, Ward JR, Lowe W. Concurrent medical disease in work-related carpal tunnel disease. *Arch Intern Med.* 1998;158:1506–12.
32. Ferry S, Pritchard T, Keenan J, et al. Estimating the prevalence of delayed median nerve conduction in the general population. *Br J Rheumatol.* 1998;37(6):630–5.
33. Leigh JP, Miller TR. Occupational illness with two national data sets. *Int J Occup Environ Health.* April–June 1998;4(2):99–130.
34. *Carpal Tunnel Syndrome, Report 34.* Available at: http://bewell.healthgate.com/hic/wcon/wcon-34.asp. Accessed March 12, 2000.
35. Brooks P. Repetitive strain injury does not exist as a separate medical condition. *Br Med J.* 1993;307:1298.
36. Lohr S. Vigorous defense stalls injury claims on repetitive strain. *New York Times.* May 29, 1995; First Business page.
37. Greening J, Lynn B. Vibration sense in the upper limb in patients with repetitive strain injury and a group of at-risk office workers. *Int Arch Occup Environ Health.* 1998;71:29–34.
38. Quinet RJ, Halder NM. Diagnosis and treatment of backache. *Semin Arthritis Rheum.* 1979;8:261–87.
39. Waddell G. A new clinical model for the treatment of low back pain. *Spine.* 1987;12:632.
40. Crown S. Psychologic aspects of low back pain. *Rheumatol Rehabil.* 1978;17:114–24.
41. Hammacher DP and Associates. External analgesics. *NARD J.* 1997;139(1):55–6.
42. Oddis CV. New perspectives on osteoarthritis. *Am J Med.* 1996;100(suppl 2A):10S–15S.
43. Altman RD, Aven A, Holmberg CE, et al. Capsaicin cream 0.025% as monotherapy for osteoarthritis: a double-blind study. *Semin Arthritis Rheum.* 1994;6(suppl 3):25–33.
44. Hecker-Kia A, Kolkenbrock H, Orgel D, et al. Substance P induces the secretion of gelatinase A from human synovial fibroblasts. *Eur J Clin Chem Biochem.* 1997;35:655–60.
45. Harris ED Jr. Rheumatoid arthritis: pathophysiology and implications for therapy. *N Engl J Med.* 1990;322:1277–89.
46. Department of Health and Human Services. External analgesics drug products for over-the-counter human use: tentative final monograph. *Federal Register.* 1983;48(27):5852–69.
47. Buschbacher RM. Rehabilitation of musculoskeletal disorders: the sports medicine approach. In: Buschbacher RM, ed. *Principles of Musculoskeletal Rehabilitation.* Boston: Andover Medical Publishers; 1994: 25–40.
48. Sherman M. Which treatment to recommend? Hot or cold. *Am Pharm.* 1980; NS20:46–9.
49. Heng MCY. Local necrosis and interstitial nephritis due to topical methyl salicylate and menthol. *Cutis.* 1987;39:442–4.
50. Department of Health, Education and Welfare. External analgesics drug products for over-the-counter human use; establishment of a monograph and notice of proposed rulemaking. *Federal Register.* 1979;44(234):68831–9866.
51. Gossel TA. External analgesics. *US Pharm.* 1987;12(8):26, 28, 30, 35, 36, 105.
52. Swinyard EA, Pathak MA. Locally acting drugs—surface acting drugs: irritants. In: Goodman AG, Goodman LS, Rall TW, et al., eds. *The Pharmacological Basis of Therapeutics.* 7th ed. New York: Macmillan Publishing; 1985:950–1.
53. Post BS. Effect of percutaneous medication on muscle tissue: an electromyographic study. *Arch Phys Med Rehabil.* 1961;42:791–8.
54. Aviado DM, ed. Drugs administrated systemically and counterirritants. In: *Krantz and Carr's Pharmacological Principles of Medical Practice.* 8th ed. Baltimore: Williams & Wilkins; 1972:891–93.
55. Lewis DW, Verhonick PJ. Thermography of analgesics/rubefacients. *Appl Radiol.* 1977;6(2):114–8.
56. Hong C-Z, Shellock FG. Effects of a topically applied counterirritant (Eucalyptamint) on cutaneous blood flow and on skin and muscle temperatures: a placebo-controlled study. *Am J Phys Med Rehabil.* 1991;70:29–33.
57. Danon A, Ben-Shimon S, Ben-Zvi Z. Effect of exercise and heat exposure on percutaneous absorption of methyl salicylate. *Eur J Clin Pharmacol.* 1986;31:49–52.
58. Mustard. In: Olin BR, ed. *The Lawrence Review of Natural Products.* St. Louis: Facts and Comparisons Division, JP Lippincott; February 1992.
59. Strong ammonia solution. In: Reynolds JEF, ed. *Martindale—The Extra Pharmacopoeia.* 31st ed. London: The Royal Pharmaceutical Society; 1996:1674.3.
60. Clark GS IV. Methyl salicylate or oil of wintergreen. *Perfumer Flavorist.* 1999;24:5, 6, 8, 10, 11.
61. Cross SE, Anderson L, Roberts MS. Topical penetration of commercial salicylate esters and salts using human isolated skin and clinical microdialysis studies. *Br J Clin Pharmacol.* 1998;46:29–35.
62. Roberts MS, Favretto WA, Mayer A, et al. Topical bioavailability of methyl salicylate. *Aust N Z J Med.* 1982;12:303–5.
63. Morra P, Bartle WR, Walker SE, et al. Serum concentrations of salicylic acid following topically applied salicylate derivatives. *Ann Pharmacother.* 1996;30:935–40.
64. Methyl salicylate. In: Budavari S, ed. *The Merck Index.* 12th ed. Rahway, NJ: Merck Research Laboratories; 1996:6200.
65. Trapnell K. Salicylate intoxication. *J Am Pharm Assoc.* 1976;16:147.
66. Methyl salicylate. In: Reynolds JEF, ed. *Martindale—The Extra Pharmacopoeia.* 31st ed. London: The Royal Pharmaceutical Society; 1996: 62.2.
67. Chan TUK. The risk of severe cation. *J Am Pharm Assoc.* 1976;16:147.
66. Methyl salicylate. In: Reynolds JEF, ed. *Martindale—The Extra Phar-*

macopoeia. 31st ed. London: The Royal Pharmaceutical Society; 1996: 62.2.

67. Chan TUK. The risk of severe salicylate poisoning following the ingestion of topical medicaments or aspirin. *Postgrad Med J.* 1996;72: 109–12.
68. Littleton F Jr. Warfarin and topical salicylates [letter]. *JAMA.* 1990; 263:2888.
69. Yip ASB, Chow WH, Tai YT, et al. Adverse effect of topical methylsalicylate ointment on warfarin anticoagulation: an unrecognized potential hazard. *Postgrad Med J.* 1990;66:367–9.
70. Turpentine oil. In: Reynolds JEF, ed. *Martindale—The Extra Pharmacopoeia.* 31st ed. London: The Royal Pharmaceutical Society; 1996: 1764.1.
71. Centers for Disease Control and Prevention. Self-treatment with herbal and other plant-derived remedies—Rural Mississippi, 1993. *MMWR Morbid Mortal Wkly Rev.* 1995;44:204–7.
72. Green BG. Menthol inhibits the perception of warmth. *Physiol Behav.* 1986;38:833–8.
73. Schafer K, Braun HA, Rempe L. Discharge pattern analysis suggests existence of a low-threshold calcium channel in cold receptors. *Experientia.* 1991;47:47–50.
74. Eccles R. Menthol and related cooling compounds. *J Pharm Pharmacol.* 1994;46:618–30.
75. Menthol. In: Reynolds JEF, ed. *Martindale—The Extra Pharmacopoeia.* 29th ed. London: The Pharmaceutical Press; 1989:1586.
76. Fisher AA. Reactions to menthol. *Cutis.* 1986;38:17–8.
77. Blondeel A, Oleffe J, Achten G. Contact allergy in 330 dermatological patients. *Contact Derm.* 1978;4(5):270–6.
78. Spurlock BW, Dailey TM. Shortness of (fresh) breath: toothpaste-induced bronchospasm [letter]. *N Engl J Med.* 1990;323:1845–6.
79. Wilkinson SM, Beck MH. Allergic contact dermatitis from menthol in peppermint. *Contact Derm.* 1994;30:42–3.
80. Phalen WJ III. Over-the-counter dangers camphor poisoning. *Pediatrics.* 1976;57:428–31.
81. Gossel TA. Camphorated oil. *US Pharm.* 1983;8(4):12, 14, 16.
82. Siegel E, Wason S. Camphor toxicity. *Pediatr Clin North Am.* 1986;33: 375–9.
83. Committee on Drugs. Camphor revisited: focus on toxicity. *Pediatrics.* 1994;94:127–8.
84. Department of Health and Human Services. External analgesic drug products for over-the-counter human use; reopening of the administrative record. *Federal Register.* 1980;45(189):63878–9.
85. Nastruzzi C, Esposito E, Pastesini C, et al. Comparative study on the release kinetics of methyl-nicotinate from topic formulations. *Int J Pharm.* 1993;90:43–50.
86. Wilkin JK, Forther G, Reinhardt LA, et al. Prostaglandins and nicotinate-provoked increase in cutaneous blood flow. *Clin Pharmacol Ther.* 1985:38:273–7.
87. Guy RH, Tur E, Bjerke S, et al. Are there age and racial differences to methyl nicotinate-induced vasodilatation in human skin? *J Am Acad Dermatol.* 1985;12:1001–6.
88. Anderson KE, Maibach HI. Black and white human skin differences. *J Am Acad Dermatol.* 1979;1:276–82.
89. Bernstein JE, Swift RM, Soltani K, et al. Inhibition of axon reflux vasodilation by topically applied capsaicin. *J Invest Dermatol.* 1981;76: 394–5.
90. Bernstein JE. Capsaicin in dermatologic disease. *Semin Dermatol.* 1988;7:304–9.
91. Lembeck F, Donnerer J, Colpaert FC. Increase of substance P in primary afferent nerves during chronic pain. *Neuropeptides.* 1981; 1:175–80.
92. Fitzgerald M. Capsaicin and sensory neurons—a review. *Pain.* 1983; 15:109–30.
93. Watson CPN. Topical capsaicin as an adjuvant analgesic. *J Pain Symptom Manage.* 1994;9:425–33.
94. Deal CL, Schnitzer TJ, Lipstein E, et al. Treatment of arthritis with topical capsaicin: a double-blind trial (subset analysis of data). *Clin Ther.* 1991;13:383–95.
95. McCarthy GM, McCarthy DJ. Effect of topical capsaicin in the therapy of painful osteoarthritis of the hands. *J Rheumatol.* 1992;19:604–7.
96. Altman RD, Gottlieb NL, Howell DS, eds. Neuropeptides, capsaicin and musculoskeletal pain. *Semin Rheum Arthritis.* 1994;6(suppl 3):1–51.
97. Degim LT, Uslu A, Hadgrafi J, et al. The effects of azone and capsaicin on the permeation of naproxen through human skin. *Int J Pharmaceut.* 1999;179:21–5.
98. Patel S, Wiggins J. Eucalyptus oil poisoning. *Arch Dis Child.* 1980;55: 405–6.
99. Department of Health and Human Services. Status of certain over-the-counter drug category II and III active ingredients: final rule. *Federal Register.* 1990;55(216):46914–8.
100. Heritage Eucalyptamint-2000 arthritis pain relief gel debuting in June. *FDC Reports—The Tan Sheet.* 1999;7(15):8.
101. Rabinowitz JL, Feldman E, Weinberger A, et al. Comparative tissue absorption of oral ^{14}C aspirin and topical triethanolamine ^{14}C salicylate in human and canine knee joints. *J Clin Pharmacol.* 1982;22:42–8.
102. Politino V, Smith SL, Waggoner WC. A clinical study of topical 10% trolamine salicylate for relief of delayed-onset exercise-induced arthralgia. *Curr Ther Res.* 1985;38:321–7.
103. Hill DW, Richardson JD. Effectiveness of 10% trolamine salicylate cream on muscular soreness induced by a reproducible program of weight training. *J Orthop Sports Phys Training.* 1989;11:19–23.
104. Hochberg FH, Lavih P, Portnoy R, et al. Topical therapy of localized inflammation in musicians: a clinical evaluation of Aspercreme® versus placebo. In: *Medical Problems of Performing Artists.* Philadelphia: Hanley and Belfus; 1988:9–14.
105. Thompson Medical asks FDA to reopen administrative record. *FDC Reports—The Tan Sheet.* 1994;2(19):25.
106. Rothacker DQ, Lee I, Littlejohn TW III. Topical NSAIDs for musculoskeletal conditions. A review of the literature effectiveness of a single topical application of 10% trolamine salicylate cream in the symptomatic treatment of osteoarthritis. *J Clin Rheumatol.* 1998;4 : 6–12.
107. Heyneman CA. Topical nonsteroidal anti-inflammatory drugs for acute soft tissue injuries. *Ann Pharmacother.* 1995;29:780–2.
108. Memeo A, Garofoli F, Peretti G. Evaluation of the efficacy and tolerability of a new topical formulation of flurbiprofen in acute soft tissue injuries. *Drug Invest.* 1992;4(5):441–9.
109. O'Callaghan CA, Andrews PA, Ogg CS. Renal disease and use of topical non-steroidal anti-flammatory drugs. *Br Med J.* 1994;308:110–1.
110. Evans JMM, McMahon AD, McGilchrist MM, et al. Topical non-steroidal anti-inflammatory drugs and admission to hospital for upper gastrointestinal bleeding and perforation: a record linkage case-control study. *Br Med J.* 1995;311:22–6.
111. Fourtillan JB, Girault J. Piroxicam plasma concentrations following repeated topical application of a piroxicam 0.5% gel. *Drug Invest.* 1992;4(5):435–40.
112. Vaile JH, Davis P. Topical NSAIDs for musculoskeletal conditions. A review of the literature. *Drugs.* 1998;56:783–9.
113. Moore RA, Tramer MR, Carroll D, et al. Quantitative systematic review of topically applied non-steroidal anti-inflammatory drugs. *Br Med J.* 1998;316:333–8.
114. Eccles M, Freemantle N, Mason J. North of England evidence based guideline development project: summary guideline for non-steroidal anti-inflammatory drugs versus basic analgesia in treating the pain of degenerative arthritis. *Br Med J.* 1998;317:526–30.
115. Weisman MN, Furst DE, Paulus HE. FDA arthritis advisory committee meeting: analgesics guidelines, topical NSAIDs. *Arthritis Rheum.* 1995;34:931.
116. Carr DS, Bennett TA. A review of recent dermatologicals. *Pharm Times.* 1991;57(3):112–9.
117. Nairn JG. Lotions. In: Hoover JE, ed. *Remington: The Science and Practice of Pharmacy.* 19th ed. Easton, PA.: Mack Publishing; 1995:1518–9.
118. Block LH. Ointments. In: Hoover JE, ed. *Remington: The Science and Practice of Pharmacy.* 19th ed. Easton, Penn.: Mack Publishing; 1995: 1585–91.
119. Arnica. In: Hebel SK, ed. *The Review of Natural Products.* St. Louis: Facts and Comparisons; October 1998.
120. Calendula. In: Olin BR, ed. *The Lawrence Review of Natural Products.* St. Louis: Facts and Comparisons; January 1995.

121. SAMe: S-adenosylmethionine [Alternative Therapies]. *Am J Health-Syst Pharm.* January 2000;57:119–123.

Additional Readings

Bernstein JE. Capsaicin in dermatologic disease. *Semin Dermatol.* 1988; 7:304–9.

Watson CPN. Topical capsaicin as an adjuvant analgesic. *J Pain Symptom Manage.* 1994;9:425–33.

Bernstein JE, Bickers DR, Dahl MV, et al. Treatment of chronic post-herpetic neuralgia with topical capsaicin. *J Am Acad Dermatol.* 1987;17:93–6.

Watson CPN, Tyler KL, Bickers DR, et al. A randomized vehicle-controlled trial of topical capsaicin in the treatment of post-herpetic neuralgia. *Clin Ther.* 1993;15:510–26.

Ellis CN, Berberian B, Sulica VI, et al. A double-blind evaluation of topical capsaicin in pruritic psoriasis. *J Am Acad Dermatol.* 1993;29:438–42.

Dini D, Bertelli G, Gozza A, et al. Treatment of the post-mastectomy pain syndrome with topical capsaicin. *Pain.* 1993;54:223–6.

Cheshire WP, Snyder CR. Treatment of reflex sympathetic dystrophy with topical capsaicin. *Pain.* 1990;42:307–11.

Ross DR, Varipapa RJ. Treatment of painful diabetic neuropathy with topical capsaicin [Letter]. *N Engl J Med.* 1989;321:474–5.

Weintraub M, Golik A, Rublo A. Capsaicin for treatment of post-traumatic amputation stump pain [Letter]. *Lancet.* 1990; 336: 1003–004.

Rayner HC, Atkins RC, Westerman RA. Relief of local stump pain by capsaicin cream [Letter]. *Lancet.* 1989; 336: 1276–77.

Breneman DL, Cardone JS, Blumsack RF, et al. Topical capsaicin for treatment of hemodialysis-related pruritus *J Am Acad Dermatol.* 1992;26:91–4.

Wallengren J, Klinker M. Successful treatment of notalgia paresthetica with topical capsaicin: vehicle-controlled, double-blind crossover study. *J Am Acad Dermatol.* 1995;32:287–9.

Muhiddin KA, Gallen IW, Harries S, et al. The use of capsaicin cream in a case of erythromelalgia. *Postgrad Med J.* 1994;70:841–3.

Fusco DM, Alessandri M. Analgesic effect of capsaicin in idiopathic trigeminal neuralgia. *Anesth Anal.* 1992;74:375–7.

McCarty DJ, Csuka M, McCarthy G, et al. Treatment of pain due to fibromyalgia with topical capsaicin: A pilot study. *Semin Arthritis Rheum.* 1994;6 (suppl 3):41–7.

Donofrio PD and the Capsaicin Study Group. Treatment of painful diabetic neuropathy with topical capsaicin. A muticenter, double-blind vehicle controlled study. *Arch Intern Med.* 1991;151:2225–9.

Dailey GE III and the Capsaicin Study Group. Effect of treatment with capsaicin on daily activities of patients with painful diabetic neuropathy. *Diabetes Care.* 1992;15:159–65.

Tandan R, Lewis GA, Krusinski PB, et al. Topical 0.075% capsaicin in painful diabetic neuropathy. I. A controlled study with long-term follow-up. *Diabetes Care.* 1992;15:8–15.

Morgenlander JC, Hurwitz BJ, Massey EW. Capsaicin for the treatment of pain in Guillain-Barré syndrome. *Ann Neurol.* 1990;28:199.

Section III

Reproductive and Genital Disorders

CHAPTER 6

Vaginal and Vulvovaginal Disorders

Leslie A. Shimp

Chapter 6 at a Glance

Vaginal symptoms are among the most common health concerns of women who are of reproductive age and older. The symptoms may be experienced by women who are married or single, sexually active or sexually abstinent, and premenopausal or postmenopausal.[1] It has been estimated that more than 25% of women's visits to sexually transmitted disease (STD) clinics are related to infectious vaginitis or vulvovaginitis.[2] In addition, approximately 10% of office visits to primary care providers are in response to vaginal symptoms.[3] About 40% of women who experience vaginal symptoms have some type of vaginal infection. The three most common vaginal infections are bacterial vaginosis, trichomoniasis, and vulvovaginal candidiasis (VVC). Bacterial vaginosis (the commonly accepted term for noninflammatory vaginal infections) is the most common type, affecting 33% to 52% of women with vulvovaginal symptoms; VVC accounts for about 20% to 25% of infections, and

Editor's Note: This chapter is based, in part, on the 11th edition chapter titled "Vaginal and Menstrual Products," which was written by Leslie A. Shimp and Constance M. Fleming.

trichomoniasis accounts for about 7% to 14%. Infections may also be mixed, with more than one causative organism, and vaginal symptoms may be noninfectious (e.g., atrophic vaginitis, allergic or chemical dermatologic reaction).[1,2]

Common symptoms of vaginitis may include vaginal discharge, pruritus (itching), irritation, soreness, dysuria (pain on urination), and dyspareunia (pain during sexual intercourse).[2] Unfortunately, although each of the most common vaginal infections has its own characteristic signs and symptoms, distinguishing one infection from another is often difficult for clinicians. Symptoms may be similar for different infections, and characteristic symptoms are often absent in patients.[4,5] Vaginal infections are generally perceived as minor health problems. However, recently, bacterial vaginosis has been linked to pelvic inflammatory disease (PID),[6] and both bacterial vaginosis and trichomoniasis have been linked to an increased risk for premature birth and a greater risk for acquiring human immunodeficiency virus (HIV) from an infected partner.[7,8] In view of the large number of women seeking diagnosis and treatment for vaginal infections and the approval of vaginal antifungal compounds for nonprescription use, it is imperative that pharmacists understand the therapeutic management of these three vaginal infections.

Besides VVC, women are able to self-treat vaginal dryness. Many women also use douches for routine vaginal hygiene. Unfortunately, women are not always knowledgeable about normal vaginal health and the consequences of improper douching methods. Therefore, women (as consumers) and pharmacists (as health care providers) need to understand vaginal health to make informed and appropriate decisions about self-care for vaginal symptoms and vaginal hygiene.

Anatomy and Physiology of the Vagina

The vagina, often referred to as the female genital tract or birth canal, extends 7 to 9 cm in length from the vestibule to the cervix of the uterus. The anatomic position of the vagina is dorsal to the urinary bladder and ventral to the rectum. The lower end of the vagina is encompassed by paired masses of erectile tissue on either side of the vaginal opening. The vagina itself is void of glands; most lubrication comes from glands found in the cervix.[9]

The mature vagina is colonized by a variety of organisms, including certain species of *Lactobacillus*, *Streptococcus*, and *Staphylococcus*. *Candida albicans* may also be isolated in the absence of active infection in about 20% of women. The usual ratio of anaerobic to aerobic bacteria is 5 : 1. Various factors determine the number and type of endogenous organisms, including vaginal pH, glycogen concentration, and glucose content. The normal vagina has an acidic pH (usually between 3.5 and 4.5). This relatively acid environment is maintained by lactic acid production from bacteria and vaginal epithelial cells that use glycogen and glucose as substrates. *Lactobacillus* species aid both in maintaining a low pH (lactic acid production) and in preventing overgrowth by potential vaginal pathogens (production of hydrogen peroxide).

The healthy vagina is cleansed daily by secretions that lubricate the vaginal tract. The normal vaginal discharge, referred to as leukorrhea, consists of about 1.5 g of vaginal fluid daily, which is odorless and clear or white. This discharge, which consists of endocervical mucus, endogenous vaginal flora, and epithelial cells,[10] is a normal physiologic response to vaginal irritants, including feminine hygiene deodorant products, vaginal douches and other cleansing products, contraceptive products and devices, or tampons. In addition, an increase in mucus production is normal during ovulation, sexual excitement, or emotional flares.

In summary, normal vaginal physiologic mechanisms maintain an environment that discourages the overgrowth of pathogenic organisms. When this environment is altered, the potential for infection is increased.

This environment is often altered during perimenopause and menopause by the decline in estrogen levels. This decline affects many tissues because estrogen receptors are located throughout the body. Some degree of estrogen-deprivation symptoms are experienced by almost all perimenopausal and postmenopausal women. The most common symptoms are hot flashes, sleep disturbances, and vaginal dryness. Emotional symptoms may also be present, although clinical trials have not been able to demonstrate that either menopause or decreased estrogen levels are a cause of emotional disturbances.[11]

Bacterial Vaginosis

Epidemiology of Bacterial Vaginosis

Bacterial vaginosis affects approximately one-third of women with vaginal symptoms.[1] It is unclear whether bacterial vaginosis is sexually transmitted. The risk for bacterial vaginosis is increased with a new sexual partner, and the occurrence of bacterial vaginosis has been linked to the risk for several sexually transmitted diseases (e.g., *Chlamydia pneumoniae, Neisseria gonorrhoeae*).[1] Another predisposing factors is the use of an intrauterine device (IUD).[1]

Etiology of Bacterial Vaginosis

Historically, bacterial vaginosis has been referred to by several names, including "nonspecific vaginitis," *Haemophilus* vaginitis, and *Gardnerella* vaginitis. The organisms responsible for this infection are not well defined. However, bacterial vaginosis is the result of a change in normal vaginal flora with an increase in *G. vaginalis* and several anaerobes (e.g., *Peptostreptococcus, Mobiluncus, Bacteroides*) and a decrease in lactobacilli.[1,2] Women lacking lactobacilli, particularly lactobacilli that produce hydrogen peroxide, are more likely to develop bacterial vaginosis.[1]

Signs and Symptoms of Bacterial Vaginosis

Half of the women with bacterial vaginosis are asymptomatic. Common symptoms include a vaginal discharge with a "fishy" odor, itching, and an increased quantity of discharge (colored white, yellow, green, or gray).[1] The hallmark symptom of a fishy odor is the result of aromatic amines produced by the change in vaginal organisms; it is most prominent during menses and following intercourse with exposure to alkaline semen.

Complications of Bacterial Vaginosis

In general, bacterial vaginosis is benign, rarely resulting in adverse health outcomes. However, it may be associated with PID, preterm labor and premature rupture of the fetal membranes, and urinary tract infections.[4]

Treatment of Bacterial Vaginosis

Treatment of bacterial vaginosis requires prescription medications. The routine treatment of sexual partners is not warranted for this vaginal infection.

Trichomoniasis

Epidemiology of Trichomoniasis

Trichomoniasis is primarily a disease of young women; two-thirds of cases occur in women 30 years of age or younger.[12] Other predisposing factors are multiple sex partners, a new sexual partner, and the presence of other STDs. Approximately 30% of women with *Trichomonas* vaginitis have another STD.

Etiology of Trichomoniasis

Trichomoniasis is caused by the protozoa *Trichomonas vaginalis* and is classified as an STD. Physician visits in the United States for trichomoniasis have declined by 40% over the past two decades; this decline follows a similar trend worldwide.[12]

Signs and Symptoms of Trichomoniasis

Between 50% and 75% of women complain of a profuse vaginal discharge that is often thin and frothy or foamy. This discharge may be white, yellow, or gray and occasionally may be malodorous ("fishy"). Less frequently, women report lower abdominal pain, pruritus, and/or fever. These symptoms most commonly occur during or immediately following menstruation.[1,2,4] However, between 10% and 50% of women are asymptomatic.[2]

Treatment of Trichomoniasis

As with bacterial vaginosis, trichomoniasis requires treatment with prescription medications. Successful treatment requires concurrent treatment of sexual partners of patients with trichomoniasis.

Vulvovaginal Candidiasis

Epidemiology of Vulvovaginal Candidiasis

Approximately 25% of women with vaginal symptoms have VVC. About 75% of women experience at least one candidal vaginal infection during their childbearing years, and up to 40% experience at least one subsequent infection. Approximately 50% of women attending college have had a physician-diagnosed episode of VVC, also referred to as "yeast infection" and "moniliasis," by 25 years of age.[13] However, only a small percentage of women (less than 5%) experience recurrent VVC.[2,14]

A number of physiologic and behavioral factors have been studied as possible risk factors for VVC. These factors include pregnancy, use of estrogen-containing oral contraceptives, use of an IUD, use of barrier contraceptives, diabetes mellitus, diet (rich in sugars or yeast), treatment with broad-spectrum antibiotics or immunosuppressant drugs, HIV infection, tight-fitting clothing (e.g., pantyhose), gastrointestinal (GI) colonization, and sexual activity (frequent intercourse or receptive oral sex).[1,2,14–16]

Estrogens are thought to maintain the glycogen content and thickness of vaginal epithelial cells and, thus, to ensure the integrity of the protective lining of the vaginal tract.[17] The vagina may be more susceptible to candidal infections during pregnancy or use of estrogen-containing oral contraceptives or postmenopausal estrogen replacement therapy. This susceptibility may be because estrogen increases the glycogen content of the vagina or alters immune function, thus decreasing the ability of cells to resist infection. In addition, *Candida* organisms contain estrogen and progesterone receptors that, when stimulated, result in their proliferation.[14] However, studies[18] do not support an increased risk for candidal infections with low-dose oral contraceptives, and studies on risk during pregnancy are inconsistent. Vaginal pH increases during menstruation, and this increase may predispose menstruating women to cyclic fungal vaginal infections. Conversely, at menopause, the decrease in glycogen leads to a decrease in lactic acid and an increase in vaginal pH that can alter vaginal ecology and may predispose to vaginal infections.

Women with diabetes mellitus are known to be at greater risk for skin and vaginal candidal infections, particularly if glycemic control is poor.

Studies associating the higher levels of urinary sugar with the greater risk for candidal vaginal infections have suggested that diet is an important factor. Foods shown to produce elevated urinary sugar are milk (more than 1 quart per day), yogurt, cottage cheese, and artificial sweeteners. More studies are needed to determine the importance of diet as a risk factor for candidal vaginal infections. Paradoxically, it has been suggested that consumption of yogurt may have a potential prophylactic benefit against VVC.[19]

A number of patients (25% to 70% in several studies) report developing candidal vaginal infections during or just after treatment with broad-spectrum antibiotics such as tetracycline, ampicillin/amoxicillin, and cephalosporins.[18,20] The proposed mechanism is a decrease in normal vaginal flora, especially lactobacilli, allowing an overgrowth of *Candida* organisms. However, neither an increase in vaginal *Candida* organisms nor a decrease in lactobacilli occurs in all women who have taken antibiotics. Most women who demonstrate an increase in *Candida* organisms in the vagina are asymptomatic. Nonetheless, a subgroup of patients may be susceptible to VVC following exposure to systemic antibiotics.

Patients who are taking systemic corticosteroid, antineoplastic, or immunosuppressant drugs may be at increased risk for developing candidal infections. This risk is well known for certain patient populations, such as recipients of an organ transplant and patients with acquired immunodeficiency syndrome (AIDS).

Studies do not demonstrate a consistent association between tight-fitting, nonabsorbent clothing or pantyhose and vaginal candidal infections. Clothing of this type may increase risk by creating a warm and moist environment.

A GI reservoir of *Candida* organisms with the transfer of the organism from the rectum to the vagina was thought to explain recurrent vaginal candidal infections in some patients. However, further studies found that vaginal infections recurred even though rectal cultures for *Candida* organisms were decreased or negative, following oral antifungal therapy. It has been suggested that simultaneous oral and vaginal antifungal therapy may provide better cure rates; however, long-term studies are needed.

One study found that the frequency of sexual intercourse was related to the likelihood of candidal vaginal infections. The author suggested that sexual intercourse may facilitate movement of *Candida* organisms into the vagina and cause minor vaginal trauma that results in an increased risk for vaginitis. It is also possible that greater exposure to semen may increase the risk for VVC as seminal fluid promotes mycelial formation and increases the virulence of *Candida* organisms.[16] There is also some evidence suggesting an increase in risk associated with receptive oral sex.[1] The treatment of candidal vaginal infections does not, however, include treatment of the male partner. No controlled studies have shown that treatment of male partners prevents recurrence of candidal vaginal infections in women.

Despite the association of *Candida* vulvovaginitis to the above risk factors, none of the risk factors is consistently associated with symptomatic candidal vaginitis. The presence of these risk factors does not clearly establish an increased likelihood of VVC in a patient with vaginal symptoms. Most women with sporadic and infrequent candidal vaginitis do not have a readily apparent "cause" for the infection.[13] In addition, modification of factors linked to VVC is not warranted for most patients.[1]

Etiology of Vulvovaginal Candidiasis

Candida fungi are the causative organisms of this vaginal infection; about 80% to 90% of cases are caused by *C. albicans*.[15] The incidence of non–*C. albicans* infections has increased in the past two decades, and *C. tropicalis* and *C. glabrata* now account for a significant minority of candidal vaginal infections.[12]

Signs and Symptoms of Vulvovaginal Candidiasis

The characteristic symptoms of VVC are intense pruritus; a thick, whitish vaginal discharge (often referred to as "curd-like" or "cottage cheese–like") with no offensive odor; and vulvar or vaginal erythema.[2,4] Symptoms of vaginal fungal infection often occur the week before menses and improve with the onset of menses.

Although itching and the characteristic discharge are the usual symptoms of a candidal vaginal infection, itching is not specific to VVC. For many patients with a candidal infection, the vaginal discharge is minimal or does not conform to the characteristic discharge.[18] Most symptomatic women experience vaginal or vulvar pruritus and/or irritation, but fewer than one-half report a vaginal discharge and few report an odor to the discharge. The symptom most apt to differentiate a candidal vaginal infection from that of bacterial vaginosis and trichomoniasis is the absence of an offensive odor of the vaginal discharge.[21] Urinary tract symptoms (e.g., frequency, dysuria) are infrequent symptoms of candidal infections.[2,5]

Treatment of Vulvovaginal Candidiasis

VVC is the second most common type of vaginal infection. The treatment of this disorder, including lost productivity, is estimated to cost approximately $1 billion annually.[18]

Treatment Outcomes

The goal of therapy for vaginal fungal infections is eradication of the infection (i.e., cure of the patient) and reestablishment of normal vaginal flora. A single course of drug therapy is effective in achieving these goals for virtually all patients. However, a small percentage of patients will experience persistent or recurrent infections and will require prolonged therapy or higher doses of medication.

General Treatment Approach

Self-treatment of VVC with nonprescription antifungal therapy can be appropriate for some patients, whereas others should be referred for assessment and treatment by a

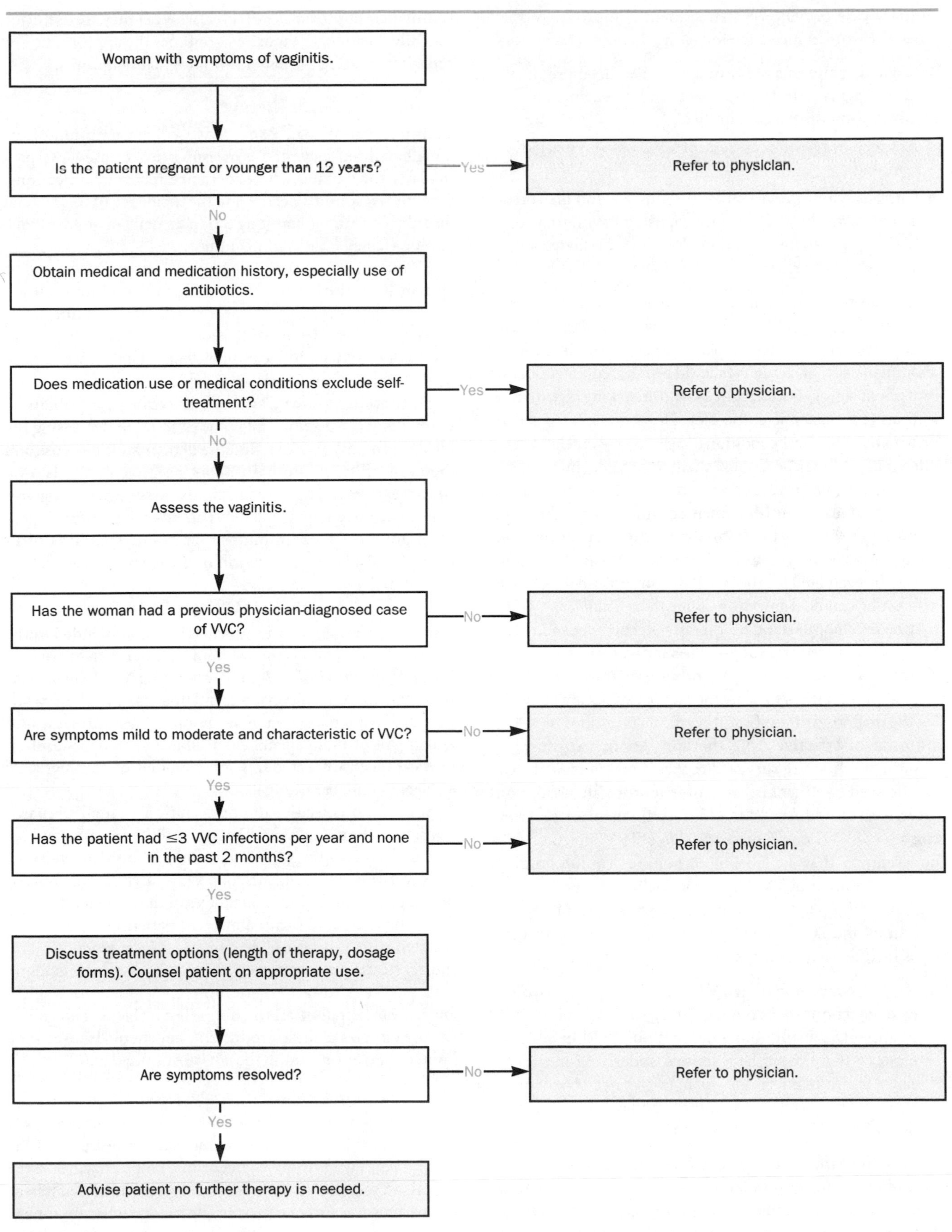

Figure 6–1 Self-care of vulvovaginal candidiasis.

primary care provider. Self-treatment is most appropriate when the woman meets the following three criteria:

- Vaginal symptoms are infrequent (i.e., no more than three vaginal infections per year and no vaginal infection within the past 2 months).
- At least one previous episode of VVC was physician diagnosed.
- Current symptoms are mild to moderate and are consistent with the characteristic signs and symptoms of VVC—in particular, a nonmalodorous discharge and an absence of urinary tract symptoms.

Self-treatment is inappropriate for women who are pregnant and for girls younger than 12 years. Similarly, patients with concurrent symptoms, such as fever or pain in the lower abdomen, back, or shoulder, should be referred for evaluation by a physician, as should patients who are taking certain medications (e.g., systemic corticosteroids, antineoplastic agents) or who have medical conditions (e.g., diabetes mellitus, HIV infection) that may predispose them to candidal infections.

By definition, recurrent VVC occurs when a woman experiences at least four (documented) infections within a 12-month period.[22] Self-treatment is not appropriate for recurrent vaginal symptoms. Patients with such symptoms should be evaluated for the possibility of a mixed infection or a strain of candidal infection other than *C. albicans*, which may be resistant to standard therapy. Recurrent candidal infections often require long-term suppressive prophylactic therapy. Repeated use of the nonprescription antifungal vaginal preparations for chronic vaginal symptoms may delay the diagnosis of important medical conditions or the institution of effective drug therapy. About two-thirds of physicians who were surveyed reported seeing patients who had delayed treatment because of inappropriate use of nonprescription products.[20] In addition, frequent or recurrent episodes of VVC may be an early sign of HIV infection. FDA now requires that the labeling of nonprescription products for the treatment of VVC infection include a statement that indicates the possible association between recurrent candidal infections and HIV. The warnings section of these medications includes statements similar to the one that follows:

> If your symptoms return within 2 months or if you have infections that do not clear up easily with proper treatment, consult your doctor. You could be pregnant, or there could be a serious underlying medical cause for your infections, such as diabetes or a damaged immune system (including damage from infection with HIV, the virus that causes AIDS).

Preventive measures are not a standard part of therapy for vaginal fungal infections. However, women with such infections that are not responsive to antifungal therapy may try dietary changes, nondrug measures, or alteration in other drug therapy known to be a risk factor for VVC. A 3- to 4-month trial of these approaches will reveal whether they are useful for individual patients.[1] Figure 6–1 outlines the appropriate approach to treating the patient with vaginal symptoms.

Nonpharmacologic Therapy

Consumption of yogurt and decreased consumption of sucrose have been suggested as measures to decrease VVC, particularly for women who experience recurrent infections. One study[19] found a decrease in the incidence of this vaginal disorder in women ingesting 8 ounces daily of yogurt (containing viable *L. acidophilus* cultures).

Home remedies such as vaginal douches of yogurt or vinegar have also been used to treat this condition but are generally not effective.[17] However, use of a sodium bicarbonate sitz bath may provide prompt relief of vulvar irritation associated with a candidal vaginal infection before benefit from an antifungal agent.[13]

Discontinuing a drug known to increase susceptibility to vaginal fungal infections might be effective in decreasing the incidence of this disorder. Because of their long-term use and the availability of alternative contraceptive methods, oral contraceptives might be discontinued to see whether the frequency of infections is altered. Patients taking broad-spectrum antibiotics or immunosuppressants should consult their physician before discontinuing these medications.

Pharmacologic Therapy (Vaginal Antifungals)

Currently, an imidazole product is the recommended initial therapy for VVC. Four topical imidazole derivatives are now available in the United States for treating VVC: butoconazole, clotrimazole, miconazole, and tioconazole. These products are available as vaginal creams, suppositories, and tablets. All of these agents are available as nonprescription medications. (See Table 6–1 for examples of commercially available vaginal antifungals.)

Several nonspecific, nonprescription vaginal preparations, including Vagisil and Yeast-Gard (benzocaine and resorcinol) and Vaginex (tripelennamine), are also available. However, use of these agents for VVC is rarely, if ever, appropriate, given the obvious advantages of the azole antifungals, including superior efficacy, improved patient compliance associated with ease of use, less frequent local reactions, and shorter treatment durations. The nonspecific products, along with medicated douches, are more appropriate for vaginal and vulvar irritation and itching. (See Table 6–2 for additional examples of these products.) They should be used for a limited time or only upon the advice of a physician.

Mechanism of Action

The major antifungal effect of the imidazole compounds is accomplished by altering the membrane permeability of the fungi. These agents inhibit cytochrome P-450 enzymes in the fungal cell membrane, thereby decreasing synthesis of the essential fungal sterol ergosterol. The reduced membrane ergosterol content is accompanied by a corresponding increase in lanosterol-like methylated sterols. These lanosterol-like sterols cause structural damage to fungal membranes, resulting in the loss of normal membrane function.

Pharmacokinetics

The topical vaginal imidazole preparations are not appreciably absorbed. Studies of butoconazole and clotrimazole found that about 5% and between 3% and 10% of a vaginal dose were systemically absorbed, respectively. Fungicidal clotrimazole concentrations were detectable in the vaginal fluid for up to 3 days after a single 500-mg intravaginal dose.[23] A study[24] of intravaginally administered radiolabeled miconazole demonstrated that approximately 1% of the dose was excreted in the urine and that the radioactivity of whole blood was too low for measurement.

Indications

Nonprescription imidazoles are FDA-approved for local treatment of VVC and for relief of external vulvar itching and irritation associated with the infection.

Dosage/Administration Guidelines

Studies have shown the imidazoles to be equally effective, with effectiveness rates of approximately 85% to 90%.[10,17] Different treatment durations have been studied. Today, the 7-day regimens of clotrimazole and miconazole, the 3-day regimens of butoconazole and miconazole, and the 1-day regimen of tioconazole are available without a prescription. Table 6–1 lists the recommended nonprescription dosage regimens for products containing these ingredients. Information on currently available prescription and nonprescription products and regimens for acute infections, recurrent infections, and prophylactic therapy is presented in several reviews.[1,4,18]

Table 6–3 describes the proper procedure for administering vaginal antifungals.

Adverse Effects

Side effects from topical therapy are minimal. Topical imidazoles are associated with vulvovaginal burning, itching, and irritation in about 7% of patients.[25] These side effects are more likely to occur with the initial application of the vaginal preparation and are similar to symptoms of the vaginal infection. Abdominal cramps (3%) plus penile irritation and allergic reactions (3% to 7%) are uncommon; headache may occur in up to 9% of women.[1]

Table 6–1

Selected Vaginal Antifungal Products and Their Dosages

Trade Name	Primary Ingredient	Dosage
Femstat 3 Cream	Butoconazole nitrate 2%	Insert cream into vagina once daily for 3 days; apply to vulva twice daily as needed for itching
Gyne-Lotrimin Cream	Clotrimazole 1%	Insert cream into vagina once daily for 7 days; apply to vulva twice daily as needed for itching
Gyne-Lotrimin 3 Combination Pack	Cream: clotrimazole 1%; tablet: clotrimazole 200 mg	Apply cream to vulva twice daily as needed for itching; insert tablet into vagina once daily for 3 days
Gyne-Lotrimin Suppositories	Clotrimazole 100 mg	Insert suppository into vagina once daily for 7 days
Gyne-Lotrimin 3 Suppositories	Clotrimazole 200 mg	Insert suppository into vagina once daily for 3 days
Monistat 3 Cream	Miconazole nitrate 4%	Insert cream into vagina once daily for 3 days; apply to vulva twice daily as needed for itching
Monistat 3 Combination Pack	Cream: miconazole nitrate 2%; suppository: miconazole nitrate 200 mg	Apply cream to vulva twice daily as needed for itching; insert suppository into vagina once daily for 3 days
Monistat 7 Suppository	Miconazole nitrate 100 mg	Insert suppository into vagina once daily for 7 days
Monistat 7 Cream	Miconazole nitrate 2%	Insert cream into vagina once daily for 7 days; apply to vulva twice daily as needed for itching
Monistat 7 Combination Pack	Cream: miconazole nitrate 2%; suppository: miconazole nitrate 200 mg	Apply cream to vulva twice daily as needed for itching; insert suppository into vagina once daily for 7 days
Mycelex-3 Cream	Butoconazole nitrate 2%	Insert cream into vagina once daily for 3 days; apply to vulva twice daily as needed for itching
Mycelex-7 Cream	Clotrimazole 1%	Insert cream into vagina once daily for 7 days; apply to vulva twice daily as needed for itching
Mycelex-7 Suppositories	Clotrimazole 1%	Insert suppository into vagina once daily for 7 days
Vagistat-1 Ointment	Tioconazole 6.5%	Insert ointment into vagina once daily for 1 day

Table 6–2

Selected Products for Vaginal Itching and Irritation

Trade Name	Primary Ingredients
Benzocaine Products[a]	
Lanacane Creme	Benzocaine 6%; benzethonium chloride 0.1%
Vagisil Cream	Benzocaine 5%
Vagisil Maximum Strength	Benzocaine 20%
Vagi-Gard Cream	Benzocaine 5%; benzalkonium chloride 0.13%
Hydrocortisone Products[b]	
Cortef Feminine Itch Cream	Hydrocortisone 0.5%
Gyne-cort Cream	Hydrocortisone 0.5%
Gyne-cort Extra Strength Cream 10	Hydrocortisone 1%
Massengill Medicated Towelette	Hydrocortisone 0.5%
Povidone–Iodine Products	
Betadine Medicated Douche Concentrate	Povidone-iodine 0.3% (when diluted)
Betadine Medicated Suppository[c]	Povidone-iodine 10%
Betadine Premixed Medicated Disposable Douche	Povidone-iodine 0.3% (in disposable bottles)
Massengill Medicated Disposable Douche	Povidone-iodine 0.3%
Summer's Eve Special Care Medicated Douche	Povidone-iodine 0.3%
Vagi-Gard Medicated Douche Concentrate	Povidone iodine 0.3% (when diluted)
Other Products	
Summer's Eve Feminine Powder[d]	Cornstarch, aloe, mineral oil
Vaginex[e]	Tripelennamine
Vagisil Feminine Powder[d]	Cornstarch, aloe, mineral oil
Yeast-Gard Suppository[f]	*Pulsatilla* (28x); *Candida albicans* (28x)
Yeast-X Suppository[g]	*Pulsatilla* (28x)

[a] Apply benzocaine products externally.
[b] Apply hydrocortisone products externally; avoid prolonged use; may use concomitantly with antifungal products.
[c] Use one povidone–iodoine suppository nightly for 7 days.
[d] Apply feminine powders externally to absorb moisture.
[e] Apply Vaginex externally 3 to 4 times daily.
[f] Use one Yeast-Gard suppository daily for 7 days.
[g] Use one Yeast-X suppository daily as needed.

Contraindications/Precautions/Warnings

Aside from an allergy to the imidazoles, there are no contraindications to use of the vaginal imidazoles.

Special Population Considerations

Self-treatment of VVC is not appropriate for girls who are younger than 12 years. This disorder is rare in premenarchal girls and warrants clinician evaluation.

The topical imidazole antifungals are generally safe for use during pregnancy. Clotrimazole is the preferred agent for use during pregnancy. (This agent has a Pregnancy Category B rating.) Treatment regimens of 6 to 7 days with these agents provide good effectiveness without risk to the fetus.[1] However, self-treatment during pregnancy is not appropriate. Clinician assessment is important to ascertain lack of complications (e.g., elevated blood sugar) and to assess for other vaginal organisms, because bacterial vaginosis and trichomoniasis have the potential for adverse pregnancy outcomes.

Product Selection Guidelines

Selection of cream, tablet, or suppository formulations can be left to patient preference. Studies have found that women who have previously experienced VVC prefer shorter courses of therapy than do women who have not had a prior infection; physicians also tend to prefer longer courses of therapy.[1] If vulvar symptoms are significant, a cream preparation or the combination of a cream with vaginal suppositories or tablets is preferred so that vulvar application can accompany intravaginal administration.

Table 6–3

Guidelines for Applying Vaginal Antifungal Products

1. Start treatment at night before going to bed. Lying down will reduce leakage of the product from the vagina.
2. Wash the entire vaginal area with mild soap and water, and dry completely before applying the product.
3. To open the tube, unscrew the cap; place the cap upside down on the end of the tube. Push down firmly until the seal is broken. (For vaginal tablets/suppositories, remove the protective wrapper.)

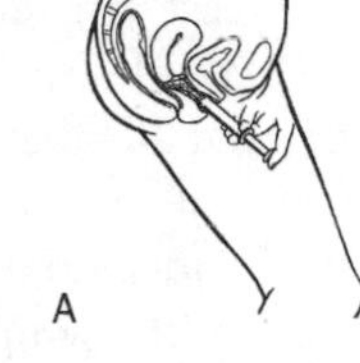

4. Attach the applicator to the tube by turning the applicator clockwise. (For vaginal tablets/suppositories, place the product into the end of the applicator barrel.)
5. Squeeze the tube from the bottom to force the cream into the applicator. Squeeze until the inside piece of the applicator is pushed out as far as possible and the applicator is completely filled with cream. Remove the applicator from the tube.
6. While standing with your feet slightly apart and your knees bent as shown in drawing A or while lying on your back with your knees bent as shown in drawing B, gently insert the applicator into the vagina as far as it will go comfortably.
7. Push the inside piece of the applicator in and place the cream as far back in the vagina as possible. (To deposit vaginal tablets/suppositories, insert the applicator into the vagina and press the plunger until it stops.)
8. Remove the applicator from the vagina.
9. After use, recap the tube (if using cream). Then clean the applicator by pulling the two pieces apart and washing them with soap and warm water.
10. If desired, wear a sanitary pad to absorb leakage of the vaginal antifungal. Do not use a tampon to absorb leakage.
11. Continue using the product for the length of time specified in the product instructions. Use the product on consecutive days, even during menstrual flow.

B

Alternative Remedies

An alternative approach to treating VVC is the use of *Lactobacillus* preparations. The rationale for use of the *Lactobacillus* preparations is to reestablish normal vaginal flora and to inhibit overgrowth of *Candida* organisms.

Gentian violet (a dye) is an old treatment for VVC that is generally used today as a therapy for resistant candidal infections. However, it is available on the nonprescription market and can be used as topical therapy; a tampon can be soaked in the dye and inserted into the vagina. The tampon is left in the vagina for several hours or overnight. Often a single application is adequate, but a treated tampons can be used once or twice a day for up to 5 consecutive days. The major disadvantage to use of gentian violet is that it stains fabrics and can stain skin.[26]

Patient Assessment of Vulvovaginal Candidiasis

As noted previously, differentiating vaginal infections on the basis of reported signs and symptoms is difficult. However, given the availability of nonprescription topical vaginal antifungal preparations and the cost and inconvenience of physician evaluation, many patients prefer to self-treat empirically for presumed VVC. Pharmacists can advise patients when it is appropriate to self-treat for vaginal symptoms and when physician evaluation, including pelvic examination and laboratory examination of vaginal secretions, is indicated.

Most episodes of VVC are uncomplicated and can be effectively treated by topical antifungal agents.[13] In particular, women who experience episodes that are sporadic and uncomplicated (i.e., healthy women who are not immunocompromised and have no predisposing drug therapy) and women who predictably experience VVC following a course of antibiotic therapy are the best candidates for self-treatment.[13,18]

In one study that examined physician attitude toward the availability of nonprescription antifungals, more than 40% of physicians stated they would encourage patients who had previously experienced a diagnosed candidal vaginal infection to self-assess and self-treat similar subsequent vaginal symptoms.[20] One study of more than 250 university students found that 70% of the women had self-diagnosed and treated what they believed to be a case of VVC, and 93% reported that their infection was cured.[27] However, 20% of women who reported self-diagnosing a candidal vaginal infection had never been treated for VVC by a physician or nurse practitioner.

One of the most important aspects of advising patients who are considering self-treatment of vaginal symptoms is being sure that they have previously had a clinician-diagnosed candidal vaginal infection. Given the remarkable lack of consistency of signs and symptoms between patients, it is important for a woman to know how vaginal fungal infections present for her. To emphasize this point, a study found that, when women who had previously had diagnosed VVC read a description of a woman with classic symptoms of the infection, only 35% could accurately recognize the case description as a candidal vaginal infection.[28]

Asking the patient the following questions will help elicit the information needed to accurately assess the signs and symptoms, and to recommend the appropriate treatment approach.

Q~ What symptoms are you currently experiencing? Are you experiencing an abnormal vaginal discharge? Is your vaginal discharge discolored or accompanied by itching and burning or by an abnormal odor? Are the symptoms the same as or different from symptoms you experienced during previous (at least one clinician-diagnosed) vaginal fungal infections?

A~ *Identify the typical signs and symptoms of VVC. (See the section "Signs and Symptoms of Vulvovaginal*

Candidiasis.") Strongly suspect a vaginal fungal infection if the characteristic symptoms of VVC are described, especially the absence of an unpleasant odor to vaginal secretions, or if the symptoms are similar to those associated with a previous, diagnosed episode of VVC.

Q~ How would you rate the severity of your symptoms?

A~ Recommend self-treatment if the symptoms are mild to moderate. For local symptoms that are more intense or bothersome, recommend a longer course of therapy (i.e., 7-day therapy) and adjunctive measures (e.g., sodium bicarbonate sitz bath) to help alleviate vulvar symptoms until the antifungal agent reduces the number of yeast organisms.[13] If symptoms are severe, particularly those that are localized (e.g., bladder symptoms, feeling "ill"), or if the patient has not had a previous, diagnosed episode of VVC, refer the patient to a physician.

Q~ What medication(s) are you currently taking? Are you taking (or have you recently taken) an antibiotic, oral contraceptives, corticosteroids, or cancer chemotherapy?

A~ Refer a patient taking any immunosuppressant known to be a risk factor for VVC to a physician for evaluation.

Q~ What medication(s) or other treatments (e.g., douching) have you used to manage or alleviate your symptoms (for prior episodes or during this episode)? How long ago did the previous episode occur?

A~ If the new episode has occurred within 2 months of a previous episode, refer the patient to a physician for treatment of possible recurrent or resistant VVC. If the previous episode was longer than 2 months ago but self-treatment of current symptoms has been ineffective, determine whether the patient used the products correctly. Then counsel as needed. For untreated new episodes occurring longer than 2 months after a previous episode, consider previous successful treatments and the patient's preferred dosage forms when recommending a product.

Q~ Do you have diabetes mellitus or HIV infection or AIDS? Are you pregnant?

A~ If the patient has diabetes or HIV infection or AIDs, refer the patient for medical treatment and evaluation of glycemic control. Refer pregnant patients to a physician because these women may need longer courses of therapy than those available for nonprescription antifungals.[18]

Q~ Are there any factors that seem to predispose you to develop candidal vaginitis?

A~ Use the patient's description of "causative" agents to help confirm the assessment of VVC and to provide clues as to how to prevent these infections. Refer any patient with frequent episodes for evaluation of recurrent VVC.

Patient Counseling for Vulvovaginal Candidiasis

The pharmacist should explain to the patient that a short course of a nonprescription vaginal antifungal product will kill the "yeast" organisms that caused the infection. The pharmacist should also review label instructions with the patient, stressing that the antifungal is applied only once a day for the length of time specified on the label. Next the pharmacist should advise the patient when symptomatic relief will begin and that the symptoms should be resolved by the end of the product-specified duration of therapy. The patient should also be advised of signs and symptoms that indicate medical attention is needed. The box "Patient Education for Vulvovaginal Candidiasis" lists specific information to provide patients.

Evaluation of Patient Outcomes for Vulvovaginal Candidiasis

Symptoms of VVC should improve within 2 to 3 days of initiation of therapy and should resolve within 1 week. The length of treatment (particularly for 1- to 3-day treatments) does not directly correspond to the time of resolution of symptoms.

Follow-up with a phone call allows the pharmacist to discuss treatment effectiveness (continued or altered symptoms) and the importance of adherence to the course of treatment. Persistent symptoms or new-onset symptoms that are incompatible with VVC are reasons for advising the patient to see a clinician.

Atrophic Vaginitis

Epidemiology of Atrophic Vaginitis

Atrophic vaginitis is inflammation of the vagina related to atrophy of the vaginal mucosa that is secondary to decreased estrogen levels. Symptomatic atrophic vaginitis is relatively uncommon among postmenopausal and lactating women. However, dyspareunia, a symptom sometimes related to inadequate vaginal lubrication or atrophic vaginitis, appears more common. In one primary care study, 46% of sexually active women reported dyspareunia; other studies reported a prevalence of 17% to 34% (a result of varying definitions of dyspareunia).[29]

Etiology of Atrophic Vaginitis

During menopause, the postpartum period, and breast-feeding, vaginal lubrication declines secondary to a decrease in

Patient Education for Vulvovaginal Candidiasis

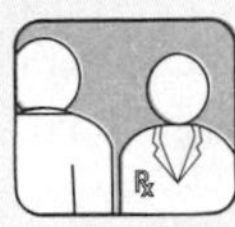

The objectives of self-treatment are to eradicate the vaginal fungal infection and to reestablish normal vaginal flora. For most patients, carefully following the product instructions and the self-care measures listed below will help ensure optimal therapeutic outcomes.

Nondrug Measures

- If significant irritation of the vulva is present, use a sodium bicarbonate sitz bath to provide relief and to give the antifungal agent time to become effective.
- If you have recurrent infections, try eating yogurt and decreasing sugar in your diet to see whether these measures help.

Nonprescription Medications

- Insert the antifungal product into the vagina once a day, preferably at bedtime to avoid leakage from the vagina. If desired, use a sanitary pad to avoid staining of underwear.
- See Table 6–3 for instructions on administering vaginal antifungals. Expect significant relief of symptoms within 24 to 48 hours. Some relief is often apparent within hours after the first dose.
- Continue the therapy for the recommended length of time even if the symptoms are gone. Stopping treatment early is one of the most common reasons for recurrence of vaginal symptoms and, possibly, occurrence of resistant organisms.
- Note that vaginal antifungals can be used during a menstrual period. If desired, wait and treat the infection after the period ends. Do not, however, interrupt a course of therapy because your period begins.
- Do not use tampons while using a vaginal antifungal product.
- Although side effects are uncommon, note that the first dose of the antifungal may cause some vaginal burning and irritation and that a few women (about 1 in 10) experience a headache.
- Refrain from sexual intercourse during treatment with the vaginal antifungals. Note that vaginal antifungals can damage latex condoms and diaphragms and may result in unreliable contraceptive effects. Do not use these contraceptives during therapy or for 3 days after therapy because the drug remains in the vagina for several days.
- Do not use vaginal antifungals if you meet any of the following criteria:
  —You are under age 12 years.
  —You are pregnant.
  —You have diabetes mellitus, are HIV positive or have AIDS, or have impaired immune function.
- If you are breast-feeding, consult a physician before using a vaginal antifungal.

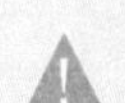

Seek medical attention if symptoms do not improve within 3 days or if symptoms persist beyond 7 days.

Seek medical attention if vaginal symptoms worsen or change, especially if the vaginal secretions become malodorous, frothy, or discolored or if other symptoms (e.g., abdominal tenderness) occur. These events may indicate that the *Candida* ("yeast") organisms are resistant to the nonprescription therapy or that another type of vaginal infection is present.

estrogen levels. Women may experience atrophic vaginitis and associated dyspareunia during these intervals.[30]

Signs and Symptoms of Atrophic Vaginitis

Symptoms of atrophic vaginitis include vaginal irritation, burning, itching, and dyspareunia. The most common cause of secondary superficial dyspareunia is a lack of adequate vaginal lubrication.[30]

Treatment of Vaginal Dryness Secondary to Atrophic Vaginitis

Self-treatment of atrophic vaginitis is limited to alleviating the primary symptom, vaginal dryness, with lubricants. Preventing the vaginal dryness would require prescription hormones, a measure often recommended for women at menopause. Women who are breast-feeding or have recently given childbirth usually have only temporary declines in estrogen levels. Vaginal lubricants may be needed only until estrogen levels return to normal.

Treatment Outcomes

The goal of therapy is to reduce or eliminate the symptoms of vaginal dryness, burning, and itching. If vaginal dryness causes discomfort during or interferes with sexual intercourse, a second goal of treatment is elimination of dyspareunia. Many women are likely to be inadequately treating dyspareunia given the apparent lack of knowledge about personal lubricant products.[29]

General Treatment Approach

Vaginal dryness can often be treated with nonprescription topical lubricants, such as those listed in Table 6–4. One study found that about half the women with vaginal dryness

Case Study 6–1

Patient Complaint/History

Sumona, a 34-year-old female, enters the pharmacy and requests advice on the use of a nonprescription vaginal antifungal product. Yesterday she developed a clumpy white vaginal discharge and intense vulvar itching. The patient thinks she has a "yeast" infection. She has selected Monistat 3 (200-mg) vaginal suppositories for purchase. Aside from the following symptoms, she feels fine. She is not having any discomfort with urination, nor is she having any abdominal symptoms. Further, the vaginal discharge is not malodorous.

During further conversation with the pharmacist, Sumona explains that her physician prescribed Monistat 7 suppositories for a couple of previous yeast infections that occurred about 2 years ago. Because she expects her period in the next several days, the patient asks about using suppositories during her menses.

Sumona is in good general health with no chronic medical problems. Her patient profile reveals seasonal allergic rhinitis and intermittent sinusitis but no drug allergies. She is currently taking chlorpheniramine 4 mg at bedtime or twice a day as needed; Ortho-Novum 1/35 21 1 tablet daily for 21 days (7 days off); and Sudafed 30–60 mg four times a day as needed. In addition, she began taking amoxicillin 500 mg three times a day for a sinus infection about 5 days ago; the antibiotic will be continued for another 5 days.

Clinical Considerations/Strategies

Readers can use the following considerations/strategies to determine whether treatment of this patient's disorder with nonprescription medications is warranted:

- Assess the appropriateness of self-treatment of the vaginal symptoms: Are the symptoms similar to those that the patient experienced previously? Are they consistent with VVC?
- Assess the appropriateness of the patient-selected dosage form.
- Discuss with the patient her possible risk factors for VVC.

Patient Counseling/Education

Readers can use the following strategies to develop a patient counseling/education plan that will ensure optimal therapeutic outcomes:

- Explain when to expect symptomatic relief and when a physician's evaluation is needed.
- Explain the optimal use of the vaginal antifungal agent and the potential side effects of this therapy.

had tried "something," including substances such as butter, baby oil, and petroleum jelly (Vaseline), before seeking medical attention.[31] Among women with dyspareunia in one primary care study,[29] 10% had tried a nonprescription analgesic and 62% had done nothing; there was little use of personal lubricant products.

Self-treatment is appropriate when the symptoms are mild to moderate and are confined to the vaginal area. Self-treatment is most appropriate for women who have previously been able to maintain adequate vaginal lubrication. A clinician should evaluate severe vaginal dryness or dyspareunia. Women with symptoms that are not localized should also be referred for medical evaluation. Figure 6–2 outlines the treatment of vaginal dryness associated with atrophic vaginitis.

Pharmacologic Therapy (Vaginal Lubricants)

A number of water-soluble products for vaginal lubrication (e.g., Gyne-Moistrin, K-Y Jelly, and Replens) are available on the nonprescription market. Personal lubricant products act to temporarily moisten vaginal tissues. These products provide short-term improvement in atrophic vaginal symptoms, such as relief from burning and itching. Personal lubricants can also provide adequate vaginal lubrication to facilitate sexual intercourse.

Vaseline should not be used because it is difficult to remove from the vagina. If the patient is using a latex condom or di-

Table 6–4

Selected Vaginal Lubricants

Trade Name	Primary Ingredients
Astroglide	Glycerin; propylene glycol
K-Y Jelly	Glycerin; hydroxyethylcellulose
K-Y Liquid	Glycerin; propylene glycol
K-Y Long Lasting Vaginal[a] Moisturizer Gel	Glycerin; mineral oil; hydrogenated palm oil; glyceride
Lubrin Suppositories	Caprylic/capric triglyceride; glycerin
Moist Again Vaginal Moisturizing Gel	Aloe vera; glycerin
Replens Gel	Glycerin; propylene glycol; mineral oil
Vagisil Intimate Moisturizer Lotion[a]	Glycerin; propylene glycol
Women's Health Formula Lubricating Gel	Chlorhexidine gluconate; glycerin
Wondergel Personal Liquid Gel	Glycerin; propylene glycol

[a] Fragrance-free product.

aphragm, only water-soluble lubricants should be used because other products may impair the efficacy of these contraceptive methods. Water-soluble lubricant gels can be applied both externally and internally. Initially, the patient should be instructed to use a liberal quantity of lubricant (up to 2 tablespoons) and then to tailor the quantity and frequency of use to her specific needs. If the patient is treating dyspareunia, the lubricant should be applied to both the vaginal opening and the penis. If the use of nonprescription lubricants does not produce adequate benefit or is aesthetically unappealing to the patient, she should be referred for medical evaluation.

Patient Assessment of Atrophic Vaginitis

When discussing symptoms of vaginal dryness, patient assessment should include obtaining a description of symptoms (including the association with sexual intercourse) and their severity, as well as information about whether the woman has recently given birth, is lactating, or is perimenopausal or postmenopausal. The pharmacist should question patients about the use of any vaginal or feminine hygiene products because such products may cause or worsen vaginal irritation and dyspareunia. Asking the patient the following questions will help elicit the information needed to accurately assess the disorder and to recommend the appropriate treatment approach.

Q~ What symptoms are you experiencing? Have you experienced vaginal dryness, burning, or itching (without discharge) and/or difficult or painful sexual intercourse?

A~ Strongly suspect atrophic vaginitis or vaginal dryness if the patient has these symptoms.

Q~ How severe are the symptoms?

A~ If the symptoms are severe, refer the patient to a physician.

Q~ Do any of the following situations apply to you: menopause (natural or surgical), recent childbirth, or breast-feeding?

A~ If either situation is applicable, advise the patient that a decrease in estrogen levels is probably causing the symptoms. Recommend a vaginal lubricant.

Patient Counseling for Atrophic Vaginitis

The pharmacist should stress the short-term nature of atrophic vaginitis to women who are breast-feeding or who re-

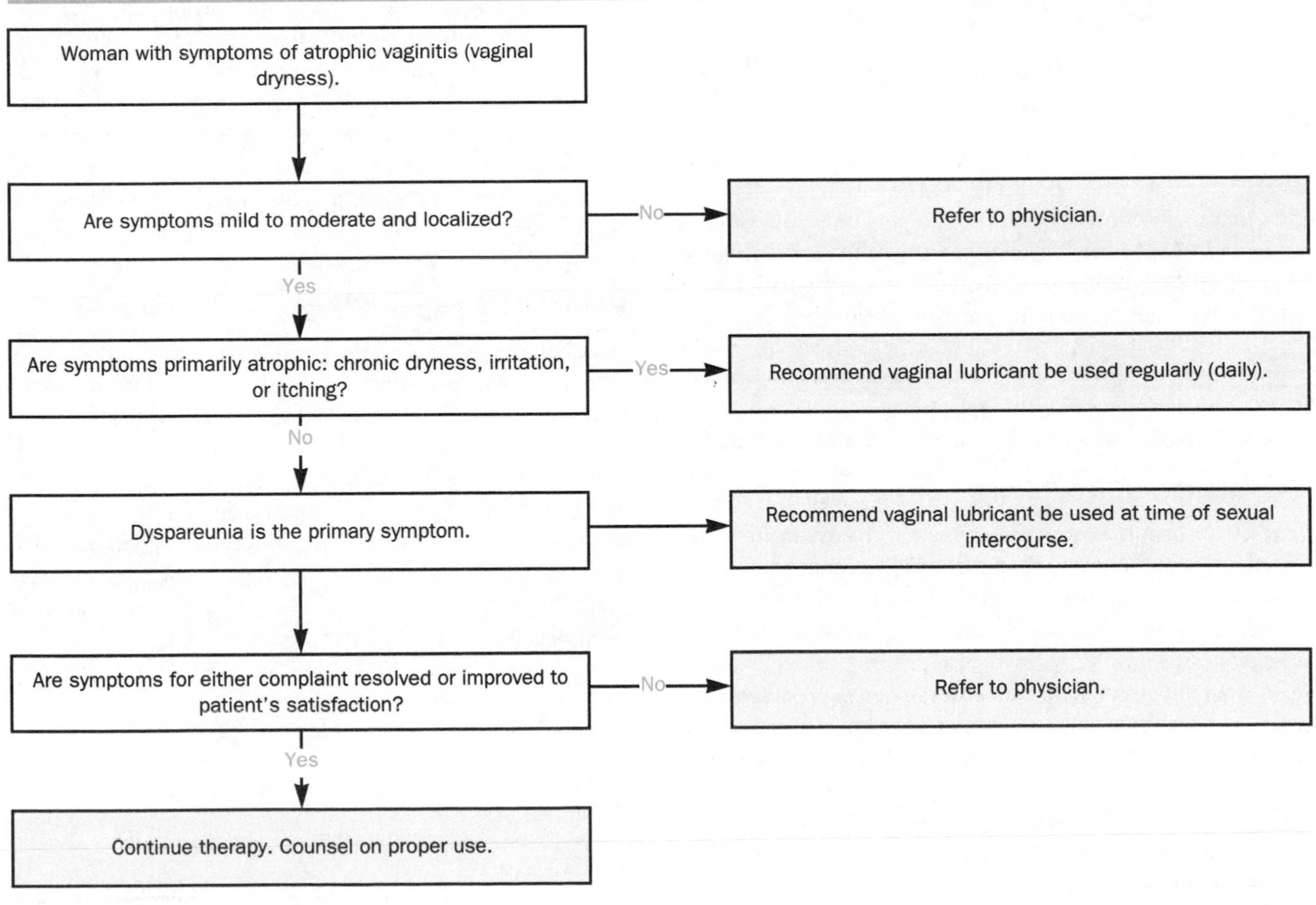

Figure 6–2 Self-care of atrophic vaginitis.

Patient Education for Atrophic Vaginitis

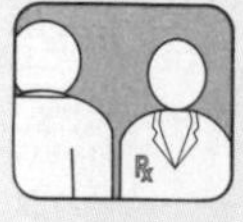

The objective of self-treatment with vaginal lubricants is to relieve vaginal dryness or pain during sexual intercourse related to atrophic vaginitis. For most patients, carefully following product instructions and the self-care measures listed below will help ensure optimal therapeutic outcomes.

- Apply the vaginal lubricant as frequently as needed for relief of atrophic symptoms or inadequate vaginal lubrication.
- Begin treatment of atrophic symptoms with a liberal quantity of lubricant (2 tablespoons); tailor subsequent doses to the quantity and frequency of application needed to provide relief.
- If using lubricants to facilitate sexual intercourse, apply the lubricant to the vagina, particularly at the vaginal opening, and to the penis.
- If desired, use a sanitary napkin to avoid staining of underwear.

Relief of symptoms can be apparent within hours after the first dose. Regular application of a lubricant can reverse atrophic symptoms to some extent. If no improvement is noticeable within a week or if symptoms worsen, see a physician for medical evaluation.

cently gave birth. Women who are perimenopausal or postmenopausal should know that long-term treatment with vaginal lubricants may be necessary. In either case, the pharmacist should explain the proper use of the lubricants for treatment of vaginal dryness or dyspareunia. The box "Patient Education for Atrophic Vaginitis" lists specific information to provide patients.

Evaluation of Patient Outcomes for Atrophic Vaginitis

Symptoms of atrophic vaginitis should improve within a week. The pharmacist should advise the patient to call to discuss treatment effectiveness if she has any questions or concerns and to call after 1 week of treatment to report progress in resolution of the symptoms. Symptoms that persist after 1 week of treatment require medical evaluation.

Vaginal Douching

Prevalence of Douching

Studies confirm that douching remains a relatively common practice, given that more than half of all women douche regularly or intermittently.[32] The National Survey of Family Growth reported that douching rates in 1988 were similar in all age groups among women of reproductive age.[33] However, douching rates were influenced by race, geographic region, socioeconomic status, and education. In one study, race was the most important predictor of douching practices; two-thirds of African American women douched compared with one-third of Caucasian women.[33] Geographic region was another strong predictor of douching, with women living in the South being more likely to douche than are women in other regions of the United States. Both education and socioeconomic status were inversely related to the practice of douching.

The most frequent reason stated for douching is to achieve good vaginal hygiene. Because vaginal douches mechanically irrigate the vagina, thus clearing away mucus and other accumulated debris, they may be used as cosmetic cleansing agents. Women who commonly douche may do so after their menstrual period, after using various contraceptive jellies and creams, or after sexual intercourse to clear out accumulations of vaginal discharge. Some may douche simply to feel clean and refreshed. How often women douche for nontherapeutic purposes is unknown. Some nonprescription douche products recommend douching no more than twice weekly.

Potential Adverse Effects of Douching

Studies have not proven douching to be either safe or desirable. Frequent douching may lead to an increased risk for PID, sterility, and/or ectopic pregnancy.[33] Additional problems include irritation or sensitization from douche ingredients and disruption of normal vaginal flora and vaginal pH. The possibility of local irritation, sensitization, and contact dermatitis exists with many antimicrobial agents found in douches. Douching may alter the vaginal chemical environment, leading to an increased risk for acquiring an STD or cervical cancer. Manufacturers recommend that women who suspect that they have PID or any STD should stop douching and immediately consult a physician.

Povidone-iodine (e.g., Betadine) has a greater potential than acetic acid douches to reduce total bacteria but may allow pathogenic species to proliferate, increasing the risk for vaginal infection.[34] Although few allergic reactions have been reported with intravaginal povidone-iodine, it may be systemically absorbed and should not be used by individuals allergic to iodine-containing products. Absorption poses a particular hazard to pregnant women in whom repeated vaginal applications may result in iodine-induced goiter and hypothyroidism in the fetus.[35,36] Table 6–2 lists examples of douche products that contain povidone-iodine. Numerous nonmedicated douches are also available.

Proper Use of Douche Equipment

Two types of syringes are available for douching purposes: the douche bag and the bulb douche syringes. The douche bag (fountain syringe or folding feminine syringe) holds 1 to 2 quarts of fluid and comes with tubing and a shut-off valve. Two types of tips are supplied: one for enema use (the shorter rectal nozzle) and one for douching. The two tips are not interchangeable; vaginal infections may occur if the rectal tip is also used for douching.

Bulb douche syringes are available as both disposable and nondisposable products. The nondisposable units hold 8 to 16 ounces of fluid, whereas the disposable units contain 3 to 9 ounces. The flow rate is regulated by the amount of hand pressure exerted when the bulb is squeezed. Gentle pressure is recommended because excess pressure may force fluid through the cervix and cause inflammation. Instructions for the proper use of these devices are found in Table 6–5.

Table 6–5

Administration Guidelines for Douches

Bulb Douche Syringe Method

1. Choose a douching position that is comfortable for you. Two positions are recommended: (a) sitting on the toilet or (b) standing in the shower. Whichever you choose, remember that douching is easier when you are relaxed.
2. Gently insert the nozzle about 3 inches into your vagina. Avoid closing the lips of the vagina.
3. Squeeze bottle gently, letting the solution cleanse the vagina and then flow freely from the body.
4. After douching, throw away bottle and nozzle.

Douche Bag Method

1. Fill the douche bag with the prescribed solution or with a warm water and vinegar solution.
2. Lie back in the tub with knees bent. Place the douche bag about 1 foot above the height of your hips. Do not place it or hang it any higher because such height will cause the pressure of fluid entering the vagina to be too high.
3. Insert the nozzle several inches into the vagina. Aim the nozzle up and back toward the small of the back. While holding the labia closed around the nozzle, release the clamp slowly to allow fluid to enter the vagina. Rotate the tip and allow fluid to enter the vagina until the vagina feels full. Stop the flow of fluid; then hold the fluid in the vagina for about 30 to 60 seconds. Release and allow the fluid to flow out; repeat until the douche bag is empty.

Patient Assessment of Douching

Pharmacists should discuss with a woman her reasons for douching. Women should be informed that douching is not necessary for cleansing of the vagina and that potential adverse consequences of douching exist. Douching for routine cosmetic purposes should be discouraged. An alternative cleansing method for vaginal and perineal areas should be suggested, such as gently washing the vagina and the vulvar, perineal, and anal regions with the fingers using lukewarm water and mild soap.[37] If a woman is douching to prevent or treat symptoms of a vaginal infection (e.g., an abnormal vaginal discharge), she should be counseled about more effective therapy or should be referred for medical evaluation, as appropriate. Douching is occasionally recommended by a prescriber.

Patient Education for Douching

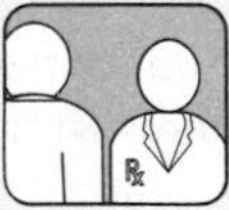

Improper methods of douching or too frequent douching can cause vaginal irritation and contact dermatitis. Such practices can also increase the risk for pelvic inflammatory disease, ectopic pregnancy, and sterility. For most patients, strictly following the product instructions and the self-care measures listed below will help to avoid these problems.

- Keep all douche equipment clean.
- Use lukewarm water to dilute products.
- Follow the appropriate instructions in Table 6–5 for the method of douching being used.
- Never instill a douche with forceful pressure.
- Do not use these products for birth control.
- Do not douche until at least 8 hours after intercourse during which a diaphragm, cervical cap, or contraceptive jelly, cream, or foam was used.
- Do not douche 24 to 48 hours before any gynecologic examination.
- Do not douche during pregnancy unless under the advice and supervision of your physician.
- Use douches only as directed for routine cleansing.
- Do not douche more often than twice a week, except on the advice of your doctor.

If vaginal dryness or irritation occurs, discontinue use of the douche.

Patient Counseling for Douching

The pharmacist should instruct patients for whom douches have been prescribed or those who insist on douching for other reasons on how to use these products safely, appropriately, and effectively. The box "Patient Education for Douching" lists specific information to provide these patients.

CONCLUSIONS

Women often have concerns about vaginal health and hygiene. Some vaginal and vulvovaginal disorders are self-treatable. Pharmacists can help women decide when self-treatment is appropriate and can recommend safe and effective pharmacologic and nonpharmacologic self-treatments.

VVC is the only vaginal infection amenable to treatment with nonprescription products. Differentiating symptoms of vaginal infections can be difficult. Therefore, it is important that women who self-treat vaginal infections have had a previous physician-diagnosed episode of VVC so that they know what symptoms indicate VVC. The nonprescription imidazole vaginal antifungals are equally effective in treating VVC.

At menopause, during the postpartum period, and during breast-feeding, vaginal lubrication declines secondary to a decrease in estrogen levels. Atrophic vaginitis and associated dyspareunia are often associated with the decline in estrogen. Nonprescription vaginal lubricants are useful in treating simple vaginal dryness. The best candidates for using the lubricants are women who previously had adequate vaginal lubrication and who may be experiencing temporary vaginal dryness. Significant atrophic symptoms or dyspareunia resulting from causes other than simple vaginal dryness are more appropriately referred for evaluation and prescribed therapy (e.g., hormone replacement therapy).

Douching is still a relatively common hygienic practice. However, studies have not proven this practice to be either safe or effective. Frequent douching may lead to an increased risk for PID, sterility, and/or ectopic pregnancy. If patients insist on douching, the pharmacist should counsel them on the proper methods and frequency of douching.

References

1. Reed BD. Vaginitis. In: Sloane PD, Slatt LM, Curtis P, et al. *Essentials of Family Medicine.* 3rd ed. Baltimore: William & Wilkins; 1998.
2. Sobel JD. Vulvovaginitis. *Dermatol Clin.* 1992;10:339–59.
3. Paavonen J, Stamm WE. Lower genital tract infections in women. *Infect Dis Clin North Am.* 1987;1:179–98.
4. Reed BD, Eyler A. Vaginal infections: Diagnosis and management. *Am Fam Physician.* 1993;47:1805–16.
5. Schaaf VM, Pérez-Stable EJ, Borchardt K. The limited value of symptoms and signs in the diagnosis of vaginal infections. *Arch Intern Med.* 1990;150:1929–33.
6. Sweet RL. Role of bacterial vaginosis in pelvic inflammatory diseases. *Clin Infect Dis.* 1995;20(suppl 2):S271–5.
7. Laga M, Manoka AT, Kivuvu M, et al. Non-ulcerative sexually transmitted diseases as risk factors for HIV-1 transmission in women: Result from a cohort study. *AIDS.* 1993;7:95–102.
8. Hillier SL, Nugent RP, Eschenbach DA, et al. Association between bacterial vaginosis and preterm delivery of a low birth-weight infant. *N Engl J Med.* 1995;333:1737–42.
9. Tortora GJ, Grabowski SR. *Principles of Anatomy and Physiology.* 7th ed. New York: Harper Collins College Publishers; 1993:943–5.
10. Eschenbach DA. Vaginal infection. *Clin Obstet Gynecol.* 1983;26:186–202.
11. Smith MA, Shimp LA. Estrogen replacement therapy. In: Rosenfeld JA, ed. *Women's Health in Primary Care.* Baltimore: Williams & Wilkins; 1997.
12. Kent HL. Epidemiology of vaginitis. *Am J Obstet Gynecol.* 1991;165:1168–76.
13. Sobel JD, Faro S, Force RW, et al. VVC: Epidemiologic, diagnostic, and therapeutic considerations. *Am J Obstet Gynecol.* 1998;178:203–11.
14. Reed BD. Risk factors for *Candida* vulvovaginitis. *Obstet Gynecol Surv.* 1992;47:551–60.
15. Haynes DG. Vaginitis. In: Rosenfeld JA, ed. *Women's Health in Primary Care.* Baltimore: Williams & Wilkins; 1997.
16. Foxman B. The epidemiology of VVC: Risk factors. *Am J Public Health.* 1990;80:329–31.
17. Rein MF. Vulvovaginitis and cervicitis. In: Mandell GL, Douglas RG, Bennett JE, eds. *Principles and Practice of Infectious Diseases.* New York: Churchill Livingstone; 1990:953–65.
18. Sobel JD. *Candida* vulvovaginitis. *Sem Dermatol.* 1996;15:17–28.
19. Hilton E, Isenberg HD, Alperstein P, et al. Ingestion of yogurt containing *Lactobacillus acidophilus* as prophylaxis for candidal vaginitis. *Ann Intern Med.* 1992;116:353–7.
20. ACOG Technical Bulletin (No. 226). Vaginitis. *Int J Gynaecol Obstet.* 1996;54:293–302.
21. Koff E, Rierdan J, Stubbs ML. Conceptions and misconceptions of the menstrual cycle. *Women Health.* 1990;16:119–36.
22. Sobel JD. Pathogenesis and treatment of recurrent VVC. *Clin Infect Dis.* 1992;14(suppl 1):S148–53.
23. Ritter W, Patzschke K, Krause U, et al. Pharmacokinetic fundamentals of vaginal treatment with clotrimazole. *Chemotherapy.* 1982;28(suppl 1):37–42.
24. Abrams LS, Weintraub HS. Disposition of radioactivity following intravaginal administration of ^{3}H-miconazole nitrate. *Am J Obstet Gynecol.* 1983;147:970–1.
25. Ernest JM. Topical antifungal agents. *Obstet Gynecol Clin North Am.* 1992;19:587–607.
26. Suess JA, Holzman C. Vulvar and vaginal disease. In: Smith MA, Shimp LA, eds. *20 Common Problems in Women's Health Care.* Stamford, CT: Appleton & Lange; 1999.
27. Lipsky MS, Taylor C. The use of over-the-counter antifungal vaginitis preparations by college students. *Fam Med.* 1996;28:493–5.
28. Ferris DG, Dekle C, Litaker MS. Women's use of over-the-counter antifungal medications for gynecologic symptoms. *J Fam Prac.* 1996;42:595–600.
29. Jamieson DJ, Steege JF. The prevalence of dysmenorrhea, dyspareunia, pelvic pain, and irritable bowel syndrome in primary care practices. *Obstet Gynecol.* 1996;87:55–8.
30. Gass ML, Rebar RW. Management of problems during menopause. *Compr Ther.* 1990;16:3–10.
31. Sarazin SK, Seymour SF. Causes and treatment options for women with dyspareunia. *Nurse Pract.* 1991;16:30–41.
32. Rosenberg MJ, Phillips RS, Holmes MD. Vaginal douching. Who and why? *J Reprod Med.* 1991;36:753–8.
33. Aral SO, Mosher WD, Cates W Jr. Vaginal douching among women of reproductive age in the United States: 1988. *Am J Public Health.* 1992;82:210–4.
34. Onderdonk AB, Delaney ML, Hinkson PL, et al. Quantitative and qualitative effects of douche preparations on vaginal microflora. *Obstet Gynecol.* 1992;80:333–8.
35. Safran M, Braverman LE. Effect of chronic douching with polyvinylpyrrolidone-iodine on iodine absorption and thyroid function. *Obstet Gynecol.* 1982;60:35–40.
36. Mahillon I, Peers W, Bourdoux P, et al. Effect of vaginal douching with povidone-iodine during early pregnancy on the iodine supply to mother and fetus. *Biol Neonate.* 1989;56:210–7.
37. McGowan L. Peritonitis following the vaginal douche and a proposed alternative. *Am J Obstet Gynecol.* 1965;90:506–9.

CHAPTER 7

Disorders Related to Menstruation

Leslie A. Shimp

Chapter 7 at a Glance

The menstrual cycle is a regular physiologic event for women, beginning during adolescence and usually continuing through late middle age. During the menstrual cycle, some women experience unpleasant symptoms, such as abdominal pain and cramping, irritability, and fluid retention. Unfortunately, women are not always knowledgeable about the menstrual cycle: One study[1] of college-aged women found that 30% could not explain why menstruation occurred. In addition, women are now able to self-treat for two common menstrual disorders: primary dysmenorrhea and premenstrual syndrome. Many women use nonprescription products and seek advice from a pharmacist on how best to manage symptoms of these disorders. Therefore, women, as consumers, and pharmacists, as health care providers, need to understand the menstrual cycle to make informed and appropriate decisions about self-care. The pharmacist should also be familiar with common menstrual symptoms and disorders, as well as with the risks associated with the misuse of menstrual products (e.g., toxic shock syndrome).

Editor's Note: This chapter is based, in part, on the 11th edition chapter titled "Vaginal and Menstrual Products," which was written by Leslie A. Shimp and Constance M. Fleming.

Physiology of the Menstrual Cycle

Menstruation results from the monthly cycling of female reproductive hormones. A single menstrual cycle is the time between the onset of one menstrual flow (menstruation or menses) and the beginning of the next.

The average age at which menarche (the initial menstrual cycle) occurs in U.S. women is 12.5 years; however, menarche may occur as early as age 9 years or as late as age 17 years. The onset of menstruation may be influenced by race, genetic factors, nutritional status, exercise intensity, and psychologic factors. Two of the earliest signs of puberty among females are a growth spurt and the beginning of breast development. On average, a 2-year lag period exists between the beginning of breast development and menarche.[2]

The menstrual cycle results from the hormonal activity of the hypothalamus, pituitary gland, and ovaries (hypothalamic–pituitary–ovarian axis). The arcuate nuclei of the hypothalamus play an important role in regulating the menstrual cycle by producing gonadotropin-releasing hormone (GnRH). Low levels of estradiol and progesterone, which occur at the end of the previous menstrual cycle, stimulate the hypothalamus to release GnRH, which is then immediately transported to the anterior pituitary. GnRH stimulates pituitary gonadotroph cells to synthesize and secrete luteinizing

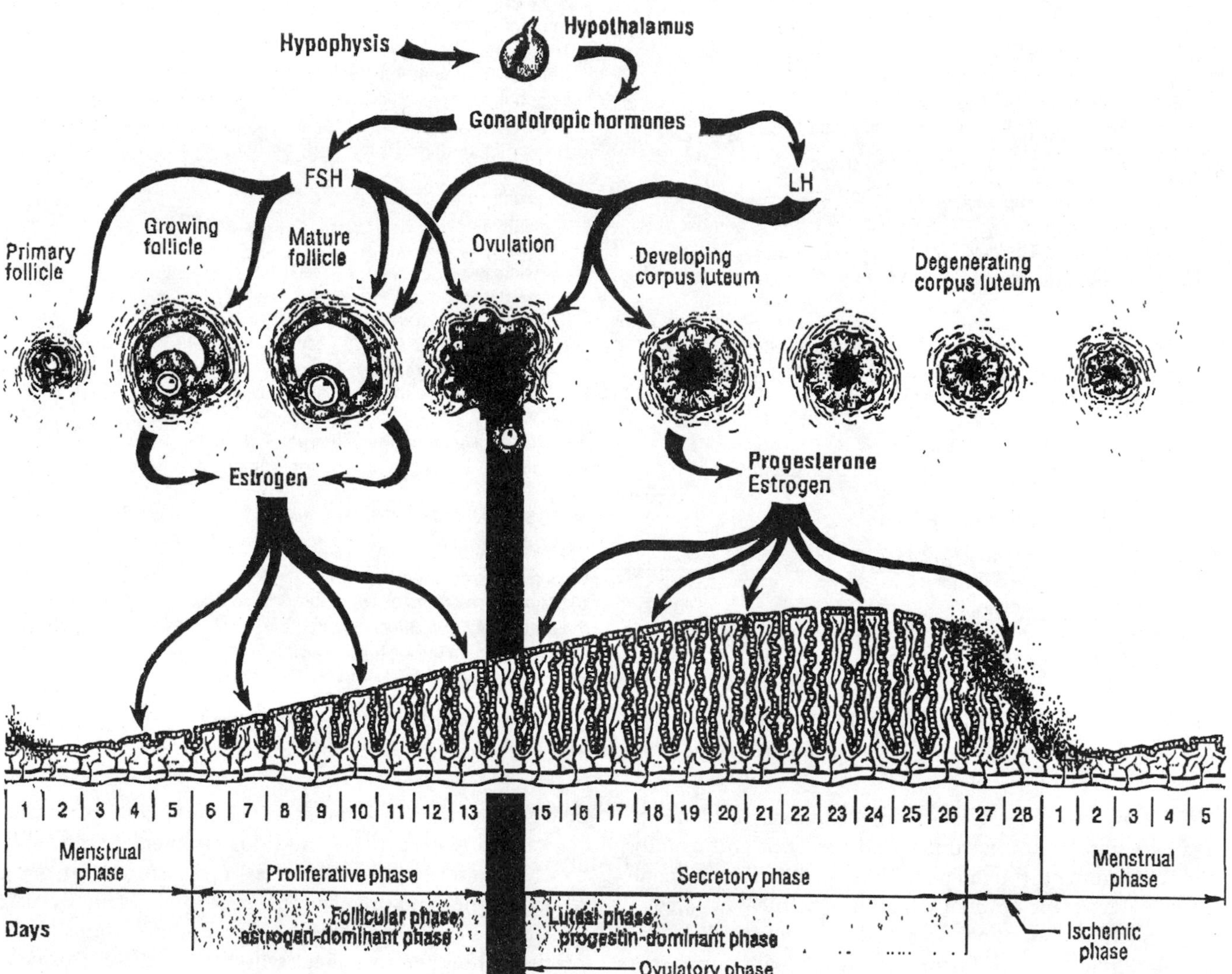

Figure 7–1 Schematic drawing illustrating the interrelations of the hypothalamus, hypophysis (pituitary gland), ovaries, and endometrium. One complete menstrual cycle and the beginning of another are shown. Changes in the ovaries, called the ovarian cycle, are promoted by the gonadotropic hormones, FSH, and LH. Hormones from the ovaries (estrogens and progesterone) then promote changes in the structure and function of the endometrium. Thus, the cyclical activity of the ovary is intimately linked with changes in the uterus. Reprinted from: Moore KL. *The Developing Human*. 2nd ed. Philadelphia: WB Saunders; 1977; used with permission.

hormone (LH) and follicle-stimulating hormone (FSH). FSH stimulates a group of ovarian follicles to mature. These maturing follicles then begin to secrete the estrogen estradiol, which influences follicular development and promotes the growth of the uterine endometrium. In addition, the increasing estradiol levels promote the midcycle surge in LH from the pituitary gland. This LH surge stimulates the cells of the graafian follicles to secrete progesterone, which helps to maintain the endometrial lining and to inhibit hormonal secretions of the hypothalamus and pituitary gland.

Two principal reproductive events, each hormonally controlled, occur during each menstrual cycle. The first event is the maturation and release of an ovum (egg) from the ovaries; the second is the preparation of the endometrial lining of the uterus for the implantation of a fertilized ovum.[3]

The average menstrual cycle lasts 28 days; the normal range for cycle length is 21 to 35 days.[4] The first day of the menstrual flow is called day 1 of the cycle. Menses usually last 4 to 6 days (plus or minus 2 days). Most of the blood loss occurs during days 1 and 2.[5,6] The major components of menstrual fluid are endometrial cellular debris and blood. Average blood loss is 30 to 35 mL (range 20 to 80 mL) per cycle. A loss of more than 80 mL per cycle is considered abnormal.

The events of the menstrual cycle can be described in phases that reflect changes either in the ovary (follicular/ovulatory and luteal phases) or in the uterine endometrium (menstrual/proliferative and secretory phases). The follicular/ovulatory phase correlates with the menstrual/proliferative phase, and the luteal phase correlates with the secretory phase. Figure 7–1 presents a graphic display of the events of the normal menstrual cycle.

Cycle day 1 (the first day of menstrual blood flow) is the beginning of the follicular phase in the ovary and of the menstrual/proliferative phase in the uterus. The follicular phase, during which the final maturation of a single dominant follicle occurs, is quite variable in length; it lasts an average of 14 days but can range in length between 7 and 22 days.

By about cycle day 7, a single ovarian follicle becomes dominant. Once it is mature and capable of ovulation, this follicle is known as the graafian follicle. The ovulatory phase of the cycle is approximately 3 days in length. During this phase, the LH surge (a 36- to 48-hour period when several large waves or pulses of LH are released) occurs. The LH surge catalyzes the final steps in the maturation of the ovum as well as stimulates the production of prostaglandins and proteolytic enzymes, which are necessary for ovulation (release of a mature ovum). During the LH surge, levels of estradiol decrease, sometimes accompanied by midcycle endometrial bleeding. Ovulation typically occurs within 24 hours after the LH surge. Ovulation releases 5 to 10 mL of follicular fluid, which contains the oocyte mass; this event may cause abdominal pain (mittelschmerz) for some women.[2,3]

The luteal phase is the time between ovulation and the beginning of menstrual blood flow. The luteal phase is more constant in length, averaging 13 to 14 days (plus or minus 2 days). After the graafian follicle ruptures, it is referred to as the corpus luteum. The duration of the luteal phase is consistent with the functional period (about 10 to 12 days) of the corpus luteum, during which time the corpus luteum secretes progesterone, estradiol, and androgens. The increased levels of estrogen and progesterone alter uterine endometrial lining; glands mature, proliferate, and become secretory in nature (secretory phase) as the uterus prepares for the implantation of a fertilized egg. Progesterone and estrogen levels reach their peaks in the middle of the luteal phase, whereas levels of LH and FSH decline in response to the increase in these two hormones. If pregnancy occurs, human chorionic gonadotropin released by the developing embryo supports the function of the corpus luteum until the placenta develops enough to begin secreting estrogen and progesterone. If pregnancy does not occur, the corpus luteum ceases to function. Then estrogen and progesterone levels decline, causing the endometrial lining of the uterus to become edematous and necrotic. The decrease in progesterone also allows prostaglandin synthesis. Following prostaglandin-initiated vasoconstriction and uterine contractions, the sloughing of the outer two endometrial layers occurs. The decline in estrogen and progesterone results in an increase in GnRH and in the renewed production of LH and FSH, which begins a new menstrual cycle.[2,3]

Dysmenorrhea

Dysmenorrhea (difficult or painful menstruation)[7] is one of the most common gynecologic problems in the United States. Dysmenorrhea is divided into primary and secondary disease. Primary dysmenorrhea is idiopathic and is associated with cramp-like abdominal pain at the time of menstruation with no identifiable organic pelvic disease. Occurring most often in young women, it usually develops within 6 to 12 months of menarche and generally affects women during their teenage years and early 20s. Primary dysmenorrhea occurs only during ovulatory cycles; therefore, its prevalence increases between early adolescence and older adolescence as the regularity of ovulation increases.

Secondary dysmenorrhea is usually associated with pelvic pathology. Possible causes include endometriosis (presence of functioning endometrial tissue in places where it is not normally found), pelvic inflammatory disease (PID), ovarian cysts, benign uterine tumors, endometrial cancer, adhesions, cervical stenosis (a narrowing of the cervix), and congenital abnormalities. Secondary dysmenorrhea may also be caused by the presence of intrauterine devices.[2] Because symptoms of dysmenorrhea are similar to those of endometriosis, ectopic pregnancy, and PID, physician evaluation is necessary to rule out the presence of secondary causes of dysmenorrhea. Secondary dysmenorrhea is suggested if dysmenorrhea initially appears years after menarche (at 20 years of age or older); if dysmenorrhea occurs throughout the duration of menstrual flow (for more than 2 to 3 days); or if the patient experiences irregular menstrual cycles, has menorrhagia (abnormally profuse menstrual flow), or has a history of PID or infertility.[6]

Epidemiology of Primary Dysmenorrhea

Dysmenorrhea occurs in approximately 30% to 60% of all women of reproductive age, but prevalence is higher (about 60% to 79%) in adolescent women.[5,8] Analysis of specific adolescent age groups shows that approximately 48% of 12-year-olds experience dysmenorrhea, and approximately 79% of 18-year-olds experience it.[8] Its prevalence decreases after 30 to 35 years of age.[9]

Severe pain is less common (7% to 15% of women). Dysmenorrhea may lead to lost productivity; one study[10] reported that 8% of women with dysmenorrhea reported missing one or more days of work per month because of dysmenorrhea. This dysfunction translates into an estimated 650 million work hours lost per year at a cost in excess of $3 billion in lost productivity. Similarly, 51% to 54% of adolescent girls report missing school or work regularly because of dysmenorrhea.[8]

Etiology of Primary Dysmenorrhea

The cause of primary dysmenorrhea is excessive contractions of the uterus.[8] Evidence suggests that primary dysmenorrhea is related to prostaglandin levels. Both the endometrium and the myometrium of the uterus have the capacity to synthesize prostaglandins. Prostaglandin levels in the endometrium and menstrual fluid of women with primary dysmenorrhea have been found to be elevated. Researchers have reported prostaglandin serum levels to be 5 to 13 times greater in women with dysmenorrhea than in women without dysmenorrhea. The symptoms of primary dysmenorrhea are very similar to those produced by the administration of a prostaglandin to induce labor. Finally, administration of prostaglandin synthesis inhibitors, such as nonsalicylate nonsteroidal anti-inflammatory drugs (NSAIDs) has been shown to reduce the symptoms of dysmenorrhea.[9] The nonprescription nonsalicylate NSAIDs include ibuprofen, ketoprofen, and naproxen.

Pathophysiology of Primary Dysmenorrhea

Prostaglandin serum levels rise as progesterone levels decrease during the luteal phase of the menstrual cycle. Concurrently, the levels of prostacyclin (a smooth-muscle relaxant) decrease. This combination of biochemical events can lead to strong uterine contractions and significant vasoconstriction, resulting in uterine hypoxia (a deficiency of oxygen reaching body tissues) and pain in some women.[9] Several physiologic changes have been identified that contribute to the development of this pain: an elevation of myometrial resting tone, an elevation of contractile myometrial pressure, and an increased frequency of uterine contractions. During normal menses, contraction pressure is 50 to 80 mm Hg, each contraction lasts about 15 to 30 seconds, and about one to four contractions occur every 10 minutes. These normal contractions help to expel menstrual fluids. With dysmenorrhea, however, contraction pressure can exceed 400 mm Hg, contractions may last longer than 90 seconds, and the time between contractions may be less than 15 seconds.[6] Both the intrauterine pressure and the number of uterine contractions have been shown to be directly related to the pain of dysmenorrhea because both effects produce tissue hypoxia from a decrease in blood flow.[9]

In a subset of women with primary dysmenorrhea, prostaglandin levels were not found to be elevated, and the administration of prostaglandin synthesis inhibitors did not alleviate their pain. One hypothesis suggests that leukotrienes, which, like prostaglandins, are formed from arachidonic acid, may cause the pain. Leukotrienes induce uterine contractions and vasoconstriction similar to the action of prostaglandins. In addition, some evidence exists that vasopressin (a substance that can produce dysrhythmic uterine contractions) may also be involved in the etiology of primary dysmenorrhea.[9]

A number of factors have been associated with the occurrence or severity of primary dysmenorrhea. As mentioned previously, primary dysmenorrhea is most common in young women and less so in women beyond the late 20s. This decrease in incidence and severity may be related to pregnancy, because, during late pregnancy, uterine adrenergic nerves virtually disappear and only a portion regenerate after childbirth.[7]

Signs and Symptoms of Primary Dysmenorrhea

Primary dysmenorrhea pain lasts from a few hours to between 48 and 72 hours.[9] Although it is experienced as lower midabdominal or suprapubic pain, which is cramping in nature, the pain may radiate to the lower back and upper thighs. Symptoms such as nausea, vomiting, fatigue, weakness, nervousness, dizziness, diarrhea, and headache may accompany the pain.[2,4,8] Even moderately severe symptoms (symptoms that might keep a woman home from work or cause a girl to miss school) can be self-managed if the patient responds to nonprescription doses of a nonsalicylate NSAID.

Treatment of Primary Dysmenorrhea

Many women feel that they are able to self-treat dysmenorrhea with over-the-counter (OTC) products. In one recent study[11] 66% of women with dysmenorrhea did not see a clinician despite having moderate to severe symptoms, and 92% were satisfied with self-treatment. A number of women, 38% to 80% in various studies, use nonprescription medications as self-treatment for dysmenorrhea symptoms.[8,10] A large percentage (61% to 70%) of adolescents also use medication to manage dysmenorrhea.[8] The three most commonly used nonprescription analgesic medications are acetaminophen, aspirin, and ibuprofen. A study of adult women found 48% used ibuprofen, 16% aspirin, and 15% acetaminophen.[10] A similar study[8] of adolescents (average age of 16 years) found that many more adolescents used acetaminophen than ibuprofen: Ninety-five percent reported using acetaminophen, 55% aspirin, and 42% ibuprofen. (Some girls used more than one agent). Obviously, in many cases, both girls and women are self-medicating with acetaminophen and aspirin, agents that are less effective than nonsalicylate NSAIDs for treating dysmenorrhea. In addition, aspirin is not recommended for use by adolescents because of its association with Reye's syndrome.[8] Furthermore, an evaluation of the doses and regimens used by adolescents showed that most girls tended not to use the maximum dosage recommended on nonprescription labels; only 31% took the recommended single dose (one to two pills) at the maximum suggested frequency of use (three to four times daily). A significant difference was found in the duration of discomfort between users who took recommended doses when compared with those who took less, suggesting that adolescents may be experiencing discomfort from dysmenorrhea that could be relieved by more appropriate selection and dosage of nonprescription medications.[8]

Treatment Outcomes

The goal of treating primary dysmenorrhea is to provide relief from or a significant improvement in symptoms so as to limit discomfort and the disruption of usual activities.

General Treatment Approach

For some of the many adolescent girls and women who experience primary dysmenorrhea, the pain, abdominal cramping, and associated symptoms interfere with school, work, and other activities. However, essentially all patients can be provided adequate relief of symptoms either by nonprescription or prescription drug therapy. Treatment can include nonpharmacologic measures, such as use of heating pads, increased exercise, and other lifestyle modifications. These measures serve as adjuncts to drug therapy and are rarely adequate as sole therapy for primary dysmenorrhea. Figure 7–2 presents an algorithm for the management of primary dysmenorrhea.

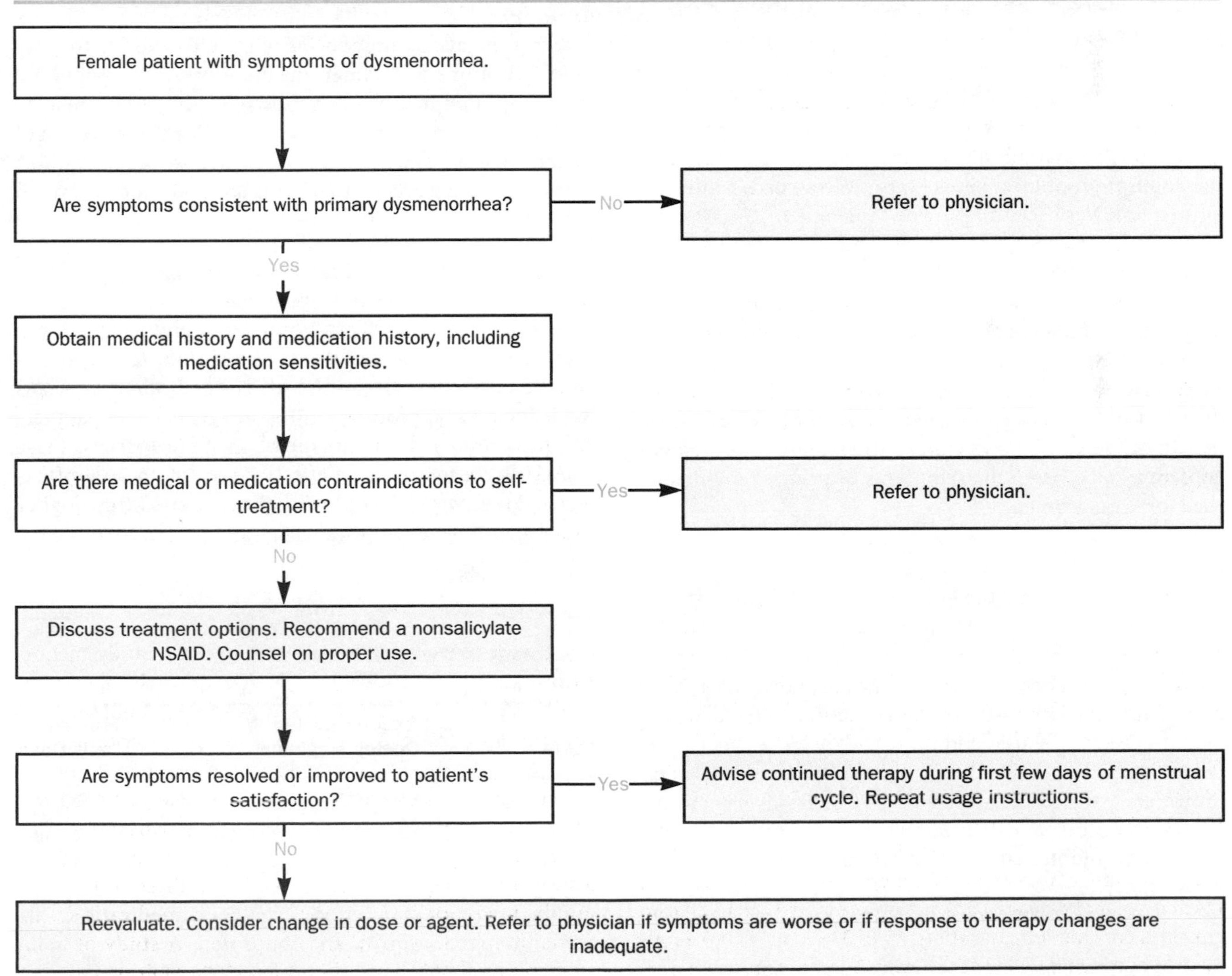

Figure 7–2 Self-care of primary dysmenorrhea.

The patient with more severe dysmenorrhea or with dysmenorrhea that does not respond to therapy with nonprescription internal analgesics should be referred to her primary care provider. A trial with other prescription NSAIDs or therapy with an oral contraceptive may be prescribed. Approximately 80% to 90% of women with dysmenorrhea can be successfully treated with NSAIDs, oral contraceptives, or a combination.

The pharmacist should be aware of other conditions that cause alterations in menstrual cycling. These conditions include amenorrhea (the absence or abnormal cessation of menses), menorrhagia, and dysfunctional uterine bleeding (a syndrome of irregular menses with periods of prolonged, heavy menstrual flow alternating with amenorrhea). None of these conditions is amenable to self-treatment; the patient should be advised to seek medical evaluation. Midcycle bleeding (spotting) is a relatively common phenomenon. This type of intermenstrual bleeding, which may be accompanied by short-lived abdominal pain, is typically caused by the decrease in ovarian estrogen production that occurs at midcycle. Bleeding of this type is self-limited and does not require therapy.[12]

Nonpharmacologic Therapy

Although nonpharmacologic therapy is not the principal therapy for primary dysmenorrhea, some women find that the application of local heat (e.g., a heating pad) to the abdomen or lower back can provide some relief.

Lifestyle alterations may alleviate symptoms to varying degrees. Smoking tobacco or consuming excessive amounts of ethyl alcohol has been associated with more severe dysmenorrhea. The severity reportedly increases with the number of cigarettes smoked per day. The basis for this effect is unknown, but it has been hypothesized that nicotine-induced vasoconstriction is involved.[13] Evidence regarding the benefit of exercise is conflicting. Participation in regular exercise may also lessen the symptoms of primary dysmenorrhea for some women.[2,9,13]

Pharmacologic Therapy

Unfortunately, despite the efficacy of drug therapy with aspirin, acetaminophen, or nonsalicylate NSAIDs, many women with dysmenorrhea remain untreated or are inadequately treated. They continue to experience the pain and activity limitations imposed by this condition.[7] The following sections outline the uses and properties of these agents. The reader is referred to Chapter 3, "Headache and Muscle and Joint Pain," for further discussion of their adverse effects, contraindications, and drug interactions. Chapter 3 also provides a table of internal analgesic products that are commercially available.

Aspirin

Aspirin may be adequate for treating mild symptoms of dysmenorrhea. However, in low doses, aspirin has only a limited effect on prostaglandin synthesis and is, therefore, only moderately effective in treating women with more than minimal symptoms of dysmenorrhea.

Dosage/Administration Guidelines When used for menstrual discomfort, the adult dosing of aspirin is 650 to 1000 mg every 4 to 6 hours as needed, not to exceed 4000 mg per day. (See Table 7–1.) Aspirin is best taken with food or with a full glass of water.

Drug–Drug Interactions Clinically significant aspirin–drug interactions occur with anticoagulants, methotrexate, valproate, probenecid, phenytoin, oral hypoglycemics, and high doses of antacids (e.g., 60 to 120 mL of an aluminum–magnesium hydroxide suspension).

Contraindications Patients who are allergic or intolerant to aspirin should not use this agent. Disease states that are relative contraindications to aspirin therapy include peptic ulcer disease, gastritis, bleeding disorders, asthma, or renal insufficiency. In addition, adolescent girls should not use aspirin because of the potential for Reye's syndrome.

Acetaminophen

Like aspirin, acetaminophen may be adequate for treating mild symptoms of dysmenorrhea only. Acetaminophen, which has a minimal effect on prostaglandins, is known to be less effective than a nonsalicylate NSAID for the treatment of dysmenorrhea.[8] The adult dosing for menstrual discomfort is 650 to 1000 mg every 4 to 6 hours as needed, not to exceed 4000 mg per day. (See Table 7–1.)

Nonsalicylate Nonsteroidal Anti-Inflammatory Agents

Three nonsalicylate NSAIDs are available as nonprescription products: ibuprofen 200 mg, naproxen sodium 220 mg, and ketoprofen 12.5 mg. All of these agents belong to the proprionic acid derivative class of NSAIDs, which some clinicians feel is the most appropriate group of agents for initial therapy for primary dysmenorrhea.[4] In clinical trials, these NSAIDs were found to be effective in 66% to 90% of patients. However, clinical trial doses were often higher (ibuprofen 400 mg four times daily, ketoprofen 50 to 100 mg

Table 7–1

Treatment of Dysmenorrhea with Nonprescription Products

Agent	Recommended Dosing Regimen	Maximum Daily Dose
Acetaminophen	650–1000 mg every 4–6 hours	4000 mg
Aspirin	650–1000 mg every 4–6 hours	4000 mg
Ibuprofen	200–400 mg every 4–6 hours	1200 mg
Ketoprofen	12.5–25 mg every 4–8 hours; not more than 25 mg within 4–6 hours	75 mg
Naproxen sodium	220–440 mg initially; then 220 mg every 8–12 hours	660 mg

four times daily, and naproxen sodium 275 mg four times daily) than the labeled nonprescription doses.[9,14]

Mechanism of Action/Indication Nonsalicylate NSAIDs are the principal nonprescription agents for treating primary dysmenorrhea. These agents inhibit the production and action of prostaglandins.

Dosage/Administration Guidelines Therapy with nonsalicylate NSAIDs should begin at the onset of pain; there is no proven value to beginning therapy in anticipation of dysmenorrhea.[4] If the possibility of pregnancy exists, then therapy should be initiated only after menses begin. Pharmacists should explain to patients that the NSAID is used as much to prevent cramps as to relieve pain. Optimal pain relief is achieved when these agents are taken on a scheduled rather than on an as-needed basis. Therefore, ibuprofen should be taken every 4 to 6 hours, ketoprofen every 4 to 8 hours, and naproxen sodium every 8 to 12 hours for the first 48 to 72 hours of menstrual flow because that time frame correlates with maximum prostaglandin release.[9] The recommended regimen of ibuprofen for treating primary dysmenorrhea is 400 mg taken initially and every 6 hours thereafter as needed. However, 200 mg taken every 4 to 6 hours may be used at first; if it is not effective, 400 mg taken every 6 hours should be recommended, not to exceed 1200 mg per day. The nonprescription dosage of naproxen sodium recommended for dysmenorrhea is 220 to 440 mg taken initially followed by 220 mg every 8 to 12 hours, not to exceed 660 mg per day. The labeled nonprescription dose of ketoprofen is 12.5 to 25 mg taken initially and then every 4 to 8 hours, not to exceed 75 mg per day or 25 mg within any 4- to 6-hour period.

A patient with dysmenorrhea may respond better to one nonsalicylate NSAID than to another. If an adequate dose (or the maximum nonprescription dose) of one agent does not provide adequate benefit, then switching to another agent is recommended. A plateau to the analgesic effect exists for most of these NSAIDs so that further dose increases do not provide more benefit but instead may increase the risk of adverse drug effects.[4] Therapy with nonsalicylate NSAIDs should be undertaken for three to six menstrual cycles, with changes in the agent, dosage, or both before a judgment is made as to the effectiveness of these agents for a particular patient.

Adverse Effects Each nonsalicylate NSAID has a somewhat individual side-effect profile. Naproxen sodium is more likely to cause drowsiness, shortness of breath, and tinnitus (noise in the ears) than is either ibuprofen or ketoprofen. Ketoprofen and naproxen are associated with a greater incidence of fluid retention, constipation, and headache than is ibuprofen. Further, ketoprofen is more likely to cause gas/bloating, diarrhea, or nervousness/irritability than is either ibuprofen or naproxen. Side effects from a few days of use are limited. Side effects most commonly associated with short-term nonsalicylate NSAID therapy include gastrointestinal (GI) symptoms (e.g., upset stomach, vomiting, heartburn, abdominal pain, diarrhea, constipation, and anorexia) and side effects of the central nervous system (e.g., headache and dizziness). The GI side effects may be decreased by taking the drugs with food.

Drug-Drug Interactions As with aspirin, nonsalicylate NSAIDs should not be recommended as self-treatment agents for women taking anticoagulants (warfarin or heparin) because the NSAID-induced inhibition of platelets and possibly even GI irritation/bleeding are hazardous to patients taking anticoagulants. These NSAIDs may also cause fluid retention. Women taking antihypertensives or having conditions that may be aggravated by fluid retention (e.g., congestive heart failure, asthma) should be monitored for a reversal of control of hypertension or for a worsening of these conditions. Finally, nonsalicylate NSAIDs may increase the serum concentration of lithium, and women taking this agent should not self-treat with this type of NSAID.

Contraindications/Precautions/Warnings Relative contraindications to using nonsalicylate NSAIDs include a history of allergy to aspirin, with such manifestations as bronchospastic reaction, urticaria, or angioedema (an allergic skin reaction characterized by patches of circumscribed swelling involving the skin, mucous membranes, and sometime the viscera), or an allergy to any other NSAID. Other contraindications include active GI disease (e.g., peptic ulcer disease, gastroesophageal reflux disease, or ulcerative colitis), and bleeding disorders.[9]

Product Selection Guidelines

Nonsalicylate NSAIDs are the preferred analgesic for treating primary dysmenorrhea. Selection of one of these agents should be based on cost and the patient's preference for the number of doses and the number of tablets to take. Product selection should also be based on the side-effect and drug-interaction profile of the individual nonsalicylate NSAIDs. Patients who already have problems with fluid retention should avoid ketoprofen and naproxen. Acetaminophen may provide some relief for patients who are allergic to aspirin or who are intolerant to the GI and platelet-inhibition side effects of aspirin and the nonsalicylate NSAIDs.

Patient Assessment of Primary Dysmenorrhea

Before recommending any product to a patient experiencing symptoms of dysmenorrhea, the pharmacist should establish the onset of pain in relation to the onset of menses. Primary dysmenorrhea produces abdominal and lower back pain that begins within 1 to 2 days before the onset of menses and ceases during the first several days of menstrual blood flow. Most commonly, primary dysmenorrhea occurs during the first 3 days of menses. Pain that does not follow this pattern or that is severe or different in character from pain occurring during previous menstrual cycles should be evaluated by a physician.

Case Study 7–1

Patient Complaint/History

Lashana, a 27-year-old female, comes to the pharmacy counter and asks whether Advil or Aleve is better for dysmenorrhea. She reveals that in her late teens a physician diagnosed her as having dysmenorrhea.

The patient's symptoms, which include severe cramping, backache, and diarrhea, usually occur when her period begins and last about 2 days. After she married and began taking "the Pill," her symptoms improved a great deal. However, she recently stopped taking the oral contraceptive because she and her husband want to start a family. Since then, she has experienced symptoms of dysmenorrhea every month. Further, because of menstrual cramps, she has missed 2 days of work in each of the past 2 months.

Lashana recently saw her nurse clinician who confirmed that the symptoms were consistent with dysmenorrhea and who added that their intensity would most likely diminish following a pregnancy. Until she becomes pregnant, the patient wants to take something to relieve the symptoms and avoid missing work.

Lashana is in good general health. Her patient profile shows an allergy to sulfa drugs, which is manifested as hives. Minor medical problems include mild acne for which she applies erythromycin topical solution 2% once daily at bedtime. The recently discontinued contraceptive is listed as Brevicon 21 day.

Clinical Considerations/Strategies

Readers can use the following considerations/strategies to determine whether treatment of the patient's condition with nonprescription medications is warranted:

- Determine the patient's suitability for self-treatment.
- Determine patient factors and/or preferences that might influence product selection.
- Develop a protocol for the management of patients with dysmenorrhea who are ambulatory. Include initial drug selection, initial dose selection, dose modifications, possible switch to another nonsalicylate NSAID, and medical referral.

Patient Education/Counseling

Readers can use the following strategies to develop a patient education/counseling plan that will ensure optimal therapeutic outcomes:

- Explain the optimal use of a nonsalicylate NSAID for the use of dysmenorrhea.
- Explain the expected outcomes of therapy.
- Advise the patient of the conditions that indicate medical attention is appropriate.

Asking the patient the following questions will help elicit the information needed to accurately assess the disorder and to recommend the appropriate treatment approach.

Q~ What symptoms are you currently experiencing? When do your symptoms occur in relation to the beginning of your menstrual period? How severe are your symptoms?

A~ *Identify the common symptoms of primary dysmenorrhea. (See the section "Signs and Symptoms of Primary Dysmenorrhea.")* If the symptoms occur within 2 days before menses through the first few days of menses, strongly suspect primary dysmenorrhea.

Q~ Are these symptoms the same as or different from symptoms you have experienced in previous menstrual cycles?

A~ If the patient describes an increase in pain intensity, a difference in the timing in relation to menses, or an additional symptom, refer the patient to a physician for evaluation.

Q~ What medication(s) or other treatments (e.g., local heat) have you used to manage or alleviate your symptoms during previous episodes or this episode? Will you describe how you use those medications? For example, how many tablets do you use for a dose? How often do you take the medication? Do you use the medication regularly (i.e., every so many hours) or just as you need it for pain?

A~ If appropriate for the medication being used, adjust the dosage to achieve maximum pain relief. Advise the patient to take analgesics on a scheduled rather than on an as-needed basis. If aspirin or acetaminophen is being taken, explain that nonsalicylate NSAIDs are the most appropriate nonprescription therapy for primary dysmenorrhea because of their ability to reduce prostaglandin levels, which are the cause of dysmenorrhea pain.

Q~ What medication(s) are you currently taking? Are you allergic or hypersensitive to any drugs? If yes, which one(s)?

A~ *Identify potential drug interactions for the nonprescription analgesics. (See the section "Treatment of Primary Dysmenorrhea.")* If the patient is taking medications that could interact with one or more of the nonprescription agents, recommend the appropriate analgesic, if possible, or refer the patient to a physician. Do not recommend aspirin or nonsalicylate NSAIDs if the patient has asthma or a history of sensitivity to these agents.

Q~ Do you have anemia, asthma, congestive heart failure, hypertension, or an inflammatory or ulcerative GI disease, such as peptic ulcer disease, Crohn's disease, or ulcerative colitis?

A~ Advise a patient with any of these medical conditions to consult a physician before using a nonprescription nonsalicylate NSAID.

Patient Counseling for Primary Dysmenorrhea

It is important that adolescents and young women who experience dysmenorrhea symptoms be educated about this condition and that they realize it can be treated with products that can provide symptomatic relief. They should also be reassured about the prevalence or "normality" of primary dysmenorrhea. Those patients who wish to use internal analgesics for pain control should be advised that any of the nonprescription nonsalicylate NSAIDs can be appropriate for initial therapy but that not all women will respond to these agents. If response to the first agent is not adequate, the other nonsalicylate NSAIDs should be tried before a physician is consulted. The pharmacist should explain the proper use of these agents, as well as their potential adverse effects. The box "Patient Education for Primary Dysmenorrhea" lists specific information to provide patients.

Evaluation of Patient Outcomes for Primary Dysmenorrhea

Patient monitoring is accomplished by having the patient report whether the symptoms are resolved. Symptoms should improve within an hour or so of taking an analgesic. The optimal effect of drug therapy may not be seen, however, until the woman has used the medication on a scheduled basis. The pharmacist should follow up with a phone call to discuss treatment effectiveness (i.e., continued or altered symptoms) and the importance of scheduled dosing. The pharmacist can also inquire about the dose of medication being taken and can discuss an adequate dose. Persistent symptoms are reasons for advising the patient to try another nonprescription nonsalicylate NSAID or to see a clinician.

Premenstrual Syndrome (PMS)

PMS can be defined as a cyclic disorder composed of a combination of physical and emotional (mood) changes that occur during the luteal phase of the menstrual cycle, improve

Patient Education for Primary Dysmenorrhea

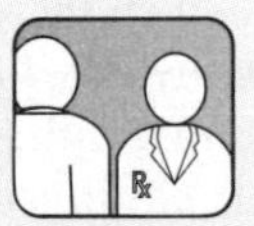

The objective of self-treatment is to relieve or significantly improve symptoms of dysmenorrhea so as to limit discomfort and the disruption of usual activities. For most patients, carefully following product instructions and the self-care measures listed below will help ensure optimal therapeutic outcomes.

Nondrug Measures

- If effective, apply heat to the abdomen, using a heating pad or hot-water bottle.
- Stop smoking cigarettes.
- Limit intake of alcoholic beverages at the time of menses.
- Participate in regular exercise if it lessens the symptoms.

Nonprescription Medications

- Note that the nonsalicylate NSAID nonprescription medications (ibuprofen, ketoprofen, and naproxen sodium) are the best type of nonprescription medication to treat primary dysmenorrhea. These medications stop or prevent the strong contractions (cramping) of the uterus.
- Start taking the medication when the menstrual period begins or when menstrual pain or other symptoms begin. Take the medication regularly, that is, according to the product instructions instead of just when the symptoms are "bad."
- See Table 7–1 for recommended dosages of the nonprescription nonsalicylate NSAIDs.
- Take a nonsalicylate NSAID with food to limit the most common side effects: upset stomach, heartburn, diarrhea or constipation, headache, and dizziness.
- Do not take nonsalicylate NSAIDs if you are allergic to aspirin or a nonsalicylate NSAID, or if you have peptic ulcer disease, gastroesophageal reflux disease, colitis, or any bleeding disorder.
- If you have hypertension, asthma, or congestive heart failure, watch for early symptoms that the nonsalicylate NSAID is causing fluid retention.
- Do not take a nonsalicylate NSAID if you are also taking anticoagulants or lithium.

⚠ If abdominal pain occurs at times other than just before or during the first few days of a menstrual period, seek medical attention.

⚠ Seek medical attention if the pain intensity increases or if new symptoms occur.

significantly or disappear within the first several days of menstrual flow, and are absent during the first week following menses.

Epidemiology of Premenstrual Syndrome

Approximately 80% of women experience some physical or mood changes before the onset of menses.[15] These changes are regarded as part of the normal menstrual cycle and are referred to medically as molimina. Sixty-six percent of women report positive changes, such as increased energy, creativity, and work productivity. Few women who experience premenstrual symptoms experience a decline in their ability to function normally. The majority of women with premenstrual symptoms experience only mild, primarily physical symptoms that do not interfere with their lives. An estimated 20% to 40% of women with premenstrual symptoms—particularly emotional symptoms—experience some difficulty during the premenstrual interval, but only 3% to 8% report symptoms that interfere with relationships, lifestyle, or work.[15,16] This severity of symptoms indicates a more severe form of PMS called premenstrual dysphoric disorder (PMDD). PMS can occur any time after menarche but occurs only during ovulatory cycles. Symptoms disappear during events that interrupt ovulation such as pregnancy, and breast-feeding will also cause symptoms to disappear. Women are most commonly in their late 20s or in the third or fourth decade of life when PMS is diagnosed. Some women report a worsening of symptoms over time, but PMS symptoms disappear at menopause.[17]

Etiology of Premenstrual Syndrome

Many biophysiologic and endocrinologic theories have been developed to explain the etiology of PMS, but its cause remains unknown. Nonetheless, a variety of therapies paralleling these theories has been advocated.

Progesterone Deficiency

One of the more publicized theories has been the progesterone-deficiency theory. However, inadequate progesterone levels have not been clearly demonstrated as an etiologic factor, and well-controlled clinical trials have not shown a benefit from progesterone therapy.[18] The American College of Obstetrics and Gynecology states, "The use of progesterone in treating PMS should be discouraged."[15] Similarly, neither aldosterone nor prolactin levels have been found to be different in control subjects versus symptomatic patients.[18]

Pyridoxine Deficiency

Another popular theory hypothesizes that a deficiency of pyridoxine (vitamin B_6) might occur, thereby causing altered estrogen levels, and it suggests that pyridoxine might be an effective treatment for PMS. However, no evidence exists for altered pyridoxine absorption or metabolism. Still, one study[19] reported a high percentage (60%) of physicians prescribed vitamins for women with premenstrual symptoms, and a significant number (40%) of patients had taken pyridoxine. Pyridoxine supplementation is not without risk. High doses (2 to 6 g daily) have been associated with developing peripheral neuropathy (an abnormal, usually degenerative state of the peripheral nervous system). Risk of neuropathy can occur with daily doses greater than 200 mg, although with lower doses the neuropathy is usually reversible.[20]

Prostaglandin Deficiency

The relationship of prostaglandins and PMS has been explored. Yet another theory is that PMS is caused by a prostaglandin E_1 deficiency. Accordingly, evening primrose oil (efamol), which contains 72% γ linoleic acid (a prostaglandin E_1 precursor), has been advocated for treating PMS. Controlled trials did not confirm a benefit, and use of this agent is not warranted. Prostaglandin inhibitors (e.g., NSAIDs) have also been studied for treating PMS. Although nonsalicylate NSAIDs can reduce some of the physical symptoms (e.g., headache, dizziness) associated with PMS, emotional symptoms are essentially unaffected. Their benefit is believed to be due largely to the coexistence in subjects of dysmenorrhea and PMS.[18,21]

Dietary Effects

Nutritional theories have been postulated for the etiology of PMS. Although the benefit of nutritional therapy for PMS is unproven, many clinicians recommend a balanced diet combined with avoiding salty foods and simple sugars (which aggravate fluid retention) as well as caffeine (which increases irritability). Cravings for foods high in carbohydrates (e.g., chips and cookies) are not uncommon in women with PMS. High-carbohydrate foods contain the serotonin precursor tryptophan. Decreases in serotonin are thought to be related to PMS, and it is known that serotonin reuptake inhibitor medications are effective in treating PMDD. One study of a carbohydrate-rich beverage, which increased tryptophan levels, demonstrated an improvement in mood scores (depression, tension, anger, confusion) for women with PMDD without psychiatric illness.[22] Consuming foods that are rich in carbohydrates and low in protein during the premenstrual interval may reduce symptoms.[18]

Hormonal Effects

Exogenous hormones can cause PMS-like symptoms. Women taking either oral contraceptives or postmenopausal hormone replacement therapy may experience adverse effects similar to PMS symptoms as a result of the alteration in hormone levels.

Pathophysiology of Premenstrual Syndrome

None of the symptoms of PMS or PMDD is unique to these conditions; however, the occurrence of symptoms and their fluctuation with the phases of the menstrual cycle are diagnostic. The current consensus is that normal ovarian function (and the consequent fluctuation of estrogen and progesterone levels) causes the symptoms of PMS and PMDD.[16] The fluctuation of hormones also causes changes in levels of central nervous system neurotransmitters. Therefore, treatment of symptoms severe enough to warrant drug therapy (e.g., PMDD) is based on medications that affect the levels of serotonin and γ-butyric acid or that suppress ovulation or interrupt hormonal cycling.

Signs and Symptoms of Premenstrual Syndrome

Common symptoms include minor weight gain, abdominal bloating, mild fatigue, and irritability. Table 7–2 lists other common symptoms of PMS and the percentage of women experiencing them.[15] Women with PMDD experience significant symptoms that can impair personal relationships and the ability to function well at work. The criteria for the diagnosis of PMDD are shown in Table 7–3.[18] A woman with PMS or PMDD should experience essentially a symptom-free interval during days 4 to 12 of her menstrual cycle. Her symptoms during the late luteal phase (last 7 days of the cycle) should be at least 30% worse than those she experiences during the mid-follicular phase (days 3 to 9 of the menstrual cycle).[15] A daily rating of symptoms for several cycles is used to establish a diagnosis. In addition, a woman should have experienced these types of symptoms during most menstrual cycles over the past year.

Lack of a symptom-free interval suggests that the patient has a psychiatric disorder (e.g., anxiety or panic disorder) or a medical condition (e.g., perimenopause) rather than PMS.

Table 7–2

Common Symptoms of Premenstrual Syndrome

Symptom	% Women with PMS Showing Symptom
Behavioral	
Fatigue	92
Irritability	91
Labile mood with alternating sadness and anger	81
Depression	80
Oversensitivity	69
Crying spells	65
Social withdrawal	65
Forgetfulness	56
Difficulty concentrating	47
Physical	
Abdominal bloating	90
Breast tenderness	85
Acne	71
Appetite changes and food cravings	70
Swelling of the extremities	67
Headache	60
Gastrointestinal upset	48

Source: Reference 15; used with permission.

Table 7–3

Diagnostic Criteria for Premenstrual Dysphoric Disorder (PMDD)

On prospective evaluation of patient symptom charting for two to three menstrual cycles, five (or more) of the following symptoms are present during the last week of the luteal phase, and they are absent postmenstrually. At least one of the symptoms *must* be 1, 2, 3, or 4:

1. Markedly depressed mood, feelings of hopelessness, or self-deprecating thoughts.
2. Marked anxiety, tension, feeling of being "keyed up" or "on edge."
3. Marked affective lability (e.g., feeling suddenly sad or tearful or increased sensitivity to rejection).
4. Persistent and marked anger, irritability, or increase in interpersonal conflicts.
5. Decreased interest in usual activities (e.g., work, school, friends, hobbies).
6. Subjective sense of difficulty in concentrating.
7. Lethargy, easy fatigability, or marked lack of energy.
8. Marked change in appetite, overeating, or specific food cravings.
9. Hypersomnia or insomnia.
10. A subjective sense of being overwhelmed or out of control.
11. Other physical symptoms, such as breast tenderness or swelling, headaches, joint or muscle pain, sensation of "bloating," weight gain.

The symptoms *must* markedly interfere with work or school or with usual social activities and relationships with others (e.g., avoidance of social activities, decreased productivity, and decreased efficiency at work or school).

The disturbances *must not* be an exacerbation of the symptoms of another disorder (e.g., major depressive disorder, panic disorder, dysthymic disorder, or a personality disorder).

Source: American Psychiatric Association. *Diagnostic and Statistical Manual, Fourth Edition.* Washington DC: American Psychiatric Association, 1994; adapted with permission.

Treatment of Premenstrual Syndrome

PMS is a multisymptom disorder, involving behavioral and physical symptoms. Internal analgesics at the dosages listed in Table 7–1 are appropriate for treating the headache that some women report with more common symptoms of PMS. This section discusses several nonprescription agents shown to be effective in treating physical and/or behavioral symptoms of PMS. A single-therapeutic agent is unlikely to address all symptoms; thus, specific agents should be selected to address the patient's major symptoms.

Treatment Outcomes

Two outcomes are desirable for women with PMS or PMDD. The first outcome is an understanding of PMS: Knowledge of this disorder can allow a woman to exert some control over her symptoms and to limit the influence of this condition on her social and occupational functioning. The second desirable outcome is symptom improvement or resolution. Because of the variety of symptoms, the focus should be to relieve the most bothersome symptoms; multiple agents may be required.

General Treatment Approach

The initial treatment of PMS symptoms is generally conservative, consisting of education and nondrug measures such as dietary modifications, physical exercise, and stress management. Women with symptoms of PMS should be educated about the syndrome and encouraged to elicit family support and understanding.

For symptoms that are not responsive to nondrug therapy, several nonprescription agents that are relatively nontoxic might be suggested. These agents include calcium, magnesium, vitamin E, and pyridoxine. Use of a nonprescription diuretic may prove helpful for women with fluid retention. It is not uncommon for women with PMS-type symptoms to self-medicate. Prescription drug therapy should be considered if the treatments outlined in Figure 7–3 fail or if the patient suffers from severe PMS or PMDD. Prescription therapy includes psychotropic medications (e.g., alprazolam, selective serotonin reuptake inhibitors) and menstrual cycle modifiers (e.g., oral contraceptives, danazol, GnRH agonists). Selective serotonin reuptake inhibitors have been demonstrated in a number of clinical trials to be efficacious in treating women with PMDD and are now considered the treatment of choice for this severe form of PMS.[16]

Nonpharmacologic Therapy

Psychologic nondrug measures include avoiding stress, developing effective coping mechanisms for managing stress, and learning relaxation techniques. Participating in regular aerobic exercise is beneficial for some women. Suggested dietary modifications for the luteal phase are (1) lowering or eliminating intake of salt, caffeine, chocolate, and alcohol-containing beverages and (2) increasing the consumption of carbohydrates.[16]

Pharmacologic Therapy

One study[23] of more than 1000 women ages 21 to 64 years, found that 42% of women who stated they had PMS-type symptoms (feeling more emotional, bloating, food cravings, pain) took medication for their symptoms; 80% were taking a nonprescription product. Among women taking a nonprescription product, the medications most commonly cited were Midol (24% of women), acetaminophen (19%), ibuprofen (16%), and Pamprin (14%).

Calcium

A recent well-designed trial studied the effect of calcium (600 mg twice daily) in 466 women with moderate-to-severe PMS.[24] Symptoms were significantly reduced by the second month of therapy; by the third month, calcium had reduced overall symptoms by 48%. The reduction in symptoms occurred for emotional (e.g., mood swings, depression, anger); behavioral (e.g., food cravings); and physical symptoms (e.g., fluid retention, breast tenderness, backaches, and abdominal cramping). More than 50% of the women taking calcium had a greater than 50% improvement in symptoms; 29% had a greater than 75% improvement in symptoms. Few women experienced adverse effects from calcium, five withdrew from the study because of nausea, and one woman each in the calcium and placebo group developed kidney stones. The dose of calcium used in the trial is consistent with the recommended daily calcium intake for women of reproductive age.

Magnesium

One small trial has shown that magnesium (360 mg daily administered during the luteal phase) can relieve affective symptoms of PMS.[25] It has been hypothesized that magnesium deficiency may lead to PMS-type symptoms (e.g., irritability), and low magnesium levels in red blood cells have been found in women with PMS.[25] The dose of magnesium used in the trial was similar to the recommended dietary allowance for magnesium for women (280 to 300 mg). Side effects from magnesium are uncommon; diarrhea is the most common side effect from oral magnesium.

Vitamin E

Vitamin E (400 IU daily) is sometimes recommended for the symptom of breast tenderness. However, data on its effectiveness are unconvincing.[18] Adverse effects are unlikely at this dose of vitamin E.

Pyridoxine

A recent meta-analysis[20] of nine trials of pyridoxine for PMS symptoms found that the vitamin is likely to be beneficial for the treatment of overall PMS symptoms (odds ratio 2.32; 95% confidence interval [CI] 1.95 to 2.54) such as mastalgia (breast pain), irritability, fatigue, bloating, and tension. This vitamin was also beneficial for symptoms of depression (odds ratio 2.12; 95% CI 1.8 to 2.48). However, this meta-analysis was not able to show a dose–response correlation. It is recommended that the daily dose of pyridoxine be limited to 100 mg daily because of the potential for neuropathy at higher doses. Symptoms of this toxicity include paresthesia (a sensation of pricking, tingling, or creeping on the skin), bone pain, muscle weakness, and hyperesthesia (stinging, burning, itching sensations).[26]

Diuretics

One of the most common premenstrual complaints is fluid accumulation, particularly abdominal bloating. However, a

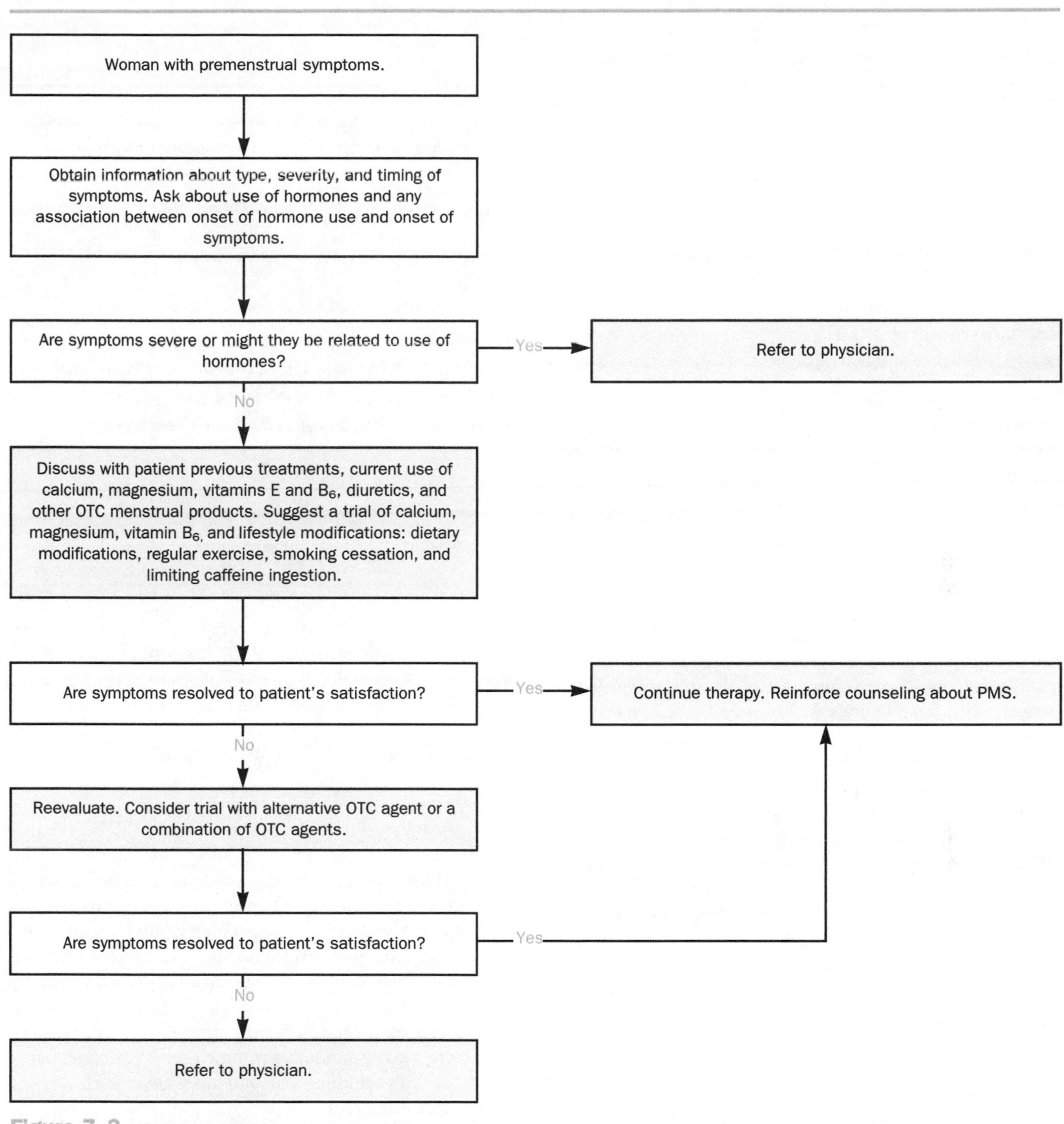

Figure 7–3 Self-care of premenstrual syndrome.

distinction must be made between fluid redistribution and fluid retention (detected by weight gain). The bloating and swelling observed with PMS are primarily a fluid shift; therefore, diuretics, indicated for relieving fluid retention, are unlikely to be helpful for most PMS patients.[17,18]

The Food and Drug Administration (FDA) has examined the usefulness and safety of nonprescription diuretics to relieve water retention, weight gain, bloating, swelling, and a full feeling. Three nonprescription diuretics—ammonium chloride, caffeine, and pamabrom—are contained in commercially available menstrual products. (See Table 7–4.) Ammonium chloride is an acid-forming salt with a short duration of effect; it is taken in oral doses of up to 3 g per day (divided into three doses) for no more than 6 consecutive

Table 7–4

Selected Menstrual Products

Trade Name	Primary Ingredients
Diurex PMS	Pamabrom 25 mg; acetaminophen 500 mg; pyrilamine maleate 15 mg
Diurex Maximum Relief Water Caplets[a–e]	Pamabrom 50 mg
Diurex-2 Water Pills[a–d]	Pamabrom 25 mg; magnesium salicylate tetrahydrate 202 mg; calcium carbonate; calcium sulfate
Midol Maximum Strength Multisymptom Menstrual Formula Caplets[a,c]	Caffeine 60 mg; acetaminophen 500 mg; pyrilamine maleate 15 mg
Midol Maximum Strength PMS Caplets	Pamabrom 25 mg; acetaminophen 500 mg; pyrilamine maleate 15 mg
Midol Teen Caplets[a,c,d]	Pamabrom 25 mg; acetaminophen 400 mg
Pamprin Maximum Pain Relief Caplets[d]	Pamabrom 25 mg; magnesium salicylate 250 mg; acetaminophen 250 mg
Pamprin Multisymptom Caplets/Tablets[c,d]	Pamabrom 25 mg; acetaminophen 500 mg; pyrilamine maleate 15 mg
Premsyn PMS Caplets	Pamabrom 25 mg; acetaminophen 500 mg; pyrilamine maleate 15 mg

[a] Sodium-free product.
[b] Preservative-free product.
[c] Aspirin-free product.
[d] Caffeine-free product.
[e] Sucrose-free product.

days. Larger doses of ammonium chloride (4 to 12 g per day) can produce significant adverse effects of the GI and central nervous systems. Ammonium chloride is contraindicated in patients with renal or liver impairment because metabolic acidosis may result.

Caffeine, a xanthine, promotes diuresis by inhibiting the renal tubular reabsorption of sodium and water. It is safe and effective as a diuretic in dosages of 100 to 200 mg every 3 to 4 hours. Tolerance to the diuretic effect may occur. Caffeine may cause anxiety, restlessness, or insomnia (if taken within several hours of bedtime). Additive side effects (nervousness, irritability, nausea, or tachycardia) might occur if other caffeine-containing beverages, foods, or medications are consumed concurrently. This agent may not be an appropriate choice for a woman who experiences irritability as a PMS symptom. Caffeine may also cause GI irritation, so patients with a history of peptic ulcer disease should avoid it. Patients taking monoamine oxidase inhibitors or other xanthine medications (e.g., theophylline, aminophylline, oxtriphylline, or dyphylline) should avoid diuretics that contain caffeine.

Pamabrom, a derivative of theophylline, is contained in combination products (along with analgesics and antihistamines) and is marketed for the treatment of PMS. It is taken in doses of up to 200 mg per day (50 mg four times daily).

Combination Products

Several nonprescription products are marketed for women with PMS-type symptoms. Two of the most commonly used products are Midol and Pamprin (acetaminophen, pamabrom, and pyrilamine). Pain is a relatively uncommon feature of PMS, and no evidence exists that the sedative effect of an antihistamine will provide benefit to women experiencing the emotional symptoms of PMS. Therefore, pharmacists should not recommend these types of nonprescription products. More definitive agents, such as those previously discussed, or referral for prescription drug therapy are more appropriate therapeutic recommendations.

Product Selection Guidelines

Calcium, magnesium, or pyridoxine should be recommended for the initial treatment of PMS symptoms. If the initial selected agent provides inadequate relief, another agent or a combination of two or all three agents may be tried. Women who experience bloating might try pamabrom or caffeine. However, distinguishing fluid retention from fluid redistribution is useful in determining whether a nonprescription diuretic will be beneficial. Caffeine may not be a good choice for women who experience irritability during their menstrual cycle. Both xanthine agents (caffeine, pamabrom) are contraindicated in patients who have a history of peptic ulcer disease or who are taking monoamine oxidase inhibitors or other xanthine medications (e.g., theophylline, aminophylline, oxtriphylline, dyphylline).

Patient Assessment of Premenstrual Syndrome

The pharmacist should obtain a complete description of the patient's symptoms and their timing to determine whether the patient has PMS, PMDD, or another disorder with PMS-type symptoms. The severity of PMS symptoms is another factor in ruling self-treatment in or out. As with any disorder, the pharmacist should explore the use of medications

Case Study 7–2

Eugenia is a 44-year-old woman who is experiencing some premenstrual symptoms: abdominal bloating, irritability, breast tenderness, food cravings, and fatigue. She reports that she has really noticed these symptoms over the past 4 to 6 months and that they occur during the week before her menstrual period. She describes them as bothersome but not incapacitating. She would like to know if there are any nonprescription products that she can use for relief of these symptoms.

A check of her prescription profile shows that she is not taking any prescription medications on a regular basis. Over the past year she used antibiotics twice, and she had a prescription for lorazepam (Ativan) about 6 months ago but she has not had it refilled recently.

On questioning her, the pharmacist learns that she takes several vitamins daily, including a multiple vitamin with minerals (Unicap M; 30 mg vitamin E, 60 mg calcium, no magnesium), vitamin C 250 mg, and vitamin E 400 IU. She also occasionally takes ibuprofen for headaches or muscle aches and famotidine (Pepcid AC) for heartburn.

Clinical Considerations/Strategies

Readers can use the following considerations/strategies to determine whether treatment of the patient's condition with nonprescription medications is warranted:

- Determine the patient's suitability for self-treatment.
- Recommend nonpharmacologic measures for the appropriate PMS symptoms.
- Develop a protocol for the management of patients with mild symptoms of PMS. Include initial drug selection, initial dose selection, dose modifications, possible switch to another OTC agent, and medical referral.

Patient Education/Counseling

Readers can use the following strategies to develop a patient education/counseling plan that will ensure optimal therapeutic outcomes:

- Educate the patient about PMS.
- Explain nonpharmacologic measures that can alleviate some PMS symptoms.
- Explain the optimal use of nonprescription agents for PMS symptoms.
- Explain the expected outcomes of therapy.
- Advise the patient of the conditions that indicate medical attention is appropriate.

that might cause the symptoms or that might potentially interact with nonprescription agents used to treat PMS. Previous treatments of the symptoms should also be explored. Asking the patient the following questions will help elicit the information needed to accurately assess the disorder and to recommend the appropriate treatment approach.

Q~ What symptoms are you currently experiencing? Have you experienced one or more of the following symptoms just before your menstrual period: mood swings, depression, anger, irritability, tension, fatigue, forgetfulness, confusion, difficulty concentrating, food craving, abdominal bloating, or breast tenderness? Describe the severity of your symptoms.

A~ If the patient describes the typical symptoms of PMS listed above, educate her about the disorder. Then recommend a trial of nonpharmacologic treatment for mild-to-moderate symptoms. Refer women with more severe symptoms to a physician for more definitive treatment.

Q~ At what time in the menstrual cycle do your symptoms occur? Are these symptoms the same as or different from symptoms you have experienced in previous menstrual cycles?

A~ *Identify the correlation of PMS or PMDD symptoms with the menstrual cycle. (See the section "Signs and Symptoms of Premenstrual Syndrome.")* If the timing of the symptoms suggests a disorder other than PMS or PMDD, or if the symptoms have changed, refer the patient to a physician. Otherwise, strongly suspect PMS or PMDD.

Q~ What medication(s) are you currently taking?

A~ *Identify medications that can cause PMS-like symptoms. (See the section "Etiology of Premenstrual Syndrome.")* If the patient is taking any of these medications, refer the patient to a physician for evaluation of whether the symptoms are drug induced.

Q~ What medication(s) or other treatments (e.g., diet or exercise) have you tried to manage or to alleviate your symptoms? Are you allergic or hypersensitive to any drugs? If yes, which one(s)?

A~ Recommend lifestyle modifications and exercise as an initial treatment unless the patient has tried these measures and found them ineffective. Explore with the patient the use of nonprescription agents. If a product is recommended, discuss with the patient the doses suggested from clinical trials and dosage limitations. Avoid recommending agents to which the patient has a history of sensitivity or intolerable side effects.

Patient Counseling for Premenstrual Syndrome

Educating women who experience PMS about this disorder, especially about the timing of symptoms and what might control them, can increase compliance with recommended therapies. The pharmacist should be prepared to discuss treatment of behavioral as well as physical symptoms of mild-to-moderate PMS. If the patient wishes to use nonprescription medications or vitamins, the pharmacist should explain the proper use and potential adverse effects of these agents. The patient should also be advised that treatment measures must be implemented during every menstrual cycle because it may take several cycles for symptomatic relief to occur. The box "Patient Education for Premenstrual Syndrome" lists specific information to provide patients.

Evaluation of Patient Outcomes for Premenstrual Syndrome

Patient monitoring is accomplished by having the patient report whether the symptoms are resolved. It may take several menstrual cycles to ascertain if lifestyle changes or nonprescription therapies are reducing the symptoms of PMS. Follow-up with a phone call allows the pharmacist to discuss treatment effectiveness (continued or altered symptoms) and to clarify information or to answer any patient questions. Reasons for advising the patient to see a clinician are either persistent symptoms or symptoms that the patient reports to be disruptive to personal relationships or to the patient's ability to engage in usual activities or to function productively at work.

Menstrual Products and Toxic Shock Syndrome

Tampons are intravaginal inserts made of cellulose, cotton, or synthetic materials that are designed to absorb menstrual and other vaginal discharges. Both the composition of tampons and their high absorbency have been associated with toxic shock syndrome (TSS).[27] In an effort to decrease the likelihood of TSS, tampon manufacturers have altered the composition and lowered the absorbency of these products.[27] In addition, FDA changed the requirement for the labeling of tampons so that terms such as *regular* and *super*, which are used to indicate the absorbency of tampons, have a uniform meaning and indicate a specific range of fluid absorbed per tampon.[28]

Toxic shock syndrome was a term originally coined by Todd and co-workers in 1978 to describe a severe multisys-

Patient Education for Premenstrual Syndrome

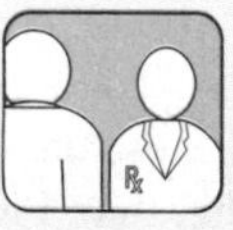

The objective of self-treatment is to achieve relief from or significant improvement in symptoms so as to limit discomfort, distress, and the disruption of personal relationships or usual activities. For most patients, carefully following product instructions and the self-care measures listed below will help ensure optimal therapeutic outcomes.

Nondrug Measures

- Try to avoid stress, develop effective coping mechanisms for managing stress, and learn relaxation techniques.
- If possible, participate in regular aerobic exercise.
- During the 7 to 14 days before your menstrual period, reduce or eliminate intake of salt, caffeine, chocolate, and alcoholic beverages. Eating foods rich in carbohydrates and low in protein during the premenstrual interval may also reduce symptoms.

Nonprescription Medications

- Note that nonprescription medications and lifestyle modifications may not improve symptoms for all women and that it may take several months to determine whether these therapies are working.
- Note that therapy with one nonprescription medication may improve only some of the symptoms; several medications may be needed for optimal symptom control.
- Follow the guidelines below for the agents that best control your symptoms:
  - —Take 1200 mg of calcium daily in divided doses. Take no more than 500 mg at one time. Note that calcium may cause stomach upset or constipation.
  - —Take 360 mg of magnesium daily during the premenstrual interval only. Note that magnesium may cause diarrhea.
  - —Take 400 IU of vitamin E daily.
  - —Take 100 mg of pyridoxine (vitamin B_6) daily. Do not exceed this daily dosage.
- Note that neurologic symptoms caused by vitamin B_6 toxicity may occur.

If you are taking vitamin B_6 and develop symptoms, such as a sensation of pricking, tingling, or creeping on the skin; bone pain; muscle weakness; and stinging, burning, or itching sensations, stop taking the vitamin and seek medical attention.

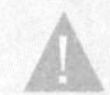

If the symptoms of premenstrual syndrome do not improve or if they worsen, seek medical attention.

tem illness characterized by high fever, profound hypotension, severe diarrhea, mental confusion, renal failure, erythroderma, and skin desquamation.[29] In 1980, these symptoms were recognized as affecting a relatively large number of young, previously healthy, menstruating women, and the term *toxic shock syndrome* was applied to their illness. Table 7–5 shows the Centers for Disease Control and Prevention's case definition of TSS.[30]

Epidemiology of Toxic Shock Syndrome

TSS is commonly divided into menstrual and nonmenstrual cases; nonmenstrual TSS is much less common, accounting for only about one-third of TSS cases. Currently, the incidence of TSS in the United States is low; in 1997 the Centers for Disease Control and Prevention recorded only 157 cases.[31]

Menstrual TSS has been found to affect primarily young women between 15 to 19 years of age. One reason for the greater incidence in young women is the absence of preexisting antibodies to the TSS toxin. By age 20 to 25 years of age, more than 90% of both men and women have detectable antibodies to this toxin.[29] However, in almost all cases of TSS, an absent or low titer of antibody to toxic shock syndrome toxin 1 (TSST-1), an exotoxin that causes TSS, has been found.[32]

Table 7–5

CDC[a] Case Definition of Toxic Shock Syndrome

- Fever: temperature ≥102°F (38.9°C)
- Rash: diffuse macular erythroderma
- Desquamation: 1–2 weeks after onset of illness, particularly on palms and soles
- Hypotension: systolic blood pressure ≤90 mm Hg, orthostatic drop in diastolic ≥15 mm Hg; orthostatic syncope or dizziness
- Involvement of three or more of the following organ systems:
  —Gastrointestinal: vomiting or diarrhea at onset of illness
  —Muscular: severe myalgia or twice-normal creatine phosphokinase
  —Mucous membranes: vaginal, oropharyngeal, or conjunctival hyperemia
  —Renal: twice-normal blood urea nitrogen or creatinine or pyuria (more than 5 white blood cells in a high-power field)
  —Hepatic: twice-normal bilirubin or transaminases
  —Hematologic: platelets <1,000,000/mm^3
- Central nervous system: disorientation or alterations in consciousness without focal neurologic signs when fever and hypotension are absent
- Negative results on the following tests, if obtained:
  —Blood, throat, or cerebrospinal fluid cultures (blood culture may be positive for *S. aureus*)
  —Serologic tests for Rocky Mountain spotted fever, leptospirosis, or measles

[a] Centers for Disease Control and Prevention.

Risk factors for menstrual TSS have been identified. The strongest predictor of risk is the use of tampons. One study[30] found that women who use tampons have a 33-fold greater risk for TSS. A case–control study[28] from 1986 to 1987 found that the use of all major tampon brands was associated with the increased risk, although the risk varied by the brand of tampon. The risk also varied with the absorbency of the tampon: Two studies[28] found that for every 1-g increase in absorbency, the risk for TSS increased 34% to 37%. Additionally, the occurrence of TSS has been related to tampon composition, which can alter the presence of several factors (e.g., oxygen, magnesium, and glucose) that can influence the production of toxin by *Staphylococcus aureus*.[29] Since the early 1980s, when the association between tampon usage and TSS was first noted, the absorbency and composition of tampons have changed dramatically. Nonetheless, the risk for TSS continues to be greater in tampon users than in other individuals, and the greatest risk is associated with the use of higher-absorbency tampons. Finally, patterns of tampon use may affect the risk for TSS. Continuous use of tampons for at least 1 day of menses has been shown to correlate with an increased risk for menstrual TSS.[27]

Besides tampons, the risk for TSS has been associated with the use of all barrier contraceptives, including diaphragms, cervical caps, and cervical sponges. This risk has been calculated to be about 10 to 12 times greater for women who use these forms of contraception than for women who do not. Neither oral contraceptive use nor use of an intrauterine device has been related to the development of TSS.[32]

Etiology of Toxic Shock Syndrome

TSS is a severe, life-threatening disease known to result from infections (at any site) with toxin-producing strains of *S. aureus*. TSS is essentially a consequence of the systemic effects of the exotoxin TSST-1. The effects of TSST-1 are caused by both the direct effects of the toxin and by the toxin's ability to induce production of two cytokines.

Signs and Symptoms of Toxic Shock Syndrome

The clinical manifestations of TSS characteristically evolve quite rapidly. Within 8 to 12 hours an individual can move from a state of good health to full-blown TSS, which includes high fever, myalgias,, vomiting and diarrhea, erythroderma, decreased urine output, severe hypotension, and shock.[29,30] Multisystem organ involvement typically occurs in TSS. Myalgias, muscle weakness, arthralgias, and GI symptoms (vomiting, diarrhea, and abdominal pain) typically occur early in the illness and affect almost all patients. Neurologic manifestations occur in almost all cases. Encephalopathy from cerebral edema can be manifested as headache, confusion, agitation, lethargy, and seizures. Both acute renal failure and adult respiratory distress syndrome are also common in this condition.

Dermatologic manifestations are characteristic of TSS;

both the early rash and subsequent skin desquamation are required for a definite diagnosis. The early rash is often described as a sunburn-like, diffuse, macular erythroderma that is not pruritic. It usually appears on the lower abdomen and thighs but may involve the perineum, torso, or extremities. It usually disappears after 3 days, and about 1 to 3 weeks later, desquamation of the skin on the patient's soles and palms begins. A second rash that exhibits erythema, pruritis, and maculopapules (discolored conical elevations of the skin) occurs in more than 50% of patients. Telogen effluvium, a late dermatologic manifestation that is a common and nonspecific reaction to severe sepsis and stress, may also be seen. Telogen effluvium describes the loss of hair, nails, or both, which can occur after 4 to 16 weeks; growth is restored in 5 to 6 months.[30]

Prevention of Toxic Shock Syndrome

Women can reduce the risk of TSS to zero by using sanitary pads instead of tampons during their menstrual cycle. If this measure is not feasible, women who use tampons can reduce the risk by following the guidelines in the box "Patient Education for Toxic Shock Syndrome."

Women who have had TSS are at higher risk for recurrent episodes, especially during the first year after the illness, because it takes at least that long for protective antibodies to reappear. Prevention of TSS for these patients includes avoiding tampons; administering oral antistaphylococcal antibiotics during menses until the TSST-1 titer rises;[30] and using nonbarrier forms of contraception, at least until the TSST-1 titers rise.[32]

Patient Assessment of Toxic Shock Syndrome

Obtaining prompt medical attention is a very important aspect of care for patients with symptoms consistent with TSS. A pharmacist can be alert to symptoms of TSS when patients seek nonprescription therapy for a severe "flu" (e.g., fever, vomiting, diarrhea, dizziness) or an unusual skin rash that occurs in conjunction with the previously described symptoms. Asking the patient the following questions will help elicit the information needed to determine whether the patient has TSS.

Q~ What symptoms are you currently experiencing? Are you experiencing a high fever, dizziness, nausea, vomiting, diarrhea, sunburn-like rash, muscle aches, and/or mental confusion?

A~ If the patient is an adolescent or young woman who describes symptoms similar to those above, ask specifically whether a rash appeared in conjunction with the symptoms and whether severe dizziness or faintness is present. The latter may indicate hypotension.

Q~ What is the relationship between the onset of these symptoms and your menstrual period? Do you use menstrual pads or tampons? Which contraceptive method do you use?

A~ If the symptoms appear to be related to the menstrual cycle and the use of tampons, strongly suspect TSS and refer the patient for immediate medical attention. Note that certain forms of contraception also increase the risk of TSS.

Patient Education for Toxic Shock Syndrome

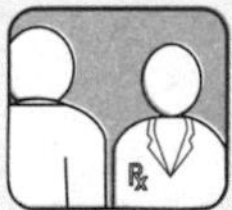

The objective of self-treatment is to reduce the risk of developing toxic shock syndrome associated with the use of tampons or contraceptive devices. For most patients, carefully following product instructions and the self-care measures listed below will help ensure optimal therapeutic outcomes.

- To reduce the risk to almost zero, use sanitary pads instead of tampons during your period.
- To lower the risk while using tampons, use the lowest-absorbency tampons compatible with your needs. Also, alternate the use of menstrual pads (e.g., at night) with the use of tampons.
- Change tampons four to six times a day.
- Wash your hands with soap before inserting anything into the vagina (e.g., a tampon, a diaphragm, a contraceptive sponge, or a vaginal medication).
- Do not leave a contraceptive sponge, a diaphragm, or a cervical cap in place in the vagina longer than recommended; do not use any of them during a menstrual period.
- Do not use tampons, contraceptive sponges, or a cervical cap during the first 12 weeks after childbirth. It may be best to avoid using a diaphragm as well.
- Read the insert on toxic shock syndrome enclosed in the tampon package, and familiarize yourself with the early symptoms of this disorder. These symptoms include a high fever, muscle aches, a sunburn-like rash appearing after a day or two, weakness, fatigue, nausea, vomiting, and diarrhea.

⚠ If you develop the symptoms above, remove the tampon immediately and seek emergency medical treatment.[29] If left untreated, toxic shock syndrome can cause dizziness, faintness, shock, and even death.

Patient Counseling for Toxic Shock Syndrome

The pharmacist should be able to counsel patients about the prevention of TSS as outlined in the box "Patient Education for Toxic Shock Syndrome." The pharmacist should emphasize, however, that the risk for this condition is quite small. If a patient presents with early symptoms of TSS, the pharmacist should encourage her to remove the tampon or contraceptive device and to seek emergency medical treatment.[29] In severe cases, TSS can cause dizziness, faintness, shock, and even death.

CONCLUSION

Menstrual health concerns and symptoms are common among healthy women who are ambulatory. Several important and common symptoms can be appropriately and safely self-treated by many women. Pharmacists can help women to decide when self-treatment is appropriate, recommend effective nonprescription therapy, and advise the patient about safe and effective nonpharmacologic therapies. The pharmacist must also be able to identify symptomatic patients who should be referred to their primary care provider.

Dysmenorrhea is one of the most common gynecologic problems in the United States. It occurs in approximately 30% to 60% of women of reproductive age, but its prevalence is higher (about 60% to 79%) in adolescent women. The principal agents for the treatment of primary dysmenorrhea are nonsalicylate NSAIDs. In clinical trials, these agents were found to be effective in 66% to 90% of patients. Therapy with a nonsalicylate NSAID should begin at the onset of pain; there is no proven value to beginning therapy in anticipation of dysmenorrhea. The NSAID is used as much to prevent cramps as to relieve pain. Optimal pain relief is achieved when these agents are taken on a scheduled rather than on an as-needed basis.

Approximately 80% of women experience some physical or mood changes before the onset of menses. PMS can be defined as a cyclic disorder composed of a combination of physical, behavioral, and emotional (mood) changes that occur during the luteal phase of the menstrual cycle. The majority of women with premenstrual symptoms experience only mild, primarily physical symptoms that do not interfere with their lives. A more severe form of PMS is PMDD. Women with PMDD experience significant symptoms that can impair personal relationships and the ability to function well at work.

TSS is a severe, life-threatening disease that has been linked to tampon use. To lower the risk for TSS while using tampons, women should use the lowest-absorbency tampons compatible with their needs and should alternate the use of menstrual pads (e.g., at night) with the use of tampons.

References

1. Koff E, Rierdan J, Stubbs ML. Conceptions and misconceptions of the menstrual cycle. *Women Health.* 1990;16:119–36.
2. Neinstein LS. Menstrual problems in adolescents. *Med Clin North Am.* 1990;74:1181–203.
3. Espey LL, Halim IA. Characteristics and control of the normal menstrual cycle. *Obstet Gynecol Clin North Am.* 1990;17:275–98.
4. Osathanondh R. Dysmenorrhea. *Curr Ther Endocrinol Metab.* 1997;6: 246–51.
5. Harlow SD, Park M. A longitudinal study of risk factors for the occurrence, duration, and severity of menstrual cramps in a cohort of college women. *Br J Obstet Gynaecol.* 1996;103:1134–42.
6. Johnson J. Level of knowledge among adolescent girls regarding effective treatment for dysmenorrhea. *J Adolesc Health Care.* 1988;9: 398–402.
7. Jensen DV, Andersen KB, Wagner G. Prostaglandins in the menstrual cycle of women. *Dan Med Bull.* 1987;34:178–81.
8. Campbell MA, McGrath PJ. Use of medication by adolescents for the management of menstrual discomfort. *Arch Pediatr Adolesc Med.* 1997;151:905–13.
9. Dawood MY. Dysmenorrhea. *Clin Obstet Gynecol.* 1990;33:168–78.
10. Jamieson DJ, Steege JF. The prevalence of dysmenorrhea, dyspareunia, pelvic pain, and irritable bowel syndrome in primary care practices. *Obstet Gynecol.* 1996;87:55–8.
11. Hewison A, van den Akker OB. Dysmenorrhea, menstrual attitude, and GP consultation. *Brit J Nurs.* 1996;5:480–4.
12. Sundell G, Milsom I, Andersch B. Factors influencing the prevalence and severity of dysmenorrhea in young women. *Br J Obstet Gynaecol.* 1990;97:588–94.
13. Kauppila A, Puolakka J, Ylikorkala O. The relief of primary dysmenorrhea by ketoprofen and indomethacin. *Prostaglandins.* 1979;18:647–53.
14. Field CS. Dysfunctional uterine bleeding. *Prim Care.* 1988;15:561–74.
15. ACOG Committee Opinion. Premenstrual syndrome. *Int J Gynaecol Obstet.* 1995;50:80–4.
16. Korzekwa MI, Steiner M. Premenstrual syndromes. *Clin Obstet Gynecol.* 1997;40:564–76.
17. Severino SK, Moline ML. Premenstrual syndrome. Identification and management. *Drugs.* 1995;49:71–82.
18. Barnhart KT, Freeman EW, Sondheimer SJ. A clinician's guide to the premenstrual syndrome. *Med Clin North Am.* 1995;79:1457–72.
19. Kendall KE, Schnurr PP. The effects of vitamin B_6 supplementation on premenstrual symptoms. *Obstet Gynecol.* 1987;70:145–9.
20. Wyatt KM, Dimmock PW, Jones PW, et al. Efficacy of vitamin B_6 in the treatment of premenstrual syndrome: Systematic review. *Br Med J.* 1999;318:1375–81.
21. Mortola JF. A risk–benefit appraisal of drugs used in the management of premenstrual syndrome. *Drug Safety.* 1994;10:160–9.
22. Sayegh R, Wurtman J, Spiers P, et al. The effect of a carbohydrate-rich beverage on mood, appetite, and cognitive function in women with premenstrual syndrome. *Obstet Gynecol.* 1995;86:520–8.
23. Singh B, Berman BM, Simpson RL, et al. Incidence of premenstrual syndrome and remedy usage: A national probability sample study. *Altern Ther Health Med.* 1998;4:75–9.
24. Thys-Jacobs S, Starkey P, Bernstein D, et al. Calcium carbonate and the premenstrual syndrome: Effect on premenstrual and menstrual symptoms. *Am J Obstet Gynecol.* 1998;179:444–52.
25. Facchinetti F, Borella P, Sances G, et al. Oral magnesium successfully relieves premenstrual mood changes. *Obstet Gynecol.* 1991;78:177–81.
26. Dalton K, Dalton MJ. Characteristics of pyridoxine overdose neuropathy syndrome. *Acta Neurol Scand.* 1987;76:8–11.
27. Reingold AL, Broome CV, Gaventa S, et al. Risk factors for menstrual toxic shock syndrome: Results of a multistate case–control study. *Rev Infect Dis.* 1989;2(suppl 1):S35–41.
28. Nightingale SL. New requirements for tampon labeling. *Am Fam Physician.* 1990;41:999–1000.
29. Reingold AL. Toxic shock syndrome: An update. *Am J Obstet Gynecol.* 1991;165:1236–9.
30. Freedman JD, Beer DJ. Expanding perspectives on the toxic shock syndrome. *Adv Intern Med.* 1991;36:363–97.
31. Centers for Disease Control and Prevention. Summary of notifiable diseases, United States 1997. *MMWR.* 1998;46:1–80.
32. Schwartz B, Gaventa S, Broome CV, et al. Nonmenstrual toxic shock syndrome associated with barrier contraceptives: Report of a case–control study. *Rev Infect Dis.* 1989;11(suppl 1):S43–9.

CHAPTER 8

Prevention of Unintended Pregnancy and Sexually Transmitted Diseases

Louise Parent-Stevens and David L. Lourwood

Chapter 8 at a Glance

Unprotected sexual activity can result in unintended pregnancy, sexually transmitted diseases (STDs), or both and can exact a high physical, psychologic, and financial toll on those affected. This chapter reviews the two adverse outcomes and discusses how nonprescription contraceptive products or methods, when properly used, can guard against the risks of unprotected sex.

Unintended Pregnancy

Throughout history, people have sought ways to control their fertility so they can choose the number and timing of their pregnancies. As knowledge of reproductive physiology has evolved, a wider variety of safe and reliable methods of contraception has been developed.

According to the 1995 National Survey of Family Growth (NSFG) of 15- to 44-year-old U.S. women, 20% of women relied on a nonprescription method of contraception, 18.9% used male condoms, 1.3% used spermicides, and approximately 2% relied on periodic abstinence. Slightly less than 10% of subjects reported using two or more methods, with condoms as the most common component of a multiple contraceptive regimen. Overall, 94.8% of the sexually active women reported using some form of birth control.[1]

In the United States and worldwide, reliance on nonprescription methods of contraception is widespread. The fact that such products are accessible and relatively inexpensive makes them very important for those who do not have access to family-planning services, who choose not to use physicians or clinics, or who are unable or unwilling to use prescription contraceptives. Even if a prescription product is chosen as the primary contraceptive method, low-cost and low-risk nonprescription methods may be appropriate at different times during a person's sexually active life.

Editor's Note: This chapter is based, in part, on the 11th edition chapter titled "Contraceptive Methods and Products," which was written by Louise Parent-Stevens and David L. Lourwood.

Epidemiology of Unintended Pregnancy

The consistent and proper use of contraceptives, whether prescription or nonprescription, significantly reduces the incidence of unintended pregnancies. However, a recent survey of women with unintended pregnancies found that more than half had been using a method of contraception during the month in which they conceived.[2] Given that close to 50% of pregnancies in the United States are unintended, apparently much more attention needs to be paid to family planning and contraceptive counseling.[2]

Of particular concern is the high risk of pregnancy in the adolescent population. The 1995 Youth Risk Behavior Survey found that slightly more than half of students in grades 9 through 12 had experienced sexual intercourse.[3] Of sexually active teenagers, 7% report using no method of contraception despite being sexually active.[1] The teenage pregnancy rate in the United States (9.6% of 15- to 19-year-olds) is high compared with that in other developed countries.[4]

Etiology of Unintended Pregnancy

Contraceptives work by preventing egg fertilization. (See Chapter 7, "Disorders Related to Menstruation," for a discussion of the reproductive process.) Pregnancy can result only when a viable egg is available for fertilization by a sperm. It is estimated that there is a 4- to 5-day window around the time of ovulation when conception can occur. The estimated risk of pregnancy from an unprotected coital act at the middle of the menstrual cycle is 17% to 30%.[5] Pregnancy can occur even with the use of contraceptive products if the product is used incorrectly or if a product fails (e.g., condom breakage).

According to one study, the average U.S. teenager has unprotected intercourse for an average of 1 year before seeking contraceptive advice.[6] The reasons adolescents delay seeking contraceptive advice include fear about perceived dangers of contraceptives, fear of parental discovery, and belief that they cannot get pregnant because of their young age or low frequency of intercourse.[7] However, 50% of all adolescent pregnancies occur within the first 6 months after the initiation of sexual intercourse, with 20% occurring during the first month.[8] Of teenage pregnancies, 78% are unintended.[2] Often the young woman does not use contraceptives until after she becomes pregnant. Clearly, efforts to disseminate accurate reproductive information as well as to provide access to contraceptive products are vital when addressing this serious public health problem.

Prevention of Unintended Pregnancy

No method of birth control is perfect. Contraceptive choices may change during a person's sexually active life. Major points to consider in selecting a contraceptive method should include safety, effectiveness, accessibility, and acceptability of each method to each sexual partner.

Safety factors to consider in choosing a method of contraception include the risk of side effects, including the potential for method-associated adverse effects on future fertility as well as on the fetus if unintended conception should occur.

The effectiveness of a contraceptive method is reported in two ways: the accidental pregnancy rate in the first year of *perfect* use (method-related failure rate) and in the first year of *typical* use (use-related failure rate). (See Table 8–1.) The lowest expected rate—that of perfect use—is very difficult to measure and indicates the method's theoretical effectiveness. It assumes accurate and consistent use of the method every time intercourse occurs. The more realistic rate of typical use includes pregnancies that may have occurred because of inconsistent or improper use of the method. Reported use-related failure rates may vary, depending on the population studied. Effectiveness increases the longer a particular method is used. Declining fertility in a population of older users may contribute to increased effectiveness rates. In addition, couples who use contraception to prevent pregnancy have fewer failures than those who use contraceptives to space the births of their children.[9]

The percentage of people who continue with a given contraceptive method after a year of use is an indication of the method's acceptability. (See Table 8–1.) Important factors in determining a method's acceptability include user's religious beliefs and future reproductive plans, partner's supportiveness, complexity of method use, degree of interruption of spontaneity, "messiness," and cost. To help their patients make informed decisions, pharmacists should be aware of the safety, effectiveness, accessibility, acceptability, and relative cost of the different contraceptive methods. The algorithm in Figure 8–1 can assist the pharmacist in making appropriate contraceptive recommendations.

Nonprescription Contraceptive Products

Nonprescription contraceptive products vary in effectiveness as protection both against unintended pregnancy and against sexually transmitted diseases. The types of nonprescription contraceptive products include the male condom, the female condom, vaginal spermicides, and the contraceptive sponge.

Male Condoms

Condoms—also known as rubbers, sheaths, prophylactics, safes, skins, or pros—are the most important barrier contraceptive device in an era of infectious STDs. According to the NSFG, condom users grew from 5.1 million in 1988 to 7.9 million in 1995, a 20% increase.[1] Apart from its role as a contraceptive, its importance in disease prevention is second only to that of abstinence.

Composition/Features The condom was originally described in the 16th century by Fallopius as a linen sheath used to protect the wearer from syphilis.[11] Current-day materials, which include latex, polyurethane, and lamb cecum (natural membrane, or skin), are much more comfortable for users and their partners.

Table 8–1

First-Year Failure/Continuation Rates of Various Contraceptive Methods[a,b]

Method (1)	% Who Experience Accidental Pregnancy in First Year of Use: Typical Use[b] (2)	Perfect Use[c] (3)	% Who Continue Using Contraceptive Method for One Year[a] (4)
Chance[d]	85	—	—
Spermicides[e]	26	6	40
Withdrawal	19	4	—
Natural family planning (Periodic abstinence)	25	—	63
Calendar (rhythm) method	—	9	—
Cervical mucus (ovulation) method	—	3	—
Symptothermal method[f]	—	2	—
Basal body temperature (postovulation) method	—	1	—
Cervical cap[g]			
Parous women	40	26	42
Nulliparous women	20	9	56
Diaphragm[g]	20	6	56
Sponge[h]			
Parous women	36	26	45
Nulliparous women	18	9	58
Condom[i]			
Male	14	3	61
Female	25[j]	5	56
Prescription Methods	≤5	≤1.5	≥70
Sterilization			
Female	0.5	0.5	100
Male	0.15	0.10	100

[a] Percentage of couples who in attempting to avoid pregnancy continue to use a method for 1 year.

[b] Among typical couples who initiate use of a method (not necessarily for the first time), the percentage who experience an accidental pregnancy during the first year if they do not stop use for any other reason.

[c] Among couples who initiate use of a method (not necessarily for the first time) and who use it perfectly (both consistently and correctly), the percentage who experience an accidental pregnancy during the first year if they do not stop use for any other reason.

[d] The percentages failing in columns (2) and (3) are based on data from populations in which contraception is not used and from women who cease using contraception to become pregnant. Among such populations, about 89% become pregnant within 1 year. This estimate was lowered slightly (to 85%) to represent the percentage who would become pregnant within 1 year among women now relying on reversible methods of contraception if they abandoned contraception altogether.

[e] Foams, gels, vaginal suppositories, and vaginal film.

[f] Cervical mucus (ovulation) method supplemented by calendar in the preovulatory phase and by BBT in the postovulatory phase.

[g] With spermicidal cream or jelly.

[h] Data accumulated before product was withdrawn from market in 1995; product to be reintroduced in 1999.

[i] Without spermicides. Extrapolated from 6-month failure rates.

[j] Extrapolated from 6-month failure rates

Source: Adapted from pages 216–7 of reference 10; used with permission.

Latex condoms come in various colors, styles, shapes, and thicknesses (ranging from 0.03 mm to approximately 0.11 mm). Other features include reservoir tips, ribs, studs, and lubrication. Spermicide-treated condoms are also available, but the amount of spermicide present is much less than that of a vaginal spermicide.[12]

One brand of polyurethane condom has been available for several years, and others not yet on the market have been

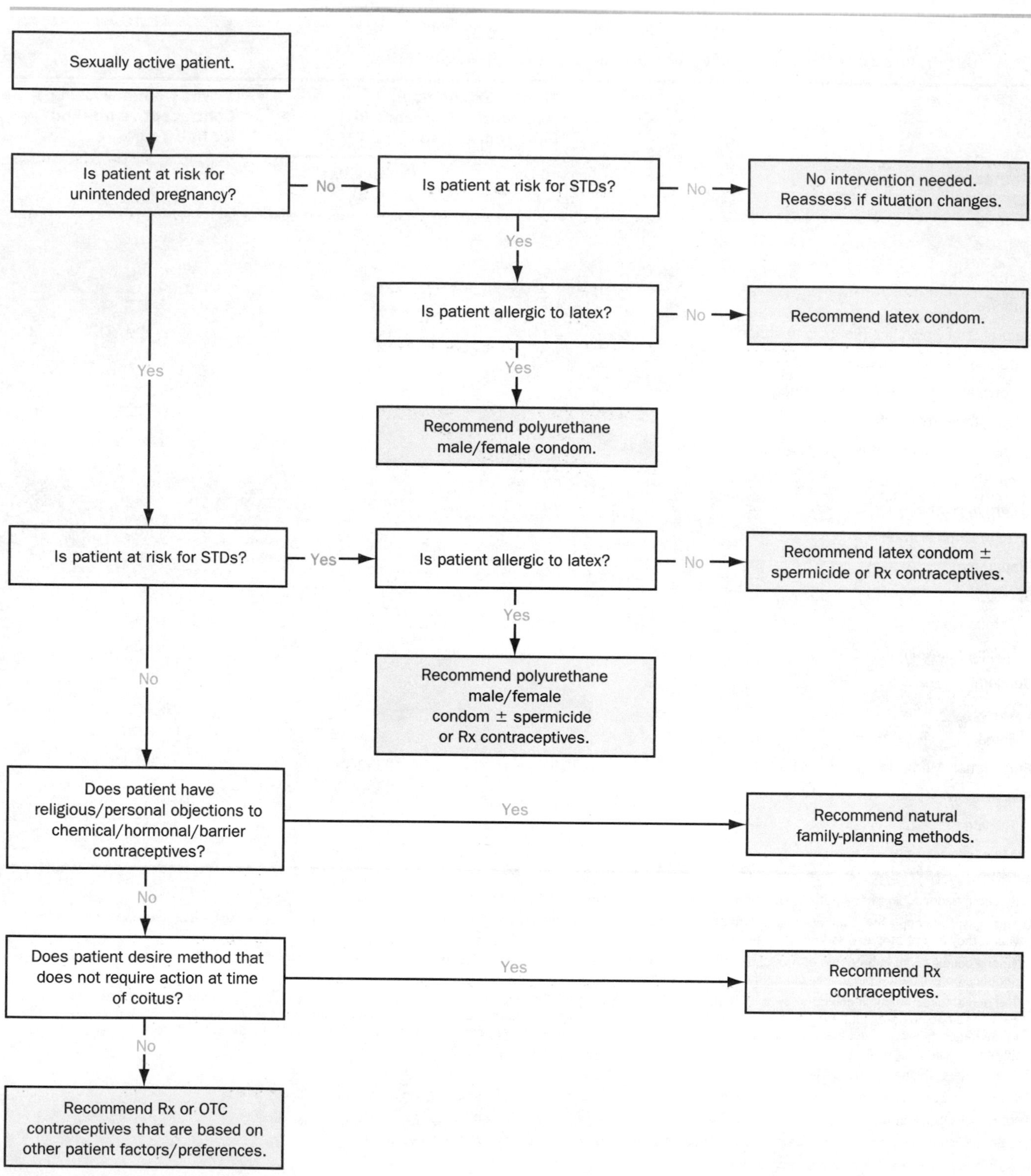

Figure 8–1 Self-care of unintended pregnancy and sexually transmitted diseases.

approved by the Food and Drug Administration (FDA). The polyurethane condom conducts heat well, comes prelubricated, and is not subject to degradation by oil-based products.[13] However, it is not as stretchy and is more expensive than latex condoms.

Condoms made from lamb cecum are labeled only for pregnancy prevention because the presence of pores in the membrane may allow the passage of viral organisms, including human immunodeficiency virus (HIV) and hepatitis B virus.[14] They conduct heat well and are very strong. They are also more expensive than latex condoms. Only a few brands of natural membrane condoms are on the market. Table 8–2 lists examples of each type of condom.

Effectiveness Since 1976, condom quality has been under the purview of the FDA. The Center for Devices and Radiological Health is responsible for monitoring the quality of domestically produced as well as imported condoms. The testing program was expanded in 1987 because of concerns about protection from acquired immunodeficiency syndrome (AIDS). The United States uses a water-leak test as the standard. The failure rate per batch is not to exceed 4 condoms per 1000. Of batches that met the quality guidelines, the average failure rate was 2.3 per 1000 tested. Another test is the air-burst test in which the condom is slowly inflated to its breaking point. Regular-size condoms must be able to hold 16 liters of air, and large-size condoms must hold approximately 10% more. A given lot fails if more than 1.5% of condoms fail the air-burst test.[12]

The true incidence of condom breakage is unknown, and breakage rates from studies vary widely, ranging from 0.41% to 12.9%.[15–18] In some studies, however, a limited group of study patients reported multiple incidences of breakage, indicating that breakage may be related as much to the individual user as it is to manufacturing defects.[15,18,19] Behaviors that have been associated with an increased risk of condom breakage are (1) incorrect placement of the condom, (2) use of an oil-based lubricant, (3) reuse of condoms, and (4) increased duration and intensity of coitus. One study found a higher incidence of breakage in the first five uses, indicating that correct use may improve with experience.[15] Past use of condoms without breakage problems indicates a decreased likelihood of condom breaks.[19] One study found that using additional lubrication with lubricated condoms increased the likelihood of condom slippage, leading to the possible spillage of semen. However, another study found that use of an additional water-based lubricant was associated with decreased breakage rates but no increase in condom slippage rates.[20,21] Initial studies with the polyurethane condom suggest that it has a breakage rate similar to that of the latex condom,[13] but a recent study found a significantly higher breakage and slippage rate for the polyurethane condom when compared to the latex condom.[22]

The use-related failure rate for condoms is approximately 14 pregnancies per 100 women during the first year of use. (See Table 8–1.) Efficacy of condoms does appear to improve, however, with increasing duration of use; one study found a pregnancy rate of only 0.6% in experienced users.[23]

Table 8–2

Selected Male Condoms

Trade Name	Product Features
Polyurethane Condoms	
Avanti	Lubricated
Avanti Super Thin	Lubricated
Natural Membrane Condoms	
Fourex	With or without spermicidal lubricant
Kling · Tite Naturalamb	With or without spermicidal lubricant
Naturalamb	With or without spermicidal lubricant
Latex Condoms	
Class Act Ribbed and Sensitive	Reservoir end; with or without spermicidal lubricant; ribbed surface
LifeStyles: Assorted Colors, Form Fitting, or Studded	Colored; contour shaped; or rubber studded
Ramses Extra Strength	Reservoir end; spermicidal lubricant
Ramses Ultra Thin	Reservoir end; spermicidal lubricant; smooth or ribbed surface
Sheik Exita Extra	Reservoir end; spermicidal lubricant; ribbed surface
Sheik Fiesta	Reservoir end; lubricant; ribbed surface
Sheik Super Thin	Reservoir end; with or without spermicide lubricant; smooth or ribbed surface
Trojan-Enz Large	Reservoir end; with or without spermicidal lubricant; large size
Trojan Magnum	Reservoir end; with or without spermicidal lubricant; large size
Trojan Plus 2 Ultra Fit	Reservoir end; spermicidal lubricant; contoured shape
Trojan Ribbed	Reservoir end; with or without spermicidal lubricant; ribbed/textured surface
Trojan Shared Sensation	Flared end with reservoir tip; with or without spermicidal lubricant; textured surface with bumps and ribs
Trojan Ultra Pleasure	Bulbous-shaped reservoir end; with or without spermicidal lubricant

The most common cause of use-related failure with condoms, as with all other contraceptive methods, is the lack of consistent, proper use. Spermicide-treated condoms have not been shown to be more efficacious at preventing pregnancy than nontreated condoms.[12]

Usage/Storage Guidelines Proper use of condoms is essential to their preventing pregnancy. (See Table 8–3 for usage guidelines.) Patients using the polyurethane condom should be advised that it is not as elastic as the latex condom and will not fit as snugly. Also it does not have a reservoir tip, so a space must be left at the tip as when using a non–reservoir-tipped latex condom.

If the latex condom user wants a lubricant, the pharmacist must stress the importance of using lubricants that do not harm or weaken the strength and integrity of the condom. Table 8–4 lists lubricants that are safe or unsafe to use with latex condoms.

Excessive heat or overexposure to ozone at levels found in some metropolitan areas will rapidly decrease the integrity of the latex; consequently, condoms should be kept in their sealed packages until time of use. Pharmacists should emphasize that packaged condoms must be protected from light and excessive heat. The shelf life of condoms under optimal conditions, as packaged by the manufacturers, is 3 to 5 years. As of March 1998, the FDA requires that latex condoms be labeled with an expiration date.[24] Even for condoms within their expiration date, the user should always check for discoloration, brittleness, or stickiness and should discard condoms displaying any of these characteristics.

Adverse Effects The most frequent complaint is decreased sensitivity of the glans penis and decreased sexual pleasure for the male. Latex allergy is becoming a more common problem with condoms. An estimated 1% to 2% of the population and a higher percentage of health care workers may be sensitized to latex.[25] These patients may develop contact dermatitis from using latex condoms. This condition, which may occur in the male or female partner, may be characterized by immediate localized itching and swelling (urticarial reaction) or by a delayed eczematous reaction. In patients with severe sensitivity, the reaction may spread beyond the area of physical contact with the latex.[26] Spermicide-treated condoms may enhance latex allergy or cause sensitivity reactions because of the spermicide itself.[12]

Table 8–3

Usage Guidelines for Male Condoms

- Use only condoms that are fresh (not previously opened), that are within their expiration date, and that have been stored in a dry, cool place (not a wallet or car glove compartment).
- Do *not* attempt to test the condom for leaks before using; this test only increases the risk of tearing.
- Condoms occasionally break. Have a vaginal spermicidal product (foam or jelly) available, and insert it as soon as possible if a condom break or spill occurs.
- Be aware that long fingernails or jewelry may easily tear condoms.
- As shown in drawing A, unroll the condom onto the erect penis before the penis comes into any contact with the vagina. If you start to put the condom on backward, discard that condom and use a fresh one.
- If you are not using a reservoir-tipped condom, leave 1/2 inch of space between the end of the condom and the tip of the penis by pinching the top of the condom as you unroll it. (See drawing B.) This method leaves space for the ejaculate as shown in drawing C and decreases the risk of breakage.
- If your partner has vaginal dryness, use additional lubrication, if desired. This step will help decrease the risk of tears and breakage. Use only water-based lubricants; oil-based lubricants weaken condoms and increase the chance of breakage. Spermicidal agents may be used as lubricants with condoms and may also increase the effectiveness of the condom. See Table 8–4 for a list of safe and unsafe lubricants.
- After ejaculation, withdraw the penis immediately. To prevent the condom from slipping off, especially if you have used additional lubrication, hold on to the rim of the condom as you withdraw.
- Check the condom for tears and then discard.
- If a tear has occurred, immediately insert spermicidal foam or jelly containing a high concentration of spermicide into the vagina. Do not use suppositories or a vaginal film in these cases, as the delay time for dissolution may decrease the product's efficacy.

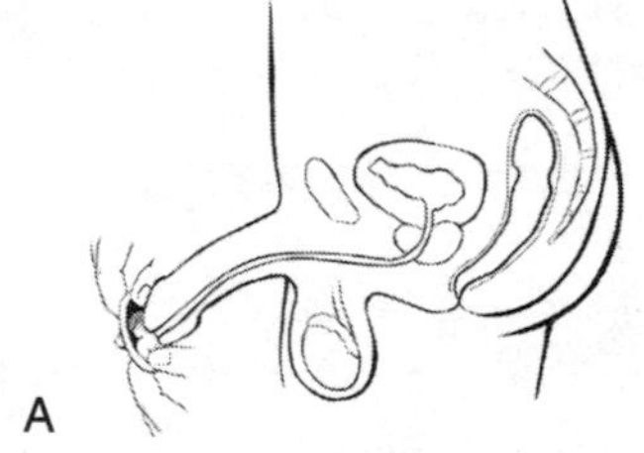

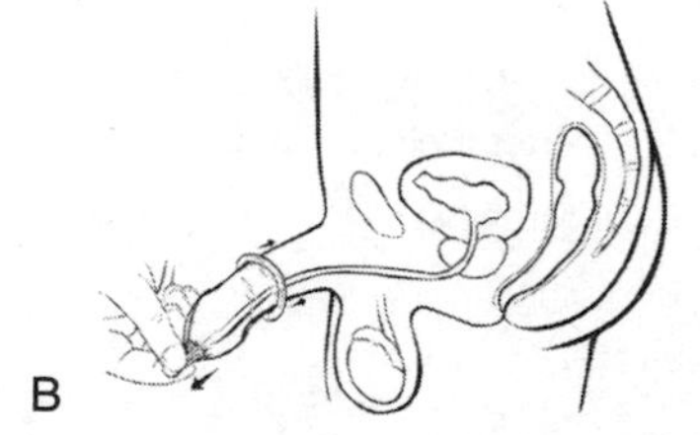

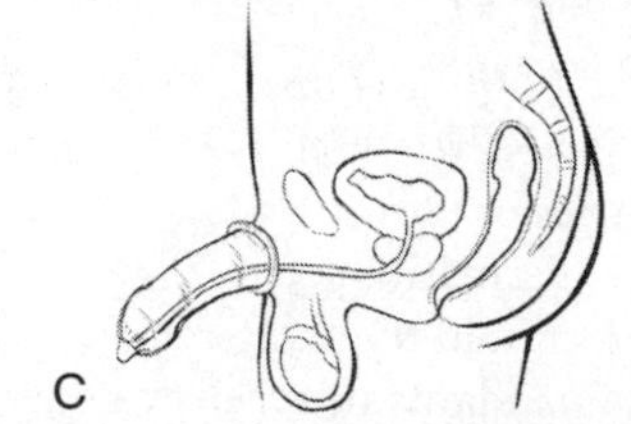

Table 8–4

Lubricants/Products That Are Safe or Unsafe to Use with Latex Condoms

Safe
Aloe-9
Aqua-Lube
Aqua Lube Plus (spermicidal)
Astroglide
Carbowax
Contraceptive foams (e.g., Emko, Delfen, Koromex)
Contraceptive gels (e.g., Prepair, Contraceptrol)
Duragel
Egg white
ForPlay Lubricant
Glycerin (USP)
H-R Lubricating Jelly
Intercept
Koromex Gel
Lubafax
Lubrin Insert
Norform Insert
Ortho-Gynol
Personal Lubricant
Prepair Lubricant
Probe
Saliva
Semicid
Silicones DC 360
Transi-Lube
Water
Unsafe
Baby oils
Burn ointments
Coconut oil/butter
Edible oils (e.g., olive, peanut, corn, sunflower)
Hemorrhoidal ointments
Insect repellents
Margarine/dairy butter
Mineral oil
Palm oil
Petroleum jelly (e.g., Vaseline)
Rubbing alcohol
Suntan oil
Vaginal creams (e.g., Monistat, Estrace, Femstat, Vagisil, Premarin, Rendell's Cone, Pharmatext Ovule)
Some sexual lubricants (e.g., Elbow Grease, Hot Elbow Grease, Shaft)

Source: Page 158 of reference 10; used with permission.

Product Selection Guidelines For most people, condoms are an effective, acceptable, inexpensive, safe, and nontoxic method of birth control. Before recommending a latex condom, pharmacists should ask patients if they can wear rubber gloves or blow up a balloon without itching occurring. If contact dermatitis secondary to latex condoms develops, the patient should try a different brand. The sensitizers are usually antioxidants or accelerators used in processing the rubber. Because different manufacturers use different processes, changing brands may alleviate the problem. In one study, reactions in patients who are allergic to latex ranged from 0% to 76%, depending on the brand.[27] If switching brands does not eliminate the irritation, the patient may use polyurethane or lamb cecum condoms—if the patient recognizes their limitations in preventing STDs. Also, some patients may be sensitized to components of the lubricant or spermicide. Changing brands or using a condom without spermicide may resolve the problem.

The use of very thin condoms, ridged condoms, polyurethane condoms or—in a monogamous relationship with an HIV-negative individual—natural membrane condoms, may alleviate complaints of decreased sensitivity.

Female Condom

Although the FDA approved the female condom in 1993, only one product—the Reality condom—is currently available.

Composition/Features The Reality condom is made of polyurethane rather than latex. It is prelubricated, comes with additional lubricant, and resists degradation by oil-based lubricants. The female condom consists of an outer ring, a sheath or pouch that fits over the vaginal mucosa, and an inner ring that secures the sheath by fitting like a diaphragm over the cervix. The female condom is designed for one-time use only.

Effectiveness The 6-month pregnancy failure rate among all users of the female condom is 12.4%, similar to that for users of diaphragms and cervical caps; among perfect users, however, the 6-month pregnancy failure rate has been documented as low as 2.6%. The extrapolated annual pregnancy failure rate for the female condom is 25% for all users and 5% for perfect users.[28] (See Table 8–1.) A reduced chance of breakage when compared to latex condoms has been reported.[29]

Usage/Storage Guidelines Table 8–5 provides step-by-step instructions for the proper use of the female condom. The condom may be inserted up to 8 hours before intercourse, but it is effective immediately on insertion.

Fresh condoms can be stored at room temperature in their unopened package. Before inserting the female condom, the woman should ensure that the product is within its expiration date.

Adverse Effects Vaginal irritation and increased noise ("squeaking") are the most common complaints about the female condom. Additional lubrication may resolve these problems. Some women may complain of decreased sensation or discomfort caused by the outer ring during intercourse.

Product Selection Guidelines The female condom provides a way for women to protect themselves against pregnancy. It is thinner than many latex condoms and has a lower breakage rate than the male condom.[29] Compared to vaginal spermicides, the female condom can be inserted much earlier before intercourse and is less messy to use. However, some women find the female condom cumbersome and unattractive.

Vaginal Spermicides

Vaginal spermicides use surface-active agents to immobilize (kill) sperm. For gels and foams, the spermicide vehicle also acts as a physical barrier against sperm. The effective spermicides include nonoxynol-9, octoxynol-9, and menfegol. Nearly all currently available products use nonoxynol-9. No products containing menfegol are currently marketed in the United States; however, several are available in Asia.

Dosage Forms The vehicles for vaginal spermicides include gels, foams, suppositories, and film. Although the onset and duration of action varies for the dosage forms, the woman should delay douching for at least 6 hours after intercourse no matter which dosage form she uses. The following sections discuss the advantages and disadvantages of each dosage form.

Vaginal Gels Some gels (jellies) are labeled for use only in conjunction with a diaphragm or cervical cap. When selecting a vaginal jelly to use without a diaphragm or cervical cap, the person should be careful to choose a product with a higher concentration of spermicide, not one that has a lower concentration and was designed to use with barrier methods. Products with a higher concentration of spermicide may be used alone or with a diaphragm or cervical cap.

People must pay strict attention to directions for using each product; some require two full applicators, whereas others require only one for an effective dose. For convenience, applicators may be prefilled before use. Prefilled unit-dose applicators are also available commercially.

Vaginal Foams Vaginal foams come in canisters or in prefilled applicators. They distribute more evenly and adhere better to the cervical area and vaginal walls but provide less lubrication compared with jellies. Because it may be difficult for a woman to identify when the canister of foam is nearly empty, a new canister should always be available.

Vaginal Suppositories Vaginal suppositories are solid or semisolid dosage forms that are activated by moisture in the woman's vaginal tract. Some occasions may exist when the suppository will not completely dissolve, resulting in an unpleasant, gritty sensation. As with other medicated suppositories, the woman may forget to unwrap the product or may choose the wrong orifice for insertion, so the pharmacist

Table 8–5

Usage Guidelines for Female Condoms

- Remove the condom from the package. As shown in drawing A, one end of the condom is closed to form a pouch.
- Gently rub the sides together to evenly distribute the lubricant. If needed, use additional lubrication at this point.
- Add a drop of lubricant on the outside of the pouch to improve the ease of insertion. Oil- or water-based lubricants can be used with this condom.
- To place the pouch properly, grasp the inner ring between the thumb and middle finger of one hand. Place the index finger on the sheath between the other two fingers. (See drawing B.)
- Be careful that sharp fingernails or jewelry do not tear the condom.
- As shown in drawing C, squeeze the inner ring. Then insert the condom into the vagina as far as possible.
- Be sure that the inner ring is placed beyond the pubic bone, that the pouch is not twisted, and that the outer ring is outside the vagina. (See drawing D.)
- During intercourse, make sure that the penis enters the vagina inside the pouch and that the outer ring remains outside the vagina.
- If desired, add more lubricant during intercourse, without removing the condom.
- As shown in drawing E, remove the pouch before standing by twisting the outer ring and pulling gently.
- Discard the used condom in a trash can, not a toilet.
- Insert a new condom for each act of intercourse.
- Do not use a male condom with the female condom. The increased friction could cause displacement of the female condom.

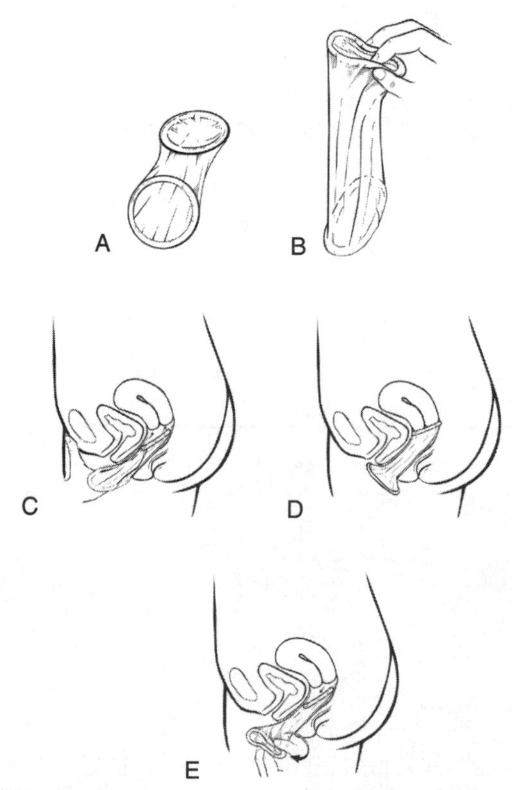

should make certain that she understands the directions. Vaginal suppositories do not require refrigeration, although in warmer climates, refrigeration may be desirable to prevent softening of the suppository.[30]

Vaginal Contraceptive Film Vaginal contraceptive film has been available in the United States since 1987. The film contains 28% nonoxynol-9 as its active ingredient and is available in packets of 3, 6, or 12 paper-thin 2-inch-square sheets. Other spermicidal films are under development. The film is activated by vaginal secretions. Patients should be advised not to place the film over the penis for insertion. This method does not ensure proper placement and does not allow adequate time for dissolution. In one comparison of spermicide dosage formulations, the film was widely preferred. It was rated the most difficult to use; however, this difficulty decreased with continued use.[30]

Effectiveness Spermicides used alone have a relatively high failure rate among typical first-year users (see Table 8–1). Of these products, vaginal foam appears to be a most effective form of spermicide dosage when it is used consistently and properly.[31] Some felt that suppositories are less efficacious than other spermicide dosage forms because of the potential for inadequate dissolution of the insert.[32] Efficacy improves greatly if spermicides are used in conjunction with barrier methods such as diaphragms, cervical caps, or condoms.

Administration Guidelines Table 8–6 provides guidelines for the proper administration of vaginal spermicides.

Adverse Effects Although allergic reactions are rare, either partner may experience such reactions to spermicides. Couples having oral–genital sex may find the taste of some products unpleasant. Very frequent use or use of high-concentration products may irritate or damage the vaginal and cervical epithelium.[33] Some people are concerned about a possible association between spermicide use and birth defects or miscarriage. However, a meta-analysis of available studies concluded that no increased risk of birth defects can be attributed to spermicides.[34]

Product Selection Guidelines The relatively low effectiveness of spermicides when used alone is their major disadvantage. However, studies suggest that simultaneous use of condoms and spermicides can lead to pregnancy prevention similar to that of oral contraceptives and intrauterine devices (IUDs).[35] The availability and ease of use of spermicides make them (1) a good backup method for women who use oral contraceptives and (2) useful for women with newly inserted IUDs. Spermicides are not recommended for women with anatomic abnormalities that would preclude proper placement of the spermicide near the cervical opening.

Product selection depends on the individual. Suppositories are generally not recommended, especially as a single-entity contraceptive, because more efficacious vaginal spermicides are available. One study of spermicide formulations found that gel use was associated with excessive lubrication and that women compensated by using less than a full dose, which may decrease product effectiveness.[30] If a patient complains of excessive lubrication, an alternate vehicle, such as foam or film, should be recommended. (See Table 8–7 for examples of each type of vaginal spermicide.)

Contraceptive Sponge

The FDA approved the contraceptive sponge in 1983 but its manufacturer withdrew it from the market in 1995 for financial reasons. In 1999, another manufacturer acquired product rights and plans to reintroduce it to the United States.

Composition/Features The contraceptive sponge is a small, circular, disposable sponge that is 2.5 cm thick and 5.5 cm in diameter and is made of polyurethane permeated with 1 g of nonoxynol-9. The sponge is believed to act as a contraceptive in three ways: (1) by serving as a mechanical barrier, (2) by the direct action of the spermicide, and (3) by absorbing semen.

Effectiveness Typical failure rates for the contraceptive sponge range from 13.4 to 28.3 pregnancies per 100 women in the first year of use.[36] Women who have previously given birth (parous women) have a significantly higher pregnancy rate while using the sponge as compared to women who have never given birth (nulliparous women). This higher pregnancy rate may be related to poor fit in women who have delivered vaginally.

Usage/Storage Guidelines A woman must be able to locate her cervix and must be comfortable in doing so to correctly place the sponge. Table 8–6 provides instructions for properly using this product. However, the sponge may become dislodged during intercourse.

Removing the sponge is facilitated by a woven polyester loop attached to the convex side. Some women have difficulty removing the sponge, and it has been known to fragment on removal. The sponge should be stored in its unopened package in a cool place and used before its expiration date.

Adverse Effects A relative risk of 7.8 to 40 times baseline for toxic shock syndrome from the contraceptive sponge—about the same magnitude as that for tampon users—has been identified by the Centers for Disease Control and Prevention.[37] Women should take special care to wash their hands before inserting the sponge, should not use the sponge during menstruation or postpartum, and should not exceed the 24-hour maximum recommended retention time. Women should also be advised to make sure that the entire sponge is removed, because fragments left in the vagina may serve as a focus for infection. Some studies have reported a small increase in the incidence of vaginal fungal infections among sponge users.[38] Frequent sponge use may also be associated with an increased incidence of vaginal and cervical ulcers.[35]

Product Selection Guidelines The contraceptive sponge is convenient, safe, and portable. Contraindications for use in-

Table 8–6

Administration Guidelines for Vaginal Spermicides and the Contraceptive Sponge

Dosage Form	Application Method	Onset/Duration of Action	Application Time Before Intercouse	Reapplication Requirements
Vaginal gel alone[a]	Insert full dose near cervix	Effective immediately/ Lasts 1 hour	Up to 30–60 minutes	For each coital act
Vaginal gel used with diaphragm/cervical cap[a]	Fill barrier device one-third full with gel and place near cervix; leave barrier in place for at least 6 hours	Effective immediately/ Diaphragm: lasts 6 hours; cervical cap: lasts 48 hours	Up to 1 hour	Diaphragm: for each coital act that occurs within 6 hours of initial insertion of device, reapply spermicide; for coitus after 6 hours of initial insertion, remove and wash device, fill with new spermicide, and reinsert device. Cervical cap: remove and wash device and reapply spermicide for each coital act that occurs 48 hours after initial insertion of device
Vaginal foam[a]	Insert full dose near cervix	Effective immediately/ Lasts 1 hour	Up to 1 hour	For each coital act
Vaginal suppository[a]	Insert suppository near cervix	Effective in 10–15 minutes/Lasts 1 hour	10–15 minutes	For each coital act
Vaginal contraceptive film[a]	Drape film over fingertip; place film near cervix	Effective in 15 minutes/Lasts 2 hours	15 minutes	For each coital act
Contraceptive sponge[a]	Moisten sponge with 2 tbsp (1 oz) of water; insert so that concave side covers cervix; leave in place for at least 6–8 hours after coitus	Effective immediately/ Lasts 24 hours	Up to 24 hours	Insert new sponge for coitus that occurs ≥24 hours after insertion of initial device

[a] Delay douching for at least 6 hours after the last coital act.

clude spermicide sensitivity, anatomic abnormalities of the vagina, and a history of toxic shock syndrome. At this time, it may be prudent not to routinely recommend the contraceptive sponge to parous women because of possible problems with vaginal fit.

Pharmacoeconomics of Contraceptive Products

Unintended pregnancies can provide significant social and economic burdens both on the people involved and on society. Medical costs for unintended pregnancies can be significant. The annual cost for teenage unintended births is more than $1.3 billion.[39] Induced and spontaneous abortions add another $180 million. Family support programs, such as Medicaid, Food Stamps, and Aid to Families with Dependent Children, add even more costs. In 1990, the total annualized costs for teenage childbearing were more than $25 billion.[39] Applying the concepts of pharmacoeconomics to contraception can be different from that seen with other drug products. The costs of the different contraceptive methods vary. If one assumes 100 acts of intercourse annually, product costs can range from approximately $30 to $100 for the male latex condom, $35 to $100 for spermicides, and $170 for the female condom.[40] Use of more than one method is often recommended to increase the potential for preventing unintended pregnancies and STDs; the cost of combination methods are additive. However, compared to the overall costs of prescription methods for contraception, which include the physician and office fees as well as the cost of the prescription itself, nonprescription products are generally less expensive.

Studies have demonstrated that all forms of contraceptives are cost-effective when viewed against the costs of unintended pregnancy.[39,41] As a result, part of the pharmacist's role may be to educate third-party payers and patients that the up-front acquisition costs of contraceptives must be examined from the standpoint of that product's ability to provide economic savings and societal benefits.

Natural Contraceptive Methods

Some individuals use contraceptive methods that do not rely on the presence of a chemical or barrier to prevent conception. These methods include natural family planning, lactational infertility, home ovulation prediction tests, and withdrawal. Many couples like the fact that these methods produce no chemical risk to the fertility or health of the cou-

Table 8–7

Selected Vaginal Spermicides

Trade Name	Spermicide
Spermicidal Foams	
Emko	Nonoxynol-9, 12%
Koromex	Nonoxynol-9, 12.5%
Ortho Options Delfen	Nonoxynol-9, 12.5%
Spermicidal Gels/Jellies	
K-Y Plus Lubricating	Nonoxynol-9, 2.2%
Koromex/Koromex Crystal Clear	Nonoxynol-9, 3%
Ortho Options Conceptrol	Nonoxynol-9, 4%
Ortho Options Gynol II	Nonoxynol-9, 2%
Ortho Options Gynol II Extra Strength	Nonoxynol-9, 3%
Ortho Options Ortho-Gynol	Octoxynol-9, 1%
Shur Seal	Nonoxynol-9, 2%
Spermicidal Suppositories	
CarePlus	Nonoxynol-9, 100 mg
Encare	Nonoxynol-9, 100 mg
Koromex Inserts	Nonoxynol-9, 125 mg (5%)
Ortho Options Conceptrol Inserts	Nonoxynol-9, 100 mg
Semicid Inserts	Nonoxynol-9, 100 mg
Spermicidal Film	
VCF Vaginal Contraceptive Film	Nonoxynol-9, 28%

ple (or to the fetus, should pregnancy occur). For others, these methods are used for financial or religious reasons. In some cases, lack of access to or knowledge of other methods of contraceptive is the reason for their use.

Natural Family Planning

Natural family-planning methods, also called periodic abstinence, rhythm, or fertility-awareness methods, use various techniques to determine a woman's period of fertility. The information provided by these techniques helps pinpoint the time of ovulation and the optimal time for conception. Natural family-planning methods have the positive effect of encouraging communication within a relationship and may be the only truly shared contraceptive method. As the only method of contraception approved by the Roman Catholic Church, it is widely used around the world.

Although no chemicals are present when a couple uses natural family planning, a potential risk does exist for abnormal pregnancy outcomes, such as birth defects or fetal wastage, should a couple conceive unintentionally. This risk is related to the possible association of such a conception with aged gametes (either sperm or ovum). Comparative studies have found a relative risk of 1.0 to 5.2 for birth defects or spontaneous abortion among those couples practicing natural family planning at the time of conception. At present, however, the evidence is not conclusive for an increased risk of abnormal pregnancy outcomes. This controversial issue may become clearer as surveillance continues.[42] (See Chapter 7, "Disorders Related to Menstruation," for a review of menstrual physiology and biochemistry.)

Natural family planning can be divided into four methods: calendar, basal body temperature (BBT), cervical mucus, and symptothermal. Each method requires the woman to keep detailed records of her menstrual cycles and other symptoms associated with cyclical hormonal levels. The data acquired, such as BBT or the character and quantity of cervical mucus, are recorded on detailed monthly charts. After a period of instruction and with the information provided by charts from several months, a woman is usually able to predict her most fertile time. With this information, a couple can choose to abstain from sexual intercourse during that period if they want to avoid pregnancy.[43]

Calendar Method The calendar method (also known as the rhythm method) is based on records of monthly menstrual cycle lengths. The estimated day of ovulation, considered to be 14 ± 2 days before the onset of menstruation, is used to determine the woman's fertile period, which is calculated on the basis of estimates of the viable life of ova and sperm.[44] The fertilizable life of the ovum (egg) is estimated to be from 6 to 24 hours following ovulation, as measured by peaks in estrogen and luteinizing hormone. Sperm is considered to be viable for 48 to 72 hours. Table 8–8 gives calculations for fertility based on 12 months of cycle charts.

Basal Body Temperature Method In the BBT method, the woman measures and charts her body temperature every morning. She takes her temperature with a mercury or electronic digital thermometer that is calibrated in increments of 0.1°F (0.05°C). Such a thermometer allows her to detect small changes in body temperature. She must obtain her temperature before embarking on *any* physical activity (i.e., she must check her temperature before getting out of bed) and must obtain it at the same time every day. Oral or rectal temperature may be used, but each woman should use only one method (site) consistently.

The charts help estimate the time of ovulation because the BBT usually drops 12 to 24 hours before ovulation and then rises sharply over a 24- to 48-hour period to between 0.4°F and 1.0°F (0.2°C and 0.5°C) above the lowest point (the *nadir*).[43–45] (See Figure 8–2.) This sharp rise, called the *thermal shift*, is caused by high progesterone levels. The *safe* (infertile) *period* is considered to begin after 3 days of postnadir temperature elevation and to last until the start of the next menstrual cycle. Because this method is not absolutely accurate in predicting when ovulation occurs, the postmenstrual or preovulatory safe period is difficult to determine. Thus women who engage in unprotected intercourse during this period have a higher pregnancy rate.

Electronic digital thermometers are more accurate than mercury thermometers and have a shorter recording time (45 to 90 seconds). Because the activity of shaking down a

Case Study 8–1

Patient Complaint/History

Leigh, a 27-year-old woman, has been looking at the display of contraceptive products for some time. When approached by the pharmacist, she admits that she is looking for a product to use during sexual intercourse. During further conversation, she reveals that she and her boyfriend have a monogamous relationship. Her boyfriend, however, refuses to use a male condom; he insists that intercourse "doesn't feel the same" when he uses a condom.

The patient's profile shows that she has a history of hypertension, which has been treated for the past 3 years with nifedipine sustained-release tablets of 90 mg once daily.

Clinical Considerations/Strategies

Readers can use the following considerations or strategies to determine whether use of nonprescription products is warranted in this patient:

- Assess the patient's desires and priorities for prevention of pregnancy versus protection from STDs.
- Assess the patient's experience with various contraceptive methods.
- Elicit the patient's opinion of which contraceptive methods are acceptable to her and her partner.
- Suggest contraceptive methods other than condoms for this patient's needs.
- Consider any disease-related contraindications and potential acceptance by the patient and her sexual partner.

Patient Education/Counseling

Readers can use the following strategies to develop a patient education/counseling plan that will help ensure optimal outcomes:

- Develop a patient education plan that will optimize successful use of the recommended contraceptive product(s).

thermometer may cause the woman's body temperature to change, mercury thermometers must be shaken down each night rather than immediately before use in the morning.

For patients who feel that they may have difficulty interpreting shifts in their BBT, a computerized monitor, the Bioself Fertility Indicator, registers and stores the BBTs. The monitor uses the collected data to indicate periods of infertility, fertility, and high fertility. It has a six-cycle memory, and printouts of stored temperatures are available from the manufacturer. However, this product is only as good as the information it records. A woman must still take her temperature at the same time every morning before any physical activity. Anything that affects her BBT will interfere with the computer's ability to generate an accurate indicator of her fertility levels. (See Chapter 43, "Home Testing and Monitoring Devices," for further discussion of this product.)

Poor correlation of the thermal shift with ovulation reduces the accuracy of the BBT method. Furthermore, some women have monophasic menstrual cycles and do not have a definite or significant temperature dip or rise. Stress, fever, lactation, and use of an electric blanket may affect BBT. Also, temperature changes are difficult to interpret just before and during menopause.[45] Use of medications, such as phenothiazines and aspirin, may alter body temperature.[46] At such times, it is best for couples whose religious beliefs do not preclude doing so to use one or more alternative methods of contraception.

Cervical Mucus Method The cervical mucus method is based on the rather consistent changes in cervical mucus that take place during a normal menstrual cycle. Every day, the woman observes the mucus at the vaginal orifice; she charts its character and the amount produced. After menstruation, most women notice a sensation of dryness at the vaginal orifice on some days. As estrogen levels rise, the cervical mucus increases in quantity and in elasticity and becomes clear, resembling raw egg white.[43–45] The peak symptom, the last day of the clear, stretchy, estrogenic mucus, has been shown to be within a day of ovulation for most women. With the postovulatory rise in progesterone, the mucus becomes thick and sticky or is absent. The woman is considered fertile from the first day after menstruation on which mucus is detected until 72 hours after the appearance of the peak symptom. (See Table 8–9.) With experience, a woman learns to differentiate other vaginal secretions, such as an infectious discharge or seminal fluid, from normal mucus. Most women can learn this method after three cycles. The average number of days of abstinence required per cycle is 17.[43] This method of natural family planning is preferred over the BBT method for postpartum lactating women and those women nearing menopause. Women who use this method are also apt to detect abnormalities in their normal mucus patterns that may be caused by infections. Thus they are able to seek early treatment. Women should be informed that vaginal foams, gels, creams, and douches will interfere with cervical mucus.

Symptothermal Method The symptothermal method combines BBT charting with notations of other cyclical signs of ovulation. These signs might include breast tenderness, intermenstrual pain (mittelschmerz), labial edema, peak symptom cervical mucus, and changes in the character and position of the cervix. Most studies of this method's effectiveness use the thermal shift (the temperature rise after the nadir) of the BBT method to determine the postovulatory

Table 8–8

Fertility Intervals Based on Calendar or Rhythm Method[a]

No. of Days in Shortest Cycle	First Fertile (Unsafe) Day	No. of Days in Longest Cycle	Last Fertile (Unsafe) Day
21[b]	3rd day	21	10th day
22	4th	22	11th
23	5th	23	12th
24	6th	24	13th
25	7th	25	14th
26	8th	26	15th
27	9th	27	16th
28	10th	28	17th
29	11th	29	18th
30	12th	30	19th
31	13th	31	20th
32	14th	32	21st
33	15th	33	22nd
34	16th	34	23rd
35	17th	35	24th

[a] Based on 12-month record of a woman's cycle. Subtract 18 days from the shortest cycle to determine the first fertile day; subtract 11 days from longest cycle to determine the last fertile day.

[b] Day 1, first day of menstrual bleeding.

Source: Page 341 of reference 10; used with permission.

safe period, as well as the cervical mucus or calendar method to determine the end of the preovulatory or postmenstrual infertile period.[45]

Other Natural Contraceptive Methods

Less-effective methods of natural contraception include lactational infertility, withdrawal, and use of home tests for ovulation prediction. Although health care or family-planning professionals do not consider douching to be a contraceptive method, some individuals may use douches as a sole means of contraception.

Lactational Infertility In many developing countries, breast-feeding is used as a contraceptive method for spacing the birth of children. When the infant receives only breast milk and the mother has not menstruated, protection against conception may persist for up to 6 months. However, if breast-feedings are supplemented with feedings by bottle, lactational amenorrhea may not be a reliable form of contraception. Milk extraction through a breast pump does not inhibit the return of fertility.[47] Although menstrual periods in lactating women may be anovulatory, ovulation may occur before the return of menses. In general, if a breast-feeding woman is sexually active, she should use other contraceptive measures no later than 5 weeks postpartum.[44]

Home Tests for Ovulation Prediction Ovulation prediction tests, which are designed to aid couples in conceiving, detect the surge in luteinizing hormone (LH) that occurs shortly before ovulation. (See Chapter 43, "Home Testing and Monitoring Devices.") These kits detect an increase in urinary excretion of LH, which usually occurs 8 to 40 hours before

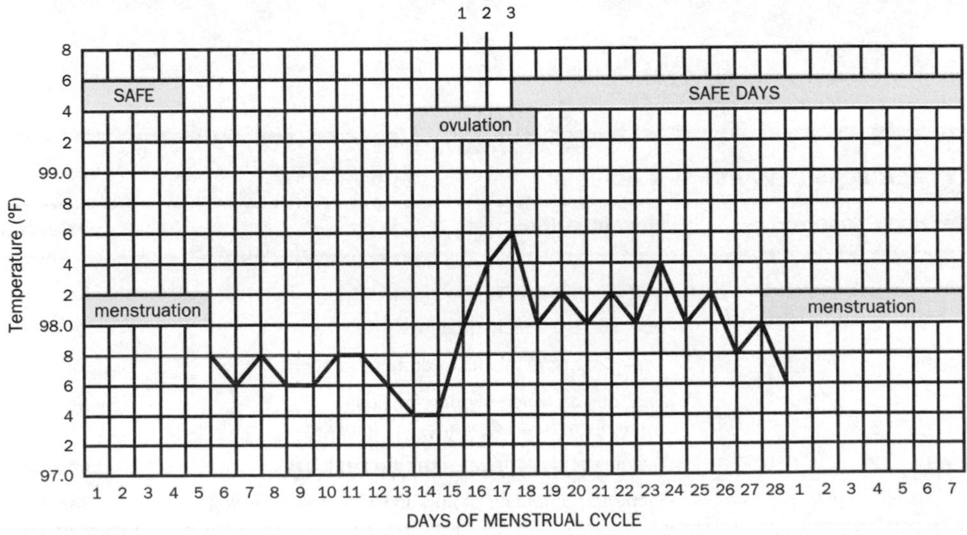

Figure 8–2 Basal body temperature variations during a model menstrual cycle. Source: Page 343 of reference 10; used with permission.

actual ovulation. Because the life expectancy of sperm may be longer than 72 hours, these ovulation predictors do not give warning of impending ovulation with enough accuracy to be effective contraceptive agents when used alone.

Withdrawal Coitus interruptus (withdrawal) is used intentionally by only a small percentage of couples in the United States.[1] The practice involves coital activity until ejaculation is imminent, followed by withdrawal of the stimulated penis and ejaculation away from the vagina or vulva. Method failures (pregnancy even when the method is used correctly and consistently) are due in part because involuntary pre-ejaculation secretions may contain millions of sperm. Disadvantages of this method include a higher pregnancy rate, a lack of protection against STDs, the requirement of considerable self-control by the man, and the potential for diminished pleasure for the couple because of interrupted lovemaking. Although this method should not be recommended, it is better than no contraceptive method.

Douching Vaginal douches should *never* be considered a method of contraception. Under favorable conditions in the female reproductive tract, active sperm have been found in the cervical crypts and oviducts within 5 minutes after ejaculation.[44] Postcoital douching has no effect in removing sperm from the upper reproductive tract and could, in fact, force or propel sperm higher up in the tract. (See Chapter 7, "Disorders Related to Menstruation.")

Effectiveness of Natural Contraceptive Methods

Overall, the pregnancy rate for natural family planning methods is approximately 25%. The calendar method is considered the least effective of these methods, primarily because of natural variations in the length of a woman's normal menstrual cycle. Although it is still widely used as a sole contraceptive method, such reliance results in many unintended pregnancies as shown in Table 8–1.[43,44] Consequently, family planners do not recommend its use as the sole method of contraception but suggest instead using the calendar method in conjunction with other methods of natural family planning. Natural family-planning methods that specifically identify preovulatory or postovulatory changes, such as BBT, cervical mucus, and symptothermal methods, have much better outcomes. Table 8–1 shows that combinations of these methods have good predicted effectiveness; with perfect use, the annual failure rate is 2%.

For a woman who is breast-feeding an infant almost exclusively, studies have reported pregnancy rates of 0.5% to 1.5% for the 6-month period following delivery. However, once supplemental feedings begin, the efficacy rate falls significantly.[47] Efficacy rates on using home ovulation predictors are not available; however, assuming correct use, an efficacy rate similar to that seen with BBT monitoring could be expected. For couples who rely on withdrawal, accidental pregnancy rates are in the range of 19 pregnancies per 100 couples in the first year of use.[40]

Patient Assessment of Unintended Pregnancy

Before advising a patient on contraception, the pharmacist must first identify the patient's level of knowledge about contraceptive methods. Patients who prefer natural family-planning methods must understand the reproductive cycle before using these methods effectively. Patients who prefer nonprescription contraceptive products must know how to use them properly and must be prepared to use them with every act of intercourse. The pharmacist should identify the patient's preferences for products or methods on the basis of timing or on the basis of religious or cultural practices. Asking the patient the following questions will help elicit the information needed to recommend the appropriate contraceptive method or product.

Table 8–9

Summary of Cervical Mucus (Ovulation) Method of Contraception

Approximate Cycle Day: Phase	How Identified	Intercourse Allowed?
1–5: Menstruation[a]	Menstrual bleeding	No
6–9: Dry days	Absence of cervical mucus	On alternate nights only
10: Fecund period begins	Onset of sticky mucus secretion	No
16: Peak fecund day	Last day on which slippery mucus (resembling raw egg white) is observed	No
20: Fecund period ends	Evening of the 4th day after the peak day	After the fecund period ends
20–29: Safe period	From end of fecund period until onset of bleeding	Yes

[a] The cycle begins on the first day of menstruation.

Source: Page 337 of reference 10; used with permission.

Q~ Have you discussed contraception and sexual health matters with your physician or another health care provider?

A~ The response will reveal the patient's level of knowledge about contraception. Drawing on such knowledge, either initiate a full discussion of contraception or reinforce and enhance the patient's current knowledge.

Q~ What type of contraceptive method are you using now? What contraceptive products have you used before?

A~ If the patient has used contraceptive products, determine which products are possible alternatives.

Q~ What do you like or dislike about your current or previous contraceptive method? What does your partner like or dislike about your current or previous contraceptive method?

A~ Both partners' acceptance of a contraceptive method, especially one that involves use during sexual intercourse, is vital in preventing an unintended pregnancy. *Identify the adverse effects for each contraceptive method discussed in the section "Nonprescription Contraceptive Products," and recommend alternative nonprescription products for each method.*

Q~ Do you belong to a religious faith that has specific guidelines concerning family planning?

A~ Tailor the possible selection of contraceptives to those that meet the patient's specific guidelines.

Q~ Do you have children already? Do you want additional children?

A~ Recommend a contraceptive method that is based on the patient's preferences as to efficacy.

Patient Counseling for Unintended Pregnancy

Pharmacists should thoroughly familiarize themselves with the proper use of currently available nonprescription contraceptive products and should provide opportunities for consultation with patients by removing barriers that may prevent dialogue. Contraceptive products and information should be available in an area where the patient can browse and where the pharmacist can easily interact with the patient, such as next to or directly in front of the prescription counter. A private area for education and counseling is important if adequate discussion is to take place. The box "Patient Education for Unintended Pregnancy" lists specific information to provide patients.

Special efforts should be made to offer contraceptive information and services to adolescents. This population group is especially likely to be uninformed or misinformed about reproductive matters. Those pharmacists who are uncomfortable discussing reproductive health with young people should refer adolescents to a clinic that specializes in services to young people, if one is available. Adolescents need clear, accurate information on all aspects of reproductive health. The pharmacist should keep in mind that printed instructions are often written above the reading level of most adolescents (as well as of many adults); therefore, verbal instructions are very important.[48] Nonprescription methods that are particularly useful for the sometimes impulsive adolescent might include condoms and contraceptive foam in prefilled applicators.

The diaphragm, cervical cap, or natural family-planning methods may be an acceptable approach to contraception for a couple in a stable relationship. The first two methods require special fitting. Natural family-planning methods, especially the BBT and cervical mucus methods, require extensive training and support from health care professionals who have experience and training with these methods. The pharmacist should be supportive and available to answer questions regarding such techniques. Besides stocking spermicidal products, BBT thermometers, and monitoring charts, the pharmacist may serve as a referral center for those patients who want to use these methods of family planning. A pharmacist with the proper training might consider counseling patients on natural family planning as a unique practice possibility.

Sexually Transmitted Diseases

Besides the risk of unintended pregnancy, sexually active persons who do not use appropriate means of contraception place themselves at significant risk for acquiring a sexually transmitted disease (STD). More than 20 STDs are known, both bacterial and viral, and some may have severe, long-standing consequences on the health and reproductive capabilities of those infected. This chapter discusses only the most common STDs.

The probability of unprotected sexual intercourse leading to an STD is quite different from the risk of unintended pregnancy. The risk of unintended pregnancy varies throughout the menstrual cycle. The risk of developing an STD depends on several factors: the risk of having intercourse with an infected person, the potential for transmission of a specific STD, and the gender of the infected person. As an example, the potential of developing gonorrhea after a single unprotected sex act is 25% for men and 50% for women.[5] Often adolescents engage in risky behavior because they perceive themselves to be immune to contracting AIDS. Education of this population must include the real probability that risky sexual behavior may lead to acquiring this deadly disease.

Epidemiology of Sexually Transmitted Diseases

It is noteworthy that the number and seriousness of STDs continue to grow. In fact, a recent study revealed that most STDs occur in individuals who are under 25 years old.[49] The rate of several STDs is known to increase in adolescents and then to decrease steadily in older adults. These STDs include syphilis, gonorrhea, vaginitis, and pelvic inflammatory disease (PID). The rate of cases of each of these STDs has demonstrated a predilection for persons of lower socioeconomic status. Many STDs have been stated to follow a "biological sexism."[5] When disease severity is compared in women and men, women have been noted to suffer more long-term consequences: PID, infertility, ectopic pregnancy, chronic pelvic pain, and cervical cancer. In addition, because initial symptoms are less often recognized as serious by women, a higher proportion of early STDs go unreported. Many women will wait until later in the course of the disease to seek medical attention.[5]

Because of the profound effect on the immune system that is seen secondary to HIV infection, many STDs may be potentiated by co-infection with HIV. STDs that produce a vaginal or urethral discharge (gonorrhea, chlamydia, and trichomoniasis) have also been associated with higher levels of potential HIV infectivity.[50] Statistics for the occurrence of each STD are given in the individual discussions of STDs.

Etiology and Transmission of Sexually Transmitted Diseases

STDs may be caused by several bacteria and viruses. The specific causative organism for each condition is identified in the individual discussions of STDs.

An important risk to understand is the correlation between infections caused by HIV and by other STDs. Organisms that cause genital ulcers (herpes, syphilis, and chancroid) are known to be highly correlated with the transmission and acquisition of HIV.[50]

The known routes of transmission of AIDS are (1) blood and blood products (through transfusions, the sharing of contaminated needles and syringes, and accidental contamination from needle sticks); (2) mucous membrane exposures

Patient Education for Unintended Pregnancy

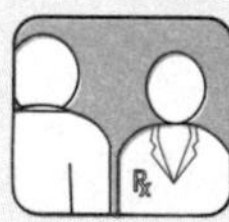

Pregnancy can result from any act of sexual intercourse. The objective of self-care is to prevent pregnancy by using nonprescription contraceptive products or natural contraceptive methods. For most patients, carefully following the instructions for contraceptive products or natural contraceptive methods, as well as the self-care measures listed below, will help prevent unintended pregnancy.

Nonprescription Contraceptive Products

- If relying on nonprescription contraceptive products, use the chosen product with every act of sexual intercourse.
- If latex male condoms cause an allergic reaction, first change to a different brand. If allergic reactions still occur, and if sexually transmitted diseases are not a concern, polyurethane or lamb cecum condoms are options.
- See Table 8–3 for instructions on the proper use of male condoms.
- If the female condom causes vaginal irritation or squeaking, apply additional lubrication.
- See Table 8–5 for instructions on the proper use of the female condom.
- Do not use vaginal spermicides if you have vaginal abnormalities that will not allow proper placement of the spermicide near the cervical opening.
- See Table 8–6 for instructions on the proper use of vaginal spermicides.
- If a nonprescription contraceptive product causes side effects or is difficult to use, do not just stop using the product. Talk to a physician or pharmacist about other contraceptive methods.

Natural Contraceptive Methods

- Natural family-planning specialists do not recommend the calendar method as the sole contraceptive method. To decrease the chance of pregnancy, combine the calendar method with family-planning methods that identify preovulatory or postovulatory changes, such as the basal body temperature, cervical mucus, or symptothermal methods.
- See Table 8–8 for instructions on calculating fertility intervals using the calendar method.
- See Table 8–9 for a summary of the cervical mucus method.
- For maximum protection, use both the basal body temperature and the cervical mucus methods, or use both the cervical mucus and symptothermal methods.
- Be aware that the methods of lactation infertility, home ovulation prediction tests, and withdrawal are not accurate enough to be the sole means of contraception.
- Be aware that douching is not a method of contraception.

(saliva, seminal fluid, and vaginal fluids, including menstrual blood); and (3) perinatal and peripartum transmission to infants. In the United States, at least 53% of HIV infections are transmitted through heterosexual or homosexual intercourse.[51] High-risk behavior is unprotected sex with an infected individual or with an individual whose sexual history and STD status is unknown to his or her partner. Table 8–10 provides a list of safer sex options, as well as of high-risk sexual activities.

Common Sexually Transmitted Diseases

The most common STDs include chlamydia, nongonococcal urethritis, gonorrhea, herpes infection, syphilis, hepatitis B, trichomoniasis, bacterial vaginosis, and chancroid.

Table 8–10

Safer Sex Options for Physical Intimacy

Safe Options
Massage
Hugging
Body rubbing
Dry kissing
Masturbation
Hand-to-genital touching (hand job) or mutual masturbation
Erotic books and movies
All sexual activities when both partners are monogamous, trustworthy, and known by testing to be free of HIV
Possibly Safe Options
Wet kissing with no broken skin, cracked lips, or damaged mouth tissue
Vaginal or rectal intercourse using latex or synthetic condom correctly
Oral sex on a man using a latex or synthetic condom
Oral sex on a woman using a latex or synthetic barrier such as a female condom, dental dam, or modified male condom, especially if she does not have her period or a vaginal infection with discharge
All sexual activities when both partners are in a long-term monogamous relationship and trust each other
Unsafe Options (in the absence of HIV testing and of trust and monogamy)
Any vaginal or rectal intercourse without a latex or synthetic condom
Oral sex on a man without a latex or synthetic condom
Oral sex on a woman without a latex or synthetic barrier such as a female condom, dental dam, or modified male condom, especially if she is having her period or has a vaginal infection with discharge
Semen in the mouth
Oral–anal contact
Sharing sex toys or douching equipment
Blood contact of any kind, including menstrual blood, or any sex that causes tissue damage or bleeding

Source: Page 55 of reference 10; used with permission.

AIDS

The incidence of AIDS is increasing almost exponentially. As many as 31 million patients have been infected with HIV as of late 1997. Of those infected, about one-third of all cases are reported in women, with sexual intercourse with an infected partner being the cause of most of these infections.[52] About 25% of women with AIDS are 20 to 29 years old, suggesting that many were infected in their teen years.[53]

The clinical presentation of AIDS varies from patient to patient. In its earliest phases, the disease may resemble other viral infections. Patients may present with fever, enlarged lymph nodes, and sore throat. Many patients may also present with a reddened maculopapular rash. Approximately 5% of patients infected with HIV will develop AIDS within 3 years; 20% will develop AIDS within 5 years. The average time to development of AIDS or an opportunistic infection is 10 years.[54] Opportunistic bacterial, viral, and parasitic infections may occur readily in the patient with AIDS and will often be the cause of death.

Studies have examined several contraceptive methods for their utility in preventing the spread of HIV infections. Male condoms remain the "gold standard" for this prophylactic measure.[55] (See the section "Prevention of Sexually Transmitted Diseases.")

Chlamydia

Chlamydia is now the most commonly occurring STD in the United States. In 1997, the reported number of cases of genital chlamydia infections was more than 500,000, a rate of 207 per 100,000 individuals. For women, the overall reported rate (335.8 per 100,000) was approximately five times that noted in men (70.4 per 100,000).[56] Chlamydia is an obligate intracellular parasite that often does not present immediate symptoms in the female but may lead to PID, infertility, and chronic pelvic pain. As many as 3 million cases of chlamydia infection may occur in women annually.[23] Women infected with chlamydia most often present with a mucopurulent discharge from the cervix. Unfortunately, many women do not recognize this discharge as abnormal.

Chlamydia may be transmitted by a pregnant woman to the fetus and may result in neonatal infections such as ophthalmia (severe conjunctivitis) or pneumonia.

Nongonococcal Urethritis

Men often present with nongonococcal urethritis (NGU). This infection is caused by chlamydia in up to 50% of cases, yet may also be caused by other sexually transmittable organisms such as *Ureaplasma urealyticum*, *Trichomonas vaginalis*, and herpes simplex virus. NGU is believed to occur more often than gonorrhea in men, with more than 2 million cases estimated to occur annually.[23] Symptoms in men include dysuria (difficult or painful urination), urinary frequency, and mucoid to purulent urethral discharge. It is important to realize that many men have asymptomatic infections. Several complications, including urethral strictures (lesions that narrow the urethra) and epididymitis (inflammation of the elongated structure that stores sperm), may occur in a male with untreated NGU. As listed above for chlamydia, NGU may be transmitted to female sexual partners with complications.

Gonorrhea

Gonorrhea remains a major STD in the United States with approximately 600,000 cases reported annually. After unreported cases are added, an estimated 1.5 million cases of gonorrhea occur annually.[23] In 1997, the gonorrhea rate had declined slightly from 127.3 cases per 100,000 population to 125.4 in men. The rate had a slight increase in women from 118.8 cases per 100,000 population to 119.3.[56] As a result, gonorrhea remains the second most common STD noted in the United States. Males who are symptomatic will present with dysuria, increased urinary frequency, and a purulent urethral discharge. Women with gonorrhea may have an abnormal vaginal discharge, abnormal menses, or dysuria. Gonorrhea may also present in the pharynx and the anus. Pharyngeal involvement will most often present as acute pharyngitis. Anal disease will produce symptoms of diarrhea, tenesmus (painful spasms of the anal sphincter), or constipation. Up to one-fourth of men infected with gonorrhea and as many as three-fourths of women may be asymptomatic.

Up to 40% of untreated women with gonorrhea may develop PID, and the risk of tubal infertility increases with each episode of PID.[5] Men, when untreated, are at increased risk for epididymitis, urethral stricture, and sterility.[23] In both sexes, gonorrhea may disseminate to involve the skeletal, cardiovascular, and nervous systems. Gonorrhea may also be transmitted to newborns who may present with ophthalmia neonatorum (inflammation of the conjunctiva that occurs in the first 10 days of life), scalp abscesses (at the site of fetal monitors), rhinitis, and anorectal infections. Finally, HIV infection may be associated with gonorrhea.

If one or both sexual partners are infected with gonorrhea, both partners should abstain from sexual activity until they have been treated.

Herpes Infection

Herpes genitalis is caused by herpes simplex virus types 1 or 2, both of which are DNA viruses that cannot be clinically distinguished. Type 2 infection is more common in genital infections. Symptomatic primary disease may affect as many as 200,000 people each year.[57] Recurrent infections are much more common, with as many as 40 million Americans being infected. Of importance, most people with herpes infections are asymptomatic, yet are capable of transmitting the infection.

Both sexes may present with single or multiple vesicles, which are usually quite pruritic. These vesicles, which may appear anywhere on the genitalia, spontaneously rupture to form a shallow ulcer that may be quite painful. Lesions then spontaneously resolve with minimal scarring. First, or primary, clinical infections often take longer to heal and are more often symptomatic. Subsequent, or recurrent, infections are usually milder and resolve quicker. Recurrent infections may be asymptomatic in some individuals. Drug therapy for herpes does not cure the STD; rather, treatment only relieves the symptoms and hastens healing of the ulcers. Thus, patients with herpetic genital infections remain infectious all their lives. Patients are most infectious at the time ulcers are present. In addition, as mentioned above, NGU may be a frequent complication of genital herpes infections in men.

Genital herpes has been associated with an increased risk for contracting HIV infections. Because this risk is especially high when ulcers are present, patients with herpes should avoid sexual activity during such times.

Syphilis

Syphilis, an acute and chronic infectious disease caused by *Treponema palladium*, currently affects 20,000 persons each year in the United States, with a higher prevalence among persons in the lower socioeconomic strata.[23] During the 1980s, syphilis reached its highest level in the past 40 years. Recent syphilis outbreaks have been associated with the exchange of sex for drugs, particularly crack cocaine.

Symptoms of syphilis vary according to the stage of the disease. Primary syphilis presents with a classic chancre, which is a painless, indurated ulcer located at the site of exposure. Any genital lesions should be suspected of indicating syphilis. In men, this chancre may appear on the penis; in women, the chancre may be difficult to see because it is found on the internal structures of the genital tract. Chancres may also appear inside the anus, in the pharynx, on the lips, or on the fingers of infected individuals.

The secondary stage of syphilis may present as a highly variable skin rash. Mucus patches, condylomata lata (flat, wartlike outgrowths in the anal or genital region; lymphadenopathy (enlarged lymph nodes); and alopecia (hair loss) are also common. Latent syphilis is asymptomatic. Patients who are untreated may present with sequelae of late disease, including localized gumma (infectious, nodular, inflammatory lesion) formation; neurosyphilis (infection of the central nervous system); and cardiovascular disease.

Genital ulcerations may be associated with, and facilitate spread of, HIV infections. Thus, obtaining an HIV test may be warranted. Patients with syphilis should avoid sexual activity until they and their sexual partners are cured.

Hepatitis B

Hepatitis B, an inflammation of the liver caused by a viral infection, is not often thought of as an STD. Yet it can often be transmitted by sexual activity. An estimated 5% to 20% of the U.S. population may show evidence of past hepatitis B, and 70,000 to 120,000 new cases are transmitted sexually each year.[5] Heterosexual intercourse is now the predominant mode of hepatitis B transmission.

Most hepatitis B infections are asymptomatic. Symptoms, when noted, may include a serum sickness–like prodrome, which includes skin eruptions, urticaria (eruptions of itching wheals), arthralgia (severe joint pain), and arthritis; lassitude; anorexia; nausea; vomiting; headache; fever; dark urine; jaundice (yellow coloration of skin, eyes, and deeper tissues); and moderate liver enlargement with tenderness. Long-term complications of hepatitis B can include chronic, persistent, and active hepatitis; cirrhosis (a progressive liver disease associated with function failure of liver cells and interference with blood flow in the liver); hepatocellular carcinoma; hepatic failure; and death. Because of these risks, all young, sexually active adults should be encouraged to seek out vaccination for hepatitis B.

Trichomoniasis

Trichomoniasis is predominantly noted as a vaginal infection and is the most readily curable STD. An estimated 3 million women may be infected with trichomoniasis each year.[56] The infection usually presents with a frothy, excessive vaginal discharge; other symptoms include erythema, edema, and pruritus of the external genitalia. Also, dysuria and dyspareunia (painful sexual intercourse) may be common. In some women, however, trichomoniasis may be asymptomatic. Men rarely exhibit symptoms but may present with urethritis (inflammation of the urethra), balanitis (inflammation of the penis), or cutaneous lesions on the penis. It is important to realize that symptomatology alone will not distinguish the etiology of the disease.

Complications of trichomoniasis include common recurrent infections and infections secondary to excoriations. Increased risk of PID, low birth weight, and premature birth may occur.

Patients with trichomoniasis should not resume sexual relations until they and their partners have been treated.

Bacterial Vaginosis

Bacterial vaginosis (BV) is a syndrome caused by several species of vaginal bacteria, including *Gardnerella vaginalis*, *Mycoplasma hominis*, and various anaerobes such as *Mobiluncus*. Although BV is associated with having multiple sexual partners, it is unclear whether BV results in acquisition of a sexually transmissible pathogen.[58] Common symptoms include an excessive or malodorous vaginal discharge. Erythema, edema, and pruritus of the external genitalia may also occur. Recurrent infections may be common in untreated patients, as may be secondary infections resulting from excoriations. An increased risk of PID and premature childbirth may be common in patients with BV.

Chancroid

Chancroid is caused by *Haemophilus ducreyi*, a gram-negative rod that is often noted to occur in small clusters along with strands of mucus. Chancroid is a well-established potentiating cause of HIV transmission. Although the overall incidence of chancroid remains small in developed nations, it is frequently seen in developing nations. The disease has been reported to be endemic in various parts of the United

Case Study 8–2

Patient Complaint/History

Gina, a 22-year-old woman, comes to the pharmacy counter holding a tube of Monistat 7 vaginal cream and a box of spermicide-treated latex condoms. In the past few months, the patient has purchased the vaginal cream on several occasions. A quick review of her pharmacy profile shows that the following prescription was filled the previous week: Acyclovir 200 mg, one capsule five times daily for 5 days.

In response to questions about her symptoms, Gina describes intense vaginal itching but denies any vaginal discharge. She says that the itching, which has occurred numerous times, usually occurs after intercourse but not after every act of intercourse. Her sexual partner has no symptoms. Gina also says that the itching, which she usually treats with the Monistat 7 vaginal cream, resolves in a day or so. Once when she was unable to obtain the product, the itching resolved within 2 days without treatment.

The patient and her partner use either latex condoms or vaginal spermicides for contraception; however, when she has an outbreak of genital herpes, they always use latex condoms.

Clinical Considerations/Strategies

Readers can use the following considerations or strategies to determine whether use of nonprescription products is warranted in this patient:

- Assess the appropriateness of Monistat 7 vaginal cream for treatment of the vaginal itching.
- Assess alternative causes, other than candidal vaginitis, of the vaginal itching.
- Assess the contraceptive needs of this patient and her partner.
- Suggest an alternative contraceptive product that will meet their needs for prevention of pregnancy and STDs.

Patient Education/Counseling

Readers can use the following strategies to develop a patient education/counseling plan that will help ensure optimal outcomes:

- Develop a patient education plan that will optimize proper and consistent use of the recommended contraceptive product.

States.[56] Women who become infected with chancroid are often asymptomatic. In men, a single painful ulcer with erythematous edges is noted. The ulcer may be necrotic. Painful lymphadenopathy along the inguinal distribution is noted in half of cases. This distribution may rupture in up to 60% of cases.[5]

Prevention of Sexually Transmitted Diseases

The only sure way to guard against AIDS infection through sexual contact is to abstain from sex or to remain in a mutually monogamous relationship with an uninfected individual. If neither action is feasible, the next best option is to use latex (not natural membrane) condoms for any oral, anal, or vaginal intercourse. Most data indicate that the male condom can protect against HIV transmission, and some authorities believe the female condom may provide similar protection.[59] However, the high failure and pregnancy rates of 25% reported with the female condom strongly suggest a lack of adequate protection against STDs. In populations at risk, individuals who consistently use male condoms have demonstrated a significantly lower seroconversion rate (an indicator of infection with the AIDS virus) than those who do not use condoms or who use them inconsistently.[60,61]

It is very important to emphasize that condom use does not guarantee safety because condoms can break.[16,17] Laboratory data are being accumulated that suggest the spermicide nonoxynol-9 in proper concentrations may be somewhat effective in killing the AIDS virus and might offer additional protection when used with condoms.[60] However, as stated previously, recent data have indicated that spermicide-mediated vulvovaginal microabrasions could increase a woman's susceptibility to HIV. Although the quality of the data to date is questionable, women with compromised vulvar and vaginal tissue may be at an increased risk for susceptibility to HIV.[62] Timing is important in the proper use of the male condom. Patients must realize that seminal fluid can leak from the erect penis in some men. This preejaculatory fluid can contain HIV, other pathogens, and viable sperm.[63,64] Thus, for proper use in safer sex, the condom must be placed on the penis well before contact is made with the partner's mouth, vagina, anus, or any broken skin.

In the past, spermicides have been recommended to aid in preventing STD transmission. Recent data indicate that spermicides may alter vaginal flora and may be responsible for vulvovaginal microabrasions that might actually increase the risk of infecting the patient.[55] As a result, it may be appropriate to recommend avoiding routine spermicidal use.

Other contraceptive methods have also been studied for their efficacy in preventing transmission of AIDS.[59,65,66] However, as indicated in Table 8–11, the use of other nonprescription barrier methods (e.g., the diaphragm and cervical cap) has thus far shown limited protection against AIDS as well as against other STDs.[5,67] The same is true for hormonal contraceptives, such as oral contraceptives and parenteral products (e.g., depot medroxyprogesterone acetate and levonorgestrel implants). It is important to keep in mind that some STDs, such as syphilis and herpes, may be spread through external skin lesions. Condoms and spermicides may not be effective in preventing these types of infection.

Because compliance with the safer sex practices listed in Table 8–11, especially with regard to condom use, is poor even among those at risk, other behavioral factors aimed at lowering risk should be stressed.[68] These behavioral factors include changes in lifestyle and sexual practices.

Table 8–11

Effects of Contraceptives on Bacterial and Viral STDs

Contraceptive Method	Bacterial STD	Viral STD
Latex male condoms	Protective	Protective
Polyurethane male condoms	Probably protective	Probably protective
Natural membrane condoms	Protective	Possibly not protective
Female condom	Possibly protective against recurrent vaginal trichomoniasis	Possibly protective
Spermicides	Protective against cervical gonorrhea and chlamydia	Undetermined in vivo
Diaphragms	Protective against cervical infection: associated with vaginal anaerobic overgrowth	Protective against cervical infection
Hormonal	Associated with increased cervical chlamydia, protective against symptomatic PID	Not protective
Intrauterine device	Associated with PID in first month after insertion	Not protective
Natural family planning	Not protective	Not protective

Source: Reference 67; used with permission.

Patient Assessment of Risk for Sexually Transmitted Diseases

Before recommending a method to prevent STDs, including contraceptive products, the pharmacist must first determine the patient's risk for acquiring an STD. If the patient has an untreated STD, the pharmacist should refer the patient immediately to a physician. Asking the patient the following questions will help elicit the information needed to recommend the appropriate preventive measures.

Q~ Are you in a mutually monogamous relationship now?

A~ The patient's response will determine the relationship's level of risk. *Identify preventive measures for STDs. (See the section "Prevention of Sexually Transmitted Diseases.")* Advise a patient in a unilaterally monogamous relationship to be tested for STDs and to take appropriate preventive measures during intercourse.

Q~ Do you or your partner currently have or have either had in the past a sexually transmitted disease?

A~ If either partner currently has an STD, determine whether the disease is being treated. If so, recommend preventive measures appropriate for the particular STD. If the STD is not being treated, advise the infected partner to seek treatment. Also advise the other partner to be tested for STDs. If protective measures are not being taken, recommend the appropriate measures. Past infections indicate a risk for STDs; recommend that the partners use preventive measures even if neither is currently infected.

Q~ If you or your partner were previously in other relationships, have you both been examined or tested for sexually transmitted diseases?

A~ If the sexual partners have not been tested for STDs and if the STD status of their previous partners is unknown, advise the present partners to be tested. Also recommend they take preventive measures during intercourse until their STD status is known.

Q~ Do you know what your risks are for being infected with the virus that causes AIDs or with other sexually transmitted diseases?

A~ *Identify the risk factors for contracting AIDS. (See the section "AIDS.")* If the patient is unaware of the risk factors for STDs, provide the appropriate information.

Q~ How do you protect yourself from sexually transmitted diseases, including AIDs?

A~ If the patient's protection methods are nonexistent or inadequate, recommend the appropriate preventive measures.

Patient Counseling for Sexually Transmitted Diseases

Given the prevalence of these diseases and the fact that more than 1 million Americans are HIV-positive, the prevention of STDs must be a priority. As health care practitioners in a

Patient Education for Sexually Transmitted Diseases

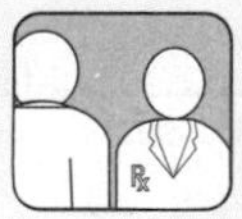

The number and seriousness of sexually transmitted diseases (STDs) continue to grow, with most of these diseases occurring in people younger than 25 years old. Women have a higher risk of contracting STDs and suffer more long-term consequences, such as pelvic inflammatory disease, infertility, ectopic pregnancy, chronic pelvic pain, and cervical cancer.

The objective of self-care for all sexually active persons is to prevent the contraction of STDs or, if a disease is already contracted, to prevent its transmission to sexual partners. For most patients, carefully following the measures listed below will help to achieve the objective.

- To decrease chances of contracting a STD, avoid having intercourse with an infected person or with someone whose sexual history and STD status are unknown.
- Syphilis, herpes, and chancroid may be spread through skin ulcers; consequently, condoms and spermicides may not prevent transmission of these diseases. Avoid intercourse with people who have herpes, especially when ulcers are present. Avoid intercourse with people who have syphilis or chancroid until they are cured.
- If you have or your partner has syphilis, gonorrhea, or trichomoniasis, abstain from intercourse until both of you are treated.
- To decrease the chances of contracting AIDS, do not share needles and syringes with anyone. Also avoid intercourse with people who have genital ulcers (herpes, syphilis, chancroid) or are known to have gonorrhea.

⚠ Abstaining from intercourse or having a mutually monogamous relationship with an uninfected partner is the best way to prevent AIDs and other STDs. If these measures are not feasible, use latex condoms for oral, anal, and vaginal intercourse; avoid the unsafe sex options listed in Table 8–10.

position to offer much-needed health information, pharmacists must keep abreast of all aspects of the prevention and treatment of STDs, especially with respect to AIDS.

Different patients will accept differing levels of self-risk to satisfy their personal needs. Part of the pharmacist's role can be to aid the patient in realizing that using proper contraceptive choices can reduce the risk associated with sexual intimacy. Latex condom use should be stressed as a method of disease prevention for all patients at risk for STDs, including those who currently use prescription methods of birth control (e.g., oral contraceptives or the intrauterine device). The box "Patient Education for Sexually Transmitted Diseases" lists specific information to provide patients.

CONCLUSIONS

Unintended pregnancy and STDs, which are potential adverse outcomes of unprotected sexual intercourse, continue to be a major public health issue in the United States. Proper counseling from the pharmacist may aid in preventing both of these problems. It is essential that patients understand the need for appropriate contraceptive measures not only to prevent unintended pregnancy but also to reduce the risk of STDs.

Not many decisions in life are more personal or more important than the choice of a contraceptive method. Optimally, both sexual partners should make the decision. Because no single method is likely to be suitable throughout a person's reproductive life, it is important for all options to be presented in a clear and nonjudgmental manner. All sexually active individuals who are not in a mutually monogamous relationship should be aware that they must protect themselves and their partners from AIDS and other STDs. They should choose a contraceptive method accordingly.

References

1. Piccinino LJ, Mosher WD. Trends in contraceptive use in the United States: 1982–1995. *Fam Plann Perspect.* 1998;30:4–10,46.
2. Henshaw SK. Unintended pregnancy in the United States. *Fam Plann Perspect.* 1998;30:24–9,46.
3. Warren CW, Santelli JS, Everett SA, et al. Sexual behavior among U.S. high school students, 1990–1995. *Fam Plann Perspect.* 1998;30:170–2, 200.
4. Spitz AM, Velebil P, Koonin LM, et al. Pregnancy, abortion, and birth rates among U.S. adolescents—1980, 1985, and 1990. *JAMA.* 1996;275;989–94.
5. Cates W. Reproductive tract infections. In: Hatcher RA, Trussell J, Stewart F, et al., eds. *Contraceptive Technology.* 17th rev ed. New York: Ardent Media; 1998:179–210.
6. Forrest JD, Singh S. The sexual and reproductive behavior of American women, 1982–1988. *Fam Plann Perspect.* 1990;22:206–14.
7. Zabin LS, Stark HA, Emerson MR. Reasons for delay in contraceptive clinic utilization: adolescent clinic and nonclinic populations compared. *J Adolesc Health.* 1991;12:225.
8. Zabin LS, Kantner JF, Zelnik M. The risk of adolescent pregnancy in the first months of intercourse. *Fam Plann Perspect.* 1979;11:215–22.
9. Schirm AL, Trussell J, Menker J, et al. Contraceptive failure in the United States: the impact of social, economic and demographic factors. *Fam Plann Perspect.* 1982;14:68–94.
10. Hatcher RA, Trussell J, Stewart F, et al., eds. *Contraceptive Technology.* 17th rev ed. New York: Ardent Media; 1998:55, 158, 216–7, 337, 341, 343.
11. Eichhorst BC. Contraception. *Prim Care.* 1988;15:437–9.
12. Anon. Condoms get better. *Consumer Reports.* 1999;64:46–9.
13. Rosenberg MJ, Waugh MS, Solomon HM, et al. The male polyurethane condom: a review of current knowledge. *Contraception.* 1996;53: 141–6.
14. Minuk GY, Bohme CE, Bowen TJ. Condoms and hepatitis B virus infection. *Ann Intern Med.* 1986;104:584.
15. Rosenberg MJ, Waugh MS. Latex condom breakage and slippage in a controlled clinical trial. *Contraception.* 1997;56:17–21.
16. Gotzsche PC, Hording M. Condoms to prevent HIV transmission do not imply truly safe sex. *Scand J Infect Dis.* 1988;20:233–4.
17. van Griensven GJ, de Vroome EM, Tielman RA, et al. Failure rate of condoms during anogenital intercourse in homosexual men. *Genitourin Med.* 1988;64:344–6.
18. Russell-Brown P, Piedrahita C, Foldesy R, et al. Comparison of condom breakage during human use with performance in laboratory testing. *Contraception.* 1992;45:429–37.
19. Steiner M, Piedrahita C, Glover L, et al. Can condom users likely to experience condom failure be identified? *Fam Plann Perspect.* 1993; 25: 220–3, 226.
20. Trussell J, Warner DL, Hatcher RA. Condom slippage and breakage rates. *Fam Plann Perspect.* 1992;24:20–3.
21. Gabbay M, Gibbs A. Does additional lubrication reduce condom failure? *Contraception.* 1996;53:155–8.
22. Freziers RG, Walsh TL, Nelson AL, et al. Breakage and acceptability of a polyurethane condom: a randomized, controlled study. *Fam Plann Perspect.* 1998;30:73–8.
23. Cates W Jr, Stone KM. Family planning, sexually transmitted diseases, and contraceptive choices: a literature update—part I. *Fam Plann Perspect.* 1992;24:75–84.
24. FDA. Latex condoms; user labeling; expiration date. *Fed Reg.* 1997;62: 187.
25. Liss GM, Sussman GL. Latex sensitization: occupational versus general population prevalence rates. *Am J Ind Med.* 1999;35:196–200.
26. Levy DA, Khouaders S, Leynadier F. Allergy to latex condoms. *Allergy.* 1998;53:1107–8.
27. Turjanmaa K, Reunala T. Condoms as a source of latex allergen and cause of contact urticaria. *Contact Dermatitis.* 1989;20:360–4.
28. Trussell J, Sturgeon K, Strickler J, et al. Comparative contraceptive efficacy of the female condom and other barrier methods. *Fam Plann Perspect.* 1994;26: –72.
29. Stewart F. Vaginal barriers: the diaphragm, contraceptive sponge, cervical cap, and female condom. In: Hatcher, RA, Trussell J, Stewart F, et al., eds. *Contraceptive Technology.* 17th rev ed. New York: Ardent Media; 1998:371–404.
30. Coggins C, Elias CJ, Atisook R, et al. Women's preferences regarding the formulation of over-the-counter vaginal spermicides. *AIDS.* 1998;12: 1389–91.
31. Mears E. Chemical contraception trial: II. *J Reprod Fertil.* 1962;4: 337–43.
32. Cates W, Raymond EG. Vaginal spermicides. In: Hatcher, RA, Trussell J, Stewart F, et al., eds. *Contraceptive Technology.* 17th rev ed. New York: Ardent Media; 1998:357–69.
33. Poindexter AN, Levine H, Sangi-Haghpeykar H, et al. Comparison of spermicides on vulvar, vaginal, and cervical mucosa. *Contraception.* 1996;53:147–53.
34. Einarson TR, Korn G, Mattice D, et al. Maternal spermicide use and adverse reproductive outcome: a meta-analysis. *Am J Obstet Gynecol.* 1990;162:655–60.
35. Kestelman P, Trussell J. Efficacy of the simultaneous use of condoms and spermicides. *Fam Plann Perspect.* 1991;23:226–7, 232.
36. McIntyre SL, Higgins JE. Parity and use-effectiveness with the contraceptive sponge. *Am J Obstet Gynecol.* 1986;155:796–801.
37. Faich G, Pearson K, Fleming D, et al. Toxic shock syndrome and the vaginal contraceptive sponge. *JAMA.* 1986;255:216–8.
38. Rosenberg MJ, Rojanapithayakorn W, Feldblum PJ, et al. Effect of the contraceptive sponge on chlamydia infection, gonorrhea, and candidiasis: a comparative clinical trial. *JAMA.* 1987;257:2308–12.

39. Trussell J, Koenig J, Stewart F, et al. Medical care cost savings from adolescent contraceptive use. *Fam Plann Perspect.* 1997;29 : 248–55, 295.
40. Trussell J, Kowal D. The essentials of contraception: efficacy, safety, and personal considerations. In: Hatcher RA, Trussell J, Stewart F, et al. eds. *Contraceptive Technology.* 17th rev ed. New York: Ardent Media; 1998: 211–48.
41. Trussell J, Leveque JA, Koenig JD, et al. The economic value of contraception: a comparison of 15 methods. *Am J Public Health.* 1995;85 : 494–503.
42. Gray RH, Kambic RT. Epidemiological studies of natural family planning. *Hum Reprod.* 1988;3:693.
43. Brown JB, Blackwell LF, Billings JJ, et al. Natural family planning. *Am J Obstet Gynecol.* 1987;157(pt 2):1082–9.
44. Klaus H. Natural family planning: a review. *Obstet Gynecol Survey.* 1982;37:128–50.
45. Gross BA. Natural family planning indicators of ovulation [invited review]. *Clin Reprod Fertil.* 1987;5:91.
46. Frazier JL, Schumock GT. Drug-induced alterations in body temperature. *P&T.* 1991; 16:164, 271–5.
47. Kennedy KI, Trussell J. Postpartum contraception and lactation. In: Hatcher RA, Trussell J, Stewart F, et al., eds. *Contraceptive Technology.* 17th rev ed. New York: Ardent Media; 1998:589–614.
48. Richwald GA, Wamsley MA, Coulson AH, et al. Are condom instructions readable? Results of a readability study. *Public Health Rep.* 1988;103:355–9.
49. Cates W. Contraception, unintended pregnancies, and sexually transmitted diseases: why isn't a simple solution possible. *Am J Epidemiol.* 1996;143 : 311–8.
50. Wasserheit JN. Epidemiological synergy: interrelationships between human immunodeficiency virus infection and other sexually transmitted diseases. *Sex Transm Dis.* 1992;19:61–77.
51. Centers for Disease Control and Prevention. Contraceptive method and condom use among women at risk for HIV infection and other sexually transmitted diseases—selected U.S. sites, 1993–1994. *MMWR Morb Mortal Wkly Rep.* 1996;45:820–3.
52. Karon JM, Rosenberg PS, McQuillan G, et al. Prevalence of HIV infection in the United States 1984–92. *JAMA.* 1996;276:126–31.
53. Centers for Disease Control and Prevention. *HIV/AIDS Surveillance Report.* 1998;10(2):1–43.
54. Mu-oz A, Wang MC, Bass S, et al. Acquired immunodeficiency syndrome (AIDS)-free time after human immunodeficiency virus type 1 (HIV-1) seroconversion in homosexual men. *Am J Epidemiol.* 1989;130: 530–9.
55. Howe HE, Minkoff HL, Duerr AC. Contraceptives and HIV. *AIDS.* 1994;8:861–71.
56. Division of STD Prevention, Centers for Disease Control and Prevention. *Sexually Transmitted Disease Surveillance, 1997.* Atlanta: US Department of Health and Human Services, Public Health Service; September 1998.
57. Hooten TM, Scholes D, Hughes JP, et al. A prospective study of risk factors for symptomatic urinary tract infection in young women. *N Engl J Med.* 1996;335:468–74.
58. Centers for Disease Control and Prevention. 1998 guidelines for sexually transmitted diseases. *MMWR Morbid Mortal Weekly Rep.* 1998 : 47(RR–1):1–118.
59. Guest F. HIV/AIDS and reproductive health. In: Hatcher RA, Trussell J, Stewart F, et al., eds. *Contraceptive Technology.* 17th rev ed. New York: Ardent Media; 1998: 141–78.
60. Feldblum PJ, Fortney JA. Condoms, spermicides, and the transmission of human immunodeficiency virus: a review of the literature. *Am J Public Health.* 1988;78:52–4.
61. Darrow WW. Condom use and use-effectiveness in high-risk populations. *Sex Transm Dis.* 1989;16:157–9.
62. Kreiss J, Ngugi E, Holmes K, et al. Efficacy of nonoxynol-9 contraceptive sponge use in preventing heterosexual acquisition of HIV in Nairobi prostitutes. *JAMA.* 1992;268:477–82.
63. Ilaria G, Jacobs JL, Polsky B, et al. Detection of HIV-1 DNA sequences in pre-ejaculatory fluid. *Lancet.* 1992; 340:1469.
64. Pudney J, Oneta M, Mayer K, et al. Pre-ejaculatory fluid as potential vector for sexual transmission of HIV-1. *Lancet.* 1992;340:1470.
65. Deneberg R. Female sex hormones and HIV. *AIDS Clin Care.* 1993;5: 69–71,76.
66. Clemetson DB, Moss GB, Willerford DM, et al. Detection of HIV DNA in cervical and vaginal secretions: prevalence and correlates among women in Nairobi, Kenya. *JAMA.* 1993;269:2860–4.
67. Cates W. Contraception, unintended pregnancies, and sexually transmitted diseases: why isn't a simple solution possible? *Am J Epidemiol.* 1996;143:313.
68. Henry K, Osterholm MT. Reduction of HIV transmission by use of condoms. *Am J Public Health.* 1988;78:1244.

SECTION IV

RESPIRATORY DISORDERS

CHAPTER 9

Disorders Related to Cold and Allergy

Karen J. Tietze

Chapter 9 at a Glance

Pharmacists have an important role both in triage and in evaluating the appropriateness of self-care drug and nondrug interventions. Among the most common nonprescription medications used to self-medicate are those that treat cough, the common cold, and seasonal and perennial allergic rhinitis. This chapter reviews the role of nonprescription medications in managing these disorders.

Editor's Note: This chapter is based, in part, on the 11th edition chapter titled "Cold, Cough, and Allergy Products," which was written by Karen J. Tietze.

Anatomy and Physiology of the Respiratory System

The respiratory system is divided into (1) the upper respiratory system, which filters, warms, and humidifies inspired air, and (2) the lower respiratory system, which directs the air flow and participates in gas exchange.

Each breath passes from the nasal passages to the throat, larynx, trachea, bronchi, and lungs (in that order). Gas exchange takes place at the cellular level in tiny air sacs (alveoli) of the lung. The nose, which is part of the upper respiratory system, contains the olfactory apparatus, many arteriovenous anastomoses, and the cavernous sinusoids. Vibrissae (coarse hairs) line the nostrils and remove large particles from inspired air. Each nostril ends in a cavity that is divided horizontally into three turbinates. The mucous layer covering the turbinates traps particles that have greater mass and momentum than air and, therefore, cannot change direction fast enough to avoid the trap. Inspired air is warmed and humidified by the large nasal surface area and the blood flow.

Sensory, cholinergic, and sympathetic nerves innervate the nose. Sensory fibers respond to mechanical and thermal stimuli and to mediators such as histamine and bradykinin. Cholinergic and sympathetic nerves innervate glands and the arteries that supply the glands. Sympathetic nerves also innervate veins and venules. Cholinergic stimulation dilates and sympathetic stimulation constricts arterial blood flow. The cavernous sinusoids contain erectile tissue that engorges when the sympathetic tone is reduced or when the cholinergic system is stimulated. The sensory, cholinergic, and sympathetic nerves also respond to a variety of neuropeptide neurotransmitters.

The pharynx is divided into the nasopharynx, oropharynx, and hypopharynx. It connects the nasal cavities to the larynx and esophagus. Four pairs of sinus cavities (paranasal sinuses) drain posteriorly into the pharynx, lighten the cranium, and serve as resonating chambers for speech. The nasopharynx contains the pharyngeal tonsils (adenoids) and is connected to the middle ears through eustachian tubes. Closed 99% of the time, these tubes open during swallowing, thereby equilibrating atmospheric and middle ear pressure. The palatine tonsils are located in the oropharynx, and the vocal cords and epiglottis are located in the larynx.

The respiratory mucosa, a specialized membrane, lines the surfaces of the upper and lower respiratory tracts, including the sinuses. The respiratory mucosa contains ciliated and nonciliated epithelial, goblet, and basal cells as well as mucus-secreting glands. The glands secrete a variety of enzymes, immunoglobulins, and other immunomodulatory factors. A double fluid layer covers the respiratory mucosa. Outermost is a thick, sticky layer that traps dust, bacteria, viruses, and other foreign materials. Innermost is a thinner, more aqueous layer in which ciliated epithelial cells beat in a synchronized, wavelike pattern, thus sweeping the thicker outer layer toward the larynx where the mucus is swallowed. The interstitial tissue contains lymphocytes, fibroblasts, and mast cells. Mast cells are located close to nerves and blood vessels and are clustered in the epithelium just beneath the basement membrane.

Cough

Cough is the most common symptom for which patients seek medical care.[1] Americans spend about $500 million annually on antitussives.[2] Coughing irritates the throat and chest, interferes with work and sleep, and generates concern over what illness the cough may portend.

Epidemiology/Etiology of Cough

Cough is a symptom of diverse infectious and noninfectious disorders. Each of these disorders has its own epidemiology. (See the section "Epidemiology of the Common Cold," for example.) Cough is classified as either acute (e.g., the cough has a duration of 3 weeks or less), or chronic (e.g., the cough's duration is longer than 3 weeks).[3] Viral infections of the upper respiratory tract and, less commonly, pulmonary emboli and pneumonia cause acute cough. Chronic cough, reported by 14% to 23% of adults,[4] is often a symptom of postnasal drip syndrome that is secondary to sinusitis or rhinitis, asthma, bronchitis, gastroesophageal reflux disease, and congestive heart failure.[5] Patients with lung disorders (e.g., emphysema, idiopathic pulmonary fibrosis, lung cancer, and dust diseases—farmer's lung, silicosis, asbestosis, pneumoconiosis) may have a chronic cough as well.

Chronic cough can be linked to smoking. Among smokers, 25% who smoke one-half pack per day and more than 50% of those who smoke more than two packs per day report chronic cough.[4,6]

A few drugs can cause cough. Angiotensin-converting enzyme (ACE) inhibitors cause cough in 10% of patients,[7] and systemic and ophthalmic β-adrenergic blockers may cause cough in patients with obstructive airway diseases.

In children, a cough may be a symptom of viral or bacterial respiratory infection, heart disease, foreign body aspiration, aspiration caused by poor coordination of sucking and swallowing, or esophageal motility disorders.[8]

Physiology of Cough

Cough is an important defensive reflex of the respiratory tract. A cough starts with a deep inspiration followed by closure of the glottis and forceful contraction of the chest wall, abdominal wall, and diaphragmatic muscles against the closed glottis. When the glottis opens, high expiratory velocities propel mucus, cellular debris, and foreign material from the lower respiratory system. The central cough control center, located in the medulla but separate from the respiratory control center, coordinates the complex cough response.

Signs and Symptoms of Cough

Coughs are described as productive or nonproductive. A productive cough (e.g., a wet or "chesty" cough) expels secretions from the lower respiratory tract that, if retained, could impair ventilation and the lungs' ability to resist infection. The secretions may be clear (e.g., bronchitis), purulent (e.g., bacterial infection), discolored (e.g., yellow with inflammatory disorders), or malodorous (e.g., anaerobic bacterial infection). A nonproductive cough (e.g., a dry or "hacking" cough) serves no useful physiologic purpose. Nonproductive coughs are caused by viral respiratory tract infections, atypical bacterial infections, gastroesophageal reflux disease, cardiac disease, and some drugs. Table 9–1 lists the signs and symptoms of illness associated with chronic cough.

Complications of Cough

Complications secondary to high intrathoracic pressures and expiratory velocities are common regardless of the cause or type of cough.[8] Common complications include exhaustion, insomnia, musculoskeletal pain, hoarseness, excessive perspiration, and urinary incontinence. Less-common complications include cardiac dysrhythmias, syncope, stroke, and rib fractures.

Treatment of Cough

Treatment Outcomes

The goals of therapy are to improve patient comfort and relieve the cough.

General Treatment Approach

Choosing a medication for self-care of cough depends on the nature of the cough.[9] (See Figure 9–1.) Cough suppressants, medications that increase the cough threshold, are the drugs of choice for nonproductive coughs.

Expectorants, which are medications that increase bronchial secretion and facilitate its removal, are the drugs of choice for irritative nonproductive coughs and for cough that expels thick, tenacious secretions from the lungs with difficulty. Water cannot be incorporated into previously formed mucus, but less-viscid secretions are formed if the patient is well hydrated.

Products containing both an expectorant and a cough suppressant are irrational and should be avoided. The expectorant increases secretions of the lower respiratory tract, but the cough suppressant decreases the cough threshold. Lower respiratory tract secretions may be retained, which may lead to potentially adverse consequences (e.g., infection, airway obstruction).

Exclusions to self-care with nonprescription medications include coughs that produce thick yellow or green phlegm, fever higher than 101.5°F, unintended weight loss, drenching nighttime sweats, hemoptysis, foreign object aspiration, a history of symptoms suggestive of chronic underlying disease states associated with cough, suspected drug-associated cough, worsening symptoms during self-treatment, and development of new symptoms during self-treatment for cough.

Nonpharmacologic Therapy

Cool-mist vaporizers or humidifiers provide increased humidity that may soothe irritated airways and decrease cough. However, high humidity may accelerate mold growth and worsen either allergies or asthma. Cool-mist vaporizers are preferable to warm-mist vaporizers because they eliminate the risk of scalding if they are tipped over. Hard candies and other lozenges soothe throat irritation and may decrease coughing.

Pharmacologic Therapy

Table 9–2 lists examples of products that contain oral antitussives, topical antitussives, and expectorants. Properties of the specific agents are discussed below.

Antitussives

Nonprescription cough suppressants approved by the Food and Drug Administration (FDA) include codeine, dextromethorphan, and diphenhydramine.

Table 9–1

Signs and Symptoms of Diseases Associated with Chronic Cough

Disease	Signs and Symptoms
Viral upper respiratory tract infection	Sneezing, rhinorrhea, low-grade temperature
Lower respiratory tract infection	Temperature >101.5°F; thick, purulent, discolored phlegm; drenching sweats in bed at night
Postnasal drip	Mucus drainage from nose or frequent clearing of throat
Asthma	Wheezing or chest tightness, coughing predominantly at night, cough in response to exposure to specific irritants such as dust, smoke, or pollen
Gastroesophageal reflux disease	Heartburn, worsening of symptoms when supine, improvement with antacids or histamine$_2$-receptor blocker
Chronic pulmonary obstructive disease	Productive cough most days of the month at least 3 months of the year for at least 2 consecutive years
Congestive heart failure	Fatigue, edema, breathlessness

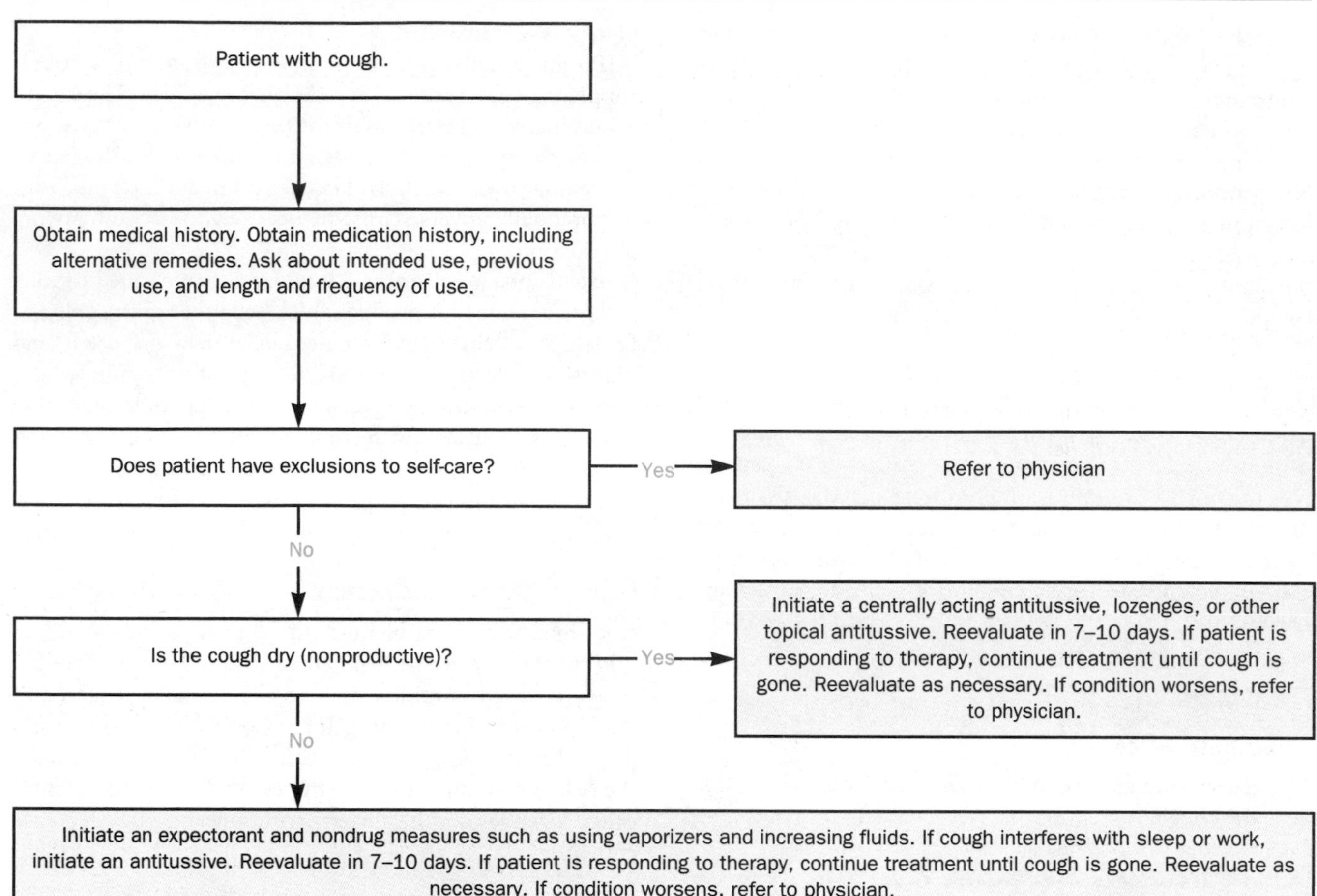

Figure 9–1 Self-care of cough. Adapted from reference 9.

Codeine Codeine is the gold standard antitussive.

Mechanism of Action Codeine, the methyl ether of morphine, acts centrally on the respiratory centers in the medulla and nucleus tractus solaris to increase the cough threshold.

Pharmacokinetics Codeine is well absorbed orally with a 15- to 30-minute onset of action and a 4- to 6-hour duration of effect; the elimination half-life is 2.5 to 3 hours. This agent is hepatically metabolized to norcodeine and morphine; morphine may be the active antitussive. Approximately 3% to 16% of codeine is eliminated unchanged in the urine.[10]

Indications Codeine is indicated for the suppression of cough caused by chemical or mechanical respiratory tract irritation. Although codeine is the gold standard antitussive, recent evidence suggests that this agent is not effective for acute coughs associated with the common cold or other infections of the upper respiratory tract.[11,12]

Dosage/Administration Guidelines Table 9–3 lists FDA-approved dosages of codeine.[13–15] The frequency of chronic cough decreases linearly with doses varying between 7.5 and 60 mg per day.[16] The efficacy and the safety of codeine in children are not well documented; pediatric dosage guidelines are extrapolated from the adult literature.[17] Reduced doses are appropriate for the very young, the elderly, and the debilitated.

Adverse Effects Usual antitussive codeine dosages have low toxicity and little risk of addiction. The lethal overdose in adults is 0.5 to 1 g, with death from marked respiratory depression and cardiopulmonary collapse. The most common side effects associated with antitussive dosages are nausea, vomiting, sedation, dizziness, and constipation.

Drug–Drug Interactions Concomitant use of codeine and central nervous system depressants (e.g., barbiturates, sedatives, and alcohol) causes additive CNS depression.

Contraindications/Precautions/Warnings Codeine is contraindicated in people with known hypersensitivity to it and during labor when a premature birth is anticipated. Patients with impaired respiratory reserve (e.g., asthma, chronic obstructive pulmonary disease) or preexisting respiratory

Table 9–2

Selected Products for Cough

Trade Name	Primary Ingredients
Single-Entity Cough Suppressants	
Benylin Adult Cough Formula Liquid[a,b]	Dextromethorphan hydrobromide 15 mg/5 mL
Benylin Pediatric Cough Formula Liquid[a,c]	Dextromethorphan hydrobromide 7.5 mg/5 mL
Robitussin Cough Calmers Lozenges	Dextromethorphan hydrobromide 5 mg
Robitussin Maximum Strength Cough Liquid	Dextromethorphan hydrobromide 15 mg/5 mL
Robitussin Pediatric Cough Liquid[c]	Dextromethorphan hydrobromide 7.5 mg/5 mL
St. Joseph Cough Suppressant for Children Syrup[a,c]	Dextromethorphan hydrobromide 7.5 mg/5 mL
Sucrets 4-Hour Cough Suppressant Lozenges	Dextromethorphan hydrobromide 15 mg
Vicks 44 Soothing Cough Relief Liquid[d]	Dextromethorphan hydrobromide 10 mg/5 mL
Single-Entity Expectorant Products	
Robitussin Syrup	Guaifenesin 100 mg/5 mL
Combination Cold and Cough Products	
Alka-Seltzer Plus Cold & Cough Medicine Effervescent Tablets	Phenylpropanolamine bitartrate 20 mg; chlorpheniramine maleate 2 mg; aspirin 325 mg; dextromethorphan hydrobromide 10 mg
Alka-Seltzer Plus Cold & Cough Medicine Liqui-Gels[e]	Pseudoephedrine HCl 30 mg; chlorpheniramine maleate 2 mg; acetaminophen 325 mg; dextromethorphan hydrobromide 10 mg
Alka-Seltzer Plus Flu & Body Aches Liqui-Gels[e]	Pseudoephedrine HCl 30 mg; acetaminophen 325 mg; dextromethorphan hydrobromide 10 mg
Comtrex Maximum Strength Cold & Flu Relief Non-Drowsy Liqui-Gels[e,f]	Phenylpropanolamine HCl 12.5 mg; acetaminophen 500 mg; dextromethorphan hydrobromide 15 mg
Comtrex Day and Night Maximum Strength Cold and Flu Relief Caplets/Tablets[e]	Day: Pseudoephedrine HCl 30 mg; acetaminophen 500 mg; dextromethorphan hydrobromide 15 mg Night: Pseudoephedrine HCl 30 mg; chlorpheniramine maleate 2 mg; acetaminophen 500 mg; dextromethorphan hydrobromide 15 mg
Comtrex Maximum Strength Cold/Flu Relief Liqui-Gels[a,f]	Phenylpropanolamine HCl 12.5 mg; chlorpheniramine maleate 2 mg; acetaminophen 500 mg; dextromethorphan hydrobromide 15 mg
Contac Non-Drowsy Caplets	Pseudoephedrine HCl 30 mg; acetaminophen 325 mg; dextromethorphan hydrobromide 15 mg
Contac Severe Cold & Flu Maximum Strength Caplets	Phenylpropanolamine 12.5 mg; chlorpheniramine maleate 2 mg; acetaminophen 500 mg; dextromethorphan hydrobromide 15 mg
Coricidin HBP Cough & Cold Tablets	Chlorpheniramine maleate 4 mg; dextromethorphan hydrobromide 30 mg
Dimetapp Cold & Cough Maximum Strength Liqui-Gels	Phenylpropanolamine 25 mg; brompheniramine maleate 4 mg; dextromethorphan hydrobromide 20 mg
Novahistine DH Liquid	Pseudoephedrine HCl 30 mg/5 mL; chlorpheniramine maleate 2 mg/5 mL; codeine phosphate 10 mg/5 mL
PediaCare Cough-Cold Liquid[a,c,e]	Pseudoephedrine HCl 15 mg/5 mL; chlorpheniramine maleate 1 mg/5 mL; dextromethorphan hydrobromide 5 mg/5 mL
Pediacare Infants' Decongestant Plus Cough Drops[a,c,e,g]	Pseudoephedrine HCl 7.5 mg/0.8 mL; dextromethorphan hydrobromide 2.5 mg/0.8 mL
Robitussin Night-Time Cold Softgel[e]	Pseudoephedrine HCl 30 mg; doxylamine succinate 6.25 mg; acetaminophen 325 mg; dextromethorphan hydrobromide 15 mg
Robitussin PE Syrup	Pseudoephedrine HCl 30 mg/5 mL; guaifenesin 100 mg/5 mL
Robitussin Pediatric Night Relief Liquid[c]	Pseudoephedrine HCl 15 mg/5 mL; chlorpheniramine maleate 1 mg/5 mL; dextromethorphan hydrobromide 7.5 mg/5 mL
Robitussin Severe Congestion Liqui-Gels	Pseudoephedrine HCl 30 mg; guaifenesin 200 mg
Sudafed Severe Cold Caplets/Tablets	Pseudoephedrine HCl 30 mg; acetaminophen 500 mg; dextromethorphan hydrobromide 15 mg

(continued)

Table 9–2

Selected Products for Cough (continued)

Trade Name	Primary Ingredients
TheraFlu, Cold & Cough Medicine NightTime Individual Packet	Pseudoephedrine HCl 60 mg; chlorpheniramine maleate 4 mg; acetaminophen 1000 mg; dextromethorphan hydrobromide 30 mg
TheraFlu Maximum Strength Non-Drowsy Caplets[e]	Pseudoephedrine HCl 30 mg; acetaminophen 500 mg; dextromethorphan hydrobromide 15 mg
Triaminic AM, Non-Drowsy Cough & Decongestant Syrup[a,c,g]	Pseudoephedrine HCl 15 mg/5 mL; dextromethorphan hydrobromide 7.5 mg/5 mL
Triaminic DM Cough Relief Syrup[a,c,d]	Phenylpropanolamine HCl 6.25 mg/5 mL; dextromethorphan hydrobromide 5 mg/5 mL
Triaminic Expectorant, Chest & Head Congestion Liquid[a,c,d]	Phenylpropanolamine HCl 6.25 mg/5 mL; guaifenesin 50 mg/5 mL
Triaminic Sore Throat, Throat Pain & Cough Liquid[a,c]	Pseudoephedrine HCl 15 mg/5 mL; acetaminophen 160 mg/5 mL; dextromethorphan hydrobromide 7.5 mg/5 mL
Tylenol Cold Multi-Symptom Caplets or Tablets	Pseudoephedrine HCl 30 mg; chlorpheniramine maleate 2 mg; acetaminophen 325 mg; dextromethorphan hydrobromide 15 mg
Tylenol Cold No Drowsiness Gelcaps or Caplets[b,e]	Pseudoephedrine HCl 30 mg; acetaminophen 325 mg; dextromethorphan hydrobromide 15 mg
Tylenol Children's Cold Plus Cough Chewable Tablets[c,e,f]	Pseudoephedrine HCl 7.5 mg; chlorpheniramine maleate 0.5 mg; acetaminophen 80 mg; dextromethorphan hydrobromide 2.5 mg
Tylenol Cough Multi-Symptom Liquid[d]	Acetaminophen 650 mg/15 mL; dextromethorphan hydrobromide 30 mg/15 mL
Vicks 44M Soothing Cough, Cold & Flu Relief Liquid[d,e]	Pseudoephedrine HCl 15 mg/5 mL; chlorpheniramine maleate 1 mg/5 mL; acetaminophen 162.5 mg/5 mL; dextromethorphan hydrobromide 7.5 mg/5 mL
Vicks DayQuil Multi-Symptom Cold & Flu Relief LiquiCaps[b,d,e]	Pseudoephedrine HCl 30 mg; acetaminophen 250 mg; dextromethorphan hydrobromide 10 mg
Vicks NyQuil Children's Cold & Cough Relief Liquid[a,c,d,e]	Pseudoephedrine HCl 30 mg/15 mL; chlorpheniramine maleate 2 mg/15 mL; dextromethorphan hydrobromide 15 mg/15 mL
Vicks NyQuil Multi-Symptom Cold & Flu Relief Liquid[d,e]	Pseudoephedrine HCl 60 mg/30 mL; doxylamine succinate 12.5 mg/30 mL; acetaminophen 1000 mg/30 mL; dextromethorphan hydrobromide 30 mg/30 mL
Topical Antitussives	
Mentholatum Ointment	Camphor 9%; natural menthol 1.3%
Mentholatum Cherry Chest Rub for Kids	Camphor 4.7%; natural menthol 2.6%; eucalyptus oil 1.2%
Vicks VapoRub Ointment	Camphor 4.8%; menthol 2.6%
Vicks VapoSteam Liquid	Camphor 6.2%; menthol

[a] Alcohol-free product.
[b] Sucrose-free product.
[c] Pediatric formulation.
[d] Sulfite-free product.
[e] Aspirin-free product.
[f] Sodium-free product.
[g] Dye-free product.

depression; patients who are addicted individuals; and patients who receive other respiratory depressants or sedatives including alcohol should use codeine with caution. Codeine is a Pregnancy Category C drug and should be used during pregnancy only if the potential benefits outweigh the risks. Women should not breast-feed while taking codeine.

Dextromethorphan Dextromethorphan is the methylated dextrorotatory analogue of levorphanol.

Mechanism of Action Dextromethorphan, a nonopioid, has no analgesic, sedative, respiratory depressant, or addictive properties at usual antitussive doses. Considered ap-

Table 9–3

Dosage Guidelines for Nonprescription Oral Antitussives and Expectorants

Drug	Dosage (Maximum Daily Dosage)		
	Adults	Children 6–<12 Years	Children 2–<6 years
Codeine[a,b]	10–20 mg every 4–6 hours (120 mg)	5–10 mg every 4–6 hours (60 mg)	1 mg/kg/day in 4 equal doses or by ABW[c]
Dextromethorphan	10–20 mg every 4–8 hours or 30 mg every 8 hours (120 mg)	5–10 mg every 4 hours or 15 mg every 6–8 hours (60 mg)	2.5 mg every 4 hours or 7.5 mg every 8 hours (30 mg)
Diphenhydramine	25 mg every 4–6 hours (100 mg)	12.5 mg every 6 hours (50 mg)	6.25 mg every 6 hours (25 mg)
Guaifenesin	100–400 mg every 4 hours (2.4 g)	100–200 mg every 4 hours (1.2 g)	50–100 mg every 4 hours (600 mg)

[a] Codeine is not recommended for use in children younger than 2 years. These children may be more susceptible to the respiratory depressant effects of codeine, including respiratory arrest, coma, and death.

[b] The FDA recommends that the labels on nonprescription agents containing codeine not give dosage information for children younger than 6 years.

[c] Codeine may be dosed by actual body weight (ABW): 2 years of age (ABW of 12 kg) = 3 mg every 4–6 hours (maximum: 12 mg); 3 years of age (ABW of 14 kg) = 3.5 mg every 4–6 hours (maximum: 14 mg); 4 years of age (ABW of 16 kg) = 4 mg every 4–6 hours (maximum: 16 mg); 5 years of age (ABW of 18 kg) = 4.5 mg every 4-6 hours (maximum: 18 mg). A dispensing device such as a dropper calibrated for age or weight should be dispensed along with the product when it is intended for use in children 2 to under 6 years of age to prevent possible overdose because of improperly measuring the dose.

Source: References 13–15.

proximately equipotent with codeine, dextromethorphan acts centrally on the respiratory centers in the medulla and nucleus tractus solaris to increase the cough threshold.

Pharmacokinetics Dextromethorphan is well absorbed orally with a 15- to 30-minute onset of action and a 3- to 6-hour duration of effect. Dextromethorphan exhibits polymorphic metabolism, with a usual elimination half-life of 1.2 to 2.2 hours. However, the half-life may be as long as 45 hours in persons with a poor metabolism phenotype.[18]

Indications Dextromethorphan is indicated to suppress a cough associated with allergy or the common cold in adults and children age 2 years or older.

Dosage/Administration Guidelines Table 9–3 cites the FDA-approved dosages for dextromethorphan.[13–15]

Adverse Effects Dextromethorphan has a wide margin of safety, but it does have neurologic, cardiovascular, and gastrointestinal side effects that are dose related. Dextromethorphan overdoses cause confusion, excitation, nervousness, and irritability; respiratory depression may occur with very high doses. Reports exist of limited and sporadic recreational abuse of dextromethorphan as a "kick-inducer."[18,19] Abuse of this agent may also be associated with psychosis and mania.[20]

Contraindications/Precautions/Warnings Patients who have known hypersensitivity to dextromethorphan or who have a prior history of dextromethorphan dependence should not take it. If the patient takes monoamine oxidase inhibitors (MAOIs), dextromethorphan should not be administered for at least 14 days after the MAOIs are halted. Dextromethorphan is a Pregnancy Category C drug. It is not known whether dextromethorphan is excreted in breast milk.

Drug-Drug Interactions Additive depression of the central nervous system occurs with alcohol, antihistamines, and psychotropic medications. Dextromethorphan blocks serotonin reuptake; the combination of MAOIs and dextromethorphan may cause serotonergic syndrome (increased blood pressure, hyperpyrexia, arrhythmias, and myoclonus).

Diphenhydramine Diphenhydramine is a sedating (first-generation) nonselective antihistamine. Although diphenhydramine is an FDA-approved antitussive, it is not considered a first-line antitussive.

Mechanism of Action Diphenhydramine acts on the respiratory centers in the medulla and nucleus tractus solaris to increase the cough threshold. It is indicated to control coughs that result from colds or allergy.

Pharmacokinetics Diphenhydramine is well absorbed following oral administration with a bioavailability of 40% to 70% and an onset of action of about 15 minutes.[21,22] The volume of distribution, 3.3 to 4.5 L/kg in Caucasians, is greater in Asians and in those with chronic liver disease.[23,24] Diphenhydramine is hepatically metabolized to n-dealkylated and acidic metabolites with a clearance of 0.4 to 0.7 L/hour/kg.[22] Less than 4% is excreted unchanged in the urine.

Dosage/Administration Guidelines The antitussive dose is lower than the antihistaminic dose. Table 9–3 lists the FDA-approved dosages of diphenhydramine.[13–15]

Adverse Effects The side effects of diphenhydramine include drowsiness, disturbed coordination, blurred vision, respiratory depression, urinary retention, dry mouth, and dry respiratory secretions. Reports have described acute dystonic reactions such as oculogyric crisis (rotation of the eyeballs), torticollis (contraction of neck muscles), and catatonia-like states, as well as allergic and photoallergic reactions.

Drug–Drug Interactions Diphenhydramine potentiates the depressant effects of narcotics, nonnarcotic analgesics, benzodiazepines, tranquilizers, and alcohol on the central nervous system and intensifies the anticholinergic effect of MAOIs and other antimuscarinics.

Contraindications/Precautions/Warnings Diphenhydramine should be used with caution in patients with a history of narrow-angle glaucoma, stenosing peptic ulcer, pyloroduodenal obstruction, symptomatic prostatic hypertrophy, bladder-neck obstruction, asthma and other lower respiratory disease, elevated intraocular pressure, hyperthyroidism, cardiovascular disease, or hypertension. The elderly are more likely to experience dizziness, excessive sedation, syncope, confusion, and hypotension with diphenhydramine than will the general population. Children and the elderly may experience paradoxical excitation, restlessness, and irritability. Diphenhydramine is a Pregnancy Class B drug. It is excreted in breast milk and may cause unusual excitation and irritability in the infant; it may decrease the flow of milk.

Expectorants (Guaifenesin)

Guaifenesin (glyceryl guaiacolate) is the only FDA-approved nonprescription expectorant.[13–15] Terpin hydrate, potassium iodide (saturated solution), and iodinated glycerol have been used as expectorants in the past, but evidence of their efficacy is absent.[25] Diverse substances (e.g., chloroform, iodides, ipecac fluid extract, ammonium chloride, benzoin preparations, camphor, eucalyptus oil, horehound, peppermint oil, menthol, pine tar preparations, and sodium citrate) have been used as expectorants. Although present in many nonprescription products, these substances are considered inactive ingredients.

Mechanism of Action Guaifenesin loosens and thins lower respiratory tract secretions and makes minimally productive coughs more productive.

Pharmacokinetics The pharmacokinetics of guaifenesin is not known.

Indications Guaifenesin is indicated for the symptomatic relief of ineffective productive coughs; however, few data support its efficacy.

Dosage/Administration Guidelines Table 9–3 lists FDA-approved dosages of guaifenesin.[13–15]

Adverse Effects Guaifenesin is generally well tolerated, but its side effects may include nausea, vomiting, dizziness, headache, rash, diarrhea, drowsiness, and stomach pain.

Drug–Test Interactions There are no reported drug interactions with guaifenesin; however, this agent interferes with the urinary 5-hydroxyindoleacetic acid and vanillylmandelic acid lab tests.[26]

Contraindications/Precautions/Warnings Guaifenesin is contraindicated in persons with a known hypersensitivity to the drug.

Topical Antitussives

Volatile oils (e.g., camphor, menthol, and eucalyptus), which are common in many cough and cold preparations, impart a strong medicinal odor to medications and may have topical antitussive, analgesic, anesthetic, and antipruritic activity. Camphor and menthol are the only two topical antitussives approved by the FDA.[13,14]

Mechanism of Action Although the mechanism of action is not well described, inhaled vapors stimulate sensory nerve endings within the nose and mucosa, creating a local anesthetic sensation and a sense of improved airflow. However, little objective evidence exists of clinical efficacy.

Indications Both ointments and steam inhalant forms of topical antitussives have been approved for soothing cough.

Dosage/Administration Guidelines Topical antitussive ointments contain camphor (4.7% to 5.3%) or menthol (2.6% to 2.8%), steam inhalants contain 6.2% camphor or 3.2% menthol, and each lozenge contains 5 mg to 10 mg menthol. Many lozenges and compressed tablet formulations contain one or more of the volatile oils.[13,14] Table 9–4 provides administration guidelines for these agents. (See Table 9–2 for examples of commercially available products.)

Adverse Effects Ointments and solutions containing camphor or menthol are toxic if ingested. Toxicities include burning sensations in the mouth, nausea and vomiting, epigastric distress, restlessness, excitation, delirium, seizures, and death. Ingestion of as little as four teaspoonfuls of products containing 5% camphor may be lethal for children.[27] Products with better risk:benefit ratios are preferred, especially for children.

Alternative Remedies

The book *PDR® for Herbal Medications* lists more than 100 products for cough.[28] (See Chapter 45, "Herbal Remedies," for a more detailed discussion of these types of products.) Common herbal antitussives include slippery elm (*Ulmus*

Table 9–4

Administration Guidelines for Nonprescription Topical Antitussives (Adults and Children 2–<12 Years[a])

Drug	Administration
Camphor ointment, 4.7%–5.3%	Rub on the throat and chest as a thick layer. Application may be repeated up to 3 times/day or as directed by a physician.
Menthol ointment, 2.6%–2.8%	Rub on the throat and chest as a thick layer. Application may be repeated up to 3 times/day or as directed by a physician.
Menthol lozenges, 5–10 mg	Allow lozenge or tablet to dissolve slowly in the mouth. Repeat hourly or as needed or as directed by a physician.
Camphor for steam inhalation, 6.2%	Add 1 tablespoon of solution per quart of water directly to the water in a hot steam vaporizer, bowl, or washbasin; or add 1.5 teaspoons of solution per pint of water to an open container of boiling water. Breathe in the medicated vapors. Repeat up to 3 times/day or as directed by a physician.
Menthol for steam inhalation, 3.2%	Add 1 tablespoon of solution per quart of water directly to the water in a hot steam vaporizer, bowl, or washbasin; or add 1.5 teaspoons of solution per pint of water to an open container of boiling water. Breathe in the medicated vapors. Repeat up to 3 times/day or as directed by a physician.

[a] For children age 2 years or younger, consult a physician.

Source: References 13 and 14.

Case Study 9–1

Patient Complaint/History

Rita, a 32-year-old woman, presents to the pharmacist with a cough. She says that she was in her usual state of health until yesterday when she developed muscle aches, cough, and fever. The cough is a dry, "hacking" cough that interrupts her sleep. Her temperature last night was 99.6°F (37.6°C). She still feels hot but has not taken her temperature today. Both of her school-aged children (ages 9 and 7 years) had similar symptoms last week. The patient has seasonal allergies but no other known chronic diseases. She has no known drug allergies. Her only prescription medication is Claritin-D, which she takes daily in the spring. Her routine nonprescription medications include multivitamins with iron (one tablet daily for 5 years) and calcium carbonate (600 mg three times daily with meals for 5 years). Codeine-containing cough syrups have worked well for Rita in the past. She selects the following nonprescription medication: Contac Night Cold and Flu caplets.

Clinical Considerations/Strategies

Readers can use the following considerations/strategies to determine whether treatment of this patient's disorder with nonprescription medication is warranted:

- Characterize the patient's cough on the basis of symptoms and of medical and medication history.
- Evaluate the patient's choice of medication.
- Identify which, if any, of the active ingredients in the patient's medication will contribute to symptomatic relief. If necessary, propose a more appropriate formulation.

Patient Education/Counseling

Readers can use the following strategies to develop a patient education/counseling plan that will ensure optimal therapeutic outcomes:

- Optimize the patient's understanding of the source of her illness.
- If nondrug measures are appropriate, advise the patient on which ones to use.
- If a nonprescription medication is recommended, counsel the patient on its use, possible adverse effects, warnings, and cautions.
- If symptoms get worse or new ones arise, advise the patient to see a doctor.

fulva) and plantain (*Plantago lanceolata*). Each contains mucilage, which may soothe the alimentary canal. There is little evidence that these remedies are effective; however, there are no reported health hazards.

Numerous homeopathic remedies are available for a cough (e.g., *Bryonia, Rumex,* Arsenicum, Phosphorus, *Pulsatilla, Lachesis, Ipecacuanha,* Antimonium tartaricum, *Rhus toxicodendron*, and Kali carbonicum). (See Chapter 46,

"Homeopathic Remedies," for a discussion of these remedies.) There is little evidence from controlled clinical trials that these remedies are effective.

Patient Assessment of Cough

Before recommending any treatment, the pharmacist will need to know how long the patient has been coughing, whether the cough is productive, and whether it is associated with a chronic illness. It is also important to obtain a list of all the patient's current medications to identify possible drug–drug or drug–disease interactions. In addition, the pharmacist should find out how the patient has treated the current cough as well as previous coughs, and whether these treatments were satisfactory and/or effective. Asking the patient the following questions will help elicit the information needed to accurately assess the disorder and to recommend the appropriate treatment approach.

Q~ How long have you been coughing?

A~ *Identify the criteria for chronic cough. (See the section "Epidemiology/Etiology of Cough.")* Refer the patient to a physician if the cough is chronic or has persisted longer than 7 to 10 days despite self-treatment with nonprescription medications.

Q~ Are you coughing up mucus?

A~ If mucus is associated with the cough, ask the patient to describe its color, consistency, odor, and amount. Also ask if the mucus contains blood. *Identify the characteristics of mucus that indicate medical referral is necessary. (See the section "Signs and Symptoms of Cough.")* If self-treatment is appropriate, recommend medications specific to the type (productive, nonproductive) of cough.

Q~ Do you smoke?

A~ If the cough is related to smoking, refer the patient to a physician. Such coughs should not be self-treated with cough suppressants and/or expectorants.

Q~ Do you have other symptoms? Has a physician diagnosed you as having a cough-associated illness? Do you have a history of cough-associated illness?

A~ *Identify symptoms that indicate a cough-associated illness. (See Table 9–1.)* If the patient has a history or chronic symptoms of one of these illnesses, refer the patient to a physician.

Q~ What medications are you taking? Do you have a history of allergy or adverse reactions to prescription or nonprescription medications?

A~ *Identify medications that can induce cough. (See the section "Epidemiology/Etiology of Cough.")* If drug-induced cough is suspected, refer the patient to a physician. The physician will determine whether the cough is drug induced and, if needed, how medications should be adjusted.

Q~ How have you treated previous coughs?

A~ Consider the patient's satisfaction or dissatisfaction with specific products when recommending nonprescription medications.

Patient Counseling for Cough

The pharmacist should explain to the patient the appropriate drug and nondrug measures for treating the patient's type of cough. After recommending a product, the pharmacist should fully explain the dosage guidelines and the possible side effects, interactions, and precautions or warnings. The patient needs to know the symptoms that indicate self-treatment should be discontinued and medical care sought. If the patient has an underlying medical disorder, the pharmacist should explain which nonprescription medications are contraindicated and what symptoms indicate the need to see a physician. The box "Patient Education for Cough" lists specific information to provide patients.

Evaluation of Patient Outcomes for Cough

For most patients, the initial nonprescription drug therapy should relieve the symptoms in 7 to 10 days. If, at follow-up, the cough has improved, the pharmacist should advise the patient to continue the therapy until the cough is resolved. If the patient's symptoms have worsened or the patient has developed other exclusions to self-care, medical referral is necessary.

Common Cold

The common cold is a self-limited viral infection of the upper respiratory tract. These viral infections cause about half of all illnesses in adults and about three-quarters of all illnesses in young infants.[29,30] Although patients often self-medicate their colds with nonprescription drugs, the common cold cannot be prevented or cured. Antibiotics, which are often prescribed for colds, are ineffective against viral infections.

Epidemiology of the Common Cold

The highest incidence of the common cold occurs in preschool children, who typically have 5 to 7 colds per year but may have as many as 12 colds annually, especially if they attend daycare.[31] Adults typically have 2 to 3 colds per year but may have more if they live with or frequently encounter preschool or school-aged children.

Although colds occur throughout the year, the respiratory virus "season" starts in August to September and peaks in

Patient Education for Cough

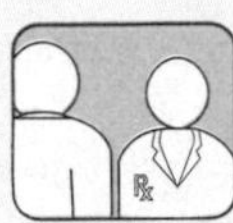

The primary objective of self-treatment is to reduce the number and severity of cough episodes, which, in turn, will help the patient feel better during the day and sleep better at night. The second objective is to prevent complications such as exhaustion, insomnia, muscle or bone pain, hoarseness, excessive perspiring, and loss of bladder control. For most patients, carefully following product instructions and the self-care measures listed below will help ensure optimal therapeutic outcomes.

Nondrug Measures

- Note that the following measures may provide relief for or speed up recovery from a cough:
  —Getting adequate rest may speed up recovery from the cough.
  —Increased humidification with cool-mist vaporizers may soothe irritated airways.
  —Slowly dissolving hard candies or other lozenges in the mouth, gargling with salt water, or drinking fruit juices may soothe an irritated throat.
- Note that staying well-hydrated by drinking plenty of fluids may thin respiratory secretions and make them easier to cough up. Drink more fluids unless your physician advises otherwise.

Nonprescription Medications

- Ask a pharmacist to help you select a nonprescription cough medication based on the type of cough:
  —Cough suppressants, such as codeine, dextromethorphan, and diphenhydramine, are usually recommended for nonproductive (dry) coughs. These medications inhibit coughing.
  —Cough suppressants are sometimes recommended for nighttime treatment of productive (wet) coughs.
  —An expectorant such as guaifenesin is recommended for productive coughs when the respiratory secretions are hard to cough up. These medications loosen mucus so that it is easier to cough up.
- If you have asthma, chronic obstructive pulmonary disease, or congestive heart failure, do not use nonprescription cough medications unless a physician recommends them.

Codeine

- Do not take codeine
  —If you are pregnant unless a physician recommends the medication.
  —During labor if a premature birth is anticipated.
  —If you are breast-feeding.
  —If you are allergic to codeine or a similar medication.
  —When you drink alcohol or take other medications that cause drowsiness, such as antihistamines or other narcotics.
- Even recommended doses of codeine may cause nausea, vomiting, drowsiness, dizziness, and constipation. While taking this medication, do not drive a vehicle, operate machinery, or engage in other activities requiring mental alertness.

Dextromethorphan

- Do not use dextromethorphan
  —If you are allergic to this medication.
  —If you have a history of dextromethorphan dependency.
  —If you are pregnant unless a physician recommends such use.
  —If you are breast-feeding.
- Separate doses of dextromethorphan and a monoamine oxidase inhibitor such as phenelzine or tranylcypromine by at least 14 days.
- Note that even recommended dosages of dextromethorphan can upset your stomach.

Diphenhydramine

- Do not use diphenhydramine
  —If you have any of the following medical conditions: history of narrow-angle glaucoma, stenosing peptic ulcer, pyloroduodenal obstruction, symptomatic prostatic hypertrophy, bladder-neck obstruction, asthma and other lower respiratory disease, elevated intraocular pressure, hyperthyroidism, cardiovascular disease, or hypertension. Check with a physician before using this medication.
  —If you are breast-feeding. It may decrease the flow of breast milk and may cause unusual excitation and irritability in your infant.
  —When you drink alcohol or take other medications that cause drowsiness, such as codeine, other narcotics, or tranquilizers.
- Even recommended doses of diphenhydramine cause drowsiness and impair mental alertness. While taking this medication, do not drive a vehicle, operate machinery, or engage in other activities that require alertness.
- Note that diphenhydramine is likely to cause dizziness, excessive sedation, fainting, confusion, and decreased blood pressure in the elderly.
- Note also that diphenhydramine may cause excitation, restlessness, and irritability in the elderly or children.

(continued)

Patient Education for Cough (continued)

Guaifenesin

- Do not take guaifenesin
  - —If you are allergic to this medication.
  - —If your cough is persistent or lasts longer than 3 weeks.
  - —If you are pregnant unless your physician recommends such use.
- Even recommended doses of guaifenesin cause drowsiness and impairs mental alertness. While taking this medication, do not drive a vehicle, operate machinery, or engage in other activities that require alertness.

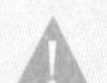

Seek medical attention in the following situations:

—The cough symptoms worsen, or you cough up blood, develop a fever higher than 101.5°F, or have chest pain or shortness of breath.

—The cough does not improve in 7 to 10 days.

—The cough persists longer than 3 weeks, even if it has responded to nonprescription medications.

April to May.[32] Smoking, poor nutrition, increased population density, and chronic (e.g., 1 month or more) psychologic stress increase susceptibility to the common cold.[32–35] Contrary to common belief, cold environments and sudden chilling do not increase susceptibility to viral upper respiratory infections.[36,37]

Etiology of the Common Cold

Viruses that infect ciliated epithelial mucosal cells in the upper respiratory tract cause the common cold. Rhinoviruses, which are the most common pathogens with more than 100 serotypes, cause 50% to 60% of all adult colds.[38,39] Other important pathogens of the common cold include respiratory syncytial virus (RSV), which is an important pathogen in children, and coronaviruses. Some pathogens (e.g., influenza viruses, parainfluenza viruses, adenoviruses, enterovirus, rubeola, rubella, and varicella) cause respiratory symptoms that are similar to those of the common cold. Double viral infection and bacterial co-infection (usually with group A β-hemolytic streptococci) occur but are rare.[38]

Viral contact with the nasal mucosa or conjunctiva initiates the infection. The most efficient mode of transmission is hand-to-hand contact with someone who has viral-laden nasal secretions on their hands. Patients then touch their noses or eyes with their hands and inoculate themselves. Less-efficient modes of transmission are by inhaling small- and large-particle viral aerosols and by handling viral-laden inanimate surfaces (e.g., doorknobs, telephones) followed by self-inoculation.[31] Viral transmission during brief (e.g., less than 72 hours) person-to-person contact is not common.[40]

Pathophysiology of the Common Cold

Infection begins when the virus attaches to a cell surface glycoprotein receptor on a nasopharyngeal epithelial cell. Binding initiates a series of biochemical and immunologic events that generate inflammatory mediators.[41] These substances induce various local reactions, including increased vascular permeability and glandular secretion, inflammatory cell infiltration, and neural pathway stimulation.[41] Histamine and other mast cell mediators have little, if any, role in the viral inflammatory response. Bradykinins cause nasal stuffiness, rhinorrhea, and sore throat.[42] Interleukins may be responsible for enhanced vascular permeability, inflammatory cell recruitment, and release of additional pro-inflammatory mediators. Nasal fluid hypersecretion, which is caused by inflammatory mediators and parasympathetic nervous system reflex mechanisms, is watery. Parasympathetic pathways are also involved in sneezing.[43]Viscid purulent glandular secretions that are not under the control of the parasympathetic nervous system are produced later in the cold.[44]

Signs and Symptoms of the Common Cold

The sequence of symptoms is the same regardless of the infecting virus; however, the timing, frequency, and severity vary with the virus.[45] Symptoms typically appear 1 to 3 days after infection. Sore throat is the first symptom to appear, followed by nasal symptoms (congestion, rhinorrhea), sneezing, and cough. Next come chills, headache, malaise, myalgia, or low-grade fever.[45] The sore throat resolves quickly. Nasal symptoms dominate by day two or three and cough dominates by day four or five. Cough is an infrequent symptom (e.g., less than 20%) except for infection with respiratory syncytial virus, which causes cough in more than 60% of those infected.[45] Symptoms persist for 1 to 2 weeks. Signs and symptoms of the common cold and influenza can be confused. (See Table 9–5 for common symptoms of respiratory tract illnesses other than the common cold.)

Complications of the Common Cold

Virus-induced, nasal inflammatory changes may spread to contiguous structures such as the sinuses, eustachian tubes, and lower respiratory tract. Complications include sinusitis,

Table 9–5

Symptoms Suggestive of Respiratory Illnesses Other Than the Common Cold

Illness	Signs and Symptoms
Otitis media	Ear popping, ear fullness, otalgia, otorrhea, hearing loss, dizziness
Bacterial throat infection	Sore throat, fever, and tender anterior cervical adenopathy
Sinusitis	Tenderness over the sinuses, facial pain aggravated by Valsalva's maneuver or postural changes, fever >101.5°F, tooth pain, upper respiratory tract symptoms for >7 days with poor response to decongestants
Pneumonia or bronchitis	Chest tightness, wheezing, dyspnea, productive cough, persistent fever
Allergic rhinitis	Watery eyes; itchy nose, eyes, or throat; congestion or clear rhinorrhea
Influenza	Myalgia, arthralgia, fever, sore throat, nonproductive cough
Asthma	Cough, dyspnea, wheezing

Source: Reference 47.

eustachian tube obstruction, middle ear effusions, bronchitis, bacterial pneumonia, other bacterial infections, exacerbations of asthma, and exacerbations of chronic obstructive pulmonary disease.

Treatment of the Common Cold

Treatment Outcomes

There is no known cure for the common cold. The goals of therapy are to reduce the symptoms and to help the patient feel and function better.

General Treatment Approach

The mainstays of therapy remain rest and an adequate fluid intake. Otherwise, treatment is symptom specific. Most cold symptoms are present sometime during the course of the cold; however, they appear, peak, and resolve at different times.[40] When self-treatment with nonprescription medications is the appropriate choice, the recommendation of particular medications will depend on the symptoms the patient exhibits and considers most bothersome.[46] (See the algorithm in Figure 9–2.) Single-entity products enable the patient to maximally treat a specific symptom. Combination products are convenient, but this convenience must be weighed against the risks from taking unnecessary drugs.

Pharyngitis is treated with anesthetic lozenges or sprays and with systemic analgesics.

Nasal congestion is treated with topical or oral adrenergic agonist decongestants.

Rhinorrhea is multifactorial and only partially treatable with available medications. Histamine is not involved in the pathogenesis of rhinorrhea. However, antihistamines with anticholinergic properties (sedating antihistamines) and the prescription anticholinergic drug ipratropium bromide both decrease rhinorrhea by about 30%.[44,47–49]

Sneezing is a common but minor symptom. Sedating antihistamines may reduce sneezing.

Cough secondary to postnasal drip usually is self-limiting and needs no treatment. Although nonspecific cough suppression with codeine or dextromethorphan is frequently recommended, neither drug has been proven effective in natural colds.[50,51] Similarly, guaifenesin has not been proven effective in natural colds.[52]

The exclusions to self-care of cough apply to self-care of the common cold. (See the section "General Treatment Approach" under "Treatment of Cough.") In addition, patients with multiple medical problems; chronic diseases (asthma, chronic obstructive pulmonary disease, congestive heart failure, diabetes mellitus); and chronic immunosuppression from either a disease state such as AIDS or chronic immunosuppressive drug therapy (e.g., corticosteroids or cyclosporin), along with the frail elderly, are at risk and should be excluded. Patients with hypertension, ischemic heart disease, coronary artery disease, hyperthyroidism, diabetes mellitus, increased intraocular pressure, or prostatic hypertrophy should use decongestants only with the advice of a physician.

Nonpharmacologic Therapy

Nondrug therapy includes increased fluid intake, adequate rest, a nutritious diet as tolerated, increased humidification with cool mist vaporizers or steamy showers, saline gargle, and nasal irrigation. Simple, inexpensive remedies such as tea with lemon and honey, chicken soup, and hot broths are soothing and increase fluid intake. Saline nasal sprays or drops soothe irritated mucosal membranes and loosen encrusted mucus.

Nondrug therapy for infants includes clearing the nasal passageways with a bulb syringe, positioning the infant in an upright position to enhance drainage, maintaining an adequate fluid intake, increasing the humidity of inspired air, and irrigating the nose with saline drops.

Pharmacologic Therapy

Decongestants are the mainstay of therapy for the common cold. When patients are feverish (cold is rarely associated with a fever above 100°F [37.8°C]), a nonprescription analgesic/antipyretic (aspirin, acetaminophen, ibuprofen, naproxen, or ketoprofen) is an effective treatment. Cough, when present, is usually nonproductive and may be treated with antitussives. (See the section "Antitussives" under "Treatment of Cough.") Sore throats are treated with lozenges, gargles, and anesthetics (e.g., benzocaine and dyclonine).

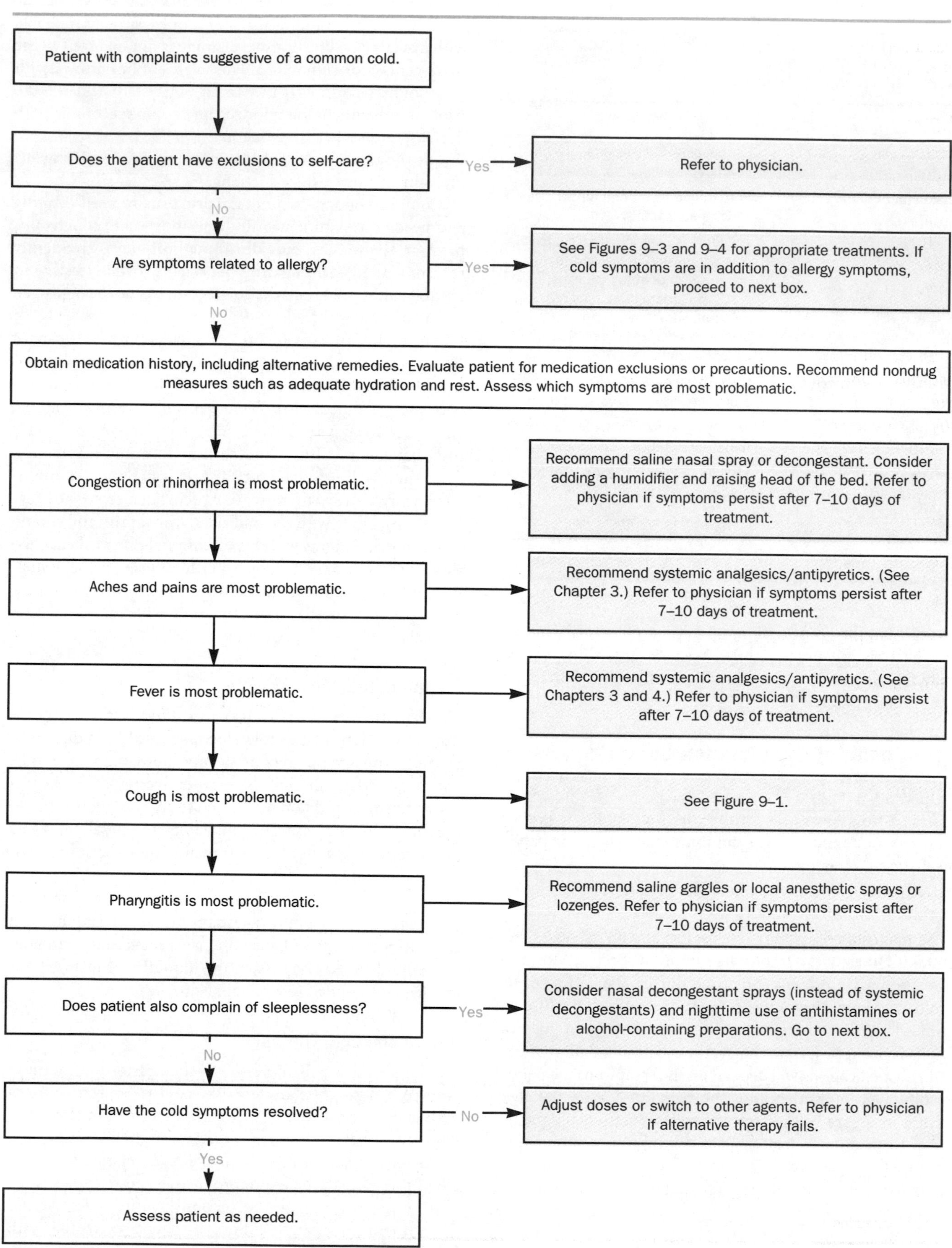

Figure 9–2 Self-care of the common cold. Adapted from reference 46.

Decongestants

Nasal decongestants specifically treat sinus and nasal stuffiness caused by colds, allergy, and hay fever.

Mechanism of Action Decongestants are α-adrenergic agonists (sympathomimetics). Stimulation of α-adrenergic receptors constricts blood vessels throughout the body, reduces the supply of blood to the nose, decreases the amount of blood in the sinusoid vessels, and decreases mucosal edema.[53]

If decongestants bind directly to α-adrenergic receptors, they are classified as direct acting; if they are taken up into prejunctional nerve terminals where they displace norepinephrine from storage vesicles, they are classified as indirect acting. Some drugs have mixed actions. Phenylephrine, oxymetazoline, and tetrahydrozoline are examples of direct-acting decongestants; ephedrine, pseudoephedrine, and phenylpropanolamine are among the indirect- or mixed-acting decongestants.[54] In general, indirect-acting sympathomimetics have the slowest onset and longest duration of action; however, tachyphylaxis (rapid resistance) develops as stored neurotransmitter is depleted.

Indications Decongestants are indicated for the temporary relief of nasal and eustachian tube congestion; phenylpropanolamine is also indicated as an oral anorexiant.

Dosage/Administration Guidelines Tables 9–6 and 9–7 list the FDA-approved dosages of decongestants.[55,56]

Decongestants are marketed in systemic and topical (intranasal and ophthalmic) dosage formulations. Nonprescription systemic decongestants include phenylpropanolamine and pseudoephedrine. Nonprescription ophthalmic decongestants include naphazoline, oxymetazoline, phenylephrine, and tetrahydrozoline. (See Chapter 22, "Ophthalmic Disorders," for a detailed discussion of these agents.) Nonprescription intranasal decongestants (sprays and drops) include short-acting (4–6 hours) decongestants (ephedrine, epinephrine, naphazoline, phenylephrine, and tetrahydrozoline); intermediate-acting (8–10 hours) decongestants (xylometazoline); and long-acting decongestants (oxymetazoline). Desoxyephedrine and propylhexedrine are available as nonprescription nasal inhalers.

The advantages and disadvantages of each dosage form must be weighed during product selection. Sprays are simple to use and are relatively inexpensive. They also have fast onset of action and cover a large surface area. Their disadvantages include the high risk of aspiration of nasal mucus into the bottle, a tendency for the bottle tip to become clogged, and imprecise dosage. Metered pump sprays, however, deliver a more precise dose.

Drops are preferred for small children, but they are awkward to use, cover a limited area of nasal mucosa, and pass easily into the larynx. There is also a high risk of the dropper contaminating medication in the bottle.

Inhalers are small and unobtrusive, which makes them easy to handle and carry. However, an unobstructed airway and sufficient airflow are needed to distribute the drug to nasal mucosa. Further, inhaler products lose efficacy after 2 to 3 months even when tightly capped.

Overdosage Overdoses of systemic decongestants may result in cardiovascular collapse, shock, and coma; there is no specific antidote.

Adverse Effects Because topical decongestants are minimally absorbed, systemic side effects are generally infrequent and mild. More common problems include propellant- or vehicle-associated local irritation and trauma from the dosage administration device. Local side effects also include burning, stinging, sneezing, and local dryness. Rhinitis medicamentosa (rebound congestion) occurs when topical decongestants are administered longer than 3 to 5 days. The classic rhinitis medicamentosa symptom is nasal congestion despite frequent use of the topical decongestant. Rebound congestion is more common with short-acting topical decongestants. Treatment consists of slowly withdrawing the topical decongestant (one nostril at a time); replacing the decongestant with topical normal saline, which soothes the irritated nasal mucosa; and, if needed, using topical corticosteroids and systemic decongestants.[57] The mucous membrane returns to normal 1 to 2 weeks after discontinuing the topical decongestant.

Systemic decongestants have short half-lives because of their rapid metabolism by monoamine oxidase and catechol-*o*-methyltransferase in the gastrointestinal mucosa, liver, and other tissues.

Table 9–6

Dosage Guidelines for Nonprescription Systemic Nasal Decongestants

	Dosage (Maximum Daily Dosage)		
Drug	**Adults ≥ 12 years**	**Children 6–<12 years**	**Children 2–<6 years**
Phenylpropanolamine	25 mg every 4 hours, or 50 mg every 8 hours (150 mg)	12.5 mg every 4 hours, or 25 mg every 8 hours (75 mg)	6.25 mg every 4 hours, or 12.5 mg every 8 hours (37.5 mg)
Pseudoephedrine	60 mg every 4–6 hours (240 mg)	30 mg every 4–6 hours (120 mg)	15 mg every 4–6 hours (60 mg)

Source: References 55 and 56.

Table 9–7

Dosage Guidelines for Topical Nasal Decongestants

Drug	Concentration	Adults ≥12 years	Children 6–<12 years	Children[a] 2–<6 years
L-Desoxyephedrine	NA	1–2 inhalations not more often than every 2 hours	—[b]	—[b]
Ephedrine	0.5%	2–3 drops/sprays not more often than every 4 hours	1–2 drops/sprays not more often than every 4 hours	—[c]
Naphazoline	0.05%	1–2 drops/sprays not more often than every 6 hours	—[d]	—[d]
	0.025%	1–2 drops/sprays not more often than every 6 hours	1–2 drops/sprays not more often than every 6 hours	—[e]
Oxymetazoline	0.05%	2–3 drops/sprays twice daily in am and pm	2–3 drops/sprays twice daily in am and pm	—[f]
	0.025%	2–3 drops/sprays twice daily in am and pm	2–3 drops/sprays twice daily in am and pm	2–3 drops twice daily in am and pm
Phenylephrine	1%	2–3 drops/sprays not more often than every 4 hours	—[g]	—[g]
	0.5%	2–3 drops/sprays not more often than every 4 hours	—[h]	—[h]
	0.25%	2–3 drops/sprays not more often than every 4 hours	2–3 drops/sprays not more often than every 4 hours	—[i]
	0.125%	2–3 drops/sprays not more often than every 4 hours	2–3 drops/sprays not more often than every 4 hours	2–3 drops not more often than every 4 hours
Propylhexedrine	NA	2 inhalations not more often than every 2 hours	2 inhalations not more often than every 2 hours	—[j]
Tetrahydrozoline	0.1%	2–4 drops not more often than every 3hours	2–4 drops not more often than every 3 hours	—[k]
	0.05%	2–4 drops not more often than every 3 hours	2–4 drops not more often than every 3 hours	2–3 drops not more often than every 3 hours
Xylometazoline	0.1%	2–3 drops/sprays not more often than every 8–10 hours	—[l]	—[l]
	0.05%	2–3 drops/sprays every 8–10 hours	2–3 drops/sprays every 8–10 hours	2–3 drops every 8–10 hours

NA = Not applicable.

[a] No recommended dosage exists for children under age 2 years except under the advice and supervision of a physician.

Except under the advice a physician, the following drugs or drug concentrations are not recommended for children under the specified ages:

[b] L-Desoxyephedrine: <6 years

[c] Ephedrine: <6 years

[d] Naphazoline 0.05%: <12 years

[e] Naphazoline 0.025%: <6 years

[f] Oxymetazoline 0.05%: <6 years

[g] Phenylephrine 1%: <12 years

[h] Phenylephrine 0.5%: <12 years

[i] Phenylephrine 0.25%: <6 years

[jj] Propylhexedrine: <6 years

[k] Tetrahydrozoline 0.1%: <6 years

[l] Xylometazoline 0.1%: <12 years

Source: References 55 and 56.

Adverse effects include cardiovascular stimulation (elevated blood pressure, tachycardia, palpitation, arrhythmias) and central nervous system stimulation (restlessness, insomnia, anxiety, tremors, fear, hallucinations). Children and the elderly are more likely to have adverse effects.

Drug-Drug Interactions Decongestants interact with numerous drugs. Monoamine oxidase inhibitors (MAOIs), including the antibiotic furazolidone and the anticancer drug procarbazine, interact with indirect or mixed decongestants to increase blood pressure. Blood pressure increases when methyldopa is combined with epinephrine, phenylephrine, ephedrine, phenylpropanolamine, and pseudoephedrine. Tricyclic antidepressants increase blood pressure when combined with direct-acting decongestants and decrease the sensitivity to indirect-acting decongestants. Urinary acidifiers (ammonium chloride, potassium phosphate, sodium acid phosphate) enhance the elimination of ephedrine and pseudoephedrine, whereas urinary alkalinizers (potassium acetate, sodium acetate, sodium bicarbonate, sodium citrate, sodium lactate, tromethamine) decrease the elimination of ephedrine and pseudoephedrine.

Contraindications/Precautions/Warnings Decongestants are contraindicated in patients who have a history of hypersensitivity or idiosyncratic reaction to a decongestant and in patients receiving concomitant MAOIs. Some decongestants are contraindicated in children of varying ages. (See the footnotes in Table 9–7.) Product labels and inserts also carry this information.

Decongestants may exacerbate diseases that are sensitive to adrenergic stimulation, such as hypertension, hyperthyroidism, diabetes mellitus, coronary heart disease, ischemic heart disease, elevated intraocular pressure, and prostatic hypertrophy. Patients with hypertension should use decongestants only with medical advice. No clear evidence exists that any one agent is safer in patients with hypertension. Decongestants (phenylephrine, phenylpropanolamine, and pseudoephedrine) may enter breast milk and, therefore, are contraindicated in nursing mothers.

Product Selection Guidelines The duration of treatment and the presence of concomitant disease will determine which product is selected. Patients with the common cold may require only short-term treatment, but patients with perennial allergic rhinitis (PAR) or seasonal allergic rhinitis (SAR) will require treatment for extended periods.

Although nasal sprays are simple and easy to use, they cannot be used longer than 3 to 5 days without risk of rebound congestion. Nasal polyps, enlarged turbinates, abnormalities such as septal deviation and blockage from head injury reduce, if not prevent, the efficacy of topical dosage forms. Topical drugs (e.g., intranasal, ophthalmic) work locally but have little effect on systemic symptoms.

Prolonged use of systemic decongestants is relatively safe. Short-acting products may be safer for patients with cardiovascular disease because an adverse reaction would be of short duration.

Product selection should be based on the patient's symptoms, concomitant illnesses, and preferences. Table 9–8 lists examples of products that treat nasal congestion.

Antihistamines

Nonprescription sedating antihistamines may decrease the rhinorrhea associated with the common cold by about 30%. These antihistamines may also reduce sneezing. (For a detailed discussion of these agents, see the section "Antihistamines" under "Treatment of Allergic Rhinitis.")

Systemic Analgesics

Systemic analgesics are effective for aches and fever that are sometimes associated with cold. (For discussions of these agents, see Chapter 3, "Headache and Muscle and Joint Pain," and Chapter 4, "Fever.")

Local Anesthetics and Antiseptics

Lozenges, troches, mouthwashes, and sprays containing local anesthetics (benzocaine, dyclonine hydrochloride) are available for the temporary relief of sore throats. Table 9–9 lists examples of these types of products. Local anesthetic products may be used every 3 to 4 hours. Some products contain local antiseptics (cetylpyridinium chloride, hexylresorcinol) and/or counterirritants (menthol, camphor). Local antiseptics are not effective for viral infections, and the clinical efficacy of counterirritants is not well documented.

Lozenges and troches should be slowly dissolved in the mouth without biting or chewing. Patients should not exceed the recommended dose or use the medication longer than recommended. Local anesthetics numb the mouth and tongue; patients should avoid eating or drinking as long as the numbness persists. Nondrug alternatives include hard candy, warm saline gargles, and fruit juices. Patients with sore throats that are severe or persist after several days should be referred to their physician. Sore throats associated with fever, headache, nausea, or vomiting also require medical attention.

Alternative Remedies

Numerous alternative remedies are marketed to treat the common cold. Echinacea, zinc, ephedra (ma huang), goldenseal (*Hydrastis canadensis*), and vitamin C are among the most popular alternative remedies. (For a detailed discussion of these types of remedies, see Chapter 45, "Herbal Remedies.")

Echinacea is purported to be a "natural antibiotic" that enhances the immune system.[58] Formulations include single-entity and combination hydroalcoholic extracts, capsules, teas, and soups. The efficacy of marketed products is unproven. Echinacea should not be used longer than a few weeks at a time. It also should not be taken by breast-feeding or pregnant women or given to children younger than 2 years.

Zinc purportedly blocks the adhesion of human rhinovirus to the nasal epithelium, thereby modestly decreasing the severity and duration of the infection.[59] Dosage formulations include tablets, capsules, chewing gums, and lozenges. The efficacy of zinc ion salts is unclear despite at least eight clinical trials involving U.S. adults.[60] Half of the clinical trials showed some efficacy, but numerous study design issues prevent definitive conclusions. Efficacy has not been demonstrated in children.[61] Clinical trials that showed some efficacy in adults used zinc gluconate lozenges containing at least 13.3 mg elemental zinc and followed a rigorous drug administration schedule. Therapy began within 24 to 48 hours of symptom onset, and the patient took zinc lozenges every 2

Table 9–8

Selected Products for Nasal Congestion

Trade Name	Primary Ingredients
Topical Decongestants	
Afrin 12-Hour Nasal Spray/Drops/Pump Spray	Oxymetazoline HCl 0.05%
Afrin Allergy Nasal Spray	Phenylephrine HCl 0.5%
Benzedrex Nasal Inhaler	Propylhexedrine 250 mg
Dristan Nasal Spray	Phenylephrine HCl 0.5%
Dristan 12-Hour Nasal Spray	Oxymetazoline HCl 0.05%
4-Way Fast-Acting or Menthol Nasal Spray	Phenylephrine HCl 0.5%; naphazoline HCl 0.05%
4-Way Long-Lasting 12-Hour Relief Nasal Spray	Oxymetazoline HCl 0.05%
Little Noses Decongestant Nasal Drops[a]	Phenylephrine HCl 0.125%
Neo-Synephrine 12-Hour Nasal Spray	Oxymetazoline HCl 0.05%
Neo-Synephrine Nasal Drops/Spray	Phenylephrine HCl 0.25%; 0.05% or 1%
Otrivin Nasal Drops/Spray[b]	Xylometazoline HCl 0.1%
Otrivin Pediatric Nasal Drops[a, b]	Xylometazoline HCl 0.05%
Privine Nasal Drops/Spray[b]	Naphazoline HCl 0.05%
Vicks Sinex Nasal Spray[b]	Phenylephrine HCl 0.5%
Vicks Sinex 12-Hour Nasal Spray[b]	Oxymetazoline HCl 0.05%
Vicks Vapor Inhaler[b]	Levodesoxyephedrine 50 mg/inhaler
Oral Decongestants	
Dimetapp Decongestant Non-Drowsy Liqui-Gels	Pseudoephedrine HCl 30 mg
Dimetapp Pediatric Decongestant Drops	Pseudoephedrine HCl 7.5 mg/0.8 mL
Drixoral Nasal Decongestant Non-Drowsy Formula Timed-Release Tablets	Pseudoephedrine sulfate 12 mg
PediaCare Infants' Decongestant Drops[a,c]	Pseudoephedrine HCl 7.5 mg/0.8 mL
Sudafed Tablets[a]	Pseudoephedrine HCl 30 or 60 mg
Sudafed 12-Hour Extended Release Caplets[d]	Pseudoephedrine HCl 120 mg
Sudafed 24-Hour Timed-Release Tablets	Pseudoephedrine HCl 240 mg (controlled release: 180 mg; immediate release: 60 mg)
Sudafed Children's Nasal Decongestant Liquid[a,c,e]	Pseudoephedrine HCl 15 mg/5 mL
Sudafed Children's Nasal Decongestant Chewable Tablets[a,e]	Pseudoephedrine HCl 15 mg
Sudafed Pediatric Nasal Decongestant Drops[a,c,e,f]	Pseudoephedrine HCl 7.5 mg/0.8 mL
Triaminic Infant Oral Decongestant Drops[a,b,c,f]	Pseudoephedrine HCl 7.5 mg/0.8 mL

[a] Pediatric formulation.
[b] Sulfite-free product.
[c] Alcohol-free product.
[d] Sodium-free product.
[e] Sucrose-free product.
[f] Dye-free product.

waking hours for the duration of the cold.[60,62] Gastrointestinal side effects (e.g., nausea, upset, bitter taste) are common. The lozenge should be allowed to dissolve slowly in the mouth. Because citrus-containing juices chelate zinc, they should be avoided for 1 hour after ingestion of the lozenge.

Ephedra (ma huang), which is an herbal product containing ephedrine and other sympathomimetic derivatives such as norpseudoephedrine (also called cathine, a major alkaloid of khat), is widely marketed for treating the common cold. Ephedrine has a lower potency, a longer duration of action, and a more-pronounced central stimulatory action than that of epinephrine; tachyphylaxis and dependence can develop. Heart palpitations, heart attacks, psychosis, and strokes have been reported in patients taking ephedra. The amount of ac-

Table 9–9

Selected Products for Sore Throat

Trade Name	Primary Ingredients[a]
Cepacol Sore Throat Maximum Strength Lozenges[b]	Benzocaine 10 mg; menthol 2–3.6 mg (concentration varies with product flavor); cetylpyridinium chloride
Cepacol Maximum Strength Sore Throat Pump Spray[c]	Dyclonine HCl 0.1%; cetylpyridinium chloride
Cepastat Extra Strength Sore Throat Lozenges[c]	Phenol 29 mg; eucalyptus oil; menthol
Cepastat Sore Throat Lozenges[c]	Phenol 14.5 mg; menthol
Halls Juniors Sugar-Free Cough Drops[c]	Menthol 2.5 mg
Halls Mentho-Lyptus Cough Suppressant Drops	Menthol 6–12 mg (concentration varies with product flavor)
Halls Mentho-Lyptus Sugar-Free Cough Suppressant Drops[c]	Menthol 5–6 mg (concentration varies with product flavor)
Luden's Lozenges	Menthol 2 mg
Luden's Maximum Strength Lozenges	Menthol 10 mg
N'Ice Sore Throat & Cough Lozenges[c]	Menthol 5 mg
Ricola Sugar-Free Herb Throat Drops[b,c]	Menthol 1.1–4.8 mg (concentration varies with product flavor)
Ricola Echinacea Throat Lozenges[b]	Menthol 2.7–4.5 mg (concentration varies with product flavor)
Robitussin Cough Drops/Liquid Center Cough Drops	Menthol 7.4–10 mg (concentration varies with product flavor); eucalyptus oil
Sucrets Children's Sore Throat Lozenges	Dyclonine HCl 1.2 mg
Sucrets Maximum Strength Sore Throat Lozenges	Dyclonine HCl 3 mg
Sucrets Original Mint Sore Throat Lozenges	Hexylresorcinol 2.4 mg
Tylenol Sore Throat Liquids	Acetaminophen 1000 mg
Vicks Chloraseptic Sore Throat Spray[c]	Phenol 1.4%
Vicks Chloraseptic Sore Throat Lozenges[b]	Menthol 10 mg; benzocaine 6 mg
Vicks Cough Drops[b]	Menthol 1.7–3.3 mg (concentration varies with product flavor)

[a] Primary ingredients include local anesthetics and antibacterials. Menthol is also considered a local antitussive.

[b] Sodium-free product.

[c] Sucrose-free product.

tive chemical varies unpredictably in the natural products. The efficacy of marketed products is unknown. Ephedra is contraindicated in the same conditions as other sympathomimetic amines.

Goldenseal is an alkaloid-containing herbal product (e.g., hydrastine and berberine). The alkaloids may have modest astringent and antiseptic properties. Formulations include tablets, capsules, tinctures, and powdered teas. Goldenseal is used to treat the sore throat associated with the common cold. The efficacy of marketed products is unknown. Goldenseal should not be used longer than 3 weeks at a time, nor should it be taken by children younger than 2 years or by pregnant or breast-feeding women.

Vitamin C supplementation does not reduce the number of cold episodes in the general population.[63,64] Large doses (e.g., 1 g per day or more) of vitamin C started early in the course of the common cold may decrease the duration of illness slightly (less than 1 day) and may reduce the severity of illness by about 22%.[65] The clinical significance and risk:benefit ratio of these effects are debatable. Patients who have known vitamin C deficiency or who experience extreme physiologic stress (e.g., military troops in harsh environmental conditions) may benefit from high-dose vitamin C supplementation.[66] Doses of 4 g per day or greater are associated with diarrhea and other gastrointestinal symptoms in otherwise healthy individuals.[67]

Patient Assessment of the Common Cold

The pharmacist should ask the patient what symptoms are most troublesome. If questions about the patient's medical history or medication use do not reveal exclusions to self-treatment, the pharmacist should recommend medications that target the specific symptoms. The patient should also be asked about self-treatments of the current and previous colds and about the effectiveness of the treatments. Asking the patient the following questions will help elicit the information needed to accurately assess the disorder and to recommend the appropriate treatment approach.

Q~ What symptom or combination of symptoms is the most distressing?

A~ *Identify the signs and symptoms of the common cold and the course of their development. (See the section "Signs and Symptoms of the Common Cold.") Identify also signs and symptoms that suggest a respiratory illness other than the common cold. (See Table 9–5.)* If the patient's medical history suggests a respiratory illness other than the common cold or a complication from a common cold, refer the patient to a physician. If the symptoms indicate a cold, recommend medications that target the patient's symptoms but do not contain unnecessary drugs and their inherent unnecessary risks.

Q~ Do you have a history of allergy or adverse reactions to any nonprescription or prescription medication?

A~ If applicable, use the patient's allergy and adverse drug reaction histories to recommend an appropriate medication while minimizing the risk of medication allergies or adverse drug reactions.

Q~ Do you have other medical problems?

A~ *Identify underlying illnesses that may exclude self-care of the common cold. (See the section "General Treatment Approach" under "Treatment of the Common Cold.")* Refer patients with any of these illnesses to a physician for evaluation and treatment of the cold.

Q~ What nonprescription and prescription medications are you taking? Have you had any adverse reactions to nonprescription and prescription medications?

A~ *Identify possible drug–drug interactions and adverse effects for nonprescription antihistamines and decongestants. (See the section "Decongestants" under "Treatment of the Common Cold" and the section "Antihistamines" under "Treatment of Allergic Rhinitis.")* Refer to a physician those patients whose current or past medication use indicates potential problems.

Q~ How have you treated previous colds?

A~ Consider the patient's satisfaction or dissatisfaction with specific products when recommending specific products.

Patient Counseling for the Common Cold

Nondrug measures are often very effective in relieving the discomfort of cold symptoms. The pharmacist should explain the appropriate measures for the patient's particular symptoms. For patients who prefer self-medication, the pharmacist should explain the purpose of each medication and counsel the patient to take the appropriate medication as symptoms appear. Patients need an explanation of the medications' possible side effects, interactions, and precautions/warnings. Finally, the pharmacist should describe the signs and symptoms that indicate the disorder is worsening and that medical care should be sought. The box "Patient Education for the Common Cold" lists specific information to provide patients.

Evaluation of Patient Outcomes for the Common Cold

For most patients, initial therapy using nonprescription drugs relieves symptoms of the common cold in 7 to 10 days. After this time frame, the pharmacist should follow up, with either a telephone call or a scheduled appointment, the outcome of the recommended therapy. If symptoms are not resolved, the pharmacist should adjust current medications to maximum effective dosages, recommend a different medication, or refer the patient to a physician. If the patient exhibits any of the warning signs or symptoms listed in the box "Patient Education for the Common Cold," medical referral is necessary.

Allergic Rhinitis

Allergic rhinitis, a systemic disease with prominent nasal symptoms, affects 20% to 25% of the U.S. population.[68,69] Annual direct costs (e.g., medications, office visits) and indirect costs (e.g., lost school and work days) are approximately \$2 billion[67] and \$4 billion, respectively.[70] Impaired quality of life creates additional significant, but yet-to-be quantified, intangible costs.[71–73]

Epidemiology of Allergic Rhinitis

Allergic rhinitis is classified as seasonal (seasonal allergic rhinitis or SAR) or perennial (perennial allergic rhinitis or PAR) depending on the timing and duration of symptoms. Symptoms of both types of allergic rhinitis generally begin during childhood. Repetitive and predictable seasonal symptoms characterize SAR, whereas symptoms that persist throughout the year without any obvious seasonal pattern characterize PAR. Symptoms of PAR overlap those of many nonallergic rhinitis disorders (e.g., vasomotor rhinitis, nonallergic rhinitis with eosinophilia syndrome); successful therapy requires careful diagnostic evaluation. Many patients experience relatively severe seasonal symptoms superimposed on more moderate perennial symptoms.

Etiology of Allergic Rhinitis

Allergic rhinitis is triggered by aeroallergens (airborne environmental allergens). Common outdoor aeroallergens include pollen and mold spores, though less-common, insect-pollinated plant triggers have been documented.[74] Common indoor aeroallergens include house dust mites, cockroaches, mold spores, cigarette smoke, and pet danders. Occupational aeroallergens include wool dust, latex, resins, biological enzymes, organic dusts (e.g., flour), and various chemicals (e.g., isocyanate, glutaraldehyde).

Patient Education for the Common Cold

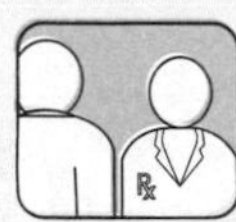

The objectives of self-treatment are to (1) reduce the patient's symptoms, (2) improve the patient's sense of well-being and function, and (3) prevent the spread of the disease. For most patients, carefully following product instructions and the self-care measures listed below will help ensure optimal therapeutic outcomes.

Nondrug Measures

- To prevent spreading a cold to others, wash your hands before touching other people or the objects they have touched.
- Note that the following measures may provide relief for or speed up recovery from a cold:
  —Getting adequate rest may help you recover more quickly.
  —Drinking more fluids may loosen mucus and promote sinus drainage.
  —Sucking on hard candy, gargling with salt water, or drinking fruit juices may soothe a sore throat.

Nonprescription Medications

- Ask a pharmacist to help select medications that target the most bothersome symptoms.

Sore Throat and Cough

- Sore throat may be treated with anesthetic lozenges or sprays and/or systemic analgesics:
  —Allow lozenges or troches to dissolve slowly in the mouth; do not chew or bite the lozenge or troche.
  —Benzocaine and dyclonine may numb the mouth and tongue. If these effects occur, do not eat or drink until they go away.
- Note that cough related to a runny nose (postnasal drip) is treated with decongestants.

Rhinorrhea (Runny Nose) and Sneezing

- See the box "Patient Education for Allergic Rhinitis" for treatment of rhinorrhea (runny nose) and sneezing.

Nasal Congestion

- Nasal congestion may be treated with topical or systemic decongestants:
  —Do not touch the tips of spray or dropper bottles with the hands. Do not rinse droppers.
  —Do not use topical nasal decongestants longer than 3 to 5 days.
- Note the following side effects for decongestants:
  —The most common side effects caused by systemic decongestants include cardiovascular stimulation (elevated blood pressure, rapid heart rate, palpitations, arrhythmias) and central nervous system stimulation (restlessness, tremor, insomnia, anxiety, tremors, fear, hallucinations).
  —Topical decongestants may cause any of the side effects listed for systemic decongestants; however, less of the topical medication gets into the body so side effects are less common. Topical decongestants may irritate the nose or the bottle tip can injure the nose if used forcefully.
- Note the following precautions for use of decongestants in persons with other medical conditions:
  —Persons with hypertension should use decongestants only with medical advice.
  —Persons with hyperthyroidism, coronary heart disease, ischemic heart disease, intraocular pressure, or prostatic hypertrophy may experience worsening symptoms of their underlying disease if they take decongestants.
  —Persons with diabetes mellitus may need to adjust their dose of insulin if they take decongestants. Blood sugar levels need to be monitored closely.
- Note the following drug interactions for decongestants:
  —Persons taking monoamine oxidase inhibitors, including the antibiotic furazolidone and the anticancer drug procarbazine, should not take indirect acting or mixed decongestants.
  —Persons taking rauwolfia alkaloids, methyldopa, and tricyclic antidepressants should use direct and indirect acting decongestants with caution. These medications interact with decongestants to increase blood pressure, sometimes to the point of causing strokes. Tricyclic antidepressants may increase or decrease blood pressure, depending on the specific decongestant.
  —Medications that decrease the pH of urine increase the elimination of ephedrine and pseudoephedrine.
  —Medications that increase the pH of urine decrease the elimination of ephedrine and pseudoephedrine.

Seek medical attention for the following situations:
—A sore throat persists after several days, is severe, or is associated with persistent fever, headache, or nausea or vomiting.
—A cough does not improve after 7 to 10 days.
—Your symptoms worsen while taking nonprescription medications.
—You develop signs and symptoms of bacterial infections (thick, opaque nasal or respiratory secretions, fever higher than 101.5°F, shortness of breath, chest congestion, wheezing, rash, or significant ear pain).

Pathophysiology of Allergic Rhinitis

The pathogenesis of allergic rhinitis is complex, involving histamine and numerous other preformed (heparin, tryptan, kininogenase, tumor necrosis factor-2, interleukins) and newly formed (prostaglandins, leukotrienes) cell-derived inflammatory mediators.[75] Mast cell-derived mediators predominate, but granulocytes also generate inflammatory mediators. Histamine, released from mast cells, is one of the most important mediators. Histamine causes itching, pain, paroxysmal sneezing, vasodilation, and plasma exudation.

The four phases of response to an allergen include the sensitization phase, the early-phase, the cellular recruitment phase, and the late-phase.[75,76] Initial allergen exposure stimulates β-cell–mediated immunoglobulin E (IgE) production (sensitization phase). Subsequent allergen exposure results in a rapid release of preformed mast cell mediators and triggers the production of additional mediators (early-phase response), causing itching, sneezing, and discomfort within minutes of allergen exposure. Inflammatory granulocytes and mast cells infiltrate the mucosa during the cellular recruitment phase. The late-phase response, a perpetual inflammatory response, begins several hours after allergen exposure. Late-phase response symptoms include mucus hypersecretion secondary to submucosal gland hypertrophy and congestion. Continued persistent inflammation "primes" the tissue resulting in a lower threshold for allergic- and nonallergic-mediated (e.g., cold air, cigarette smoke, strong odors) triggers.

Signs and Symptoms of Allergic Rhinitis

Symptoms of allergic rhinitis include itching of the eyes, nose, and palate; bursts of repetitive sneezing; profuse watery rhinorrhea; postnasal drip; nasal congestion; and red, irritated eyes with conjunctival injection (prominent conjunctival blood vessels). Systemic symptoms include fatigue, irritability, malaise, and mood and cognitive impairment. Patients may have signs or symptoms of concomitant allergic disorders such as eczema or asthma.

On physical examination, the nasal mucosa is engorged and varies in color from pale pink to blue-gray. The posterior pharynx may have a cobblestone appearance. The patient may have "allergic shiners" (dark circles under the eyes secondary to venous congestion); the "allergic crease" (a horizontal crease just above the bulbar portion of the nose secondary to the "allergic salute"—rubbing of the tip of the nose upward with the palm of the hand); the "allergic gape" (open-mouth breathing secondary to the nasal obstruction); and "Dennie's lines" (wrinkles beneath the lower eyelids).[77]

Complications of Allergic Rhinitis

Complications of allergic rhinitis in adults and children include sinusitis, otitis media, nasal polyps, sleep apnea, hyposmia (diminished sense of smell), and asthma.[78] Children may have delayed speech development and facial and dental abnormalities.[78]

Treatment of Allergic Rhinitis

Nonprescription allergy medications relieve and control symptoms of both SAR and PAR. Treatment of PAR is, by necessity, long term, whereas patients with SAR may need medications only during peak pollen or mold seasons.

Treatment Outcomes

Allergic rhinitis cannot be cured. The goals of therapy are to reduce symptoms and improve the patient's functional status and sense of well-being. Treatment is individualized to provide optimal symptomatic relief and control of symptoms.

General Treatment Approach

Allergic rhinitis is treated in three steps: allergen avoidance, pharmacotherapy, and allergen immunotherapy. Each step is maximized before going on to the next intervention. Patient education is an important part of all three steps. The algorithms in Figures 9–3 and 9–4 outline the self-treatment of SAR and PAR, respectively.

Patients with a history of nonallergic rhinitis should be discouraged from self-medicating. (See the section "Patient Assessment of Allergic Rhinitis" for indicators of this disorder.) Other exclusions to self-treatment include patients with symptoms of otitis media or sinusitis, or those with symptoms suggestive of a lower respiratory tract problem such as pneumonia, bronchitis, or asthma. (See Table 9–5 for symptoms of these disorders.)

Nonpharmacologic Therapy

Allergen avoidance is the primary nonpharmacologic measure for allergic rhinitis. The mechanism of avoidance depends on the specific allergen. House dust mites (*Dermatophagoides* spp.) are found in all but the driest regions of the United States and thrive in warm (65°F to 70°F), humid (more than 50%) household environments. The main allergen is a fecal glycoprotein, but other mite proteins and proteases are also allergenic.[79] Avoidance measures try to reduce the mite population (e.g., lower household humidity to less than 40%, apply acaricides) and reduce environmental dust, especially in the patient's bedroom (e.g., by removing carpets, upholstered furniture, stuffed animals, bookshelves, etc.). Encasing the mattress, box springs, and pillows with mite-impermeable materials reduces the mite population in bedding. Bedding that cannot be encased is washed at least weekly in hot (130°F) water.

Outdoor mold spores are prevalent in late summer and fall, especially on calm, clear, dry days. *Alternaria* and *Cladosporium* are the most common outdoor mold allergens; *Penicillium* and *Aspergillus* are the most common indoor molds. Avoiding activities that disturb decaying plant material (e.g., raking leaves) will lessen exposure to outdoor mold. Indoor mold exposure is minimized by lowering household humidity, removing houseplants, venting food preparation areas and bathrooms, repairing damp basements, and frequently applying fungicide to obviously moldy areas.

Cat-derived allergens (proteins secreted through sebaceous glands in the skin) are small and light, and they stay airborne for several hours. Cat allergens can be found in the house months after the cat is gone. Ideally, cats should be completely removed from the indoor environment. However, bathing the cat weekly may reduce the allergen load if the patient chooses to keep the pet and live with allergy symptoms.

Cockroaches are major urban allergens. Pesticides reduce the allergen load, but infestations in multiple family dwellings are difficult to eliminate.

Trees typically pollinate in March and April, grasses in May and June, and ragweed in mid-August to the first frost in the fall. Avoiding outdoor activities when pollen counts are high plus closing house and car windows will keep pollen exposure to a minimum. Pollen counts (the number of pollen grains per cubic meter per 24 hours) help patients plan outdoor activities. Low pollen counts (1 to 15 grains/m^3 per 24 hours depending on the specific pollen) are associated with symptoms in very sensitive patients. Most patients are symptomatic when pollen counts are very high (more than 200 to 1500 grains/m^3 per 24 hours, depending on the specific pollen). Pollen counts are the highest early in the morning and in the evening and are the lowest after rainstorms clear the air.

High efficiency particulate air (HEPA) filters remove pollen, mold spores, and cat allergens from household air, but they do not remove fecal particles from house dust mites, which settle to the floor too quickly to be removed. Vacuum cleaners with HEPA filters may reduce airborne allergens. HEPA filtration systems are expensive and not effective for all patients. Patients should be encouraged to rent a HEPA filtration device before investing in freestanding or permanently installed systems.

Pharmacologic Therapy

Pharmacotherapy is symptom specific[80,81] and depends on the severity of the illness. Medications should be used regularly rather than episodically. There is no single ideal medication; combination drug regimens are common. Patients with SAR should start pharmacotherapy at least 1 week before symptoms usually appear.[82,83] Patients with PAR should begin taking medication before known exposures, when possible.

Therapy is initiated by targeting a single drug at the dominant symptom.[80,84] Drugs with different mechanisms of action or different delivery systems are added if the single drug therapy does not provide adequate relief or if the symptoms are already moderately severe, particularly intense, or long lasting. Patients who respond poorly to treatment should be assessed to determine whether they are complying with avoidance strategies and medication regimens; the diagnosis may need to be reconsidered.

Regimens combining antihistamines and decongestants are effective for most symptoms. Antihistamines are effective for itching, sneezing, and rhinorrhea, while decongestants work well for nasal congestion. Topically applied medications act locally but have little, if any, effect elsewhere. Intranasal cromolyn may help if intranasal and systemic antihistamines fail. Prescription intranasal corticosteroids may help if intranasal cromolyn fails. A physician might order a short course of systemic corticosteroids (e.g., prednisone 20 mg daily for 5 days) to control severe symptoms while another drug therapy is being initiated. If all else fails, allergy immunotherapy is indicated.

The role of the sedating (first-generation) antihistamines is controversial. Sedating antihistamines are effective, readily available without a prescription, and relatively inexpensive. However, all sedating antihistamines impair performance and should be used with caution. Some health care professionals advocate using only nonsedating antihistamines.

Nasal wetting agents (e.g., saline, propylene, and polyethylene glycol sprays) may relieve nasal mucosal irritation and dryness, thus decreasing nasal stuffiness, rhinorrhea, and sneezing. These agents also aid in the removal of dried, encrusted, or thick mucus from the nose. Nasal wetting agents have no significant side effects. (For examples of these agents, see Table 9–10.)

Several treatment choices are available for pregnant women. Intranasal cromolyn is the initial drug of choice.[85] An intranasal corticosteroid may be used if cromolyn is ineffective. An approved antihistamine (chlorpheniramine) or decongestant (pseudoephedrine) may be used for intermittent symptoms.

Several treatment choices are available for children.[86] Mast cell stabilizers and intranasal corticosteroids are safe and effective, but they may be difficult for children to administer by themselves. Nonsedating antihistamines are generally the preferred initial treatment. Systemic corticosteroids and topical decongestants should be avoided, if possible.

Immunotherapy consists of a series of subcutaneous injections with patient-specific allergens. Injections are given weekly, with the concentrations of allergen gradually increasing. The maintenance dose is generally reached within 4 to 8 months. Maintenance injections are repeated every 3 to 4 weeks for 3 to 5 years.

Immunotherapy is indicated for patients who fail to respond to maximal pharmacotherapy or who cannot tolerate or comply with pharmacotherapy. Immunotherapy is most effective for pollen-related allergens. The exact mechanism of action is not known but may involve changes in serum antibodies and the T-lymphocyte response.[87] Relative contraindications to immunotherapy include autoimmune disease, unstable coronary artery disease, unstable asthma, and concurrent drug therapy for β-adrenergic blocking.[88]

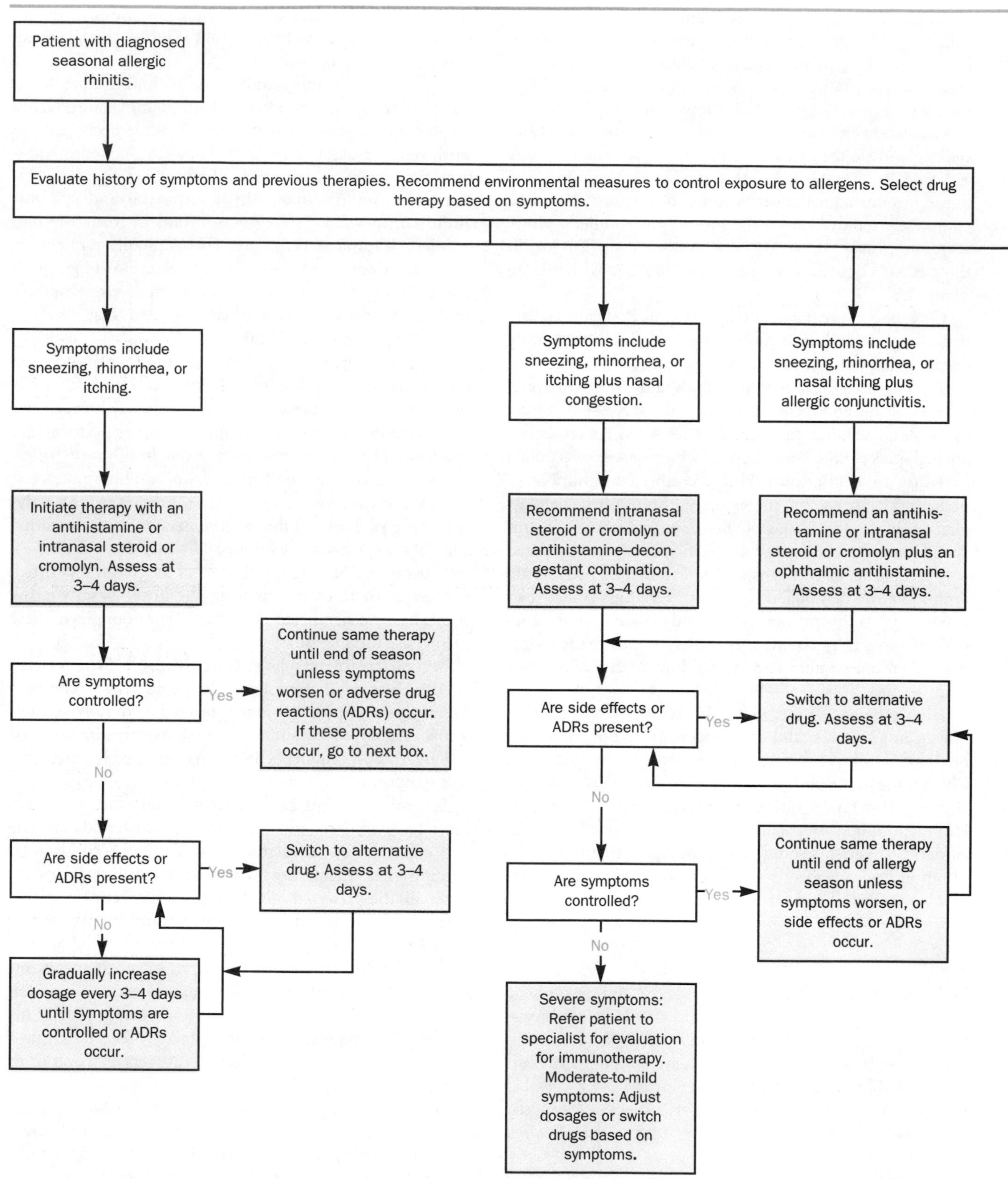

Figure 9–3 Self-care of seasonal allergic rhinitis. Adapted from reference 84.

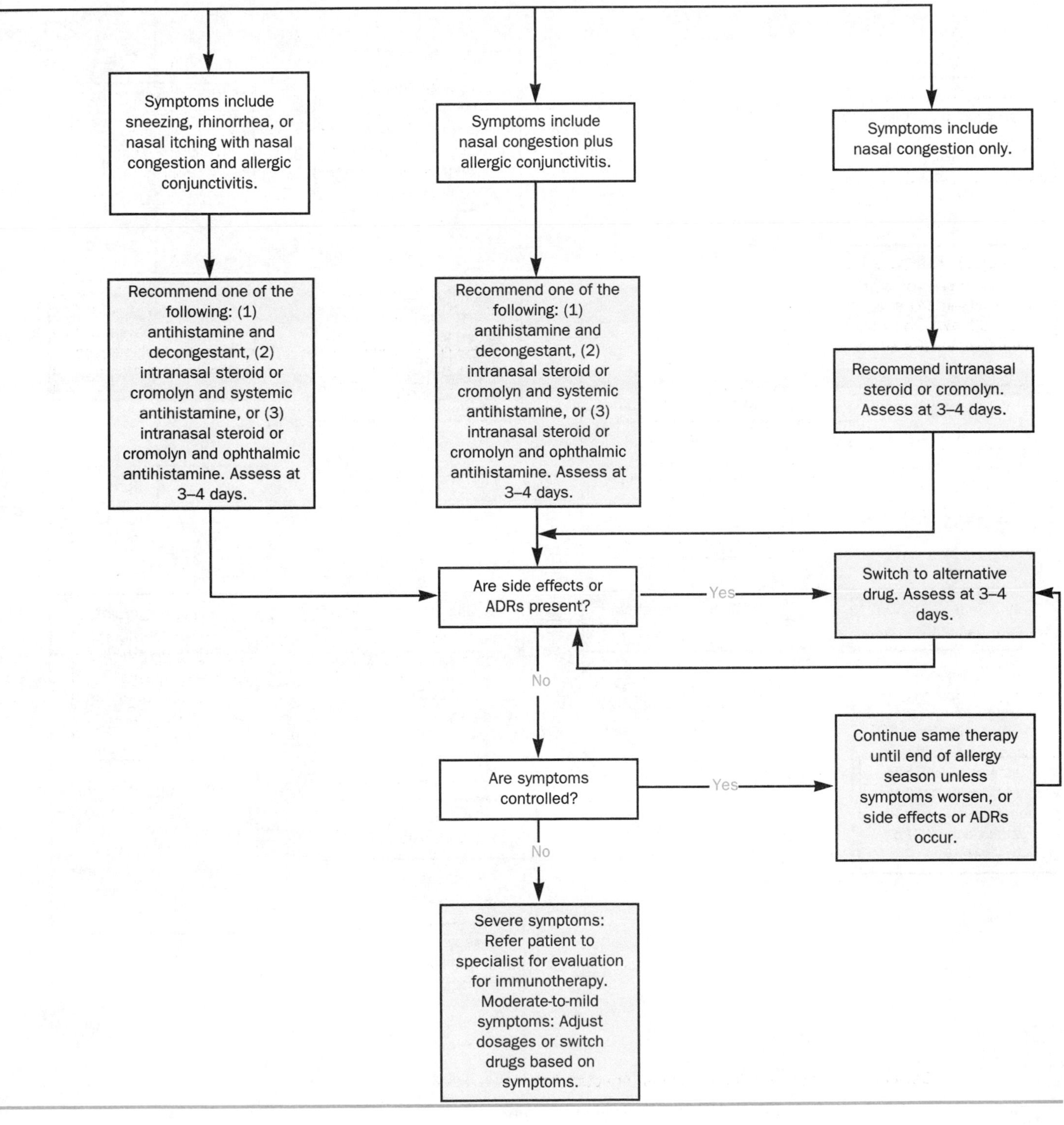
Symptoms include sneezing, rhinorrhea, or nasal itching with nasal congestion and allergic conjunctivitis.
Symptoms include nasal congestion plus allergic conjunctivitis.
Symptoms include nasal congestion only.
Recommend one of the following: (1) antihistamine and decongestant, (2) intranasal steroid or cromolyn and systemic antihistamine, or (3) intranasal steroid or cromolyn and ophthalmic antihistamine. Assess at 3–4 days.
Recommend one of the following: (1) antihistamine and decongestant, (2) intranasal steroid or cromolyn and systemic antihistamine, or (3) intranasal steroid or cromolyn and ophthalmic antihistamine. Assess at 3–4 days.
Recommend intranasal steroid or cromolyn. Assess at 3–4 days.
Are side effects or ADRs present?
Yes
Switch to alternative drug. Assess at 3–4 days.
No
Are symptoms controlled?
Yes
Continue same therapy until end of allergy season unless symptoms worsen, or side effects or ADRs occur.
No
Severe symptoms: Refer patient to specialist for evaluation for immunotherapy. Moderate-to-mild symptoms: Adjust dosages or switch drugs based on symptoms.

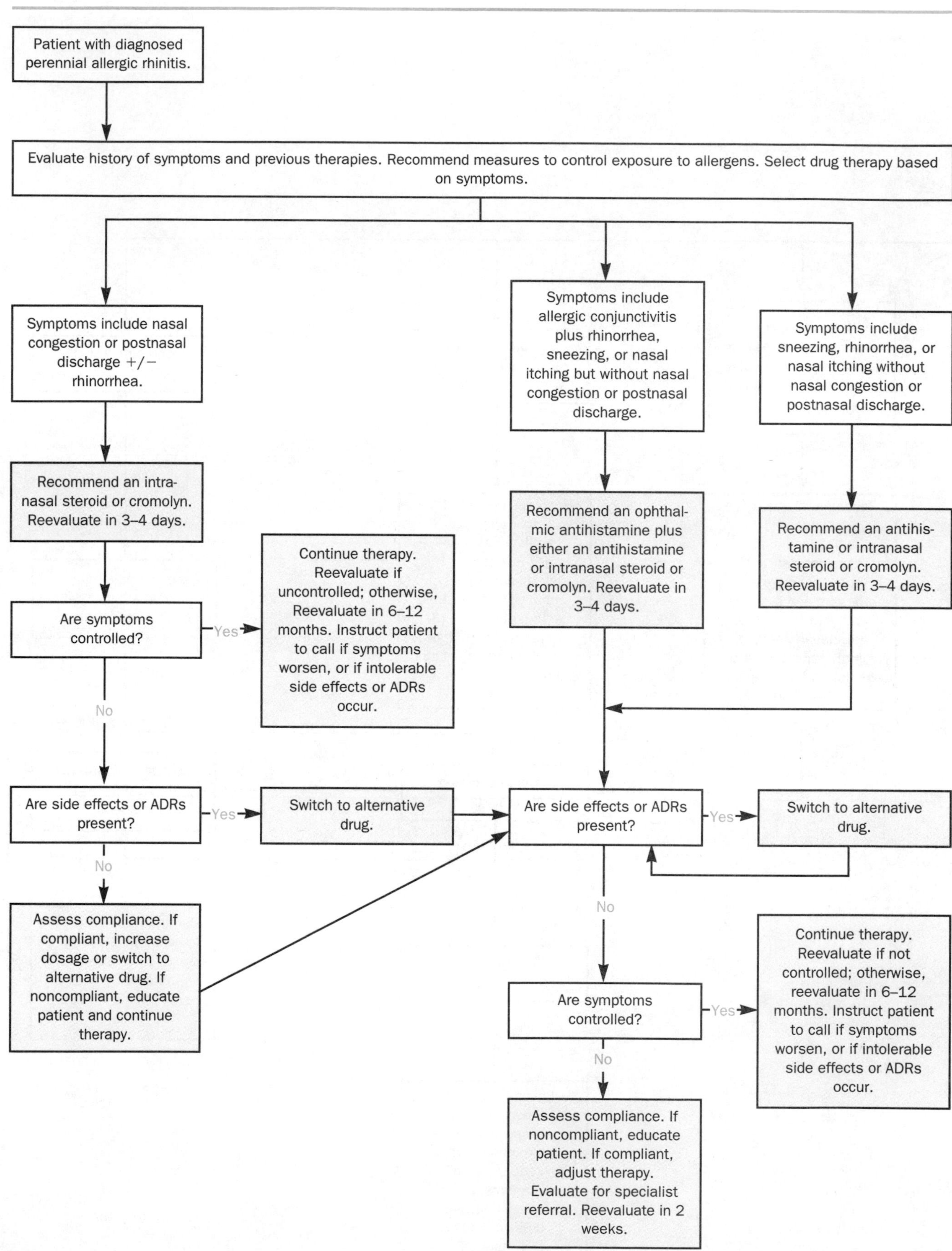

Figure 9–4 Self-care of perennial allergic rhinitis. Adapted from reference 80.

Table 9–10

Selected Saline Nasal Products

Trade Name	Primary Ingredients
Ayr Gel	Sodium chloride 0.5%
Ayr Drops/Spray	Sodium chloride 0.65%
4-Way Saline Moisturizing Mist Spray	Sodium chloride; glycerin; polysorbate 80
HuMIST Saline Spray[a]	Sodium chloride 0.65%
Ocean Spray[a]	Sodium chloride 0.65%
Pediamist Pump Spray[b]	Sodium chloride 0.5%
Pretz Solution/Spray[a]	Sodium chloride 0.75%; glycerin 3%

[a] Sulfite-free product.

[b] Pediatric formulation.

Immunotherapy is also contraindicated for children younger than 5 years and for women who are pregnant. Although immunotherapy should not be initiated during pregnancy, maintenance therapy may be continued.[88]

Antihistamines

Mechanism of Action Antihistamines compete with histamine at central and peripheral histamine$_1$ receptor sites, thereby preventing the histamine–receptor interaction and subsequent release of mediators. Older antihistamines do not prevent the release of mast cell or circulating basophil mediators and will not reverse histamine-related symptoms that are already present. Newer antihistamines inhibit the release of mast cell mediators and may decrease cellular recruitment.

Antihistamines are classified as sedating (first-generation, nonselective) or nonsedating (second-generation, peripherally selective). The nonsedating antihistamines (acrivastin, azelastine, cetirizine, fexofenadine, ketotifen, and loratadine) are prescription medications. Differences between the types of antihistamines relate to the rapidity and degree to which they penetrate the blood–brain barrier as well as to their receptor specificity.[89,90] Sedating antihistamines are highly lipophilic molecules that readily cross the blood–brain barrier. Nonsedating antihistamines, which are large protein-bound lipophobic molecules with charged side chains, do not readily cross the blood–brain barrier. Both types of antihistamines are highly selective for histamine$_1$ receptors, but have little effect on histamine$_2$ or histamine$_3$ receptors. The sedating and some of the nonsedating antihistamines may also activate cholinergic, 5-hydroxytryptamine (serotonin), and α-adrenergic receptors.

Each chemical class differs slightly in terms of its activity and its side-effect profile. For example, the alkylamines are among the most active antihistamines and are less sedative than other sedating antihistamines. Chemical class differences make it plausible to suggest switching to a new class of drugs if the patient has a less-than-optimal response to one type of antihistamine.

Pharmacokinetics The pharmacokinetics of the sedating antihistamines are not well characterized.[90] Most antihistamines appear to be well absorbed after oral administration, with time-to-peak plasma concentrations in the 1.5- to 3-hour range for chlorpheniramine, hydroxyzine, and diphenhydramine. Protein binding is in the range of 78% to 99%. Antihistamines are metabolized in the liver by the hepatic microsomal mixed-function oxygenase system with significant first-pass metabolism. Half-lives range from approximately 9 hours for diphenhydramine to 28 hours for chlorpheniramine.

Indications Antihistamines are indicated for relief of symptoms of allergic rhinitis (e.g., itching, sneezing, and rhinorrhea) and other types of immediate hypersensitivity reactions. They are also used as sedatives, antiemetics, antitussives, antiparkinsonism agents, and antimotion-sickness agents. An unapproved indication is chronic idiopathic urticaria.

Dosage/Administration Guidelines Table 9–11 lists common dosages for selected systemic and topical antihistamines.[91]

Overdosage Overdoses of sedating antihistamines are characterized by excessive histamine$_1$ receptor and cholinoreceptor blockade and by α-adrenergic and serotonergic activity.[92] Central nervous system (CNS) symptoms (e.g., toxic psychosis, hallucinations, agitation, lethargy, tremor, insomnia, tonic-clonic seizures) predominate, with children more sensitive to the CNS excitatory effects and adults more likely to experience CNS depression. Peripheral symptoms include tachycardia, hyperpyrexia, mydriasis, vasodilation, decreased exocrine secretion, urinary retention, decreased gastrointestinal motility, dystonic reactions, rhabdomyolysis, and cardiac tachyarrhythmias and conduction abnormalities including torsades de pointes (a dysrhythmia).[93]

Adverse Effects The side-effect profile of the systemic antihistamines depends on the receptor activity, chemical structure, and lipophilicity of the drug.[94,95] Side effects associated with cholinergic blockage include dryness of the eyes, mouth, and nose; blurred vision; urinary hesitancy and retention; constipation; and tachycardia. High doses may cause nervousness, tremor, insomnia, agitation, and irritability. CNS stimulatory effects include anxiety, hallucinations, appetite stimulation, muscle dyskinesias, and activation of epileptogenic foci.

CNS depressive effects include sedation and impaired performance (impaired driving performance, poor work performance, reduced coordination, reduced motor skills, and impaired information processing).[96] Performance may be impaired in the absence of sedation and may persist the morning after a nighttime dose. CNS effects vary among the antihistamines. The alkylamines (brompheniramine and

Table 9–11

Dosage Guidelines for Systemic Nonprescription Antihistamines

	Dosage (Maximum Daily Dosage)	
Drug	**Adults (≥12 years)**	**Children[a]**
Brompheniramine	4 mg every 4–6 hours (24 mg)	6–<12 years: 2 mg every 4–6 hours (12 mg) 2–<6 years: 1 mg every 4–6 hours (6 mg)
Chlorcycline hydrochloride	25 mg every 6–8 hours (75 mg)	6–<12 years: 12.5 mg every 6–8 hours (37.5 mg) 2–<6 years: 6.25 mg every 6–8 hours (18.75 mg)
Chlorpheniramine maleate	4 mg every 4–6 hours (24 mg)	6–<12 years: 2 mg every 4–6 hours (12 mg) 2–<6 years: 1 mg every 4–6 hours (6 mg)
Dexbrompheniramine maleate	2 mg every 4–6 hours (12 mg)	6–<12 years: 1 mg every 4–6 hours (6 mg) 2–<6 years: 0.5 mg every 4–6 hours (3 mg)
Dexchlorpheniramine maleate	2 mg every 4–6 hours (12 mg)	6–<12 years: 1 mg every 4–6 hours (6 mg) 2–<6 years: 0.56 mg every 4–6 hours (3 mg)
Diphenhydramine citrate	38–76 mg every 4–6 hours (456 mg)	6–<12 years: 19–38 mg every 4–6 hours (228 mg) 2–<6 years: 9.5 mg every 4–6 hours (57 mg)
Diphenhydramine hydrochloride	25-50 mg every 6–8 hours (300 mg)	6–<12 years: 12.5–25 mg every 4–6 hours (150 mg) 2–<6 years: 6.25 mg every 4–6 hours (37.5 mg)
Doxylamine succinate	7.5–12.5 mg every 4–6 hours (75 mg)	6–<12 years: 3.75–6.25 mg every 4–6 hours (37.5 mg) 2–<6 years: 1.9–3.125 mg every 4–6 hours (18.75 mg)
Phenindamine tartrate	25 mg every 4–6 hours (150 mg)	6–<12 years: 12.5 mg every 4–6 hours (75 mg) 2–<6 years: 6.25 mg every 4–6 hours (37.5 mg)
Pyrilamine maleate	25–50 mg every 6–8 hours (200 mg)	6–<12 years: 12.5–25 mg every 6–8 hours (100 mg) 2–<6 years: 6.25–12.5 mg every 6–8 hours (50 mg)
Thonzylamine hydrochloride	50–100 mg every 4–6 hours (600 mg)	6–<12 years: 25–50 mg every 4–6 hours (300 mg) 2–<6 years: 12.5–25 mg every 4–6 hours (150 mg)
Triprolidine hydrochloride	2.5 mg every 4–6 hours (10 mg)	6–<12 years: 1.25 mg every 4–6 hours (5 mg) 4–<6 years: 0.93 mg every 4–6 hours (3.744 mg) 2–<4 years: 0.625 mg every 4–6 hours (2.5 mg) Infants 4 months–<2 years: 0.313 mg every 4–6 hours (1.252 mg)

[a] With the exception of triprolidine hydrochloride, these products are not recommended for children under age 2 years except under the advice and supervision of a physician.

Source: Reference 91.

chlorpheniramine) are considered the least sedating of the sedating antihistamines. The nonsedating antihistamines are less impairing than the sedating antihistamines but are not free of these adverse effects.[97,98]

Side effects reported with ocular antihistamines include burning, stinging, itching, foreign body sensation, dry eye, hyperemia, and lid edema. Ocular antihistamines should be used with caution in patients with a history of narrow-angle glaucoma.

Drug–Drug Interactions Alcohol, sedatives, and other CNS depressants increase the depressive effects of sedating antihistamines. Monoamine oxidase inhibitors (MAOIs) prolong and intensify the anticholinergic and CNS depressive effects of sedating antihistamines. Hypotension may also occur with MAOIs and dexchlorpheniramine. Chlorpheniramine inhibits phenytoin metabolism and may increase phenytoin serum concentration, resulting in more phenytoin side effects or adverse reactions. All antihistamines decrease or prevent immediate dermal reactivity and should be discontinued at least 4 days before scheduled tests for skin allergies.

Contraindications/Precautions/Warnings The sedating antihistamines are contraindicated for patients with a history of hypersensitivity to the drug or similar chemical structure, for newborns or premature infants, for nursing mothers, and for patients with narrow-angle glaucoma. They are also contraindicated for patients with stenosing peptic ulcer, symptomatic prostatic hypertrophy, bladder neck obstruction, and pyloroduodenal obstruction, and for patients taking MAOIs.

Patients with lower respiratory tract diseases (e.g., asthma, emphysema, chronic bronchitis) should use sedating antihistamines with caution, as should any patient in a situation requiring mental alertness. Patients will be impaired even if they do not feel drowsy or if they have taken the dose the evening before. The sedating antihistamines are photosensitizing drugs. Patients should be advised to use sunscreens and wear protective clothing.

Children and the elderly may experience paradoxical excitation with sedating antihistamines. The elderly are more likely than younger adults to have CNS depressive side effects and hypotension with all sedating antihistamines.

Product Selection Guidelines The side effects of and the patient's response to antihistamines determine which product to choose. The nonprescription medications are first generation antihistamines, and all are sedating. The alkylamines (chlorpheniramine, brompheniramine, and pheniramine) are the least sedating, whereas the ethanolamines (diphenhydramine, doxylamine, and phenyltoloxamine) are the most sedating. Second-generation antihistamines are nonsedating, are available only by prescription, and are more expensive than nonprescription (first-generation) antihistamines. (See Table 9–12 for examples of commercially available nonprescription antihistamines.)

Some patients report that antihistamines are less effective after prolonged use. This decline is most likely not true tol-

Table 9–12

Selected Products for Allergic Rhinitis

Trade Name	Primary Ingredients
Single-Entity Antihistamine Products	
Aler-Dryl Caplets	Diphenhydramine HCl 50 mg
Benadryl Allergy Tablets	Diphenhydramine HCl 25 mg
Benadryl Allergy Capsules[a]	Diphenhydramine HCl 25 mg
Benadryl Allergy Dye-Free Liquid[b,c]	Diphenhydramine HCl 12.5 mg/5 mL
Chlor-Trimeton 12-Hour Allergy Tablets	Chlorpheniramine maleate 12 mg
Dimetane Allergy Extentabs Timed-Release Tablets	Brompheniramine maleate 12 mg
Dimetapp Allergy Children's Elixir[d]	Brompheniramine maleate 2 mg/5 mL
Dimetapp Allergy Liqui-Gels/Tablets	Brompheniramine maleate 4 mg
Tavist-1 Antihistamine Tablets[a]	Clemastine fumarate 1.34 mg
Combination Antihistamine–Analgesic Products	
Coricidin HBP Cold & Flu Tablets[e]	Chlorpheniramine maleate 2 mg; acetaminophen 325 mg
Coricidin HBP Night Time Liquid[e]	Brompheniramine maleate 12.5 mg; acetaminophen 325 mg
Combination Antihistamine–Decongestant Products	
Actifed Tablets	Pseudoephedrine HCl 60 mg; triprolidine HCl 2.5 mg
Actifed Allergy Daytime/Nighttime Caplets	Daytime: Pseudoephedrine HCl 30 mg Nighttime: Pseudoephedrine HCl 30 mg; diphenhydramine HCl 25 mg
Benadryl Allergy/Congestion Tablets	Pseudoephedrine HCl 60 mg; diphenhydramine HCl 25 mg
Chlor-Trimeton 12-Hour Allergy D Tablets	Pseudoephedrine sulfate 120 mg; chlorpheniramine maleate 8 mg
Contac 12-Hour Cold Maximum Strength Caplets	Phenylpropanolamine HCl 75 mg; chlorpheniramine maleate 12 mg
Dimetapp Cold & Allergy Quick Dissolve Tablets[e]	Phenylpropanolamine HCl 6.25 mg; brompheniramine maleate 1 mg
Drixoral Cold & Allergy Timed-Release Tablets	Pseudoephedrine sulfate 120 mg; dexbrompheniramine maleate 6 mg
Novahistine Elixir[f]	Phenylephrine HCl 5 mg/5 mL; chlorpheniramine maleate 2 mg/5 mL
Tavist D Antihistamine/Nasal Decongestant Extended Release Caplets[a,c]	Phenylpropanolamine HCl 75 mg; clemastine fumarate 1.34 mg
Triaminic, Cold & Allergy Syrup[b,d,g]	Phenylpropanolamine HCl 6.25 mg/5 mL; chlorpheniramine maleate 1 mg/5 mL

[a] Sodium-free product.
[b] Alcohol-free product.
[c] Dye-free product.
[d] Pediatric formulation.
[e] Aspirin-free product.
[f] Sucrose-free product.
[g] Sulfite-free product.

erance; rather it stems from (1) patient noncompliance, (2) an increase in antigen exposure, (3) the worsening of the disease, (4) the limited effectiveness of antihistamines in severe disease, or (5) the development of similar symptoms from unrelated diseases. Although antihistamines induce their own metabolism, tolerance has not been clinically demonstrated. Nevertheless, some clinicians still recommend trying different structural classes of drugs when patients report a lack of response.

Nonprescription Category B sedating antihistamines include chlorpheniramine and diphenhydramine. Prescription Category B sedating antihistamines include azatadine, cetirizine, clemastine, cyproheptadine, dexchlorpheniramine, and loratadine. Sedating antihistamines in Category C (available only by prescription) include azelastine, hydroxyzine, and promethazine. The sedating antihistamines in Category B are preferred because experience with the drugs is extensive.[99] Although individual risk:benefit decisions must be considered, chlorpheniramine is the preferred antihistamine during pregnancy.[85]

Cromolyn

Mechanism of Action Cromolyn stabilizes mast cells, thereby preventing mediator release. Although the precise mechanism of action is not yet known, cromolyn probably prevents the influx of calcium ion into mast cells.[100] Cromolyn protects mast cells from immune-mediated (i.e., antigen–antibody) and nonimmune-mediated (e.g., cold air, hyperventilation, and exercise) triggers.

Pharmacokinetics Less than 7% of an intranasal cromolyn dose is absorbed systemically,[89] and what little is absorbed has no systemic activity. The absorbed drug is rapidly excreted unchanged in the urine and bile with a half-life of 1 to 2 hours. Cromolyn that is swallowed is excreted unchanged in the feces.

Indications Intranasal cromolyn is indicated for preventing and treating allergic rhinitis.

Dosage/Administration Guidelines The recommended dose is one spray in each nostril three to six times daily at regular intervals. Treatment is more effective if started before seasonal symptoms begin. It may take 3 to 7 days for its initial efficacy to become apparent and 2 to 4 weeks of continued therapy before it reaches the maximal therapeutic benefit.

Adverse Effects Sneezing is the most common side effect reported for intranasal cromolyn. Other side effects include nasal stinging and burning.

Drug–Drug Interactions No drug interactions are reported with intranasal cromolyn.

Contraindications/Precautions/Warnings Cromolyn has a wide margin of safety and is safe to use during pregnancy, in the elderly, and in children age 6 years or older. Intranasal cromolyn is not indicated for children age 5 years or younger or for anyone with a history of hypersensitivity to cromolyn or related drugs.

Decongestants

For a detailed discussion of these agents, see the section "Decongestants" under "Treatment of the Common Cold."

Alternative Remedies

Numerous alternative remedies and self-diagnostic kits for allergic rhinitis are marketed directly to consumers. No scientific evidence exists that any of the alternative self-diagnostic tests (hair analysis, bioresonance diagnostics, autohomologous immune therapy, antigen leukocyte cellular antibody tests, etc.) are of value.[101]

Ephedra (ma huang) and feverfew are commonly suggested alternative remedies. Parthenolide, feverfew's biologically active component, may have anti-inflammatory properties. However, the safety and efficacy of feverfew in allergic rhinitis are not known. Common side effects include mouth ulcers and gastrointestinal upset. (For a further discussion of these types of products, see Chapter 45, "Herbal Remedies.")

Homeopathic practitioners stress avoidance techniques but limit symptomatic treatment.[102] Symptom-specific homeopathic remedies include sabadilla for nasal and ocular symptoms (red watery eyes), wyethia for itching, and many of the same products recommended for the common cold. (For a further discussion of these types of products, see Chapter 46, "Homeopathic Remedies.")

Patient Assessment of Allergic Rhinitis

Asking the patient for a detailed description of the symptoms is the first step in determining whether the patient has a common cold or rhinitis related to other causes. The patient's medical history and medication use (previous and current) may reveal disorders associated with noninfectious allergic rhinitis. The patient should be asked about the following indicators of noninfectious allergic rhinitis:

- Recent use of topical nasal decongestants for longer than 3 to 5 days.
- History of poor response to decongestant/antihistamine therapy.
- Symptoms that began during pregnancy.
- Symptoms that are unilateral.
- Presence of anatomic abnormalities such as nasal polyps, deviated septum, or adenoid hypertrophy.
- Elderly patient.
- Recent history of facial or head trauma.
- History of cocaine abuse.
- Use of medications that cause nasal congestion (e.g., β-adrenergic blockers, ACE inhibitors, chlorpromazine, clonidine, reserpine, hydralazine, oral contraceptives,

Case Study 9–2

Patient Complaint/History

Edward, a 23-year-old man, presents to the pharmacist with symptoms of allergic rhinitis, which include moderate nasal congestion with watery rhinorrhea; sneezing paroxysms; itchy nose; itchy throat; and itchy, puffy, red eyes. He has had similar symptoms every fall since he was a teenager, but the symptoms seem to be much more severe this year. He feels better when he works in his air-conditioned office and worse when he is at home with the windows open or when he is outdoors. Edward has no known drug allergies. He has a history of repeated sinus infections for which he usually takes Bactrim DS. He selects the following nonprescription medications for his allergic rhinitis symptoms: Neo-Synephrine 0.5% nasal spray, Neo-Synephrine 1% ophthalmic solution, and generic chlorpheniramine tablets.

Clinical Considerations/Strategies

Readers can use the following considerations/strategies to determine whether treatment of this patient's disorder with nonprescription medications is warranted:

- Assess the appropriateness of the antihistamine.
- Assess the appropriateness of the ophthalmic solution and nasal spray.
- Identify which drugs, if any, will have little effect on the patient's symptoms.
- Suggest a more effective combination of nonprescription medications to treat allergic rhinitis.

Patient Education/Counseling

Readers can use the following strategies to develop a patient education/counseling plan that will ensure optimal therapeutic outcomes:

- Inform the patient about ways to avoid allergens (pollen) in and out of the home.
- Explain any changes made in the treatment regimen.
- Tell the patient how to use medication and adjust dosage, if necessary.
- Encourage compliance with antibiotic regimens.
- Explain the value of skin testing and possible immunotherapy, and refer the patient to an allergist.

aspirin or other nonsteroidal anti-inflammatory drugs).[103]

The medical history may uncover other respiratory illnesses that may complicate treatment of allergic rhinitis. The patient's current medication use will also alert the pharmacist to possible interactions with nonprescription allergy medications. The pharmacist should also ask whether nonprescription products used to treat episodic or chronic rhinitis were effective and without adverse effects.

Asking the patient the following questions will help elicit the information needed to accurately assess the disorder and to recommend the appropriate treatment approach.

Q~ What are your symptoms, and how frequently do they occur?

A~ *Identify the signs and symptoms of the common cold and compare with those of allergic rhinitis. (See the sections that discuss signs and symptoms of these disorders.)* It can be difficult to distinguish between symptoms of these disorders. Recommend appropriate medications based on verification of the patient's signs and symptoms.

Q~ Does the patient have a history of or symptoms suggestive of nonallergic rhinitis as described previously?

A~ If yes, refer the patient to a physician.

Q~ Do you have other medical problems?

A~ *Identify the exclusions to self-care of allergic rhinitis. (See the section "General Treatment Approach" under "Treatment of Allergic Rhinitis.")* If any of the exclusions apply to the patient, refer the patient to a physician.

Q~ What medications are you taking? Do you have a history of allergy or adverse reactions to any nonprescription or prescription medication?

A~ *Identify the possible drug–drug and drug–disease interactions and contraindications for nonprescription allergy medications. (See the discussion of these agents under "Treatment of Allergic Rhinitis.")* Using the patient's medication history, recommend an allergy medication. If the history precludes use of nonprescription allergy medications, refer the patient to a physician.

Q~ How have you treated past allergy symptoms?

A~ Consider the patient's satisfaction or dissatisfaction with specific products when recommending nonprescription medications.

Patient Counseling for Allergic Rhinitis

The pharmacist should stress that the best method of treating allergic rhinitis is to avoid allergens. Many patients, however, have no control over their working environment or are

Patient Education for Allergic Rhinitis

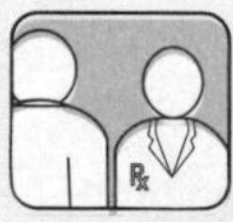

The primary objective of self-treatment is to prevent or reduce symptoms, which, in turn, will improve the patient's function and sense of well-being. If supervised by a physician, prescription antihistamines are the preferred initial treatment for children. For some patients, prescribed short-course oral corticosteroids may help control symptoms while other therapy is initiated or when symptoms are especially severe For most patients, carefully following instructions for nonprescription allergy medications and the self-care measures listed below will help ensure optimal therapeutic outcomes.

Nondrug Measures

- Note that avoidance of allergens is important regardless of whether allergy medications are being taken.
- For symptoms that develop mainly when outdoors
  —Shut the house and car windows on days with high counts of pollen (spring/summer) or mold (late summer/fall).
  —Try not to do yard work or engage in outdoor sports.
- For symptoms that occur mainly when indoors
  —Try to remove the source (cats, dust mites, tobacco smoke, and molds) of the symptoms from the house.
  —Use a HEPA filter to remove mold and pollen from the air in the home. This filter does not, however, remove the dust mite allergens.
  —Reducing the humidity in a home will reduce molds. Lower settings on humidifiers, repair damp basements, vent kitchens and bathrooms, and remove houseplants.

Nonprescription Medications

- Ask a pharmacist for help in selecting an allergy medication that treats the most bothersome symptoms. If needed, additional medications can be added for other symptoms:
  —Antihistamines are effective for itching, sneezing, and rhinorrhea but have little effect on nasal congestion.
  —Decongestants, are effective for nasal congestion but have little effect on other symptoms.
  —Combination therapy with an antihistamine and a decongestant is common.
  —Intranasal and ocular medications reduce nasal and eye symptoms, respectively, but have little effect on other symptoms.
- Allergy medications are more effective if they are used regularly rather than episodically.
  —If you have seasonal allergies, start allergy medications at least 1 week before symptoms are expected to begin.
  —If you have perennial allergies, take allergy medications before exposure to intermittent allergens.

Rhinorrhea (Runny Nose) and Sneezing

- Note that many factors cause a runny nose. Nonprescription antihistamines or prescription medications only partially treat this symptom. Because nonprescription antihistamines may make you very drowsy, the potential benefits of the medication must be weighed against the potential risks.
- Note that sneezing may be treated with nonprescription antihistamines. Sneezing is a common but rarely bothersome symptom. The potential benefits of using these medications must be weighed against the potential risks.
- Antihistamines are the preferred initial treatment for runny nose and sneezing in persons who are not pregnant. These medications may cause drowsiness and impair mental alertness though. These effects impair mental alertness even if drowsiness is not felt or the dose was taken the prior evening. While taking these medications, do not drive a vehicle, operate machinery, or engage in other activities that require alertness.
- Note that nasal saline solutions may relieve nasal mucosal irritation and dryness and aid in the removal of dried encrusted or thick mucus from the nose.
- Note that intranasal cromolyn is the preferred initial drug of choice during pregnancy. This medication is not absorbed into the body. The most common side effects include nasal stinging and burning.
- Note the following side effects for antihistamines:
  —Nonprescription antihistamines may cause sensitivity to sunlight. Use sunscreens and wear protective clothing when you are outdoors.
  —Children and the elderly may experience unexpected excitement with antihistamines. Because the elderly are more sensitive to the effects these medications have on the central nervous system and the heart, they may better tolerate lower doses.
- Do not use antihistamines
  —If you are allergic to antihistamines or similar medications.
  —If you are breast-feeding.
- Do not give antihistamines to newborns or premature infants unless directed to do by a physician.
- Note the following precautions for use of nonprescription antihistamines in persons with the described medical conditions:
  —Persons with narrow-angle glaucoma, stenosing peptic ulcer, symptomatic prostatic hypertrophy, bladder neck ob-

struction, or pyloroduodenal obstruction should not use these medications.

—Persons with lower respiratory tract disease (e.g., asthma, emphysema, and chronic bronchitis) should use these medications with caution.

- Note that nonprescription antihistamines interact with the following drugs:

—Alcohol, sedatives, and other central nervous depressants may cause additive depressive effects of the central nervous system when taken with nonprescription antihistamines.

—Monoamine oxidase inhibitors prolong and intensify some of the side effects of the nonprescription antihistamines.

—Decreased blood pressure may occur when monoamine oxidase inhibitors are taken with dexchlorpheniramine.

—Chlorpheniramine may increase the side effects of phenytoin.

Nasal Congestion

- See the box "Patient Education for the Common Cold" for information about relieving nasal congestion.

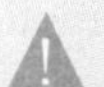

Seek medical attention in the following situations:

—Your allergy symptoms do not improve while taking nonprescription medications.

—Your symptoms worsen while taking nonprescription medications.

—You develop signs or symptoms of secondary bacterial infections (thick, opaque nasal or respiratory secretions, fever higher than 101.5°F, shortness of breath, chest congestion, wheezing, significant ear pain, rash).

unable to implement all the preventive measures at home. These patients usually rely on allergy medications for symptom control. The pharmacist should advise the patient about proper use of the recommended medications and about their possible adverse effects, any drug–drug and drug–disease interactions, and other precautions and warnings. The pharmacist should also describe the signs and symptoms that indicate the disorder has progressed to the point where medical care is needed. The box "Patient Education for Allergic Rhinitis" lists specific information to provide patients.

Evaluation of Patient Outcomes for Allergic Rhinitis

Many patients achieve symptomatic relief with initial nonprescription drug therapy in 3 to 4 days. After this time frame, the pharmacist should follow up, with a telephone call or a scheduled appointment, the outcome of the recommended therapy. Second-line treatment for patients who do not achieve this objective includes (1) increasing current medications to maximally effective dosages, (2) changing to a different medication or dosage formulation, or (3) referring the patient to a physician. Patients who develop any of the warning signs or symptoms listed in the box "Patient Education for Allergic Rhinitis" should be referred to a physician.

CONCLUSIONS

The common cold is a viral infection whose symptoms are similar to those of influenza and allergic rhinitis. General therapeutic measures include rest and an adequate fluid intake. Treatment is symptomatic and targeted at the most bothersome symptoms. Sore throat or pharyngitis is treated with topical anesthetics, systemic analgesics, or both. Nasal congestion is treated with topical or systemic decongestants. Rhinorrhea is partially amenable to treatment with first-generation antihistamines. Sneezing is treated with first-generation antihistamines. Cough secondary to postnasal drip is treated with decongestants.

Patients who will require evaluation and treatment by a physician include those with complications of the common cold; those with multiple medical problems, chronic pulmonary or cardiac disease, and immunosuppression; and the frail elderly.

Allergic rhinitis is a systemic disease characterized by rhinorrhea, nasal congestion, sneezing, and nasal pruritus. Therapy is sequential and consists of allergen avoidance, pharmacotherapy, and allergen immunotherapy. Patient education is an important component of all these steps.

In the pharmacotherapy stage, medications are taken regularly rather than episodically. No single medication is ideal. Combination drug regimens are common, especially for more severe disease. Initially, monotherapy is targeted at the dominant symptom. Other drugs are added if monotherapy is inadequate. The pharmacist may recommend a multiple-drug formulation if the patient presents with moderately severe, particularly intense, or long-lasting symptoms, or if the patient is at risk from exacerbation of an underlying disease.

Patients who will require evaluation and treatment by a physician include those with symptoms suggestive of nonallergic rhinitis, otitis media, sinusitis, or lower respiratory tract problems such as pneumonia, asthma, or bronchitis. Patients who fail to respond to nonprescription medications should also be evaluated by a physician.

Antihistamines are very effective for itching, sneezing, and rhinorrhea, but they are not an effective treatment for nasal congestion. Decongestants are very effective for nasal congestion, but they are not effective treatment for other symptoms. Topical (intranasal or ophthalmic) drug therapy may provide effective treatment for localized symptoms but will not treat other symptoms.

Nonsedating antihistamines are generally the preferred initial treatment for children. Because the elderly tend to have more adverse effects from allergic rhinitis medications, they may respond well with fewer adverse effects to lower initial dosages.

Patients who do not respond well should be asked about their allergen avoidance strategies and medication compliance. Treatment options include adjusting dosages, changing to drugs with different mechanisms of action, and using combination drug therapy. Medical referral may be appropriate.

References

1. Schappert SM. Ambulatory care visits to physician offices, hospital outpatient departments, and emergency departments: United States, 1995. In: *Vital and Health Statistics*, Series 13, No. 129. U.S. Department of Health and Human Services; June 1997:13. DHSS Publication 97–1790.
2. Corrao WM. Chronic cough: an approach to management. *Compr Ther.* 1986;12(7):14–9.
3. Irwin RS, Rosen MJ, Braman SS. Cough. A comprehensive review. *Arch Intern Med.* 1977;137(9):1186–91.
4. Wynder EL, Lemon FR, Mantel N. Epidemiology of persistent cough. *Am Rev Resp Dis.* 1965;91(5):679–700.
5. Smyrnios NA, Irwin RS, Curley FJ. Chronic cough with a history of excessive sputum production: the spectrum and frequency of causes, key components of the diagnostic evaluation, and outcome of specific therapy. *Chest.* 1995;108(4):991–7.
6. Di Pede C, Viegi G, Quackenboss JJ, et al. Respiratory symptoms and risk factors in an Arizona population sample of Anglo and Mexican-American whites. *Chest.* 1991;99(4):916–22.
7. Overlack A. ACE inhibitor-induced cough and bronchospasm. *Drug Safety.* 1996;15(1):72–8.
8. Irwin RS, Boulet L-P, Cloutier MM, et al. Managing cough as a defense mechanism and as a symptom. A consensus panel report of the American College of Chest Physicians. *Chest.* 1998;114(2 suppl):133S–81S.
9. Self-care of coughing. In: Albrant, DH, ed. *The American Pharmaceutical Association Drug Treatment Protocols.* Washington, DC: American Pharmaceutical Association; 1999:395–400.
10. Reisine T, Pasternak G. Opioid analgesics and antagonists. In: Hardman JG, Limbird E, Molinoff PR, Ruddon RW, Gilman AG, eds. *The Pharmacological Basis of Therapeutics.* 9th ed. New York: McGraw-Hill. 1996;521–55.
11. Freestone C, Eccles R. Assessment of the antitussive efficacy of codeine in cough associated with common cold. *J Pharm Pharmacol.* 1997;49(10):1045–9.
12. Eccles R. Codeine, cough, and upper respiratory infection. *Pulm Pharmacol.* 1996;9(5–6):293–7.
13. Cold, cough, allergy, bronchodilator, and antiasthmatic drug products for over-the-counter human use; final monograph for OTC antitussive drug products: final rule. *Federal Register.* August 1987;52: 30042–57.
14. Cold, cough, allergy, bronchodilator, and antiasthmatic drug products for over-the-counter human use; amendment of final monograph for OTC antitussive drug products. *Federal Register.* October 1993;58: 54232–6.
15. Cold, cough, allergy, bronchodilator, and antiasthmatic drug products for over-the-counter human use; expectorant drug products for over-the-counter human use; final monograph. *Federal Register.* February 1989;54:8494–509.
16. Sevelius H, McCoy JF, Colmore JP. Dose response to codeine in patients with chronic cough. *Clin Pharmacol Ther.* 1971;12(3):449–55.
17. Use of codeine- and dextromethorphan-containing cough remedies in children. *Pediatrics.* 1997;99(6):918–20.
18. Bem JL, Peck R. Dextromethorphan: an overview of safety issues. *Drug Safety.* 1992;7(3):190–9.
19. Murray S, Brewerton T. Abuse of over-the-counter dextromethorphan by teenagers. *South Med J.* 1993;86(10):1151–3.
20. Schadel M, Sellers EM. Psychosis with Vicks Formula 44-D abuse. *Can Med Assoc J.* 1992;147(6):843–4.
21. Paton DM, Webster DR. Clinical pharmacokinetics of H_1-receptor antagonists (the antihistamines). *Clin Pharmcokinet.* 1985;10(6):477–97.
22. Blyden GT, Greenblatt DJ, Scavone JM, et al. Pharmacokinetics of diphenhydramine and a demethylated metabolite following intravenous and oral administration. *J Clin Pharmacol.* 1986;26(7):529–33.
23. Meredith CG, Christian CD, Johnson RF, et al. Diphenhydramine disposition in chronic liver disease. *Clin Pharmacol Ther.* 1984; 35(4):474–9.
24. Spector R, Choudhury AK, Chiang C-K, et al. Diphenhydramine in Orientals and Caucasians. *Clin Pharmacol Ther.* 1980;28(2):229–34.
25. Irwin RS, Curley FJ, Bennett FM. Appropriate use of antitussives and protrussives. *Drugs.* 1993;46(1):80–91.
26. Pedersen AT, Batsakis JG, Vanselow NA, et al. False-positive tests for urinary 5-hydroxyindoleacetic acid: error in laboratory determinations caused by glyceryl guaiacolate. *JAMA.* 1970;211(7):1184–6.
27. Camphor revisited: focus on toxicity: Committee on Drugs. *Pediatrics.* 1994;94(1):127–8.
28. Fleming T, ed. *PDR® for Herbal Medications.* 1998. Montvale, NJ: Medical Economics Company, Inc.
29. Dingle JH, Dingle GF, Jordan WS Jr. Common respiratory diseases. In: *Illness in the Home: A Study of 25,000 Illnesses in a Group of Cleveland Families.* Cleveland, Ohio: Press of Western Reserve University. 1964: 33–9.
30. Gwaltney JM Jr, Hendley JO, Simon G, et al. Rhinovirus infections in an industrial population: I. The occurrence of illness. *N Engl J Med.* 1966;275(23):1261–8.
31. Turner RB. Epidemiology, pathogenesis, and treatment of the common cold. *Ann Allergy Asthma Immunol.* 1997;78(6):531–40.
32. Cohen S, Doyle WJ, Skoner DP, et al. Social ties and susceptibility to the common cold. *JAMA.* 1997;277(24):1940–44.
33. Cohen S, Tyrrell DAJ, Russell MAH, et al. Smoking, alcohol consumption, and susceptibility to the common cold. *Am J Public Health.* 1993;83(9):1277–83.
34. Cohen S, Tyrrell DAJ, Smith AP. Psychological stress and susceptibility to the common cold. *N Engl J Med.* 1991;325(9):606–12.
35. Cohen S, Frank E, Doyle WJ, et al. Types of stressors that increase susceptibility to the common cold in healthy adults. *Health Psychol.* 1998;17(3):214–23.
36. Paul JH, Freese HL. An epidemiological and bacteriological study of the "common cold" in an isolated arctic community (Spitsbergen). *Am J Hyg.* 1933;17(5):517–35.
37. Douglas RG, Lindgren KM, Couch RB. Exposure to cold environment and rhinovirus common cold. *N Engl J Med.* 1968;279(14):742–7.
38. Makela MJ, Puhakka T, Ruuskanen O, et al. Viruses and bacteria in the etiology of the common cold. *J Clin Microbiol.* 1998;36(2):539–42.
39. Monto AS. Studies of the community and family: acute respiratory illnesses and infections. *Epidemiol Rev.* 1994;16(2):351–73.
40. D'Alessio DJ, Meschievitz CK, Peterson JA, et al. Short-duration exposure and the transmission of rhinoviral colds. *J Infect Dis.* 1984;150(2):189–94.
41. Fireman P. Pathophysiology and pharmacotherapy of common upper respiratory diseases. *Pharmacotherapy.* 1993;13(6 Pt 2):101S–9S.
42. Proud D, Reynolds CJ, Lacapra S, et al. Nasal provocation with bradykinin induces symptoms of rhinitis and a sore throat. *Am Rev Resp Dis.* 1988;137(3):613–6.
43. Leung AKC, Robson WLM. Sneezing. *J Otolaryngol.* 1994;23(2):125–9.
44. Ostberg B, Winther B, Borum P, et al. Common cold and high-dose ipratropium bromide: use of anticholinergic medication as an indicator of reflex-mediated hypersecretion. *Rhinology.* 1997;35(2):58–62.
45. Tyrrell DAJ, Cohen S, Schlarb JE. Signs and symptoms in common colds. *Epidemiol Infect.* 1993;111:143–56.
46. Self-care of the common cold. In: Albrant DH, ed. *The American Pharmaceutical Association Drug Treatment Protocols.* Washington, DC: American Pharmaceutical Association. August; 1999:381–93.

47. Viral upper respiratory tract infection in adults. *Postgrad Med.* 1998;103(1):71–80.
48. Gwaltney JM Jr, Park J, Paul RA, et al. Randomized controlled trial of clemastine fumarate for treatment of experimental rhinovirus colds. *Clin Infect Dis.* 1996;22(4):656–62.
49. Turner RB, Sperber SJ, Sorrentino JV, et al. Effectiveness of clemastine fumarate for treatment of rhinorrhea and sneezing associated with the common cold. *Clin Infect Dis.* 1997;25(4):824–30.
50. Korppi M, Laurikainen K, Pietikainen M, et al. Antitussives in the treatment of acute transient cough in children. *Acta Paediatr Scand.* 1991;80(10):969–71.
51. Tukiainen H, Karttunen P, Silvasti M, et al. The treatment of acute transient cough: a placebo-controlled comparison of dextromethorphan and dextromethorphan-beta 2-sympathomimetic combination. *Eur J Respir Dis.* 1986;69(2):95–9.
52. Kuhn JJ, Hendley JO, Adams KF, et al. Antitussive effect of guaifenesin in young adults with natural colds. *Chest.* 1982;82(6):713–8.
53. Lefkowitz RJ, Hoffman BB, Taylor P. Neurotransmission: the autonomic and somatic motor nervous systems. In: Hardman JG, Limbird E, Molinoff PB, Ruddon RW, Gilman AG, eds. *The Pharmacological Basis of Therapeutics.* 9th ed. New York: McGraw-Hill. 1996;105–39.
54. Johnson DA, Hricik JG. The pharmacology of alpha-adrenergic decongestants. *Pharmacotherapy.* 1993;13(6 Pt 2):110S–15S.
55. Establishment of a monograph for OTC cold, cough, allergy, bronchodilator, and antiasthmatic products. *Federal Register.* September 1976;41:38312–424.
56. Cold, cough, allergy, bronchodilator, and antiasthmatic drug products for over-the-counter human use; Final monograph for OTC nasal decongestant drug products. *Federal Register.* August 1994;1–48.
57. Black MJ, Remsen KA. Rhinitis medicamentosa. *Can Med Assoc J.* 1980;122:881–4. 58. Tyler VE. *The Honest Herbal.* 3rd ed. New York: Pharmaceutical Products Press. 1993;115–7.
59. Garland ML, Hagmeyer KO. The role of zinc lozenges in treatment of the common cold. *Ann Pharmacotherapy.* 1998;32(1):63–9.
60. Jackson JL, Peterson C, Lesho E. A meta-analysis of zinc salts lozenges and the common cold. *Arch Intern Med.* 1997;157(20):2373–6.
61. Macknin ML, Piedmonte M, Calendine C, et al. Zinc gluconate lozenges for treating the common cold in children. *JAMA.* 1998; 279(24):1962–7.
62. Marshall S. Zinc gluconate and the common cold. *Can Fam Physician.* 1998;44:1037–42.
63. Chalmers TC. Effects of ascorbic acid on the common cold. *Am J Med.* 1975;58(4):532–6.
64. Hemila H. Vitamin C intake and susceptibility to the common cold. *Br J Nutr.* 1997(1);77:59–72.
65. Hemila H. Does vitamin C alleviate the symptoms of the common cold? A review of current evidence. *Scand J Infect Dis.* 1994;26(1):1–6.
66. Hemila H. Vitamin C and common cold incidence: a review of studies with subjects under heavy physical stress. *Int J Sport Med.* 1996;17(5):379–83.
67. Cathcart RF. Vitamin C, titrating to bowel tolerance, anascorbemia, and acute induced scurvy. *Med Hypotheses.* 1981;7(11):1359–76.
68. Ferguson BJ. Cost-effective pharmacotherapy for allergic rhinitis. *Otolaryngol Clin North Am.* 1998;31(1):91–110.
69. Sibbald B, Rink E. Epidemiology of seasonal and perennial rhinitis: clinical presentation and medical history. *Thorax.* 1991;46(12): 895–901.
70. Fireman P. Treatment of allergic rhinitis: effect on occupation productivity and work force costs. *Allergy Asthma Proc.* 1997;18(2):63–7.
71. Reilly MC, Tanner A, Meltzer EO. Work, classroom, and activity impairment instruments. Validation studies in allergic rhinitis. *Clin Drug Invest.* 1996;11(5):278–88.
72. Bousquet J, Bullinger M, Fayol C, et al. Assessment of quality of life in patients with perennial allergic rhinitis with the French version of the SF-36 Health Status Questionnaire. *J Allergy Clin Immunol.* 1994;94(2 Pt 1):182–8.
73. Bousquet J, Knani J, Dhivert H, et al. Quality of life in asthma. I. Internal consistency and validity of the SF-36 questionnaire. *Am J Resp Crit Care Med.* 1994;149(2 Pt 1):371–5.
74. McSharry C. Oilseed rape sensitivity. *Clin Exp Allergy.* 1997;27(2): 125–7.
75. Baraniuk JN. Pathogenesis of allergic rhinitis. *J Allergy Clin Immunol.* 1997;99(2):S763–72.
76. The impact of allergic rhinitis on quality of life and other airway diseases. Summary of a European conference. *Allergy.* 1998;53(41 suppl):1–31.
77. Urval KR. Overview of diagnosis and management of allergic rhinitis. *Primary Care.* 1998;25(3):649–62.
78. Fireman P. Treatment strategies designed to minimize medical complications of allergic rhinitis. *Am J Rhinol.* 1997;11(2):95–102.
79. Sporik R, Platts-Mills TAE. Epidemiology of dust-mite-related disease. *Exp Appl Acarol.* 1992;16:141–51.
80. Management of perennial allergic rhintis. In: Albrant, DH, ed. *The American Pharmaceutical Association Drug Treatment Protocols.* Washington, DC: American Pharmaceutical Association; 1999:351–8.
81. International Rhinitis Management Working Group. International consensus report on the diagnosis and management of rhinitis. *Allergy.* 1994;49(19 suppl):1–34.
82. Wong L, Hendeles, L, Weinberger M. Pharmacologic prophylaxis of allergic rhinitis: relative efficacy of hydroxyzine and chlorpheniramine. *J Allergy Clin Immunol.* 1981;67(3):223–8.
83. Juniper EF, Guyatt GH, O'Byrne PM, et al. Aqueous beclomethasone dipropionate nasal spray: regular versus "as required" use in the treatment of seasonal allergic rhinitis. *J Allergy Clin Immunol.* 1990;86(3 Pt 1):380–6.
84. Management of seasonal allergic rhinitis. In: Albrant DH, ed. *The American Pharmaceutical Association Drug Treatment Protocols.* Washington, DC: American Pharmaceutical Association. 1999:359–66.
85. Schatz M, Petitti D. Antihistamines and pregnancy (editorial). *Ann Allergy Asthma Immunol.* 1997;78(2):157–9.
86. Meltzer EO. Treatment options for the child with allergic rhinitis. *Clin Pediatr.* 1998;37(1):1–10.
87. Durham SR. New insights into the mechanisms of immunotherapy. *Eur Arch Otorhinolaryngol.* 1995;252(suppl 1):S64–7.
88. Guidelines to minimize the risk from systemic reactions caused by immunotherapy with allergen extracts. *J Allergy Clin Immunol.* 1994;93(5):811–2.
89. Meltzer EO. An overview of current pharmacology in perennial rhinitis. *J Allergy Clin Immunol.* 1995;95(5 Pt 2):1097–110.
90. Simons FER, Simons KJ. The pharmacology and use of H_1-receptor-antagonist drugs. *N Engl J Med.* 1994;330(23):1663–70.
91. Cold, cough, allergy, bronchodilator, and antiasthmatic drug products for over-the-counter human use; final monograph for OTC antihistamine drug products. *Federal Register.* December 1992;57:58356–76.
92. Cetaruk EW, Aaron CK. Hazards of nonprescription medications. *Emerg Med Clin North Am.* 1994;12(2):483–510.
93. Woosley RL. Cardiac actions of antihistamines. *Annu Rev Pharmacol Toxicol.* 1996;36:233–52.
94. Aaronson DW. Side effects of rhinitis medications. *J Allergy Clin Immunol.* 1998;101(2 Pt 2):S379–81.
95. Milgrom H, Bender B. Adverse effects of medications for rhinitis. *Ann Allergy Asthma Immunol.* 1997;78(5):439–46.
96. Storms WW. Treatment of allergic rhinitis: effects of allergic rhinitis and antihistamines on performance. *Allergy Asthma Proc.* 1997;18(2):59–61.
97. Horak F, Stubner UP. Comparative tolerability of second generation antihistamines. *Drug Safety.* 1999;20(5):385–401.
98. O'Hanlon JF, Ramackers JG. Antihistamine effect on actual driving performance in a standard test: a summary of Dutch experience, 1989–94. *Allergy.* 1995;50(3):234–42.
99. Mazzotta P, Loebstein R, Koren G. Treating allergic rhinitis in pregnancy. Safety considerations. *Drug Safety.* 1999;20(4):371–5.
100. Foreman JC, Garland LG. Cromoglycate and other antiallergic drugs: a possible mechanism of action. *Br Med J.* 1976;1(6013);820–1.
101. Rusznak G, Davies RJ. ABC of allergies: diagnosing allergy. *Br Med J.* 1998;316(7132):686–9.
102. Cummings S, Ullman D. *Everybody's Guide to Homeopathic Medicines.* 3rd ed. New York: Jeremy P Tarcher/Putnam. 1977;224–41.
103. Mackay IS, Durham SR. ABC of allergies: perennial rhinitis. *Br Med J.* 1998;316(7135):917–20.

CHAPTER 10

Asthma

Dennis M. Williams and Timothy H. Self

Chapter 10 at a Glance

The National Heart, Lung, and Blood Institute estimates that the total cost of asthma exceeds $12 billion annually.[1] These costs include emergency department visits and hospitalizations, as well as losses associated with work and school absences resulting from asthma exacerbations. Clearly, poorly controlled asthma is costly to the health care system. In contrast to many other chronic diseases, improvements in asthma control can result in immediate and significant reductions in costs and can significantly enhance the patient's quality of life.

Although nonprescription pharmacologic therapies for asthma are limited to two agents, the market for nonprescription asthma therapies exceeds $80 million annually.[2] Because asthma is a life-threatening condition, a decision to self-medicate should be made in conjunction with a knowledgeable health professional. For example, assisting patients in the assessment of symptoms and the need for referral to another health professional for diagnosis is an important role for the pharmacist. Numerous studies[3–11] have documented the value of pharmacist services in improving asthma control.

Epidemiology of Asthma

Asthma affects approximately 15 million people in the United States, including 5 million children.[12] Symptomatic asthma is more common in children, with the age of onset being younger than 10 years for 50% of all subjects. The prevalence rate is slightly higher in males until puberty, at which time the gender ratio is approximately equal. Often, symptoms significantly decrease in severity as patients age, so the overall prognosis for children who develop asthma is good. Longitudinal studies[13] indicate that 50% to 70% of children with asthma have a permanent or temporary symptom-free remission by adulthood. However, 30% of children with asthma continue to have chronic symptoms into adulthood. Asthma is present in 3.8% of men and 7.1% of women older than 65 years.[14]

The prevalence and severity of asthma have increased over the past 20 years.[15] Nearly 500,000 hospitalizations are reported annually, and asthma represents the fourth leading cause in limiting activities of normal daily living. Mortality has steadily increased over the past two decades with 5434

Editor's Note: This chapter is based, in part, on the 11th edition chapter titled "Asthma Products," which was written by Dennis M. Williams and Timothy H. Self.

deaths reported in 1997.[16] The cause of the increase in mortality is multifactorial, but the increase has been greater in elderly and urban populations. Lack of access to medical care is a contributing factor. Among persons ages 15 to 44 years, African Americans have a death rate five times that of Caucasians.

Anatomy and Physiology of the Respiratory System

The respiratory system, which comprises the upper and lower respiratory tracts, consists of a series of airways, starting with the nose and mouth and leading ultimately to the terminal air sacs or alveoli. The oral and nasal passages lead to the pharynx, which branches out into the esophagus and the trachea. The trachea divides into the two large mainstem bronchi that supply air to the lungs. Each bronchus progressively divides into smaller airways (bronchioles), leading through the alveolar ducts to the alveoli. Layers of smooth muscle are wrapped around the airways; the number of muscle layers decreases as the airways progress toward the alveoli. As an airway branches, the walls become progressively thinner. At the level of the alveoli, only a thin layer of cells surrounded by pulmonary capillaries remains.

The nasal cavities are lined with highly vascular mucous membranes, mucus-producing goblet cells, and ciliated epithelial cells. Inspired air is conditioned en route to the alveoli. Dust particles, bacteria, and other foreign matter are trapped in the mucus and propelled toward the pharynx by the wavelike movement of the nasal cilia. The humidification and filtration processes continue as air passes through the trachea, bronchi, and bronchioles.

Bronchial smooth muscle tone and secretion of mucus are under neural and humoral control.[17] (See Figure 10–1.) Afferent nerves leading from irritant receptors in the mucosal epithelium produce reflex bronchoconstriction, increased production of mucus, and cough through cholinergic innervation of bronchial smooth muscle and goblet cells from the vagus nerve. Smooth muscle of the airway is only sparsely innervated by the adrenergic system; however, β-adrenergic receptors are prominent in smooth muscle. α-Adrenergic stimulation produces vascular smooth muscle contraction, and β_2-adrenergic stimulation produces smooth muscle relaxation. The nonadrenergic, noncholinergic (NANC) nervous system is the principal inhibitory system of the airways, thus counteracting the cholinergic excitatory system.[18] Stimulation of the NANC system through the vagus nerve primarily produces bronchodilation but can also produce bronchoconstriction. NANC neurotransmission is mediated by neuropeptides, which have not been conclusively identi-

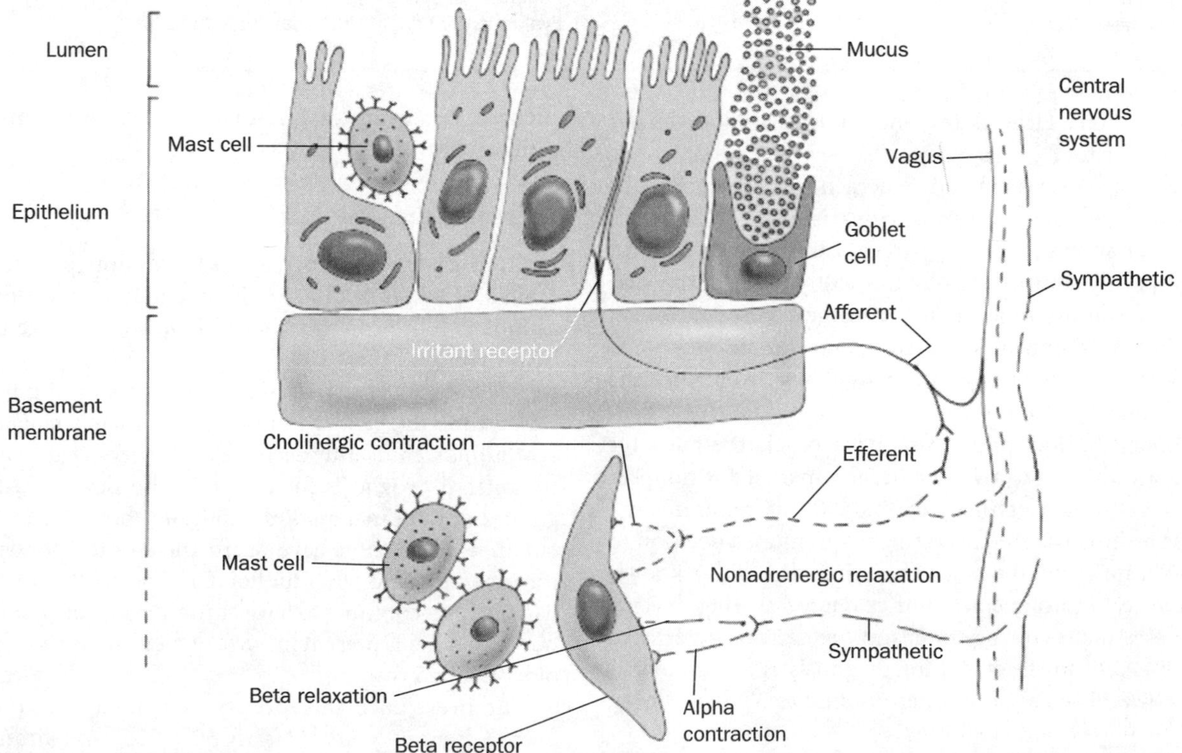

Figure 10–1 Innervation of the airways by the sympathetic, cholinergic, and nonadrenergic inhibitory systems. Mast cell concentration increases from the epithelial lumen to the submucosa. Adapted with permission from Dipiro J, Talbert RL, Yee GC, et al., eds. *Pharmacotherapy: A Pathophysiologic Approach*. 2nd ed. New York: Elsevier Publishing; 1992:410.

fied. It appears that a vasoactive intestinal peptide acts as an inhibitory transmitter (resulting in smooth muscle relaxation) and that substance P acts as an excitatory transmitter.[18] Under normal circumstances, all of these systems assist in maintaining normal bronchomotor tone.

Respiration is the exchange of gases between the alveoli and capillary blood. The process of respiration occurs by passive diffusion as gases move from areas of higher to lower concentration. Inspired oxygen passes across the alveolar walls into the capillaries, whereas carbon dioxide diffuses from the blood and is expired. Oxygenated blood returns through the pulmonary vein to the left side of the heart, where it is pumped through the aorta to carry oxygen to other organs.

The lungs are essentially elastic air sacs suspended in the airtight thoracic cavity. The movable walls of this cavity are formed by the sternum (breastbone), ribs, and diaphragm. The ribs are attached to the spinal vertebrae, and they join at the sternum. Inspiration occurs through two simultaneous mechanisms. The diaphragm, a dome-shaped muscle (when relaxed) that extends upward into the thoracic cavity, contracts. As it contracts, the diaphragm becomes flattened and moves downward into the abdomen, thereby increasing the longitudinal size of the thoracic cavity. Simultaneous contraction of the external intercostal muscles raises the ribs, causing an elevation and forward movement of the sternum plus an increase in the diameter of the chest cavity. Internal pressure in the thoracic cavity is less than the atmospheric pressure; therefore, air flows in and the lungs expand. Expiration results from relaxation of the ventilatory muscles and from the elastic recoil force of the alveoli and airways.

Etiology of Asthma

The precise etiology of asthma is not known; however, epidemiologic studies[13] in families and twins suggest a genetic component. Atopy is the strongest identified predisposing factor in developing asthma. An estimated 30% to 50% of the population is atopic, although the prevalence of asthma is much lower. Atopy in parents and children predicts an increased risk of developing asthma but is not essential; further, not all allergic patients develop asthma.[13] Another important risk factor for the development of asthma is childhood exposure to tobacco smoke from parents.[19]

Several causal factors that sensitize the airways and lead to the onset of asthma have been identified. The most frequent and important ones are indoor allergens, including house-dust mites, furred animals, and fungi. These allergens sensitize the individual, resulting in the production of immunoglobulin E antibodies. Other factors may play a role in asthma development, although the association is unclear. These factors include exposure to outdoor allergens, including dust, pollens, occupational exposures, and drug or food additives.[13]

Although underlying lung pathology is common to all patients with asthma, patients often differ in susceptibility to various asthma triggers. Once patients have been sensitized, they are susceptible to asthma triggers. Asthma is generally exacerbated by respiratory tract infections (primarily viral); inhaled allergens; inhaled air pollutants; smoking (active and passive); exercise; or occupational and industrial irritants, sulfites, or drugs. An identifiable allergen is the major precipitating factor in 35% to 55% of the population with asthma, and respiratory infections are a major factor in about 40%.[13]

From 2% to 28% of patients with asthma will have bronchospasm induced by aspirin.[19,20] A cross-sensitivity may exist with other nonsteroidal anti-inflammatory drugs (NSAIDs) (e.g., ibuprofen, ketoprofen, and naproxen). Patients should be cautioned that some nonprescription allergy, cough/cold, and analgesic preparations contain aspirin. Aspirin-sensitive patients can usually take acetaminophen as an analgesic.[20] Some patients may be aspirin sensitive and may not be aware of the problem because of infrequent aspirin use.

Pathophysiology of Asthma

According to the expert panel report of the National Asthma Education and Prevention Program (NAEPP), asthma is a chronic inflammatory disorder of the airways in which many cells and cellular elements play a role, particularly mast cells, eosinophils, T lymphocytes, macrophages, neutrophils, and epithelial cells.[19] In susceptible individuals, this inflammation causes recurrent episodes of wheezing, breathlessness, chest tightness, and coughing, frequently at night or in the early morning. These episodes are usually associated with widespread but variable airflow obstruction that is often reversible either spontaneously or with treatment. The inflammation also causes an associated increase in the existing bronchial hyperresponsiveness to a variety of stimuli. Recent evidence suggests that permanent changes, which are consistent with fibrosis, may occur in the subbasement membrane in some patients with asthma, and those changes may contribute to persistent airflow obstruction.[21]

Asthma is a chronic inflammatory disease of the airways that is characterized by recurrent exacerbations. The airways of the asthma patient are hyperresponsive, which is exhibited as an exaggerated bronchoconstrictor response to various stimuli. The inflammation contributes to bronchial hyperresponsiveness, airflow limitation, respiratory symptoms, and the chronicity of asthma.[19] Limitation of airflow in asthma is caused by obstruction of airflow. Permanent obstruction may occur because of airway remodeling.

Although the cellular defect in asthma is still unknown, it is now recognized that unchecked inflammation of the airways is the principal cause of their excessive reactivity to various triggering events.[18,19,22] This bronchial hyperresponsiveness (BHR) is characterized by (1) smooth muscle contraction (bronchoconstriction), (2) hypersecretion of mucus, (3) mucosal edema, and (4) epithelial desquamation. (See Figure 10–2). Inflammation in asthma is characterized

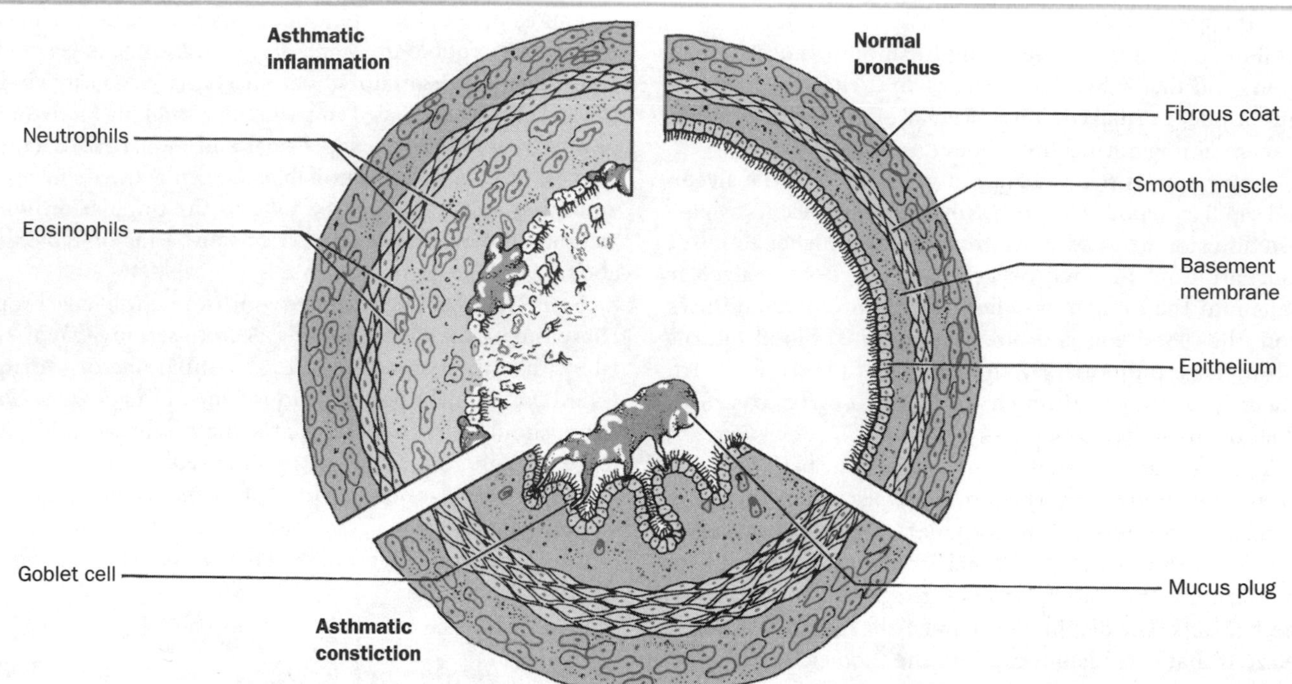

Figure 10–2 Representative illustration of the pathology found in the asthmatic bronchus compared with a normal bronchus (upper right section). Each section demonstrates how the lumen is narrowed. Edema of the basement membrane, mucus plugging, smooth muscle hypertrophy, and construction contribute (lower section). Inflammatory cells producing epithelial desquamation fill the airway lumen with cellular debris and expose the airway smooth muscles to other mediators (upper left section). Adapted with permission from Dipiro J, Talbert RL, Yee GC, et al., eds. *Pharmacotherapy: A Pathophysiologic Approach*. 2nd ed. New York: Elsevier Science Publishing; 1992:409.

by submucosal infiltration of eosinophils and lymphocytes, with epithelial shedding and hyperplasia of the basement membrane.[22] On exposure to a trigger, activated mast cells degranulate and release preformed mediators such as histamine; eosinophil chemotactic factor; platelet-activating factor; prostaglandins; and leukotrienes C-4, D-4, and E-4. These various mediators are responsible for producing bronchoconstriction; stimulating secretion of mucus; increasing vascular permeability; and attracting and activating eosinophils, neutrophils, and lymphocytes.[18] Within 5 minutes of inhaling a specific allergen, patients with asthma demonstrate a drop in pulmonary function that reaches a nadir in 10 to 20 minutes and then spontaneously improves within 1 hour. This airflow obstruction results from the release of mediators described above and is known as the early asthmatic response (EAR).

Many patients with asthma will undergo a second response 4 to 12 hours later, and that response may persist for 2 to 4 hours. The response is known as the late asthmatic response (LAR). Eosinophils and other cells that are activated during the EAR release toxins such as major basic protein, which can desquamate epithelium. The lymphocytes release cytokines capable of retaining and priming eosinophils in the airways as well as amplifying the effects of other mediators.[22]

The LAR occurs after inflammatory cells infiltrate the airways and is associated with an increase in BHR that does not occur with EAR alone. Drugs that effectively block the LAR prevent the increase in BHR and, with chronic use, can lower BHR. Because the LAR is associated with an influx of inflammatory mediators, agents that only influence EAR (e.g., β agonists) have no significant effect on BHR or the LAR. (See Table 10–1).

The bronchial smooth muscle hypertrophy, goblet cell hypertrophy, and excessive production of mucus are secondary to the ongoing inflammatory process. Imbalances in neural control of the airways are likely to play a role in amplifying the inflammation and bronchoconstriction.[19]

The clinical severity of asthma correlates with the degree of BHR; further, acute exacerbations are associated with an increase in BHR.[23] The degree of BHR can be measured with a number of pharmacologic (histamine, methacholine), physical (cold air or hypertonic saline), or physiologic (exercise or eucapnic hyperventilation of dry air) stimuli. Patients inhale increasing concentrations of either histamine or methacholine, and spirometric measurements are made after each increment. The provocative dose or concentration that produces a 20% drop in forced expiratory volume exhaled in 1 second (FEV_1) is calculated, and that value is used as a measure of airway reactivity.[23] A lower provocative dose indicates greater BHR.

Historically, asthma has been diagnosed by reversibility testing (defined as at least a 15% improvement in FEV_1 fol-

Table 10–1

Phase Activity of Asthma Medications

Medication	EAR	LAR
β_2 Agonist	+	–[a]
Theophylline	+	–
Steroids	–	+
Cromolyn	+	+
Nedocromil	+	+
Anticholinergics	+	–
H_1 Antihistamines	–	–

Key:

Early asthmatic response (EAR).

Late asthmatic response (LAR).

+ means medication inhibits this response.

– means medication does not inhibit this response.

[a] Long-acting β_2 agonists may inhibit the LAR.

Source: Lipworth BJ, McDevitt DG, *Br J Clin Pharmacol.* 1992;33:129–38.

Twentyman OP, Finnerty JP, Harns F, et al. *Lancet.* 1990;336:1338–42.

lowing treatment with a bronchodilator) during spirometry. Bronchoprovocation challenges can be useful for patients who have normal spirometry on examination but have a history consistent with asthma. Spirometry often does not correlate with BHR, so bronchoprovocation is a more sensitive indicator of airway inflammation.

BHR increases following allergen exposure, viral respiratory tract infections, and environmental exposure to pollutants. It decreases as a result of allergen avoidance and therapy with certain anti-inflammatory drugs. A positive bronchoprovocation challenge is consistent with asthma; [23] however, it can also occur with other conditions (i.e., cystic fibrosis, chronic obstructive lung disease, and allergic rhinitis). The degree of BHR is typically greater in asthma. Studies demonstrate a good correlation between the number of various inflammatory cells and desquamated epithelial cells and the degree of BHR.[19]

Finally, although the airflow limitation caused by asthma has traditionally been considered completely reversible, it is now apparent that some patients develop irreversible airflow limitation over a period of several years. This irreversibility is most likely related to airway wall remodeling and associated with an accumulation of inflammatory cells, edema, fibrosis, and changes in elastic properties.[21]

Signs and Symptoms of Asthma

Common symptoms of asthma are cough, wheezing, dyspnea, and chest tightness. These symptoms may be present in various combinations in individual asthma patients. The classic symptom of asthma is wheezing (a fine whistling sound) on expiration; in more severe obstruction, wheezing may occur on inspiration as well. Coughing caused by stimulation of the irritant receptors is common. Chronic cough may be the only presenting symptom in some patients with asthma. About 30% to 50% of patients with asthma complain of excessive sputum production. The sputum is usually yellowish and, on microscopic examination, eosinophils may be abundant.

By definition, asthma is episodic in nature. Periods of airway obstruction may last from a few minutes to several days. The severity of obstruction is highly variable, producing mild symptoms or rapidly progressing to respiratory failure. Patients with more severe disease may have continuous symptoms that require chronic medication for control; others may have normal pulmonary function between episodes and may require only periodic medication.

Classification of Asthma

Patients with asthma are classified according to severity of the disease.[19] (See Table 10–2.) The categories are mild intermittent, mild persistent, moderate persistent, and severe persistent. The classification is based on the frequency and extent of symptoms, as well as on objective assessment of lung function. Because asthma is highly variable, a patient's classification may change over time.

Treatment of Asthma

To improve recognition, awareness, and management of asthma, the National Heart, Lung, and Blood Institute initiated the NAEPP in 1989. The most recent document published through this program, titled "Expert Panel Report 2: Guidelines for the Diagnosis and Management of Asthma (EPR 2)" was published in February 1997.[19] This report, as well as a companion publication referred to as the practical guide,[24] are valuable resources for clinicians who provide care for patients with asthma. It can be obtained from the National Heart, Lung, and Blood Institute Information Center (fax 301-251-1223) or from the Internet at www.nhlbi.nih.gov/guidelines/asthma/asthgdln.htm. The practical guide includes numerous tools that can be used in educating patients, teaching skills, and developing self-management plans. Despite the lack of preferred asthma medications as nonprescription therapies, many opportunities are available for pharmacists to provide care for the patient with asthma.

Treatment Outcomes

To assist with the appropriate treatment plan for a specific asthma patient, the pharmacist must consider the goals of treatment, the severity of the disease, the specific characteristics of each patient, the patient's medical history, and the benefits and risks of the various drug classes for asthma treatment. The goals of asthma management include the following:[19]

Table 10–2

Classification System for Asthma Severity

	Clinical Features before Treatment		
Severity	**Days with Symptoms**	**Nights with Symptoms**	**PEF or FEV/PEF (%)**
STEP 4 Severe Persistent	Continual	Frequent	≤60/>30
STEP 3 Moderate Persistent	Daily	≥5/month	>60–<80/>30
STEP 2 Mild Persistent	3–6/week	3–4/month	≥80/20–30
STEP 1 Mild Intermittent	≤2/week	≤2/month	≥80/<20

Key: PEF = peak expiratory flow; FEV = forced expiratory volume.

- Preventing chronic asthma symptoms during the day and night.
- Preventing hospitalizations and emergency department visits from asthma exacerbations.
- Maintaining normal activity levels.
- Having normal or near-normal lung function.
- Being satisfied with asthma care received.
- Having no or minimal side effects from optimal pharmacotherapy.

In addition to the general goals, the patient should be asked to identify any other personal goals that he or she would like to achieve with good asthma control.

General Treatment Approach

Pharmacists can improve asthma care and outcomes. Undertreatment and suboptimal therapy have been identified as major contributors to morbidity and mortality from asthma. Many patients are not prescribed, or do not adhere to, appropriate anti-inflammatory therapies. Thus, written asthma management plans are underused.[25]

A report from the National Heart, Lung, and Blood Institute published in 1995 and titled *The Role of the Pharmacist in Improving Asthma Care*[26] describes numerous areas of involvement for the pharmacist, including these:

- Educating patients about asthma medications.
- Instructing patients in proper inhalation techniques.
- Monitoring medication use and refill intervals to identify patients with poorly controlled asthma.
- Referring patients for appropriate care.
- Assisting patients in using peak flow meters properly.
- Assisting patients in incorporating peak flow monitoring into a self-management plan that is designed in collaboration with a physician.
- Helping patients discharged from hospitals to understand their asthma management plan.

Pharmacists can also collaborate with other health professionals to ensure optimal asthma outcomes for the patient. Pharmacotherapy recommendations consistent with EPR 2 should be made. Such activities represent the core of an asthma disease management program that is provided by a pharmacist, and they should be the primary focus of pharmaceutical care for the asthma patient.

Further, optimal asthma care requires attention to the four major components of management: education, environmental control, self-monitoring, and pharmacotherapy. The first three management strategies are discussed in the following section "Nonpharmacologic Therapy." A brief discussion of severity-based pharmacologic therapy and exercise-induced asthma is provided here.

The goals of pharmacologic therapy are to prevent and control asthma symptoms, to reduce the frequency and severity of exacerbations, and to reverse airflow obstruction. Asthma medications are classified according to their role as long-term control therapies or quick-relief agents.

Long-term control therapies are used on a chronic basis to maintain control of persistent asthma. They include anti-inflammatory agents, long-acting bronchodilators, and leukotriene modifiers. Although many agents may possess anti-inflammatory activity, EPR 2 defines anti-inflammatory agents as those that reduce markers of airway inflammation in tissue or secretion. This classification includes corticosteroids and nonsteroidal anti-inflammatory asthma agents (e.g., cromolyn and nedocromil).

Pharmacologic therapy is often required to achieve the goals of asthma management. Although mild, intermittent asthma symptoms may be managed with a nonprescription asthma medication, when pharmacologic therapy for asthma is indicated, most patients should be treated with a prescription medication. The algorithms in Figures 10–3 and 10–4 summarize long-term treatment of all severity levels of asthma.[19]

To gain control of asthma, the clinician may start treatment at the appropriate severity level and may gradually increase the intensity of therapy if control is not achieved. A

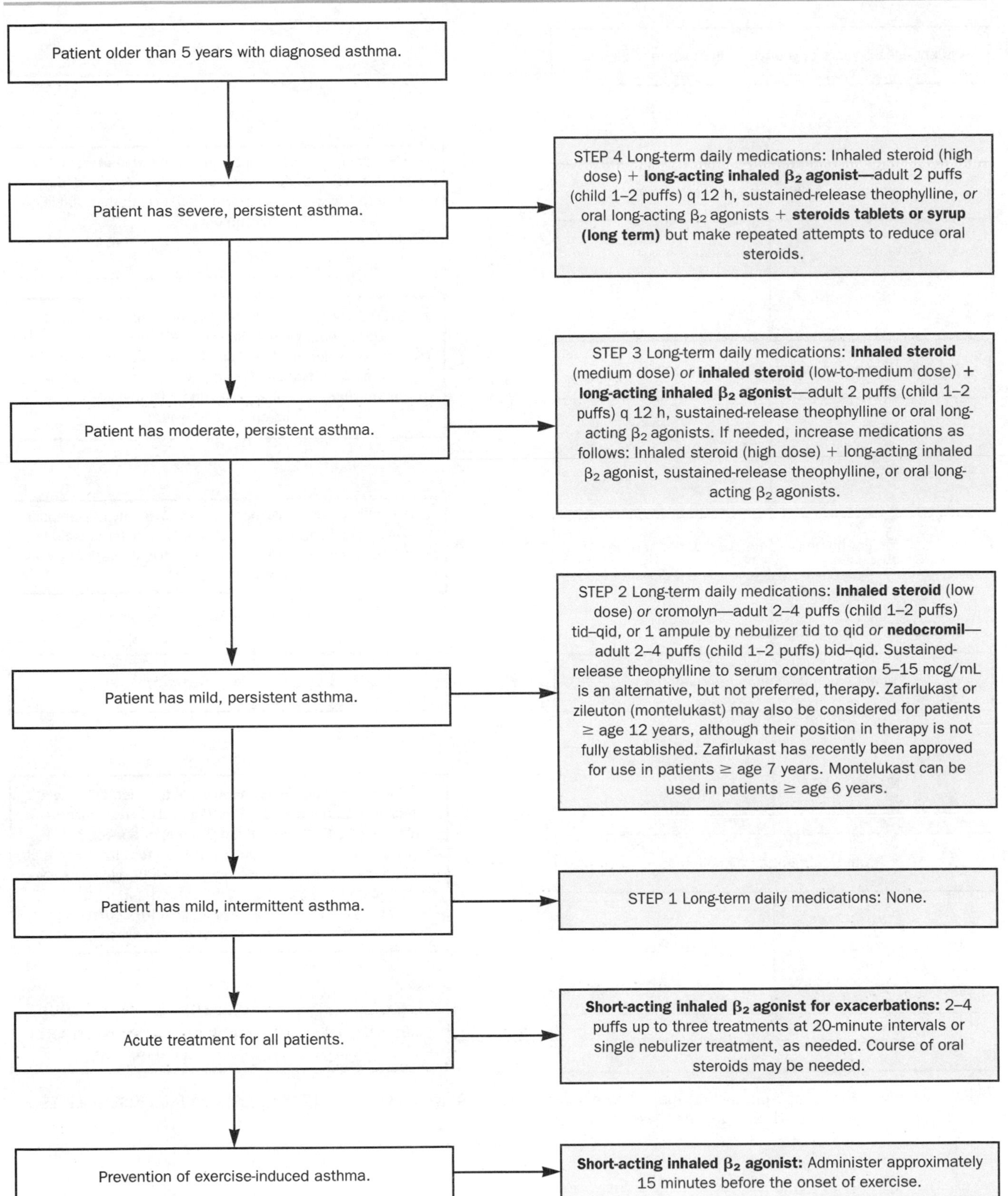

Figure 10–3 Stepwise approach to managing asthma in patients older than 5 years. Adapted from Reference 19. Note: Bold text indicates preferred therapy.

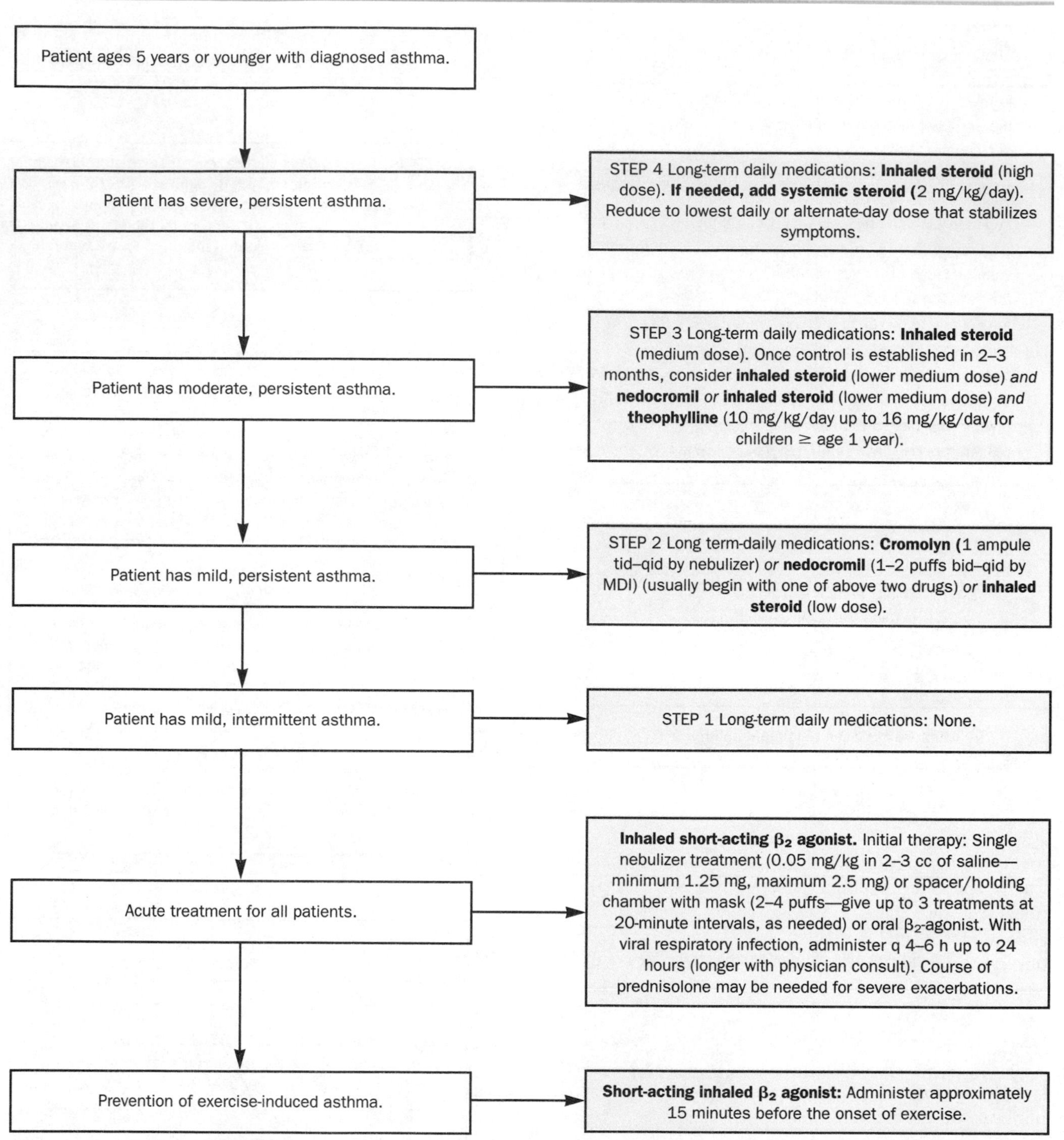

Figure 10–4 Stepwise approach to managing asthma in patients ages 5 years or younger. Adapted from Reference 19. Note: Bold text indicates preferred therapy.

common and cost-effective approach to achieving rapid control is to use a 1-week course of systemic corticosteroids (e.g., prednisone) while concurrently starting inhaled anti-inflammatory therapy at low to medium doses. An alternative approach that is often preferred is to initiate therapy with higher doses of inhaled corticosteroids and to step down treatment once control is achieved. Continual monitoring is required with either method to determine improvements in symptoms and lung function.

Asthma is a variable disorder and may improve spontaneously or as a result of therapy. Specifically, chronic treatment with anti-inflammatory therapy may reduce the severity of asthma. When asthma control is achieved and maintained for at least 3 months, it is reasonable to attempt

Case Study 10–1

Patient Complaint/History

Pernell, a 35-year-old man who has asthma, selects two Primatene Mist inhalers from the shelf and proceeds to the checkout counter. While checking out, he casually mentions to the pharmacist that his current asthma medication "doesn't work very well" and that using the Primatene Mist along with his prescription asthma medication provides the greatest relief.

The patient, who was diagnosed with asthma at age 10 years, has no other significant medical history. His patient profile lists the following current medications: Proventil (albuterol) inhaler one to two puffs q6h prn and Azmacort (triamcinolone) inhaler two puffs qid. The profile also shows that the patient has been using at least two Proventil inhalers per month for the past 5 months and that he has not had the prescription for Azmacort filled in the past 3 months. When asked to check his PEF, the patient reports that it is 65% of his baseline value.

Clinical Considerations/Strategies

Readers can use the following considerations/strategies to determine whether treatment of the patient's condition with nonprescription medications is warranted.

- Assess the patient's symptoms and the status of his asthma control.
- Assess the patient's compliance with the regimen of prescribed asthma medications.
- Consider referring the patient to his local primary care physician.
- Advise the patient whether it is appropriate to use a nonprescription inhaler under the current circumstances.

Patient Education/Counseling

Readers can use the following strategies to develop a patient education/counseling plan that will ensure optimal therapeutic outcomes:

- Counsel the patient on how to identify factors that precipitate asthma attacks.
- Reinforce the proper technique in administering inhalers.
- Ensure that the patient understands the disease and what constitutes appropriate therapy. For example, use illustrations and diagrams of normal and asthmatic lungs (inflammation).
- Explain the importance of strict compliance with the prescribed regimen, with emphasis on the long-term control therapy (which will not provide instant relief).
- Explain the limitations of nonprescription inhalers in treating asthma.
- Determine the proper role, if any, of adjunctive therapy with nonprescription asthma medications.
- Ensure that the patient knows when to contact a physician about his asthma management program.

to identify the minimum therapy required to maintain control by gradually reducing doses or by discontinuing medication. Step-down therapy must be done in a stepwise fashion, and symptoms and lung function must be closely monitored during the process. This approach should help reduce the occurrence of side effects and enhance patient compliance.

Exercise-induced asthma may be prevented or minimized by modifying the exercise regimen or by using inhaled β_2 agonists or other therapies to prevent the symptoms. Patients with exercise-induced asthma may minimize the adverse effect of exercise by choosing exercises that are conducted in warm and humid areas (e.g., swimming), by extending their warm-up period, by increasing their fitness level, by refraining from food ingestion 2 hours before exercise, or by wearing a face mask. Short-acting β_2-agonist therapy should generally be administered approximately 15 minutes before the onset of exercise. However, ephedrine and epinephrine are banned by the U.S. Olympic Committee. The committee allows inhalation therapy with β_2-selective agonists (e.g., albuterol, bitolterol, pirbuterol, procaterol, and terbutaline), cromolyn, ipratropium, and corticosteroids; it also allows oral therapy with theophylline, guaifenesin, and pyrilamine maleate.[27] The patient or health care providers may consult with the committee to determine the current status of accepted drug use in amateur competitive athletic competition (800-233-0393). The rules of the National Collegiate Association of America and other national and international sports rules are generally consistent with guidelines established by the U.S. Olympic Committee. Nonprescription asthma therapies contain either epinephrine (in the inhaled form) or ephedrine (orally). Several years ago,[28] FDA removed from the market those theophylline-containing products that were available without a prescription. In November 1994, an FDA advisory committee considered the approval of cromolyn sodium and albuterol (in a dry powder formulation) for nonprescription use.[29] However, no products were recommended for a switch to nonprescription status.

Self-treatment with nonprescription asthma drugs is not appropriate if the symptoms are new or a physician has not diagnosed the patient as having asthma. Medical referral for evaluation is essential in both cases.

The pharmacist may consider using a nonprescription asthma drug if the previous situations do not apply and if the patient (1) has never been to an emergency room or been hospitalized for asthma treatment, (2) is not currently receiving prescription asthma medications, and (3) does not have any of the following conditions:

- Hypertension.
- Diabetes.
- Uncontrolled thyroid disease.
- Heart disease.
- Difficulty in urinating because of an enlarged prostate.

Nonpharmacologic Therapy

As mentioned previously, pharmacists can provide valuable services to the asthma patient by addressing the primary components of management other than medications. Patient education and avoidance of asthma triggers are important strategies in the management of all asthma patients. Pharmacists can also assist the patient in self-management and in monitoring activities.

Patient Education

Education of the asthma patient is an essential component of success and should be provided at every step of asthma care. The literature supports the use of asthma patient education as a cost-effective strategy for adults and children.[30,31] Key educational topics include (1) the basic facts about asthma, (2) the role of medications, (3) the proper use of inhalation and monitoring devices, (4) the avoidance of allergens, and (5) the use of self-management and action plans. Written and verbal educational approaches can be used. Group education sessions can be beneficial but should not replace individual education provided by the clinician. It is also important to involve family members in the educational sessions because they will likely play a role if successful control is to be achieved. In addition to education about asthma and the medications, the patient should be taught skills that are important in asthma self-management, including the use of long-term therapies, action plans, and appropriate monitoring of his or her condition.[24]

Environmental Control

It is important to identify and minimize exposures to various triggers and to control other factors that can aggravate asthma symptoms. Avoidance strategies should eliminate or minimize exposure to known asthma triggers for the individual patient. A careful medical history should be taken to identify problems with common triggers. The various factors that should be investigated are summarized in Table 10–3.[19] A visit to the patient's home is an excellent method of assessing exposure to potential triggers, and it would enhance the clinician's relationship with the patient. When a potential trigger is identified for a patient's asthma, the pharmacist can recommend measures in Table 10–3 that are specific for the

Table 10–3

Control Measures for Factors Contributing to Asthma Severity

Contributing Factor	Control Measures: Instructions to Patients
Inhalant allergens (furred animals, house-dust mites, cockroaches, indoor fungi, outdoor allergens)	Review strategies to minimize/avoid exposure to specific allergen.
Tobacco smoke	Strongly advise patient and others living in the home to *stop smoking*. Discuss ways to reduce exposure to other sources of tobacco smoke, such as from day-care providers and the workplace.
Other irritants (indoor/outdoor pollution, fumes, strong odors	Discuss ways to reduce exposure to irritants.
Rhinitis	Treat with intranasal steroids; antihistamine/decongestant combinations may also be used.
Sinusitis	Use medical measures to promote drainage; antibiotic therapy is appropriate when complicating acute bacterial infection is present.
Gastroesophageal reflux	Do not eat within 3 hours of bedtime, keep head of bed elevated 6 to 8 inches, and use appropriate medications (e.g., H_2 antagonist).
Sulfite sensitivity	Avoid shrimp and other seafood; dried/packaged fruit; processed potatoes; beer, wines, and other fermented beverages; salads and salad bar ingredients; guacamole and other dips; pickled vegetables; processed, preserved, and "ready-to-eat" foods and beverages. Check medication labels for sulfites.
Medication interactions	Avoid β blockers (including ophthalmologic preparations). If previous reaction (e.g., anaphylaxis, bronchospasm) with aspirin has been reported, avoid salicylates and other NSAIDs. Usually safe alternatives are acetaminophen or salsalate.
Occupational exposures (irritant gases, dusts, fumes)	Discuss with asthma patients the importance of avoidance, ventilation, respiratory protection, and a tobacco smoke-free environment. If occupationally induced asthma, recommend complete cessation of exposure to initiating agent. Obtain permission from patient before contacting management or on-site health professionals about work-place exposure.
Viral respiratory infections	Give annual influenza vaccinations to patients with persistent asthma.

patient and that can be reasonably accomplished. (See Chapter 9, "Disorders Related to Cold and Allergy," for measures on avoiding specific allergens.)

Self-Monitoring

It is extremely important to recognize that delay in seeking medical care is a major contributing factor to asthma mortality. Subjective symptoms of wheezing and dyspnea are poor measures of lung function in certain patients who have an altered perception of asthma symptoms. EPR 2 recommends home monitoring of peak expiratory flow (PEF) in patients with labile or severe persistent asthma.[19]

Various brands of peak flow meters are available, but they all work similarly to achieve the same objective: to determine either the PEF or the maximum rate of air flow during forced expiration. PEF correlates well with a patient's FEV_1 and provides an objective at-home measurement of airway obstruction. These devices are to asthma patients what home blood pressure monitors are to hypertensive patients and what blood glucose meters are to diabetic patients. An example of improper technique using a peak flow meter has been reported.[32]The patient can accelerate airflow by inadvertently spitting into the meter, which will result in a large, false increase in PEF. This maneuver can be avoided by placing the mouthpiece of the peak flow meter well into the mouth. Patients should be instructed about the home use of a peak flow meter so therapy can be initiated as soon as significant obstruction is measured. (See Table 10–4.) If as-needed or chronic medications do not abate the asthma attack, the patient should be instructed to seek medical attention early.

Pharmacologic Therapy

The use of nonprescription medications for managing asthma symptoms is controversial.[33] The pulmonary–allergy advisory committee to the Food and Drug Administration (FDA) has stated that "although the bronchodilators are generally safe for OTC [over-the-counter] use at recommended dosage and are effective in relieving the shortness of breath caused by bronchospasm, . . . it is emphasized that these preparations should not be used unless a diagnosis of asthma has been made by a physician and a dosage schedule of the OTC medication has been established by a physician. Patients with asthma may also require prescription drugs which may have serious dangers and side effects and there is, then, an added need for continued medical supervision."[34]

It is pertinent to note that EPR 2 recommends the use of selective β_2 agonists when therapy is indicated.

The pharmacist should be actively involved in the patient's process of deciding to use nonprescription medications. It is extremely important for the pharmacist to determine the pattern of use for patients using nonprescription bronchodilator inhalers. If the underlying disease is asthma, self-treatment may delay necessary medical care and may result in resistant, acute, and severe asthma attacks. Patients with symptoms that occur more often than one to two times weekly, or with nocturnal asthma, should be *strongly encouraged* to seek medical advice and to consider using a home peak flow meter for a more objective assessment. Symptoms that require short-acting inhaled β agonist use more than twice weekly—other than for prevention of exercise-induced symptoms—indicate the need for assessment and long-term control therapy. (See Figures 10–3 and 10–4.)

Nonprescription medications are clearly reserved for patients with mild, intermittent symptoms. Even in this situation, many clinicians prefer to recommend a prescription, short-acting, inhaled, and selective β_2 agonist (e.g., albuterol) because of the product's longer duration of effect and its potential for fewer adverse effects. Prescription therapy with an as-needed selective β_2-agonist inhaler or chronic use of one of the anti-inflammatory medications (e.g., inhaled corticosteroids or cromolyn) should be instituted if nonprescription drug therapy does not provide adequate symptomatic relief. The nonprescription, as well as some prescription, β agonists also influence other adrenergic receptors. (See Table 10–5.) The α-adrenergic stimulation produces bronchoconstriction, vasoconstriction, urinary retention, and mydriasis, which are not beneficial in asthma. Stimulating β_1 receptors results in increased cardiovascular inotropic and chronotropic activity. β_2 agonists relieve spasms of bronchial smooth muscle caused

Table 10–4

Guidelines for Using Peak Flow Meters

1. Set the meter indicator on the bottom of the scale before each forced expiration.
2. (If possible) Take all measurements while standing.
3. Make sure that the hole in the back of the meter is not covered.
4. Take a deep breath and fill up the lungs completely.
5. Seal the lips tightly around the mouthpiece as shown in the drawing. Do not let any air leak out.
6. Rest the mouthpiece on the tongue, but do not obstruct the opening of the mouthpiece with the tongue.
7. Exhale as hard and fast as you can.
8. Record the best of three efforts as the peak flow value.

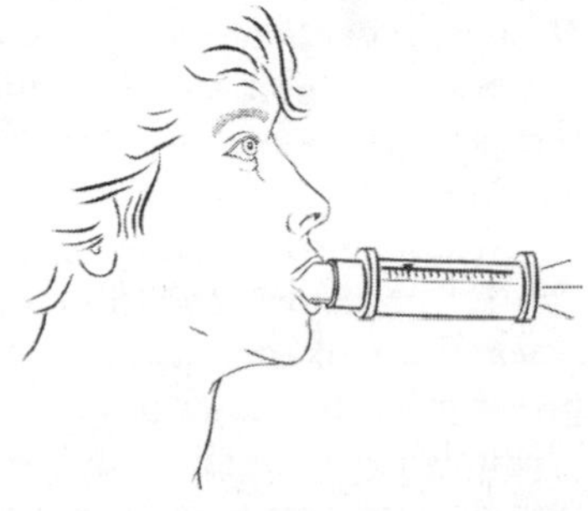

Table 10–5

Selected Characteristics of Bronchodilator Drugs

Drug	Route of Administration	Availability	Pharmacologic Activity				Duration of Action (hours)
			Sympathomimetic			Anticholinergic	
			Alpha	*Beta$_1$*	*Beta$_2$*		
Albuterol[a]	Inhalation	Rx		+	+++		3–6
	Oral: tablets	Rx		+	+++		5–8
Atropine	Inhalation	Rx	—	—	—	+++	<1
Bitolterol[a]	Inhalation	Rx		+	+++		4–6
Epinephrine[a]	Inhalation	OTC	+++	+++	+++		0.5
	Subcutaneous	Rx	+++	+++	+++		1–4
Ephedrine	Oral: syrup, capsules, tablets	OTC	+++	++	++		3–5
	Intramuscular, subcutaneous	Rx	+++	++	++		
Ipratropium	Inhalation	Rx	—	—	—	+++	4–6
Isoproterenol[a]	Inhalation	Rx		+++	+++		
	Sublingual	Rx		+++	+++		1–2
Isoetharine[a]	Inhalation	Rx		++	+++		1–3
Metaproterenol[a]	Inhalation	Rx		+++	+++		2–4
	Oral: tablets, syrup	Rx		+++	+++		
Pirbuterol[a]	Inhalation	Rx		+	+++		4–6
Salmeterol	Inhalation	Rx		+	+++	—	12
Terbutaline[a]	Inhalation	Rx		+	+++		3–6
	Oral: tablet	Rx		+	+++		4–8
	Subcutaneous	Rx		+	+++		
Theophylline[b] (various salts) (sustained release)	Oral: liquid, tablets	Rx	+	++	++		Various

Rx = prescription; OTC = over the counter, nonprescription

+ indicates relative intensity of effect.

[a] Inhalation confers more bronchial activity than systemic administration.

[b] Although theophylline is not a sympathomimetic drug, it causes the release of endogenous catecholamines.

by the EAR. When β_2 receptors are stimulated by sympathomimetic amines, the enzyme adenylate cyclase is stimulated, which then produces an increased intracellular concentration of cyclic adenosine monophosphate. In the airways, this increased production results in smooth muscle relaxation, prejunctional inhibition of cholinergic neurotransmission, increased mucociliary clearance, reduced mucosal edema, and inhibition of mast cell mediator release.[18]

Because current asthma management emphasizes using anti-inflammatory medications as first-line therapy for persistent forms of asthma, the utility of currently available nonprescription therapies has been appropriately questioned. The only apparent clinically relevant effect of nonprescription asthma agents is bronchodilation. Nonprescription bronchodilator therapy is essentially symptomatic treatment for asthma.

Historically, many clinicians have recommended that patients use a short-acting β_2 agonist before other inhaled, nonbronchodilator medications to improve pulmonary delivery of the agents and to reduce the potential for side effects. This practice is no longer recommended because no evidence is available that these benefits exist, and it is a potential source of confusion for the patient because β_2 agonists are advocated for as-needed use only.

Epinephrine

FDA has classified the following agents as Category I: epinephrine, epinephrine bitartrate, and epinephrine hydrochloride (racemic) in pressurized, metered-dose aerosol dosage forms and aqueous solutions equivalent to 1% epinephrine for use with hand-held rubber-bulb nebulizers. (See Table 10–6 for examples of commercially available products.) The inhaled epinephrine product has been available since 1963. However, worldwide phase out of chlorofluorocarbon (CFC) use will affect current epinephrine-containing metered-dose inhalers (MDIs). Although MDIs have been granted a medical exemption that allows continuing CFC use, this exemption will likely not be continued beyond 2005. It is unclear whether the manufacturers of epinephrine-containing products will pursue approval of a product with an alternative propellant or an alternative delivery system. Alternative delivery devices have also been developed as a result of the CFC phase out.

Mechanism of Action As previously described, epinephrine has equipotent α-, β_1-, and β_2-agonist effects, all of which are dose dependent. These effects are terminated as sympathetic nerve endings and surrounding tissues take up the drug. Epinephrine is metabolized in the nerve endings by monoamine oxidase and in the tissues by catechol-*O*-methyltransferase (COMT). Epinephrine is ineffective when taken by mouth because nearly complete metabolism by COMT and sulfatase occurs in the gastrointestinal tract and the liver. The peak effect of epinephrine aerosol for inhalation occurs within 5 to 10 minutes after use; the duration of action is less than 30 minutes.

Indications Inhaled epinephrine is indicated for the temporary relief of shortness of breath, chest tightness, and wheezing caused by asthma. For many years, subcutaneous epinephrine was the gold standard of treatment for acute bronchospasm. Its use has declined greatly because use of selective inhaled β_2 agonists increased during the 1980s. Although the various epinephrine-containing products differ slightly in the dose delivered, no significant difference exists between prescription and nonprescription epinephrine inhalation products. However, inhalation of inhaled, selective β_2 agonists is considered the therapy of first choice for acute asthma symptoms.[19]

Dosage/Administration Guidelines A single inhalation from epinephrine-containing inhalers contains the equivalent of 0.16 to 0.25 mg of epinephrine base.[29] For adults and for children ages 4 years and older, the dosage recommendation adopted for metered-dose delivery systems is one inhalation followed by a second inhalation if symptoms have not been relieved after at least 1 minute;[35] usage should not be repeated for at least 3 hours.

Table 10–7 describes the proper technique for MDI administration. The open- or closed-mouth method is acceptable. Because of the prevalence of suboptimal MDI technique, many patients may use or need spacers or holding chambers (e.g., Aerochamber or InspirEase) in conjunction with MDIs.

Spacers or extender devices used with MDIs can improve delivery of the drug to the airways. The distance between the inhaler mouthpiece and the mouth allows the CFC to evaporate, resulting in smaller droplet sizes and greater lung deposition. Use of a spacer also lessens impaction of the drug on the oropharynx and thereby decreases the incidence of oral candidiasis that can occur with regular use of a corticosteroid.

The Aerochamber and InspirEase are examples of holding chambers that provide the patient with feedback on the appropriate rate of inhalation. If a whistle is heard on inhalation, it indicates that the patient inhaled too quickly. These devices also have inhalation valves to minimize drug loss from the device until the patient is ready to inhale, obviating the need for good hand–lung coordination.

When an aqueous solution at a concentration equivalent to 1% epinephrine base is used with a hand-held rubber-bulb nebulizer, the inhalation dosage for adults and for children ages 4 years or older is one to three inhalations no more often than every 3 hours. For children younger than 4 years, no dosage recommendations exist, and the physician should be consulted. The solution should not be used if it is brown or cloudy. An adult should supervise the use of these products by children to avoid underuse or overuse.

The inhalation technique for dry powder inhalers (turbuhaler, diskhaler, discus) is significantly different from that for MDIs. Most importantly, a rapid, deep inhalation is required. Currently, there are no dry powder inhaler products available as nonprescription.

Adverse Effects Adverse effects related to epinephrine (e.g., tachycardia, cardiac arrhythmia, hypertension, tremor, and anxiety) are almost always associated with the parenteral route of administration. These effects would not generally be expected by the inhalation route except in an overdose situation. Some patients may tend to overuse these products, particularly when relief of symptoms does not occur.

Table 10–6

Selected Asthma Inhalant Products

Trade Name	Primary Ingredients
Asthma Haler	Epinephrine 0.22 mg/spray
Asthma Nefrin Solution for Nebulization[a]	Epinephrine 2.25% base (as racemic epinephrine HCl)
Broncho Saline Solution[a,b]	
Bronchaid Mist and Refill Inhaler[b,c]	Epinephrine 0.25 mg base/spray (as nitrate and HCl salts)
Bronkaid Mist Suspension Inhaler	Epinephrine bitartrate 7 mg/mL
Primatene Mist Inhaler	Epinephrine 5.5 mg/mL

[a] Alcohol-free product.

[b] Sulfite-free product.

[c] Sodium-free product.

Table 10–7

Guidelines for Using Metered-Dose Inhalers

Administration of Doses

1. Remove dust cap from inhaler.
2. Shake canister to distribute drug particles evenly throughout the suspension.
3. Position inhaler with mouthpiece at the bottom.
4. Tilt head back slightly.
5. Breathe out slowly.
6. Close lips on inhaler as shown in drawing A or hold inhaler 1 to 2 inches from open mouth as shown in drawing B. The open-mouth method has been recommended because it may decrease the amount of medication adhering to the back of the throat. (Both methods are equally effective. Ask your pharmacist to select the best technique for your clinical situation.)
7. Actuate while inhaling slowly and deeply. The slower the breath, the greater is the likelihood that the drug will reach the smaller airways.
8. If needed, use a holding chamber to help you inhale properly as shown in drawing C. Actuate the MDI once, and inhale the drug immediately after actuating the aerosol into the device.
9. If a whistle is heard on inhalation, inhalation was too quick.
10. Hold breath as long as possible, up to 10 seconds; then breathe out slowly. These actions increase the amount of drug retained in the airways.
11. Wait 30 seconds to 1 minute before administering second inhalation. This wait allows the bronchodilator to work and may increase delivery of the drug to the airways with subsequent inhalations. Note: Expect relief of symptoms within 5 to 15 minutes. Seek medical attention if symptomatic relief takes longer than 20 minutes.
12. If steroid inhaler is being used, rinse mouth after use.

Care/Disposal of Canister

- Wash the inhaler mouthpiece daily with warm water to prevent clogging; keep the mouthpiece free of particles.
- Routinely clean and air dry inhaler devices.
- Keep the dust cap over the mouthpiece of the inhaler to prevent small objects from becoming trapped in the mouthpiece and possibly aspirated.
- Do not puncture the unit. The contents are under pressure.
- Note that canisters left in freezing temperatures will release large aerosol particles after actuation. Allow the canister to come to room temperature (59°F to 86°F [15°C to 30°C]) before use.
- Do not store the canister near heat (greater than 120°F [greater than 48.9°C]) or open flames.
- Do not discard canisters into fires or incinerators.

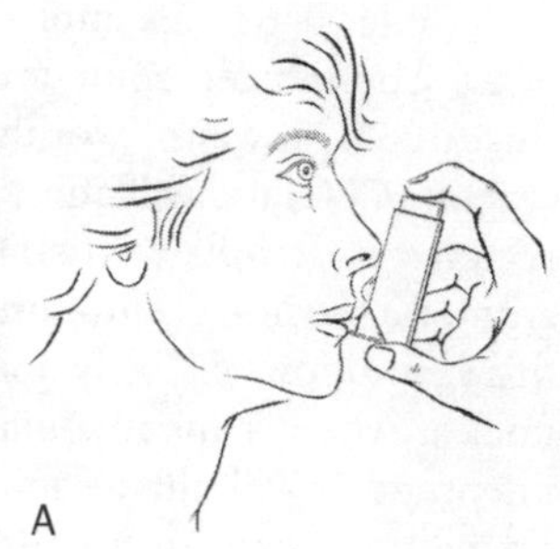
A

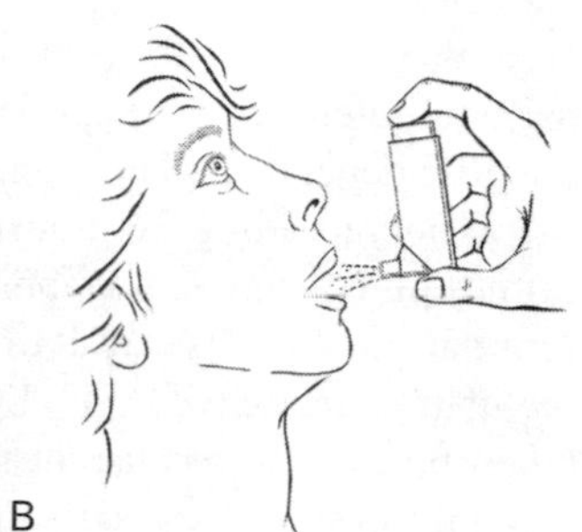
B

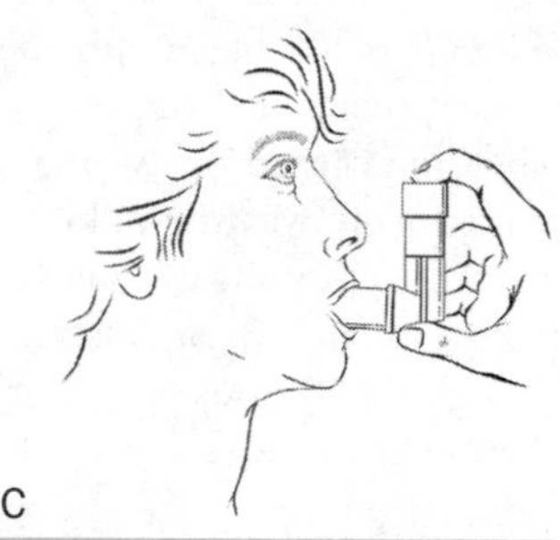
C

Drug–Drug Interactions Clinically significant interactions with epinephrine are rare because of its delivery by inhalation and its relatively short duration. Concomitant therapy with β blockers will reduce the bronchodilator response to epinephrine.

Contraindications Epinephrine products should not be used unless (1) a physician has made a diagnosis of asthma, (2) the patient has never been hospitalized for asthma, and (3) no other medications are being taken for asthma unless directed by a physician.[35] Patients with preexisting disease or conditions—such as heart disease (e.g., coronary artery disease, heart failure, or cardiac rhythm disturbance), high blood pressure, thyroid disease, diabetes, or difficulty in urinating because of enlargement of the prostate—should avoid self-treatment with these products except under the advice and supervision of a physician.[35] In addition, patients taking a prescription medication for hypertension or depression should consult their physician or pharmacist before using the epinephrine products.[35]

Precautions/Warnings Epinephrine products require statements that warn against exceeding the recommended dosages unless directed by a physician. The following warnings must appear in boldface type on the package labeling:

> Do not continue to use this product, but seek medical assistance immediately if symptoms are not relieved within 20 minutes or become worse. Patients should be warned that excessive use of epinephrine-containing products may cause nervousness, rapid heart beat, and possibly adverse effects on the heart. Epinephrine may increase certain symptoms of Parkinson's disease such as tremor and rigidity.[27]

Many clinicians consider the nonselective adrenergic properties and short duration of action of epinephrine to be adequate reasons not to recommend these products. The short duration of action may increase the potential for abuse of epinephrine-containing products. In recent years, awareness of safety issues with nonprescription asthma inhalers has increased as a result of a celebrity model's death.[36] The death was actually related to inadequate asthma therapy, thereby highlighting the fact that nonprescription asthma products are not appropriate in most cases. These issues severely limit the utility of inhaled epinephrine products in asthma management.

Special Population Considerations Elderly patients may have altered pharmacodynamic and pharmacokinetic responses to asthma medications. Some investigators[37] have reported decreased β-agonist activity in elderly patients as a result of (1) decreased receptor number, (2) decreased receptor affinity, or (3) altered biochemical pathways. Because most of the receptor studies have been in vitro or in vivo on cardiovascular and endocrine receptors, the effect of aging on β receptors in the lungs is largely unknown. These patients are also particularly sensitive to adrenergic stimulants.

With the currently available asthma therapies, it is neither reasonable nor prudent to use a nonprescription asthma medication in a pregnant or lactating patient. Optimal asthma treatment strategies during pregnancy are similar to those used for nonpregnant patients.

Asthma worsening has been reported to be associated with the menstrual cycle. Premenstrual or perimenstrual asthma is not uncommon, although the basis is not well understood. A careful history may indicate this problem, and appropriate measures can be taken to improve control.

Ephedrine

Ephedrine as an oral therapy for asthma has been available since 1954. The status of ephedrine as a nonprescription asthma therapy is also controversial because increasing reports indicate that ephedrine is being diverted for use in the illegal production of methamphetamine. Ephedrine is available as a base, as hydrochloride and sulfate salts, and as racemic ephedrine hydrochloride. This agent has been used as a precursor compound in producing methamphetamine and methcathinone, both of which are controlled substances with the potential for abuse. Like amphetamines, ephedrine produces the release of catecholamines in the central nervous system (CNS). Ephedrine, caffeine, and phenylpropanolamine are common ingredients in drugs manufactured to physically resemble amphetamine-containing dosage forms.

In November 1994, all sales of single-entity ephedrine products became subject to the record-keeping and reporting requirements of the 1988 Chemical Diversion and Trafficking Act.[38] Purchase of an ephedrine product requires the buyer's signature and two forms of identification. Sales records should be kept for 4 years and are subject to inspection by the Drug Enforcement Administration.

FDA continues to review whether nonprescription ephedrine products should remain on the market. In 1995, a Notice of Proposed Rulemaking challenged its continuing availability on the basis of reports about large-scale diversion for illicit use, information about harmful effects, and consensus from two FDA committees that the potential for misuse and abuse outweighed any benefit when used as a nonprescription bronchodilator.[39] Then, in 1999, FDA published a notice under the Controlled Substances Act inviting comments on a proposal that would classify ephedrine as a Schedule IV compound according to its CNS effects, its dependence and abuse potential, and its therapeutic usefulness.[40] Nonetheless, ephedrine remains available on the market in the United States and its status is unchanged. (See Table 10–8 for examples of commercially available products.)

Mechanism of Action Ephedrine has equivalent α, β_1, and β_2 activity. Those effects are primarily produced indirectly through the release of norepinephrine from sympathetic nerve endings. The peak bronchodilation effect from orally administered ephedrine occurs in 1 hour and lasts about 5 hours. Tachyphylaxis or tolerance may develop with long-term use. Ephedrine is predominantly eliminated unchanged in urine. Although the average elimination half-life is 6 hours, the half-life is decreased by urinary acidification and is increased by urinary alkalinization.

Indications Ephedrine is useful for treating only mild forms of seasonal or chronic asthma. FDA has also approved ephedrine for enuresis, hypotension, nasal congestion, penile erection, rhinorrhea, and sinusitis.

Dosage/Administration Guidelines Ephedrine sulfate is available on a nonprescription basis for use as a single entity in a 25 mg capsule and a syrup. The dosage recommendation for ephedrine in adults and children older than 12 years is 12.5 to 25 mg every 4 hours, not to exceed 150 mg in 24 hours.[29] For children ages 6 to 12 years, the recommended dosage is one-half to one tablet every 3 to 5 hours, depending on the specific combination product. The American Medical Association suggests 3 mg/kg per day divided into four to six doses. The manufacturers suggest that a physician be consulted for use of ephedrine in children younger than 6 years. The maximum daily dosage recommended for adults is 150 mg per day.

Table 10–8

Selected Oral Asthma Products

Trade Name	Primary Ingredients
Bronkaid Dual Action Caplets[a]	Ephedrine 25 mg (as sulfate); guaifenesin 400 mg
Dynafed Two-Way Tablets	Ephedrine 25 mg (as HCl); guaifenesin 200 mg
Mini Two-Way Action Tablets	Ephedrine 25 mg (as HCl); guaifenesin 200 mg
Primatene Tablets	Ephedrine 12.5 mg (as HCl); guaifenesin 200 mg

[a] Sodium-free product.

Adverse Effects The principal adverse effects of ephedrine are CNS stimulation, sleeplessness, nausea, loss of appetite, tremors, tachycardia, and urinary retention. To prevent insomnia, the patient should take ephedrine a few hours before bedtime. Reports indicate that chronic ephedrine overdosage may result in either severe cardiac toxicity or psychosis.[41,42]

Drug–Drug Interactions Severe hypertension could develop in a patient who has been receiving ephedrine while taking a monoamine oxidase inhibitor (MAOI). The MAOI decreases the degradation and increases the storage of norepinephrine. Blood pressure may also be increased if ephedrine is taken with clonidine, procarbazine, furazolidone, and selegiline. Further, ephedrine may increase the effect of ergotamine on the heart and blood vessels[27] and may decrease the blood pressure–lowering ability of guanethidine.

Potential toxicities associated with ephedrine use are numerous. Serious and life-threatening toxicities may occur and may involve the cardiovascular system, CNS, and gastrointestinal tract. Reported problems include cardiac dysrhythmias, cardiac arrest, myocardial infarct, psychosis, and mental confusion.

As an example of the potential risks from ephedrine-containing products, during a 2-year period from 1993 to 1995, the Texas Department of Health received 500 reports of adverse events in people who took dietary supplements containing ephedrine or associated alkaloids. The events ranged from tremor and headache to strokes, myocardial infarct, chest pain, seizures, and death (eight reports).[43]

The effects of ephedrine may be minimized if it is taken with methyldopa or reserpine. In addition, tricyclic antidepressants may partially block the action of ephedrine.[27] Because of alkalinization of the urine, the concentrations of ephedrine may be increased with concomitant administration of acetazolamide, dichlorphenamide, or a large dose of sodium bicarbonate. The risk–benefit profile of ephedrine is poor and limits the clinical utility of ephedrine-containing products.

Contraindications FDA considers nonprescription ephedrine to be a safe and effective bronchodilator. However, the drug is not to be used unless a physician has made a diagnosis of asthma, the patient has never been hospitalized for asthma, and no other medications are being taken for asthma unless directed by a physician. Patients with heart disease, high blood pressure, thyroid disease, diabetes, or difficulty in urinating as a result of an enlarged prostate should avoid self-treatment with these products except under the advice and supervision of a physician. In addition, patients taking a prescription antihypertensive or antidepressant drug should consult their physician or pharmacist before using the products.

Precautions/Warnings The labeling requirements for ephedrine-containing products include a warning statement against exceeding the recommended dosage unless directed by a physician. If symptoms are not relieved within 1 hour or become worse, the patient should discontinue using the product and should consult a physician immediately.[35]

Long-term use of sympathomimetic agents may produce minor degrees of tolerance or tachyphylaxis. Down regulation (decreased number) and a decreased affinity at the β_2 receptor may develop.[44] A plateau response is reached within 2 to 8 weeks with no further deterioration; the duration of action is affected more than the intensity of effect.[44] The clinical consequence of tolerance appears minor in that β_2 receptors in the airways are not as susceptible to tolerance as are other β_2 receptors.[45] However, shorter-acting adrenergic agents, such as epinephrine or ephedrine, may be more likely to result in overuse because of tolerance.

Special Population Considerations All patients are susceptible to the adverse effects and toxicities from ephedrine. However, elderly patients may have altered pharmacodynamic and pharmacokinetic responses to asthma medications. Some investigators have reported decreased β agonist activity in elderly patients as a result of decreased receptor number, decreased receptor affinity, or altered biochemical pathways.[37] Because most of the receptor studies have been in vitro or in vivo on cardiovascular and endocrine receptors, the effect of aging on β receptors in the lungs is largely unknown. Elderly patients, however, are particularly sensitive to adrenergic stimulants.

With the currently available asthma therapies, it is neither reasonable nor prudent to use a nonprescription asthma medication in a pregnant or lactating patient. Optimal asthma treatment strategies during pregnancy are similar to those used for nonpregnant patients. Asthma worsening has been reported to be associated with the menstrual cycle. Premenstrual or perimenstrual asthma is not uncommon, although the basis is not well understood. A careful history may indicate this problem, and appropriate measures can be taken to improve control.

Other Therapies

Antihistamines Because histamine produces bronchospasm, inflammation, and edema, antihistamines have a benefit for the asthma patient, although they should not be considered as primary therapy.[46] Perhaps the most important point is that good control of concurrent allergic rhinitis helps control asthma, whereas poorly controlled allergic rhinitis may worsen asthma. The strongest evidence suggesting that therapeutic agents for rhinitis may improve asthma control exists for nasal corticosteroids; however, antihistamines may be beneficial as well. Some of the second-generation antihistamines, such as cetirizine and azelastine, also have anti-inflammatory activity unrelated to their antihistamine activity.[46] These newer agents are lipophobic, do not cross the blood–brain barrier, act more peripherally, and, therefore, produce less sedation than the first-generation antihistamines. Further information on available nonprescription antihistamines can be found in Chapter 9, "Disorders Related to Cold and Allergy."

Another issue related to the use of antihistamines by the patient with asthma has changed substantially in recent years. Historically, these agents were felt to be contraindicated in asthma patients because of the potential for excessive drying of the secretions of mucus that are secondary to anticholinergic side effects. With the introduction of less-sedating antihistamines (fexofenadine and loratadine) that may possess some mild direct antiasthma activity, this concern was reconsidered. The current prevailing opinion is that antihistamines are not contraindicated and may offer modest benefit for the patient with asthma and associated allergies (e.g., allergic rhinitis). Although the labeling of most prescription and nonprescription antihistamine products still contains warnings about their use in patients with asthma, these products are generally considered safe. However, one report suggests that many pharmacists still advise asthma patients to avoid antihistamines.[47] In this survey, only 17% of pharmacists felt that antihistamines pose no problems for asthma patients.

Expectorants Many asthma products contain an expectorant, usually guaifenesin. At proper doses, guaifenesin, is considered to be a safe and effective expectorant. Other nonprescription expectorants, however, are probably no more effective than is adequate hydration of the patient and are, therefore, of questionable clinical value. Iodide was previously considered an effective expectorant, but because of concern about toxicity, an FDA advisory panel has recommended that iodide-containing products (expectorants) be restricted to prescription status. FDA also states that, unless ordered by a physician, guaifenesin should not be taken for a persistent or chronic cough that occurs with asthma or is accompanied by excessive sputum.[35] A change in production of mucus may be a sign of worsening asthma or infection, and this change requires medical evaluation rather than self-assessment and self-treatment. Further information on expectorants can be found in Chapter 9, "Disorders Related to Cold and Allergy."

Antitussives Coughing is the major mechanism for physiologic host defense and for removing bronchial secretions and plugs of mucus. Antitussives should generally not be used for asthma because a productive cough has a highly useful effect. The reflex cough induced by bronchospasm is often relieved by bronchodilators, not antitussives. However, nonprescription antitussives, such as codeine and dextromethorphan, have been used in asthma products in the past.

According to FDA, codeine should not be taken by patients with a chronic pulmonary disease or shortness of breath unless directed by a physician.[35] Similarly, dextromethorphan should not be used without a physician's prescription if a cough persists longer than 1 week; tends to recur; or is accompanied by fever, rash, or persistent headache.[35] Further information on antitussives can be found in Chapter 9, "Disorders Related to Cold and Allergy."

Therapeutic Comparisons

No clinically useful pharmacotherapeutic comparisons are available between the various therapies used as nonprescription asthma therapies.

Product Selection Guidelines

Although many geriatric patients exhibit adequate MDI technique, the percentage of elderly patients who are unable to perform correctly most of the steps required for proper inhaler use is likely greater than that of younger adult patients. Reasons for the elderly patients' inappropriate inhaler technique include arthritis, decreased muscle strength, dementia, inability to read or comprehend the instructions, and/or inadequate previous patient education on inhaler technique. One-third of elderly patients may not have sufficient hand strength to actuate the inhaler.[48] Specialized inhaler instruction should be repeatedly given to the elderly patient. Spacers or nebulizers should be used with elderly patients who are unable to use inhalers correctly.

Many children younger than 5 years will not be able to use an MDI correctly; they may need nebulizers to administer their medication. Some studies suggest that children as young as 2 and 3 years can learn to use a spacer device.[49] An MDI attached to a spacer device is more convenient than a nebulizer and can be mastered by some preschool-age asthma patients. Children older than 8 years can generally use an inhaler without a spacer. The child's technique should be assessed often, and the need for a spacer should be ascertained. Among children who previously showed good administration technique, 30% were found to develop an incorrect technique over time.[50] Holding chamber-type spacers are preferred for patients with technique difficulty. Spacer devices with whistles may help a child learn the appropriate rate for breathing during an inhalation.

Pharmacoeconomics

No pharmacoeconomics data are available for comparing the use of nonprescription asthma therapies with the stepwise therapy recommended by EPR 2. Such comparisons are inappropriate because nonprescription therapy use should be limited to patients with infrequent and mild symptoms of asthma.

Alternative Remedies

Despite the lack of scientific support, many individuals in the United States use alternative therapies. The prevalence of herbal medicine use among the general population is estimated at 3%.[51] In selected chronic conditions, use may be higher. These agents are not currently regulated by FDA because they are dietary supplements protected under the Dietary Supplement Health and Education Act of 1994. Thus, standardized evaluation of the products is lacking.

The recent popularity of alternative therapies and herbal products has affected asthma therapy. In general, alternative therapies do not have an established scientific basis for their use in asthma. Some examples of methods that have been used in asthma treatment are acupuncture, homeopathy, and Ayurvedic medicine (e.g., transcendental meditation, herbs, and yoga). Specific herbal medicines have been touted for their benefits in asthma. Ephedrine is a primary component in ephedra and ma huang. (See Chapter 45, "Herbal

Remedies," for discussion of these substances.) Additionally, coffee or black tea is suggested as useful self-treatments for asthma.

A comprehensive review of numerous acupuncture trials concluded that the effectiveness of this method of asthma treatment was not established.[52] Similarly, the value of homeopathy is currently unproven,[53] and claims about herbal medicine are not substantiated.[54]

In a study involving a cohort of 601 asthma patients, the prevalence of use of herbal medicines, coffee or black tea, or nonprescription asthma medications was 16.3%.[55] More specifically, 7.7% used herbal medicines, and 6% used either coffee or black tea as asthma therapies. Further analysis of these data showed an increased risk of hospitalization with herbal product use (odds ratio 2.5) and with coffee or black tea use (odds ratio 3.1). The authors[55] suggested that this risk may be related to a delay in using more efficacious therapies.

Patient Assessment of Asthma

The pharmacist's assessment of the patient with asthma should include a review of the common signs and symptoms of the condition, as well as a physical assessment for objective findings. A comprehensive medication history is essential.

Physical Assessment and Evaluation Tools

The initial assessment of asthma involves a medical history, physical examination, and spirometry.[19] As with other diseases, medical diagnosis of asthma is essential to rule out other causes of pulmonary symptoms, such as physical obstruction from a tumor, congestive heart failure, and chronic bronchitis. For example, a patient may develop new pulmonary symptoms associated with hypertension or heart disease. A patient who awakens in the middle of the night with dyspnea and cough resulting from pulmonary edema ("cardiac asthma") may have congestive heart failure. As another example, shortness of breath and chest pain in women taking oral contraceptives may be signs of pulmonary emboli rather than asthma. Such patients should be referred to a physician immediately. Patients with chronic bronchitis and emphysema experience some symptoms similar to those associated with asthma. However, those symptoms are usually continuous, not episodic, and should not be treated with nonprescription drugs except under a physician's direction.

Asthma is frequently unrecognized, especially in children, and, therefore, goes untreated. Pharmacists can play a major role in identifying potential patients with asthma and in referring them for appropriate care. Symptoms such as recurrent wheezing, periods of dyspnea, coughing, chest tightness, and repeated respiratory tract infections warrant additional assessments to determine whether asthma is present. In some cases, however, the patients themselves make the diagnosis of asthma after several episodes of intermittent shortness of breath and wheezing. Many patients have mild asthma that does not progress. In others, the condition may worsen and may be accompanied by dyspnea and wheezing, cough, tachycardia, retraction of the sternocleidomastoid muscle, apprehension, chest distention, tenacious sputum, and flaring nostrils. Sinus tachycardia with a pulse rate up to 120 beats per minute is a very common finding, as is sternocleidomastoid muscle retraction in patients with severe airway obstruction.[17]

If a diagnosis of asthma has been previously established, it is important to determine the frequency and severity of symptoms and to ascertain which self-treatment approaches have already been attempted. Patients need immediate medical intervention if shortness of breath makes them unable to complete a full sentence without stopping, if discomfort persists while they are at rest after using a bronchodilator, or if the bronchodilator does not completely relieve their symptoms. If a bronchodilator is being used but the dyspnea becomes worse, a severe attack may be imminent or already in progress. The patient should see a physician immediately. Patients who have progressive dyspnea and wheezing and who are dependent on nonprescription products may be in danger of severe pulmonary obstruction, which may require treatment in a hospital.

Spirometry, or pulmonary function testing, provides objective data about lung function and is useful in the initial assessment and ongoing monitoring of asthma. Although most spirometry is performed by a medical specialist, some pharmacists have developed limited spirometry testing programs in collaboration with other clinicians. Patients may have normal tests of the spirometric pulmonary function between episodes, but many patients with asthma have increased bronchomotor tone, which is readily reversed with a bronchodilator drug. During attacks, patients with asthma demonstrate a marked decrease in all measures of expiratory flow rate and often complain of tightness in their chest and of dyspnea.

Medication Assessment

Once the assessment of asthma has been confirmed, the pharmacist should ask the patient a series of questions to gather the necessary information for product choice and to determine whether the patient needs medical attention. The patient's pharmacy profile and use of other nonprescription medications must then be reviewed for (1) drugs that interact with any of the products available in the nonprescription drugs and (2) any allergies or hypersensitivities to the nonprescription products, including aspirin or other NSAIDs. Specific patient factors (e.g., age, pregnancy, lactation, and finances) need to be considered. The patient's compliance with other medications may also be determined from the pharmacy profile. A comprehensive medication history should be collected for all new patients. Periodic updates of medication use should be performed for established patients. These histories should include prescription medications, nonprescription medications, and alternative therapies.

Asking the patient the following questions will help elicit the information needed to distinguish asthma from other pulmonary conditions and to recommend the appropriate treatment approach.

The initial question should be "Has a physician diagnosed your condition as asthma?" If the patient answers, "No," then the pharmacist should proceed with questions for undiagnosed asthma. If the patient answers, "Yes," the pharmacist should ask the questions for diagnosed asthma.

Undiagnosed Asthma

These questions may be helpful in initially assessing the presence of asthma. Using the responses, the pharmacist may refer the patient to another health care provider for diagnosis and treatment.

Q~ Have you experienced a sudden, severe, or recurrent episode of coughing and a wheezing (whistling) sound while breathing out?

A~ If yes, consider asthma as a possible cause, and refer the patient to a physician. Ask the remaining questions to pinpoint possible triggers for asthma.

Q~ Do you experience colds that go to your chest or take more than 10 days to resolve?

A~ If yes, asthma triggered by upper respiratory viral infections may be indicated.

Q~ Do you have coughing, wheezing, or shortness of breath at a particular time each year?

A~ If yes, suspect asthma triggered by outdoor allergens.

Q~ Do you experience coughing, wheezing, or shortness of breath when exposed to certain things (e.g., house dust, animals, tobacco smoke, or perfumes)?

A~ If yes, suspect asthma triggered by allergens or irritants.

Q~ Have you used a medication to ease breathing? How often?

A~ Advise a patient who frequently uses nonprescription asthma medications that a physician should evaluate the asthma.

Q~ Do your symptoms improve with the medication?

A~ If yes and if the medication is used less than two times a week, suspect mild, intermittent asthma.

Q~ During the past month, have you experienced coughing, wheezing, or shortness of breath at any of the following times: during the night, in the early morning, or after running or other physical activity?

A~ Note that asthma symptoms typically occur in this pattern and should be evaluated. Suspect exercise-induced asthma if the symptoms occur after physical exertion.

Diagnosed Asthma

Q~ Are you under the care of a physician?

A~ If no, strongly encourage the patient to see a physician. Emphasize the life-threatening nature of asthma.

Q~ What is bothering you the most about your asthma?

A~ Identify patient concerns, as well as frequency and severity of asthma attacks. This information will be helpful in the assessment.

Q~ Do you have other medical problems such as heart disease, seizures, high blood pressure, hyperthyroidism, or diabetes?

A~ Advise a patient with one of those conditions that management of the asthma with nonprescription asthma medications is not appropriate.

Q~ What prescription or nonprescription medications are you currently taking?

A~ *Identify possible drug interactions with nonprescription asthma medications. (See the sections "Drug–Drug Interactions" under "Pharmacologic Therapy.")* Determine whether any of the patient's medications are known to interact with nonprescription asthma medications.

Q~ How often do you take your medication?

A~ Using the frequency of dosing, determine whether the patient is complying with the medication regimen or whether additional intervention is needed.

Q~ Has your asthma medication caused you any problems?

A~ If yes, determine whether side effects or toxicity is present.

Q~ Has your asthma been better or worse recently (or since your last visit)?

A~ If the asthma has worsened despite patient compliance with the therapy, consider referral or modification of the therapy.

Q~ Have you experienced problems with coughing, wheezing, shortness of breath, or chest tightness during the day or night? Have you had any episodes where your asthma was a lot worse than usual? Have you missed work or school or had to limit your activities? Have you been to the emergency department or hospital because of your asthma?

A~ If yes to any of these questions, refer the patient to a physician for evaluation of possible worsening of the condition or of problems with asthma medications.

Case Study 10–2

Patient Complaint/History

The mother of a 7-year-old boy named Jamie purchases Pedia Care Cough-Cold Formula in a liquid dosage form and then asks to speak to a pharmacist. She explains her concerns about her son's frequent "summer colds," which are characterized by wheezing, chest congestion, and a dry cough. She notes that he often has to stop to "catch his breath" during physical activities, especially during soccer practice.

During further discussion, the pharmacist determines that Jamie is in good general health and that his current medications include only a children's chewable vitamin taken once daily. Further, the mother has seasonal allergies and the father is a heavy cigarette smoker.

Clinical Considerations/Strategies

Readers can use the following considerations/strategies to determine whether treatment of the patient's condition with nonprescription medications is warranted:

- Further assess the nature of the summer colds and any correlation between the symptoms and potential causal factors.
- Determine whether the patient has any allergies to drugs, foods, or other substances.
- Determine whether the patient's difficulty in breathing follows any predictable pattern or frequency of occurrence.
- Determine whether the difficulty in breathing has ever required a visit to a physician or hospital emergency room.
- Identify which nonprescription medication, if any, might be appropriate for providing some symptomatic relief.
- Suggest a response to the mother's choice of nonprescription medication, taking into consideration the indications for the decongestant, antihistamine, and antitussive contained in the selected medication.
- Identify any warnings, precautions, or adverse effects associated with the use of the selected medication.
- In the presence of a strong suspicion of asthma, refer the patient to a physician for diagnosis.

Patient Education/Counseling

Readers can use the following strategies to develop a patient education/counseling plan that will ensure optimal therapeutic outcomes:

- Ensure that the mother knows when to contact a physician about the symptoms.
- Address the issue of the father's cigarette smoking as a confounding factor.
- Determine the proper role of adjunctive nonprescription drug therapy.
- Explain the proper selection and use of nonprescription drug therapy.

Patient Counseling for Asthma

Patients with asthma will benefit from participation in their care through self-management. All clinicians involved in the care of the asthma patient should jointly develop—in consultation with the patient—a written, individualized, daily self-management plan. This plan includes the goals of asthma therapy, as well as the allergen avoidance strategies to be practiced, the peak flow monitoring to be performed, and the regimens for long-term control therapies. Additionally, the pharmacist should provide a written action plan to help patients manage asthma symptoms and exacerbations. Action plans are implemented when the patient exhibits a change in symptoms or a decline in peak respiratory flow.

Action plans are individualized for the specific patient according to the usual symptoms, time course, and comfort with adjusting medications. Three typical strategies are increased use of the short-acting inhaled β_2 agonists, increased (doubling) of inhaled corticosteroid doses for several days, and short courses of oral corticosteroids for 4 to 10 days. The use of action plans has been proven beneficial in preventing work and school absences, emergency room visits, and hospitalizations.

Periodic assessment and ongoing monitoring of these strategies are also required. When patients obtain refills for long-term control therapies, pharmacists can question them about asthma control and the need to use the action plan. Regular or frequent use of an action plan may suggest a need to reevaluate and to modify the daily self-management plan.

The counseling of patients is an art that must be practiced. Asthma patients can have significant concerns and fears about their condition. It is essential for the pharmacist to use active listening and to demonstrate concern for the patient.

When counseling asthma patients, the pharmacist should provide general information about the use and storage of medications as well as pertinent pharmacologic information about a patient's particular medication. Explaining the proper use of peak flow meters and, if appropriate, inhalers and spacer devices is another important service. Evidence suggests that the performance accuracy and durability of spacer devices vary; therefore, the pharmacist should evaluate individual products before recommending their use.[56]

Delivery of therapeutic agents to the airway is challenging. MDIs deliver approximately 10% to 25% of the labeled dose to the lower airway; therefore, it is essential that proper technique be used. In a classic study, correct inhaler technique deposited only about 8.8% of inhaled particles from an aerosol into the lungs.[57] Incorrect inhaler technique, which can reduce drug delivery and efficacy, can result from incorrect or conflicting instruction, lack of instruction, and patient confusion and forgetfulness. Several reports suggest that knowledge about correct MDI technique among health professionals is lacking.[58–60] Education of patients and health care practitioners, as well as evaluation programs on proper inhaler technique and use of spacers, can improve therapeutic response.

Up to 89% of patients using inhalers do not perform all of the drug administration steps correctly.[57] Results from two evaluations revealed that 50% to 79% of nonpulmonary physicians, 35% to 53% of medical residents, 71% of pharmacists, 43% of nurses, and 8% of respiratory technicians did not perform or identify at least four of the steps required for correct inhaler usage.[59,60] The number and nature of specific steps taught by various health care practitioners may also differ. Currently, both the closed- and open-mouth techniques are taught. However, manufacturers' package instructions are for the closed-mouth technique. Many health practitioners instruct patients on only the basic steps; others include specific, complete instructions on every aspect of inhaler use. As a result of this inconsistency in education, patients may be confused on how to use inhalers.

Investigators have found that patients perform inhaler technique better when they receive written and verbal education.[61] Yet 87% of patients visiting a community pharmacy did not receive any verbal education on inhaler use.[62] In addition, a patient's inhaler technique may actually worsen over time. Therefore, repeated patient education and assessment of inhaler technique are strongly encouraged.

To educate patients adequately on inhaler use, pharmacists should provide demonstrations of correct technique along with both written and verbal instructions.[63] Patients should then demonstrate their inhaler technique to the phar-

Patient Education for Asthma

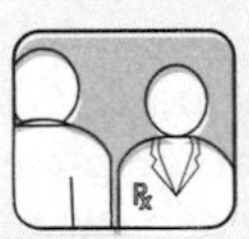

The objectives of self-treatment with nonprescription asthma medications are to (1) prevent or control asthma symptoms, (2) reduce frequency and severity of exacerbations, and (3) reverse obstruction of airflow. For most patients with mild, intermittent asthma, carefully following product instructions and the self-care measures listed below will help ensure optimal therapeutic outcomes.

Nondrug Measures

- Identify and reduce exposures to relevant allergens and irritants that increase asthma symptoms. (See Table 10–3.)
- Control other conditions and factors that you know worsen your symptoms.
- Take the following precautions if you have exercise-induced asthma:
  - —Choose exercises, such as swimming, that are conducted in warm, humid areas.
  - —Extend the warm-up period.
  - —Increase your fitness level.
  - —Eat at least 2 hours before exercise.
  - —If needed, wear a face mask.
- Use a peak flow meter to monitor your asthma. (See Table 10–4 for instructions on proper use.)

Nonprescription Medications

- If you are using a nonprescription asthma inhaler, check with your pharmacist or physician periodically to ensure that you are using it correctly. (See Table 10–7 for instructions on proper use.)
- If you are allergic to aspirin, check the ingredients on nonprescription allergy, cough/cold, and analgesic (pain relieving) products. For relief of minor pain, take acetaminophen. Note that use of other nonprescription analgesics (ibuprofen, ketoprofen, and naproxen) may cause an asthma attack if you are sensitive to aspirin.
- If you exercise, take your asthma medication approximately 15 minutes before you begin exercising.

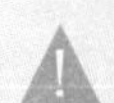

Contact a physician if your symptoms worsen or you are using your asthma medication more frequently.

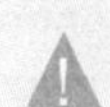

Contact a health care practitioner if you experience decreased responsiveness to a drug. This decrease may indicate a worsening of the asthma.

Seek immediate medical intervention if you experience any of the following:

- —Inability to complete a full sentence without stopping.
- —Persistent discomfort after using a bronchodilator even while at rest.
- —Incomplete relief of symptoms after using a bronchodilator.
- —Response to β_2 agonist that lasts less than 4 hours.
- —Worsening of dyspnea after using a bronchodilator.

macist. Resources such as videotaped demonstrations are available from several pharmaceutical manufacturers.

The box "Patient Education for Asthma" lists specific information to provide patients about this disorder and its management with nonprescription medications and nondrug measures.

Evaluation of Patient Outcomes for Asthma

Ongoing monitoring by the clinician is essential to determine whether goals of asthma management are being met. These parameters include monitoring for signs and symptoms of asthma, lung function, quality of life, occurrences of exacerbations, pharmacotherapy, and patient satisfaction with care. Additional parameters to monitor include days absent from school or work, emergency room visits, and hospitalizations caused by asthma. Monitoring of these areas allows the pharmacist to assess outcomes and to determine whether the goals of asthma management are being met. In addition to several subjective assessments, the expert panel recommends the use of spirometry (e.g., pulmonary function tests) initially to assess asthma and periodically to determine maintenance of airway function. An excessive or increasing pattern use of β-agonist MDIs is a sign of poorly controlled asthma and has been associated with an increase in asthma mortality.[64] Pharmacists should monitor the use of β agonists by patients with asthma because chronic, excessive use or increasing requirements can be a warning sign of poorly controlled asthma. In addition, asthma deaths have occurred both outside and inside the hospital, indicating that failure to appreciate the severity of illness may lead to inadequate therapy.

The patient plays an important role in ongoing monitoring as well. Patients should be taught to recognize symptoms of asthma and evidence of poorly controlled asthma. Additionally, periodic monitoring of lung function through measurement of PEF can be performed by the patient and can provide important information about asthma control. Peak flow monitoring can be a useful tool for short-term or long-term monitoring, or during exacerbations.[19] Short-term monitoring can be used to determine the patient's personal best value or to evaluate the relationship between lung function and exposure to potential asthma triggers. Long-term monitoring is helpful for many patients with persistent asthma that is moderate to severe. Such monitoring can be used to evaluate response to therapy, or to detect early changes in PEF that may signal an exacerbation. This strategy is particularly important in asthma patients who are known to have a poor perception of changes in lung function. Short-term monitoring of peak flows may necessitate two to four measurements each day to determine the patient's personal best and to assess variability throughout the day. When long-term self-monitoring is used, the peak flow should be taken in the morning before using any bronchodilator medication. Finally, peak flow monitoring during an acute exacerbation can provide information about the severity of the episode and can help assess the response to therapeutic strategies that are implemented.

The NAEPP's expert panel recommends in EPR-2 that the patient and the physician determine the patient's best peak flow value. Once this value has been adequately determined, the "three-zone" system may be used to relate peak flow readings to asthma management. (See Table 10–9.) However, this color-coded scheme, which uses a traffic light analogy, should serve as a guideline only: The patient and his or her physician should individualize the system by defining the peak flow values for each zone that will provide optimal therapy for the patient. A key point in peak flow monitoring is to establish the patient's baseline because this value represents a more practical parameter than a population value. Until the patient's best peak flow value is determined (e.g., typically after a few weeks of optimal therapy), the use of population averages (based on age, height, and gender) is helpful.[24] An example of an action plan developed for a patient is described in Figure 10–5.

CONCLUSIONS

Asthma is a chronic inflammatory disease of the airways that requires continuous care. Asthma therapy is directed at preventing severe attacks and at normalizing an asthma patient's lifestyle. Treatment involves pharmacologic and nonpharmacologic strategies. Nonprescription medications currently available for managing asthma are suited only for managing mild, infrequent symptoms. Asthma medications are classified as long-term control therapies or as quick-relief agents.

Pharmacists can play a major role in facilitating optimal control of asthma. Pharmaceutical care for asthma patients

Table 10–9

Three-Zone System of Asthma Management

Zone	Peak Flow Values	Patient Guideline
Green	≥80% to 100% of the patient's personal best, or the predicted flow value indicated by a standard chart	*Go!* Continue regular activity and regular asthma maintenance therapy.
Yellow	50% to 79% of the patient's personal best, or the predicted flow value indicated by a standard chart	*Caution!* Patient may require additional medication or increase in regular maintenance therapy.
Red	<50% of the patient's personal best, or the predicted flow value indicated by a standard chart	*Stop!* Initiate action plan (inhaled medication or prednisone) immediately.

ASTHMA ACTION PLAN

Patient Name:________________________________ Date:________________________________

Predicted or personal best (circle one) peak flow:________________________________

Peak Flow: ____ to ____ *Green Zone Action Steps*

CONTROLLED: No symptoms, able to do usual activities.

1. Avoid triggers that cause your asthma to be worse.
2. Monitor peak flow each morning and after quick-relief medication (record as instructed).
3. Take your daily green zone medications for long-term control as described.

Peak Flow: ____ to ____ *Yellow Zone Action Steps*

CAUTION: Increased asthma symptoms, usual activities limited, increased need for quick-relief medication Take action to get your asthma under control.

1. Take your quick-relief medication:
   - Albuterol MDI 2 puffs.
   - Albuterol nebulizer treatment.
   - Other ________________________________
2. Measure your peak flow 20 minutes after using above medication:
   - If peak flow is in the green zone, continue regular medication, and monitor peak flow twice daily for 2 days.
   - If peak flow is still in yellow zone,

     —Use albuterol MDI 2 puffs 3 times daily.

     —Use albuterol nebulizer treatment every 6 hours.

     —Increase inhaled anti-inflammatory to ________________.

     —Use prednisone ____ mg ____ times/day for 5 days.

     —Monitor peak flow twice daily for 5 days.

Peak Flow: ____ to ____ *Red Zone Action Steps*

EMERGENCY: Symptoms for more than 24 hours, medications not helping, very short of breath, usual activities severely limited.

1. Take your quick-relief medication IMMEDIATELY:
   - Albuterol MDI 2 puffs.
   - Albuterol nebulizer treatment.
   - Prednisone ____ mg ____ times/day for 5 days.
   - Other ________________________________
2. Measure your peak flow 20 minutes after using medication:
   - If peak flow is in green or yellow zone, follow steps above.
   - If peak flow is still in red zone,

     —Use albuterol MDI 2 puffs 3 times daily.

     —Use albuterol nebulizer treatment every 6 hours.

     —Increase inhaled anti-inflammatory to ________________.

     —Contact physician immediately by phone.

ALWAYS call your doctor to notify him or her of your red zone event!

Physician Name: ________________________________

Pharmacist Name: ________________________________

Physician Number: ________________________________

Pharmacy Number: ________________________________

Figure 10–5 Patient's asthma action plan.

involves a multifaceted approach of education, counseling, instruction, monitoring, and encouragement. Because most therapies for asthma are delivered through inhalation, patient education and instruction about techniques in using various inhalation devices are important. Asthma self-management by the patient is an essential component of optimal care. Patients should have written self-management and action plans.

References

1. National Heart, Lung, and Blood Institute. *Morbidity and Mortality: 1996 Chartbook on Cardiovascular, Lung and Blood Diseases.* Rockville, MD: National Institutes of Health; May 1996.
2. No-Scrip Meds Don't Help Matters. Available at: www.nydailynews.com/archives/98_022598/news/49476.htm. Accessed March 22, 2000.
3. Kelso TM, Abou-Shala N, Heilker GM, et al. Comprehensive long-term management program for asthma: effect on outcomes in adult African-Americans. *Am J Med Sci.* 1996;311:272–80.
4. Kelso TM, Self TH, Rumbak MJ, et al. Educational and long-term therapeutic intervention in the ED: effect on outcomes in adult indigent minority asthmatics. *Am J Emerg Med.* 1995;13:632–7.
5. Im JH. Evaluation of the effectiveness of an asthma clinic managed by an ambulatory care pharmacist. *Calif J Hosp Pharm.* 1993;5:5–6.
6. Pauley TR, Magee MJ, Cury JD. Pharmacist-managed, physician-directed asthma management program reduces emergency department visits. *Ann Pharmacother.* 1995;29:5–9.
7. Diamond S, Chapman K. The impact of a nationally coordinated pharmacy-based asthma education intervention. *Am J Respir Crit Care Med.* 1999;159(No. 3 pt 2):A242.
8. Cheng B, Paulson Y, Wan H, et al. Evaluation of the long-term outcome of adult patients managed by a pharmacist-run asthma program in a health maintenance organization. *J Allergy Clin Immunol.* 1999;103:2.
9. Wan H, Kurohara M. Utilization outcomes evaluation of a clinical pharmacist run adult asthma management program. *J Allergy Clin Immunol.* 1999;103:18.
10. McGill KA, Sorkness CA, Decker CA, et al. Improved asthma outcomes in Head Start children using pharmacist asthma counselors. *Am J Respir Crit Care Med.* 1997;155:A202.
11. Knoell DL, Pierson JF, Marsh CB, et al. Measurement of outcomes in adults receiving pharmaceutical care in a comprehensive asthma outpatient clinic. *Pharmacotherapy.* 1998;18:365–74.
12. National Heart, Lung, and Blood Institute. *Fiscal Year 1997 Fact Book.* Rockville, MD: National Institutes of Health; February 1998.
13. National Heart, Lung, and Blood Institute. *Global Initiative for Asthma.* Pub No. 95–3659. Bethesda, MD: US Department of Health and Human Services; 1995.
14. Burrows B, Barbee RA, Cline MG, et al. Characteristics of asthma among elderly adults in a sample of the general population. *Chest.* 1991;100:935–42.
15. Centers for Disease Control and Prevention. CDC surveillance summaries, April 24, 1998. *Morbid Mortal Wkly Rep MMWR.* 1998;47(No. SS-1).
16. *National Vital Statistics Report.* 1998;47(14). Available at: www.cdc.gov/nchswww/fastats/asthma/htm. Accessed March 22, 2000.
17. Kelly HW, Kamada AK. Asthma. In: DiPiro JT, Talbert RL, Yee GC, et al., eds. *Pharmacotherapy: A Pathophysiologic Approach.* 4th ed. Stamford, Conn: Appleton & Lange; 1999:430–59.
18. Kaliner MA, Barnes PJ, Persson CGA. *Asthma: Its Pathology and Treatment.* New York: Marcel Dekker; 1991.
19. *Clinical Practice Guidelines. Expert Panel Report 2: Guidelines for the Diagnosis and Management of Asthma.* NIH Publication 97-4051. Rockville, MD: National Heart, Lung, and Blood Institute; April 1997.
20. Slepian IK, Mathews KP, McLean JA. Aspirin-sensitive asthma. *Chest.* 1985;87:386–91.
21. Fish JE, Peters SP. Airway remodeling and persistent airway obstruction in asthma. *J Allergy Clin Immunol.* 1999;104:509–16.
22. Barnes PJ. A new approach to the treatment of asthma. *N Engl J Med.* 1989;321:1517–27.
23. Hargreave FE, Gibson PG, Ramsdale EH. Airway hyperresponsiveness, airway inflammation, and asthma. *Immunol Allergy Clin North Am.* 1990;10:439–48.
24. *Practical Guide for the Diagnosis and Management of Asthma.* NIH Pub No. 97-4053. Rockville, MD: National Heart, Lung, and Blood Institute; October 1997. Available at: www.nhlbi.nih.gov/health/prof/lung/asthma/practgde.htm. Accessed March 22, 2000.
25. Hartert TV, Windom HH, Peebles RS, et al. Inadequate outpatient medical therapy for patients with asthma admitted to two urban hospitals. *Am J Med.* 1996;100:386–94.
26. National Heart, Lung, and Blood Institute, National Asthma Education and Prevention Program. *The Role of the Pharmacist in Improving Asthma Care.* NIH Pub No. 95–3280. Bethesda, MD: US Department of Health and Human Services; 1995.
27. *USP DI 2000: Advice for the Patient.* Vol II. Englewood, CO: Micromedex 2000.
28. Cold, cough, allergy, bronchodilator, and antiasthmatic drug products for over-the-counter human use; combination bronchodilator drug products containing theophylline; final rule. *Federal Register.* 1995;60:38636–42.
29. The news this week. *FDC Reports—The Tan Sheet.* 1994;2(47):5–7.
30. Wilson SR, Scamagas P, German DF, et al. A controlled trial of two forms of self-management education for adults with asthma. *Am J Med.* 1993;94:564–76.
31. Abramson MJ, Puy RM, Weiner JM. Is allergen immunotherapy effective in asthma? A meta-analysis of randomized controlled trials. *Am J Respir Crit Care Med.* 1995;151:969–74.
32. Strayhorn V, Leeper K, Tolley E, et al. Elevation of peak expiratory flow by a "spitting" manuever: measured with five peak flow meters. *Chest.* 1998;113:1134–6.
33. Gibson P, Henry D, Francis L, et al. Association between availability of non-prescription beta$_2$ agonist inhalers and undertreatment of asthma. *Br Med J.* 1993;306:1514–8.
34. Report of the FDA advisory review panel on OTC cold, cough, allergy, bronchodilator, and antiasthma drug products. *Federal Register.* 1976;41:38312.
35. Cold, cough, allergy, bronchodilator, and antiasthma drug products for over-the-counter human use. *Federal Register.* 1991;56:190–7.
36. Gorman C. Asthma! The hidden killer. *Time.* August 7, 1995;146(6):56.
37. Vestal RE, Wood AJJ, Shand DG. Reduced β-adrenoceptor sensitivity in the elderly. *Clin Pharmacol Ther.* 1979;26:181–6.
38. New reporting requirements for ephedrine take effect. *Am J Health Syst Pharm.* 1995;52:10.
39. Cold, cough, allergy, bronchodilator, and antiasthmatic drug products for over-the-counter human use; proposed amendment of monograph for OTC bronchodilator drug products. *Federal Register.* 1995;60:38643–47.
40. World Health Organization scheduling recommendations for ephedrine, dihydroetorphine, remifentanil, and certain isomers. *Federal Register.* 1999:64:1629–34.
41. Van Mieghem W, Stevens E, Cosemans J. Ephedrine-induced cardiopathy. *Br Med J.* 1978;1:816.
42. Roxanas MG, Spalding J. Ephedrine abuse psychosis. *Med J Aust.* 1977;2:639–40.
43. Adverse events associated with ephedrine-containing products—Texas, December 1993–September 1995. *Morbid Mortal Wkly Rep MMWR.* 1996;45:689–92.
44. Kelly HW. New beta$_2$-adrenergic agonist aerosols. *Clin Pharm.* 1985;4:393–403.
45. Lipworth BJ, Struthers AD, McDevitt DG. Tachyphylaxis to systemic but not to airway response during prolonged therapy with high dose inhaled salbutamol in patients with asthma. *Am Rev Respir Dis.* 1989;140:586–92.
46. Holgate ST, Finnerty JP. Antihistamines in asthma. *J Allergy Clin Immunol.* 1989;83:537–47.
47. Lantner R, Tobin MC. Pharmacist advice to asthmatics regarding antihistamine use. *Ann Allergy.* 1991;66:411–3.
48. Armitage JM, Williams SJ. Inhaler technique in the elderly. *Age Ageing.* 1988;17:275–8.

49. Croft RD. 2 year old asthmatics can learn to operate a tube spacer by copying their mothers. *Arch Dis Child.* 1989;64:742.
50. Lee H, Evans HE. Evaluation of inhalation aids of metered-dose inhalers in asthmatic children. *Chest.* 1987;91:366–9.
51. Eisenberg DM, Kessler RC, Foster C, et al. Unconventional medicine in the United States: prevalence, costs, and patterns of use. *N Engl J Med.* 1993;328:246–52.
52. Kleijnen J, ter Riet G, Knipschild P. Acupuncture and asthma: a review of controlled trials. *Thorax.* 1991;46:799–802.
53. Reilly DT, Taylor MA, McSharry C, et al. Is homeopathy a placebo response? Controlled trial of homeopathic potency, with pollen in hayfever as model. *Lancet.* 1986;2:881–6.
54. Ziment I, Stein M. Inappropriate and unusual remedies. In: Weiss EB, Stein M, eds. *Bronchial Asthma.* Boston: Little, Brown, and Company; 1993:1145–51.
55. Blanc PD, Kuschner WG, Katz PP, et al. Use of herbal products, coffee or black tea, and over-the-counter medications as self-treatments among adults with asthma. *J Allergy Clin Immunol.* 1997;100:789–91.
56. Jackson AC. Accuracy, reproducibility, and variability of portable peak flowmeters. *Chest.* 1995;107:648–51.
57. Newman SP, Pavia D, Moren F, et al. Deposition of pressurized aerosols in the human respiratory tract. *Thorax.* 1981;36:52–5.
58. Kelly HW. Correct aerosol medication use and the health professions: who will teach the teachers? *Chest.* 1993;104:1648–9.
59. Kesten S, Zive K, Chapman KR. Pharmacist knowledge and ability to use inhaled medication delivery systems. *Chest.* 1993;104:1737–42.
60. Interiano B, Guntupalli KK. Metered dose inhalers: do health providers know what to teach? *Arch Intern Med.* 1993;153:81–5.
61. Guidry GG, Brown WD, Stogner SW, et al. Incorrect use of metered-dose inhalers by medical personnel. *Chest.* 1992;101:31–3.
62. Mickle TR, Self TH, Farr GE, et al. Evaluation of pharmacists' practice in patient education when dispensing a metered-dose inhaler. *DICP.* 1990;24:927–30.
63. Self TH, Brooks JB, Lieberman P, et al. The value of demonstration and role of the pharmacist in teaching the correct use of pressurized bronchodilators. *Can Med Assoc J.* 1983;128:129–31.
64. Spitzer WO, Suissa S, Ernst P, et al. The use of beta agonists and the risk of death and near death from asthma. *N Engl J Med.* 1992;326:501–6.

SECTION V

GASTROINTESTINAL DISORDERS

CHAPTER 11

Acid–Peptic Disorders and Intestinal Gas

Robert P. Henderson

Chapter 11 at a Glance

In the United States, 25% of adults report having at least one episode of dyspepsia in an average 2-week period.[1] The underlying conditions responsible for this complaint range from mild "heartburn" caused by gastric reflux to serious gastrointestinal (GI) disorders that require medical attention. Self-care is an important part of managing upper abdominal pain and discomfort, as seen by the popularity of antacids, antireflux agents, and antiflatulents. Patients will frequently pursue self-treatment initially rather than seek medical care, thus underscoring the importance of involving the pharmacist.

Total sales of nonprescription drugs have consistently

Editor's Note: This chapter is based, in part, on the 11th edition chapter titled "Acid–Peptic Products," which was written by Julianne B. Pinson and C. Wayne Weart.

grown, estimated at more than $16 billion in 1997.[2] The nonprescription market grew by approximately 5% from 1997 to 1998, and the top five categories of products include antacids and antiflatulents.[3]

Antacids are useful for the short-term relief of indigestion, heartburn, and symptoms associated with gastroesophageal reflux disease (GERD) and with peptic ulcer disease (PUD). The availability of nonprescription histamine$_2$-receptor antagonists (H_2RAs) has broadened the scope of self-care of GI complaints. It is important that the pharmacist be able to distinguish between patients who can be appropriately self-treated and those who need additional medical attention. The pharmacist should then be able to recommend appropriate nonprescription products for patients with mild GI complaints.

Anatomy and Physiology of the Upper Gastrointestinal System

An understanding of the physiology of the esophagus, stomach, and duodenum is essential to understanding the pathophysiology and pharmacotherapy of upper GI disorders.

The esophagus serves as a conduit between the pharynx and the stomach and is closed at both ends by the upper esophageal sphincter and the lower esophageal sphincter (LES). The LES is an area of specialized smooth muscle located at the lower end of the esophagus, about 2 to 5 cm above the junction where the stomach meets the esophagus. When at rest, the LES is contracted, preventing the passage of stomach contents into the esophagus. When swallowing occurs, the LES relaxes and allows food to pass into the stomach.

The anatomic and functionally distinct regions of the stomach are the cardia, fundus, body, and antrum. The cardia contains mucus-secreting cells. The body and fundus account for 80% to 90% of the stomach's mass and contain parietal cells (responsible for hydrochloric acid and intrinsic factor secretion that is necessary for vitamin B_{12} absorption) and chief cells (responsible for pepsinogen secretion). The antrum contains G cells, which are responsible for gastrin secretion.

Regulation of Gastric Acid Secretion

Gastric acid and pepsin are powerful proteolytic substances that hydrolyze protein and other foods so they can be absorbed by the intestine. In addition, gastric acid kills most bacteria in the stomach.

Parietal cells have receptors for histamine, acetylcholine, and gastrin, all of which can induce gastric acid secretion. When any of these substances comes into contact with its receptors on the parietal cell, intracellular calcium and cyclic adenosine monophosphate (cAMP) concentrations increase.[4] The increased levels of calcium and cAMP activate a unique proton pump, adenosine triphosphatase, found only on the membranes of parietal cells. When stimulated, the proton pump secretes hydrogen ions in the stomach lumen in exchange for potassium. The proton pump can be stimulated directly by calcium and cAMP and indirectly by histamine, acetylcholine, and gastrin. Thus, the proton pump is the final common pathway for acid secretion from these stimuli.

The parietal cells serve as the target for pharmacologic inhibition of acid secretion. Anticholinergic agents inhibit acid secretion by occupying the acetylcholine receptor. H_2RAs reduce acid secretion by blocking the histamine$_2$ receptors. Proton pump inhibitors abolish acid secretion regardless of the stimulus because the proton pump is the final step in acid secretion.

Pepsinogen is released by the chief cells of the body, and fundus is released by vagal stimulation (acetylcholine) and histamine. In the presence of acid, pepsinogen is hydrolyzed to the active proteolytic enzyme pepsin. Pepsin is active when the pH ranges from 1.8 to 3.5 and is inactivated when the pH exceeds 5.[5]

Gastric acid secretion occurs continuously; however, the rate and amount secreted depend on whether the stomach has been stimulated or is in the basal state, when no stimuli are present. Both basal and stimulated acid outputs vary considerably among individuals and are generally higher in men than in women. Basal acid secretion follows a circadian rhythm, with peak secretion occurring in the evening and with lowest secretion in the morning.[5]

Mucosal Defense Mechanisms

The gastric mucosa is equipped to withstand the acidic environment of the stomach through a combination of defense and repair mechanisms that are collectively called the gastric mucosal barrier. Gastric epithelial cells secrete mucus and bicarbonate that help to protect the mucosa from damage. Mucus and bicarbonate serve as a barrier to limit penetration of hydrogen ions across the gastric mucosa ("back-diffusion"). Rapid gastric mucosal blood flow allows (1) removal of hydrogen ions that cross the gastric mucosa and (2) rapid healing in the presence of damage. If this blood flow is compromised, the risk of mucosal damage is increased. When damage does occur, the epithelial cells have a special ability to repair themselves quickly through rapid cell turnover. This process, known as restitution or reconstitution, is aided by the delivery of oxygen and other nutrients to the cells by the mucosal blood supply.[4]

Prostaglandins, such as prostaglandin E_2, are synthesized by the gastric mucosa and work to enhance its protective mechanisms. Prostaglandins inhibit gastric acid secretion from the parietal cells, increase mucus and bicarbonate secretion from the epithelial cells, and help maintain mucosal blood flow.

Esophageal defense mechanisms differ from those of the stomach. The factors that normally protect the esophagus from acid reflux include (1) barriers that limit the rate of reflux, (2) clearance mechanisms that limit the duration of contact of refluxate with the epithelium, and (3) esophageal mucosal resistance that minimizes epithelial damage from noxious gastric contents.[6] The gastroduodenal epithelium rapidly repairs mucosal injury (rapid restitution), thus allowing cell replication. The esophagus does not undergo a rapid repair process. Once injury occurs to the esophageal mucosa, cell replication takes from days to weeks for complete healing to occur.[7]

The maintenance of normal mucosal defense mechanisms protects the esophagus, stomach, and duodenum from acid and pepsin. When this barrier is disrupted, however, acid and pepsin predominate; then mucosal injury and ulceration occur. Although acid and pepsin play a critical role in the pathogenesis of acid–peptic diseases, a breakdown in mucosal defense is equally important in determining whether disease will occur. Normally, these protective mechanisms counteract aggressive forces on the gastric mucosa. Ulceration typically develops when there is a deficiency in protective factors or an excess in aggressive factors.

Gastroesophageal Reflux Disease

The reflux of gastric contents into the esophagus, or GERD, is generally a benign physiologic process that occurs in normal individuals. Most of these episodes do not cause mucosal damage to the esophagus.

Epidemiology of Gastroesophageal Reflux Disease

It has been estimated that up to 50% of the population will experience occasional episodes of reflux and that approximately 7% experience it daily. Among the U.S. population, 10% to 20% experience GERD that is serious enough to require medication.[8,9] Among pregnant women, 30% to 50% have symptomatic gastroesophageal reflux, and approximately 25% complain of heartburn daily. Gastroesophageal reflux occurs commonly in infants and children. Most patients with GERD have only mild and sporadic symptoms. Accordingly, most patients do not seek medical attention from a physician but rather seek symptomatic relief from antacid products.

Etiology of Gastroesophageal Reflux Disease

GERD is caused by retrograde flow of gastric contents into the esophagus. The acidic contents damage tissue of the esophagus, oropharynx, larynx, and respiratory system.[6] What distinguishes patients with GERD from those with normal physiologic reflux is the frequency and duration of reflux episodes, which can result in related signs and symptoms and/or esophageal tissue damage.

Pathophysiology of Gastroesophageal Reflux Disease

The pathogenesis of GERD can be described as an imbalance between aggressive and protective factors. The aggressive side of this balance is determined by the noxious quality of the gastric contents that reflux into the esophagus. Most patients with GERD secrete normal or greater than normal amounts of gastric acid; thus they have acid reflux.

The major barrier that prevents the passage of stomach contents into the esophagus is the LES. Normal individuals experience transient relaxation of the LES multiple times throughout the day. Patients with GERD, however, tend to have more episodes of transient relaxation of the LES and, thus, reflux more often than healthy individuals do. Many patients with GERD also have a weak, or hypotonic, LES.[6,9] In such patients, the high pressure in the stomach creates enough force to overcome the LES strength, allowing reflux to occur. Many factors may promote reflux by reducing LES tone, delaying gastric emptying, increasing acid secretion, or impairing the gastroesophageal pressure gradient. (See Table 11–1.)

After reflux occurs, the symptoms and degree of damage depend on the duration of contact between the gastric contents and the esophageal mucosa. The esophagus normally clears the refluxate by one to two peristaltic contractions induced by swallowing. Gravity hastens this process when the patient is upright, but it does not operate when the patient is lying down. The residual acid refluxate in the esophagus is then neutralized by bicarbonate-rich saliva that has been swallowed. A defect in one or both of these processes may lead to increased contact time with refluxed material and to the development of esophagitis. These mechanisms are impaired during sleep, when there is neither swallowing nor salivation and when clearance by gravity is not operative. Thus, prolonged acid exposure may occur during sleep and predispose patients to esophagitis.[6,9] Esophageal damage caused by reflux occurs more often in the elderly. Saliva production diminishes with age, and reduced esophageal motility impairs clearance of refluxed material.[9,10]

Helicobacter pylori is a known cause of chronic gastritis and PUD; however, its role in the pathogenesis of GERD is the subject of current study and controversy. Evidence indicates that *H. pylori* has little or no role in the development of GERD and may not require eradication, except in conjunction with gastritis and PUD.[11]

Signs and Symptoms of Gastroesophageal Reflux Disease

The most common form of GERD is reflux esophagitis, which develops when the acidic contents of the stomach make prolonged contact with esophageal tissue. This contact may produce a broad range of damage, such as inflammation, hyperplasia, esophageal erosions, or ulcerations.[6] Heartburn, or pyrosis, occurs in more than half of the pa-

Table 11–1

Factors That Promote Gastroesophageal Reflux Disease

Factors That Reduce LES Tone

Foods
Chocolates
Fatty foods
Garlic
Onions
Spearmint
Peppermint

Drugs/Substances
α-Adrenergic antagonists
Anticholinergic agents
Barbiturates
β_2-Agonists
Calcium channel antagonists
Cholecystokinin
Diazepam
Dopamine
Ethanol
Estrogen
Gastric acid
Glucagon
Meperidine
Morphine
Nitrates
Progesterone
Prostaglandins (E_1, E_2, and A_2)
Secretin
Somatostatin
Serotonin
Theophylline
Tricyclic antidepressants
Vasoactive intestinal peptide

Other Factors
Smoking (Nicotine)

Factors That Delay Gastric Emptying
Anticholinergic medications
Overeating
Motility disorders

Direct Irritant Effect on Gastric/Esophageal Mucosa

Foods
Spicy foods
Orange juice
Tomato juice
Coffee

Drugs
Alendronate
Aspirin/NSAIDs
Iron
Potassium
Quinidine
Tetracycline
Zidovudine

Factors/Conditions Associated with Increased Acid Secretion
Duodenal ulcers
Endocrine adenomas
Smoking
Zollinger–Ellison syndrome

Impaired Gastroesophageal Pressure Gradient
Bending over
Exercise
Obesity
Straining during bowel movement
Supine body position
Tight-fitting clothing

Sources: References 6, 8, and 9.

tients with this disorder and is usually described as a burning sensation or pain located in the lower chest (substernal area). The pain may radiate up into the chest, into the back, and, less often, into the throat. Most patients complain of heartburn soon after meals and on lying down at bedtime; they may be awakened from sleep because of the pain. It may also occur as the patient bends or stoops over and after some forms of exercise. Some patients have brief episodes of heartburn that are readily relieved by antacids or simple dietary measures; others have persistent and severe symptoms that disrupt their daily lives.

Some patients with GERD may complain of chest pain that is not typical of heartburn and is difficult to distinguish from anginal chest pain caused by ischemic heart disease.[6] Like anginal pain, this atypical chest pain may be sharp or dull and may radiate widely, extending into the neck or arms. Severe, crushing chest pain—especially if accompanied by sweating—strongly suggests ischemic pain and possibly myocardial infarction, which requires immediate medical attention. Pain that is exacerbated by physical activity or exercise, but that subsides with rest or nitroglycerin, is consistent with anginal pain rather than with GERD. Other symptoms of reflux disease may occur with or without heartburn and may include dysphagia, odynophagia, hypersalivation, and regurgitation of liquid into the mouth. Patients complain of an acid, burning, or bitter taste and may refer to this problem as "sour stomach." Patients with delayed gastric emptying often complain of bloating, early satiety, belching, and nausea.

Complications of Gastroesophageal Reflux Disease

Complications of GERD include acute and chronic bleeding from esophageal ulcers, esophageal strictures, and extra esophageal manifestations. Dysphagia, a sensation of slow or blocked passage of food from the mouth to the esophagus, may indicate an esophageal stricture (narrowing of the esophageal lumen), cancer, or motility disorder. Odynophagia, or pain on swallowing, usually suggests severe mucosal damage in the esophagus. Extra esophageal manifestations include pulmonary complications that result from the aspiration of refluxed material into the upper airways and lungs and that can produce hoarseness, cough, laryngitis, bronchitis, pneumonia, chest pain, and nonallergic asthma. Approximately 10% to 15% of patients with erosive esophagitis develop Barrett's esophagus.[6] Barrett's esophagus is associated with midesophageal strictures, esophageal ulcers, and histologic changes in the lower esophageal mucosa that may become cancerous in 5% to 10% of patients, usually by the time of diagnosis.[8,9] Approximately one-third of all esophageal cancers are linked with Barrett's esophagitis. The incidence of esophageal cancer, especially adenocarcinoma, has risen rapidly over the past few decades.[12] Additional evidence shows that a strong association exists between gastroesophageal reflux and the risk of esophageal cancer, regardless of the presence of Barrett's esophagus.[13] Any patient presenting with a history of bleeding, possibly from the esophagus or stomach, should be referred immediately to a physician.

Treatment of Gastroesophageal Reflux Disease

The pharmacist will often be the first health care professional encountered by patients with GERD, because most patients do not seek professional help until they have severe symptoms.[8] Thus, the pharmacist has a special opportunity and responsibility to ensure that patients' symptoms are appropriate for self-medication and to recommend the appropriate treatments.

Treatment Outcomes

The goals of therapy for GERD are to (1) reduce or eliminate symptoms, (2) reduce or eliminate the occurrence of reflux, (3) limit or prevent damage to the esophagus, and (4) prevent complications and recurrences of GERD.

General Treatment Approach

The overall management of GERD may be viewed as a stepped-care approach as outlined in Figure 11–1.[9] The management of mild heartburn with nonpharmacologic measures and antacids or with nonprescription H_2RAs forms the basis for accomplishing the treatment outcomes. These measures may help to alleviate symptoms in patients but cannot be expected to heal patients with damaged esophageal mucosa or to prevent complications.[8,9]

The fundamental premise of controlling the symptoms and allowing healing to occur is to decrease the exposure to the acidic refluxate. This control is best achieved by increasing the intragastric pH above 4 for as long as possible.[7] Because a causal relationship appears to exist between reflux and esophageal adenocarcinoma, the treatment used should progress rapidly toward prescription antisecretory agents if not controlled adequately by nonprescription medications.[13] If antacids or H_2RAs are recommended in any of these situations and if the patient does not experience prompt relief, the pharmacist should refer the patient to a physician for further evaluation. Similarly, patients with symptoms that are relieved by these products but that frequently recur probably warrant medical attention.

Antacids and nonprescription H_2RAs are useful for patients who need symptomatic relief for mild-to-moderate GERD. These agents reduce the aggressive factors in GERD by neutralizing gastric acid and by increasing the pH of refluxed gastric contents. As a result, the refluxed contents are not as damaging to the esophageal mucosa. Antacids also strengthen defensive forces because gastric alkalinization increases LES pressure. The nonprescription H_2RAs are indicated for relieving heartburn, acid indigestion, and sour stomach for preventing these symptoms, which are brought on by consuming food and beverages.

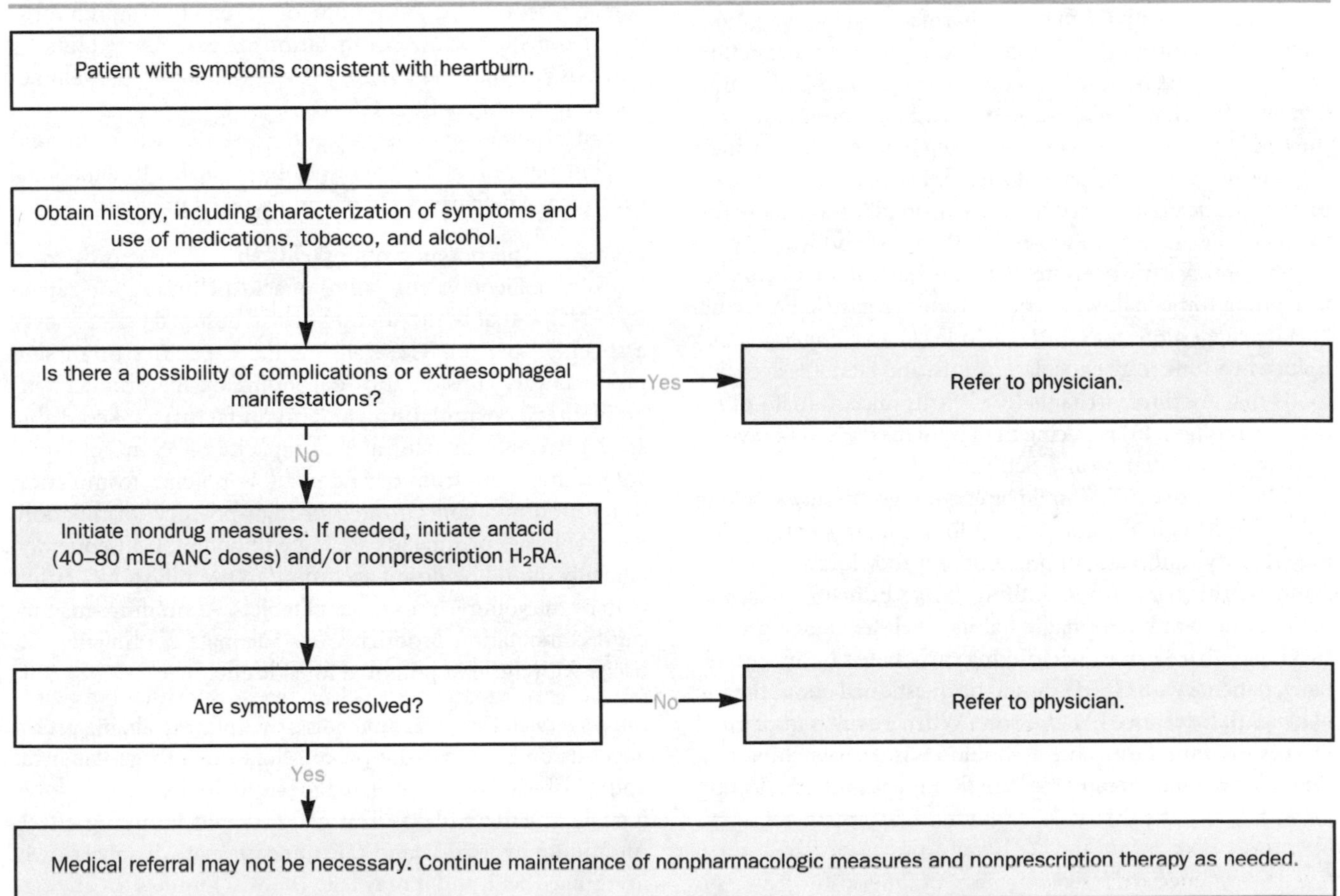

Figure 11–1 Self-care of gastroesophageal reflux disease.

Moderate-to-severe GERD may require high doses of prescription H_2RAs or proton pump inhibitors because damaged mucosa in the esophagus is more difficult to heal than that in the duodenum. Some patients may benefit from adding a prokinetic agent that stimulates esophageal motility, such as cisapride, metoclopramide, or bethanechol chloride. Patients with recurring disease require maintenance therapy with full doses of H_2RAs, proton pump inhibitors, or antireflux surgery to restore competence of the LES.

Any patient who describes complications from GERD or angina-like symptoms should be referred to a physician for evaluation. Because of the relationship of reflux and associated complications, including the risk of cancer, patients whose treatment outcomes are not accomplished with nonpharmacologic and nonprescription therapy should be referred to a primary care provider as soon as possible.

Nonpharmacologic Therapy

Dietary and lifestyle modifications are considered a cornerstone of therapy for GERD. Some patients with mild GERD can be managed with such measures alone and without pharmacologic intervention. Those who respond to antacids or nonprescription H_2RAs should still be educated about lifestyle modifications because such changes may significantly reduce or eliminate symptoms.

For patients with GERD, nonpharmacologic interventions attempt to reduce or eliminate factors that promote reflux. Nocturnal reflux is more likely during sleep because of recumbency.[6,9] Patients should be instructed to elevate the head of the bed at least 6 inches either by using blocks or by placing a foam wedge under the patient's head. Patients should not try to raise the head of the bed by sleeping on pillows because this practice will cause them to bend at the waist and will actually increase intragastric pressure. Eating no later than 3 hours before going to bed allows adequate time for gastric emptying. Dietary suggestions for GERD include (1) avoiding foods that reduce LES tone (e.g., chocolate, mints, and fats), (2) avoiding foods that are direct irritants (e.g., citrus juice, tomato products, and coffee), (3) reducing the size of meals, and (4) avoiding lying down after meals. (See Table 11–1.)

Patients with GERD should be encouraged to stop smoking and to limit their alcohol intake. Obese patients with GERD may have symptomatic improvement if they lose weight and avoid wearing tight-fitting clothing. It may be helpful to advise patients to avoid aerophagic habits, such as chewing gum, sucking on hard candy, or drinking carbonated beverages. Finally, patients with GERD should be questioned about the use of drugs that decrease LES pressure. When a drug is implicated in causing reflux, the patient should consider switching to a drug with similar therapeutic benefit but without an effect on the LES.

Pharmacologic Therapy

Antacids

Four primary neutralizing compounds are found in antacid products: sodium bicarbonate, calcium carbonate, aluminum salts (hydroxide, phosphate), and magnesium salts (hydroxide, chloride). All antacid products contain at least one of these ingredients, which differ significantly in potency, GI side effects, systemic complications, and drug interactions. Most of these properties are determined by the metal cation of the antacid and by the degree of its systemic absorption.

Mechanism of Action All antacids are basic compounds that react with gastric acid to form a salt and water. Antacids neutralize existing gastric acid; they do not affect the amount or rate of gastric acid secreted. Antacids increase pH in both the stomach and the duodenal bulb, with a greater effect on duodenal pH than on gastric pH. Antacids do not neutralize all stomach acid; with usual therapeutic doses, they do not raise and cannot maintain gastric pH above 4 to 5.[14] However, when the pH is increased from 1.3 to 2.3, 90% of acid is neutralized; at a pH of 3.3, 99% is neutralized.[14]

Antacids also inhibit the conversion of pepsinogen to pepsin, which depends on the degree of acid neutralization. Pepsin is most active at a pH of 1.8 to 3, and progressive inhibition occurs as gastric pH increases.[4,15] At a pH of 4 or greater, pepsin activity is completely inhibited. Additionally, aluminum-containing antacids have been reported to bind pepsin.[14]

Aluminum antacids appear to delay gastric emptying, presumably because the aluminum ion relaxes the smooth muscle of the stomach. Alkalinization of gastric contents by antacids generally increases LES tone, which may partially account for their benefit in GERD.

Antacids may have healing and protective actions beyond and independent of their neutralizing capacities by enhancing the mucosal defense mechanisms discussed previously.[16]

Potency The potency of antacids should be expressed in terms of milliequivalent (mEq) of acid-neutralization capacity (ANC)—that is, the amount of acid buffered per dose over a specified period. The neutralizing capacities of antacid products vary considerably, depending on the product's ingredient(s), formulation, and manufacturer. (See Table 11–2.) Because the neutralizing capacity of 15 mL of liquid antacid may vary from 6 mEq in a low-potency formulation to 60 mEq in a concentrated or high-potency formulation, equal volumes of antacids are not equipotent. Consequently, antacids should be dosed according to the mEq ANC rather than by the volume or number of tablets. Aluminum–magnesium combination products offer adequate neutralizing capacity with the least potential for side effects.

Pharmacokinetics An antacid's onset of neutralizing action depends on how fast the product dissolves in gastric acid. Sodium bicarbonate and magnesium hydroxide dissolve quickly at gastric pH and provide a rapid buffering effect. Aluminum hydroxide and calcium carbonate dissolve slowly in stomach acid, and it may take 10 to 30 minutes for any significant neutralization to take place. Antacid suspensions generally dissolve more easily in gastric acid than do tablets or powders.

Table 11–2

Comparison of Selected Antacid Suspension and Tablet Product Formulations[a]

Antacid Suspension	mEq ANC per mL[b]	Equivalent Volume[c]	Antacid Tablet	mEq ANC per tablet[b]	Equivalent No. Tablets[c]
Riopan Extra Strength	6	13.3	Maalox TC	28	3
Extra Strength Maalox Plus	5.8	13.8	Riopan Plus 2	30	3
Maalox-TC	5.44	14.7	Extra Strength Maalox	23.4	4
Mylanta II	5.08	15.7	Mylanta II	23	4
Gelusil-II	4.8	16.7	Gelusil-II	21	4
Camalox	3.7	21.6	Camalox	18	5
ALternaGEL	3.2	25	Amphojel (600 mg)	16	5
Riopan Plus	3	26.7	Riopan Plus	13.5	6
Milk of Magnesia	2.8	28.6	Temp	14.4	6
Maalox	2.66	30	Tums E-X	15	6
Mylanta	2.54	31.5	Basaljel	13	7
Di-Gel	2.45	32.7	Mylanta	11.5	7
Gelusil	2.4	33.3	Maalox Plus	11.4	7
Basaljel	2.4	33.3	Tums	10	8
Titralac Plus	2.2	36.4	Gelusil	11	8
Kolantyl Gel	2.1	38.1	Maalox	9.7	9
Amphojel	2	40	Rolaids Sodium-Free	8.5	10
Gaviscon	0.8	100	Titralac	7.5	11
			Gaviscon	0.5	160

[a] Products are listed in order of decreasing strength per ANC.

[b] Acid-neutralizing capacity (ANC), as stated by the product's manufacturer.

[c] Equivalent volumes (mL) or number of tablets calculated to provide 80 mEq ANC.

An antacid's duration of action depends on how long the product remains in the stomach, which is determined by gastric emptying time. If taken on an empty stomach, antacids are rapidly emptied from the stomach and have a duration of action of only 20 to 40 minutes.[17] However, gastric emptying is greatly slowed by the presence of food; thus, antacids taken after meals leave the stomach more slowly. When taken 1 hour after meals, antacids may neutralize acid for up to 3 hours. Sodium bicarbonate and magnesium hydroxide have the shortest duration of neutralizing action, whereas aluminum hydroxide and calcium carbonate have the longest. Combination aluminum–magnesium antacids have an intermediate duration of neutralizing action.

Indications The Food and Drug Administration (FDA) has approved antacids as safe and effective (Category I) for treating heartburn, sour stomach, and acid indigestion. Clinical evidence as to the benefits of antacids in treating GERD, however, provides conflicting results. At least three controlled studies found antacids superior to placebo for symptomatic relief, but two studies failed to find a significant benefit of antacids over placebo.[9,18] In patients whose symptoms are relieved by antacids, relief usually occurs rapidly, within 5 to 15 minutes after administration. Relief can be expected to last from 1 to 3 hours, depending on the gastric emptying rate.

Patients often take antacids for numerous GI complaints besides heartburn, sour stomach, or acid indigestion. One of the most common reasons people take antacids is for relief of symptoms associated with overeating or excessive indulgence in alcohol. FDA has endorsed the use of antacids to relieve symptoms associated with overindulgence in food and drink.[19] Thus, along with indications for heartburn, sour stomach, and acid indigestion, antacid product labeling may include the statement "and upset stomach associated with these symptoms" or "associated with overindulgence in food and drink." FDA has also approved antacid–acetaminophen combination products for the relief of symptoms associated with hangover or overindulgence in food and drink. All combination products for hangover that contain both an antacid and caffeine are considered by FDA as Category II products (not generally recognized as safe and effective).[19]

Dosage/Administration Guidelines Because antacids have a short duration of action, patients taking such agents for GERD may need to take four to five doses throughout the day for adequate symptomatic relief, but the agents cannot be expected to neutralize acid adequately throughout the night. In addition, antacids do not adequately affect the volume of acid secretion or heal eroded esophageal mucosa.[7,18]

Patients seeking relief from GERD with antacid therapy have used numerous dosage regimens. Treatment ranging from high doses of liquid aluminum–magnesium antacids (80 to 160 mEq ANC given seven times daily) to low doses of antacid tablets (14 to 30 mEq ANC/tablet taken as needed) have been reported to provide symptomatic relief.[14,18] Given this variability, it is reasonable to advise patients to begin with 40 to 80 mEq as needed for symptoms. If necessary, doses may be titrated to a scheduled regimen, such as 40 to 80 mEq after meals and at bedtime. Patients should not take more than 500 to 600 mEq per day nor take antacids longer than 2 weeks.

Adverse Effects Although only small amounts of antacids are absorbed in the small intestine, the risk of toxicity from all antacids exists for patients with impaired renal function. Certain antacids pose other risks for specific population groups.

Magnesium The oxide, hydroxide, carbonate, and trisilicate forms of magnesium salts have antacid properties. The hydroxide salt of magnesium is used most often and produces a potent, short-acting neutralizing action. Most of the magnesium chloride formed reacts with bicarbonate in the small intestine, minimizing the risk of systemic alkalosis (increased systemic pH). However, about 5% to 10% of the magnesium chloride is absorbed and rapidly excreted by the kidneys in patients with normal renal function. The risk of cation absorption and toxicity is significant only in patients with impaired renal function. The ANC of magnesium salts is greater than that of aluminum hydroxide but is less than that of sodium bicarbonate and calcium carbonate.

The most frequent and limiting side effect of magnesium-containing antacids is dose-related diarrhea. Magnesium hydroxide that does not react with gastric acid is converted in the small intestine into poorly absorbed magnesium salts, causing an osmotic gradient that is at least partially responsible for the diarrhea associated with magnesium. The incidence of diarrhea from magnesium ranges from 4% in patients taking low-dose antacids (144 mEq per day) to 76% in patients taking higher doses (1064 mEq per day). Diarrhea caused by magnesium does not usually involve abdominal cramps or nocturnal bowel movements. Efforts to minimize this diarrhea include using combination aluminum–magnesium antacid products or alternating aluminum–magnesium therapy with an aluminum-only antacid.

Magnesium toxicity from antacids is rare, occurring primarily in patients with significant renal failure in which it can produce life-threatening complications. Magnesium is a strong central nervous system (CNS) depressant. Severe hypermagnesemia can cause depressed reflexes, muscle paralysis, nausea, vomiting, hypotension, respiratory depression, severe cardiac depression that is manifested clinically as hypotension and bradyarrhythmias, coma, and even death. Considering these risks, magnesium antacids should not be used in patients with marked renal failure (i.e., those with creatinine clearance of less than 30 mL/minute). If they are taken, oral doses of magnesium exceeding 50 mEq per day should be used cautiously and only under the supervision of a primary care provider.

Aluminum Antacids Aluminum hydroxide dissolves slowly in the stomach, where it reacts with gastric acid to form aluminum chloride and water. In the small intestine, aluminum chloride reacts with bicarbonate to form a series of poorly absorbed basic aluminum salts. Because most of the aluminum chloride reacts with intestinal bicarbonate, very little endogenous bicarbonate is left over, and systemic alkalosis is a minimal risk.

The most frequent side effect of aluminum-containing antacids is constipation. Antacids containing aluminum hydroxide have been reported to cause intestinal obstruction, hemorrhoids, fissures, and fecal impaction.[20] Patients predisposed to obstruction include those with reduced bowel motility, dehydration, and fluid restriction. Constipation from aluminum is dose related but can be managed with stool softeners or laxatives or with combination aluminum–magnesium antacids.

Although the formation of insoluble salts limits aluminum absorption, about 17% to 30% of the aluminum chloride formed is absorbed.[20] In patients with normal renal function, this aluminum chloride is rapidly excreted by the kidneys. However, patients who have impaired renal function and who take aluminum antacids chronically may fail to clear the aluminum, resulting in hyperaluminemia and in accumulation of aluminum in other tissues.

Aluminum may be administered in several different salt forms (hydroxide, carbonate, phosphate, or aminoacetate); the hydroxide salt is the most potent buffer and is used most often. In comparison with magnesium hydroxide, calcium carbonate, and sodium bicarbonate, however, aluminum hydroxide has a relatively low ANC.

Available aluminum-containing antacids, except for aluminum phosphate, bind phosphate in the gut, forming insoluble phosphate salts that are excreted in the feces. The result is reduced intestinal phosphate absorption. This effect is beneficial in patients who have chronic renal failure and who have increased serum levels of phosphorous. However, use of aluminum-containing antacids as phosphate binders in patients with renal failure is associated with serious risks. Elevated aluminum concentrations have been reported in the bone, muscle, and brain tissue of such patients.[16]

In patients with normal renal function, reducing phosphate absorption caused by aluminum antacids may lead to clinically significant phosphate depletion. Phosphorous depletion is characterized by anorexia, malaise, and muscle weakness. If severe and prolonged, it may lead to osteomalacia, osteoporosis, and fractures. Although uncommon, phosphorous depletion may occur as early as the second week of therapy and may occur in some patients with dosages of aluminum hydroxide as low as 30 mL three times daily. Other patients at risk for hypophosphatemia include the elderly, alcoholics, and people with diarrhea or malabsorption syndromes.

Aluminum–Magnesium Combinations Many commercially available antacid products contain a mixture of aluminum and magnesium. Because constipation from aluminum and diarrhea from magnesium are dose related, combining these two agents allows for potent ANC with lower doses of each agent. In theory, the constipating effect of aluminum should balance the diarrheal effect of magnesium, and vice versa. However, the optimal ratio between magnesium and aluminum to achieve this balance has not been found in any commercially available product. Diarrhea appears to be the predominant effect, regardless of the ratio, with up to three-fourths of patients taking these combination products experiencing diarrhea; constipation is rarely reported.

The risk of side effects other than those affecting the GI system are not reduced with combination products. To the contrary, the presence of both salts introduces the possibility of side effects from absorption of two cations. Thus, patients taking combination products may experience hypermagnesemia, aluminum intoxication, hypophosphatemia, or metabolic alkalosis. As with either agent alone, these risks appear to be of concern primarily in patients with reduced renal function.

Magaldrate is a chemical mixture of aluminum and magnesium hydroxides that converts to aluminum and magnesium ions in hydrochloric acid. Magaldrate has a lower ANC than does a physical mixture of aluminum and magnesium hydroxides. Because the presence of aluminum is not readily recognized from the term *magaldrate,* the pharmacist should take care not to recommend magaldrate as a non–aluminum-containing product.

Calcium Carbonate Calcium carbonate dissolves more slowly in the stomach than sodium bicarbonate does, but it produces a potent and more prolonged neutralization of gastric acid. It reacts with gastric acid to produce calcium chloride, carbon dioxide, and water. Unlike sodium chloride, which is formed from the reaction of sodium bicarbonate and gastric acid, about 90% of calcium chloride reacts with bicarbonate in the small intestine to form insoluble calcium salts. Because these calcium salts are excreted in the feces and are not absorbed, calcium carbonate is considered a nonsystemic antacid. However, about 10% of the calcium chloride does not react with intestinal bicarbonate; thus, a small percentage of leftover endogenous calcium is reabsorbed into the systemic circulation.

Although a minimal (10%) amount of calcium does not react with intestinal bicarbonate and is absorbed systemically, enough may be absorbed after several days of high-dose antacid ingestion to cause or exacerbate hypercalcemia. Hypercalcemia is characterized by neurologic symptoms, renal calculi, and reduced renal function. These side effects are rare in healthy patients, and they do not appear to occur in patients with normal renal function if daily consumption of calcium carbonate is less than 20 g. However, patients with impaired renal function may develop hypercalcemia from as little as 4 g per day.

Calcium carbonate has been noted to cause acid rebound, which is a sustained hypersecretion of gastric acid after antacid has been emptied from the stomach. Increased gastric acid secretion begins within 2 hours after administration of calcium carbonate and may last for 3 to 5 hours. This effect has been reported after large doses (4 to 8 g) as well as after single, small doses (500 mg). Acid rebound caused by calcium carbonate is particularly pronounced after meals.[14] The mechanism for this effect is not well defined but may be related to a local effect of calcium ions on gastric mucosa in addition to hypergastrinemia.[21] Despite evidence that acid rebound occurs, there is no evidence that it is clinically significant. Acid rebound has not been shown to delay ulcer healing, and no studies suggest that calcium carbonate is inferior to other antacids in treating of acid–peptic disorders.

Sodium Bicarbonate Sodium bicarbonate is widely available in the form of baking soda and is an active component in some nonprescription combination products (e.g., Alka-Seltzer). It is a potent, highly soluble compound that reacts almost instantaneously with acid in the stomach to produce sodium chloride, carbon dioxide, and water. Sodium bicarbonate differs from other antacids in that it has the capability of being absorbed into the systemic circulation and can alter systemic pH. When sodium bicarbonate is taken orally, gastric acid is neutralized by exogenous antacid instead of by endogenous bicarbonate in the intestinal lumen. Because sodium chloride does not react with bicarbonate in the small intestine, this endogenous bicarbonate is "left over" in the small intestine, where it is absorbed into the systemic circulation. Thus, the amount of sodium bicarbonate taken orally equals the amount that is absorbed into the blood. In patients with normal renal function, this excess bicarbonate is rapidly excreted by the kidneys. However, in patients with poor renal function, sodium bicarbonate can accumulate and cause a clinically significant metabolic alkalosis, or it can offset the metabolic acidosis of renal failure.

A particular form of systemic alkalosis is the milk-alkali syndrome, which can occur whenever high intake of calcium combines with any factor producing alkalosis. Sodium bicarbonate can cause (1) alkalosis when ingested alone and (2) the milk-alkali syndrome when ingested chronically with calcium. The milk-alkali syndrome may still be important in pregnant women, for whom milk or calcium intake is emphasized, as well as in postmenopausal women taking large doses of supplemental calcium salts. Calcium carbonate as the sole source of both calcium and alkali may also cause this adverse effect when taken chronically. Other risk factors for developing the syndrome include factors that may worsen or prolong alkalosis, such as vomiting, gastric aspiration, hypokalemia, and dehydration.

Milk-alkali syndrome may include symptoms of hypercalcemia, alkalosis, irritability, headache, vertigo, nausea, vomiting, weakness, and myalgia. If calcium and alkali ingestion continue, neurologic symptoms (e.g., memory loss, personality changes, lethargy, stupor, coma) and renal dysfunction may develop.[14]

Sodium bicarbonate can also cause sodium overload, resulting in fluid retention, weight gain, edema, congestive heart failure, renal failure, and cirrhosis in patients on low-salt diets. Each gram of sodium bicarbonate contains 12 mEq of sodium, delivering large quantities of sodium into the systemic circulation with normal doses.

Because of the risks of systemic alkalosis and sodium overload, sodium bicarbonate should be used, if at all, only for short-term relief of indigestion brought on by consuming food and beverages. It is contraindicated for chronic use.

Effect of Additional Ingredients Most antacid products contain excipient ingredients that may be clinically important in certain patients. In addition, many products contain ingredients that do not have antacid properties but that are used by manufacturers to meet special advertising claims.

Some antacids contain considerable amounts of sugars or saccharin. When taken occasionally or in small doses, the sugar content is not great enough to cause clinical problems. However, when taken in large amounts over long periods, enough sugar may be ingested to alter glucose control in patients with diabetes. The pharmacist should consider the sugar content when recommending an antacid for diabetic patients. Unfortunately, this information is not required to be listed on the product labeling.

Most antacids contain sodium, but the amount differs considerably among products. Because of the risks of sodium to certain patients, the sodium content in antacids has been reduced significantly when compared with the past, and many products have been developed that contain either less than 0.04 mEq (1 mg) sodium per 5 mL or no sodium at all. These products should be used by patients with hypertension, congestive heart failure, renal failure, edema, or cirrhosis and by patients on salt-restricted diets. The usual amount of sodium allowed in sodium-restricted diets is 2 to 4 g per day. Antacids containing more than 5 mEq (115 mg) sodium in the total daily dose should not be recommended without first consulting with the patient's primary care provider. Antacids containing sodium bicarbonate have the largest quantities of sodium and should not be used in such patients.

Simethicone See the discussion of simethicone in the section "Treatment of Intestinal Gas."

Alginic Acid Alginic acid is combined with sodium bicarbonate and other antacids in several commercial products. The addition of alginic acid to antacids appears to be effective in relieving symptoms of GERD. Some studies suggest that this combination is superior to antacids alone, although FDA considers alginic acid to be of questionable value.[6,9,18] Alginic acid works by reacting with sodium bicarbonate and saliva to form a viscous solution of sodium alginate. This viscous solution floats on the surface of gastric contents so that, when reflux occurs, sodium alginate rather than acid is refluxed and irritation is minimized. When using antacid–alginic acid combination tablets, patients should understand that the tablets must be chewed to be effective and should be followed by a glass of water so that the viscous foam (sodium alginate) can float on water in the stomach. In addition, patients should be aware that the formulation works only when they are in the upright position and, therefore, must not be taken at bedtime or just before they lie down.

The use of alginic acid–containing products is not indicated for acid–peptic diseases other than GERD because the amount of antacid ingredients included does not provide sufficient ANC to be useful.

Drug–Drug Interactions Antacid–drug interactions have been reported with more than 30 classes of drugs. Although most of these interactions are not clinically important, some may be significant enough to result in clinical treatment failures with one or both drugs. (See Table 11–3.)

Antacids interact with drugs by a variety of mechanisms. Intraluminal interactions occur when an antacid chelates another drug or adsorbs another drug onto its surface.[22] Antacids can interfere with the absorption and elimination of drugs by increasing gastric pH and urine pH, respectively. Although all antacids may interact in these ways, some antacids are more likely to cause these changes than are others. Factors that influence whether an antacid interacts with another drug include the valence of the cation in the antacid, the dose used, the chronicity of dosing, and, most important, the timing of the administration of the antacid in relation to the other drug. As a rule, doses of antacids and tetracyclines, iron, and digoxin should be separated by at least 2 hours, whereas doses of antacids and fluoroquinolone antibiotics should be separated by 4 to 6 hours. If the fluoroquinolone dose cannot be spaced as recommended, it should be taken first followed by the antacid dose at least 2 hours later.

Special Population Considerations As with other medications, use of antacids in the elderly, children, or pregnant or breast-feeding women should be evaluated carefully.

Geriatric Patients Selection of an antacid product for an elderly patient should be guided by the same principles used in choosing antacids for any patient population. However, the pharmacist should realize that elderly patients are less likely to tolerate a large sodium load, more likely to experience side effects from antacids, and more likely to be taking a drug that can interact with antacids. Because constipation is a troublesome and frequent occurrence in elderly patients, magnesium-containing antacids should be recommended if the patient does not have severe renal impairment. Antacids containing only aluminum hydroxide are not good choices for elderly patients with constipation and can cause hypophosphatemia and resultant bone changes in this population. However, these patients may be more likely to have

Table 11–3

Antacid–Drug Interactions

Drug	Antacids: Al	Mg	Al–Mg	$CaCO_3$	$NaHCO_3$	Effect	Mechanism	Clinical Implication
Allopurinol	√					↓ absorption in 3 patients on chronic hemodialysis with failure to reduce uric acid	Unknown	Monitor patient for ↓ allopurinol response. Separate doses by ≥2 hours
Amphetamine					√	↓ urinary excretion, allowing potential for retention & intoxication	↓ renal clearance caused by ↑ urine pH	Avoid concurrent use
Antibiotics								
Nitrofurantoin	√					↓ rate & extent of absorption		Separate doses by ≥2 hours
Tetracycline and quinolones	√	√	√	√		↓ absorption (up to 90%), resulting in ↓ serum & urine concentrations	Chelation	May result in treatment failures. Separate doses by ≥2 hours, preferably 4–6 hours
Anticoagulants		√				↑ absorption of dicumarol by 50%; no effect on warfarin absorption	Chelation	Patients needing antacids & anticoagulants should receive warfarin
Anticonvulsants								
Phenytoin		√	√			↓ rate & extent of absorption with large doses of antacid; no effect with small doses	Unknown	Monitor phenytoin effects/levels
Valproic acid	√	√	√			↑ absorption by 12%	Unknown	Potential for valproic acid toxicity
β-Blockers								
Propranolol	√					↓ bioavailability by 50% in 4 of 5 subjects; no effect in another study	Delay in gastric emptying	Clinical significance of long-term therapy not assessed
Metoprolol			√			↑ bioavailability by 25% after single dose in 6 healthy volunteers	Interference with first-pass metabolism	Probably not significant
Atenolol	√		√	√		↓ bioavailability from 37%–51%		May be clinically significant; separate doses by at least 1 hour
Benzodiazepines							Unknown	May result in sedative effect. Important only in acute anxiety with single doses, not in chronic dosing
Diazepam	√					↑ absorption & ↑ sedative effects; ↓ rate, but not extent, of absorption		
Chlordiazepoxide		√				↓ rate, but not extent, of absorption		
Clorazepate			√			↓ rate & extent of absorption		
Captopril			√			↓ absorption by 42% in 10 healthy volunteers	Unknown	No evidence of compromised efficacy
Chlorpromazine			√			↓ absorption & serum concentration; ↓ therapeutic response reported	Adsorption	Monitor for ↓ therapeutic response. Separate doses by ≥2 hours
Corticosteroids							Adsorption	Evidence conflicting & clinical significance questionable
Dexamethasone		√				↓ absorption		
Prednisone	√		√			↓absorption in one study, but not confirmed		

(continued)

Table 11–3

Antacid–Drug Interactions (continued)

Drug	Antacids					Effect	Mechanism	Clinical Implication
	Al	Mg	Al–Mg	$CaCO_3$	$NaHCO_3$			
Digoxin	√	√	√			↓ absorption of digoxin up to 30% in some reports, but no effect in others; may be more likely to occur with tablets than capsules	Adsorption	Clinical significance uncertain; monitor patients for ↓ digoxin effect when antacids are given concurrently; space doses to avoid possible interaction
H_2RAs						↓ absorption & peak concentration; by 10%–40% clinical failures not reported	Adsorption	Separate doses by at least 1–2 hours
Cimetidine	√							
Ranitidine	√		√					
Famotidine		√						
Nizatidine		√						
Iron	√	√		√	√	↓ absorption by 50%–60%	↓ iron solubility due to chelation or ↑ gastric pH	May interfere with patient's response to iron replacement therapy; separate doses by ≥2 hours
Isoniazid	√	√				↓ absorption, particularly with aluminum antacids	Delayed gastric emptying caused by aluminum	Separate doses by ≥1 hour
Ketoconazole	√		√		√	↓ ketoconazole absorption	↑ gastric pH	Separate doses by ≥2 hours
Levodopa			√			↑ absorption in some patients, but effect is variable	↑ gastric emptying caused by antacids, thus more levodopa delivered to small intestine for absorption	May be clinically useful in certain patients with delayed gastric emptying; monitor patient response when adding or stopping antacid
NSAIDs								
Aspirin		√	√			↓ serum concentrations by 30%–70%	↑ renal clearance due to ↑urine pH	Monitor serum salicylate levels & observe symptoms when sustained levels are important (e.g., rheumatoid arthritis, SLE)
Enteric-coated aspirin						Premature rupture of enteric coating & dissolution in the stomach	↑ gastric pH	Separate doses in patients at risk for NSAID gastropathy
Indomethacin		√	√					
Naproxen			√					
Diflunisal	√		√			Delayed absorption & possible ↓ peak concentrations	Adsorption	Not clinically important
Pseudoephedrine						↑ rate, but not extent, of absorption in 6 healthy volunteers		Clinical significance unknown
Quinidine		√	√	√	√	↑ serum concentrations; toxicity has been reported	↓ renal clearance caused by ↑ urine pH	Use with caution; monitor levels & patient response
Sodium polystyrene sulfonate		√	√	√		Metabolic alkalosis	Antacid binds resin instead of intestinal HCO_3, resulting in ↑ reabsorption of HCO_3	Concurrent use may be dangerous; separate doses by ≥2 hours
Sucralfate						↓ dissolution & possible	↑ gastric pH	Separate doses by ≥30 minutes

Key: √ indicates interactions reported in humans. However, interactions may be likely with other antacids in which interactions are not yet reported. ↑ = increased; ↓ = decreased.

Source: Reference 15 and the following: Gugler R, Allgayer H. *Clin Pharmacokin*. 1990;18:210–9; Gibaldi M, Grundhofer B, Levy G. *Clin Pharmacol Ther*. 1974;16:520–5; and Hansten PD, Horn JR. *Drug Interactions*. 6th ed. Philadelphia: Lea & Febiger; 1997.

diarrhea from magnesium or calcium carbonate antacids, and fluid–electrolyte disturbances are more dangerous in elderly patients than in younger patients.

Pregnant/Lactating Patients Because of the incidence of gastroesophageal reflux in pregnant women, they often seek advice from the pharmacist about the safe use of antacids. Heartburn in pregnancy occurs most commonly in the third trimester and is a recurrent problem for 45% to 85% of women.[23] Antacids have not produced teratogenic effects and are generally considered safe in pregnancy as long as chronic high doses are avoided. There have been reports of magnesium-, calcium-, or aluminum-containing antacids causing hypermagnesemia, hypomagnesemia, hypercalcemia, and increased tendon reflexes in fetuses and neonates whose mothers were chronically using these antacids in high doses.[23,24] In addition, it is best not to recommend sodium bicarbonate to pregnant women because of the risks of systemic alkalosis and the sodium load leading to edema and weight gain.

Concerning lactation, neither aluminum nor magnesium hydroxide enters breast milk significantly, and no problems have been reported in lactating women.[25] Data regarding the safety of taking alginic acid or simethicone while breastfeeding, however, are not available.

In addition, data regarding the safety of alginic acid when taken by pregnant women are not available.

Pediatric Patients Signs and symptoms of GERD in pediatric patients include vomiting, chest pain, irritability, feeding refusal, belching, hoarseness, hiccups, and apnea.[26] Antacids, with or without alginic acid, have been widely used in pediatric patients for this disorder as well as for esophagitis (inflammation of the esophagus) and PUD.[26] Despite the widespread use of antacids, however, their safety in pediatric patients has not been clearly established. Rickets documented in infants was attributed to phosphate depletion resulting from the prolonged use of aluminum-containing antacids.[27]

Many cases of reflux in infants are benign, but important complications can occur, including failure to thrive, esophageal strictures, Barrett's esophagus, intraesophageal polyps, and associated pulmonary diseases. Considering the serious nature of these complications and the inability of pharmacists to assess such problems, as well as the potential for harmful effects, any parents or caregivers who are seeking to use antacids for infants or children should be advised to consult the children's physicians or pediatricians for further evaluation.

Product Selection Guidelines When an antacid is to be used, selection of a particular product should be guided by consideration of the chemical properties of the ingredients, adverse effects, potency, formulation, taste, drug interactions, and cost. High-potency antacids are generally preferred because smaller amounts can neutralize large amounts of gastric acid, thereby reducing the amount of medication the patient must take. Care should be taken to select a formulation that is palatable to the patient because a product that tastes good is almost a prerequisite to successful antacid therapy. Unfortunately, clear guidelines for palatability do not exist; the patient's personal history of antacid use may be the best indicator of what he or she considers acceptable.

Chemical Properties Before selecting an antacid for a patient, the pharmacist should consider contents, including sodium, lactose, potassium, magnesium, and sugar. In general, all antacids pose a risk of systemic side effects or electrolyte imbalances in patients with chronic renal failure, as already mentioned. Lactose content should be evaluated when choosing an antacid for patients with lactose intolerance, whereas sugar content is important to evaluate for diabetic patients.

Patients complaining of constipation, which is common in elderly patients, or hemorrhoids should be given antacids containing magnesium or magnesium–aluminum combinations. Conversely, patients with a history of diarrhea (e.g., Crohn's disease, irritable bowel syndrome) should avoid magnesium-containing antacids and may best be treated with aluminum-only antacids.

The pharmacist should carefully review the patient's medication history when selecting an antacid product. However, the most significant drug interactions (i.e., tetracycline, fluoroquinolones) have been reported with aluminum–magnesium combinations as well as with calcium-containing antacids.

Cost Another consideration in antacid product selection is cost. Although most antacids are relatively inexpensive, the cost may vary considerably when the ANC of each is compared. The cost should be calculated for equipotent not equivolume quantities.

Dosage Forms The formulation of an antacid is important for neutralizing capacity as well as for patient acceptance and compliance. The most popular antacid formulations—liquids (suspensions) and tablets—differ significantly with regard to neutralizing capacity and patient acceptance. Antacid suspensions are more potent than tablets of the same antacid on a milligram-for-milligram basis.

Despite the higher potency, many patients find liquid antacids unpalatable or cumbersome and prefer to take tablets. Some patients may prefer to alternate tablets during the day at work with liquids at night at home. Patients should be instructed to chew antacid tablets thoroughly and to follow with a full glass of water to ensure maximum therapeutic benefit.

Other formulations of antacids include lozenges, chewing gums with antacid coating, and effervescent tablets and powders to be dissolved in water. These formulations do not offer any advantages over liquids and tablets in either neutralizing capacity or patient acceptance. (See Table 11–4 for examples of commercially available antacids and their dosage forms.)

Table 11–4

Selected Antacid Products

Trade Name	Primary Ingredients
Single-Entity Magnesium Products	
Mag-Ox 400 Tablets[a–c]	Magnesium oxide 400 mg
Phillips' Milk of Magnesia Chewable Tablets	Magnesium hydroxide 311 mg
Phillips' Milk of Magnesia Suspension Concentrate[d]	Magnesium hydroxide 800 mg/5 mL
Phillips' Milk of Magnesia Suspension	Magnesium hydroxide 400 mg/5 mL
Uro-Mag Capsules	Magnesium oxide 140 mg
Single-Entity Aluminum Products	
ALternaGEL Liquid[c,e]	Aluminum hydroxide 600 mg/5 mL
Alu-Cap Capsules	Aluminum hydroxide 400 mg
Alu-Tab Tablets	Aluminum hydroxide 500 mg
Amphojel Tablets	Aluminum hydroxide 300 mg; 600 mg
Amphojel Original/Peppermint Suspension	Aluminum hydroxide 320 mg/5 mL
Basaljel Capsules/Tablets	Aluminum hydroxide 500 mg
Basaljel Suspension	Aluminum hydroxide 400 mg/5 mL
Aluminum–Magnesium Combination Products	
Maalox Suspension[a–c,e,f]	Aluminum hydroxide 225 mg/5 mL; magnesium hydroxide 200 mg/5 mL
Maalox Therapeutic Concentrate Suspension[a–c,f]	Aluminum hydroxide 600 mg/5 mL; magnesium hydroxide 300 mg/5 mL
Riopan Suspension	Magaldrate 108 mg/mL
Single-Entity Calcium Carbonate Products	
Amitone Chewable Tablets[e]	Calcium carbonate 350 mg
Chooz Gum[e]	Calcium carbonate 500 mg
Mylanta Children's Upset Stomach Relief Liquid[g]	Calcium carbonate 400 mg/5 mL
Mylanta Children's Upset Stomach Relief, Flavored Chewable Tablets[g]	Calcium carbonate 400 mg
Tums E-X Extra Strength, Flavored Chewable Tablets	Calcium carbonate 750 mg
Tums E-X Sugar Free Chewable Tablets	Calcium carbonate 750 mg
Tums Ultra, Flavored Chewable Tablets	Calcium carbonate 1000 mg
Tums, Flavored Chewable Tablets	Calcium carbonate 500 mg
Single-Entity Sodium Bicarbonate Products	
Alka-Seltzer Flavored Effervescent Tablets[e]	Sodium bicarbonate 1700 mg; aspirin 325 mg
Antacid–Alginic Acid Combination Products	
Gaviscon Chewable Tablets[a,b]	Aluminum hydroxide 80 mg; magnesium trisilicate 20 mg; sodium bicarbonate 70 mg; alginic acid
Gaviscon Extra Strength Chewable Tablets[a,b]	Aluminum hydroxide 160 mg; magnesium carbonate 105 mg; sodium bicarbonate; alginic acid
Gaviscon Extra Strength Suspension[a–c,f]	Aluminum hydroxide 508 mg/10 mL; magnesium carbonate 475 mg/10 mL; sodium alginate
Gaviscon Suspension[b,c,f]	Aluminum hydroxide 95 mg/15 mL; magnesium carbonate 358 mg/15 mL; sodium alginate
Gaviscon-2 Chewable Tablets[a,b]	Aluminum hydroxide 160 mg; magnesium trisilicate 40 mg; sodium bicarbonate 140 mg; alginic acid 400 mg

Table 11–4

Selected Antacid Products (continued)

Trade Name	Primary Ingredients
Antacid–Simethicone Combination Products	
Riopan Plus Suspension	Magaldrate 540 mg/5 mL; simethicone 40 mg/5 mL
Riopan Plus Chewable Tablets	Magaldrate 480 mg; simethicone 20 mg
Riopan Plus Double Strength Chewable Tablets	Magaldrate 1080 mg; simethicone 20 mg
Riopan Plus Double Strength Flavored Suspension	Magaldrate 1080 mg/5 mL; simethicone 40 mg/5 mL
Tums Anti-Gas/Antacid Chewable Tablets	Calcium carbonate 500 mg; simethicone 20 mg
Other Antacids	
Mylanta Gelcaps	Calcium carbonate 311 mg; magnesium carbonate 232 mg
Mylanta Double Strength Chewable Tablets	Calcium carbonate 700 mg; magnesium hydroxide 300 mg
Mylanta Regular Strength Chewable Tablets	Calcium carbonate 350 mg; magnesium hydroxide 150 mg
Rolaids Fruit-Flavored Chewable Tablets[e]	Calcium carbonate 550 mg; magnesium salts 110 mg
Rolaids Peppermint/Spearmint Chewable Tablets[e]	Calcium carbonate 550 mg; magnesium salts 110 mg
XS Hangover Relief Liquid	Calcium carbonate 350 mg/15 mL; magnesium trisilicate 750 mg/15 mL; acetaminophen 1000 mg/15 mL; caffeine 125 mg/15 mL

[a] Dye-free product.
[b] Lactose-free product.
[c] Sucrose-free product.
[d] Alcohol-free product.
[e] Sodium-free product.
[f] Sulfite-free product.
[g] Pediatric formulation.

Palatability Because antacids often must be taken frequently and in large amounts, their taste, or palatability, is a critical factor in determining patient compliance. Taste tests have been performed without finding any overwhelming favorites, and much individual variation exists. In one comparison, 14 aluminum–magnesium antacid suspensions were evaluated for smell, taste, texture, and aftertaste.[28] Overall palatability was highest for Mylanta Cherry Creme and Mylanta Double Strength Cool Mint Creme, whereas Riopan Plus 2 and Di-Gel Lemon Orange were ranked lowest. Unfortunately, it is unlikely that any scientific study can resolve the issue of taste for all patients because taste preference is an individual matter.

General recommendations for improving taste tolerability of antacids include refrigerating the product and using high-potency liquid antacids, which can be taken in smaller quantities. However, patients should be advised not to freeze antacid suspensions because freezing may result in coarse particles that are less reactive to acid. Some patients may prefer flavored tablets if an equivalent neutralizing capacity can be provided with a reasonable number of tablets.

Histamine$_2$-Receptor Antagonists

H_2RAs that are currently available for prescription and nonprescription use in the United States include cimetidine, ranitidine, famotidine, and nizatidine.[29,30] They differ in potency, chemical structure, adverse effects, and ability to cause drug interactions. Famotidine is the most potent, followed by nizatidine, ranitidine, and cimetidine.

Mechanism of Action H_2 antagonists competitively and reversibly bind to the H_2 receptor of the parietal cells, causing a dose-dependent inhibition of gastric acid secretion. Although all phases of acid secretion are suppressed, H_2RAs generally inhibit basal and nocturnal acid secretion to a greater extent than meal-stimulated acid secretion. By decreasing gastric acid secretion, H_2RAs reduce the damaging potential of refluxed gastric contents. H_2RAs do not strengthen LES tone or reduce the frequency of reflux episodes. However, this effect is not reliable throughout a 24-hour period in all patients because of the cholinergic and gastrin pathways involved in regulating acid secretion.[7]

Antisecretory activity usually begins within 1 hour of administration and persists for 6 to 12 hours.[30] The duration of antisecretory effect reported for oral nonprescription doses of cimetidine (200 mg) and famotidine (10 mg) is 6 hours and 8 to 10 hours, respectively. The duration of this effect for oral nonprescription doses of ranitidine (75 mg) and nizatidine (75 mg) is approximately 6 to 8 hours. Both the degree and the duration of acid suppression achieved with H_2RAs depend on the dose. Therefore, both the reduction in acid output and the duration of effect are significantly lower with nonprescription doses of H_2RAs than with prescription doses of these agents.

Pharmacokinetics The pharmacokinetic profiles of the H_2RAs are very similar in healthy, normal volunteers. (See Table 11–5.) These drugs are rapidly absorbed from the small intestine, with peak concentrations occurring from 1 to 3 hours after oral administration. Their bioavailability is not affected by food but may be reduced modestly by antacids.[15,31] For all H_2RAs, elimination occurs by a combination of renal and hepatic metabolism, with renal elimination being the most important for nizatidine. Although prescription doses of H_2RAs must be reduced in patients with renal impairment and/or in patients who are elderly, this reduction is not required for approved nonprescription doses. Dosage adjustment is not necessary in patients with liver disease who have normal renal function.

Indications The nonprescription H_2RAs ranitidine, cimetidine, famotidine, and nizatidine are indicated to relieve heartburn, acid indigestion, and sour stomach and to prevent these symptoms, which are brought on by consuming food and beverages. The nonprescription H_2RA regimens cannot be expected to heal esophageal erosions.

According to pharmacokinetic parameters and clinical experience with these agents, some symptomatic relief should be expected promptly with antacid administration, whereas H_2RAs may not offer relief for 1 to 2 hours after administration.

Dosage/Administration Guidelines The oral doses approved for nonprescription use—famotidine 10 mg (up to 20 mg per day), cimetidine 200 mg (up to 400 mg per day), ranitidine 75 mg (up to 150 mg per day), and nizatidine 75 mg (up to 150 mg per day)—are substantially lower than those indicated to manage PUD and GERD that involves more than intermittent, mild heartburn.

Patients may take 1 tablet when symptoms occur or, if symptoms are anticipated, 1 hour before a meal. These medications should not be taken longer than 2 weeks unless a physician is supervising their long-term use.

Overdosage The toxic-to-therapeutic dose ratio for all four H_2RAs appears to be very high. Ingestion of up to 10 to 20 g of cimetidine has caused only minimal and transient adverse

Table 11–5

Comparison of Nonprescription H_2-Receptor Antagonists

	Cimetidine (Tagamet-HB)	Ranitidine (Zantac-75)	Nizatidine (Axid AR)	Famotidine (Pepcid-AC)
Nonprescription dosage form	100 mg tablet	75 mg tablet	75 mg tablet	10 mg tablet
Relative potency	14–8	4–8	—	20–50
Oral bioavailability	60%–80%	50%–60%	90%–100%	40%–50%
Elimination half-life	1.5–2.5 hours	2–3 hours	1–2 hours	2.5–4 hours
Urinary excretion of oral dose	50%	30%	>90%	30%
Dosages[a]	200 mg bid prn, up to twice daily	75 mg bid prn, up to twice daily	75 mg bid prn, up to twice daily	10 mg bid prn, up to twice daily
Mechanisms/potential for drug interactions				
Inhibit cP450 enzymes[b]	+++	+	—	—
Increase gastric pH[c]	+	+	+	+
Change renal elimination[d]	+++	++	—	—
Inhibit gastric alcohol dehydrogenase[e]	+	+	+	—

Key:

+ indicates degree of potential for drug interactions.

– indicates no potential for drug interactions.

[a] Dosages are for relief and prevention of heartburn, sour stomach, acid indigestion.

[b] Monitor serum levels and adverse effects if cimetidine is given with theophylline, phenytoin, or warfarin. Use caution if cimetidine is administered with tricyclic antidepressants, lidocaine, quinidine, benzodiazepines, or tacrine.

[c] H_2RAs may significantly decrease bioavailability of itraconazole, ketoconazole, enoxacin, and cefpodoxime proxetil. Avoid concomitant administration or administer antibiotic when antisecretory effect of H_2RA is lowest.

[d] Avoid concomitant administration of cimetidine and ranitidine with procainamide, or monitor levels of procainamide and *N*-acetylprocainamide.

[e] H_2RAs may increase alcohol concentrations slightly, but clinical significance appears to be minimal.

effects. However, serious CNS effects have been reported after acute ingestion of 20 to 40 g of cimetidine, and deaths have been reported in adults who ingested more than 40 g.[14] There is limited experience with ranitidine overdose, but acute ingestion of up to 18 g has not caused serious toxicity. Famotidine overdose has not been documented, and no evidence exists of serious toxicity in patients receiving more than 800 mg famotidine daily for hypersecretory conditions.[14] To date, there is very little information on nizatidine overdose in humans.

Adverse Effects H_2RAs rarely cause serious side effects with an overall incidence of side effects of less than 3%.[4] The most common adverse effects reported with standard doses of H_2RAs are headache, drowsiness, constipation, diarrhea, nausea, vomiting, and abdominal pain/discomfort.[4,5,23] Despite a clinical impression that CNS reactions occur more often with cimetidine, no evidence exists that such effects are more common with one H_2RA than with another. Serious CNS reactions, including confusion, dizziness, agitation, and hallucinations, have occurred with all the H_2RAs but are extremely rare in patients who are ambulatory. Hematologic effects, such as thrombocytopenia, leukopenia, neutropenia, and anemia, have been reported with all H_2RAs as has mild and reversible elevations in hepatic aminotransferase enzymes. The incidence of these reactions is very low, however.[4,5] Small reductions in blood pressure and heart rate have been reported with oral H_2RAs, but clinically important hypotension and bradycardia are generally associated with rapid intravenous infusions of these drugs.

Cimetidine is unique among the H_2RAs in its ability to cause impotence and gynecomastia. These antiandrogenic effects result from the ability of cimetidine to displace dihydrotestosterone from androgen-binding sites and to inhibit the cytochrome P-450 metabolism of estradiol.[3,4] However, this effect occurs primarily in men who receive large doses (more than 3 g per day) for hypersecretory conditions. The effect is reversible on discontinuation or on changing to another H_2RA. These reactions would be highly unlikely from cimetidine doses approved for nonprescription use.

The extensive safety profile of prescription doses of H_2RAs suggests that the lower nonprescription doses will be well tolerated and safe. The most frequent adverse effects reported by patients receiving such drugs in nonprescription doses include headache, dizziness, nausea, and diarrhea.

Drug–Drug Interactions Of the H_2RAs, cimetidine has the greatest potential to interact with other drugs. (See Table 11–2.) Because cimetidine binds to several isoenzymes (CYP 3A4, 2D6, 1A2, and 2C9) of the cytochrome P-450 enzyme system, it impairs the hepatic metabolism of drugs that are normally cleared by this system.[32] In adults with normal re-

Case Study 11–1

Patient Complaint/History

Marjorie, a 24-year-old overweight woman, presents to the pharmacist with a complaint of substernal pain that has been present for the past 2 weeks. During questioning about the pain, the pharmacist learns that it occurs after meals and when the patient lies down. The patient reports that she takes two Tums tablets at each episode of pain.

In response to questions about her diet, the patient reveals that she often eats fast foods, usually eats a Milky Way candy bar after dinner, and drinks one cup of coffee in the morning as well as several glasses of fruit juice during the day. Further, she is often so tired after work that she goes to sleep 30 minutes after dinner.

The patient's other current medications include Centrum 1 tablet daily every morning and Monistat 7 a full applicator at bedtime for 7 days (she is currently on day 3 of therapy). She is allergic to penicillin. The patient smokes one pack of cigarettes a day and occasionally drinks beer.

Clinical Considerations/Strategies

Readers can use the following clinical considerations/strategies to determine whether treatment with nonprescription products is warranted:

- Assess the possible causes of the substernal pain.
- Recommend dietary and lifestyle changes to decrease the pain.
- Assess the appropriateness of self-medication with a nonprescription H_2RA. If appropriate, recommend the most appropriate agent.
- Determine the appropriate response to the clinical situation.

Patient Education/Counseling

Readers can use the following strategies to develop a patient education/counseling plan that will help ensure optimal therapeutic outcomes:

- Explain the importance of dietary and lifestyle modifications.
- Explain the proper use of the recommended nonprescription medications.
- Advise the patient of signs and symptoms that require medical attention.

nal function, cimetidine doses lower than 400 mg per day do not generally cause clinically important increases in serum concentrations of other drugs.[31] However, even small increases in concentrations of drugs that are eliminated by nonlinear kinetics and/or have a narrow therapeutic range may be important. In this regard, concomitant administration of cimetidine is of particular concern with theophylline, phenytoin, and warfarin.

However, the potential for adverse clinical consequences exists, particularly in elderly patients whose renal function may be declining and who are likely to be taking multiple medications. The potential for drug interactions will be magnified if patients exceed the recommended dosage. Accordingly, the product label for nonprescription cimetidine includes a warning for patients who take theophylline, phenytoin, or warfarin to consult a physician before taking the product. When cimetidine is added or stopped in a patient receiving one of these drugs, theophylline or phenytoin levels and international normalized ratios (warfarin) should be monitored and doses should be adjusted accordingly. Other drugs whose metabolism may be inhibited by cimetidine include the tricyclic antidepressants, ketoconazole, itraconazole, benzodiazepines, β-blockers, calcium channel blockers, lidocaine, and quinidine.[15,31]

Although ranitidine also binds to cytochrome P-450 enzymes, it does so with much less affinity than cimetidine does; therefore, the potential for drug interactions is much lower. Famotidine and nizatidine do not bind appreciably to the system and, therefore, do not inhibit the metabolism of other drugs.

Cimetidine, ranitidine, and nizatidine have been shown to inhibit gastric alcohol dehydrogenase, the enzyme responsible for the first-pass metabolism of alcohol. Famotidine does not inhibit this enzyme. FDA's Advisory Committee on Gastrointestinal Drugs concluded that a labeling change for the H_2RAs was not necessary at this time because the elevations in blood alcohol concentrations have yet to be proven to be clinically significant.[33]

Precautions/Warnings The potential for undertreatment of PUD or esophagitis exists because the H_2RAs may provide pain relief without actually healing existing mucosal damage. However, this concern is neither new nor unusual to H_2RAs because patients with dyspeptic symptoms have had the option to self-medicate with antacids for years. The product labeling for H_2RAs, like that for antacids, recommends that they not be taken longer than 2 weeks without consulting a physician. If these recommendations are followed, a 2-week delay in diagnosis is not likely to affect the prognosis of gastric cancer or other acid–peptic disorders.

Pharmacoeconomics The availability of nonprescription H_2RAs offers the convenient option of self-care for patients with dyspeptic symptoms and may especially benefit patients in underserved areas where a shortage of health care providers exists. Significant cost savings may be seen in the form of reducing physician visits and avoiding fees for dispensing prescriptions. Overall, the extensive safety record of the H_2RAs supports the shift to nonprescription status.

Pharmacists have a special opportunity to minimize the risk of using these agents by recognizing and triaging patients who are at risk for serious GI disease, guiding patients at risk for cimetidine–drug interactions to other agents, and counseling/educating patients about the appropriate use of these agents.

Special Population Considerations Although nonprescription H_2RAs have been available only since 1995 and 1996, the long clinical history of their prescription counterparts can be used to establish safety and effectiveness for most special population groups.

Geriatric Patients Elderly patients with acid–peptic complaints may be safely treated with nonprescription H_2RAs. Despite clinical impressions that adverse CNS effects occur more often in this population, no evidence supports this idea in patients who are ambulatory.[4] The nonprescription doses of H_2RAs are low enough that dosage reductions are not necessary to compensate for age-related reductions in elimination and metabolism. The most important concern is that elderly patients are more likely to be taking medications that interact with cimetidine.

Pregnant/Lactating Patients Data from controlled studies are limited concerning the safety of H_2RA use in pregnancy. Cimetidine readily crosses the placenta and in one study produced antiandrogenic effects and feminization of male rat pups who were exposed in utero.[23,24,34] However, data collected by the manufacturer in pregnant women receiving prescription doses of cimetidine failed to reveal any teratogenic effects, nor have teratogenic effects been reported with ranitidine or famotidine.[34] Clinical experience with nizatidine is too limited to draw any conclusions, but data in animals do not suggest any adverse effects. Cimetidine, ranitidine, and famotidine have received FDA's Pregnancy Category B rating, whereas nizatidine has a Pregnancy Category C rating.[20] Despite H_2RAs' apparent safety, more clinical experience is available from using antacids in pregnancy than from using H_2RAs. For this reason, pregnant women seeking a nonprescription product for an acid–peptic disorder should be directed to use antacids rather than H_2RAs unless a health care provider has instructed her otherwise.

Although cimetidine is concentrated in breast milk, adverse effects on breast-feeding newborns have not been observed, and the American Academy of Pediatrics considers cimetidine compatible with breast-feeding.[35] Famotidine, ranitidine, and nizatidine have also been shown to concentrate in human breast milk.

Pediatric Patients Ranitidine, cimetidine, and famotidine have all been shown to be effective and have been used to treat acid–peptic disorders in infants and children.[36] However, the nonprescription H_2RAs are not available in liquid formulations. These products should not be used in children younger than 12 years unless directed by a physician.

Product Selection Guidelines Currently, no data support either superior efficacy or the side-effects profile of one H_2RA over another when used for heartburn, acid indigestion, and sour stomach. The duration of acid suppression reported for cimetidine 200 mg (6 hours) may be shorter than that of the other nonprescription H_2RAs. Whether this difference is clinically important is unknown.

Although significant drug–drug interactions at low doses of cimetidine are unlikely, patients receiving medications that have known interactions with cimetidine may be better managed with famotidine, ranitidine, or nizatidine. Elderly patients are more likely to be taking drugs that might interact with cimetidine.

The nonprescription H_2RAs are substantially less expensive than the prescription H_2RAs, but some patients may still prefer the prescription ones because many managed care reimbursement schemes will not cover the cost of nonprescription medications. No significant cost difference exists among the nonprescription H_2RAs. Table 11–6 lists examples of commercially available products.

Alternative Remedies

Nearly one-third of Americans use practices of alternative medicine, including herbal remedies. The market for herbal products has increased in recent years. However, it is difficult to track sales because these products are included in different categories, such as dietary supplements and vitamins.[3] It is important to recognize that several herbal remedies are available and claim to improve GI function and to treat several disorders, including dyspepsia and intestinal gas.[37,38] (See Table 11–7.) In addition, a need exists for controlled clinical trials to evaluate the place in therapy, if any, that these agents may have. The most comprehensive listing of information on herbals, many of which are not available in the United States, can be found in the German E Commission monographs.[39] (See Chapter 45, "Herbal Remedies," for further discussion of these types of remedies.)

Table 11–6

Histamine$_2$-Receptor Antagonist Products

Trade Name	Primary Ingredients
Axid AR Tablets	Nitazidine 75 mg
Mylanta AR Tablets	Famotidine 10 mg
Pepcid AC Tablets	Famotidine 10 mg
Tagamet HB 200 Tablets[a–c]	Cimetidine 200 mg
Zantac 75 Tablets[b,c]	Ranitidine HCl 84 mg (equivalent to ranitidine 75 mg)

[a] Dye-free product.

[b] Sodium-free product.

[c] Sucrose-free product.

Table 11–7

Herbal Remedies Claimed to Be Useful for Indigestion, Heartburn, and Peptic Ulcer Disease

Carminatives[a]	**Cholagogues[b]**
Peppermint (*Mentha x piperita* L.)	Turmeric (*Curcuma domestica* Val.)
Chamomile (*Matricaria recruita* L.)	Boldo (*Peumus boldus* Mol.)
Minor Carminative Herbs	Dandelion (*Taraxacum officinale* Weber)
Anise (*Pimpinella anisum* L.)	**Peptic Ulcer Disease**
Caraway (*Carum carvi* L.)	Licorice (*Glycyrrhiza glabra* L.)
Coriander (*Coriandrum sativum* L.)	Deglycyrrhizinated licorice
Fennel (*Foeniculum vulgare* Mill.)	Ginger
Calamus (*Acoru calamus* L.)	

[a] Defined as an agent that relieves flatus, but current usage attributes a wider range of action to these agents.

[b] Used for dyspepsia that is attributed to inadequate flow of bile. They supposedly act to empty the gall bladder (cholekinetics), to stimulate production of bile (chloleretics), or both.

Source: References 36 and 37.

Patient Assessment of Gastroesophageal Reflux Disease

Patients presenting with dyspeptic symptoms should be carefully questioned to rule out pain related to ischemic heart disease, complications of GERD, PUD, or other serious conditions that warrant medical attention. Once serious disorders and complications have been ruled out, the pharmacist should assess whether the patient's symptoms are related to minor acid–peptic disorders such as heartburn or acid indigestion. To this end, the pharmacist should ask the patient about the relationship of the pain to consumption of food and alcoholic beverages. Postural effects on the pain should also be explored, as well as medication use. Patients who describe symptoms of uncomplicated heartburn are appropriate candidates for self-treatment with nonpharmacologic actions (lifestyle modification) and with nonprescription acid–peptic products. Asking the patient the following questions will help elicit the information needed to accurately assess the disorder and to recommend the appropriate treatment approach.

Q~ Are you having pain or discomfort in your abdomen or chest? If so, can you describe it?

A~ *Identify characteristic symptoms of ischemic pain versus those of pain associated with GERD. (See the section "Signs and Symptoms of Gastroesophageal Reflux Disease.")* Check the patient's medication profile for calcium channel antagonists, nitrates, and/or β-blockers. If ischemic pain is clearly evident or if the type of pain cannot be determined, refer the patient for immediate medical evaluation.

Q~ Do you experience the pain or discomfort immediately after meals or several hours later?

A~ If the pain coincides with meals, strongly suspect GERD and continue the evaluation.

Q~ Are there any other signs and symptoms that accompany this pain or discomfort?

A~ *Identify signs and symptoms of GERD complications. (See the section "Complications of Gastroesophageal Reflux Disease.")* If the patient describes any of these manifestations, refer the patient to a physician.

Q~ Is it worse when you lie down? When you bend over?

A~ If either position worsens the pain, strongly suspect GERD and continue the evaluation.

Q~ Is the pain or discomfort relieved by food? Do certain foods, coffee, or carbonated beverages make it worse? When do you normally eat?

A~ *Identify foods and beverages known to promote GERD. (See Table 11–1.)* If foods worsen the symptoms, strongly suspect GERD. If food relieves the pain, refer the patient for evaluation of PUD.

Q~ Have you had any difficulty or pain when swallowing?

A~ If yes, refer the patient to a physician for evaluation of GERD complications.

Q~ Do you drink alcohol? How much? Is the pain or discomfort worse after drinking alcohol?

A~ If alcohol worsens the symptoms, strongly suspect GERD.

Q~ Have you coughed up any blood?

A~ If yes, refer the patient immediately to a physician.

Q~ Have you taken antacids or H_2RAs for the pain?

A~ If either of these GERD treatments were taken for the recommended duration of use without providing any relief, refer the patient to a physician for evaluation.

Q~ Are you taking any prescription medications or nonprescription medications other than antacids or H_2RAs?

A~ *Identify medications that can promote GERD. (See Table 11–1.)* If the patient is taking a prescription drug known to promote GERD, refer the patient to a physician for possible medication adjustments. If nonprescription medications are a possible cause, recommend alternative products.

Patient Counseling for Gastroesophageal Reflux Disease

Pharmacists should tailor the counseling provided to any patient by using their perception of the patient's knowledge and understanding of his or her condition. Maintaining a professional, yet personable demeanor will facilitate counseling and will impart to the patient an impression of confidence and compassion. The patient should view the pharmacist as capable of handling information discreetly and confidentially. Patients should be told that the primary aim of nonprescription medication use in treating acid–peptic disorders is to provide symptomatic relief. Patients should be told that if symptoms persist or nonprescription medications are needed beyond a 2-week period, they should be evaluated by a physician. They should also be told that the use of nonprescription drugs, in conjunction with prescription medications, should be guided by the advice of a physician. The box "Patient Education for Gastroesophageal Reflux Disease" lists specific information to provide patients.

Evaluation of Patient Outcomes for Gastroesophageal Reflux Disease

The pharmacist should ask the patient to return after 2 weeks of self-treatment for reevaluation. If the progression of symptoms indicates complicated GERD, the patient should seek medical attention. Patients who achieve symptomatic relief should be advised to continue the nonpharmacologic measures and to use the nonprescription medications as needed.

Peptic Ulcer Disease

PUD is a group of chronic disorders characterized by ulcerating mucosal lesions in the upper GI tract with a lifetime prevalence of 5% to 10% in the general population.[4–6] The most common sites of PUD are the duodenum and the stomach. Peptic ulcer is typically a recurrent disease, with 50% to 90% of patients who have a duodenal ulcer having a recurrence within 1 year of diagnosis; the relapse rate is lower for gastric ulcer.

Etiology of Peptic Ulcer Disease

The two most important factors that disturb the gastric mucosal barrier and thus promote ulcer development are *H. pylori* and nonsteroidal anti-inflammatory drugs (NSAIDs). *H.*

Patient Education for Gastroesophageal Reflux Disease

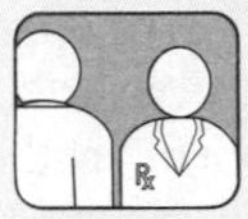

The objectives of self-treatment of GERD are to (1) reduce or eliminate symptoms, (2) reduce or eliminate the occurrence of reflux, (3) limit or prevent damage to the esophagus, and (4) prevent complications and recurrences of GERD. For most patients, carefully following product instructions and the self-care measures listed below will help ensure optimal therapeutic outcomes.

Nondrug Measures

- If possible, do not take aspirin or NSAIDs.
- Do not eat within 3 hours of going to bed. Also, elevate the head of the bed 6 to 8 inches with blocks.
- Eat smaller meals and do not lie down for approximately 3 hours after eating.
- Avoid smoking, caffeine, alcohol, and foods that exacerbate symptoms of GERD.
- Do not wear tight-fitting clothing.
- If needed, lose weight.

Nonprescription Medications

Note that antacids and H_2RAs work very differently to relieve symptoms of GERD. Antacids provide faster relief, whereas H_2RAs take longer to work but provide longer relief per dose.

Antacids

- Take 40 to 80 mEq as needed. Taking scheduled doses immediately after meals and at bedtime may bring greater relief.
- Do not take more than 500 to 600 mEq of antacid per day. Do not take these medications for longer than 2 weeks.
- Chew antacid or antacid–alginic acid tablets thoroughly, and then drink a full glass of water. Dissolve effervescent tablets completely in water; wait until the bubbles subside before drinking the liquid.
- For products containing alginic acid, drink a glass of water after taking it and wait 1 to 2 hours before lying down or going to bed. For best results, take this product during the daytime.
- If constipation or diarrhea occurs, seek advice on switching antacids.
- If you are on a low-salt diet, take only products with a low sodium content. If you have renal or cardiac disease, take products with low potassium and/or magnesium content. Ask your pharmacist for help in selecting the appropriate products.
- Liquid antacids are stronger than antacid tablets. Take antacid tablets during the day at work and liquid antacids at night.
- Take antacids at least 2 hours apart from interacting drugs, such as tetracyclines, iron, and digoxin.
- When possible, take antacids and fluoroquinolone antibiotics 4 to 6 hours apart. If doses are spaced only 2 hours apart, take the fluoroquinolone first.

Histamine$_2$-Receptor Anatagonists

- H_2RAs are not antacids, and they work differently to relieve acid-related symptoms. Moreover, nonprescription H_2RAs are the same medications as prescription H_2RAs but are simply lower doses.
- See Table 11–5 for dosing information.
- If you anticipate heartburn or indigestion, take one dose of any of the H_2RAs 1 hour before eating.
- Do not take H_2RAs longer than 2 weeks unless a physician supervises such use.
- Do not give H_2RAs to children younger than 12 years, pregnant women, or lactating women without the advice of a physician.
- Note that nonprescription doses of H_2RAs may cause headache, dizziness, nausea, and diarrhea.
- If you are taking phenytoin, theophylline, or warfarin, consult a physician before taking cimetidine. Famotidine, ranitidine, or nizatidine are safe alternatives.

Seek medical attention if

—Symptoms of GERD persist after 2 weeks of treatment with antacids or H_2RAs.

—Symptoms such as difficulty in swallowing or persistent abdominal pain occur while taking H_2RAs.

Seek medical attention immediately if chest pain occurs, particularly tight, "vise-like" pain or discomfort that may radiate to the neck, shoulder, or left arm.

pylori may largely account for the recurrent nature of the disease if not properly treated or if reacquired. *H. pylori* eradication reduces ulcer recurrence to less than 10% or eliminates recurrence in some cases.[4,5,40] Unless reinfection occurs, it is rare for an ulcer to recur once the organism has been eradicated. Reinfection in some cases may result from different strains of *H. pylori*, which are obtained from sources such as family members, environmental reservoirs, and endoscopic equipment.[40]

Drug-induced gastroduodenal damage is common and can result in significant morbidity. Drugs such as methotrexate, cyclophosphamide, azathioprine, erythromycin, iron salts, corticosteroids, and potassium chloride can cause gastroduodenal damage or ulceration; however, the drugs most frequently associated with this condition are NSAIDs. NSAIDs are the most common cause of ulcers in patients who are not infected with *H. pylori*. An estimated 20 million Americans use NSAIDs chronically. The incidence of ulcers is approximately 15% to 20% in patients taking NSAIDs for osteoarthritis or rheumatoid arthritis.[5,41] Prolonged ingestion of NSAIDs is a major cause of gastric ulcers, and more than 10% of patients receiving NSAIDs have endoscopically verified peptic ulcers. The risk of developing NSAID-induced ulcers and/or complications increases with advancing age, previous history of peptic ulcer or GI bleeding, higher doses of NSAIDs, concomitant cardiovascular disease, and concomitant use of corticosteroids or anticoagulants.[4,41]

Pathophysiology of Peptic Ulcer Disease

PUD is a chronic inflammatory condition involving a group of disorders characterized by ulceration in regions of the upper GI tract where parietal cells secrete pepsin and hydrochloric acid. The most common sites are the duodenum and the stomach where the major forms are duodenal and gastric ulceration.

Signs and Symptoms of Peptic Ulcer Disease

Patients with PUD can be asymptomatic or can experience any of the following symptoms: anorexia, nausea, vomiting, belching and bloating, and heartburn or epigastric pain. The most frequent symptom is epigastric pain (in the upper abdomen). About 50% to 80% of patients with ulcers report being awakened with pain at night, usually between midnight and 3:00 am, when gastric acid secretion is maximal and food that could buffer the acid is absent. Patients with duodenal ulcers usually describe epigastric pain or tenderness as burning, gnawing, and aching between the xiphoid and umbilicus, which is often relieved with food intake or antacids. Gastric ulcer typically involves diffuse pain over the midepigastrium and may be worsened by food. Very poor correlation exists between symptoms and ulceration, and it should be emphasized that some patients have a "silent ulcer" and do not experience symptoms with active ulcer disease, especially with recurrences. This "silence" is especially true of patients with NSAID-associated ulcers, more than half of whom are asymptomatic.

Complications of Peptic Ulcer Disease

The most common complication of PUD is bleeding, which occurs in about 20% of all patients.[4] Signs of blood loss can be obvious or subtle. Vomited blood or black material that looks like coffee grounds (hematemesis) indicates blood loss from an upper GI lesion, whether esophageal or gastroduodenal in origin. Red blood in the stool indicates a source of blood near the rectum and is commonly associated with hemorrhoids. If stools are reported as black or tarry and foul smelling (melena), then the locus of bleeding can be upper or lower but not in immediate proximity to the rectal area. Patients with significant blood loss may complain of lightheadedness, dizziness, or syncope.

Many NSAID-induced ulcers and ulcers in the elderly bleed without any prior symptoms. Therefore, the presence or absence of pain is not reliable in the diagnosis or assessment of healing with therapy in PUD. Other major complications include perforation, penetration, and gastric outlet obstruction.

Treatment of Peptic Ulcer Disease

A physician must diagnose PUD before the pharmacist assists a patient with its treatment. Patients who present with any of the following complaints or complications should be referred to a physician whether PUD is diagnosed or suspected:

- Known allergy to H_2RAs.
- Possibility of being pregnant.
- Severe abdominal or back pain.
- Unexplained weight loss.
- Syncope or dizziness.
- Abdominal pain or heartburn that is unresponsive to 2 weeks of therapy with antacids or nonprescription H_2RAs or that recurs soon after cessation of therapy.
- Chest pain that is indistinguishable from heartburn.
- Difficulty or pain on swallowing.
- Presence or history of vomiting blood.
- Black, tarry bowel movements (if not taking iron or bismuth subsalicylate).
- Fever (temperature greater than 100°F, [37.8°C]).
- Blood in urine.
- Elderly patients taking NSAIDs with risk factors for NSAID-induced ulceration and complications.
- Children younger than 12 years.

Treatment Outcomes

The goals of adjuvant therapy of PUD with nonprescription medications are to (1) control pain with antacids and (2) use bismuth subsalicylate to help in eradicating *H. pylori*. Use of these medications should, however, be approved by a physician within the context of the entire prescription drug regimen accompanying nonprescription medications.

General Treatment Approach

Prescription antisecretory drugs (H_2RAs and proton pump inhibitors) are used in PUD; however, antacids are commonly used for pain control on an as-needed basis. Sucralfate is as effective as the H_2RAs in healing and reducing recurrence rates of duodenal ulcers but is not approved for healing or maintenance of gastric ulcers. Ulcer healing may also be accomplished with proton pump inhibitors, which tend to achieve faster symptomatic relief and healing rates than H_2RAs.

It is generally recognized that patients with an ulcer from an infection of *H. pylori* should be treated with antibiotics in addition to antisecretory agents, regardless of whether the patients are suffering from the initial presentation of the disease or from a recurrence.[42] The best combination of drugs is a continuing subject of debate, but eradication rates of 80% to greater than 90% can be achieved with appropriate therapy. Eradication rates of 90% or higher have been documented with triple- and quadruple-therapy regimens.[17,43] These regimens combine antisecretory drugs, such as H_2RAs or proton pump inhibitors, and antibiotics with or without bismuth subsalicylate. Successful eradication of *H. pylori* modestly reduces time to ulcer healing, enhances healing of refractory ulcers, and substantially reduces the rate of ulcer recurrence.

Pharmacologic Therapy

Adjuvant Antacid Therapy

Antacids can provide symptomatic relief and can heal peptic ulcers, although it is no longer common to find them used as sole therapy because of the inconvenience of the regimens used, palatability, and adverse effects. However, antacids are still widely used on an as-needed basis for symptom control.

A regimen that administers antacids several times between meals and at bedtime maximizes the buffering ability of the antacid at the times of greatest acid output. Standard high-dose regimens for healing ulcers are 80 to 160 mEq ANC, usually 30 mL, taken 1 and 3 hours after meals and at bedtime. When given 1 and 3 hours after meals, antacids will neutralize acid for approximately 2 hours. In this way, the gastric pH is continuously elevated throughout the day.

Whether antacids relieve ulcer pain better than a placebo does has been difficult to determine from clinical trials. A significant problem in interpreting results of these trials is the large placebo response (up to 50%) observed in patients.[4] Accordingly, some ulcer patients report significant pain relief from antacids whereas others do not.

When antacids are recommended for supplemental pain relief, patients should be advised to take doses providing 40 to 80 mEq neutralizing capacity. These doses may be taken on an as-needed basis and may be titrated upward if needed. Most patients will need supplemental antacids for pain relief only for the first 7 to 14 days of treatment. Pharmacists should base selection of an antacid on the detailed discussion of these agents in the section "Antacids" under "Treatment of Gastroesophageal Reflux Disease."

Bismuth

Bismuth compounds have been used to treat various GI disorders for more than 200 years. Bismuth subsalicylate (BSS), sold as Pepto Bismol, is the only nonprescription bismuth compound available in the United States. BSS was once called an antacid but has no measurable ANC.

Mechanism of Action Bismuth compounds have recently attracted attention because of their ability to suppress *H. pylori* infection and their potential for cytoprotection. Although BSS has been shown to coat the mucosal lining in animals, it does not appear to form a protective coating in human mucosa and is not recognized as a gastric mucosal protectant. It is generally believed that the benefit of BSS in treating peptic ulcers is derived almost entirely from its ability to suppress *H. pylori.*

Indications Currently, BSS is indicated only for common diarrhea, traveler's diarrhea, and occasional relief of upset stomach or upper GI symptoms. As mentioned, it is also used with prescription antisecretory and antibiotic regimens to eradicate *H. pylori.*

Dosage/Administration Guidelines The recommended dosage varies according to the strength of the BSS product selected, the patient's age, and the indication.

Adverse Effects The major concern with the chronic use of the bismuth salts is the potential for systemic bismuth absorption and toxicity, the primary manifestation of which is neurotoxicity. Reports of bismuth neurotoxicity are rare and have mostly been related to other bismuth salts, such as the subnitrate and the subgallate forms, which are rarely used. Bismuth compounds react with hydrogen sulfide to produce bismuth sulfide, a highly insoluble black salt responsible for the darkening of the tongue or for grayish-black stools.[4] This side effect should not be confused with melena, in which the stools become black and tarry because of GI blood loss.

Special Population Considerations Symptoms of PUD in elderly patients can be very different from those seen in younger patients and can be quite misleading. Many elderly patients with ulcers, as well as most patients with NSAID-induced ulcers, have no symptoms at all. The pharmacist should not expect the elderly patient with an ulcer to complain of classic burning epigastric pain. If symptoms are present, they are more likely to be vague abdominal discomfort, weakness, dizziness, anorexia, and severe weight loss. An adequate drug history, especially with regard to NSAID use, should be obtained. If the pharmacist cannot determine that the symptoms are related to overeating, eating spicy foods, or experiencing occasional reflux, it is wise to refer the elderly patient to a physician for further evaluation.

Patient Assessment of Peptic Ulcer Disease

To differentiate between GERD and PUD, the pharmacist should ask the patient the questions listed in the section "Patient Assessment of Gastroesophageal Reflux Disease." Finding out whether a family history of PUD exists will also help in assessing the patient's disorder. If PUD has been diag-

Case Study 11–2

Patient Complaint/History

Reba, a 46-year-old female, presents to the pharmacist with a complaint of fatigue. She goes on to explain that for the past week she has been unable to perform her usual daily half-mile swim. Two weeks ago, she noticed a dull ache in her upper abdomen that was more pronounced at night and when she was hungry. The pain caused her to eat more often, increasing her weight by 4 pounds. Reba's sister, who has a duodenal ulcer, recommended ALternaGEL for the stomach pain. Since taking the ALternaGEL, the patient has felt the stomach pain only at night.

Questions about the patient's lifestyle and dietary habits reveal that she smokes a pack of cigarettes a day, drinks a glass of wine with dinner every night, and drinks four cups of coffee during the day. When asked about the presence of other medical conditions, the patient explains that she was diagnosed with osteoarthritis of the right knee 5 years ago and that she has had occasional constipation for the past week. Her current medications include Motrin 400 mg every 6 hours as needed for pain; Fer-In-Sol 60 mg 1 capsule daily every morning; Centrum once daily every morning; Aristospan 10 mg intra-articular once a month; Ex-Lax 90 mg 1 tablet as needed for constipation; and ALternaGEL 30 mL 4 times a day as needed for pain.

Clinical Considerations/Strategies

Readers can use the following clinical considerations/strategies to determine whether treatment with nonprescription products is warranted:

- Assess the possible causes of the fatigue and abdominal pain.
- Assess the appropriateness of treating the pain with ALternaGEL.
- Assess the effect of cigarette smoking, alcohol, and caffeine on this patient's condition.
- Determine the appropriate response to the clinical situation.

Patient Education/Counseling

Readers can use the following strategies to develop a patient education/counseling plan that will help ensure optimal therapeutic outcomes:

- Explain the importance of smoking cessation and dietary modifications.
- Advise the patient of signs and symptoms that require medical attention.

nosed, the pharmacist should find out which treatments have been prescribed and whether the patient has other medical conditions. The patient should also be questioned about the presence of symptoms that indicate complications of PUD. Asking the patient the following additional questions will help elicit the information needed to accurately assess the disorder and to recommend the appropriate treatment approach.

Q~ Have you or has anyone in your family ever had an ulcer?

A~ If a family history of ulcers exists, strongly suspect the patient has an ulcer and continue with the assessment.

Q~ Do you have any medical problems such as diabetes or kidney or heart disease? Are you currently under a physician's care for any medical conditions?

A~ If the patient has any of the specific diseases listed, strongly suspect that their symptoms are mimicking gastric pain or that they are contributing to the development of GI problems. Refer the patient to a physician for evaluation.

Q~ Have you recently taken aspirin, naproxen sodium, ketoprofen, or ibuprofen-containing products?

A~ If the patient has taken NSAIDs, determine whether the use has been sufficient to cause PUD. Advise the patient to check labels of combination nonprescription products for NSAIDs. Refer elderly patients or those deemed at high risk for an NSAID-induced ulcer to a physician for medical evaluation.

Q~ Have you experienced any nausea and vomiting? If so, have you vomited blood or black material that looks like coffee grounds? Have you noticed red blood in the stool, or have the stools been black or tarry?

A~ *Identify symptoms of bleeding ulcers. (See the section "Complications of Peptic Ulcer Disease.")* If such symptoms are described, refer the patient to a physician.

Q~ Have you seen a physician about these symptoms? If so, what did the physician tell you to do? Are you on any special diet or do you have any dietary restrictions?

A~ Determine whether dietary restrictions affect selection of nonprescription drug treatments. Also, determine whether the physician's instructions preclude the use of nonprescription drug treatments.

Q~ What prescription and nonprescription drugs do you regularly take?

A~ *Identify medications that can interact with antacids or H_2RAs. (See Table 11–3 and the section "Histamine$_2$-Receptor Antagonists.")* Base any product recommendations, if appropriate, on potential drug interactions or duplication of therapy.

Patient Counseling for Peptic Ulcer Disease

The pharmacist should stress that adjuvant therapy with antacids usually lasts only 7 to 14 days. The patient should be encouraged to continue treatment for the prescribed length of time whether the symptoms have resolved or not. If the pharmacist explains that continued pain in the first phases of treatment is not uncommon, that explanation may prevent premature termination of therapy. The patient should also receive the counseling information for antacids listed in the box "Patient Education for Gastroesophageal Reflux Disease."

Patients taking BSS for suppression of *H. pylori* should be advised to follow the physician's recommended dosages. They should be warned that this agent can cause darkening of the tongue or grayish-black stools.

Evaluation of Patient Outcomes for Peptic Ulcer Disease

The pharmacist should ask the patient to return for reevaluation after 2 weeks of self-treatment with antacids. If no pain control has been achieved, the patient should seek medical attention. Patients who achieve symptomatic relief should be advised to consult their physician about discontinuing the antacid therapy.

Other Acid–Peptic Disorders

Gastritis

The term *gastritis* is often used vaguely in reference to conditions involving the stomach and inflammation of the gastric mucosa. The classification of gastritis is a subject of controversy and can be based on (1) the acuteness or chronicity of the clinical manifestations, (2) histologic features, (3) anatomic distribution, or (4) proposed mechanism of pathogenesis.[44] Several infectious causes of gastritis with *H. pylori* are recognized as the most common. Gastritis is commonly caused by alcohol and NSAIDs as previously discussed in the section "Etiology of Peptic Ulcer Disease"; therefore, use of alcohol and, if possible, NSAIDs should be discontinued. Antacids and nonprescription H_2RAs may be used for relief of gastritis symptoms, but they are not drugs of choice. Depending on the etiology of the gastritis, prescription drug therapy will typically be implemented.

Nonulcer Dyspepsia

Dyspepsia is a vague term that clinicians and patients use to describe any abdominal discomfort, including epigastric pain, heartburn, nausea, bloating, belching, and indigestion. Patients are said to have nonulcer dyspepsia (NUD) when they present with symptoms that prompt a clinician to believe an ulcer is present but when no ulcer is found on eval uation. Thus, by definition, NUD requires exclusion of an ulcer, which requires diagnosis by a physician. A patient diagnosed with NUD may use antacids for symptoms of dyspepsia. (See the section "Antacids" under "Treatment of Gastroesophageal Reflux Disease" and the box "Patient Education for Gastroesophageal Reflux Disease.") Prescription antisecretory drugs will typically be used, however.

Intestinal Gas

A common patient complaint heard by pharmacists is that of intestinal gas. Despite the frequency of this problem, the pathogenesis is poorly understood and treatment is not satisfactory.

Etiology of Intestinal Gas

The formation of intestinal gas can be affected by several factors.[45,46] Malabsorption disorders, such as lactose intolerance, or gastric motility disorders can increase intestinal gas. Foods such as legumes (beans); items that contain indigestible carbohydrates (e.g., asparagus, broccoli, brussels sprouts, cabbage, cauliflower, celery, corn, lettuce, onions, potatoes, and some cereals or grains); fatty foods; carbonated beverages; and sweeteners (e.g., fructose or sorbitol) can increase intestinal gas production. Some antibiotics can also contribute by altering the balance of colonic bacteria that are responsible for gas production.

Pathophysiology/Signs and Symptoms of Intestinal Gas

Intestinal gas is formed mostly by anaerobic fermentation of carbohydrates by colonic bacteria, which produce various gases such as hydrogen, carbon dioxide, methane, and trace gases. Additional common sources of gas include swallowed air and the secretion of carbon dioxide in the duodenum as bicarbonate to neutralize gastric acid.

Symptoms of intestinal gas may present as excessive belching, abdominal discomfort or cramping, bloating, audible bowel sounds, and/or flatulence.

Treatment of Intestinal Gas

Treatment Outcomes

The goals of therapy are to (1) reduce the consequences of painful or troublesome intestinal gas and (2) reduce the production of painful or troublesome intestinal gas. Elimination of intestinal gas is not realistic, taking into account that a certain amount of intestinal gas production is normal.

General Treatment Approach

Identification of the underlying cause of intestinal gas will guide treatment decisions. (See Figure 11–2). Inquiry into the patient's diet can often lead to appropriate suggestions in attempting to reduce the problem. Although several antiflatulent products are available for nonprescription use, their use is largely empiric, and evidence supporting their benefit is limited.

Nonpharmacologic Therapy

Patients may benefit from dietary modification. Reducing the consumption of legumes, carbohydrates, carbonated beverages, and fatty foods may be appropriate depending on the patient's history.

Pharmacologic Therapy

Simethicone and activated charcoal are promoted as relieving intestinal gas after it has formed. α-Galactosidase and lactase enzymes are taken with foods to prevent gas from forming.

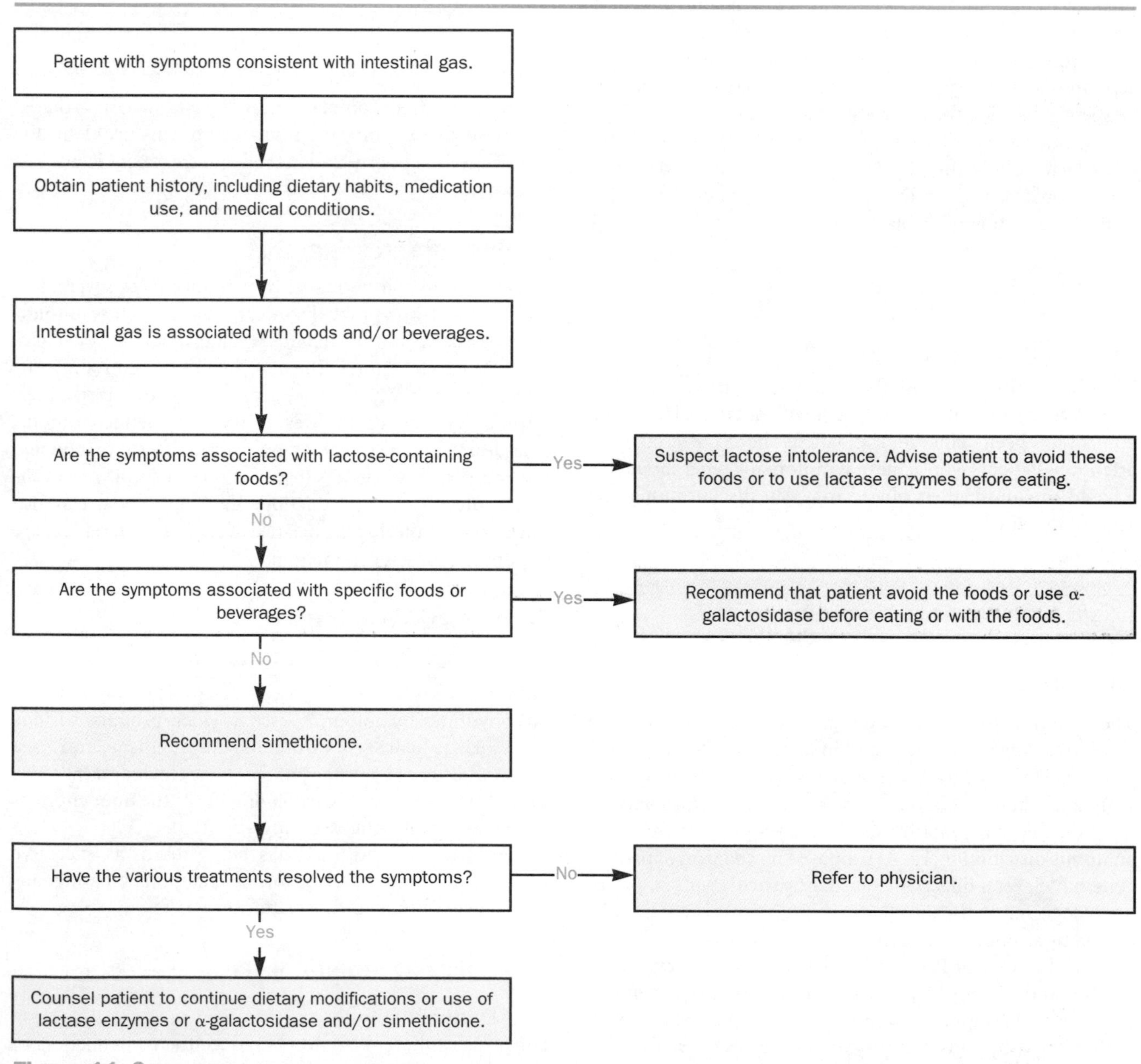

Figure 11–2 Self-care of intestinal gas.

Simethicone

Simethicone, a mixture of inert silicon polymers, is used as a defoaming agent to relieve gas.

Mechanism of Action Simethicone acts in the stomach and intestine to reduce the surface tension of gas bubbles embedded in mucus in the GI tract. As surface tension changes, the gas bubbles are broken or coalesced so that they can be eliminated more easily by belching or passing flatus.[20]

Indications FDA considers simethicone safe and effective as an antiflatulent agent, but simethicone has no activity as an antacid. The ability of simethicone to reduce intestinal gas is questionable. Nonetheless, the use of simethicone may be encouraged on a trial basis as some patients subjectively report benefit from it.

Dosage/Administration Guidelines Patients should follow the label instructions for dosages. Many antacid products contain a combination of simethicone and antacids. However, use of both agents is often unnecessary, and the efficacy of such combination products has not been well studied. Further, antiflatulent products usually contain a higher concentration of simethicone than that of the combination products.

Adverse Effects Because it is not absorbed from the GI tract, simethicone has no known systemic side effects and its safety has been well documented.

Special Population Considerations Several pediatric formulations of simethicone are indicated for the relief of intestinal gas. These products, which contain 40 mg simethicone per 0.6 mL suspension, are often promoted and used to relieve gas associated with colic. Earlier studies found simethicone to be beneficial in infantile colic, but deficiencies in the study designs limit the validity of their conclusions. More recent, carefully controlled trials have not found simethicone superior to a placebo for intestinal gas and/or infantile colic.[47] Although its efficacy is questionable, simethicone is not absorbed from the GI tract and is considered safe for use in infants and children.[14,20]

There are no reports linking simethicone to congenital defects.[34] Simethicone is a Pregnancy Category C drug.

Activated Charcoal

Although activated charcoal is promoted for relief of intestinal gas, it is neither approved nor shown to be effective for this indication. This substance also has poor palatability. Table 11–8, however, lists examples of commercially available products.

α-Galactosidase

Another product approved for use as an antiflatulent is Beano, a solution of the enzyme α-galactosidase.

Mechanism of Action α-galactosidase, which is derived from the *Aspergillus niger* mold and is classified as a food, is said to hydrolyze oligosaccharides into their component parts before they can be metabolized by colonic bacteria.[19,48]

Table 11–8

Selected Antiflatulent Products

Trade Name	Primary Ingredients
Single-Entity Simethicone Products	
Alka-Seltzer Gas Relief Gelcaps	Simethicone 125 mg
Gas-X Extra Strength Chewable Tablets[a]	Simethicone 125 mg
Gas-X Extra Strength Softgels[b]	Simethicone 125 mg
Gas-X Extra Strength Suspension	Simethicone 50 mg/5 mL
Mylanta Gas Relief Chewable Tablets	Simethicone 80 mg
Mylanta Gas Relief Maximum Strength Gelcaps	Simethicone 62.5 mg
Mylanta Gas Relief Maximum Strength Chewable Tablets	Simethicone 125 mg
Mylicon Infant's Drops[c]	Simethicone 40 mg/0.6 mL
Phazyme Gas Relief Drops[c]	Simethicone 40 mg/0.6 mL
Phazyme Gas Relief Extra Softgels	Simethicone 125 mg
Phazyme Gas Relief Maximum Strength Chewable Tablets/Softgels	Simethicone 166 mg
Phazyme Gas Relief Maximum Strength Liquid	Simethicone 62.5 mg/5 mL
Activated Charcoal Products	
Activated Charcoal Tablets[d]	Activated charcoal 250 mg
CharcoCaps Capsules[a,b,d]	Activated charcoal 260 mg
α-Galactosidase Products	
Beano Tablets/Drops	α-Galactosidase enzyme

[a] Sodium-free product.
[b] Sucrose-free product.
[c] Pediatric-formulation.
[d] Dye-free product.

Indications Because high-fiber foods contain large amounts of oligosaccharides, Beano is recommended as a prophylactic treatment of intestinal gas symptoms produced by high-fiber diets (e.g., whole grains, lentils, broccoli, peas, cabbage). Controlled trials have found α-galactosidase to significantly reduce flatulence in patients fed oligosaccharide-containing foods.[48] However, patient numbers have been limited, and evidence for this product's efficacy is far from conclusive.

Dosage/Administration Guidelines The recommended dose is about five drops added to each serving of the problem food (usually two to three servings per meal) or three tablets per meal. A five-drop dose or one tablet contains 150 units of galactosidase. The solution should be added after the food has cooled because food temperatures higher than 130°F may inactivate the enzyme.

Adverse Effects The safety of α-galactosidase also remains to be determined. Although this enzyme has been used in food processing for years and is regarded as safe by FDA, the amount contained in Beano is probably much greater than that in processed foods. One patient developed an intestinal perforation after taking Beano for several weeks, but a causal relationship was not established and there have been no similar reports. Because the enzyme produces galactose, patients with galactosemia should not use this product. Similarly, diabetic patients should be cautioned about the use of the enzyme, which may produce 2 to 6 g of carbohydrates per 100 g of food. Allergic symptoms are also possible in patients allergic to molds.

Special Population Considerations The safety and efficacy of α-galactosidase have not been evaluated in infants and children. Therefore, this product should not be used in pediatric patients until data are available to support such use.

Lactase Enzymes

See Chapter 13, "Diarrhca," for discussion of these agents.

Product Selection Guidelines

Because α-galactosidase is intended for use as a preventive measure, patients experiencing symptoms of gas who need immediate relief or patients who cannot associate their symptoms with certain foods will be better managed with simethicone. Patients who anticipate gas from certain foods may add α-galactosidase to their food for prophylaxis, or they may prefer to have simethicone on hand to take as needed. If used on a regular basis, α-galactosidase is more cost-effective than simethicone. Finally, because α-galactosidase produces carbohydrates, patients with galactosemia or diabetes mellitus should avoid this product and should use simethicone instead. (See Table 11–8 for examples of commercially available products.)

Patient Assessment of Intestinal Gas

When a patient complains of intestinal gas, it is important to try to discern the causes, duration, and frequency of the symptoms. Items noted that produce relief may provide clues as to the cause. A thorough review of dietary habits, medical problems, and use of prescription and nonprescription medications may provide other clues. Asking the patient the following questions will help elicit the information needed to accurately assess the cause of the complaint and to recommend the appropriate treatment approach.

Q~ What symptoms are you having?

A~ *Identify the typical signs and symptoms of intestinal gas. (See the section "Pathophysiology/Signs and Symptoms of Intestinal Gas.")* If the patient describes symptoms consistent with PUD or NSAID-induced gastropathy, refer the patient to a physician. Otherwise, proceed with the assessment of causes of the symptoms.

Q~ Does anything seem to cause or relieve the symptoms?

A~ If the patient correlates the symptoms with certain foods, recommend at least the temporary discontinuation of the suspected foods to delineate the cause.

Q~ What medications are you taking?

A~ If the patient is taking an antibiotic, explain that the medication could be causing the symptoms and that they should be resolved once the therapy is concluded.

Q~ Do you have any medical conditions?

A~ *Identify medical conditions that can cause intestinal gas. (See the section "Etiology of Intestinal Gas.")* If the patient has one of these conditions, explain how they affect the GI system. If the cause of the symptoms cannot be determined, refer the patient to a physician.

Patient Counseling for Intestinal Gas

Avoidance of foods or other substances that cause intestinal gas is the best advice to give patients suffering from this disorder. This advice is often difficult to follow, causing patients to resort to pharmacologic agents. The pharmacist should explain the proper use of these medications and should warn the patient of possible adverse effects. The box "Patient Education for Intestinal Gas" lists specific information to provide patients.

Evaluation of Patient Outcomes for Intestinal Gas

The pharmacist should ask the patient to return after 1 week of self-treatment with either dietary measures or with nonprescription antiflatulents or digestive enzymes. If symptoms persist or have worsened, the patient should seek medical attention. Patients who achieve symptomatic relief should be advised to continue the self-care measures as needed.

CONCLUSIONS

The safe and effective use of acid–peptic products starts with the pharmacist's ability to distinguish between patients who are appropriate for self-treatment and those who need to be referred to a health care provider. The pharmacist should take care in selecting a safe acid–peptic product for a particular patient by evaluating a patient's symptoms, age, history, concomitant disease states, and concomitant medications.

To date, no evidence supports the superior efficacy of antacids or nonprescription H_2RAs for heartburn, sour stomach, or indigestion. Until such data are available, the choice of agents for such indications may best be dictated by practical issues, such as ease of use, frequency of administra-

Patient Education for Intestinal Gas

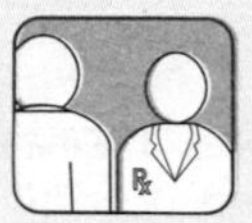

The objectives of self-treatment are to (1) reduce the symptoms of intestinal gas and (2) reduce the chance of its recurrence. For most patients, carefully following product instructions and the self-care measures listed below will help ensure optimal therapeutic outcomes.

Nondrug Measures

- If possible, avoid foods known to cause intestinal gas.
- Avoid activities known to introduce gas into the digestive system such as drinking carbonated beverages.

Nonprescription Medications

- Note that lactase enzymes and α-galactosidase should be taken with foods to prevent intestinal gas from forming.
- Note that simethicone is used to treat intestinal gas after it has occurred.

α-Galactosidase

- If using drops, add three to eight drops to the first bite of the offending food after it has cooled. High temperatures (greater than 130°F) may inactivate the enzyme.
- Do not cook with this product.
- If using tablets, swallow, chew, or crumble two to three tablets with the first bite of problem foods. If needed, use more tablets for larger meals. (One tablet is equivalent to five drops of α-galactosidase solution [150 units galactosidase].)

Lactase Enzymes

- If using drops, add three to four drops to dairy products or take with milk at mealtimes.
- If using tablets, swallow or chew one or two tablets before eating dairy products.

Simethicone

- For adults, take one tablet after meals and at bedtime. Do not take more than 500 mg simethicone per 24 hours.
- For infants younger than 2 years, give 0.3 mL four times daily after meals and at bedtime. To ease administration, mix the suspension with 1 ounce of cool water, infant formula, or other liquid.
- For children older than 2 years, give 0.6 mL four times daily after meals and at bedtime.

tion, duration of effect, potential for adverse effects, and cost. Many patients will prefer H_2RAs because they are easier to use, more palatable, and less likely to cause troublesome GI side effects than are antacids. However, antacids provide faster symptomatic relief and are substantially less expensive than H_2RAs. Patients who may be taking a medication that has the potential to interact with cimetidine should instead take famotidine, ranitidine, or nizatidine. The pharmacist should instruct the patient not to take the product longer than 2 weeks, at which time the patient should be referred to a health care provider if symptoms persist.

Knowledge of GI diseases is advancing rapidly, and changing with it is the role of antacids and antisecretory agents (i.e., H_2RAs). As the association of *H. pylori* with acid–peptic disorders grows stronger, the roles of acid neutralization and suppression become secondary to eradication of *H. pylori* with antibiotics. Antacids continue to be used widely for short-term relief of mild GI complaints; however, nonprescription H_2RAs have affected the popularity of antacids for such indications. To continue the safe and effective use of acid–peptic products, pharmacists should understand the value of these agents in relation to other therapies for acid–peptic disorders and should be informed of advances that affect the use of these products.

References

1. Gonzalez ER, Grillo JA. Over-the-counter histamine$_2$-blocker therapy. *Ann Pharmacother.* 1994;28:392–5.
2. OTC retail sales (1964–1997): sources AC Nielsen 1992–1997. Available at http://www.ndmainfo.org/facts/factsretail.html. Accessed September 1999.
3. Levy S, Breu J. The OTC/HBC market. *Drug Topics.* July 19, 1999:32,41.
4. Del Valle J, Cohen H, Laine L, et al. Acid–peptic disorders. In: Yamada T, Alpers DH, Owyang C, eds. *Textbook of Gastroenterology.* 3rd ed. Philadelphia: JB Lippincott; 1999:1370–1444.
5. Berardi RR. Peptic ulcer disease. In: DePiro JT, Talbert RL, Yee GC, et al., eds. *Pharmacotherapy: A Pathophysiologic Approach.* 4th ed. Stamford, CT: Appleton & Lange Publishing Co; 1999:548–70.
6. Orlando RC. Reflux esophagitis. In: Yamada T, Alpers DH, Owyang C, eds. *Textbook of Gastroenterology.* 3rd ed. Philadelphia: JB Lippincott; 1999:1235–63.
7. Hunt RH. Importance of pH control in the management of GERD. *Arch Intern Med.* 1999;159:649–57.
8. Kahrilas PJ. Gastroesophageal reflux disease and its complications. In: Feldman M, Scharschmidt BF, Sleisinger MH, eds. *Sleisinger and Fordtran's: Gastrointestinal and Liver Disease: Pathophysiology/Diagnosis/Management.* 6th ed. Philadelphia: Saunders; 1998:498–517.
9. Williams DB. Gastroesophageal reflux disease. In: DePiro JT, Talbert RL, Yee GC, et al, eds. *Pharmacotherapy: A Pathophysiologic Approach.* 4th ed. Stamford, CT: Appleton & Lange Publishing Co; 1999:532–47.
10. Ferriolli E, Oliveira RB, Matsuda NM, et al. Aging, esophageal motility, and gastroesophageal reflux. *J Am Geriatr Soc.* 1998;46:1534–7.
11. Labenz J. Does *Helicobacter pylori* affect the management of gastroesophageal reflux disease? *Am J Gastroenterol.* 1999;94:867–9.

12. Cohen S, Parkman HP. Heartburn—a serious symptom. *N Eng J Med.* 1999;340:878–9.
13. Lagergren J, Bergstrom R, Lindgren A, et al. Symptomatic gastroesophageal reflux as a risk factor for esophageal adenocarcinoma. *N Eng J Med.* 1999;11:825–31.
14. McEvoy GI, Litvak K, Welsh OH, eds. *AHFS Drug Information.* Bethesda, MD: American Society of Health-System Pharmacists; 1998.
15. Tatro DS, ed. *Drug Interaction Facts.* St Louis: JB Lippincott, Facts and Comparisons Division; 1998.
16. Piper DW. A comparative overview of the adverse effects of antiulcer drugs. *Drug Safety.* 1995;12:120–38.
17. Howden CW, Hunt RH. Guidelines for the management of *Helicobacter pylori* infection. *Am J Gastroenterol.* 1998;93:2330–8.
18. Ching CK, Lam SK. Antacids. Indications and limitations. *Drugs.* 1994;47:305–17.
19. FDA changes approach to hangovers. *NDMA Executive Newsletter.* 1992 January;1–92:1–2.
20. Hebel SK, ed. *Drug Facts & Comparisons.* St Louis: JB Lippincott; 1999.
21. Hade JE, Spiro HM. Calcium and acid rebound: a reappraisal. *J Clin Gastroenterol.* 1992;15:37–44.
22. Welage LS, Berardi RR. Drug interactions with antiulcer agents: considerations in the treatment of acid–peptic disease. *J Pharm Pract.* 1994;7: 177–95.
23. Broussard CN, Richter JE. Treating gastro-esophageal reflux disease during pregnancy and lactation: what are the safest therapy options? *Drug Safety.* 1998;19:325–37.
24. Smallwood RA, Berlin RG, Castagnoli N, et al. Safety of acid-suppressing drugs. *Dig Dis Sci.* 1995;40(2 suppl):63S–80S.
25. Smallwood RA, et al. Safety of acid-suppressing drugs. *Dig Dis Sci.* 1995;40 (suppl):63S–80S.
26. Glassman M, George E, Grill B. Gastroesophageal reflux in children. Clinical manifestations, diagnosis, and therapy. *Gastroenterol Clin North Am.* 1995;24:71–98.
27. Pivnick EK, Kerr NC, Kaufman RA, et al. Rickets secondary to phosphate depletion. A sequela of antacid use in infancy. *Clin Pediatr.* 1995;34:73–8.
28. Bahal-O'Mara N, Force RW, Nahata MC. Palatability of 14 over-the-counter antacids. *Am Pharm.* 1994;34:31–5.
29. *PDR for Nonprescription Drugs and Dietary Supplements.* Montvale, NJ: Medical Economics Company; 1999.
30. Marsh TD. Nonprescription H_2-receptor antagonists. *J Am Pharm Assoc.* 1997;37:552–6.
31. Hansten PD, Horn JR, eds. *Drug Interactions & Updates Quarterly 13.* Vancouver, Wash: Applied Therapeutics; 1997.
32. Michalets EL. Update: clinically significant cytochrome P-450 drug interactions. *Pharmacotherapy.* 1998;18:84–112.
33. H_2 blocker interaction with alcohol is not clinically significant. *FDC Rep Pink Sheet.* March 22, 1993;55:10–1.
34. Briggs GG, Freeman RK, Yaffe SJ. *Drugs in Pregnancy and Lactation.* 5th ed. Baltimore: Williams & Wilkins; 1998.
35. American Academy of Pediatrics, Committee on Drugs. The transfer of drugs and other chemicals into human milk. *Pediatrics.* 1994;93:137–50.
36. Kelly DA. Do H_2 receptor antagonists have a therapeutic role in childhood? *J Pediatr Gastroenterol.* 1994;19:270–6.
37. Indigestion—dyspepsia. In: Robbers JE, Tyler VE, eds. *Tylers Herbs of Choice. The Therapeutic Use of Phytomedicinals.* New York: Haworth Press; 1999;65–88.
38. Murray WJ. Herbal medications for gastrointestinal problems. In: Miller LG, Murray WJ, eds. *Herbal Medicinals. A Clinicians Guide.* New York: Hayworth Press; 1998:79–93.
39. Blumenthal M, Busse WR, Goldberg A, et al., eds. *The Complete German Commission E Monographs. Therapeutic Guide to Herbal Medicines. Americana Botanical Council.* Boston: Integrative Medicine Communications; 1998.
40. Abu-Mahfouz MZ, Prasad VM, Sautograde P, et al. *Helicobacter pylori* recurrence after successful eradication: 5 year follow-up in the United States. *Am J Gastroenterol.* 1997;92:2025–7.
41. Lanza FL. A guideline for the treatment and prevention of NSAID-induced ulcers. *Am J Gastroenterol.* 1998;93:2037–45.
42. Drea EJ. Evaluation of outcomes achieved through peptic ulcer disease state management. *Am J Managed Care.* 1998;4:S272–9.
43. Salcedo JA, Al-Kawas F. Treatment of *Helicobacter pylori* infection. *Arch Intern Med.* 1998;158:842–51.
44. Friedman LS, Peterson WL. Peptic ulcer and related disorders. In: Fauci AS, Braunwald E, Isselbacher KJ, et al, eds. *Harrison's Principles of Internal Medicine.* 14th ed. New York: McGraw-Hill; 1998:1596–616.
45. Rao SSC. Belching, bloating, and flatulence. How to help patients who have troublesome abdominal gas. *Postgrad Med.* 1997;101:263–8.
46. Clearfield HR. Clinical intestinal gas syndromes. *Prim Care.* 1996; 23:621–8.
47. Metcalf TJ, Irons TG, Sher LD, et al. Simethicone in the treatment of infant colic: a randomized, placebo-controlled, multicenter trial. *Pediatrics.* 1994;94:29–34.
48. Ganiats TG, Norcross WA, Halverson AL, et al. Does Beano prevent gas? A double-blind crossover study of oral α-galactosidase to treat dietary oligosaccharide intolerance. *J Fam Pract.* 1994;39:441–5.

CHAPTER 12

Constipation

Clarence E. Curry Jr. and Demetris M. Butler

Chapter 12 at a Glance

Extensive media advertising suggests that having clockwork-like bowel movements somehow enhances physical well-being and social acceptability. Constipation is seen by many as a frequent interruption in the "good life," and nonprescription laxatives are often used as the cure-all. Laxative products are purchased in a variety of places, and their use is common. Overall laxative sales in the United States during 1996 amounted to more than $678 million.[1]

Constipation is generally defined as a decrease in the frequency of fecal elimination and is characterized by the difficult passage of hard, dry stools. It usually results from the abnormally slow movement of feces through the colon with a resultant accumulation in the descending colon. Patients might describe it as (1) straining to have a stool; (2) the passage of hard, dry stool; and (3) feelings of incomplete bowel evacuation.

By definition, a laxative facilitates the passage and elimination of feces from the large intestine (colon) and rectum. Despite numerous recognized indications for when to use laxatives, many people use them inappropriately to alleviate what they consider to be constipation.

Editor's Note: This chapter is based, in part, on the 11th edition chapter titled "Laxative Products," which was written by Clarence E. Curry Jr. and Demetris Tatum-Butler.

Epidemiology of Constipation

Constipation occurs throughout the age continuum and in both men and women. It is reported to occur more often in women than in men.[2] There appears to be an increased prevalence of this disorder among people ages 65 years and older, making it a common complaint.[3,4] Constipation is also a common complaint during pregnancy. One study showed a 31% incidence of constipation in pregnancy, and 65% of the women were self-treating with either diet or laxatives and without professional advice.[5]

Anatomy and Physiology of the Gastrointestinal Tract

The digestive and absorptive functions of the gastrointestinal (GI) system involve the intestinal smooth muscle, visceral reflexes, and GI hormones. (See Figure 12–1.) Nearly all absorption of solids (greater than 94%) occurs in the small intestine; relatively little occurs in the stomach.

The function of the colon is to allow for the orderly elim-

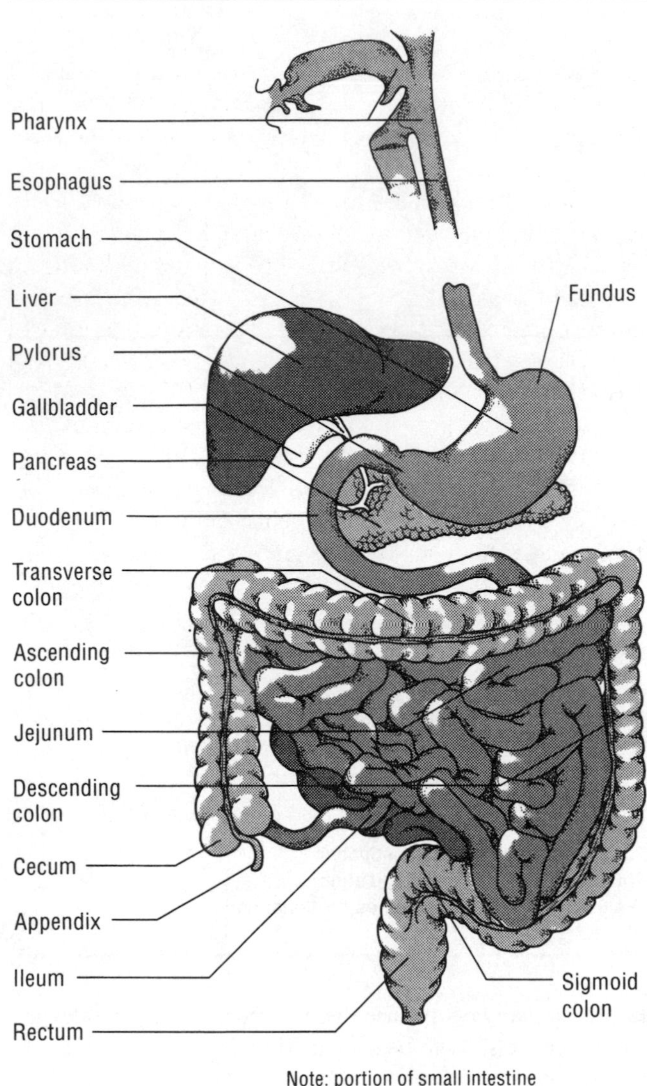

Figure 12–1 Anatomy of the digestive system.

ination from the body of nonabsorbed food products, desquamated cells from the gut lumen, and detoxified and metabolic end products. The colon functions to conserve fluid and electrolytes so that the quantity that is eliminated represents about 10% of what was presented to it in a 24-hour period. In addition, the colon has the capacity (as does the kidney) to absorb certain electrolytes because of differences in osmotic pressure. If approximately 6 L of fluid per day are ingested and supplied by secretions of the GI tract, then about 1.5%, or 90 mL, will be excreted with the feces.

Tonic contractions of the stomach churn and knead food, and large peristaltic waves start at the fundus and move food toward the duodenum. Autonomic reflexes or a hormonal link between the duodenum and the stomach regulates the time it takes the stomach contents to empty into the duodenum. Carbohydrates are emptied from the stomach most rapidly, proteins more slowly, and fats are emptied the slowest. Vagotomy and fear tend to lengthen gastric emptying time; excitement generally shortens it. Most factors that increase gastric emptying time also inhibit the secretion of hydrochloric acid and pepsin. When the osmotic pressure of the stomach contents is higher or lower than that of the plasma, gastric emptying time is increased until isotonicity is achieved.

The mixture and passage of the contents of the small and large intestines are the result of four muscular movements: pendular, segmental, peristaltic, and vermiform (wormlike). Pendular movements result from contractions of the longitudinal muscles of the intestine, which pass up and down small segments of the gut at the rate of about 10 contractions per minute. Pendular movements mix rather than propel the contents. Segmental movements result from contractions of the circular muscles and occur at about the same rate as pendular movements. Their primary function is also mixing. Pendular and segmental movements are caused by the intrinsic contractility of smooth muscle and occur in the absence of innervation of intestinal tissue.

Peristaltic movements propel intestinal contents by circular contractions that form behind a point of stimulation and pass along the GI tract toward the rectum. The contraction rate ranges from 2 to 20 cm per second. These contractions require an intact mysenteric (Auerbach's) nerve plexus, which apparently is located in the intestinal mucosa. Peristaltic waves move the intestinal contents through the small intestine in about 3.5 hours. Vermiform movements occur mainly in the large intestine and are caused by the contraction of several centimeters of the colonic smooth muscle at one time. In the cecum and ascending colon, the contents retain a fluid consistency, and peristaltic and antiperistaltic waves occur frequently. However, the activity of the transverse, descending, and sigmoid segments of the colon is very irregular, and there—through further water absorption—the contents become semisolid.

Three or four times a day, a strong peristaltic wave (mass movement) propels the contents about one-third (38 cm) the length of the colon. When initiated by a meal, the mass movement is referred to as the gastrocolic reflex. This normal reflex seems to be associated with the entrance of food into the stomach and the subsequent distention of the stomach, and it is very strong in infants. The sigmoid colon serves as a storage place for fecal matter until defecation. The GI tract normally functions involuntarily in a coordinated manner.

The act of defecation involves multiple physiologic processes, but it is basically the rectal passage of accumulated fecal material. The fecal material from the sigmoid colon is propelled into the rectum by a mass peristaltic movement, which often occurs at breakfast time in people with normal eating habits. This movement results in a desire to defecate because somatic impulses are sent to the defecation center in the sacral spinal cord. The defecation center then sends impulses to the internal anal sphincter, causing it to relax; this relaxation causes intra-abdominal pressure to increase as the muscles of the abdominal wall tighten, and a Valsalva maneuver forces the stool down. Voluntary relaxation of the external anal sphincter occurs, followed by elevation of the pelvic diaphragm, which lifts the anal sphincter over the fecal mass, allowing the mass to be expelled. Defecation, a spinal reflex, either is voluntarily inhibited by keeping the external sphincter contracted or is facilitated by relaxing the sphincter and contracting the abdominal muscles. Children usually defecate after meals; in adults, however, habits and cultural factors may determine the "proper" time for defecation.

Etiology of Constipation

Causes of constipation are numerous and include various medical conditions and medications, psychologic and physiologic conditions, and lifestyle characteristics. Some population groups are more susceptible to developing constipation as a result of one or more of the defined causes.

Disease-Induced Constipation

Constipation of recent onset suggests a possible organic or drug-induced cause. (See Tables 12–1 and 12–2.) Constipation of organic origin may be caused by numerous pathologic conditions, including hypothyroidism, megacolon, stricture, lesions (benign or malignant), or diabetes mellitus. Constipation is often a problem in patients with ulcerative colitis that is limited to the rectum. When such patients experience diarrhea, the use of antidiarrheal agents can result in colonic dilation and in the accumulation of hard stool in an area of bowel not affected by disease.[6] Irritable bowel syndrome (IBS) is a frequent cause of constipation. Although it occurs in men and women, it is reported more often in women. One variant of IBS is a constipation-predominant type characterized by abdominal pain, nausea, bloating and gas.[7] Laxatives should not be encouraged in such cases; instead, referral for proper diagnosis and medical treatment is appropriate.

Painful lesions of the anal canal, such as ulcers, fissures, and thrombosed hemorrhoidal veins, can lead to constipation if individuals suppress defecation to avoid pain. Pain from various causes, including gallbladder disease, appendicitis, and regional ileitis, may inhibit GI reflexes, leading to functional and acute symptomatology.

Table 12–1

Selected Conditions Associated with Constipation

Metabolic Disorders	**Disorders of the Large Intestine, Rectum, and Anus**
Diabetic ketoacidosis	Stenotic obstruction
Diabetic neuropathy	Hernias
Hypokalemia	Tumors
Amyloidosis	Chronic amebiasis
Porphyria	Corrosive enemas
Uremia	Diverticulitis
Endocrine Disorders	Ischemic colitis
Hypercalcemia: pseudohypoparathyroidism, hyperparathyroidism, milk–alkali syndrome, carcinomatosis	Strictures
Hypothyroidism	Irritable bowel syndrome
Panhypopituitarism	Internal rectal prolapse
Pheochromocytoma	Rectocele
Neurologic Disorders	Surgical stricture (end-to-end [EEA] anastomosis)
Aganglionosis, or Hirschsprung's disease	Ulcerative proctitis
Autonomic neuropathy: paraneoplastic, pseudo-obstruction	Lesions of the pelvic floor
Chagas' disease	Anal fissure
Ganglioneuromatosis	Mucosal prolapse
Cauda equina tumor	**Muscular Disorders**
Multiple sclerosis	Dermatomyositis
Shy–Drager syndrome	Myotonic dystrophy
Cerebrovascular accidents	Segmental dilatation of the colon
Parkinson's disease	Systemic sclerosis
Tumors	

Source: References 8 and 9.

Table 12–2

Drugs That May Induce Constipation

Analgesics (including nonsteroidal anti-inflammatory drugs)
Antacids (e.g., calcium and aluminum compounds, bismuth)
Anticholinergics (e.g., benztropine)
Anticonvulsants (e.g., carbamazepine)
Antidepressants (e.g., amitriptyline)
Antimotility (e.g., diphenoxylate, loperamide)
Barium sulfate
Benzodiazepines (especially alprazolam and estazolam)
Calcium channel blockers (e.g., verapamil)
Diuretics (e.g., thiazide-type)
Excessive laxative use
Ganglionic blockers (trimethaphan camphorsulfonate)
Hematinics (especially iron)
Hyperlidemia agents (e.g., cholestyramine, pravastatin, simvastatin)
Hypotensives (e.g., angiotensin-converting enzyme inhibitors, β-blockers)
Monoamine oxidase inhibitors (e.g., phenelzine)
Opiates (e.g., morphine, codeine)
Parasympatholytics (e.g., atropine)
Parkinsonism agents (e.g., bromocriptine)
Psychotherapeutic drugs (e.g., phenothiazines, butyrophenones)
Polystyrene sodium sulfonate
Vinca alkaloids (e.g., vincristine)

Source: References 8, 9, and 10.

Drug-Induced Constipation

Drugs with constipating side effects (e.g., calcium- or aluminum-containing antacids, narcotic analgesics, and drugs with anticholinergic activity) may counteract the therapeutic effects of laxatives or may require their use. Tricyclic antidepressants (e.g., amitriptyline, imipramine, amoxapine, and others) and certain calcium channel blockers (e.g., verapamil) are two frequently used groups of prescription drugs that have persistently caused constipation in many patients.

A clinical condition known as the narcotic bowel syndrome is characterized by chronic abdominal pain, nausea and vomiting, abdominal distention, and constipation. When narcotics are discontinued and narcotic bowel syndrome does not abate, patients may require therapy to achieve symptom resolution with clonidine.[11] Such a condition might occur in a cancer patient or in other patients who require chronic administration of large doses of narcotics. Some drugs, such as magnesium-containing antacids, prostaglandins (e.g., misoprostol), and antiadrenergic drugs (e.g., carvedilol), may produce laxative side effects (e.g., diarrhea).

Psychogenic Causes

Constipation can also be related to psychologic conditions. Depression, eating disorders such as anorexia nervosa, and conscious efforts to withhold stool are frequently responsible for the presence of constipation.

Lifestyle Factors

Eating a low-fiber diet can lead to constipation. Dietary fiber dissolves or swells in the intestinal fluid, which increases the bulk of the fecal mass and, in turn, aids in stimulating peristalsis and eliminating stools. Increasing dietary fiber and reducing consumption of soft foods and foods that harden stools (e.g., processed cheese) are effective treatments for constipation in most individuals. Some foods generally considered high in fiber, such as cereals, could actually contribute to constipation because of the processed sugar they contain. Fruits and vegetables, which provide roughage if cooked properly, provide little roughage if they are overcooked. Patients should be advised of these facts so that improper selection or preparation of foods does not cause them to abandon a healthful, high-fiber diet.

Inadequate intake of fluids can also cause constipation. Intestinal fluids are essential in the normal GI mechanisms for eliminating stools and must be replenished from dietary sources. Gravity and good abdominal muscle tone also aid in proper bowel function. Exercise increases muscle tone and promotes bowel motility. Sedentary or immobile patients are prime candidates for constipation.

Avoiding the urge to empty the bowel can eventually lead to constipation. If patients ignore or suppress this stimulus, rectal muscles can lose tonicity and become less effective in eliminating stool. Nerve pathways may degenerate and stop sending the signal to defecate. Bowel retraining will be needed to establish a pattern of regular bowel movements.

Constipation in the Elderly

Constipation in the elderly is often associated with a prolonged transit time through the colon and a decreased perception of the need to defecate, which is frequently precipitated by conditions such as neuromuscular disorders, confusion, and depression.[3,12,13] In addition, geriatric patients tend to have multiple diseases and to take multiple medications, some of which may contribute to developing constipation and, in some cases, chronic constipation. Such agents include sedatives; hypnotics; antispasmodics; antidepressants; antipsychotics; calcium-, aluminum-, and iron-containing products; and calcium channel blockers.[12] The elderly often abuse stimulant laxatives in an attempt to regulate bowel activity, which paradoxically leads to constipation.

Lifestyle factors that increase the chance of constipation in elderly patients include failure to establish a schedule for bowel movements, insufficient fluid and/or fiber intake, and immobility. Immobility increases the risk for developing constipation because walking has a positive impact on gut peristalsis. Dietary issues related to the development of constipation include insufficient fluid intake, low fiber content of the diet, excessive ingestion of foods (e.g., processed cheese) that harden stools, a diet consisting mainly of soft foods, or poor chewing of food. If any of these factors exist, the pharmacist should consider corrective action in the patient's lifestyle or current drug therapy before recommending a laxative.

Constipation in Children

A number of factors can alter a child's bowel habits, including emotional distress, febrile illness, family conflict, dietary changes (e.g., switching from human to cow milk), or environmental changes such as a move or recent travel. The pharmacist must consider these factors when determining whether constipation exists.[14,15] Idiopathic constipation often begins in childhood or adolescence.

Constipation in Women

Constipation in women can be caused by hormonal changes or slower gut transit times.[8] Pregnancy is a common cause of constipation in women. The increasing size of the uterus causes compression of the colon, thereby affecting the emptying of fecal material. However, the primary reason is probably a reduction in intestinal muscle tone, which contributes to a decrease in peristalsis.[8] In addition, prenatal vitamin and mineral supplements that contain iron and calcium tend to be constipating.

Pathophysiology of the Lower Gastrointestinal Tract

Alteration in motor activities is responsible for various disorders in the small intestine. Distention or irritation of the small intestine can cause nausea and vomiting; the duodenum is most sensitive to irritation. Motility in the small intestine is intensified when the mucosa is irritated by bacterial toxins, chemical or physical irritants, and mechanical obstruction.

As mentioned previously, the pain from anal ulcers and fissures and from thrombosed hemorrhoidal veins can induce spasms of the anal sphincter, which often result in reflexive suppression of defecation and then lead to constipation. Pain from other causes, such as gallbladder disease, appendicitis, and regional ileitis, may inhibit GI reflexes. As a result, functional obstruction may occur in the small intestine and, with it, symptoms of acute intestinal blockage.

Large masses of fecal material tend to accumulate in a greatly dilated rectum, especially in older people. Ignoring or suppressing the urge to defecate may cause the loss of tonicity in the rectal musculature. Loss of tonicity may also be caused by degeneration of nerve pathways concerned with defecation reflexes.

The normal rectal mucosa is relatively insensitive to cutting or burning. However, when it is inflamed, it becomes highly sensitive to all stimuli, including those acting on the receptors mediating the stretch reflex. A constant urge to defecate in the absence of appreciable material in the rectum may occur with an inflamed rectal mucosa.

Signs and Symptoms of Constipation

If a decrease in frequency of bowel movements or if difficult passage of hard stools does occur, other symptoms of varying degrees of severity may develop, including anorexia, dull headache, lassitude, low back pain, abdominal distention, and lower abdominal distress. Abdominal discomfort and an inadequate response to increasing varieties and dosages of laxatives are common complaints.

The frequency of bowel movements in humans generally ranges from three times a day to three times a week.[16] Individuals in the latter category are usually symptom free and do not have any specific abnormality related to their individual pattern of defecation. Therefore, constipation cannot be defined solely in terms of the number of bowel movements in any given period. Regularity is what is "regular" or typical for the individual who experiences none of the classic symptoms of constipation.

Bowel movement patterns vary widely in children, and constipation can be a complex problem that is often difficult to detect and manage. Infants and children appear to show a decreasing frequency of bowel movements with increasing age. Normally, neonates may pass more than four bowel movements a day during the first week of life. This number declines to approximately one to two bowel movements a day by age 4 years. Constipation can occur in infants who have one to two daily bowel movements and is often unrecognized as such. Infants whose frequency of bowel movements is less than average in the first weeks of life may be prone to developing chronic constipation in later years.[17,18]

Complications of Constipation

Elderly patients often strain to pass hard stools, which may predispose them to serious complications, including cardiovascular problems and hemorrhoids. Because defecation has been found to alter hemodynamics, straining to defecate may result in blood pressure surges or cardiac rhythm disturbances. In patients who had previously experienced a myocardial infarct, straining to defecate has resulted in death from emboli, ventricular rupture, and cardiogenic shock.

Treatment of Constipation

Constipation is a symptom that can result from various conditions such as a poor diet, inadequate fluid intake, a sedentary lifestyle, changes in environment, medication use, or some underlying disease process. The patient should attempt nondrug measures initially to relieve constipation and to aid in preventing recurrences. Constipation associated with an underlying medical condition or with the use of medications should be referred to a physician to evaluate the need for medical treatment or to discontinue constipating medications.

At minimum, successful therapy for constipation should return the patient to the preconstipation frequency of stool, consistency of stool, and quantity of stool. Pharmacotherapy should restore usual function using the lowest effective dosage without producing adverse effects.

Treatment Outcomes

The primary goals of treatment are (1) to relieve constipation and reestablish normal bowel function, (2) to establish dietary and exercise habits that will prevent recurrences, (3) to promote the safe and effective use of laxative products, and (4) to avoid the overuse of laxative products.

General Treatment Approach

In general, constipation should be initially managed with adjustments in the diet to include foods high in fiber content and an increase in fluid intake, accompanied by some form of exercise. Pharmacologic intervention can be used in conjunction with lifestyle modifications if more immediate relief is desired. Laxatives should be selected according to the age and health status of the patient as well as the mechanism of action of the individual product. Treatment with laxatives should be short term (i.e., less than 1 week) to preserve the normal physiologic functioning of the gut. Most patients who develop constipation will self-medicate and will consult a healthcare provider only after a nonprescription preparation or dietary manipulation has failed. Treatment success is enhanced when likely causes of constipation have been identified and when therapeutic modalities are tailored to the individual. The treatment algorithm in Figure 12–2 provides a systematic approach to the self-care of constipation.[19]

Self-treatment should not be attempted if any of the following conditions are present:

- Marked abdominal pain or significant distention or cramping.
- Marked or unexplained flatulence.
- Fever.
- Nausea and/or vomiting.
- Paraplegia or quadriplegia.
- Daily laxative use.
- Unexplained changes in bowel habits, especially if accompanied by weight loss.
- Blood in stool, or dark or tarry stool.
- Change in the caliber of stool (i.e., pencil thin).
- Any bowel symptoms that persist for 2 weeks or recur over a period of at least 3 months.
- Any bowel symptoms that recur after previous dietary or lifestyle changes or laxative use.
- History of inflammatory bowel disease.

Nonpharmacologic Therapy

Constipation that does not have an organic etiology can often be alleviated with lifestyle modifications such as increased fiber in the diet, adequate fluid intake, and exercise. It is commonly thought that increasing dietary fiber enhances regularity; fiber improves bowel function by adding bulk and softening the stool. Both insoluble fiber (e.g., whole grain breads, prunes, raisins, and corn) and soluble fiber (e.g., beans, oat bran, barley, peas, carrots, citrus fruits, and apples) have been thought to be instrumental in this regard. (See Table 12–3.) Including bran, fruits, and vegetables in the diet should increase dietary fiber. However, the pharmacist should advise patients that increasing bran in the diet may lead to erratic bowel habits, flatulence, and abdominal discomfort during the first few weeks. Pharmacists should suggest that excess bran be avoided in patients with hypocalcemia or low serum iron, as well as in patients who are confined to bed.[13,20] While this approach is useful for many people, it is not a panacea for all cases of constipation. Some people simply do not respond to the addition of fiber.

In conjunction with fiber, an increase in the intake of fluids, especially water, helps alleviate constipation in most patients. Recommendations for daily fluid consumption vary widely and range from 32 to 128 ounces. Most investigators think the additional fluid expands and softens the fiber, thereby leading to improved stool evacuation, but microbial action on the fiber may account for the improved evacuation.[23] As with adults, increasing both fluids and the bulk content of the child's diet may improve bowel habits and may decrease frequency of constipation. Simply increasing the amount of fluid or sugar in the formula may be corrective during the first few months of life. Once solid foods are introduced, better results are obtained by adding or increasing the amounts of high-fiber cereal, vegetables, and fruits. Sugar-water solutions (fruit juice or soda) often diminish the child's appetite for solid foods and should be administered in moderation. The child should be encouraged to drink water, and excessive milk intake should not be considered a substitute for water. Unbuttered popcorn is a good bulk-containing snack for children.

Because constipation often afflicts sedentary persons, the importance of exercise to the body cannot be discounted. While any concentrated regular exercise is good, aerobic exercise is best. Regular walking, running, or swimming, among other forms of exercise, may help to alleviate constipation.

Finally, for those people who achieve a beneficial effect from one of these measures, heeding the urge to pass the stool is paramount or the ultimate result will be the same as before. When such measures prove ineffective, however, a laxative may be indicated.

Pharmacologic Therapy

The ideal laxative would (1) be nonirritating and nontoxic, (2) act only on the descending and sigmoid colon, and (3)

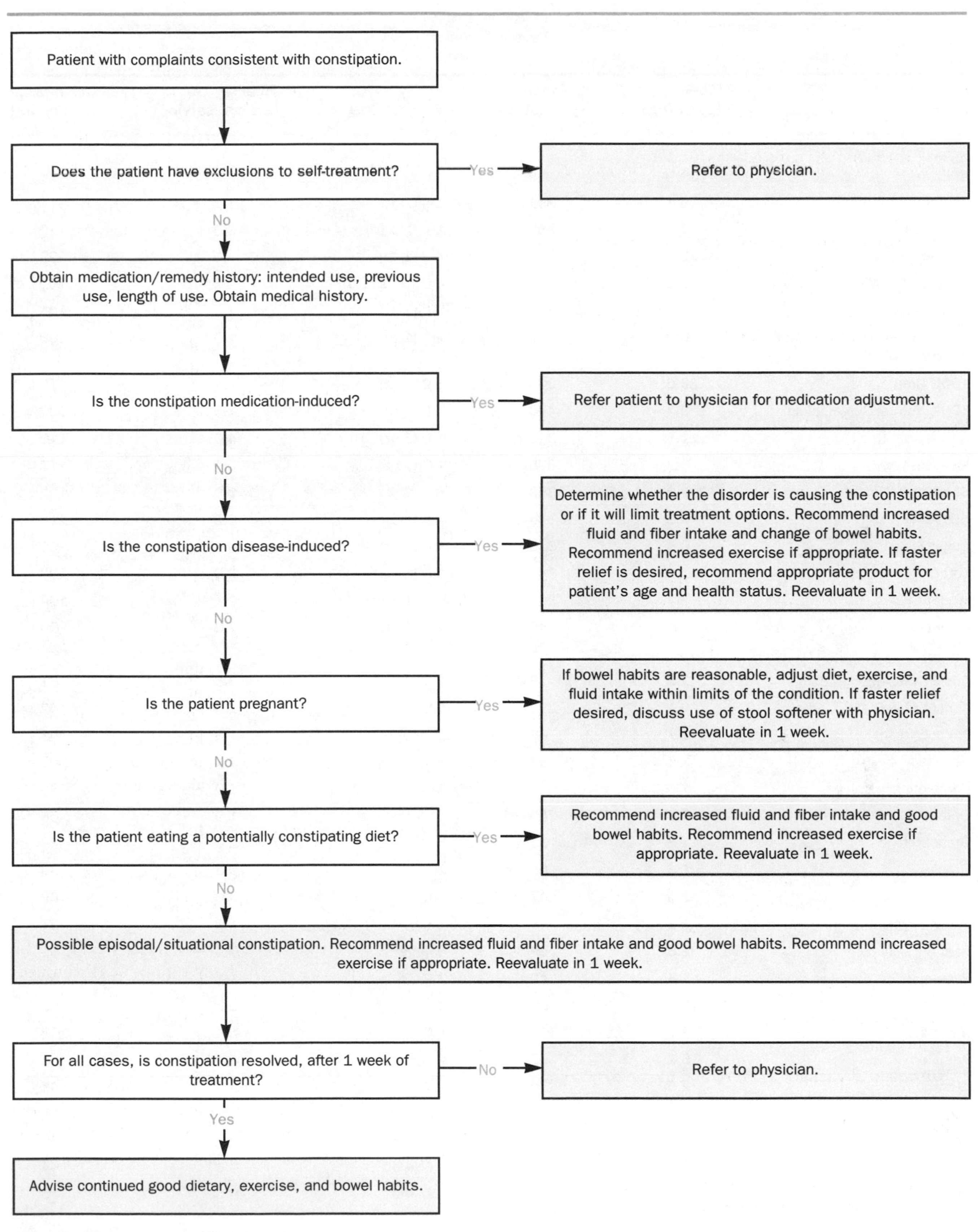

Figure 12–2 Self-care of constipation.

Table 12–3

Dietary Fiber Table[a]

Food	Fiber (g/100 g)	Calories (per 100 g)	Serving Size	Fiber (grams/serving)	Calories per Serving
Breakfast Cereals					
All-Bran	29.9	249	⅓ C (1 oz)	8.5	71
Cheerios-type	3.8	391	1 ¼ C (1 oz)	1.1	111
Cornflakes	1.1	389	1 ¼ C (1 oz)	0.3	110
40% Bran-type	13.4	325	¾ C (1 oz)	4.0	93
Frosted-Mini Wheats	7.6	359	4 biscuits (1 oz)	2.1	102
Grape-Nuts	4.8	357	¼ C (1 oz)	1.4	101
Oatmeal, regular, quick, and instant, cooked	0.9	62	¾ C (1 oz)	1.6	108
100% Bran	29.6	269	½ C (1 oz)	8.4	76
100% Natural Cereal, plain	3.7	470	¼ C (1 oz)	1.0	133
Raisin Bran-type	11.3	312	¾ C (1 oz)	4.0	115
Rice Krispies	0.2	395	1 C (1 oz)	0.1	112
Shredded Wheat	9.3	359	⅔ C (1 oz)	2.6	102
Special K	0.8	390	1 ⅓ C (1 oz)	0.2	111
Sugar Smacks	0.9	373	¾ C (1 oz)	0.4	106
Total	7.2	352	1 C (1 oz)	2.0	100
Wheat Chex	7.4	367	⅔ C (1 ⅓ oz)	2.1	104
Wheaties	7.0	349	1 C (1 oz)	2.0	99
Fruits					
Apple (w/skin)	2.5	59	1 med	3.5	81
Apricot (dried)	8.1	238	5 halves	1.4	42
Apricot (fresh)	1.7	48	3 med	1.8	51
Banana	2.1	92	1 med	2.4	105
Cantaloupe	1.0	24	¼ melon	1.0	30
Dates	7.6	275	3	1.9	68
Grapefruit	1.3	32	½	1.6	38
Grapes	1.3	63	20	0.6	30
Orange	2.0	47	1	2.6	62
Peach (w/skin)	2.1	43	1	1.9	37
Pear (w/skin)	2.8	59	½ large	3.1	61
Pineapple	1.4	49	½ C	1.1	39
Prunes	11.9	239	3	3.0	60
Raisins	8.7	300	¼ C	3.1	108
Raspberries	5.1	57	½ C	3.1	35
Strawberries	2.0	30	1 C	3.0	45
Juices					
Apple	0.3	47	½ C (4 oz)	0.4	56
Grape	0.5	51	½ C (4 oz)	0.6	64
Orange	0.4	45	½ C (4 oz)	0.5	56

Table 12–3

Dietary Fiber Table (continued)

Food	Fiber (g/100 g)	Calories (per 100 g)	Serving Size	Fiber (grams/serving)	Calories per Serving
Vegetables					
Cooked					
Asparagus, cut	1.5	20	½ C	1.0	15
Beans, string, green	2.6	25	½ C	1.6	16
Broccoli	2.8	26	½ C	2.2	20
Brussels sprouts	3.0	36	½ C	2.3	28
Cabbage, white & red	2.0	20	½ C	1.4	15
Carrots	3.0	31	½ C	2.3	24
Cauliflower	1.7	22	½ C	1.1	14
Corn, canned	2.8	83	½ C	2.9	87
Kale, leaves	2.6	34	½ C	1.4	22
Peas	4.5	71	½ C	3.6	57
Potato (w/skin)	1.7	93	1 med	2.5	106
Spinach	2.3	23	½ C	2.1	21
Sweet potatoes	2.4	141	½ med	1.7	80
Raw					
Bean sprout, soy	2.6	46	½ C	1.5	13
Cucumber	0.8	15	½ C	0.4	8
Lettuce, sliced	1.5	12	1 C	0.9	7
Mushrooms, sliced	2.5	28	½ C	0.9	10
Onions, sliced	1.3	23	½ C	0.8	33
Tomato	1.5	22	1 med	1.5	20
Spinach	4.0	26	1 C	1.2	8
Legumes					
Baked beans, tomato sauce	7.3	121	½ C	8.8	155
Dried peas, cooked	4.7	115	½ C	4.7	115
Kidney beans, cooked	7.9	118	½ C	7.3	110
Lentils, cooked	3.7	97	½ C	3.7	97
Navy beans, cooked	6.3	118	½ C	6.0	112
Breads and Flours					
Bagels	1.1	264	1 bagel	0.6	145
Bran muffins	6.3	263	1 muffin	2.5	104
Crisp bread, rye	14.9	376	2 crackers	2.0	50
Pita bread (5-inch)	0.9	273	1 piece	0.4	123
Pumpernickel bread	3.2	207	1 slice	1.0	66
White bread	1.6	279	1 slice	0.4	78
Whole wheat bread	5.7	243	1 slice	1.4	61
Pasta and Rice (Cooked)					
Macaroni	0.8	111	1 C	1.0	144
Rice, brown	1.2	119	½ C	1.0	97
Rice, polished	0.3	109	½ C	0.2	82
Spaghetti (regular)	0.8	111	1 C	1.1	155
Spaghetti (whole wheat)	2.8	111	1 C	3.9	155

Key: C = cup; med = medium; oz = ounce.

[a] The values presented are literature-derived averages. Also, cereals vary greatly in their fiber content, so consumers should read labels to determine fiber content per serving.

Source: References 21 and 22.

produce a normally formed stool within a few hours, after which its action would cease and normal bowel activity would resume. Because a laxative that precisely meets these criteria is not currently available, proper selection of a laxative depends on the etiology of the constipation.

Laxative drugs have been classified according to their chemical structure, site of action, intensity of action, or mechanism of action. The most meaningful classification is the mechanism of action, whereby laxatives are classified as bulk forming, emollient, lubricant, saline, hyperosmotic, or stimulant. (See Table 12–4.)

Bulk-Forming Laxatives

Most bulk-forming laxatives are derived from agar, plantago (psyllium) seed, kelp (alginates), and plant gums (e.g., tragacanth, chondrus, and karaya [*Sterculia*]). The synthetic cellulose derivatives—methylcellulose and carboxymethyl cellulose sodium—are being used more frequently. These synthetic colloidal materials have a high degree of uniformity and can be readily compressed into tablets.

Mechanism of Action Because they most closely approximate the physiologic mechanism in promoting evacuation, bulk-forming products are the recommended choice as initial therapy for most forms of constipation. Such laxatives are natural and semisynthetic hydrophilic polysaccharides and cellulose derivatives that dissolve or swell in the intestinal fluid, thereby forming emollient gels that facilitate passage of the intestinal contents and that stimulate peristalsis. Calcium polycarbophil, the calcium salt of a synthetic polyacrylic resin, has a marked capacity for binding water and is a quite useful agent of this class. Another bulk-forming laxative, malt soup extract, is obtained from barley and contains maltose protein, potassium, and amylolytic enzymes. An interesting aspect of this agent is that it reduces fecal pH, which may contribute to its laxative activity.

Pharmacokinetics The hydrophilic colloid bulk laxatives are not absorbed systemically and do not seem to interfere with the absorption of nutrients. The usual onset of action is from 12 to 24 hours but may be delayed as long as 72 hours.

Indications Bulk-forming laxatives are indicated as short-term therapy to relieve constipation, and they may be indicated for (1) people on low-residue diets that cannot be corrected; (2) postpartum women; (3) elderly patients; and (4) patients with colostomies, irritable bowel syndrome, or diverticular disease. They are also indicated prophylactically in patients who should refrain from straining during a bowel movement.

Dosage/Administration Guidelines Dosages vary for the bulk-forming laxatives according to the type of product. Table 12–4 lists dosing information for the various agents.

Overdosage Exceeding the recommended doses for a bulk-forming agent could lead to increased amounts of flatulence and to obstruction if appropriate fluid intake is not maintained.

Adverse Effects Esophageal obstruction has occurred in elderly persons, in patients who have difficulty swallowing, and in patients with strictures of the esophagus after they ingested a bulk laxative that had been chewed or taken in dry form. Symptoms of esophageal obstruction include chest pain, vomiting, excessive salivation, and an inhibited swallowing reflex that may precipitate choking. There have also been reports of acute bronchospasm associated with the inhalation of dry hydrophilic mucilloid, as well as of hypersensitivity reactions characterized by anaphylaxis.[24]

Drug–Drug Interactions Concurrent use of cellulose bulk-forming agents with oral anticoagulants, digitalis glycosides, or salicylates may reduce the desired effect of the co-administered medications because of physical binding or other mechanisms, which hinder absorption. The use of oral tetracylines with calcium polycarbophil may decrease absorption because of the possible formation of nonabsorbable calcium complexes. Patients should not take calcium polycarbophil within 1 to 2 hours of taking tetracyclines.

Contraindications Because of the danger of fecal impaction or intestinal obstruction, individuals with intestinal ulcerations, stenosis, or disabling adhesions should not take bulk-forming laxatives. Diarrhea, abdominal discomfort, flatulence, and excessive loss of fluid can also occur. However, when taken properly, these agents have few systemic side effects because they are not absorbed.

Bulk-forming laxatives may be inappropriate for patients who must severely restrict their fluid intake, such as those with significant renal dysfunction. Patients who have demonstrated a previous hypersensitivity or who may be susceptible to an allergic reaction should not take bulk-forming laxatives, especially psyllium.

Precautions/Warning Caution should be exercised when recommending a bulk-forming laxative product for children under age 6 years. Failure to consume sufficient fluid with a bulk laxative decreases drug efficacy and may result in intestinal or esophageal obstruction. The maximum calcium content of calcium polycarbophil is approximately 150 mg (7.6 mEq) per tablet. Susceptible patients who ingest the recommended therapeutic doses of calcium polycarbophil may increase the risk of hypercalcemia, so such patients should use caution. The U.S. recommended daily allowance of calcium is 1000 to 1300 mg for adults. (See Chapter 19, "Nutritional Deficiencies.") A recent conference of the National Institutes of Health indicated that up to 2000 mg per day of calcium—from all sources—appears safe for most individuals.[25]

The dextrose content of some of the commercial products should be evaluated before use by diabetic patients and other patients on carbohydrate-restricted diets. Further, sugar-free, bulk-forming agents that contain aspartame should be avoided by patients suffering from phenylketonuria.

Emollient Laxatives

Emollient laxative agents include docusate sodium (formerly known as dioctyl sodium sulfosuccinate), docusate calcium, and docusate potassium.

Table 12–4

Classification and Properties of Laxatives

Agent	Dosage Form	Daily Dosage Range		Site of Action	Approximate Onset of Action	Systemic Absorption
		Adult	Pediatric (age, years)			
Bulk-Forming						
Methylcellulose	Solid	4–6 g	1–1.5 g (>6)	Small and large intestines	12–72 hours	No
Carboxymethyl cellulose sodium	Solid	4–6 g	1–1.5 g (>6)	Small and large intestines	12–72 hours	No (laxative); Yes (sodium)
Malt soup extract	Solid, liquid, powder	12–64 g	6–32 mL (1 mo–2 years)	Small and large intestines	12–72 hours	—
Polycarbophil	Solid	1–6 g	0.5–1.0 g (<2) 1–1.5 g (2–5) 1.5–3.0 g (6–12)	Small and large intestines	12–72 hours	No
Plantago seeds	Solid	2.5–30 g	1.25–15 g (>6)	Small and large intestines	12–72 hours	No
Emollient						
Docusate calcium	Solid	0.05–0.36 g	0.02–0.05 g (<2) 0.05–0.150 g (≥2)	Small and large intestines	12–72 hours	Yes
Docusate sodium	Solid	0.05–0.36 g	0.02–0.05 g (<2) 0.05–0.15 g (≥2)	Small and large intestines	12–72 hours	Yes
	Liquid	50–240 mg	10–40 mg (<3) 20–60 mg (3–6) 40–120 mg (6–12)	—	—	—
Docusate potassium	Solid	100–300 mg	100 mg (≥6) at bedtime	Colon	2–15 minutes	—
Lubricant						
Mineral oil	Liquid (oral)	14–45 mL	10–15 mL (>6)	Colon	6–8 hours	Yes, a minimal amount
Saline						
Magnesium citrate	Liquid	240 mL	0.5 mL/kg	Small and large intestines	0.5–3 hours	Yes
Magnesium hydroxide	Liquid	15–40 mL	0.5 mL/kg	Small and large intestines	0.5–3 hours	
Magnesium sulfate	Solid	10–30 g	2.5–5.0 g (2–5) 5.0–10.0 g (≥6)	Small and large intestines	0.5–3 hours	Yes
Dibasic sodium phosphate	Solid (oral) Solid (rectal)	1.9–3.8 g 3.8 g	¼ adult dose (5–10) ½ adult dose (≥10) ½ adult dose (>2)	Small and large intestines Colon (rectal)	0.5–3 hours 2–15 minutes	Yes
Monobasic sodium phosphate	Solid (oral)	8.3–16.6 g	¼ adult dose (5–10) ½ adult dose (≥10)	Small and large intestines	0.5–3 hours	Yes
	Solid (rectal)	16.6 g	½ adult dose (>2)	Colon	2–15 minutes	
Sodium biphosphate	Solid (oral)	9.6–19.2 g	¼ adult dose (5–10) ½ adult dose (≥10)	Small and large intestines	0.5–3 hours	Yes
	Solid (rectal)	19.2 g	½ adult dose (>2) intestines	Small and large	2–15 minutes	—
Hyperosmotic						
Glycerin	Solid (rectal)	3 g	1–1.5 g (<6)	Colon	0.25–1 hour	—
	Liquid (rectal)	Not recommended	1–1.5 g/kg or 40 g/m^2	—	—	—

(continued)

Table 12–4

Classification and Properties of Laxatives (continued)

Agent	Dosage Form	Daily Dosage Range		Site of Action	Approximate Onset of Action	Systemic Absorption
		Adult	Pediatric (age, years)			
Stimulant						
Anthraquinones	Solid	0.12–0.25 g	Not recommended (<6)	Colon	8–12 hours	Yes
Aloe		120–220 mg (≥15)	80–120 mg (8–14)			
Cascara sagrada	Fluidextract (aromatic)	2–6 mL	½ adult dose (2–11)	Colon	6–8 hours	Yes
	Solid	0.3–1.0 g (daily)	Consult physician (<2)			
Senna	Solid	0.5–2.0 g	⅛ adult dose (>2)	Colon	6–10 hours	Yes
	Fluidextract	2.0 mL				
	Syrup	8.0 mL	¼ adult dose (1–6)			
	Fruit extract	3.4–4.0 mL	½ adult dose			
	Suppository	1 at bedtime	½ adult dose (children >60 lb)			
Calcium salt of sennosides A and B	Solid	12–24 mg	20 mg (≥6) at bedtime	Colon	6–10 hours	Yes
Diphenylmethane Stimulants						
Bisacodyl	Solid (oral)	10–30 mg	5–10 mg (>6)	Colon	6–10 hours	Yes
	Solid (rectal)	10 mg	5 mg (<2) 10 mg (≥2)	Colon	15–60 minutes	Yes
Phenolphthalein	Solid	0.03–0.27 g	Not recommended (<2) 0.015–0.020 g (2–6) 0.03–0.06 g (>6)	Colon	6–8 hours	Yes
	Liquid	60–194 mg at bedtime	1 mg/kg or 30 mg/m²	—	—	—
Miscellaneous						
Castor oil	Liquid	15–60 mL	1–5 mL (<2) 5–15 mL (2–12)	Small intestines	2–6 hours	Yes

Mechanism of Action Emollient laxatives are anionic surfactants. When administered orally, they increase the wetting efficiency of intestinal fluid and facilitate admixture of aqueous and fatty substances to soften the fecal mass. This product is commonly known as a stool softener.

Pharmacokinetics Docusate has an onset of action after oral administration of between 24 and 72 hours, and the effect lasts about 72 hours. As a result, fecal-softening emollient laxatives are usually effective in 1 to 2 days but may take as long as 3 to 5 days in some individuals. These agents are thought not to be appreciably absorbed from the gastrointestinal tract. In addition, docusate does not retard absorption of nutrients from the intestinal tract.

Indications Orally administered emollient laxatives are best suited to prevent constipation and are of little or no value in treating long-standing constipation, especially in patients who are elderly or debilitated. Thus, their value when used in proper doses is more prophylactic than therapeutic. Emollient laxatives may be used for up to 1 week without consulting a physician. Emollient laxatives are indicated to soften and inhibit painful elimination of stool when the patient has acute perianal disease or when it is desirable for the patient to avoid straining at the stool (e.g., after rectal or abdominal surgery, labor and delivery, or myocardial infarct). The patient should increase fluid intake to facilitate softening stools.

Patients with abdominal hernia, severe hypertension, or cardiovascular disease should not strain to defecate, nor should patients who are immediately postpartum or who have undergone or are about to undergo surgery for hemorrhoids or other anorectal disorders. An emollient or fecal-softening laxative is indicated in such cases.

Dosage/Administration Guidelines Table 12–4 lists dosing information for emollient laxative agents. Children younger than 6 years should not use emollient laxatives except as prescribed by a physician.

Overdosage Although overdosage of docusate may result in weakness, sweating, muscle cramps, and an irregular heartbeat, it is unlikely to be life-threatening.

Adverse Effects Docusate can potentially cause diarrhea and mild abdominal cramping.

Drug–Drug Interactions Emollient laxatives facilitate the absorption of other poorly absorbed substances such as mineral oil and may increase the toxicity of these substances.[26] Docusate and its congeners are claimed to be nonabsorbable, relatively nontoxic, and pharmacologically inert. However, it has been postulated that the detergent (surfactant) properties of docusate facilitate transport of other substances across cell membranes. Consequently, an advisory panel of the Food and Drug Administration (FDA) recommended that these laxatives carry the following warning statement: "Do not take this product if you are presently taking a prescription drug or mineral oil."[27]

With the exception of combining docusate with mineral oil, which should be avoided as previously indicated, no additional drug interactions of clinical significance are noted.

Contraindications/Precautions/Warnings Emollient laxative use should be avoided if nausea and vomiting; symptoms of appendicitis (e.g., abdominal pain, nausea, and vomiting); or undetermined abdominal pain exist.

Lubricant Laxatives

Liquid petrolatum (mineral oil) is the only nonprescription lubricant laxative.

Mechanism of Action Mineral oil and certain digestible plant oils such as olive oil soften fecal contents by coating them, thus preventing colonic absorption of fecal water. Emulsified products are used to increase palatability. There is little difference in their cathartic efficacy although emulsions of mineral oil penetrate and soften fecal matter more effectively than nonemulsified preparations.

Pharmacokinetics The onset of action of mineral oil is about 6 to 8 hours after oral administration and 5 to 15 minutes after rectal administration. Doses of emulsified mineral oil have an absorption rate of between 30% and 60%. Nonemulsified mineral oil is minimally absorbed after oral or rectal doses.

Indications Liquid petrolatum is beneficial when used judiciously in cases requiring the maintenance of a soft stool to avoid straining (e.g., when there has been hernia, aneurysm, hypertension, myocardial infarct, or cerebrovascular accident, or after a hemorrhoidectomy or abdominal surgery). However, routine use of liquid laxatives in these cases is probably not indicated; instead, stool softeners such as docusate sodium are probably better agents for preventing constipation.

Dosage/Administration Guidelines Table 12–4 lists dosing information for mineral oil. This laxative should not be given to children younger than 6 years.

Overdosage Excessive dosage of mineral oil increases the possibility of loss of fat-soluble nutrients from the GI tract and enhances the likelihood of product aspiration and anal leakage.

Adverse Effects The adverse effects and toxicity of mineral oil are associated with repeated and prolonged use. Significant absorption of mineral oil may occur, especially if emulsified products are used. The oil droplets may reach the mesenteric lymph nodes and may also be present in the intestinal mucosa, liver, and spleen, where they elicit a typical foreign-body reaction.

Lipid pneumonia may result from the oral ingestion and subsequent aspiration of mineral oil, especially when the patient reclines. The pharynx may become coated with the oil, and droplets may reach the trachea and the posterior part of the lower lobes of the lungs. Because aspiration into the lungs is possible, mineral oil should not be administered at bedtime or to patients who are very young, elderly, or debilitated.

When a patient takes large doses of mineral oil, the oil may leak through the anal sphincter and produce anal pruritus (pruritus ani), cryptitis, or other perianal conditions. The patient can avoid this leakage by reducing or dividing the dose, or by using a stable emulsion of mineral oil. Because surfactants tend to increase the absorption of otherwise "nonabsorbable" drugs, the patient must not take mineral oil with emollient fecal softeners.[28] The patient should also avoid prolonged use.

Drug–Drug Interactions The role of mineral oil in impairing the absorption of fat-soluble nutrients is uncertain. Mineral oil may impair the absorption of vitamins A, D, E, and K; then impaired vitamin D absorption may affect the absorption of calcium and phosphates. Patients should not take mineral oil with meals because it may delay gastric emptying. Additionally, it should not be given to pregnant women because it can decrease the availability of vitamin K to the fetus. Patients taking oral anticoagulants should use mineral oil with caution because the potentially decreased absorption of vitamin K may increase the blood-thinning property of the anticoagulant. As indicated, mineral oil may reduce the absorption of oral anticoagulants, oral contraceptives, and digitalis glycosides. Its absorption may be enhanced when used concomitantly with docusate.

Contraindications/Precautions/Warnings Mineral oil is contraindicated if a patient is bedridden and if any of the following are present: appendicitis or its symptoms, undiagnosed rectal bleeding, dysphagia.

Special Population Considerations Mineral oil must be used with care, if at all, by elderly patients. Mineral oil is not recommended for elderly patients who are bedridden because they are especially prone to the potential development of lipid pneumonia as a result of aspiration of the mineral oil droplets.

Case Study 12–1

Patient Complaint/History

Quentin, a 68-year-old man who retired 2 years ago from his job as a landscaper, walks up to the pharmacy counter with two products in hand: Fleet Mineral Oil Enema and Kondremul. He explains that he is having a difficult time deciding between the two products. He also notes that he cannot remember being constipated since he became an adult. For occasional constipation during adolescence, his mother always gave him mineral oil. "It always seemed to work," he says.

During questioning about his symptoms, the patient remarks that he should have come to the pharmacy 4 days ago. However, thinking that a good night's sleep would solve the problem, he picked up Benadryl capsules at a convenience store and has taken them for 3 nights. The patient reports that he is sleeping well but has had only one small bowel movement in 9 days.

The patient profile lists gouty arthritis, hypertension, and hyperlipidemia as chronic medical conditions for which the patient takes Capoten 25 mg twice a day, colchicine 0.6 mg twice a day, and Pravachol 10 mg twice a day, which was begun 3 weeks earlier. The patient has no known allergies.

Clinical Considerations/Strategies

Readers can use the following considerations/strategies to determine whether treatment of the patient's condition with nonprescription medications is warranted:

- Determine whether this patient has constipation.
- Assess the appropriateness of the active ingredient (mineral oil) in the patient-selected nonprescription products.
- Assess the appropriateness of the dosage forms selected by the patient.
- Assess the usefulness of dietary and lifestyle changes.
- Consider the patient's age as a factor in recommending a nonprescription product.
- Assess whether the patient's current drug therapy could play a role in developing constipation.

Patient Education/Counseling

Readers can use the following strategies to develop a patient education/counseling plan that will help ensure optimal therapeutic outcomes:

- Explain the importance of the dietary and lifestyle modifications.
- Explain the proper use of the recommended nonprescription medications.
- Explain the signs and symptoms that warrant medical attention.

Saline Laxatives

Saline laxative agents include magnesium citrate, magnesium hydroxide, magnesium sulfate, dibasic sodium phosphate, monobasic sodium phosphate, and sodium biphosphate.

Mechanism of Action The active constituents of saline laxatives (also referred to as osmotics) are relatively nonabsorbable cations and anions such as magnesium and sulfate ions. Sulfate salts are considered to be the most potent of this category of laxatives. The wall of the small intestine, which acts as a semipermeable membrane to the magnesium, sulfate, tartrate, phosphate, and citrate ions, retains the highly osmotic ions in the intestine. The presence of these ions draws water into the intestine, causing an increase in intraluminal pressure. This increased pressure exerts a mechanical stimulus that increases intestinal motility.

However, different mechanisms that are independent of the osmotic effect may be partially responsible for the laxative properties of the salts. Saline laxatives produce a complex series of reactions, both secretory and motor, on the GI tract. For example, the action of magnesium sulfate on the GI tract is similar to that of cholecystokinin–pancreozymin. There is evidence that this hormone is released from the intestinal mucosa when saline laxatives are administered.[28] This release, in turn, favors accumulation of fluid and electrolytes within the intestinal lumen.

Pharmacokinetics Saline laxatives have an onset of action of between 30 minutes and 3 hours for oral doses and between 2 and 5 minutes for rectal doses. Up to 20% of an orally administered dose may be absorbed.

Indications Saline laxatives are indicated for use only when acute evacuation of the bowel is required, as when preparing for endoscopic examination or when eliminating drugs in suspected poisonings. Saline laxatives have no place in the long-term management of constipation.

In some cases of food or drug poisoning, saline laxatives are used in purging doses. Magnesium sulfate is recommended except in cases of depressed central nervous system (CNS) activity or renal dysfunction. Liquid preparations may be more palatable if chilled before administration, but chilling is not possible in acute medical emergencies. In these situations, magnesium sulfate may be given in an oral dose of 20 to 40 g in 240 mL of water.

Dosage/Administration Guidelines Table 12–4 lists dosing information for saline laxative agents. Rectal agents should not be used in children younger than 2 years. Oral products should not be used in children younger than 5 years.

Overdosage Any of the magnesium-containing saline laxatives are capable of leading to hypermagnesemia in both adults and children. Hypotension, muscle weakness, and electrocardiographic changes may indicate a toxic effect of magnesium. In addition, excessive levels of serum magnesium exert a depressant effect on the CNS and neuromuscular activity. Phosphate laxatives can be troublesome when dosed excessively. An overdose of a sodium phosphate enema led to a coma in one elderly patient as a result of hyperphosphatemia and hypocalcemia.[29] It is very important to monitor dosages of these products in any patient who has renal impairment.

Adverse Effects In some cases, the choice of a saline laxative may result in serious adverse effects. As much as 20% of the administered magnesium ion may be absorbed from magnesium salts. If renal function is normal, the absorbed ion can be eliminated without consequence. However, if renal function is markedly impaired, or if the patient is a newborn or is elderly, toxic concentrations of the magnesium ion could accumulate with resulting intoxication.[30] Other adverse effects include abdominal cramping, excessive diuresis, nausea, vomiting, and dehydration.

Drug-Drug Interactions Saline laxatives can interact with oral anticoagulants, digitalis glycosides, and some phenothiazines (especially, chlorpromazine). Magnesium-containing laxatives may interfere with the absorption of oral tetracycline products. If used concurrently with a magnesium saline laxative, sodium polystyrene sulfonate may bind with magnesium and lead to systemic alkalosis.

Contraindications/Precautions/Warnings Saline laxatives are contraindicated in patients with ileostomy or colostomy, dehydration syndromes or renal function impairment, or congestive heart failure.

Phosphate salts are available in oral and rectal dosage forms. The typical oral dose contains 96.5 mEq of sodium and, therefore, should be administered with caution to patients on sodium-restricted diets. When phosphate salts are given as an enema, up to 10% or more of the sodium content may be absorbed. Rectal phosphate products are used to prepare the bowel for a barium enema and for eliminating fecal impaction. However, cathartics containing sodium may be toxic to individuals with edema, congestive heart disease, or renal failure; phosphates will accumulate with impaired renal function and should be avoided in such patients. Because dehydration may occur with the repeated use of hypertonic solutions of saline cathartics, patients who cannot tolerate fluid loss should not use phosphate salts. In patients who are not fluid restricted, oral phosphate salts should be followed by at least one full glass of water to prevent dehydration.

Special Population Considerations Use of saline laxatives is of special concern in pregnant women and children younger than 2 years. Saline products, which contain sodium, may promote sodium retention and edema. Patients who are pregnant and who are suspected of using these products should be monitored for serum sodium increases and for weight gain. Very young children may develop electrolyte abnormalities, such as hypocalcemia, tetany, hypernatremia, dehydration, and hyperphosphatemia. Electrolyte levels in these patients require careful monitoring.

Hyperosmotic Laxatives

Glycerin is the primary example of a hyperosmotic laxative.

Mechanism of Action Glycerin's laxative capability is caused by combining an osmotic effect with the local irritant effect of sodium stearate. The combination acts by drawing water into the rectum to stimulate a bowel movement.

Pharmacokinetics Glycerin is poorly absorbed after rectal administration. Use of glycerin suppositories in infants and adults usually produces a bowel movement within 30 minutes.

Indications Glycerin has been available for many years in suppository form to be used for lower bowel evacuation.

Dosage/Administration Guidelines Table 12–4 lists dosing information for glycerin. The customary rectal dose of glycerin considered to be safe and effective for adults and children older than 6 years is 3 g. Use of liquid glycerin as an enema is not recommended in adults and older children; such use may cause considerable rectal irritation. For infants and children younger than 6 years, the dose is 1 to 1.5 g as a suppository.[27]

Overdosage Overdosage with glycerin might cause additional rectal irritation, but would not be expected to lead to serious sequelae.

Adverse Effects Adverse reactions and side effects from glycerin suppositories are minimal. Some rectal irritation may occur. The irritation can be attributed to the sodium stearate component of the suppository.

Drug-Drug Interactions Interactions between glycerin and other drugs are not clinically important.

Contraindications/Precautions/Warnings Use of glycerin may be inappropriate in patients with a previous condition involving rectal irritation. Chronic use or overuse may lead to reduced serum potassium concentrations.

Special Population Considerations In infants, the physical manipulation and insertion of a solid rectal mass, such as a glycerin suppository, will usually initiate the reflex to defecate.

Stimulant Laxatives

Stimulant laxatives are conveniently classified according to their chemical structure and pharmacologic activity. Anthraquinone laxatives include aloe, cascara sagrada, casanthranol, senna, aloin, danthron, rhubarb, and frangula. The drugs of choice in this group are the cascara, casanthranol, and senna compounds. The pharmacist should not recommend rhubarb, aloe, and aloin, which are very irritating. Danthron, a breakdown product of the glycosides of senna, was withdrawn from the market in 1987 because of its tendency to produce liver tumors in rats.

The most commonly used diphenylmethane laxatives have been bisacodyl and phenolphthalein. However, after a review of reports of the development of carcinogenic tumors and genetic damage in rats, FDA recently determined that phenolphthalein posed a risk, and FDA placed it on the list of misbranded substances.[31] Castor oil is the third category of stimulant laxative.

Mechanism of Action Stimulant laxatives are thought to increase the propulsive peristaltic activity of the intestine by local irritation of the mucosa or by a more selective action on the intramural nerve plexus of intestinal smooth muscle, thus increasing motility. It has been suggested that these laxative products stimulate secretion of water and electrolytes in either the small or large intestine or both, depending on the specific laxative.[32] Intensity of action is proportional to dosage, but individually effective doses vary.

The precise mechanism by which anthraquinones increase peristalsis is unknown. Preparations of senna, however, are more potent than those of cascara and can produce considerably more abdominal cramping.

Bisacodyl acts in the colon on contact with the mucosal nerve plexus. Stimulation is segmented and axonal, producing contractions of the entire colon. Bisacodyl's action is independent of intestinal tone, and the drug is minimally absorbed systemically (approximately 5%).[33]

Castor oil's laxative action is produced by ricinoleic acid, which is produced when castor oil is hydrolyzed in the small intestine by pancreatic lipase. Its exact mechanism of action is unknown. However, its laxative effect appears to depend primarily on cyclic adenosine monophosphate–mediated fluid secretion and not on an increased peristalsis caused by the irritant effect of ricinoleic acid.[34]

Pharmacokinetics Anthraquinone derivatives used orally have an onset of action of between 6 and 12 hours. The action of these agents may be prolonged up to 72 hours in some cases. The cathartic activity of anthraquinones is limited primarily to the colon. Anthraquinones usually produce their action 8 to 12 hours after administration but may require up to 24 hours. The properties of each anthraquinone laxative vary somewhat, depending on the anthraquinone content and the speed with which the active principles are liberated. The anthraquinones are hydrolyzed by colonic bacteria into active compounds and are minimally absorbed.

Bisacodyl has an oral onset of action of between 15 to 60 minutes. It is minimally absorbed whether given by oral or rectal administration. Action on the small intestine is negligible. A soft, formed stool is usually produced 6 to 10 hours after oral administration and 15 to 60 minutes after rectal administration.

Castor oil has an oral onset of action of about 2 to 6 hours. It is metabolized to ricinoleic acid, which is absorbed to a small extent. Castor oil, a glyceride, is probably metabolized like other fatty acids. Because the main site of action is the small intestine, its prolonged use may result in excessive loss of fluid, electrolytes, and nutrients. Castor oil is most effective when administered on an empty stomach.

Indications Stimulant laxatives, such as castor oil and bisacodyl, are often used before radiologic or endoscopic examination of the GI tract and before GI surgery, when thorough evacuation of the bowel is crucial. Bisacodyl may be administered orally or rectally and may be used in combination with or instead of an enema or suppository for emptying the colon and rectum before proctologic or colonic examination or GI surgery. Bisacodyl is effective in patients with colostomies, and it may reduce or eliminate the need for irrigations.

Dosage/Administration Guidelines In general, stimulant laxatives may be used as initial drug therapy in patients with simple constipation, but they should not be used for more than 1 week. The dose should be within the recommended dosage range listed in Table 12–4. However, listed doses and dosage ranges are only guides when determining the optimal individual dose.

The liquid preparations of cascara sagrada are more reliable than the solid forms. Aromatic cascara sagrada fluid extract is less active and less bitter than cascara sagrada fluid extract. Magnesium oxide, used in preparing aromatic cascara fluid extract, removes some of the bitter and irritating principles from the crude drug.

Overdosage Stimulants, especially anthraquinones, in overdoses may lead to sudden vomiting, nausea, diarrhea, or severe abdominal cramping and may require prompt medical attention.

Adverse Effects Major hazards of stimulant laxative use are severe cramping, electrolyte and fluid deficiencies, enteric loss of protein, malabsorption resulting from excessive hypermotility and catharsis, and hypokalemia. Stimulant laxatives are effective but should be recommended cautiously. Because the intensity of their activity is proportional to the dose used, a large enough dose of any stimulant laxative can produce unwanted and sometimes dangerous adverse effects. Nevertheless, these laxatives are frequently used by those who self-medicate for constipation. Stimulant laxatives are often abused; such abuse can lead to "cathartic colon," a poorly functioning colon. (See the box "A Word about Laxative Abuse.") Patients should be advised that the dose might need to be individualized to obtain the appropriate effect.

The prolonged use of anthraquinone laxatives, especially cascara sagrada, can result in a harmless, reversible melanotic pigmentation of the colonic mucosa (melanosis coli), which is usually found on sigmoidoscopy, colonoscopy, or rectal biopsy.

A Word about Laxative Abuse

Routine, chronic use of most laxative preparations is considered laxative abuse and should be avoided if at all possible. The laxative abuser is not always elderly. Some adolescents, college students, and young adults (especially women) may use laxatives for weight control.[35,36] Such abuse is often part of a pattern of "purging behavior," which may also include self-induced vomiting. These individuals may suffer from bulimia nervosa or anorexia nervosa.[37]

Excessive use of laxatives can cause diarrhea and vomiting, leading to fluid and electrolyte losses, especially hypokalemia, which may result in a general loss of tone of smooth and striated muscle. Clinical features of laxative abuse include (1) factitious diarrhea; (2) electrolyte imbalance (e.g., hypokalemia, hypocalcemia, and hypermagnesemia); (3) osteomalacia; (4) protein-losing enteropathy (intestinal disease); (5) steatorrhea; (6) cathartic colon; and (7) liver disease.

Cathartic colon, which develops after years of laxative abuse, is difficult to diagnose. In a study of seven hospitalized female patients who were ages 26 to 65 years, the chief admitting complaints were abdominal pain and diarrhea, the number of hospital admissions ranged from 2 to 11, and the total number of days spent in the hospital ranged from 58 to 202.[38] The diagnosis of laxative abuse was difficult because the patients invariably denied taking laxatives, and none of the colonic tissue characteristics usually associated with excessive laxative use was observed on sigmoidoscopy or radiologic examination. With such patients, psychiatric intervention provided the only viable means to establish patient actions.

Diarrhea can be a serious consequence of the overuse of laxative products, especially stimulant laxatives. The prolonged misuse of laxatives can produce morbid anatomic changes in the colon.[38] The anatomic changes often seen include mucosal inflammation, loss of intrinsic innervation, atrophy of smooth muscle coats, and pigmentation of the colon. Such changes seem to occur when using laxatives regularly for many years. Cases may be characterized by a pendulous transverse colon, a highly dilated sigmoid section, thin muscle layers, and excess adipose tissue, which indicates some tissue atrophy.

Laxative abuse can usually be classified as either habitual or surreptitious. The habitual abuser often believes that a daily bowel movement is a necessity and uses a laxative to accomplish this end. Such patients may freely admit to this practice because they believe regular laxative use to be entirely correct and natural. Conversely, surreptitious abuse is similar to other illnesses. Surreptitious abusers tend to manifest various psychiatric disturbances. Confronting this type of abuser does not usually help resolve the problem, and psychiatric intervention should be encouraged. To assess the abuser, the pharmacist must include effective detection methods in the diagnostic process. The diagnosis may include a stool osmolarity test to detect salines and a colonoscopy to detect melanosis coli. Urine samples may be analyzed for the presence of the most commonly used laxatives.[39]

Once the abuse has been adequately substantiated, it may be possible to (1) wean the patient off the laxative before permanent bowel damage occurs and (2) regularize the patient's bowel habits with a high-fiber diet supplemented by bulk-forming laxatives as needed. After an abuser is withdrawn from one or more laxatives, several months may be required to retrain the bowel to work in regular, unaided function. Affected patients should be educated about laxative abuse. The information provided should describe types of laxatives and their harmful effects. Patients should be advised that constipation, weight gain, bloating, or abdominal distention may occur following the end of laxative abuse. These patients should be encouraged to exercise, increase dietary fiber, and maintain adequate fluid intake. The pharmacist should also encourage them to discuss their attitudes about laxative abuse and should be prepared to answer any questions that arise in such discussions.

Adverse effects of diphenylmethanes, which come with chronic, regular use (abuse), include metabolic acidosis or alkalosis, hypocalcemia, tetany, loss of enteric protein, and malabsorption. The suppository form may produce a burning sensation in the rectum. No systemic or adverse effects on the liver, kidney, or hematopoietic system have been observed following administration.

Drug–Drug Interactions/Diagnostic Test Interference The administration of bisacodyl tablets within 1 hour of antacids, cimetidine, famotidine, ranitidine, or milk results in rapid erosion of the enteric coating, which may lead to gastric or duodenal irritation. Enteric-coated bisacodyl tablets prevent irritation of the gastric mucosa and, therefore, should not be broken, crushed, chewed, or administered with agents that increase gastric pH such as antacids, histamine$_2$-receptor antagonists, or proton pump inhibitors.

Senna may color urine pink to red, red to violet, or red to brown, thus affecting the accurate interpretation of the phenolsulfonphthalein test.

Contraindications/Precautions/Warnings Patients with undiagnosed rectal bleeding or signs of intestinal obstruction should not use stimulant laxatives. Pregnant women should also avoid these agents.

Stimulant laxatives should be used with caution when symptoms of appendicitis are present, and they should not be used at all when the diagnosis of appendicitis is made. All stimulant laxatives may produce griping, colic, increased mucus secretion, and, in some people, excessive evacuation of fluid. Chrysophanic acid, a component of rhubarb and senna that is excreted in urine, colors acidic urine yellowish-brown and colors alkaline urine reddish-violet. The pharmacist should warn patients that a number of prescription and nonprescription medications as well as some foods will produce either alkaline or acidic urine and that the use of senna may lead to urine discoloration. Because a laxative effect occurs quickly, castor oil should not be given at bedtime.

Special Population Considerations Because the active principles of anthraquinones are absorbed from the GI tract, they subsequently appear in body secretions, including human milk. However, the practical significance of this event in nursing infants is poorly defined. After taking a senna-based laxative, postpartum patients have reported a brown discoloration of breast milk and subsequent catharsis by their nursing infants. A study with breast-feeding women who were constipated postpartum and who received a senna laxative reported that 17% of their infants experienced diarrhea.[5]

Combination Products

Many combination laxative products are available. (See Table 12–5.) Companies attempt to take advantage of multiple mechanisms of action and other factors to create a product that better meets the criteria for an ideal laxative. Several combination products contain a stimulant product and a second entity. Emollient laxatives do not stimulate bowel movements when used alone but do achieve this purpose when combined with stimulant laxatives. A popular combination is docusate sodium with casanthrol, which makes the best use of both cathartic action and stool softening effect.

In many cases of fecal impaction, a solution of docusate is often added to the enema fluid. Mineral oil has been combined with cascara and other stimulants to produce an often-used product. What may seem to be an unlikely combination—milk of magnesia and mineral oil—has been available for years in a popular formulation (Haley's M-O). Some products incorporate senna with psyllium. The desired effect is that the senna will act quickly, and the bulk-forming agents will continue to help the bowel function beyond the initial movement. Additional combination oral products exist and include various agents such as psyllium, bisacodyl, or docusate as the principal ingredient and glycerin as an adjunctive agent. It is unlikely that the contributing effect of glycerin is significant to the overall laxative action of the product. The amount of glycerin necessary to produce laxation orally would lead to appreciable glycerin absorption from the small intestine.

Because a common ingredient to most combination products is a stimulant, it is important to remember that combining laxative entities will have the potential for greater adverse impact if administration and dosing guidelines are not closely followed. If a stimulant and a stool softener are combined, the potential for adversity depends largely on the stimulant. However, if a stimulant and a saline are combined, a greater potential exists for adverse effects to occur because both agents have significant effects on the intestine.

Prep kits are designed for use to prepare the bowel for endoscopic examination or surgery. (See Table 12–5.) The kit usually contains separate dosages of the specific laxatives rather than a single dosage form containing all the ingredients. Although a patient may experience adverse effects from prep kits, they are intended for a single use before a procedure, unlike the usual treatment for constipation.

Pharmacotherapeutic Comparison

Head-to-head comparison studies solely among nonprescription laxatives are largely unavailable. Much of what is practiced has been gained through observation following laxative use. One study has suggested that psyllium is superior to docusate in treating chronic constipation. The multisite, randomized, and double-blind parallel design study of 170 subjects with chronic idiopathic constipation concluded that psyllium showed superior action to docusate for softening stools because it increased stool water content and exhibited greater overall laxative efficacy.[40] If used properly, a bulk-forming product should soften the stool by its normal action. Because both a traditional stool softener and a bulk-forming agent take about the same length of time to work, a bulk-forming agent may be the correct choice for some patients who require stool softening.

Very few new entity laxative products have been introduced into the marketplace in recent years. Most principal ingredients were brought into being before the current era of rigorous comparative studies. Patients popularly use stimulants and saline-type laxatives, but the continued practice of recommending a laxative on the basis of the lowest ability to produce significant untoward effect remains an important concept.

Product Selection Guidelines

When considering the use of any laxative to treat constipation, the pharmacist should remember that normal defecation empties only the rectum and the descending and sigmoid branches of the colon. The preparation chosen should duplicate the normal physiologic process as nearly as possible. Most stimulant products have the potential to promote catharsis—that is, a complete emptying of the entire colon. However, the laxative user who is unaware of this effect may take another laxative dose on the first or second post-laxative day, thereby maintaining a completely empty colon. Thus, when it is necessary to use a laxative to treat constipation, the recommended initial choice is most often a bulk-forming product. Mineral oil can cause malabsorption of fat-soluble vitamins or lipid pneumonia if it is aspirated, so its use should be avoided. (See Table 12–5 for examples of commercially available laxatives.)

Acute constipation is the primary indication for self-treatment with a nonprescription laxative. However, nonprescription laxative products are also prescribed or indicated for patients preparing for diagnostic GI procedures and radiography. A physician should supervise the use of laxatives (1) during treatment for perianal disease (preoperatively or post-

Table 12–5

Selected Laxative Products

Trade Name	Primary Ingredients
Bulk-Forming Laxatives	
Citrucel Powder	Methylcellulose 2 g/tablespoon
Citrucel Sugar Free Powder[a]	Methylcellulose 2 g/tablespoon
FiberCon Tablets[a–c]	Calcium polycarbophil 625 mg
Konsyl Powder[a]	Psyllium mucilloid 100%
Maltsupex Liquid	Barley malt extract 750 mg/tablespoon
Metamucil Fiber Wafer[b,c]	Psyllium hydrophilic mucilloid 3.4 g/2 wafers
Metamucil Original Texture, Powder[c]	Psyllium hydrophilic mucilloid 3.4 g/tablespoon
Metamucil Original Texture, Regular Flavor Powder[c]	Psyllium hydrophilic mucilloid 3.4 g/teaspoon
Metamucil Smooth Texture, Orange Flavor Powder[c]	Psyllium hydrophilic mucilloid 3.4 g/tablespoon
Metamucil Smooth Texture, Sugar Free Orange Flavor Powder/Individual Packets[a,c]	Psyllium hydrophilic mucilloid 3.4 g/teaspoon
Mitrolan Chewable Tablets[d]	Calcium polycarbophil 500 mg
Perdiem Fiber Granules	Psyllium 4 g/teaspoon
Serutan Granules	Psyllium hydrophilic mucilloid 2.5 mg/teaspoon
Emollient Laxatives	
Colace Liquid[c,e]	Docusate sodium 50 mg/5 mL
Colace Capsules	Docusate sodium 50 mg; 100 mg
Correctol Stool Softener Sofgels	Docusate sodium 100 mg
Ex-Lax Stool Softener Caplets[a,c]	Docusate sodium 100 mg
Lubricant Laxatives	
Fleet Mineral Oil Enema	Mineral oil 100%
Fleet Mineral Oil Oral Lubricant Liquid[c–f]	Mineral oil 100%
Kondremul Emulsion[d]	Mineral oil 55%
Saline Laxatives	
Citroma Solution	Magnesium citrate 1.74 g/oz
Fleet Ready-to-Use Enema	Monobasic sodium phosphate 19 g/118 mL; dibasic sodium phosphate 7 g/118 mL
Fleet Ready-to-Use Enema for Children[g]	Monobasic sodium phosphate 9.5 g/59 mL; dibasic sodium phosphate 3.5 g/59 mL
Phillips' Milk of Magnesia Concentrate Suspension[c,f]	Magnesium hydroxide 800 mg/5 mL
Phillips' Milk of Magnesia Suspension[c,f]	Magnesium hydroxide 400 mg/5 mL
Hyperosmotic Laxatives	
Fleet Babylax Liquid	Glycerin
Fleet Glycerin Suppository (Adult/Child Size)	Glycerin
Fleet Glycerin Rectal Applicators Liquid	Glycerin 7.5 mL
Stimulant Laxatives	
Correctol Caplets/Tablets	Bisacodyl 5 mg
Correctol Herbal Tea	Senna (total sennosides), 30 mg/teabag
Dulcolax Tablets[d]	Bisacodyl 5 mg
Ex-Lax Gentle Nature Natural Tablets	Sennosides A and B 20 mg
Ex-Lax Maximum Strength Tablets	Sennosides 25 mg

(continued)

Table 12–5

Selected Laxative Products (continued)

Trade Name	Primary Ingredients
Stimulant Laxatives (continued)	
Ex-Lax Regular Strength Chocolate Tablets[d]	Sennosides 15 mg
Feen-A-Mint Tablets	Bisacodyl 5 mg
Fleet Laxative Suppository	Bisacodyl 10 mg
Fleet Laxative Tablets	Bisacodyl 5 mg
Neoloid Oil	Castor oil 36.4%
Purge Liquid[a,c,e]	Castor oil 95%
Senokot Tablets	Senna concentrate 8.6 mg sennosides
Senokot Children's Syrup[f,g]	Senna concentrate 8.8 mg/5 mL sennosides
X-Prep Liquid	Senna concentrate 3.7 g/75 mL standardized extract of senna fruit
Combination Laxatives	
Fleet Bisacodyl Enema[d]	Bisacodyl 10 mg; glycerin
Haleys M-O Flavored or Regular Emulsion[c,f]	Mineral oil 1.25 mg/5mL; magnesium hydroxide 301 mg/5mL
Innerclean Herbal Cut Plants/Tablets	Senna leaves; psyllium seed husks; buckthorn bark
Perdiem Granules	Senna (cassia pod concentrate) 0.74 g/teaspoon; psyllium 3.25 g/teaspoon
Phospho-soda Buffered Liquid	Monobasic sodium phosphate 2.4 g/5 mL (sodium 550 mg/5 mL); dibasic sodium phosphate 0.9 g/5 mL; glycerin
Senokot-S Tablets	Senna concentrate 8.6 mg sennosides; docusate sodium 50 mg
Sof-lax Overnight Gelcaps	Casanthranol 30 mg; docusate sodium 100 mg; glycerin
Surfak Liqui-gels[c,d]	Docusate calcium 240 mg; glycerin
Bowel Evacuant Kits	
Evac-Q-Kwik System Liquid/Suppository/Tablets[a]	Tablets: bisacodyl 15 mg/3 tablets; suppository: bisacodyl 10 mg; liquid: magnesium citrate 25 mEq/30 mL
Fleet Prep Kit 1	Tablets: bisacodyl 20 mg/4 tablets; suppository: bisacodyl 10 mg; liquid: sodium phosphate oral solution 45 mL (total sodium 495 mg/45 mL); glycerin
Fleet Prep Kit 2[e]	Tablets: bisacodyl 20 mg/4 tablets; liquid: sodium phosphate oral solution 45 mL; glycerin; enema: liquid castile soap 9 mL
Fleet Prep Kit 3	Tablets: bisacodyl 20 mg/4 tablets; enema: bisacodyl 10 mg; glycerin; liquid: sodium phosphate oral solution 45 mL

[a] Sucrose-free product.
[b] Dye-free product.
[c] Lactose-free product.
[d] Sodium-free product.
[e] Sulfite-free product.
[f] Alcohol-free product.
[g] Pediatric formulation.

operatively), (2) during conditions in which straining is undesirable (e.g., postoperative or postmyocardial infarct), or (3) for chronic constipation. Although bulk-forming and emollient laxatives may be suitable for such problems, therapy in these situations is highly individualized.

Guidelines for Use in Underlying Pathology The pharmacist should exercise caution when recommending magnesium-containing products to patients with renal failure because of the risk of hypermagnesemia. The pharmacist should be similarly cautious when recommending sodium-containing products to patients with cardiovascular disease because of the potential for sodium overload. As a rule, laxative products whose maximum daily dose contains more than 345 mg (15 mEq) of sodium, 975 mg (25 mEq) of potassium, 600 mg (50 mEq) of magnesium, or 1800 mg (90 mEq) of calcium should not be used in kidney or liver disease, heart failure, hypertension, or other conditions requiring sodium, potassium, magnesium, or calcium restriction.

Any product containing dextrose should be used with caution in labile diabetic patients because glycemic control may be lost, and products containing aspartame should be avoided in patients with phenylketonuria.

Guidelines for Use in Children Laxatives are often given to children according to what the parents believe should be normal bowel habits. As a result, indiscriminate use of laxatives may occur. The pharmacist should always consider a child's age when recommending laxative products. The route of administration and the taste of oral products may be especially significant in children. The use of laxatives may be avoided in older children if they are encouraged to establish a regular pattern of bowel movements and adhere to suggested dietary guidelines.

If medications are indicated in children younger than 5 years, glycerin suppositories may initiate the defecation reflex with an onset usually within 15 to 60 minutes. Malt soup extract is relatively safe for infants younger than 2 months. Breast-fed infants may receive 6 to 10 mL in 2 to 4 ounces of water or fruit juice twice daily. Bottle-fed infants may receive 7.5 to 32 mL in a day's total formula, or 5 to 10 mL every second feeding. Dark corn syrup (1 to 2 teaspoons per feeding) or milk of magnesia (beginning with ½ teaspoon) may be useful for fecal impaction. Bisacodyl may be used for moderate to severe constipation. In general, stimulants should probably be avoided, as should excessive use of enemas. Enemas are not usually recommended for children under age 2 years. Senna and mineral oil should be administered only on the advice of a physician. When successful bowel evacuation cannot be achieved with oral supplementation or enemas, pediatricians may prescribe a balanced polyethylene glycol–electrolyte solution (e.g., Golytely or Colyte) to be administered orally. (See Chapter 13, "Diarrhea," for discussion of electrolyte solutions.) Children may find such a solution more palatable if it is chilled.[41]

Guidelines for Use in the Elderly Prolonged and excessive laxative use is not uncommon in the elderly. The colon in the elderly can lack normal tone, resulting in an overreliance on oral laxatives or rectal enemas. Many elderly patients have been laxative dependent for many years. However, because of the physiologic effects of chronic laxative use on the intestine, laxative dependency is often difficult to manage. Laxative preparations can also increase the rate at which other drugs pass through the GI tract by increasing GI motility, which then decreases absorption and the effectiveness of concurrently administered medications.

Elderly patients are particularly sensitive to shifts in fluid and electrolytes. Use of any laxative that alters the fluid and electrolyte balance, particularly saline-type laxatives, may be inappropriate in certain elderly patients. Such laxatives can place patients—particularly those who are on diuretics or have decreased fluid intake—at risk for adverse effects.

It has been suggested that an acute episode of constipation be treated with plain water or saline enemas.[13,20] Soapsuds enemas should be avoided because they can be irritating and can cause serious complications.[13,42] Sodium phosphate and biphosphate enemas are effective. Polyethylene glycol–electrolyte solutions, commonly used as bowel preparations for GI procedures, have been safely used for acute management of constipation in elderly patients who suffer from cardiac or renal disease.[13] For elderly patients requiring laxatives, bulk-forming agents are generally preferred; onset is usually in 2 to 3 days. Sugar-free products (e.g., Konsyl, Serutan, and various Metamucil products) are recommended for diabetic patients.[13] Glycerin suppositories and orally administered lactulose are safe and have been used successfully in elderly patients;[13] lactulose may be of particular benefit to those who are bedridden.[13] Some health care providers may recommend chronic stimulant laxatives in certain situations, but these products should not be generally recommended in all elderly patients. Recommendations of laxative use in this population should be patient specific because the elderly have complicating pathology and multiple disease states and these patients are often vulnerable to medications. Even though bulk-forming agents are often successfully used in this population, a complete and thorough history should aid in selecting the most-appropriate product.

Guidelines for Use in Pregnancy Most types of laxatives appear to be effective during pregnancy. Laxatives may have to be administered postpartum to reestablish normal bowel function that may have been lost because of perineal pain. Other indications include ileus secondary to colonic dilatation in a decompressed abdomen, laxness of the anal sphincter and abdominal musculature, low fluid intake, and administration of enemas during labor. In addition, hemorrhoids in the period after delivery may be aggravated, if not caused, by constipation. In some instances, the pharmacist should consult with the woman's health care provider before recommending a laxative, especially if any doubt exists regarding the provider's desire for the patient to have a laxative.

Because of the potential for adverse effects such as (1) decreased vitamin absorption caused by mineral oil, (2) premature labor brought on by the irritant effects of castor oil, or (3) possible dangerous electrolyte imbalances with osmotic agents, pregnant women are probably best treated with bulk-formers or emollient laxatives. Although stimulant laxatives should generally be avoided during pregnancy, one source suggests that some stimulants may be acceptable for use during the lactation period.[43] Senna and related anthraquinones have been used during breast-feeding despite a lack of information regarding their concentration in breast milk. Bisacodyl appears in breast milk in trace amounts but may not pose problems for the infant.[43] If these products are used, the infant should be carefully observed for diarrhea. Saline cathartics should probably be avoided during pregnancy and lactation because appreciable GI absorption can occur in the mother. Toxicity occurring from excessive use of a saline cathartic such as magnesium sulfate could be significant, considering that such toxicity could result in diarrhea, drowsiness, respiratory difficulty, and hypotonia.

Guidelines for Selecting Dosage Forms Laxative products are available in a wide array of dosage forms, most of them for oral use. This variety probably yields the most benefits for pediatric and geriatric patients. Many of the dosage forms

Case Study 12–2

Patient Complaint/History

Aja, a 34-year-old mother of two small children (ages 2 and 5 years), is 7 months pregnant. Her managed care plan requires that she obtain any chronic or long-term medication (more than a month's supply) from a mail-order program. Because the patient obtains her prenatal vitamins by mail order, she calls the hotline counseling number for advice about her constipation. She asks, "What nonprescription product should I take to relieve my constipation? I've been having a bowel movement about every 4 or 5 days, and it's difficult to pass. I have some milk of magnesia with cascara. Is it all right to use it?"

The patient's profile lists iron deficiency anemia and irritable bowel syndrome as current medical conditions. Current medications include Natalins 1 tablet daily and Vitron-C 1 tablet twice a day with meals. The patient has no known allergies.

Clinical Considerations/Strategies

Readers can use the following considerations/strategies to determine whether treatment of the patient's condition with nonprescription medications is warranted:

- Determine whether this patient has simple constipation.
- Assess whether the patient's current drug therapy could play a role in developing constipation.
- Assess the usefulness of dietary and lifestyle changes.
- Assess the appropriateness of the laxative products that the patient has at home.
- Recommend appropriate nonprescription medications to manage this patient's constipation.

Patient Education/Counseling

Readers can use the following strategies to develop a patient education/counseling plan that will help ensure optimal therapeutic outcomes:

- Explain the importance of dietary and lifestyle modifications.
- Explain the proper use of the recommended nonprescription medication.
- Explain the signs/symptoms that warrant medical attention.

enhance patient acceptability and perhaps make laxative use more pleasant. However, laxatives available as chewing gum, wafers, effervescent granules, and chocolate tablets may not be thought of as drug products and thus are more likely to be misused and abused. Enemas and suppositories are dosage forms often used for laxative administration.

Enemas Routine use of laxative enemas includes preparing patients for surgery, child delivery, and GI radiologic or endoscopic examination as well as treating certain cases of constipation. The enema fluid determines the mechanism by which evacuation is produced. Tap water and normal saline create bulk by an osmotic volume effect; vegetable oils lubricate, soften, and facilitate the passage of hardened fecal matter; and soapsuds produce defecation by their irritant action. However, prolonged rectal irritation may occur after soap enemas and may result in proctitis or colitis.[44] Therefore, soap enemas are not recommended.

The popular sodium phosphate–sodium biphosphate enemas (e.g., Fleet) fall into the category of saline laxatives. They are usually effective evacuants in preparing patients for surgical, diagnostic, or other procedures involving the bowel. These agents are more efficient and effective than tap water, soapsuds, or saline enemas. Because they can alter fluid and electrolyte balance significantly if used on a prolonged basis, chronic use of these products is not warranted in the control of constipation.

A properly administered enema cleans only the distal colon, most nearly approximating a normal bowel movement. Proper administration requires that the diagnosis, the enema fluid, and the technique of administration be correct. Improperly administered, an enema can produce fluid and electrolyte imbalances. Enema fluids have caused mucosal changes or spasm of the intestinal wall. Water intoxication has resulted from the use of tap water or soapsuds enemas in the presence of megacolon. A misdirected or inadequately lubricated nozzle may cause abrasion of the anal canal and rectal wall or may cause colonic perforation.

Patients should be advised to follow all directions carefully when using these products. The patient should lie or be placed either on the left side with knees bent or in the knee-to-chest position. If the patient is in a sitting position, use of an enema clears only the rectum of fecal material. The solution should be allowed to flow into the rectum slowly; if the patient is uncomfortable, the flow is probably too fast. One pint (500 mL) or less of properly introduced fluid usually produces adequate evacuation if it is retained until definite lower abdominal cramping is felt. As long as 1 hour may be needed for the entire procedure.

Suppositories Bisacodyl suppositories are promoted as replacements for enemas when the distal colon requires cleaning. Suppositories that contain bisacodyl are promoted for postoperative, antepartum, and postpartum care and are adequate in preparing for proctosigmoidoscopy. Although bisacodyl suppositories are prescribed and are used more often than other suppositories, some clinicians still prefer enemas as agents for cleaning the lower bowel.

Liquids Liquid formulations of emollients may be made more palatable if mixed with juices or milk. The most commonly used products containing castor oil are the more palatable emulsions. When plain castor oil is used, it may be administered with fruit juice or a carbonated beverage to mask its unpleasant taste. Chilling the oral form of a sodium phosphate–type product or taking it with ice seems to make it more palatable. Palatability may be improved by drinking the product with a citrus fruit juice or with a citrus-flavored carbonated beverage.

Pharmacoeconomics

A recent comprehensive review by the United Kingdom's National Health Service states, "There have been very few economic evaluations of either laxative treatment or the prevention of constipation."[45] It continues, "The relative cost-effectiveness of different laxative classes will depend on the results of comparisons between different laxative preparations, and this information is, by and large, unavailable."

Individual products vary widely in cost. The variation is evident in brand versus generic and in well-known versus lesser-known manufacturers. This kind of variation exists among all of the major categories and for most of the principal active ingredients. Some products, such as citrate of magnesia, despite a relatively low cost (perhaps, $2.00 per 240 mL) of purchase, have a relatively high cost per dose when compared with most laxatives. Although it is cheap to purchase, only one dose is available per unit as opposed to most of the other available products having multiple dosages per unit of sale. Of course, cost per dose becomes an issue only if the product is used frequently versus the occasional use intended.

Cost of therapy can be an important issue when the therapy is warranted. It seems reasonable to assume that laxative expenditures may be artificially elevated because of the presumed poor use of nonpharmacologic measures. However, the application of potentially useful lifestyle changes may reduce the need for laxative purchases and, correspondingly, lower overall cost to the patient. Of course, the most effective treatment for constipation is the one that provides for normal or close to normal bowel function without causing untoward effects. Nonpharmacologic measures, when appropriately followed, have the potential to fulfill this criterion in many constipated patients.

Alternative Remedies

Constipation is frequently treated with herbal products.[19,46] (See Table 12–6.) Although many of the stimulant and bulk-forming laxatives that are commercially available are derived from plants, some consumers prefer to use a "more natural" version of these products. Consumers are cautioned that FDA does not regulate these products and that the manufacturers are not required to provide information on how to use the products safely and effectively. Although such products are considered dietary substances and not "medications," they can potentially interact with prescription medications.

Table 12–6

Popular Herbs That May Act as Laxatives or Cathartics

Herb
Aloe (*Aloe vera*)
Cascara sagrada bark (*Rhamnus purshiana*)
Chicory (*Cichorium intybus*)
Dandelion (*Taraxacum officinale*)
Dong quai (*Angelica seninsis*)
Feverfew (*Tanacetum parthenium*)
Fo-ti (*Polygonum multiflorum*)
Kelp (seaweed/algae)
Licorice (*Glycyrrhiza glabra*)
Prune concentrate (*Prunus domestica*)
Rose hips (*Rosa* sp.)
Sarsaparilla (*Menispermum canadense*)
Senna leaves (*Cassia* sp.)
Yellow dock (*Rumex crispus*)

Source: References 19 and 46.

Patients should be encouraged to consult a physician or pharmacist for advice on the safe use of these products.

Patient Assessment of Constipation

The pharmacist should obtain as much lifestyle and medical information as possible before making any recommendations for preventing or treating constipation. Appropriate information allows the pharmacist to make rational recommendations that are based on knowledge of the patient, the problem, and the product, as well as on the pharmacist's own judgment and experience. Evaluation of all drug use is critical in selecting appropriate laxatives.

A patient who presents with constipation should initially be evaluated for any signs of significant gastrointestinal problems that may warrant medical evaluation, such as severe abdominal pain, nausea and vomiting, or rectal bleeding. The pharmacist must recognize the situations in which laxative use is inappropriate. For example, laxatives are not recommended to treat constipation associated with intestinal pathology or secondary to laxative abuse unless bowel retraining has been successful. Laxatives also are not a cure for functional constipation and, therefore, are of only secondary importance in treating this condition. Attention should be directed first to questions relating to diet, fluid intake, physical activity, and any underlying pathology that may be producing constipation as a symptom.

Patients should then be questioned regarding the characteristics of bowel movements including the size, color, and texture of stools as well as the frequency of elimination. Additional assessment should include questions about use of medications, both prescription and nonprescription, as well as previous laxative use. Adequate patient assessment is essential to effective management of constipation. For geriatric patients without a history of constipation, a thorough investigation should be conducted to determine whether acute cases of constipation have resulted from new or old diseases or from the use of medications. When information is insufficient to assess the cause of the symptoms or any doubt exists regarding the patient's disease status, medical referral is appropriate.

Asking the patient the following questions will help elicit the information needed to accurately assess the disorder and to determine the appropriate treatment approach.

Q~ Why do you feel you need a laxative?

A~ If the laxative is to be used in preparation for a GI exam, verify that the patient has seen a gastroenterologist and received instructions to make this purchase. If the patient thinks he or she has constipation, ask about the symptoms. If the rationale for use is unclear, try to clarify the situation.

Q~ Are you experiencing or have you experienced abdominal discomfort or pain, bloating, weight loss, nausea, or vomiting?

A~ If yes, refer the patient to a physician. (See the "General Treatment Approach" for a list of other exclusions to self-treatment.) If no, ask about the presence of other symptoms and about any preexisting disease and its treatment. Evaluate the response carefully. Any patient who has an established disease or surgery affecting the GI tract presents a particular concern because laxative products very possibly may affect the patient's condition adversely.

Q~ How often do you normally have a bowel movement? Have you noticed a change in frequency? How would you describe your bowel movements? Has the nature of your bowel movements recently changed in any way?

A~ To determine whether constipation is present, evaluate the patient's description of frequency of bowel movements, consistency of the stool, difficulty in elimination, and accompanying symptoms. If necessary, ask the patient to clarify descriptive terms to ensure an accurate translation of the symptoms.

Q~ Has the appearance of your stools changed? In what way?

A~ *Identify stool characteristics that require medical referral. (See the section "General Treatment Approach.")* If the stools have such characteristics, refer the patient to a physician.

Q~ How long has constipation been a problem?

A~ If the constipation is long-standing, find out how often and for how long the patient has used laxatives and whether the patient is having other symptoms. Refer the patient to a physician if symptoms of underlying pathology are present.

Q~ Have you attempted to relieve the constipation by eating more cereals, bread with a high-fiber content, fruits, or vegetables?

A~ If the patient's diet is low in fiber, advise eating more of the high-fiber foods listed in Table 12–3. (See the food guide pyramid in Chapter 19, "Nutritional Deficiencies," for recommended daily servings of food groups.) Explain that it may take 3 or more days for the dietary changes to relieve constipation.

Q~ How much physical exercise do you get?

A~ If the patient describes a sedentary lifestyle, advise increasing physical activity. (See the section "Nonpharmacologic Therapy.") Advise the patient that his or her physical conditioning will determine how soon this lifestyle change produces an effect.

Q~ How many glasses of water or other fluids do you drink each day?

A~ If fluid intake is inadequate, advise the patient to drink more fluids. (See the section "Nonpharmacologic Therapy.") Advise the patient that increased fluid intake may help relieve the constipation in 2 or more days.

Q~ Have you previously used laxatives to relieve constipation?

A~ From the patient's history of laxative use, determine the frequency and severity of constipation, previous patterns of medication use, effective or ineffective products, and use of home remedies. Use the findings to recommend either self-treatment or medical referral. (See the section "General Treatment Approach" for exclusions to self-treatment.)

Q~ Are you using a laxative medication or herbal laxative now?

A~ If the patient is using a laxative without effect, recommend another product if self-treatment is appropriate.

Q~ How often and how long have you used a laxative?

A~ If the laxative use has exceeded product recommendations, caution the patient that such use can cause laxative dependence or other adverse effects, depending on the type of laxative being used.

Q~ Have you had any unwanted effects from laxatives, such as diarrhea or stomach pain?

A~ If yes, find out which types of laxatives caused the adverse effects; then recommend a different type.

Q~ Are you currently taking any medication other than laxatives? If so, what prescription and nonprescription medications are you currently taking?

A~ *Identify medications that cause constipation. (See Table 12–2.)* If the patient is taking a prescription medication known to cause constipation, contact the prescriber or refer the patient for possible medication adjustment. If the medication history does not indicate use of constipating drugs, recommend a laxative product that will not interact with the patient's medications.

Q~ Are you allergic to any medication?

A~ Do not neglect to record known allergies for patients who request a laxative consultation. Monitor any patient who takes any laxative to determine whether a heretofore unsuspected allergic reaction to a product has occurred.

Patient Counseling for Constipation

Because laxative products are both widely used and abused, the pharmacist can provide a valuable service by educating patients about the appropriate use of laxatives. Proper education about laxative products and wise advice on product selection and use are particularly crucial for the elderly patient. Before recommending a laxative product, however, the pharmacist should first discuss with the patient the nondrug measures for treating constipation. Pregnant women, especially, should be counseled on proper diet, adequate fluid intake, and reasonable exercise. Patients may not understand how these factors affect the development of constipation and how they can return a person to a relatively normal state of bowel function without laxative use. If a laxative is needed, the pharmacist should explain why a particular type of laxative is appropriate for the present situation, how to use the laxative, what adverse effects could occur, and what precautions to take. The box "Patient Education for Constipation" lists specific information to provide patients.

Patient Education for Constipation

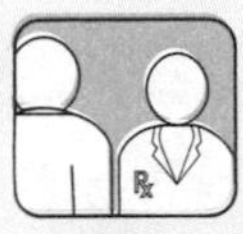

The objectives of self-treatment are to relieve constipation and restore "normal" bowel functioning by implementing (1) dietary and lifestyle measures and/or (2) the safe use of laxative products. For most patients, carefully following the product instructions and the self-care measures listed below will help ensure optimal therapeutic outcomes.

Nondrug Measures

- Use natural methods such as a high-fiber diet, adequate fluid intake, and exercise to foster regular bowel movements.
- Increase dietary fiber by eating foods containing wheat grains, oats, fruits, and vegetables.
- Avoid constipating foods such as processed cheeses and concentrated sweets.
- Drink plenty of fluids (four to six 8-ounce glasses a day) to aid in stool softening and to facilitate fecal evacuation.
- Develop and maintain a routine exercise program. Walking can be beneficial if your cardiovascular system is healthy and if you have no other apparent health risks.
- Establish a regular pattern for bathroom visits. Do not delay responding to the urge to defecate; allow adequate time for elimination in a relaxed, unhurried atmosphere.
- Maintain general emotional well-being and avoid stressful situations.

Nonprescription Medications

- Do not routinely take laxatives if your bowel habits are interrupted for a day or two, or to routinely "clean your system."
- Do not give laxatives to children younger than 6 years unless prescribed by a physician.
- If you have kidney or liver disease; heart failure; hypertension; or other conditions requiring sodium, potassium, magnesium, or calcium restriction, do not use laxative products whose maximum daily dose contains more than 345 mg (15 mEq) of sodium, 975 mg (25 mEq) of potassium, 600 mg (50 mEq) of magnesium, or 1800 mg (90 mEq) of calcium.
- Consult your physician before using laxatives if you currently have or have a history of any of the following conditions: colectomy, ileostomy, diabetes, heart disease, kidney disease, or swallowing difficulties.
- Consult a physician or pharmacist before using a laxative product if you are taking anticoagulants (blood thinners), digoxin (a heart medicine), sodium polystyrene sulfonate (a treatment for high potassium levels), or tetracycline antibiotics.
- Avoid taking laxatives within 2 hours of taking other medications.
- Do not take laxatives longer than 1 week. Consult a doctor if symptoms of constipation persist.
- Take laxatives at bedtime, especially if more than 6 to 8 hours is required to produce results.

(continued)

Patient Education for Constipation (continued)

- Discard any medications that are outdated, that appear to have been tampered with, or that have an unusual appearance.

Bulk-Forming Laxatives

- Unless a rapid effect, such as cleaning out the bowel for a diagnostic procedure or X-ray is needed, take a bulk-forming laxative. Be sure to drink at least 8 ounces of fluids with each dose to prevent intestinal obstruction.
- Use bulk-forming laxatives with caution if you are diabetic or are on a carbohydrate-restricted diet. These laxatives have a high caloric content per dose and contain the sweetener dextrose.
- Do not give sugar-free, bulk-forming products to patients with phenylketonuria. Such products may contain aspartame, which contributes excessive levels of phenylalanine, an amino acid these patients cannot metabolize.

Lubricant Laxatives

- Do not give mineral oil to children younger than 6 years, pregnant patients, elderly patients, or patients taking anticoagulants.
- Do not take mineral oil with emollient laxatives.
- To avoid delaying the absorption of foods, nutrients, and vitamins, do not take mineral oil within 2 hours of eating.

Saline Laxatives

- Take saline laxatives on an empty stomach; the presence of food will delay action.
- Do not take saline laxatives every day.
- Do not give these laxatives orally to children younger than 6 years or rectally to infants younger than 2 years.

Stimulant Laxatives

- Do not use castor oil to treat constipation except under the advice of a physician.

⚠ Do not take laxatives if you have any symptoms of appendicitis (abdominal pain, nausea, vomiting), rectal bleeding, painful anal or rectal conditions, bloating, or cramping. See a physician immediately.

⚠ If symptoms are unrelieved by nondrug measures or by 1 week of laxative treatment, see a physician. Chronic constipation may be a symptom of an underlying medical condition.

Evaluation of Patient Outcomes for Constipation

Constipation often presents with a great degree of variability among individuals. Although a decrease in frequency of bowel movements is typically associated with constipation, difficulty in passing stools and a decrease in the amount passed are also common complaints. The type, severity, and chronicity of symptoms are an important determinant in selecting the most appropriate treatment modality. Once therapy has been selected, effectiveness is determined by how rapidly constipation is relieved and to what degree normal bowel habits have been restored.

For acute constipation, dietary changes and exercise or the use of bulk-forming laxatives may take several days to weeks to provide relief. Stimulant laxatives usually provide results within 24 hours; osmotic laxatives provide more immediate relief, usually within 15 minutes to 3 hours for oral preparations. Laxative enemas, often used when fecal impaction accompanies constipation, can produce evacuation within minutes. If initial treatment is ineffective, therapy should be repeated according to product-specific directions. If an adequate response is not achieved after a short period of time, usually within 1 week, chronic constipation should be considered and the patient should be evaluated by a physician.

Self-medication with laxatives can be safe and effective if used as directed and not excessively. Close monitoring of the frequency and duration of laxative use can be beneficial in determining whether normal bowel habits are actually reestablished between bouts of constipation or if a more severe condition exists. If a laxative must be continued for an extended period such as in chronic constipation, bulk-forming agents are preferred. However, the need for frequent laxative use should be discussed with a physician, because this may be a sign of (1) a more severe form of constipation, (2) a side effect of a medication, or (3) an underlying medical problem. Overuse or extended use of some laxatives can alter the normal physiologic functioning of the gut and may lead to a dependence on laxatives for bowel function. Adhering to a diet high in fiber and drinking plenty of fluids can aid in preventing constipation and should be continued even during periods when bowel habits are normal.

Any signs of appendicitis, blood in the stool, severe abdominal pain, nausea and vomiting, or hypersensitivity reactions that occur during the course of treatment should be reported immediately to a physician. An increase in dietary fiber or use of a bulk-forming laxative may cause an increase in flatulence or bloating that typically resolves after several days of continuous use and that is not usually a cause for concern.

CONCLUSIONS

The widespread misuse and abuse of nonprescription laxatives is evidence of the need for professional consultation and patient education. Successful treatment of constipation depends on careful identification of the cause. To determine whether self-treatment or medical referral is indicated, the pharmacist needs to know the case history and current symptoms, as well as the patient's reason for purchasing a laxative. What is perceived as constipation varies from person to person; therefore, careful questioning about frequency of bowel movements and stool characteristics is vital in determining whether constipation is present. If the case history discloses a sudden change in bowel habits that has persisted for 2 weeks, the pharmacist should refer the patient to a physician immediately.

If the constipation can be treated without physician intervention, the pharmacist must have knowledge of nondrug measures and of the many available laxative products. For most cases of simple constipation, proper diet, exercise, and adequate fluid intake will be helpful. Patient factors (i.e., consideration for age, pregnancy, etc.) must be considered when evaluating a person for potential laxative use. Patient preferences such as dosage form and palatability issues should be considered when recommending a laxative agent so as to ensure good adherence and a short treatment period. Therapy with any laxative product should be limited in most cases to short-term use (1 week). If no relief has been achieved after 1 week of proper laxative therapy, use of the product should be discontinued and a physician consulted.

Overall, laxative cost is variable. Concomitant use of nonpharmacologic measures may lead to lower cost of laxative product therapy for the patient with simple constipation.

References

1. Snyder K. The state of the o-t-c marketplace. *Drug Topics.* June 1997;141:82–90.
2. Harari D, Gurwitz JH, Avorn J, et al. Bowel habit in relation to age and gender: findings from the National Health Interview. *Arch Intern Med.* 1996;156:315–20.
3. Talley NJ, Fleming KC, O'Keefe EA, et al. Constipation in an elderly community: a study of prevalence and potential risk factors. *Am J Gastroenterol.* 1996;91:19–25.
4. Campbell AJ, Busby WJ, Horwath CC. Factors associated with constipation in a community based sample of people aged 70 years and over. *J Epidemiol Community Health.* 1993;47:23–6.
5. Greenhalf JO, Leonard HS. Laxatives in the treatment of constipation of pregnant and breast feeding mothers. *Practitioner.* 1973;210:259.
6. Gattuso JM, Kamm MA. Review article: the management of constipation in adults. *Aliment Pharmacol Ther.* 1993;7:487–500.
7. Talley NJ, Zinsmeister AR, Melton LJ. Irritable bowel syndrome in a community: symptoms subgroups, risk factors, and health care utilization. *Am J Epidemiol.* 1995;142:76–83.
8. Cummings JH. Constipation. In: Misiewicz JJ, Pounder RE, Venables CW, eds. *Diseases of the Gut and Pancreas.* 2nd ed. Oxford, England: Blackwell Scientific Publications; 1994:51–70.
9. Lennard-Jones JE. Constipation. In: Feldman M, Scharschmidt BF, Sleisenger MH, eds. *Sleisenger & Fordtran's Gastrointestinal and Liver Disease: Pathophysiology, Diagnosis, Management.* 6th ed. Philadelphia: WB Saunders Company; 1998:174–97.
10. Hogue VW. Diarrhea and constipation. In: Herfindal ET, Gourley DR, eds. *Textbook of Therapeutics: Drug and Disease Management.* 6th ed. Baltimore: Williams and Wilkins; 1996:517–31.
11. Wong V, Sobala G, Losowsky M. A case of narcotic bowel syndrome successfully treated with clonidine. *Postgrad Med J.* 1994;70:138–40.
12. Wald AW. Constipation and fecal incontinence in the elderly. *Semin Gastr Dis.* 1994;5:179–88.
13. Rosseau P. Treatment of constipation in the elderly. *Postgrad Med.* 1988;83:339–40, 343–5, 349.
14. Nowicki MJ, Bishop PR. Organic causes of constipation in infants and children. *Pediatric Annals.* 1999;28:293–300.
15. Loening-Baucke V. Constipation in children. *Curr Opinion Pediatr.* 1994;6:556–61.
16. Connell AM, Hilton C, Irvine G, et al. Variation of bowel habit in 2 population samples. *Br Med J.* 1965;2:1095.
17. Felt B, Wise CG, Olson A, et al. Guideline for the management of pediatric idiopathic constipation and soiling. *Arch Pediatr Adolesc Med.* 1999;153:380–5
18. Murphy SM. Constipation. In: Walker WA, Durie PR, Hamilton JR, et al. eds. *Pediatric Gastrointestinal Disease: Pathophysiology, Diagnosis, Management.* 2nd ed. St. Louis: Mosby-Year Book; 1996:293–321.
19. Self-care for constipation. In: Albrant DH, ed. *The American Pharmaceutical Association Drug Treatment Protocols.* Washington, DC: American Pharmaceutical Association; 1999.
20. Brandt LJ. *Gastrointestinal Disorders of the Elderly.* New York: Raven Press; 1984:261–367.
21. Lanza E, Butrum RR. A critical review of food fiber analysis and data. *J Am Diet Assoc.* 1986;86:732–43.
22. Williams CL. Importance of dietary fiber in childhood. *J Am Diet Assoc.* 1995;95:1140–7.
23. Cummings JH. Fermentation in the human large intestine: evidence and implications for health. *Lancet.* 1983;1:1206.
24. Vaswani SK, Hamilton RG, Valentine MD, et al. Psyllium laxative-induced anaphylaxis, asthma, and rhinitis. *Allergy.* 1996;51:266–8.
25. National Institutes of Health. *Optimal calcium intake* [abstract]. National Institutes of Health Consensus Development Conference Statement. September 1994.
26. Wald A. Constipation in elderly patients: pathogenesis and management. *Drugs and Aging.* 1993; 3:220–31.
27. Proposed monograph of the panel on the safety and efficacy of laxatives, antidiarrheals, antiemetics, and emetics. Part II. *Federal Register.* 1975;40:12907, 12911–2.
28. Gattuso JM, Kamm MA. Adverse effects of drugs used in the management of constipation and diarrhea. *Drug Safety.* 1994;10:47–65.
29. Knobel B, Petechenko P. Hyperphosphatemic hypocalcemic coma caused by hypertonic sodium phosphate (fleet) enema intoxication. *J Clin Gastroenterol.* 1996;23:217–9.
30. Mofenson HC, Caraccio TR. Magnesium intoxication in a neonate from oral magnesium hydroxide laxatives. *J Toxicol Clin Toxicol.* 1991;29:215–22.
31. Laxative drug products for over-the-counter human use. *Federal Register.* 1999;64:4535–40.
32. Muller-Lissner SA. Adverse effects of laxatives: fact and fiction. *Pharmacology.* 1993;47(suppl 1):138–45.
33. Brunton LL. Agents affecting gastrointestinal water flux and motility, digestants, and bile acids. In: Gilman AG, Hardman JG, Limbird LE, et al., eds. *The Pharmacological Basis of Therapeutics.* 9th ed. New York: Pergamon Press; 1996:923.
34. Binder HJ, Dobbins JW, Whiting DS. Evidence against importance of altered mucosal permeability in ricinoleic acid induced fluid secretion. *Gastroenterology.* 1977;72:1029.

35. Pryor T, Wiederman MW, McGilley B. Laxative abuse among women with eating disorders: an indication of psychopathology? *Int J Eat Disord.* 1996;20:13–8.
36. Hall RC, Blakey RE, Hall AK. Bulimia nervosa: four uncommon subtypes. *Psychomatics.* 1992;33:428–36.
37. Babb RR. Constipation and laxative abuse. *West J Med.* 1975;122:93.
38. Baker EH, Sandle GI. Complications of laxative abuse. *Annu Rev Med.* 1996;47:127–34.
39. Stolk LM, Hoogtanders K. Detection of laxative abuse by urine analysis with HPLC and diode array detection. *Pharm World Sci.* 1999;21:40–3.
40. McRorie JW, Daggy BP, Morel JG, et al. Psyllium is superior to docusate sodium for treatment of chronic constipation. *Ailment Pharmacol Ther.* 1998;12:491–7.
41. Loening-Baucke V. Management of chronic constipation in infants and toddlers. *Am Fam Physician.* 1994;49:2397–406.
42. Rosseau P. No soapsuds enemas. *Postgrad Med.* 1988;83:352–3.
43. Briggs GG, Freeman RK, Yaffe SJ. *Drugs in Pregnancy and Lactation.* 5th ed. Baltimore: Williams & Wilkins; 1998.
44. Longe RL, DiPiro JT. Diarrhea and constipation. In: DiPiro JT, Talbert RL, Yee GC, et al., eds. *Pharmacotherapy: A Pathophysiologic Approach.* 4th ed. Baltimore: Appleton and Lange; 1999:780.
45. Pettigrew M, Watt I, Sheldon T. Systematic review of the effectiveness of laxatives in the elderly. *Health Technol Assess.* 1997;1:1–52.
46. Tyler VE. *The Honest Herbal. A Sensible Guide to the Use of Herbs and Related Remedies.* 3rd ed. Binghamton, NY: Pharmaceutical Products Press; 1993:27, 89, 113, 136, 189.

CHAPTER 13

Diarrhea

R. Leon Longe

Chapter 13 at a Glance

Diarrhea is a symptom characterized by abnormal frequency or consistency of stools. The normal frequency of bowel movements varies with each individual. Some healthy adults have as many as three well-formed stools a day; others defecate once every 2 or more days. Except for vegetarians, who consume a fiber-rich diet and thus may produce daily stools of more than 300 g, the mean daily fecal weight loss is 100 to 150 g. An increase to 200 to 300 g may be interpreted as diarrhea. Disruption of intestinal water absorption of even a few hundred milliliters may bring on diarrhea.

The etiology of diarrhea is different in Third World countries versus developed countries. In the United States, viral and food-borne diarrheal illnesses are frequent causes. Of the defined causes in the United States, Norwalk and rotavirus groups account for many gastrointestinal diarrheas.[1] However, the majority of causes cannot be determined. In Third World countries, poor sanitation and poor hygiene lead to infectious causes of diarrhea including parasites, bacteria, and viruses. Bacterial causes are as common as viral infections in these countries.

Food-borne bacterial infection has become a public health problem traced to poor sanitary conditions in meat processing plants and various retail outlets (e.g., grocery stores, drive-in restaurants). A major public health issue is *Escherichia coli* 0157:H7 contamination of food, especially undercooked hamburger.

Day care centers, nursing homes, prisons, multifamily dwellings, and other congregate environments contribute to the spread of such illnesses. Infectious illnesses that are related to acquired immunodeficiency syndrome (AIDs) have become a leading cause for diarrhea, especially in homosexual men.

Epidemiology of Diarrhea

As noted previously, diarrhea is not a disorder but a symptom of an underlying pathology or infection. The epidemiology, therefore, is related to the causes of diarrhea, as are the specific signs and symptoms. The section "Etiology of

Editor's Note: This chapter is based, in part, on the 11th edition chapter titled "Antidiarrheal Products," which was written by R. Leon Longe.

Diarrhea" correlates the various causes with their epidemiology and manifestation. Because episodes of diarrhea are often not reported, the exact epidemiology of the various causes is usually underestimated.

Children have a higher incidence of diarrhea and its complications than do adults. In the United States, about 3 million children are stricken each year at an estimated direct cost of $400 million. About 55,000 of these children need hospitalization. Most have a complete recovery but some die of complications.[2,3] In Third World countries, about 5 million children die annually from complications of acute diarrhea.

Anatomy and Physiology of the Intestines

The intestines consist of layers of smooth muscle and various glandular cells. Active contractions of the various muscles control intestinal tone. The glandular cells are actively and passively involved in maintaining normal secretory and absorptive functions. The small intestine has three anatomic divisions: the duodenum, jejunum, and ileum. It begins at the pylorus of the stomach and ends at the cecum. The digestive process begins in the mouth, but the small intestine is the primary site of digestion, absorption of nutrients, and retention of waste material.

A mucous layer protects and lubricates the walls of the intestine. Mucus is released from goblet cells interspersed among the enterocytes (columnar epithelial cells) in the intestine. Local irritation (from foods, stimulant cathartics, or stress) increases secretion. The mucus is more viscous in the upper portion of the small intestine than it is in the colon. It forms a protective physical barrier to the intestinal lining, thus reducing contact with irritating substances, bacteria, and viruses. The alkalinity of the mucus contributes further to protecting the intestinal lining as it neutralizes acidic dietary and bacterial products.

Smooth muscles and intrinsic nerves maintain normal intestinal motility and peristalsis. The vagus and parasympathetic pelvic nerves stimulate intestinal motility and secretion, whereas sympathetic innervation inhibits these activities.

Normally, about 9 L of digestive fluid enter the gastrointestinal (GI) tract daily. Of this fluid, 2 L comes from ingested foods and liquids; the remainder comes from normal GI secretions. The small intestine reabsorbs 8 L of the digestive fluid. The large intestine reabsorbs about 850 mL of the remaining liter, leaving about 150 mL to be excreted in the stool each day.

Approximately 3 to 5 L of stomach fluid, containing electrolytes and nutrients, enter the small intestine every 24 hours. Reabsorption reduces the quantity that reaches the large intestine as chyme (an isotonic semiliquid substance), which consists primarily of unabsorbed, undigested food residue; nutrients; electrolytes; water; and bacteria. Ileal chyme has an average electrolyte content per liter of 140 mEq sodium, 70 mEq bicarbonate, 60 mEq chloride, and 8 mEq potassium. Stool electrolyte content per liter is 90 mEq potassium, 40 mEq sodium, 30 mEq bicarbonate, and 15 mEq chloride.

The colon, which is about 1.5 m long, is composed of the cecum, ascending colon, transverse colon, descending colon, and sigmoid colon. Its two primary functions are absorption and storage. The first two-thirds of the colon facilitates absorption, and the remaining one-third functions as a storage area. The proximal half (ascending and transverse parts) of the colon reduces chyme to a semisolid substance called feces, or stool. Stool is a 75% water and 25% solid material; it contains unabsorbed food residue and minerals, bacteria, desquamated epithelial cells, and a small quantity of electrolytes.

In the colon, bacteria produce enzymes necessary to degrade waste products, synthesize certain vitamins, and generate ammonia. *Bacteroides* species and anaerobic Lactobacillus species make up much of the colonic bacterial flora. Organisms such as *Enterobacteriaceae* species (e.g., *E. coli*), hemolytic *Streptococcus, Clostridium* species, and yeasts may also be present in the colon but may represent only a small portion of the normal flora. Many factors such as diet, intestinal pH, coexisting disease, and drugs may influence the relative proportion of these organisms. If such potential pathogens are allowed to overgrow or if their normal balance is disrupted, they may cause serious symptoms and complications.

Etiology of Diarrhea

Diarrhea may be acute or chronic in nature. Usually, acute diarrheal episodes are self-limiting and subside within 72 hours of onset. Chronic diarrhea indicates an illness lasting at least a month. Acute diarrheal illnesses generally can be managed with fluid–electrolyte, dietary, and nonprescription treatment. However, chronic diarrheal illnesses need medical care and, therefore, are outside the scope of this book. The reader is referred to other standard pharmacy textbooks for information about chronic diarrhea.

Acute diarrhea is characterized by a sudden onset of abnormally frequent, watery stools lasting less than 14 days and may be accompanied by weakness, flatulence, abdominal pain, fever, and vomiting. The following discussions of causative agents describe specific characteristics of the resultant diarrhea. Acute diarrhea may be caused by infectious organisms, poisoning, medications, or intolerance of certain foods. Various nongastrointestinal acute or chronic illnesses can also cause acute diarrhea. Many cases of mild-to-moderate diarrhea are viral and more severe diarrhea is generally bacterial.

Food-Borne or Water-Borne Infectious Organisms

Bacteria, protozoa, and viruses cause infectious diarrheas. Table 13–1 highlights these diarrheas and their treatment. The specific causative agent is often not readily identifiable. The pathogens commonly responsible for producing diarrhea in the United States are *Shigella* sp., *Salmonella* sp.,

Table 13–1

Infectious Diarrheas and Their Treatment

Type	History	Symptoms	Treatment	Usual Prognosis
Bacterial				
Salmonella sp.	Ingestion of improperly cooked or refrigerated poultry and dairy products, immunocompromised host	Onset of 12–24 hours, diarrhea, fever, and chills	Fluid and electrolytes; antibiotics (fluoroquinolone, tmp/smx)	Self-limiting
Shigella sp.	Ingestion of contaminated vegetables or water, immunocompromised host	Onset of 24–48 hours, nausea, vomiting, diarrhea	Fluid and electrolytes; antibiotics (fluoroquinolone, tmp/smx)	Self-limiting
Enterotoxigenic *Escherichia coli* (traveler's diarrhea)	Ingestion of contaminated food or water, recent travel outside the United States or to a U.S. border area	Onset of 8–72 hours, watery diarrhea, fever, abdominal cramps	Fluid and electrolytes; in moderate or severe cases, antibiotics (fluoroquinolone, tmp/smx)	Self-limiting
Campylobacter jejuni	Ingestion of contaminated water, fecal–oral route, immunocompromised host	Nausea, vomiting, headache, malaise, fever, watery diarrhea	Fluid and electrolytes; in severe or persistent diarrhea, antibiotics (erythromycin, fluoroquinolone)	Self-limiting
Clostridium difficile	Antibiotic-associated diarrhea	Watery or mucoid diarrhea, high fever, cramping	Water and electrolytes; discontinuation of offending agent; oral metronidazole, oral vancomycin, bacitracin, cholestyramine	Good, if treated
Staphylococcus aureus	Ingestion of improperly cooked or stored food	Nausea, vomiting, watery diarrhea	Fluid and electrolytes; no antibiotics	Self-limiting
Protozoal				
Giardia lamblia	Ingestion of water contaminated with human or animal feces, travel outside the United States, immunocompromised host (AIDS)	Chronic watery diarrhea	Metronidazole, quinacrine	Good, if treated
Cryptosporidia	Travel outside the United States, AIDS, immunocompromised host	Chronic watery diarrhea	Fluid and electrolytes	Self-limiting, except in AIDS or other immunocompromised patients
Entamoeba histolytica	Travel outside the United States, fecal-soiled food or water, immunocompromised host	Chronic watery diarrhea	Fluid and electrolytes; metronidazole followed by iodoquinol	Good, except for immunocompromised patients
Viral				
Rotaviruses	Infects infants, fecal–oral spread	Vomiting, fever, nausea, acute watery diarrhea	Vigorous fluid and electrolyte replacement; no antibiotics	Self-limiting
Norwalk	Infects all ages	"24-hour flu," vomiting, nausea, headache, myalgia, fever, watery diarrhea	Fluid and electrolytes; no antibiotics	Self-limiting

Key: tmp/smx = trimethoprim–sulfamethoxazole.

Campylobacter sp., *Staphylococcus* sp., *Bacillus cereus,* and Norwalk viruses. Some organisms cause diarrhea through an enterotoxin (toxigenic *E. coli* and *Staphylococcus aureus*). Others (*Shigella, Salmonella, Yersinia, Campylobacter jejuni,* and invasive *E. coli*) directly invade the mucosal epithelial cells. Patients with diarrhea caused by toxin-producing agents have a watery diarrhea, which primarily involves the small intestine. Such patients experience an abrupt onset of large-volume watery stools, upper abdominal pain, nausea, vomiting, cramps, and possibly a low-grade fever. If the large intestine is the site of attack, invasive organisms produce a dysentery-like (bloody diarrhea) syndrome. This syndrome is characterized by fever, abdominal cramps, tenesmus (straining), and the frequent passage of small-volume stools that may contain blood and mucus.

An attentive and thorough history regarding food intake before the onset of diarrhea is essential in identifying a probable cause. For example, *Staphylococcus aureus* grows rapidly in food (especially salads, custard, sausage, ham, dairy products, and poultry), producing a toxin. Upon ingestion, the enterotoxin provokes an attack of nausea and vomiting with diarrhea within 6 hours. In contrast, the incubation period for *Salmonella,* which harbors on raw foods and particularly on eggs, is 12 to 24 hours. These microbes invade the mucosal layer to disrupt absorptive-secretory mechanisms. Fever, malaise, muscle aches, and profound epigastric or periumbilical discomfort with severe anorexia suggest an infectious, inflammatory disease of the large intestine. Abdominal pain, vomiting, and diarrhea suggest viral gastroenteritis, and symptoms usually persist for 2 to 3 days before gradually subsiding.

Campylobacter species is another cause of acute bacterial diarrhea. With an onset of 2 to 4 days, the diarrhea is usually limited to 1 week. If supportive therapy fails to manage symptoms, erythromycin 500 mg twice daily for 5 days may be used to eradicate the organism.[4] *Yersinia enterocolitica* and *Yersinia pseudotuberculosis* are isolates of bacterial diarrhea, and symptoms of this self-limiting infectious process may persist for 1 to 3 weeks.

The acute diarrhea that may develop among tourists visiting foreign countries or U.S. border areas with warm climates and poor sanitation is usually caused by bacterial enteropathogens.[5] Enterotoxigenic *E. coli* is a common infecting organism in traveler's diarrhea, which is a secretory diarrhea acquired, for the most part, through contaminated food or water. The causative organism is found most often on foods such as fruits, vegetables, raw meat, and seafood and less commonly in the local water, including ice cubes. After ingestion, the bacteria produces two plasmid-mediated enterotoxins, known as heat-labile toxin and heat-stable toxin. These toxins cause a diarrheal disorder characterized by a sudden onset of loose stools (usually within 3 to 7 days of arrival), nausea, occasional vomiting, abdominal cramping, bloating, malaise, and possibly a low-grade fever. Traveler's diarrhea is also a self-limiting illness; patients may experience between three and eight (or more) watery stools per day, and symptoms usually subside over 3 to 5 days.

Infectious diarrhea is treated with fluid and electrolytes. (See the section "Fluid and Electrolyte Management" under "Treatment of Diarrhea.") Often the illness is self-limiting, and normal function of the alimentary tract is often restored with or without additional treatment in 24 to 72 hours. If the patient has a moderate or severe case of infectious diarrhea, a physician may prescribe a specific anti-infective such as metronidazole, trimethoprim–sulfamethoxazole, or one of the fluoroquinolones.

Viral Gastroenteritis

Diarrhea is a common complaint in infants and young children. The etiology may be difficult to determine, but the illness is often caused by a viral infection of the intestinal tract. A hallmark feature of viral diarrhea is vomiting.

Rotaviruses can cause up to 50% of infantile gastroenteritis. Children ages 3 to 24 months have the highest incidence of this viral infection. Respiratory illnesses such as otitis media or tonsillitis may occur concurrently. The peak infectious period is during the winter months (November to February). Spread is by the fecal–oral route. Clinical features include a 12- to 48-hour incubation period, followed by vomiting, watery diarrhea, and a low-grade fever. The illness tends to be self-limiting, lasting 5 to 8 days, and treatment is usually restricted to fluid and electrolyte therapy.[6]

Norwalk viruses have also been implicated in children and adults, with signs and symptoms resembling those of rotaviruses. The diarrhea with vomiting is sudden, often accompanied by a low-grade fever, malaise, mild nausea, and abdominal cramps, and usually lasts 1 to 2 days. The virus is usually transmitted by contaminated water or food. Community-wide outbreaks may result when municipal water supplies become contaminated.

Protozoal Diarrhea

Giardia lamblia and *Entamoeba histolytica* are protozoa associated with acute diarrhea. *Giardia* is an infection of the small intestine commonly involving children, travelers, or institutionalized patients, as well as hikers who drink from streams or ponds. Diarrhea that occurs after travel to a mountainous or recreational water area is suggestive of infection with *Giardia.* Symptoms may be absent or mild. Following a 1- to 3-day incubation, symptoms may include sudden onset of watery stool, abdominal cramps, flatulence, and epigastric pain. *Giardia* should be suspected in patients not responding to empiric antibiotic therapy and in whom diarrhea persists longer than 14 days. Quinacrine 100 mg taken orally three times a day for 5 to 7 days is effective therapy in adults, but metronidazole 250 mg taken orally three times a day for 5 days is equally effective and is better tolerated.[4]

E. histolytica causes amebiasis in areas with poor sanitation and among travelers, migrant workers, and institutionalized patients.The illness is characterized by severe crampy pain, tenesmus, and dysentery within 3 to 10 days of infection. Patients with mild-to-moderate symptoms should be given metronidazole, 750 mg three times a day for 10 days, followed by iodoquinol, 650 mg three times a day for 20 days.[4]

Drug-Induced Diarrhea

All antibiotics can produce adverse GI symptoms, but severity depends largely on the specific antibiotic, its spectrum, and the dose and duration of therapy. Commonly prescribed antibiotics that have a broad spectrum of activity against aerobic and anaerobic organisms (e.g., ampicillin and numerous other penicillins, clindamycin, erythromycin, azithromycin, clarithromycin, trimethoprim–sulfamethoxazole, the tetracyclines, the fluoroquinolones, and the cephalosporins) can produce diarrhea as a side effect.

Antibiotic-associated diarrhea (AAD) may be caused by an overgrowth of an antibiotic-resistant bacterial or fungal strain or of toxin-producing *Clostridium difficile*. Intestinal microorganisms other than *C. difficile* that tend to proliferate during antibiotic therapy include *S. aureus, Pseudomonas aeruginosa, Streptococcus faecalis, Candida albicans,* and selected species of *Salmonella* and *Proteus.* Any antibiotic can cause AAD, and the disease can begin during or several weeks after treatment. AAD may be self-limiting with antibiotic discontinuation.

C. difficile may also cause antibiotic-associated pseudomembranous colitis. Although *C. difficile* produces at least two identified toxins (A and B), enterotoxin A is the primary cause of diarrhea. Enteric isolation precautions are recommended because these bacteria can be spread to other individuals. The diagnosis is suggested by a test for the toxins in the stool, although the toxins have been found in patients without AAD. The watery or greenish-mucoid diarrhea usually starts during antibiotic treatment, but it can begin up to 4 weeks after the antibiotic has been discontinued. The offending antibiotic must be discontinued and *C. difficile* eradicated. Relapses are common and can be treated with the same antibiotic if the microorganisms have been shown to be susceptible. Oral vancomycin 125 mg four times daily for 10 to 14 days or oral metronidazole 500 mg three times a day for 10 to 14 days is usually prescribed for adults. Metronidazole is the preferred initial antibiotic because it is less expensive than vancomycin and patients do not develop vancomycin-resistant *Enterococcus.* Treatment in children is less well defined. Bacitracin or rifampin may be used in treatment failure. Exchange resins, such as cholestyramine, bind the toxins but do not eradicate *C. difficile* and so are used to treat only mild cases.

Medications such as laxatives, misoprostol, olsalazine, anticancer agents, quinidine, and colchicine may cause diarrhea. Drugs that cause the retention of electrolytes and water in the intestinal lumen (e.g., mannitol, sorbitol, and lactulose) may produce a hyperosmolar, osmotic diarrhea. Certain antacid laxative preparations containing magnesium may induce diarrhea, depending on the dose taken and the individual's susceptibility. Drugs that affect the autonomic control of normal intestinal motility, such as certain antihypertensive agents with sympatholytic activity (e.g., guanethidine, methyldopa, and reserpine), may also cause diarrhea. Generalized cramping and diarrhea may follow the use of a prokinetic drug such as bethanecol, metoclopramide, or cisapride.

AIDS-Associated Diarrhea

Patients with AIDS and individuals infected with human immunodeficiency virus (HIV) are known to be susceptible to many intestinal infections that produce diarrhea as one of the manifestations. An estimated 80% of AIDS patients will experience a diarrheal infection at some time in their illness. These immunocompromised patients may be infected with bacteria, fungi, parasites, viruses, and protozoal organisms. Common stool isolates are *Cryptosporidium, C. difficile, Isospora belli, G. lamblia,* and *E. histolytica.*[4]

Fever and a sudden onset of explosive watery stool begin after a 1- to 3-day incubation. Abdominal cramps also frequently occur. No currently available antimicrobial is effective in diarrhea caused by *Cryptosporidium. Isospora* infections are managed with trimethoprim–sulfamethoxazole. Quinacrine and metronidazole are the treatments of choice for proven *G. lamblia* diarrhea in adults and older children. For empiric therapy of suspected giardiasis, metronidazole may offer advantages relative to its tolerability, side-effect profile, and effects on other causes of persistent diarrhea.

Food-Induced Diarrhea

Food intolerance can provoke diarrhea and may result from a food allergy or from ingesting foods that are excessively fatty or spicy or that contain a high amount of roughage or many seeds. For patients with diverticulosis, avoiding food with seeds is the most effective measure.

Carbohydrates in the diet commonly include the disaccharides, lactose and sucrose, which are normally hydrolyzed to monosaccharides by the enzyme lactase. When these disaccharides are not hydrolyzed, they pool in the lumen of the intestine, where they not only ferment but also produce an osmotic imbalance and pH change. The resultant hyperosmolarity draws fluid into the intestinal lumen, causing diarrhea. Lactase enzymatic activity may be reduced in intestinal disorders such as infectious diarrhea and GI allergy. Acute viral diarrhea may cause a temporary milk intolerance in all ages. Infants born with a lactase deficiency and adults who develop one are intolerant of whole milk and milk-based products. Thus, milk and ice cream may be particularly problematic because of the lactose content. Lactase enzyme products are effective treatments for some patients. (See the section "Digestive Enzymes" under "Treatment of Diarrhea.")

Pathophysiology of Diarrhea

Variability in the causes of diarrhea makes identification of the pathophysiologic mechanisms difficult. The etiology, and subsequently the pathophysiology, can be determined by a thorough medical history in most cases. However, a complete medical assessment, including clinical laboratory evaluation, may be required to identify the cause in a subset of patients with severe or persistent diarrhea.

The development of diarrhea may involve four general pathophysiologic mechanisms: decreased absorption, increased secretion, excessive exudation, and motility alterations. These mechanisms are classified into four clinical groups: osmotic, secretory, exudative, and motility disorder. Table 13–2 correlates the clinical groups and mechanism with their most common causes. The common mechanisms of acute diarrhea are osmotic and secretory, whereas altered motility and decreased absorption are common mechanisms for chronic diarrheal illnesses.

A balance between absorption and secretion is maintained during normal functioning of the intestines. Water absorption in the intestines is passive and depends on the electrolytes and selected solutes (i.e., sodium chloride, glucose, small peptides, and amino acids). As these substances are absorbed, water accompanies their movement to maintain an isotonic state. Generally, 1 L of water is absorbed with about 150 mEq of sodium chloride. Secretory mechanisms are also at work balancing iso-osmotic pressure.[7]

Several intestinal ion-transport mechanisms (diffusion, active transport, and solvent drag) regulate the normal transfer of electrolytes and other solutes and play a primary role in maintaining the balance between absorption and secretion. Sodium transport is the primary ion-transport mechanism that controls water movement. Enterocytes have an active sodium–potassium adenosine triphosphatase pump throughout the intestines. This pump moves sodium into the enterocyte and potassium out of it. Other transport mechanisms are the cotransport of sodium–glucose and sodium–amino acids into the enterocyte and the sodium luminal exchange mechanism. Chloride movement maintains electrical neutrality. Chloride is transferred from the interstitial space into the enterocyte and is secreted into the intestinal lumen. Chloride secretion is an energy-dependent transfer. Chloride also moves from the intestinal lumen in exchange for bicarbonate.

Various intracellular and extracellular regulators (e.g., cyclic adenosine monophosphate, calmodulin, hormones, and neurotransmitters) can modify the normal functioning of intestinal ion transport.[8] Hormones such as vasopressin, atrial natriuretic factor, aldosterone, and glucocorticoids have variable effects on various intestinal segments. For example, glucocorticoids enhance sodium absorption in the small intestine and colon, and aldosterone enhances sodium absorption in the colon. Neurotransmitters (e.g., acetylcholine, serotonin, somatostatin) have either absorptive or secretory effects. Acetylcholine has primarily secretory effects, whereas somatostatin has absorptive effects.

Stool characteristics give valuable information about diarrhea. For example, undigested food particles in the stool suggest small bowel disease; black, tarry stools may indicate GI bleeding; and red stools suggest possible lower bowel or hemorrhoidal bleeding or perhaps simply the recent ingestion of red food (e.g., beets) or of drug products (e.g., rifampin). Diarrhea originating from the small intestine is characterized by a marked outpouring of fluid high in potassium and bicarbonate. Passage of many, small-volume stools suggests diarrhea with a colonic disorder. Yellowish stools may suggest the presence of bilirubin and a potentially serious pathology of the liver. Whitish tint stool suggest a fat malabsorption disease. Patients who have stool containing blood or mucus need medical evaluation.

Table 13–2

Clinical Classification of Diarrhea

Type	Mechanism	Causes
Osmotic	Unabsorbed solute	Lactase deficit, magnesium antacid excess
Secretory	Increased secretion of electrolytes	*Escherichia coli* infection, ileal resection, thyroid cancer
Exudative	Defective absorption, outpouring of mucus and/or blood	Ulcerative colitis, Crohn's disease, dysentery, leukemia
Motility disorder	Decreased contact time	Irritable bowel syndrome, diabetic neuropathy

Complications of Diarrhea

Fluid and electrolyte imbalance is the major complication of diarrheal illnesses. Certain age groups are at risk of dehydration, specifically infants, young children, and the elderly. Certain medical conditions can increase the risk of dehydration. Patients who have multiple chronic medical conditions, such as diabetes mellitus or severe cardiovascular or renal diseases, might need to be referred to medical care. Patients receiving cancer treatment, recipients of organ transplant, patients with AIDS, and other immunocompromised patients also need medical evaluation. Pregnancy can be a potential barrier to self-care medication unless approved by a physician.

Most patients with acute diarrhea can be managed with self-care measures. Assessing the degree of dehydration is the key decision for self-care versus medical referral. In children, particularly infants, acute diarrhea may cause severe and possibly dangerous dehydration and electrolyte imbalance; children age 2 years or less are likely to suffer complications requiring hospitalization. In newborns, water may make up 75% of total body weight; water loss in severe diarrhea may be 10% or more of body weight. After 8 to 10 bowel movements within a 24-hour period, a 2-month-old infant could lose enough fluid to cause circulatory collapse and renal failure. Moderate-to-severe diarrhea in infants requires evaluation by a physician. Other groups at risk of dehydration are elderly (older than 70 years) and immunocompromised patients (AIDS, cancer).

The specific signs and symptoms of dehydration associated with diarrhea are related to the etiology and degree of fluid and electrolyte losses. (See Table 13–3.) An abnormal increase of bowel movements both in frequency and consistency of stools determines the degree of dehydration.

Depending on the degree of dehydration the signs and symptoms include dizziness, thirst, confusion, lethargy, fatigue, low blood pressure, rapid pulse, and cool, sweaty skin. Depending on the etiology other findings are fever, vomiting, nausea, muscle aches, abdominal cramping, bloody or mucoid stools, and weight loss. If the diarrhea is secondary to another illness such as hyperthyroidism, then many other disease-specific signs and symptoms will be present.

High fever (greater than 101°F [38°C]) is a sentinel finding for medical referral. An accurate assessment of fluid balance is a change in body weight; however, the patient seldom knows the exact premorbid weight for comparison. As detailed in Table 13–3, the signs and symptoms of mild dehydration (fewer than 3 loose stools per day) are (1) normal blood pressure and no drop in blood pressure upon standing, (2) afebrile or low grade fever, (3) a slight thirst, and (4) dry mouth (especially under the tongue). Moderate (4 to 5 loose stools per day) dehydration findings are (1) skin tenting with poor turgor, (2) normal blood pressure with mild

Table 13–3

Oral Rehydration and Dietary Management of Acute Diarrhea

	Mild Diarrhea (Self-treatable)	Moderate Diarrhea (Self-treatable)	Severe Diarrhea (Non-self-treatable)
Degree of dehydration	3%–5%	6%–9%	>10%
Signs of dehydration[a]	Slightly dry buccal mucous membranes, increased thirst	Sunken eyes, sunken fontanelle, loss of skin turgor, dry buccal mucous membranes	Same signs of moderate dehydration with one of the following: rapid thready pulse, cyanosis, cold extremities, rapid breathing, lethargy, coma
Number of unformed stools/day	<3	4–5	6–9
Other signs/symptoms of diarrhea	Afebrile or low-grade fever, normal blood pressure, no orthostatic changes in blood pressure/pulse without orthostatic-related symptoms	Fever >101°F (38°C), normal blood pressure lying down, mild orthostatic blood pressure/pulse changes with no or mild orthostatic-related symptoms	Fever >101°F (38°C), low blood pressure, dizziness, severe abdominal pain
Rehydration therapy	≤5 years: ORS 50 mL/kg within 4 hours	≤5 years: ORS 100 mL/kg within 4 hours	≤5 years: Give IV fluids (lactated Ringer's solution) until pulse/perfusion/mental status return to normal
	>5 years: ORS 2 L within 4 hours	>5 years: ORS 2–4 L within 4 hours	>5 years: IV fluid/electrolytes
Maintenance therapy	≤5 years: 10 mL/kg or ½–1 cup of ORS for each diarrheal stool	≤5 years: 10 mL/kg or ½–1 cup of ORS for each diarrheal stool	≤5 years: IV fluids
	>5 years: replace ongoing losses of body fluids/electrolytes	>5 years: replace ongoing losses of body fluids/electrolytes	>5 years: replace ongoing losses of body fluids/electrolytes
Dietary therapy[b]	Infants: human milk feeding, half- or full-strength lactose-containing milk, or undiluted lactose-free formula	Infants: human milk feeding, half- or full-strength lactose-containing milk, or undiluted lactose-free formula	Infants: human milk feeding, half- or full-strength lactose-containing milk, or undiluted lactose-free formula
	Children/adults: sport drinks, diluted juices, salty crackers, soups/broths until diarrhea stops	Children/adults: sport drinks, diluted juices, salty crackers, soups/broths until diarrhea stops	Children/adults: sport drinks, diluted juices, salty crackers, soups/broths until diarrhea stops

Key: ORS = oral rehydration solution; IV = intravenous.

[a] If no signs of dehydration are present, rehydration therapy is not required. Maintenance therapy and replacement of stool losses should be undertaken.

[b] Infants and children who receive solid food can continue their usual diet, but should avoid foods high in simple sugars and fats.

Source: References 6, 9, and 10.

drop in blood pressure with standing, and (3) dry buccal mucous membranes. With severe dehydration (more than 6 loose stools per day), the patient shows the following signs of hypoperfusion (i.e., shock related to decreased circulating blood): lethargy; altered mental state (e.g., confusion); extremely poor skin turgor and prolonged tenting; orthostatic hypotension with tachycardia; oliguria; metabolic acidosis; slow capillary refill in the fingernail bed; and cool, clammy skin. The pharmacist should ask the patient about vomiting, high (greater than 101°F [38°C]) and/or prolonged fever, and the nature and amount of fluid intake, which may further contribute to the dehydration.

Treatment of Diarrhea

Treatment Outcomes

The goals of self-treatment are to (1) assess and correct the fluid and electrolyte loss and the acid-base disturbance; (2) manage the diet; (3) manage concurrent diseases (e.g., diabetes mellitus); (4) provide symptomatic relief; and (5) identify and treat the cause, if possible. Symptomatic relief and correcting fluid and electrolyte loss are generally adequate for mild-to-moderate diarrhea that is only temporary, self-limiting, and uncomplicated. Severe diarrhea must be treated by a physician.

General Treatment Approach

Initial management should focus on fluid and electrolyte replacement by administering commercially available oral solutions (e.g., Pedialyte) in adequate doses. (See Table 13–4.) A variety of common household fluid oral solutions may be used for this purpose. (See Table 13–5.) Simultaneously, symptomatic relief can be achieved by having carefully selected patients use various nonprescription antidiarrheal drugs such as loperamide. Lactose-containing products and fatty foods may not be tolerated in some patients. If not dehydrated and otherwise healthy, patients should consume a liquid diet with salty crackers for the first 24 hours, then should advance to an easily digestible, low-residue diet such as bananas, crackers, yogurt, potatoes, and rice.

Immediate referral is required if the patient has a high fever (greater than 101°F [38°C]), severe dehyration, protracted vomiting, chronic diarrhea, and stools that contain blood or mucus. Severe abdominal pain in any patient is also included. Medical referral is also indicated for the elderly (age 70 years or older) and children age 3 years or younger. Medical referral is needed for patients with multiple chronic conditions such as diabetes mellitus or severe cardiovascular or renal diseases. Immunocompromised patients, such as organ transplant recipients, individuals with AIDS, or individuals undergoing cancer treatment, need medical evaluation of their diarrhea. Pregnant women should consult a physician before self-treating diarrhea.

Nonpharmacologic Therapy

Simultaneous implementation of oral rehydration and specific dietary measures is appropriate for treating all diarrheal illness. Implementing preventive measures can prevent recurrences of these illnesses.

Table 13–4

Selected Oral Rehydration Products

Trade Name	Osmolarity	Calories	Carbohydrate	Electrolytes
WHO-ORS	333 mOsm/L	85 Cal/L	Glucose 20 g/L	Sodium 90 mEq/L; chloride 80 mEq/L; citrate 30 mEq/L; potassium 20 mEq/L
Infalyte Solution[a,b]	200 mOsm/L	126 Cal/L	Rice syrup solids 30 g/L	Sodium 50 mEq/L; chloride 45 mEq/L; citrate 34 mEq/L; potassium 25 mEq/L
Kaolectrolyte Packets[b-d]	—	22 Cal/L	Dextrose 5 g/L per packet	Sodium 50 mEq/L; chloride 40 mEq/L; citrate 30 mEq/L; potassium 20 mEq/L
Pedialyte[d]	249 mOsm/L	100 Cal/L	Dextrose 20 g/L; fructose 5 g/L	Sodium 45 mEq/L; chloride 35 mEq/L; citrate 30 mEq/L; potassium 20 mEq/L
Pedialyte Freezer Pops[c,d]	—	6.25 Cal	Dextrose 25 g/L	Sodium 45 mEq/L; chloride 35 mEq/L; citrate 30 mEq/L; potassium 20 mEq/L
Rehydralyte Solution	304 mOsm/L	100 Cal/L	Dextrose 25 g/L	Sodium 75 mEq/L; chloride 65 mEq/L; citrate 30 mEq/L; potassium 20 mEq/L
Revital Ice Freezer Pops[d]	—	12 Cal	Crystalline fructose 30 g/L	Sodium 45 mEq/L; chloride 35 mEq/L; citrate 30 mEq/L; potassium 20 mEq/L

[a] Dye-free product.

[b] Lactose-free product.

[c] Pediatric formulation.

[d] Phenylalanine-containing product.

Table 13–5

Comparison of Electrolyte–Glucose Concentrations of Household Fluids

Clear Liquids	Sodium (mEq/L)	Potassium (mEq/L)	Bicarbonate (mEq/L)	Glucose (g/L)	Osmolarity (mM/L)
Cola	2	0.1	13	50–150 glucose and fructose	550
Ginger ale	3	1	4	50–150 glucose and fructose	540
Apple juice	3	20	0	100–150 glucose and fructose	700
Chicken broth	250	5	0	0	450
Tea	0	0	0	0	5
Gatorade	20	3	3	45 glucose and other sugars	330

Source: Page 6 of reference 9.

Fluid and Electrolyte Management

The algorithms in Figures 13–1 and 13–2 outline the management of fluid and electrolytes according to the degree of dehydration and the age of the patient. Depending on the patient's fluid and electrolyte state, treatment may be carried out in two phases: rehydration, followed by maintenance therapy. Rehydration replaces lost water and electrolytes to restore the normal body composition. After rehydration therapy is completed, electrolyte solutions are given to maintain the normal body composition. If the patient is not dehydrated, only maintenance of fluid and electrolytes (i.e., replacement of losses) is needed. (See Table 13–3.)

Correction of fluid loss and electrolyte imbalances is very important. The secretory and absorptive mechanisms appear to function separately; therefore, an oral sugar–electrolyte solution can be absorbed during diarrhea.[11,12] In mild-to-moderate diarrhea, pharmacists can safely prescribe oral fluids. Mild diarrhea is three or fewer stools per day with minimal symptoms; moderate diarrhea is up to six stools per day; severe diarrhea is more than six stools per day with dehydration symptoms.

In developing countries, the World Health Organization (WHO) recommends an oral replacement fluid that contains the following per liter: glucose 20 g, sodium 90 mEq, potassium 20 mEq, citrate 30 mEq, and chloride 80 mEq.[9] The WHO oral rehydration solution (WHO-ORS) was developed to manage cholera diarrhea, which occurs rarely in the United States. Several such products are available in the United States, but they differ slightly from the WHO-ORS. (See Table 13–4.) The American Academy of Pediatrics (AAP) recommends that oral solutions have not more than 75 to 90 mEq/L of sodium for rehydration and 40 to 60 mEq/L of sodium for maintenance. To lessen the risk of carbohydrate-induced osmotic diarrhea, the ratio of carbohydrate to sodium should not exceed 2 : 1. Commercial ORS products are convenient and safe because they are premixed.

Although oral rehydration therapy (ORT) has saved millions of infants and children in developing countries, it has not been the primary therapeutic method for managing acute diarrhea in the United States for several reasons: Administration is labor intensive; parents must be carefully educated to follow instructions in preparation and administration; and if the child is hospitalized, parents expect intravenous therapy. However, intravenous therapy also has risks, such as phlebitis, infection, and fluid–electrolyte imbalance, and it is more expensive. By eliminating or reducing hospital costs, ORT may have an important cost-effective benefit.

The Centers for Disease Control and Prevention (CDC) and the AAP published recommendations addressing management of diarrhea in infants and children.[9,10] Managing acute diarrhea in such patients requires fluid–electrolyte rehydration and maintenance and nutritional therapy.

After the degree of dehydration is determined, treatment of children is carried out in two phases: rehydration and maintenance with nutritional support. For mild dehydration, an ORS is given at 50 mL/kg over a 4-hour period. For example, a 20-kg mildly dehydrated child should receive a total volume of 1000 mL over 4 hours. After 1 to 2 hours, the hydration status should be reassessed; if the patient remains dehydrated, rehydration should continue. For moderate dehydration, the ORS should be given as it is for mild dehydration but should be increased to 100 mL/kg over 4 hours. For severe dehydration, intravenous rehydration should be administered. Once the patient can tolerate oral therapy, the ORS can be used to replace intravenous therapy. For a child without evidence of dehydration, the caregiver should give ORS at 10 mL/kg for each loose stool or could simply continue the child's usual age-appropriate diet and fluid intake. A child who is vomiting may tolerate 1 teaspoon every few minutes. Table 13–3 outlines rehydration and maintenance therapy for adults and children age 5 years or older.

Dietary Management

Nondehydrated, otherwise healthy patients should consume a liquid diet of sport drinks or diluted fruit juices with salty crackers until the diarrhea subsides. Pharmacists should advise the patient to avoid fatty, spicy, or other foods that cause GI upset.

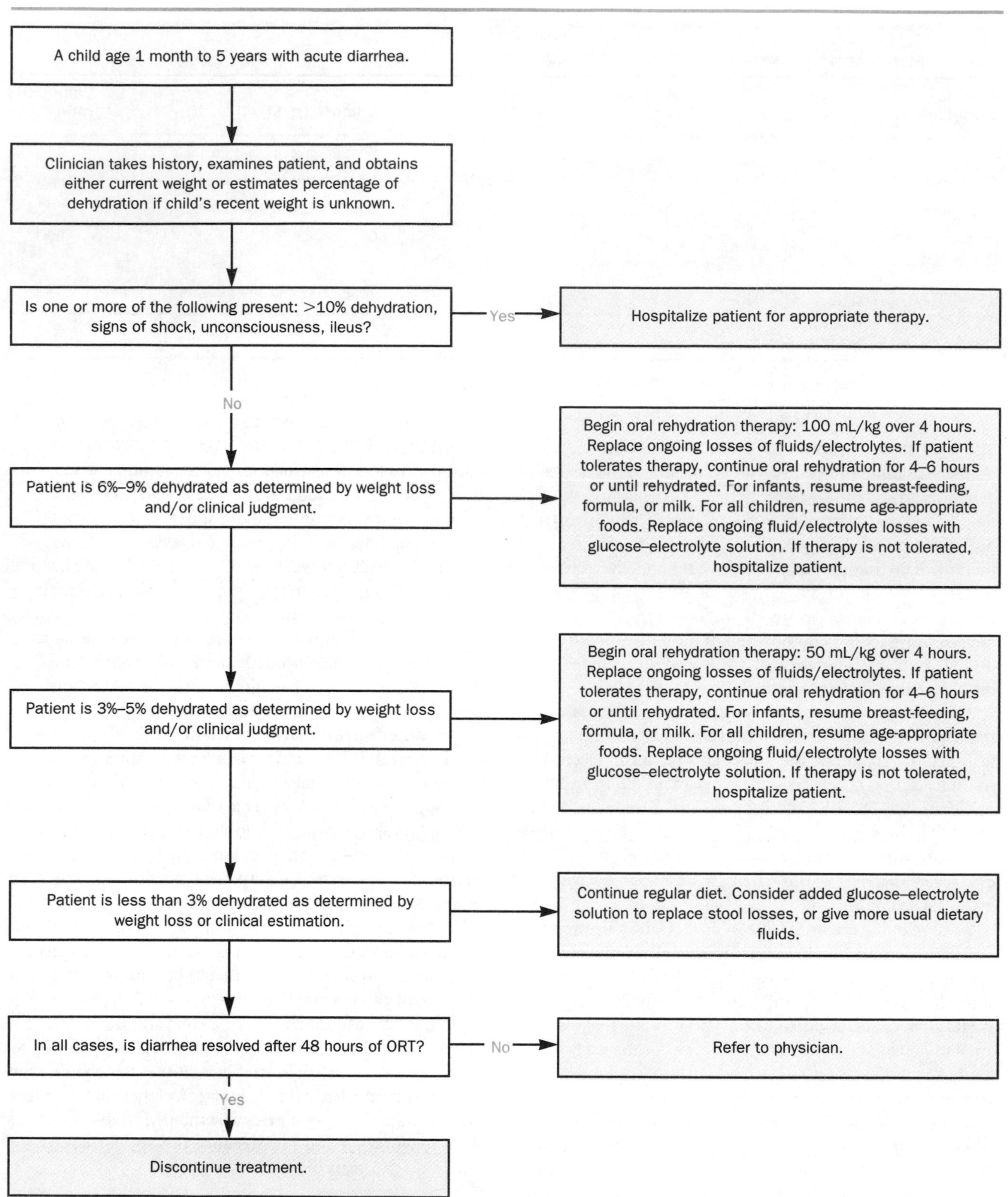

Figure 13–1 Self-care of diarrhea in children ages 1 month to 5 years. Adapted from reference 10.

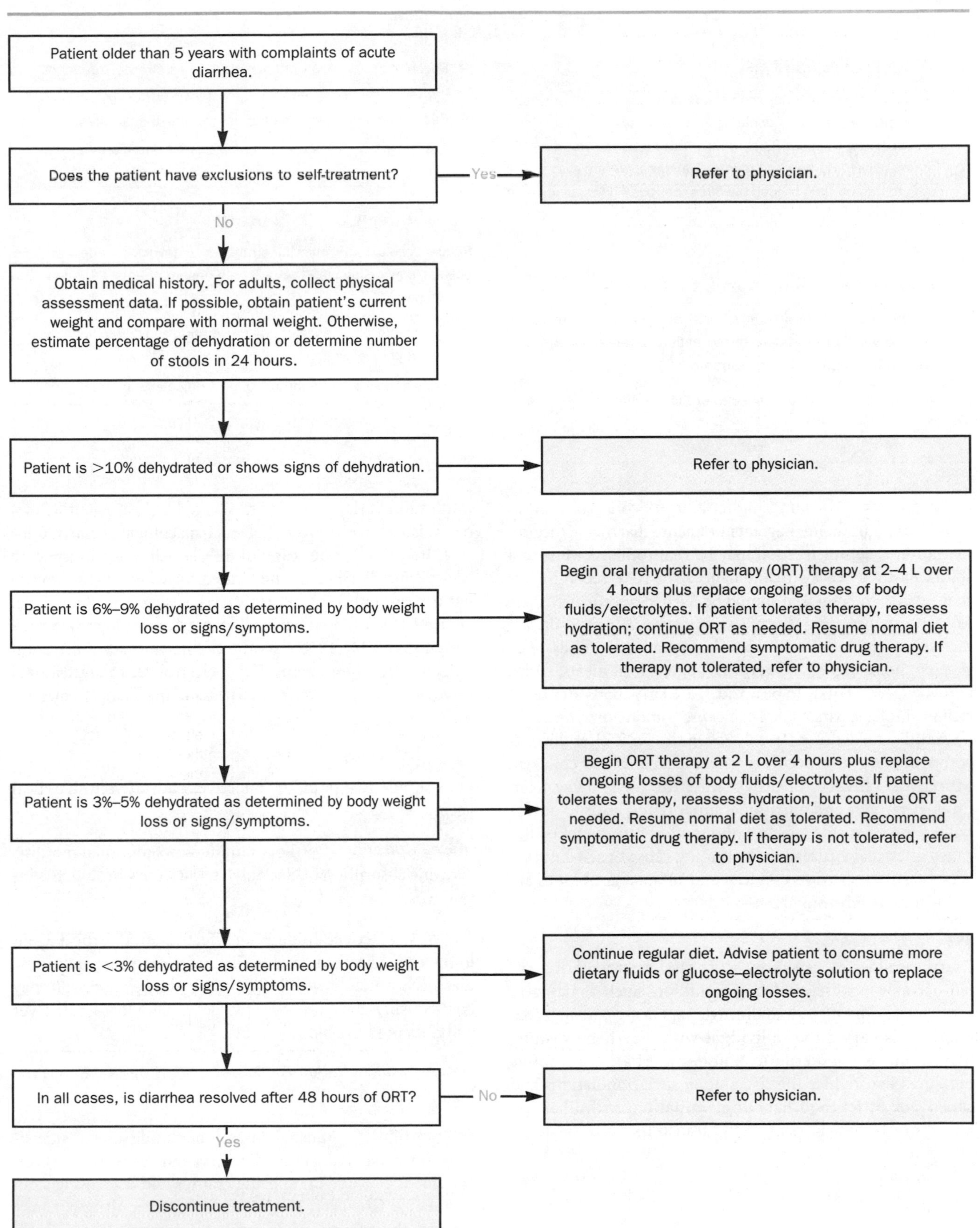

Figure 13–2 Self-care of acute diarrhea in children age 5 years or older, adolescents, and adults.

Case Study 13–1

Patient Complaint/History

Fezan, a 45-year-old man, complains of sudden onset of watery diarrhea, nausea, and vomiting. He has had a fever of 99°F (37°C) during the past 8 hours for which he has been taking acetaminophen. He has had four to five loose, watery stools. The patient has no drug or food allergies, nor does he regularly take any medications.

Clinical Considerations/Strategies

Readers can use the following considerations/strategies to determine whether treatment of the patient's condition with nonprescription medications is warranted:

- Assess the possible cause(s) of the diarrhea.
- Recommend an appropriate fluid and electrolyte treatment that is based on the degree of dehydration.
- Recommend dietary measures for treating the diarrhea.
- Assess the benefits and risks of treating the diarrhea with loperamide.

Patient Counseling/Education

Readers can use the following strategies to develop a patient education/counseling plan that will help ensure optimal therapeutic outcomes:

- Explain the importance of oral rehydration and dietary therapy as the primary treatment of diarrhea.
- Explain the role of nonprescription medications in treating diarrhea.

For infants and young children, dietary concerns need to be addressed in the management of acute diarrhea. Once rehydration is complete, food may be reintroduced while oral solutions are given for maintenance. The AAP recommends that infants and children should be fed age-appropriate diets as soon as rehydration therapy is completed. For children, the diet should include complex carbohydrate-rich foods (e.g., rice, potatoes, bread, and cereals), yogurt, lean meats, fruits, and vegetables. Foods to be avoided are fatty foods and those rich in simple sugars, which can cause osmotic diarrhea.

Antidiarrheal drugs have not been shown to alter the outcomes of acute nonspecific diarrhea in infants and children. Moreover, reliance on drugs shifts the focus away from fluid–electrolyte and nutritional support and leads to potentially dangerous side effects without additional benefits. Because intestinal viruses are the leading cause of self-limiting acute gastroenteritis in children and infants, antibiotics are not routinely recommended.

Preventive Measures

Diarrheal illnesses, especially acute viral gastroenteritis, often occur in congregate living conditions such as day care centers and nursing homes through person-to-person transmission. Isolating the individual with diarrhea, washing hands, and using sterile techniques are basic preventive measures that reduce the risk among such populations and caregivers. Strict food handling, sanitation, and other hygienic practices help control the transmission of bacterial and other infectious agents. For traveler's diarrhea, bismuth subsalicylate prophylaxis is recommended for short-term use in high-risk areas.

Pharmacologic Therapy

Some health care providers recommend loperamide or adsorbents for acute diarrhea. Except for loperamide and bismuth subsalicylate used in traveler's diarrhea, scientific evidence is lacking to prove that pharmacologic agents reduce stool frequency or duration of disease. Although most acute nonspecific diarrhea in the United States is self-limiting in nature, nonprescription antidiarrheals may provide relief and will usually do no harm when used according to label instructions. Table 13–6 lists the dosage and administration guidelines for these agents. Fluid, electrolyte, and nutritional therapies remain the most important components to managing diarrhea.

Loperamide

Loperamide is a popular, effective, and safe antidiarrheal agent.

Mechanism of Action Loperamide slows intestinal motility, allowing absorption of electrolytes and water through the intestine.

Indications Loperamide is an effective antidiarrheal agent in traveler's diarrhea, nonspecific acute diarrhea, or chronic diarrhea associated with inflammatory bowel disease. It may be used when the patient is afebrile or has a low-grade fever and does not have bloody stools.

Dosage/Administration Guidelines See Table 13–6 for dosing information.

Adverse Effects At usual doses, loperamide has few side effects other than occasional dizziness and constipation. Loperamide is effective in relieving cramps and decreasing stool frequency. However, like all antiperistaltic drugs, it may worsen the effects of invasive (enteroinvasive *E. coli*, *Salmonella*, *Shigella*, *C. jejuni*) or inflammatory (*C. difficile*) bacterial infection and may cause toxic megacolon in antibiotic-induced diarrhea or pseudomembranous colitis.

Table 13–6

Recommended Dosages of Antidiarrheal Agents for Acute Diarrhea

Medication	Dosage Forms	Adult Dosages	Pediatric Dosages	Duration of Use
Loperamide	Caplets (2 mg), liquid (1 mg/5 mL)	4 mg initially, then 2 mg after each loose stool; do not exceed 16 mg/day	Consult product instructions; not recommended for children <6 years except under physician supervision	48 hours
Adsorbents				
Attapulgite	Tablets, caplets, liquids, suspensions	30–120 mL or 2 tablets after each loose stool	Children >6 years: 10–20 mL; not recommended for children <6 years except under physician supervision	48 hours
Kaolin–pectin mixture	Liquids, suspensions	15–30 mL after each loose stool up to 8 doses/24 hours	—	48 hours
Polycarbophil	Tablets	2 tablets 4 times/day or after each loose stool up to 6 g/day; dose may be repeated every 30 minutes until maximum dosage reached	Children 6–12 years: 2 tablets 3 times/day up to 3 g/day; children 2 to <6 years: 1 tablet 2 times/day; not recommended for children <2 years except under physician supervision	48 hours
Bismuth subsalicylate	Tablets (262 mg), caplets (262 mg), liquids (262 mg/15 mL; 525 mg/15 mL)	2 tablets every hour up to 16 tablets or 30 mL every 30–60 minutes up to 240 mL/day	Check product instructions; not recommended for children <2 years except under physician supervision	48 hours
Digestive enzymes	Chewable tablets, caplets, liquids	5–15 drops placed in or taken with dairy product; 1–3 tablets or 1–2 capsules with first bite of dairy product	Same as adult dosage	Take with each consumption of dairy product

Drug–Drug Interactions Drug interactions are rarely reported for loperamide. It can, however, potentiate (increase) the effects of central nervous system depressants.

Contraindications/Precautions/Warnings Loperamide should be used with caution in patients with fecal leukocytes, high fever, or bloody diarrhea (dysentery).

Adsorbents

Nonprescription GI adsorbents (attapulgite, kaolin, and pectin) are generally used to treat mild nonspecific acute diarrhea. Because large doses are generally used, commercially available products are formulated as flavored liquid suspensions to improve palatability.

Mechanism of Action Adsorption by these agents is not selective. When given orally, they may adsorb nutrients and digestive enzymes as well as toxins, bacteria, and various noxious materials in the GI tract. They may also adsorb drugs in the GI tract.

Dosage/Administration Guidelines See Table 13–6 for dosing information.

Adverse Effects Because there is negligible systemic absorption of the adsorbent drug, the infrequent side effects associated with adsorbents include constipation, bloating, and fullness.

Drug–Drug Interactions Although the systemic absorption of an orally administered drug from the GI tract is expected to be compromised during a diarrheal episode, the concomitant administration of an antidiarrheal adsorbent may further hamper absorption. A change in the dose or dosage interval may be required, depending on the medication involved, the usual rate and site of absorption, and the absolute necessity of getting specific and consistent blood levels of the drug. Sometimes, administering the drug parenterally might be better (if available by injection) until the diarrheal episode is over and the adsorbent drugs are discontinued. Decreased gastrointestinal absorption of clindamycin, tetracyclines, digoxin, and penicillamine has been reported with the use of adsorbents.

Polycarbophil

Polycarbophil is a bulk laxative that is also effective in treating diarrhea. (See Chapter 12, "Constipation," for a discussion of this agent's laxative properties.)

Mechanism of Action The absorbent polycarbophil can absorb up to 60 times its original weight in water.

Indications Because of its absorptive properties, polycarbophil has been recommended in treating both diarrhea and constipation.

Case Study 13–2

Patient Complaint/History

Ivana, a 21-year-old female college student, presents to the pharmacist with complaints of about three watery loose stools per day for 2 days along with abdominal cramps. Unable to keep down her breakfast of a bowl of cereal, she has not tried to eat anything else. She is not dizzy, does not feel faint, and is afebrile.

Ivana is currently on day 5 of a 10-day course of amoxicillin. When asked about her current medication use, she admits to taking a tablespoon of Kaopectate a couple of hours earlier and to taking ibuprofen for muscle aches.

Clinical Considerations/Strategies

Readers can use the following considerations/strategies to determine whether treatment of the patient's condition with nonprescription medications is warranted:

- Assess the possible cause(s) of the diarrhea.
- Recommend an appropriate fluid and electrolyte treatment that is based on the degree of dehydration.
- Recommend dietary measures for treating the diarrhea.
- Assess the appropriateness of treating her diarrhea with an absorbent.

Patient Education/Counseling

Readers can use the following strategies to develop a patient education/counseling plan that will help ensure optimal therapeutic outcomes:

- Explain possible drug interactions of all antidiarrheal agents.
- Review product labels with the patient to familiarize her with the type of information presented.

Dosage/Administration Guidelines See Table 13–6 for dosing information.

Adverse Effects Polycarbophil is metabolically inert, and no systemic toxicity has been shown. Side effects, which are mild and infrequent, include dose-related epigastric pain and bloating.

Drug–Drug Interactions Polycarbophil is reported to decrease absorption of warfarin, digoxin, tetracycline, and ciprofloxacin.

Bismuth Subsalicylate

Bismuth subsalicylate (BSS), another therapeutically versatile agent, is the only nonprescription bismuth compound available in the United States.

Mechanism of Action BSS is reported to have an antisecretory mechanism, to bind bacterial toxins, and to have anti-inflammatory and antibacterial properties.

Indications BSS is indicated for symptomatic relief of mild, nonspecific diarrhea; for indigestion; for treatment and prevention of traveler's diarrhea; and as adjuvant to antibiotics for treating *Helicobacter pylori*-associated peptic ulcer disease. Chapter 11, "Acid–Peptic Disorders and Intestinal Gas," discusses BSS's role in treating acid–peptic disorders.

Dosage/Administration Guidelines See Table 13–6 for dosing information.

Adverse Effects BSS dosage forms contain various amounts of salicylate. Methylsalicylate (oil of wintergreen) is used as a flavoring agent in the suspension dosage form and the original tablets. The suspension dosage form (262 mg/15 mL) contains 130 mg of salicylate, whereas the original tablets (262 mg) contain 102 mg of salicylate. The caplets (262 mg) and cherry-flavored tablets (262 mg) contain 99 mg of salicylate. If patients are taking aspirin or other salicylate-containing drugs, toxic levels of salicylate may be reached even if the patient follows dosing directions on the label for each drug. Thus, patients who are sensitive to aspirin (because of asthmatic bronchospasm) should not use BSS.

Children and teenagers who have or are recovering from chicken pox or flu are at risk of aspirin-induced Reye's syndrome, a rare but serious illness, and should not use BSS. In susceptible patients, salicylate-induced gout attacks have occurred.

Harmless black-stained stool may occur, which should not be confused with melena; harmless darkening of the tongue may occur as well. Mild tinnitus is a side effect that may be associated with moderate-to-severe salicylate toxicity. If diarrhea is seen with high fever or continues beyond 48 hours, the patient should seek medical care.

Contraindications/Precautions/Warnings The product is contraindicated for nursing or pregnant women without medical advice. Bismuth is radiopaque and may interfere with radiographic intestinal studies.

Drug–Drug Interactions BSS may interact adversely with oral anticoagulants, methotrexate, probenecid, and any other drug that potentially interacts with aspirin. Also, salicylate may exert an antiplatelet effect.

Digestive Enzymes

For patients with lactase gastrointestinal enzyme deficiency, lactase enzymes are available as SureLac, Lactaid, Dairy Ease, and Lactrase. (See Table 13–7 for other commercially avail-

Table 13–7

Selected Lactase Enzyme Products

Trade Name	Primary Ingredient
Dairy Ease Drops	Lactase enzyme
Dairy Ease Caplets	Lactase enzyme 3000 FCC units
Dairy Ease Chewable Tablets	Lactase enzyme 3000 FCC units
Lactaid Caplets[a]	Lactase enzyme 3000 FCC units
Lactaid Drops[a,b]	Lactase enzyme
Lactaid Extra Strength Caplets[a]	Lactase enzyme 4500 FCC units
Lactaid Ultra Caplets	Lactase enzyme 9000 FCC units
Lactrase Capsules	Lactase enzyme 250 mg
SureLac Chewable Tablets	Lactase enzyme 3000 FCC units

[a] Dye-free product.

[b] Sucrose-free product.

Table 13–8

Selected Antidiarrheal Products

Trade Name	Primary Ingredient
Loperamide-Containing Products	
Imodium A-D Liquid[a]	Loperamide HCl 1 mg/5mL
Imodium A-D Caplets[a]	Loperamide HCl 2 mg
Imodium Advanced Chewable Tablets	Loperamide HCl 2 mg; simethicone 125 mg
Kao-Paverin Caps	Loperamide HCl 2 mg
Adsorbents	
Donnagel Suspension	Attapulgite 600 mg/15mL
Donnagel Chewable Tablets	Attapulgite 600 mg
Kao-Paverin Liquid	Pectin 65 mg/15 mL; kaolin 3 g/15 mL; bismuth subsalicylate 250 mg/15 mL
Kaopectate Liquid[a,b]	Attapulgite 750 mg/15mL
Kaopectate Caplets	Attapulgite 750 mg
Kaopectate Children's Liquid[a-c]	Attapulgite 375 mg/7.5 mL
Pepto-Bismol Caplets[a]	Bismuth subsalicylate 262 mg
Pepto-Bismol Maximum Strength Liquid[a,b,d]	Bismuth subsalicylate 525 mg/15 mL
Pepto-Bismol Original Strength Liquid[a,b,d]	Bismuth subsalicylate 262 mg/15 mL
Pepto-Bismol Chewable Tablets[a]	Bismuth subsalicylate 262 mg
Rheaban Caplets	Activated attapulgite 750 mg
Polycarbophil-Containing Products	
Equalactin Chewable Tablets	Polycarbophil 500 mg
Mitrolan Chewable Tablets	Polycarbophil 500 mg

[a] Lactose-free product.

[b] Sulfite-free product.

[c] Pediatric formulation.

[d] Sucrose-free product.

able products.) These preparations may be added (as drops) to milk products or taken (as tablets) with milk at mealtimes to prevent osmotic diarrhea.

Product Selection Guidelines

For children, self-treatment is limited to treating dehydration with oral rehydration solutions. If such solutions are ineffective, a physician must be consulted. Selection of an antidiarrheal product should be based on patient factors such as the etiology of the diarrhea, if known; the potential interactions with prescribed medications; and the applicable contraindications. Table 13–6 is a quick reference for tailoring selection of an agent to a patient's particular medical history.

A patient's preference for a particular dosage form or a product that requires fewer doses is another selection criterion. Table 13–8 lists the dosage forms and primary ingredients of selected commercially available antidiarrheal agents.

Patient Assessment of Diarrhea

To evaluate a patient with diarrhea, the pharmacist differentiates symptoms and makes clinical judgments. This triage function is based on the patient's responses to questions designed to help determine the cause of the specific signs and symptoms and their severity and characteristics. The patient's susceptibility to complications should also be determined. The duration of illness (acute versus chronic), presence of high fever, presence of protracted vomiting, presence of abdominal pain in patients older than age 50 years, and presence of blood or mucus in the stool are important assessment criteria. Chronic diarrhea or the presence of any of the other factors precludes self-treatment. If these factors are not present, the degree of dehydration is the next important assessment. The initial assessment of a pediatric patient should also determine the degree of dehydration and plausible causes. The common symptoms of acute gastroenteritis (e.g., vomiting, loose stools, and fever) are nonspecific findings associated with many other childhood diseases (e.g., acute otitis media, bacterial sepsis, meningitis, pneumonia, and urinary tract infections). This information is key to recommending a proper course of action, which may include self-treatment or referral to a health care provider. A complete medication history must be assessed before a product is selected.

Physical assessment of a patient with complaints of diarrhea can provide definitive information as to the presence of diarrhea and, if present, its severity. The abdomen of a patient with diarrhea shows hyperactive bowel sounds and generalized or local tenderness in moderate diarrhea. (See Table 13–3.) In severe diarrhea, the bowel sounds may be absent or hypoactive. Vital signs (e.g., pulse, temperature, respiration, blood pressure) are important indicators of illness severity and should be routinely measured. A high fever (greater than

101°F [38°C]) suggests a severe infectious disease and requires immediate medical referral. Checking skin turgor and degree of oral saliva will help decide the degree of dehydration. (See Table 13–3.) A change in body weight is a key indicator of a change in body fluid load and should be routinely monitored along with the frequency and number of bowel movements.

Severe dehydration includes complaints of dizziness, fainting, or near fainting. Symptoms may also include postural (orthostatic) hypotension, defined as a drop in the systolic and/or diastolic pressure by greater than 15 to 20 mm Hg on moving from a lying to an upright position. Normally, the diastolic pressure remains the same or slightly increases and the systolic pressure drops slightly on arising. If the blood pressure drops, the pulse should be checked simultaneously; the pulse rate should increase as the blood pressure drops. Failure of the pulse to rise could suggest that the problem is neurogenic (e.g., diabetic patients with peripheral neuropathy) or that the patient is taking a β-blocker. The presence of orthostatic hypotension suggests that the patient has lost one or more liters of vascular volume and should be referred for medical care.

Special populations that require medical referral include those age 70 years or older, children age 3 years or younger, and pregnant patients. Other high-risk populations include those with multiple medical chronic medical conditions or immunocompromised patients.

Uncomplicated healthy patients usually improve from the diarrhea within 24 to 48 hours. If the condition remains the same or worsens after 48 hours of onset, medical referral is necessary.

Performing a physical assessment and asking the patient the following questions will help elicit the information needed to assess the problem accurately and to recommend the appropriate treatment approach.

Q~ How long have you (or the patient) had diarrhea? Was the onset of diarrhea sudden? How often do the episodes of diarrhea occur?

A~ *Identify the criteria for chronic and acute diarrhea. (See the section "Etiology of Diarrhea.")* Recommend the appropriate self-treatment for acute diarrhea. (See the section "Treatment of Diarrhea.") Refer patients with chronic diarrhea to a physician.

Q~ How old are you? (Or, if a child is the patient, how old is your child?) Do you (or the patient) have potentially complicating conditions?

A~ *Identify the types of patients most at risk for developing dehydration. (See the section "Complications of Diarrhea.")* Also, see the following question.

Q~ Is the diarrhea associated with other symptoms such as fever, severe weakness, severe loss of appetite, persistent vomiting, dizziness, mental confusion, or abdominal pain?

A~ *Identify the signs and symptoms of the three classifications of dehydration. (See Table 13–3.)* Recommend an appropriate treatment that is based on a patient's symptoms.

Q~ What is the character of the stool? Do the stools contain blood or mucus?

A~ Refer patients with blood or mucus in the stool to a physician. (See the section "Pathophysiology of Diarrhea" for a description of other characteristics of stool and their possible relationship to diarrhea.)

Q~ Has your (or the patient's) diet changed recently?

A~ *Identify the types of food that can induce diarrhea. (See the section "Food-Induced Diarrhea" under "Etiology of Diarrhea.")* Recommend the appropriate treatment if a patient's description of a dietary change implicates food intolerance.

Q~ Can you relate the onset of diarrhea to a specific cause such as a particular meal?

A~ *Identify the possible causes of food-related diarrhea. (See Table 13–1 and the section "Food-Induced Diarrhea" under "Etiology of Diarrhea.")* If the diarrhea coincides with a meal, recommend an appropriate treatment that is based on the patient's description of food intake and the onset of diarrhea.

Q~ Have you (or the patient) recently traveled to a foreign country or to a mountainous or recreational water area of the United States?

A~ *Identify the causative agents for diarrhea associated with travel. (See Table 13–1 and the section "Food-Borne or Water-Borne Infectious Organisms.")* Recommend an appropriate treatment that is based on the patient's description of activities coinciding with the diarrhea.

Q~ Have you (or the patient) taken antibiotics in the past month? What medications do you (or the patient) routinely take?

A~ *Identify medications that can induce diarrhea. (See the section "Drug-Induced Diarrhea" under "Etiology of Diarrhea.")* If an antibiotic or other prescription medication is being taken, refer the patient to a physician. If a nonprescription medication is being taken, advise the patient to stop taking the medication, unless a physician approved such use. Then recommend an alternative treatment or product.

Patient Counseling for Diarrhea

Patients with diarrhea may focus on the need for a nonprescription medication to stop the frequent bowel movements. The pharmacist should remind them that most episodes of acute diarrhea stop after 48 hours and that preventing dehydration is the most important component of treating the problem. Counseling on the two-step treatment of dehydration and the need for dietary management should follow. For infants and children, educating parents on the appropriate use of an ORS and of dietary management is very important preventive care. For families with infants, the CDC recommends a home supply of ORS because early administration of an ORS at home is vital if hospitalization is to be avoided.

If a nonspecific antidiarrheal is recommended, the pharmacist should review label instructions with the patient. The pharmacist should stress an appropriate dosage that is based on the patient's age, the maximum number of doses per 24 hours, and the auxiliary administration instructions. The pharmacist should also explain potential drug interactions, side effects, contraindications, and the maximum duration of treatment before seeking medical help. The box "Patient Education for Diarrhea" lists specific information to provide patients.

Evaluation of Patient Outcomes for Diarrhea

Many patients have mild-to-moderate distress, and the illness is generally self-limiting within 48 hours. Mild-to-moderate diarrhea is managed with oral rehydration therapy, symptomatic drug therapy, and diet changes. The primary monitoring parameter is checking for dehydration by measuring body weight, vital signs, and mental alertness. With effective symptomatic relief, the patient can expect reduced frequency and normal consistency of stools, as well as relief of generalized symptoms such as lethargy and abdominal pain. As the diarrheal episode clears, the appetite will return to normal and the diet can be advanced to a regular diet.

Medical referral is necessary if any of the following occur before or during treatment: high fever, worsening illness, blood or mucoid stools, diarrhea continuing beyond 48 hours, or signs of worsening dehydration (e.g., low blood pressure, rapid pulse, mental confusion). Also, medical referral is advised for infants, young children, the frail elderly, and patients with chronic illness at risk from secondary complications (e.g., diabetes mellitus).

Patient Education for Diarrhea

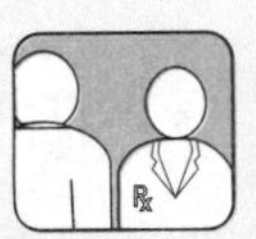

The primary objective of self-treatment is to prevent excessive fluid and electrolyte losses. Secondary objectives are to (1) relieve the symptoms; (2) manage the diet to avoid making the diarrhea worse; (3) identify and treat the cause, if known; and (4) manage secondary conditions, such as diabetes mellitus. For most patients, carefully following product instructions and the self-care measures listed below will help ensure optimal outcomes.

Nondrug Measures

Infants and Children Ages 5 Years and Younger

- For moderate diarrhea indicated by four to five unformed bowel movements per day, give the child or infant an oral rehydration solution at a volume of 100 mL/kg of body weight over 2 to 4 hours. Continue to give the solution for the next 4 to 6 hours or until the child is rehydrated.
- For mild diarrhea (three or fewer unformed bowel movements per day), give the child or infant an oral rehydration solution at a volume of 50 mL/kg of body weight over 2 to 4 hours. Continue to give the solution for the next 4 to 6 hours or until the child is rehydrated.
- If the child is vomiting, give 1 teaspoonful of oral rehydration solution every few minutes.
- If the child is not dehydrated, give 10 mL/kg or ½ to 1 cup of the oral rehydration solution for each bowel movement.
- After the child is rehydrated, reintroduce food appropriate for the child's age while also administering oral solutions as maintenance therapy.
  - —If breast-feeding an infant with diarrhea, continue the breast-feeding. If the infant is bottle fed, consult your doctor or pediatrician about substituting a milk-based formula with a lactose-free formula.
  - —Give children complex carbohydrate-rich foods (e.g., rice, potatoes, bread, and cereals), yogurt, lean meats, fruits, and vegetables. Do not give them fatty foods or sugary foods. Sugary foods can cause osmotic diarrhea.
- As maintenance therapy, administer 10 mL/kg or ½ to 1 cup of the oral rehydration solution for each subsequent unformed bowel movement.

Adults and Children Ages 5 Years and Older

- For moderate dehydration indicated by a 6% to 9% drop in body weight, drink 2 to 4 liters of an oral rehydration solution over 4 hours.
- For mild dehydration indicated by a 3% to 5% loss of body weight, drink 2 liters of an oral rehydration solution over 4 hours.
- If not dehydrated, drink ½ to 1 cup of oral rehydration solution or fluids with each unformed bowel movement.
- If you have no medical conditions, consume sport drinks, diluted juices, salty crackers, soups, and broths until the diarrhea stops.

(continued)

Patient Education for Diarrhea (continued)

Nonprescription Medications

- See Table 13–6 for dosages of loperamide, attapulgite, kaolin–pectin mixture, and polycarbophil.

Loperamide

- Be aware that loperamide can cause dizziness and constipation.
- Do not take this agent if you are taking sedatives, antianxiety drugs, or other antidepressants.
- Do not give this agent to children age 2 years or younger.
- If loperamide is not effective in treating your diarrhea, check with your doctor or pharmacist about using a different nonprescription medication. You may have a bacterial diarrhea or pseudomembranous colitis, conditions that loperamide cannot treat.

Attapulgite and Kaolin–Pectin Mixture

- Be aware that attapulgite and kaolin–pectin products can cause constipation on rare occasions.
- Do not take these agents if you are taking an antibiotic or digoxin.
- Do not give these agents to children age 2 years or younger.

Polycarbophil

- Be aware that polycarbophil can cause bloating and constipation.
- Do not give this agent to children age 2 years or younger.
- Do not take this agent if you are taking warfarin, digoxin, tetracycline, or ciprofloxin.

Bismuth Subsalicylate

- Be aware that bismuth subsalicylate can cause a dark discoloration of the tongue and stool.
- Do not take this agent if you are taking tetracyclines or uricosurics.
- Do not give this agent to children age 2 years or younger.
- Do not give this agent to children or teenagers who have or are recovering from influenza or chicken pox. Reye's syndrome (a rare, but serious, condition) could occur.
- Do not take this agent if you are sensitive to aspirin, have a history of gastrointestinal bleeding, or have a history of problems with blood coagulation.

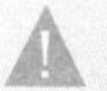
If the diarrhea has not resolved after 72 hours of initial treatment, see your doctor.

Monitor for excessive number of bowel movements, signs of dehydration, high fever, or blood in the stool. If any of these complications are present, see your doctor.

CONCLUSIONS

Diarrhea is often considered a trivial disorder, but it can be a symptom of a more serious underlying disease. The condition can be either acute or chronic. Acute diarrhea is characterized by a sudden onset of loose stools in a previously healthy patient. Chronic diarrhea is characterized by persistent or recurrent episodes of loose stools accompanied by anorexia, weight loss, and weakness. Simple diarrhea can usually be treated by supportive care and/or a nonprescription drug or oral hydration product.

The debilitating effect of persistent diarrhea is caused largely by loss of water through excretion resulting in an imbalance of both fluids and electrolytes. Replacing these important substances is an integral part of diarrhea therapy, particularly in infants, children, and frail elderly patients. This replacement can be accomplished with appropriate intravenous fluids or with oral glucose–electrolyte formulations.

Patients who appear volume depleted, weak, dizzy, or hypotensive should be referred to a health care provider, as should all patients with severely acute, uncontrolled, or chronic complaints involving the GI tract. For minor acute problems such as food or drink intolerance, however, relief may be provided by a nonprescription product such as loperamide.

References

1. Glass RI, Kilgore PE, Holman RC, et al. The epidemiology of rotavirus diarrhea in the United States: surveillance and estimates of disease burden. *J Infect Dis.* 1996;174(suppl 1):S5–S11.
2. Matson DO, Estes MK. Impact of rotavirus infections at a large pediatric hospital. *J Infect Dis.* 1990;162:598–604.
3. Liddle JL, Burgess MA, Gilbert GL, et al. Rotavirus gastroenteritis: impact on young children, their families, and the health care system. *Med J Australia.* 1997;167:304–7.
4. Gilbert DN, Moellering RC, Sande MA. *The Sanford Guide to Antimicrobial Therapy.* 29th ed. Hyde Park, VT: Antimicrobial Therapy; 1999: 11–4, 88.
5. Advice for Travelers. *Med Lett.* 1999;41:39–42.
6. Dupont HL. Guidelines on acute infectious diarrhea in adults. *Am J Gastro.* 1997;1962–75.
7. Gray GM. Acute diarrhea. In: Dale DC, Federman DD, eds. *Scientific American Medicine.* New York: Scientific American; 1992:1–16.
8. Field M, Rao MC, Chang EB. Intestinal electrolyte transport and diarrheal disease. *N Engl J Med.* 1989;321(pt 1):800–6.
9. Centers for Disease Control and Prevention. The management of acute diarrhea in children: oral rehydration, maintenance, and nutritional therapy. *MMWR Morb Mortal Wkly Rep.* 1992;41(RR-16):1–20.
10. American Academy of Pediatrics. Practice Parameters: the management of acute gastroenteritis in young children. *Pediatrics.* 1996;97:424–34.
11. Pizarro D, Posada G, Sands L, et al. Rice-based oral electrolyte solutions for the management of infantile diarrhea. *N Engl J Med.* 1991;324: 517–21.
12. Avery ME, Snyder JD. Oral therapy for acute diarrhea. *N Engl J Med.* 1990;323:891–4.

CHAPTER 14

Anorectal Disorders

Eddie L. Boyd and Rosemary R. Berardi

Chapter 14 at a Glance

Anorectal disorders involve the perianal area, the anal canal, and the lower rectum. Patients with these conditions may complain of anorectal bleeding, pain, burning, itching, discomfort, seepage, protrusion, swelling, irritation, inflammation, swelling, changes in bowel patterns, or any combination thereof.[1] Many of these signs and symptoms are associated with hemorrhoids, but they may also be related to other anorectal disorders such as an anal fissure, fistula, abscess, or malignant neoplasm.[1] Most signs and symptoms can be self-treated; however, some are not amenable to self-treatment and require medical attention. The pharmacist should carefully evaluate all anorectal signs and symptoms reported by patients and should recommend self-treatment, if appropriate, or consultation with a physician. Numerous nonprescription products are available for the symptomatic treatment of anorectal disorders. This chapter focuses on self-treating hemorrhoids and on recognizing anorectal signs and symptoms that require referral to a physician.

Epidemiology of Hemorrhoids

Hemorrhoids (also known as piles) are abnormally large, bulging, symptomatic conglomerates of hemorrhoidal vessels, supporting tissues, and overlying mucous membranes or skin in the anorectal region. About 10% to 15% of the adult population in the United States complain of anorectal signs and symptoms that they attribute to hemorrhoids.[2] The

Editor's Note: This chapter is based, in part, on the 11th edition chapter titled "Hemorrhoidal Products," which was written by Benjamin Hodes.

prevalence of hemorrhoids increases with advancing age and peaks in individuals between 45 and 65 years of age.[2] Men appear to suffer from hemorrhoids more often than women.[3,4] Although epidemiologic data are lacking, the incidence of hemorrhoids among pregnant women, however, appears to be much higher than for nonpregnant women of similar child-bearing age.[3] In the United States, Caucasians self-report symptoms attributed to hemorrhoids 1.5 times more often than African Americans.[3] More than 3.5 million individuals, approximately one-third of those who complain of hemorrhoidal-like symptoms, visit a physician annually for treatment.[4]

Anatomy and Physiology of the Anorectal Area

Anorectal disorders occur in the perianal area, the anal canal, and the lower portion of the rectum. (See Figure 14–1.) The perianal area (about 7 cm in diameter) is the portion of the skin and buttocks immediately surrounding the anus. The presence of sensory nerve endings makes this area very sensitive to pain. Perianal tissue differs from most other skin tissue in that it is normally more moist than exposed skin in other areas of the body.

The anal canal (about 2.5 cm long) is the channel connecting the end of the gastrointestinal tract (rectum) with the outside of the body. The lower two-thirds of the canal is covered by modified anal skin, which is structurally similar to the skin covering other parts of the body. The canal contains sensory nerve endings as well as pressure receptors, which allow for the perception of distention pain. Two powerful sphincter muscles encircle the anal canal and control the passage of fecal material. The external sphincter, located at the bottom of the anal canal, is a voluntary muscle. The internal sphincter, which allows passage from the rectum into the anal canal, is an involuntary muscle. Both sphincters lie under the tissues of the anal canal and extend downward (vertically around the anal canal). Under normal conditions, the external sphincter is closed and prevents the involuntary passage of feces or discharges.

In healthy individuals, the skin covering the anal canal serves as a barrier against absorption of substances into the body. Therefore, treatment applied to this area may manifest primarily local (topical) effects. If disease is present, either loss of the protective barrier or breaks in the surface may alter the absorptive character of skin covering the canal, thereby diminishing the skin's protective capabilities. The point in the mid-upper anal canal at which the skin lining changes to mucous membrane is the dentate or pectinate line, also known as the anorectal line.

The rectum (about 12 to 15 cm long) lies above the anal canal and extends from the anorectal line to the sigmoid colon. It is lined with a semipermeable mucous membrane, is highly vascularized, and contains no sensory pain fibers. Like the anal canal, the rectum contains pressure receptors and a mucous membrane that protects the body from invasion by bacteria present in feces. Investigators commonly distinguish between the rectal mucosa and anal mucosa; they consider the anorectal line to be the upper end of the anal canal. In this chapter, we will consider the mucosal region to be the beginning of the rectal area.

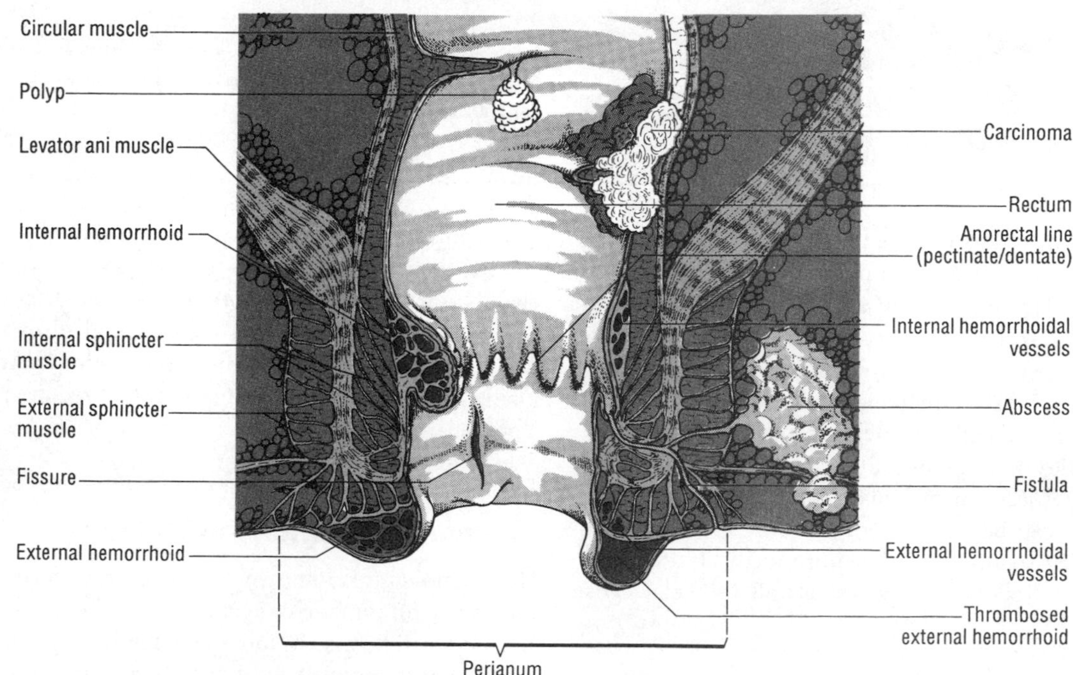

Figure 14–1 Disorders of the anorectal area.

The most prominent parts of the vasculature in the region above and below the anorectal line are three hemorrhoidal arteries and their accompanying veins. Arteries and veins lying above the anorectal line are referred to as internal; those below the anorectal line are referred to as external. Because of the plexus of hemorrhoidal vessels located beneath the rectal mucosa and the path followed by blood returning to the heart through the hemorrhoidal veins, substances absorbed through the rectal mucous membranes may enter the systemic circulation without passing through the liver. It is important to consider this fact when evaluating the potential systemic toxic effects of rectally administered medications.

Etiology of Hemorrhoids

Many factors have been implicated in the etiology and pathogenesis of hemorrhoids, including heredity, erect posture, pregnancy, prolonged standing or sitting, lack of dietary bulk, constipation, diarrhea, and heavy lifting with straining. Symptomatic hemorrhoids appear to develop only in susceptible individuals. Although data are conflicting, heredity may play an important role; also socioeconomic and cultural factors (e.g., diet and lifestyle) may precipitate hemorrhoid formation.[3] Although most evidence points to a lack of relationship between dietary fiber intake and the formation of hemorrhoids, a preliminary study suggests that an increase in fiber for more than 15 days did decrease bleeding from internal hemorrhoids.[5] However, other studies have not confirmed these results. Bowel habits, such as straining at defecation or prolonged sitting on the toilet during bowel movements, may increase pressure within the hemorrhoidal vessels and precipitate the formation of hemorrhoids.[3] Alternatively, constipation has been reported to follow the onset of hemorrhoidal symptoms and may improve with prolapse.[3,6] These data suggest that hemorrhoids can cause constipation rather than constipation causing hemorrhoids. Recent studies indicate that diarrhea may also be a risk factor for hemorrhoids.[7,8] Further, the gravid uterus may increase pressure in the hemorrhoidal veins and contribute to forming hemorrhoids during pregnancy.

Pathophysiology of Hemorrhoids and Other Anorectal Disorders

The most widely accepted pathogenic theory is that hemorrhoids (vascular cushions) are a part of the normal anatomy and are located circumferentially around the anal canal above the dentate line. These cushions are present at birth in three discrete masses and, by partially occluding the anus, contribute to continence. The cushions, which contain blood vessels, smooth muscle, and supportive connective tissue, project into the lumen where they are subject to downward pressure during defecation. In younger individuals, the muscle fibers anchor the cushions and support the venous sinusoidal vessels. However, with increasing age, the muscle fibers become attenuated; then the cushions slide, become congested, bleed, and eventually prolapse.[2,3] Physiologic vulnerability and high-resting anal pressure are both common denominators in developing hemorrhoids.[3]

Types of Hemorrhoids

Hemorrhoids are classified according to their location, leading to two major types of hemorrhoids: internal and external. (See Figure 14–1.) Frequently, internal and external hemorrhoids are present in the same individual.

Internal Hemorrhoids

Internal hemorrhoids occur above the anorectal line, are covered with anal mucosa (simple columnar epithelium), and lack sensory innervation.[9] They are further classified according to the three primary hemorrhoid locations (e.g., left lateral, right posterior, or right anterior).[10] The end branches of the superior and middle hemorrhoidal arteries terminate in the submucosa above the dentate line with an anterior and posterior branch on the right and a single lateral branch on the left. Internal hemorrhoids are designated using a four-degree system: (1) first-degree hemorrhoids do not move from the anal canal, (2) second-degree hemorrhoids can descend into the anal canal and return spontaneously, (3) third-degree hemorrhoids can be returned manually into the anus, and (4) fourth-degree hemorrhoids are prolapsed and cannot be reintroduced into the anus.

External Hemorrhoids

External hemorrhoids are dilations of the inferior (external) hemorrhoidal plexus. They lie below the dentate (pectinate) line and are covered with anoderm (the epithelial lining of the anal canal) and perianal skin. Because the two plexus (internal and external) freely form anastomoses, many patients have a combination of both types (interoexternal or mixed hemorrhoids).[2] External hemorrhoids are frequently seen as bluish lumps at the anal verge (the external or distal boundary of the anal canal). The blue color may be caused by thrombosed veins in the complex. Symptoms of thrombosed external hemorrhoids range from minimal discomfort to severe pain.[10]

Other Anorectal Disorders

Potentially serious anorectal disorders, including abscesses, fistulas, fissures, tumors, polyps, and inflammatory bowel disease, may present with hemorrhoidal-like symptoms and should not be self-treated. Patients should be referred to a physician if any of the following conditions are suspected.

Abscess

An abscess is a painful swelling in the perianal or anal canal area caused by a bacterial (primarily staphylococcal) infection and resulting in the formation of a localized area of pus. Perianal abscesses, the most common anorectal abscess, lie just beneath the perianal skin. Fever is common with large abscesses.[2]

Anal Fistula

An anal fistula is a hollow fibrous tract lined by granulation tissue that usually has an opening (primary or internal) inside the anal canal or rectum and that includes one or more orifices (secondary or external) in the perianal skin. An anal fistula often results from an anorectal abscess.[2]

Anal Fissure

An anal fissure is a slit-like ulcer in the anal canal lining, which may be painful and may exist alone or in conjunction with hemorrhoids. It sometimes causes bleeding (as evidenced by a few spots of bright red blood on toilet tissue). Other symptoms may include a mass at the anus (sentinel pile), scant mucoid discharge, and itching.[2]

Malignant Neoplasm

Malignant neoplasm is a serious disease, most often presenting with nonspecific symptoms of rectal bleeding (most common), anal pain, and a sensation of a rectal mass.[2] Other symptoms may include a change in bowel habits, diarrhea, constipation, discharge, and itching. Squamous cell or epidermoid carcinomas are the most prevalent anal cancers.[2,11]

Polyps

Polyps are benign or malignant rectal tumors characterized by bleeding, a mass protruding through the anus (rare), or a feeling of fullness or pressure in the rectum.

Signs and Symptoms of Hemorrhoids and Other Anorectal Disorders

The Food and Drug Administration (FDA) Advisory Panel reviewed anorectal nonprescription medications and identified these signs and symptoms of anorectal disorders: itching, irritation, burning, inflammation, swelling, discomfort, pain, bleeding, seepage, protrusion, thrombosis, changes in bowel habits, or any combination thereof.[1] Itching, irritation, burning, inflammation, and swelling are usually considered common signs and symptoms of minor anorectal disorders. By contrast, pain, bleeding, seepage, protrusion, and thrombosis may indicate a more serious condition not amenable to self-treatment.

Itching

Itching, or pruritus, is caused by mild stimulation of the sensory nerve fibers and is associated with many anorectal disorders, including hemorrhoids. Itching is the most common symptom of these disorders and may be secondary to swelling, irritation caused by dietary factors, parasitic diseases (e.g., pinworm), or moisture in the anal area.[1] Pruritus ani refers to persistent itching in the anal and perianal regions that occurs even in the presence of good hygiene. Itching is typically associated with hemorrhoids when there is mucus discharge from prolapsing internal hemorrhoids. Sensitivity to fabrics, detergents, and dyes and perfumes in toilet tissue are common causes of itching. Fungal infections, parasites, allergies, and associated anorectal pathologic lesions may also cause itching. Oral broad-spectrum antibiotic therapy may trigger itching in the anorectal area as a result of infection secondary to the overgrowth of nonsusceptible organisms, particularly fungi. On rare occasions, itching may have psychological origins.

Burning

Burning, a common symptom of anorectal disorders, suggests a somewhat greater degree of irritation of the anorectal sensory nerves than that associated with itching. The burning sensation may range from a feeling of warmth to a feeling of intense heat and may be constant or associated with defecation. This symptom is often associated with hemorrhoids.

Inflammation/Swelling

Trauma, allergy, or infection often causes inflammation, a tissue reaction distinguished by heat, redness or discoloration, pain, and swelling. Swelling is caused by an accumulation of excess fluid associated with engorged hemorrhoids or hemorrhoidal tissue. The inflammation itself, but not the underlying causes, may be relieved by self-treatment.

Discomfort

Discomfort in the anorectal area may result from burning, itching, pain, inflammation, or swelling.[1]

Pain

Pain may result from an intensely uncomfortable stimulation of the sensory nerve fibers of the anorectal area. Inflammation or irritation tends to cause minor pain. Internal hemorrhoids are above the dentate line and are usually painless. In contrast, patients with acutely thrombosed external hemorrhoids will complain primarily of pain. Pain may also be associated with an abscess, fissure, fistula, or malignant neoplasm of the anorectum.

Bleeding

Painless bleeding during defecation is a common symptom of hemorrhoids.[9] Bleeding is almost always associated with internal hemorrhoids and is most often described as either a bright red spot or streak on the toilet tissue or dripping into the toilet bowl. Bleeding most often occurs at the end of defecation, is separate from the stool, and usually does not occur apart from defecation.[12] Bleeding usually occurs late in the course of thrombosed external hemorrhoids after the overlying perianal skin ulcerates. Because it may indicate the presence of serious anorectal disorders such as abscess, fistula, fissure, or malignancy, or because it may result from intestinal diseases such as inflammatory bowel disease or diverticulitis, bleeding should not be self-treated.

Seepage

An anal sphincter that does not close completely may cause seepage, which is the involuntary passage of fecal material or

Case Study 14–1

Patient Complaint/History

Andrew, a 55-year-old man, presents to the pharmacist complaining of irritation and itching in the rectal area. The patient asks if Anusol-HC cream is "any good." When questioned about his symptoms, Andrew responds that he has not noticed any swelling or soreness in the rectal area, but did notice "red blood" in the toilet a couple of days ago. He tells the pharmacist that when sitting for prolonged periods of time, he has a sense of discomfort (burning and itching) in the rectal area. The medication profile indicates that Andrew takes Dyazide for mild hypertension; Synthroid, because his thyroid gland was removed about 30 years ago for cancer; Metamucil to increase dietary fiber; and Dulcolax tablets for constipation. The patient, whose job requires that he stand most of the day and lift heavy boxes, took two Dulcolax last week for constipation.

Clinical Considerations/Strategies

Readers can use the following considerations/strategies to determine whether treating the patient's condition with nonprescription medications is warranted:

- Assess the possible cause(s) of the patient's anorectal symptoms.
- Determine the appropriateness of treatment with Anusol-HC cream.
- Recommend, if appropriate, a nonprescription medication treatment regimen for the rectal irritation, itching, and bleeding.
- Assess the possible adverse effects associated with the nonprescription medication, if recommended.

Patient Education/Counseling

Readers can use the following strategies to develop a patient education/counseling plan that will ensure optimal therapeutic outcomes:

- Ensure that the patient understands when and how to apply the recommended nonprescription medication, if appropriate.
- Ensure that the patient knows whether the self-treatment regimen (if recommended) was successful and when to contact a physician.

mucus. Seepage may include the discharge of pus from a fistula or feces through a fistula that connects the rectum to the anal canal.[1] A patient with seepage should be referred to a physician and should not be self-treated.

Protrusion

Protrusion (prolapse), a frequent sign or symptom of uncomplicated internal and internal/external hemorrhoids (mixed hemorrhoids), is defined as the projection of hemorrhoidal or rectal tissue outside the anal canal. The rectal protrusion may vary in size and usually appears after defecation, prolonged standing, or unusual physical exertion.[2] It is painless except when thrombosis, infection, or ulceration is present. Strangulation of a protruding hemorrhoid by the anal sphincter may lead to thrombosis. Additionally, when contraction of the anal sphincter interferes with blood flow from a prolapsed interior mixed hemorrhoid, a painful lump may develop, also resulting in thrombosis. If, by using digital manipulation, this prolapsed hemorrhoid is returned to an area above the anal sphincter before thrombosis occurs, the pain and lump usually disappear. However, when defecation occurs, both the pain and the lump are likely to recur. Permanently prolapsed internal hemorrhoids cause a mucoid discharge, which, in turn, may lead to perianal irritation, itching, pain, and swelling. Self-treatment is not appropriate and should not be encouraged.

Thrombosis

Thrombosis is a common manifestation of hemorrhoids. Painful symptoms from a thrombosed external hemorrhoid are most acute during the first 48 to 72 hours, with symptoms usually resolving over a 7- to 10-day period. If a thrombosed hemorrhoid persists, ulcers or gangrene may develop on its surface and may cause bleeding, especially when the patient defecates. If the thrombosed hemorrhoid resides entirely above the anorectal line (a pure internal hemorrhoid), minimal pain may exist because this area lacks sensory nerves. Patients are likely to be unaware that such a hemorrhoid is present unless they have sudden changes in bowel habits.

Treatment of Hemorrhoids

Treatment Outcomes

The major goal of treating anorectal disorders is to alleviate symptoms and to prevent complications that may lead to adverse consequences for the patient. The outcome of self-treatment should be to control anorectal itching, burning, inflammation, swelling, and discomfort.

General Treatment Approach

Figure 14–2 presents an algorithm for treating patients with hemorrhoids. If the patient has self-treatable signs and symp-

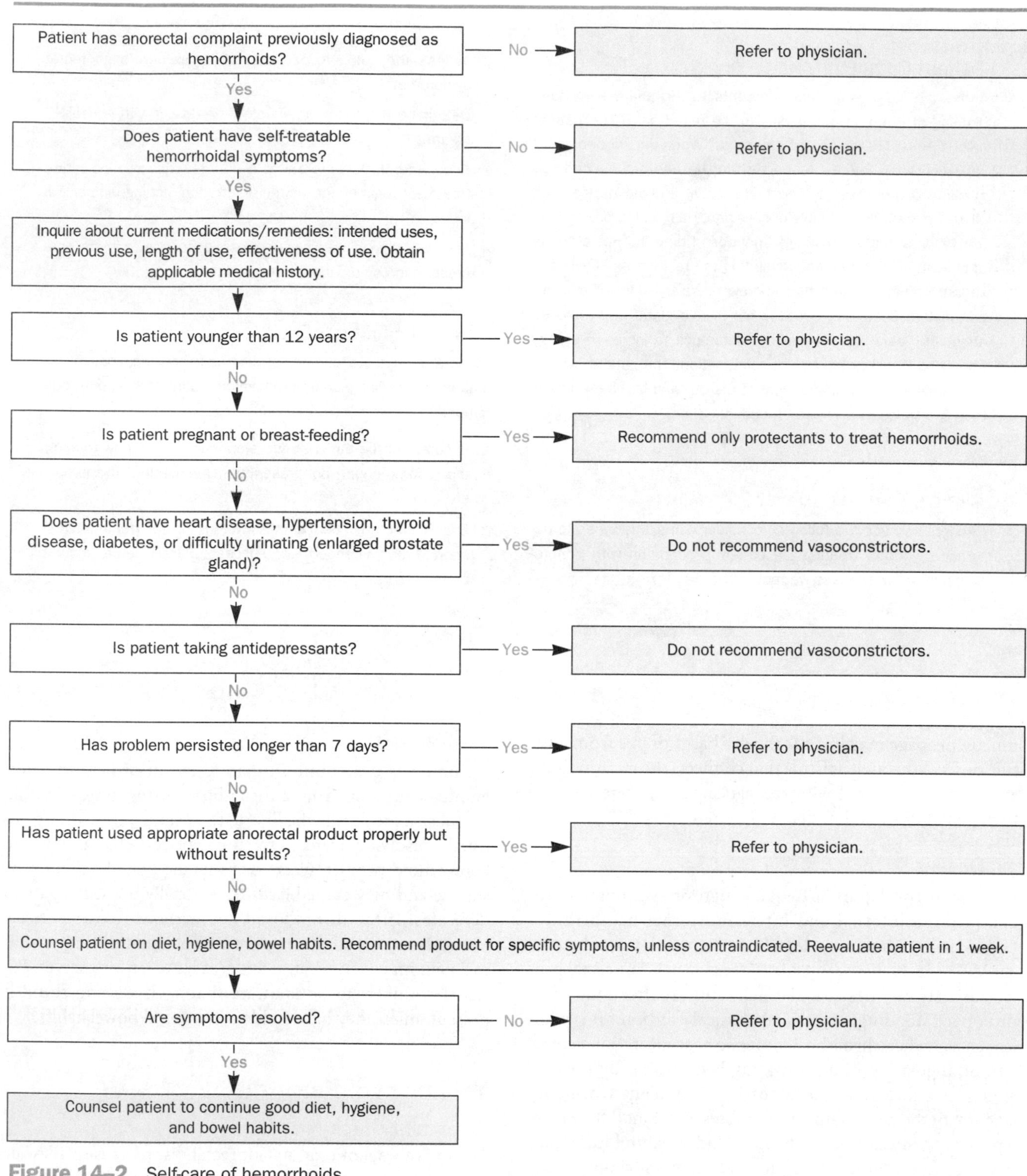

Figure 14–2 Self-care of hemorrhoids.

toms of hemorrhoids, the pharmacist should recommend appropriate nonpharmacologic measures and a nonprescription preparation that contains a medication to treat that specific symptom (e.g., topical corticosteroids for the temporary relief of itching). The patient should be advised to maintain a well-balanced diet (preferably high in fiber and bulk) and good perianal hygiene, as well as to avoid prolonged sitting on the toilet. The pharmacist should counsel the patient as to how and when to apply the topical anorectal product. If alarm symptoms develop (e.g., blood in the stool, severe pain) or if symptoms do not resolve after 7 days, the patient should be advised to seek medical attention. If the symptoms resolve, the patient should be encouraged to maintain the well-balanced diet, good personal hygiene, and good bowel habits.

Women who are pregnant or nursing mothers should use protectants only intrarectally. Patients with high blood pressure, cardiac disease, diabetes, hyperthyroidism, or urination problems caused by enlargement of the prostate gland should not use anorectal products containing vasoconstrictors. Additionally, patients taking monoamine oxidase inhibitors, tricyclic antidepressants, or antihypertensive agents should not use topical vasoconstrictors.

As mentioned previously, exclusions to self-treatment include potentially serious anorectal disorders such as abscesses, fistulas, fissures, tumors, polyps, and inflammatory bowel disease, as well as anorectal disorders that have been previously diagnosed and treated by a physician. Patients with anorectal pain, bleeding, seepage, protrusion, and thrombosis or with initially more severe itching, burning, inflammation, swelling, and discomfort should also be referred to a physician. Patients with anorectal disorders, including hemorrhoids, who are younger than 12 years of age should be immediately referred to a physician. Finally, patients with minor symptoms that are unresponsive to 7 days of self-treatment should consult a physician.

Nonpharmacologic Therapy

Nondrug measures for treating hemorrhoids range from dietary measures to hygiene practices to methods for removing the hemorrhoids.

Dietary Measures

Small symptomatic hemorrhoids can be treated with a high-fiber diet with or without bulk agents. Increasing fiber, bulk, and fluid intake in the diet may reduce or prevent straining at defecation and may permit the passage of softer stools.

Defecation Time

Avoiding prolonged sitting (no more than 5 minutes) on the toilet in an attempt to defecate may reduce straining and the associated increased pressure on hemorrhoidal vessels.

Anal Hygiene

Good anal hygiene helps relieve anorectal symptoms and may prevent recurrence of perianal itching. The patient should cleanse the anorectal area regularly and after each bowel movement by using a mild, unscented soap and water or, more practically, by using commercially available hygienic and lubricated wipes or pads.

Sitz Baths

Sitz baths promote good hygiene and often relieve hemorrhoidal symptoms, especially after bowel movements. Patients should sit in warm water (110°F to 115°F [43.3°C to 46.1°C]) two to three times a day for about 15 minutes. Plastic sitz tubs that fit over the toilet rim are convenient, easily cleaned, and available at pharmacies and from medical supply vendors.

Surgery

Large and prolapsed hemorrhoids are often treated with surgery. The procedure involves excising one or more of the three hemorrhoidal masses (hemorrhoidectomy).

Nonsurgical Procedures

Nonsurgical procedures include injection of sclerosing agents, rubber band ligation, dilation of the anal canal and lower rectum, cryosurgery, electrocoagulation, infrared photocoagulation, bipolar diathermy, and local anal hypothermia with a frozen finger.[13,14]

Pharmacologic Therapy

The following nonprescription pharmacologic agents are used to relieve the symptoms of anorectal disorders: local anesthetics, vasoconstrictors, protectants, astringents, keratolytics, analgesics/anesthetics/antipruritics, and corticosteroids. The following discussion summarizes the use, risks, and efficacy of these agents when used topically to treat anorectal disorders. Table 14–1 provides FDA-approved dosages for anorectal drug products.[15]

Local Anesthetics

The following local anesthetics have met the FDA safety and efficacy standards for use in anorectal preparations: benzocaine, benzyl alcohol, dyclonine, lidocaine, pramoxine, and tetracaine.

Mechanism of Action/Indications Local anesthetics temporarily relieve itching, irritation, burning, discomfort, and pain by reversibly blocking the transmission of nerve impulses. Use of these products should be limited to the perianal region or the lower anal canal because the rectum is not innervated with sensory nerve fibers. The local anesthetic effect may mask the pain of a more severe anorectal disorder.

Adverse Effects Local anesthetics may be rapidly absorbed through the rectal mucosa and may cause potentially toxic systemic effects. However, absorption through the perianal skin is usually minimal unless the skin is abraded. Local anesthetics may produce local allergic reactions (e.g., burning and itching), which are indistinguishable from the anorectal symptoms being treated. Systemic reactions can also occur. Individuals who have had a previous adverse reaction to such agents should not use them. Adverse effects are rare with pramoxine hydrochloride, which exhibits less cross-sensitivity because—unlike the other local anesthetics—it is not chemically derived from lidocaine or procaine.[17]

Contraindications/Precautions/Warnings Anorectal preparations that contain local anesthetics must carry a warning that allergic reactions may occur in some individuals. If the symptoms being treated do not subside or if redness, irritation, swelling, pain, or other symptoms develop or increase, the user should discontinue use and should consult a physician.

Table 14–1

Dosage and Administration Guidelines for Anorectal Products

Ingredient	Concentration per Dosage Unit (%)	Frequency of Use
Local Anesthetics		
Benzocaine	5–20	Up to 6 times/day; not to exceed 24 g/day
Benzyl alcohol	1–4	Up to 6 times/day; not to exceed 480 mg/day
Dibucaine, dibucaine hydrochloride	0.25–1	Up to 3–4 times/day
Dyclonine hydrochloride	0.5–1	Up to 6 times/day; not to exceed 100 mg/day
Lidocaine	2–5	Up to 6 times/day; not to exceed 500 mg/day
Pramoxine chloride[a]	1	Up to 5 times/day; not to exceed 100 mg/day
Tetracaine, tetracaine hydrochloride	0.5–1	Up to 6 times/day; not to exceed 100 mg/day
Vasoconstrictors		
Ephedrine	0.1–1.25	Up to 4 times/day; not to exceed 100 mg/day
Epinephrine hydrochloride/Epinephrine base	0.005–0.01	Up to 4 times/day; not to exceed 800 mg/day
Phenylephrine hydrochloride	0.25	Up to 4 times/day; not to exceed 2 mg/day
Protectants		
Aluminum hydroxide gel, cocoa butter, glycerin, hard fat, kaolin, lanolin, mineral oil, white petrolatum, petrolatum, shark liver oil, zinc oxide, topical starch	See footnote b	Petrolatum/white petrolatum: as often as needed; other protectants: up to 6 times/day or after each bowel movement
Astringents		
Calamine, zinc oxide	5–25	Up to 6 times/day or after each bowel movement
Witch hazel	10–50	Up to 6 times/day or after each bowel movement
Keratolytics		
Alcloxa	0.2–2	Up to 6 times/day
Resorcinol	1–3	Up to 6 times/day
Analgesics/Anesthetics/Antipruritics		
Menthol	0.1–1	Up to 6 times/day
Juniper tar	1–5	Up to 6 times/day
Camphor	0.1–3	Up to 6 times/day
Corticosteroids		
Hydrocortisone	0.25–1	Up to 3–4 times/day

[a] External dosage forms may include aerosol foams, ointments, creams, and jellies (water-miscible base).

[b] If a single protectant ingredient is used, it must compose at least 50% of the product. Aqueous solutions of glycerin cannot contain less than 20% or more than 45% glycerin (weight-to-weight). (See Table 14–2 for concentrations of protectants used in combination products.)

Source: References 15 and 16.

Vasoconstrictors

Vasoconstrictors are chemical agents structurally related to the naturally occurring catecholamines, epinephrine and norepinephrine. Four topical vasoconstrictors—ephedrine sulfate, epinephrine hydrochloride, epinephrine base, and phenylephrine hydrochloride—are FDA-approved.

Mechanism of Action When applied topically to the anorectal area, vasoconstrictors stimulate the alpha-adrenergic receptors in the vascular beds, thus causing constriction of the arterioles and a resultant modest and transient reduction of swelling. These agents relieve itching, discomfort, and irritation, in part because they produce a slight anesthetic effect by an unknown mechanism. Although studies have demonstrated that locally applied vasoconstrictors promptly alter the blood supply to the mucosa, the FDA does not recognize or approve of the use of such agents to control minor bleeding.[1]

Ephedrine sulfate, which is readily absorbed through

mucous membranes in the rectum, has a more prolonged effect than epinephrine and acts on both alpha- and beta-adrenergic receptors. When ephedrine is applied to the perianal area, its onset of action ranges from a few seconds to 1 minute; its duration of action is between 2 and 3 hours.

Epinephrine hydrochloride and epinephrine base are effective only when used externally, because epinephrine is inactivated at the pH of the rectum (which ranges from neutral to basic). Epinephrine is absorbed from the mucous membranes (none of which are in the perianal area) and acts on both alpha- and beta-adrenergic receptors.

Phenylephrine hydrochloride reduces congestion in the anorectal area and is believed to relieve itching caused by histamine release. It acts primarily on the alpha-adrenergic receptors and produces vasoconstriction by a direct effect on receptors rather than by norepinephrine displacement.

Indications Ephedrine sulfate, epinephrine hydrochloride, epinephrine base, and phenylephrine hydrochloride, when used externally, are FDA-approved for itching, discomfort, swelling, and irritation. Ephedrine sulfate and phenylephrine hydrochloride are recommended for internal (intrarectal) use. However, data are insufficient to establish the safety and effectiveness of epinephrine base and epinephrine hydrochloride for intrarectal use.

Adverse Effects Topical ephedrine sulfate may cause nervousness, tremor, sleeplessness, nausea, and loss of appetite. If these symptoms persist or become worse, a physician should be consulted. The FDA has concluded that potentially serious adverse effects, including elevation of blood pressure, nervousness, tremor, sleeplessness, aggravation of symptoms of hyperthyroidism, and risk of cardiac arrhythmias, are less likely to occur with topical vasoconstrictors when used in recommended dosages.

Drug–Drug Interactions The hypertensive effects of ephedrine are potentiated by monoamine oxidase inhibitors and tricyclic antidepressants only when ephedrine is inserted in the anorectal canal. Adverse effects may occur with concomitant administration of antihypertensive medications and vasoconstrictors. Patients taking these prescription medications should consult a physician before using vasoconstrictors.

Contraindications/Precautions/Warnings Patients with diabetes, hyperthyroidism, hypertension, and difficulty urinating because of an enlarged prostate should not use these agents without first consulting a physician because of the slight possibility of systemic adverse effects from topical application of vasoconstrictors.

Protectants

The protectant drug class includes absorbents, adsorbents, demulcents, and emollients. Specific agents include aluminum hydroxide gel, cocoa butter, glycerin, hard fat, kaolin, lanolin, mineral oil, white petrolatum, petrolatum, shark liver oil, zinc oxide, and topical starch. Many substances classified as protectants are used as vehicles, bases, and carriers of pharmacologically active substances (e.g., vasoconstrictors and local anesthetics). One of the following criteria must be met to justify a claim for a protective effect: (1) at least one protectant must be present in at least 50% concentration; or (2) a combination of two, but no more than four, protectants must be present for a combined concentration of at least 50%.[1] As discussed further in the section "Combination Products," protectant ingredients that are limited to concentrations of less than 50% may be used in combination with other protectants.[1]

Glycerin is FDA-approved in an aqueous solution so that the final product contains not less than 10% and not more than 45% glycerin (weight-to-weight). Any combination product containing glycerin must contain at least this minimum amount of glycerin.[16] Hard fat is defined according to the official *National Formulary* monograph and according to the FDA's designation of "hard fat" in the monograph of nonprescription anorectal drug products and includes Witepsol ingredients (cocoa butter substitutes, hydrogenated cocoglycerides, and hydrogenated palm kernel glycerides).[18]

Mechanism of Action/Indications By forming a physical barrier on the skin, protectants prevent irritation of the anorectal area and water loss from the stratum corneum. Protecting the perianal area from irritants such as fecal matter reduces irritation, itching, burning, and discomfort.

All of the above protectants are recommended for external and internal (intrarectal) use with the exception of glycerin, which is recommended for external use only.

Adverse Effects Little or no absorption of protectants occurs; therefore, adverse reactions to protectants as a class are minimal. Wool (lanolin) alcohols may cause allergies and are probably responsible for most cases of lanolin allergy.

Contraindications/Precautions/Warnings Anorectal preparations containing aluminum hydroxide gel and kaolin are required to contain a warning to remove petrolatum or greasy ointment before applying the products because those products interfere with the ability of aluminum hydroxide gel and kaolin to adhere properly to the skin.

Astringents

Astringents used in anorectal preparations include calamine, zinc oxide, and witch hazel.

Mechanism of Action/Indications Astringents are applied to the skin of mucous membranes for a local and limited effect. They act by coagulating the protein in the skin cells, thereby protecting the underlying tissue while decreasing cell volume. Zinc, a heavy metal, acts as a protein precipitate and provides an astringent effect. When appropriately used, astringents contribute to drying by decreasing mucus and other secretions. This drying effect helps relieve local anorectal irritation, discomfort, itching, and burning.

Calamine and zinc oxide are recommended for both external and internal anorectal disorders, whereas witch hazel is recommended for external use only. Witch hazel's effectiveness is primarily attributed to its alcohol content (14%).

Calamine and zinc oxide, in concentrations of 5% to 25%, are safe and effective when applied up to six times a day or after each bowel movement.[16] Witch hazel (hamamelis water), in a concentration of 10% to 50%, is safe and effective when applied up to six times a day or after each bowel movement. Witch hazel is incorporated into several commercially available rectal pads or wipes that are advertised as being useful for hemorrhoids. Recommended products should be limited to those containing the appropriate concentration of an astringent.

Adverse Effects Adverse reactions to the topical use of calamine, zinc oxide, and witch hazel are rare.

Keratolytics

The two FDA-approved keratolytics for use in anorectal preparations are aluminum chlorhydroxy allantoinate (alcloxa) and resorcinol.

Mechanism of Action/Indications Keratolytics cause desquamation and debridement or sloughing of epidermal surface cells. By fostering cell turnover and loosening surface cells, keratolytics may help expose underlying tissue to therapeutic agents. Keratolytics, when used externally, are somewhat useful in reducing itching and discomfort, but their exact mechanism of action is not known. Because mucous membranes contain no keratin layer, the intrarectal use of keratolytics is not justified and may be harmful.

Adverse Effects The labels of nonprescription preparations containing resorcinol must warn against use on an open wound near the anus because of the potential for severe allergic reactions.

Contraindications/Precautions/Warnings Anorectal preparations that contain resorcinol must list the following warning: "Certain persons can develop allergic reactions to ingredients in this product. If the symptom being treated does not subside or if redness, irritation, swelling, pain, or other symptoms develop or increase, discontinue use and consult a physician."

Analgesics/Anesthetics/Antipruritics

To promote consistency, the FDA has redesignated several ingredients as either "analgesic, anesthetic, or antipruritic" that were formerly classified as "counterirritants."[15] This nomenclature was adopted to conform with the FDA's pharmacologic designations of the active ingredients, despite the inherent redundancy of the terms *anesthetic* and *antipruritic* as defined in this chapter. The ingredients in anorectal preparations that fall in this new classification are menthol, juniper tar, and camphor.

Mechanism of Action/Indications Menthol, juniper tar, and camphor are safe and effective when used externally in the perirectal area to relieve pain, discomfort, and burning. Such agents relieve those symptoms by depressing cutaneous sensory receptors. The agents should not be used internally because the rectum has no identifiable nerve fibers.

Adverse Effects Anorectal preparations containing menthol must list the following warning: "Certain persons can develop allergic reactions to ingredients in this product. If the symptom being treated does not subside or if redness, irritation, swelling, pain, or other symptoms develop or increase, discontinue use and consult a physician."

Corticosteroids

Hydrocortisone is the topical corticosteroid contained in most anorectal preparations.

Mechanism of Action/Indications Topical hydrocortisone acts as a vasoconstrictor and antipruritic. This agent has the potential to reduce itching and pain by producing lysosomal membrane stabilization and antimitotic activity. Nonprescription topical hydrocortisone is safe and effective for the temporary relief of minor external anal itching caused by minor irritation or rash.

Adverse Effects Hydrocortisone may mask the symptoms of bacterial and fungal infections.

Combination Products

Federal regulations state that a nonprescription product may combine two or more safe and effective active ingredients and may generally be recognized as safe and effective when (1) each active ingredient contributes to the claimed effect; (2) the combination of active ingredients does not decrease the safety or effectiveness of any individual active ingredients; and (3) the combination, when listing adequate directions for use and warning against unsafe use, provides rational, concurrent therapy for a significant proportion of the target population.[16] The FDA placed the restrictions listed in Table 14–2 on nonprescription anorectal preparations containing combinations.

Because some self-treatable anorectal disorders may have concurrent symptoms, combination preparations are reasonable. However, there is no evidence that an anorectal preparation with combined active ingredients is any more effective than a preparation with a therapeutic amount of a single ingredient. Theoretically, restricting the number of ingredients in the anorectal preparation should decrease the risk of interactions and of altering the product's effectiveness.

Laxatives

To prevent straining during defecation, some patients may require the addition of a bulk-forming (e.g., psyllium) or emollient (e.g., docusate) laxative in addition to a high-fiber diet and adequate fluid intake.[2,12] (See Chapter 12, "Constipation.") Patients with symptomatic hemorrhoids may experience a significant reduction in pain and bleeding within a few weeks after beginning regular use of a bulk laxative. However, excessive dietary fiber and bulk-forming laxatives may cause diarrhea.

Table 14–2

FDA Restrictions for Combination Nonprescription Anorectal Preparations

The FDA allows the following combinations of ingredients in nonprescription anorectal preparations.

- 2, 3, or 4 protectants composing at least 50% of weight of final product[a–e]
- 1 local anesthetic; vasoconstrictor; astringent; or keratolytic or analgesic/anesthetic/antipruritic; ± 1–4 protectants
- 1 local anesthetic + 1 vasoconstrictor, astringent, or keratolytic ± 1–4 protectants
- 1 local anesthetic + 1 vasoconstrictor + 1 astringent ± 1–4 protectants
- 1 local anesthetic + 1 astringent + 1 keratolytic ± 1–4 protectants
- 1 vasoconstrictor + 1 astringent ± 1–4 protectants
- 1 vasoconstrictor + 1 analgesic/anesthetic/antipruritic + 1 astringent ± 1–4 protectants
- 1 single analgesic/anesthetic/antipruritic + 1 keratolytic ± 1 astringent ± 1–4 protectants
- 1 astringent + 1 keratolytic ± 1–4 protectants

[a] Aluminum hydroxide gel and kaolin may not be combined with cocoa butter, cod liver oil, hard fat, lanolin, mineral oil, shark liver oil, petrolatum, and white petrolatum because petrolatum and greasy ointments may prevent aluminum hydroxide gel and kaolin from adhering to the skin and providing a protective function.[1,16]

[b] Any protectant ingredient, except cod liver oil, shark liver oil, and glycerin, included in a combination must contribute at least 12.5 % by weight.

[c] When included in a combination product, glycerin must compose at least 10% of the product.

[d] If calamine and zinc oxide are included in a combination product, their concentrations are limited to 5% to 25% (weight-to-weight) per dosage units. When used as protectants in a combination product, these agents can be combined with only other protectant ingredients.

[e] When used as protectants in combination products, cod liver oil and shark liver oil can be combined with only other protectant ingredients. If either cod liver oil or shark liver oil is included in a combination protectant product, the product must contain an amount of the oil that provides a daily dose of no more than 10,000 USP units of vitamin A and 400 USP units of cholecalciferol (vitamin D_3).[1]

Product Selection Guidelines

Table 14–3 contains examples of products the pharmacist can recommend on the basis of patient factors or preferences.

Patient Factors Knowledge of a patient's present medical condition, medical history, medication profile, and socioeconomic status is necessary to determine how an individual may respond to self-treatment. The pharmacist should decide on a suitable anorectal product, if any, while taking into account the following: (1) what other diseases the patient may have; (2) what medications the patient may be taking; (3) whether the patient is able to apply or insert the medication (physical, mental, and emotional limitations); and (4) any other factors, such as diet, daily activities, or cost of the product, that may affect treatment. Pregnant and breast-feeding women should use only those products recommended for external use except for the recommended protectants, which may be used internally. Children younger than 12 years with hemorrhoids or any other anorectal disorder should be referred to a physician.

Patient Preferences The FDA does not require in situ testing of anorectal products in the manufacturer's final dosage form. Thus, therapeutic differences among various dosage forms, if any, are not known. Products containing FDA-approved ingredients in appropriate dosages are probably therapeutically similar when used to treat indicated anorectal signs and symptoms. Whatever differences exist are most likely related to individual patient preference for a specific dosage form.

Medications used to treat symptomatic anorectal disorders are available in many different dosage forms. Ointments, creams, suppositories, gels, and foams are available for intrarectal use. Applicators, pile pipes (intrarectal applicator), or fingers are used to facilitate applying the preparations. Creams, ointments, gels, pastes, liquids, and foams are used externally. Although considerable pharmaceutical differences exist among ointments, creams, pastes, and gels, the therapeutic differences do not appear to be clinically important. This discussion uses the term *ointment* to refer to all semisolid preparations designed for intrarectal or external use in the anorectal area. Suppositories are considered to be a solid dosage form that differs very little from semisolid vehicle formulations. The primary function of an ointment is to provide a vehicle for the safe and efficient delivery of the active ingredients, yet some ointments also possess inherent protectant and emollient properties.

When used externally, the ointment should be applied as a thin covering to the perianal area and the anal canal. When used intrarectally, the ointment may be inserted using an intrarectal applicator or a finger. Intrarectal applicators are preferred to digital application because the drug product can be introduced into the rectal mucosa where the desired effect on a minor hemorrhoid may be needed and where the finger cannot reach. An intrarectal applicator should have lateral openings, as well as a hole in the tip, in order to facilitate application in the most efficient manner and to permit the drug product to cover the greatest area of rectal mucosa. The intrarectal applicator should be lubricated before insertion by spreading ointment around the applicator tip.

The lubricating effect of a suppository may ease straining at defecation, thereby easing or alleviating hemorrhoidal symptoms. However, suppositories should not be recommended as an initial dosage form when treating anorectal symptoms because they may leave the affected anal region and may ascend into the rectum and lower colon when the patient is in a prone position. If the patient remains prone after inserting a suppository or an ointment, the active ingredients may not distribute evenly over the rectal mucosa.

Table 14–3

Selected Products for Hemorrhoids

Trade Name	Primary Ingredients
Local Anesthetics[a]	
Anusol Ointment	Pramoxine HCl 1%; zinc oxide 12.5%; mineral oil; cocoa butter; kaolin; peruvian balsam
Anusol Suppositories	Benzyl alcohol; topical starch 51%
Fleet Pain-Relief Pads	Pramoxine HCl 1%; glycerin 12%
Lanacane Crème	Benzocaine 6%; zinc oxide; glycerin
Lanacane Maximum Strength Cream	Benzocaine 20%; dimethicone; mineral oil
Nupercainal Ointment	Dibucaine 1%; lanolin; white petrolatum; light mineral oil
Procto Foam Non-Steroid	Pramoxine HCl 1%
Tronolane Cream	Pramoxine HCl 1%; zinc oxide; glycerin
Tronothane Hydrochloride Cream	Pramoxine HCl 1%; glycerin
Tucks Clear Gel	Benzyl alcohol; witch hazel 50%; glycerin 10%
Vasoconstrictors[b]	
Hemorid for Women Suppositories	Phenylephrine HC1 0.25%; zinc oxide 231 mg; hard fat 88.25%
Hemorid for Women Cream/Ointment	Phenylephrine HCl 0.25%; pramoxine HCl 1%; petrolatum; mineral oil
Pazo Ointment	Ephedrine sulfate 0.2%; camphor 2%; zinc oxide 5%; lanolin; petrolatum
Preparation H Ointment	Phenylephrine HCl 0.25%; petrolatum 71.9%; mineral oil 4%; shark liver oil 3%; lanolin; glycerin
Preparation H Cream	Phenylephrine HCl 0.250%; petrolatum 18%; glycerin 12%; shark liver oil 3%; lanolin
Preparation H Suppositories	Phenylephrine HCl 0.25%; cocoa butter 79%; shark liver oil 3%
Skin Protectants	
Balneol Lotion	Mineral oil; lanolin oil
Rectacaine Ointment	Petrolatum 71.9%; mineral oil 14%; shark liver oil 3%; glycerin
Hydrocortisone Products	
Anusol-HC	Hydrocortisone acetate (equivalent to hydrocortisone 1%)
Cortaid Intensive Therapy Cream	Hydrocortisone 1%
Preparation H Hydrocortisone 1% Cream	Hydrocortisone 1%
Miscellaneous Combination Products[c]	
Calmol 4 Suppositories	Zinc oxide 10%; cocoa butter 80%
Fleet Medicated Pads	Witch hazel 50%; glycerin 10%
Nupercainal Suppositories	Zinc oxide 0.25 g; cocoa butter 2.1 g
Tronolane Suppositories	Zinc oxide 5%; hard fat 95%
Tucks Pads	Witch hazel 50%; glycerin

[a] Products do not contain vasoconstrictors but may contain protectants and astringents.

[b] Products may also contain local anesthetics, protectants, and astringents.

[c] Products contain astringents and protectants.

Suppositories are relatively slow acting because they must melt to release the active ingredients. Foam products offer no proven advantage over ointments. Foams should, theoretically, provide more rapid release of active ingredients. However, the foam may not remain in the affected area, and the size of the foam bubbles determines the concentration of the active ingredient.

Alternative Remedies

Alternative treatments for hemorrhoids include herbal and homeopathic products, as well as various home remedies.

Herbal Remedies

Herbal remedies that have been used to treat hemorrhoids include aloe, cat's claw, chestnut, comfrey, corn cockle, indigo, marijuana, mullein, passion flower, Peru balsam, plantain, quinine, St. John's wort, storax, and witch hazel.[19–23] Table 14–4 summarizes the use, risks, and effectiveness of these herbal remedies in treating anorectal disorders. Other herbs, including manna *(Fraxinus ornus)*, senna leaf *(Cassia senna, C. angustifolia)*, black psyllium seed *(Plantago psyllium, P. indica)*, blonde psyllium seed *(Plantaginis ovata semen)*, and blonde psyllium seed husk *(Plantaginis ovata testa)*, have been approved by the German Commission E for treating hemorrhoids because of their laxative effects (assuming that easier passage of stool is desirable).[19] Additionally, butcher's broom *(Ruscus aculeatus)*, and sweet clover *(Melilotus officinalis, M. altissimus)* are approved as supportive therapy for itching and burning associated with hemorrhoids. Semisolid preparations made from poplar bud *(Populus canadensis)* are approved because they are thought to aid wound healing. (See Chapter 45, "Herbal Remedies," for further discussion of these types of remedies.)

Homeopathic Remedies

Homeopathic remedies used for treating a painful attack of acute hemorrhoids include the venom of a South American snake *(Lachesis mutus)*, hydrochloric acid, horse chestnut *(Aesculus hipposcastanum)*, and Caltha alpina *(Arnica montana)*.[24–27] The following homeopathic remedies have been used for symptomatic relief of chronic hemorrhoids, including heaviness in the pelvis, sporadic hemorrhages, and pruritis: stone root *(Collinsonia canadensis)*, witch hazel *(Hamamelis virginiana)*, graphite, potassium carbonate, fluoric acid, and nitric acid. Additionally, basic remedies like sulfur, calcium fluoride, club moss *(Lycopodium clavatum)*, strychnine, and sepia (dried brownish-black substance from the cuttlefish) have been used for chronic conditions.[26] No comment can be made regarding the effectiveness of such remedies. However, they may be safe because of the dilutions required in homeopathic medicine. (See Chapter 46, "Homeopathic Remedies," for further discussion of these types of remedies.)

Home Remedies

One study involving African Americans showed they had used the following substances to treat hemorrhoids: butter, flour, kerosene, lard, olive oil, snuff, turpentine, and Vicks VapoRub.[28] Kerosene and turpentine are irritating and should not be used for this purpose. No data exist to support the efficacy of any of these home remedies.

Patient Assessment of Hemorrhoids

To accurately assess whether a patient's anorectal condition is self-treatable, the pharmacist should obtain a thorough description of the signs and symptoms. If the condition is self-treatable, a thorough medical history, including use of prescription and nonprescription medications, is needed before recommending a nonprescription anorectal preparation. The pharmacist should ask about the patient's dietary habits and possible use of alternative remedies. Asking the patient the following questions will help elicit the information needed to accurately assess the disorder and to recommend the appropriate treatment approach.

Case Study 14–2

Patient Complaint/History

Frieda, a 23-year-old woman who is 7 months pregnant, presents to the pharmacist complaining of rectal itching. When questioned about additional symptoms, the patient responds that she has not noticed any pain, burning, swelling, or soreness in the rectal area. She admits she occasionally strains during bowel movements. Her job as a secretary requires that she sit for long periods of time. In response to queries about current medication use, Frieda reports that she takes Stuartnatal Plus, ferrous sulfate, and docusate sodium daily.

Clinical Considerations/Strategies

Readers can use the following considerations/strategies to determine whether treating the patient's condition with nonprescription medications is warranted:

- Assess the possible cause(s) of the rectal itching.
- Recommend an appropriate regimen of nonprescription medication treatment.
- Recommend an appropriate plan of nonpharmacologic treatment.
- Assess the possible adverse effects associated with the recommended nonprescription medication.

Patient Education/Counseling

Readers can use the following strategies to develop a patient education/counseling plan that will help ensure optimal therapeutic outcomes:

- Ensure that the patient understands when and how to apply the recommended nonprescription medication.
- Ensure that the patient knows whether the self-treatment regimen was successful and when to contact a physician.

Table 14–4

Herbal Remedies Used to Treat Anorectal Disorders

Herb (Scientific Name)	Uses	Risks	Effectiveness as Hemorrhoid Treatment
Aloe *(Aloe vera, A. perryi, A. barbadensis, A. vulgaris, A. ferox)*	Drastic laxative that may cause severe cramping and diarrhea. Treatment based on constipation as cause of hemorrhoids.	Use not recommended, especially in pregnant patients.	Not proven.
Cat's claw *(Uncaria tomentosa, U. guianensis)*	Astringent and antidiarrheal tea from bark used to treat hemorrhoids, diverticulitis, colitis, peptic ulcers, gastritis, parasites, and leaky bowel syndrome.	None reported.	Not proven.
Chestnut *(Aesculus hippocastanum, A. californica, A. glabra)*	Horse chestnut *(A. hippocastanum)* seed extracts used to treat hemorrhoids, varicose veins, and other venous disorders.	Toxic, especially in children. Not recommended for internal use.	Experiments show aescin causes vein contraction, which supports use in managing hemorrhoids and varicose veins. The FDA, however, has classified herb as unsafe.
Comfrey *(Symphytum officinale, S. asperum, S. tuberosum)*	Claimed to heal hemorrhoids and gastric ulcers. Poultices of leaves/roots used to treat burns, sprains, swelling, and bruises. Anti-inflammatory activity attributed to allantoin and rosmarinic acid.	Several reports of veno-occlusive disease when taken orally.	Not currently recommended for use.
Corn cockle *(Agrostemma githago)*	Roots used to treat hemorrhoids.	Possible systemic poisoning from the saponins: *githagin* and *agrostemmic acid.* Hogs have died from eating the roots.	Poisonous. Do not use as a medication.
Indigo *(Indigofera spp.)*	Used to treat numerous ailments ranging from hemorrhoids to scorpion bites.	Some species may be toxic.	Not proven.
Mullein *(Verbascum thapsus, V. phlomoides, V. thapsiforme)*	Used to treat hemorrhoids, burns, bruises, gout, numerous respiratory problems. Saponins, mucilage, tannins in leaves/flowers probably contribute to soothing topical effect.	Long history of herbal use. No toxicity reported.	FDA Category II: generally not safe and effective for treatment of anorectal disorders.
Passion flower *(Passiflora spp. primarily P. incarnata)*	Used to treat many disorders including inflamed hemorrhoids, burns, asthma. Passion flower extracts used for sedative effects.	No significant toxicity reported. Large doses of extract may cause central nervous system depression.	Not proven for topical or oral use.
Peru balsam *(Myroxylon pereirae)*	Used topically to treat hemorrhoids (as a suppository) and wounds.	Contact dermatitis occurs frequently.	Initially placed in Category III (as a wound-healing agent for anorectal disorders), later removed from anorectal products because of insufficient data to establish effectiveness.

Table 14–4

Herbal Remedies Used to Treat Anorectal Disorders (continued)

Herb (Scientific Name)	Uses	Risks	Effectiveness as Hemorrhoid Treatment
Plantain *(Plantago lanceolata, P. major, P. psyllium, P. arenatia)*	Pulverized seeds of plantain are mixed with oil and applied topically to inflamed sites. Seeds and refined colloid commonly used in commercial bulk laxative preparations. Psyllium is a bulk laxative and has shown some success in treating anal fissures and hemorrhoids.	At one time, psyllium preparations sold in health food stores were found to contain digitalis. Drug interactions reported between oral psyllium and oral lithium or carbamazepine.	Psyllium-containing preparations appear to reduce bleeding and pain of hemorrhoids during defecation.
Quinine *(Cinchona succirubra)*	Bark extracts used to treat hemorrhoids, manage varicose veins, stimulate hair growth. Quinine/urea hydrochloride mixture used as sclerosing agent in treating internal hemorrhoids and varicose veins.	Chronic ingestion/absorption may lead to cinchonism (severe headache, abdominal pain, convulsions, visual disturbances, and blindness, as well as to paralysis, collapse, and auditory disturbances such as tinnitus). No risks associated with use as a sclerosing agent.	Not recommended for treating hemorrhoids.
St. John's wort *(Hypericum perforatum)*	Olive oil extract of fresh flowers used topically to treat hemorrhoids.	Volatile oil of St. John's wort is an irritant.	Not proven.
Storax *(Liquidamber orientalis, L. styraciflua)*	Storax is one ingredient in compound tincture of benzoin, which has been used to treat hemorrhoids. Tannin-rich leaves used to treat diarrhea.	No significant toxicity reported.	Not proven.
Witch hazel *(Hamamelis virginiana)*	More than 30 traditional uses, including treatment of hemorrhoids, burns, cancer, colds, and fever.	No significant toxicity reported.	FDA-approved for treatment of anorectal disorders.

Source: References 19–23.

Q~ What are your symptoms? Has your condition been diagnosed by a physician? If yes, how do your current symptoms differ from those of the diagnosed condition?

A~ *Identify which symptoms are self-treatable and which indicate a potentially serious medical problem that should be referred to a physician. (See the section "Signs and Symptoms of Hemorrhoids and Other Anorectal Disorders.")* If a patient is under medical supervision for a similar condition, consult with the physician or advise the patient to do so.

Q~ How long have you had these symptoms? Do they recur? If so, when?

A~ *Identify the time frame and criteria that indicate an acute temporary anorectal problem versus a long-standing or serious problem.* If the patient's problem is not acute and temporary, refer the patient to a physician.

Q~ What improves or worsens your symptoms? Are your symptoms associated with straining during a bowel movement, constipation, or diarrhea?

A~ *Identify the factors that can precipitate or alleviate symptoms of hemorrhoids. (See the section "Etiology of Hemorrhoids.")*

Q~ Have you noticed any bleeding? If so, describe the color and amount of blood.

A~ *Identify which anorectal disorders cause bleeding. Determine the potential consequences of the bleeding. (See the section "Signs and Symptoms of Hemorrhoids and Anorectal Disorders.")* Refer patients with anorectal bleeding to a physician immediately.

Q~ (If the patient is a woman of child-bearing age) Are you now or have you recently been pregnant?

A~ Hemorrhoids occur frequently during pregnancy. *Identify which ingredients are appropriate for external and intrarectal use in pregnant or breast-feeding women. (See the section "General Treatment Approach.")*

Q~ What nondrug measures have you used to treat your symptoms?

A~ *Identify the appropriate nondrug measures for the patient's symptoms. (See the section "Nonpharmacologic Therapy.")* Explain to the patient how these measures can help relieve the symptoms.

Q~ Have you recently changed your diet or the amount of fluid you ingest?

A~ *Identify dietary changes that will help relieve symptoms of hemorrhoids. (See the section "Nonpharmacologic Therapy.")* Explain to the patient how these factors can affect the symptoms.

Q~ Have you used or do you currently use any nonprescription or prescription medications for these symptoms? Do you take laxatives regularly? If so, which ones do you use and how often do you take them?

A~ *Identify possible drug–drug interactions for anorectal preparations. Identify the role of laxatives in treating hemorrhoids. (See the section "Pharmacologic Therapy.")* If the patient's medication history indicates possible interactions, refer the patient to a physician.

Q~ Have you tried any herbal products or home remedies to treat these symptoms?

A~ *Identify which alternative remedies pose risks to the patient. (See Table 14–4.)* Determine whether the patient is receptive to using traditional nonprescription medications.

Q~ Do you have any other medical conditions such as heart failure, liver disease, inflammatory diseases of the intestine, or varicose veins?

A~ *Identify which disorders rule out self-treatment of hemorrhoids. (See the section "Pharmacologic Therapy.")* Refer patients with these disorders to a physician.

Patient Counseling for Hemorrhoids

The pharmacist should advise the patient that maintaining good overall health care, consuming sufficient dietary fiber and fluids, and maintaining proper perianal hygiene are essential in preventing and alleviating constipation, straining, and anorectal symptoms. The patient should then be instructed on how to distinguish between minor symptoms of hemorrhoids and those that require medical treatment.

The pharmacist should advise the patient to use products containing the least number of ingredients to minimize undesirable effects and to maximize effectiveness. The best product to recommend is one that contains a single or appropriate combination of ingredients in safe and effective dosages and in a dosage form acceptable to the patient.

The pharmacist should instruct the patient on using anorectal products, including specific directions on how to (1) insert an ointment with an intrarectal applicator, (2) insert a suppository, or (3) apply a foam product. Finally, the pharmacist should explain precautions in selecting and using anorectal products. The box "Patient Education for Hemorrhoids" lists specific information to provide patients.

Evaluation of Patient Outcomes for Hemorrhoids

The most important outcome of self-treatment of anorectal disorders is to relieve symptoms and to prevent complications that may lead to more serious consequences. Patients who self-treat the minor symptoms of anorectal itching, burning, pain, swelling, irritation, and discomfort should be advised that symptoms should improve within 7 days. However, if seepage, bleeding, black tarry stools, protrusion, or severe pain occurs, or if symptoms worsen, the patient should discontinue nonprescription treatment and should contact a physician as soon as possible.

CONCLUSIONS

Pharmacists can play an important role in the self-treatment of anorectal disorders by assisting the patient to select an appropriate product, by providing instructions for nonpharmacologic and nonprescription pharmacologic approaches to treatment, and by advising the patient when to consult a physician. Self-treatment of anorectal disorders should be limited to patients with minor symptoms such as burning, itching, pain, discomfort, swelling, and irritation. If serious signs and symptoms, such as seepage, bleeding, black tarry stools, protrusion, or severe pain, are present, the pharmacist should advise the patient to consult a physician. The pharmacist should recommend only products containing active ingredients approved for anorectal use (local anesthetics, keratolytics, protectants, analgesics, antipruritics, vasoconstrictors, and astringents). Pregnant and breast-feeding women should use only products recommended for external use (except for acceptable protectants), and children younger than 12 years with anorectal disorders should be referred to a physician. If self-treatment does not improve the anorectal condition in 7 days, or if the condition worsens, the patient should be advised to seek medical attention.

Patient Education for Hemorrhoids

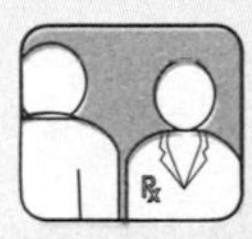

The objectives of self-treatment are to (1) alleviate the symptoms of hemorrhoids and (2) prevent complications that may lead to more serious consequences. Nonprescription anorectal preparations are intended to provide temporary relief of minor symptoms such as burning, itching, mild pain, swelling, irritation, and mild discomfort. For most patients, carefully following product instructions and the self-care measures listed below will help ensure optimal therapeutic outcomes.

Nondrug Measures

- Increase the amount of fiber and fluids in the diet to reduce or prevent straining during bowel movements.
- Avoid sitting on the toilet for long periods.
- Clean the perianal area after a bowel movement with a moistened, unscented, and uncolored toilet tissue or a wipe.
- Before applying the medication, wash the perianal area with mild soap and warm water, rinse thoroughly, and gently dry by patting or blotting with toilet tissue or a soft cloth.
- If desired, use a sitz bath for managing mild symptoms of uncomplicated anorectal disease.
- Advise the patient to avoid using laxatives regularly to prevent constipation. Laxatives are intended for the occasional treatment of constipation.

Nonprescription Medications

- Use anorectal products after, rather than before, bowel movements to obtain maximum benefit.
- Anorectal products contain local anesthetics; vasoconstrictors; protectants; analgesics/anesthetics/antipruritics; astringents; and keratolytics. With the help of a pharmacist, select a product that contains only the ingredients needed to relieve your specific symptoms.
- See Table 14–1 for recommended dosages of anorectal products.
- Do not use suppositories as the primary treatment for hemorrhoids.
- Use only vasoconstrictors (ephedrine and phenylephrine), protectants, and astringents (calamine and zinc oxide) inside the rectum.
- If you have cardiovascular disease, diabetes, hypertension, or hyperthyroidism, or if you experience difficulty urinating, do not use a topical anorectal product containing a vasoconstrictor.
- If you are taking prescription medications to treat hypertension or depression, do not use an anorectal product containing a vasoconstrictor without consulting a physician. Avoid medications that cause constipation, if possible.
- Be aware that anorectal products containing ephedrine sulfate may cause nervousness, tremor, sleeplessness, nausea, and loss of appetite.
- Apply products to the external perianal area sparingly.
- Before applying anorectal products containing aluminum hydroxide gel or kaolin, clean the perianal area, being sure to remove any previously used petrolatum-containing or greasy ointment.

⚠ Stop using the anorectal product and contact a physician immediately if insertion of a product into the rectum causes pain.

⚠ Contact a physician if symptoms of hemorrhoids worsen or do not improve after 7 days of self-treatment.

⚠ Be aware that certain people may develop allergic or hypersensitivity reactions to anorectal products containing recommended concentrations of approved ingredients. Discontinue use of the product and contact a physician immediately if redness, irritation, swelling, pain, or any other sign or symptom develops or worsens.

⚠ If seepage of feces, bleeding, black tarry stools, protrusion of hemorrhoids, or severe pain or discomfort occurs, contact a physician immediately.

References

1. Anorectal drug products for over-the-counter human use; establishment of a monograph. *Federal Register.* 1980;45:35576–7.
2. Schrock TR. Examination and diseases of the anorectum. In: Feldman M, Scharschmidt BF, Sleisenger MH, eds: *Sleisenger & Fordtran's Gastrointestinal and Liver Disease: Pathophysiology/Diagnosis/Management.* 6th ed. Philadelphia: WB Saunders; 1998:1960–76.
3. Loder PB, Kamn MA, Nicholls RJ, et al. Haemorrhoids: pathology, pathophysiology and aetiology. *Br J Sur.* 1994;81:946–54.
4. Parks AG. Hemorrhoids. *Practitioner* 1962;189:309–16.
5. Perez-Miranda M, Gomez-Cedenilla A, Leon-Columbo T, et al. Effect of fiber supplements on internal bleeding hemorrhoids. *Hepato-Gastroenterology* 1996;43:1504–7.
6. Gibbons CP, Bannister JJ, Read NW. Role of constipation and anal hypertonia in the pathogenesis of hemorrhoids. *Br J Sur.* 1988;75:656–60.
7. Johanson JF. Association of hemorrhoidal disease with diarrheal disorders. *Dis Colon Rectum.* 1997;40:215–21.
8. Johanson JF, Sonnenberg A. Constipation is not a risk factor for hemorrhoids: a case-control study of potential etiological agents. *Am J Gastroenterol.* 1994;1981–6.

9. Janicke DM, Pundt MR. Anorectal disorders. *Emergency Med Clinics of North America.* 1996;14:757–88.
10. Nagle D, Rolandelli RH. Primary care office management of perianal and anal disease. *Gastroenterology.* 1996;23:609–20.
11. Benninga MA, Wijers GB, van der Hoeven CW. Manometry, profilometry, and endosonography: normal physiology and anatomy of the anal canal in healthy children. *J Pediatr Gastroenterol Nutr.* 1994;18:68–77.
12. Barnett JL, Raper SE. Anorectal diseases. In: Yamada T, Alpers DH, Powell DW, et al., eds: *Textbook of Gastroenterology.* 3rd ed. Philadelphia: JB Lippincott Co; 1999.
13. Johanson JF, Rimm A. Optimal nonsurgical treatment of hemorrhoids: a comparative analysis of infrared coagulation, rubber band ligation, and injection sclerotherapy. *Am J Gastroentrol.* 1992;87:1601–6.
14. El Ashaal Y, Chandran V, Prem V, et al. Short note: local anal hypothermia with a frozen finger: a treatment for acute painful prolapsed piles. *Br J Sur.* 1998;85:520–1.
15. Anorectal drug products for over-the-counter human use: tentative final monograph. *Federal Register.* 1988;53:30756–8.
16. Anorectal drug products for over-the-counter human use: final monograph. *Federal Register.* 1990;55:31776–6.
17. Fisher AA. Allergic reactions to topical (surface) anesthetics with reference to the safety of tronothane (pramocaine hydrochloride). *Curtis.* 1980;6:584–92.
18. *United States Pharmacopeia/National Formulary.* USP 23/NF 18. Hard fat. United States Pharmacopeial Convention: Rockville, MD; 1995:2246.
19. Blumenthal M. *The Complete German Commission E Monographs—Therapeutic Guide to Herbal Medicines.* 1st ed. American Botanical Council: Austin, TX;1998:190–2.
20. DerMarderosian A. *Facts and Comparisons—The Review of Natural Products* [quarterly subscription service]. St Louis: Facts and Comparisons.
21. Gruenwald J, Brendler T, Jaenicke C., eds. *PDR for Herbal Medicine.* 1st ed. Montvale, NJ: Medical Economics Co; 1998:985–6;1015–6.
22. Tyler VE. *The Honest Herbal—A Sensible Guide to the Use of Herbs and Related Remedies.* 3rd ed. New York: Pharmaceutical Products Press; 1993:275–6.
23. Pittler, MH, Ernst E. Horse-Chestnut seed extract for chronic venous insufficiency: a criteria-based systemic review. *Arch Derm.* 1998;134:1356–60.
24. Downey P. *Homeopathy for the Primary Health Care Team.* 1st ed. Oxford: Butterworth-Heinemann; 1997:99–100.
25. Leckridge B. *Homeopathy in Primary Care.* 1st ed. New York: Churchill Livingstone; 1997:142,191–2.
26. Jouanny J. *The Essentials of Homeopathic Therapeutics.* Lyon, France: Laboratories Boiron; 1985:255–61.
27. *The Homeopathic Pharmacopoeia of the United States.* 8th ed. Boston: American Institute of Homeopathy; 1978.
28. Boyd EL, Shimp LA, Hackney ML. *Home Remedies and the Black Elderly.* Ann Arbor: University of Michigan; 1984:19–22.

CHAPTER 15

Pinworm Infection

Kathryn K. Bucci and Gary A. Goforth

Chapter 15 at a Glance

Parasitic helminths (worm) and protozoa (e.g., *Giardia intestinalis*) infections cause significant morbidity and mortality worldwide.[1] This discussion will focus on enterobiasis (pinworm) detection and management because it is the most common worm infestation in the United States and the only helminthic infection that should be treated with nonprescription medications.[2]

Worms that infect humans can be divided into three groups: (1) endemic nematode (roundworm) infections, which include enterobiasis, ascariasis, anisakiasis, trichinosis, and infections caused by whipworms and hookworms; (2) cestodes (tapeworms); and (3) trematodes (flukes). A parasitic protozoa, *G. intestinalis* (formerly *G. lamblia*), represents the most common cause of parasitic diarrhea in the United States.[1] (See Chapter 13, "Diarrhea.")

Helminthic infections can be serious, but they are not generally widespread in the United States and therefore do not pose a major societal threat. However, the incidence of helminthic infections may exceed 90% in areas with insufficient sanitation, unclean water, suboptimal waste disposal, and poor control of rodents and insects, particularly in areas with poor economic conditions or inadequate preventive medicine practices.[3] Immigration has escalated the spread of helminthic infections, which may produce serious health problems, particularly in tropical regions. Such infections reduce resistance to disease, impair physical development in children, decrease occupational productivity, and result in the general debilitation of large populations.

Worm infections are primarily parasitic. The use of immunosuppressive drugs and the spread of acquired immunodeficiency syndrome (AIDS) are resulting in infections by previously unfamiliar parasites. Table 15–1 shows selected human worm infections, their sources, common signs and symptoms, and treatment options.[3–10]

Epidemiology of Pinworm Infection

Enterobiasis is commonly called pinworm, seatworm, or threadworm infection. Intestinal infection in humans is caused by *Enterobius vermicularis.* Unlike many helminthic infections, enterobiasis is not limited to rural and poverty-stricken areas; it occurs in urban communities and infects individuals from all socioeconomic groups. *E. vermicularis* is most commonly found in temperate climates but is widely distributed and is especially prevalent among schoolchildren.

The estimated prevalence of pinworm infection in the United States is 20 to 42 million cases, with the greatest infection rate found in children ages 5 to 15 years. Parents and siblings will likely become infected if one child in the household is infected.[11]

Etiology of Pinworm Infection

The most common route of transmission of pinworms is probably the direct anus-to-mouth transfer of eggs when

Editor's Note: This chapter is based, in part, on the 11th edition chapter titled "Anthelmintic Products," which was written by Kathryn K. Bucci.

Table 15–1

Common Human Helminthic Infections in the United States

Organism	Common Name	Source of Infection	Signs and Symptoms	Treatment
Nematodes (Roundworms)				
Ancylostoma duodenale, Necator americanus	Hookworm	Penetration of intact skin by larvae.	Erythematous maculopapular rash and edema with severe itching for several days. Lesions commonly between toes (ground itch). Passage of long worm (15 cm) in stool. Major clinical manifestation is iron deficiency anemia.	Adult/pediatric doses: Mebendazole (Vermox) 100 mg bid × 3 days or 500 mg once. Pyrantel pamoate[a] 11 mg/kg or 5 mg/pound (maximum: 1 g) × 3 days. Albendazole[a] (Albenza) 400 mg once. Correct anemia (if present) with oral iron supplements.
Ascaris lumbricoides	Roundworm	Ingestion of soil containing mature eggs.	Many patients asymptomatic. Vague abdominal discomfort and abdominal colic common. Children: fever, weight loss, failure to grow. Intestinal obstruction that may lead to intestinal perforation, suppurative cholangitis, cholecystitis, liver abscess, pancreatitis, appendicitis, peritonitis. Cough and possible coughing up of larvae.	Adult/pediatric doses: Mebendazole (Vermox) 100 mg bid × 3 days or 500 mg once. Pyrantel pamoate[a] 11 mg/kg or 5 mg/pound (maximum: 1 g) once. Albendazole[a] (Albenza) 400 mg once. (See text for discussion of pyrantel pamoate.)
Enterobius vermicularis	Pinworm	Ingestion of eggs from fecal contamination of hands, food, clothing, and bedding. Reinfection is common.	Minor infections asymptomatic. Most frequent: irritating itch in perianal and perineal regions, usually at night. Children: nervousness, inability to concentrate, lack of appetite.	Adult/pediatric doses: Pyrantel pamoate 11 mg/kg or 5 mg/pound once (maximum: 1 g). Mebendazole (Vermox) 100 mg once; repeat in 2 weeks. Albendazole[a] (Albenza) 400 mg once; repeat in 2 weeks. (See text for discussion of pyrantel pamoate.)
Strongyloides stercoralis	Strongyloidiasis	Skin penetration by filariform larvae in fecally contaminated moist soil.	One-third of patients asymptomatic. Skin penetration: pruritic, maculopapular rash or migrating linear urticaria. Pulmonary migration: cough, shortness of breath, wheezing, fever, transient pulmonary infiltrates, eosinophilia. Intestinal stage: abdominal pain, diarrhea, vomiting, malabsorption, weight loss, steatorrhea.	Adult/pediatric doses: Ivermectin[b] 200 mcg/kg/day × 1–2 days. If patient immunocompromised or disease disseminated, prolonged or repeated therapy may be necessary. Thiabendazole[c] 50 mg/kg/day in 2 doses (maximum: 3 g/day) × 2 days.
Trichinella spiralis	Trichinosis	Ingestion of raw/rare meat containing infective, encysted larvae in striated muscle of wild animals or domestic pigs.	Light infection (<10 larvae): subclinical. Moderate infection (50–500 larvae): nausea, abdominal cramps, loss of appetite, vomiting, mild fever, diarrhea or constipation, headache, dizziness, weakness. Severe infection (>1000 larvae): severe diarrhea, seizures, encephalitis, coma, respiratory distress, myocarditis, anemia, muscular swelling.	Adult/pediatric doses: Prednisone 40–60 mg/day for severe symptoms plus mebendazole[a] (Vermox) 50 mg/kg/day × 14 days. Albendazole may also be effective.

Table 15–1

Common Human Helminthic Infections in the United States (continued)

Organism	Common Name	Source of Infection	Signs and Symptoms	Treatment
Trichuris trichiura	Whipworm	Ingestion of eggs in feces-contaminated soil, food, or water.	Patients may be asymptomatic. Trauma to intestinal epithelium/submucosa: chronic blood in the stool, resulting in anemia. Secondary bacterial infection: colitis, proctitis, or, in extreme cases, rectal prolapse. Possible insomnia, loss of appetite, urticaria, flatulence, prolonged diarrhea.	Adult/pediatric doses: Mebendazole (Vermox) 100 mg bid × 3 days or 500 mg once. Albendazole (Albenza) 400 mg once. Extended 3-day albendazole therapy may be necessary for severe infections.
Trematodes (Flukes)				
Clonorchis sinensis	Chinese or oriental liver fluke	*C. sinensis*: ingestion of raw fish (endemic in countries such as Japan).	Majority of patients asymptomatic. Mild infections: persistent episodic upper abdominal pain. Possible dyspepsia, flatulence, diarrhea, poor appetite, and weight loss.	Adult/pediatric dose: Praziquantel (Biltricide) 75 mg/kg/day in 3 doses × 1 day.
Opisthorchis viverrini, Opisthorchis felineus	Southeast Asian liver fluke	*O. viverrini/felineus*: contraction from dogs, cats, many fish-eating mammals. Humans are accidental host.		Adult dose: Albendazole (Albenza) 10 mg/kg × 7 days (alternative therapy for *C. sinensis* only).
Paragonimus westermani	Lung fluke	Ingestion of larval-infected crabs or crayfish.	Light infections may be asymptomatic. Invasion and migration (acute) phase: diarrhea, abdominal pain, urticaria, fever, chest pain, cough, dyspnea, malaise, and night sweats. Chronic symptoms include dry cough that becomes productive. Extrapulmonary disease: possible seizures, impaired vision, bloody diarrhea.	Adult/pediatric doses: Praziquantel (Biltricide) 75 mg/kg/day divided into 3 doses × 2 days. Bithionol 30–50 mg/kg on alternate days × 10–15 doses.
Cestodes (Tapeworms)				
Diphyllobothrium latum	Fish tapeworm	Ingestion of raw or inadequately cooked freshwater fish.	Often asymptomatic. Possible: abdominal pain, sensation of "something moving inside," bloating, sore gums, allergic symptoms, headache, appetite change. Rarely: intestinal obstruction, diarrhea, megaloblastic anemia, thrombocytopenia, mild leukopenia.	Adult/pediatric dose: Praziquantel[a] 5–10 mg/kg once.
Taenia saginata	Beef tapeworm	Ingestion of poorly cooked, egg-contaminated beef.	No characteristic symptoms. Digestive upset, diarrhea, anemia, dizziness, allergic symptoms, morning abdominal pain may vary with degree of infestation. Rarely: intestinal, appendiceal, biliary, or pancreatic obstruction; acute surgical abdomen.	Adult/pediatric doses: Praziquantel[a] 5–10 mg/kg once.
T. solium	Pork tapeworm	Ingestion of poorly cooked infected pork.	Similar to beef tapeworm. Cysticercosis involving lungs, brain, eye, connective tissue.	Adult/pediatric dose: Praziquantel[a] 5–10 mg/kg once.

(continued)

Table 15–1

Common Human Helminthic Infections in the United States (continued)

Organism	Common Name	Source of Infection	Signs and Symptoms	Treatment
Echinococcus granulosus	Hydatid cyst (unilocular)	Ingestion of embryonated eggs in feces of infected dogs or wild carnivores.	Most patients asymptomatic. Cysts discovered incidentally in liver, lungs, muscle, bones, kidney, spleen, eye, and brain. Symptoms from expanding cysts: occasional traumatic/surgical rupture of cysts with peritonitis, allergic manifestations including anaphylaxis.	Adult dose: Albendazole (Albenza) 400 mg bid × 28 days, repeated as necessary. Pediatric dose: Albendazole (Albenza) 15 mg/kg/day × 28 days, repeated as necessary. Some patients may benefit from or require surgical resection of cysts.

[a] Drugs are FDA-approved, but they are considered investigational for this indication.

[b] Ivermectin is not FDA-approved for treating disseminated disease; thiabendazole may be preferred.

[c] Because of the greater incidence of side effects at higher doses, the thiabendazole dosages may be toxic for adult and pediatric patients and may need to be decreased.

Source: References 1, 3–10.

children use contaminated fingers to handle and ingest food. Reinfection may readily occur because eggs are often found under the fingernails of infected children who have scratched the anal area. Eggs dislodged from the perianal region into the environment may survive for as long as 3 weeks and can be inhaled or swallowed if they become airborne. Eggs may be spread by house dust, from the coats of pets, or through contact with contaminated objects such as bedding, cups and utensils, toothpaste, and doorknobs.[12]

Pathophysiology of Pinworm Infection

The female adult pinworm is about 10 mm long, is light yellowish-white, and has a pin-shaped and pointed tail (from which the name is derived).[2,13] Adult worms inhabit the first portion, or ileocecum, of the large intestine and seldom cause damage to the intestinal wall. The mature female usually stores approximately 11,000 eggs in her body. She then migrates down the colon and out the anus, deposits the sticky eggs in the perianal region, and dies. If the eggs are not washed off, they hatch within a few hours, and the larvae may return to the large intestine (retroinfection).[13] Alternatively, the eggs can be transferred to the mouth, most commonly on the fingers of a child who scratches the anal area, and the cycle begins again. Within 2 to 6 weeks of egg infestation, the larvae are released and mature into gravid females that migrate to the anal area and discharge eggs, thus continuing the cycle.

Signs and Symptoms of Pinworm Infection

The first indication of helminthic infection may be a worm passed with a stool; often, however, such worms are not detected because vegetable material, mucus strands, or other artifacts may look like worms. Patients with minor enterobiasis infections may be asymptomatic. Major infections may produce symptoms that range from abdominal discomfort to severe pain, insomnia, nervousness, inability to concentrate, loss of appetite and nausea (rather than an increase in hunger, as was commonly believed), diarrhea, and intractable localized itching.[13] The most frequent symptom is usually an irritating perianal or perineal itch that typically occurs at night when the female deposits eggs.

Perianal itching is a symptom of many conditions and is often mistakenly attributed to pinworm infection.[14] Seborrheic dermatitis, atopic eczema, tinea cruris, psoriasis, lichen planus, and neurodermatitis may also produce severe perianal itching. An allergic or contact dermatitis may result from soaps or ointments used by a patient attempting to alleviate pinworm infestation symptoms. Ointments containing topical anesthetics are well-known sensitizers and should be suspected of contributing to the problem. Other parasitic infestations that induce itching, such as scabies and pediculosis pubis, may involve the perianal skin in addition to larger areas of the body. Candidiasis may be the cause of pruritus ani, especially in patients with diabetes mellitus or a suppressed immune system. Other causes of pruritus include excessive sweating during hot weather or excessive vaginal discharge and urinary incontinence in women.

Physical signs and symptoms are not the only misery-inducing effects of enterobiasis. Parents are often dismayed to find worms near the anus of a child, and this psychologic trauma or "pinworm neurosis" must be considered a harmful effect of enterobiasis. Patients need to be assured that pinworms are common and that no social stigma is attached to their occurrence.[2]

Case Study 15–1

Patient Complaint/History

A mother presents to the pharmacist with her 5-year-old daughter and asks for assistance in selecting a product to stop the child's itching. The mother explains that the child has intense perianal itching, especially at night, and has not been sleeping well. Physical observation reveals that the child seems exceptionally fidgety.

Clinical Considerations/Strategies

Readers can use the following considerations/strategies to determine whether treating the patient's condition with nonprescription medication is warranted:

- Ask the mother whether other family members or close personal contacts have similar symptoms.
- Ask the mother whether she has seen worms in the child's stool.
- Determine the child's age and weight.

Patient Education/Counseling

Readers can use the following strategies to develop a patient education/counseling plan that will help ensure optimal therapeutic outcomes:

- Explain the proper administration and possible adverse effects of the recommended product.
- After reassuring the mother that pinworms are common, explain the treatment method for family members and methods to prevent reinfection.

Case Study 15–2

Patient Complaint/History

JS, a 30-year-old male refugee, recently arrived in the United States. He presents to the pharmacist and asks assistance in selecting a product for treating "worms." The patient says he noticed a large worm (about 6 inches) in his stool today and has experienced a nonproductive cough and mild abdominal pain over the past week. When questioned about prior treatment for parasitic infections, he says a medical missionary team provided deworming medicine to his entire family 1 year ago, but he has not received any treatment since then.

Clinical Considerations/Strategies

Readers can use the following considerations/strategies to determine whether treatment of the patient's condition with nonprescription medication is warranted:

- Determine how the family obtained food for their usual daily meals and what hygienic measures were taken to minimize food contamination. Ask what type of fertilizer was used (e.g., human, pig).
- Determine whether family members or others eating in the same household have had similar symptoms.
- Determine whether the patient or family members (especially children) have lost weight or whether other symptoms are present.
- Determine the appropriate approach to treating the patient.

Complications of Pinworm Infection

Scratching to relieve the itching from pinworm infection may lead to a secondary bacterial infection of the perianal and perineal regions. Pinworms may cause vulvovaginitis and, occasionally, enter the female genital tract, where they can become encapsulated within the uterus or fallopian tubules. They may migrate into the peritoneal cavity and form granulomas.[11,13] Parasitic infections may impair fertility and, during pregnancy, may (1) injure the mother's health, (2) injure the fetus, (3) induce premature labor and delivery, and (4) infect the neonate. A physician must consider the risks and benefits to both mother and fetus when planning treatment.

Treatment of Pinworm Infection

Treatment Outcomes

The goal of therapy is to eradicate pinworms from the patient and the household, thereby preventing reinfection.

General Treatment Approach

Pinworm infection management includes drug treatment for the patient and prevention of reinfection, as well as drug treatment for every household member. Strict hygiene (e.g., washing linens, disinfecting toilet seats, etc.) is an integral part of the treatment. The algorithm in Figure 15–1 outlines treatment of this infection.

Exclusions to self-treatment include helminthic infections other than pinworms, pregnancy, liver disease, anemia, and hypersensitivity to pyrantel pamoate. In addition, children under 2 years of age or weighing less than 25 pounds are excluded, unless a physician has already recommended the nonprescription treatment.[15,16]

Nonpharmacologic Therapy

Once a pinworm infection is confirmed, the patient or caregiver should follow the nondrug measures in Table 15–2 to prevent family and household infections and reinfections. The transmission of other helminthic infections can be prevented by (1) avoiding undercooked beef, pork, and fish (especially fish from areas where marine mammals are present); (2) eating sushi from a reputable establishment and avoiding sushi prepared at home; (3) avoiding walking barefoot in areas prone to hookworms; and (4) avoiding swimming or wading in areas that are conducive to swimmers' itch. Pharmacists are in an ideal position to inform patients of behaviors that may increase their risk of helminthic infections.

Pharmacologic Therapy

At one time, gentian violet was the only nonprescription medication available to treat pinworm infections. The Food

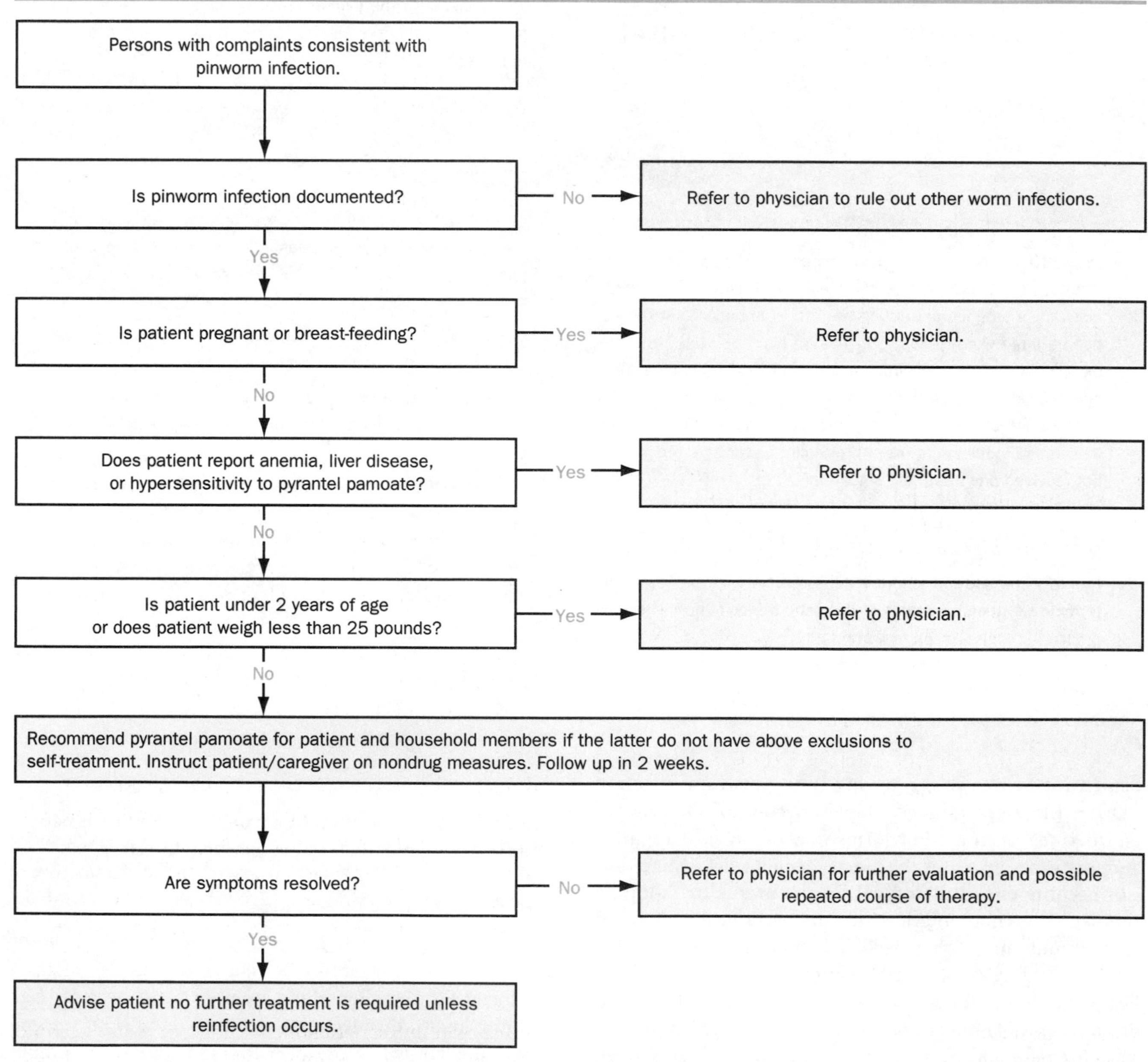

Figure 15–1 Self-care of pinworm infection.

Table 15–2

Nondrug and Preventive Measures for Treating Pinworm Infection

- Wash the bed linens, bedclothes, towels, and underwear of the infected individual and of the entire family in hot water daily during the treatment period. Do not shake these items; shaking can spread eggs into the air.
- Have the infected individual take daily morning showers to remove eggs deposited in the perianal region during the night.
- Use disinfectants on toilet seats and bathtubs daily during the treatment period.
- Daily vacuum (do not sweep) the area around beds, curtains, and elsewhere in the bedroom where the concentration of eggs is likely to be the greatest. Wet-mopping before or instead of vacuuming may limit the spread of pinworm eggs into the air.
- Wear close fitting shorts under one-piece pajamas at night to prevent migration of worms from the perianal and perineal regions.
- After an infected child uses the toilet, scrub the child's fingers with soap and a brush. Trim the child's nails regularly to prevent the harboring of eggs and autoinoculation (hand-to-mouth reinfection). Wash hands frequently, especially before meals and after using the toilet.

Source: References 2, 12, and 17.

and Drug Administration (FDA) has declared gentian violet a "nonmonograph ingredient," and as such, it can no longer be marketed as an anthelmintic.[2]

Pyrantel Pamoate

Pyrantel pamoate was first used in veterinary practice as a broad-spectrum drug for pinworms, roundworms, and hookworms. Because of its effectiveness and lack of toxicity, it has become an important drug for treating certain helminthic infections in humans.[15]

Pyrantel pamoate may be used as a self-medication to treat pinworms; the cure rate is reported to be 90% to 100%.[15] Although the product is readily available, helminthic infections other than those caused by pinworms should be diagnosed and treated by a physician.

Mechanism of Action Pyrantel pamoate is a depolarizing neuromuscular agent that paralyzes and kills the worms. It is poorly absorbed and 50% of the drug is excreted unchanged in the feces.

Indications Pyrantel pamoate is effective in treating enterobiasis (pinworm), *Ascaris lumbricoides* (roundworm), *Ancylostoma duodenale* (hookworm), *Necator americanus* (hookworm), and *Trichostrongylus orientalis* (hairworm).[16]

Dosage/Administration Guidelines A single oral dose of pyrantel pamoate (capsule, liquid, caplet) is based on body weight (5 mg per pound or 11 mg/kg). A maximum single dose of 1 g is recommended. The recommended dosage is the same for infants under 2 years of age or children weighing less than 25 pounds; however, they should not be treated without first consulting a health care provider.[16,18] The product includes a schedule of recommended dosage that is based on body weight and should not be exceeded. If necessary, the dose may be repeated in 2 weeks under the direction of a physician.

The drug may be taken at any time of the day, with or without meals. A special diet, fasting, or purgation before administering pyrantel pamoate is not necessary. The liquid formulation, containing 50 mg/mL, should be shaken well before the dose is measured.

Adverse Effects Side effects are uncommon with this medication. However, a patient who experiences severe or persistent abdominal cramps, nausea, vomiting, anorexia, diarrhea, headache, drowsiness, or dizziness after taking this medication should consult a physician.

Drug–Drug Interactions Anthelmintic piperazine (Vermizine) and pyrantel pamoate have antagonistic mechanisms of action; therefore, concomitant administration is not recommended.[17]

Contraindications/Precautions/Warnings Pyrantel pamoate is contraindicated in patients with hypersensitivity to the drug. Patients with preexisting liver dysfunction, severe malnutrition, or anemia should not self-medicate without first consulting a health care provider.[15] Pyrantel pamoate has never been studied in pregnant women, and it should be used during pregnancy only when clearly indicated.[15,16] Pregnant women should self-medicate only under the direction of a health care provider.

Prescription Medications

Pyrantel pamoate is the drug of choice in treating pinworms. Two prescription alternatives are mebendazole (Vermox), 100 mg taken once, then repeated in 2 weeks, as well as albendazole (Albenza), 400 mg taken once, then repeated in 2 weeks. Albendazole is approved to treat other helminthic infections, but FDA considers it an investigational drug when used to treat pinworms.[4] Household members should be treated because they may also be infected and can act as a reservoir to reinfect others.[5]

Product Selection Guidelines

Pyrantel pamoate is a safe and effective treatment for pinworms. It is the only agent approved for self-treatment of pinworm infection. The several brands of pyrantel pamoate listed in Table 15–3 are comparatively priced and are generally less expensive than prescription treatment (e.g., Vermox). Pharmacoeconomic studies of anthelmintics are not available.

Patient Assessment of Pinworm Infection

The use of nonprescription medications for the treatment of helminthic infections is limited, given the one nonprescription anthelmintic currently on the market (pyrantel pamoate) is indicated only for pinworms. Despite this limi-

Table 15–3

Selected Anthelmintic Products

Trade Name	Primary Ingredient
PinRid Capsule/Softgel	Pyrantel pamoate 180 mg (equals 62.5 mg pyrantel base)
PinRid Liquid	Pyrantel pamoate 50 mg/mL
Pin-X Liquid	Pyrantel pamoate 50 mg/mL
Pyrantel Pamoate Suspension	Pyrantel pamoate 50 mg/mL
Reese's Pinworm Caplet	Pyrantel pamoate 180 mg (equals 62.5 mg pyrantel base)
Reese's Pinworm Liquid	Pyrantel pamoate 50 mg/mL

tation, the pharmacist is often the first person contacted when a patient suspects a helminthic infection and thus should know the signs, symptoms, and complications of common helminthic infections. (See Table 15–1.) All health care providers must be factual and sensitive because most people find the thought of a worm infection disturbing.

The pharmacist should determine whether the pinworm infection has been confirmed before recommending treatment. The presence of pinworms can be determined by either of two methods. One method is to cover the end of a cotton swab or tongue depressor with tape (sticky side out), to apply it to the perianal area, and to examine the tape under a microscope to confirm the presence or absence of eggs. Egg collection can be done at home, but inspection and evaluation must be done in a laboratory or health care provider's office. Another method frequently used by parents is to visually inspect the child's anal area with a flashlight an hour or more after the child has gone to bed. Female pinworms can be seen emerging from the anus to deposit their eggs. This second method is preferable because the chance of injury to the child is small and the method does not require a trip to the doctor.[2,13]

Asking the patient the following questions will help elicit the information needed to accurately assess the disorder and to recommend the appropriate treatment approach.

Q~ For whom is the medication?

A~ A parent or caregiver may be seeking treatment for a child. Tailor further questions and advice for the actual patient.

Q~ What are the child's or your symptoms?

A~ *Identify the classic symptoms of pinworm infection. (See the section "Signs and Symptoms of Pinworm Infection.")* Determine whether the patient's symptoms are typical for pinworm infection.

Q~ Why do you think your child or you might have worms? Have you seen any worms in the stool?

A~ If a suspected worm was seen in stools, advise the patient/caregiver to put the sample, if saved, in a container with tap water and to take it to a health care provider for identification. Give instructions for other methods of confirming pinworm infection.

Q~ How long have the symptoms been present?

A~ *Identify the length of time that indicates a first occurrence as opposed to a recurrence of an earlier infection. (See the section "Pathophysiology of Pinworm Infection.")* If the response indicates a recurrent infection, refer the patient to a physician.

Q~ Are other family members or close contacts also infected?

A~ *Identify the appropriate hygiene methods to take if a pinworm infection is confirmed. (See Table 15–2.)* Advise the patient/caregiver that the whole family should be treated. Stress to the patient/caregiver the importance of these measures in preventing reinfection.

Q~ Has a physician been seen for this problem? Has the problem occurred in the past? How was it treated? Did the treatment work?

A~ Responses to these questions help determine whether medical referral is necessary. If dangerous or dubious treatments were tried for previous infections, caution against such remedies.

Q~ If not an adult, what is the age and approximate weight of the patient?

A~ *Identify the criteria for treating children without consulting a physician. Use an arbitrary body weight to calculate a child's dose of pyrantel pamoate. (See the section "Dosage/Administration Guidelines.")* If the child does not meet the criteria, advise the caregiver to take the child to a physician.

Q~ Are you taking medications to treat this problem or other medical conditions?

A~ *Identify possible drug–drug interactions and contraindications for pyrantel pamoate. (See the sections "Drug–Drug Interactions" and "Contraindications/Precautions/Warnings".)* If the patient's medical/medication history indicates possible problems, refer the patient to a physician.

Q~ Is the patient pregnant or breast-feeding?

A~ If yes, refer the patient to a physician. A physician must consider the treatment's risks and benefits to both mother and fetus.

Q~ Has the patient traveled outside the United States? If so, where and when?

A~ Advise the patient that worm infections are prevalent in some countries. Recommend that the patient contact the Centers for Disease Control and Prevention Web site (www.cdc.gov/travel) for precautions to take during travel.

Patient Education for Pinworm Infection

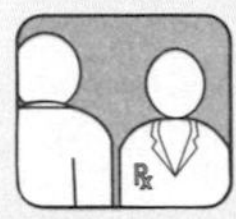

The objectives of self-treatment are to (1) eradicate pinworms in the infected patient, (2) prevent reinfection, and (3) prevent transmission of the infection to others. For most patients, carefully following product instructions and the self-care measures listed below will help ensure optimal therapeutic outcomes.

Nondrug Measures

- See Table 15–2 for nondrug/preventive measures.

Nonprescription Medications

- Read the package insert information carefully; this information will help prevent reinfection or transmission of the infection.
- Consult a physician before giving the medication to a person with liver disease or anemia, to a child under age 2 and/or weighing less than 25 pounds, or to a woman who is pregnant or breast-feeding.
- Treat all household members to ensure elimination of the infection. Consult a physician if household members meet the criteria discussed previously.
- Take only one dose as shown on the dosing schedule included with this product. For adults and children over 2 years old the dosing is the same: 11 mg/kg or 5 mg per pound orally. The maximum dose is 1 g.
- If desired, take the drug with food, milk, or fruit juices on an empty stomach any time during the day. The liquid formulation may be mixed with milk or fruit juice.
- Shake the liquid formulation well, and use a measuring spoon to ensure an accurate dose.
- Be aware that fasting, laxatives, special diets, or purging is not necessary to aid treatment.

⚠ If abdominal cramps, nausea, vomiting, anorexia, rash, diarrhea, headache, drowsiness, or dizziness occur and persist after taking the medication, consult a physician.

⚠ If symptoms of the pinworm infection persist, contact a physician to determine whether a second dose is indicated.

Patient Counseling for Pinworm Infection

Before recommending treatment, the pharmacist should explain how to confirm a pinworm infection and ask the patient/caregiver to return to the pharmacy once the infection is confirmed. The pharmacist should then review the package insert material for pyrantel pamoate with the patient/caregiver. This material explains the pinworm life cycle, symptoms of pinworm infection, and methods of transmitting the infection. The pharmacist should calculate the doses for the patient and all family members, being sure to emphasize the need to treat the whole family. The patient/caregiver should be advised to implement strict hygienic measures to prevent reinfection or transmission of the infection to other family members. The box "Patient Education for Pinworm Infection" lists specific information to provide the patient/caregiver.

Evaluation of Patient Outcomes for Pinworm Infection

The patient/caregiver should return in 2 weeks for a follow-up evaluation. If symptoms of the infection persist, the patient should see a physician. A second dose of pyrantel pamoate may be needed. If hygienic measures are not being followed, the pharmacist should again stress their importance in preventing reinfection.

CONCLUSIONS

The pharmacist should be familiar with common helminthic infections, their symptoms, and their treatment. Pinworm infection is the only helminthic infection that should be treated with a nonprescription drug, although pyrantel pamoate is a secondary drug in treating other helminthic infections. Self-medication should be discouraged for all helminthic infections other than pinworm. Clinical manifestations of these parasitic diseases characterize many other illnesses and attempting self-diagnosis not only is difficult but may also result in neglect of a more serious condition. The availability of effective, relatively safe, easy-to-take prescription drugs that can eradicate many helminthic infections should be reason enough to avoid self-medication. The pharmacist should encourage the patient/caregiver to consult a physician for treatment when helminths other than pinworms are suspected.

References

1. Liu LX, Weller PF. Antiparasitic drugs. *N Engl J Med.* 1996; 334:1178–84.
2. Van Riper G. Pyrantel pamoate for pinworm infestation. *Am Pharm.* 1993;33(2):43–5.
3. Schmidt GD, Roberts LS. *Foundations of Parasitology.* 2nd ed. St. Louis: C.V. Mosby; 1981:2,448,473.

4. Anon. Drugs for parasitic infections. *Med Lett Drugs Ther.* 1998;40:1–2.
5. Mishriki YY. Dealing with the unexpected nematode. *Postgrad Med.* 1997;102:37–8.
6. Summer L, Johnson CA. Ascariasis. *Am Fam Physician.* 1990;42: 999–1002.
7. Owen RL. Parasitic diseases. In: Sleisenger MH, Fordtran JS, eds. *Gastrointestinal diseases: Pathohysiology, Diagnosis, Management.* 5th ed. Philadelphia: WB Saunders; 1993;1207–8.
8. Khuroo MS. Ascariasis. *Gastroenterol Clin North Am.* 1996;25:553–77.
9. Harinasuta T, Pungpak S, Keystone JS. Trematode infections. Opisthorchiasis, Clonorchiasis, Fascioliasis, and Paragonimiasis. *Infect Dis Clin North Am.* 1993;7:699–716.
10. Strickland GT. *Hunter's Tropical Medicine.* 7th ed., Philadelphia: WB Saunders; 1991:706–710, 756–61, 834–45.
11. Hamblin J. Pinworms in pregnancy. *J Am Board Fam Pract.* 1995;8:321–4.
12. Jones JE. Pinworms. *Am Fam Physician.* 1988;8:159–64.
13. Junkett G. Common intestinal helminths. *Am Fam Physician.* 1995;52: 2039–48.
14. Schrock TL. Diseases of the anorectum. In: Sleisenger MH, Fordtran JS, eds. *Gastrointestinal Disease: Pathophysiology, Diagnosis, Management.* 5th ed. Philadelphia: W.B. Saunders; 1993:1505–6.
15. Hardman JG, Limbird LE, Molinoff PB, et al., eds. *Goodman and Gilman's The Pharmacological Basis of Therapeutics.* 9th ed. New York: Pergamon Press; 1996:1022.
16. American Society of Health-System Pharmacists. *American Hospital Formulary Service (AHFS) 1999.* Bethesda, MD: American Society of Health-System Pharmacists, Inc; 1999:61–2.
17. American Society of Hospital Pharmacists. *Medication Teaching Manual: The Guide to Patient Drug Information.* 6th ed. Bethesda, MD: American Society of Hospital Pharmacists; 1994:383.
18. Barone MA. *The Harriet Lane Handbook.* 14th ed. By The Johns Hopkins Hospital. St. Louis: Mosby-Year Book, Inc; 1996:625.

CHAPTER 16

Nausea and Vomiting

Jenifer C. Jennings and Gary M. Oderda

Chapter 16 at a Glance

Severe nausea and the realization that one is about to vomit are two of the more common unpleasant symptoms an individual may experience. Nausea and vomiting are symptoms associated with many medical disorders. Nonprescription antiemetics are used to prevent or control the symptoms of nausea and vomiting that are primarily caused by motion sickness, pregnancy, and mild infectious diseases. Some nonprescription antiemetics are promoted for the relief of vague symptoms such as "upset stomach," indigestion, and distention associated with food overindulgence. However, their value in treating these complaints is not well documented.

Nausea and vomiting associated with radiation therapy; cancer chemotherapy; and serious metabolic, central nervous system (CNS), gastrointestinal (GI), and endocrine disorders are not covered in this chapter because they are not appropriate conditions for self-medication. Instead, they require appropriate management by a health care provider.

Editor's Note: This chapter is based, in part, on the 11th edition chapter titled "Emetic and Antiemetic Products," which was written by Gary M. Oderda and Jenifer Jennings.

Epidemiology of Nausea and Vomiting

Nausea and vomiting are common complaints in both adults and children. Acute transient attacks of vomiting in association with diarrhea are very common. This symptom is often observed with viral gastroenteritis, a common acute infectious disease that is usually harmless and self-limiting and that may affect any age group.

Physiology of the Vomiting Process

Vomiting is a complex process that involves both the CNS and the GI tracts. Nausea, an unpleasant sensation that is vaguely associated with the epigastrium and abdomen, usually precedes vomiting. Retching is a strong, involuntary, and unsuccessful effort to vomit. Regurgitation is the casting up of stomach contents without oral expulsion.

The essential area for coordinating vomiting is located in the medulla. This vomiting coordinating circuitry has been referred to as the vomiting center. Vomiting related to the following are received by this coordinating circuitry: (1) psychogenic vomiting from the cerebral cortex and limbic system; (2) motion and space sickness from vestibular and visual afferents; (3) GI tract disturbance including food poisoning, cancer chemotherapy, and radiation; (4) pregnancy; (5) postoperative vomiting; (6) miscellaneous problems including vomiting from heart, glossopharyngeal, and trigeminal afferents; and (7) blood poisoning involving the area postrema of the medulla (the chemoreceptor trigger zone).[1] Neurotransmitters and receptors of major importance involved in eliciting vomiting include dopamine D_2, histamine type 1, muscarinic cholinergic receptors, adrenergic type 2 receptors, and serotonin receptors.[1]

Vomiting begins with a deep inspiration, the closing of the glottis, and the depression of the soft palate. A forceful contraction of the diaphragm and abdominal musculature occurs, producing an increase in intrathoracic and intra-abdominal pressure that compresses the stomach and raises esophageal pressure. The stomach and esophageal musculature relax, and the positive intrathoracic and intra-abdominal pressure moves stomach contents into the esophagus and mouth. Several cycles of reflux into the esophagus occur before actual vomiting begins. Vomitus is expelled from the esophagus by a combination of increased intrathoracic pressure and reverse peristaltic waves. Normally, the glottis closes off the trachea and prevents the vomitus from entering the airway; however, aspiration of the vomitus can occur in patients with CNS depression or with an absent or impaired gag reflex.

Overstimulation of the labyrinth (inner ear) apparatus produces the nausea and vomiting of motion sickness. The three semicircular canals in the labyrinth on each side of the head are responsible for maintaining equilibrium. Postural adjustments are made when the brain receives nervous impulses initiated by the movement of fluid in the canals. Motion sickness may be produced by unusual motion patterns in which the head is rotated on two axes simultaneously. Mechanisms other than stimulation of the semicircular canals are also important. Erroneous interpretation of visual stimuli by stationary subjects, which occurs when watching a film taken from a roller coaster or an airplane performing aerobatics or when extending the head upward while standing on a rotating platform, can produce motion sickness. Some individuals are more tolerant of the effect of a particular type of motion, but no one is immune. Individuals can vary in their susceptibility to various kinds of motions, such as flying and boat riding. But regardless of the type of stimulus-producing event, motion sickness is much easier to prevent than to treat once it has already begun.

Etiology of Nausea and Vomiting

Vomiting (emesis) can be caused by many stimuli: travel (i.e., motion sickness), pregnancy, drug therapy, stress, viral gastroenteritis, overeating, food poisoning, bulimia, distension, diseases, and other factors. Most minor nausea and vomiting, such as may occur with motion sickness or overeating, are self-limiting symptoms that require minimal therapy. Table 16–1 lists the primary causes of nausea and vomiting.[2,3] The section "General Treatment Approach" discusses some of these underlying causes in more detail.

Table 16–1

Primary Causes of Nausea and Vomiting

Primary Causes of Nausea and Vomiting
Visceral Afferent Stimulation
Mechanical Obstruction
Gastric outlet obstruction (i.e., peptic ulcer disease, gastric carcinoma, pancreatic disease)
Small intestinal obstruction
Motility Disorders
Gastroparesis (i.e., diabetes, drug-induced, postviral)
Chronic intestinal pseudo-obstruction
Irritable bowel syndrome
Anorexia nervosa
Idiopathic gastric stasis
Peritoneal Irritation
Appendicitis
Bacterial peritonitis
Infections
Viral gastroenteritis (i.e., Norwalk virus, rotavirus)
Food poisoning (i.e., toxins from *Bacillus cereus, Staphylococcus aureus, Clostridium perfringens*)
Hepatitis A or B
Acute systemic infections
Topical Gastrointestinal Irritants
Alcohol
Nonsteroidal anti-inflammatory drugs (NSAIDs)
Antibiotics
Other
Cardiac disease (i.e., myocardial infarction, congestive heart failure)
Urologic disease (i.e., stones, pyelonephritis)
CNS Disorders
Vestibular Disorders
Labyrinthitis
Ménière's syndrome
Motion sickness
Increased Intracranial Pressure
CNS tumor
Subdural or subarachnoid hemorrhage
Infections
Meningitis
Encephalitis
Psychogenic
Anticipatory vomiting
Bulimia
Psychiatric disorders
Other CNS Disorders
Migraine headache

Table 16–1

Primary Causes of Nausea and Vomiting (continued)

Irritation of Chemoreceptor Trigger Zone
Initiated/Withdrawn Drugs
Cytotoxic chemotherapy
Opiates
Theophylline toxicity
Digitalis toxicity
Antibiotics
Radiation therapy
Drug withdrawal (i.e., opiates, benzodiazepines)
Systemic Disorders
Diabetes (i.e., diabetic ketoacidosis)
Renal disease (i.e., uremia)
Adrenocortical crisis (i.e., Addison's disease)
Pregnancy

Complications of Nausea and Vomiting

Vomiting may produce complications that include dehydration, aspiration, malnutrition, electrolyte and acid–base abnormalities, and Mallory–Weiss syndrome tears of the esophagus resulting in blood in the vomitus. Dehydration and electrolyte imbalances are major concerns with vomiting. Signs and symptoms of dehydration include dry mouth, excessive thirst, little or no urination, dizziness, and lightheadedness.

Treatment of Nausea and Vomiting

Over-the-counter (OTC) antiemetic medications are suitable to relieve the symptoms of occasional self-limiting nausea and vomiting. Antiemetic medications may be given to prevent or control symptoms. Available products for self-medication include antacids, histamine$_2$-receptor antagonists, antihistamines, and phosphorated carbohydrate solutions. Oral rehydration solutions (ORSs) are available for treating dehydration that can result from prolonged vomiting.

Treatment Outcomes

The treatment of nausea and vomiting should focus on identifying and correcting the underlying cause. Most cases of acute vomiting require no specific treatment because they are mild and self-limiting, resolve spontaneously, and require only symptomatic treatment. However, more severe acute vomiting necessitates referral and may require hospitalization.

The cause and severity of the nausea and vomiting determine the outcomes of pharmacologic or nonpharmacologic therapy. Depending on etiology, symptomatic relief may not be possible until the underlying cause has been identified and controlled or eliminated. In other situations, self-care may offer improvement in symptoms and the patient's overall well-being.

General Treatment Approach

The algorithms in Figures 16–1 and 16–2 outline the self-care of nausea and vomiting in adults and children, respectively. The following considerations of nausea and vomiting associated with special population groups and certain etiologies are important in determining the appropriate use of an antiemetic product.

Nausea and Vomiting in Children

Vomiting in newborns can result from a number of serious abnormalities, including obstruction of the GI tract, neurologic disorders, and neuromuscular control disorders. It may rapidly lead to acid–base disturbances and dehydration. Dehydration and electrolyte disturbances occur more often in children and, if not appropriately managed, may result in death. Thus, referral to a health care provider is always recommended for further evaluation of any vomiting in newborns.

Regurgitation or spitting up, whereby milk appears to spill gently from the mouth, is common in infants. Often the causes are simple, such as overfeeding, feeding too rapidly, burping ineffectively, swallowing air, and laying the infant down after feeding, as well as immaturity of the esophageal sphincters. Regurgitation generally should not cause concern and does not require medical attention.

A more common cause of vomiting in children is acute viral gastroenteritis. However, acute onset of vomiting in children can be secondary to head trauma, toxic ingestion, CNS infection, and GI obstruction. Treatment of gastroenteritis is directed primarily at preventing and correcting dehydration and electrolyte disturbances. Lost fluids should generally be replaced within 24 hours. An ORS may be used in mild cases. If severe diarrhea or vomiting persists for more than 24 to 48 hours, the child should be referred to a health care provider for evaluation and for parenteral fluid and electrolyte replacement.[4]

The use of antiemetics in children is controversial, in part, because most antiemetic studies have been conducted with adult patients. Some clinicians question the wisdom and value of treating children with antiemetics in an acute, self-limiting disorder. It is suggested that vomiting in gastroenteritis is a host defense process that sheds the pathogen and should, therefore, not be suppressed. However, recurrent or protracted vomiting can lead to marked dehydration and electrolyte imbalance that cannot be ignored, especially in small children. The patient should be observed for the following signs of dehydration: dry oral mucous membranes; sunken eyes, with or without sunken fontanel; decreased urine output (i.e., no wetting for 8 to 12 hours or more); no tears when crying; decreased skin turgor with tenting; weight

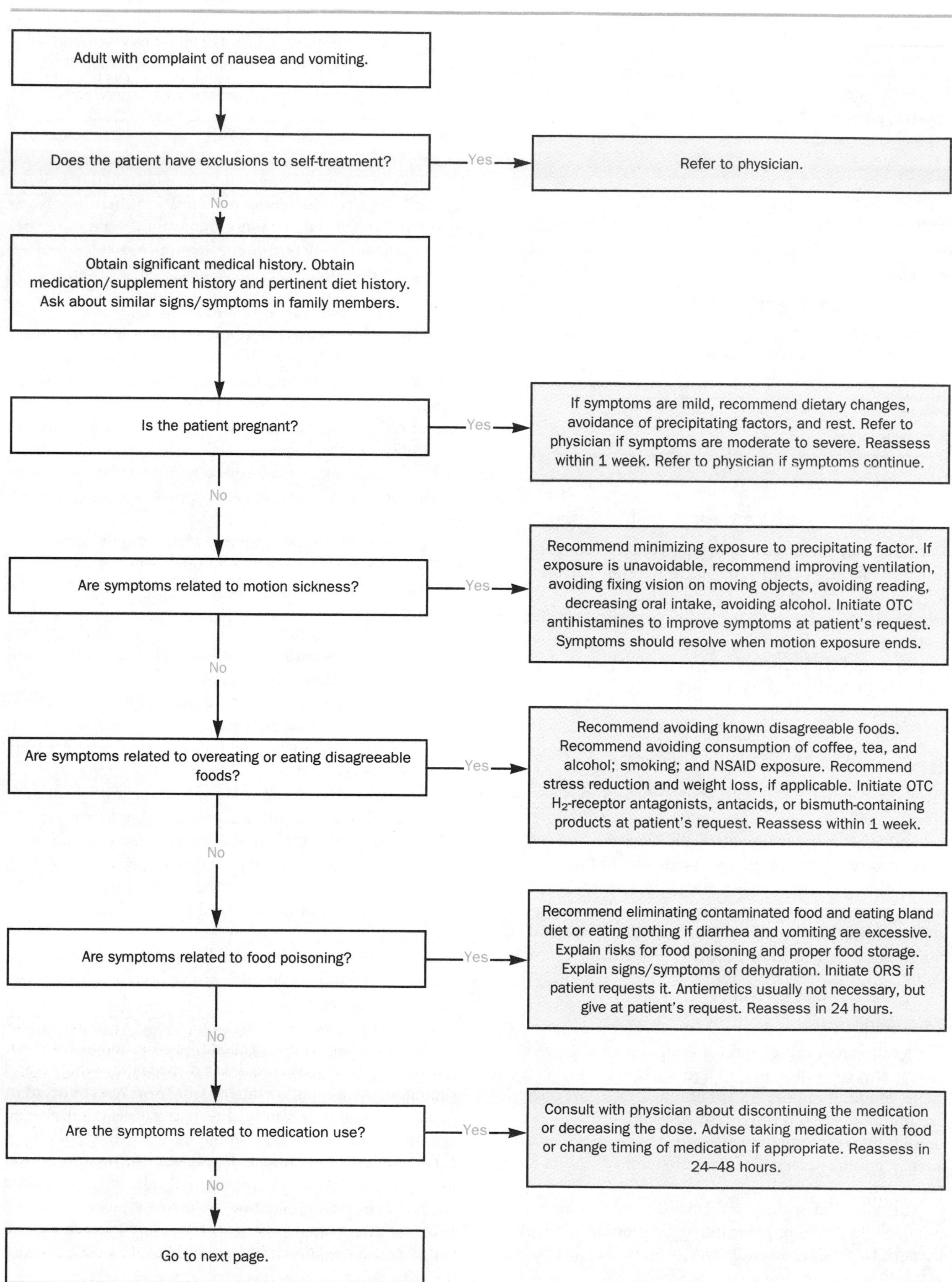

Adult with complaint of nausea and vomiting.
Does the patient have exclusions to self-treatment?
Yes
Refer to physician.
No
Obtain significant medical history. Obtain medication/supplement history and pertinent diet history. Ask about similar signs/symptoms in family members.
Is the patient pregnant?
Yes
If symptoms are mild, recommend dietary changes, avoidance of precipitating factors, and rest. Refer to physician if symptoms are moderate to severe. Reassess within 1 week. Refer to physician if symptoms continue.
No
Are symptoms related to motion sickness?
Yes
Recommend minimizing exposure to precipitating factor. If exposure is unavoidable, recommend improving ventilation, avoiding fixing vision on moving objects, avoiding reading, decreasing oral intake, avoiding alcohol. Initiate OTC antihistamines to improve symptoms at patient's request. Symptoms should resolve when motion exposure ends.
No
Are symptoms related to overeating or eating disagreeable foods?
Yes
Recommend avoiding known disagreeable foods. Recommend avoiding consumption of coffee, tea, and alcohol; smoking; and NSAID exposure. Recommend stress reduction and weight loss, if applicable. Initiate OTC H_2-receptor antagonists, antacids, or bismuth-containing products at patient's request. Reassess within 1 week.
No
Are symptoms related to food poisoning?
Yes
Recommend eliminating contaminated food and eating bland diet or eating nothing if diarrhea and vomiting are excessive. Explain risks for food poisoning and proper food storage. Explain signs/symptoms of dehydration. Initiate ORS if patient requests it. Antiemetics usually not necessary, but give at patient's request. Reassess in 24 hours.
No
Are the symptoms related to medication use?
Yes
Consult with physician about discontinuing the medication or decreasing the dose. Advise taking medication with food or change timing of medication if appropriate. Reassess in 24–48 hours.
No
Go to next page.

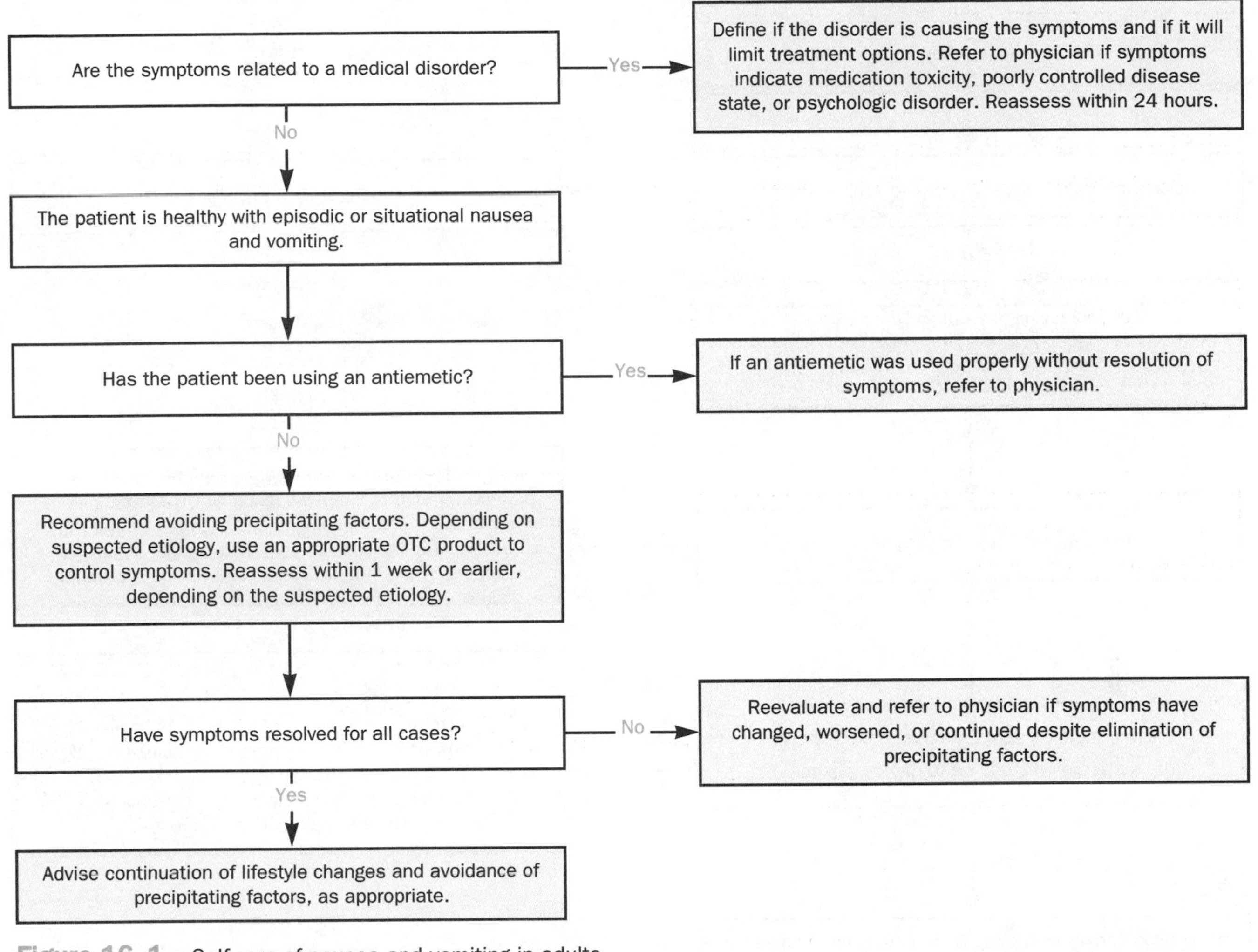

Figure 16–1 Self-care of nausea and vomiting in adults.

loss; and unusual listlessness, sleepiness, or tiredness.[5] If any of these signs are present, the child should be referred to a health care provider.

When a child experiences nausea and vomiting, the child's health care provider should be contacted if the following exist:

- The child is younger than 1 year.
- The child refuses to drink.
- Urination has not occurred in the past 8 to 12 hours.
- The child appears lethargic or is crying.
- Weight loss or dehydration occurs.
- Vomiting occurs with each feeding.
- Vomiting is repeatedly projectile.
- Vomitus contains red, black, or green fluid.
- Vomiting is associated with diarrhea, distended abdomen, fever, or severe headache.
- Vomiting occurs following a head injury.
- Poisoning is suspected.
- Vomiting occurs with recurrent, severe, acute abdominal pain.

Nausea and Vomiting during Pregnancy

Nausea, with or without vomiting, may be one of the earliest symptoms of pregnancy. A woman who experiences nausea and vomiting, and who has no other symptoms except a missed menstrual period and perhaps weight gain, should be referred for a pregnancy test and follow-up. Women who report nausea and vomiting during pregnancy generally suffer from these symptoms in the early part of the day—hence, the term "morning sickness." However, some pregnant women experience the symptoms in the afternoon or evening; a small number of women experience morning sickness throughout the day.

Nausea and vomiting during the first trimester of pregnancy is often worrisome to the patient. The symptoms, which may be mild to severe, should be taken seriously and the patient reassured. However, because teratogenicity is a

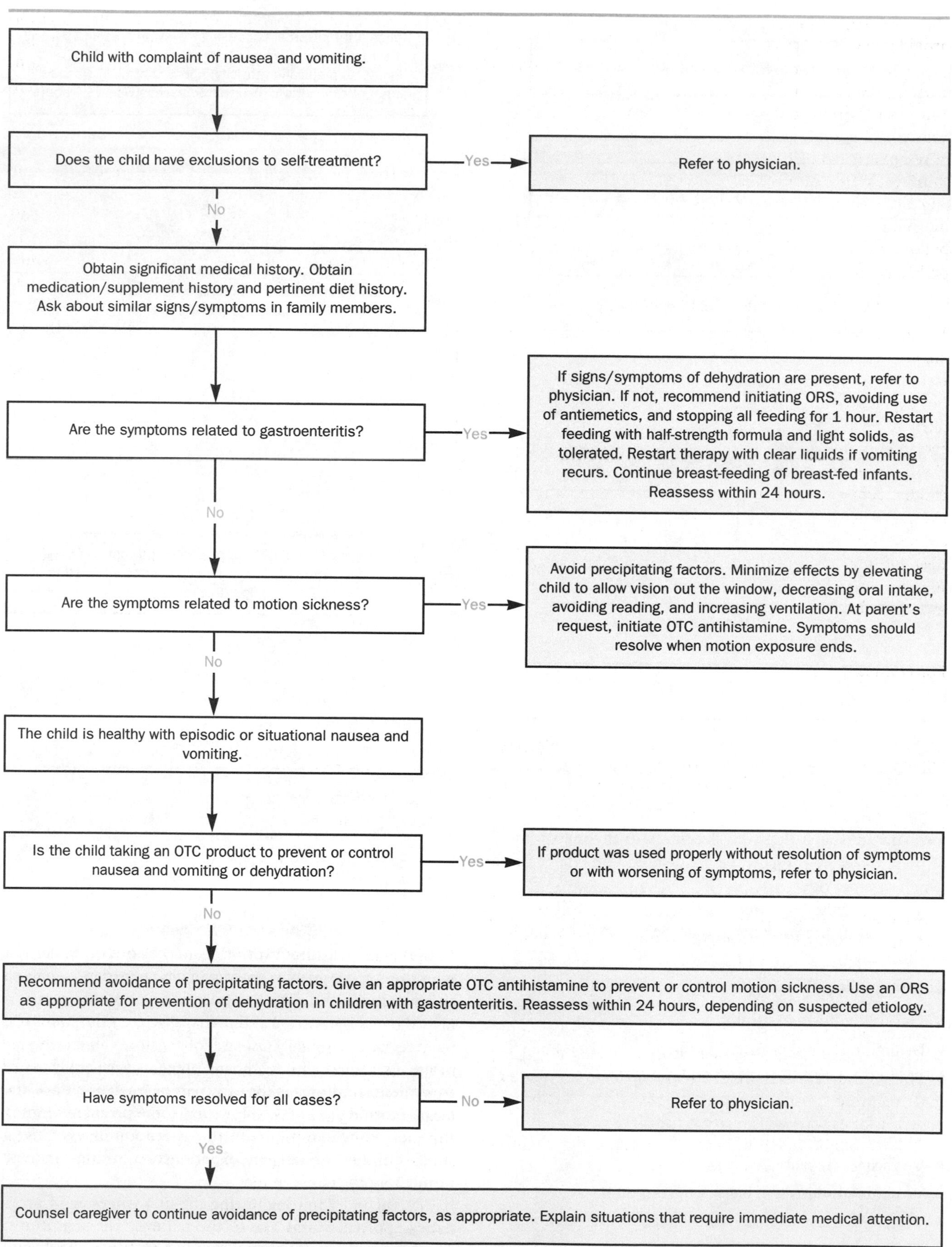

Figure 16–2 Self-care of nausea and vomiting in children.

major consideration during pregnancy, most health care providers are reluctant to prescribe any medication for a pregnant woman unless it is absolutely necessary. Indications for nonprescription antiemetics approved by the Food and Drug Administration (FDA) do not include treating nausea and vomiting associated with pregnancy. A number of nonpharmacologic approaches can be recommended instead, including eating small, frequent meals; lowering the fat content of meals; ingesting crackers before arising in the morning; lying down; and avoiding precipitating factors. If nausea, vomiting, or both continue despite such measures, a patient should be referred to her health care provider.[6]

Nausea and Vomiting Related to Motion Sickness

Motion sickness occurs when visual and vestibular stimuli are not in accord. The symptoms consist of pallor, yawning, restlessness, nausea, and then vomiting. Although anyone can experience motion sickness, some individuals are more likely to be affected, and susceptibility appears to vary with age. Infants are generally least likely to experience it, whereas children ages 2 to 12 years are more likely to do so. In young children, placing the child in a car seat may minimize motion sickness associated with car travel. The resulting elevation and position are sufficient to allow vision out the front window and may prevent the disorder. Antihistamines are the primary nonprescription agents used to prevent or control motion sickness.

Nausea and Vomiting Related to Overeating

For complaints of nausea associated with excessive or disagreeable food or beverage intake, avoidance or moderation of consumption may prove beneficial. Otherwise, antacids, bismuth-containing products, and histamine$_2$-receptor antagonists are indicated for the relief of heartburn, indigestion, and upset stomach associated with dietary overindulgence. (See Chapter 11, "Acid–Peptic Disorders and Intestinal Gas.")

Nausea and Vomiting Related to Food Poisoning

Signs and symptoms associated with food poisoning usually include vomiting in addition to diarrhea, abdominal cramps, and possible fever.[4] Symptomatic treatment, which is often recommended, consists of fluid and electrolyte replacement, dietary modification, and antidiarrheal products when appropriate. A diet of clear liquids and simple carbohydrates is recommended for the first 24 hours. The patient can return to a regular diet when it can be tolerated.[7] Food poisoning typically resolves within 24 to 36 hours. However, if symptoms continue beyond this period, referral to a health care provider for evaluation is recommended.[2]

The use of nonprescription antidiarrheal agents for infectious diarrhea is not appropriate without a specific medical recommendation.[7] (See Chapter 13, "Diarrhea.")

Drug-Induced Nausea and Vomiting

Many medications, such as cancer chemotherapeutic agents, narcotics, antibiotics, and estrogens, are known to cause nausea and vomiting as an adverse side effect. Other medications, such as digitalis or theophylline, may produce nausea and vomiting as a sign of toxicity. In these situations, nonprescription antiemetics are not indicated. The patient should instead be referred to a health care provider.

Psychogenic/Pathology-Induced Nausea and Vomiting

Bulimia (binge–purge behavior) is a psychologic disorder in which patients attempt to control their weight by repeated vomiting and the chronic use of emetics. These patients should be referred for medical and psychologic management of the underlying problems. Patients with other chronic medical conditions such as diabetes (which could be affected by the lack of adequate nutritional intake or by missed doses of medication) should also be referred to their health care providers.

Signs and symptoms or medical conditions associated with nausea and vomiting that necessitate referral to a health care provider for evaluation and treatment include the following:

- Blood in the vomitus.
- Abdominal pain or distention.
- Projectile vomiting or prolonged nausea and vomiting (more than 24 to 48 hours), especially for children younger than 1 year.
- Dehydration.
- Weight loss of more than 5% of body weight.
- Fever.
- Severe headache.
- Change in behavior or alertness.
- Pregnancy.
- Presence of diabetes or other medical conditions that may be affected by lack of nutritional intake or missed doses of oral medications.
- Recent trauma, particularly a significant head injury.
- Suspected poisoning.

Nonpharmacologic Therapy

In addition to the nondrug measures discussed above for nausea and vomiting associated with pregnancy, motion sickness, and overeating, acupressure wristbands are used to treat these symptoms. The use of acupressure therapy to treat nausea and vomiting is based on the ancient Chinese theory of the vital force, Chi. For centuries, the Chinese have used stimulation of the Neiguan—or Pericardium 6 (P6)—point, located on the inner forearm just above the wrist, to relieve the signs and symptoms of nausea and vomiting. Several studies[8–10] have investigated the use of acupressure therapy in this regard. These studies suggest a beneficial effect and have resulted in the availability of acupressure wristbands such as SeaBands and Travel Aides, which are marketed to prevent motion sickness. Controlled studies have also demonstrated a positive patient response in suppressing pregnancy-related nausea and vomiting.[8–10] Acupressure wristbands offer an alternative to the pharmacologic management of nausea and vomiting and should be considered by patients who wish to avoid the adverse effects associated with antihistamines.

Another device that stimulates the P6 point became available in 1999. ReliefBand NST (Nerve Stimulation Technology) is FDA-approved for nonprescription use in treating nausea and vomiting related to motion sickness, including air sickness, car sickness, and sea sickness.[11]

Although several theories have been proposed, the exact mechanism of action for the ReliefBand is unknown.[12] The device is believed to stimulate the P6 acupuncture point using electricity to exert its effect. Studies using P6 point acupressure[12] or P6 acustimulation[13] have shown positive results in relieving experimentally induced motion sickness. ReliefBand was also found to have positive results in controlling sea sickness among cruise ship passengers. No adverse reactions to the device were reported by the passengers.[14] However, a few patients in other clinical trials experienced a mild, transient rash at the application site following use of ReliefBand.[15]

The ReliefBand can be used before the onset of anticipated motion sickness or when symptoms are first noticed. In contrast, nonprescription antiemetics such as dimenhydrinate must be taken at least 30 to 60 minutes before beginning the activity that causes motion sickness. Antiemetic drugs can also cause drowsiness, which may not be acceptable to some travelers. ReliefBand can be used concomitantly with antiemetics.[11]

Pharmacologic Therapy

Selection of a nonprescription medication to treat nausea and vomiting is determined by their potential cause. The myriad causes of nausea and vomiting account for numerous medications used to treat these symptoms.

Antacids

Antacids neutralize gastric acidity, increasing the pH of the stomach and duodenum. Antacids are indicated for complaints of heartburn, dyspepsia, acid indigestion, and the symptomatic relief of upset stomach associated with gastric acidity. For relief of such symptoms, the patient should take 15 mL of most antacids 30 minutes after meals and at bedtime. Because antacids may impair the absorption of many medications, patients should be counseled not to take potentially interacting oral medications within 1 to 2 hours of the antacid dose. The available nonprescription antacid products contain various combinations of ingredients, such as magnesium hydroxide, aluminum hydroxide, calcium carbonate, and magnesium carbonate. (See Chapter 11, "Acid–Peptic Disorders and Intestinal Gas," for a thorough review of antacid pharmacotherapy.)

Histamine$_2$-Receptor Antagonists

Histamine$_2$-receptor antagonists provide symptomatic relief of heartburn, dyspepsia, and indigestion by inhibiting the secretion of gastric acid. FDA has approved lower nonprescription doses of such agents for these acid–peptic indications. (See Chapter 11, "Acid–Peptic Disorders and Intestinal Gas" for a thorough review of these agents.)

Antihistamines

Antihistamines are the primary nonprescription agents used as antiemetics. These agents include meclizine, cyclizine, dimenhydrinate, doxylamine, and diphenhydramine. Meclizine and cyclizine are members of the piperazine group of antihistamine compounds. Doxylamine, diphenhydramine, and dimenhydrinate are antihistamines of the ethanolamine class. Table 16–2 lists examples of commercially available products containing these agents.

Mechanism of Action Antihistamines depress labyrinth excitability and, therefore, are effective—to varying degrees—for the prevention and control of motion sickness.

Indications The available preparations of nonprescription antihistamines are classified as safe and effective for preventing and treating nausea, vomiting, or dizziness associated with motion sickness.

Dosage/Administration Guidelines Antihistamines should be taken at least 30 to 60 minutes before departure for travel and should be continued during travel. Table 16–3 lists dosages for these agents.

Table 16–2

Selected Antiemetic Products

Trade Name	Primary Ingredients
Bonine Chewable Tablets	Meclizine HCl 25 mg
Dramamine Chewable Tablets[a,b]	Dimenhydrinate 50 mg
Dramamine Children's Liquid[a,c,d,e]	Dimenhydrinate 12.5 mg/5 mL
Dramamine Less Drowsy Formula Tablets[b]	Meclizine HCl 25 mg
Dramamine Original Formula Tablets[b]	Dimenhydrinate 50 mg
Emetrol Cherry or Lemon Mint Liquid[c]	Phosphoric acid 21.5 g/5 mL; dextrose 1.87 g/5 mL; fructose 1.87 g/5 mL
Nauzene Tablets[b,f,g]	Diphenhydramine HCl 25 mg
Rekematol Anti-Nausea Liquid[a,c,d,f]	Phosphoric acid 21.5 mg/5 mL; dextrose 1.87 g/5 mL; levulose 1.87 g/5 mL

[a] Lactose-free product.
[b] Sodium-free product.
[c] Alcohol-free product.
[d] Sulfite-free product.
[e] Pediatric formulation.
[f] Dye-free product.
[g] Sucrose-free product.

Table 16–3

Dosage Guidelines for Antiemetic Antihistamines[a]

		Pediatric Dosages	
Agent	**Adult Dosages**	**Children 6–<12 years**	**Children 2–<6 years**
Meclizine	25–50 mg once daily; not to exceed 50 mg in 24 hours	Not recommended	Not recommended
Cyclizine	50 mg every 4–6 hours; not to exceed 200 mg in 24 hours	25 mg every 6–8 hours; not to exceed 75 mg in 24 hours	Not recommended
Diphenhydramine	25–50 mg every 4–6 hours; not to exceed 300 mg in 24 hours	(>20 pounds or 9.1 kg) 12.5–25 mg every 4–6 hours; not to exceed 150 mg in 24 hours	6.25 mg every 4–6 hours; not to exceed 37.5 mg in 24 hours
Dimenhydrinate	50–100 mg every 4–6 hours; not to exceed 400 mg in 24 hours	25–50 mg every 6–8 hours; not to exceed 150 mg in 24 hours	12.5–25 mg every 6–8 hours; not to exceed 75 mg in 24 hours

[a] Take antihistamines at least 30 to 60 minutes before travel; continue taking them during travel.

Adverse Effects Drowsiness with therapeutic doses of antihistamines can occur and is the most common side effect. Patients should be cautioned not to drive a vehicle, operate hazardous machinery, or engage in tasks requiring a high degree of mental alertness and physical dexterity while using these products. In large doses, these agents may also produce anticholinergic adverse effects, including blurred vision, dry mouth, and urinary retention.

Drug–Drug Interactions The effects of antihistamines are additive to those of other CNS depressants, such as alcohol, tranquilizers, hypnotics, and sedatives.

Contraindications/Precautions/Warnings Antihistamines should be used with caution in patients with asthma, narrow-angle glaucoma, obstructive disease of the GI or genitourinary tracts, or benign prostatic hypertrophy.[16]

Special Population Considerations In 1965, FDA required that products containing meclizine and cyclizine carry a warning against their use during pregnancy. This warning was based on animal studies and anecdotal case reports, which suggested that the drugs might have teratogenic potential. Subsequent epidemiologic studies of pregnant women have not shown an increase in fetal deaths or in malformations with exposure to these drugs during the first trimester;[17] therefore, the warning regarding possible teratogenic effects during pregnancy is not required. However, none of these agents has an FDA-approved indication for managing the nausea and vomiting associated with pregnancy. All antihistamines appear to have a low risk of teratogenicity but should be reserved for pregnant women who have severe nausea and vomiting that are unresponsive to nonpharmacologic measures.[18] Pregnant women should always consult their health care providers before taking any medication.

Doxylamine was originally in the combination product Bendectin, which contained doxylamine 10 mg and pyridoxine 10 mg. (See the section "Pyridoxine.") Although FDA had approved this product for treating nausea and vomiting in pregnancy, its manufacturer withdrew Bendectin from the market in 1983 because of the high cost of defending against lawsuits that claimed birth defects occurred in infants whose mothers had taken the drug. However, the ingredients—doxylamine and pyridoxine—remain available as nonprescription products, and many health care providers continue to recommend these agents for pregnant women whose nausea and vomiting do not respond to nonpharmacologic management. Doxylamine and pyridoxine are not considered to be teratogenic.

Pyridoxine

Pyridoxine (vitamin B_6) is a water-soluble B complex vitamin that is essential in the human diet. Uncontrolled studies in the 1940s suggested that pyridoxine might be effective in treating nausea and vomiting associated with pregnancy. Although the American Medical Association Council on Drugs stated in 1979 that no conclusive evidence existed that pyridoxine was effective for this indication, a more recent controlled study,[19] using 25 mg of pyridoxine given orally every 8 hours, produced significant improvement in women who complained of severe nausea and vomiting during pregnancy. The specific mechanism of action of pyridoxine is unknown.[17] As noted previously, pyridoxine was included in the formulation of Bendectin, which was withdrawn from the market in 1983.

Phosphorated Carbohydrate Solution

Phosphorated carbohydrate solution is a mixture of levulose (fructose), dextrose (glucose), and phosphoric acid. (See Table 16–2 for examples of commercially available products.) Phosphoric acid is added to adjust the pH of the commercial product to between 1.5 and 1.6.

Mechanism of Action Theoretically, phosphorated carbohydrate solutions have the potential to inhibit gastric emptying and to reduce gastric tone through the high osmotic pressure exerted by the solution of simple sugars.

Indications Phosphorated carbohydrate solution is indicated for nausea and vomiting associated with upset stomach caused by viral gastroenteritis, food indiscretions, and emotional upset. This hyperosmolar carbohydrate product has been used in attempts to alleviate the nausea and vomiting associated with pregnancy. This product, however, shows no advantage over other products for this problem.

Dosage/Administration Guidelines The usual adult dosage of phosphorated carbohydrate solution is 15 to 30 mL (1 to 2 tablespoons) at 15-minute intervals until vomiting ceases. No more than five doses should be taken in 1 hour. The solution should not be diluted, and the patient should not consume other liquids for 15 minutes after taking a dose. If vomiting does not cease after five doses, a health care provider should be contacted.

Adverse Effects Large doses of fructose may cause abdominal pain and diarrhea. Thus, phosphorated carbohydrate solution should not be used by individuals with hereditary fructose intolerance. Practitioners should be aware of the product's high glucose content and of associated problems in people with diabetes.

Bismuth Salts

Bismuth salts have been used for centuries for various GI complaints, such as upset stomach, indigestion, nausea, and diarrhea. Bismuth subsalicylate (Pepto-Bismol) is available as a nonprescription suspension and as a chewable tablet to relieve nausea associated with dyspepsia, heartburn, and fullness (gas) caused by overindulgence in food and drink. Bismuth is proposed to act by coating the gastric mucosa. Bismuth salts are poorly absorbed from the GI tract, although the amount of bismuth subsalicylate included in nonprescription preparations may lead to the absorption of some salicylate. In patients who are taking other salicylate-containing products or who have renal insufficiency, salicylate levels may be increased. Patients taking bismuth-containing products should be counseled that the mouth, tongue, and stool might temporarily appear gray-black or black. Also, patients should avoid bismuth subsalicylate if they are taking medications that may interact adversely with salicylates. Bismuth subsalicylate should *never* be recommended for children with viral influenza or chicken pox because of concern about development of Reye's syndrome. (See Chapter 11, "Acid–Peptic Disorders and Intestinal Gas" for further discussion of this agent.)

Oral Rehydration Solutions

Dehydration secondary to vomiting and diarrhea is a result of a net loss of extracellular fluid that is composed of sodium, chloride, potassium, water, and bicarbonate. Replacement of fluid should mimic extracellular fluid losses. Because active glucose absorption in the small bowel promotes sodium absorption, oral rehydration therapy is based on using glucose to increase sodium absorption and to allow for rapid replacement of extracellular fluid.[20] ORSs contain electrolyte mixtures; available solutions include Pedialyte, Ricelyte, Infalyte, Rehydralyte, Resol, and Naturalyte. (See Chapter 13, "Diarrhea," for more information about these products and treatment of dehydration.)

Although they are not as osmotically or chemically balanced, the patient can drink gelatin water, sports drinks, fruit juices, and carbonated beverages. However, even if such products are adequate energy sources, they are too low in sodium, potassium, and chloride to produce a rapid and significant therapeutic response to severe dehydration with electrolyte depletion. Use of homemade sugar-water or salt-water solutions should be discouraged.

For a child who is vomiting, the fluid should be given very slowly, starting with 5 to 10 mL every 10 minutes. The quantity of fluid may be increased as tolerated. If vomiting and diarrhea stop after 12 to 24 hours of clear liquids, the child should be gradually returned to a regular diet over the next 2 or 3 days.[4]

Product Selection Guidelines

Antacids, histamine$_2$-receptor antagonists, and bismuth subsalicylate are appropriate for treating nausea related to overeating or eating disagreeable foods. Patients taking medications that can interact with salicylates should not take bismuth subsalicylate. Children and teenagers recovering from chicken pox or viral influenza should not take this agent either. Chapter 11, "Acid–Peptic Disorders and Intestinal Gas," discusses possible drug interactions with antacids and H_2-receptor antagonists.

Vomiting related to food poisoning or other self-limiting causes should be treated with ORSs to prevent dehydration and electrolyte disturbances. The inability to eat or drink because of nausea could also cause dehydration. The same treatment is appropriate in this case.

Nonprescription antihistamines and phosphorated carbohydrate solutions are suitable to prevent or control self-limiting nausea and vomiting such as that associated with motion sickness or overindulgence in food and drink. Patients with hereditary fructose intolerance, however, should not take phosphorated carbohydrate solutions.

Patient Assessment of Nausea and Vomiting

Vomiting is a symptom produced not only by benign processes but also by serious illnesses. Complications can result from vomiting. Physical assessment of the patient can help to determine whether some of the complications listed in the section "Complications of Nausea and Vomiting" have occurred. The physical assessment should include the patient's general appearance, mental status, volume status, and the presence of any abdominal pain. Assessing whether the patient has a fever or recent weight loss is also pertinent.

A major concern with vomiting is the loss of fluids and the inability to eat or drink. This situation can result in dehydration and electrolyte disturbances. Self-care is inappropriate for patients with dehydration, severe anorexia, weight loss, or a poor nutritional status. Patients should be evaluated for dehydration if they have severe vomiting or diarrhea that persists for more than 24 hours in children or 48 hours in adults.[4,5]

Case Study 16–1

Patient Complaint/History

The parent of a 2-year-old girl, Tess, asks the pharmacist questions about managing the child's nausea and vomiting, which started the night before. During questioning of the parent about the child's symptoms, the pharmacist learns that Tess refused to eat lunch and dinner on the previous day and began vomiting around bedtime. Six episodes of vomiting occurred during the period from bedtime until this morning. The child was able to drink small amounts of liquids between episodes of vomiting. The parent requests a recommendation for a nonprescription antiemetic.

During the interview, the pharmacist determines that the child has no medical problems and takes no chronic medications. Although the child occasionally receives acetaminophen as needed, she has not taken it in the past 24 hours because her temperature is 98.6°F (37°C).

Clinical Considerations/Strategies

Readers can use the following considerations/strategies to determine whether treatment of the patient's condition with nonprescription medications is warranted:

- Assess the appropriateness of giving the child an antiemetic. If appropriate, recommend a nonprescription product.
- Assess the need for medical referral.
- Recommend the appropriate steps in managing this child's nausea and vomiting.

Patient Education/Counseling

Readers can use the following strategies to develop a patient education/counseling plan that will help ensure optimal therapeutic outcomes:

- Explain proper use of the recommended nonprescription antiemetic.
- Explain which signs/symptoms require medical referral.

Evaluation of concurrent signs and symptoms is useful in determining the potential cause of vomiting. Preexisting disease is also an important factor to rule out. Detailed information about the patient's medical history related to the GI tract is especially helpful to determine potential causes.

Pharmacists should be aware that some patients might use nonprescription antiemetics to self-treat the early stages of a serious illness. Many patients choose to self-medicate their nausea and vomiting with various nonprescription products to avoid a medical office visit. However, the pharmacist should be cautious about recommending self-medication for these symptoms and should ask appropriate questions to determine whether referral to a health care provider is indicated.

Asking the patient the following questions will help elicit the information needed to accurately assess the cause of the symptoms and to recommend the appropriate treatment approach.

Q~ For whom is the medication intended? (If for someone else) How old is the patient?

A~ Base the appropriateness of self-treatment and the type of self-care on the patient's age.

Q~ How long has the nausea or vomiting been present?

A~ Refer cases of chronic or prolonged nausea and vomiting (longer than 24 to 48 hours), especially in children younger than 1 year, to a physician.

Q~ Do you know what caused the nausea and vomiting? Are you pregnant? Do you have diabetes or other medical problems?

A~ Refer cases of nausea and vomiting secondary to a poorly controlled medical condition for immediate medical attention. Recommend nondrug measures to pregnant patients. For situational cases of vomiting, such as motion sickness, recommend an appropriate self-treatment.

Q~ What medications are you currently taking?

A~ *Identify medications that can cause nausea and vomiting. (See Table 16–1.)* If the patient is taking any of these medications, consult with the physician about discontinuing the medication or decreasing the dose. If appropriate, advise the patient to take medication with food or to change the timing of doses.

Q~ What foods or liquids have you recently consumed?

A~ If food poisoning is suspected and the symptoms have been present for less than 36 hours, recommend the appropriate self-treatment. (See the section "Nausea and Vomiting Related to Food Poisoning.") For symptoms of food poisoning that have persisted for longer than 36 hours, refer the patient to a physician.

Q~ Have you noted other signs or symptoms, such as diarrhea, abdominal pain, headache, fever, weight loss, muscle pain, visual changes, altered behavior, or pain outside the abdominal area? Have you noted blood in the vomitus or stool?

A~ For cases of nausea and vomiting associated with diarrhea, suspect viral gastroenteritis and recommend appropriate self-treatment if other more serious symptoms are absent. Refer to a physician the cases of nausea and vomiting associated with any of the other symptoms listed above.

Patient Education for Nausea and Vomiting

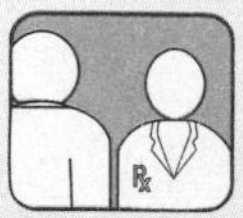

The objectives of self-treatment are (1) to prevent or control symptoms of occasional mild, self-limiting nausea and vomiting, (2) to improve the symptoms and the patient's overall sense of well-being, and (3) to avoid unnecessary emergency health care visits. For most patients, carefully following product instructions and the self-care measures listed below will help ensure optimal therapeutic outcomes.

Nondrug Measures

- To prevent "morning sickness," eat small, frequent meals that are low in fat content. Also try eating crackers before getting up in the morning. Try lying down to relieve the symptoms once they occur.
- To prevent motion sickness in young children, place them in a car seat that allows them to see out the front window. Try acupressure wristbands to prevent motion sickness in adults or in older children.
- To prevent nausea associated with overeating, avoid foods or beverages known to cause nausea; consume other foods and beverages in moderation.

Nonprescription Medications

Antacids, Histamine$_2$-Receptor Antagonists, or Bismuth Subsalicylate

- Take antacids, histamine$_2$-receptor antagonists (ranitidine, famotidine, cimetidine, or nizatidine), or bismuth subsalicylate (Pepto-Bismol) for nausea caused by overeating. Follow product instructions for dosages.
- Do not take bismuth subsalicylate if you are taking medications that interact with salicylates.
- Do not give bismuth subsalicylate to children or teenagers who have viral influenza or chicken pox. Reye's syndrome, a rare but potentially fatal condition, could occur.

Phosphorated Carbohydrate Solution

- Take phosphorated carbohydrate solutions for nausea and vomiting associated with upset stomach caused by viral gastroenteritis, food indiscretions, and emotional upset. (See Table 16–2 for brand-name products.)
- Give 1 to 2 tablespoons of the solution to adults at 15-minute intervals until vomiting stops. Do not give more than five doses in 1 hour.
- Do not dilute the solution, and do not allow the patient to consume other liquids for 15 minutes after taking a dose.
- Do not take this product if you have hereditary fructose intolerance.
- If you have diabetes, consult your physician before taking this product.

Antihistamines

- Take antihistamines for self-treatment of nausea and vomiting caused by motion sickness.
- To prevent motion sickness, take antihistamines at least 30 to 60 minutes before departure for travel. Continue taking the medication during travel. Follow the dosage guidelines in Table 16–3.
- Avoid driving or operating hazardous machinery or engaging in tasks requiring a high degree of mental alertness while using antihistamines. Drowsiness is the most common adverse effect of these medications.
- If you have asthma, narrow-angle glaucoma, obstructive disease of the GI or genitourinary tract, or benign prostatic hypertrophy, consult a physician before using antihistamines.
- Be aware that antihistamines can increase the sedative effects of alcohol, tranquilizers, hypnotics, and sedatives.

Oral Rehydration Solutions

- If needed, take an oral rehydration solution to prevent dehydration secondary to vomiting and diarrhea.

Seek medical attention if vomiting does not stop after five doses of a phosphorated carbohydrate solution.

Seek medical attention if any of the following signs and symptoms or medical conditions are associated with the nausea and vomiting:

—Blood in the vomitus.

—Abdominal pain or distention.

—Projectile vomiting or prolonged nausea and vomiting (more than 24 to 48 hours), especially in children younger than 1 year.

—Dehydration.

—Weight loss of more than 5% of body weight.

—Fever.

—Severe headache.

—Change in behavior or alertness.

—Pregnancy.

—Presence of diabetes or other medical conditions that may be affected by lack of nutritional intake or by missed doses of oral medications.

—Recent trauma, particularly a significant head injury.

—Suspected poisoning.

Patient Counseling for Nausea and Vomiting

The pharmacist should stress that treatment of nausea and vomiting should focus on identifying and, if possible, correcting the underlying cause. Patients prone to overeating, bulimia, or motion sickness should, when possible, avoid these behaviors or situations that cause nausea and vomiting. The patient should be advised that most cases of acute vomiting require only symptomatic treatment because they are self-limiting and will resolve spontaneously. If the cause of the symptoms is known and if self-treatment is appropriate, the pharmacist should explain the proper use of the recommended product. Patient counseling should include information about possible adverse effects as well as signs and symptoms that indicate medical attention is required. The box "Patient Education for Nausea and Vomiting" lists specific information to provide patients.

Evaluation of Patient Outcomes for Nausea and Vomiting

A follow-up assessment of the patient should occur within 24 hours of the initial encounter to determine whether symptoms have improved, changed, or worsened. Prolonged nausea and vomiting (longer than 24 to 48 hours) or a change or worsening of symptoms requires immediate referral to a health care provider.

CONCLUSIONS

Because nausea and vomiting are symptoms of an underlying disorder, treatment should focus on identifying and correcting the underlying cause. Nonprescription antiemetic medications are suitable for preventing and controlling the symptoms of occasional self-limiting nausea and vomiting. Food overindulgence, food poisoning, and motion sickness can cause self-limiting cases of these symptoms.

The loss of fluids and the inability to eat or drink because of nausea and vomiting can result in dehydration and electrolyte disturbances. This primary complication of nausea and vomiting should be treated with ORSs.

References

1. Miller AD. Central mechanisms of vomiting. *Dig Dis Sci.* 1999;44:39S–43S.
2. McQuaid KR. Alimentary tract. In: Tierny LM, McPhee SJ, Papadakis MA, eds. *Current Medical Diagnosis and Treatment.* 36th ed. Stamford, CT: Appleton & Lange; 1997:519–606.
3. McQuaid Taylor AT, Holland EG. Nausea and vomiting. In: Dipiro JT, Talbert RT, Yee GC, et al., eds. *Pharmacotherapy: A Pathophysiologic Approach.* 3rd ed. Stamford, CT: Appleton & Lange; 1996:751–65.
4. Brownlee HJ. Family practitioner's guide to patient self-treatment of acute diarrhea. *Am J Med.* 1990;88:27S–9S.
5. Jospe N, Forbes G. Fluids and electrolytes—clinical aspects. *Pediatr Rev.* 1996;17:395–403.
6. Kousen M. Treatment of nausea and vomiting in pregnancy. *Am Fam Physician.* 1993;48:1279–83.
7. Johnson PC, Ericsson CD. Acute diarrhea in developed countries. *Am J Med.* 1990;88(suppl 6A):5S–9S.
8. Hyde E. Acupressure therapy for morning sickness. A controlled clinical trial. *J Nurse Midwifery.* 1989;34:171–8.
9. DeAloysio D, Penachioni P. Morning sickness control in early pregnancy by Neiguan point acupressure. *Obstet Gynecol.* 1992;80:852–4.
10. Stainton MC, Neff EJ. The efficacy of SeaBands for the control of nausea and vomiting in pregnancy. *Health Care Women Int.* 1994;15:563–75.
11. Newton GD, McCullough JA, Pray WS, et al. New OTC drugs and devices 1999: A selective review. *J Am Pharm Assoc.* 2000:49(2):225–6.
12. Hu S, Stritzel R, Chandler A, Stern R. P6 acupressure reduces symptoms of vection induced motion sickness. *Aviat Space Eviron Med.* 1995;66:631–4.
13. Hu S, Stern R, Koch K. Electrical acustimulation relieves vection-induced motion sickness. *Gastroent.* 1992;102:1854–8.
14. Bertolucci L, DiDario B. Efficacy of a portable acustimulation device in controlling seasickness. *Aviat Space Environ Med.* 1995;66:1155–7.
15. Dundee J, Yang J, McMillan C. Non-invasive stimulation of the P6 (Neiguan) antiemetic acupuncture point in cancer chemotherapy. *J R Soc Med.* 1991;84:210–2.
16. Mitchelson F. Pharmacological agents affecting emesis. A review. *Drugs.* 1992;43:295–315.
17. Shapiro S, Heinonen OP, Siskind V, et al. Antenatal drug exposure to doxylamine succinate and dicyclomine hydrochloride (Bendectin) in relation to congenital malformations, perinatal mortality rate, birth weight, and intelligence quotient score. *Am J Obstet Gynecol.* 1977;128:480–5.
18. Leathem AM. Safety and efficacy of antiemetics used to treat nausea and vomiting in pregnancy. *Clin Pharm.* 1986;5:660–8.
19. Sahakian V, Rouse D, Sipes S, et al. Vitamin B_6 is effective therapy for nausea and vomiting of pregnancy: a randomized, double-blind placebo-controlled study. *Obstet Gynecol.* 1991;78:33–6.
20. Balisteri WF. Oral rehydration in acute infantile diarrhea. *Am J Med.* 1990;88:30S–3S.

CHAPTER 17

Poisoning

Gary M. Oderda

Chapter 17 at a Glance

Poisoning is a common and potentially life-threatening condition in both children and adults. The body attempts to rid itself of a variety of toxins and poisons by inducing vomiting. Nonprescription emetic medications are also used to induce vomiting. These agents are intended primarily for the treatment of poisoning.

Epidemiology of Poisoning

Unintentional poisonings occur most often in children younger than 5 years of age. Such events are a leading cause of injury-related hospitalizations in preschoolers, even though fatalities among preschoolers have declined significantly during the past 30 years. During 1997, 66 poison centers throughout the United States, serving a population of 267.6 million, submitted 2,192,088 cases to the American Association of Poison Control Centers' (AAPCC) Toxic Exposure Surveillance System (TESS).[1] The majority of the poison exposures (52.5%) and deaths (3.2%) occurred in children younger than 6 years of age.[1] Although poison-related deaths in children have declined by 90% since the 1960s, poison ingestion remains a common pediatric health concern, requiring significant expenditures of health care dollars for inpatient and outpatient care.

Etiology of Poisoning

Poisoning can occur from thousands of chemicals and products from different routes of exposure, such as oral ingestion and inhalation. Chemicals used in occupational settings, household cleaning supplies, cosmetics and personal care products, automotive supplies such as gasoline or antifreeze, pesticides, and medications are some of the most common sources of poisoning.

Signs and Symptoms of Poisoning

The signs and symptoms of poisoning can affect every organ system and can range in severity from mild to life threatening. Variable manifestations result from the number of poisonous agents and the different routes of exposure. Because of delays in absorption and the need for some agents, such as methanol, to be metabolized to produce toxicity, patients may be asymptomatic for a period of time and then go on to develop severe toxicity.

Editor's Note: This chapter is based, in part, on the 11th edition chapter titled "Emetic and Antiemetic Products," which was written by Gary M. Oderda and Jenifer C. Jennings.

Treatment of Poisoning

A poison center should be contacted in all cases in which poisoning is suspected. The poison center staff will help the pharmacist determine whether self-treatment is appropriate. (See the section "Patient Assessment of Poisoning" for the type of information needed to determine the appropriate treatment approach.)

Treatment Outcomes

Emetics are used in acute poisoning episodes to remove potentially toxic agents from the gastrointestinal (GI) tract. The goal of therapy is to decrease the amount of the toxic substance that is absorbed. The ideal treatment outcome is to prevent further progression of toxicity and to prevent mortality, serious morbidity, and sequelae.

General Treatment Approach

Treatment of poisoning depends primarily on basic management principles such as preventing absorption and providing supportive care. Support of vital functions, especially respiratory and cardiovascular, is critical. Treatment of specific signs and symptoms such as seizures is also important, as are other specific actions, including emptying the stomach and administering agents such as adsorbents, cathartics, or antidotes. Stomach contents may be removed by mechanical lavage or administration of an emetic, such as ipecac syrup. Both types of treatment are more effective if undertaken shortly after ingestion of the poison. However, these treatments supplement symptomatic and supportive care, which is the mainstay of successfully managing the poisoned patient. Figure 17–1 outlines an appropriate process for self-care of poisoning.

Exclusions to Self-Treatment with Emetics

Use of emetics for poisonings that involve certain substances or patients in certain physical states can do more harm than good. A brief discussion of such substances and the signs and symptoms that preclude self-treatment follows. In general, all ingestions in which moderate-to-severe toxicity is possible must be referred to an emergency treatment facility.

Use of emetics in cases of acute overdose of antiemetic medications is controversial. A theoretical concern exists that if an emetic is not given soon after the antiemetic has been ingested, a significant emetic failure rate may result. In practice, using emetics in such cases does not appear to be a problem.[2]

Presence of Central Nervous System Effects

Efforts to induce vomiting should not be attempted in patients who are lethargic, somnolent, or comatose because those patients are at high risk of aspirating gastric contents while vomiting. A high risk of aspiration also exists if vomiting occurs when seizures are present. Similarly, emetics are generally not recommended when patients have taken agents that may produce a rapid decrease in the level of consciousness (e.g., antidepressants) or may rapidly produce seizures (e.g., camphor or amphetamines). The stimulation of vomiting may enhance the epileptogenic potential of the poison.

Ingestion of Caustic Substances

Patients who have ingested a caustic substance should *not* be made to vomit. Caustic agents are strong acids or bases that can severely burn the mucous membranes of the GI tract, including the mouth, esophagus, and stomach. Should vomiting occur, the esophagus and oral cavity would be reexposed to the caustic agent and more damage could occur. In addition, if the esophagus is already damaged, the force of vomiting could cause esophageal or gastric perforation.

When ingestion of a caustic agent is suspected, the patient—if conscious and able to drink—should immediately be given water or milk to dilute the agent. Attempts to neutralize the agent using an acid or base would generate heat and produce more serious injury and must, therefore, be avoided. Most patients who have ingested a caustic agent should be immediately referred to a medical facility.

Ingestion of Hydrocarbons

Patients who have ingested aliphatic hydrocarbons (e.g., kerosene, gasoline, or furniture polish) traditionally have not been given emetics because induced vomiting was thought to increase the likelihood of pulmonary aspiration, leading to alveolar irritation and pneumonitis. Studies have since shown that aspiration is not likely to occur when vomiting is induced. However, emptying the stomach of aliphatic hydrocarbons is generally not necessary and should not be done outside of an emergency care facility.

Nonpharmacologic Therapy

Gastric lavage is a procedure in which a tube is placed into the stomach through the mouth or nose and the esophagus. Normal saline is then instilled into the tube, allowed to mix with stomach contents, and removed by suction or aspiration. Gastric lavage is reserved for use in health care facilities. During 1997, gastric lavage was used in 53,342 of the patients reported to the AAPCC TESS data collection system.[1] This number represents 2.4% of all reported patients.

Vomiting can be mechanically induced by giving the patient fluids and then manually stimulating the gag reflex at the back of the throat with either a blunt object or a finger. The percentage of people who vomit following this procedure is low, however, and the mean volume of vomitus is small compared with that induced by ipecac syrup.[3] Thus, lack of efficacy and potential injury to the patient preclude the use of mechanically induced vomiting.

Pharmacologic Therapy

Ipecac syrup, an emetic, is the only appropriate agent for self-treatment of poisoning to induce vomiting. Use of home remedies for emesis should be discouraged. Activated charcoal, an adsorbent, is another nonprescription agent for treating poisoning; however, it is used primarily in health

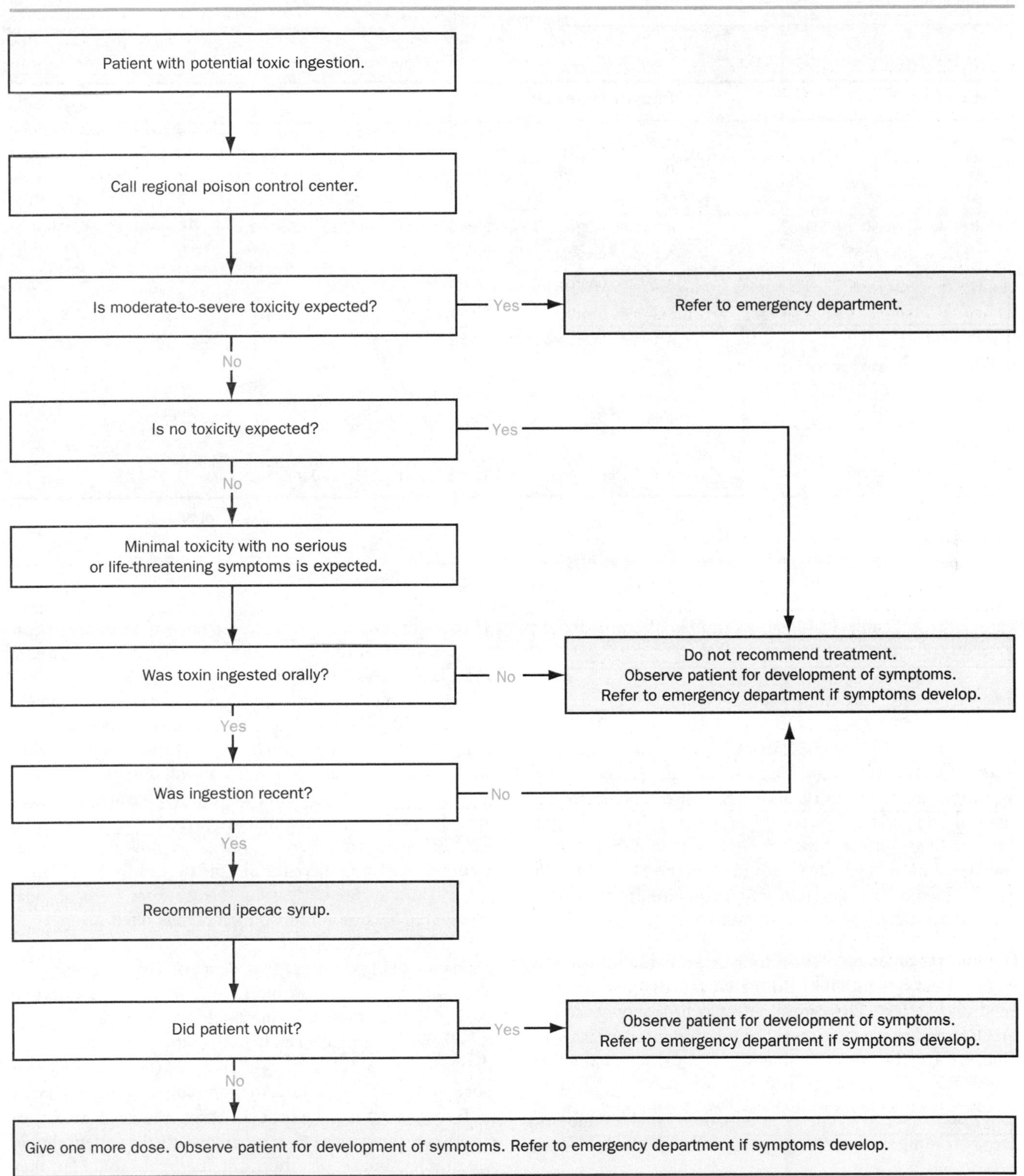

Figure 17–1 Self-care of poisoning.

Table 17–1

Selected Nonprescription Agents for Treating Poisoning

Trade Name	Primary Ingredients
Emetics	
Ipecac Syrup	Powdered ipecac
Activated Charcoal Products	
Actidose-Aqua Liquid	Activated charcoal 15 g/72 mL, 25 g/120 mL, 50 g/240 mL
CharcoAid G Granules[a,b]	Activated charcoal 15 g/120 mL
Insta-Char Cherry Flavored Suspension	Activated charcoal 25 g/120 mL, 50 g/240 mL
Insta-Char Unflavored Suspension	Activated charcoal 50 g/240 mL
Liqui Char	Activated charcoal 25 g/120 mL
Activated Charcoal–Cathartic Products	
Actidose with Sorbitol Liquid	Activated charcoal 25 g/120 mL, 50 g/240 mL, sorbitol
Insta-Char and Cherry Flavored Suspension with Sorbitol	Activated charcoal 25 g/120 mL, 50 g/240 mL, sorbitol 25 g/120 mL, 50 g/240 mL
Liqui Char with Sorbitol	Activated charcoal 25 g/120 mL, sorbitol 27 g/120 mL

[a] Dye-free product.

[b] Sucrose-free product.

care settings. Table 17–1 lists examples of commercially available products.

Emetic Treatment with Ipecac Syrup

Of the 2,192,088 cases reported to TESS during 1997, ipecac syrup was used in 32,098 cases.[1] This number represents 1.5% of all reported human exposures. This percentage has steadily decreased from 1983, when 13.4% of all reported human poison exposure received ipecac syrup. Ipecac syrup is the emetic of choice, however. It is prepared from ipecac powder, a natural product derived from the plant *Cephaelis ipecacuanha* or *C. acuminata*, and it contains approximately 2.1 g of powdered ipecac per 30 mL.

Mechanism of Action Vomiting is probably induced by both a local irritant effect on the GI mucosa and a central medullary effect. The central effect is probably caused by emetine and cephaeline, two alkaloids present in ipecac. (See Chapter 16, "Nausea and Vomiting," for discussion of the physiology of vomiting.)

Indication Syrup of ipecac is approved by the Food and Drug Administration (FDA) as an emetic for use in some poisonings.

Dosage/Administration Guidelines For children 1 year of age or older, the recommended dose of ipecac syrup is 15 mL (1 tablespoon). This dose can be repeated once if vomiting has not occurred within 20 minutes. Children from age 6 months to 1 year may be given 5 to 10 mL (1 to 2 teaspoons). Although home use of ipecac in children younger than 1 year of age is controversial, the product has been shown to be safe and effective.[4] For adolescents and adults, the initial dose is 15 to 30 mL, and it can be repeated once, if necessary. Ipecac syrup is highly effective at inducing vomiting when 15 mL or more is given.[5]

Fluid administration is generally recommended immediately after the ipecac dose. Children should receive 4 to 8 ounces of fluid; adults should receive 12 to 16 ounces. One study[6] of adult volunteers given a 15-mL dose of ipecac suggests that it takes longer to induce vomiting when milk is given after the ipecac than when water is given. However, two studies[7,8] of overdosed children given either milk or water after ipecac showed no difference in time needed for vomiting to occur. Thus, the use of clear fluids (e.g., water, juice, or soda) is preferred because administration of milk offers no apparent advantages over that of clear fluids. Also, milk may obscure examination of the vomitus for evidence of tablets and capsules. Vomiting should occur within 15 to 20 minutes. If it does not, the initial dose of ipecac syrup should be repeated.

Whether fluids are given before or after ipecac or whether the fluids are tepid (104°F or 40°C) or cold (50°F or 10°C) does not appear to affect the time for vomiting to occur in adults.[9]

If the patient is to be brought to an emergency facility or health care provider's office for follow-up, the patient should vomit into a bucket or other container that should be taken to the treatment facility so the vomitus can be inspected for evidence of the poison.

Adverse Effects Toxicity following administration of ipecac syrup is rare. After therapeutic doses are given, diarrhea and slight depression of the central nervous system (CNS) are common; mild GI upset may last for several hours following emesis. Clinical experience has shown that ingestion of 30 mL of ipecac syrup (the largest amount available without a prescription in a single unit of purchase) is safe in children older than 1 year of age. The death of a 14-month-old child following the administration of less than 30 mL given for an ingestion of amaryllis leaves was not a direct result of the pharmacologic effects of ipecac but rather resulted from a congenital anomaly.[10] In larger chronic doses, ipecac is cardiotoxic and may cause hypotension, bradycardia, atrial fibrillation, ventricular fibrillation, and death.[11] A fatal intracerebral hemorrhage was reported in an 84-year-old woman given a therapeutic dose of ipecac syrup and activated charcoal following a nontoxic dose of boric acid.[12]

Fluidextract of ipecac is 14 times stronger than ipecac syrup and should no longer be found in any pharmacy. Severe toxicity and death have occurred when fluidextract of ipecac was given by mistake.[13]

Inappropriate Use of Ipecac Several cases of chronic ipecac poisoning by proxy have been reported. In those cases, parents had repeatedly given ipecac syrup to their children and had sought medical attention for the children's repeated vomiting.[14] This situation has been described as a form of Munchausen syndrome by proxy.[14] Most patients demonstrated recurrent GI effects, including grossly bloody stools, and other effects such as cardiomyopathy.[14]

Pharmacists must be aware that ipecac syrup is used inappropriately by some bulimic patients to remove food from the stomach and to lose weight. This practice is particularly dangerous because it brings about a drug-induced fluid and electrolyte imbalance and cardiotoxicity. However, the abuse problem does not warrant removing 1-ounce (30-mL) bottles of ipecac syrup from nonprescription status.[15] Pharmacists should question any person buying ipecac syrup regularly to be certain it is being purchased for its appropriate use, and they should view with suspicion frequent purchases by the same person.

Drug–Drug Interactions The only potential drug interaction with ipecac syrup involves activated charcoal. Activated charcoal is used as an adsorbent in many poisoning cases. When it is administered with ipecac, the concern has been that the ipecac may be adsorbed by the charcoal, thus delaying or preventing emesis. In addition, the adsorptive capacity of the charcoal could be reduced. However, a prospective study[16] allayed these concerns. In fact, no scientific evidence supports the fact that administering ipecac syrup at the same time as, or after, activated charcoal inhibits vomiting. This combination is not recommended, however, because patients given ipecac are very likely to vomit the activated charcoal.

Use of Outdated Ipecac Using drugs beyond their stated expiration date is generally not recommended. If, however, parents have an expired container of ipecac syrup and it is the only ipecac available, should it be used? A study[17] demonstrated no difference in the percentage of patients who vomited or in the amount of time lapsed before vomiting when ipecac was used by the expiration date as opposed to after that date. The ipecac used in this study ranged from 1 month to 16 years beyond the expiration date.

Unacceptable Emetic Methods

Vomiting may be induced in numerous ways. Home remedies (emetics) other than ipecac, however, produce unpredictable results, are often ineffective, are sometimes dangerous, and, thus, are not recommended.

Liquid dishwashing detergent, which contains anionic and nonionic surfactants, has been studied as an emetic agent.[18] Its effectiveness could not be determined because many patients refused to drink any or all of it. However, those who did drink most of the administered solution vomited.

Salt water is an unpalatable, unreliable, and potentially dangerous emetic. Salt solutions may be quite toxic because of sodium absorption. Severe hypernatremia may result, and the use of salt as an emetic has produced fatalities in children and adults.[19,20] It is estimated that 1 tablespoon (15 mL) of salt contains about 250 mEq of sodium. If retained and absorbed, this amount could raise the serum sodium level by 25 mEq/L in a healthy 3-year-old child with an estimated total body water of 10 L. Thus, salt water should *not* be used under any circumstances.

Mustard water is an unreliable and unpalatable emetic that should not be recommended.

Copper sulfate has been used as an emetic. It acts by producing direct gastric irritation that leads to direct stimulation of the vomiting center. According to the available data, copper sulfate is an effective emetic. However, concerns about copper absorption and its potential toxicity[21] preclude recommending this agent to induce emesis.

Apomorphine, an opiate analogue, produces rapid emesis. However, it is available only by prescription and must be given parenterally. Apomorphine may produce or worsen CNS and respiratory depression. Naloxone given intravenously can usually reverse those effects. In several cases, however, significant respiratory and/or CNS depression that is unresponsive to naloxone has developed in patients given apomorphine.[22]

Sticking the finger down the patient's throat to stimulate gagging is also ineffective and potentially harmful.

Treatment with Activated Charcoal and Cathartics

As shown in Figure 17–2, the use of ipecac syrup in poison management over the past 15 years has decreased significantly, whereas the use of activated charcoal has dramatically increased.[1] Because ipecac syrup is used primarily in children in the home, some of the decrease in ipecac use reflects the decrease in the percentage of children younger than 6 years of age in the TESS system (64% in 1983, 52.5% in 1977).[1]

Mechanism of Action Activated charcoal is an effective adsorbent for most drugs and chemicals.

Indications Activated charcoal is FDA-approved for use as an emergency antidote in the treatment of poisoning.

Dosage/Administration Guidelines Activated charcoal is usually administered as a water slurry of 60 to 100 g of activated charcoal for adults or 15 to 30 g of activated charcoal for children in a minimum of 8 ounces of water. A larger dose of charcoal may require more than 8 ounces of water to

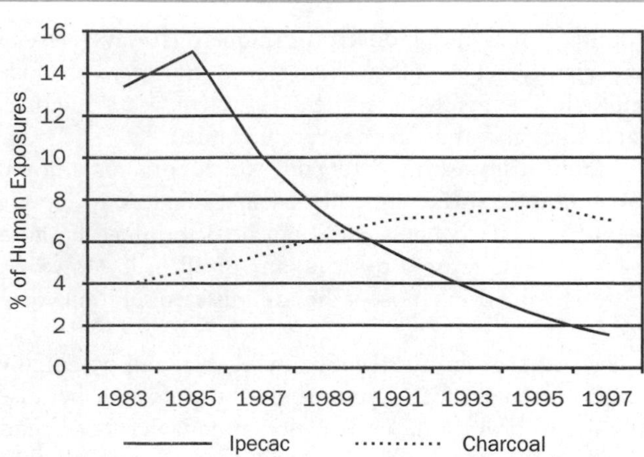

Figure 17–2 Use of ipecac and activated charcoal in poisoned patients, 1983–1997. Reprinted with permission from reference 1.

yield the proper consistency for administration orally or by gastric tube. The slurry can be prepared by adding water to a container with activated charcoal and shaking it. Because measuring the correct amount of charcoal is difficult, preweighed packages are available.

Activated charcoal products that are premixed with water, sorbitol (for catharsis), or water and carboxymethylcellulose are also commercially available. (See Table 17–1.) When multiple doses of activated charcoal are given, a cathartic should be given only with the first dose. Pharmacists should check premixed charcoal products to see if they contain sorbitol. If they do, other cathartics should not be given, and the sorbitol-containing product should be given only initially. If the activated charcoal does not contain sorbitol, a single dose of a saline cathartic, such as magnesium sulfate or magnesium citrate, may be administered after charcoal administration if bowel sounds are present. This process speeds elimination of the charcoal drug complex through the GI tract.

Optimally, activated charcoal should be given as soon as possible after ingestion of the poison. However, it has sometimes been shown to be effective even when administration has been delayed by several hours. No maximum dose limit is given because no systemic toxicity exists. Repeat doses of activated charcoal may be recommended to interrupt enterohepatic recycling of some drugs (e.g., phenobarbital or theophylline) secreted into the GI tract. Contrary to popular belief, burnt toast is not a substitute for activated charcoal and is not indicated in the treatment of poisoning.

Although not effective for all ingestions, activated charcoal can reduce absorption of many poisons, such as analgesics (e.g., salicylates, acetaminophen, or propoxyphene), sedatives, hypnotics, and tricyclic antidepressants.[23] (See Table 17–2.) In the past, a "universal antidote" mixture of activated charcoal, magnesium oxide, and tannic acid was used. However, this combination is ineffective.

Table 17–2

Compounds That Effectively Bind Activated Charcoal in the GI Tract

Well Adsorbed	Moderately Adsorbed
Alphatoxins	Aspirin and other salicylates
Amphetamines	DDT
Antidepressants	Disopyramide
Antiepileptics	Kerosene, benzene, dichloroethane
Antihistamines	Malathion
Atropine	Mexiletine
Barbiturates	NSAIDs
Benzodiazepines	Paracetamol (acetaminophen)
β-Blocking agents	PCBs
Chloroquine and primaquine	Phenol
Cimetidine	Syrup of ipecac
Dapsone	Tolbutamide, chlorpropamide, carbutamide, tolazamide
Dextropropoxyphene and other opioids	**Poorly or Clinically Inadequately Adsorbed**
Digitalis glycosides	Cyanide
Ergot alkaloids	Ethanol
Furosemide	Ethylene glycol
Glibenclamide and glipizide	Iron
Glutethimide	Lithium
Indomethacin	Methanol
Meprobabate	Strong acids and alkali
Nefopam	
Phenothiazines	
Phenylbutazone	
Phenylpropanolamine	
Piroxicam	
Quinidine and quinine	
Strychnine	
Tetracycline	
Theophylline	

Adverse Effects The most common adverse effects of activated charcoal are vomiting and black stools. When given with sorbitol, diarrhea, abdominal cramps, and electrolyte abnormalities may be seen.

Pharmacotherapeutic Comparison of Poisoning Treatments

The comparative efficacy of methods to treat poisoning is an important factor in determining which method to recommend. Studies have compared the use of ipecac with gastric lavage and the use of activated charcoal with both methods of GI decontamination.

Ipecac versus Gastric Lavage Several studies have compared the efficacy of ipecac treatment and gastric lavage in removing gastric contents. One study[24] found ipecac to be superior in removing salicylates from 20 patients who were 12 to 20 months of age; another study[25] found it superior in removing a toxic dose of aspirin from two adults. A third study[26] determined that ipecac was three times as effective as gastric lavage when treatment was delayed. However, prospective studies[27–30] using markers, including thiamine, technetium-99m, and cyanocobalamin, in overdosed patients found that gastric lavage was superior to induced emesis. Concerns relating to methodologic interpretation leave study results unresolved.

Saetta and Aminton[31] found intragastric solids remaining in 38.5% of patients who vomited following administration of ipecac syrup and in 88.2% of patients following gastric lavage. In a follow-up study, however, when Saetta et al.[32] administered barium-impregnated polyethylene pellets to poisoned patients immediately before gastric lavage or ipecac syrup, 58.5% of the pellets were retained following ipecac syrup as compared with 51.5% following gastric lavage. Moreover, the number of pellets in the small intestine at the end of the procedure was greater in both the ipecac and gastric lavage groups than it was in an untreated control group. These studies, thus, suggest that neither ipecac nor gastric lavage is solely effective in emptying the stomach and that, in fact, both procedures may enhance movement of gastric contents into the small intestine. This finding reinforces the importance of administering activated charcoal to poisoned patients.

In general, ipecac syrup, when used with appropriate instruction and follow-up, is the only safe and effective in-home method of induced emesis. Not only can it prevent emergency room visits, but also in those cases when treatment in the hospital is necessary, it allows for earlier administration and vomiting. In the hospital setting, however, both induced emesis and gastric lavage are often used. Most hospitals prefer lavage over ipecac, particularly for adults; others have stopped using GI decontamination in favor of activated charcoal alone.

Activated Charcoal versus Gastrointestinal Decontamination

The possible benefits of ipecac or gastric lavage over activated charcoal in preventing absorption from the GI tract and toxicity are unclear. Two studies[33,34] in human volunteers used near-therapeutic doses of drugs or simulated drug overdoses. Two other studies[35,36] used a prospective clinic-trial design to compare use of activated charcoal alone with that of activated charcoal plus either gastric lavage or ipecac in overdose patients treated in an emergency room. In general, both pairs of studies showed no added benefit of gastric lavage or ipecac plus activated charcoal over charcoal alone in hospital-treated patients. Kulig et al.[35] did show a benefit for early gastric lavage (within 1 hour of the exposure) and activated charcoal when compared with activated charcoal alone. In the home, however, activated charcoal is not a viable substitute for ipecac syrup because it is difficult for parents to administer a therapeutic dose to children successfully. Ipecac syrup is intended primarily for patients who will be treated at home and for pediatric patients treated in a hospital setting who will not be given activated charcoal.

These recommendations are consistent with a recent series of position statements published by the American Academy of Clinical Toxicology and the European Association of Poison Control Centers and Clinical Toxicologists. Their conclusions include the following: (1) No evidence from clinical studies shows that ipecac improves the outcome of poisoned patients, and its routine recommendation in the emergency department should be abandoned.[37] (2) The administration of activated charcoal may be considered if a patient has ingested a potentially toxic amount of a poison (which is known to be adsorbed to charcoal) up to 1 hour previously; insufficient data support or exclude its use after 1 hour of ingestion.[38]

Product Selection Guidelines

Although activated charcoal products are available as nonprescription medications, ipecac syrup is the preferred self-treatment for poisoning of minimal toxicity in children.

Pharmacoeconomics of Poisoning Management

Data are not available to adequately describe the pharmacoeconomics of poisoning management. Indirect data do exist that allow general conclusions regarding the value of poison centers and home therapy for poisoning. For every dollar spent on poison center services, $8 in savings is realized.[39] A significant portion of the cost savings results from managing and observing patients at home who use agents such as ipecac syrup that reduce transport and emergency treatment costs.

Patient Assessment of Poisoning

Assessment of poisoned patients is the same as that for patients involved in other medical emergencies. The most important areas to address are listed below. Some of these measures apply to assessment in a nonhospital setting; others do not.

- Check whether the airway is open.
- Check whether the patient is breathing. If so, check whether the patient is adequately oxygenated.
- Check whether blood circulation is affected. Specifically, determine whether the patient (1) is hypotensive

or hypertensive, (2) is exhibiting bradycardia or tachycardia, or (3) is having ventricular arrhythmias.

- Check whether the patient's mental status is altered. Specifically, determine whether the patient (1) is in a coma or stupor, (2) is exhibiting hypothermia or hyperthermia, (3) is having seizures, or (4) is agitated.

It is often difficult to decide whether a patient should be referred directly to an emergency treatment facility, be given a nonprescription emetic and managed at home, or be given no treatment. Because poison centers have specialized resources not usually available to pharmacists in general practice and have considerable experience in dealing with poisoned patients, this decision must involve the poison center. Patients can call the poison center directly, or the pharmacist can call for the patient. Knowing the telephone number of the nearest poison center is critical because guidance from a poison center must always be obtained.

Obtaining a reliable history, identifying the agent, and accurately assessing the patient's condition are critical steps in determining appropriate treatment for a poisoned patient. All ingestions in which moderate-to-severe toxicity is possible must be referred to an emergency treatment facility. If minimal toxicity (no serious or life-threatening symptoms) is anticipated, the administration of a nonprescription emetic at home by a competent adult may be all that is necessary. Many ingestions reported to poison control centers fall into this category. For example, a child who ingests aspirin at 150 to 300 mg/kg of body weight can usually be treated at home by emesis induced with ipecac syrup and appropriate follow-up by center staff members. If an emetic is indicated, the pharmacist should also determine whether any contraindications exist to its use and whether the emetic can be administered safely outside an emergency treatment facility. (See the section "Exclusions to Self-Treatment with Emetics.")

If a patient asks to purchase ipecac syrup, the pharmacist must find out whether the ipecac is for acute use. Asking the patient the following questions will help elicit this information, as well as the information needed to interact effectively with staff members at the poison center and to determine the appropriate treatment approach.

Patient's Name and Location

Q~ Who will be taking the medication? Do you want the emetic for immediate or possible future emergency use? If for immediate use, have you spoken to a poison center?

A~ In cases of immediate poisoning, obtain the information solicited in the following questions. Contact a poison control center if the patient has not done so. Obtain the patient's and, if applicable, the caregiver's name, location, and telephone number so that poison center staff can follow up with the patient.

Patient's Age and Weight

Q~ What is the patient's age and weight?

A~ Obtain the patient's weight so that the toxicity of an agent can be determined on a dose-per-body-weight (mg/kg) basis. Determine whether self-treatment is appropriate based on the severity of toxicity. Obtain the patient's age to help determine the appropriateness of use and the appropriate dose of an emetic.

Name and Amount of Poison Ingested

Q~ What substance was taken?

A~ Obtain the name of the ingested substance from the patient or caregiver. If possible, check the product label or container to identify the substance and the amount of each ingredient. Call the manufacturer or distributor if necessary to obtain this information. Investigate the potential toxicity of each ingredient.

Amount of Poison Ingested

Q~ How much of the substance was taken?

A~ If the amount ingested is difficult to determine, as in the case of poisoning in children, base decisions on observed behavior, such as actually seeing the amount that the child took, or other objective information, such as pill counts. In the absence of reliable information, assume that a toxic dose was taken if the agent taken is potentially toxic.

Time Since Ingestion

Q~ How long ago did the ingestion occur?

A~ Based on the time of ingestion, determine whether a substantial amount of the ingested substance remains in the stomach. Emetics are usually most effective if given within 1 hour of the time of ingestion.

Prior Treatment of Poisoning

Q~ Has the patient already been given something for the ingestion?

A~ Determine whether first aid or another procedure such as those discussed in the section "Unacceptable Emetic Methods" has been performed.

Signs and Symptoms

Q~ What symptoms is the patient showing? Is the patient conscious and alert?

A~ *Identify the signs and symptoms that preclude self-treatment with an emetic. (See the section "Exclusions to Self-Treatment with Emetics.")* If the patient shows any of those signs and symptoms, refer the patient to a physician or emergency department for immediate treatment.

Other Illnesses or Medication Use

Q~ Does the patient have any chronic or acute illnesses that may affect the poisoning? Is the patient taking any nonprescription or prescription medications?

A~ Consider the effect of preexisting illnesses or therapeutic prescription or nonprescription medications on the toxicity expected from the ingested poison or on recommendations for therapy. (See the section "Exclusions to Self-Treatment with Emetics.") Consider also the degree of use of a medication. For example, patients who chronically take theophylline would have a higher risk of toxicity from an additional dose than would individuals who take the single acute dose of theophylline.

Case Study 17–1

Patient Complaint/History

The parents of an 18-month-old boy, Roberto, call the pharmacy because they found their son with an open bottle of Robitussin DM. They want to know whether the child's ingestion of the medication could cause problems and what they should do. When asked about the amount of medication ingested, the parents respond they are not sure. They report Roberto seems drowsy but it is also his usual nap time.

Clinical Considerations/Strategies

Readers can use the following considerations/strategies to determine whether treatment of the patient's condition with nonprescription medications is warranted:

- Obtain additional history on the medication exposure, including the time of the exposure, other specific symptoms, and an estimate of the amount of medication ingested.
- Contact the nearest poison control center to obtain a consultation.
- Assess the appropriateness of the parents observing the child at home, administering ipecac syrup, or taking the child to a health care facility. After assessing these alternatives, provide the parents with the appropriate recommendation(s).
- After resolution of the acute episode, develop an educational program that will help the parents prevent future drug or poison exposures.

Patient Education for Poisoning

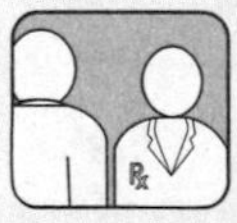

The objectives of self-treatment are (1) to prevent absorption of potentially toxic agents in the GI tract through induction of vomiting and (2) to treat patients with minimally toxic ingestions at home under supervision of a poison center. For most patients, carefully following product instructions and the self-care measures listed below will help ensure optimal therapeutic outcomes.

Treatment with Ipecac Syrup

- Take ipecac syrup to produce vomiting and to remove stomach contents.
- Expect vomiting to occur 15 to 20 minutes after administration.
- Give ipecac syrup according to the following dosage guidelines. Repeat the dose once if vomiting does not occur 20 minutes after administration.
  - —Children 6 months to 1 year: 5 to 10 mL.
  - —Children 1 year or older: 15 mL.
  - —Adolescents and adults: 15 to 30 mL.
- Give ipecac with additional liquids. Clear liquids such as water, juice, or soda are preferable to milk.
- Be aware that ipecac can cause drowsiness, diarrhea, and continued vomiting.
- Do not give ipecac syrup and activated charcoal at the same time. The charcoal will adsorb the ipecac, and vomiting will not occur.
- Do not give this medication to patients
  - —Who are lethargic or comatose or who are having seizures.
  - —Who have taken caustic substances or hydrocarbons such as gasoline or kerosene.
  - —Who have taken medications that may produce a rapid decline in consciousness or may produce seizures.

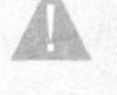
Consult the regional poison center or a physician if the patient becomes symptomatic.

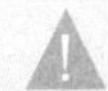
Transport the patient to an emergency department if significant symptoms develop.

Patient Counseling for Poisoning

When a patient purchases ipecac for a possible future ingestion, the pharmacist should discuss poison prevention with the patient, distribute poison prevention materials, and provide the telephone number of the nearest poison control center. Additionally, the purchaser should be advised that, whenever possible, ipecac syrup should not be given without first consulting a poison control center staff member, pharmacist, or health care provider.

Patients purchasing ipecac for immediate use that has been deemed appropriate by the poison control center should be counseled on the appropriate use of the emetic. The pharmacist should also explain the agent's potential adverse effects, as well as signs and symptoms that indicate medical attention should be sought. The box "Patient Education for Poisoning" lists specific information to provide patients or caregivers.

Evaluation of Patient Outcomes for Poisoning

The patient should be contacted 20 minutes after ipecac administration to find out whether vomiting has occurred. At least one additional contact should be made to determine whether the patient has become symptomatic. The time of the second call depends on what has been ingested, how rapidly it is absorbed, and how long it takes for symptoms to develop.

CONCLUSIONS

Although poisoning is common in adults and children, it is a potentially life-threatening disorder. A regional poison control center should be contacted in all cases of suspected poisoning. If a patient shows potentially life-threatening clinical effects (e.g., convulsions, coma, respiratory depression), transportation to an emergency department should be arranged immediately by using the emergency 911 system. For poisonings that involve minimal toxicity (i.e., no serious or life-threatening symptoms), administration of ipecac syrup by a competent adult is appropriate.

References

1. Litovitz TL, Klein-Schwartz W, Dyer KS, et al. 1997 annual report of the American Association of Poison Control Centers Toxic Exposure Surveillance System. *Am J Emerg Med.* 1998;16:443–97.
2. Manoguerra AS, Krenzelok EP. Rapid emesis from high dose ipecac syrup in adults and children intoxicated with antiemetics and other drugs. *Am J Hosp Pharm.* 1978;35:1360–2.
3. Dabbous IA, Bergman AB, Robertson WO, et al. The ineffectiveness of mechanically induced vomiting. *J Pediatr.* 1965;66:952–4.
4. Litovitz T, Klein-Schwartz W, Oderda GM, et al. Ipecac administration in children younger than 1 year of age. *Pediatrics.* 1985;76:761–4.
5. Robertson WO. Syrup of ipecac—a fast or slow emetic? *Am J Dis Child.* 1962;103:136–9.
6. Varipapa RJ, Oderda GM. Effect of milk on ipecac induced emesis. *N Engl J Med.* 1977;296:112–3.
7. Grbcich PA, Lacouture PG, Lewander WJ, et al. Effect of milk on ipecac-induced emesis. *J Pediatr.* 1987;110:973–5.
8. Klein-Schwartz W, Litovitz T, Oderda GM, et al. The effect of milk on ipecac-induced emesis. *J Toxicol Clin Toxicol.* 1991;29:505–11.
9. Spigiel RW, Abdouch I, Munn D. The effect of temperature of concurrently administered fluid on the onset of ipecac induced emesis. *Clin Toxicol.* 1979;14:281–4.
10. Robertson WO. Syrup of ipecac associated fatality: a case report. *Vet Hum Toxicol.* 1979;21:87–9.
11. McLeod J. Ipecac intoxication—use of a cardiac pacemaker in management. *N Engl J Med.* 1963;268:146–7.
12. Klein-Schwartz W, Gorman RL, Oderda GM, et al. Ipecac use in the elderly: the unanswered question. *Ann Emerg Med.* 1984;13:1152–4.
13. Smith DM, Smith RR. Acute ipecac poisoning: report of a fatal case and review of the literature. *N Engl J Med.* 1961;265:523–5.
14. Johnson JE, Carpenter BL, Benton J, et al. Hemorrhagic colitis and pseudomelanosis coli in ipecac ingestion by proxy. *J Pediatr Gastroenterol Nutr.* 1991;12:501–6.
15. Litovitz T. In defense of retaining ipecac syrup as an over-the-counter drug. *Pediatrics.* 1986;82:514–6.
16. Freedman GE, Pasternak S, Krenzelok EP. A clinical trial using ipecac and activated charcoal concurrently. *Ann Emerg Med.* 1987;16:164–6.
17. Grbcich PA, Lacouture PG, Kresel JJ, et al. Expired ipecac syrup efficacy. *Pediatrics.* 1986;78:1085–9.
18. Geisecker DR, Troutman WG. Emergency induction of emesis using liquid detergent product: a report of 15 cases. *Clin Toxicol.* 1981;18:277–82.
19. Barer J, Hill LL, Hill RM, et al. Fatal poisoning from salt used as an emetic. *Am J Dis Child.* 1973;125:889–90.
20. DeGenaro F, Nyhan W. Salt—a dangerous antidote. *J Pediatr.* 1971;78:1048–49.
21. Stein RS, Jenkins D, Korns ME. Death after cupric sulfate as emetic [letter]. *JAMA.* 1976;235:801.
22. Schofferman J. A clinical comparison of ipecac and apomorphine use in adults. *J Am Coll Emerg Phys.* 1976;5:22–5.
23. Neuvonen PJ, Olkolla KT. Oral activated charcoal in the treatment of intoxications: role of single and repeated doses. *Med Toxicol.* 1988;3:33–58.
24. Boxer L, Anderson FP, Rowe DS. Comparison of ipecac induced emesis with gastric lavage in the treatment of acute salicylate ingestion. *J Pediatr.* 1969;74:800–3.
25. Goldstein L. Emesis vs lavage for drug ingestion. *JAMA.* 1969;208:2162.
26. Arnold F Jr, Hodges JB, Barta RA, et al. Evaluation of the efficacy of lavage and induced emesis in treatment of salicylate poisoning. *Pediatrics.* 1959;23:286–301.
27. Auerbach PS, Osterloh J, Braun O, et al. Efficacy of gastric emptying: gastric lavage versus emesis induced with ipecac. *Ann Emerg Med.* 1986;15:692–8.
28. Vasquez TE, Evans DG, Ashburn WL. Efficacy of syrup of ipecac-induced emesis for emptying gastric contents. *Clin Nucl Med.* 1988;13:638–9.
29. Tandberg D, Diven GB, McLeod JW. Ipecac-induced emesis versus gastric lavage: a controlled study in normal adults. *Am J Emerg Med.* 1986;4:205–9.
30. Litovitz T. Emesis versus lavage for poisoning victims. *Am J Emerg Med.* 1986;4:294–5.
31. Saetta JP, Aminton DN. Residual gastric content after gastric lavage and ipecacuanha-induced emesis in self-poisoned patients. *J R Soc Med.* 1991;84:35–8.
32. Saetta JP, March S, Gaunt ME, et al. Gastric emptying procedures in the self-poisoned patients: are we forcing gastric contents beyond the pylorus? *J R Soc Med.* 1991;82:274–6.
33. Curtis RA, Barone J, Giacona N. Efficacy of ipecac and activated charcoal/cathartic. Prevention on salicylate absorption in a simulated overdose. *Arch Intern Med.* 1984;144:48–52.
34. Neuvonen PJ, Vartiainen M, Tokola O. Comparison of activated charcoal and ipecac syrup in prevention of drug absorption. *Eur J Clin Pharmacol.* 1983;24:557–62.
35. Kulig K, Bar-Or D, Cantrill SV, et al. Management of acutely poisoned patients without gastric emptying. *Ann Emerg Med.* 1985;14:562–7.

36. Merigian KS, Woodard M, Hedges JR, et al. Prospective evaluation of gastric emptying in the self-poisoned patient. *Am J Emerg Med.* 1990;8: 479–83.
37. American Academy of Clinical Toxicology and the European Association of Poison Control Centers and Clinical Toxicologists. Position statement: ipecac syrup. *J Toxicol Clin Toxicol.* 1997;35: 699–709.
38. American Academy of Clinical Toxicology and the European Association of Poison Control Centers and Clinical Toxicologists. Position statement: single dose activated charcoal. *J Toxicol Clin Toxicol.* 1997; 35:721–41.
39. Miller T, Lestina DC. Costs of poisoning in the United States and savings from poison control centers. A benefit–cost analysis. *Ann Emerg Med.* 1997;29:239–45.

CHAPTER 18

Ostomy Care and Supplies

Michael L. Kleinberg and Melvin F. Baron

Chapter 18 at a Glance

An ostomy is the surgical formation of an opening or outlet through the abdominal wall for the purpose of eliminating waste. It is usually made by bringing the colon, small intestine, or ureters through the abdominal wall. The opening of the ostomy is called the stoma.

The creation of an ostomy leads to a dramatic change in the manner in which one performs a basic bodily function. Ostomy surgery interrupts the major functions of the digestive system: digesting and absorbing foodstuffs, absorbing water, and eliminating waste. Thus, it is not uncommon for many health care professionals and patients to view the procedure with apprehension. An understanding of improvements in surgical procedures, ostomy products, and outcomes can allay much of a patient's fear and anxiety. Moreover, ostomy patients and those involved with their care must realize that optimal outcomes will be achieved only if products selected for use during initial hospitalization are modified (1) as the stoma heals and (2) in response to changing medical and physical circumstances.

Prevalence of Ostomies

In North America, approximately 1 million individuals have established ostomies, and an estimated 90,000 new ostomies are created annually. The U.S. Centers for Disease Control

Editor's Note: This chapter is based, in part, on the 11th edition chapter titled "Ostomy Care Products," which was written by Michael L. Kleinberg.

and Prevention reports that 9% of the users of home health care are age 65 years or older and have either an ostomy or an indwelling catheter.[1] The number of ostomies performed in other population groups is not available, but they are performed in individuals of all ages and for many reasons, both congenital and acquired.

Indications for Ostomies

Ostomies may be permanent or temporary, and they are performed in individuals of all ages, from neonates to the elderly. Reasons for performing ostomies include congenital anomalies, a wide range of acquired conditions (e.g., inflammatory bowel disease, cancer, radiation damage), and trauma.[2,3] The type of ostomy the surgeon performs depends on the condition being treated.

The indications for performing an ileostomy include ulcerative colitis, Crohn's disease, trauma, cancer, familial polyposis, and necrotizing enterocolitis. The two most common disorders leading to ileostomy surgery—ulcerative colitis and Crohn's disease—are inflammatory conditions that affect the intestines: (1) ulcerative colitis affects the large intestine and rectum, and (2) Crohn's disease may involve any part of the gastrointestinal tract.

Major indications for a colostomy include obstruction of the colon or rectum, cancer of the colon or rectum, genetic malformation, diverticular disease, trauma, radiation colitis, and loss of anal muscular control. The most common reasons for colostomy surgery are (1) cancer of the colon or rectum and (2) diverticulitis. In some cases, a temporary colostomy may be performed to protect areas of the colon that have been surgically repaired. Healing of a diseased or damaged bowel may take several weeks, months, or years, but eventually the colon and rectum are reconnected and bowel continuity is restored. Figure 18–1 shows the location of various types of colostomies and indicates whether they are permanent or temporary.

Urinary diversions are performed to correct bladder loss or dysfunction, which are usually caused by cancer, neurogenic bladder, or genetic malformation.

Types of Ostomies

The three basic types of ostomics arc (1) ileostomy, in which the entire colon and possibly part of the ileum are removed; (2) colostomy (the most common type of ostomy), in which the colon may be partially removed; and (3) urinary diver-

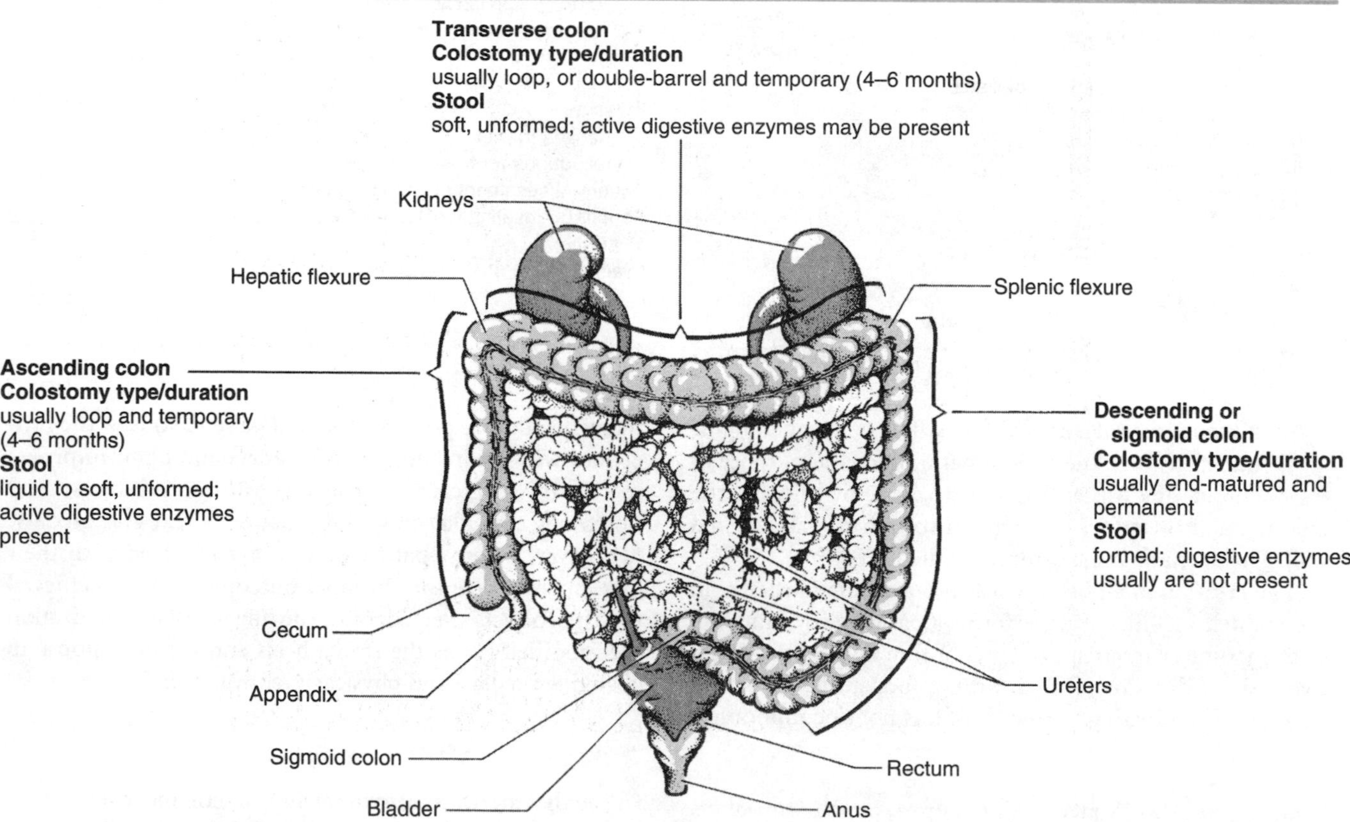

Figure 18–1 Anatomic drawing of the lower digestive and urinary tracts, which depicts the location and permanence of colostomies. Adapted with permission from *Am J Nurs.* 1977;77:443.

sion, in which the bladder or normal structures may be removed or bypassed. Each type of ostomy has several variations depending on the location of the stoma or whether the procedure renders a patient continent. The following discussion of the types of ostomies is supported by illustrations in Figure 18–2.

Ileostomy

An ileostomy is a surgically created opening in the abdomen through which the end of the ileum is brought to the surface of the skin. (See Figure 18–2A.) Initially, the discharge is liquid, but as the ileum adapts, it assumes some of the absorptive functions of the colon and the discharge may become

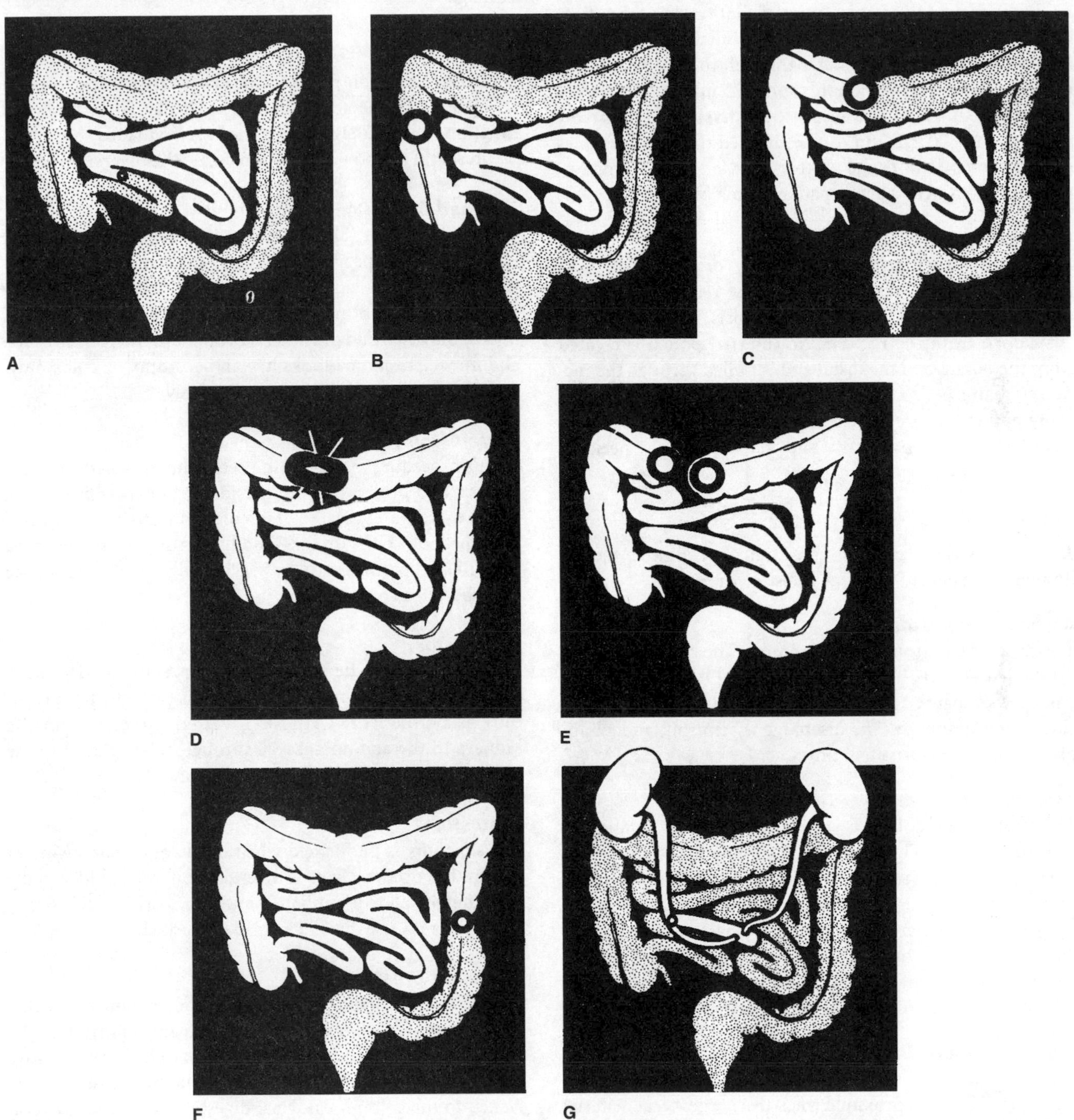

Figure 18–2A–G Types of ostomies: A, ileostomy; B, ascending colostomy; C, transverse colostomy; D, loop ostomy; E, double-barrel colostomy; F, descending or sigmoid colostomy; G, ileal conduit. Adapted with permission from the *Hollister Ostomy Reference Chart*. Liberty, IL: Hollister, Inc (all rights reserved); 1980; and Wuest JR. *J Am Pharm Assoc.* 1975;NS15:626.

semisoft. The discharge is continuous, often odorous, and contains intestinal enzymes that may irritate the peristomal skin.

Continent Ileostomy

Several types of continent ileostomies exist. An internal pouch is created from the ileum, and an intussusception (a slipping of a length of intestine into an adjacent portion) of the bowel is used to create a "nipple" that renders the patient continent for stool and flatus. The pouch is periodically emptied by inserting a catheter through the nipple into the pouch. At first, the pouch holds about 75 mL, but it stretches with use so that at 6 months postoperatively, it comfortably holds 600 to 800 mL and can be drained three to five times daily. Patients do not need to wear an external pouching system, but often wear a gauze pad or stoma cap.

Ileoanal Reservoir

Also called restorative proctocolectomy, or an S pouch or a J pouch, an ileoanal reservoir spares the rectum of patients with ulcerative colitis or familial polyposis. Diseased mucosa is stripped from the rectum. An internal pouch is created from the ileum, and the distal end is pulled through the rectum and attached. Thus, the sphincter is preserved, and ostomy appliances are unnecessary. Patients will have more frequent bowel movements and may experience perianal skin irritation.

Colostomy

A colostomy is the creation of a surgical opening in the abdomen using part of the large intestine or colon.

Ascending Colostomy

This type of colostomy is uncommon. The ascending colon is retained, but the rest of the large bowel is removed or bypassed. (See Figure 18–2B.) The stoma is usually on the right side of the abdomen. The discharge is semisoft, and an appliance must be worn at all times.

Transverse Colostomy

The transverse colon is the site of most temporary colostomies. (See Figure 18–2C.) An opening is created on the right side of the transverse colon. A loop of the transverse colon is lifted through the abdominal incision, and a rod or bridge (which is removed after a few days) is placed under the loop to give it support. The discharge is usually semiliquid or very soft, malodorous, and irritating to peristomal skin. An appliance must be worn at all times.

Loop and Double-Barrel Transverse Colostomies

Loop colostomies have one opening, but two tracks. (See Figure 18–2D.) The proximal track discharges fecal material (generally semisoft), and the distal track secretes small amounts of mucus. An appliance must be worn at all times. A double-barrel transverse colostomy has two openings. (See Figure 18–2E.)

Descending and Sigmoid Colostomies

Descending and sigmoid colostomies are fairly common and generally are on the left side of the abdomen. (See Figure 18–2F.) They can be made as single- or double-barrel openings. The fecal discharge has a pasty consistency and can often be regulated by irrigation, therefore, an appliance may not be needed. However, many patients prefer an appliance to irrigation.

Urinary Diversions

A urinary diversion provides for eliminating urine through an opening in the abdominal wall. Urinary stomas should function immediately following surgery. Mucous shreds will be present if the bowel is used to create the diversion.

Ileal and Colon Conduits

The ileal conduit (also known as "Brickers Loop") is the most common type of urinary diversion. (See Figure 18–2G.) After the bladder is removed, ileal and colon conduits are created by implanting the ureters into an isolated loop of bowel, the distal end of which is brought to the surface of the abdomen. The stoma looks like an ileostomy or colostomy. An appliance must be worn continuously.

Ureterostomy

In this procedure, one or both ureters are detached from the bladder and brought to the outside of the abdominal wall, where a stoma is created. This procedure is used less frequently because the ureters tend to narrow unless they have been dilated permanently by previous disease. An appliance must be worn continuously.

Nephrostomy

A nephrostomy is often a temporary procedure used to manage ureter obstruction. When cancer is present, the procedure is permanent. Urine is diverted directly from the kidneys to the abdominal wall through tubes placed in the kidneys. An appliance must be worn continuously.

Cystostomy

A cystostomy is performed when blockage or narrowing of the urethra occurs. Urine is diverted from the bladder to the abdominal wall. An appliance must be worn continuously. An infant may use diapers instead of a pouch.

Continent Urostomy

An Indiana pouch is a type of continent urostomy in which a pouch is created from part of the cecum and a portion of the ileum is brought through the abdominal wall. The ureters are attached to the cecum pouch. The remaining ileum is reattached to the colon for normal digestive flow. The ileocecal valve is left intact and regulates the emptying of urine into the pouch. The pouch is emptied by insertion of a catheter several times daily. An appliance is not necessary. Most patients wear a gauze pad or stoma cap.

Case Study 18–1

Patient Complaint/History

Euri, a 57-year-old man, presents to the pharmacist with a complaint of severe itching of the skin. During questioning of the patient, the pharmacist learns that Euri was diagnosed with diverticulitis 10 years ago and had a sigmoid colostomy 2 years ago. The patient noticed severe itching around the stoma a couple of days earlier for which he is applying Benadryl cream. He also noticed loose, black stools for which he takes Pepto-Bismol. Physical observation of the stoma reveals that it is red and slightly swollen around the faceplate. The patient, who wears a close-ended, one-piece, flushable appliance, reports that he is diligent about replacing the appliance each morning and each night at bedtime.

Euri's current medication regimen includes Biaxin 500 mg once every 12 hours for 14 days for a sinus infection (he is on day 6 of therapy); Claritin 10 mg once a day; Tylenol 500 mg once every six hours for pain; Benadryl cream 2% as needed for itching; and Pepto-Bismol 30 mL three to four times a day.

Clinical Considerations/Strategies

Readers can use the following considerations/strategies to determine whether treatment of the patient's condition with nonprescription medications is warranted:

- Assess the possible causes of the severe itching.
- Assess the possible causes of the diarrhea and black stools.
- Determine the appropriate response to the clinical situation.

Patient Education/Counseling

Readers can use the following strategies to develop a patient education/counseling plan that will help ensure optimal therapeutic outcomes:

- Explain the importance of nonpharmacologic treatment.
- Ensure that the patient knows when to contact a health care provider.

Pathophysiologic Consequences of Ostomies

The major pathophysiologic consequence of an ostomy is fluid and electrolyte imbalance, which is most problematic in patients with a liquid or semisoft stoma discharge, such as ileostomies or ascending and transverse colostomies. Patients with these types of ostomies must maintain adequate fluid intake to compensate for loss of the absorptive function of the colon and loss of ileocecal valve function. Patients with ileostomies lose about 500 to 700 mL of fluid daily through the stoma compared with a loss of 100 to 200 mL daily by individuals with a normally functioning colon.[4] During illnesses, patients with ileostomies, especially infants, are particularly vulnerable to fluid and electrolyte imbalance that can lead to vomiting and diarrhea. They should be counseled regarding common signs and symptoms of imbalance. (See Table 18–1.)

Patients with urostomy, ileostomy, or ascending colostomy must include an adequate amount of fluid in their diets to prevent the precipitation of crystals or kidney stones in the urine. They also may have an increased incidence of gallbladder stone formation. Patients with urostomies should adjust their diet to produce an acidic urine, thus reducing the risk of infection and crystal formation around the stoma. These patients are at risk of urine reflux into the stoma, which increases the risk of infection and skin breakdown.

Because the gastrointestinal tract is the site of nutrient absorption, some patients with ostomies may experience defi-

Table 18–1

Signs and Symptoms of Fluid and Electrolyte Imbalance

Adults	Infants
Increased thirst	Depressed fontanelle
Dry mouth and mucous membranes	Lethargy
Orthostatic hypotension	Sunken eyes
Decreased urine volume	Weak cry
Increased urine concentration (dark in color)	Decreased frequency of wet diaper
Sunken eyes	Increased urine concentration (dark in color)
Extreme weakness	
Flaccid muscles	
Diminished reflexes	
Muscle cramps (abdominal and leg)	
Lethargy	
Tingling or cramping in feet and hands	
Confusion	
Nausea and vomiting	
Shortness of breath	

Source: References 4–6.

ciencies. For example, iron and vitamins D_2 and D_3 are absorbed in the small intestine; riboflavin is absorbed in the upper gastrointestinal tract; vitamin B_{12} is absorbed in the terminal ileum; phytonadione is absorbed in the proximal small intestine; menadione is absorbed in the distal small intestine; and calcium, pyridoxine, pantothenic acid, biotin, choline, inositol, carnitine, vitamins C and E, and thiamine are absorbed in various sites within the intestinal tract (specific sites not identified). Vitamin A deficiency may be seen in individuals with disease of the terminal ileum (e.g., Crohn's disease). Hypophosphatemia and hypomagnesemia are present in individuals with calcium deficiency caused by malabsorption. In addition, copper deficiency, which interferes with the absorption of iron, has been reported in individuals who have undergone intestinal bypass surgery. Folic acid absorption requires interaction with enzymes present in the upper part of the jejunum; therefore, most absorption of folic acid takes place in the proximal part of the small intestine.[7–10] The effect of ostomy surgery on absorption of vitamins and minerals has not been well studied; patients with ileostomies or colostomies should be monitored for signs and symptoms of deficiencies.

Complications of Ostomies

Ostomy patients may experience both psychologic and physical complications. The pharmacist should be prepared to address these complications or to refer patients to their physician or a Wound Ostomy and Continence Nurse (WOCN), previously known as an enterostomal therapy nurse. WOCNs are often based in hospitals or home health care agencies.

To alleviate any anxiety, patients should receive a thorough explanation before surgery describing what procedure will be performed, what to expect during the postsurgical recovery period, and what appliances and supplies the patient will use. The pharmacist can use the following information on potential complications to assist patients who seek advice after their surgery.

Psychologic Complications

Some patients fear they will not be able to continue their former job, participate in sports, perform sexually, or have children. These patients need reassurance that an ostomy will not impair their ability to carry out such activities.

Physiologic Complications

The normal stoma is shiny, wet, and either dark pink or red. The stoma does not contain nerve fibers, so it does not transmit pain or other sensations. In an adult, the stoma size is usually ¾ to 2 inches, depending on the portion of the bowel or urinary tract used. The stoma gradually shrinks after surgery and reaches its permanent size within several months. Problems related to the stoma and the skin surrounding it can occur. Other physiologic complications involve digestive and other bodily processes.

Skin Irritation

Output from the intestines or kidneys can irritate the skin around the stoma. Ostomy appliances and accessories can also irritate skin either from materials used in their composition or from poor-fitting appliances.

Alkaline Dermatitis Alkaline dermatitis occurs in patients with urinary diversions because of the alkaline nature of the output. The skin around the stoma may feel gritty, like sandpaper. Alkaline dermatitis is a major cause of blood in the pouch because it renders the stoma extremely friable. Dissolving urine crystals on the stoma will minimize the risk of irritation. A cloth soaked with a solution of one-third white

Case Study 18–2

Patient Complaint/History

Clarissa, a 66-year-old woman with a urinary diversion, presents to her pharmacist with a complaint of increased urine output necessitating more frequent emptying of her pouch. A review of the patient's medication profile reveals that Lasix 40-mg daily was recently prescribed for treatment of high blood pressure. The pharmacist, asking open-ended questions, also determines that Clarissa is taking Tums for stomach distress and multiple vitamins that have a high vitamin-B complex. She also complains of a strange odor in her pouch.

Clinical Considerations/Strategies

Readers can use the following considerations/strategies to determine whether treatment of the patient's condition with another nonprescription medication is warranted:

- Assess the possible cause of the increased urine output.
- Assess the possible causes of the odor in her pouch.
- Determine the appropriate response to the clinical situation.

Patient Education/Counseling

Readers can use the following strategies to develop a patient education/counseling plan that will help ensure optimal therapeutic outcomes:

- Explain the importance of using the recommended nonprescription medication.
- Explain the effects her medication and vitamins are having on her condition.
- Ensure that the patient knows when to contact a health care provider.

vinegar to two-thirds water is applied for 5 to 10 minutes to the stoma at least once weekly before putting on the appliance. Patients who use a two-piece system can apply the solution as often as three to four times daily. The vinegar may cause the stoma to blanch, but blanching is not indicative of damage.

Treatment is acidification of the urine. Patients should avoid alkaline ash foods, such as citrus fruits and juices, which, although acidic when consumed, are excreted in alkaline form. Ascorbic acid and cranberry juice acidify the urine. Increasing fluid intake to between 2 and 3 quarts daily may reduce alkalinity. Use of a urinary appliance with an antireflux feature is also suggested.

Contact Dermatitis Contact dermatitis is characterized by burning, stinging, itching, and red or denuded skin. This complication usually results from an allergic reaction to the appliance or an accessory. Patch-testing patients who have a history of allergy, reaction to adhesive tape, eczema, or psoriasis and those who have very fair skin will identify the allergen. Patients exhibiting a sensitivity may need to change products. A pouch cover may be helpful if the allergy is to the pouch itself. Special precautions are necessary in patients with a latex allergy. Upon request, manufacturers will provide written information regarding the natural latex rubber content of their products and packaging. In some cases, the latex source is a dry, natural latex rubber, which is used to seal blister packs that contain nonlatex products.

Excoriation Excoriation is caused by abrasion of the epidermis by digestive enzymes. The abraded area may bleed and is painful when touched and when applying the appliance. Excoriation occurs when an improper pouch is worn, when the pouch opening is too big, or when the pouch has leaked and has not been promptly replaced. These problems can allow the output to come in contact with the skin. The output produced by patients with ileostomies is particularly irritating. The patient should be referred to a physician or WOCN for treatment. After treatment, a skin barrier and pouch may be applied. The pouch should be changed more often to reduce the risk of irritation. Treatment should be continued until the skin is clear.

Hyperplasia Hyperplasia (an overgrowth of skin) occurs when the faceplate opening is too large. There is no pain in the early stages, but later the affected skin cells multiply and cause agonizing pain. The condition resembles a mucosal polyp. Treatment entails ensuring that the pouch has the correct size opening and that the seal is secure. Other management approaches include cauterization using silver nitrate sticks and surgical removal.

Mechanical Irritation Mechanical irritation is caused by a poorly fitting appliance, a skin barrier, a stoma that is difficult to access, or tight-fitting clothing. Poorly fitting appliances can be corrected by measuring the stoma before each purchase of supplies, selecting a skin barrier of the proper size, and adjusting the size of the skin barrier opening, if necessary. Patients experiencing mechanical irritation should be encouraged to contact a WOCN.

Skin Stripping Skin stripping refers to pulling off the top layer of the skin. The skin around the stoma may be irritated by using too strong an adhesive or by removing the skin barrier in a rough manner. The skin barrier should be removed by pushing the skin away from the barrier, not by pulling the barrier away from the skin.

Stenosis Stenosis of the stoma results from the formation of scar tissue. Excessive scar tissue usually is caused by improper surgical construction, postoperative ischemia, active disease, or alkaline stomatitis or dermatitis. Although dilation of the stoma is often advocated to prevent or palliate this problem, the only cure is revision of the stoma.

Excessive Sweating Sweating under the pouch can decrease wearing time and cause monilial infection. A skin sealant or cement plus a belt may be necessary to hold the appliance in place. Purchasing or making a cover or bib to keep the pouch material from touching the skin can alleviate discomfort from perspiration underneath the collection pouch.

Folliculitis

Folliculitis, an inflammation of the hair follicles, is characterized by redness at the base of the hair folliculus around the stoma. Aggressive removal of any adhesive around the stoma can lead to removal of hairs, resulting in irritation and infection. Using an electric razor to shave the areas on which adhesive will be applied can prevent folliculitis. If needed, a corticosteroid spray will relieve the inflammation.

Infection

With the possible exception of patients with Crohn's disease or ruptured diverticulitis, or those undergoing radiation, patients with ostomies do not have more frequent infections than patients without ostomies. In some cases, however, infections under the appliance faceplate can be problematic. Monilial infection may be a problem in patients who wear appliances continuously. A dark, warm, moist environment promotes the growth of *Candida* species. The primary symptom is itching. If the infection is allowed to continue unchecked, the skin will become denuded, the faceplate will not stick, and additional skin irritation will result from the output.

If the skin is indurated, swollen, and red, it may need incision and draining. Culture and susceptibility testing should be performed and an appropriate antibiotic should be prescribed for topical use, systemic use, or both. Patients should be encouraged to contact a WOCN for assistance. Minor monilial infections may be treated with nystatin powder or 2% miconazole powder. For more advanced cases, a corticosteroid spray should be applied, followed by an antifungal powder. Excess powder should be brushed off before the pouch is applied. Antifungal preparations are generally used every other day and for 1 week after the skin has become clear. When treating monilial infections it is important to ascertain whether the patient is taking antibiotics. Any antibiotic, but especially a broad-spectrum agent, changes the flora of the skin, and the entrenched monilia can become difficult to eradicate. It is often helpful to continue using nystatin powder or 2% miconazole powder for 1 month after the monilial infection is gone in ostomy patients being treated with antibiotics.

Constipation

Constipation is caused by the regular use of constipating analgesics or other medications or by a patient's eating

Table 18–2

Effects of Food on Stoma Output

Foods That Thicken Stool	Foods That Cause Urine Odor
Applesauce	Asparagus
Bananas	Seafood
Bread	Some spices
Buttermilk	**Foods That Combat Urine Odor**
Cheese	Buttermilk
Marshmallows	Cranberry juice
Milk, boiled	Yogurt
Pasta	**Foods That Cause Gas**
Peanut butter, creamy	Beans (dried, string, or baked)
Potatoes	Beer
Pretzels	Cabbage-family vegetables (onions, cabbage, brussels sprouts, broccoli, cauliflower)
Rice	Carbonated beverages
Tapioca	Corn
Toast	Cucumbers
Yogurt	Dairy products
Foods That Loosen Stool	Mushrooms
Beer and other alcoholic beverages	Peas
Chocolate	Radishes
Dried or string beans	Spinach
Fried foods	**Foods That Color Stool**
Greasy foods	Beets
Highly spiced foods	Berries
Leafy green vegetables (lettuce, broccoli, spinach)	Chocolate
Prune or grape juice	Fats
Raw fruits (except bananas)	Fish
Raw vegetables	Meat (large amounts of red)
Foods That Cause Stool Odor	Milk
Asparagus	Red Jello
Beans	Vegetables
Cabbage-family vegetables (onions, cabbage, brussels sprouts, broccoli, cauliflower)	
Cheese	
Eggs	
Fish	
Garlic	
Some spices	
Turnips	

Source: References 4, 6, 11–13.

Table 18–3

High-Fiber Foods

Apple skins	Hot dogs
Apricots	Mushrooms
Asparagus	Nuts
Beans and lentils	Oranges and orange rinds
Bologna	Pineapples
Bran	Popcorn
Celery	Potato peels
Chinese vegetables	Raisins
Coconut	Raw vegetables
Corn	Sausage
Dried figs	Seeds
Grapefruits	Shrimp
Grapes	Tomatoes

Source: References 4–6.

habits. Patients should be encouraged to avoid the foods listed in Table 18–2 that can thicken the stool. Constipation may be a problem in patients with descending and sigmoid colostomies. Treatment depends on the cause and may include dietary changes or medication adjustment.

Diarrhea

Certain foods can cause diarrhea in ostomy patients. (See Table 18–2.) Other gut pathology or obstruction caused by a food bolus can also cause diarrhea. Medications, influenza, and food poisoning are other potential causes. Diarrhea is a special problem in patients with ileostomies and ascending colostomies, whose capacity for fluid and electrolyte reabsorption is impaired.

Eliminating the cause of diarrhea is the best management strategy. Patients should avoid foods in Table 18–2 that cause loose stools as well as high-fiber foods such as those listed in Table 18–3. They should instead eat bland foods and drink commercially available high-energy sports drinks. *Lactobacillus* preparations may be helpful for treating antibiotic-induced diarrhea. Some patients may require intravenous fluids. Patients must be aware of the risks of diarrhea so that they can seek medical treatment before dehydration occurs.

Odor or Intestinal Gas

Intestinal gas may be related to food. Eliminating from the diet those foods that cause gas may solve the problem. (See Table 18–2.) Odor can be the result of poor hygiene or leakage, failure to properly connect the pouch to the skin barrier, or use of a pouch with small holes that allow gas to escape. The pharmacist should review proper care and connection of the appliance with patients who are concerned about odor. Oral deodorants are also available that will act in the digestive system to eliminate odors from digested foods. (See Table 18–4.)

Peristomal Hernia

A peristomal hernia is a protrusion of the colon or ileum into the subcutaneous layers of the skin around the stoma. Various factors can cause this complication. Modification of the pouching equipment or technique, clothing, or diet may help alleviate a peristomal hernia. Surgery may be required in some cases.

Fistula

A fistula is a formation of an opening from inside the body to the skin. This complication is most often a manifestation of inflammatory bowel disease. Other causes include cancer, abscess formation, foreign body retention, radiation, tuberculosis, and trauma.

Prolapse

Prolapse is a telescoping of the bowel through the stoma. This problem results when the opening in the abdominal wall is too large. Women with ileostomies may experience prolapse of the ileostomy during pregnancy. Other causes include inadequate fixation of the bowel to the abdominal wall, poorly developed fascial support, or increased abdominal

Table 18–4

Oral Deodorants

Type	Effects	Contraindications/Guidelines for Use
Activated charcoal	Reduces fecal odor; darkens stool	Large doses can interfere with vitamin absorption.
Chlorophyllin copper complex	Reduces fecal and urinary odor; turns stool dark green; may cause temporary, slight diarrhea	Should not be used in children younger than aged 12 years; effective dose is usually 100–200 mg daily.
Bismuth subgallate	Reduces fecal odor; reduces flatus; thickens stool; turns stool dark green-black	Excessively large doses may cause heavy metal toxicity; may cause shadows on abdominal films; may interfere with absorption of anticoagulants and antibiotics. Product is contraindicated in patients with renal failure; initial recommended dose is 1 to 2 tablets 2 to 4 times daily, then titrated to the lowest effective dose (e.g., 1 to 2 tablets daily).

Source: Reference 4; used with permission.

pressure associated with tumors, coughing, or crying (the latter being of special concern in infants). The danger of prolapse is the resultant decrease in blood supply to the bowel outside the abdominal cavity.

A prolapse may be reduced by the patient's lying on the back and applying continuous pressure against the most distal part of the stoma. Once the prolapse is reduced, rigid ring appliances should be avoided because of the risk of strangulation; the appliance may need to be resized. In some cases, surgical correction may be required.

Retraction

Retraction, a recession of the stoma to a subnormal length, is caused by several factors. Active Crohn's disease and weight gain may lead to this damage of the skin surface. If it is not severe, a convex pouching system may be adequate. In other cases, treatment may require surgical correction.

Organic Impotence

Organic impotence results from a radical resection of the rectum or bladder. Male patients who are impotent should be referred to a urologist for assistance in regaining erectile function.

Management of Ostomies

Management Outcomes

The ideal ostomy system should be leakproof, odorproof, comfortable, easily manipulated, inconspicuous, safe, and as inexpensive as possible. The pharmacist, in conjunction with other health care providers such as a physician and WOCN, can facilitate the patient's achieving these outcomes.

General Management Approach

Patients are most likely to achieve optimal outcomes if an appliance is properly fitted and the stoma is appropriately cared for. The pharmacist should always be aware of the sensitive nature of the topic and ensure that privacy is respected during all discussions. Failure to provide a comfortable environment in which to discuss problems, concerns, and alternatives may cause patients to avoid such discussions and may result in less than optimal outcomes. Follow-up assessment and care may be by telephone, by scheduled appointment, or during routine visits to purchase supplies or medications.

Frequent changes in appliance and accessory types should signal a potential problem, as should the use of multiple products intended for the same purpose. In many cases, patients may be referred to a physician or a WOCN for follow-up of problems identified by the pharmacist. Physiologic complications such as impotence; peristomal hernia; and stenosis, prolapse, retraction, or excoriation of the stoma require medical referral. There are some cases, however, in which self-care is appropriate, particularly by experienced ostomy patients. Self-care for constipation and diarrhea, as outlined in Figures 18–3 and 18–4, are two such cases.

The presence of an ostomy and its location should always be noted on the patient's profile so that medication-related risks can be minimized. It is helpful to maintain a record of current and past ostomy products used by the patient and any problems experienced. This information can be useful in making future recommendations.

Use of Ostomy Supplies

The stoma appliance and accessory industry is highly specialized and is rapidly changing in an effort to improve designs, which has resulted in a wide choice of appliances and accessories. Although the ideal ostomy system should be leakproof, odorproof, comfortable, easily manipulated, inconspicuous, safe, and as inexpensive as possible, no one appliance meets all of these criteria.

Ostomy Appliances

The appliance is an extremely important aspect of the ostomy patient's well-being. The patient has lost a normal body function; the appliance takes over that lost function and almost becomes a part of the body. It is common for ostomy needs to be difficult or embarrassing for patients and their families to discuss, especially during the first several weeks or months after surgery.

Adult and adolescent patients must be taught self-care skills to maintain the stoma, including (1) sizing the stoma, (2) cutting a pouch or skin barrier to fit the stoma, (3) cleaning the skin, (4) applying the pouch, (5) applying paste or powder if necessary, (6) removing the pouch, and (7) emptying the pouch. Patients must be prepared for discharge from the stoma at any time during the pouch-changing procedure.

Types of Pouches The surgical technique used to create the stoma influences the pouching equipment required, the complexity of the pouching procedure, and the risks of stomal and peristomal complications (e.g., necrosis, stenosis, hernia). In the past, most ostomy appliances were reusable. The advantages of reusable appliances were their durability, availability in numerous configurations, and relatively low cost. Their disadvantages were that they required cleaning before each use, and that they were heavy, tended to retain odor, and often required a separate skin barrier.

Most ostomy patients are now fitted with odorproof, lightweight, disposable appliances. Most appliances incorporate a skin barrier in each flange, which eliminates the need for a separate skin barrier. Disposable equipment is available in one- and two-piece systems. (See Figure 18–5.) The two-piece system allows patients to center the flange easily and to change the pouch, if desired, without having to remove the flange from the skin. It is easy to apply and is generally more pliable and adaptable to different abdominal contours.

Although appliances are available for infants, some ostomies are managed with a diaper instead. If a diaper is used, care must taken to avoid skin irritation from a caustic effluent.

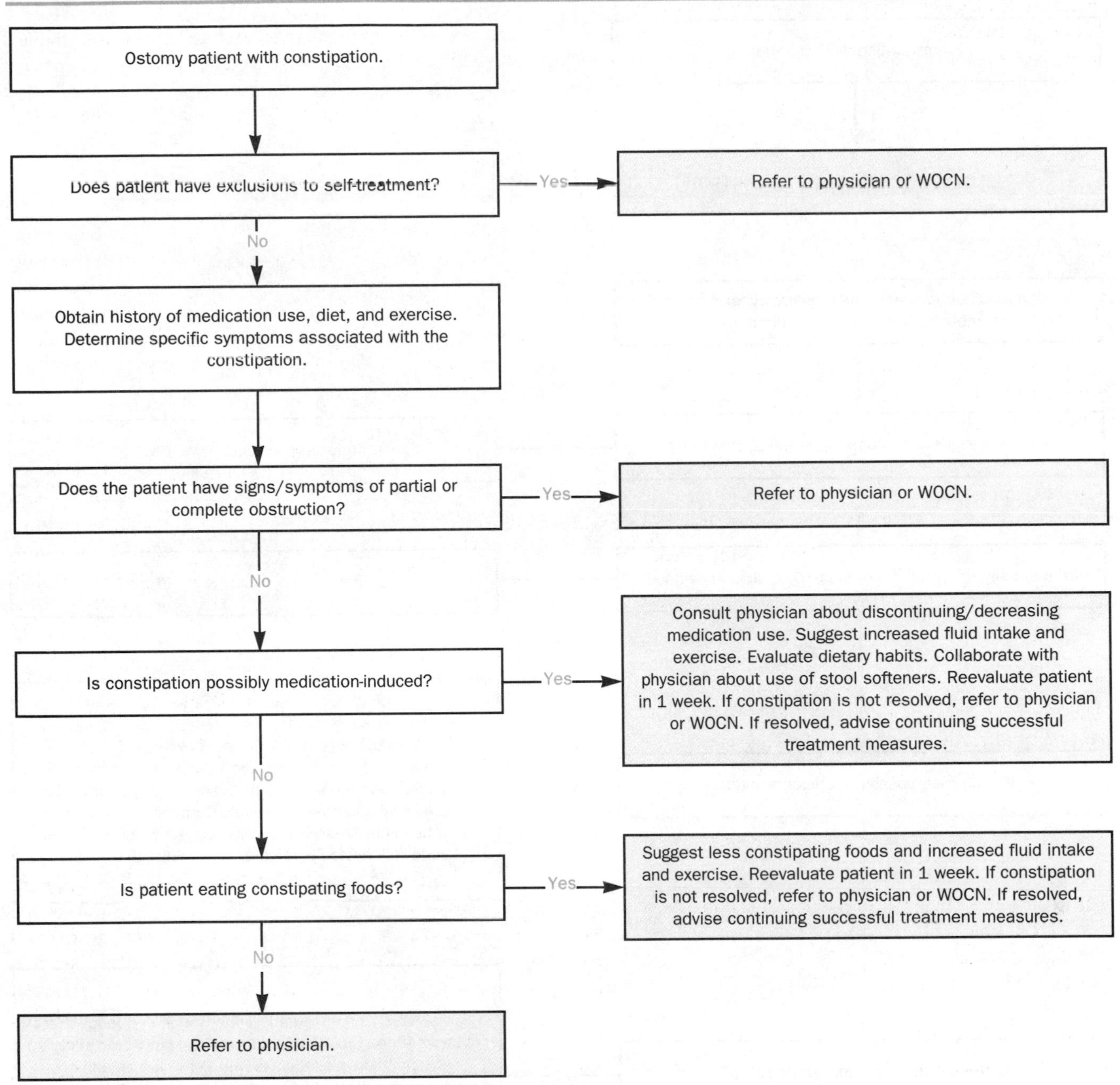

Figure 18–3 Self-care for ostomy patients with constipation.

Newer, one-piece convexity pouches are available with oval openings that fit flush with the skin, which allows the contents to flow into the pouch without leaking onto the skin. Flushable one-piece pouches are available for use by patients with colostomies. These pouches are not practical for patients with ileostomies or urostomies, however, because of the frequency of output.

Both one- and two-piece systems are available in drainable, closed-end, and urostomy styles. Drainable styles are used when bowel regulation cannot be established, and they allow for easy and frequent emptying. Closed-end systems are used by patients who have regulated colostomies and who routinely irrigate the ostomy to remove output. No output from the stoma occurs between irrigations. Urostomy systems allow a constant output of urine and easy emptying throughout the day through a narrow valve opening.

Fitting and Application Reusable and disposable appliances are available in transparent and opaque styles and in various sizes. The pouch opening may be cut to fit or presized. If they are cut to fit, the stoma pattern is traced onto the skin bar-

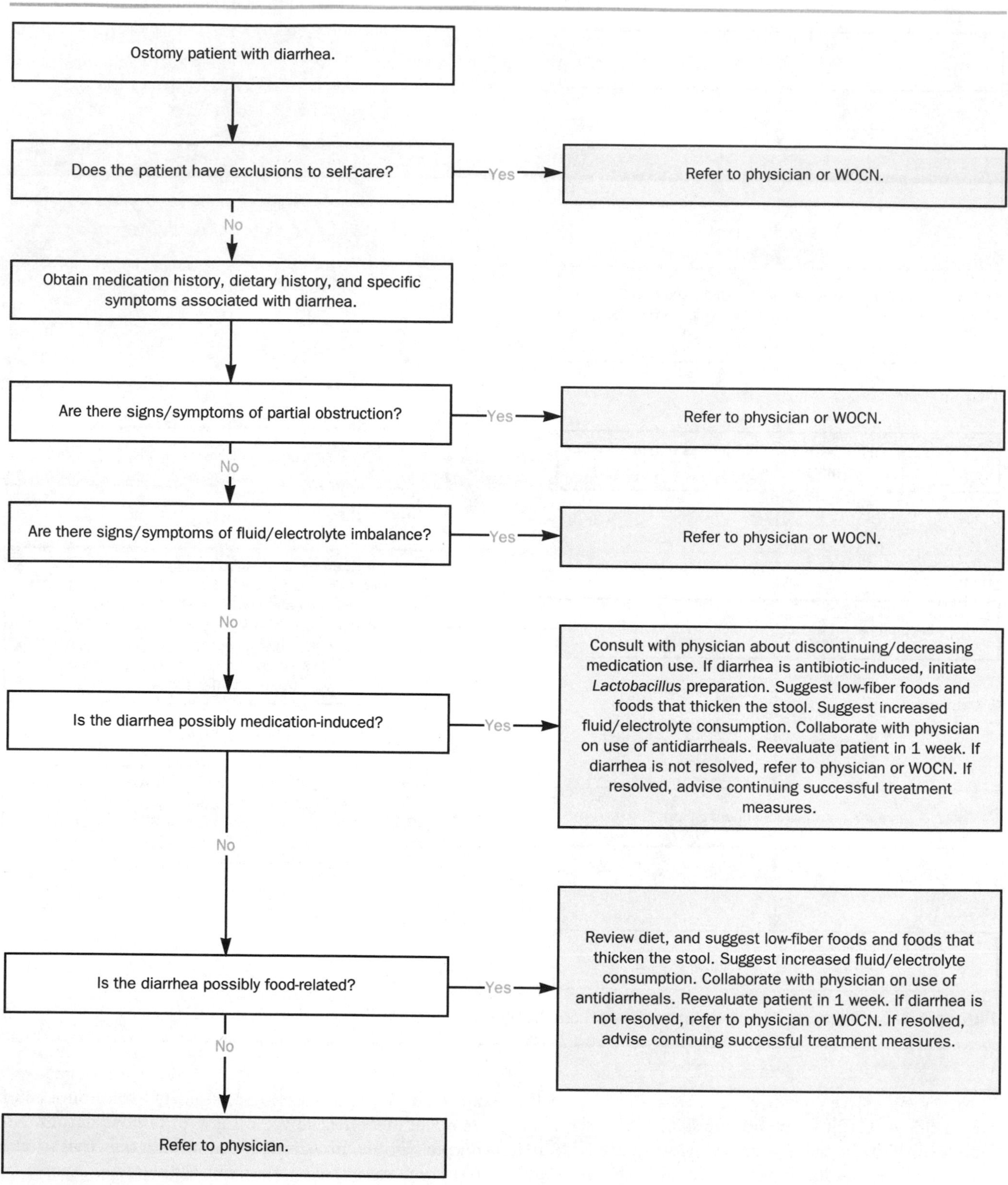

Figure 18–4 Self-care for ostomy patients with diarrhea.

rier–wafer surface of the pouch and then cut out before being applied.

Measuring the stoma to determine the proper fit of an appliance is an important part of ostomy care. The diameter of the round stoma is measured at the base, where the mucosa meets the skin, which is considered the widest measurement. Oval stomas should be measured at both their widest and narrowest diameters. A stoma may swell if the appliance fits

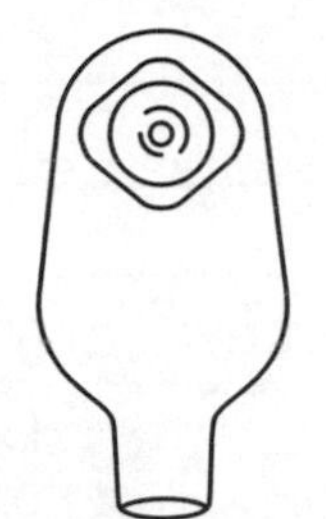

Drainable
A wide opening at the tail for draining fecal discharge.

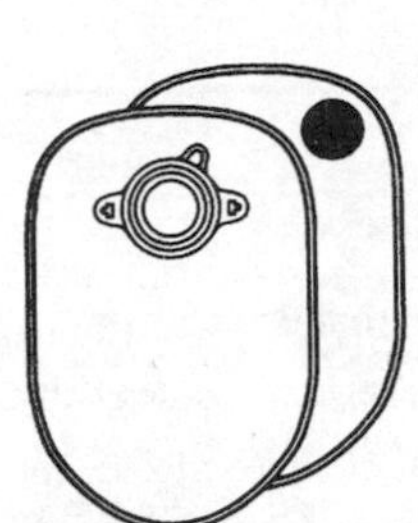

Closed-End
No opening for drainage. One-piece systems with skin barrier attached may be precut or have starter openings.

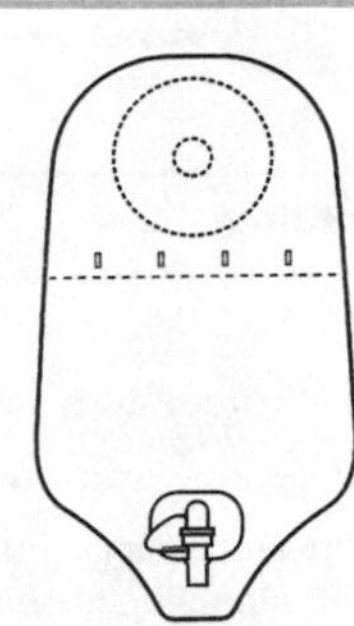

Urostomy
Narrow valve opening for urine or liquid drainage.

A Basic design of one-piece systems

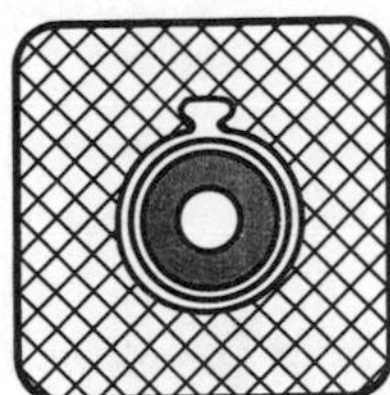

Barrier
Skin barrier with flange.

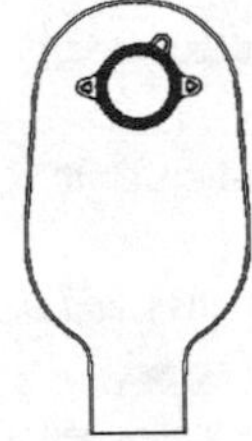

Drainable
Wide opening at the tail for draining fecal discharge.

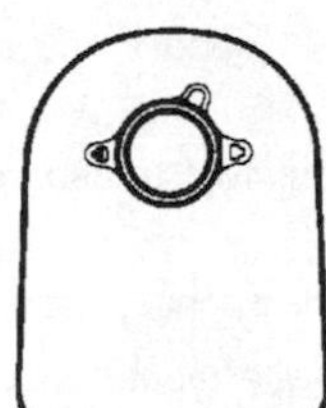

Closed-End
No opening for drainage.

B Basic design of two-piece systems

Figure 18–5 Types of ostomy appliances: A, one-piece system; B, two-piece system. Illustrations courtesy of ConvaTec, a Division of Bristol-Myers Squibb Canada, Inc., Skillman, NJ.

too tightly or slips, or if the patient falls or experiences a hard blow to the stoma.

Other considerations in fitting the appliance include body contour, stoma location, skin creases and scars, and type of ostomy. The lack of uniformity in types of ostomies and ostomy equipment makes it difficult to give standard instructions for application. Also, the stoma and the contour of the area that surrounds it change over time, which necessitates continuous adjustments to appliances and accessories. In general, when a rigid barrier is used, the opening should provide a clearance of 1 to 2 mm around the stoma. Less clearance (0 to 1 mm) is required when using a flexible barrier. A WOCN is an excellent source of assistance in custom fitting these appliances.

Wearing Time To prevent leakage, the pouch should be emptied when it is one-third to one-half full. With a two-piece system, the closed-end pouch is simply removed from the flange for easy emptying. Some patients who use the two-piece system will alternate the use of two pouches. The full pouch is removed, replaced by a second pouch, emptied, washed, and then reused when the second pouch is changed. One-piece closed-end systems are removed and disposed of once or twice daily; those that can be drained can be left in place as long as they are comfortable and there is no leakage. The flange and skin barrier may be left in place for 3 to 7 days, depending on the condition of the skin and skin barrier. Although activities such as swimming or playing tennis may decrease the wear time of the pouch, this decreased time should not discourage participation in physical activities. New pouch adhesives can effectively keep the system in place during such activities. However, because water will not enter the stoma, it is not necessary to cover it while swimming, bathing, or showering.

Product Selection Guidelines The selection of products must be tailored to the patient's activity level and, if present, specific disabilities. Some systems require manipulation that may not be possible for an individual with arthritis to perform. Special products are also available to assist a patient who has poor vision. In general, patients with visual or physical impairments will do best with two-piece systems because they are precut or prefitted and require minimal manipulation. Other options include the use of waterproof materials or a stoma cover. Selection of these and other options depends on how the stoma functions. Table 18–5 lists examples of commercially available appliances.

No particular device will prevent patients with Alzheimer's disease from reaching and dislodging it. It may be helpful to dress such patients in garments that make it difficult for the patient to reach the appliance.

Ostomy Accessories

Belts Special belts that attach to various appliances give additional support. Not all ostomy patients need to wear belts. Indications for their use are a deeply convex faceplate, poor wearing time, activity level (especially in children), heavy perspiration, and personal preference. Some patients may find that wearing a belt for just a few hours after changing their appliance helps the adhesive to adhere, which thus increases wear time and decreases the risk of leakage. Belts may cause skin ulcers if worn too tight. To be effective, the belt must be kept even with the belt hooks. If the belt slips up around the waist, it may cause poor adherence and, possibly, a cut of the stoma. Women may find that pantyhose or a panty girdle are excellent alternatives to a belt.

Skin Barriers, Powders, and Pastes Skin barriers, powders, and pastes are available for special skin problems. (See Table 18–6.) Skin barriers are intended to protect the skin immediately adjacent to the stoma from stoma discharge and to serve as the means to attach a pouching system. They correct imperfections in skin surface, which allows the appliance to fit securely. Powders are used on weeping skin. Pastes (which are not a glue but have a pasty consistency) are used to seal around the stoma and to fill creases in the skin. These products are generally required only by patients who have problems with leakage or who have uneven skin contours. Pastes produce a flat surface for application of other skin barriers.

Table 18–5

Selected Ostomy Pouches and Belts

Trade Name	Product Features
One-Piece Ileostomy and/or Colostomy Pouches	
Bard Medical Closed-End Adhesive Colostomy Pouches	Odorproof; rustle free; extra gauge; rounded corners
Bard Medical Drainable Adhesive Ileostomy Pouches	Odorproof; rustle free; extra gauge; regular size available in plain or wide opening
Coloplast Small Drainable One-Piece Pouches/ Coloplast Standard Drainable One-Piece Pouches	Odorproof film and simple integral closure; stoma opening sizes: 0.75–1.625 inches (small); stoma opening sizes: 0.75–2.375 inches (standard)
Hollister Karaya Seal Drainable Pouches	Karaya five-seal ring and microporous adhesive; stoma opening sizes: 1–2 inches and 1–3 inches
Nu-Flex Adult Oval or Round Drainable Pouches	Transparent; stoma opening sizes: 0.5–2 inches (round) and 0.75 inch × 1.5 inches to 2.25 inches × 3.75 inches trim to fit (oval)
Sheer Plus Drainable Pouches	Clear or opaque; one piece; 4-inch × 4-inch adhesive face plate on free-floating collar with barrier; odor proof; Pre-Fit or Trim 'n' Fit openings
Two-Piece Ileostomy and/or Colostomy Pouches	
Coloplast Small Drainable Two-Piece Pouches/ Coloplast Standard Drainable Two-Piece Pouches	Opaque (small); opaque or transparent (standard)
Hollister Adhesive Drainable Pouches	Standard adhesive; transparent odor-barrier film; stoma opening sizes: 1–3 inches
Nu-Self Adult or Brief Drainable Pouches	Opaque; stoma opening sizes: 0.5–2 inches and 3.5 inches; adhesive foam pad
Perma-Type Colostomy or Ileostomy Pouches	High-quality white rubber; may be worn 1–3 weeks without changing; appliance may be emptied with a turn of the white plastic valve; stomal opening available in round, oval, or irregular shape, as well as various sizes, including larger special-order; six disc convexities available
Permettes	Three-ply; semidisposable; opaque white, vinyl pouch for colostomy or ileostomy; for use with almost any two-piece appliance
Torbot Plastic Pouches, Opaque White	Lined; heavy duty; odorproof; reusable; average life of 2 weeks
Torbot Plastic Pouches, Transparent	Lightweight, clear vinyl; reusable; average life of 1 week
Torbot Rubber Pouches	Recommended for use by ostomates with loose drainage; high-quality butyl rubber; for longer term usage; available in black or white, folded or welded seam, and lightweight or medium weight
VPI Non-Adhesive Colostomy Systems	Reusable system; for single patient use only; closed-end set includes pouches, o-ring seal, and belt; open-end set includes pouches, o-ring seal, belt, and drain tail closure; flange sizes: 1⅞ inches, 2 inches, 2⅜ inches, 2⅞ inches
VPI Non-Adhesive Ileostomy Systems	Reusable system; for single patient use only; set includes pouch, o-ring seal, belt, and drain tail closure
One-Piece Urostomy Pouches and Bags	
Nu-Flex Adult Oval or Round Urinary Pouches	Transparent; 3.5-inch adhesive foam pad (round); stoma opening sizes: 0.5–2 inches (round) and 0.75 inch × 1.5 inches to 2.25 inches × 3.75 inches trim to fit (oval)
Nu-Flex Brief or Mini Urinary Pouches	Transparent; 3-inch adhesive foam pad; stoma opening sizes: 0.5–2 inches
Two-Piece Urostomy Pouches	
Coloplast Small Urostomy Two-Piece Pouches/ Coloplast Standard Urostomy Two-Piece Pouches	Antireflux valve; transparent; stoma opening sizes: up to 1.75 inches (small); up to 2 inches (standard)
Hollister Urostomy Pouches	Karaya five-seal ring; standard adhesive; transparent odor-barrier film; stoma opening sizes: 1–2 inches
Perma-Type UR&V Ileal Bladder or Ureterostomy	High-quality white rubber; may be worn 1–3 weeks without changing; appliance may be emptied with a turn of the white plastic valve; stomal opening available in round, oval, or irregular shape, as well as various sizes, including larger special-order; six disc convexities available
Torbot PeeWees Pediatric Urine Collection	Nonsterile or sterile

Table 18–5

Selected Ostomy Pouches and Belts (continued)

Trade Name	Product Features
Two-Piece Urostomy Pouches (continued)	
Torbot Plastic Urinary Pouches, Opaque White	Lined, heavy duty; odorproof; reusable; average life of 2 weeks; small, narrower spout for special urinal outlet
Torbot Plastic Urinary Pouches, Transparent	Lightweight, clear vinyl; includes small spout fitted for urinal valve and stem; reusable; average life of 1 week
VPI Non-Adhesive Urostomy Systems	Reusable system; for single patient use only; set includes pouch, o-ring seal, and belt
Belts	
Cool Comfort Nu-Support Belts	Lightweight, ventilated elastic; hinged horizontally for contoured fit; standard pouch opening: 2³/₈ inches, custom openings available by request; belt sizes: 16–27 inches, 28–52 inches
Torbot Belts	Elastic web (width from 1¹/₈–4¹/₂ inches); Reliabelt (5-inch width): small, medium, large; rubber: adjustable, for wet environment; versatile (2-inch or 3-inch width)

Table 18–6

Selected Ostomy Skin Barriers, Adhesives, and Solvents

Trade Name	Ingredients
Skin Barriers	
Bard Medical Protective Barrier Film Wipes	Isopropanol; butyl methacrylate; dimethyl phthalate
Carbo Zinc	Karaya powder; zinc oxide; corn starch; petrolatum
Nu-Hope Labs Barrier #54	Karaya; pectin
Skin-Prep Protective Dressing	Isopropyl alcohol; butyl ester of PVM/MA copolymer; acetyl tributyl citrate
Triple Care Cream	Water; petrolatum; zinc oxide; cetearyl alcohol; PEG–40 castor oil; polysorbate 20; octyl palmitate; sodium cetearyl sulfate; octyl stearate; dioctyl adipate; vitamin E acetate; methylparaben; allantoin; clove oil; *o*-phenylphenol; aloe
Triple Care Extra Protective Cream	Petrolatum; zinc oxide; karaya; water; carboxymethylcellulose sodium; methyl glucose dioleate; mineral oil; glycerin; triethanolamine; chloroxylenol; tocopheryl acetate; butylparaben
Uni-Salve Ointment	Petrolatum; benzethonium chloride; chloroxylenol; propylparaben; butylated hydroxyanisole; fragrance; vitamin A palmitate; vegetable oil; vitamin D3; D&C green #6
Skin Adhesives	
A-Ds Transdermal Patch	Medical grade adhesive
Blanchard Karaya Wafers	Karaya gum powder 70%; glycerin 30%
Lan-Tex Disks	Hydrophilic polymer combined with synthetic rubber polymer
Mastisol	Gum mastic
Nu-Hope Adhesive	Natural rubber; hexane
Smith & Nephew Skin-Bond Cement	Natural rubber; hexane; fillers
Solvents	
Remove Adhesive Remover	C10–11 isoparaffin; dipropylene glycol methyl ether; aloe extract; benzyl alcohol; fragrance
Torbot Adhesive Remover	Naphtha petroleum
Uni-Solve Adhesive Remover	Isopropyl alcohol; C10–11 isoparaffin; dipropylene glycol methyl ether; aloe extract; fragrance

Solid skin barriers are preattached to the pouch (one-piece system) or provided separately (two-piece system) and may be custom cut (sizable) or precut (presized). Some manufacturers will custom cut the barriers; however, in most cases, the patient or WOCN modifies the barrier to fit the stoma. The opening in the skin barrier should match the size and shape of the stoma. To create a skin barrier, the patient should apply a bead of skin barrier paste around the stoma or directly to the edge of the skin barrier, apply the skin barrier to wrinkle-free skin, and then press the skin barrier around the stoma to improve adherence.

Solid skin barriers may melt if exposed to high temperatures. Therefore, during the summer and especially when traveling, the solid skin barrier should be put in an insulated box (ice is not required) to minimize the risk of melting.

Cleansing and Special Skin Care Products The stoma and surrounding skin are best cleansed with plain water. If soap is used, it should be rinsed off thoroughly and the skin dried before a new pouching system is applied. Use of moisturizers and lanolin-containing products should be avoided because they prevent the pouching system from adhering to the skin.

Adhesives Adhesives, in the form of cements or tapes, are used to keep the pouch in place. Hypoallergenic tape may be used to support the appliance. A strip may be applied across the top, bottom, and sides of the flange, with half on the flange and half on the skin. Waterproof tape may be used during swimming or bathing. Solvents are available to remove adhesive residue.

Irrigating Sets In patients who are candidates for irrigation, control can be maintained without a pouch. Irrigation is similar to performing an enema at the site of the stoma. Water or another solution is inserted into the bowel through the stoma. The bowel then expands, causing peristalsis and elimination of waste through the stoma. A good candidate for irrigation is an adult patient who has a colostomy distal to the splenic flexure and who does not have a history of irritable bowel syndrome, is not undergoing chemotherapy, or does not have a disabling handicap. For the process to be safe and effective, the patient should use a colostomy irrigation set, rather than a standard enema set.

Frequency of irrigation depends somewhat on a patient's normal bowel habits. After achieving control, the patient may wear a security pouch or a piece of gauze, a stoma cover, or a cap over the stoma. Irrigation is not necessary for health; it is merely one method of colostomy management. Patients should use this procedure only if instructed to do so by a physician or WOCN.

Deodorizers When pouches are properly fitted, disposable, and odorproof, deodorizers are not required as often as they are with reusable systems. In most cases, regular changing of the appliance is all that is needed to prevent odor. Oral deodorizers (internal, or systemic) or those inserted into the pouch (external, or local) can be used to reduce stool odor. Oral deodorizers, which are most often used by patients with colostomies, include bismuth subgallate and chlorophyllin copper complex. Activated charcoal can also be used. (See Table 18–4.) Liquid concentrates are available as companion products to most ostomy devices; they can be placed directly into the pouch to neutralize odor. A common household remedy is to add one capful of mouthwash to the pouch. Specially formulated bathroom sprays are also available. Patients sometimes place aspirin tablets in the pouch to control odor, but this practice should not be used because aspirin may irritate the stoma and cause ulceration.

In addition to local methods of odor control, devices are available that fit directly on the pouch to filter and control gas and odors. One such commercial device is a charcoal filter.

Changes in Diet

Diet does not generally play an important role in ostomy management. Most patients can eat a liberal diet, including all the foods they ate before surgery—if the foods are chewed well. However, it is wise to remain on a diet low in fiber for the first 6 weeks after surgery to allow the intestine to heal and swelling to resolve. A regular diet can be resumed after that time.

The effects of various foods on stoma output are summarized in Table 18–2. Patients with a urostomy may want to avoid foods that cause odor. Patients who irrigate their colostomies should avoid foods that cause loose stools. (This problem varies among individuals.) Because patients have no control over gas passage, patients with fecal ostomies may prefer to reduce their intake of gas-forming foods. Products such as α-D-galactosidase may be used to control gas. (See Chapter 11, "Acid–Peptic Disorders and Intestinal Gas," for a discussion of this agent.) Patients with ileostomies are more prone to intestinal obstruction from high-fiber foods eaten in large quantities or exclusive of other foods. (See Table 18–3.) Chewing high-fiber foods well and eating them in small amounts and with other types of food will help prevent food blockage. The patient should be instructed how to manage food blockage, should it occur. Table 18–7 lists signs and symptoms of blockage, and Table18–8 describes its management.[4]

Precautions for Medication Use

Because part or all of the colon is removed and intestinal transit time may be altered, the patient may experience adverse effects from taking prescription or nonprescription medications, or the medications may be ineffective. Table 18–9 lists a broad selection of medications and their potential to cause adverse effects, which vary with different dosage forms. Ostomy patients should be instructed to check the pouch for undissolved tablets or tablet fragments whenever they take solid oral medications. Coated or sustained-release

Table 18–7

Signs and Symptoms of Intestinal Obstruction

Partial Obstruction	Complete Obstruction
Cramping abdominal pain	Absence of output (urine and fecal)
Watery output with foul odor	Severe cramping pain
Abdominal distention (possible)	Abdominal distention
Stomal swelling (possible)	Stomal swelling
Nausea and vomiting (possible)	Nausea and vomiting
	Decreased pulse rate
	Fever (possible)

Source: References 4, 5.

Table 18–8

Conservative Management of Food Blockage

1. Sit in warm tub bath to relax abdominal muscles.
2. Massage the peristomal area while in the knee-to-chest position to attempt dislodgement of fibrous mass.
3. If stoma is swollen, remove pouch and replace with a pouch that has a larger stoma opening.
4. If able to tolerate fluids (i.e., not vomiting) and passing stool, increase intake of fluid and electrolytes, but avoid solid foods. Drink one glass of liquid each time pouch is emptied. Juices such as grape juice exert a mild cathartic effect.
5. If vomiting, not passing stool, or both, do not take liquids or solid food orally.
6. Notify the physician or WOCN if any of the following develops:
   —Stool output stops (complete blockage).
   —Conservative measures (listed above) fail to resolve symptoms.
   —Signs of partial obstruction persist. (See Table 18–7.)
   —Inability to tolerate fluids or replace fluids and electrolytes occurs.
   —Signs and symptoms of fluid and electrolyte imbalance occur. (See Table 18–2.)

Source: Reference 4; reprinted with permission.

preparations may pass through the intestinal tract without being absorbed; thus patients may receive a subtherapeutic dose. Liquid preparations or preparations that are crushed or chewed before swallowing are preferred.

Patients must be careful when taking antibiotics, diuretics, and laxatives. Antibiotics may alter the normal flora of the intestinal tract, causing diarrhea or fungal infection of the skin surrounding the stoma. Antidiarrheal and antimotility drugs may reduce ileal output. Sulfa drugs should be used with caution because crystallization in the kidney may occur more often in patients who have difficulty with fluid balance. To minimize this problem, patients should increase fluid intake and should not acidify the urine. In patients who have had an ileostomy and whose fluid and electrolyte balance is more difficult to maintain, diuretics should be given with care because additional loss of fluid may cause dehydration and electrolyte imbalance.

Patients with colostomies may use laxatives, but only under close supervision. Such patients tend to have problems of obstruction, and the laxative may cause perforation. If the patient is constipated, the pharmacist may recommend a stool softener. Both prokinetic agents (e.g., metoclopramide, cisapride) and antacids should be taken with caution. Products that contain calcium may cause calcium stones in patients with a urostomy; products containing magnesium may cause diarrhea in patients with an ileostomy; and aluminum products may cause constipation in patients with a colostomy.

To alleviate anxiety, the pharmacist should counsel the patient about medications that may discolor the feces. Some of these medications and the discoloration they cause are listed in Table 18–10.

Patient Assessment of Ostomy Care

In most cases, ostomy surgery necessitates the use of an appliance designed to collect the waste material normally eliminated through the bowel or bladder. Because each ostomy patient is different, one patient may benefit from a particular type of appliance, accessory, or procedure whereas another may develop problems with it. Moreover, appliance needs may change over time. An appliance, accessory, or procedure that previously produced ideal outcomes may no longer be appropriate because of changes in body contour caused by aging, pregnancy, weight change, or concurrent medical conditions.

Patients who have an ostomy are often apprehensive about how the surgery will proceed, how to manage the ostomy, and how they will be perceived by others. A patient's self-image may also be affected. Therefore, a special effort should be made to ensure the patient's privacy and to gain the patient's confidence during the assessment encounter.

Asking the patient the following questions will help elicit the information needed to accurately asses an ostomy patient's physical needs.

Q~ What type of ostomy do you have? Is it permanent or temporary? Where is it located?

A~ The type of ostomy will determine the appliance requirements. (See the section "Ostomy Appliances" under "Management of Ostomies.") The type of problems that might occur and their management often depend on the location of the ostomy. (See the section "Complications of Ostomies.")

Table 18–9

Effect of Common Medications in Patients with Ostomy

Medication	Type of Ostomy			
	Distal Colostomy	**Transverse Colostomy**	**Ileostomy**	**Urostomy**
Analgesics				
Narcotic analgesics	Possible adverse effects	Possible adverse effects	Possible adverse effects	Probably no adverse effects
Nonsteroidal anti-inflammatory drugs	Possible adverse effects	Possible adverse effects	Possible adverse effects	Possible adverse effects
Salicylates (aspirin)	Possible adverse effects	Possible adverse effects	Possible adverse effects	Possible adverse effects
Antacids				
Aluminum-hydroxide antacids	Possible adverse effects	Possible adverse effects	Possible adverse effects	Possible adverse effects
Calcium-containing antacids	Possible adverse effects	Possible adverse effects	Probably no adverse effects	Avoid; harmful
Magnesium-containing antacids	Probably no adverse effects	Probably no adverse effects	Avoid; harmful	Probably no adverse effects
Sodium bicarbonate	Probably no adverse effects	Probably no adverse effects	Probably no adverse effects	Avoid; harmful
Antibiotics				
Broad-spectrum antibiotics	Possible adverse effects	Possible adverse effects	Possible adverse effects	Possible adverse effects
Sulfa antibiotics	Possible adverse effects	Possible adverse effects	Possible adverse effects	Possible adverse effects
Anticholinergics				
Antiparkinsonism drugs	Possible adverse effects	Possible adverse effects	Possible adverse effects	Possible adverse effects
Antihistamines	Possible adverse effects	Possible adverse effects	Possible adverse effects	Possible adverse effects
Phenothiazines	Possible adverse effects	Possible adverse effects	Possible adverse effects	Possible adverse effects
Tricyclic antidepressants	Possible adverse effects	Possible adverse effects	Possible adverse effects	Possible adverse effects
Laxatives				
Stimulant laxatives	Possible adverse effects	Possible adverse effects	Avoid; harmful	Probably no adverse effects
Stool softeners	Probably no adverse effects	Probably no adverse effects	Possible adverse effects	Probably no adverse effects
Vitamins				
Multiple vitamins	Probably no adverse effects	Probably no adverse effects	Probably no adverse effects	Benign side effects
Vitamin C	Probably no adverse effects	Probably no adverse effects	Possible adverse effects	Possible adverse effects
Other Compounds				
Alcohol	Probably no adverse effects	Probably no adverse effects	Probably no adverse effects	Probably no adverse effects
Antidiarrheal agents	Probably no adverse effects	Probably no adverse effects	Probably no adverse effects	Possible adverse effects
Corticosteroids	Probably no adverse effects	Probably no adverse effects	Possible adverse effects	Possible adverse effects
Diuretics	Probably no adverse effects	Probably no adverse effects	Possible adverse effects	Benign side effects
Oral contraceptives	Probably no adverse effects	Probably no adverse effects	Possibly ineffective	Probably no adverse effects
Salt substitutes	Probably no adverse effects	Probably no adverse effects	Possible adverse effects	Probably no adverse effects
Dosage Forms				
Chewable tablets	Probably no adverse effects	Probably no adverse effects	Probably no adverse effects	Probably no adverse effects
Enteric coated	Probably no adverse effects	Possibly ineffective	Avoid; ineffective	Probably no adverse effects
Gelatin capsules	Probably no adverse effects	Probably no adverse effects	Possibly ineffective	Probably no adverse effects
Liquid medication	Probably no adverse effects	Probably no adverse effects	Probably no adverse effects	Probably no adverse effects
Suppositories	Possibly ineffective	Avoid; ineffective	Avoid; ineffective	Probably no adverse effects
Sustained-release	Probably no adverse effects	Possibly ineffective	Avoid; ineffective	Probably no adverse effects
Uncoated tablets	Probably no adverse effects	Probably no adverse effects	Probably no adverse effects	Probably no adverse effects

Source: Reference 14; used with permission.

Table 18–10

Selected Drugs That Discolor Feces and Urine

Drugs That Discolor Feces

Black
Acetazolamide
Aluminum hydroxide
Aminophylline
Amphetamine
Amphotericin B[a]
Anticoagulants[a]
Aspirin[a]
Barium
Bismuth
Charcoal
Chloramphenicol
Chlorpropamide
Cholestyramine
Clindamycin
Corticosteroids
Cyclophosphamide
Cytarabine
Digitalis
Ethacrynic acid
Fluorouracil
Hydralazine
Iodide-containing drugs
Iron
Levodopa
Melphalan
Methotrexate
Nitrates
Nonsteroidal anti-inflammatory drugs[a]
Phenylephrine
Potassium salts[a]
Procarbazine
Sulfonamides
Tetracycline
Thallium
Theophylline
Thiotepa[a]

Blue
Chloramphenicol
Methylene blue

Gray
Colchicine

Green
Chlorophyllin copper complex
Indomethacin
Iron
Medroxyprogesterone
Pancrelipase

Green-Gray
Oral antibiotics

Orange-Red
Phenazopyridine
Rifampin
Rifapentine

Orange-Brown
Rifabutin

Pink-Red
Anticoagulants[a]
Aspirin[a]
Barium
Cefdinir[b]
Nonsteroidal anti-inflammatory drugs[a]
Tetracycline syrup

Red to Brown-Black
Clofazimine

White or Speckled
Aluminum hydroxide
Barium
Oral antibiotics

Yellow or Yellow-Green
Senna

Drugs That Discolor Urine

Black
Cascara
Ferrous salts
Phenacetin

Blue or Green
Amitriptyline
Cimetidine (injection)
Flutamide
Methocarbamol
Mitoxantrone
Promethazine (injection)
Propofol (injection)
Triamterene

Dark
Metronidazole
Phenacetin

Orange
Chlorzoxazone
Phenazopyridine
Warfarin[a]

Orange-Red
Phenazopyridine
Rifampin

Pink-Red
Phenothiazines
Phenytoin

Purplish-Red
Chlorzoxazone

Red
Daunorubicin
Dimethylsulfoxide (DMSO)
Doxorubicin
Idarubicin

Red-Brown
Aloe
Levodopa
Methyldopa
Phenothiazines
Phenytoin
Warfarin[a]

Violet
Senna

Yellow
Aloe
Riboflavin
Vitamin B_{12}

Yellow-Brown
Cascara
Nitrofurantoin
Senna
Sulfonamides

Yellow-Orange
Vitamin A

Yellow-Pink
Cascara

[a] Discoloration may be caused by bleeding.
[b] Discoloration caused by nonabsorbable complex between cefdinir or metabolites and iron in the gastrointestinal tract.
Source: References 15–18.

Q~ What is the appearance of your stoma?

A~ *Identify the appearance of the normal stoma. (See the section "Physiologic Complications.")* Refer the patient to a physician if the stoma looks abnormal.

Q~ How long have you had the ostomy?

A~ If the ostomy was not performed recently, the stoma and surrounding area may have changed since the first fitting. Assist the patient in selecting appliances or accessories to compensate for the changes. (See the section "Use of Ostomy Supplies.")

Q~ Do you have leakage around your appliance?

A~ Determine whether the appliance is the wrong size for the stoma or is the wrong type for the discharge. If poor adhesion seems to be the problem, find out how the patient is applying the skin barrier. Recommend solutions or alternative appliances for these problems. (See the sections "Ostomy Appliances" and "Ostomy Accessories.") If excoriated skin is present, refer the patient to a physician.

Q~ Why did you need an ostomy?

A~ Knowing why ostomy surgery was indicated can help the pharmacist identify non-ostomy issues that should be addressed. (See the section "Indications for Ostomies.")

Q~ What type of appliance are you using?

A~ Determine what type of surgery was performed. If the bowel is affected, find out whether bowel output is regulated or unregulated. Using this information, determine whether the patient is using the right appliance. (See the section "Ostomy Appliances.") Instruct a patient who is purchasing a type of appliance different from that previously worn to thoroughly remove all adhesive residue before changing appliances. The adhesion or wearing time of the new product may be affected if the residue is not removed.

Q~ What accessories do you use?

A~ When advising a patient on ostomy accessories, try to keep the number of products to a minimum. (See the section "Ostomy Accessories.")

Q~ What is the stoma size?

A~ Correctly measuring the stoma diameter is vital to achieving a good fit of the appliance whether it is presized or sized after purchase. (See the section "Ostomy Appliances.") If a patient complains of a swollen stoma and denies trauma to the stoma, recommend a pouch with a larger stoma opening.

Q~ Do you have problems with the skin surrounding the stoma?

A~ *Identify common causes of skin irritation around the stoma. (See the section "Physiologic Complications.")* Drawing on a patient's particular complaint, recommend appropriate measures to alleviate the irritation.

Q~ Who is responsible for changing the appliance? Does the responsible person have any physical disabilities that should be considered, such as arthritis or reduced eyesight?

A~ Tailor selection of a pouching system to the limitations of the patient or caregiver. (See the section "Product Selection Guidelines" under "Ostomy Appliances.")

Q~ Have you noticed any change in the contents of your fecal discharge or urinary output?

A~ Refer patients with such changes to a physician or WOCN for evaluation.

Q~ What kinds of prescription or nonprescription products are you taking?

A~ *Identify medications that can cause adverse effects in ostomy patients or can be rendered ineffective. (See Table 18–9 and the section "Precautions for Medication Use" under "Management of Ostomies.")* If patients are taking such medications, refer them to a physician or WOCN for evaluation. Advise the patient about medications that can discolor the feces or urine. (See Table 18–10.)

Patient Counseling for Ostomy Care

The pharmaceutical care needs of a patient with an ostomy include procurement and distribution of ostomy supplies and selection of appropriate products. Monitoring a patient's management of the ostomy and counseling on special needs (e.g., skin care, diet, fluid intake, and drug therapy) are other important components of pharmaceutical care for these patients.

When counseling an ostomy patient, the pharmacist should provide services in a sensitive and caring manner. An ostomy patient's self-esteem is often damaged; therefore, when assisting a patient with ostomy needs, the pharmacist must take special care to avoid verbal or facial expressions that might convey negative feelings regarding the procedure. Peer support can be especially helpful to such patients; therefore, the pharmacist should consider providing patients with a list of local and national ostomy associations, as well as a list of product manufacturers who can supply information about product use. (See Table 18–11.)

The patient should be encouraged to express problems and concerns so that the pharmacist can better assess the patient's ability to achieve self-treatment objectives. Moreover, the pharmacist must maintain an awareness of the patient's

Case Study 18–3

Patient Complaint/History

Hubert, a 32-year-old man, presents to the pharmacist with a complaint of skin irritation around an ileostomy; he says that he has had several bouts of skin irritation in the past 2 months. The patient reveals that 10 years ago he was diagnosed with Crohn's disease, which was treated with prednisone and sulfasalazine. About 2 years ago, he was hospitalized for an acute exacerbation of the condition. Following a diagnosis of partial obstruction of the small bowel at the terminal ileum, the patient received an ileostomy.

When asked about his appliance and ostomy-cleaning regimen, Hubert explains that he empties his open-ended, two-piece appliance four times a day. He also applies a skin paste barrier and skin barrier wafer weekly; he ran out of the custom-cut material and has been using a precut wafer for the past 2 weeks. He cleans the stoma with Dial soap once a week when he changes the wafer.

For the past 6 months, Hubert has been taking the following allergy medications: Beconase AQ two puffs intranasally once in the morning and once in the evening, Chlor-Trimeton 12 mg daily. He has no known drug allergies.

Clinical Considerations/Strategies

Readers can use the following considerations/strategies to determine whether treatment of the patient's condition with nonprescription medications is warranted:

- Assess the appropriateness of the patient's ostomy cleaning regimen.
- Assess the advantages of a two-piece ostomy appliance.
- Assess the absorption of the oral medications.

Patient Education/Counseling

Readers can use the following strategies to develop a patient education/counseling plan that will help ensure optimal therapeutic outcomes:

- Explain the importance of a rigorous ostomy cleaning regimen.
- Explain the proper use of the recommended cleaning products.

Table 18–11

Sources of Ostomy Support and Information

Organization/Manufacturer	Telephone Number	Web Site[a]
American Cancer Society	800-ACS-2345	www.cancer.org
Coloplast Group	800-237-4555 770-281-8400	www.coloplast.com
ConvaTec	800-422-8811	www.convatec.com
Crohn's and Colitis Foundation of America, Inc.	800-343-3637	www.ccfa.org
Cymed Ostomy Company	800-582-0707	www.cymed-ostomy.com
Dansac (Importer is Incutech, Inc.)	800-699-4232	www.incutech.com www.dansac.dk
Hollister Inc.	800-323-4060	www.hollister.com
Hy-Tape Corp.	800-248-0101	www.hytape.com
International Ostomy Association	44 1189 391537 (United Kingdom) 847-823-6312 (United States)	www.ostomyinternational.org
Marlen Manufacturing	212-292-7060	www.marlenmfg.com
Nu-Hope Laboratories, Inc.	800-899-5017	www.nu-hope.com
Options Ostomy Support Barrier, Inc.	800-736-6555	www.options-ostomy.com
Torbot Group, Inc.	800-545-4254	None
United Ostomy Association, Inc.	800-826-0826	www.uoa.org
United Ostomy Association of Canada, Inc.	416-595-5452 888-969-9698	www3.ns.sympatico.ca/canada.ostomy
VPI, A Cook Group Company	800-843-4851	www.grii.com
Wound Ostomy and Continence Nurses Society (WOCN)	888-224-WOCN	www.wocn.org

[a] Some Web sites may copyright their information. People who access a site should read and follow the instructions in the copyright statement if one is given.

Patient Education for Ostomy Care

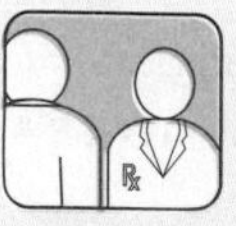

The objectives of self-care of ostomies are to (1) understand how the stoma functions and how to manage it, (2) understand the proper use of appliances and accessories and avoid complications that result from improper use, and (3) reduce the risk of other types of complications. For most patients, carefully following the product instructions and the self-care measures listed below will help ensure optimal therapeutic outcomes.

Appliance Selection and Use

- Use only the type of appliance system recommended for your type of ostomy.
- If the appliance no longer fits well, consult your pharmacist or WOCN before changing to a different type of appliance.
- Do not consider skin irritation to be inevitable; identify the cause and treat as soon as it occurs.
- If possible, identify the cause for leakage around the appliance and correct immediately. Consult your pharmacist, physician, or WOCN if you cannot determine the cause.
- Establish a routine for ostomy care. Keep the routine simple; use as few accessories as possible.

Effects of Medication Use

- Use caution with coated or sustained-release medications; liquid, crushed, or chewed medications are preferred.
- Use caution when taking antibiotics and diuretics. Antibiotics can cause diarrhea or fungal infections of the skin around the stoma. Diuretics can cause dehydration or electrolyte imbalance in individuals with ileostomies.
- Use caution when taking laxatives, antidiarrheals, or other medications that alter gastrointestinal motility. Laxatives can increase fecal output in individuals with ileostomies, whereas antidiarrheals decrease the fecal output.
- Know which medications will discolor the urine or feces. (See Table 18–10.)

Complications

- To prevent urine crystals from forming and causing skin irritation, apply a cloth soaked with a solution of one-third white vinegar to two-thirds water for 5 to 10 minutes to the stoma at least once weekly before putting on the appliance. If you use a two-piece system, apply the solution as often as three to four times daily. The vinegar may cause the stoma to turn white, but this effect does not indicate the stoma is being harmed.
- Consult your pharmacist about using nonprescription medications to treat diarrhea or constipation. Return for reevaluation of the problem after 1 week of treatment.

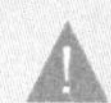

See your physician if you experience any of the following complications:
—Depression and anxiety.
—Sexual dysfunction.
—Abdominal pain.
—Narrowing of the stoma.
—A bulge near the stoma.
—An extension of the bowel through the stoma.
—Recession of the stoma to a subnormal length.
—Bleeding from or around the stoma.
—Pain when touching the skin around the stoma or when applying the appliance.
—Overgrowth of the skin around the stoma.

special needs when managing conditions unrelated to the ostomy. The box "Patient Education for Ostomy Care" lists specific information to provide patients with ostomies.

Evaluation of Patient Outcomes for Ostomy Care

Evaluating patient outcomes should occur each time a patient purchases a new appliance or accessories. The pharmacist should ask patients whether the old appliance had caused any problems other than those related to an aged appliance. If other problems have occurred, the pharmacist should explore the causes and should recommend solutions or refer the patient to a physician or WOCN. The pharmacist should take advantage of patient encounters to ask whether the patient has experienced problems with any special needs (listed earlier in this chapter). If needed, the pharmacist should repeat instructions for preventing these types of problems.

CONCLUSIONS

With proper instructions and equipment, ostomy patients can lead normal, healthy lives. Pharmacists can help by giving patients information about treatment and ostomy supply services and by referring patients to a WOCN when appropriate.

References

1. Dey AN. Characteristics of elderly home health care users: data from the 1994 National Home and Hospice Survey, advance data from vital and

health statistics; No. 279. Hyattsville, MD: National Center for Health Statistics; September 26, 1996.

2. Garvin G. Caring for children with ostomies. *Nurs Clin North Amer.* 1994;29:645–54.
3. Bryant RA. Ostomy patient management: care that engenders adaptation. *Cancer Invest.* 1993;11:565–77.
4. Hampton BG, Bryant RA. Ostomies and continent diversions. St. Louis: Mosby–Year Book; 1992.
5. Chapman GM, Sinclair L, Langevin JM. *A Patient Handbook for the Ileoanal Reservoir Procedure.* Princeton, NJ: ConvaTec, a Division of Bristol-Myers Squibb Canada, Inc.
6. Krenta KS. *Living with Confidence after Ileostomy Surgery.* Princeton, NJ: ConvaTec, a Bristol-Myers Squibb Company; 1998.
7. Hillman RS. Hematopoietic agents: growth factors, minerals, and vitamins. In: Hardman JG, Limbird LE, eds. *Goodman and Gilman's The Pharmacological Basis of Therapeutics.* 9th ed. New York: McGraw-Hill; 1996:1311–40.
8. Marcus R. Agents affecting calcification and bone turnover: calcium, phosphate, parathyroid hormone, vitamin D, calcitonin, and other compounds. In: Hardman JG, Limbird LE, eds. *Goodman and Gilman's The Pharmacological Basis of Therapeutics.* 9th ed. New York: McGraw-Hill; 1996:1519–46.
9. Marcus R, Coulston AM. Water-soluble vitamins: the vitamin B complex and ascorbic acid. In: Hardman JG, Limbird LE, eds. *Goodman and Gilman's The Pharmacological Basis of Therapeutics.* 9th ed. New York: McGraw-Hill; 1996:1555–72.
10. Marcus R, Coulston AM. Fat-soluble vitamins: vitamins A, K, and E. In: Hardman JG, Limbird LE, eds. *Goodman and Gilman's The Pharmacological Basis of Therapeutics.* 9th ed. New York: McGraw-Hill; 1996: 1573–90.
11. *Patient Education Series: Managing Your Colostomy.* Libertyville, IL: Hollister Inc; 1997.
12. Krenta KS. *Living with Confidence after Urostomy Surgery.* Princeton, NJ: ConvaTec, a Bristol-Myers Squibb Co; 1998.
13. Krenta KS. *Living with Confidence after Colostomy Surgery.* Princeton, NJ: ConvaTec, a Bristol-Myers Squibb Co; 1998.
14. *A Professional's Guide for Counseling Ostomy Patients.* Princeton, NJ: ConvaTec, a Bristol-Myers Squibb Co; January 1998.
15. Knoben JE, Anderson PO. *Handbook of Clinical Drug Data.* 7th ed. Hamilton, IL: Drug Intelligence Publications, Inc; 1993.
16. Allen J, Burson SC. Drug discoloration of the urine. Document 150907. Stockton, CA: *Pharmacist's Letter*; September 1999.
17. *Physicians' Desk Reference Electronic Library.* Montvale, NJ: Medical Economics Company; 1999.
18. Fecal discoloration induced by drugs, chemicals, and disease states. In: Gelman CR, Rumack BH, Hutchison TA, eds. *DRUGDEX System.* Englewood, NJ: MICROMEDEX, Inc; 1999.

Section VI

Disorders Related to Nutrition

CHAPTER 19

Nutritional Deficiencies

Loyd V. Allen Jr. and Andrew Glasnapp

Chapter 19 at a Glance

Vitamins are potent organic compounds (exclusive of protein, carbohydrate, and fat) that are essential for growth, maintenance, and reproduction. Vitamins are classified as fat soluble or water soluble. Because most vitamins (except vitamin D) cannot be synthesized by the body in sufficient quantities to meet metabolic needs, they must be supplied by food or supplementation. Vitamins are widely consumed by the American public, accounting for annual sales in excess of $3 billion.[1,2]

In most cases, the typical American diet does not need supplementation, although an estimated one-third of Americans consume vitamin supplements daily.[3] Nutrition experts agree that foods are the preferred source of vitamins and minerals and that most individuals can easily meet their requirements by eating a balanced diet. There is less agreement, however, about the extent to which the U.S. population consumes a balanced diet. Some believe that most Americans receive adequate levels of vitamins and minerals from their usual diet; the lack of deficiency symptoms supports this position. But certain people (e.g., elderly persons, smokers, nursing home patients, and teenagers) are less likely to consume the recommended daily allowances (US RDAs) of all vitamins and minerals. Primary attention should be directed toward improving the diet; under some circumstances, however, a supplement is appropriate.

The issue of who would benefit from supplements, however, is complex. One of the greatest dangers of food fads, high-potency supplements, and large doses of single vitamins is that they are sometimes used in place of sound medical care. The false hope of superior health or freedom from disease may attract desperate or uninformed individuals who have cancer, heart disease, arthritis, or other serious illnesses and may place them at greater risk because it causes them to delay seeking and receiving appropriate medical attention.

Guidelines for optimum nutrition are provided by two organizations: the Food and Nutrition Board of the National Research Council–National Academy of Sciences and the Food and Drug Administration (FDA).

Epidemiology/Etiology of Nutritional Deficiencies

The primary causes of malnutrition include starvation, disease-related factors, eating disorders, alcoholism, and food fads. Certain segments of the population are predisposed to vitamin deficiencies because of the following pathophysiologic, physiologic, behavioral, or economic situations:

- Iatrogenic situations: patients using oral contraceptives and estrogen, patients on prolonged broad-spectrum antibiotics or prolonged parenteral nutrition.

Editor's Note: This chapter is based, in part, on the 11th edition chapter titled "Nutritional Products," which was written by Loyd V. Allen Jr.

- Inadequate dietary intake: patients who are alcoholics or who are impoverished, elderly patients on severe calorie-restricted diets or fad diets, or patients with eating disorders.
- Increased metabolic requirements: women who are pregnant or lactating; women of childbearing age who have regular menstrual blood loss; infants; children undergoing periods of accelerated growth; or patients with major surgery, cancer, severe injury, infection, or trauma.
- Poor absorption: patients who are elderly; or patients with conditions such as prolonged diarrhea, severe gastrointestinal (GI) disorders or malignancy, surgical removal of a section of the GI tract, celiac disease, obstructive jaundice, or cystic fibrosis.

Epidemiologic surveys have shown that school children, factory workers, business people, and farmers are less likely to be poorly nourished. The causes of nutritional deficiency in the elderly may be related to disease, malabsorption, physiologic changes of the GI tract, mastication difficulty, or loss of perception (taste, smell, or sight). Other factors include social isolation, fear for personal safety, lack of knowledge about an adequate diet, poverty, alcoholism, and drug abuse.

Pathophysiology of Nutritional Deficiencies

A comprehensive discussion of the pathophysiology of vitamin and mineral deficiencies is outside the scope of this book. The reader is referred to standard medical and nutrition textbooks for such information.

Signs and Symptoms of Nutritional Deficiencies

The signs and symptoms of vitamin and mineral deficiencies are discussed in the individual micronutrient sections.

Complications of Nutritional Deficiencies

Poor nutrition increases the risks of cancer, infection, and complications from surgery and chemotherapy. Wound-healing time and mortality may be increased. The conditions associated with severe malnutrition include marasmus, kwashiorkor, and mixed malnutrition. Marasmus is caused by inadequate total caloric dietary intake and presents as decreased fat deposits, decreased muscle mass, and cachexia (profound state of ill health or malnutrition)—primarily in infants or children. Kwashiorkor is caused by inadequate dietary intake of protein and is characterized by edema and decreased serum protein levels, including hypoalbuminemia (abnormally low serum levels of albumin). Mixed malnutrition is caused by inadequate dietary intake of calories and protein; it exhibits features of both marasmus and kwashiorkor.

The evolution of vitamin deficiency may include several stages.[4] (See Table 19–1.)

Table 19–1

Stages in the Evolution of a Vitamin Deficiency

Stages	Effects
Preliminary	Decreased tissue stores, decreased urinary excretion
Biochemical	Reduced enzyme activity, negligible urinary excretion
Physiologic	Malaise, weight loss, insomnia, impaired psychologic functions
Clinical	Increased nonspecific symptoms, appearance of clinical signs
Anatomic	Clear specific symptoms, pathologic tissue changes that may be fatal

Treatment of Nutritional Deficiencies

Supplemental nutritional products should be used as adjuncts to a regular diet and not as substitutes for food. Often, individuals who request a nutritional supplement have self-diagnosed their condition. However, although dietary supplements can be obtained without a prescription, they are complex agents with specific indications, and medical assessment should precede their use. The pharmacist should not be reluctant to consult a dietitian or physician concerning nutritional supplementation and should refer patients when necessary.

Health care professionals often recommend general nutritional supplements or, in the case of certain disease states, specific nutritional supplements (e.g., for renal compromised patients and those with lactose intolerance).

Treatment Outcomes

The goal of self-treatment with nutritional products is to prevent nutritional deficiencies or to maintain the present nutritional status.

General Treatment Approach

If a patient's diet is not providing the required levels of micronutrients, supplementation with vitamins and minerals is appropriate, as long as the patient has no underlying pathology and is not taking megadoses of the micronutrients. A once daily multivitamin should suffice in most cases.

Other patients may also need supplemental macronutrients (fat, protein, carbohydrate) because they are unable to consume all the nutrients they need by mouth. Enteral dietary supplements provide those macronutrients, as well as electrolytes and some micronutrients. Some patients may have a temporary medical condition, such as dental problems, which interferes with ingestion of whole foods. Others may have serious illnesses that require feeding by tubes. Although enteral dietary supplements are available without a prescription, a physician or home health care agency should supervise tube feedings.

Nonpharmacologic Therapy

The best method to avoid nutritional deficiencies is to eat the appropriate number of servings of food groups each day. The Food Guide Pyramid, developed by the U.S. Department of Agriculture and shown in Figure 19–1, illustrates the different food groups. The largest group (breads, cereals, rice, and pasta) should provide 6 to 11 servings daily; next, the fruit group should provide 2 to 4 servings, and the vegetable group should provide 3 to 5 servings. Protein from meats, eggs, and nuts should provide 2 to 3 servings, and milk and dairy products should provide 2 to 3 servings. Fats, oils, and sweets should be used sparingly. Patients should be urged to select a variety of foods within the groups to ensure adequate nutrition.

Pharmacologic Therapy

Vitamins, minerals, and enteral nutritional supplements are FDA-approved nonprescription nutritional supplements. The average American consuming an average diet, however, does not need vitamin supplementation. Some claim that everyone would benefit from supplements, but a general lack of knowledge concerning the risks and benefits of megadose vitamin therapy leads others to argue that vitamin supplements are unnecessary and that megavitamin therapy is even dangerous. The truth probably lies closer to the second claim. Some segments of the population may benefit from supplemental multivitamins, but most others do not.

Although there are specific situations in which high doses of specific vitamins were reported as being of therapeutic benefit, the claims of megavitamin enthusiasts have not been objectively confirmed. In those cases, vitamins are actually being used as drugs for treatment and not as a supplement for prevention or maintenance. Furthermore, prolonged ingestion of vitamins has not been tested for safety. Some vitamins, such as A, D, niacin, and pyridoxine, are known to be toxic in high doses. Thus, patients should be cautioned against initiating high-dose self-medication with vitamins. Pharmacists should discourage chronic ingestion of large doses of any drug, including vitamins, for relief of a relatively mild or self-limiting condition.

Vitamins

Vitamins are used both as dietary supplements and as therapeutic agents to treat deficiencies or other pathologic conditions. Recommended daily allowances, or US RDAs, are the levels of daily intake of essential nutrients that, according to scientific data available in 1989, the Food and Nutrition Board judged to be adequate to meet the known nutrient needs of most healthy people. (See Table 19–2.) The US RDA is two standard deviations above the minimal daily requirement, which is the amount of a vitamin necessary to prevent deficiency of that vitamin in the U.S. population. The US RDAs are currently being reviewed and will eventually be replaced by a new set of recommended nutrient intakes called

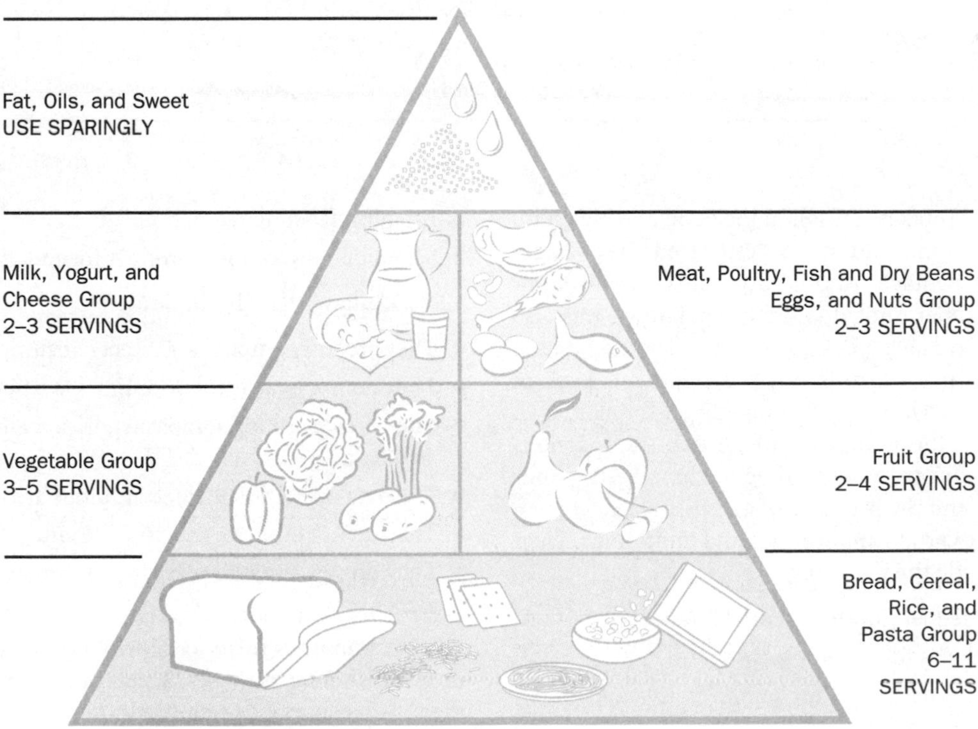

Figure 19–1 The Food Guide Pyramid.

Table 19–2

Food and Nutrition Board, National Academy of Sciences–National Research Council's Recommended Dietary

Category	Age (year) or Condition	Weight[b] (kg)	Weight[b] (lb)	Height[b] (cm)	Height[b] (in)	Protein (g)	Fat-Soluble Vitamins: Vitamin A (mcg RE)[c]	Vitamin D (mcg)[d]	Vitamin E (mg α-TE)[e]	Vitamin K (mcg)	Vitamin C (mg)	Thiamine (B_1) (mg)
Infants	0.0–0.5	6	13	60	24	13	375	7.5	3	5	30	0.3
	0.5–1.0	9	20	71	28	14	375	10	4	10	35	0.4
Children	1–3	13	29	90	35	16	400	10	6	15	40	0.7
	4–6	20	44	112	44	24	500	10	7	20	45	0.9
	7–10	28	62	132	52	28	700	10	7	30	45	1.0
Males	11–14	45	99	157	62	45	1000	10	10	45	50	1.3
	15–18	66	145	176	69	59	1000	10	10	65	60	1.5
	19–24	72	160	177	70	58	1000	10	10	70	60	1.5
	25–50	79	174	176	70	63	1000	5	10	80	60	1.5
	51+	77	170	173	68	63	1000	5	10	80	60	1.2
Females	11–14	46	101	157	62	46	800	10	8	45	50	1.1
	15–18	55	120	163	64	44	800	10	8	55	60	1.1
	19–24	58	128	164	65	46	800	10	8	60	60	1.1
	25–50	63	138	163	64	50	800	5	8	65	60	1.1
	51+	65	143	160	63	50	800	5	8	65	60	1.0
Pregnant						60	800	10	10	65	70	1.5
Lactating	1st 6 months					65	1300	10	12	65	95	1.6
	2nd 6 months					62	1200	10	11	65	90	1.6

[a] The allowances, expressed as average daily intakes over time, are intended to provide for individual variations among most normal people as they live in the United States under usual environmental stresses. Diets should be based on a variety of common foods in order to provide other nutrients for which human requirements have been less well defined.

[b] The use of these figures does not imply that the height-to-weight ratios are ideal.

[c] RE = retinol equivalents. One RE = 1 mcg retinol or 6 mcg β-carotene. One IU = 0.3 mcg retinol or 0.6 β-carotene.

Dietary Reference Intakes (DRIs). In the Food and Nutrition Board's 1989 recommendations, an "estimated safe and adequate daily dietary intake" of other nutrients for which human requirements are not quantitatively known was also promulgated. (See Table 19–3.) These data should be used merely as guidelines for nutritional assessment. Lack of knowledge prevents US RDAs from being set for all known nutrients. Further, the application of US RDAs to individuals may require adjustment according to climate, strenuous physical activity, and the presence of a disease state.

US RDAs have certain applications and limitations. Their applications include the following:

- Evaluate the adequacy of the national food supply.
- Establish standards for menu planning.
- Establish nutritional policy for public institutions/organizations and hospitals.
- Evaluate diets in food-consumption studies.
- Develop materials for nutritional education.
- Establish labeling regulations.
- Set guidelines for food product formulation.

US RDAs have these limitations:

- They are too complex for direct consumer use.
- They do not state ideal or optimal levels of intake.
- The allowances for some categories are based on limited data.
- The data on some nutrients in foods are limited.
- They do not evaluate nutritional status.
- They do not apply to seriously ill or malnourished patients.

FDA publishes a less-comprehensive set of values to be used for labeling purposes. These values, formerly known as the U.S. recommended daily allowances (US RDAs), are included in Table 19–4. US RDAs are now called U.S. reference daily intakes (US RDIs). Other associated terminology includes daily reference values and percentage of daily value

Allowances (RDA),[a] Revised 1989

Water-Soluble Vitamins					Minerals						
Riboflavin (B_2) (mg)	Niacin (B_3) (mg NE)[f]	Pyridoxine (B_6) (mg)	Folic acid (folate) (mg)	Cyanocobalamin (B_{12}) (mcg)	Calcium (mg)	Phosphorus (mg)	Magnesium (mg)	Iron (mg)	Zinc (mg)	Iodine (mcg)	Selenium (mcg)
0.4	5	0.3	25	0.3	400	300	40	6	5	40	10
0.5	6	0.6	35	0.5	600	500	60	10	5	50	15
0.8	9	1.0	50	0.7	800	800	80	10	10	70	20
1.1	12	1.1	75	1.0	800	800	120	10	10	90	20
1.2	13	1.4	100	1.4	800	800	170	10	10	120	30
1.5	17	1.7	150	2.0	1200	1200	270	12	15	150	40
1.8	20	2.0	200	2.0	1200	1200	400	12	15	150	50
1.7	19	2.0	200	2.0	1200	1200	350	10	15	150	70
1.7	19	2.0	200	2.0	800	800	350	10	15	150	70
1.3	15	1.4	150	2.0	1200	1200	280	15	12	150	45
1.3	15	1.5	180	2.0	1200	1200	300	15	12	150	50
1.3	15	1.6	180	2.0	1200	1200	280	15	12	150	55
1.3	15	1.6	180	2.0	800	800	280	15	12	150	55
1.2	13	1.6	180	2.0	800	800	280	10	12	150	55
1.6	17	2.2	400	2.2	1200	1200	320	30	15	175	65
1.8	20	2.1	280	2.6	1200	1200	355	15	19	200	75
1.7	20	2.1	260	2.6	1200	1200	340	15	16	200	75

[d] As cholecalciferol; 10 mcg cholecalciferol = 400 IU of vitamin D.

[e] α-TE = α-tocopherol equivalents. 1 mg *d*-α-tocopherol = 1 mg α-TE = 1.49 IU.

[f] NE = niacin equivalent, equal to 1 mg of niacin or 60 mg of dietary tryptophan.

Source: Reference 5; adapted with permission.

(%DV). The nutrition labeling of a dietary supplement or of a vitamin or mineral is a box with the heading "Supplement Facts." In addition to information on serving size and servings per container, the label lists all required nutrients that are present in the dietary supplement in significant amounts and the %DV where a reference has been established. It also lists all other dietary ingredients present in the product, including botanicals and amino acids, for which no %DV has been established. Percentages of daily value may be expressed to the nearest whole number except that "less than 1%" may be used in place of "0%" when the material is present in a quantity greater than zero.

The percentage of daily value is based on US RDI values for adults and for children age 4 years or older, unless the product is designed for children younger than 4 years, for pregnant women, or for lactating women. These groups will be specified in a separate column. Pharmacists may find US RDI values useful for patient discussions.

US RDAs provided in this chapter are primarily for infants, children, adult men and women, and pregnant and lactating women. (See Table 19–2.) Resource information is available from several standard textbooks and reference books about nutrition and pharmacy.[5–10] The discussion of product forms is primarily limited to the items available for nonprescription oral administration.

Frequently, "natural" vitamin products are supplemented with synthetic vitamins. For example, because the amount of ascorbic acid that can be acquired from rose hips (the fleshy fruit of a rose) is relatively small, synthetic ascorbic acid is added to prevent too large a tablet size. However, this addition may not be noted on the label, and the price of the partially natural product is often considerably higher than that for the completely synthetic, but equally effective, product. Patients should be informed that the body cannot distinguish between a vitamin molecule derived from a synthetic source and one derived from a natural source and that synthetic vitamins are absorbed the same as the more-expensive "natural" vitamins.

Table 19-3

Estimated Safe and Adequate Daily Dietary Intakes of Selected Vitamins and Minerals[a]

		Vitamins		Trace Elements[b]				
Category	**Age (year)**	**Biotin (mcg)**	**Panto-thenic Acid (mg)**	**Copper (mg)**	**Manganese (mg)**	**Fluoride (mg)**	**Chromium (mcg)**	**Molybdenum (mcg)**
Infants	0–0.5	10	3	0.4–0.6	0.3–0.6	0.1–0.5	10–40	15–30
	0.5–1	15	3	0.6–0.7	0.6–1.0	0.2–1.0	20–60	20–40
Children and adolescents	1–3	20	3	0.7–1.0	1.0–1.5	0.5–1.5	20–80	25–50
	4–6	25	3–4	1.0–1.5	1.5–2.0	1.0–2.5	30–120	30–75
	7–10	30	4–5	1.0–2.0	2.0–3.0	1.5–2.5	50–200	50–150
	11+	30–100	4–7	1.5–2.5	2.0–5.0	1.5–2.5	50–200	75–250
Adults		30–100	4–7	1.5–3.0	2.0–5.0	1.5–4.0	50–200	75–250

[a] Because less information exists on which to base allowances, these figures are not given in Table 19–2 and are provided here in the form of ranges of recommended intakes.

[b] Because the toxic levels for many trace elements may be only several times the usual intakes, the upper levels for the trace elements given in the table should not be habitually exceeded.

Source: Reference 5; used with permission.

Vitamins are grouped in two broad classifications: fat soluble and water soluble. Vitamins A, D, E, and K are fat-soluble vitamins. They are soluble in lipids and are usually absorbed along with chylomicrons into the lymphatic system of the small intestine, where they pass into the general circulation. Their absorption is facilitated by bile. These vitamins are stored in body tissues, and may be toxic when excessive quantities are ingested. Deficiencies occur when fat intake is limited or fat absorption is compromised. Drugs that affect lipid absorption, such as cholestyramine (which binds bile acids and thereby hinders lipid emulsification) and mineral oil (which increases fecal elimination of lipids), may precipitate such a deficiency.

Vitamin C and the vitamin B complex (riboflavin, thiamine, pyridoxine, B_{12} [cyanocobalamin], niacin, pantothenic acid, biotin, and folic acid) are water-soluble vitamins.

As dietary supplements, vitamins are usually dosed at 50% to 150% of the US RDI. As therapeutic agents, vitamins should be recommended only by physicians according to specific medical indications. Typically, therapeutic doses should not exceed 2 to 10 times the US RDA, depending on the vitamin.

Vitamin A The designation *vitamin A* refers to a group of compounds essential for vision, growth, reproduction, cellular differentiation and proliferation, and integrity of the immune system. A number of names and forms exist of vitamin A, including the retinoids (e.g., retinoic acid) and the carotenoids (e.g., β-carotene). The term *retinoid* is also used to refer to this very large group of compounds, some of which are without vitamin A activity. Biochemical changes occur in the retinoids and carotenoids during absorption in the intestine to form active compounds.

More than 90% of the body's supply of vitamin A is stored in the liver, and those reserves are usually sufficient for several months to a year. Infants and young children are more susceptible to vitamin A deficiency because they have not established the necessary reserves.

Vitamin A is measured in international units (IUs); 1 IU equals 0.3 mcg of retinol, 0.6 mcg of β-carotene, or 1.2 mcg of other carotenoids. The retinol equivalent (RE) has been recommended by the Food and Nutrition Board as a way to determine the amount of absorption of the carotenoids, as well as their degree of conversion to vitamin A in the body. In the RE system, 1 RE equals 1 mcg of retinol, 6 mcg of β-carotene, and 12 mcg of other carotenoids. This system is appropriate because retinol is assumed to be completely absorbed from the GI tract, whereas carotenes are only about one-third absorbed. Thus, because only about half of the absorbed β-carotene is converted to retinol, only one-sixth of the intake is actually used by the body. Similarly, because one-fourth of the other carotenoids is converted to retinol, only one-twelfth of the intake is available.

Function Vitamin A is essential for normal growth and reproduction, normal skeletal and tooth development, and proper functioning of most organs of the body, notably the specialized functions involving the conjunctiva, retina, and cornea of the eye. It is thus indicated in preventing and treating symptoms of vitamin A deficiency, such as xerophthalmia (dry eye) and nyctalopia (night blindness). The synthesis of the glycoproteins necessary to maintain normal epithelial cell mucous secretions requires vitamin A, which is also vital to the body's defense against bacterial infections in the upper respiratory system.

Table 19–4

U.S. Recommended Daily Allowances (US RDAs) for Labeling Purposes

	Unit	Infants	Children <4 Years	Adults and Children ≥4 Years	Pregnant and Lactating Women
Vitamin A	IU	1500	2500	5000	8000
Vitamin D	IU	400	400	400	400
Vitamin E	IU	5	10	30	30
Ascorbic acid	mg	35	40	60	60
Folic acid	mg	0.1	0.2	0.4	0.8
Thiamine	mg	0.5	0.7	1.5	1.7
Riboflavin	mg	0.6	0.8	1.7	2.0
Niacin	mg	8	9	20	20
Pyridoxine	mg	0.4	0.7	2	2.5
Cyanocobalamin	mcg	2	3	6	8
Biotin	mg	0.05	0.15	0.3	0.3
Pantothenic acid	mg	3	5	10	10
Calcium	g	0.6	0.8	1.0	1.3
Phosphorus	g	0.5	0.8	1.0	1.3
Iodine	mcg	45	70	150	150
Iron	mg	15	10	18	18
Magnesium	mg	70	200	400	450
Manganese[a]	mg	0.5	1.0	4.0	4.0
Copper	mg	0.6	1.0	2.0	2.0
Zinc	mg	5	8	15	15
Protein	g	—	20 (28)[b]	45 (65)[b]	—

[a] Proposed US RDA.

[b] Values in parentheses are US RDAs when the protein efficiency ratio (PER) is less than that of casein. The other values are used when the PER is equal to or greater than that of casein. No claim may be made for a protein with a PER equal to or less than 20% that of casein.

Source: Reference 5; used with permission.

One of the most encouraging developments in vitamin research has been the discovery that vitamin A analogues show promise in preventing and treating certain cancers and in treating certain skin disorders. It has long been known that vitamin A deficiency in animals leads to preneoplastic conditions of epithelial tissues such as hyperkeratosis and metaplasia. Systemic administration of high doses of vitamin A may retard the development of these precancerous lesions. Experimental results also suggest that certain systemic retinoids may be useful in treating acne, psoriasis, and other skin conditions characterized by hyperkeratosis. Topical retinoic acid (Retin-A) and systemic isotretinoin (Accutane) may be used to treat acne vulgaris.

Dietary Sources The primary dietary source of vitamin A is the carotenoids, which are synthesized by plants and converted in the body into vitamin A. Vitamin A and carotenoids, which are fat soluble, are found mainly in fatty foods. Good sources are fish, butter, cream, eggs, milk, and organ meats. Carotenoids are the yellow-orange pigments of carrots, squash, and pumpkin; they are also present in many dark, leafy vegetables. However, the color intensity of a vegetable is not a reliable indicator of its vitamin A content.

Deficiency Vitamin A deficiency is rare in well-nourished populations and develops slowly because of body stores. It is most common in poorly nourished children younger than 5 years. Serum levels usually remain normal until the liver reserve becomes highly depleted. Deficiency occurs when vitamin A plasma levels fall below 10 mcg/dL. (Normal blood levels range from 20 to 80 mcg/dL.) Conditions such as cancer, tuberculosis, pneumonia, chronic nephritis, urinary tract infections, and prostate disease may cause excessive excretion of vitamin A. Conditions in which there is fat malabsorption (e.g., celiac disease, short gut syndrome, obstructive jaundice, cystic fibrosis, and cirrhosis of the liver) may impair vitamin A absorption. Neomycin or cholestyramine may cause significant malabsorption of vitamin A and other fat-soluble vitamins and may precipitate deficiencies with long-term use. In the United States, vitamin A deficiency occurs more often from diseases of fat malabsorption than from malnutrition.

One of the earliest symptoms of vitamin A deficiency is night blindness, caused by failure of the retina to obtain adequate supplies of retinol for the formation of rhodopsin. If the situation is not reversed, it may be rapidly followed by structural changes in the retina and xerosis (abnormal dryness) of the conjunctiva. Bitot's spots (small patches of bubbles that resemble tiny drops of meringue) may appear on the conjunctiva, which may look dry and opaque; then photophobia (light sensitivity) may occur. If the deficiency continues, xerosis of the cornea occurs, followed by corneal distortion. The loss of continuity of the surface epithelium, with formation of a noninflammatory ulcer and infiltration of the stroma, can lead to softening of the cornea, alteration of the iris, and permanent loss of vision.

Other characteristic clinical findings of a deficiency disorder include increased susceptibility to infection, follicular hyperkeratosis, loss of appetite, impaired taste and smell, impaired equilibrium, and an increase in cerebrospinal fluid pressure. Some of these findings may be masked by concurrent deficiencies of other nutrients. Notable, however, is the drying and hyperkeratinization of the skin, which predisposes patients to infections. The integrity of epithelial tissues depends on vitamin A activity.

Dose/US RDA The usual requirements for vitamin A are supplied by an adequate diet. The use of supplemental vitamin A would be appropriate in treating vitamin A deficiency and as prophylaxis in at-risk patients during times of increased requirements (e.g., infancy, pregnancy, or lactation). Dietary intake of vitamin A should be estimated when determining the dose for administration. Vitamin A is usually administered orally.

The US RDA values published by the Food and Nutrition Board express the potency of vitamin A in terms of an RE. Thus, the US RDA in adult men and women is 1000 and 800 mcg RE, respectively. The US RDI still retains the IU as a measure of potency, so the US RDI for adults is 5000 IU, which is equivalent to 1000 RE. This dosage is increased to 8000 IU for pregnant and lactating women and is decreased to 2500 IU for children younger than 4 years and to 1500 IU for infants. (See Table 19–4.) There does not appear to be a special requirement for vitamin A for the elderly. If the pharmacist determines that a vitamin A supplement is appropriate, the recommendation should be a nonprescription multiple vitamin that contains no more than the US RDA of vitamin A. High-dose vitamin A therapy should be undertaken only with close medical supervision. Tables 19–2, 19–3, and 19–4 show the requirements for children.

Adverse Effects Because vitamin A is stored in the body, high doses of it can lead to a toxic syndrome known as hypervitaminosis A. The incidence of hypervitaminosis A is increasing because of publicity regarding the potential application of vitamin A in cancer and skin disorders. A single dose (2,000,000 IU, or 400,000 RE) may precipitate acute toxicity 4 to 8 hours after ingestion. Chronic daily ingestion of at least 25,000 IU of vitamin A, a dose readily available to the public, has resulted in toxicity in children. Headache is a predominant symptom, but it may be accompanied by diplopia (double vision), nausea, vomiting, vertigo, or drowsiness. Fatigue, malaise, and lethargy are also common symptoms. Abdominal upset, bone and joint pain, throbbing headaches, insomnia, restlessness, night sweats, loss of body hair, brittle nails, exophthalmos (abnormal protrusion of the eyeball), rough and scaly skin, peripheral edema, and mouth fissures may occur as well. Treatment consists of discontinuing vitamin A supplementation, and the prognosis is good. β-carotene does not produce toxicity rapidly because its conversion to vitamin A is slow. However, eating large amounts of carrots daily may result in carotenemia, which can produce a yellow skin hue. Pregnant women or women of childbearing age who are not using contraception should avoid vitamin A doses above the US RDA because of a teratogenic risk.

Drug–Drug Interactions Large doses of vitamin A may increase the hypoprothrombinemic effect of warfarin. Thus, the recommended dose of vitamin A supplements should not be exceeded, and cholestyramine or mineral oil (nonabsorbed), which may reduce the absorption of vitamin A, should not be used for a prolonged period while using these supplements. Additionally, oral contraceptive use may increase plasma levels of vitamin A.

Vitamin D (Calciferol) A number of chemicals are associated with vitamin D activity. Table 19–5 lists the structurally similar chemicals and their metabolites for which vitamin D is the collective name. Cholecalciferol (vitamin D_3) is the naturally occurring form of vitamin D. It is synthesized in the skin from endogenous or dietary cholesterol on exposure to UV radiation (sunlight). Ergocalciferol, which differs structurally only slightly from cholecalciferol, is of dietary importance. Ergocalciferol and cholecalciferol are equipotent.

Activation of vitamin D requires both the liver and the kidney. One metabolite, 25-hydroxycholecalciferol, is formed by the liver and then hydroxylated by the kidney to its most active form, 1,25-dihydroxycholecalciferol. Its deficiency explains why hypocalcemia occurs in patients with renal failure, and why some patients fail to respond even to massive doses of vitamin D_3. Administration of 1,25-dihydroxycholecalciferol (available as calcitriol) to those patients has been successful, whereas supplementation with 25-hydroxycholecalciferol is sufficient in patients with hepatic failure.

Function Vitamin D, which has properties of both hormones and vitamins, is necessary for the proper formation of bone and for mineral homeostasis. It is closely involved with parathyroid hormone, phosphate, and calcitonin in the homeostasis of serum calcium.

Table 19–5

Chemicals that Have Vitamin D Activity

Activity Ratio	Name	Synonyms	
1	Vitamin D_3	Cholecalciferol	Calciol
2–5	25-Hydroxyvitamin D_3	25-Hydroxycholecalciferol	Calcifediol
10	1,25-Dihydroxyvitamin D_3	1,25-Dihydroxycholecalciferol	Calcitriol
1	Vitamin D_2	Ergocalciferol, Ergocalciol	Ercalciol
2–5	25-Hydroxyvitamin D_2	25-Hydroxyergocalciferol	Ercalcidiol
10	1,25-Dihydroxyvitamin D_2	1,25-Dihydroxyergocalciferol	Ercalcitriol

Dietary Sources Milk and milk products are the major sources of preformed vitamin D in the United States because milk is routinely supplemented with 400 IU of vitamin D per quart. Eggs and animal livers are also rich in vitamin D; fish, beef, and butter are additional natural sources. Vitamin D is stable, and normal food processing does not appear to alter its activity.

Deficiency Vitamin D deficiency may result from the following: dietary deficiency; GI disorder (hepatobiliary disease, malabsorption, or chronic pancreatitis); acidosis; chronic renal failure; hereditary disorders of vitamin D metabolism; phosphate depletion; renal tubular disorders; poisoning from lead, cadmium, or outdated tetracycline; or prolonged parenteral nutrition without proper vitamin D supplementation.

The signs and symptoms of vitamin D deficiency diseases are reflected as calcium abnormalities, specifically those involved with bone formation. The classic deficiency state is rickets. Vitamin D increases calcium and phosphate absorption from the small intestine, mobilizes calcium from bone, permits normal bone mineralization, improves renal absorption of calcium, and maintains serum calcium and phosphorus levels. As serum calcium and inorganic phosphate decrease, compensatory mechanisms attempt to increase the calcium. Parathyroid hormone secretion increases, possibly leading to secondary hyperparathyroidism. If physiologic mechanisms fail to make the appropriate adjustments in levels of calcium and phosphorus, demineralization of bone will ensue to maintain essential plasma calcium levels. During growth, demineralization leads to a failure of bone matrix mineralization. In adults, it may lead to severe osteomalacia. The epiphyseal plate may widen because of the failure of calcification combined with weight load on the softened structures during growth. As a result, rickets is manifested by soft bones and deformed joints. The diagnosis is made radiologically by observing the bone deformities. The lack of adequate calcium in muscle tissue results in tetany.

The incidence of rickets in the United States is low, but the increasing popularity of vegetarian diets has led to rickets in some children who abstain from milk and in infants breastfed by mothers who do not drink milk, who fail to take prenatal vitamins, or who otherwise receive inadequate intake of vitamin D. A deficiency of vitamin D may result in liver disease or myopathy because of decreased muscle phosphate.

Osteomalacia may develop in elderly people because of the following: vitamin D deficiency (malabsorption syndromes, inadequate diet or sunlight, gastrectomy, laxative abuse, and pancreatic insufficiency); anticonvulsant, cholestyramine, or glucocorticoid therapy; liver disease; chronic renal failure; hypoparathyroidism; postmenopausal endocrine changes; and/or cadmium and strontium toxicity. In adults, bone fractures may result from the bone loss that accompanies hypocalcemia.

Dose/US RDA Most people obtain the US RDA of vitamin D from dietary sources and exposure to sunlight. (See Tables 19–2 and 19–4.) People regularly exposed to sunlight will generally have no dietary requirement for vitamin D. However, a substantial part of the U.S. population is exposed to very little sunlight, especially during the winter.

If a patient asks for a vitamin D supplement and if the pharmacist determines that the need is based on poor dietary intake or on indoor confinement, a multivitamin supplement containing no more than 100 IU of vitamin D may be recommended. Liquid preparations that contain vitamin D should be measured carefully, particularly when given to infants. The pharmacist should refer patients who request therapeutic doses of vitamin D to a physician. The pharmacist should encourage patients using a prescription vitamin D product to see their physician regularly.

Vitamin D is included in most multivitamin preparations. Two active metabolites, 25-hydroxycholecalciferol (calcifediol) and 1,25-dihydroxycholecalciferol (calcitriol), are available by prescription for use in patients with hypocalcemia associated with hepatic or renal failure, respectively. The former compound has a longer half-life but is less potent. Dihydrotachysterol, which is available by prescription, is also useful in renal failure because it does not require metabolic activation by the kidneys.

Large daily doses of vitamin D (1000 to 4000 IU) are prescribed for the treatment of rickets. Calcitriol (0.25 to 1 mcg per day) is often prescribed for adults with osteomalacia caused by renal disease.

Adverse Effects Taking five or more times the US RDA of vitamin D may lead to adverse effects, including hypercalcemia, hypercalciuria, polyuria, nephrocalcinosis, renal failure, metastatic calcification, and kidney stones. Daily doses exceeding 400 IU (25 mcg of cholecalciferol) are not advisable. In infants, as little as 1800 IU of vitamin D per day may inhibit growth.

The more common symptoms of hypervitaminosis D are anorexia, nausea, weakness, weight loss, polyuria, constipation, vague aches, stiffness, soft tissue calcification, nephrocalcinosis, hypertension, anemia, hypercalcemia, acidosis, and irreversible renal failure. If patients do not know their recent serum calcium level, they should consult a physician.

Drug–Drug Interactions Concurrent drug therapy must be closely monitored because vitamin D may interact with other drugs. Phosphate in chronically used drugs, such as certain laxatives, may lower the calcium level and contribute to a vitamin D deficiency. Some antacids may interfere with vitamin D absorption. In particular, patients with renal problems should use caution in taking antacids. The pharmacist should advise patients with severe renal problems to select antacids for the specific ingredients they contain. Patients may choose aluminum-containing antacids because they bind phosphates, or calcium-containing antacids because they help increase serum calcium levels. However, patients should avoid magnesium-containing antacids because magnesium tends to accumulate to toxic levels in renal disease. Cholestyramine and mineral oil may reduce the amount of vitamin D absorbed, so patients should avoid their prolonged use. Phenytoin or barbiturates may decrease the half-life of vitamin D.

Vitamin E (Tocopherol) Vitamin E is present in all cell membranes. The term *vitamin E* refers to a series of eight compounds. The tocopherols and the tocotrienols are naturally occurring compounds in plants. The most active of these compounds, α-tocopherol, is used to calculate the vitamin E content of food.

The following equivalents can be used to estimate the total α-tocopherol equivalents (α-TEs) of diets containing only natural forms of vitamin E. To use the table below, the reader should multiply the number of milligrams of vitamin E in the diet by the number in the factor column. One α-TE equals 1.49 IU.

Item	*Factor*
β-tocopherol	0.5
γ-tocopherol	0.1
α-tocotrienol	0.3
all-rac-α-tocopherol	0.74

Function All its metabolic roles are not completely understood, but vitamin E functions primarily as an antioxidant in protecting cellular membranes from oxidative damage or destruction. This process may be aided by selenium and ascorbic acid. Vitamin E may also have a role in heme biosynthesis, steroid metabolism, and collagen formation.

Dietary Sources Foods rich in vitamin E include vegetable oils, margarines (made from plant oils), green vegetables, nuts, wheat germ, and whole grains. Refining grains removes much of the vitamin. Meats, fruits, and milk contain very little vitamin E.

Deficiency Vitamin E deficiency is extremely rare but may occur in two groups: premature, very low birth-weight infants or patients who do not absorb fat normally, such as children with cystic fibrosis. Neurologic abnormalities responsive to supplemental vitamin E have been reported in some patients with biliary disease and cystic fibrosis. Patients with those conditions should receive vitamin E supplements.

Symptoms of vitamin E deficiency include edema, hemolytic anemia, reticulocytosis, and thrombocytosis. That deficiency is cleared by a vitamin E supplement. In adults, the primary signs of vitamin E deficiency are reproductive failure and neurologic abnormalities. Signs or tests include increased hemolysis of red blood cells, creatinuria, and smooth muscle deposits of brown pigment. Evidence for deposition of ceroid (age) pigments, creatinuria, altered erythropoiesis, and myopathy have been found in patients with vitamin E deficiency secondary to steatorrhea.

Dose/US RDA The average daily diet contains approximately 3 to 15 mg of vitamin E; therefore, large doses (i.e., about 100 mg per day) are not necessary unless the patient is experiencing malabsorption. Doses of 300 to 400 mg per day have been prescribed for claudication (lameness), angina, diabetes, and Parkinson's disease, with inconclusive results.

Vitamin E requirements may vary in proportion to the amount of polyunsaturated fatty acids in the diet. Although the polyunsaturated fatty acid content of the U.S. diet has increased in recent years, the plant oils responsible for the increase are rich in tocopherol. It has been theorized that, with the increasing oxidant insult to the environment in the form of atmospheric pollutants, people should increase their intake of vitamin E. However, the lack of evidence of deficiency at the present intake supports the current adult US RDA of 8 to 10 mg per day.

Adverse Effects Vitamin E is relatively nontoxic. Most adults tolerate 100 to 1000 IU daily without adverse effects, but the hazards of long-term, high-dose therapy are unknown.

Drug–Drug Interactions Vitamin E has been reported to enhance warfarin anticoagulation. The pharmacist should caution patients taking oral anticoagulants to avoid vitamin E in large doses. Vitamin E should not be taken at the same time as iron; studies of supplementation in infant formulas containing iron and vitamin E show that blood tocopherol levels do not increase.

Vitamin K Phytonadione (vitamin K_1) is present in many vegetables. Menaquinone (vitamin K_2) is a product of bacterial metabolism, and the colonic bacteria may be able to synthesize about 2 mcg/kg of body weight per day of the vitamin. Menadione (vitamin K_3) is a synthetic compound that is two to three times as potent as the natural vitamin K. At least five proteins in the body depend on vitamin K for hepatic synthesis, including Factors II (prothrombin), VII, IX, and X of the plasma clotting cascade.

Function Vitamin K has two roles in normal physiology. First, it promotes the synthesis of clotting factors II, VII, XI, and X in the liver. Second, it activates these factors, along with the anticoagulation proteins C and S. The clotting factors remain inactive in the liver in the presence of coumarin or in the absence of vitamin K. When vitamin K is present, it enables the enzyme system to convert terminal glutamic acid residues on the clotting factors to γ-carboxyglutamyl residues in the completed protein, thus allowing the clotting factors to bind Ca++ and further bind to the phospholipids necessary for the clotting residue.

Dietary Sources Sources of vitamin K include pork liver and vegetables such as spinach, kale, cabbage, and cauliflower. Food composition tables and product labels may not list vitamin K content because it is not precisely known.

Deficiency Deficiencies do not readily occur because normal U.S. diets contain 300 to 500 mcg of vitamin K daily, so there is a low incidence of deficiency among healthy, well-nourished individuals. Moreover, microbiologic flora of the normal gut synthesize enough menaquinones to supply a significant part of the body's requirement for vitamin K. However, because the absorption of vitamin K requires bile in the small intestine, anything that interferes with bile production or secretion may contribute to a vitamin K deficiency. Malabsorption syndromes and bowel resections may decrease vitamin K absorption. Liver disease may also cause symptoms of vitamin K deficiency if hepatic production of the prothrombin clotting factor is decreased. Other potential causes of deficiency include breast-feeding of newborns; regional enteritis; blind loop syndrome; ulcerative colitis; and chronic, broad-spectrum antibiotic therapy. A deficiency may be evidenced by defective blood coagulation with hemorrhage and may be demonstrated by a prolonged prothrombin time.

Dose/US RDA The 1989 US RDA values included vitamin K for the first time: 65 mcg per day for adult women and 80 mcg per day for adult men. For minor bleeding, 1 to 5 mg of vitamin K is given daily; for a major hemorrhage, 20 mg is given. The cause of the deficiency and the severity of bleeding will determine whether oral administration is adequate. Vitamin K_1 (phytonadione) is routinely given to neonates at birth (one dose of 1 mg) to prevent hemorrhaging. This dosage is necessary because placental transport of vitamin K is low and the neonate has yet to acquire the intestinal microflora that produce the vitamin.

Only a small number of available nonprescription products contain vitamin K.

Adverse Effects Even in large amounts over an extended period, vitamin K does not produce toxic manifestations. However, administration of menadione may cause hemolytic anemia, hyperbilirubinemia, and kernicterus in the newborn as a result of interaction with sulfhydryl groups.

Drug–Drug Interactions In addition to agents such as cholestyramine resins and mineral oil, which interfere with the absorption of all fat-soluble vitamins, the oral anticoagulants are antagonists of vitamin K. Dietary amounts of vitamin K (near the US RDA value) do not usually interfere with coumarin anticoagulant activity, but an interaction with the 5-mg therapeutic dose of warfarin sodium (Coumadin) may be significant.

Long-term, broad-spectrum antibiotic therapy may initiate a vitamin K deficiency by decreasing gut flora. However, this interaction is not usually seen if dietary intake is normal. In large quantities, vitamins A and E may interfere with the absorption or metabolism of vitamin K.

Ascorbic Acid (Vitamin C) Ascorbic acid is the most easily destroyed of all the vitamins. A relatively simple compound, it is a powerful reducing agent that serves to protect the capillary basement membrane. As a nutrient, ascorbic acid is necessary to form collagen and to serve as a water-soluble antioxidant.

Function Ascorbic acid, which must be ingested because it is not produced in the body, is necessary for the biosynthesis of hydroxyproline, a precursor of collagen, osteoid, and dentin. It also assists in the absorption of nonheme iron from food by reducing the ferric iron in the stomach and by combining in complex formation with ions that remain solubilized in the alkaline pH of the duodenum.

Ascorbic acid has been promoted to prevent the common cold and to attenuate symptoms should a cold occur, but such claims are largely unsupported by well-designed and controlled clinical studies. It has been suggested that a decreased recovery time from cold sores, an increased healing rate of pressure sores, and a decreased incidence of rectal polyps may occur following administration of ascorbic acid. There are conflicting data, however, concerning the ability of ascorbic acid to lower cholesterol levels in hyper-cholesterolemic patients.

Dietary Sources Ascorbic acid has been called the "fresh-food" vitamin, and most of the daily intake is derived from the vegetable and fruit groups. Sources relatively high in vitamin C content include green and red peppers, collard greens, broccoli, spinach, tomatoes, potatoes, strawberries, oranges, and other citrus fruits. Meat, fish, poultry, eggs, and dairy products contain some vitamin C, but it is generally absent in grains.

Deficiency Characteristics of ascorbic acid deficiency include malaise, weakness, capillary hemorrhages and petechiae, hyperkeratotic follicles (corkscrew hairs), swollen hemorrhagic gums, and bone changes. A deficiency may also impair wound healing. A profound dietary deficiency can eventually lead to scurvy, producing widespread capillary hemorrhaging and a weakening of collagenous structures.

Scurvy, the classical deficiency state, is rare in the United States. It develops only when there is chronically inadequate nutritional consumption of ascorbic acid. Infants who are fed artificial formulas without vitamin supplements may develop symptoms of scurvy. In adults, however, scurvy would not occur for 3 to 5 months after all ascorbic acid consumption was stopped.

Several other uses of ascorbic acid are worthy of mention. For example, ascorbic acid supplementation in institutionalized elderly patients, among whom marginal ascorbic acid deficiencies have been reported, may measurably improve their general health and well-being. Such supplementation may also benefit smokers and women taking oral contraceptives, in whom lower than normal levels of ascorbic acid (and several other vitamins) have been noted. Ascorbic acid can also be used to increase iron absorption because it can form a soluble iron chelate and can inhibit the oxidation of ferrous to ferric iron, although this increase is generally not necessary for patients taking adequate iron supplementation.

Dose/US RDA Pharmacists are rarely confronted with overt symptoms of ascorbic acid deficiency. Only 10 mg per day of ascorbic acid prevents scurvy; a normal diet containing fresh fruits and vegetables contains many times this amount. The US RDA of ascorbic acid for most adults is 60 mg per day. The apparent average daily intake of vitamin C in the United States is about 77 mg for women and 109 mg for men, although losses during cooking may decrease the actual amount ingested. About 200 mg per day will saturate the body; most of a dose above this level will be excreted.

Most multivitamin supplements contain 60 to 100 mg of ascorbic acid, an appropriate level to consume if supplements are required. Doses of more than 200 mg are rarely indicated. In patients with a severe vitamin C deficiency, as evidenced by clinical signs of deficiency, 300 mg of ascorbic acid per day is recommended to replenish body stores. Infants who do not have ascorbic acid supplements in their formula should receive 35 to 50 mg per day; those who are breast-fed by well-nourished mothers will receive a sufficient amount. The Food and Nutrition Board recommends that smokers ingest at least 100 mg of supplemental vitamin C per day to compensate for an increased ascorbic acid metabolism and the lower levels of ascorbic acid in the body. If a supplement is warranted, the pharmacist may recommend a multivitamin product containing 60 to 100 mg of ascorbic acid.

Adverse Effects The pharmacist is urged to weigh the relative risks and benefits of ascorbic acid therapy. Short-term use to promote healing or for serious disorders such as rectal polyps may warrant a trial of ascorbic acid with medical supervision. Megadoses, however, may be harmful in certain circumstances, and the expense and potential risks of ingesting large quantities of the vitamin over the long term may be questionable for a seemingly minor beneficial effect on the common cold, a self-limiting condition. While the incidence of toxicity with ascorbic acid is low, ascorbic acid toxicity may increase oxalate excretion, produce nephrolithiasis, and lead to hemolysis in patients deficient in glucose 6-phosphate dehydrogenase. Rebound scurvy occurred upon sudden withdrawal of ascorbic acid in infants whose mothers took megadoses of vitamin C during pregnancy.

Drug–Drug Interactions When the urine is acidified, acidic drugs are reabsorbed more readily from the tubules, resulting in higher, more prolonged blood levels. Conversely, basic drugs such as tricyclic antidepressants and amphetamines may be excreted more rapidly from acidified urine, and their effect may be reduced by ascorbic acid therapy. The clinical significance of the effects of ascorbic acid on the reabsorption and elimination of acidic and basic drugs is controversial because the ascorbic acid–induced decrease in urine pH has been shown to be small. Nevertheless, patients should be monitored if they are on medications eliminated by renal excretion and if they initiate megadose ascorbic acid therapy. Cholestyramine may bind ascorbic acid, reducing not only ascorbic acid absorption but also the bile acid–binding capacity of cholestyramine. Therefore, administration of the two should be separated. Ascorbic acid may increase the serum levels of estrogens and reduce the anticoagulant action of warfarin.

Cyanocobalamin (Vitamin B_{12}) Cyanocobalamin contains a single atom of cobalt and is the most complex vitamin molecule. It is available in the body as methylcobalamin, hydroxocobalamin, and adenosylcobalamin, all designated as "Acobalamins." The term *vitamin B_{12}* refers to all cobalamins that have vitamin activity in humans. Cyanocobalamin, the common pharmaceutical form of the vitamin, is one of two commercially available forms and is the most stable; however, it is present in only small amounts in the body.

Function Vitamin B_{12} is active in all cells, especially those in the bone marrow, the central nervous system (CNS), and the GI tract. It is also involved in fat, protein, and carbohydrate metabolism. A cobalamin coenzyme functions in the synthesis of DNA and in the synthesis and transfer of single-carbon units (e.g., the methyl group in the synthesis of methionine and choline). Vitamin B_{12} participates in methylation reactions and cell division, usually in concert with folic acid. It is necessary for the metabolism of folates; therefore, a folate deficiency may be observed as a feature of vitamin B_{12} deficiency. Vitamin B_{12} is also necessary for the metabolism of lipids and the formation of myelin.

Dietary Sources Vitamin B_{12} is produced almost exclusively by microorganisms, which accounts for its presence in animal protein (meats, oysters, and clams). It may be found in small amounts in the root nodules of legumes and in selected vegetables and fruits, again because of the presence of microorganisms.

Deficiency In healthy individuals who have not restricted their diets, cyanocobalamin levels are maintained by the body. Vitamin B_{12} deficiency may be caused by poor absorption or utilization, or by an increased requirement or excretion of this vitamin. Because vitamin B_{12} is conserved by the body, it requires approximately 3 years for the deficiency to develop. In patients with malabsorption (ileal diseases or resection), the reabsorption phase of the enterohepatic cycle is affected, and the deficiency may occur much earlier.

Because of the general lack of vitamin B_{12} in vegetables, vegetarians who consume no animal products are at risk for developing a vitamin B_{12} deficiency, including infants breast-fed by vegetarian mothers. Strict vegetarians should consider taking vitamin B_{12} supplements or should adjust their diet to include fermented foods, such as soy sauce, that contain the vitamin. Certain drugs such as neomycin may impair absorption of vitamin B_{12}.

The symptoms of a vitamin B_{12} deficiency mimic those of a folate deficiency and are manifested in organ systems with rapidly duplicating cells. Thus, one effect of such a deficiency on the hematopoietic system is macrocytic anemia. The GI tract is also affected, with glossitis and epithelial changes occurring along the entire digestive tract. Some people lack the glycoprotein (intrinsic factor) necessary for the gastric absorption of vitamin B_{12}, which results in pernicious anemia. Because vitamin B_{12} is necessary for the maintenance of myelin, deficiency states produce many neurologic symptoms: paresthesia, unsteadiness, poor muscular coordination, mental confusion, agitation, hallucinations, and overt psychosis. Other clinical manifestations of cyanocobalamin deficiency include macrocytic megaloblastic anemia, atrophic gastritis, achlorhydria, peripheral neuropathy, spinal cord degeneration, and dementia.

The pharmacist should caution patients that an accurate diagnosis of the causes of a suspected anemia is essential in selecting effective treatment. For example, anemia resulting from a folic acid deficiency should be treated with folic acid, pernicious anemia should be treated with vitamin B_{12}, and iron deficiency anemia should be treated with iron. The pharmacist should discourage use of a "shotgun" antianemia preparation that contains multiple hematinic factors.

Dose/US RDA The US RDA for vitamin B_{12} is 2 mcg for adults. Requirements increase to 2.2 mcg during pregnancy and to 2.6 mcg during lactation. Oral forms can be used if the deficiency is nutritionally based; intramuscular or subcutaneous administration is necessary for deficiencies caused by malabsorption.

Hydroxocobalamin is a longer-acting form equal in hematopoietic effect to cyanocobalamin. Because it is more extensively bound to proteins at the site of injection and to plasma proteins, renal excretion is slower; thus the vitamin remains in the body for a longer period.

Adverse Effects Excessive doses have not resulted in toxicity, nor has any benefit been reported from nondeficient patients taking large quantities of the vitamin.

Drug–Drug Interactions No drug interactions have been reported for cyanocobalamin.

Folic Acid (Pteroylglutamic Acid, Folacin) The term *folacin* is used as a generic term to designate folic acid, pteroylglutamic acid, and other similar-acting compounds. Current guidelines for terminology are that *folate* and *folic acid* are preferred synonyms for *pteroylglutamate* and *pteroylglutamic acid.* Because *folates* can be used in a generic sense referring to the above, the term *folacin* should not be used.

Function Folates are reduced in vivo to the bioactive form, tetrahydrofolic acid, and are involved in the biosynthesis of purine, pyrimidine, serine, methionine, and choline. Folic acid is further biotransformed in the body and is involved in DNA synthesis and in maturation and cell production activities. The function of folic acid is closely related to that of vitamin B_{12}. A folic acid deficiency can occur as a consequence of a vitamin B_{12} deficiency.

Dietary Sources Folates are present in nearly all natural foods. Primary sources in the diet include liver, lean beef, veal, yeast, leafy vegetables, legumes, some fruits, eggs, and whole-grain cereals. The diet should include some foods that require little cooking, however, because folates are heat labile and the folic acid content of food depends on how the food is processed. Canning, long exposure to heat, and extensive refining may destroy 50% to 100% of the naturally occurring folic acid.

Deficiency The requirements for folic acid are related to the metabolic rate and cell turnover. Thus, increased amounts of folic acid are needed during pregnancy, lactation, and infancy, as well as for infection, hemolytic anemias and blood loss (in which red blood cell production must be increased to replenish blood supply), and hypermetabolic states such as hyperthyroidism. Rheumatoid arthritis may also increase folic acid requirements.

Causes of folic acid deficiency include alcoholism, malabsorption, food faddism, liver disease, and iatrogenic forms associated with the administration of various therapeutic agents.

A deficiency of folic acid results in impaired cell division and protein synthesis. Symptoms of folic acid deficiency are similar to those of vitamin B_{12} deficiency, including sore mouth, diarrhea, and CNS symptoms such as irritability and forgetfulness. The most common laboratory feature of folic acid deficiency is megaloblastic anemia, an anemia characterized by large erythroblasts circulating in the blood.

Because vitamin B_{12} is essential for the metabolism of folates, a megaloblastic anemia responsive to folic acid administration is a feature of pernicious anemia. Folic acid given without vitamin B_{12} to patients with pernicious anemia will correct the anemia but will have no effect on the more insidious damage to the CNS, symptoms of which include lack of coordination, impaired sense of position, and various behavioral disturbances. Because of the potential for folic acid to mask the signs, but not the progression, of pernicious anemia (which is caused by a vitamin B_{12} deficiency), products containing more than 0.8 mg of folic acid per dose are available only by prescription. Pharmacists should refer all patients with suspected anemias for medical consultation.

Dose/US RDA The US RDA for folic acid is 200 mcg for most adult men and 180 mcg for most adult women, increasing to 400 mcg during pregnancy. Folic acid supplementation starting before pregnancy, if possible, is now recommended to prevent neural tube defects, one of the most common severe congenital malformations.

The oral dose of folic acid for correction of a deficiency is usually 1 mg per day, particularly if the deficiency occurs with conditions that may increase the folate requirement or suppress red blood cell formation (e.g., pregnancy, hypermetabolic states, alcoholism, or hemolytic anemia). Doses larger than 1 mg per day are not necessary except in some life-threatening hematologic diseases. Maintenance therapy for deficiencies may be stopped after 1 to 4 months if the diet contains at least one fresh fruit or vegetable daily. For chronic malabsorption diseases, folic acid treatment may be lifelong and parenteral doses may be required.

Adverse Effects Folic acid toxicity is virtually nonexistent because of folic acid's water solubility and rapid excretion. Up to 15 mg have been given daily without toxic effect.

Drug–Drug Interactions Several drugs taken chronically may increase the need for folic acid. Phenytoin and possibly other related anticonvulsants may inhibit folic acid absorption, leading to megaloblastic anemia. This problem is further complicated because folic acid supplementation may decrease serum phenytoin levels and complicate seizure control. The pharmacist should note when folic acid is prescribed to patients whose medication records indicate concurrent phenytoin therapy.

Trimethoprim may act as a weak folic acid antagonist in humans. Megaloblastic anemia may be precipitated in patients who possess a relatively low folic acid level at the onset of trimethoprim therapy; however, this problem is rarely seen in most patients using trimethoprim. Pyrimethamine, which is related to trimethoprim, may induce megaloblastic anemia in large doses. The mechanism of pyrimethamine's folic acid antagonism is inhibition of active tetrahydrofolate production. Methotrexate is also a folic acid antagonist, so patients on maintenance regimens for psoriasis or rheumatoid arthritis should be questioned carefully if they request folic acid supplements.

Niacin (Nicotinic Acid) The physiologically active form of niacin is nicotinamide. Niacin and niacinamide (nicotinic acid amide) are constituents of the coenzymes nicotinamide adenine dinucleotide and nicotinamide adenine dinucleotide phosphate.

Function The niacin coenzymes are electron transfer agents; that is, they accept or donate hydrogen in the aerobic respiration of all body cells. Niacin is unusual as a vitamin in that humans can synthesize it from dietary tryptophan, with about 60 mg of tryptophan being equivalent to 1 mg of niacin. Most individuals receive about 50% of their niacin requirement from tryptophan-containing proteins and the rest as preformed niacin or niacinamide. In therapeutic doses, niacin will lower triglycerides and low-density lipoprotein cholesterol by mechanisms unrelated to its function as an essential micronutrient.

Dietary Sources Niacin is present in most foods, including lean meats, fish, liver, cold cereals, whole grains, green vegetables, and legumes.

Deficiency Clinical findings of niacin deficiency include the three "Ds" of *d*ermatitis, *d*iarrhea, and *d*ementia, often accompanied by neuropathy, glossitis, stomatitis, and proctitis. The classical and only described niacin deficiency state is pellagra (the name given to symptomatic niacin deficiency). Pellagra is rare, occurring most often in alcoholics, poorly nourished elderly persons, and individuals on bizarre diets. It may occur in areas where much corn is eaten because niacin in corn may be bound to undigestible constituents, making it unavailable. Other causes of pellagra include isoniazid therapy and decreased tryptophan conversion, as in Hartnup disease and carcinoid tumors. The main body systems affected are the CNS, the skin, and the GI tract. Symptoms involving the CNS include peripheral neuropathy, myelopathy, and encephalopathy. Mania may occur. Seizures and coma precede death. Before the cause of CNS manifestations of niacin deficiency was discovered, many psychiatric admissions were occasioned by symptoms of niacin deficiency. Both niacin and niacinamide are effective in treating pellagra.

Niacin-deficient patients manifest a characteristic rash. The skin over the face and on pressure points may become thickened or hyperpigmented, or it may appear burned. Secondary infections may occur in such lesions. The entire GI tract is generally affected, with angular fissures around the mouth, atrophy of the epithelium, a beefy-red color of the tongue, and hypertrophy of the papillae. Inflammation of the small intestine may be associated with episodes of occult bleeding and/or diarrhea.

An individual's niacin status can be estimated by measuring the urinary levels of niacin metabolites. Low values together with symptoms point to a diagnosis of pellagra.

Dose/US RDA The US RDA of niacin is 19 mg for most adult men and 15 mg for most adult women. As previously noted, 1 mg of niacin is equivalent to 60 mg of dietary tryptophan. Niacin requirements are increased when the patient has an acute illness; when the patient is convalescing after a severe injury, infection, or burns; when the patient has substantially increased either caloric expenditure or dietary caloric intake; or when the patient has a low tryptophan intake (e.g., a low-protein diet or a high intake of corn as a staple in the diet).

Treatment of pellagra involves the ingestion of 300 to 500 mg of niacinamide daily in divided doses. Because other nutritional deficiencies may be present, treatment may include the other B vitamins, vitamin A, and iron.

Niacin has been used in daily dosages of 1 to 2 g three times per day, up to 8 g per day, to treat hypercholesterolemia and hyperlipidemias. Niacin treatment increases beneficial high-density lipoprotein cholesterol and decreases levels of potentially harmful triglycerides, total cholesterol, and low-density lipoprotein cholesterol. Niacin treatment of hyperlipidemias requires close medical supervision for evidence of effectiveness and manifestations of drug-induced toxicity.

Niacin and niacinamide are available as tablets and capsules in strengths ranging from 25 to 500 mg and in both regular and timed-release products. They are also available in elixir form (50 mg/5 mL), as well as in many combination products. Prenatal multivitamins may contain up to 20 mg of niacin.

Adverse Effects Niacin toxicity can involve GI symptoms (e.g., nausea, vomiting, and diarrhea), hepatotoxicity, skin lesions, tachycardia, hypertension, and flushing. Doses of niacin in excess of 1 g per day may result in flushing and burning sensations. High doses may cause significant and potentially serious adverse effects. Chronic high-dose usage may lead to hyper-keratotic pigmented skin lesions.

Patients should be forewarned that niacin may cause flushing and a sensation of warmth, especially around the face, neck, and ears. This reaction, which many people experience especially upon initiation of therapy, may be diminished if they take 325 mg of aspirin or 200 mg of ibuprofen 30 minutes before the niacin dose, provided there are no contraindications. Itching or tingling and headache may also occur. All these effects will usually subside or decrease in intensity with continued therapy. If niacin causes GI upset, it should be taken with meals.

Niacinamide does not produce the discomforting flushing associated with therapeutic doses of niacin; however, it also does not have a beneficial lowering effect on plasma lipids.

Drug–Drug Interactions Niacin has decreased the effect of oral hypoglycemics and may inhibit the uricosuric effects of sulfinpyrazone and probenecid. It may also cause an increased risk for myopathy with lovastatin—and possibly with other hepatic hydroxymethylglutaryl coenzyme A (HMG-CoA) reductase inhibitors. It has an additive vasodilating effect with adrenergic blocking agents and may contribute to postural hypotension.

Contraindications Because of the adverse effects on the GI tract, high doses of niacin are contraindicated in patients with gastritis or peptic ulcer disease. Niacin can provoke the release of histamine, so its use in patients with asthma should be undertaken carefully. Niacin may also impair liver function, as evidenced by cholestatic jaundice, and it can disturb glucose tolerance and cause hyperuricemia. If niacin and niacinamide are used in high doses, laboratory parameters suggested by the potential side effects should be followed.

Pantothenic Acid Pantothenic acid is a water-soluble vitamin of the B-complex family. Only the dextrorotatory isomer has biologic activity.

Function Pantothenic acid is a precursor of coenzyme A (CoA), a product that is active in many biologic reactions and that plays a primary role in cholesterol, steroid, and fatty acid synthesis. Pantothenic acid is important for acetylation reactions and the formation of citric acid for the Krebs cycle; it is crucial in the intraneuronal synthesis of acetylcholine. It is also important in gluconeogenesis; in the synthesis and degradation of fatty acids; in the synthesis of sterols, steroid hormones, and porphyrins; in the release of energy from carbohydrates; and in acylation reactions.

Dietary Sources Pantothenic acid is widely distributed in plant and animal tissues. Sources include meat, liver, milk, eggs, vegetables, cereal grains, and legumes.

Deficiency Because pantothenic acid is contained in many foods, deficiency states are rare and hard to detect. In malabsorption syndromes, it is difficult to separate pantothenic acid deficiency symptoms from symptoms of other deficiencies. Symptoms of pantothenic acid deficiency include the following: somnolence, fatigue, headache, cardiovascular instability, GI complaints, changes in disposition, increased susceptibility to infections, and paresthesia of hands and/or feet followed by hyperreflexia and muscular weakness in the legs. Administration of pharmacologic doses of pantothenic acid reverses these symptoms and has even been used to eliminate burning feet syndrome.

Dose/US RDA The Food and Nutrition Board does not list a US RDA value for this vitamin but estimates a safe and adequate daily intake to be 4 to 7 mg for adults.

Adverse Effects Pantothenic acid is generally considered nontoxic, even in large doses. Doses as high as 10 g of calcium pantothenate daily have been given to young men for 6 weeks with no toxic symptoms. However, ingestion of more than 20 g has been reported to result in diarrhea and water retention. Dexpanthenol may prolong bleeding time in hemophiliacs and should be used with extreme caution.

Drug–Drug Interactions The miotic effects of anticholinesterase ophthalmic preparations (echothiophate iodide, isoflurophate) may be potentiated (increased) by pantothenic acid.

Pyridoxine (Vitamin B_6) This water-soluble vitamin exists in three forms: pyridoxine (vitamin B_6), pyridoxal, and pyridoxamine. Although all three forms are equally effective in nutrition, pyridoxine hydrochloride is the form most often used in vitamin formulations.

Function Pyridoxine serves as a cofactor for more than 60 enzymes, including decarboxylases, synthetases, transaminases, and hydroxylases. It is important in heme production and in the conversion of oxalate to glycine.

Dietary Sources Foods rich in pyridoxine include meats, cereals, lentils, nuts, and some fruits and vegetables (e.g., bananas, avocados, and potatoes). Cooking destroys some of

Case Study 19–1

Patient Complaint/History

Patrick, a 45-year-old stock market analyst on the fast track, is a confident individual, who says he thrives on his work pressure and many community activities. The 6-foot 11-inch, 195-pound analyst enjoys playing baseball and basketball with his children; he also enjoys golfing and fishing. He comes to the pharmacy today to ask about symptoms that occur about an hour after he takes niacin, ascorbic acid, and multivitamin supplements. He says that he becomes very flushed and red-faced; further, his face feels as though "it's on fire."

During his physical checkup performed 2 weeks earlier, Patrick's temperature (98.6°F [37.0°C]), pulse rate (73 bpm), and electrocardiogram were normal. His blood pressure was 140/90 mm Hg. Laboratory findings showed a hemoglobin level of 15 g/dL, a blood urea nitrogen (BUN) level of 10 mg/dL, a creatinine level of 1.2 mg/dL, a total cholesterol level of 300 mg/dL, a high-density lipoprotein (HDL) cholesterol level of 35 mg/dL, and a triglyceride level of 120 mg/dL.

The patient, who at that time was a heavy smoker and drank six cups of coffee a day, was diagnosed as having borderline hypertension and Type IIa hyperlipoproteinemia (excess lipoprotein in the blood). He was advised to stop smoking, to reduce his caffeine intake, and to increase his participation in sports and outdoor activities. He was also advised to reduce his intake of saturated fat and cholesterol.

Patrick immediately began to read materials about his condition. After learning that niacin is used to help lower cholesterol levels, he decided to try it. He decided that his increased participation in sports and outdoor activities warranted his taking a high-potency multivitamin. Last week, he purchased 500 mg ascorbic acid tablets (labeled as meeting USP standards), high-potency multivitamin tablets, and long-acting 500-mg niacin tablets at a health food store. Patrick has been taking one tablet of each vitamin in the morning and evening. He now wonders whether his symptoms are related to his change in lifestyle or to the vitamins.

Clinical Considerations/Strategies

Readers can use the following considerations/strategies to determine whether treatment of the patient's condition with nonprescription nutritional supplements is warranted:

- Assess the appropriateness of the multivitamin and ascorbic acid therapy.
- Assess the appropriateness of the niacin therapy.
- Discuss with the patient the possibility of seeking medical intervention in managing his hyperlipoproteinemia.
- Propose alternative products that will meet the patient's actual versus perceived needs.

Patient Education/Counseling

Readers can use the following strategies to develop a patient education/counseling plan that will help ensure optimal therapeutic outcomes:

- Support/justify changes in the patient-selected vitamin therapy.
- Explain the therapeutic regimen for the recommended product (i.e., dose, time and frequency of administration, warnings/precautions, adverse effects, and drug interactions).

the vitamin. The average U.S. diet provides slightly less than the US RDA; certain restricted diets may result in low pyridoxine intake. Infant formulas are required to contain pyridoxine hydrochloride.

Deficiency Causes of pyridoxine deficiency include alcoholism, severe diarrheal syndromes, food faddism, malabsorption syndromes, drugs (isoniazid, hydralazine, penicillamine, and cycloserine), and genetic diseases (cystathioninuria and xanthinuric aciduria).

The symptoms of severe pyridoxine deficiency in infants are convulsive disorders and irritability. Treatment with pyridoxine hydrochloride (2 mg per day for infants) generally brings the electroencephalogram back to normal and resolves clinical symptoms. Symptoms in adults whose diets are deficient in pyridoxine or who have been given a pyridoxine antagonist are difficult to distinguish from symptoms of niacin and riboflavin deficiencies. These symptoms include pellagra-like dermatitis; oral lesions; peripheral neuropathy; scaliness around the nose, mouth, and eyes; and dulling of mentation. Serious deficiency symptoms include convulsions, peripheral neuritis, and sideroblastic anemia.

Dose/US RDA The US RDA for pyridoxine is 2 mg for most adult men and 1.6 mg for most adult women. This requirement is increased to 2.2 mg during pregnancy and to 2.1 mg during lactation.

Treatment of sideroblastic anemia requires 50 to 200 mg per day of pyridoxine hydrochloride to aid in producing hemoglobin and erythrocytes. At least five pyridoxine-dependent inborn errors of metabolism have been shown to respond to large doses of pyridoxine. Pyridoxine (100 mg taken three times daily) for at least 11 weeks has been reported to relieve paresthesia and pain in the hands of patients with carpal tunnel syndrome. However, the value of such therapy has not been clearly and objectively determined.

Adverse Effects Pyridoxine may be toxic in high doses. A severe sensory neuropathy, similar to that observed with the deficiency state, has been reported when gram quantities were taken to relieve symptoms of premenstrual syndrome (PMS). Similar symptoms have been reported in women taking doses as small as 50 mg per day for PMS. Recovery occurred on withdrawal of pyridoxine but was slow.

High daily doses of pyridoxine (200 to 600 mg) have been shown to inhibit prolactin. Prenatal vitamins, which contain 1 to 10 mg per dosage unit, do not appear to have a significant antiprolactin effect. Large doses of pyridoxine may also increase the activity of plasma aminotransferase, but the consequences of this effect are unknown.

Drug–Drug Interactions Several drugs interact with pyridoxine, and it affects the action of several drugs. Isoniazid and cycloserine antagonize pyridoxine; hydralazine may have this effect as well. Perioral numbness resulting from peripheral neuropathy is a clinical manifestation of this antagonism. To overcome this problem, the patient should routinely use 50 mg per day of pyridoxine hydrochloride with isoniazid and 20 mg per day with cycloserine. Another recommended dose is 10 mg of pyridoxine for each 100 mg of isoniazid. Psychotic behavior and seizures, both produced by cycloserine, may be prevented with increased pyridoxine intake. Penicillamine may bind with pyridoxine hydrochloride, causing pyridoxine-responsive neurotoxicity. Pyridoxine may reduce the clinical effects of phenobarbital and phenytoin by reducing their serum levels.

Pyridoxine antagonizes the therapeutic action of levodopa (the biologically active form of dopa) by facilitating the transformation of levodopa into dopamine before the former can cross the blood–brain barrier and enter the CNS. The pharmacist should inform patients who take levodopa about the interaction and should advise them to avoid supplemental pyridoxine. Conversely, pyridoxine may be useful in treating patients who have overdosed on levodopa. A combination product containing levodopa and carbidopa, a peripherally acting dopa decarboxylase inhibitor, does not appear to be affected by the concurrent administration of pyridoxine.

Riboflavin (Vitamin B_2) Riboflavin occurs in the free state in foods, in combination with phosphates, or with both phosphates and proteins. The free riboflavin is released and absorbed during digestion.

Function Riboflavin is a constituent of two coenzymes: flavin adenine dinucleotide and flavin mononucleotide. It is involved in numerous oxidation and reduction reactions, including the cytochrome P-450 reductase enzyme system involved in drug metabolism. Cellular growth cannot occur without riboflavin.

Dietary Sources Primary sources of riboflavin include meats; poultry; fish; dairy products; enriched and fortified grains, cereals, and bakery products; and green vegetables such as broccoli, turnip greens, asparagus, and spinach.

Deficiency Riboflavin deficiency may occur in association with other vitamin B complex deficiency states (e.g., pellagra) or during pregnancy. Deficiencies are common in many migraine headache sufferers. Early signs of riboflavin deficiency may involve ocular symptoms as the eyes become light sensitive and easily fatigued. The patient may develop blurred vision; itching, watering, sore eyes; and increased capillarization in the cornea with a bloodshot appearance of the eye. Later clinical findings of deficiency include stomatitis, glossitis, seborrheic dermatitis, and magenta tongue.

Dose/US RDA The US RDA for riboflavin is 1.7 mg for most adult men and 1.3 mg for most adult women. The need for riboflavin appears to increase during periods of increased cell growth, such as during pregnancy and wound healing.

Riboflavin is poorly soluble. If oral absorption is poor, 25 mg of the soluble riboflavin salt may be injected intramuscularly. Riboflavin may also be given intravenously as a component of an injectable multivitamin, but the dose is relatively low (about 10 mg).

Adverse Effects/Drug–Drug Interactions The use of riboflavin may cause a yellow-orange fluorescence or discoloration of the urine. Patients who report this effect should be reassured that this color is normal.

No drug interactions have been reported for riboflavin.

Thiamine (Vitamin B_1) Thiamine, a water-soluble vitamin, is necessary for several critical functions in carbohydrate metabolism.

Function Thiamine's active form, thiamine pyrophosphate (formerly known as cocarboxylase), plays a vital role in the oxidative decarboxylation of pyruvic acid; in the formation of acetyl CoA, which enters the Krebs cycle; and in other important biochemical conversion cycles. Thiamine is also essential in neurologic function. The amount of vitamin that is required increases with increased caloric consumption.

Dietary Sources The most familiar natural thiamine source is the hull of rice grains; other sources are pork, beef, fresh peas, and beans.

Deficiency Several genetic diseases respond to the administration of thiamine. These diseases fall into the category of vitamin-responsible inborn errors of metabolism and are generally attributable to a defect in the binding of enzyme and cofactor. Large daily doses of vitamins (5 to 100 mg in the case of thiamine) saturate the enzyme system(s) and usually obviate the pathology. Examples of thiamine-responsive inborn metabolic errors are lactic acidosis caused by defective pyruvate carboxylase, branched-chain aminoacidopathy caused by defective branched-chain amino acid decarboxylase, and some cases of the Wernicke–Korsakoff syndrome caused by defective transketolase. These disorders justify the rational use of megadose thiamine therapy.

The primary causes of thiamine deficiency are generally related to inadequate diet, alcoholism, malabsorption syndromes, prolonged diarrhea, increased use (pregnancy), or food faddism.

Accordingly, thiamine deficiency in the United States is

found primarily in alcoholics, in patients with chronic diarrhea, and in patients maintained on a high carbohydrate diet. Among alcoholics, thiamine deficiency is common. Because their diet is often nutritionally deficient and unbalanced, alcohol ingestion further impairs thiamine absorption and transport across the intestine and increases the rate of destruction of thiamine diphosphate. High-dose, parenteral thiamine is commonly given to patients who are admitted to hospitals for alcohol detoxification and treatment. A vitamin supplement containing thiamine is often prescribed for the alcoholic patient.

A diet that consists chiefly of unenriched white rice and white flour, or a situation in which low dietary levels of thiamine are accompanied by the consumption of large amounts of raw fish with thiaminase-containing intestinal microbes, may also produce a thiamine deficiency. Individuals subsisting on a diet of 0.2 to 0.3 mg of thiamine per 1000 calories (slightly less than the thiamine requirement) may gradually become depleted of thiamine and may develop peripheral neuropathy. If the patient has been subsisting on substantially less than 0.2 mg of thiamine per 1000 calories, the deficiency will be more severe.

Symptoms of thiamine deficiency may become evident 3 weeks after thiamine intake is stopped. The deficiency causes cardiac dysfunction, possibly accompanied by edema, tachycardia on only minimal exertion, enlarged heart, and electrocardiographic abnormalities. The patient may have pain in the precordial or epigastric areas. Neuromuscular symptoms include paresthesia of the extremities, weakness, and atrophy.

Dose/US RDA The US RDA for most adult men and women is 1.5 mg and 1.1 mg, respectively. To treat the symptoms of heart failure caused by a thiamine deficiency, the patient should take 5 to 10 mg of thiamine three times a day. At this dosage, the failure is rapidly corrected, but the neurologic signs correct much more slowly. The daily dose of thiamine for neurologic deficits is 30 to 100 mg given parenterally for several days or until an oral diet can be started. If thiamine is mixed in a solution, the solution should be acidic because thiamine is labile at an alkaline pH.

Adverse Effects The kidney easily clears excessive thiamine intake, and oral doses of 500 mg have been found to be nontoxic. Some toxicity may exist from large doses given parenterally, however, with symptoms of itching, tingling, and pain.

Drug–Drug Interactions No drug interactions have been reported for thiamine.

Diagnostic Test Interferences Thiamine may interfere with several diagnostic tests. A false positive may occur for uric acid using the phosphotungstate method and for urobilinogen using Ehrlich's reagent. Large doses of thiamine may interfere with the spectrophotometric determination of serum theophylline concentrations.

Vitamin-Like Compounds and Pseudovitamins

Vitamin-like compounds, or pseudovitamins, are substances having a chemical structure very similar to that of vitamins but without the usual physiologic or biochemical actions; that is, they are not essential for specific body functions of growth, maintenance, and reproduction.

Bioflavonoids (Vitamin P) The term *bioflavonoids* (flavonoids) has been used to designate flavones and flavonols. Bioflavonoids are available as capsules and tablets and in combination products (both regular and sustained release) as tablets, capsules, and wafers.

Function Because no known bioflavonoid deficiency condition exists, bioflavonoids have no accepted preventive or therapeutic role in human nutrition. Their mechanism of action is unknown but has been presented as "decreasing capillary permeability and fragility."

Dietary Sources The flavonoids are widely distributed in plants and are concentrated in the skin, peel, and outer layers of fruits and vegetables.

Dose/US RDA The average daily dietary intake of flavonoids is approximately 1000 mg. Consequently, dietary supplementation using 20- to 30-mg tablets would not be significant. There is no listed US RDA for this pseudovitamin.

Adverse Effects/Drug–Drug Interactions Adverse effects and drug interactions have not been reported for bioflavonoids. Therefore, bioflavonoids have no known adverse effects.

Biotin (Vitamin H) Biotin has been included in several multivitamin preparations.

Function Biotin, a member of the B-complex group of vitamins, is required for various metabolic functions (e.g., gluconeogenesis, lipogenesis, fatty acid biosynthesis, propionate metabolism, and the catabolism of branched-chain amino acids). Nine known biotin-dependent enzymes now exist, and biotin plays an important role in fat, amino acid, and carbohydrate metabolism.

Dietary Sources Biotin is widely distributed in animal tissue and is thus present in the diet. Sources include liver, egg yolk, cauliflower, salmon, carrots, bananas, soy flour, and yeast. Colonic flora probably contribute to the amount of biotin in the body.

Deficiency Deficiency states of biotin are rare but have been associated with nausea, vomiting, lassitude, muscle pain, anorexia, anemia, and depression. Dermatitis, a grayish color of the skin, and glossitis may be among the physical findings; hypercholesterolemia and cardiac abnormalities may occur.

Biotin deficiency in humans can be caused by ingesting a large number of raw egg whites. Raw egg white contains avidin, a protein that binds biotin, thereby preventing its absorption. Biotin deficiency symptoms have been noted in patients on parenteral nutrition without biotin supplements. In pregnant women, blood biotin levels decrease as gestation progresses.

Individuals undergoing a rapid weight loss program with intense caloric restriction or those with malnutrition may not be obtaining adequate biotin and should receive supplementation.

Dose/US RDA Biotin is known to be necessary for carboxylation reactions in the body, but the nutritional requirements for this vitamin are imprecise and no US RDA has been determined for it. However, 100 to 200 mcg per day is generally considered safe and adequate.

Adverse Effects/Drug–Drug Interactions Adverse effects and drug interactions have not been reported with biotin therapy.

L-Carnitine (DL-Carnitine) Carnitine, a vitamin-like molecule, can be synthesized from lysine and methionine in the liver and kidney; thus, it is considered an essential nutrient but not necessarily a vitamin.

Function A number of actions are attributed to carnitine, including oxidation of fatty acids, promotion of certain organic acid excretions, and enhancement of the rate of oxidative phosphorylation.

L-Carnitine is required to transport long-chain fatty acids in mitochondria, which is prerequisite to their beta-oxidation, and to maintenance of energy production. Although carnitine is biosynthesized adequately by adults, newborns have a low capacity for carnitine synthesis from lysine and methionine; they may be further compromised if fed soy formulas or maintained on total parenteral nutrition with no supplemental carnitine.

Dietary Sources Dietary sources and synthesis in the liver and kidney satisfy the primary need for carnitine. Food sources include dairy products and meat, especially red meat.

Deficiency Carnitine deficiency may be evidenced by muscle weakness, cardiomyopathy, abnormal hepatic function, decreased ketogenesis, and hypoglycemia during fasting. Lipids may accumulate between muscle fibers. Rarely, valproic acid can induce carnitine deficiency; thus, carnitine is sometimes given with valproic acid particularly if there are liver function abnormalities. Also, a deficiency state may be seen in hemodialysis patients.

Dose/US RDA Human carnitine deficiency has been documented, but no US RDA has been established. Therapy for carnitine deficiency should include a pharmaceutical supplement and a high-carbohydrate, low-fat diet. L-Carnitine is available as 250-mg capsules, as 330-mg tablets, and as a liquid containing 100 mg/mL. It is present in several strengths in various combination products.

Adverse Effects/Drug–Drug Interactions L-Carnitine is without appreciable adverse effects in normal adults, and doses of 15 g per day have been well tolerated.

No drug interactions have been reported for this pseudovitamin.

Choline Choline is contained in most living cells and in foods. It is usually present in the form of phosphatidylcholine, commonly known as lecithin, and in several other phospholipids found in cell membranes. Intestinal mucosal cells and pancreatic secretions contain enzymes capable of splitting phospholipids to release choline. Choline is also found in sphingomyelin and is highly concentrated in nervous tissue.

Function Choline, a precursor in the biosynthesis of acetylcholine, is an important donor of methyl groups used in the biochemical formation of other substances in vivo. It can be biosynthesized in humans by the donation of methyl groups from methionine to ethanolamine. Further, choline and inositol are considered to be lipotropic agents (i.e., agents involved in the mobilization of lipids). They have been used to treat fatty liver and disturbed fat metabolism, but their efficacy has not been established.

Dietary Sources Although choline is found in egg yolks, cereal, fish, and meat, it is also synthesized in the body. Therefore, it is doubtful that choline is a vitamin. Choline is obtained from the diet as either choline or lecithin.

Deficiency A deficiency state has not been identified in humans, possibly because choline is readily available in the diet.

Dose/US RDA An average diet will furnish 200 to 600 mg of choline daily.

Adverse Effects/Drug–Drug Interactions The administration of large doses of lecithin has been associated with sweating, GI distress, vomiting, and diarrhea. Most adults, however, tolerate up to 20 g per day with no adverse effects. No drug interactions with lecithin have been reported.

Essential Fatty Acids (Vitamin F) The essential fatty acids are involved in properly developing various biomembranes. They are also important as precursors of prostaglandins, leukotrienes, and various hydroxy fatty acids. The polyunsaturated fatty acids regulate cell permeability to a significant degree because they are constituents of phospholipids.

Linoleic and linolenic acids are essential in human nutrition but do not meet the definition of a vitamin. They are considered macronutrients. Linoleic acid cannot be synthesized in the body and must be present in the diet. If the total dietary calories consist of 1% to 2% linoleic acid, deficiencies do not usually occur. Linoleic acid is rapidly converted to arachidonic acid, a functioning polyunsaturated fatty acid that is physiologically important. Linolenic acid has some essential fatty acid properties, but its biochemical role is not well defined. It is not a substitute for linoleic acid. Linoleic acid deficiency symptoms can include scaly skin, hair loss, and impaired wound healing.

The typical Western diet, with its heavy polyunsaturated fat and oil content, provides ample essential fatty acids; thus, deficiencies do not usually occur.

Inositol Inositol is a hexitol found in large amounts in muscle and brain tissues. It is widely distributed in nature and is also synthesized in the body. Inositol seems to be necessary for amino acid transport and for the movement of potassium and sodium, but its value in human nutrition has not been well documented. Like choline, it is considered a lipotropic agent of unproven therapeutic value.

Inositol is a sweet, water-soluble substance occurring naturally in fruits, vegetables, whole grains, meats, and milk. It is present in cells as a phosphatide, and inositol lipids appear to be involved in the calcium-mediated control of cell functions, in cell proliferation, and in the attachment of enzymes to the plasma membrane.

A normal dietary intake is approximately 1 g per day, derived primarily from plant sources. The human requirement has not been established.

Laetrile (Amygdalin, Vitamin B_{17}) Laetrile occurs naturally in almond, apricot, and peach pits and in apple seeds. Consisting of 6% cyanide by weight, it is made up of two parts glucose, one part benzaldehyde, and one part cyanide. When spelled with a capital "L," it refers to a synthetic substance that was never marketed; when spelled with a small "l," it refers to amygdalin, the product marketed by laetrile promoters as a cancer cure, and is a synonym for cyanogenic glycosides. Many toxic reactions have been reported worldwide with the ingestion of cyanogenic glycosides; cyanide poisoning has occurred with some laetrile products.

Although it is called vitamin B_{17}, laetrile contains no vitamin activity, has no nutritional or therapeutic value, and has no approved medical use. Moreover, no physiologic or biochemical abnormalities develop when the diet is deficient in laetrile. Thus, the term *vitamin B_{17}* is erroneous, misleading, and fraudulent, and it should not be used. Use by desperate and uninformed individuals may lead to critical delays in seeking and receiving appropriate medical attention.

Pangamic Acid (Vitamin B_{15}) Pangamic acid is an uncharacterized extract of the Prunus family. It is a substance or mixture of substances isolated from apricot kernels and rice bran. The unsupported claim has been that the extract provides immunization against toxic products present in the human or animal system, as well as that it produces symptomatic relief and immunity to persons afflicted with asthma, eczema, arthritis, neuritis, painful nerve and joint afflictions, and numerous other conditions. Pangamic acid is described as a poorly defined mixture of dimethylglycine and sorbitol. No studies have shown it to have any efficacy in treating any medical disorder. Pangamic acid has been categorized as a pseudovitamin, and it has no nutritional or therapeutic value.

Taurine (Aminoethanesulfonate) Along with carnitine, choline, and inositol, taurine has been referred to as a vitamin-like compound. The most common dietary source of taurine is human breast milk. It is now considered important enough to be included in human infant formulas, enteral products, and some parenteral nutritional solutions.

A unique chemical aspect of taurine is that it contains a sulfonic acid group that replaces the carboxyl group of what would otherwise be glycine. It is not incorporated into peptides, but it does participate in a few biochemical reactions. Taurine is present in most cells and exhibits a wide range of activity. Some of the physiologic functions that are affected by taurine include retinal photoreceptor activity, bile acid conjugation, white blood cell antioxidant activity, CNS neuromodulation, platelet aggregation, cardiac contractility, sperm motility, growth, and insulin activity.

Taurine, which is important in many metabolic activities, is normally biosynthesized in adequate amounts. Plasma levels of taurine normally range from 50 to 220 mcmol/L, and any excess is excreted in the urine.

Even though it is not known whether taurine is essential for humans, some concern has been expressed about the risk of taurine insufficiency in formula-fed infants—especially those born prematurely—as compared with breast-fed infants. Cow's milk contains lower levels of taurine than does human milk. No US RDA is established at this time.

Minerals

Minerals constitute about 4% of body weight. The major mineral content of the skeleton consists of calcium and phosphorus in a ratio of approximately 2 : 1. Any change of one may be reflected in changes of the other.

Minerals are present in the body in a diverse array of organic compounds (e.g., phosphoproteins, phospholipids, hemoglobin, and thyroxine) as well as in inorganic compounds (e.g., sodium chloride, potassium chloride, calcium, and phosphate), which are present as free ions. Different body tissues contain different quantities of different elements. For example, bone has a high content of calcium, phosphorus, and magnesium; soft tissue has a high quantity of potassium. Minerals function as constituents of enzymes, hormones, and vitamins. They are involved in regulating cell membrane permeability, osmotic pressure, and acid–base and water balance. In addition, certain ions act as the mediators of action potential conduction and neurotransmitter action.

A well-balanced diet is required to maintain proper mineral balance. Calcium and iron are two elements that may require particular dietary attention from normal individuals. Optimal mineral intake values for humans are still imprecise; only estimated ranges are available for trace element minerals such as chromium, fluorine, copper, manganese, and molybdenum. Those ranges are based on the mineral content of the average diet. Similarly, the possible adverse effects of long-term ingestion of high-dose mineral supplements are unknown, and high doses of one mineral can decrease the bioavailability of other minerals and even of vitamins.

Unlike vitamins, minerals exist in plants in varying amounts, according to the composition of the soil in which the plant is grown. This variability, in turn, affects the mineral content of local livestock. Mineral intake varies considerably from region to region, although the use of foods delivered from diverse geographic locations tends to minimize intake variations. Marginal deficiencies of minerals have been reported only in certain segments of the population, but the increasing use of highly refined foods, which are low in minerals, may contribute to such deficiencies.

Mineral deficiency is often difficult to evaluate. Hair analysis has received attention in recent years, and its noninvasiveness is advantageous. However, a number of factors, such as distance from the scalp where the sample was obtained, color of the hair, and the use of shampoos, sprays, and conditioners, can adversely influence the accuracy of results. The analysis for zinc and toxic minerals such as arsenic, mercury, and lead has provided interesting results, but accepted normal values have not been established in routine nutritional assessment.

Calcium The most abundant cation in the body is calcium (about 1200 g). About 99% of calcium is present in the skeleton, and the remaining 1% is present in the extracellular fluid, intracellular structures, and cell membranes. Calcium is a major component of bones and teeth. The calcium content in bone is continuously undergoing a process of resorption and formation. In elderly people, the resorption process predominates over formation, and a decrease in calcium absorption efficiency results in a gradual loss of bone (osteoporosis). This effect can be minimized by ensuring an optimal calcium intake during the formative years to develop optimal bone mass and by promoting weight-bearing exercise.

Function Calcium is important for these reasons: It activates a number of enzymes (e.g., pancreatic lipase, adenosine triphosphatase, and some proteolytic enzymes), it is required for acetylcholine synthesis, it increases cell membrane permeability, it aids in vitamin B_{12} absorption, it regulates muscle contraction and relaxation, and it catalyzes several steps in the activation of plasma clotting factors. Calcium is also necessary for the functional integrity of many cells, especially those of the neuromuscular and cardiovascular system.

The average blood level of calcium in the body is about 9.0 to 10.5 mg/dL. Three forms of calcium exist in the blood and body fluids; these forms include ionized calcium, calcium complexes with organic acids, and protein-bound calcium.

The small intestine controls calcium absorption. Patients ingesting relatively low amounts of calcium absorb proportionately more, and some patients taking large amounts of calcium excrete more as fecal calcium. Calcium requirements may increase as the consumption of protein increases.

Dietary Sources Rich dietary sources of calcium include milk and other dairy products. Teenagers experiencing rapid growth and bone maturation need to consume adequate calcium through dairy products, especially milk, or through nutritional supplements in tablet or capsule form. Adults can easily meet calcium US RDA levels by incorporating dairy products (especially low-fat and nonfat milk) into their diets. Nonfat milk contains about 300 mg of calcium per 8 oz. As an alternative, calcium supplements are essentially free of adverse effects in daily doses of less than 2 g of calcium.

Dietary factors that increase calcium absorption include certain amino acids such as lysine and arginine, vitamin D, and lactose. Dietary factors that decrease the efficiency of calcium absorption include foods with high phosphate content (e.g., unpolished rice, hexaphosphoinositol in bran, and wheat meal) and foods high in oxalate content (e.g., cocoa, soybeans, kale, and spinach). Vitamin D deficiency may also reduce the absorption and physiologic effects of calcium.

Deficiency Decreased calcium levels may have profound and diverse consequences, including convulsions, tetany, behavioral and personality disorders, mental and growth retardation, and bone deformities (the most common being rickets in children and osteomalacia in adults). Changes that occur in osteomalacia include softening of bones, rheumatic-type pain in the bones of the legs and lower back, general weakness with difficulty walking, and spontaneous fractures.

Common causes of hypocalcemia and associated skeletal disorders are as follows: malabsorption syndromes; hypoparathyroidism; vitamin D deficiency; renal failure with impaired activation of vitamin D; long-term anticonvulsant therapy (with increased breakdown of vitamin D); and decreased dietary intake of calcium, particularly during periods of growth, pregnancy, and lactation and among elderly people.

Dose/US RDA To maximize bone mass before the inevitable decline that occurs after menopause, the US RDA set values at 1200 mg per day for both women and men ages 11 to 24 years. The US RDA for adults older than 24 years is 800 mg per day. Some suggest that, for women, about 1100 mg per day before menopause and 1500 mg per day after menopause is advantageous; during pregnancy and lactation, 1200 mg per day is recommended. Weight-bearing exercise is very important in maintaining bone mass, and any program to decrease the risk for osteoporosis should include regular exercise.

Calcium is available in many salt forms without a prescription with different percentages of calcium in each, including the carbonate (40%), citrate (21%), lactate (18%), gluconate (9%), and phosphate salts (23% to 39%). Calcium carbonate and calcium phosphate salts are insoluble and should be taken with meals to enhance absorption, which depends on a low pH in the stomach. Patients requiring supplementation who have low levels of achlorhydria (gastric hydrochloric acid) or who are on histamine II (H_2) antagonists or proton pump inhibitors may need to take a soluble salt (e.g., calcium citrate, calcium lactate, or calcium gluconate). Bonemeal (mostly a calcium phosphate matrix) and oyster shell products (calcium carbonate matrix) are insoluble and require an acid pH for absorption. Products that do not disintegrate as well as others may have limited amounts of calcium available for absorption. (See Table 19–6 for examples of commercially available calcium products.)

Table 19–6

Selected Calcium Supplements

Trade Name	Primary Ingredients
Calcel Tablets[a–c]	Elemental calcium 150 mg (as gluconate, lactate, and carbonate); vitamin D 100 IU
Calci-Chew Chewable Tablets[a,d]	Elemental calcium 500 mg (as carbonate)
Caltrate 600 + D High Potency Tablets[b–d]	Elemental calcium 600 mg (as carbonate); vitamin D 200 IU
Caltrate 600 High Potency Tablets[b–d]	Elemental calcium 600 mg (as carbonate)
Chewy Bears Chewable Calcium Wafers[e]	Elemental calcium 250 mg (as carbonate and citrate)
Citracal+ D Caplets[a–d]	Elemental calcium 315 mg (as citrate); vitamin D 200 IU
Citracal Liquitab Effervescent Tablets	Elemental calcium 500 mg (as citrate)
Citron Caplets	Elemental calcium 1000 mg (as citrate carbonate)
Dical-D Tablets	Elemental calcium 117 mg; vitamin D 133 IU
Florical Tablets/Capsules[c]	Elemental calcium 145.6 mg (as carbonate and oyster shell, 346 mg)
Neo-Calglucon Syrup	Elemental calcium 115 mg/5 mL (as gluconate)
One-A-Day Calcium Plus Chewable Tablets[f]	Elemental calcium 500 mg; vitamin D 100 IU
Os-Cal 250 + Tablets[b–d]	Elemental calcium 250 mg (as oyster shell); vitamin D 125 IU
Os-Cal 500 Chewable Tablets[a,c,d,g]	Elemental calcium 500 mg (as carbonate)
Os-Cal 500 Tablets[b,d]	Elemental calcium 500 mg (as oyster shell)
Os-Cal 500 + D Tablets[b,d]	Elemental calcium 500 mg; vitamin D 125 IU
Posture Tablets	Elemental calcium 600 mg (as tribasic phosphate)
Posture-D Tablets	Elemental calcium 600 mg (as tribasic phosphate); vitamin D 125 IU
Tums 500 Chewable Tablets[b,d]	Elemental calcium 500 mg (as carbonate)
Vita-Cal Chewable Tablets[a,d]	Elemental calcium 250 mg; vitamin D 66.7 IU

[a] Dye-free product.
[b] Sodium-free product.
[c] Sucrose-free product.
[d] Lactose-free product.
[e] Pediatric formulation.
[f] Phenylalanine-containing product.
[g] Aspirin-free product.

Adverse Effects Calcium in doses greater than 2 g per day can be harmful. Large amounts taken as dietary supplements or antacids can lead to high levels of calcium in the urine and to renal stones; the latter development may result in renal damage. Hypercalcemia—with associated anorexia, nausea, vomiting, constipation, and polyuria—is also possible, particularly in patients taking high-dose vitamin D preparations. Hypercalcemia can also result in an increased deposition of calcium in soft tissue.

Drug–Drug Interactions High calcium intake levels may inhibit the absorption of iron, zinc, and other essential minerals. Corticosteroids inhibit calcium absorption from the gut, and their use has been associated with increased bone fractures and osteoporosis. The excessive ingestion of aluminum-containing antacids has been shown to result in negative calcium balances. Several other drugs, including phosphates, calcitonin, sodium sulfate, furosemide, magnesium, cholestyramine, estrogen, and some anticonvulsants, also lower calcium serum levels. Thiazide diuretics, conversely, increase serum calcium levels.

Iron Iron is widely available in the U.S. diet. Iron absorption from the intestinal tract is controlled by the body's need for iron, the intestinal lumen conditions, and the food content of the meal. Iron-deficient patients may absorb about 10% to 20% of dietary iron, and people with normal iron stores absorb about 5% to 10%.

Function Iron plays an important role in oxygen and electron transport. In the body, it is either functional or stored. Functional iron is found in hemoglobin, myoglobin, heme-containing enzymes, and transferrin, which is the transport form of iron. Stored iron is primarily found in the hemoglobin of red blood cells, which contains 60% to 70% of total body iron. The rest is stored primarily in the form of ferritin and hemosiderin and is found in the intestinal mucosa, liver, spleen, and bone marrow.

Normally, adult men have iron stores of about 50 mg/kg of body weight; women have about 35 mg/kg of body weight. The normal hemoglobin level in adult men is about 14 to 17 g/100 mL of blood; in adult women, it is 12 to 14 g/100 mL of blood.

Dietary Sources Dietary iron is available in two forms. Heme iron is found in meats and is reasonably well absorbed. Nonheme iron constitutes most of the dietary iron and is poorly absorbed. Therefore, the published values of the iron content of foods are misleading because the amount absorbed depends on the nature of the iron. The available iron content of foods is calculated by assuming that about 10% of the total iron (heme plus nonheme) is absorbable if no iron deficiency exists. In the iron-deficient state, iron absorption improves so that as much as 20% may be absorbed and used from an average diet.

Nonheme ingested iron, which is mostly in the form of ferric hydroxide, is solubilized in gastric juice to ferric chloride, is reduced to the ferrous form, and is chelated to substances such as ascorbic acid, sugars, and amino acids. Chelates have a low molecular weight and can be solubilized and absorbed before they reach the alkaline medium of the distal small intestine, where precipitation may occur. In intestinal mucosal cells, iron is stored in a protein-bound form as ferritin. As needed, it is released into the plasma, where it is oxidized to the ferric state and is bound to a β-globulin to form transferrin. When released at the spleen, liver, bone marrow, intestinal mucosa, and other iron storage sites, the iron is combined with apoferritin to form ferritin or hemosiderin. Iron is used in all cells of the body; however, most of it is incorporated into the hemoglobin of red blood cells. Iron is lost from the body by the sloughing of skin cells and GI mucosal cells; hemorrhagic loss; menstruation; and excretion of urine, sweat, and feces.

Deficiency Early symptoms of iron deficiency are vague. Weakness, lassitude, and easy fatigability cannot in themselves be easily related to iron deficiency. Other signs and symptoms of anemia include pallor, split or "spoon-shaped" nails, sore tongue, angular stomatitis, palpitation, dyspnea on exertion, and a feeling of exhaustion. Coldness and numbness of the extremities may be reported. Small red blood cells (decreased mean corpuscular volume) and low hemoglobin concentrations (decreased mean corpuscular hemoglobin concentration) characterize iron deficiency.

There are three general stages of iron deficiency:

- Iron depletion, in which iron stores are depleted and associated with plasma ferritin levels below 12 mcg/L.
- Iron-deficient erythropoiesis, in which red cell protoporphyrin levels are elevated but the hemoglobin levels are within the 95% reference range.
- Iron deficiency anemia, in which the total blood hemoglobin levels are below normal levels.

Iron deficiency anemia is a widespread clinical problem and the most common form of anemia in the United States. Although it causes few deaths, it does contribute to the poor health and suboptimal performance of many people. Iron deficiency results from inadequate diet, malabsorption, pregnancy and lactation, or blood loss. Because normal excretion of iron through the urine, feces, and skin is small, iron deficiency caused by poor diet or malabsorption may develop very slowly because iron is stored and conserved (recycled) by the body.

Despite fortification of flour and educational efforts regarding proper nutrition, iron deficiency remains a problem for certain segments of the population, especially children in poverty and women who are menstruating or pregnant. Iron supplements are routinely recommended as a component of prenatal care.

Iron deficiency is most common in the following four life periods:

- From 6 months to 4 years of age, the child obtains low iron content from cow's milk.
- During early adolescence, the youngster experiences rapid growth that entails an expanding red cell mass and the need for iron in myoglobin.
- During the female reproductive years, the woman experiences menstrual iron losses.
- During and after pregnancy, the woman faces the expanding blood volume of the mother, the demands of the fetus and placenta, and the blood losses during childbirth.

Menstruation normally results in a loss of 60 to 80 mL of blood per month and of about 1.4 mg of iron in addition to that normally lost. The daily amount required for replacement is about 0.7 to 2.3 mg of absorbed iron. The average U.S. diet contains about 5 to 7 mg of iron per 1000 calories, but only about 10% of iron in food is absorbed. If the menstrual blood loss exceeds 60 to 80 mL, supplemental iron may be desirable because the dietary requirement may be as high as 40 mg per day.

The donation of 500 mL (1 pint or unit) of blood produces a loss of approximately 250 mg of iron. This problem is not significant in healthy, well-nourished adults with adequate iron stores. However, some blood donors, especially those who donate frequently, may benefit from short-term iron replacement following blood donation.

The differential diagnosis in adults or postmenopausal women should rule out iron deficiency caused by excess blood loss associated with peptic ulcer disease, hemorrhoids, Crohn's disease, esophageal varices, intestinal parasites, regional enteritis, ulcerative colitis, cancer, and diverticulitis.

Chronic use of drugs such as salicylates, nonsteroidal anti-inflammatory drugs, reserpine, corticosteroids, warfarin, ulcerogenic drugs, and antiprothrombinemic drugs or of most drugs that treat neoplasms might indicate drug-induced blood loss. Drug-induced blood loss may occur because of irritating effects on the gastric mucosa or an indirect effect on the GI tract.

The pharmacist may sometimes ascertain the cause of the patient's condition by consulting the medication record. Medications such as aspirin or ibuprofen may not be included on a medication record. Thus, the pharmacist should routinely question the patient regarding the use of nonprescription drugs and should ascertain whether the patient's problem is chronic, whether self-treatment has been tried, and whether medical care has been sought or received. Anemia in patients other than those who are pregnant, lactating, or menstruating, or who are on a restricted diet may be a symptom of a more serious medical disorder. Pharmacists should strongly encourage such patients to seek medical attention. That intervention may prevent a more serious problem.

Pharmacists should immediately refer a patient who reports blood loss to a physician. Abnormal blood loss may be indicated by (1) vomiting blood ("coffee-ground" vomitus); (2) bright red blood in the stool or black, tarry stools; (3) large clots or an abnormally heavy flow during the menstrual period; or (4) cloudy or pink-red urine if drugs that may cause urine discoloration have been ruled out.

Blood loss, particularly through the stool, is not always obvious. Even when abnormal blood loss occurs, the patient may not notice or report it. Periodic testing using home occult blood test kits may be considered for certain high-risk or at-risk patients.

Dose/US RDA The US RDA for iron is 10 mg for adult men, 15 mg for adult women, and 30 mg for pregnant women. Most healthy individuals who self-medicate, including menstruating females, will absorb adequate iron from one 325-mg ferrous sulfate tablet per day. In a 325-mg ferrous sulfate tablet, 20% (about 60 mg) is elemental iron. In patients with iron deficiencies, 20% of the elemental iron (12 mg) may be absorbed. Because 36 to 48 mg of iron daily is enough to support maximum incorporation into red blood cells (0.3 g of hemoglobin per 100 mL of blood) and to replace iron stores, the usual therapeutic dose of two to four tablets daily for 3 months is probably reasonable in treating a deficiency. If the patient has an inadequate response or if symptoms worsen during this time, the patient should consult a physician. In cases of severe or chronic iron deficiency and when serious medical conditions have been ruled out, continuous low-maintenance doses of three to four tablets daily for approximately 3 to 6 months should normalize hemoglobin and should replace iron stores, provided there is no ongoing bleeding and the diet is adequate.

If iron supplementation is appropriate, the pharmacist may recommend which iron product is best. The choice should be based on how well the iron preparation is absorbed and tolerated, as well as on its price. Because ferrous salts are more efficiently absorbed than ferric salts, an iron product of the ferrous group is usually appropriate. Ferrous sulfate is the standard against which other iron salts are compared. The quantities of various iron salts that will provide 60 mg of elemental iron are ferrous ascorbate 437 mg, ferrous succinate 185 mg, ferrous lactate 310 mg, ferrous fumarate 183 mg, ferrous gluconate 518 mg, and ferrous sulfate 300 mg. Ferrous citrate, ferrous tartrate, ferrous pyrophosphate, and some ferric salts are not well absorbed. (See Table 19–7 for examples of commercially available iron products.)

Ferrous salts may be given in combination with ascorbic acid. At a ratio of 200 mg of ascorbic acid to 30 mg of elemental iron, the increased amount of iron absorbed validates this practice. Other agents that may help increase absorption include sugars and amino acids. Chemicals that may decrease iron absorption include phosphates in eggs, phytates in cereals, carbonates, oxalates, and tannins.

Iron is available in numerous salt forms and as immediate and controlled-release products. The enteric-coated and delayed-release products are generally more expensive but may cause fewer symptoms of gastric irritation. However, progressively less iron is absorbed as it moves from the duodenum (the site of maximum absorption) to the ileum of the small intestine; overall iron absorption is decreased by delaying the time of release.

Adverse Effects All iron products tend to irritate the GI mucosa and may produce nausea, abdominal pain, and diarrhea. These adverse effects may be minimized by reducing the dose or by giving iron with meals. However, because food may decrease the amount of iron absorbed by as much as 50%, physicians may recommend iron with instructions for between-meal dosing. It is advantageous for absorption if the patient is able to tolerate iron taken in this manner. But if nausea or diarrhea is intolerable, it is usually better for the patient to take the iron with food or to decrease the number of tablets taken per day rather than to stop taking iron supplements entirely.

A frequent side effect of iron therapy is constipation. This adverse effect has prompted the formulation of iron products that also contain a stool softener (e.g., docusate). During iron therapy, stools may become black and tarry, usually caused by unabsorbed iron. Black, tarry stools may also indicate GI blood loss and a serious GI problem. Medical referral is indicated if an underlying GI condition is suspected or if there is a history of GI disease. If the stool does not darken somewhat during iron therapy, however, the iron product may not have disintegrated properly or released the iron.

Accidental poisoning with iron occurs most often in children, who are attracted to the sugar-coated, colored tablets. It can also occur from overingestion of chewable multivitamins containing iron. Such poisoning is considered a medical emergency. As few as 15 tablets of 325-mg ferrous sulfate have been lethal to children; however, recovery has followed the ingestion of as many as 70 such tablets. The clinical outcome depends on the speed and adequacy of treatment.

Toxic ingestion of iron may be life-threatening and should be referred immediately to a poison control center or emergency medical facility. Symptoms of acute iron poisoning include pain, vomiting, diarrhea, electrolyte imbalances, and shock. In later stages, cardiovascular collapse may occur, especially if the cause has not been properly recognized and treated as a medical emergency. Treatment of iron toxicity may begin immediately at home by giving ipecac syrup to induce vomiting, but follow-up emergency room treatment with an iron chelator, such as deferoxamine (Desferal) and gastric lavage, is essential.

Table 19–7

Selected Iron Supplements

Trade Name	Primary Ingredients
Femiron Daily Iron Supplement Tablets	Elemental iron 20 mg (as fumarate)
Feosol Elixir	Elemental iron 44 mg/5 mL (as sulfate)
Feosol Tablets/Caplets	Elemental iron 65 mg and 50 mg, respectively
Fer-In-Sol Drops[a–d]	Elemental iron 15 mg/0.6 mL (as sulfate)
Fer-In-Sol Syrup[a–d]	Elemental iron 18 mg/5 mL (as sulfate)
Fergon Tablets	Elemental iron 27 mg (as gluconate)
Fero-Grad-500-Filmtabs	Elemental iron 105 mg (as sulfate); sodium ascorbate 500 mg
Ferro-Sequels Timed-Release Tablets[f]	Elemental iron 50 mg (as fumarate)
Hytinic Capsules[a,b,f]	Elemental iron 150 mg (as polysaccharide-iron complex)
Ircon Tablets	Elemental iron 200 mg (as fumarate)
Ircon FA Tablets[c]	Elemental iron 250 mg (as fumarate); folic acid 800 mcg
Irospan Tablets[f]	Elemental iron 65 mg; ascorbic acid, 150 mg
Nephro-Fer Tablets[a,e,f]	Elemental iron 115 mg (as fumarate)
Niferex-150 Capsules[b]	Elemental iron 150 mg (as polysaccharide-iron complex, as cell-contracted akaganeite)
Slow Fe Tablets[e]	Elemental iron 50 mg (as sulfate)

[a] Dye-free product.
[b] Lactose-free product.
[c] Sulfite-free product.
[d] Pediatric formulation.
[e] Sodium-free product.
[f] Sucrose-free product.

Drug–Drug Interactions Iron is chelated, or its solubility is altered, by many substances. Iron's interaction with antacids may be clinically significant. The mechanism of this interaction is probably related to the relative alkalinization of the stomach contents by an antacid that reduces the solubility of iron in the gastrointestinal fluids. The chelate of iron with an antacid is less soluble in the alkaline medium. Iron appears to chelate with several of the tetracyclines, resulting in decreased tetracycline and iron absorption. If concurrent administration of an iron salt and a tetracycline is medically unnecessary, patients should take tetracycline 3 hours after or 2 hours before iron administration.

Magnesium Magnesium, which is essential for all living cells, is the second most-plentiful cation of the intracellular fluids and the fourth most-abundant cation in the body. About 2000 mEq of magnesium are present in an average 70-kg adult, with about 50% of this in bone, about 45% as an intracellular cation, and about 1% to 5% in the extracellular fluid.

Function Magnesium is required for normal bone structure formation and the proper function of more than 300 enzymes, including those involved with adenosine triphosphatase-dependent phosphorylation, protein synthesis, and carbohydrate metabolism. Extracellular magnesium is critical to both the maintenance of nerve and muscle electrical potentials and the transmission of impulses across neuromuscular junctions.

Magnesium tends to mimic calcium in its effects on the CNS and skeletal muscle. Magnesium deficiency blunts the normal response of the parathyroid glands to hypocalcemia. Thus, tetany caused by a lack of calcium cannot be corrected with calcium unless the magnesium deficiency is also corrected.

Dietary Sources Individuals consuming natural diets should not develop magnesium deficiency because all unprocessed foods contain magnesium, albeit in widely varying amounts. Vegetables are a good source of magnesium; whole seeds such as nuts, legumes, and unmilled grains contain the highest concentrations. Processing, which leads to removal of the germ and outer layers of cereal grains, results in a loss of more than 80% of the magnesium.

Deficiency Deficiency states are usually caused by GI tract abnormalities, renal dysfunction, general malnutrition, alcoholism, and iatrogenic causes. Additionally, hypomagnesemia may result from the following: diarrhea and steatorrhea, prolonged total parenteral nutrition therapy with magnesium-free solutions, hemodialysis, diabetes mellitus, pancreatitis, diuretic-induced electrolyte imbalance, and primary aldosteronism—a condition characterized by loss of body potassium, muscular weakness, and elevated

Case Study 19–2

Patient Complaint/History

Miguel is the 14-year-old son in a migrant farm family in east Texas. He comes to the pharmacy today seeking help in relieving a recurrence of fatigue; he first experienced the fatigue last summer. At that time, he had a busy schedule, working all day and spending time with friends in the evening. His diet consisted mainly of tortillas; pinto beans; rice; and, when available, onions, garlic, and tomatoes. His daily fluid intake included several soft drinks and fruit-flavored beverages; he rarely drank milk.

Subsequently, Miguel's mother took him to the Migrant Health Care Clinic. A physical examination revealed the following: the patient's height and weight were 5 ft 8 in. and 130 lb. His temperature (98.8°F [37.1°C]), pulse rate (74 bpm), and blood pressure (110/75 mm Hg) were normal. Using a hemoglobin level of 9.5 g/dL, the physician prescribed a slow-release iron product and a multivitamin tablet, each to be taken once daily. Over the next several weeks, Miguel slowly improved. However, about 8 months after the clinic visit, his mother could no longer afford the prescription iron medication, and she purchased 325-mg ferrous sulfate tablets instead. After Miguel began taking one ferrous sulfate tablet at bedtime, he developed stomach distress for which he began taking antacids. He continued to take the multivitamin and antacids but stopped taking the ferrous sulfate. He is now experiencing fatigue again.

Clinical Considerations/Strategies

Readers can use the following considerations/strategies to determine whether treating the patient's condition with nonprescription nutritional supplements is warranted:

- Assess the appropriateness of the physician-prescribed, slow-release iron therapy in treating the iron deficiency anemia.
- Assess the appropriateness of the mother replacing the slow-release iron medication with a regimen of ferrous sulfate 325 mg one tablet daily.
- Discuss the possible etiology of the recurrence of fatigue.
- Propose an alternative therapeutic plan for the patient.
- Determine what information about the changes in the prescribed therapeutic regimen should be included in a phone conversation or letter to the patient's physician.

Patient Education/Counseling

Readers can use the following strategies to develop a patient education/counseling plan that will help ensure optimal therapeutic outcomes:

- Support/justify the changes in the prescribed therapeutic regimen.
- Explain the therapeutic regimen recommended by the pharmacist (i.e., dose, time and frequency of administration, warnings/precautions, adverse effects, and drug interactions).

blood pressure. Hypomagnesemia may also be associated with hypokalemia and hypocalcemia.

Magnesium deficiencies are rarely noted in the normal adult population because magnesium is present in most foods. Magnesium deficiency causes apathy, depression, increased CNS stimulation, delirium, and convulsions. Symptoms of hypomagnesemia may include nausea, muscle weakness, irritability, behavioral changes, and myographic changes.

Dose/US RDA The US RDA values of magnesium for men and women older than 18 years are 350 mg per day and 280 mg per day, respectively.

Adverse Effects No evidence is available to suggest that oral intake of magnesium is harmful to individuals with normal renal function. Hypermagnesemia can occur with overzealous use of magnesium sulfate (epsom salts) or magnesium hydroxide (milk of magnesia) as a laxative, or even with use of magnesium-containing antacids in patients with severe renal failure.

Hypermagnesemia may cause hypotonic (deficient), diminished, or absent deep tendon reflexes; varying degrees of muscle weakness; and complete flaccid paralysis with resultant respiratory depression, depending on the serum concentration of magnesium attained. CNS depression may result in varying degrees of lethargy and sedation, which may progress to stupor and coma, especially at high serum concentrations. Hypotension, cutaneous vasodilation, sinus bradycardia, first-degree heart block, nodal rhythms, bundle branch block, and complete heart block progressing to asystole and cardiac arrest may occur, depending on the serum concentrations.

Phosphorus Phosphorus is present throughout the body. Approximately 85% of the body's store is located in bone. About 1% of body weight, or one-fourth of the total mineral content in the body, is phosphorus. Normal plasma levels of inorganic phosphate range between 2.5 and 4.4 mg/dL.

Function Phosphorus is essential for many metabolic processes. As calcium phosphate, it serves as an integral structural component of the bone matrix and as a functional component of phospholipids, carbohydrates, nucleoproteins, and high-energy nucleotides. Plasma phosphate levels are under tight biologic control involving parathyroid hormone, calcitonin, and vitamin D. The DNA and RNA structures contain sugar-phosphate linkages. Cell membranes contain phospholipids, which regulate the transport of solutes into and out of the cell. Many metabolic processes depend on phosphorylation. The storage and controlled release of energy, which is the adenosine diphosphate–adenosine triphosphate system, involves phosphorus compounds. An important buffer system of the body consists of inorganic phosphates.

There is a reciprocal relationship between calcium and phosphorus. Both minerals are regulated partially by parathyroid hormone. Secretion of parathyroid hormone stimulates an increase in calcium levels through increased bone resorption, gut absorption, and reabsorption in renal tubules. Parathyroid hormone causes a decrease in the resorption of phosphate by the kidney. Thus, when serum calcium is high, serum phosphate is generally low, and vice versa.

Dietary Sources Phosphorus is present in nearly all foods, especially protein-rich foods and cereal grains. Milk, meat, poultry, and fish contain about half the dietary phosphorus in the U.S. diet. Other rich sources include seeds, nuts, and eggs.

Deficiency Because nearly all foods contain phosphorus, deficiency states do not usually occur unless induced. For example, patients receiving aluminum hydroxide as an antacid for prolonged periods may exhibit weakness, anorexia, malaise, pain, and bone loss. This result is because aluminum hydroxide binds phosphorus, making it unavailable for absorption because of the formation of insoluble and poorly absorbed complexes.

Dose/US RDA The US RDA for phosphorus is 800 mg for adults age 24 years or older, 1200 mg for those ages 11 to 24 years, 800 mg for children ages 1 to 10 years, and 1200 mg for women during pregnancy and lactation. In addition to being used to alleviate the deficiency state, phosphates have been used to increase tissue calcium uptake in osteomalacia and to decrease serum calcium levels in hypercalcemia. Sodium and potassium phosphate salts are available without a prescription for those requiring supplements. Products available include different salt forms and strengths of phosphorus in tablet, capsule, powder, and liquid dose forms, as well as in numerous combination products.

Adverse Effects/Drug–Drug Interactions Side effects and drug interactions have not been commonly reported with phosphorus therapy.

Trace Elements

Trace elements, which are present in minute quantities in plant and animal tissue, are considered essential for numerous physiologic processes. "Ultratrace minerals" have been defined as those elements with an estimated dietary requirement of usually less than 1 mg per day. The essential minerals include arsenic, boron, chromium, molybdenum, nickel, selenium, and silicon. Lithium and vanadium are considered probably essential minerals, but further study is required. Bromine, cadmium, fluorine, lead, and tin are considered not essential because the evidence for essentiality is inadequate. Using the amount of trace elements in the average diet, the Food and Nutrition Board has published a range of intake values for those elements thought to be safe and adequate. (See Table 19–8 for commercially available products that contain single-entity trace elements or a combination of minerals and trace elements.)

Chromium About 5 mg of chromium is present in the normal adult, and levels decline with age. Higher concentrations occur in the hair, spleen, kidney, and testes; lesser concentrations are present in the heart, pancreas, lungs, and brain.

Function Chromium is a component of glucose tolerance factor, a dietary organic chromium complex that appears to facilitate the glucose use that is apparently essential for the

Table 19–8

Selected Trace Element Supplements

Trade Name	Primary Ingredients
Chromemate Capsules	Chromium 200 mg (as polynicotinate)
Dr. Powers Colloidal Mineral Source Liquid[a]	Magnesium 100 mg/15 mL; calcium 25 mg/15 mL; potassium 10 mg/15 mL; zinc 10 mg/15 mL; manganese 5 mg/15 mL; selenium 50 mcg/15 mL; chromium 50 mcg/15 mL
Sundown Chromium Picolinate Tablets[b,c]	Chromium 200 mg (as picolinate, 1.6 mg)
Sundown Manganese Chelate Tablets[a–d]	Manganese 50 mg (as gluconate)
Sundown Mega Mineral Tablets[b,c]	Calcium 333.3 mg (as carbonate); magnesium 133.3 mg (as oxide); potassium 16.6 mg; iron 5 mg (as carbonyl); zinc 5 mg (as sulfate); manganese 0.83 mg; copper 0.66 mg; chromium 66.6 mcg (from picolinate); iodine 50 mcg; boron 33.3 mcg; molybdenum 33.3 mcg; selenium 16.6 mcg; tin 6.6 mcg; nickel 1.6 mcg; vanadium 3.3 mcg
Sundown Selenium Tablets[b,c]	Selenium 50 mg; 100 mcg
Sundown Zinc Tablets[b,c]	Zinc 10 mg; 30 mg; 50 mg; 100 mg (as gluconate and oxide)

[a] Lactose-free product.
[b] Sodium-free product.
[c] Sucrose-free product.
[d] Dye-free product.

efficient use of insulin. Fatty acid stimulation and cholesterol synthesis are attributed to chromium, as is the possible role of RNA in protein synthesis.

Chromium combined with picolinic acid (a metabolite of tryptophan) forms chromium picolinate (a form of chromium with enhanced bioavailability). Chromium picolinate, in doses of 200 mcg per day, has recently been promoted as an aid in controlling diabetes and as an aid for lowering cholesterol, producing weight loss, and increasing muscle mass.

Dietary Sources Significant amounts of chromium are present in liver, fish, whole grains, and milk. There is concern that the increasing consumption of refined foods may lead to a marginal chromium deficiency.

Deficiency Deficiency of trivalent chromium (the chemical form present in diets) is manifested by glucose intolerance, elevated circulating insulin, glycosuria, fasting hyperglycemia, elevated serum cholesterol and triglycerides, neuropathy, and encephalopathy. Impaired glucose tolerance may be a manifestation of chromium deficiency, especially in older people and in protein-calorie malnourished infants. Chromium-responsive impairment of glucose tolerance has been reported in malnourished children, in middle-aged subjects with impaired glucose tolerance, and in some but not all studies of mild diabetics. The connection between coronary heart disease and chromium stems from the fact that uncontrolled diabetes is a risk factor for coronary heart disease. The same correlation may be true for other risk factors for uncontrolled diabetes. Low chromium concentrations have been associated with juvenile diabetes and coronary artery disease. However, evaluation of chromium-deficient patients is difficult because of problems associated with total chromium analysis.

Dose/US RDA Chromium intake in the United States is low (about 50 mcg per day) compared with that of other countries. The estimated safe and adequate dietary intake for adults has been set at 50 to 200 mcg per day. Chromium has a relatively high margin of safety and is available in 1 mg tablets.

Adverse Effects Oral administration of trivalent chromium has not been reported to be toxic. However, the hexavalent forms of chromium can be toxic and carcinogenic. These forms, which are encountered through industrial exposure, may enter the body through inhalation or cutaneous absorption.

Drug–Drug Interactions Drug interactions have not been reported for chromium.

Cobalt Cobalt is an essential component of vitamin B_{12}, but ingested cyanocobalamin is metabolized in vivo to form the B_{12} coenzymes.

Function Cobalt's nutritional functions are the same as those for cyanocobalamin. (See the section "Cyanocobalamin [Vitamin B_{12}].")

Dietary Sources Cobalt is an integral part of vitamin B_{12} and, therefore, the normal dietary sources of cobalt are the same as for vitamin B_{12}. It is contained in organ meats (e.g., liver, heart, kidney, clam, and oyster) and in products naturally containing microorganisms (e.g., milk, cream, cheese, and legumes).

Deficiency No deficiency state for cobalt is reported to exist in humans.

Dose/US RDA No US RDA exists for cobalt.

Adverse Effects Large doses of cobalt may result in goiter, congestive heart failure, and myxedema. Cardiomyopathy has also been described. Cyanosis and coma may result from accidental ingestion by children.

Copper Copper ions exist in two states: the cuprous and the cupric (a potent oxidizing agent). Copper is similar to zinc in the complexes it forms with a number of the same chelating agents. Copper is found in virtually all tissues of the body, but concentrations are highest in the liver, brain, heart, and kidney.

Function Copper is essential for the proper structure and function of the CNS, and it plays a major role in iron metabolism. Ceruloplasmin, one of the copper metalloenzymes, is especially important in converting absorbed ferrous iron to transported ferric iron. Other copper-containing enzymes are cytochrome oxidase, dopamine β-hydroxylase, and superoxide dismutase.

Dietary Sources Food sources for copper include organ meats (especially liver), shellfish, chocolate, whole-grain cereals, legumes, and nuts.

Deficiency Copper deficiency is uncommon in humans even though many individuals may have lower than recommended intake. Contemporary diets provide about 1.2 mg per day for men and 0.9 mg per day for women, which is somewhat less than the estimated safe and adequate range of 1.5 to 3.0 mg per day. Deficiencies have been observed in premature infants; in severely malnourished infants fed milk-based, low-copper diets; and in patients receiving parenteral nutrition with inadequate copper.

One of the prominent features of copper deficiency is impaired iron absorption. This problem is most likely caused by the loss of activity of the copper metalloenzymes titled ferroxidase and ceruloplasmin (a protein-copper complex), which results in hypochromic anemia. In copper-deficient animals, bone cortices are fragile and thin, resulting from the failure of collagen cross-linking. Spontaneous rupture of major vessels may also be observed in deficiency states.

Wilson's disease is an inborn error of metabolism causing a failure to eliminate copper. The result is CNS, kidney, and liver damage. Acute symptoms of copper toxicity include nausea, vomiting, diarrhea, hemolysis, convulsions, and GI bleeding. Symptoms respond to treatment with penicillamine.

Dose/US RDA Adults can safely take 1.5 to 3.0 mg of copper per day; 0.7 to 2.5 mg per day is suggested for children. Copper is available in different salt forms.

Adverse Effects Copper administered orally has an emetic action, with copper sulfate doses in excess of 250 mg producing vomiting. However, copper salts should not be used for this purpose.

Drug–Drug Interactions Molybdenum, zinc, and cadmium are antagonistic to copper, and large amounts of ascorbic acid impair copper absorption. Oral contraceptives have been shown to increase serum copper at the expense of tissue levels.

Fluorine Available therapeutic forms of fluorine include sodium fluoride and acidulated phosphate fluoride (both of which are available for oral and topical administration), sodium monofluorophosphate, and stannous fluoride. Sodium fluoride contains about 45% fluoride ion, and stannous fluoride contains about 24% fluoride ion.

Function Fluoride occurs normally in bones and tooth enamel as a calcium salt. Intake of small amounts has been shown to markedly reduce tooth decay, presumably by making the enamel more resistant to the erosive action of acids produced by bacteria in the oral cavity. Fluoride has also been used in women with osteoporosis at a dose of 50 mg per day. However, this treatment may have adverse effects, so the patient must be carefully monitored.

Dietary Sources Fluoride is present in soil and water, but the content varies widely from region to region. Most municipal water supplies are fluoridated to 1 ppm of fluoride, a level that has been shown to be safe and to reduce caries in children by about 50%. Estimates of fluoride intake from food, beverages, and water vary greatly depending on the presence of fluoridated drinking water.

Deficiency Fluoride deficiency states in humans, other than potential dental decay, have not been described.

Dose/US RDA The safe and adequate estimated dose range for children is 0.5 to 2.5 mg per day and for adults is 1.5 to 4.0 mg per day. Fluoride is a normal constituent of the diet, given that it occurs in soils, water supplies, plants, and animals. Fluoride supplements should be routinely administered to children who consume water that is low in fluoride ion, such as well water. Sodium fluoride is available by prescription as oral tablets and solutions, topical solutions, and gels, as well as in combination products. Nonprescription products include topical rinses containing 0.01% to 0.02% fluoride, such as sodium fluoride.

Adverse Effects Excess fluoride can be toxic. Acute toxicity should not result from the low levels present in drinking water but may result from the administration of excessive doses of fluoride supplements. Because acute toxicity affects the GI system and the CNS, it can be life-threatening. Symptoms include salivation, abdominal pain, nausea, vomiting, diarrhea, dehydration, thirst, urticaria, muscle weakness, tremors, and (rarely) seizures. Because of the calcium-binding effect of fluoride, symptoms of calcium deficiency, including tetany, may be seen. The patient may exhibit mental irritability. Eventually, respiratory and cardiac failure may occur. The dose that causes acute toxicity in adults is approximately 5 g. Death has occurred after ingestion of 2 g in adults, but much larger overdoses have been treated successfully. In children, 0.5 g of sodium fluoride may be fatal. Treatment includes precipitation of the fluoride by using gastric lavage with 0.15% calcium hydroxide solution, intravenous glucose and saline for hydration, and treatment with calcium to prevent tetany.

Chronic fluoride toxicity is manifested as changes in the structure of bones and teeth. Bones become more dense and may be afflicted with disabling disease. Tooth enamel acquires a mottled appearance consisting of white, patchy plaques occurring with pitting brown stains. Prolonged ingestion of water that contains more than 2 ppm of fluoride has resulted in a significant incidence of mottling. Extremely large doses (e.g., 20 to 80 mg per day) have resulted in chalky, brittle bones that tend to fracture easily, a condition known as skeletal fluorosis.

Drug–Drug Interactions Fluoride causes both a decreased effect and decreased absorption when given with magnesium, aluminum, and calcium-containing products.

Iodine The thyroid gland contains about one-third of the iodine in the body, stored in the form of a complex glycoprotein, thyroglobulin. The only known function of thyroglobulin is to provide thyroxine and triiodothyronine, which are hormones that regulate the metabolic rate of cells and, therefore, influence physical and mental growth, nervous and muscle tissue function, circulatory activity, and use of nutrients.

Function Iodine is required to synthesize thyroxine and triiodothyronine and is an essential micronutrient. High concentrations of iodine inhibit the release of these hormones, and in its absence, thyroid hypertrophy occurs, resulting in goiter. However, iodine is usually present as the iodide in food and water and is sometimes organically bound to amino acids. The consumption of foods from diverse sources and the addition of iodide to table salt have essentially eliminated goiter as a health problem in the United States.

Dietary Sources The primary dietary source of iodine is iodized salt, which contains 1 part of sodium or potassium iodide per 10,000 parts (0.01%) of salt. A dose of about 95 mcg of iodine can be obtained from about one-fourth of a teaspoon of salt (1.25 g). In the United States, most of the table salt sold is iodized; however, salt used in food processing and for institutional use is not. Additional dietary sources of iodine include saltwater fish and shellfish.

Deficiency A deficiency of iodine can result in goiter; thyroidectomy may result in iodine insufficiency.

Dose/US RDA The iodine content of typical diets in the United States is still well above the US RDA value of 0.15 mg for adults. Iodine supplements are unwarranted for most individuals. Potassium iodide is available as a tablet and solution and is included in various combination products.

Adverse Effects Some individuals are allergic to iodide or to organic preparations containing iodine and may develop a rash. Symptoms of chronic iodism (iodide intoxication) include an unpleasant taste and burning in the mouth or throat, along with soreness of the teeth or gums. Increased salivation, sneezing, irritation of the eyes, and swelling of the eyelids commonly occur.

Drug–Drug Interactions Potassium iodide, when given with lithium salts, may cause additive hypothyroid effects.

Manganese Manganese can apparently substitute for magnesium in selected enzymes involved in oxidative phosphorylation.

Function Manganese is required for the utilization of glucose, the synthesis of mucopolysaccharides of cartilage, the biosynthesis of steroids, and the biologic activity of pyruvate carboxylase.

Dietary Sources Manganese is widely available in vegetables and fruits. Nuts, legumes, and whole-grain cereals are particularly good sources.

Deficiency Manganese deficiency is generally not a problem; the only theorized method of manganese deficiency is dietary.

Dose/US RDA Even though manganese is poorly absorbed after oral administration (3%), sufficient quantities are present in the average diet to maintain appropriate levels. A dose or dietary intake of 2 to 5 mg per day is considered safe and adequate; it is available as different salt forms.

Adverse Effects Toxicity is rare for orally administered manganese. It has been observed, however, from inhalation of dust and industrial fumes containing manganese.

Drug–Drug Interactions A possible antagonistic effect exists between manganese and iron, resulting in less iron absorption. Also, low iron levels may result in enhanced manganese absorption and possible toxicity.

Molybdenum Patients on long-term parenteral nutrition must be careful to avoid deficiencies of molybdenum.

Function Molybdenum can readily change its oxidation state and can act as an electron transfer agent in oxidation–reduction reactions. It may also function as an enzyme cofactor.

Dietary Sources The molybdenum content of food varies, depending on the growth environment. Milk, organ meats, beans, breads, and cereals appear to contribute the most dietary molybdenum.

Deficiency Molybdenum is a cofactor for several flavoprotein enzymes and is found in xanthine oxidase. Because xanthine oxidase is involved in the oxidation of xanthine to uric acid, high molybdenum intake has been associated with goutlike symptoms. Parenteral nutrition without molybdenum has resulted in an acquired molybdenum deficiency, which has been treated with ammonium molybdate. Symptoms of molybdenum deficiency include the following: tachycardia, tachypnea, headache, night blindness, nausea, vomiting, edema, lethargy, disorientation, hypermethioninemia, hypouricemia, hypooxypurinemia, hypouricosuria, and low urinary sulfate excretion. Also, mental disturbances may occur and may progress to coma.

Dose/US RDA The human molybdenum requirement is low (about 75 to 250 mcg per day for adults) and is easily furnished by the average diet. A safe and adequate daily dietary intake of 150 to 500 mcg has been estimated, but supplements may not be warranted.

Adverse Effects Molybdenum is relatively nontoxic.

Drug–Drug Interactions When consumed in excess, molybdenum may be antagonistic to copper, resulting in symptoms of copper deficiency. Molybdenum may increase the excretion rate of copper.

Nickel Divalent and trivalent forms of nickel are important in biologic systems. The absorption of nickel may be related to iron, but only a very low percentage is absorbed, most of it being lost in the feces.

Function It has been speculated that nickel is involved in specific metalloenzymes, but its actual activity has not been clearly delineated, even though nickel is essential.

Dietary Sources The highest concentrations of nickel are in chocolate, nuts, dried beans, peas, and grains.

Deficiency Symptoms of a deficiency state have not been documented in humans.

Dose/US RDA A safe and adequate intake of nickel is 100 to 300 mcg daily.

Adverse Effects Side effects of nickel administration can include gastrointestinal irritation and a hypersensitivity reaction.

Drug–Drug Interactions No drug interactions have been reported for nickel.

Selenium Selenium is present in all tissues. Selenium is generally incorporated into organic compounds involving amino acids such as methionine or cysteine. Selenium compounds are about 80% absorbed. The highest concentrations are in the kidneys and liver; the lowest are in the lungs and brain. The kidney is the primary route of excretion.

Function Many selenium compounds are analogous to sulfur compounds. Glutathione peroxidase, a selenoenzyme, is important in the destruction of inflammatory hydroperoxides.

Dietary Sources Dietary sources of selenium include meat, seafoods, and some cereal grains. Vegetables and fruits contain little of this element. The selenium content of foods depends on the soils in which the plants are grown.

Deficiency Selenium is an essential trace element in humans, but deficiencies are not common in the general population. Selenium deficiency has been reported in patients with alcoholic cirrhosis, probably resulting from an insufficient diet or the altered metabolism of selenium. It has been rarely reported in patients on long-term parenteral nutrition.

Limited evidence in humans suggests that deficiency results in cardiomyopathy, muscle pain, and abnormal nail beds. Epidemiologic studies suggest that cancer and heart disease may be common in areas of low selenium availability. Keshan disease has been shown to respond to selenium.

Dose/US RDA The US RDA for selenium is 70 mcg for adult men and 50 to 55 mcg for adult women. Selenium is included in some multivitamin and mineral preparations. Doses in excess of 200 mcg per day are not recommended.

Adverse Effects Toxic effects of selenium include loss of hair and nails, skin lesions, and CNS and teeth involvement. Selenium toxicity may be evidenced by growth retardation, muscular weakness, infertility, focal hepatic necrosis, dysphagia, dysphonia, bronchopneumonia, and respiratory failure.

Drug–Drug Interactions The possibility of an interaction exists between selenium and any nutrient that is involved in antioxidant/pro-oxidant cell balance (i.e., the requirement of selenium is inversely proportional to antioxidant intake). A positive interaction might be the protection against mercury, cadmium, and silver.

Silicon Little is known about the absorption, distribution, metabolism, and excretion of silicon.

Function Silicon apparently functions in the development and maintenance of connective tissue. It is required for collagen biosynthesis and for the mineralization process in bone calcification.

Dietary Sources Silicon is obtained from foods of plant origin, especially cereal products, root vegetables, and unrefined grains of high fiber content. The role of silicon in human nutrition, if any, is unknown at present.

Deficiency Silicon deficiency states in humans have not been described.

Dose/US RDA The daily requirement of silicon has not been established, and the best product form for silicon administration has not been determined.

Adverse Effects When taken orally, silicon is essentially nontoxic. This lack of toxicity is evidenced by the administration of silicon-containing magnesium trisilicate (a nonprescription antacid that has been available for more than 40 years without apparent toxic effects) and by the ingestion of simethicone (a common anti-gas ingredient in many nonprescription antacids).

Drug–Drug Interactions The absorption and metabolism of silicon may be altered by fiber, molybdenum, magnesium, and fluoride. Possible interactions related to the silicate form (magnesium trisilicate) may be (1) decreased effects of digoxin, tetracycline, and ticlopidine hydrochloride and (2) increased effects of sulfonylurea and quinidine.

Tin Tin may be involved in growth and reproductive functions, but evidence of its necessity is lacking. A deficiency state for tin has not been described in humans. Adequate quantities of tin are apparently obtained from the diet.

Vanadium The most important forms of vanadium in biologic systems are the tetravalent and pentavalent states. The tetravalent form easily complexes with other substances, such as transferrin or hemoglobin, to stabilize it against oxidation.

Function Vanadium may be involved in functions related to growth and reproduction; however, the evidence of its necessity is not well established.

Dietary Sources Shellfish, mushrooms, parsley, and some spices (e.g., dill seed and black pepper) are rich in vanadium.

Deficiency Vanadium is presumed essential, but a deficiency state has not been confirmed. It is obtained in sufficient quantities in the diet.

Dose/US RDA A daily dose of 10 to 100 mcg is considered safe and adequate.

Adverse Effects Toxicity can occur through excessive dietary intake. Symptoms include diarrhea, anorexia, depressed growth, and neurotoxicity. Vanadium toxicity may be diminished by administration of ascorbic acid, ethylenediaminetetraacetic acid, chromium, protein, ferrous iron, chloride, and possibly aluminum hydroxide.

Drug–Drug Interactions No drug interactions have been reported for vanadium.

Zinc Zinc is an integral part of at least 70 metalloenzymes, including carbonic anhydrase, lactic dehydrogenase, alkaline phosphatase, carboxypeptidase, aminopeptidase, and alcohol dehydrogenase.

Function Zinc is a cofactor in the synthesis of DNA and RNA. It is involved in the mobilization of vitamin A from the liver and in the enhancement of follicle-stimulating hormone and luteinizing hormone. Zinc is essential for normal cellular immune functions and for spermatogenesis and normal testicular function. It is important in the stabilization of membrane structure.

The divalent ion is most commonly found and used in the body. Zinc has a relatively rapid turnover rate, and the body pool appears to be about 2 to 3 g. Zinc is efficiently regulated in the body.

Dietary Sources Most dietary zinc (about 70%) is derived from animal products. Good sources of zinc include oysters; liver; high-protein foods such as beef, lamb, pork, legumes, and peanuts; and whole-grain cereals.

Deficiency Although zinc deficiencies are not widespread in the United States, marginally low zinc values have been associated with growth retardation in children, slow wound healing in adults, birth defects, and problems in childbirth. Additional symptoms include loss of appetite, skin changes, and immunologic abnormalities. Symptoms may also include alopecia, behavioral disturbances, night blindness, impaired taste and smell, delayed sexual maturation, hypogonadism, and hypospermia.

Malabsorption syndromes, infection, myocardial infarct, major surgery, alcoholism, liver cirrhosis, pregnancy, lactation, and high-fiber diets rich in phytate predispose an individual to a suboptimal zinc status. Zinc depletion is relatively rare but may be seen in patients on long-term parenteral nutrition and in patients with GI tract abnormalities, such as fistulas and high-output diarrhea.

Zinc deficiencies adversely affect DNA, RNA, carbohydrate, and protein metabolism. Iron supplements decrease zinc absorption just as zinc supplements decrease iron absorption, probably resulting from competition for the same transport system. If these minerals are taken with a meal, the adverse interaction is less pronounced. Vegetarian diets, despite their high fiber content, do not result in low plasma zinc levels. In patients with impaired wound healing, zinc supplementation may be marginally beneficial.

Dose/US RDA The US RDA for zinc is 15 mg and 12 mg for adult men and women, respectively. The US RDA for infants is 5 mg and for children is 10 mg. Typical Western diets supply 10 to 15 mg of zinc per day. Because zinc is only 10% to 40% absorbed from the GI tract, ingestion of the 220-mg dose form of zinc sulfate (50 mg of elemental zinc) will supply 5 to 20 mg of zinc. Treatment of suspected deficiencies usually involves administration of 150 mg of elemental zinc in three divided doses daily. At these dosages, copper deficiency may be induced, so it has been suggested that the elemental zinc dosage be limited to 40 mg per day if therapy with zinc is going to be chronic.

Patients with large GI losses through fistulas, ostomies, or stool require larger supplemental doses of zinc. Chronic ingestion of more than 15 mg per day of elemental zinc is not recommended without adequate medical supervision.

Adverse Effects Because the ingestion of 2 g or more of zinc sulfate has resulted in GI irritation and vomiting, zinc can be taken with food. However, dairy and bran products, as well as foods high in calcium, phosphorus, or phytate, may decrease absorption of zinc. Zinc is also toxic, although the emetic effect that occurs after consumption of large amounts may minimize problems with accidental overdose. Reported signs of zinc toxicity in humans include vomiting, dehydration, muscle incoordination, dizziness, and abdominal pain.

Drug–Drug Interactions High intake of zinc may decrease copper levels (in fact, zinc is used to decrease copper absorption in Wilson's disease), and zinc may decrease tetracycline absorption.

Enteral Nutritional Supplements

More than 100 commercial preparations are currently available for enteral feeding. (See Table 19–9 for examples of these preparations.) Some are designed for general nutrition; others are designed for specific metabolic or clinical conditions. In addition to the various vitamins and minerals previously discussed in this chapter, the bulk volume/weight of these supplements consists primarily of proteins, carbohydrates, and lipids (fats, oils). Chapter 20, "Infant Nutrition and Special Nutritional Needs," has detailed information on infant nutrition.

In addition to oral nutritional supplementation, enteral nutrition is being increasingly used in patients who cannot ingest or digest sufficient amounts of food. For some patients, this impairment is temporary; for others, long-term use of these supplements is necessary. The pharmacist can assist patients or caregivers in selecting the appropriate formulation on the basis of the type of underlying pathology.

The advances in products specifically designed for enteral use and the availability of sophisticated formulas, small-bore nasogastric tubes, and constant-infusion delivery systems have lead to a resurgence of interest in enteral nutrition. The popularity of this mode of feeding has increased significantly in recent years in the hospital, home, and long-term care settings.

Enteral nutrition is defined as providing liquid nutrients by tube or by mouth into the GI tract. It is the desired method of feeding patients whose ability to ingest adequate nutrients by mouth is impaired but who have a functional GI tract. Its advantages over parenteral feeding include preservation of the structure and function of the GI tract, more efficient use of nutrients, decreased incidence of infections and metabolic complications, and decreased cost. Enteral foods are not diet foods or health food supplements and are not intended for that purpose.

Currently, enteral feeding devices (tubes) are divided into two major categories: those entering the GI tract through the nose (nasogastric or nasoantral tubes) and those entering through the abdominal wall (gastrostomies, duodenostomies, or jejunostomies). Most tubes are made of either silicone or polyurethane. The nasogastric and nasoantral tubes are between 30 and 43 inches long, with diameters from 5 to 16 French scale. The longer tubes are for nasoduodenal or nasojejunal feeding. The small diameter of these tubes often results in clogging, especially when medications are added to enteral liquids and administered through the tubes. Gastrostomy and jejunostomy tubes are of a larger diameter (16 to 24 French scale) and do not tend to clog. These tubes also allow quicker and easier administration of medications and feeding preparations. The newer percutaneous endoscopic gastrostomy tubes are increasingly popular because they are easier to place in patients, even on an outpatient basis.

Table 19-9

Selected Enteral Nutritional Supplements

Trade Name	Calories (per mL)	Protein (g)	Carbohydrate (g)	Fat (g)
Boost Liquid[a]	1.01	43	173	17.6
Boost Plus Liquid[a,b]	1.52	61	190	57
Citrotein Powder[a,c]	0.67	41	122	1.6
Compleat Pediatric Liquid[a,d]	1	38	126	39
Criticare HN	1.06	38	220	5.3
DiabetiSource Liquid[a,e]	1	50	90	49
Ensure Liquid[a]	1.06	9/8 fl oz	40/8 fl oz	6/8 fl oz
Ensure Pudding	250/5 oz can	7/5 oz can	34/5 oz can	10/5 oz can
Ensure Light Liquid[a]	0.84	10/8 fl oz	33/8 fl oz	3/8 fl oz
Ensure Plus Liquid[a]	1.5	13/8 fl oz	47.3/8 fl oz	12.6/8 fl oz
Ensure Plus HN Liquid[a]	1.5	14.8/8 fl oz	47.3/8 fl oz	11.8/8 fl oz
Fibersource Liquid[a]	1.2	43	170	39
Forta Shake Powder	140/1.4 oz mix	9/1.4 oz mix	24/1.4 oz mix	<1/1.4 oz mix
Isocal Liquid[a,c,e,f]	1.06	34	135	44
Jevity Liquid[a]	1.06	10.5/8 fl oz	36.4/8 fl oz	8.2/8 fl oz
Jevity Plus Liquid[a,e]	1.2	13.2/8 fl oz	41.1/8 fl oz	9.3/8 fl oz
Microlipid Emulsion[a,c,e–g]	4.5		510	
Moducal Powder[a,c–e]	3.8/g	0.95/g		
Nepro Liquid[a]	2	16.6/8 fl oz	52.8/8 fl oz	22.7/8 fl oz
Osmolite	1.06	37.1	151.1	34.7
Pro Mod Powder	28/6.6 g (scoop)	5/6.6 g (scoop)	0.67/6.6 g (scoop)	0.6/6.6 g (scoop)
Pulmocare	1.5	62.6	105.7	93.3
Resource Diabetic Liquid[a,e]	1.06	63	99	47
Resource Just for Kids Liquid[a,d]	1	30	110	50
Sustacal Pudding	1.69/g	6.8/5 oz	32/5 oz	9.5/5 oz
Sustacal Basic Liquid[a,c]	1.06	38	146	38
Sustacal Plus Liquid[a,c]	1.52	61	190	57

[a] Lactose-free product.
[b] Geriatric formulation.
[c] Cholesterol-free product.
[d] Pediatric formulation.
[e] Sucrose-free product.
[f] Dye-free product.
[g] Sodium-free product.

Classification of Enteral Nutrition Products Preparations for enteral feeding may be classified according to clinical indications or to composition of the products.

Clinical Indications Method Using the clinical indications method, enteral feeding products are classified as natural foods, polymeric solutions, monomeric solutions, solutions for specific metabolic needs, modular solutions, and hydration solutions.

Natural foods include blenderized foods either commercially available or prepared at home. Polymeric solutions contain macronutrients in the form of proteins, triglycerides, and carbohydrate polymers. The protein is obtained from casein, lactalbumin, whey, or egg white or from a combination of those. It is also present in the carbohydrates, from glucose polymers such as starch or its hydrolysates, and in the fats, from vegetable sources such as corn oil, safflower oil, sunflower oil, or others.

Monomeric solutions require less digestion because they contain protein in the form of peptides and/or free amino acids, which are derived from the hydrolysis of casein, whey, and other proteins. Carbohydrates are in the form of partially hydrolyzed starch (maltodextrins and glucose oligosaccharides), and the fat is often a mixture of medium and long-chain triglycerides. Monomeric solutions are lactose free and do not contain fiber. Solutions for specific metabolic needs include branched-chain amino acid solutions, essential amino acid solutions, high-fat/low-carbohydrate solutions, and immune-modulating solutions. Modular solutions are designed to provide macronutrients or micronutrients singly or in combination for specialized formulas for both oral and enteral feedings. Hydration solutions are designed primarily to provide fluid and minerals for therapeutic purposes or to prevent dehydration.

Specialty formulations include puddings (Sustacal Pudding), predigested/hydrolyzed formulas (Criticare HN), low-carbohydrate formulas (Pulmocare), low-protein formulas (Amin-Aid), isotonic formulas (Osmolite), clear liquid formulas (Citrotein), nutrient-dense products, and modular products (Moducal).

Product Composition Method Enteral preparations classified according to composition are either supplemental or complete, with general and specialized applications. Supplemental products of protein-calorie formulas are used only as adjuncts to a regular diet because they are not nutritionally complete.

Complete formulas can be used orally or as tube feedings, and may be used as sole dietary intake (if the patient's electrolytes are monitored) or as supplementation. These products may contain ingredients that make them appropriate for special needs. Several such products (Instant Breakfast, Sustacal, and Meritene) are milk based; others (Compleat-B and Gerber Meat Base Formula) have a mixed-food base. Another type supplies (1) protein in the form of crystalline amino acids or protein hydrolysate, (2) carbohydrate in the form of oligosaccharides or disaccharides, and (3) vitamins and minerals in the form of individual chemicals. These last products are chemically defined diets, also known as "elemental diets"; examples include Vivonex and Jejunal. Some other complete products (Precision LR and Portagen) are only partly chemically defined.

Nearly all elemental diets have low-fat content and contain electrolytes, minerals, trace elements, and water- and fat-soluble vitamins. All chemically based products require little or no digestion, are absorbed over a short distance in the small intestine, and have low residue. These attributes mean that the number and volume of the stools are reduced, making these products appropriate for patients who had ileostomies or colostomies and who wish to decrease fecal output. The low-residue products may also facilitate the care of elderly patients with stool incontinence or patients with brain damage from strokes, congenital defects, or retardation. Because of the ease of absorption and the low fecal residues, these products are often used in postoperative care, in treating GI disease, and in treating neoplastic disease in which tissue breakdown is extensive.

Administration and Monitoring Guidelines Supplemental and complete formulas are available in several forms, including those that must be diluted with water or milk and those that are ready to use. The extent of dilution is based on the amount of nutrients needed and the amount that can be tolerated. Adults will not generally tolerate preparations of more than 25% weight per volume (w/v), which generally delivers 1.0 cal/mL. The maximum concentration for infants is 12% w/v, which generally delivers 0.5 cal/mL. Infants should generally be started on a concentration of 7 to 7.5% w/v, increasing to 12% over 4 to 5 days as tolerated. For children older than 10 months, 15% w/v formulas may be initiated, with gradual increases to 25%. Higher concentrations may cause osmotic diarrhea.

If the preparations are taken orally, 100 to 150 mL should be ingested at one time. Over the course of a day, 2000 mL of most preparations provide about 2000 calories. If the patient is tube fed, 40 to 60 mL of the product per hour may be given initially. Once opened, the container should be kept cold to prevent bacterial growth, and all prepared products remaining after 24 hours should be discarded. Tubing should be rinsed three times a day with water. If diarrhea, nausea, or distention occurs, the diet should be withheld for 24 hours and then gradually resumed. For elderly or unconscious people or for patients who recently had surgery, elevating the head of the bed is advisable during administration to avoid aspiration.

Pharmacists should store supplemental formula products at temperatures under 75° F (23.8° C) and should check expiration dates before dispensing.

Patients must be monitored for biochemical abnormalities, electrolyte values, and adequate nutrition and hydration. Urine and blood glucose concentrations can be monitored. Patients with diabetes may require increased insulin doses. Edema may be precipitated or aggravated in patients with protein-calorie malnutrition or cardiac, renal, or hepatic disease because of the relatively high sodium content of the elemental diets. Some commercially available nutritional products (e.g., Ensure and Ensure Plus) are a source of vitamin K supplementation, which may interfere with oral anticoagulant therapy. Tube feedings have been shown to interfere with the absorption of phenytoin administered through the tube. This interaction can be avoided by flushing the tube with saline (or water) before and after phenytoin and by waiting 15 minutes both before and after the dose is given.

Product Selection Guidelines

For most patients concerned about their nutritional status, a once daily multivitamin is the appropriate recommendation if a deficiency is not suspected. If a patient's diet lacks servings from some of the basic food groups, the pharmacist should recommend supplements to cover the nutrients in the missing food groups.

Women with heavy menstrual flow who describe symptoms of iron deficiency need only an iron supplement unless they describe symptoms of other nutrient deficiencies. Pregnant or breast-feeding women need additional intake of pyridoxine. The pharmacist should find out whether a physician recommended such supplementation.

Underlying pathology usually determines the selection of an enteral nutritional supplement. Milk-free supplements (Nutramigen, Mull-Soy) are appropriate for patients who have a milk allergy or lactose malabsorption. A low protein and electrolyte formula (Controlyte) is the best selection for patients with acute or chronic renal failure. Because of decreased fecal output, elemental diets (Vivonex and Jejunal) are appropriate for patients who had ileostomies or colostomies, for elderly patients with stool incontinence, or for patients with brain damage from strokes, congenital defects, or retardation. These products are also appropriate for use in caring for patients postoperatively, in treating GI disease, and in treating neoplastic disease in which tissue breakdown is extensive.

Patient Assessment of Nutritional Deficiencies

Assessing a patient's nutritional status is difficult in the ambulatory environment. Clinical impressions about nutrition are often erroneous because the stages between well-nourished and poorly nourished states are not readily evident. There are guidelines, however, that may help to provide a more objective assessment of a patient's nutritional status. Pharmacists should know which population groups tend to be poorly nourished, exercise good observational skills, and know which questions yield helpful information. By asking key questions, the pharmacist may detect cultural, physical, environmental, and social conditions that may suggest inadequate vitamin intake. The more specific the information obtained from the patient, the more helpful the pharmacist can be in determining the need for nutritional supplementation. Questions about foods generally not included in the diet and about previous treatment of similar symptoms may also be important.

Although most assessment measures are beyond the scope of routine pharmacy practice, the pharmacist must observe the status of the patient. For example, a patient's fingernails may indicate malnutrition if they lose their luster and become dark at the upper ends. The texture, amount, and appearance of the hair may indicate the patient's nutritional status. The eyes, particularly the conjunctiva, may indicate vitamin A and iron deficiencies. The mouth may show stomatitis, glossitis, or hypertrophic or pale gums. The number and general condition of the teeth may reflect the patient's choice of food. Visible goiter, poor skin color and texture, obesity or thinness relative to bone structure, and the presence of edema may also be indications of malnutrition. The pharmacist should be able to recognize overt but nonspecific symptoms of vitamin and mineral deficiencies where prompt physician referral may be crucial.

Checking a patient's medication history is important because of the numerous potential drug–micronutrient interactions. (See Table 19–10.) It is also the pharmacist's responsibility to refer patients with a suspected serious illness to a physician. Just as nutritional deficiencies may lead to disease, disease may lead to nutritional deficiencies. Patients may present with one or more deficiencies, which may be very difficult to identify. Rarely in the United States do

Table 19–10

Micronutrient–Drug and Micronutrient–Micronutrient Interactions

Micronutrient	Drug/Micronutrient	Effect	Precautionary Measures
Vitamins			
Vitamins A, E, K (large doses)	Warfarin	↑ anticoagulation	Take only recommended US RDAs
Vitamins A, E, D, K	Cholestyramine or mineral oil (nonabsorbed)	Possible ↓ vitamin absorption	Avoid prolonged use of cholestyramine or mineral oil
Vitamin A	Oral contraceptives	Possible ↑ plasma levels of vitamin A	
Vitamin D	Phosphate in chronically used drugs (e.g., certain laxatives)	Possible ↓ calcium levels; vitamin D deficiency	
	Phenytoin or barbiturates	Possible ↓ half-life of vitamin D	
Vitamin E	Iron	↓ vitamin E absorption	Separate doses of iron and vitamin E
Vitamin K	Broad-spectrum antibiotics (long-term therapy)	Vitamin K deficiency induced by ↓ gut flora	Ensure normal dietary intake of vitamin K
	Vitamins A and E (large doses)	↓ absorption/metabolism of vitamin K	Take only recommended US RDAs of all vitamins

(continued)

Table 19–10

Micronutrient–Drug and Micronutrient–Micronutrient Interactions (continued)

Micronutrient	Drug/Micronutrient	Effect	Precautionary Measures
Vitamin C	Medications eliminated by renal excretion	Possible ↑ effect of acidic drugs and ↓ effect of basic drugs (amphetamines, tricyclic antidepressants)	Monitor patients on these medications who are also taking megadoses of vitamin C
	Cholestyramine	↓ absorption of vitamin C; ↓ bile acid–binding capacity of cholestyramine	Separate doses of the two agents
	Estrogens	Possible ↑ serum levels of estrogens	
	Warfarin	↓ anticoagulation	
Folic acid	Phenytoin and possibly other related anticonvulsants (chronic use)	Possible inhibited folic acid absorption, leading to megaloblastic anemia. Subsequent ↑ folic acid supplementation may decrease serum phenytoin levels and complicate seizure control	
	Trimethoprim	Weak folic acid antagonism; ↓ activity/effectiveness	Although rare, megaloblastic anemia may occur in patients with low folic acid level at onset of trimethoprim therapy
	Pyrimethamine (large doses)	Possible megaloblastic anemia	
	Methotrexate	Folic acid antagonism; ↓ activity/effectiveness	Monitor use of folic acid in patients on maintenance regimens for psoriasis or rheumatoid arthritis
Niacin	Oral hypoglycemics	↓ hypoglycemic effect	
	Sulfinpyrazone and probenecid	Possible inhibited uricosuric effects	
	Lovastatin and possibly other HMG-CoA reductase inhibitors	Possible ↑ risk for myopathy	
	Adrenergic blocking agents	Additive vasodilating effect; may contribute to postural hypotension	
Pantothenic acid	Anticholinesterase ophthalmic preparations (echothiophate iodide, isoflurophate)	Possible ↑ miotic effects	
Pyridoxine	Isoniazid, cycloserine, hydralazine	Pyridoxine antagonism, manifested as perioral numbness resulting from peripheral neuropathy	Routinely take 50 mg/day of pyridoxine hydrochloride with isoniazid, or 10 mg of pyridoxine for each 100 mg of isoniazid, and 20 mg/day with cycloserine
	Penicillamine	Possible pyridoxine-responsive neurotoxicity caused by drug binding with pyridoxine hydrochloride	
	Phenobarbital and phenytoin	↓ serum levels of the drugs	
	Levodopa	Levodopa antagonism ↓ effectiveness	Avoid supplemental pyridoxine or, if possible, substitute levodopa–carbidopa for levodopa

Table 19–10

Micronutrient–Drug and Micronutrient–Micronutrient Interactions (continued)

Micronutrient	Drug/Micronutrient	Effect	Precautionary Measures
Minerals			
Calcium	Iron, zinc, other essential minerals	Inhibited mineral absorption caused by high calcium intake	
	Corticosteroids	Inhibited calcium absorption from gut; ↑ bone fractures and osteoporosis	
	Aluminum-containing antacids (excessive ingestion)	Negative calcium balances	
	Phosphates, calcitonin, sodium sulfate, furosemide, magnesium, cholestyramine, estrogen, some anticonvulsants	↓ calcium serum levels	
	Thiazide diuretics	↑ calcium serum levels	
Iron	Antacids	↓ iron solubility and absorption	
	Tetracyclines	↓ tetracycline and iron absorption	If concurrent administration is medically necessary, take tetracycline 3 hours after or 2 hours before taking iron
Trace Elements			
Copper	Molybdenum, zinc, and cadmium	Copper antagonism	Possible competition for absorption and utilization
	Vitamin C (large doses)	Impaired copper absorption	
	Oral contraceptives	↑ serum copper levels at the expense of tissue levels	
Fluorine	Magnesium, aluminum, calcium	↓ effect and absorption of fluoride	
Iodine (potassium iodide)	Lithium salts	Possible additive hypothyroid effects	
Manganese	Iron	↓ iron absorption; low iron levels in turn may ↑ manganese absorption with possible toxicity	
Molybdenum	Copper	Possible ↑ excretion rate of copper, resulting in symptoms of copper deficiency	
Selenium	Vitamins C and E	Vitamins have heme antioxidant effects but compete at different areas in metabolic pathway	
	Mercury, cadmium, and silver	Selenium's role with glutathione peroxidase protects against these trace elements	
Silicon	Molybdenum, magnesium, fluoride, fiber	Altered absorption/metabolism of silicon	
Silicon as magnesium trisilicate	Digoxin, tetracycline, ticlopidine	↓ effects of the drugs	
	Sulfonylurea, quinidine	↑ effects of the drugs	
Zinc	Copper	Possible ↓ copper levels	
	Tetracycline	Possible ↓ tetracycline absorption	

pharmacists encounter patients with severe deficiencies resulting in diseases such as scurvy, pellagra, or kwashiorkor. However, milder forms of malnutrition may be seen.

Observing the patient's physical appearance and asking the following questions will help elicit the information needed to determine the appropriate treatment approach.

Q~ Why do you think you need a vitamin, mineral, or nutritional supplement?

A~ If a physician has not diagnosed a nutritional deficiency and if the patient does not show signs of a deficiency, encourage the patient to take only a once daily multivitamin in the recommended dosage. If the patient does show signs of a deficiency, refer the patient to a physician for evaluation.

Q~ What are your symptoms? Have they appeared suddenly or gradually?

A~ If the symptoms are severe with a sudden onset, refer the patient to a physician. For people who are just overworked or in stressful situations, recommend a once daily multivitamin taken in the recommended dosage.

Q~ What is your age and weight? Have you experienced any recent weight change?

A~ Refer patients with sudden weight gain or loss to a physician. These symptoms often indicate serious underlying pathology.

Q~ Do you eat meats, vegetables, dairy products, and grain products every day?

A~ Advise patients who are eating well-balanced meals that nutritional supplements are not needed. If only one or two food groups are supplying the daily intake, recommend a once daily multivitamin to ensure the patient is receiving sufficient vitamins and minerals.

Q~ Are you dieting, or do you have any type of dietary restrictions?

A~ If the patient describes a diet that may be detrimental to health, advise the patient to stop the diet and to see a physician for evaluation and a possible prescribed diet plan. If the patient has specific dietary restrictions, check that supplements being taken do not contain those ingredients. Then recommend a supplement that contains any nutrients their diet may be lacking.

Q~ Do you participate regularly in sports, or do you have a job requiring physical activity?

A~ Regular exercise is an important component of overall health. Advise patients with a sedentary lifestyle that walking for 30 minutes at least three times weekly can make a great difference in their health. Caution them to consult their physician before beginning an exercise program.

Q~ Do you have any chronic illness (diabetes, peptic ulcer, ulcerative colitis, or epilepsy)?

A~ If the patient has a chronic illness that may cause decreased absorption of necessary nutrients, advise the patient to consult a physician before starting a supplementation regimen.

Q~ Are you currently taking any prescription or nonprescription medications?

A~ *Identify medications that can interact with micronutrients. (See Table 19–10.)* Before recommending a nutritional supplement, determine whether any of the patient's medications could interact with a vitamin or mineral.

Q~ Are you taking, or have you recently taken, any vitamins, minerals, or nutritional supplements?

A~ Using the patient's answer, determine whether additional supplementation could cause vitamin toxicity. Consider supplemental vitamins and minerals from all sources.

Q~ Do you donate blood? How often? When did you last donate blood? Do you have a heavy menstrual flow?

A~ If the patient's response and previous description of symptoms indicate a possible iron deficiency, recommend an iron supplement. Advise the patient to return in 30 days for reevaluation unless symptoms worsen before then.

Q~ Do you smoke, or are you around smokers daily?

A~ Advise patients who smoke that smoking can decrease appetite, resulting in inadequate nutrition. If smoking is being used as a weight-loss method, encourage the patient to see a physician for evaluation and possibly a prescribed diet plan.

Q~ Do you drink alcohol? How often and how much?

A~ Advise patients who drink that alcohol decreases the appetite and can cause nutrient deficiencies. Stress the importance of a proper diet. Recommend vitamin and mineral supplementation if the patient's nutritional status warrants it.

Q~ Are you pregnant? Have you recently given birth?

A~ Advise a pregnant or breast-feeding woman that a fetus or infant puts an extra nutritional burden on the body. Explain that pyridoxine requirements in particular are increased during pregnancy and breast-feeding. Find out whether the patient's physician recommended a nutritional supplement.

Q~ Do you take oral contraceptives (birth control pills)?

A~ *Identify potential interactions between oral contraceptives and vitamin supplements. (See Table 19–10.)* Advise the patient of the effects of estrogen on vitamins. If a vitamin deficiency is possible, recommend the appropriate supplementation.

Patient Counseling for Nutritional Deficiencies

By being familiar with daily US RDAs of the various vitamins and minerals, and by knowing which natural food sources provide these US RDAs, the pharmacist may be able to educate the patient and to improve the diet so that nutritional requirements are met through food. If a supplement is needed, the pharmacist can recommend a product that will provide appropriate levels of the needed vitamins at a reasonable price.

The public is often exposed to exaggerated and fraudulent claims concerning vitamin products. The pharmacist can help to expose such claims by keeping up with medical and pharmaceutical literature and by not supporting or appearing to support the claims until they are substantiated by reliable clinical studies. Patients inquiring about such claims should be educated about the increased potential risk of the nontraditional use of vitamins. They should be told, for example, about adverse drug reactions that might occur with such products when used in alternative doses or in combination with prescription and nonprescription drug products. This advice, however, becomes difficult to give when patients purchase their nutritional supplements from health food stores or from on-line and mail-order vendors.

Patients purchasing a nonprescription liquid dietary supplement should be instructed on its proper use and storage, including dilution and preparation techniques. In addition, the pharmacist should offer to discuss with the patient possible adverse effects such as diarrhea.

The box "Patient Education for Nutritional Deficiencies" lists specific information to provide patients.

Patient Education for Nutritional Deficiencies

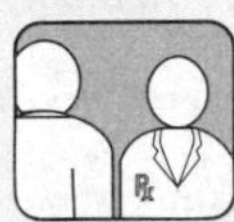

The objective of self-treatment is to prevent nutritional deficiencies or maintain the present nutritional status. For most patients, carefully following product instructions and the self-care measures listed below will help ensure optimal therapeutic outcomes.

Vitamins, Minerals, and Trace Elements

- To ensure proper nutrition, eat foods from all the basic food groups (meats, fruits and vegetables, dairy products, and grains). (See Figure 19–1.) Vitamin supplements are not a substitute for a well-balanced diet.
- Read labels on all vitamin or vitamin and mineral preparations carefully before taking them. Note the quantity of vitamins and minerals required to meet the recommended daily allowance (US RDA).
- Do not take doses of vitamins and minerals higher than the US RDAs. High doses of vitamins or minerals may be dangerous and should not be taken indiscriminately.
- Take vitamins or vitamin and mineral supplements with meals if you experience gastrointestinal symptoms.
- If desired, mix liquid vitamin and mineral supplements with food (fruit juice, milk, baby formula, or cereal).
- Be aware that iron supplements or vitamins with iron may turn stool black. This occurrence is not a cause for alarm unless it is associated with other symptoms involving the digestive system.
- As with any medicine, store vitamin and combination vitamin and mineral supplements out of the reach of children, especially if the product contains iron. Teach children that vitamins are drugs and potential poisons, and vitamins cannot be taken indiscriminately.
- Be aware that niacin-containing products may cause a flushing sensation, which should decrease in intensity with continued therapy.
- Note that riboflavin-containing products may cause a yellow fluorescence in the urine.

Do not self-medicate if you suspect a vitamin deficiency; consult a physician or pharmacist instead.

Enteral Nutrition

- For preparations taken orally, take 100 to 150 mL at one time. Over the course of a day, 2000 mL of most preparations provide about 2000 calories.
- For preparations administered by tube, give 40 to 60 mL of the product per hour initially.
- Keep opened containers cold to prevent bacterial growth; discard all remaining prepared products after 24 hours.
- Rinse tubing three times a day with water.
- If diarrhea, nausea, or abdominal distention occurs, withhold

(*continued*)

Patient Education for Nutritional Deficiencies (continued)

the preparation for 24 hours and then gradually resume feeding.

- When tube-feeding the elderly, unconscious people, or patients who have recently had surgery, elevate the head of the bed during feeding to avoid aspiration.
- Make sure patients on long-term enteral nutrition are monitored for biochemical abnormalities, electrolyte values, and adequate nutrition and hydration.
- Monitor urine and blood glucose concentrations in patients with diabetes. They may require increased insulin doses.

Evaluation of Patient Outcomes for Nutritional Deficiencies

Nutritional therapy could involve a diet based on the Food Guide Pyramid or nutritional supplements. The pharmacist should advise patients to return after 30 days of implementing nutritional therapy or sooner if the symptoms worsen. Patients whose symptoms have worsened should be referred to a physician. Patients whose symptoms have improved while taking nutritional supplements should be encouraged to eat a healthful diet and not to rely on supplements as the primary source for vitamins and minerals.

CONCLUSIONS

Pharmacists can significantly contribute to improving the nutritional status of the population by becoming familiar with the basics of nutrition, observing patients, listening to their requests, and providing general nutritional counseling. Much misinformation is being disseminated, and pharmacists are in a position to dispel myths, downplay exaggerated claims, and provide objective facts on nutritional agents such as vitamins, minerals, and nutritional supplements.

The pharmacist should not hesitate to recommend that a patient talk to a physician about starting a supplement, if it is felt that one is needed. Likewise, taking the time to counsel a patient on the food pyramid, food groups, and supplement requirements may save the patient the expense of needless products. It may also build a bridge of trust and understanding that will allow the pharmacist to help patients make wise and healthy choices.

References

1. Ehrlich FJ. Drugstores and nutrition: played right, a winning combination. *Drug Topics.* 1985;129:28–31.
2. Swain R, Kaplan B. Vitamins as therapy in the 1990s. *J Am Board Fam Pract.* 1995;8:206.
3. Olson JA. Vitamins: the tortuous path from needs to fantasies. *J Nutr.* 1994;124:1771S.
4. Marcus R, Coulston AM. In: Hardman JG, Limbird LE, eds. *Goodman and Gilman's The Pharmacological Basis of Therapeutics.* 19th ed. New York: McGraw Hill; 1996:1555.
5. Food and Nutrition Board, National Research Council. *Recommended Dietary Allowances.* 10th ed. Washington, DC: National Academy of Sciences; 1989.
6. Shils ME, Olson, JA, Shike M, eds. *Modern Nutrition in Health and Disease.* 8th ed. Philadelphia: Lea and Febiger; 1994.
7. Robinson CH, Lawler MR, Chendweth WL, Garwick AE. *Normal and Therapeutic Nutrition.* 17th ed. New York: Macmillan; 1990.
8. *American Hospital Formulary Service, 1992.* Bethesda, MD: American Society of Hospital Pharmacists; 1992.
9. *U.S. Dispensing Information.* 12th ed. Bethesda, MD: US Pharmacopoeial Convention; 1992.
10. Billups NF, Billups SM. *American Drug Index.* 35th ed. St. Louis: JB Lippincott; 1991.

CHAPTER 20

Infant Nutrition and Special Nutritional Needs

Claudia Kamper, Rosalie Sagraves, and Judi Doerr

Chapter 20 at a Glance

Breast-feeding is the desired method for feeding infants because human milk provides a nutritional source that is physiologically sound while it helps to facilitate a close bond between mother and child. Breast-feeding appears to decrease the incidence of infant allergy and illness. In addition, breast-feeding can decrease the amount of time spent in nutrition preparation, lower the cost of infant feeding, and decrease a woman's postpartum recovery time.[1–3] Because some women do not want to breast-feed or are unable to do so, commercially prepared infant formulas are a good alternative when used in developed countries. Formula use is less desirable in developing nations where inadequate sanitation and refrigeration, as well as an inability of illiterate women to follow instructions for preparing the formula, increase the risk of infant morbidity and mortality.[3]

Technical advances in the early 20th century helped popularize artificial milk feedings. Between 1930 and 1960, evaporated milk was frequently used in preparing infant formula, but by 1978 fewer than 5% of all formula-fed infants received evaporated milk formulas.[4] Between 1971 and 1982, a greater acceptance of breast-feeding in the United States resulted in a change in infant feeding patterns. During this time, breast-feeding at hospital discharge increased from 24.7% to 61.9%, and the incidence at ages 5 to 6 months increased from 5.5% to 28.8%.[5–7] In 1997, the incidence of breast-feeding early postpartum was 62%, decreasing to 26% by ages 5 to 6 months.[8]

Most women in the United States decide before or during early pregnancy whether they will breast-feed.[9] *Healthy People 2000: National Health Promotion and Disease Prevention Objectives*[8] is a national plan to improve the health of the American people, and throughout the 1990s, it published periodic status reports on progress toward its objectives. One goal of *Healthy People 2000* was to have 75% of all infants in the United States breast-fed at birth, with 50% still receiving some breast milk at age 6 months.[8] Until this goal is attained, advances in nutritional quality, safety, and convenience have established infant formulas as a good alternative to breast-feeding. The U.S. formula industry produces and sells approximately 3.6 billion 8-ounce formula equivalents annually.[10] Variations among formulas allow for product se-

---

Editor's Note: This chapter is based, in part, on the 11th edition chapter titled "Infant Formula Products," which was written by Rosalie Sagraves, Claudia Kamper, and Judi Doerr.

lection that will meet a specific infant's nutritional requirements, with variations producing differences in palatability, digestibility, sources of nutrients, and convenience of administration.

A pharmacist, in consultation with the infant's parents and physician, should be able to evaluate indications, advise on the selection of an infant formula, and help to ensure its appropriate use. A pharmacist should be knowledgeable about infant nutritional requirements, commercially prepared infant formulas, differences in formula composition, and specific uses for therapeutic formulas.

Infant Physiology and Growth

The physiology of the infant's gastrointestinal (GI) and renal systems is crucial in understanding an infant's nutritional needs. Standard growth parameters can confirm whether the nutritional needs are being met.

Physiology

Only liquid nutrition is appropriate for an infant until complex tongue movements and swallowing reflexes mature. Frequent feedings are necessary because stomach capacity of a full-term infant (38 to 42 weeks' gestation and birth weight greater than 2500 g) is only 20 to 90 mL but increases to 90 to 150 mL by age 1 month.[11]

Stomach acid and pepsin secretion peak in the newborn by day 10, decrease between days 10 and 30, and then gradually increase over year 1 of life. A full-term infant can digest most carbohydrates because intestinal enzymes, such as lactase, sucrase, maltase, isomaltase, and glucoamylase, are sufficiently mature at birth.[11] Sucrase, maltase, and isomaltase usually are fully active in preterm infants (gestational age 38 weeks or less), but lactase activity can be immature. Lactose intolerance is uncommon in full-term infants because of postnatal adaptive responses to ingested carbohydrates. Lactase activity may begin declining in African American and Asian children when they are toddlers.[12] Because amylase and lipase secretion from the pancreas does not reach adult levels until infants are approximately age 1 year, they may develop diarrhea if they cannot digest glucose polymers or starches found in certain infant formulas. Salivary amylase and lingual lipase may help to compensate for this deficiency in early infancy and among premature infants.[13]

Newborn infants exhibit low lipase concentrations and slow rates of bile salt synthesis, which are important for fat absorption.[13] This situation may result in a lower absorption of dietary fats and fat-soluble vitamins during early infancy that will improve with maturation.

Protein digestion does not differ appreciably between infants and adults. Amino acids produced by protein digestion are absorbed by active transport mechanisms that reach adult levels by age 14 weeks.[11]

The renal solute load is composed of soluble waste products (e.g., nitrogenous waste, excess electrolytes, and minerals) that the kidneys must eliminate. The potential renal solute load (PRSL) is defined as the solute load that is derived from dietary ingestion that would be excreted renally if amino acids from protein digestion were not used for growth or were eliminated by nonrenal routes.[14] The following equation can be used to calculate PRSL for breast milk or various infant formulas:

$$\text{PRSL (mOsm)} = \text{N}/28 + \text{sodium} + \text{chloride} + \text{potassium} + \text{phosphorus}_{\text{(available)}}$$

where N is the total nitrogen in milligrams and sodium, chloride, potassium, and available phosphorus are expressed in millimoles per unit volume.[14] The PRSL of an infant diet gains clinical importance in its influence on water balance when febrile illnesses occur and when diet may require supplementation with free water.[15] Further discussion of renal solute load will appear in the section "Commercial Infant Formulas" later in this chapter.

Growth

The human body exhibits standard growth and development patterns. Birth weight is determined primarily by maternal prepregnancy and pregnancy weight and by weight changes. The average birth weight for a full-term infant is approximately 3500 g (about 7½ pounds); infants born prematurely may weigh less than 1500 g (about 3⅓ pounds).[16]

After birth, a brief period of water weight loss (6% to 10%) occurs, followed by an average weight gain of 20 to 25 g per day in the first 4 months and 15 g per day in the next 8 months. Most infants can be expected to double their birth weight by age 4 months and triple it by age 12 months. From age 2 years to age 9 or 10 years, a fairly constant growth rate of about 5 pounds per year occurs. Thereafter, growth velocity increases and a major growth spurt accompanies adolescence. Height shows a pattern similar to weight; most infants increase their length by 50% in the first year, 100% in the first 4 years, and 300% by age 13 years.

Changes in body composition accompany height and weight changes. Most notably, total body water decreases as adipose tissue increases. Total body water accounts for approximately 70% of total body weight at birth and declines to 60% by age 1 year.[17]

Normal values of weight, height, and growth for infants and children are expressed in terms of percentiles for age; the reference standards most commonly used are those of the National Center for Health Statistics, a compilation of normative data from two major sources that was first available in the late 1970s.[18,19] According to these standards, most children fall between the 5th and 95th percentiles in weight, length/height, weight for length, and head circumference. Most children stay within the same percentile as they grow, but spurts and plateaus are common. If growth is not progressing as expected, particularly in the first year of life when the expected growth rate is rapid, the energy and nutrient content of an infant's diet should be evaluated. Concern for the degree to which these references are truly representative of healthy infants and children of the world, regardless of mode of infant feeding (breast milk or formula) or method of measurement, has led to the commitment to construct a new set of globally applicable reference standards, which have not yet been published.[20,21]

Infant Nutritional Standards

Acceptable growth is achieved through an adequate intake of energy, protein, carbohydrates, minerals, and vitamins. The Food and Nutrition Board of the National Research Council established recommended dietary allowances (RDAs) designed to meet the needs of most healthy infants. These general guidelines were last revised and published in 1989.[22] Currently, a new set of recommended nutrient intakes (Dietary Reference Intakes, DRIs) are being established that will replace the RDAs.[23] Table 20–1 reflects both the RDAs and the presently established DRIs. Table 20–2 contains the Food and Drug Administration (FDA) recommendations for nutrition for infants.

Energy requirements vary with age. Total energy expenditure is a combination of basal energy needs, the specific dynamic action of food (the energy required to digest food), and activity and growth. The infant's energy requirement is high in relation to body mass but declines over time. The accepted RDA for infants from birth to 6 months is 108 kcal/kg per day, whereas infants ages 6 to 12 months require a somewhat lower intake of 98 kcal/kg per day; however, some disagreement exists over direct measurements of energy expenditure.[22] One study of children ages 1.5 to 4.5 years showed direct measurements of total energy expenditure to be 10% to 12% less than the current recommendations.[24] This finding has been theorized to be related to a more sedentary lifestyle. No significant differences in energy requirements have been noted between boys and girls age 10 years or younger.

Components of a Healthful Infant Diet

Infants need the same dietary components as adults: fluids, carbohydrates, proteins, fats, and micronutrients. However, the proportions of these components differ in the infant diet.

Fluids

Water is a particularly important component of an infant's diet because water makes up a larger proportion of the infant's body composition than it does of the older person's. Water intake in the first 6 months of life is primarily derived from breast milk or formula. Both contain adequate amounts of water so that the normal, healthy infant should not need supplemental water. From ages 6 to 12 months, when solid foods are introduced, water intake remains high, because most infants' foods contain 60% to 70% or more water than that of children's or adults' foods.[25,26] Output is predominantly in renal excretion, evaporation from the skin and lungs, and, to a lesser extent, feces. Increases in water loss caused by diarrhea, fever, or unusually rapid breathing,

Table 20–1

Recommended Dietary Allowances (RDA) and Dietary Reference Intakes (DRI) of Nutrients for Full-Term Infants

	RDA/DRI	
Nutrient	**0–6 months**	**>6–12 Months**
Energy (kcal/kg/day)	108	98
Protein (g/kg/day)	2.2	1.6
Essential fatty acids		
Linoleic acid (% of kcal)[a]	2.7	2.7
Vitamins		
Vitamin A (mcg)[b]	375	375
Vitamin D (mcg)[c]	7.5/5	10/5
Vitamin E (mg)[d]	3	4
Vitamin K (mcg)	5	10
Vitamin C (mg)	30	35
Thiamine (mg)	0.3	0.4
Riboflavin (mg)	0.4	0.5
Vitamin B_6 (mg)	0.3	0.6
Vitamin B_{12} (mcg)	0.3	0.5
Niacin (mg)[e]	5	6
Folate (mcg)	25	35
Pantothenic acid (mg)[f]	2	3
Biotin (mcg)[f]	10	15
Minerals		
Calcium (mg)	400/210	600/210
Phosphorus (mg)	300/100	500/275
Magnesium (mg)	40/30	60/75
Iron (mg)	6	10
Iodine (mcg)	40	50
Zinc (mg)	5	5
Copper (mg)[e]	0.4–0.6	0.6–0.7
Manganese (mg)[f]	0.3–0.6	0.6–1
Fluoride (mg)[f]	0.1–0.5/0.01	0.2–1/0.5
Chromium (mcg)[f]	10–40	20–60
Selenium (mcg)	10	15
Molybdenum (mcg)[f]	15–30	20–40

[a] No specific recommendations for linoleic acid have been identified by the National Research Council, by the Food and Drug Administration, or by CON/AAP.

[b] Retinol equivalents (REs); 1 RE = 3.33 IU of vitamin A activity from retinol.

[c] Cholecalciferol; 10 mcg of cholecalciferol equals 400 IU of vitamin D.

[d] α-Tocopherol equivalents (α-TEs); 1 mg of d-α-tocopherol = 1 mg α-TE. The activity of α-tocopherol is 1.49 IU/mg.

[e] Niacin equivalents (NEs); 1 NE = 1 mg of niacin or 60 mg of dietary tryptophan.

[f] Estimated safe and adequate daily dietary intakes. Because little information exists on which to base allowances, some figures are provided as ranges of recommended intakes.

Source: References 22 and 23; adapted with permission.

Table 20-2

Nutritional Recommendations for Full-Term Infants (per 100 kcal)

Nutrient	FDA Regulations Minimum	FDA Regulations Maximum
Protein (g)	1.8	4.5
Fat		
(g)	3.3	6
(% calories)	30.0	—
Essential fatty acids		
Linoleic acid (g)	0.3	—
Vitamins		
Vitamin A (IU)	250	750
Vitamin D (IU)	40	100
Vitamin K (g)	4	—
Vitamin E (IU)	0.7	—
Vitamin C (mg)	40	—
B_1 (thiamine) (mcg)	40	—
B_2 (riboflavin) (mcg)	60	—
B_6 (pyridoxine) (mcg)	35	—
B_{12} (mcg)	0.15	—
Niacin (mcg)[a]	2.5	—
Folic acid (mcg)	4	—
Pantothenic acid (mcg)	300	—
Biotin (mcg)[b]	1.5	—
Choline (mg)[b]	7	—
Inositol (mg)	4	—
Minerals		
Calcium (mg)	60	—
Phosphorus (mg)	30	—
Magnesium (mg)	6	—
Iron (mg)	0.15	3
Iodine (mcg)	5.0	7.5
Zinc (mg)	0.5	—
Copper (mcg)	60	75
Manganese (mcg)	5	—
Sodium (mg)	20	60
Potassium (mg)	80	200
Chloride (mg)	55	150

[a] Includes nicotinic acid and niacinamide.

[b] Required only for infant formulas that are not milk-based.

Source: *Federal Register.* 1985;50:45106.

particularly in concert with decreased water intake, may result in significant dehydration and may be accompanied by an imbalance of electrolytes. Maintenance water or fluid needs in infancy are estimated to be approximately 100 mL/kg per day for the first 10 kg of body weight plus 50 mL/kg per day for each kilogram between 10 and 20 kg. Additional losses caused by conditions such as diarrhea, fever, and rapid breathing should be offset by fluid intake in excess of maintenance levels.

Carbohydrates

Although no RDA has been established for carbohydrates, under normal circumstances an infant can efficiently use 50% to 60% of total calories from a carbohydrate source.[27] A carbohydrate-free diet is not desirable because such a diet leads to metabolic modifications favoring fatty acid breakdown, dehydration, and tissue protein and cation loss. Fiber intake is of considerable interest because high-fiber diets have been associated with the prevention of diseases such as diverticular disease, colon cancer, and coronary heart disease. The Committee on Nutrition of the American Academy of Pediatrics (CON/AAP) favors adequate fiber intake to ensure regular stool frequency and has recommended a daily dietary fiber intake of 0.5 g/kg body weight in children ages 3 years and older.[27] Others have recommended a daily gram intake calculated using the equation age (years) plus 5.[28]

Lactose is the primary carbohydrate source in human milk and milk-based formulas. Acids and the enzyme lactase hydrolyze lactose into glucose and galactose. Disaccharide hydrolysis may be incomplete in a newborn. Because lactase activity develops late in fetal life, infants born during the seventh or eighth month of gestation may be unable to hydrolyze the same amount of lactose as full-term infants. Therefore, premature infants are relatively lactase deficient and thus are especially prone to lactose intolerance, which may be manifested by diarrhea, abdominal pain or distention, bloating, gas, and cramping.

Secondary lactase deficiency is a temporary reduction in intestinal lactase caused by gastroenteritis or malnutrition. Congenital lactase deficiency is a rare type of milk intolerance in infants that results from an inborn error of metabolism. Because of low levels of lactase in the GI tract, infants with congenital lactase deficiency and low-birth-weight (LBW) infants may be unable to metabolize the quantity of lactose found in breast milk or infant formulas. Formulas with nutrient sources other than cow milk may be used when lactose intolerance or hypersensitivity is suspected.

Protein and Amino Acids

The accepted average RDA for protein is 2.2 g/kg per day from birth to age 6 months and 1.6 g/kg per day from ages 6 months to l year.[22] Body protein increases by an average of 3.5 g per day in the first 4 months of life and by 3.1 g per day over the next 8 months, representing an overall change in body protein composition from 11% to 15%.[16]

Equally important as the overall protein intake is the amino acid composition of the protein. Amino acids can be classified as essential, nonessential, and conditionally essential. Eight amino acids (isoleucine, leucine, lysine, methionine, phenylalanine, threonine, tryptophan, and valine) are considered essential in adults because the body cannot synthesize them from precursors as it can nonessential amino acids. Conditionally essential amino acids (e.g., cysteine, taurine, tyrosine, and histidine) are nonessential but become essential because the synthesis process is impaired as a result of immaturity or the effects of disease on synthesis or interconversion. Impairment of synthesis may occur in preterm infants with immature enzyme systems.[22]

The National Research Council has accepted estimates of specific amino acid requirements from the World Health Organization and others (Table 20–3).[22] Despite similar amino acid densities and milk intakes, serum amino acid patterns in formula-fed infants tend to exceed those in infants fed human milk; however, the growth of formula-fed infants is normal.[29] Although the protein content of human milk adjusts to a growing infant's needs, the high protein needs of preterm infants are not completely met by early human milk.[30] Fortification produces reasonable plasma amino acid profiles and helps an infant meet expected intrauterine growth rates.[31–33]

Histidine is found in both human and cow milk in quantities larger than the estimated requirements. Synthesis of this amino acid becomes adequate by ages 2 to 3 months. Histidine deficiency results in poor nitrogen balance and growth. Supplemental tyrosine and cystine, as well as histidine, may be needed in the first weeks of life for the preterm infant.[22,34]

Taurine is an amino acid found in abundant quantities in breast milk.[34] It serves a major nutritional role as a protector of cell membranes by attenuating toxic substances (e.g., oxidants, secondary bile acids, and excess retinoids) and by acting as an osmoregulator.[35] Taurine is not an energy source nor is it used for protein synthesis. It is considered a conditionally essential nutrient. Taurine deficiency can result in retinal dysfunction, slow development of auditory brain stem–evoked response in preterm infants, and poor fat absorption in preterm infants and in children with cystic fibrosis. These conditions can be improved with taurine supplements. Although disagreement still exists as to the necessity of taurine supplements even in LBW infants, taurine is now added to many infant formulas to provide the same margin of physiologic safety that is provided by human milk.[36]

In evaluating the adequacy of an infant's protein intake, one must consider not only the absolute amount of protein ingested but also the growth rate of the child, the quantity of nonprotein calories and other nutrients necessary for protein synthesis, and the quality of the protein itself. Some authors have suggested that amino acid and protein requirements are more meaningful when expressed in terms of calories; therefore, requirements or supplementation levels may appear in gram per 100 kcal. In such cases, direct comparisons with RDAs expressed in gram per kilogram of body weight per day are not easily made.

Table 20–3

Estimated Amino Acid Requirements for Infants and Young Children (mg/kg/day)

Amino Acid	Infants (3–4 months old)	Children (~2 years old)
Histidine	28	—
Isoleucine	70	31
Leucine	161	73
Lysine	103	64
Methionine + cystine	58	27
Phenylalanine + tyrosine	125	69
Threonine	87	37
Tryptophan	17	12.5
Valine	93	38

Fat and Essential Fatty Acids

Fat is the most dense source of calories in the diet (9 kcal/g versus 4 kcal/g for protein and carbohydrates). It supplies approximately 40% to 50% of the energy intake of infants in developed countries.[16] Although concern exists in the adult population about dietary fat intake, and about the role of infant feeding practices and risk factors for obesity and disease in adulthood, the AAP recommends that children younger than 2 years not receive a fat-restricted diet because of the need for dietary fat in neurologic development.[37]

The diet must contain small amounts of linoleic acid, the polyunsaturated fatty acid (PUFA) that has been proven to be an essential nutrient. Linoleic acid and its derivatives, including arachidonic acid, enable optimum caloric intake and proper skin composition.[38] Linoleic acid deficiency manifests as increased metabolic rate, hair loss, drying and flaking of the skin, and impaired healing of wounds. Manifestations of essential fatty acid deficiency are generally delayed; however, rapid onset may occur in newborns with delayed provision of fat in their diets.[39] Linoleic acid represents the bulk of PUFAs in infant formulas. Generally, an intake of linoleic acid equal to 1% to 2% of total dietary calories is adequate to prevent biochemical and clinical evidence of deficiency; 4% to 5% is thought to be optimal.[40] The AAP recommends linoleic acid intakes of 300 mg/100 kcal, or approximately 3% of total calories.[40]

Micronutrients

RDAs for vitamins and minerals, including trace elements, are shown in Table 20–1. Precise needs are difficult to define and depend on energy, protein, and fat intakes and absorption. Infant formulas are generally supplemented with adequate amounts of vitamins and minerals to meet the needs of full-term infants.

For a discussion on vitamins and minerals, see Chapter 19, "Nutritional Deficiencies."

Nutritional Supplementation of the Infant Diet

No evidence exists that vitamin and mineral supplementation is necessary for formula-fed, full-term infants or for normal, breast-fed infants of well-nourished mothers.[1] Although the incidence of vitamin D deficiency rickets and iron deficiency appears relatively low in the United States, some segments of the population of term breast-fed infants may be at risk and may require supplementation.

Vitamin and mineral supplementation may be needed for preterm and LBW infants and for infants whose mothers are inadequately nourished. These infants and those with other nutritional deficiencies, malabsorptive and other chronic diseases, rare vitamin dependency conditions, inborn errors of vitamin or mineral metabolism, or deficiencies related to the intake of drugs will need vitamin and mineral supplementation directed by a physician.[41] Table 20–4 gives guidelines for supplementation.

Breast-Fed, Full-Term Infants

AAP recommends vitamin D supplementation (400 IU/day) of infants only for breast-fed infants whose mothers are vitamin D–deficient or when these infants are not exposed to adequate sunlight, because the condition of vitamin D–deficient rickets is uncommon in the United States.[1] Supplementation of vitamin D is recommended by some authors, however, for breast-fed infants as a protective measure against developing rickets.[42,43] A heightened concern has been expressed by practitioners who have treated infants with rickets who also have other risk factors for vitamin D deficiency such as increased birth order (3rd or greater), dark skin, cultural factors that minimize maternal skin exposure to sunlight, and delayed intake of dairy products in the infant or mother because of intolerance or other factors.[44–46] Mothers should be encouraged to maintain a balanced diet and to drink five to six 8-ounce glasses of milk a day while breastfeeding. If the mother cannot tolerate milk because of lactose intolerance, products that aid in lactose digestion (e.g., Lactaid, Dairy Aid, Lactogest, or Dairy Ease) or lactose-free milk are available. If she wishes not to drink milk, she should be encouraged to increase her vitamin D and calcium intake from other dietary sources or from supplements.

Vitamin A deficiency rarely occurs in breast-fed infants; therefore, vitamin A may be omitted from supplements designed to provide vitamin D for infants.

Vitamin B_{12} deficiency has been reported in breast-fed infants of strict vegetarian mothers.[47] This deficiency is also relatively rare in the United States. A malnourished nursing mother and her infant should receive multivitamin supplements containing vitamin B_{12} to prevent megaloblastic anemia.

The concentration of iron in human milk averages about 0.3 to 0.5 mg/L.[48,49] Iron is well absorbed from human milk (i.e., 50% of the iron is absorbed). Breast-fed infants rarely develop iron deficiency anemia before ages 4 to 6 months be-

Table 20–4

Guidelines for the Use of Vitamin and Mineral Supplements in Healthy Infants

	Multivitamin/ Multimineral	Vitamin D	Vitamin E[a]	Folate	Iron[b]
Full-term infants					
Breast-fed	0	±	0	0	±
Formula-fed	0	0	0	0	0
Preterm infants					
Breast-fed[c]	+	+	±	±	+
Formula-fed[c]	+	+	±	±	+
Older infants (>6 months)					
Normal	0	0	0	0	±
High-risk[d]	+	0	0	0	±

Key

+ means a supplement is usually indicated; ± means a supplement is possibly or sometimes indicated; 0 means a supplement is not usually indicated.

Not shown are vitamin K for newborn infants and fluoride in areas where there is insufficient fluoride in the water.

[a] Vitamin E should be in a form that is well absorbed by small, preterm infants. If this form of vitamin E is present in formulas, it need not be given separately to formula-fed infants. Infants fed breast milk are less susceptible to vitamin E deficiency.

[b] Iron-fortified formula and/or infant cereal is a more convenient and reliable source of iron than a supplement.

[c] Multivitamin supplements (plus added folate) are needed primarily when calorie intake is below approximately 300 kcal per day or when the infant weighs 2.5 kg; vitamin D should be supplied at least until age 6 months in breast-fed infants. Iron should be started by age 2 months.

[d] Multivitamin–mulitmineral preparations including iron are preferred to supplements containing iron alone.

Source: Adapted from *Pediatrics.* 1980;66:1017.

cause neonatal stores of iron are adequate. In a study supporting iron supplementation at age 4 months and beyond, the iron status in infants exclusively breast-fed for at least 9 months was found to be deficient (as reflected in a 20% higher incidence of anemia and a 28% higher incidence of inadequate iron stores) compared with that in formula-fed infants.[41] Consequently, in normal, breast-fed, full-term infants, after age 6 months, neonatal stores may be significantly depleted. Thus the addition of iron-enriched foods is suggested,[1] or an iron supplement (2 mg/kg per day of ferrous sulfate) may be desirable.

Cereals are generally the first nonmilk or formula food introduced into the breast-fed infant's diet. The bioavailability of the large particle, electrolytic iron powder used to fortify dry infant cereals has been shown to be substantially less than that of the ferrous sulfate iron used in milk- or soy-based formulas.[50] Additionally, cereals contain potent inhibitors of iron absorption and have been shown to be unreliable in preventing iron deficiency when infants received minimal iron from other sources.[51] Iron-fortified, wet-packed cereal and fruit combinations marketed in jars offer no exposure of the iron sulfate to oxygen until the jar is opened; therefore, oxidative rancidity is not a problem. Additionally, ascorbic acid–containing products or fruit juices containing ascorbic acid consumed along with cereals have been shown to enhance the iron absorption.[52] These products may be better sources of dietary iron supplementation than dry cereals alone.

Fluoride supplementation is currently not recommended in the infant from birth to age 6 months, and the recommended supplementation for children ages 6 months to 6 years has been decreased compared to previous recommendations because of an increased incidence of fluorosis.[53] Table 20–5 can be used to determine the proper fluoride supplementation for an infant, depending on the level of fluoride supplementation in the drinking water.

Formula-Fed, Full-Term Infants

Full-term infants who consume adequate amounts of a commercial milk-based formula that is iron-fortified do not need vitamin and mineral supplementation in the first 6 months of life.[54] An iron-fortified formula is preferred because of the concern over adequate iron stores for growing infants. Studies have shown that infants fed iron-fortified formulas do not demonstrate a difference in stool consistency, fussiness, colic, or regurgitation when compared with infants fed nonfortified formulas.[55,56]

Vitamin and mineral supplements are not needed for infants older than 6 months who receive a diet of formula, mixed feedings, and increased amounts of table food. A multivitamin with minerals may be needed, however, if the infant is at special nutritional risk. If a powdered or concentrated formula is used, fluoride supplements should be administered only if the community's drinking water contains less than 0.3 ppm of fluoride. Ready-to-use formulas are manufactured with defluoridated water and contain less than 0.3 ppm of fluoride. Therefore, if an infant fed ready-to-use formula does not drink water or juice or eat solid foods, the physician may recommend a fluoride supplement.

Table 20–5

Supplemental Fluoride Dosage Schedule (mg per day)

Age	Concentration of Fluoride in Drinking Water (ppm)[a]		
	<0.3	0.3–0.6	>0.6
Birth–6 months	0	0	0
6 months–3 years	0.25	0	0
3–6 years	0.50	0.25	0
6–16 years	1.00	0.50	0

[a] 2.2 mg sodium fluoride contains 1 mg fluoride.

Preterm Infants

Preterm infants, either breast-fed or formula-fed, need vitamin and mineral supplementation. Their nutrient needs are proportionately greater than those of full-term infants because of their more rapid growth rate, inability to ingest an adequate volume of formula or breast milk, and decreased intestinal absorption.[57,58] Until these infants can consume about 300 kcal per day or until they reach a body weight of 2.5 kg, a multivitamin supplement should be administered to provide the equivalent of the RDAs for full-term infants.

A multivitamin supplement should include vitamin E in a form well absorbed by preterm infants. Because of conflicting data from clinical studies, it may be prudent to monitor vitamin E serum concentrations and to maintain them at 1 to 3 mg/dL.[59]

Folic acid deficiency has been reported in preterm infants.[60] The instability of folic acid precludes its use in commercial liquid multivitamin and mineral preparations. Folate can be added to a multivitamin preparation to provide the RDA (Table 20–1). The shelf life of folate is 1 month, and the label should read "shake well."[57]

To minimize the possibility of hemolytic anemia in infants with insufficient vitamin E absorption, iron supplements should be withheld until the preterm infant is several weeks old. Iron is required at a dosage of 2 mg/kg per day starting by at least age 2 months, because iron is transferred from mother to fetus during the third trimester. Therefore, the iron stores of preterm infants may become depleted earlier than those of full-term infants. Iron-fortified formulas supply sufficient iron to prevent iron deficiency in preterm infants.[57]

Supplementation of calcium, phosphorus, and vitamin D in preterm infant formulas is necessary to ensure adequate bone mineralization and to prevent osteopenia and rickets.[57,58] The prevention of severe bone disease in preterm infants appears to depend both on high oral intakes of calcium and phosphorus and on the intake of at least 500 IU of vitamin D per day.[57,58] Therefore, breast-fed preterm infants should receive a special preterm infant formula that contains appropriate amounts of calcium, phosphorus, and vitamin D supplementation.[58] (See Chapter 19, "Nutritional Deficiencies.")

Infant Food Sources

Human milk and cow milk–based are the primary food sources for infants. Soy protein formulas and goat milk are alternative food sources.

Cow Milk

Cow milk is the nutrient source for milk-based infant formulas that are commercially prepared. Both human and cow milk are intricate liquids that contain more than 200 ingredients in the fat- and water-soluble fractions. Estimates of the concentrations of selected nutrients contained in pooled mature human milk and in cow milk are listed in Table 20–6.

Reduced-Fat Cow Milk

Reduced-fat milks, such as skim milk (0.1% fat), low-fat milk (1% fat), and 2% milk (2% fat), have been used to prevent obesity and atherosclerosis and to provide a "healthy diet."[61,62] However, when the low-fat diet recommended for adults is imposed on children younger than 2 years, it puts them at risk for failure to thrive.[61] CON/AAP does not recommend skim, 1%, or 2% milks during the first 12 months of life.[54] AAP's Statement on Cholesterol recommends that no restrictions should be placed on the fat and cholesterol content of the diet of infants from birth to age 2 years, a period of rapid growth and development and of high nutritional needs.[37]

Infants who receive a major percentage of their caloric intake from reduced-fat milks, such as skim, 1%, or 2% milk, may receive an exceedingly high protein intake and an inadequate intake of essential fatty acids. The maximum concentration of protein allowed in infant formulas is 4.5 g/100 kcal, but skim milk provides approximately 10 g of protein per 100 kcal and 2% milk provides nearly 7 g of protein per 100 kcal. Thus, a disadvantage of using reduced-fat milks as the only dietary source for infant nutrition is the unbalanced percentage of calories supplied from protein, fat, and carbohydrates.

It is important to recognize that, per unit volume, skim milk has a slightly higher PRSL than does whole cow milk (Table 20–7). The solute concentration is further increased by water loss during boiling.[54] Reduced-fat milks are not recommended for treating diarrhea because of the possibility of hypertonic dehydration.

Whole Cow Milk

The age at which it is appropriate to introduce unheated whole cow milk into an infant's diet is controversial. Because the concentration and bioavailability of iron in whole cow milk are low, whole cow milk has been associated with iron-

Table 20–6

Composition of Mature Human Milk and Cow Milk

Composition	Human Milk	Cow Milk
Water (mL/100 mL)	87.1	87.2
Energy (kcaL/100 mL)	69	66
Protein (g/100 mL)	1.05 ± 0.2	3.1–3.5
Casein (% protein)	40	80
Whey (% protein)	60	20
α-Lactalbumin (g/100 mL)	0.2–0.3	0.1
β-Lactoglobulin (g/100 mL)	—	0.4
Lactoferrin (g/100 mL)	0.1–0.3	trace
Secretory IgA (g/100 mL)	0.08–0.1	trace
Albumin (g/100 mL)	0.05	0.04
Fat (g/100 mL)	3.9 ± 0.4	3.8
Carbohydrate		
Lactose (g/100 mL)	7.2 ± 0.3	4.9
Electrolytes (per liter)		
Calcium (mg)	280 ± 26	1200
Phosphorus (mg)	140 ± 22	920–940
Calcium/phosphorus ratio	2:1	1.3:1
Sodium (mg)	180 ± 40	506
Potassium (mg)	525 ± 35	1570
Chloride (mg)	420 ± 60	1028–1060
Magnesium (mg)	35 ± 2	120
Sulfur (mg)	140	300
Minerals (per liter)		
Chromium (mcg)	50 ± 5	20
Manganese (mcg)	6 ± 2	20–40
Copper (mcg)	60	110
Zinc (mg)	0.5–1.4	3–5
Iodine (mcg)	110 ± 40	80
Selenium (mcg)	20 ± 5	5–50
Iron (mg)	0.3–0.5	0.5
Vitamins (per liter)		
Vitamin A (IU)	1898	1025
Thiamine (mcg)	150	370
Riboflavin (mcg)	380	1700
Niacin (mcg)	1700	900
Pyridoxine (mcg)	130	460
Pantothenate (mg)	2.6	3.6

Table 20–6

Composition of Mature Human Milk and Cow Milk (continued)

Composition	Human Milk	Cow Milk
Folic acid (mcg)	85	68
Vitamin B_{12} (mcg)	0.5	4
Vitamin C (mg)	43	17
Vitamin D (IU)	40	14
Vitamin E (mg)	2.3	0.4
Vitamin K (mcg)	2.1	17

Source: *Nutrition in Infancy and Childhood*. 5th ed. St. Louis: Times Mirror/Mosby College Publishing; 1993:90; Williams AF. *Textbook of Pediatric Nutrition*. 3rd ed. London: Churchill Livingstone; 1991:26–7; and Suskind RM, Lewinter-Suskind L. *Textbook of Pediatric Nutrition*. 2nd ed. New York: Raven Press; 1993:33–42.

Table 20–7

Potential Renal Solute Loads (PRSLs) of Selected Milks and Infant Formulas

	PRSL	
	mOsm/L	mOsm/100 kcal
Human milk	93	14
Milk-based formula	135	20
Soy-based formula	177	26
Whole cow milk	308	46
Skim cow milk	326	93
FDA upper limit for PRSL	277	41

Source: Adapted from Ziegler EE, Fomon SJ. Potential renal solute load of infant formulas. *J Nutr*. 1989;119(suppl):1785–8.

deficiency anemia.[54,63] In the past decade, convincing evidence has accumulated to indicate that iron deficiency impairs psychomotor development and cognitive function in infants.[64,65] This impairment has been observed even with relatively mild anemia. Through unknown mechanisms, whole cow milk can cause occult bleeding from the GI tract.[66] Milk-protein intolerance and/or allergy (estimated to affect 0.5% to 7.5% of the infant population in the first 2 years of life) poses another potential complication when using whole cow milk.[66,67]

More research is needed to establish a time frame for introducing whole cow milk. In 1983, CON/AAP reversed its previous recommendation concerning the introduction of whole cow milk and concluded, "If breast-feeding has been completely discontinued and infants are consuming one-third of their calories as supplemental foods consisting of a balanced mixture of cereal, vegetables, fruits, and other foods, whole milk [rather than infant formula] may be introduced."[66,68] When whole cow milk is fed with solid food, infants receive unnecessarily high intakes of protein and electrolytes, resulting in a high renal solute load.[69] Also, infants fed an infant formula for the first year of life are less likely to develop iron deficiency.[6] The current position of CON/AAP is that iron-fortified infant formula is the only acceptable alternative to breast milk. Whole cow milk and low-iron formulas are not recommended during the first year of life.[70,71]

Evaporated Milk

Evaporated milk is a sterile, convenient source of cow milk that has standardized concentrations of protein, fat, and carbohydrate. When ingested, evaporated milk produces a smaller, softer curd than that formed from boiled whole milk. Vitamin D is typically added to evaporated milk during processing, but evaporated milk formulas fail to meet recommendations for ascorbic acid, vitamin E for preterm infants, and essential fatty acids.[54,72,73]

Goat Milk

Goat milk is commercially available in powdered and evaporated forms. It contains primarily medium- and short-chain fatty acids and may be more easily digested than cow milk. Unfortified goat milk is deficient in folate and is low in iron and vitamin D. The evaporated form of Meyenberg goat milk is supplemented with vitamin D and folic acid. Powdered Meyenberg goat milk is supplemented with folic acid only and is recommended only for children older than 1 year. Because the powder formulation is not a complete formula for infants, the manufacturer recommends supplementation with vitamins.

Human Milk

Breast-feeding offers benefits other than nutrition. Besides the increased bonding between infants and their mothers, breast-feeding offers protection against infections such as GI illness and respiratory infections, allergies, and obesity. Studies have shown that breast-fed infants have a lower incidence of gastroenteritis, fewer episodes of diarrhea, and infrequent hospitalizations for GI illness.[2] Results of a study from the United Kingdom show a statistically significant reduction in GI illness in infants who were breast-fed for 13 or more weeks, regardless of the introduction of other supplements during this time, compared with infants who were entirely formula-fed.[74] Interestingly, this effect appears to be maintained beyond the period of breast-feeding and is associated with a decrease in the rate of hospital admissions.

Conflicting results have been reported regarding breast-feeding and a lower rate of respiratory infection. However, respiratory infections in breast-fed infants are likely to be less severe.[2] Overall, the advantages of breast-feeding in lessening respiratory tract infections are most notable in the first 6 months of life.[2] Protective effects of breast-feeding have been shown to decline in proportion to the degree of supplementation with formula or cow milk.

Although conflicting data have been reported regarding a protective effect of breast-feeding against acute otitis media (AOM), well-designed studies support the advantages of breast-feeding.[75] In a study in which more than 1000 infants were followed longitudinally, those exclusively breast-fed for at least 4 months developed AOM 50% as frequently as those who were not breast-fed at all, and they had 40% fewer episodes than those with supplemented breast-feeding before age 4 months.[76] No additional protective effect was seen against AOM in infants who were exclusively breast-fed for an additional 2 months. Differences in the incidence of recurrent AOM were also noted, with a cumulative recurrence rate of 10% for those exclusively breast-fed for longer than 6 months compared with 20% for those in other groups.

Conditions about which conflicting data exist concerning the effects of breast-feeding include sudden infant death syndrome, urinary tract infections, bacteremia and meningitis, allergic disease, obesity, anemia, and childhood cancer. Thus, many questions remain to be answered about the apparent protective effect of breast-feeding. What is the duration of protection after breast-feeding is discontinued? What influence does change in age have on the protective effect? How great is the interactive effect of social and demographic variables? How does the addition of solid foods to the diet of a breast-fed infant influence the protective effect? What consequence does partial formula-feeding have on the protective effect of breast-feeding? Better designed studies are needed to answer these questions and to document the protective effects of breast-feeding against a variety of infections.

Commercial Infant Formulas

In 1967, CON/AAP first published recommendations to standardize the nutrient composition of infant formulas.[77] The FDA adopted these recommendations in 1971, and AAP revised them in 1976. The FDA published rules in 1985 concerning the provision of nutrients in infant formulas.[78]

In 1978, two soy-based formulas were marketed that later were discovered to be deficient in chloride. Some children who received these formulas experienced a hypochloremic metabolic alkalosis, and some failed to grow appropriately. Follow-up studies have shown that these children may be at risk for learning disabilities and language deficits.[79,80] As a result, the U.S. Congress passed an amendment to the Federal Food, Drug, and Cosmetic Act (Infant Formula Act of 1980) that gave the FDA authority to establish quality control, to require adequate labeling, and to revise nutrient levels.[78,81]

Manufacturers of infant formulas must follow regulations and quality control measures to ensure that infant formulas contain appropriate amounts of nutrients. Suppliers of ingredients used in infant formulas must provide "needed ingredients within rigid tolerance limits of quality" and must comply with "good manufacturing practice."[15] Manufacturers may alter a formulation in response to changes in the availability of ingredients or modifications in recommended nutritional allowances, but such changes should not adversely affect the quality or consistency of the formula.[15] An accurate listing of the current ingredients and their quantities for a given formula may be obtained by directly communicating with the manufacturer.

Formula Properties

An infant formula must be free of pathogens, and its constituents must meet certain concentrations to ensure optimum nutrition.

Microbiologic Safety Guidelines of the Infant Formula Council (a voluntary, nonprofit trade association composed of companies that manufacture and market infant formulas) require liquid formulations to be free of all viable pathogens, their spores, and other organisms that may cause product degradation. To ensure that this requirement is met, manufacturers will usually sterilize liquid formulas using heat treatment and will incubate them while analyzing samples. Quality control measures help to ensure the production of a sterile product that is free of microbial effects as long as the container remains intact.[15] Manufacturers culture powdered formulas to ensure that coliforms and other pathogens are absent and that the level of other microorganisms is below the acceptable level set by government standards. The heating required during the final preparation of the infant formula (as indicated on label directions) destroys most microorganisms.[15] If microbiologic contamination occurs, the infant ingesting such a formula could develop diarrhea with subsequent fluid and electrolyte losses.

Physical Characteristics Infant formulas are emulsions of edible oils in aqueous solutions, but the separation of fat rarely occurs. When separation occurs, shaking the container can usually redisperse the fat. Redispersion may not happen if stabilizers are lacking or if the formula was stored beyond its shelf life. Liquid infant formulas may contain thickening agents, stabilizers, and emulsifiers to provide uniform consistency and to prolong stability.

Protein agglomeration may occur if storage time is excessive. This agglomeration may range from slight, grainy development through increased viscosity and formation of gels to eventual protein precipitation. Agglomeration and separation do not affect the safety or nutritional value of a formula; however, the appearance is a deterrent to its use.

Caloric Density The RDA for energy is 108 kcal/kg per day for infants from birth to age 6 months and 98 kcal/kg per day from ages 6 months to 1 year (see Table 20–6). A full-term infant should have no difficulty in consuming enough diluted formula (20 kcal/ounce or 67 kcal/100 mL) to meet these caloric needs, but a preterm or LBW (less than 2500 g) infant has a higher caloric need and may require as much as 130 kcal/kg per day. An infant recovering from illness or malnutrition will require more calories. Infant formulas with caloric densities significantly lower or higher than 67 kcal/100 mL are regarded as therapeutic formulas to be used for managing special clinical conditions and only under medical supervision.

Osmolarity and Osmolality The osmolarity of an infant formula may be expressed as the concentration of solute per unit of total volume of solution or as the number of milliosmoles of solute per liter of solution (mOsm/L). Osmolarity cannot be measured but must be calculated using the osmolality value for the solution in question.[82] The osmolarity of human milk is approximately 273 mOsm/L. CON/AAP recommends that formulas for normal infants have osmolarities no higher than 400 mOsm/L; formulas with higher osmolarities should have a warning statement on the label.[83] However, infant formulas with 67 kcal/100 mL or 80 kcal/100 mL that are routinely used to feed preterm infants have osmolalities less than or equal to 300 mOsm/kg and pose no apparent increased risk of GI mucosal injury.[84]

Osmolality may be expressed as the number of milliosmoles of solute per kilogram of solvent (mOsm/kg). "The osmolality of a formula is directly related to the concentration of molecular or ionic particles in a solution and is inversely proportional to the concentration of water in the formula."[85] The osmolality of human milk is approximately 290 mOsm/kg.[86] Osmolality is related to the carbohydrate and mineral content of the formula. For dilute solutions, little difference exists between osmolality and osmolarity. However, because infant formulas are relatively concentrated solutions, osmolarity may be approximately 80% of the osmolality.[85] Osmolality is the preferred term for reporting the osmotic activities of infant formulas because osmotic activity is a function of a solute–solvent relationship. Manufacturers report both osmolality and osmolarity.

The relationship between osmolality and caloric density is reasonably linear in formulas with caloric densities of 44 to 90 kcal/100 mL, which is the range of caloric concentrations usually fed to infants.[85] If the osmolality of a 67 kcal/100 mL formula is known, that of a formula with a caloric density between 44 and 90 kcal/100 mL can be calculated, assuming a direct proportion between osmolality and caloric density. The osmolality of a formula grows with increasing caloric content.

No meaningful difference exists in the osmolalities of the commonly used ready-to-use formulas that provide 67 kcal/100 mL. The osmolalities of reconstituted concentrated products when diluted to provide 67 kcal/100 mL are not considerably different from the osmolalities of corresponding ready-to-use products. Directions for diluting concentrated formulas must be followed exactly to prevent harmful hyperosmolar states, such as diarrhea and dehydration. Soy-protein formulas have lower osmolalities than milk-based formulas because of differences in carbohydrate sources. Whereas milk-based formulas usually contain lactose, soy-protein formulas contain sucrose or corn syrup solids.

Renal Solute Load Renal solute load is related to the protein, electrolyte, and mineral content of an infant formula. It represents the water soluble substances that must be removed by the kidneys. Table 20–7 lists PRSLs for various milks and infant formulas, and it provides a comparison with the FDA upper limits for PRSL for infant formulas.[14] Renal solute load is important because it determines the quantity of water that is excreted by the kidneys. Infants are less able to concentrate their urine than are older children and adults. Thus, feeding an infant a formula that is too concentrated may produce a hypertonic urine that may cause dehydration because of increased renal losses. Under normal conditions, infant formulas with 67 kcal/100 mL supply 1.5 mL of water per kilocalorie, an amount that provides adequate water for all losses, including urinary excretion. If an infant has a decreased water intake or an excessive loss, a diet that has a high renal solute load may stress the limited capacity of the infant's renal reabsorptive system.

Types, Uses, and Selection of Commercial Infant Formulas

Formulas for full-term infants are milk-based or milk-based with added whey protein (whey predominant). These formulas meet the minimum requirements for various nutrients per 100 kcal, as required by the FDA and deemed appropriate by CON/AAP. Other infant formulas are available for specific needs, but they should be used only on the advice of a physician. (See Table 20–8 for examples of commercially available infants' and children's formulas.)

Milk-Based Formulas A milk-based formula is prepared from nonfat cow milk, vegetable oils, and added carbohydrate (lactose). The added carbohydrate is necessary because the ratio of carbohydrate to protein in nonfat milk solids from cow milk is less than is desirable for infant formulas. Protein provides approximately 9% to 11% of calories and fat furnishes 48% to 50% of calories.[84] The most widely used vegetable oils are corn, coconut, safflower, sunflower, palm olein, and soy. Replacement of the butterfat with vegetable oils allows for better fat absorption. Vitamins and minerals are added in accordance with the guidelines established by the FDA. Milk-based formulas are available as iron-fortified (approximately 1.8 mg/100 kcal) or low-iron (approximately 0.2 to 0.7 mg/100 kcal) formulas. Similac is an example of a milk-based formula. Although Enfamil Lactofree and Similac Lactose Free are milk-based formulas, they differ from others in this group because they contain either corn syrup solids or corn syrup solids with sucrose rather than lactose as their carbohydrate source. Thus they can be used for infants with lactose intolerance.

Milk-Based Formulas with Added Whey Protein When whey is added in proper amounts to nonfat cow milk, the ratio of whey proteins to casein can be altered to approximate that of human milk. The ratio of 60% whey to 40% casein in human milk differs considerably from the ratio in cow milk, in which casein accounts for approximately 80% of the protein and whey for only 20%.[87] Minerals are removed from whey by electrodialysis or ion-exchange processes and then are re-added to the formula to approximate the mineral content of human milk. Formulas containing partially demineralized whey proteins are not nutritionally superior to milk-based formulas. The high nutritional quality and relatively low renal solute load of these formulas are assets in the therapeutic management of ill infants.

Table 20–8

Selected Infants' and Children's Formulas

Trade Name	Kcal[a] (per oz)	Protein (g/L)	Carbohydrate (g/L)	Fat (g/L)	Iron (mg/L)
Milk-Based Formulas					
Carnation Follow-Up Concentrate/Powder/ Ready-to-Feed	20	18	89.2	27.7	13
Enfamil Concentrate/Powder/Ready-to-Feed[a,b]	20	14.5	73	36	4.7
Enfamil 22 Nursette Bottle/Ready-to-Feed/Powder	22	21	79	39	13.3
Enfamil with Iron Concentrate/Powder/ Ready-to-Feed[b,c]	20	14.5	73	36	12.2
Similac Low Iron Concentrate/Powder/Ready-to-Feed	20	14	73	36.5	1.5
Similac with Iron Concentrate/Powder/Ready-to-Feed	20	14	73	36.5	12
Soy-Based Therapeutic Formulas					
Carnation Alsoy Concentrate/Powder/Ready-to-Feed	20	19	75	33.5	12.17
Enfamil Next Step Soy Concentrate[b]	20	20	68	36	12.2
Isomil Concentrate/Powder/Ready-to-Feed	20	16.6	69.6	36.9	12.2
Isomil DF Ready-to-Feed	20	18	68.3	36.9	12.2
Prosobee Concentrate/Powder/Ready-to-Feed[b,c]	20	17.3	73	37	12.2
RCF (Ross Carbohydrate Free) Concentrate	12 (diluted 1:1 with water, no carbohydrates added)	20	0.04	36	1.5
Other Therapeutic Formulas					
Carnation Good Start Concentrate/Powder/ Ready-to-Feed	20	16	74.4	34.5	10
Lofenalac Powder[b–d]	20	22	88	26	12.7
Nutramigen Concentrate/Powder/Ready-to-Feed[b–d]	20	19	74	34	12.2
Portagen Powder[b,d]	20	24	78	32	12.7
Pregestimil Powder/Nursette Bottle/Ready-to-Feed[b–d]	20	19	69	38	12.7
Similac PM 60/40 Powder	20	15	69	37.8	1.5
Formulas for Premature Infants					
Enfamil Premature Formula with Iron Nursette Bottle/ Ready-to-Feed[b,c]	20	20	75	35	12.2
Enfamil Premature Formula Nursette Bottle/ Ready-to-Feed[b,c]	24	24	90	41	14.6
Similac Special Care 24 with Iron Ready-to-Feed	24	18.3	71.7	36.7	12.2
Children's Formulas					
Kindercal Ready-to-Feed[b,d]	31.3	34	135	44	10.6
PediaSure Ready-to-Feed[d]	30	30	110	50.2	14
PediaSure with Fiber Ready-to-Feed[d]	30	30	114	50.2	14

[a] Unless noted otherwise, calorie content and other nutritional information pertain to ready-to-feed formula.

[b] Dye-free product.

[c] Sucrose-free product.

[d] Lactose-free product.

Therapeutic Formulas Therapeutic infant formulas are used on an individual basis for infants being treated by medical specialists for conditions that require dietary adjustment. Table 20–9 lists indications for using various therapeutic infant formulas; Table 20–10 lists formulas for infants who have a variety of metabolic disorders. Therapeutic formulas include soy-protein formulas, casein-based formulas, casein or whey hydrolysate–based formulas, low-sodium formulas, various formulas needed for specific medical problems, and formulas for LBW infants or for specific age groups.

Table 20–9

Indication for the Use of Therapeutic Infant Formulas

Problem	Suggested Formula	Comments
Allergy or sensitivity to cow milk protein or soy protein	Protein hydrolysate formula (e.g., Alimentum, Nutramigen, or Pregestimil)	Protein or allergy sensitivity
Biliary atresia	Portagen	Impaired digestion and absorption of long-chain fats
Carbohydrate intolerance	RCF, 3232A	Formulas are carbohydrate free, and a source of carbohydrate that the patient can tolerate can be added
Cardiac disease	Enfamil, Similac PM 60/40	Whey predominant, low electrolyte content
Celiac disease	Pregestimil or Nutramigen, followed by a soy formula and then a cow milk formula	Advance to more complete formulas as intestinal epithelium returns to normal
Constipation	Routine formula, increase sugar	Mild laxative effect
Cystic fibrosis	Portagen, Pregestimil	Impaired digestion and absorption of long-chain fats
Diarrhea		
Chronic nonspecific	Routine formula or soy formula	Appropriate distribution of calories; impaired digestion of intact protein, long-chain fats, and disaccharides
Intractable	Pregestimil, Alimentum	
Failure to thrive (e.g., when intestinal damage is suspected)	Pregestimil, Alimentum	Advance to more complete formulas as intestinal epithelium returns to normal
Gastroesophageal reflux	Routine formula	Thicken with cereal (1 tbsp/oz of formula); also try small, frequent feedings
Hepatitis		
Without liver failure	Routine formula	Impaired digestion and absorption of long-chain fats
With liver failure	Portagen	
Homocystinuria	Low methionine, Analog XMET	Low content of methionine
Lactose intolerance	Soy formula	Impaired digestion and use of lactose
Maple syrup urine disease	MSUD Diet Powder, Analog MSUD	Low content of leucine, isoleucine, and valine
Necrotizing enterocolitis (with resection)	Pregestimil (when oral feeding is resumed)	Impaired digestion
Phenylketonuria	Lofenalac, Analog XP	Low content of phenylalanine
Prematurity	Preterm infant formulas	Whey predominant, easily digestible sources of carbohydrate and fat; appropriate vitamin and mineral content
Renal insufficiency	Similac PM 60/40	Low phosphate content, low renal solute load

Source: Supplemental information extracted from Walker WA, Hendricks KM. *Manual of Pediatric Nutrition.* 2nd ed. Philadelphia: BC Decker; 1990:79.

Soy-Protein Formulas Soy-protein formulas contain methionine-fortified isolated soy protein.[54] Vegetable oils provide the fat content; corn syrup solids, corn maltodextrin, and/or sucrose supply the carbohydrate in these formulas. Vitamin K is added to provide a concentration of 8 to 11 mcg/100 kcal. Other vitamins, taurine, and carnitine (necessary for the optimal oxidation of fatty acids) are also added. Carnitine supplementation of soy-protein formulas is necessary because of carnitine's low concentrations in foods of plant origin compared with foods of animal origin.[89]

Food allergy occurs in infants because the immature digestive and metabolic processes may not be completely effective in converting dietary proteins into nonallergenic amino acids. The incidence of cow milk allergy in the first 2 years of life is estimated to be 0.5% to 7.5%.[90] The diagnosis of cow milk allergy is defined as symptomatology involving the respiratory tract, skin, or GI tract that disappears when cow milk is removed from the diet and reappears on two separate challenges when cow milk is given during a symptom-free period. Rechallenge must be done with caution.[91]

Soy-protein formulas are promoted for managing an allergy to milk or for infants suspected of having a milk allergy. However, CON/AAP recommends using protein hydrolysate formulas rather than soy-protein formulas for infants with documented clinical allergy to cow milk, soy protein, or both.[6,15,89] This recommendation is based on the concern

Table 20-10

Metabolic Formulas

Disease	Product
Glutaric aciduria type I	Glutarex-1
Glycogen storage disease type III, IV, V	ProVeMin
	RCF
Histidinemia	HIST 1
	80056-Protein Free Diet Powder
Homocystinuria	3200K-Low Methionine Diet Powder
	Hominex-1
	HOM 1
Hypercalcemia	Calciol XD
Hyperlysinemia	LYS 1
	80056-Protein Free Diet Powder
Hypermethioninemia	Hominex-1
Isovaleric acidemia	I-Valex-1
Maple syrup urine disease	MSUD Diet Powder
	MSUD 1
	Ketonex
Methylmalonic acidemia	80056-Protein Free Diet Powder
	Propimex-1
Organic acidemia	OS1
Phenylketonuria	Lofenalac
	Phenex-1
	PKU1
Propionic acidemia	80056-Protein Free Diet Powder
	Propimex-1
Tyrosinemia	3200AB-Low Phe/Tyr Diet Powder
	Tyromex-1
	TYR1
Urea cycle disorders	Cyclinex-1
	UCD1
	80056-Protein Free Diet Powder

Source: Reference 88 and *Ross Laboratories Product Handbook*. Columbus, OH: Ross Laboratories; 1992.

that infants with severe allergy to cow milk—as evidenced by severe diarrhea, vomiting, laryngeal edema, urticaria, or wheezing—have intestinal mucosal damage that is sufficient to expose them to higher concentrations of foreign protein in soy-protein formulas.[92,93] However, most infants suspected of having adverse reactions to milk-based formulas have not experienced life-threatening manifestations. These infants appear to tolerate soy-protein formulas, which are less expensive and better tasting and which have been studied more extensively than protein hydrolysate formulas.[6]

Some concerns regarding soy formulas include their high levels of protein and manganese. Absorption of manganese is enhanced in children who are iron deficient. In addition, the phytate content of soy formulas may have a negative effect on vitamin and mineral bioavailability.[94] However, on the positive side, exposure to phytoestrogens early in life may have long-term health benefits for hormone-dependent diseases.[95] More studies are needed in this area.

The soy-protein formulas available are Isomil, ProSobee, and Carnation Alsoy.[6] These formulas differ in amounts of ingredients, source of carbohydrates, and constituents of the fat source. The fat sources in Alsoy are palm olein, soy, coconut, and high-oleic safflower oils; Isomil contains high-oleic safflower, coconut, and soy oils; and ProSobee contains palm olein, soy, coconut, and high-oleic sunflower oils.

The carbohydrate source is an important factor in product selection. Isomil contains corn syrup solids and sucrose; Alsoy contains corn maltodextrin and sucrose; ProSobee contains only corn syrup solids.

Some infants with gastroenteritis develop intolerance to lactose and sucrose because of secondary lactase and sucrase deficiency. ProSobee can be used in this situation.

Soy-protein formulas are lactose free and, therefore, can be used for infants with primary lactase deficiency (e.g., galactosemia) and for those with secondary lactose intolerance resulting from enteric infection or other causes of mucosal damage.[54] Resumption of a cow milk formula is generally possible 2 to 4 weeks after cessation of diarrhea.[96] Soy-protein formulas also provide an alternative nutritional source for infants whose parents are vegetarians and do not wish to use animal protein–based formulas.

RCF (Ross Carbohydrate Free) soy-protein formula does not contain a carbohydrate source. This formula may be used in the dietary management of infants who are unable to tolerate the type or amount of carbohydrates in cow milk or other infant formulas. A physician may select a carbohydrate source (sucrose, dextrose, fructose, or glucose polymers) that can be added before feeding. RCF is for use only under medical supervision.

Isomil DF is a specific formula to manage diarrhea; it contains added dietary fiber from soy.

Infants with a family history of atopy but who have not shown clinical manifestations of allergy should drink a soy-protein formula only with caution.[89] These infants should be monitored closely for allergy to soy protein.

Soy-protein formulas should not be used for the routine feeding of preterm and LBW infants. In addition, soy-protein formulas are not recommended for infants with cystic fibrosis because these children do not use soy protein adequately, will lose substantial amounts of nitrogen in their stools, and may develop hypoproteinemia or even anasarca (generalized infiltration of edema fluid into subcutaneous connective tissue). Formula-fed infants with cystic fibrosis do well nutritionally when given an easily digested formula that contains elemental protein and medium-chain triglycerides (e.g., a casein hydrolysate–based formula). However, recent studies have shown they do equally well on regular milk-based formula.[97]

Prethickened Milk-Based Formulas Enfamil AR was developed for babies with gastroesophageal reflux. This iron-fortified formula contains a carbohydrate blend of 57% lactose, 30% rice starch, and 13% maltodextrin, as well as a high amylopectin rice starch for thickening. Enfamil AR has a normal consistency until ingested. After ingestion, the formula thickens to a viscosity ten times that of regular formula when it comes in contact with the acidic environment in the infant's stomach.

Casein Hydrolysate–Based Formulas Casein hydrolysate–based formulas are effective to nutritionally manage infants with a variety of severe GI abnormalities in which intolerance to enteral feeding and the malabsorption of standard forms of protein, fat, and carbohydrate are common. Indications for use include severe or intractable diarrhea, severe food allergies, sensitivity to intact protein, disaccharidase deficiency, intestinal resection, dysfunctional malabsorption, steatorrhea, cystic fibrosis, protein-calorie malabsorption, and severe protein-calorie malnutrition. Such formulas are also indicated during a transition from parenteral feeding to a normal diet whereby lack of enteral stimulation while receiving parenteral nutrition resulted in decreased digestive enzyme activity and nutrient absorptive area.

Use of these formulas for allergy prophylaxis remains controversial. Some studies indicate that either prolonged breastfeeding or extended use of hypoallergenic formulas along with delayed introduction of solids will help prevent allergic disease in infancy, but other studies challenge these findings.[98] To date, the effectiveness of dietary and environmental regimens in preventing allergic disease has not been conclusively proven in prospective studies. Infants with documented symptoms of clinical allergies to cow milk may benefit from a protein hydrolysate formula because approximately 15% to 50% of these infants also react to soy protein.[99]

Few data appear to support an association between colic and infant formula ingestion.[100] In selected situations, improvement has occurred when cow milk or soy protein was eliminated and a hydrolysate formula was introduced. For this reason, some experts have suggested decreasing cow milk protein, soy protein, or both in the diets of infants with moderate-to-severe colic.[101] However, in the vast majority of infants, symptoms of colic persisted after formula changes. In cases in which improvement was noted, it was difficult to attribute the improvement to a formula change.[100,101] Currently, no evidence exists to support the use of hydrolysate formulas for treating colic, restlessness, or irritability.[98] These symptoms are common in infants, but they rarely occur as a result of an immune-mediated reaction to cow milk protein.

Extensively hydrolyzed casein protein makes formulas less palatable. However, infants usually accept the feedings satisfactorily. If the formula is rejected when first offered, it may be tried again after a few hours. These products are designed to provide a sole source of nutrition for infants up to ages 4 to 6 months and to provide a primary source of nutrition through age 12 months when indicated. Extended use of hydrolysate formulas as a sole source of nutrition in children older than 6 months requires physician monitoring on a case-by-case basis.[88] Pregestimil, Nutramigen, Alimentum, and 3232A are formulas with enzymatic hydrolysates of casein as the protein source. They contain nonantigenic polypeptides with a molecular weight less than 1200 daltons;[98] therefore, they can be fed to infants who are sensitive to intact milk protein or other foods. These formulas differ from other formulas in that α-amino nitrogen is supplied by enzymatically hydrolyzed, charcoal-treated casein rather than by whole protein. Casein hydrolysate formulas are supplemented with three amino acids— L-cysteine, L-tyrosine, and L-tryptophan (Alimentum also contains L-methionine)—because the concentrations of these amino acids are reduced during charcoal treatment.

The carbohydrate sources in these formulas vary. Nutramigen contains corn syrup solids and modified corn starch; Pregestimil contains corn syrup solids, modified corn starch, and dextrose; Alimentum contains sucrose and modified tapioca starch; and 3232A contains tapioca starch as a stabilizer and no other source of carbohydrate.

Glucose polymers in corn syrup solids or modified corn starch are particularly useful in infants who have malabsorption disorders and who are frequently intolerant to lactose, sucrose, and glucose. Glucose polymers are more easily digested and tolerated by infants whose capacity to handle lactose and sucrose may be impaired.[12,87] In addition, glucose polymers are a low-osmolar form of carbohydrate and contribute little to the total osmolar load. This low-osmolar form is an advantage in infants who have intestinal disorders and who cannot tolerate the osmolar load of disaccharide- or glucose-containing elemental diets.

Medium-chain triglycerides and corn oil are the fat sources found in 3232A. Pregestimil contains the same types of fat but also contains soy and high-oleic safflower or sunflower oil. Nutramigen contains palm olein, soy, coconut, and high-oleic sunflower oils; Alimentum contains safflower and soy oil (sources of linoleic acid) in addition to medium-chain triglycerides. These triglycerides do not require emulsification with bile and are more easily hydrolyzed than long-chain fats. Shorter-chain fatty acids and medium-chain triglycerides are directly absorbed into the portal system. In addition, medium-chain triglycerides enhance the absorption of long-chain triglycerides. Formulas in which at least 40% of the fat consists of medium-chain triglycerides have been shown to relieve steatorrhea, to promote weight gain, and to improve calcium absorption in LBW infants.[102–104] Formulas in which at least 80% of the fat consists of medium-chain triglycerides improve the absorption of calcium and magnesium.[87,103,104] Diarrhea is a possible adverse effect of medium-chain triglyceride malabsorption caused by overfeeding or intestinal mucosal disease.[87]

Pregestimil is an effective nutritional source for infants with massive bowel resection (short-bowel syndrome), severe diarrhea, protein-calorie malnutrition, milk and soy-protein intolerance, transition from intravenous parenteral nutrition, GI immaturity, or cystic fibrosis. Pregestimil is also effective in the intractable diarrhea syndrome of infancy. Pregestimil should not be used routinely as a nutrient source for highly stressed LBW infants because of the increased risk of GI complications.[88]

Nutramigen is nutritionally effective for infants with severe diarrhea or GI disturbances and for infants who are allergic or intolerant to intact proteins of cow milk and other foods. In cases of galactosemia, which is a relatively rare disorder resulting from a deficiency of galactose-*l*-phosphate uridyltransferase or galactokinase, it is necessary to eliminate dietary lactose so that the body may convert glucose to the amount of galactose it requires. Infants with galactosemia may be fed formulas without lactose or sucrose (Nutramigen, Pregestimil, or ProSobee).

Alimentum is composed of hydrolyzed casein supplemented with free amino acids and a blend of medium- and long-chain triglycerides. The addition of long-chain triglycerides improves the palatability but increases the allergenic potential for infants with cow milk allergy.[105] Alimentum contains two carbohydrates (sucrose and modified tapioca starch) in lower concentrations than are found in other hydrolysate formulas. These carbohydrates are digested and absorbed by separate mechanisms (principally glucoamylase and sucrase-α-dextrinase). This formula can be used for infants with protein sensitivity, pancreatic insufficiency (e.g., caused by cystic fibrosis), or intractable diarrhea.

The fat source in 3232A, which is a monosaccharide- and disaccharide-free formula base, is 87% medium-chain triglycerides and 13% corn oil. Tapioca starch is used as a stabilizer and is the only carbohydrate in the formula base. The physician selects the carbohydrate source (e.g., sucrose, dextrose, fructose, or glucose polymers). The formula base is iron fortified and contains all essential vitamins and minerals. It can be used for infants with disaccharidase deficiencies, impaired glucose transport, or intractable diarrhea.

Amino Acid–Based Formula Occasionally, some infants are intolerant to even hydrolyzed casein, and they require an amino acid–containing formula.[12] Neocate Powder contains 100% free amino acids, as well as 35% medium-chain and 65% long-chain triglycerides. Carbohydrate sources are maltodextrin, sucrose, and corn syrup solids. Neocate is available in orange or pineapple flavors.[12] EleCare is another product with free amino acids and medium- and long-chain triglycerides. The carbohydrate source is corn syrup solids. Both products provide 1 kcal/mL.

Sodium Caseinate Formula Portagen is a sodium caseinate formula. It contains corn syrup solids and sucrose as its carbohydrate sources. Medium-chain triglycerides account for 87% of its fat. It also contains higher concentrations of both lipid- and water-soluble vitamins than are found in casein hydrolysate formulas. Higher concentrations of medium-chain triglycerides and vitamins in Portagen compensate for their impaired digestion or absorption from conventional foods. Portagen has been effective in feeding infants with pancreatic insufficiency (e.g., caused by cystic fibrosis), bile acid deficiency, intestinal resection, lymphatic anomalies, and celiac disease. It can be used on a physician's recommendation as the sole dietary source for both infants and older children or as a beverage to be consumed with each meal.

Whey Hydrolysate–Based Formulas Casein hydrolysate formulas have been used for many years for infants with defects in protein digestion and with adverse reactions to intact cow milk protein. Recently, heat-treated whey protein has been used as the protein source in an infant formula (Carnation Good Start) for similar purposes. Enzymatic hydrolysates of whey contain some peptides with molecular weights greater than 2000; these peptides can increase the antigenicity of the product.[98] Anaphylactic-type reactions have been reported in patients who have severe milk allergy and who received hydrolysate formulas.[105] Therefore, whey hydrolysate–based formulas should not be used in infants with a documented immunoglobulin E (IgE)–mediated allergy to cow milk protein.[90] The effectiveness of whey hydrolysate formula in infants who have GI intolerance to cow milk but are not allergic to it suggests that whey hydrolysate formula may be an acceptable alternative to milk-based and soy-protein formulas. This product is promoted as having a pleasant taste, smell, and appearance. It may be better accepted than casein-hydrolysate formulas, which mothers and infants find noticeably different from milk-based and soy-protein formulas in appearance and taste.

Metabolic Formulas Infants with inherited metabolic disorders require specific formulas tailored to their particular conditions. Table 20–10 lists various metabolic diseases and formulas available to treat them.

Low-Birth-Weight and Preterm Formulas Because of their increased caloric needs and decreased ability to consume an adequate volume of formula, LBW infants (weight less than 2500 g) and preterm infants (gestational age less than 38 weeks, but especially less than 34 weeks) may need formulas that offer a higher caloric concentration for growth. For very low-birth-weight (VLBW; weight less than 1500 g) infants, human milk is insufficient in protein, phosphorus, and calcium.[106] The nutritional goal for preterm infants is to achieve postnatal growth that approximates the in utero growth of a normal fetus at the same postconceptional age.

No commercially available formula is completely satisfactory for LBW or VLBW infants; however, improvements in special formulas permit individualization of dietary regimens for these infants. Examples of special formulas that may be beneficial are Enfamil Premature Formula, Similac Special Care, and Similac PM 60/40. These formulas share common features, such as whey-predominant proteins, carbohydrate mixtures of lactose and corn syrup solids, and fat mixtures containing combinations of medium- and long-chain triglycerides. They may differ in electrolyte, vitamin, mineral, and caloric content. Each formula has been shown to be associated with adequate growth and metabolic stability in preterm infants. An isotonic osmolality (approximately

Case Study 20–1

Patient Complaint/History

A mother presents to the pharmacist with Jay, her 2-month-old infant son who has a 2-day history of frequent spitting up; irritability; and frequent loose, watery stools. The mother is purchasing acetaminophen for the infant's mild fever. She asks for advice on changing infant formulas because Jay is "not tolerating his formula."

In discussing the infant's symptomatology, the pharmacist determines that the infant weighs 13 pounds and that the mother administers saline nose drops and uses a nasal aspirator before the infant's feedings if he has mild-to-moderate congestion. The family has no history of food allergy or formula intolerance.

Clinical Considerations/Strategies

Readers can use the following considerations/strategies to determine the appropriate approach to this complaint:

- Determine additional questions the pharmacist should ask to give the mother appropriate advice; determine why these questions are relevant to the case.
- If the infant's pediatrician thinks the symptoms are related to a sequelae of a self-limiting viral gastroenteritis, determine strategies to consider in resuming formula feedings after resolution of the symptoms with clear liquids appropriate for the infant's age (e.g., Pedialyte, an oral electrolyte solution).
- If specialized strategies are used in resuming formula feedings, determine at what point to make the transition to the infant's usual formula.

Patient Education/Counseling

Readers can use the following strategies to develop a patient education/counseling plan that will help ensure optimal outcomes:

- Instruct the mother on techniques for preparing a powder formulation of the infant's usual formula.
- Explain the precautions for preparing powder formulations.

300 mOsm/kg of water) is maintained at a dilution of 24 kcal/ounce or 80 kcal/100 mL.[84]

Calcium and phosphorus are crucial to the development and maintenance of the human skeleton. In addition, phosphorus is an integral component of many biochemical reactions. Calcium requirements are affected by protein and phosphorus intake because of these nutrients' interactions with the renal tubular reabsorption of calcium. The recommended ratio of calcium to phosphorus is 1.3:1 for infants between birth and age 6 months and 1.2:1 for infants older than 6 months. A high phosphate intake has been associated with hypocalcemic tetany.[107,108]

Formulas designed for full-term infants are deficient in calcium and phosphorus relative to the needs of LBW or preterm infants. For these infants, additional calcium and phosphorus in special infant formulas are necessary for normal bone growth and mineralization; breast milk may also need such supplementation.[58]

Preterm and LBW infants are especially susceptible to iron deficiency anemia because they have lower iron stores. Without supplemental iron, body stores of iron in such infants will be depleted by age 2 months, in contrast to depletion at ages 4 to 6 months in full-term infants.[22] Therefore, CON/AAP recommends supplementation of elemental iron at 2 mg/kg per day of iron for infants older than 2 months.[22] Iron supplementation before age 2 months must be accompanied by ample vitamin E and PUFA additions to the diet to reduce the possibility of hemolytic anemia from vitamin E deficiency. A formula without iron is preferable for VLBW infants in the first 2 to 4 postnatal weeks to prevent decreased vitamin E serum concentrations.[109]

Nutrient-enriched postdischarge formulas are designed specifically to provide for continued catch-up growth in premature infants following hospital discharge. Similac Neosure and Enfamil 22 (both milk-based formulas) have more calories (22 kcal/ounce), protein, vitamins, and minerals than standard formulas but still less than in preterm formulas. They also contain medium-chain triglycerides.

Human Milk Fortifiers Whether human milk provides optimal nutrition for VLBW infants is a controversial issue. Mothers who deliver preterm produce milk that is higher in protein, sodium, potassium, and possibly other nutrients than the milk of mothers who deliver at term. However, it is thought that these nutrients gradually decline to levels found in mature milk at 4 to 8 weeks postdelivery.

Most of the mineral content for an infant's development is delivered through the placenta during the last 2 months of gestation. During the third trimester, the fetus receives 125 to 150 mg per day of calcium and 65 to 80 mg per day of phosphorus, which are primarily deposited in bone. Human milk, whether preterm or mature, cannot supply the amount of calcium and phosphorus needed to prevent osteopenia of prematurity.[110]

Commercial products have been developed to enhance the nutrient content of human milk. Enfamil Human Milk Fortifier is a powder that can add nutrients to human milk without displacing volume, thereby allowing for a higher intake of human milk. Similac Natural Care is a liquid that may be given alternately with human milk or mixed in various ratios with human milk. Both products are made from cow milk with a whey-to-casein ratio of 60:40 and a carbohydrate mixture of lactose and corn syrup solids. Enfamil Human Milk Fortifier contains little fat, and Similac Natural Care contains a mixture of medium- and long-chain triglycerides. Studies support adequate weight gain and nutrient retention in infants when either human milk with fortifier or preterm commercial formulas are ingested.[110–112]

Concentrated Formulas A child with special nutritional needs that exceed normal requirements may be given concentrated formula under medical supervision. Such ready-to-use formulas made from cow milk are available in concentrations of 24 kcal/ounce, and some are available in concentrations of 27 kcal/ounce. Various concentrations can be prepared from liquid concentrates or powdered products by varying the amount of water added (Tables 20–11 and 20–12). When concentrated formulas are used, the resulting increase in protein and electrolytes and the decrease in fluid require careful monitoring of the infant's fluid intake and output, weight, serum electrolytes, blood urea nitrogen, and urine-specific gravity and osmolality.[96]

Modular components are available as an alternative to formula concentration. Carbohydrates can be added in liquid or powdered form. Protein powder is available, but it should be used with caution because its use may increase the renal solute load. Fat may be added as medium-chain triglycerides (MCT Oil) for infants with fat malabsorption or intolerance. Microlipid, which is made from safflower oil, is also available as an emulsion that mixes well with formula.

Table 20–11

Dilution of Concentrated Liquid Infant Formulas[a]

Desired Caloric Concentration (kcal/oz)	Amount of Liquid Formula Concentrate (oz)	Amount of Water to Add (oz)
10	1	3
20	1	1
24	3	2
26–27	3	1.5
28–29	5	2

[a] Commercial concentrates of infant formula containing 40 kcal per fluid ounce before dilution with water.

Source: Adapted from Walker WA, Hendricks KM. *Manual of Pediatric Nutrition*. 2nd ed. St. Louis: Mosby; 1990:86.

Table 20–12

Dilution of Concentrated Powdered Infant Formulas[a]

Desired Caloric Concentration (kcal/oz)	Amount of Powdered Formula Concentrate (tbsp)[b]	Amount of Water to Add (oz)
10	1	4
20	1	2
24	3	5
28	7	10

[a] Powdered infant formulas that contain 40 kcal per level, packed tablespoonful before dilution. Because the powder displaces water and makes the volume larger and the formula more dilute, water should be added to the powder to equal the volume expected if a large volume of formula is to be prepared.

[b] 1 tbsp = 1 scoop.

Source: Adapted from Walker WA, Hendricks KM. *Manual of Pediatric Nutrition*. 2nd ed. St. Louis: Mosby; 1990:86.

Follow-up Formulas "Follow-up" or "follow-on" formulas such as Enfamil Next Step, Carnation Follow Up, and Carnation Follow Up Soy are designed for infants ages 4 to 12 months. CON/AAP, however, has stated that these formulas offer no nutritional advantage. Standard formulas are appropriate for infants up to age 12 months.[12,113]

Formula for Children Ages 1 to 10 Years PediaSure, PediaSure with Fiber, Kindercal, Nutren Jr., and Nutren Jr. with Fiber are nutritionally complete, isotonic, lactose-free enteral formulas that are designed for young children who cannot tolerate a normal diet or eat solid food. The formulas have a pleasant taste and can be used as supplements to increase caloric intake. They contain adequate amounts of calcium, phosphorus, iron, and vitamin D for this age group; the amounts contained in adult nutritional enteral products are typically inadequate for children ages 1 to 10 years.

Several therapeutic formulas have also been developed for this age group. Peptamen Junior, a peptide-based elemental formula, and Vivonex Pediatric and Neocate One+, both amino acid–based elemental formulas, are now available.

Potential Problems with Infant Formulas

As with any food, GI problems, especially diarrhea, can occur with use of infant formulas. Tooth decay and nutritional deficiencies are other potential problems.

Diarrhea Infants are particularly susceptible to dehydration because of their high metabolic rate and their ratio of surface area to weight and height. Fluid volume depletion by diarrhea may quickly (within 24 hours) produce severe dehydration with fluid and electrolyte imbalances, shock, and possible death. A common cause of diarrhea is the improper dilution of a concentrated liquid or powdered formula.

If diarrhea is a problem, the pharmacist should ascertain the severity and duration of the diarrhea, frequency of stools, and method of preparing the infant formula. If the diarrhea is serious (many more stools per day than normal) or has continued for 48 hours or more, or if the infant is clinically ill (with fever, lethargy, anorexia, irritability, dry mucous membranes, decreased urine output, or weight loss), the infant should be referred to a physician. (See Chapter 13, "Diarrhea.")

Mild diarrhea of short duration may resolve without medical measures, but the infant should be observed closely. Although improper digestion of the infant's formula may initiate diarrhea, continuing the formula while diarrhea persists may yield only marginal nutrient absorption. Temporarily (24 hours) discontinuing usual dietary intake may be helpful. Oral electrolyte replacement solutions (e.g., Pedialyte) may be used cautiously for short-term management of fluid and electrolyte loss in mild-to-moderate dehydration. However, these solutions should not be used when dehydration is severe or when persistent vomiting or diarrhea inhibits retention, thus requiring parenteral rehydration.[114] Similarly, these solutions are not intended to be used to provide adequate nutrition. A solution such as Pedialyte should not replace infant formula for the baby after diarrhea has ceased. A nutritionally adequate formula should be resumed under a physician's direction. (See Chapter 13, "Diarrhea.")

There are various recommendations for resuming formula feedings. Formula may be resumed at half strength for 24 hours and then increased to full strength over a 48-hour period. If diarrhea resumes when the formula is reintroduced, a lactose-free formula (cow milk or soy protein based) may be used at half strength for 24 hours or may be resumed at full strength. Then full-strength lactose-free formula may be used for 1 to 3 weeks (depending on the severity of the diarrhea). Finally, a milk-based formula may be resumed.[11]

Other Gastrointestinal Problems Adverse effects of formula on an infant's GI tract range from mechanical obstruction (inspissated milk curds), diarrhea, and dehydration from a hyperosmolar formula to hypersensitivity from specific milk protein. Intolerance to cow milk is associated most often with an inability to digest lactose or milk proteins. It is estimated that approximately 15% of infants in the United States are fed soy-protein formulas because of concerns about cow milk allergy or sensitivity.[6]

Hyperosmolar formulas may adversely affect LBW infants during the early neonatal period and may be a potential cause of necrotizing enterocolitis. Appropriately prepared formulas for LBW infants (20 to 24 kcal/ounce) are isotonic, with osmolalities less than or equal to 300 mOsm/kg; other infant formulas in concentrations of 20 to 24 kcal/ounce have osmolalities less than or equal to 400 mOsm/kg.

Tooth Decay Baby bottle tooth decay can occur in children who are bottle-feed beyond the typical weaning period. It is especially prevalent in children who sleep with their bottles after age 1 year or are allowed to sip a bottle frequently during the day. Caries are seen in children younger than 2 years and may involve the maxillary incisors, maxillary and mandibular first molars, or maxillary and mandibular canines. Restorative dentistry is often required and may be quite extensive, leading to the potential for difficulty in speech mastery. Methods for prevention once teeth start to erupt include substituting plain water for carbohydrate-containing formula or other drinks until weaned from the bottle during sleep, ensuring adequate fluoride intake, cleaning the baby's mouth once daily, and weaning from breast or bottle at ages 10 to 12 months.[115] Sleeping with a bottle should be actively discouraged.

Nutritional Deficiencies Generally, infant formulas have proven to be nutritionally adequate and safe. A number of past nutritional deficiencies associated with infant formulas have been corrected with appropriate supplementation procedures and technological advances in processing infant formulas. Examples of deficiencies that have occurred include the following:

- Vitamin K deficiency in infants fed certain formulas that are soy-based or are not milk-based.[116,117]
- Vitamin E deficiency and hemolytic anemia in LBW infants who received iron-fortified formulas with high concentrations of PUFAs.[57]
- Thiamine deficiency in infants fed soy-protein formulas low in thiamine.[118]
- Metabolic alkalosis in infants fed soy-protein formulas that contained low concentrations of chloride with some of these children failing to grow appropriately. Some infants may be at an increased risk for learning disabilities and deficits in language skills.[79,80]

Another potential problem is vitamin D oversupplementation or undersupplementation of infant formulas and fortified milk. Researchers who measured the vitamin D content of 5 brands of infant formulas (10 samples) determined that none of the samples had vitamin D concentrations within 20% of the labeled content.[119] None contained less than the amount of vitamin D stated on the label, but 70% of the samples contained more than 200% of the labeled amount.

Rickets can develop in VLBW infants who receive a soy-protein formula. This condition occurs because of poor calcium, phosphorus, and vitamin D absorption from the formula.[120]

Because of a concern about possible aluminum contamination of infant formulas, the Joint Expert Committee on Food Additives of the Food and Agricultural Organization of the United Nations set a maximum weekly aluminum intake for infants, children, and adults at 7000 mcg/kg.[121] Human milk typically contains less than 5 to 45 mcg of aluminum per liter, and cow milk–based formulas have concentrations of 14 to 565 mcg/L. The highest concentrations of aluminum (455 to 2346 mcg/L) have been reported in soy-based formulas because plants such as soy can receive high aluminum concentrations from soil.[121]

Preparation of Infant Formulas

Most formulas are available as liquid ready-to-use, liquid concentrate, and powdered concentrate. As the name implies, ready-to-use formulas do not require the addition of water, whereas concentrated liquid and powdered formulations typically require the mixing of equal amounts of water and concentrated liquid formula (e.g., 4 ounces water to 4 ounces formula) to prepare a 20 kcal/ounce or 67 kcal/100 mL formula. (See Table 20–11.) Most powdered formulas require adding 1 packed level measure (1 tablespoon) of powder for every 2 ounces of water to obtain a concentration of 20 kcal/ounce. (See Table 20–12.)[48,122]

Infant formula containers should be checked for expiration dates and dents before use. Unopened formula containers should be stored where they will not be subjected to extreme temperature changes.[122] Protein agglomeration is a sign of product instability that can occur if storage time is excessive. This agglomeration may range from slight, grainy development, to an increased viscosity and a gel formation, to an eventual precipitation of the product's protein. Agglomeration and separation do not affect the safety or nutritional value of a formula, but the appearance is a deterrent to its use.

Preparation Techniques When preparing an infant formula, the directions on the product container should be followed closely. If bottles with disposable plastic liners are used, the formula should not be mixed in the liner but should be prepared before the formula is poured into the liner because the bottle's measurements are only approximate.

Because infants are susceptible to infection, various methods of sterilization have been recommended for the preparation of infant formula. Several methods to discuss with parents or caregivers can be found in Table 20–13. Although not recommended by AAP, some parents use the clean technique to prepare an individual bottle of formula. If this method is used, the person preparing the formula must wash his or her hands carefully. Then all equipment for preparing formula (including cans of concentrated formula, bottles, and nipples) is washed thoroughly with detergent and hot water. Then the formula is prepared, the opened can of concentrated formula is refrigerated, and the prepared formula is heated. Formula remaining in the bottle after a feeding should be discarded. Studies have shown that the clean method of preparing formula is as safe as terminal sterilization if the water supply used for formula preparation is safe (i.e., if municipal water is available). If well water is used, it should be boiled for approximately 5 minutes before use in formula preparation.[123–125] If tap water is used, the water should run for at least 2 minutes to clear any lead that might be in the pipes, which will decrease an infant's exposure to lead.[125]

Heating infant formula, warming breast milk, or thawing frozen breast milk in a microwave oven can cause scald injuries, palatal burns in infants, and exploding containers. In addition, glass bottles can get hotter than plastic bottles, and the temperature of the milk may be uneven.[126] See the section "Patient Counseling for Infant Nutrition" for specific guidelines on using a microwave oven for formula preparation.[127]

Bottles of ready-to-use formula can be stored at room temperature, and the formula does not need to be warmed before feeding. The protective cap must be removed, and a sterile nipple must be screwed onto the bottle before feeding. The bottle should be shaken to allow for adequate formula mixing. After the infant is fed, the bottle and any unused formula should be discarded.[122] Ready-to-use formula in cans needs no preparation. The top of the can should be washed with soap and hot water, shaken to mix the formula, and opened with a clean, punch-type opener. Formula is added to one bottle for a single feeding or to the bottles needed for a full day's feeding. If the latter is done, the bottles should be covered and refrigerated until needed. Formula remaining in the can may be covered and stored in the refrigerator for as long as 48 hours. Each infant formula has specific instructions for preparation, and most formulas have symbols on the containers that can be used as guidelines in preparing formula.

Adverse Effects of Improperly Prepared or Administered Formulas The failure to properly dilute a concentrated infant formula can result in a hypertonic solution that could result in diarrhea or dehydration. In extreme cases, the ingestion of overly concentrated formula could lead to hypernatremic dehydration (induced by a deficit of water), metabolic acidosis (decreased alkalinity of the blood and tissues), and even renal failure. Overdilution can lead to water intoxication that may result in irritability, hyponatremia (low sodium levels in the blood), coma, or brain damage. Such a situation may occur when a parent or caregiver misunderstands the instructions for preparing a concentrated formula, dilutes a ready-to-use formula, or tries to make a formula last longer by diluting it further.

Parents or other caregivers may have questions about how much infant formula should be administered. Typically, a pediatrician or other health care provider will give the parents instructions on feeding; if parents did not receive such information, they should contact that individual. The following is general information about the administration of an infant formula. Typically, the recommended daily intake of a formula is age and individual-infant dependent. For example, the frequency of feeding a newborn infant may vary from every 2 hours to every 4 hours. Smaller infants usually require more frequent feedings because they have smaller stomach capacities and shorter times for emptying the stomach. Infants usually lengthen the interval between feedings to 4 hours by the time they are ages 3 to 4 weeks. Typically, infants begin to stop nighttime feedings by ages 3 to 6 weeks.[72] (See Table 20–14 for the average number of daily feedings for infants of different ages.)

By the end of the first week of life, full-term infants increase the volume of their feedings from 30 mL to between 80 and 90 mL. The amount of formula offered to a bottle-fed infant should be consistent with the RDA for energy according to age and weight. The infant should be fed on demand and should not be forced to take more formula than is desired at any one feeding. If the infant finishes a bottle and still seems hungry, another bottle should be offered. Parents should also be aware that an infant may lose weight during the first week of life, but by age 2 weeks he or she should be gaining weight. This weight gain denotes that the infant appears to be receiv-

Table 20–13

Methods for Infant Formula Preparation

Aseptic Sterilization

- When this method for infant formula preparation is selected, sterilize the bottles and the other equipment (e.g., glass measuring cup, spoons, nipples, rings, and disks) separately from the formula.[a]
- Wash hands before preparing formula and again if interrupted.
- Place all equipment in a deep pan or sterilizer, cover all equipment with tap water, and boil for 20 minutes.
- Remove all items from the pan or sterilizer with tongs, and place on a clean towel. Place the bottles and nipples on the towel with their open ends facing down.

Concentrated Liquid or Powder Formula

- While the equipment is being cleaned, boil water for the formula preparation in a clean pan or teakettle for at least 5 minutes.
- Remove the boiled water from the stove, and allow it to cool almost to room temperature with the lid left in place.

Concentrated Liquid Formula

- Wash the top of the formula can with hot water and detergent, rinse in hot running water, and dry. Shake the can, open it with a clean punch-type can opener, and mix appropriate amounts of concentrated liquid and sterilized water (according to instructions on the product label). All measurements should be made with a measuring cup for accuracy.
- Pour formula into the sterilized bottles. Place nipples, rings, and disks on the bottles.
- Tightly cover any unused formula and store in the refrigerator. Use it within 48 hours or discard.

Concentrated Powder Formula

- Wash the top of the can with hot water and detergent, rinse in hot running water, and dry.
- Open the can, and mix appropriate amounts of powder and sterilized water (according to instructions on the product label). All measurements should be made with a measuring cup for accuracy.
- Pour formula into the sterilized bottles. Place nipples, rings, and disks on the bottles.
- Tightly cover any unused formula, and store in the refrigerator. Use it within 48 hours or discard.
- Cover the can containing any remaining powder with its plastic top. Store in a cool, dry place for up to 1 month.

Ready-to-Use Formula

- Wash the top of the can with hot water and detergent, rinse in hot running water, and dry.
- Shake the can, and open it with a clean punch-type can opener. Add the amount of formula needed per feeding to a sterilized bottle. *Do not add water*. Place nipple and ring on the bottle.
- Tightly cover any formula remaining in the can. Store in the refrigerator for up to 48 hours.

All Types of Formula

- Warm the bottle to the desired temperature, and shake well before feeding. After feeding the infant, discard any formula left in the bottle, and rinse the bottle and nipple in cool water immediately.

Terminal Heating Method

- Use this method to prepare infant formula from concentrated liquid formula only.
- Wash hands before preparing formula and again if interrupted.
- Wash all needed equipment (e.g., glass measuring cup, spoon, bottles, nipples, rings, and disks) with hot water and detergent. Rinse well with hot running water.
- Wash the top of the formula can with hot water and detergent, rinse in hot running water, and dry. Shake the can, and open it with a clean punch-type can opener.
- Measure the needed amount of concentrated formula and the correct amount of water in a glass measuring cup (according to instructions on the formula label). Mix well; pour the formula into clean bottles; and attach nipples, disks, and rings. Apply rings loosely.
- Place filled bottles on a rack in a deep pan or sterilizer that contains approximately 3 inches of water. Heat water to boiling, and allow it to boil gently for 25 minutes while covered. Remove the pan from the stove.
- After the sides of the pan have cooled enough to be touched comfortably, remove the bottles. Tighten the nipple rings, and store bottles in the refrigerator until needed. Use bottles within 48 hours.
- Warm the bottle to the desired temperature, and shake well before feeding. After feeding the infant, discard any formula left in the bottle, and rinse the bottle and nipple in cool water immediately.

[a] If disposable bottle liners are used, only the nipples, rings, and screw tops of bottles need to be sterilized. The manufacturer has sterilized the bottle liners.

Source: *How to Prepare Your Baby's Infant Formula*. Evansville, IN: Mead Johnson Nutritionals; 1991; and *Feeding Baby: A Guide for New Parents*. Evansville, IN: Mead Johnson Nutritionals; 1994.

ing an appropriate amount of formula.[72] Thereafter, growth curves (weight, height, and head circumference) are used by health care professionals to determine whether an infant is growing appropriately. (See Table 20–15 for a list of typical quantities of feedings for various age groups.)

Underfeeding and overfeeding are potential problems with bottle-fed infants. Improperly preparing the infant formula can cause these problems, as can feeding too much formula. Other problems that can be associated with formula feedings are regurgitation and vomiting, loose or diarrheal stools, constipation, and colic. If an infant is regurgitating or vomiting formula, a physician should be consulted. Diarrheal stools may be caused by an improperly concentrated formula, by feeding the infant too much, or by administering

Table 20–14

Number of Daily Feedings, According to Age

Age	Average Number of Daily Feedings
Birth–1 week	6–10
1 week–1 month	6–8
1–3 months	5–6
3–4 months	4–5
4–8 months	3–4
8–12 months	3

Source: Adapted from Barness LA, Curren JS. The feeding of infants and children. In: Behrman RE, ed. *Nelson Textbook of Pediatrics*. 15th ed. Philadelphia: WB Saunders; 1996:151–65.

Table 20–15

Quantity of Milk Ingested per Feeding, According to Age

Age	Average Quantity of Milk per Feeding (oz)
Birth–2 weeks	2–3
3 weeks–2 months	4–5
2–3 months	5–6
3–4 months	6–7
5–12 months	7–8

Source: Adapted from Barness LA, Curran JS. The feeding of infants and children. In: Behrman RE, ed. *Nelson Textbook of Pediatrics*. 15th ed. Philadelphia: WB Saunders; 1996:151–65.

a formula that has been contaminated. Mild diarrhea may respond to temporarily decreasing feedings or interrupting them and to administering a balanced electrolyte product. If the infant does not respond quickly or if diarrhea is more severe, the pediatrician should be contacted. (See Chapter 13, "Diarrhea.")

Some infants may have allergies to infant formulas, especially to cow milk protein. If parents or caregivers ask about this type of allergy, the pharmacist can inform them that it is rare, 0.5% to 1.5% of children. Symptoms may involve the respiratory or GI tract. The diagnosis is usually made by observing the dissipation of symptoms in an infant who is placed on a cow milk–free formula or on breast milk.[128]

Product Selection Guidelines

For healthy, full-term infants who do not need a therapeutic formula, a milk-based formula or a milk-based formula with added whey protein is indicated. When recommending a type of formula, the pharmacist should consider the method of preparation, the parents' ability to follow directions, the parents' attitudes and preferences, and the sanitary conditions and refrigeration facilities available. Before assisting parents in selecting a therapeutic formula, the pharmacist should find out whether a pediatrician recommended the formula.

For many parents, cost may be a critical factor in selecting an infant formula. Concentrated liquids and powdered formula preparations are less expensive than ready-to-use products. Convenience is also a consideration. The preparation of powdered and concentrated liquid formulas requires more manipulative functions and more attention to aseptic technique. The formula selected should be one that is well tolerated by the infant, convenient for the parents to prepare, and priced to fit the family's budget. To simplify formula preparation when away from home, parents can select products that are available in unit-of-use packaging for ready-to-use liquids and powder packets.

Patient Assessment of Infant Nutrition

Body weight, length, and head circumference are the growth standards for determining whether infants are receiving the appropriate nutrients, are properly utilizing ingested nutrients, or both. If an infant appears to be underweight or underdeveloped, the pharmacist should advise the parent to take the infant to a physician for evaluation.

The pharmacist's primary role in infant nutrition is to assist with selection of infant formulas and to provide information about formula products and breast-feeding. Asking parents the following questions will help elicit the information needed to recommend the appropriate formula.

Q~ What form of formula (e.g., ready-to-use, liquid concentrate, powdered concentrate) will be used most often?

A~ If parents are most concerned about the cost of formulas, explain that the concentrated formulas are more economical but require more time and effort to prepare. If convenience is the primary concern, recommend a ready-to-use formula, but also advise the parents to consult their pediatrician about the need for fluoride supplementation.

Q~ Do you understand how your baby's formula should be prepared?

A~ If no, have the parent read the product instructions while in the pharmacy. Then ask whether the parent has any questions about the instructions. Also, instruct the parent on aseptic techniques for preparing infant formulas. (See Table 20–13.)

Q~ Are you aware of the adverse effects that can occur if a formula is improperly prepared or administered?

A~ If no, explain the potential adverse effects. (See the section "Adverse Effects of Improperly Prepared or Administered Formulas.")

Q~ Do you know how frequently you should feed your baby and what volume of formula to give at each feeding?

A~ If no, explain that the frequency of feedings and the amount given will vary according to the baby's age. Share the information in Tables 20–14 and 20–15 with the parent. Advise the parent to also have the baby's physician check the information.

Patient Counseling for Infant Nutrition

Parents are often bewildered by the number and variety of commercial infant formulas. Once the type of formula recommended or prescribed by the baby's physician is known, the pharmacist can steer parents to the appropriate products. If parents need further assistance with product selection, the pharmacist can recommend a product to match the parents' preferences. At these encounters, the pharmacist should make sure the parents have not forgotten how to properly prepare formulas or how much formula to give at each feeding. The box "Patient Education for Infant Nutrition" lists specific information to provide parents.

CONCLUSIONS

Infant formulas are a healthy, well-accepted alternative to breast-feeding in developed countries. Adequate growth can be achieved in infants being fed entirely by formula, or receiving formula supplementation to breast-feeding. Infant formula products are currently available that provide nutrient mixes designed for various feeding situations and disease conditions. When using an appropriately selected formula product, most infants will receive the recommended daily requirements for energy, protein, carbohydrates, fats, vitamins, and minerals. Although most full-term infants thrive on standard milk-based formulas, it is not uncommon to encounter infants with lactose intolerance or cow milk protein intolerance. Lactose-free, protein hydrolysate, and soy-protein formulas are widely available for infants who need formulas to adapt to their physiologic needs. Similarly, the special nutrient needs of preterm infants can also be met with

Patient Education for Infant Nutrition

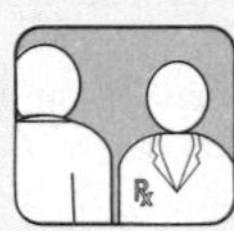

The objective of infant nutrition is to provide optimum nutrition to infants and children. Parents who carefully follow product instructions and the measures listed below will help ensure optimal outcomes.

- Before use, check unopened formula containers for dents. Do not use products if they are dented or if the expiration date has passed.
- When using concentrated powder or liquid formulas, carefully follow instructions for diluting the formula to the desired caloric concentration. (See Tables 20–11 and 20–12.) If the formula is too concentrated, the baby may have diarrhea or become dehydrated. If it is too dilute, the baby can become water intoxicated, which might lead to irritability, coma, or brain damage.
- When preparing concentrated powder, follow the technique for aseptic sterilization described in Table 20–13. Be sure to sterilize the bottles (or use sterile liners), the other equipment, and the water used to dilute the formula.
- When preparing concentrated liquid formulas, follow either the technique for aseptic sterilization or the terminal heating method as described in Table 20–13. Be sure to sterilize the bottles (or use sterile liners), the other equipment, and the water used to dilute the formula.
- When preparing ready-to-use formulas, do not add water to the formula. Follow the instructions in Table 20–13. Be sure to sterilize the bottles (or use sterile liners) and the other equipment.
- Use prepared or opened ready-to-use formula within 48 hours.
- Feed the baby according to the frequency and quantities listed in Tables 20–14 and 20–15 unless instructed otherwise by the baby's physician.
- When warming formula or breast milk in a microwave, follow the instructions below to prevent exploding containers, scalds, or burns to the baby's palate:
  —Remove the bottle cover to allow heat to escape.
  —Heat only 4 ounces or more of refrigerated milk; do not thaw frozen breast milk in a microwave.
  —Heat 4 ounces of formula on full power for no longer than 30 seconds; heat 8 ounces of formula for 45 seconds.
  —After heating the formula, replace the nipple assembly and invert the bottle ten times.
  —Test the formula's temperature by putting a few drops on your tongue or the top part of your hand. Do not feed the baby any formula unless it feels cool to the touch.

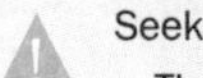

Seek medical attention if
—The baby is regurgitating or vomiting formula.
—The baby has severe diarrhea or mild diarrhea that does not respond quickly to temporary decreased feedings or to administration of a balanced electrolyte product.

formulas designed to supply the additional protein, energy, vitamins, minerals, and trace elements for a rapidly growing preterm infant with a maturing digestive capacity. Infants with very special nutrient needs can also be fed with uniquely designed formula products for inborn errors of metabolism and for other uncommon disorders. The pharmacist can play a crucial role in assisting caregivers with infant feeding, whether it be promoting education about breast-feeding, assisting with infant formula product selection, assisting with follow-up monitoring, or serving as an information resource for families regarding infant formula products.

References

1. American Academy of Pediatrics, Work Group on Breastfeeding. Breastfeeding and the use of human milk. *Pediatrics.* 1997;100:1035–9.
2. Cunningham AS, Jelliffe DB, Jelliffe EF. Breast-feeding and health in the 1980s: a global epidemiological review. *J Pediatr.* 1991;118:659–66.
3. Jason J. Breast-feeding in 1991 [editorial]. *N Engl J Med.* 1991;325: 1036–8.
4. Cone TE Jr. Infant feeding redux. *Pediatrics.* 1990;86:473–4.
5. Martinez GA, Krieger FW. 1984 milk-feeding patterns in the US. *Pediatrics.* 1985;76:1004–8.
6. Fomon SJ. Reflections on infant feeding in the 1970s and 1980s. *Am J Clin Nutr.* 1987;46(suppl 1):171–82.
7. Hoekelman RA. Highs and lows in breast-feeding rates. *Pediatr Ann.* 1992;21:615–7.
8. National Center for Health Statistics. *Healthy People 2000 Review, 1998–99.* Hyattsville, MD: Public Health Service, 1999. Library of Congress Catalog Card Number 76–641496.
9. Losch M, Dungy CI, Russel D, Dusdieker LB. Impact of attitudes on maternal decisions regarding infant feeding. *J Pediatr.* 1995;126: 507–13.
10. Filer LJ. A glimpse into the future of infant nutrition. *Pediatr Ann.* 1992;21:633–6,639.
11. Jones EG. In: Kelts DG, Jones EG, eds. *Manual of Pediatric Nutrition.* Boston: Little, Brown; 1984:17–34.
12. Redel CA, Shulman RJ. Controversies in the composition of infant formulas. *Pediatr Clin North Am.* 1994;41:909–24.
13. Werlin SL. The digestive system: exocrine pancreas. In: Behrman RE, ed. *Nelson Textbook of Pediatrics.* 15th ed. Philadelphia: WB Saunders; 1996:1119–24.
14. Fomon SJ, Ziegler EE. Renal solute load and *potential* renal solute load in infancy. *J Pediatr.* 1999;134:11–4.
15. Hansen JW, Cook DA, Cordano A, Miguel SG. Human milk substitutes. In: Tsang RC, Nichols BL, eds. *Nutrition during Infancy.* St. Louis: CV Mosby; 1988:378–98.
16. Trahms CM, Pipes PL. Growth, development and nutrition. In: Trahms CM, Pipes PL, eds. *Nutrition in Infancy and Childhood.* 6th ed. New York: McGraw-Hill; 1997:1–34.
17. Fomon SJ et al. Body composition of reference children from birth to age 10 years. *Am J Clin Nutr.* 1982;35:1169–75.
18. Hamill PV, Drizd TA, Johnson CL, et al. Physical growth: National Center for Health Statistics percentiles. *Am J Clin Nutr.* 1979;32: 607–29.
19. National Center for Health Statistics. NCHS growth curves for children, birth–18 years, 1977. *Vital and Health Statistics: Data from the National Health Survey; 165.* Series 11. DHEW Pub No. DHS 78–1650 (PHS). Hyattsville, MD: US Department of Health, Education, and Welfare, Public Health Service; November 1977.
20. Dewer KG et al. Growth of breast-fed and formula-fed infants from 0 to 18 months: the DARLING study. *Pediatrics.* 1992;89:1035–41.
21. DeOnis M, Garza C. Time for a new growth reference. *Pediatrics.* 1997;100(5). Also available at: http://www.pediatrics.org/cgi/content/full/100/5/e8.
22. Food and Nutrition Board, Commission on Life Sciences, National Research Council. *Recommended Dietary Allowances.* 10th ed. Washington, DC: National Academy Press; 1989.
23. Standing Committee on the Scientific Evaluation of Dietary Reference Intakes, Food and Nutrition Board, Institute of Medicine. *Dietary Reference Intakes for Calcium, Phosphorus, Magnesium, Vitamin D, and Fluoride.* Washington, DC: National Academy Press; 1997.
24. Davies PSW, Gregory J, White A. Energy expenditure in children aged 1.5 to 4.5 years: a comparison with current recommendations for energy intake. *Eur J Clin Nutr.* 1995;49:360–4.
25. Kliegman RM, Behrman RE. The fetus and neonatal infant: the digestive system. In: Behrman RE, ed. *Nelson Textbook of Pediatrics.* 15th ed. Philadelphia: WB Saunders; 1996:490–9.
26. Trahms CM, Pipes PL. Nutrient needs of infants and children. In: Trahms CM, Pipes PL, eds. *Nutrition in Infancy and Childhood.* 6th ed. New York: McGraw-Hill; 1997:35–67.
27. American Academy of Pediatrics, Committee on Nutrition. Carbohydrate and dietary fiber. In: Kleinman RE, ed. *Pediatric Nutrition Handbook.* 4th ed. Elk Grove Village, IL: American Academy of Pediatrics; 1998:203–11.
28. Williams CL, Bollella M, Wynder EL. A new recommendation for dietary fiber in childhood. *Pediatrics.* 1995;96(5 Pt 2):985–8.
29. Picone TA, Benson JD, Moro G, et al. Growth, serum biochemistries, and amino acids of term infants fed formulas with amino acid and protein concentrations similar to human milk. *J Pediatr Gastroenterol Nutr.* 1989;9:351–60.
30. Sanchez-Pozo A, Lopez J, Pita ML, et al. Changes in the protein fractions of human milk during lactation. *Ann Nutr Metab.* 1986;30: 15–20.
31. Polberger SKT, Axelsson IE, Raiha NCR. Amino acid concentrations in plasma and urine in very low birthweight infants fed protein-unenriched or human milk protein-enriched human milk. *Pediatrics.* 1990;86:909–15.
32. Boehm G, Borte M, Bellstedt K, et al. Protein quality of human milk fortifier in low birth weight infants: effects on growth and plasma amino acid profiles. *Eur J Pediatr.* 1993;152:1036–9.
33. Itabashi K, Hayashi T, Tsugoshi T, et al. Fortified preterm human milk for very low birth weight infants. *Early Hum Dev.* 1992;29:339–43.
34. Gaull G, Sturman JA, Raiha NCR. Development of mammalian sulfur metabolism: absence of cystathionase in human fetal tissues. *Pediatr Res.* 1972;6:538–47.
35. Chesney RW, Helma RA, Christensen M, et al. An updated view of the value of taurine in infant nutrition. *Adv Pediatr.* 1998;45:179–200.
36. Michalk DV, Tittor F, Ringeisen R, et al. The development of heart and brain function in low-birth-weight infants fed with taurine-supplemented formula. *Adv Exp Med Biol.* 1987;217:139–45.
37. Committee on Nutrition, American Academy of Pediatrics. Statement on cholesterol. *Pediatrics.* 1992;90:469–73.
38. Schlenk H. Odd numbered and new essential fatty acids. *Federal Proc.* 1972;31:1430–5.
39. Friedman ZA et al. Rapid onset of essential fatty acid deficiency in the newborn. *Pediatrics.* 1976;58:640–9.
40. Committee on Nutrition, American Academy of Pediatrics. Commentary on breast-feeding and infant formulas, including proposed standards for formulas. *Pediatrics.* 1976;57:278–85.
41. Calvo EB, Galindo AC, Aspres NB. Iron status in exclusively breast-fed infants. *Pediatrics.* 1992;90:375–9.
42. O'Connor P. Vitamin D–deficiency rickets in two breast-fed infants who were not receiving vitamin D supplementation. *Clin Pediatr.* 1971;16:361–3.
43. Fomon SJ et al. Recommendations for feeding normal infants. *Pediatrics.* 1979;63:52–9.
44. Pugliese MT et al. Nutritional rickets in suburbia. *J Am Coll Nutr.* 1998;17:637–41.
45. Sills IN et al. Vitamin D deficiency rickets. Reports of its demise are exaggerated. *Clin Pediatr.* 1994;33:491–3.
46. Daaboul J, Sanderson S, Kristensen K, Kitson H. Vitamin D deficiency in pregnant and breast-feeding women and their infants. *J Perinatol.* 1997;17:10–4.
47. Higginbottom MC, Sweetman L, Nyhan WL. A syndrome of methylmalonic aciduria, homocystinuria, megaloblastic anemia and neurologic abnormalities in a vitamin B_{12}–deficient breast-fed infant of a strict vegetarian. *N Engl J Med.* 1978;299:317–23.
48. Pipes PL. Infant feeding and nutrition. In: Trahms CM, Pipes PL, eds.

Nutrition in Infancy and Childhood. 6th ed. New York: McGraw-Hill; 1997:98–129.

49. Dallman PR. Iron, vitamin E, and folate in the preterm infant. *J Pediatr*. 1974;85:742–52.
50. Rios E. The absorption of iron as supplements in infant cereal and infant formulas. *Pediatrics*. 1975;55:686–93.
51. Walter T, Dallman PR, Pizarro F, et al. Effectiveness of iron-fortified infant cereal in prevention of iron deficiency anemia. *Pediatrics*. 1993;91:976–82.
52. Fairweather-Tait S, Fox T, Wharf SG, et al. The bioavailability of iron in different weaning foods and the enhancing effect of a fruit drink containing ascorbic acid. *Pediatr Res*. 1995;37(4 Pt 1):389–94.
53. Committee on Nutrition, American Academy of Pediatrics. Fluoride supplementation for children: interim policy recommendations. *Pediatrics*. 1995;95:777.
54. Committee on Nutrition, American Academy of Pediatrics. Formula feeding of term infants. In: Kleinman RE, ed. *Pediatric Nutrition Handbook*. 4th ed. Elk Grove Village, IL: American Academy of Pediatrics; 1998:29–42.
55. Oski FA. Iron-fortified formulas and gastrointestinal symptoms in infants: a controlled study. *Pediatrics*. 1980;66:168–70.
56. Nelson SE et al. Lack of adverse reactions to iron-fortified formula. *Pediatrics*. 1988;81:360–4.
57. Committee on Nutrition, American Academy of Pediatrics. Nutritional needs of low-birth-weight infants. *Pediatrics*. 1977;60:519–30.
58. Committee on Nutrition, American Academy of Pediatrics. Nutritional needs of low-birth-weight infants. *Pediatrics*. 1985;75:976–86.
59. Hittner HM, Godio LB, Rudolph AJ, et al. Retrolental fibroplasia: efficacy of vitamin E in a double-blind clinical study of preterm infants. *N Engl J Med*. 1981;305:1365–71.
60. Stevens D, Burman D, Strelling MK, et al. Folic acid supplementation in low birthweight infants. *Pediatrics*. 1979;64:333–5.
61. Pugliese MT. Parental health beliefs as a cause of nonorganic failure to thrive. *Pediatrics*. 1987;80:175–82.
62. Taras HL. Early childhood diet: recommendations of pediatric health care providers. *J Am Diet Assoc*. 1988;88:1417–21.
63. Committee on Nutrition, American Academy of Pediatrics. Iron fortification of infant formulas. *Pediatrics*. 1999;104:119–23.
64. Camitta B. Iron deficiency anemia. In: Behrman RE, ed. *Nelson Textbook of Pediatrics*. 15th ed. Philadelphia: WB Saunders; 1996:1387–9.
65. Gorman KS, Metallinos-Katsaras E. Nutrition and the behavior of children. In: Walker WA, Watkins JB, eds. *Nutrition in Pediatrics*. 2nd ed. Hamilton, Ontario: BC Decker; 1997:335–47.
66. Oski FA. Whole cow milk feeding between 6 and 12 months of age? Go back to 1976. *Pediatr Rev*. 1990;12:187–9.
67. Woodruff CW. Milk intolerances. *Nutr Rev*. 1976;34:33–7.
68. Committee on Nutrition, American Academy of Pediatrics. The use of whole cow's milk in infancy. *Pediatrics*. 1983;72:253–5.
69. Ziegler EE. Milk and formulas for older infants. *J Pediatr*. 1990;117(suppl):S76–9.
70. Committee on Nutrition, American Academy of Pediatrics. The use of whole cow's milk in infancy. *Pediatrics*. 1992;89:1105–9.
71. Sullivan PB. Cows' milk induced intestinal bleeding in infancy. *Arch Dis Child*. 1993;68:240–5.
72. Barness LA. Nutrition and nutritional disorders: nutritional requirements. In: Behrman RE, ed. *Nelson Textbook of Pediatrics*. 14th ed. Philadelphia: WB Saunders; 1992:105–30.
73. Committee on Nutrition, American Academy of Pediatrics. Supplemental foods for infants. In: Forbes GB, Woodruff CW, eds. *Pediatric Nutrition Handbook*. 2nd ed. Elk Grove Village, IL: American Academy of Pediatrics; 1985:28–36.
74. Forsyth JS. Is it worthwhile breast-feeding? *Eur J Clin Nutr*. 1992;46(suppl 1):S19–25.
75. Heikkinen T, Ruuskanen O. New prospects in the prevention of otitis media. *Annals Med*. 1996;28:23–30.
76. Duncan B, Ey J, Holberg CJ, et al. Exclusive breast-feeding for at least 4 months protects against otitis media. *Pediatrics*. 1993;91:867–72.
77. Committee on Nutrition, American Academy of Pediatrics. Proposed changes in Food and Drug Administration regulations concerning formula products and vitamin–mineral dietary supplements for infants. *Pediatrics*. 1967;40:916–22.
78. Food and Drug Administration. Nutrient requirements for infant formulas. *Federal Register*. 1985;50:45106–8.
79. Silver LB, Levinson RB, Laskin CR, et al. Learning disabilities as a probable consequence of using a chloride-deficient infant formula. *J Pediatr*. 1989;115:97–9.
80. Malloy MH, Graubard B, Moss H, et al. Hypochloremic metabolic alkalosis from ingestion of a chloride-deficient infant formula: outcome 9–10 years later. *Pediatrics*. 1991;87:811–22.
81. Food and Drug Administration. Infant formula: labeling requirements. *Federal Register*. 1985;50:1833–40.
82. Santeiro ML, Sagraves R, Allen LV Jr. Osmolality of small-volume iv admixtures for pediatric patients [published erratum *Am J Hosp Pharm*. 1990;47:1978]. *Am J Hosp Pharm*. 1990;47:1359–64.
83. Anderson TA, Fomon SJ, Filer LJ. Carbohydrate tolerance studies with 3-day-old infants. *J Lab Clin Med*. 1972;79:31–7.
84. *Composition of Feedings for Infants and Young Children*. Columbus, OH: Ross Laboratories; 1999.
85. Tomarelli RM. Osmolality, osmolarity, and renal solute load of infant formulas. *J Pediatr*. 1976;88:454–6.
86. Lifschitz CH. Carbohydrate needs in preterm and term newborn infants. In: Tsang RC, Nichols BL, eds. *Nutrition during Infancy*. St. Louis: CV Mosby; 1988:122–32.
87. Klish WJ. Special infant formulas. *Pediatr Rev*. 1990;12:55–62.
88. *Pediatric Products Handbook*. Evansville, IN: Mead Johnson Nutritionals; 1996.
89. Committee on Nutrition, American Academy of Pediatrics. Soy-protein formulas: recommendations for use in infant feeding. *Pediatrics*. 1983;72:359–63.
90. Merritt RJ, Carter M, Haight M, et al. Whey protein hydrolysate formula for infants with gastrointestinal intolerance to cow milk and soy protein in infant formulas. *J Pediatr Gastroenterol Nutr*. 1990;11:78–82.
91. Gerrand JW et al. Cow milk allergy: prevalence and manifestations in an unselected series of newborns. *Acta Paediatr Scand*. 1973;234(suppl):1–21.
92. Goel K, Lifshitz F, Kahn E, Teichberg S. Monosaccharide intolerance and soy-protein hypersensitivity in an infant with diarrhea. *J Pediatr*. 1978;93:617–9.
93. Powell GK. Milk- and soy-induced enterocolitis of infancy: clinical features and standardization of challenge. *J Pediatr*. 1978;93:553–60.
94. Lonnerdal B. Nutritional aspects of soy formula. *Acta Paediatr*. 1994;(suppl 402):105–8.
95. Setchell KD, Zimmer-Nechemias L, Cai J, et al. Isoflavone content of infant formula and the metabolic fate of these phytoestrogens in early life. *Am J Clin Nutr*. 1998;68(6 suppl):1453S–61S.
96. Chicago and Suburban Dietetics Association. Nutritional care of the high risk infant. In: *Manual of Clinical Dietetics*. Chicago: American Dietetics Association; 1988:115–37.
97. Ellis L, Kalnias D, Corey M, et al. Do infants with cystic fibrosis need a protein hydrolysate formula? A prospective, randomized, comparative study. *J Pediatr*. 1998;132:270–6.
98. Committee on Nutrition, American Academy of Pediatrics. Hypoallergenic infant formulas. *Pediatrics*. 1989;83:1068–9.
99. Sampson HA. Safety of casein hydrolysate formula in children with cow milk allergy. *J Pediatr*. 1991;118(suppl):520–5.
100. Barr RG, Kramer MS, Pless IB, et al. Feeding and temperament as determinants of early infant crying/fussing behavior. *Pediatrics*. 1989;84:514–21.
101. Lothe L, Lindberg T. Cow's milk whey protein elicits symptoms of infantile colic in colicky formula-fed infants: a double-blind crossover study [published erratum *Pediatrics*. 1989;84:17]. *Pediatrics*. 1989;83:262–6.
102. Andrews BF, Lorch V. Improved fat and CA absorption in LBW infants fed a medium chain triglyceride containing formula [abstract]. *Pediatr Res*. 1974;8:378.
103. Tantibhedhyangkul P, Hashim SA. Medium-chain triglyceride feeding in premature infants: effects on calcium and magnesium absorption. *Pediatrics*. 1978;61:537–45.
104. Tantibhedhyangkul P, Hashim SA. Medium-chain triglyceride feeding in premature infants: effects on fat and nitrogen absorption. *Pediatrics*. 1975;55:359–70.

105. Businco L, Contani A, Longhi MA, et al. Anaphylactic reactions to a cow's milk whey protein hydrolysate (Alfa-Ré, Nestlé) in infants with cow milk allergy. *Ann Allergy.* 1989;62:333–5.
106. Forbes GB. Is human milk the best food for low birthweight babies? *Pediatr Res.* 1978;12:434.
107. Committee on Nutrition, American Academy of Pediatrics. Calcium requirements in infancy and childhood. *Pediatrics.* 1978; 62: 826–34.
108. Mizrahi A, London RD, Gribetz D. Neonatal hypocalcemia—its causes and treatment. *N Engl J Med.* 1968; 278: 1163–5.
109. Dallman PR. Upper limits of iron in infant formulas. *J Nutr.* 1989;119(suppl):1852–4.
110. Thompson M, McClead RE. Human milk fortifiers. *J Pediatr Perinatal Nutr.* 1987;1:65–75.
111. Ehrenkranz RA, Gettner PA, Nelli CM. Nutrition balance studies in premature infants fed premature formula or fortified preterm human milk. *J Pediatr Gastroenterol Nutr.* 1989;8:58–67.
112. Kashyap S, Schulze KF, Forsyth M, et al. Growth, nutrient retention, and metabolic response of low-birth-weight infants fed supplemented and unsupplemented preterm human milk. *Am J Clin Nutr.* 1990;52: 254–62.
113. Committee on Nutrition, American Academy of Pediatrics. Follow-up or weaning formulas. *Pediatrics.* 1989;83:1067.
114. Provisional Committee on Quality Improvement, Subcommittee on Acute Gastroenteritis, American Academy of Pediatrics. Practice parameter: the management of acute gastroenteritis in young children. *Pediatrics.* 1996;97:424–33.
115. Von Burg MM, Sanders BJ, Weddell JA. Baby bottle tooth decay: a concern for all mothers. *Pediatr Nurs.* 1995;21:515–8.
116. Moss MH. Hypoprothrombinemic bleeding in a young infant: association with a soy protein formula. *Am J Dis Child.* 1969;117:540–2.
117. Goldman HI, Amadio P. Vitamin K deficiency after the newborn period. *Pediatrics.* 1969;44:745–9.
118. Cochrane WA, Collins-Williams C, Donohue WL. Superior hemorrhagic polioencephalitis (Wernicke's disease) occurring in an infant—probably due to thiamine deficiency from use of a soy bean product. *Pediatrics.* 1961;28:771–7.
119. Holick MF, Shao Q, Liu WW, Chen TC. The vitamin D content of fortified milk and infant formula. *N Engl J Med.* 1992;326:1178–81.
120. Kulkarni PB, Hall RT, Rhodes PG, et al. Rickets in very low-birth-weight infants. *J Pediatr.* 1980;96:249–52.
121. Litov RE, Sickles VS, Chan GM, et al. Plasma aluminum measurements in term infants fed human milk or a soy-based infant formula. *Pediatrics.* 1989;84:1105–7.
122. *How to Prepare Your Baby's Infant Formula.* Evansville, IN: Mead Johnson Nutritionals; 1991.
123. Hughes RB et al. Outcome of teaching clean vs terminal methods of formula preparation. *Pediatr Nurs.* 1987;13:275–6.
124. Gerber MA, Berliner BC, Karolus JJ. Sterilization of infant formula. *Clin Pediatr.* 1983;22:344–9.
125. Howard CR, Weitzman M. Breast or bottle: practical aspects of infant nutrition in the first 6 months. *Pediatr Ann.* 1992;21:619–21, 625–7, 630–1.
126. Nemethy M, Clore ER. Microwave heating of infant formula and breast milk. *J Pediatr Health Care.* 1990;4:131–5.
127. Sigman-Grant M, Bush F, Anantheswaran R. Microwave heating of infant formula: a dilemma resolved. *Pediatrics.* 1992;90:412–5.
128. Ulshen M. The digestive system: stomach and intestines. In: Behrman RE, ed. *Nelson Textbook of Pediatrics.* 15th ed. Philadelphia: WB Saunders; 1996:1088.

CHAPTER 21

Overweight and Obesity

Paul L. Doering

Chapter 21 at a Glance

Obesity is characterized by an excessive accumulation of body fat to the extent that it is thought to impair health. According to guidelines from the National Heart, Lung, and Blood Institute, an estimated 97 million adults in the United States are overweight or obese. Data from four recent federal surveys of health practices indicate that 33% to 40% of women and 20% to 24% of men are currently trying to lose weight, with an additional 28% of each group trying to maintain their weight. Among women and men trying to lose weight, their reported time on a weight-loss regimen in one year averaged 6.4 and 5.8 months, respectively, and the number of attempts to lose weight in the prior 2 years averaged 2.5 and 2.0, respectively. Studies have shown that 34% of female adolescents regarded themselves as "too fat" and that 44% were trying to lose weight. In contrast, only 15% of adolescent males thought they were too fat and 15% were trying to lose weight.[1,2]

In 1998, 45 million dieters spent $30 billion—an average of $667 each—on strategies to lose weight. Although the role of nonprescription drug products to treat obesity is somewhat limited, pharmacists can help motivate patients to set realistic, attainable weight-loss goals for themselves and to choose safe and effective weight-loss methods.

Clinical Indicators of Overweight and Obesity

Individuals are considered obese when their percentage of body fat equals or exceeds 30% of total weight in women or 25% in men. Severe obesity is characterized by a body fat content that exceeds 40% in women or 35% in men. Methods of determining percentage of body fat are either impractical for routine clinical purposes, are unreliable, or have other limitations. For these reasons, body mass index (BMI) is the most commonly used indicator for assessing over-

Editor's Note: This chapter is based, in part, on the 11th edition chapter titled "Weight Control Products," which was written by Paul L. Doering.

weight and obesity and for monitoring changes in body weight.[3] This method has replaced weight tables that were developed by the Metropolitan Life Insurance Company[4] because it correlates better with total body fat. Table 21–1 correlates BMI values with body weight and height. It also presents the two methods for calculating BMI.

For persons of average height, one BMI unit is equivalent to approximately 3.1 kg (6.8 pounds) in men and 2.6 kg (5.8 pounds) in women. In 1998, the National Heart, Lung, and Blood Institute of the National Institutes of Health, issued lower BMI values for overweight and obesity in its expert report titled *Clinical Guidelines on the Identification, Evaluation, and Treatment of Overweight and Obesity in Adults.*[3] This report defines overweight as a BMI of 25 to 29.9 and obesity as a BMI of 30 or greater. Previously, overweight was defined as a BMI value of greater than or equal to 27.9 for men and 27.3 for women. A BMI of 30 is about 13.4 kg (29.7 pounds) overweight and is equivalent to a weight of 98.6 kg (219 pounds) in a person whose height is 1.8 m (5 feet 11 inches) and equivalent to a weight of 83 kg (185 pounds) in one whose height is 1.7 m (5 feet 7 inches). According to these new definitions, the percentage of overweight adults 20 years of age or older in the United States increased from 33.4% to 54.9%.

Some clinicians use patterns of fat distribution to predict complications from excessive weight. The fat distribution after puberty characteristically differs between men and women. Women tend to store fat in the breasts, hips, and thighs; this pattern is called gynecoid distribution, or the so-called pear shape. Men tend to accumulate fat in the abdomen; this pattern is called android distribution, or the so-called apple shape. Some women, however, have an android fat distribution, and some men exhibit the gynecoid fat distribution. Android fat distribution may be more strongly associated with atherosclerosis, diabetes mellitus, and gouty arthritis than is the same degree of gynecoid fat distribution.

Waist circumference, which is positively correlated with abdominal fat content,[3] can be used to identify increased

Table 21–1

Body Weights Corresponding to Height and Body Mass Index[a]

	Body Mass Index (kg/m^2)[b]													
	19	20	21	22	23	24	25	26	27	28	29	30	35	40
Height (inches)	Body Weight (pounds)													
58	91	96	100	105	110	115	119	124	129	134	138	143	167	191
59	94	99	104	109	114	119	124	128	133	138	143	148	173	198
60	97	102	107	112	118	123	128	133	138	143	148	153	179	204
61	100	106	111	116	122	127	132	137	143	148	153	158	185	211
62	104	109	115	120	126	131	136	142	147	153	158	164	191	218
63	107	113	118	124	130	135	141	146	152	158	163	169	197	225
64	110	116	122	128	134	140	145	151	157	163	169	174	204	232
65	114	120	126	132	138	144	150	156	162	168	174	180	210	240
66	118	124	130	136	142	148	155	161	167	173	179	186	216	247
67	121	127	134	140	146	153	159	166	172	178	185	191	223	255
68	125	131	138	144	151	158	164	171	177	184	190	197	230	262
69	128	135	142	149	155	162	169	176	182	189	196	203	236	270
70	132	139	146	153	160	167	172	181	188	195	202	207	243	278
71	136	143	150	157	165	172	179	186	193	200	208	215	250	286
72	140	147	154	162	169	177	184	191	199	206	213	221	258	294
73	144	151	159	166	174	182	189	197	204	212	219	227	265	302
74	148	155	163	171	179	186	194	202	210	218	225	233	272	311
75	152	160	168	176	184	192	200	208	216	224	232	240	279	319
76	156	164	172	180	189	197	205	213	221	230	238	246	287	328

[a] To determine body mass index (BMI), find the height in the left-hand column; then move across the row to a given weight. The number at the top of the weight column is the BMI for that height and weight.

[b] BMI Calculations: Weight (kg)/height (m^2) or weight (lb)/height ($in.^2$) × 703

Source: Reference 5; used with permission.

Table 21–2

Classification of Overweight and Obesity by Body Mass Index (BMI), Waist Circumference, and Associated Disease Risk

	BMI (kg/m²)	Disease Risk[a] Relative to Normal Weight and Waist Circumference[b]	
		Men ≤102 cm, Women ≤88 cm	Men >102 cm, Women >88 cm
Underweight	<18.5	—	—
Normal	18.5–24.9	—	—
Overweight	25.0–29.9	Increased	High
Obesity, class			
I	30.0–34.9	High	Very high
II	35.0–39.9	Very high	Very high
III (Extreme obesity)	≥40	Extremely high	Extremely high

[a] Disease risk for Type 2 diabetes, hypertension, and cardiovascular disease.

[b] Increased waist circumference can also be a marker for increased risk even in patients with normal weight.

Source: Reference 3.

relative risk for complications of obesity. Men with a BMI of 25 to 34.9 and a waist circumference greater than 102 cm (greater than 40 inches) are at risk for developing complications. Women with the same BMI values and a waist circumference greater than 88 cm (greater than 35 inches) are also at risk for developing complications.[3] Table 21–2 presents the associated disease risks of abdominal fat relative to BMI.

Epidemiology of Overweight and Obesity

Overweight and obesity are especially evident in some minority groups, as well as in people with lower incomes and less education. Estimates indicate that more than half of all adult non-Hispanic African American and Mexican American women in the United States are overweight.[3]

Research data suggest a genetic relationship for overweight and obesity. A child who has one obese parent has a 40% chance of being obese; if both parents are obese, the child's chance of being obese increases to 80%. A study of obesity in twins showed a 0.86 concordance for obesity.[6] This genetic relationship is evidenced by the extraordinarily high prevalence of obesity in Native Americans, particularly in Pima Indians.

The third National Health and Nutrition Examination Survey,[3] which was conducted from 1988 to 1991, found that 54.9% of adults 20 years of age or older are overweight or obese and that adolescents are increasingly overweight (21%). The data for adolescents, based on height and weight data collected from 1490 study participants who were between ages 12 and 19 years, show a 6% increase over the second study conducted from 1976 to 1980. This disturbing trend among adults and adolescents may be attributed to a decrease in physical exercise.

Etiology of Overweight and Obesity

Excess weight results from an imbalance between caloric intake and energy expenditure. Most cases of excess weight are associated with overeating, particularly of carbohydrates or fats. The calories ingested beyond those necessary for normal energy requirements usually are deposited and stored as fat. Although the physiologic controls of caloric intake have been difficult to define, the human body is known to aggressively respond to underweight with enhanced hunger and decreased metabolic rate. The body, however, poorly counteracts the accumulation of excess weight, which may derive from the age-old struggle for survival during which the primary risk to the species is death caused by famine rather than by excessive food.

Physiologic Factors

Two areas of the hypothalamus, the satiety center and the appetite center, control eating. Destroying the satiety center leads to marked overeating with subsequent obesity; obliterating the appetite center results in emaciation. Impulses from the satiety center may inhibit feedback of the appetite center after food is ingested. The glucostatic hypothesis of appetite regulation states that hunger is related to the degree to which glucose is used by glucostat cells. When the level of glucose use is low, the inhibitory effect on the appetite center is reduced, which increases the desire for food. Conversely, when glucose levels are high, the appetite center is inhibited and the desire for food intake is reduced.

The cerebral cortex regulates how an individual responds to the appearance, aroma, and taste of food. An obese patient's responses to these stimuli may be different from those of a person of normal weight. Endogenous opioids increase food intake in animals, and naloxone (an opioid antagonist) decreases food intake in animals and obese humans. In humans, opiate receptors, which exist in the taste pathways, are believed to modulate taste. Thus, an emerging hypothesis suggests that an endogenous opioid system is involved in human perceptions of taste. Research involving the trigeminal nerve, a pathway that relays sensory input from the oral cavity to the hypothalamus, supports this system's possible role in food intake. The trigeminal circuit senses oral touch, and the excessive nibbling common to obese individuals may be caused by their greater sensitivity to this stimulus.

Genetic Factors

Although a genetic role has not been proven in human obesity, it has been indicated in animal studies. In experimental animals, genetic transmission of obesity is associated with modified organ size and composition. Human data also suggest fundamental relationships between body build and obesity. Studies[3] reveal that obese women differ from nonobese women in morphologic characteristics other than the degree of adiposity (fat deposit). Specifically, obese women are more endomorphic than nonobese women. Their abdomen mass overshadows their thoracic bulk, all their body regions are soft and round, and their hands and feet are comparatively small.

Social and Environmental Factors

Obesity may result from environmental influences such as the widespread advertising of food products. Occupational, economic, sociocultural, and lifestyle factors may also be considered as environmental influences. Today, people have numerous labor-saving devices for work and for play. Moreover, leisure-time activities often involve passive entertainment such as watching television or playing computer games, rather than participating in active sports. A sedentary life and a lack of exercise contribute to the problem of obesity.

Psychologic Factors

Obesity has a psychogenic component in most cases. Although the psychologic aspect of caloric excess is usually exemplified by compulsive overeating to replace other gratifications, other factors are involved. Decreased physical activity, a sign of mental depression, may play a role. In fact, depression may not be an incidental occurrence in obese people but one of the main reasons for their obesity.

Complications of Obesity

Being overweight or obese substantially increases the risk for weight-related health problems. People who are overweight often suffer social and economic consequences such as social stigmatization and discrimination in the workplace.[7]

Health Risks

All overweight and obese adults (18 years of age or older) with a BMI of 25 or greater are considered at risk for developing associated morbidities or diseases such as hypertension, dyslipidemia, Type 2 diabetes, coronary heart disease, stroke, gallbladder disease, osteoarthritis, sleep apnea and other respiratory problems, and certain types of cancers.[3] Treatment of patients who are overweight but not obese is recommended only when patients have two or more risk factors.[3]

Cardiovascular Disease

Cardiovascular diseases (e.g., hypertension, myocardial infarct, heart failure, and coronary artery disease) and cerebrovascular diseases (e.g., stroke) are associated with obesity. The Framingham Heart Study[8] shows evidence of sustained hypertension in overweight people. Men who do not smoke and whose body weights were more than 10% above the ideal weight had 30-year mortality rates that were 3.9 times higher than those of men of normal weight. Therefore, people who are at high risk for hypertension, such as those with a family history of youthful obesity, should consider controlling their weight and reducing their salt intake. Evidence-based recommendations of the National Heart, Lung, and Blood Institute conclude that weight loss is recommended to lower elevated blood pressure in overweight and obese patients with high blood pressure.[3]

Diabetes Mellitus

The relationship between obesity and diabetes mellitus is well documented. (See Chapter 39, "Diabetes Mellitus.") An early study revealed that 85% of patients over age 40 years who developed diabetes mellitus were overweight. Glucose intolerance commonly occurs with obesity, and relative insulin resistance is noted in obese individuals, although insulin production may be normal or high. Obesity that persists over long periods is generally (1) associated with partial exhaustion of the beta cells and a resultant hypoinsulinemia of shorter duration and (2) related to increased body fat. Weight reduction leads to improved glucose tolerance in obese patients with diabetes and to reduced hyperinsulinemia in obese patients both with and without diabetes. Losing weight may also decrease or eliminate the severity of diabetes mellitus and the need for insulin or oral antidiabetic medications.

Strong evidence from clinical trials shows that weight loss produced by lifestyle modification reduces blood glucose levels in overweight and obese people without diabetes, and that weight loss reduces blood glucose levels and hemoglobulin A_{1c} levels in some patients with Type 2 diabetes. Thus, the National Heart, Lung, and Blood Institute panel recommends weight loss to lower elevated blood glucose levels in overweight and obese patients with Type 2 diabetes.[3]

Skin Disorders

Skin disorders (including candidiasis, tinea infections, furunculosis, pruritus vulvae, and trophic ulcerations) occur more often in individuals who are obese or who have diabetes mellitus. Entrapment of moisture in skinfolds, which produces a better culture medium for some microorganisms, is a contributing factor.

Cancer

In postmenopausal women, obesity appears to be positively associated with the risk of both breast and endometrial cancers. Obesity is also associated with increased estrogen production, which is proportionately more significant in postmenopausal women, because the ovaries no longer contribute to estrogen production. The peripheral aromatization of androstenedione (a major adrenal hormone) to estrone through the aromatase reaction in adipose tissue is the principal source of estrogen in postmenopausal women; an increased rate of this reaction has been reported in obese women. Excess estrogen production predisposes women to developing breast and endometrial neoplasms.

In men, the primary risk is from cancer of the prostate, and the second is from cancer of the colon. It is unclear whether the etiology of these cancers is secondary to obesity or secondary to some dietary component associated with obesity.

Hyperlipidemia

Using a review of 22 randomized controlled trials, the National Heart, Lung, and Blood Institute panel concludes that weight loss is recommended to lower elevated levels of total cholesterol, low-density lipoprotein cholesterol, and triglycerides, and to raise low levels of high-density lipoprotein cholesterol in overweight and obese persons with dyslipidemia.[3]

Respiratory Problems

Obesity may contribute to respiratory distress, impaired gas exchange, and pulmonary embolism. Obesity alters pulmonary function, which results in reduced lung volume, hypercapnia, and pulmonary hypertension. Charles Dickens's description of Joe, the fat boy in *The Pickwick Papers*, as obese and somnolent may be the first account of this condition in literature. The pickwickian syndrome describes a person who is obese, exhibits narcoleptic behavior, and has an excessive appetite.

Other Health Risks

Although obesity is generally caused by overeating, it may mask malnutrition. An obese individual may overconsume carbohydrates and fats while omitting proteins, vitamins, and minerals from the diet.

Obesity may predispose individuals to develop gout, may aggravate degenerative joint disease (osteoarthritis) in weight-bearing joints (e.g., knees and ankles), may produce or aggravate lower back pain, and may be associated with menstrual irregularities.[3]

Data on the health effects of repeated weight gains and losses, or weight cycling, are also inconclusive. Weight cycling appears to affect energy metabolism and may result in a faster regaining of weight, but the contention that weight cycling has long-term negative effects on psychologic and physical health is unconfirmed.

Social and Economic Consequences

Obesity may create a psychologic burden and may lead to low self-esteem. Dexterity, coordination, and mobility may be impaired, which can have serious implications on the job. Among very obese individuals, weight loss has been followed by greater functional status, reduced work absenteeism, less pain, and greater social interaction.

Treatment of Overweight and Obesity

For some individuals, losing weight or maintaining a weight loss is a life-long challenge. Dietary changes and increased exercise are the preferred weight-loss therapies. Anorexiants, including nonprescription agents, should be only short-term measures unless a physician supervises the weight-loss therapy.

Treatment Outcomes

The general goals of weight loss and management are to reduce body weight and maintain the weight loss. Prevention of further weight gain is an important goal for patients who are unable to achieve significant weight reduction.[3] Patients can usually maintain a moderate weight loss over time if they continue some form of therapy.

General Treatment Approach

The initial goal of weight-loss therapy should be to reduce body weight by approximately 10 percent.[3] If a patient is successful with this first step, additional weight loss can be attempted after further assessment. Unfortunately, experience reveals that lost weight is usually regained unless a weight-management program consisting of dietary therapy, physical activity, and behavior therapy is continued indefinitely. Efforts to maintain weight loss should be put in place after 6 months of weight-loss treatment. If more weight loss is needed, another attempt at weight reduction can be made. This renewed program may require further adjustment of the diet and physical activity. The algorithm in Figure 21–1 can assist the pharmacist in recommending appropriate weight-loss measures.

Weight loss is indicated for individuals with health problems (e.g., sleep apnea, hypertension, or Type 2 diabetes mellitus) that can be lessened by weight loss. However, unsupervised weight loss is contraindicated in individuals who are severely overweight, pregnant, or lactating; are under age 18 years or over age 65 years; or have medical conditions that make such an undertaking dangerous. Young patients should be under medical supervision to ensure that diet modification does not short change them of nutrients that are essential for growth and development. A properly trained physician should supervise a multidisciplinary

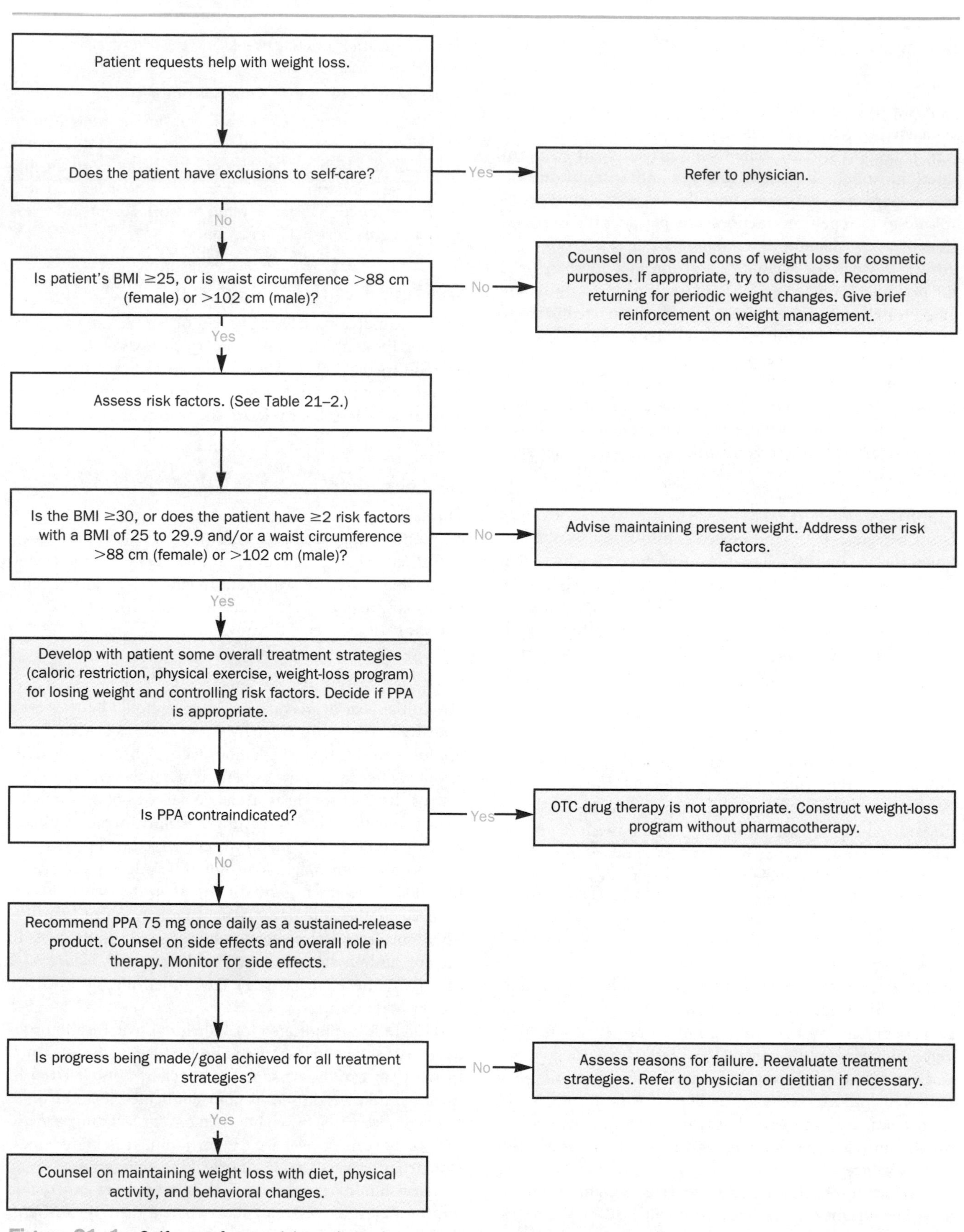

Figure 21–1 Self-care of overweight and obesity.

approach to a weight-loss process for individuals at high medical risk.

Nonpharmacologic Therapy

To avoid becoming overweight or obese, individuals must decide how much and what type of food to consume. Although physical activity alone produces less weight loss than caloric restriction, such activity is an important component of any weight-loss therapy.

Dietary Change

Dietary change is the most commonly used weight-loss strategy. Methods range from caloric restriction to changes in dietary proportions of fat, protein, and carbohydrate or use of macronutrient substitutes. Appropriate dietary programs can have positive health effects on factors other than weight loss. Short-term success for some of these methods has been documented, but information on their long-term effectiveness and safety for up to 5 years is limited. Weight loss at the end of relatively short-term programs can exceed 10% of initial body weight. However, there is a strong tendency to regain weight—as much as two-thirds of it within 1 year after completing a program and almost all of it after 5 years. Nonetheless, a small percentage of participants do maintain their weight loss over more extended periods. The duration of most dietary-change programs appears to be from several weeks to a few months. Dropout rates vary considerably but can be as high as 80%.[3]

Caloric Restriction Daily caloric allowances for moderately active individuals vary with age and sex. As a general rule, an intake of 3500 Cal (kcal) over expenditure will produce a weight gain of approximately 1 pound (0.453 kg), whereas an expenditure of 3500 Cal over intake will result in a loss of body fat of 1 pound (0.453 kg). Daily caloric intake allowances for average men (weight = 154 pounds, or 70 kg; height = 5 feet 10 inches, or 1.78 m) in a temperate climate range from 3200 Cal at age 25 years to 2550 Cal at age 65 years. Corresponding figures for average women (weight = 128 pounds, or 58 kg; height = 5 feet 4 inches, or 1.63 m) are 2300 and 1800 Cal at ages 25 and 65 years, respectively. The daily caloric requirement for women increases slightly during pregnancy (by 300 Cal) and significantly during lactation (by 500 Cal for one child and 1000 Cal for twins).[3]

A diet that is individually planned and takes into account the patient's overweight status to create a deficit of 500 to 1000 Cal/day should be an integral part of any weight-loss program.[3] Two levels of caloric restriction are commonly used. A low-calorie diet (LCD) of about 1000 to 1500 Cal per day may involve a structured commercial program with formulated and calorically defined food products or with guidelines for selecting conventional foods. A very low calorie diet (VLCD) of 800 or fewer calories per day is conducted under physician supervision and monitoring, and it should be restricted to severely overweight persons.

VLCDs and fasting are associated with numerous short-term adverse effects. Patients often report fatigue, hair loss, dizziness, and other symptoms that appear to be transitory. More serious is the increased risk for gallstones and acute gallbladder disease during severe caloric restriction.

Total fasting or semistarvation is sometimes proposed as a means of weight reduction in severely obese persons. However, starvation—either total or partial—depletes the body of some lean tissue (protein) and of essential electrolytes in addition to fat. The ketosis and ketoacidosis that result from fasting represent a significant metabolic alteration. If total fasting is used to treat obesity, then hospitalization and intensive medical supervision are recommended to deal effectively with the alteration of physiologic functions.

Altered Proportions of Food Groups High-protein, low-carbohydrate diets of 800 to 1000 Cal per day are often used in weight reduction programs. Low-carbohydrate diets have been advocated on the premise that individuals may eat as much as they desire as long as they ingest no carbohydrates. However, fat from food may be deposited as fat in the body, and proteins may be converted into fat. The excess metabolized fat may result in an increased production of ketones to the degree that ketosis, acidosis, and dehydration may occur.

Some low-carbohydrate diets recommend consumption of large quantities of fat. Although a high-fat diet may suppress fat synthesis, it does not prevent fat deposition. In addition, a high-fat diet can cause an elevation of serum lipids. Although a carbohydrate-free, high-fat diet does bring about an immediate weight reduction because of water loss (dehydration), it does not significantly affect adiposity. The "drinking-man's diet" adds alcohol to this regimen, which adds more calories and the increased liability of fat deposition. A high-meat (protein and fat), no-carbohydrate diet presents an extra burden to the kidneys because of the resultant increase in urea load. In addition, an increase in the uric acid levels in this diet may precipitate gouty arthritis in susceptible persons.

The number of injuries and deaths caused by extremely low calorie protein diets, which were once very popular in the United States, is difficult to determine. Complaints reported to the Food and Drug Administration (FDA) often included nausea, vomiting, diarrhea (from liquid preparations), constipation (from dry preparations), faintness, muscle cramps, weakness or fatigue, irritability, cold intolerance, decreased libido, amenorrhea, hair loss, dry skin, cardiac arrhythmias, recurrence of gout, dehydration, and hypokalemia. The possibility of drug–food interactions with these diets also exists. Patients who take prescription medicines such as diuretics, antihypertensives, hypoglycemic agents, insulin, adrenergics, high doses of corticosteroids, thyroid preparations other than those used in replacement therapy, and lithium should not use liquid protein diets.

A patient's age should be taken into consideration when planning extreme caloric restriction, because elderly obese persons may be more susceptible to cardiovascular stress, diabetes, and gout. Thus, the pharmacist should warn the patient not to undertake this type of diet without proper medical supervision.

A low-calorie, balanced diet containing no less than 12% to 14% protein, no more than 30% fat (preferably unsaturated), and the remainder composed of complex carbohydrates (with low amounts of sucrose) is recommended over unbalanced diets of questionable value that are also potentially dangerous.[3]

Use of Food Additives Some patients may use food additives such as artificial sweeteners and fat substitutes to reduce caloric intake. Saccharin and aspartame are the most widely used artificial sweeteners, but others are available.

Saccharin Saccharin, a sucrose substitute, is about 400 times sweeter than sucrose and contains no calories. Although it has a bitter taste to some individuals, it is the most popular artificial sweetener, especially since the nonregulated use of cyclamates was prohibited. Saccharin may have considerable importance in reducing caloric intake in some individuals. For instance, if one packet is used instead of one heaping teaspoonful of sugar to sweeten a cup of coffee, 33 Cal are removed from the diet.

Aspartame Aspartame is a synthetic dipeptide that is about 180 times as sweet as sugar. FDA has determined that it is safe as a food additive. However, patients who have phenylketonuria (i.e., cannot metabolize a metabolic product of phenylalanine) or who should avoid protein foods must be alerted that aspartame contains phenylalanine. Thus, products containing aspartame must carry the warning: "Phenylketonurics: Contains Phenylalanine." In addition, table products containing aspartame must have directions not to be used in cooking or baking (because aspartame loses its sweetness).

Other Sweeteners Fructose, sorbitol, and xylitol may be used as alternatives to saccharin, but they contain calories and should not be viewed as "sugar-free" diet items. Fructose and xylitol are sweeter than sucrose, whereas xylitol is less calorigenic and more expensive. Apparently, neither sorbitol nor xylitol causes tooth decay, and some products that contain xylitol have a pleasant taste. However, some evidence has implicated xylitol in the development of urinary tract abnormalities, kidney stones, and tumors in laboratory animals. Further tests are under way to evaluate this possibility. Ingestion of sufficient amounts of dietetic candies that contain sorbitol may result in an osmotic diarrhea in small children.

Several naturally occurring compounds show promise as substitutes for sucrose. Monellin, traumatin, and miraculin are plant proteins that are being investigated as possible sucrose substitutes.

Fat Substitutes Fat substitutes mimic the "mouth-feel" of fat but contain fewer calories. For example, Simplesse is a frozen dessert that has a blend of egg white, milk protein, or both, and is whipped to a creamlike consistency. It contains less than 1 g of fat per serving. Oatrim is a cholesterol-free fat substance designed to replace the fat in meats, cheeses, baked goods, and frozen desserts. Olestra looks and tastes like fat but is not absorbed by the body; because it is heat resistant, it can be used for cooking and frying.

Use of Low-Calorie Balanced Foods "Canned diet" products are considered as diet substitutes. One product typical of this group supplies 70 g of protein per day, an amount the manufacturer states "is the recommended daily dietary allowance of protein for normal adults." It also contains 20 g of fat and 110 g of carbohydrate in a daily ration for a total daily caloric intake of 900 Cal. Powder, granule, and liquid forms are available, as well as products that are formulated as cookies and soups.

These dietary products contain low sodium. Weight loss in the first 2 weeks is probably caused, in part, by water loss. It is questionable whether such weight loss over a short period is significant in the long-term treatment of obesity.

Pharmacists should be aware that products that substitute 900 Cal daily for a usual diet are usually effective. Moreover, it appears that any diet of 900 Cal that supplies adequate protein and lowers carbohydrate and fat intake should enable an obese patient to lose weight. Some manufacturers recommend that these products be used as substitutes for two or more meals a day, allowing the dieter to eat a "reasonable" regular meal at other times.

Many different dietary products are available in supermarkets, department stores, and other retail outlets. Some companies have developed complete lines of low-calorie products that can be used as calorie substitutes. The Slim-Fast line, for example, is heavily advertised and can be helpful to dieters who can follow the diet plan enclosed in the package.

Convenience and palatability of marketed products have improved in the past few years. Premixed liquids and easily dispersible powders have replaced older powder formulations, which required a blender to prepare the final mixture. Now, nutritional bars and other forms of calorie-substitute products are available to add variety. When used properly, Slim-Fast and similar products are efficacious and motivational in weight loss.

Commercial Weight-Loss Programs

More than 1 million people participate in weight-loss groups each week. The typical member of a commercial program is a woman between the ages 30 and 50 years who weighs 150 pounds to 176 pounds (68 kg to 80 kg). People who stay in such programs achieve modest weight losses: 4.8 to 15.6 pounds (2.2 to 7.0 kg) during the first 12 weeks and an additional 7.0 to 13.2 pounds (3.2 to 6.0 kg) during the next 12 weeks. However, fewer than 20% of participants stay in weight-loss programs long enough to lose an appreciable amount of weight.[5]

In one study of commercial weight-loss programs, men lost significantly more weight than women, people ages 21 to 51 years were slightly more successful than those on either side of that range, and people who worked outside the home fared better than those who did not.[9] In another study, encouragement from leaders and inclusion in a group were the most important factors in successful weight loss.[10] About one-third of self-help group members tend to reach their long-term goals.[5]

Many weight-loss programs include diets of 1000 to 1500 Cal per day in which projected weight loss averages 1 or 2 pounds per week (0.453 or 0.9 kg). Members usually follow a carefully controlled menu plan. In some cases, participants are required to purchase specially packaged meals that are available only from the company. These purchases usually are not reimbursable through health insurance plans. Costs for these programs vary considerably, and range from $250 to $1000 or more.

Physical Activity

An increase in physical activity is an important component of weight-loss therapy. Although most weight loss occurs because of decreased caloric intake, sustained physical activity helps prevent weight regain. The amount of weight loss that can be achieved by exercise programs alone—usually from 4 to 7 pounds (1.8 to 3.2 kg)—is more limited than the amount that can be obtained by caloric restriction. Unfortunately, data indicate that the percentage of adults who regularly exercise or play sports decreased between 1985 and 1990 among African American, Hispanic, lower-income, and unemployed persons.[5] Some patients may have underlying medical conditions, such as heart disease or severe arthritis, that might make some types of exercise ill advised.

Patients can start an exercise regimen by walking 30 minutes each day for 3 days a week and can build to 45 minutes of intense walking per day for at least 5 days a week. With this regimen, an additional expenditure of 100 to 200 Cal per day can be achieved. All adults should set a long-term goal to accumulate at least 30 minutes or more of moderate-intensity physical activity on most, and preferably all, days of the week. Other forms of physical activity can be practiced, but walking is particularly attractive because it is safe and accessible.[3] Table 21–3 lists the calories expended during 1 hour of various types of exercise.

Table 21–3

Caloric Expenditure Rates

Activity (1 hour)	Calories Expended
Bicycling (6 mph)	240
Bicycling (12 mph)	410
Cross-country skiing	700
Jogging (5.5 mph)	740
Jogging (7 mph)	920
Jumping rope	720
Running in place	650
Swimming (50 yd/minute)	500
Tennis (singles)	400
Walking (2 mph)	240
Walking (3 mph)	320
Walking (4.5 mph)	440

Behavioral Modification

Behavioral modification involves (1) identifying eating or related lifestyle behaviors to be modified, (2) setting specific behavioral goals, (3) modifying determinants of the behavior to be changed, and (4) reinforcing the desired behavior. Specific behavioral strategies include self-monitoring of both eating habits and physical activity, stress management, stimulus control, problem solving, contingency management, cognitive restructuring, and social support.[3] Behavioral modification can be undertaken through group or individual sessions, under the guidance of professional or lay personnel, or alone or in conjunction with other approaches. An emphasis on developing problem-solving skills and building social support (i.e., family, friends, group) is also important.

When used alone, a typical behavioral modification program takes about 18 weeks and can generate 1.0 to 1.5 pounds per week of weight loss. Typically about one-third of this weight will be regained at the end of 1 year, and most will be regained by 5 years after completing the program.

Pharmacologic Therapy

Weight-loss drugs approved by FDA for long-term use may be useful as an adjunct to diet and physical activity for patients with a BMI of greater than or equal to 30 and no concomitant obesity-related risk factors or diseases, as well as for patients with a BMI greater than or equal to 27 with concomitant risk factors or diseases. Using weight-loss drugs singly (not in combination) and starting with the lowest effective dose can decrease the likelihood of adverse effects from these agents.[3] The ideal appetite suppressant should have the following characteristics:[11]

- It should be safe and acceptable for long-term administration, as established by data documenting 6 months of efficacy and 2 years of safety.[11]
- It should produce a dose-related reduction in body fat.
- It should spare body protein and other body tissues.
- It should be free of significant side effects and abuse potential.

Unfortunately, no drug to date has met each of these stringent criteria.

Treatment of obesity with over-the-counter (OTC) drugs as a single strategy has limited value. All weight-loss drugs should be used with concomitant lifestyle modifications and continuous assessment of drug therapy for efficacy and safety. If a drug is efficacious in helping a patient lose and maintain weight loss and if there are no serious adverse effects, it may be continued.

In 1991, FDA issued a final rule establishing that 111 active ingredients in OTC weight-control products are not generally recognized as safe and effective.[12] The final monograph on OTC weight-control products includes only phenylpropanolamine (PPA) and benzocaine as Category I drugs.

Prescription drugs currently used in weight loss include dextroamphetamine and related drugs; mazindol, phentermine, and related drugs; sibutramine; and orlistat. The reader is directed to standard references for more information about these drugs.

Phenylpropanolamine

PPA is a sympathomimetic drug used in OTC weight control, cough/cold, nasal decongestant, and allergy drug products. It is best used by otherwise healthy but overweight patients who need help in adhering to a comprehensive weight-loss program centered around reducing caloric intake.

Similar to ephedrine, PPA stimulates both α-receptors and β-receptors and acts indirectly by releasing norepinephrine from peripheral nerve endings. PPA exerts predominantly peripheral adrenergic effects and weak stimulant actions on the central nervous system.

Indications FDA approved PPA as an appetite suppressant and as a nasal decongestant. FDA recommends that the product be used no longer than 3 months and that it be used in conjunction with a sensible weight-loss program. Product labeling stresses " . . . product's effectiveness is directly related to the degree to which you reduce your usual daily food intake." Most PPA-containing weight-loss products include a restricted-calorie diet in the package. Indeed, if the diet is followed, a patient will likely lose weight. A question remains as to what role the medication plays in helping a patient follow the diet suggestions.

Dosage/Administration Guidelines FDA permits a PPA dose of up to 25 mg in immediate-release products and up to 75 mg in sustained-release products. The maximum daily dose is set at 75 mg.[13] Self-treatment is not recommended for individuals between ages 12 and 18 years; instead, they should consult a physician before using PPA.

The adult dose of sustained-release PPA should be taken at mid-morning with a full glass of water. The immediate-release form is taken three times daily before meals.

Adverse Effects Side effects associated with PPA include nervousness, restlessness, insomnia, dizziness, perspiration, anxiety, headache, and nausea. An excessive increase in blood pressure may also occur, especially if the recommended dose is exceeded. Patients should immediately stop taking the medication if these symptoms occur during the weight-loss therapy.

Cardiovascular adverse reactions, including hypertensive episodes and stroke, have been reported following both excessive and recommended doses of products containing PPA alone or in combination with other drugs. Intracerebral hemorrhage and cerebral vasculitis have been associated with prolonged PPA use and with use at doses in excess of those recommended in package labeling. Various cardiac rhythm disturbances, myocardial infarct, and atrioventricular blockage have also been attributed to PPA.

Drug–Drug Interactions PPA is known to interact with monoamine oxidase inhibitors (MAOIs). Product labeling recommends that patients consult a physician about stopping MAOI therapy and then wait 2 weeks after stopping an MAOI before taking PPA. This time frame accounts for the prolonged pharmacodynamic effects of these drugs. Label instructions also advise that PPA should not be taken with any prescription medication except under the advice and supervision of a physician.

Contraindications/Precautions/Warnings Because PPA is found in other types of nonprescription medications, patients may receive an excessive dose of PPA. They should be warned not to take cough/cold or allergy medications containing any form of PPA or any oral nasal decongestant while taking the appetite suppressant. Patients being treated for depression, an eating disorder, enlarged prostate gland, heart disease, diabetes, thyroid disease, or any other diseases should use PPA only under a physician's supervision. Women who are pregnant or breast-feeding should also consult a physician before using PPA. Patients with high blood pressure should be advised to check their blood pressure regularly during the weight-loss therapy and to consult a physician if the values are high. Finally, PPA should not be taken by anyone who is hypersensitive to the agent.

Safety and Effectiveness Controversy has existed as to PPA's effectiveness as an anorectic agent. Early studies[11] indicated its usefulness in diminishing food intake in animals, and a qualitative difference has been reported between the anorectic activities of PPA and amphetamines. A meta-analysis of PPA clinical trials has indicated that PPA use results in weight loss in excess of placebo and somewhat less than that seen with prescription anorectics but, in any case, the weight loss was small.[14] Studies are lacking that evaluate the safety and efficacy of nonprescription anorectics beyond 12 to 14 weeks.

FDA has regularly been concerned about reports of hypertensive episodes and intracranial hemorrhage associated with the use of PPA. Despite lingering concerns, FDA has chosen not to seek removal of PPA from the market. Instead, it has proposed labeling requirements that would inform the public on when and how to use products containing PPA.[15] At the same time, nonprescription drug manufacturers have proposed a set of standards, and some companies are voluntarily including them on product labels. Additional information in the industry's proposal includes (1) the warning "If nervousness, dizziness, sleeplessness, palpitations, or headache occur, stop using this medication and consult your physician"; (2) a new, separate drug interaction for MAOIs; and (3) the warning "FDA believes that people under 18 years of age should not use an OTC weight-control drug product at all unless specifically directed by a doctor." Information in the sections

Case Study 21–1

Patient Complaint/History

Pamela, a 15-year-old high school student, and her mother approach the pharmacy counter. The mother wants to ask the pharmacist, whom she considers to be her neighborhood health expert, about the Dexatrim caplets she found in her daughter's backpack. Pamela says that she takes the diet product "to get rid of this ugly fat." The mother wants to know whether the product is addictive or otherwise harmful. According to her mother, Pamela, who is 5 feet 6 inches tall and weighs 128 pounds, is in good health except for seasonal allergies associated with certain blooming plants.

The package label identifies the diet product as Dexatrim Caffeine-Free Caplets; each caplet contains 75 mg of PPA in a sustained-release dosage form. Pamela reveals that she is also currently taking Dimetapp Allergy tablets "every so often"; the allergy medication was recommended by her pediatrician.

Clinical Considerations/Strategies

Readers can use the following considerations/strategies to determine whether treatment of the patient's condition with nonprescription medications is warranted:

- Ask the teenager why she thinks she needs to lose weight.
- Assess the teenager's self-image, and try to determine whether an underlying psychologic problem or other factors are behind her desire to lose weight. Be prepared to make appropriate referrals.
- Determine the teenager's goals or desired effects from using the appetite suppressant (e.g., weight loss or stimulant effects).
- Try to determine whether an underlying eating disorder is associated with the desire to lose weight.
- Determine whether the teenager is eating a nutritionally balanced diet and whether she has tried to lose weight by modifying her intake of high-caloric or high-fat foods, or both.
- Determine whether the teenager is experiencing adverse effects consistent with central nervous system stimulant toxicity (e.g., jitteriness, irritability, insomnia, dizziness).
- Determine whether other girls at the teenager's school are taking weight-loss products. If so, find out what products they are taking.

Patient Education/Counseling

Readers can use the following strategies to develop a patient education/counseling plan that will help ensure optimal therapeutic outcomes:

- Explain to the teenager and her mother the potential consequences of duplicating the intake of PPA, which is an active ingredient, in the allergy medication and the appetite suppressant.
- Explain to the teenager and her mother the potential consequences of taking a nonprescription product without fully understanding the potential risks and benefits of the product.
- Explain to the teenager and her mother the proper role of nonprescription products in weight-loss programs, as well as the limitations of such adjunctive products.

"Adverse Effects" and "Contraindications/Precautions/Warnings" would also be included on the label.

Product Selection Guidelines The pharmacist should point out that the choice of PPA-containing products is limited primarily to dosage forms and the number of doses. Some patients may prefer to take PPA once a day rather than three times a day. They may also prefer a particular dosage form. PPA is available in capsules, caplets, and tablets. Table 21–4 lists examples of products that contain this agent.

Benzocaine

Benzocaine was first incorporated into a weight-control preparation in 1958. Subsequently, the FDA's Advisory Review Panel on OTC Miscellaneous Internal Drug Products classified benzocaine as generally effective for short-term weight control. The panel determined that a dose of 3 to 15 mg for use in gum, lozenges, or candy just before food consumption was generally safe and effective for weight control. The theory as to how benzocaine worked was centered on its local anesthetic effects when it comes into contact with the oral mucosa, thus altering the taste of food. But the tablets and capsules of benzocaine are swallowed and, hence, do not have a local effect. The panel nevertheless included systemically acting benzocaine as a Category I active ingredient. However, the director of FDA's Monograph Review Staff does not agree with the advisory panel's assessment and has advised manufacturers of benzocaine-containing products about FDA's intent to classify the agent as an ineffective weight-loss product.[16] Citing serious design flaws in the clinical trials of oral benzocaine's efficacy, FDA has advised manufacturers that additional data from properly conducted, well-designed studies are required to provide evidence that benzocaine alone provides a statistically significant weight loss when compared with placebo. In response to this advisory letter, manufacturers have already removed benzocaine from their weight-loss products.

Nutritional Supplements

Some nonprescription appetite suppressants contain vitamins and minerals. Most well-balanced LCDs provide the

Table 21–4

Selected Appetite Suppressant Products

Trade Name	Primary Ingredient
Acutrim 16-Hour Steady Control Timed-Release Tablets	Phenylpropanolamine HCl 75 mg
Acutrim Maximum Strength Timed-Release Tablets	Phenylpropanolamine HCl 75 mg
Amfed T.D. Capsules	Phenylpropanolamine HCl 75 mg
Dexatrim Caffeine Free Extended Duration Timed-Release Tablets	Phenylpropanolamine HCl 75 mg
Dexatrim Caffeine Free Maximum Strength Timed-Release Caplets	Phenylpropanolamine HCl 75 mg
Dexatrim Caffeine Free with Vitamin C Timed-Release Caplets	Phenylpropanolamine HCl 75 mg
Dieutrim T.D. Capsules	Phenylpropanolamine HCl 75 mg
Protrim Caplets	Phenylpropanolamine HCl 37.5 mg
Protrim S.R. Caplets	Phenylpropanolamine HCl 75 mg

recommended daily allowances of vitamins and minerals. However, if a patient's diet regimen does not provide adequate levels of these substances, the pharmacist should recommend a once-daily vitamin tablet.

Use of Inappropriate Medications for Weight Loss

The desire to lose weight can lead some individuals to take drastic measures. The use of medications such as syrup of ipecac, laxatives, or diuretics to induce weight loss are among such measures.

Syrup of Ipecac Many people with eating disorders abuse syrup of ipecac to help induce vomiting. Ipecac, however, is indicated for treatment of accidental poisoning. Repeated use can weaken the heart muscle and cause cardiac arrhythmias, chest pain, respiratory difficulties, tachycardia, and cardiac arrest.

Laxatives Stimulant laxatives are the most common laxatives used by patients with eating disorders. Laxatives have little or no effect on reducing weight because the ingested calories have already been absorbed by the time a laxative takes effect. Prolonged use of laxatives can suppress the natural urge to have a bowel movement. Patients can experience severe constipation, severe abdominal pain, nausea, and vomiting. Death from electrolyte disturbances has occurred. (See Chapter 12, "Constipation," for further discussion of laxatives.)

Diuretics Diuretics are sometimes used to give the patient a feeling of weight loss. An initial weight loss may be noticed after taking a diuretic, but within a day or two, the body no longer responds to it. Electrolyte imbalances and sudden death can occur from repeated use.

Alternative Remedies

Dietary supplements, especially herbal weight-loss products, are very popular today. As evidence of safety and efficacy, proponents of these herbal remedies point to the long history of their use and to the fact that they are made of "natural" ingredients. Recently, however, FDA warned about the use of some botanical weight-loss products after receiving reports of adverse effects associated with their use.[17] In fact, Chapter 45, "Herbal Remedies," does not list any herbal products as safe and effective treatments for weight loss. Many herbal and other nutritional products do not undergo extensive premarket review of their safety or effectiveness. Reliable dosing information and monitoring advice are generally not available. Furthermore, there are no standards for potency and purity of ingredients.

Herbal Products

FDA is particularly concerned about products that contain multiple pharmacologically related ingredients, such as ma huang (*Ephedra sinica* or Chinese ephedra, a botanical source of ephedrine, pseudoephedrine, and norpseudoephedrine); guarana and kola nut (sources of caffeine); and white willow (a source of salicin). These products are touted for their stimulant effects and their ability to enhance metabolism, which leads to subsequent weight loss (so-called fat burners). As their use has expanded, however, FDA has received an increasing number of reports of adverse reactions associated with them. Reactions vary from milder effects known to be associated with sympathomimetic stimulants (e.g., nervousness, dizziness, tremor, alterations in blood pressure or heart rate, headache, and gastrointestinal distress) to chest pain, myocardial infarct, hepatitis, stroke, seizures, psychosis, or even death. Adverse reactions have been reported in young, otherwise healthy individuals as well as in patients with confounding or complicating conditions such as hypertension. In addition, a stimulant overdose syndrome has been reported in children and teenagers who have used these products.[17]

Weight loss products that are often marketed as "dieter's or slimming teas" contain a variety of strong botanical laxatives (*Cassia* species [senna], cascara sagrada [*Rhamnus purshiana*]), and diuretics. Adverse reactions reported to FDA as being associated with these products are characteristic of those seen in laxative abuse syndromes and include severe electrolyte imbalances that can lead to cardiac arrhythmia or death.

Protein-Sparing Modified Fast Diet

Promotional information on the Internet describes a particular protein-sparing modified fast diet as a "fast weight loss regimen" that consists of five servings of a powder spaced 2 to 3 hours apart. Each serving contains only 120 Cal, for a net daily caloric intake of 600 Cal. Such an extremely restricted caloric intake should never be used without medical supervision.

Chromium

Chromium is often promoted for weight loss. It is also used in the treatment of diabetes, as an ergogenic aid to increase strength and endurance, and for various other purposes. It is marketed either as a single-entity product (in oral or sublingual dosage forms) or in combination with other ingredients.

The recommended daily allowance for chromium is 50 mcg to 200 mcg; however, it is very difficult to get a valid assessment of human chromium balance. No toxicity has been reported from the oral administration of trivalent chromium salts (chromium picolinate is Cr^{+++}). In contrast, the hexavalent chromium compounds can be toxic if taken orally. In studies,[18] the median lethal dose of trivalent chromium by intravenous injection into rats varied between 10 and 30 mg/kg of body weight. Signs of toxicity from intravenous chromium chloride include nausea, vomiting, convulsions, and coma.

Chromium is considered a cofactor in maintaining normal lipid and carbohydrate metabolism. It is part of the glucose tolerance factor (GTF), which was first isolated from brewers' yeast. GTF contains one chromium atom in complex with single molecules of glycine, cysteine, and glutamic acid plus two molecules of nicotinic acid. The chromium atom is considered the active constituent of GTF. Picolinic acid, a metabolite of tryptophan, forms stable complexes with transitional metal ions such as chromium, which results in an improved bioavailability of the metal ion.

Chromium is essential for the efficient use of glucose in humans and animals. It likely plays an important role in maintaining normal glucose and lipid metabolism, but research defining its precise role is still under way. Although the medical literature contains numerous anecdotal and case reports describing the beneficial effects of GTF on glucose tolerance in patients with diabetes, few well-designed, controlled clinical trials have evaluated these effects. Even less evidence exists to support the use of chromium in weight-loss programs; its usefulness has merely been extrapolated from its apparent role in regulating glucose metabolism. Although it is probably safe, chromium is not a miracle weight-loss product.

Case Study 21–2

Patient Complaint/History

RM, a 47-year-old woman who is 5 feet 2 inches tall and weighs 182 pounds, comes to the pharmacy counter to ask about a miracle diet product. RM often asks the pharmacy staff about a new diet plan or product that she has read about. The latest product of interest purportedly allows its users to eat all they want without gaining weight. The patient remembers only that the product contains chromium.

Clinical Considerations/Strategies

Readers can use the following considerations/strategies to determine whether treatment of the patient's condition with nonprescription medications is warranted:

- Assess the patient's understanding of and expectations from medications or dietary products in producing weight loss versus traditional methods of weight loss, such as modifying eating habits, restricting high-calorie foods and snacks, decreasing consumption of high-fat foods, and exercising.
- Using typical weight standards, determine whether the patient is overweight. If she is, emphasize the health benefits of losing the extra weight.
- Determine the patient's weight loss goals.
- Assess the patient's past attempts at losing weight. Determine which methods, if any, worked well. Ask if the patient has a regular exercise program.
- Determine whether the patient has any chronic or acute illnesses and whether she is currently taking any prescription or nonprescription medications. If she is, determine whether she has consulted a physician about weight loss.

Patient Education/Counseling

Readers can use the following strategies to develop a patient education/counseling plan that will help ensure optimal therapeutic outcomes:

- Assess the patient's understanding of the role that diet and nutrition play in any weight-loss program, and stress the need for balancing caloric intake with caloric expenditure. Be prepared to refer the patient to a nutritionist or diet counselor.
- Determine whether the patient has a support group that will encourage her to adhere to a diet and maintain weight loss.
- Explain that medical evidence has not shown that taking chromium is a pharmacologically and therapeutically sound approach to weight loss. Determine whether reliable, objective published literature that is based on controlled clinical trials is available to support the safety and efficacy of such products.
- Assess whether an alternative weight-loss regimen is more appropriate.

Patient Assessment of Overweight and Obesity

When pharmacists are asked to recommend a weight-loss method or product, they should find out why the patient wants to lose weight. The reason may be immediately obvious for some patients; others may want to lose a few pounds to improve their appearance or to enhance their perception of their own good health. The pharmacist should review the patient's current prescription and nonprescription drug history and should ask about use of herbal products and other dietary supplements. Anyone with significant diseases superimposed on their obesity should be discouraged from using dietary supplements. The pharmacist should also find out what type of weight-loss methods were used previously and whether the attempts were successful so that other methods or adjunctive products may be considered, if needed.

A dieter needs support from family and friends to succeed at losing weight. It may be difficult to change eating and other behavioral habits if family members are not willing to support the dieter. Cultural differences and food preferences in different parts of the country may complicate weight-loss efforts. The pharmacist must explore the family dynamic before recommending weight-loss measures. Still, such factors should not be seen as insurmountable obstacles to weight loss.

Individuals who are within the height/weight range and are not obese but want to lose weight for other reasons (e.g., improved appearance or sense of well-being) should be advised about the difficulty of the task and about the potential adverse physical and psychologic effects.

Coupled with other information obtained during the assessment, the pharmacist can decide whether weight loss is appropriate and, if warranted, can select the type, intensity, and length of a weight-loss program. Asking the patient the following questions will help elicit the information needed to accurately assess whether a patient is overweight or obese and to recommend the appropriate treatment approach.

Q~ What is your age, height, and weight?

A~ *Identify the definitions of overweight and obesity using the BMI. (See the section "Clinical Indicators of Overweight and Obesity.")* Use the patient's information to calculate BMI and compare the calculated value with the definitions of overweight and obesity. Refer patients younger than 18 years or older than 65 years to a physician for supervision of any needed weight loss.

Q~ Why are you trying to lose weight?

A~ Refer extremely obese patients to a physician. (See Table 21–2 for criterion.) For other overweight or obese patients, continue the assessment process to determine whether exclusions to self-treatment exist or which weight-loss method to recommend. Advise underweight patients who think they need to lose weight that weight loss is not appropriate for them. Be aware that such patients may have an underlying eating disorder.

Q~ How long have you had a weight problem?

A~ Find out whether a decrease in activity level, stress, or psychologic problems may have triggered a weight gain. If the weight gain was sudden, refer patient to a physician to determine whether the weight gain is disease induced.

Q~ How many pounds overweight do you think you are?

A~ Use Table 21–1 to establish how many pounds the patient is overweight. Then help the patient set realistic weight-loss goals.

Q~ Do you have a family history of obesity? Do either of your parents have a weight problem?

A~ If a genetic component to overweight and obesity is indicated, determine whether the family supports the patient's weight loss and whether cultural preferences in foods may complicate weight-loss efforts. If family support is lacking, encourage the patient to establish a support network among friends, a community of resources, or a weight-loss program that supports safe and effective weight loss.

Q~ Do you eat a nutritionally sound diet? How much do you know about nutrition?

A~ If the patient is not knowledgeable about nutrition, advise that imbalances among the food groups can lead to malnourishment with serious consequences. Direct the patient to books or pamphlets on nutrition, or recommend consultation with a nutritionist or dietitian.

Q~ Have you consulted a physician about your desire to lose weight?

A~ If no, advise the patient to see a physician to rule out any underlying illness or complication. If the patient has not been successful losing weight in a physician-supervised weight-loss program, tactfully advise the patient that nonprescription management of obesity will probably not work either.

Q~ Are you, or have you been, on a diet to help you lose weight?

A~ If yes, and if the patient is adhering to a weight-loss diet but is not losing weight, advise the patient to see a nutritionist or dietitian for an appropriate diet. Advise the patient that nonprescription appetite suppressants work only in conjunction with restricted caloric intake.

Q~ What weight-loss preparations have you used previously? How well did they work?

A~ Consider success with previous weight-loss methods

when recommending another method. Explore how the products were used and explore ways to improve the results this time.

Q~ Do you have a regular exercise program? Does your physician recommend that you exercise?

A~ *Identify preexisting medical disorders that might make some types of exercise ill advised. (See the section "Physical Activity" under "Nonpharmacologic Therapy.")* Advise the patient to consult a physician if there is any doubt concerning the advisability of increased exercise.

Q~ Are you being treated for any chronic diseases?

A~ *Identify diseases or disorders that contraindicate the use of PPA. (See the section "Contraindications/Precautions/Warnings" under "Phenylpropanolamine.")* Advise patients with any of these conditions to use nonprescription appetite suppressants only under a physician's supervision.

Q~ What medications, both prescription and nonprescription, are you currently taking?

A~ *Identify medications that can interact with PPA. (See the section "Drug–Drug Interactions" under "Phenylpropanolamine.")* Advise patients taking these drugs to consult a physician before taking PPA. *Identify types of nonprescription medications that contain PPA. (See the section "Contraindications/Precautions/Warnings" under "Phenylpropanolamine.")* Advise the patient not to take such products while taking PPA.

Q~ Are you pregnant or lactating?

A~ *Identify the percentage of increase in calories that a pregnant or lactating woman needs. (See the section "Caloric Restriction" under "Nonpharmacologic Therapy.")* Refer a pregnant or lactating woman to a physician for specific diet recommendations that will meet the special nutritional needs of the woman and her developing baby.

Patient Counseling for Overweight and Obesity

Although the role of nonprescription appetite suppressants is limited, the pharmacist is in a key position to help people who wish to lose weight. The well-informed pharmacist can answer questions about weight-loss methods and products, help the patient set realistic weight-loss goals, and counsel

Patient Education for Overweight and Obesity

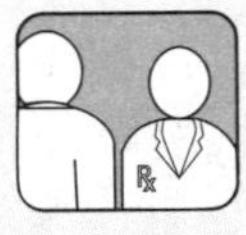

The objectives of self-treatment are to reduce body weight and maintain the weight loss over the long term. The objective for patients who are unable to lose weight is to prevent further weight gain. For most patients, carefully following product instructions and the self-care measures listed below, along with a continued adherence to a safe and effective weight-loss program, will help ensure the desired outcome.

Nondrug Measures

- Implement dietary changes, and increase physical activity to help you lose weight and establish new eating patterns.
- Eat a low-calorie, balanced diet containing no less than 12% to 14% protein, no more than 30% fat (preferably unsaturated), and the remainder composed of complex carbohydrates.
- Engage in 30 minutes or more of moderate-intensity physical activity on most—preferably all—days of the week.

Nonprescription Medications

- Do not exceed the recommended daily dosages of phenylpropanolamine (PPA). Stroke, seizure, heart attack, arrhythmia, psychosis, and death have been associated with the ingestion of PPA.
- Do not use this medication longer than 3 months.
- Do not take cough, cold, or allergy medications that contain PPA while taking the appetite suppressant.
- Do not take any prescription drug while taking the appetite suppressant, except under the advice and supervision of a physician.

Do not take PPA in the following situations:
—You are being treated for depression or an eating disorder. You have an enlarged prostate gland, heart disease, diabetes, thyroid, or any other disease. Take PPA only under the supervision of a physician.
—You have any of these symptoms: nervousness, dizziness, sleeplessness, palpitations, or headache. If any of these symptoms occur, stop taking PPA and consult your physician.
—You have high blood pressure. Check your blood pressure regularly. If it is high, consult your physician.
—You are pregnant or breast-feeding. First seek the advice of a health professional.
—You are hypersensitive to any of this product's ingredients.
—You are taking a prescription monoamine oxidase inhibitor for depression. PPA can be taken 2 weeks after you stop taking the antidepressant; however, consult your physician before discontinuing the antidepressant.

the patient on the proper use of medications and nutritional supplements. The pharmacist may refer the patient to a dietitian for evaluation and diet management and may help monitor the patient for adverse events that may occur during therapy.

When recommending a nonprescription product for weight control, the pharmacist should stress that a long-term commitment is required. The patient must change eating and exercises habits, and must realize that the product is only an adjunct to a planned weight-reduction program. The pharmacist should then advise the patient about the caloric value of various food types and the appropriate proportions for each type. If nonprescription products are recommended, the pharmacist should instruct the patient about the proper use of the product and about signs and symptoms of adverse effects. The box "Patient Education for Overweight and Obesity" lists specific information to provide patients.

Some people, especially adolescent girls, attempt weight loss when, in fact, they are already at their normal weight. By carefully monitoring all purchases of nonprescription weight-loss products, diuretics, laxatives, and ipecac, the pharmacist can spot the beginnings of an eating disorder and even take necessary steps to get help for the patient.

One of the biggest challenges for the pharmacist is answering questions about diets that patients have heard about in the media, on the Internet, or from a friend or neighbor. Such diets may appeal to patients who have failed with other weight-loss methods. Patients can fall victim to seemingly plausible but scientifically invalid concepts, such as the efficacy of a particular food or chemical to break down fat, increase metabolism, or prevent absorption. Rather than sell products of unproven efficacy or safety, the pharmacist can help patients evaluate promotional literature before they invest large sums in products that, at best, are worthless and, at worst, could cause harm. Accordingly, the pharmacist should advise patients to be wary of programs that do the following:

- Make exaggerated health claims for particular nutrients or nutrient combinations.
- Make unsubstantiated and false claims.
- Invent a physiologic process to impress the consumer.
- Use advertising hooks or gimmicks.
- Offer unorthodox treatments or diagnostic methods.
- Promise quick results for little effort by using so-called breakthrough formulas.
- Advertise their method through anecdotal data, testimonials, one-sided radio or television talk shows and infomercials, or unpublished or unscientific data.
- Preach their version of good nutrition and blame a conspiracy of organized medicine for criticizing their discovery.

CONCLUSIONS

A patient should recognize that a successful weight-reduction program includes reduced caloric intake, increased physical activity, and possibly a pharmacologic aid such as a nonprescription product. The patient should also know that the effectiveness of such a program depends largely on personal motivation, education, and acceptance of a regimen necessary to achieve long-term weight control. The pharmacist's role is to supply pertinent and accurate information regarding methods of weight loss and their relative merits. The pharmacist should advise patients about health risks of being overweight and should encourage the dieter during the difficult days ahead. The pharmacist should also help people avoid being victimized by fraudulent products and methods.

References

1. Kolbe LJ. An epidemiological surveillance system to monitor the prevalence of youth behaviors that most affect health. *Health Educ Q.* 1990;21: 44–8.
2. Remington PL, Smith MY, Williamson DF, et al. Design, characteristics, and usefulness of state-based behavioral risk factor surveillance, 1981–1987. *Public Health Rep.* 1988;103 : 366–75.
3. National Institutes of Health, National Heart, Lung and Blood Institute. *Clinical Guidelines on the Identification, Evaluation, and Treatment of Overweight and Obesity in Adults.* Bethesda, MD: National Institutes of Health; 1998.
4. 1983 Metropolitan Height and Weight Tables. In: *Statistics Bulletin.* New York: Metropolitan Life Insurance Co; 1984;64:2–9.
5. NIH Technology Assessment Conference Panel. Methods for voluntary weight loss and control. Consensus Development Conference, 30 March to 1 April 1992. *Ann Intern Med.* 1993;119(7 Part 2):764–70.
6. Stunkard AJ, Foch TT, Hrubec Z. A twin study of human obesity. *JAMA.* 1986;256:51–4.
7. Gortmaker SL, Must A, Perrin JM, et al. Social and economic consequences of overweight in adolescence and young adulthood. *N Engl J Med.* 1993;329:1008–12.
8. Kannel WB, Brand N, Skinner JJ Jr, et al. The relationship of adiposity to blood pressure and development of hypertension. The Framingham Heart Study. *Ann Intern Med.* 1967;67:48–59.
9. Stuart RB. Self-help group approach to self-management. In: Stuart RD, ed. *Behavioral Self-Management: Strategies, Techniques, and Outcomes.* New York: Brunner/Mazel; 1977:278.
10. Ashwell M, Garrow JS. A survey of three slimming and weight control organizations in the UK. *Nutrition.* 1975;29:347–56.
11. Bray GA. Use and abuse of appetite-suppressant drugs in the treatment of obesity. *Ann Intern Med.* 1993;119(7 Part 2):707–13.
12. *Federal Register.* 1996;61:5912.
13. *Federal Register.* 1982;47:8466.
14. Greenway FL. Clinical studies with phenylpropanolamine: a metananalysis. *Am J Clin Nutr.* 1992;55(1 suppl):203S–5S.
15. *Federal Register.* 1996;61:5911.
16. Gilbertson WE. *Benzocaine's Status as an OTC Active Ingredient* [FDA advisory letter]. Rockville, MD: Food and Drug Administration; April 7, 1993.
17. *FDA Medical Bulletin.* 1994;24:3.
18. Robinson CH, Lawler MR. *Normal and Therapeutic Nutrition.* 16th ed. New York: Alan R. Liss; 1980.

Section VII

Ophthalmic, Otic, and Oral Disorders

CHAPTER 22

Ophthalmic Disorders

Mark W. Swanson

Chapter 22 at a Glance

Editor's Note: This chapter is based, in part, on the 11th edition chapter titled "Ophthalmic Products," which was written by Mark W. Swanson and Jimmy D. Bartlett.

The nonprescription ophthalmic market consists of products that treat a wide range of disorders. Few population-based data are available on the epidemiology of these diverse disorders. People with such conditions are commonly seen in both the eye practitioner's office and the pharmacy. Ocular discomfort associated with dry eye may be the most common condition for which nonprescription ophthalmic products can be used. It may affect as many as 4.3 million people in the United States and 20% of all elderly people.[1]

Many common conditions causing ocular discomfort are minor and self-limiting. In some instances, however, relatively minor symptoms may be associated with severe, potentially blinding conditions. Pharmacists should be well versed in eye anatomy and physiology as well as in common ocular conditions so they can provide the best possible guidance for patients who want help in choosing between self-treatment or professional medical care.

Self-treatable ophthalmic disorders occur primarily on the eyelids; however, a few disorders of the eye surface are amenable to self-treatment. Self-care of the eye surface includes these disorders: dry eyes, allergic conjunctivitis, viral conjunctivitis, diagnosed corneal edema, presence of loose foreign debris, minor ocular irritation, and diagnosed age-related macular degeneration. Eye-surface disorders also includes the cleaning or lubricating of artificial eyes. Self-care of the eyelid covers contact dermatitis, lice infestations, hordeolum and chalazion, and blepharitis.

The pharmacist's greatest challenge in self-care of ophthalmic disorders is determining which disorder is indicated by the symptoms. For that reason, patient assessment is covered in one section: "Patient Assessment of Ophthalmic Disorders." Collective discussions of patient counseling and evaluation of patient outcomes for the various self-treatable disorders are also presented at the end of the chapter.

Eye Anatomy and Physiology

The external location and exposure of the eye make it susceptible to environmental and microbiologic contamination. However, the eye has many natural defense mechanisms to protect it against contamination, and the eyelid is one of its major protective elements. (See Figure 22–1.)

The eyelids are a multilayer tissue covered externally by the skin and internally by a thin, mucocutaneous epithelial layer: the palpebral conjunctiva. The intermediate portion of the eyelid contains glandular tissue and muscles for lid closing and opening. The five main types of glandular tissue found within the eyelid, along with conjunctival goblet cells, secrete the bulk of nonstimulated tears.

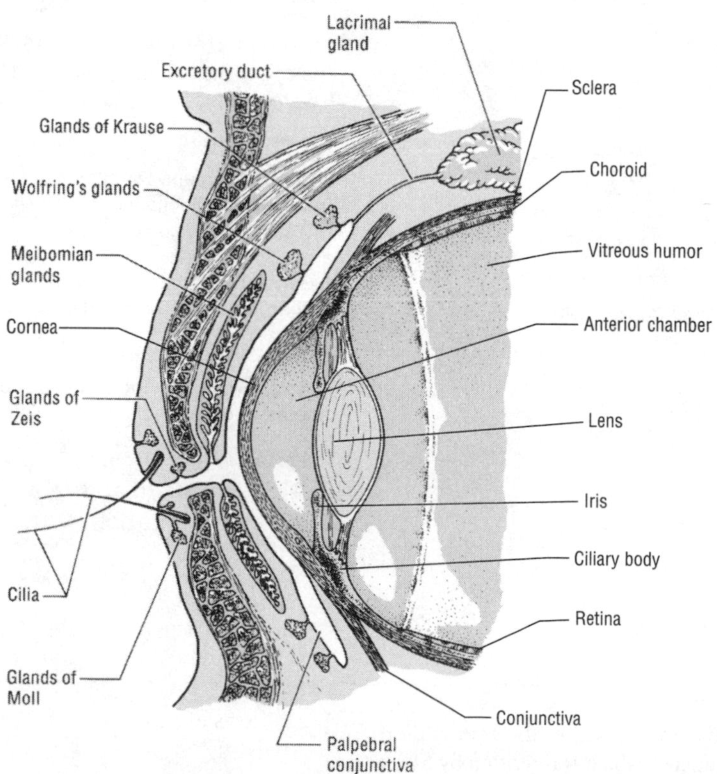

Figure 22–1 Anatomy of the eyelid and eye surface.

The eyelids primarily protect the front surface of the eye and spread the tears produced by the glandular tissue. The lids force the flow of tears toward the nose, where drainage canals are located in the upper and lower eyelids. The drainage canals converge, forming the lacrimal sac between the inner eyelid and nose. The lacrimal sac is drained by a canal opening just below the inferior turbinate of the nasal cavity. A highly vascularized epithelium lines the lacrimal drainage system, and absorption into the systemic circulation along this pathway gives rise to potential systemic effects of topically administered eye medications.[2]

The tear layer keeps the ocular surface lubricated, provides a mechanism for removing debris that touches the ocular surface, and has a potent antimicrobial action provided by specific enzymes and a number of immunoglobulins (Ig), notably IgA. The tear layer is a complex multilayer film. The outer lipid layer maintains the optical properties and reduces evaporation. The middle aqueous layer is largely responsible for the wetting properties of the tear film. The inner mucinous layer allows the aqueous and lipid layers to maintain constant adhesion across the cornea and conjunctiva. Abnormalities within any one of the tear components can result in ocular discomfort.

Tears are produced at a rate of 1 to 2 mcL/min, with a turnover of approximately 16% total volume per minute.[3,4] As much as 25% of total tear volume is lost to evaporation.[3] An ambient tear volume of approximately 7 to 10 mcL is found on the ocular surface at any point in time.[3] During episodes of ocular irritation, reflex tearing is stimulated by the lacrimal gland found underneath the outer portion of the upper eyelid, and tear production increases to more than 300% of the nonstimulated production rate.[5] Reflex tearing occurs immediately upon the instillation of a drug into the eye, diluting the drug's concentration. Studies have shown that as much as 90% of an instilled dose administered to the eye may be lost.[6]

The visible external portion of the eye is composed of the cornea and sclera. The sclera is a tough, collagenous layer that gives the eye rigidity and encases the internal eye structures. The visible sclera is covered by two epithelial layers: the episclera and the bulbar conjunctiva. The bulbar conjunctiva is contiguous with the palpebral conjunctiva at the junction between the eyelid and the ocular surface (the fornix). The episcleral and bulbar conjunctival layers contain the vascular and lymphatic systems of the anterior eye surface and are the source of visible eye redness during ocular irritation or inflammation.

The cornea is an aspherical, avascular tissue that is the principal refractive element of the eye. It is approximately 12 mm wide and 0.5 mm thick and consists of five distinct layers. The unique anatomic structure of the cornea affects drug absorption. The corneal epithelium is lipophilic and facilitates the passage of fat-soluble drugs. The corneal stroma is hydrophilic and allows the passage of water-soluble drugs. Damage to the corneal epithelium may markedly change drug absorption rates. Comparative studies with intact and compromised epithelium have shown that drug penetration into the aqueous humor may be increased by as much as threefold in corneas with compromised epithelium.[7] Corneal epithelium can be compromised by trauma, routine contact lens wear, topical ophthalmic anesthetics, and thermal or UV light exposure.

Directly behind the cornea is the anterior chamber, a cavity filled with aqueous humor. The aqueous humor maintains the normal internal eye pressure and provides nutritional support for the cornea and crystalline lens. It is produced by the ciliary body and is drained from the anterior chamber through the trabecular meshwork, which is located at the junction of the cornea and iris. During episodes of internal eye inflammation, many inflammatory cells may block the drainage system, causing the internal eye pressure to rise. Similarly, during episodes of angle-closure glaucoma, the iris physically blocks the trabecular meshwork, thereby causing an increase in intraocular pressure. Dilating of the pupil with mydriatics may precipitate the angle-closure attack. Such an attack often occurs as the pupil is returning to its normal state several hours after the mydriatic has been instilled. Any agent with anticholinergic effects has the potential to cause angle closure. The most common symptoms are brow-ache or headache, often accompanied by nausea and vomiting. These symptoms are typically severe enough to cause the individual to visit an eye doctor.

The iris is the visible colored portion of the eye. It functions in much the same way as an aperture on a camera to regulate the amount of light striking the retina. The central opening in the iris is the pupil. The pupillary diameter is controlled by two opposing muscles within the iris: the sphincter and the dilator. Prostaglandins released by the iris during episodes of inflammation may affect the sphincter muscle, resulting in constriction of the pupil. This constriction may help distinguish simple external irritation from more severe internal inflammation.

The ciliary body is bordered anteriorly by the iris and is continuous posteriorly with the choroid. Besides aqueous production, it focuses the optical mechanism (lens) for near viewing. During episodes of ocular inflammation, the ciliary muscle may begin to spasm, resulting in fluctuating vision and pain. Thus, inhibition of the ciliary muscle (cycloplegia) using anticholinergic agents is a frequent treatment during internal ocular inflammation.

The vitreous humor is the largest portion of the eye. The ubiquitous problem of floating spots in the vision ("floaters") is related to this area. Problems in this area are not susceptible to self-treatment and require professional evaluation because of the possibility of concurrent retinal problems.

The retina is responsible for the initial processing and transmission of the light signal. A number of inflammatory conditions of the retina can occur, and most have prominent symptoms. Some, however, have relatively mild symptoms mimicking common irritative conditions. Trauma, even minor, may cause the retina to separate from its underlying layer, the pigment epithelium, thereby resulting in retinal detachment. The retinal pigment epithelium provides vital vascular support to the retina. Macular degeneration, the leading cause of blindness in the United States, is directly related to atrophy in the pigment epithelium.

Dry Eye

Etiology/Signs and Symptoms of Dry Eye

Dry eye is among the most common disorders affecting the anterior eye. Dry eye is most often associated with the aging process, but it can also be caused by lid defects, loss of lid tissue turgor, Sjögren's syndrome, Bell's palsy, various collagen diseases such as rheumatoid arthritis, and systemic medications. Antihistamines, anticholinergics or drugs with anticholinergic properties (e.g., antihistamines and antidepressants), diuretics, and beta-blockers are some of the more common pharmacologic causes of dry eye. The condition may be exacerbated by environmental conditions such as dry, dusty working situations, or by heating and air conditioning systems that increase evaporation of the tears.

A white or mildly red eye characterizes this condition, and the patient may complain about a sandy, gritty feeling or a sensation that something is in the eye. Contrary to what the name suggests, dry eye is often accompanied by excess tearing. Abnormalities in the tear layer cause less than optimal lubrication of the ocular surface, thus producing more inadequate tears, and beginning a vicious cycle.

Treatment of Dry Eye

Treatment Outcomes

The goal in treating dry eye is to alleviate the dryness of the ocular surface, thereby relieving the symptoms associated with this disorder.

General Treatment Approach

The primary self-treatment for dry eye is the use of ocular lubricants. The availability of synthetic chemicals suitable for topical application to the eye has resulted in the development of various solutions (artificial tears) to help alleviate dryness of the ocular surface. Bland (nonmedicated) ophthalmic ointment is another type of ocular lubricant. Vitamin A preparations are also available for treating dry eye. Nonpharmacologic measures can increase eye comfort for patients with this disorder.

Optometrists or ophthalmologists may treat the most severe cases of dry eye with ocular inserts or sodium hyaluronate, or by occlusion of the lacrimal drainage system to increase the available tear pool.

Nonpharmacologic Therapy

The primary nondrug measure is avoiding environments that increase evaporation of the tear film. If possible, the patient should avoid dry or dusty places. Using humidifiers or repositioning work stations away from heating and air conditioning vents may help alleviate dry eyes.

Pharmacologic Therapy

Nonmedicated ointments are the mainstay of treating minor ophthalmic disorders, including dry eye. Because of the serious vision limitations this agent can cause, combination therapy of artificial tears and nonmedicated ointments is usually recommended. The effectiveness of retinol solutions in treating dry eye is still speculative.

Artificial Tear Solutions

Although science has made many advances in understanding the mechanisms involved in tear film formation, the role of tears in maintaining a normal conjunctival and corneal surface is still not completely understood. Lubricants formulated as solutions consist of preservatives, inorganic electrolytes to achieve tonicity and maintain pH, and water-soluble polymeric systems. The artificial tear products are similar, but buffering agents, preservatives, pH, and other formulation factors may vary. (See Table 22–1 for examples of these products.) One class of ophthalmic vehicles is the substituted cellulose ethers, which includes hydroxymethylcellulose (HPMC), hydroxyethylcellulose (HEC), hydroxypropylcellulose (HPC), methylcellulose, and carboxymethylcellulose. These solutions are colorless and vary in viscosity. Polyvinyl alcohol (PVA) and povidone are two other commonly used vehicles. The section "Formulation Considerations for Ocular Lubricants and Other Ophthalmic Products" discusses ophthalmic vehicles, preservatives, and excipients in greater detail.

Indications/Mechanism of Action Perhaps the most important property of the cellulose ethers in artificial tear formulations is that they stabilize the tear film, which prevents tear evaporation. Both effects are beneficial for patients with dry eye.[8] These vehicles also enhance drug action by providing increased viscosity. The increased viscosity retards drainage of the active ingredient from the eye, thus increasing the retention time of the active drug and enhancing bioavailability at the external ocular tissues. These effects generally occur without irritation or toxicity to the ocular tissues. Like the cellulose ethers, PVA also enhances stability of the tear film without causing ocular irritation or toxicity.

Povidone has surface-active properties similar to those of the cellulose ethers. This compound is thought to form a hydrophilic layer on the corneal surface, mimicking natural conjunctival mucin. This "mucomimetic" property has firmly established the role of povidone as an artificial tear formulation. Because this agent promotes wetting of the ocular surface, both mucin- and aqueous-deficient dry eyes seem to benefit from its use.

Table 22–1

Selected Ophthalmic Lubricants

Artificial Tear Solutions	
Accu-Tears PVA	Polyvinyl alcohol 1.4%; benzalkonium chloride
Adsorbotear[a]	Povidone 1.67%; hydroxyethyl cellulose 0.41%; thimerosal 0.004%
Akwa Tears[b]	Polyvinyl alcohol 1.4%; benzalkonium chloride 0.01%
AquaSite	Dextran 70, 0.1%; polycarbophil; sorbic acid 0.2%
AquaSite Preservative Free[b]	Dextran 70, 0.1%; polyethylene glycol 400, 0.2%
Bion Tears[b]	Hydroxypropyl methylcellulose 0.3%; Dextran 70, 0.1%
Celluvisc[a]	Carboxymethylcellulose sodium 1%
Computer Eye Drops	Glycerin 1%; benzalkonium chloride 0.01%
Dakrina	Polyvinyl alcohol 2.7%; povidone 2%; Busan 1507, 0.001%
Dwelle	Polyvinyl alcohol 2.7%; povidone 2%; NPX 0.001%
GenTeal Lubricant	Hydroxypropyl methylcellulose; sodium perborate
Hypo Tears	Polyvinyl alcohol 1%; polyethylene glycol 400; benzalkonium chloride 0.01%
Hypo Tears Preservative Free[b]	Polyvinyl alcohol 1%; polyethylene glycol 400
Liquifilm Tears	Polyvinyl alcohol 1.4%; chorobutanol 0.5%
Moisture Eyes	Propylene glycol 1%; glycerin 0.3%; benzalkonium chloride 0.01%
Moisture Eyes Preservative Free[b]	Propylene glycol 0.95%
Murine Tears Lubricant	Povidone 0.6%; polyvinyl alcohol 0.5%; benzalkonium chloride
Murocel Lubricant Ophthalmic	Methylcellulose 1%; propylene glycol; methylparaben 0.023%; propylparaben 0.01%
Ocucoat Lubricating	Hydroxypropyl methylcellulose 0.8%; Dextran 70, 0.1%; benzalkonium chloride 0.01%
Ocucoat PF Lubricating[b]	Hydroxypropyl methylcellulose 0.8%; Dextran 70, 0.1%
Refresh	Polyvinyl alcohol 1.4%; povidone 0.6%
Refresh Tears	Carboxymethylcellulose sodium 0.5%; Purite (stabilized oxychloro complex)
Tearisol	Hydroxypropyl methylcellulose 0.5%; benzalkonium chloride 0.01%
Tears Naturale	Hydroxypropyl methylcellulose 0.3%; Dextran 70, 0.1%; benzalkonium chloride 0.01%
Tears Naturale Free[b]	Hydroxypropyl methylcellulose 0.3%; Dextran 70, 0.1%
Tears Naturale II	Hydroxypropyl methylcellulose 0.3%; Dextran 70, 0.1%; polyquad 0.001%
Tears Plus	Polyvinyl alcohol 1.4%; povidone 0.6%; chlorobutanol 0.5%
Ultra Tears	Hydroxypropyl methylcellulose 1%; benzalkonium chloride 0.01%
Nonmedicated Ointments	
Accu-Tears	White petrolatum; light mineral oil
Akwa Tears	White petrolatum; mineral oil; lanolin
DuraTears Naturale	Petrolatum; mineral oil; lanolin
Hypo Tears	White petrolatum; light mineral oil
Lacri-Lube N.P.[b]	White petrolatum 57.3%; mineral oil 42.5%; lanolin alcohols
Lacri-Lube S.O.P.	White petrolatum 56.8%; mineral oil 42.5%; lanolin alcohols; chlorobutanol 0.5%
Moisture Eyes PM[b]	White petrolatum 80%; mineral oil 20%
Refresh P.M.[b]	White petrolatum 56.8%; mineral oil 41.5%; lanolin alcohols

[a] Product contains thimerosal.
[b] Product is preservative free.

Studies have shown that preparations without preservatives have a greater beneficial effect on the ocular surface than do those with preservatives.[9]

Dosage/Administration Guidelines Most patients with mild cases of dry eye instill drops of artificial tears once or twice per day, typically on arising in the morning and/or before bedtime.[10] (See Table 22–2.) Recommending drops twice per day is a good starting point. The viscosity of the drops, amount used, and presence of preservative can then be regulated from that point. For more severe cases, the dosage can be increased to three to four times daily, and if the patient's clinical needs and response to therapy indicate more frequent use, these solutions may be given as often as hourly.

Adverse Effects Use of ocular lubricants is a balance between the number of drops per day, the viscosity of the recommended solution, and the presence of a preservative. As the number of drops per day increases, toxicity from preservatives becomes more likely.[11]

Although PVA is compatible with many commonly used drugs and preservatives, certain compounds (including sodium bicarbonate; sodium borate; and the sulfates of sodium, potassium, and zinc) can thicken or gel solutions that contain it. For example, sodium borate is found in some extrocular irrigating solutions, or irrigants, and may react with contact lens wetting solutions containing PVA.[12] Thus, it is important to be cautious when clinically using solutions that contain PVA, which may have these other agents.

Nonmedicated Ophthalmic Ointments

The primary ingredients in available nonprescription ophthalmic ointments are white petrolatum, mineral oil, and lanolin. (See Table 22–1 for examples of these products.)

Mechanism of Action/Indications The principal advantage of nonmedicated (bland) ointments is their enhanced retention time in the eye, which appears to enhance the integrity of the tear film. Thus, both mucin- and aqueous-deficient eyes can benefit from the application of lubricating ointments.

Dosage/Administration Guidelines Ointment formulations are usually administered twice daily. (See Table 22–3.) However, depending on the patient's clinical needs and therapeutic response, ointments may be administered as often as every few hours or only occasionally, as needed. Many patients prefer to instill the ointment at bedtime to keep the eyes moist during sleep and to improve morning symptoms of dry eye.

Adverse Effects Because of the viscosity of the melted ointment base in the tear film, many patients complain of blurred vision during ointment therapy. This problem can usually be resolved by decreasing the amount of ointment instilled or by administering the ointment at bedtime. Counseling about blurred vision caused by ointments should be a routine component of dispensing.

Ointment preparations are generally nonirritating, but preservatives can be toxic to ocular tissues. Some patients develop hypersensitivity reactions, which may prompt them to discontinue therapy. Changing to nonpreserved formulations can often eliminate symptoms associated with preserved ointment products, which is particularly helpful for long-term treatment. As a rule for the treatment of dry eye, it is better to recommend nonmedicated ointments without preservatives so the patient avoids the potential problems of preserved products.

Table 22–2

Administration Guidelines for Eyedrops

1. If you have difficulty telling whether eye drops touch the eye surface, refrigerate the solution before instilling it.
2. Wash hands thoroughly.
3. Tilt head back.
4. Gently grasp lower outer eyelid below lashes, and pull eyelid away from eye to create a pouch.
5. Place dropper over eye by looking directly at it as shown in the drawing.
6. Just before applying a single drop, look up.
7. After applying the drop, look down for several seconds.
8. Release the eyelid slowly.
9. Close eyes gently for 1 to 2 minutes. Minimize blinking or squeezing the eyelid.
10. Use a finger to put gentle pressure over the opening of the tear duct.
11. Blot excessive solution from around the eye.
12. If multiple drop therapy is indicated, wait at least 5 minutes before instilling the next drop. This pause helps to ensure that the first drop is not flushed away by the second, or that the second drop is not diluted by the first.
13. If both drop and ointment therapy are indicated, instill the drops at least 10 minutes before the ointment so that the ointment does not become a barrier to the drops' penetrating the tear film or cornea.

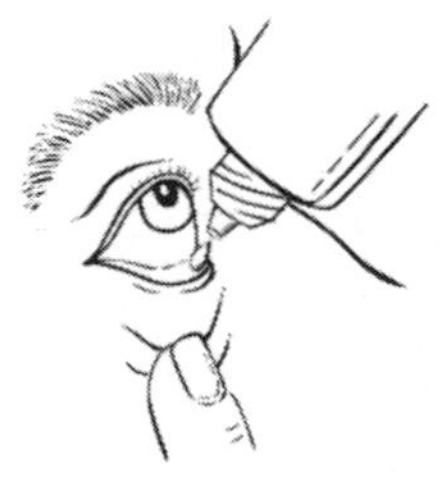

Table 22-3

Administration Guidelines for Eye Ointments

1. Wash hands thoroughly.
2. If both drop and ointment therapy are indicated, instill the drops at least 10 minutes before the ointment so that the ointment does not become a barrier to the drops' penetrating the tear film or cornea.
3. Tilt head back.
4. Gently grasp lower outer eyelid below lashes, and pull eyelid away from eye as shown in the drawing.
5. Place ointment tube over eye by looking directly at it.
6. With a sweeping motion, place 1/4- to 1/2-inch of ointment inside the lower eyelid by gently squeezing the tube.
7. Release the eyelid slowly.
8. Close eyes gently for 1 to 2 minutes.
9. Blot excessive ointment from around the eye.
10. Vision may be temporarily blurred. Avoid activities requiring good visual ability until vision clears.

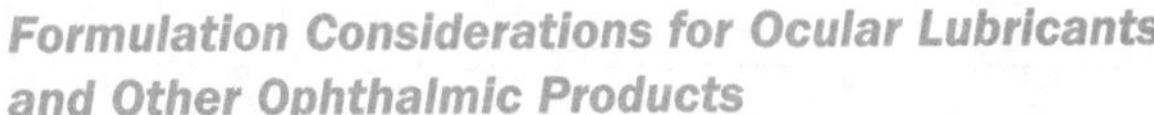

Formulation Considerations for Ocular Lubricants and Other Ophthalmic Products

Ocular lubricants as well as other nonprescription ophthalmic drugs are formulated to reduce the stinging, burning, and other side effects common with some ophthalmic drugs. Carefully controlling the pH, buffers, tonicity adjusters, and preservative systems produces a product that is comfortable to use and will, therefore, encourage adherence with the self-treatment. Drug vehicle and preservative systems are among the most important inactive ingredients of these products. Various other ingredients are often included as excipients.

Ophthalmic Vehicles Ophthalmic vehicles enhance drug action by providing increased viscosity. Because ophthalmic vehicles are more viscous than aqueous solution vehicles, the retention time of the active drug is increased, thus enhancing its bioavailability at the external ocular tissues. These polymers are generally of high molecular weight. Some of the molecules can even bind at the corneal surface to increase drug retention and stabilize the tear film.

The most commonly used ophthalmic vehicles are povidone, PVA, HPMC, and poloxamer 407. Ointments are also used as vehicles. PVA is a water-soluble viscosity enhancer commonly used in a concentration of 1.4%.[13] PVA is generally nonirritating to the eye; documentation has shown that it facilitates healing of abraded corneal epithelium.[14] Similar to PVA, HPMC is available in several molecular weights; however, HPMC 0.5% has been documented to exhibit twice the ocular retention time of polyvinyl alcohol 1.4%.[15]

Povidone is not bound to membrane surfaces and thus does not provide long-lasting viscosity enhancement beyond its normal residence time in the tears. Its viscosity does not change until near pH 1.0, at which level it doubles. Thus, the povidone molecule has no appreciable ionic character at pharmaceutical or physiologic pH values.

The first polyionic vehicle to be evaluated in the eye was poloxamer 407, a vehicle with a hydrophobic nucleus, hydrophilic end groups, and surfactant properties. Polyionic vehicles such as poloxamer 407 produce an artificial microenvironment in the tear film, which can greatly enhance the bioavailability of certain ocular drugs.[16]

Ophthalmic ointments, which are semisolids at room temperature, are produced by mixing white petrolatum and mineral oil with or without a water-miscible agent such as lanolin. The mineral oil allows the vehicle to melt at body temperature, whereas the lanolin absorbs water. This formulation allows retention of water and water-soluble drugs in the delivery system. Commercial ophthalmic ointments are generally derivatives of a hydrocarbon mixture of petrolatum 60% USP and mineral oil 40% USP. In general, ointments are well tolerated by the ocular tissues. The primary clinical purpose for an ophthalmic ointment is to increase the ocular contact time of the instilled product. The ocular contact time of an ointment vehicle is about twice as long in the blinking eye and four times as long in the nonblinking or patched eye as that of a saline vehicle.

Other commonly used vehicles are carboxymethylcellulose sodium, dextran 70, gelatin, glycerin, hydroxyethylcellulose, methylcellulose, polyethylene glycol, and propylene glycol.

Ophthalmic Preservatives Preservatives are incorporated into multidose ophthalmic products. These components are intended to destroy or limit multiplication of microorganisms inadvertently introduced into the product. Surfactants, one of the two distinct groups of preservatives, are usually bactericidal: These molecules disrupt the bacterial plasma membrane. The other group includes the metals mercury and iodine, their derivatives, and alcohols. These compounds are considered bacteriostatic if they only inhibit growth, or bactericidal if they destroy the ability of bacteria to reproduce.

Of the quaternary surfactants, benzalkonium chloride (BAK) and benzethonium chloride are preferred by many manufacturers because of their stability, excellent antimicrobial activity, and long shelf life. Unfortunately, these agents have toxic effects on both the tear film and the corneal epithelium.[17] A single drop of 0.01% BAK can break the superficial lipid layer of the tear film into numerous oil droplets. This preservative can reduce the tear film breakup time and thus may represent a poor choice for an antimicrobial preservative in artificial tear products.[18] The inclusion of BAK in artificial tear formulations does not provide protection to corneal epithelium or promote a stable oily tear surface. In actual patient use these disadvantages may become problematic only for individuals using multiple doses per day. Polyquad, a large molecular weight quaternary compound, is poorly absorbed by contact lenses and rarely results in toxicity. This compound, which was developed to avoid toxicity problems seen with BAK and chlorhexidine in contact lens solutions, is now found in a nonprescription artificial tear product.

Chlorhexidine is useful as an antimicrobial agent in the same range of concentrations as BAK, yet it is used at lower concentrations in commercial ophthalmic formulations. Because it does not alter corneal permeability to the same extent as does BAK, chlorhexidine is not as toxic to the eye.

Of the mercurial preservatives, thimerosal is less likely to degrade into toxic mercury than is either phenylmercuric acetate or phenylmercuric nitrate. Compared with BAK, which undermines tear film stability, thimerosal has no known effects on the tear film. However, some patients develop contact blepharitis or conjunctivitis after several weeks of exposure to thimerosal and must discontinue use of products that contain it. Products containing thimerosal are rapidly disappearing from the commercial marketplace.

Chlorobutanol is less effective than BAK as an antimicrobial preservative and, indeed, tends to disappear from bottles during prolonged storage.[13] However, prolonged use of chlorobutanol does not appear to produce allergic reactions.

Methylparaben and propylparaben have a long history of use in some ophthalmic medications, especially artificial tears and nonmedicated ointments. However, these preservatives are unstable at high pH and can sometimes induce allergic reactions.

Ethylenediaminetetraacetic acid (EDTA) is a chelating agent that preferentially binds and sequesters divalent cations. EDTA assists the action of thimerosal, BAK, and other agents. EDTA can sometimes induce contact allergies.[19]

Sodium perborate, which has been used extensively as a tooth-bleaching agent, has found a new application as an ophthalmic preservative. One of two so-called "disappearing preservatives," sodium perborate dissociates on contact with the eye to form hydrogen peroxide, which in turn rapidly dissociates to carbon dioxide and water. The amount of hydrogen peroxide formed is so small that it does not produce eye irritation. Purite (oxychloro complex) is also designed to dissociate on contact with the eye. After exposure to long wave-length ultraviolet light, purite reportedly dissociates to water and sodium chloride. The disappearing preservatives have the advantage of microbial protection while potentially limiting preservative toxicity.

Other common ophthalmic preservatives include cetylpyridinium chloride, phenylethyl alcohol, sodium propionate, and sorbic acid.

Ophthalmic Excipients Useful excipients are antioxidants, wetting agents, buffers, and tonicity adjusters. Antioxidants prevent or delay deterioration of products exposed to oxygen. Wetting agents reduce surface tension, allowing the drug solution to spread more easily over the ocular surface. Buffers help maintain a pH range of 6.0 to 8.0, thus promoting ocular comfort upon product instillation. Tonicity adjusters allow the medication to be isotonic with the physiologic tear film. Products in the sodium chloride equivalence range of 0.9% ± 0.2% are considered isotonic and help reduce ocular irritation and tissue damage. Solutions in the tonicity range of 0.6% to 1.8% are usually comfortable when placed on the human eye. Hypertonic solutions used for corneal edema are not well tolerated.

Product Selection Guidelines for Ocular Lubricants

In recent years, artificial tear preparations have been introduced in preservative-free formulations and more recently in so-called disappearing preservative formulations. These preparations are beneficial for patients who are sensitive to preservatives such as BAK and thimerosal. Two products, Genteal Lubricant and Refresh Tears, are uniquely formulated so that the preservative rapidly dissociates into nontoxic components on the ocular surface. Nonpreserved artificial tear preparations are available in a variety of unit-dose dispensers, and some of these products are formulated to provide electrolyte support to the damaged surface epithelium of the eye. In general, however, nonpreserved formulations have the disadvantage of increased cost compared with preserved artificial tear solutions, and they can become easily contaminated by the patient during use. Thus, the patient must follow strict hygienic procedures for self-administration and should discard any unused solution according to the manufacturer's guidelines.

Although a benefit of ophthalmic lubricant therapy is to increase the viscosity of existing tears, high viscosity alone does not necessarily provide relief for all dry eye conditions. Methylcellulose, in a concentration of 0.25% to 1.0%, was the primary cellulose ether in the first artificial tear solutions. Most contemporary artificial tear solutions incorporate other less-viscous substituted cellulose ethers, especially HEC and HPC. The latter ethers, which have emollient properties equal or superior to those of methylcellulose, can also be combined with other polymers such as PVA or povidone for use as artificial tears. PVA is generally used in a 1.4% concentration and is considerably less viscous than methylcellulose.

Clinical results and patient acceptance remain the final criteria for determining efficacy in the treatment of patients with dry eye. Importantly, no single formulation has yet been identified that will universally improve clinical signs and symptoms while maintaining patient comfort and acceptance.[12] If the patient fails to respond to initial nonprescription therapy with artificial tears or other lubricants, the appropriate strategy is to change to a different lubricant (especially one with a different polymer or preservative system), to increase the number of drops used per day, or to add an ointment at bedtime. If there is still no response, the patient should be encouraged to seek professional assessment and care from an ophthalmic practitioner.

Retinol Solution

Vitamin A deficiency can affect many epithelial-lined organs, including the eye; therefore, the topical administration of retinol (the alcohol form of vitamin A) has been advocated for treating various dry eye disorders. Unfortunately, few controlled clinical trials have been conducted to substantiate the usefulness of retinol solution in dry eye syndromes. Some preliminary studies claim possible benefits for patients with conjunctival hyperemia (increased volume of blood in the conjunctiva), superior limbic keratitis (inflammation of the cornea), superficial punctate keratitis, and giant papillary conjunctivitis. Many patients may respond favorably to solutions that contain vitamin A because these solutions have emollient qualities. Although such solutions have generally been shown to be no more effective than artificial tear preparations in routinely treating dry eye, they may be of greatest benefit in treating severe dry eye associated with glandular tissue destruction.[20] Until more definitive data become available, however, the specific benefits of topically applied vitamin A solution for treating dry eye will remain speculative. Retinol is available in nonprescription formulations, usually containing 5000 IU of vitamin A and polysorbate 80.

Allergic Conjunctivitis

Etiology/Signs and Symptoms of Allergic Conjunctivitis

The list of antigens that can cause ocular allergy is virtually endless, but the most common allergens include pollen of various types, animal dander, and topical eye preparations. Patients with ocular allergy will often report seasonal allergic rhinitis as well. Allergic conjunctivitis is characterized by a red eye with watery discharge. The hallmark symptom accompanying ocular allergy is itching. Vision is usually not impaired but may be blurred because of excessive tearing.

Treatment of Allergic Conjunctivitis

Treatment Outcomes

The goals in treating allergic conjunctivitis are to (1) remove or avoid the allergen and (2) provide symptomatic relief.

General Treatment Approach

Questioning the patient about exposure to an allergen may help identify the offending substance. Removal or avoidance of the cause is the best treatment, but ocular lubricants, ocular decongestants, ocular decongestant–antihistamine preparations, nonprescription oral antihistamines, and cold compresses will help relieve symptoms.

Nonpharmacologic Therapy

Applying cold compresses to the eyes three to four times a day will help to reduce redness and itching. Other measures include removing the offending allergen and/or avoiding exposure to allergens.

Pharmacologic Therapy

The first-line treatment of allergic conjunctivitis is to instill artifical tears as needed. (For a discussion of these agents, see the section "Treatment of Dry Eye.") If symptoms persist, the patient should switch to an ophthalmic antihistamine–decongestant product. An oral antihistamine can be added to the second regimen if needed. Medical referral is indicated if symptoms remain unresolved.

Nonprescription ophthalmic products designated specifically for treatment of allergic conjunctivitis include decongestants (vasoconstrictors, antihistamines, and decongestant–antihistamine combinations). Chapter 9, "Disorders Related to Cold and Allergy," discusses oral nonprescription antihistamines.

Ophthalmic Decongestants

Four decongestants are available in nonprescription strength for topical application to the eye: phenylephrine, naphazoline, tetrahydrozoline, and oxymetazoline. (See Table 22–4 for examples of these products.) In nonprescription ophthalmic products, phenylephrine is available in a concentration of 0.12%. Naphazoline, tetrahydrozoline, and oxymetazoline belong to the chemical structure group imidazole. As Table 22–4 shows, these agents are available as solutions in various concentrations.

Mechanism of Action/Indications Phenylephrine acts primarily on alpha-adrenergic receptors of the ophthalmic vasculature to constrict conjunctival vessels, thereby reducing eye redness. The higher concentrations of prescription forms of this agent are generally reserved for the short-term dilation needed for eye examinations. Like phenylephrine, the imidazoles have greater alpha- than beta-receptor activity and are, therefore, clinically useful in constricting conjunctival vessels. These agents have only minimal effect on underlying vessels of the episclera and sclera. Naphazoline has been documented to be effective in constricting conjunctival vessels as well as in reducing tearing and pain associated with superficial ocular inflammation.[21] Satisfactory results have similarly been obtained with tetrahydrozoline in most patients with allergic or chronic conjunctivitis. Topical treatment with oxymetazoline will improve most symptoms

Table 22–4

Selected Ophthalmic Products Containing Decongestants, Antihistamines, and/or Astringents

Trade Name	Primary Ingredients
Decongestant Products	
All Clear AR	Naphazoline HCl 0.03%; benzalkonium chloride 0.01%; polyethylene glycol 300 0.2%
Clear eyes	Naphazoline HCl, 0.012%; glycerin 0.2%; benzalkonium chloride
Murine Tears Plus	Tetrahydrozoline 0.05%; povidone 0.6%; polyvinyl alcohol 0.5%; benzalkonium chloride
Naphcon	Naphazoline HCl 0.012%; benzalkonium chloride 0.01%
Ocu Clear	Oxymetazoline HCl 0.025%; benzalkonium chloride 0.01%
Prefin Liquifilm	Phenylephrine HCl 0.12%; polyvinyl alcohol 1.4%; benzalkonium chloride 0.005%
Relief	Phenylephrine HCl 0.12%; polyvinyl alcohol 1.4%; EDTA
Vaso Clear	Naphazoline HCl 0.02%; polyvinyl alcohol; benzalkonium chloride 0.01%
Visine Advanced Relief	Tetrahydrozoline HCl 0.05%; polyethylene glycol 400, 1%; povidone 1%; Dextran 70, 0.1%; benzalkonium chloride 0.01%
Visine L.R.	Oxymetazoline HCl 0.025%; benzalkonium chloride 0.01%
Visine Original	Tetrahydrozoline HCl 0.05%; benzalkonium chloride 0.01%
Antihistamine–Decongestant Products	
Naphcon A	Pheniramine maleate 0.3%; naphazoline HCl 0.025%; benzalkonium chloride 0.01%
OcuHist	Pheniramine maleate 0.3%; naphazoline HCl 0.025%; benzalkonium chloride 0.01%
Opcon-A	Pheniramine maleate 0.315%; naphazoline HCl 0.02675%; hydroxypropyl methycellulose 0.5%; benzalkonium chloride 0.01%
Vasocon-A	Antazoline phosphate 0.5%; naphazoline HCl 0.05%; benzalkonium chloride 0.01%
Decongestant–Astringent Products	
Clear eyes ACR	Naphazoline HCl, 0.012%; zinc sulfate 0.25%; glycerin 0.2%; benzalkonium chloride
Eye-Sed	Tetrahydrozoline 0.05%; zinc sulfate 0.25%; benzalkonium chloride
Vaso Clear A	Naphazoline HCl 0.02%; zinc sulfate 0.25%; polyvinyl alcohol 0.25%; benzalkonium chloride 0.05%
Visine Allergy Relief	Tetrahydrozoline HCl 0.05%; zinc sulfate 0.25%; benzalkonium chloride 0.01%
Zincfrin	Phenylephrine 0.12%; zinc sulfate 0.25%; benzalkonium chloride 0.01%

associated with allergic or noninfectious conjunctivitis, including burning, itching, tearing, and foreign body sensation.

Dosage/Administration Guidelines See Table 22–5 for dosages of phenylephrine, naphazoline, tetrahydrozoline, and oxymetazoline.

Adverse Effects When used as directed, ocular decongestants generally do not induce ocular or systemic side effects. In fact, systemic adverse effects are extremely rare following the topical instillation of nonprescription phenylephrine for ocular decongestion.

The most important and common side effect following chronic use of phenylephrine and the imidazoles for ocular decongestion is rebound congestion of the conjunctiva, in which the conjunctival vessels become progressively more dilated with continued use of the drug. This phenomenon can create a vicious cycle in which phenylephrine is instilled to quiet an inflamed conjunctiva, which then becomes progressively more inflamed because of repeatedly instilling the medication. Patients with apparent rebound effect should be referred to professional eye care for differential diagnosis and management.

Ocular decongestants do have the potential for producing rebound conjunctival hyperemia, allergic conjunctivitis, and allergic blepharitis when used excessively or long term.[22] Rebound congestion appears to be less likely with topical ocular use of naphazoline or tetrahydrozoline, than with oxymetazoline.

The low concentrations of phenylephrine used in nonprescription topical decongestants may dilate the pupil if enough of it penetrates the corneal epithelium. Pupil dilation is not uncommon in persons who wear contact lenses and who may instill the medication following lens wear. Indiscriminate use of phenylephrine to quiet an irritated eye can induce pupillary dilation and precipitate angle-closure glaucoma in eyes predisposed with narrow anterior chamber angles. This adverse effect is more likely if the cornea is

Table 22–5

Dosage Guidelines for Ophthalmic Decongestants and Antihistamines

Agent	Nonprescription Concentration (%)	Dosage	Duration of Action (hours)	Duration of Use
Decongestant Products				
Phenylephrine	0.12	1–2 drops up to 4 times/day	0.5–1.5	All agents: 72 hours
Naphazoline	0.12, 0.02, 0.03	1–2 drops up to 4 times/day	3–4	
Oxymetazoline	0.025	1–2 drops every 6 hours	4–6	
Tetrahydrozoline	0.05	1–2 drops every 4 hours	1–4	
Antihistamine–Decongestant Products				
Pheniramine–naphazoline	0.3 (pheniramine), 0.025 (naphazoline)	1–2 drops 3–4 times/day	—	
Antazoline–naphazoline	0.5 (antazoline), 0.05 (naphazoline)	1–2 drops 3–4 times/day	—	

damaged or diseased, thereby allowing increased corneal drug penetration. Naphazoline can also alter pupil size; patients with lightly pigmented irides (e.g., blue eyes or green eyes) appear to be more sensitive to the mydriatic effect of naphazoline. Tetrahydrozoline does not appear to cause this effect. Thus, patients should be cautioned against instilling this and other ophthalmic decongestants too often.

Certain patients may experience mild, transient stinging immediately following instillation of tetrahydrozoline drops. Finally, some patients may experience epithelial xerosis (abnormal dryness) from prolonged topical instillation of local decongestants.

Drug–Drug Interactions Although not reported in the literature, certain drug–drug interactions involving low concentrations of phenylephrine and the imidazoles are theoretically possible. The pressor effects of these agents may be enhanced in patients taking atropine, tricyclic antidepressants and monoamine oxidase inhibitors, reserpine, guanethidine, or methyldopa. The drug should, therefore, be used cautiously by patients with systemic hypertension, arteriosclerosis, and other cardiovascular diseases or diabetes, or by patients taking the concomitant medications listed above. Adverse cardiovascular events are also possible when these agents are used in patients with hyperthyroidism.[23] Because of these possible adverse reactions, patients should not use phenylephrine and other ocular decongestants as ocular irrigants.

Contraindications/Precautions/Warnings Women should use ocular decongestants sparingly during pregnancy. To ensure a weakened product is not being used, patients should check expiration dates because loss of pharmacologic activity may occur without visible changes in solution color. To prolong shelf life, manufacturers often add sodium bisulfite, an antioxidant, to the phenylephrine vehicle. If offending ophthalmic signs or symptoms do not resolve within 72 hours, the patient should see an eye practitioner.

Product Selection Guidelines Although decongestants and antihistamines are the only nonprescription ophthalmic products for which product-to-product comparisons have been done, it is difficult to reach definitive conclusions regarding clinical comparisons of the available nonprescription ocular decongestants. Most of the tested preparations produce blanching of conjunctival vessels, but 0.02% naphazoline seems to produce greater blanching when compared with other nonprescription decongestants containing 0.05% tetrahydrozoline or 0.12% phenylephrine.[24] Investigators have observed no significant differences in conjunctival blanching with preparations containing naphazoline in concentrations of 0.02%, 0.05%, or 0.1%.[24] (Thus, 0.02% naphazoline is an excellent choice for nonprescription therapy of mild-to-moderate conjunctivitis that is of environmental or noninfectious origin.)

Because rebound congestion appears to be less likely following topical ocular use of naphazoline or tetrahydrozoline, these agents should generally be recommended over phenylephrine or oxymetazoline. And because it has superior documented efficacy and produces a relative lack of side effects, 0.02% naphazoline can be recommended with confidence as an ocular decongestant of choice.[23]

Ophthalmic Antihistamines

Two nonprescription antihistamines are available for topical ophthalmic use: pheniramine maleate and antazoline phosphate. Although these antihistamines are effective individually, nonprescription products containing them also contain a decongestant. The two combinations are pheniramine–naphazoline and antazoline–naphazoline. (See Table 22–4 for examples of these products.)

Mechanism of Action/Indications Pheniramine and antazoline are in different antihistamine classes, but both act as specific histamine 1 (H_1)-receptor antagonists.[25] They do, however, differ somewhat in their pharmacologic actions, both systemically and on the ocular surface. Antazoline has been shown to have some anesthetic properties, but these properties are insufficient to produce clinical effects when antazoline is used topically.[26] Pheniramine has been shown to have little effect on intraocular pressure, whereas antazoline can slightly increase it.[26] This effect is not significant during typical usage.

Topical antihistamines are indicated for rapid relief of symptoms associated with seasonal or atopic conjunctivitis. Using a decongestant with the topical antihistamines has been shown to be more effective than using either agent singly.[21,27] The Food and Drug Administration (FDA) has classified the topical antihistamines in the less-than-effective category primarily because clinical trial data on effectiveness are lacking.

Adverse Effects Burning, stinging, and discomfort on instillation are the most common side effects of ophthalmic antihistamines. Although both pheniramine and antazoline may produce stinging, pheniramine may be somewhat more comfortable. Severe side effects (death, thrombocytopenia, allergic pneumonitis) that may be associated with systemic antihistamine use have not been reported with topical ophthalmic preparations.[28–32]

Contraindications/Precautions/Warnings Ophthalmic antihistamines do have anticholinergic properties and may cause pupil dilation. Such an effect is most commonly seen in people with light-colored irides or with compromised corneas, such as contact lens wearers.[33] In susceptible patients, pupil dilation could lead to angle-closure glaucoma. Therefore, such drugs are contraindicated in people with a known risk of angle-closure glaucoma.[34] Sensitivity to one of the components is another contraindication to the use of topical antihistamines.

Alternative Remedies

The homeopathic product known as Similasan eye drops #2 is indicated for relief from itching and burning caused by allergic reactions. The active homeopathic ingredients are *Apis, Euphrasia,* and *Sabadilla.* (See Chapter 46, "Homeopathic Remedies," for further discussion of these types of products.) The efficacy of this formulation has not been demonstrated in controlled clinical trials.

Case Study 22–1

Patient Complaint/History

Lola, a 67-year-old woman, presents to the pharmacist with complaints of redness, burning, and watering of both eyes. Itching of the eyes or any discharge other than the watering is not present. She has had the symptoms, which are more severe when she arises in the morning, for several years. The symptoms, however, have recently become worse. Physical observation of the patient reveals red and teary eyes.

Lola's current medical problems include osteoarthritis, mild osteoporosis, and hypertension. She also has recurrent sinus infections associated with seasonal allergic rhinitis. Her medications include Monopril 20 mg one tablet daily; Premarin 1.25 mg one tablet daily for 21 days, off for 7 days; Os-Cal 500 one tablet daily; and Advil 200 mg two tablets prn for joint pain, headache, or vague functional aches and pain. A few days earlier, the patient selected the following nonprescription products to manage her eye symptoms: Refresh PM, Lacrilube Ophthalmic Ointment, and Visine.

Clinical Considerations/Strategies

The reader can use the following considerations/strategies to determine whether treatment of this disorder with nonprescription products is warranted:

- Determine whether the patient has used eye drops or ointment to manage previous similar eye conditions. If so, determine whether the medications were effective.
- Assess the need for an artificial tear solution.
- Assess the need for applying a lubricating ointment at bedtime.
- Assess the need for preserved versus nonpreserved solutions.
- Assess the cost-versus-benefit ratio of the selected product(s).

Patient Counseling/Education Strategies

The reader can use the following strategies to develop a patient education/counseling plan that will help ensure optimal therapeutic outcomes:

- Counsel the patient on the appropriate products for dry eye therapy and their use.
- Instruct the patient to apply the ointment only at bedtime, and provide appropriate instructions for its application.
- Explain the limited effectiveness of ophthalmic decongestants for the symptoms (i.e., discourage their use).
- Explain the chronic nature of the disorder.
- Advise the patient of the need for professional eye care if the symptoms persist.

Viral Conjunctivitis

Etiology/Signs and Symptoms of Viral Conjunctivitis

Viral conjunctivitis is the most common form of conjunctivitis. A recent cold, sore throat, or exposure to someone with "pinkeye" (viral conjunctivitis) is a common precursor of this condition. Individuals with viral conjunctivitis will usually have a pink eye with a copious amount of watery discharge. Symptoms include nondescript ocular discomfort and a mild-to-moderate sensation of a foreign object in the eye; vision may occasionally be blurred. Low-grade fever may be present, and swollen preauricular or submandibular lymph nodes may be found. If the etiology of the conjunctivitis is not clear, the patient should be referred to an optometrist or ophthalmologist.

Treatment of Viral Conjunctivitis

Treatment Outcomes

The goal in treating viral conjunctivitis is to relieve symptoms while the infection runs its course.

General Treatment Approach

Viral conjunctivitis is usually self-limiting, with symptoms resolving over 1 to 3 weeks. Treatment to relieve major symptoms should use artificial tear preparations and ocular decongestants. Because certain forms of viral conjunctivitis can be extremely contagious, nonpharmacologic hygienic measures are also important.

Nonpharmacologic Therapy

Patients with viral conjunctivitis should wash their hands after touching an infected eye and should properly dispose of tissues used to blot an infected eye. They should also avoid sharing towels or other objects that might come in contact with their infected eye.

Pharmacologic Therapy

See the section "Treatment of Dry Eye" for a discussion of artificial tear preparations. See also the section "Treatment of Allergic Conjunctivitis" for a discussion of ocular decongestants.

Corneal Edema

Etiology/Signs and Symptoms of Corneal Edema

Corneal edema may occur from various conditions, including overwear of contact lenses, surgical damage to the cornea, and inherited corneal dystrophies (a hereditary corneal degeneration). The edematous area of the cornea is often confined to the epithelium. Because fluid accumulation distorts the optical properties of the cornea, halos or starbursts around lights (with or without reduced vision) are a hallmark symptom of corneal edema. An optometrist or ophthalmologist must diagnose this disorder.

Treatment of Corneal Edema

Treatment Outcomes

The goal in treating corneal edema is to draw fluid from the cornea, thereby relieving the symptoms associated with this disorder.

General Treatment Approach

Once the initial diagnosis is established, patients can use topical hyperosmotic formulations to treat corneal edema. Of the topical ophthalmic hyperosmotic agents that are commercially available, only sodium chloride can be obtained without a prescription in both solution and ointment formulations. (See Table 22–6 for examples of these products.) Sodium chloride is available as a 2% or 5% solution, as well as a 5% ointment. First-line treatment is instilling a 2% solution four times a day. If symptoms persist, nighttime use of a 5% hyperosmotic ointment should be added to the regimen. If symptoms do not respond to the augmented treatment, the patient should switch to a 5% hyperosmotic solution and should continue nighttime use of the ointment. If symptoms still persist, medical referral is necessary.

Pharmacologic Therapy (Hyperosmotics)

Mechanism of Action

Hyperosmotic agents increase the tonicity of the tear film, thereby promoting movement of fluid from the cornea to the more highly osmotic tear film. Normal tear flow mechanisms then eliminate the excess fluid. Many patients with mild-to-moderate corneal epithelial edema may experience improved subjective comfort and vision following appropriate use of these medications.

Dosage/Administration Guidelines

Usually the patient instills one or two drops of the solution every 3 to 4 hours. (See Table 22–2.) The ointment formulation, however, requires less-frequent instillation and is usually reserved for use at bedtime to minimize symptoms of blurred vision. (See Table 22–3.) Because vision associated with edematous corneas is often worse on arising, several instillations of the solution during the first few waking hours may be helpful.

Adverse Effects

In general, the 5% concentration of sodium chloride in ointment form is the most effective to reduce corneal edema and improve vision, but it tends to cause stinging and burning. For that reason, patients often prefer the 2% concentration

Table 22-6

Selected Miscellaneous Ophthalmic Products

Trade Name	Primary Ingredients
Irrigants	
Accu-Wash	NaCl; sodium phosphate; benzalkonium chloride
Collyrium for Fresh Eyes	Boric acid; sodium borate; benzalkonium chloride
Dacriose	Sodium phosphate; NaCl; benzalkonium chloride 0.1%; EDTA 0.3%
Bausch & Lomb Eye Wash	Sodium borate; boric acid; NaCl; sorbic acid 0.1%; EDTA 0.025%
Eye Stream	Sodium acetate 0.39%; sodium citrate 0.17%; sodium hydroxide and/or hydrochloric acid; benzalkonium chloride
Lavoptik Eye Wash	Sodium phosphate; NaCl 0.49%; benzalkonium chloride 0.005%
Hyperosmotics	
Adsorbonac Solution[a]	NaCl 2% and 5%; thimerosal 0.04%
AK-NaCl Solution	NaCl 5%; methylparaben 0.023%; propylparaben 0.017%
AK-NaCl Ointment[b]	NaCl 5%; lanolin oil; mineral oil; white petrolatum
Muro 128 Solution	NaCl 2%
Muro 128 Ointment	NaCl 5%
Eyelid Scrubs	
Eye-Scrub Solution	Polyethylene glycol 200 glyceryl monotallowate; disodium laureth sulfosuccinate; cocoamidopropylamine oxide; polyethylene glycol 78 glyceryl monococoate; benzyl alcohol; EDTA
Lid Wipes-SPF Pads	Polyethylene glycol 200 glyceryl monotallowate; polyethylene glycol 80 glyceryl cocoate; laureth-23; cocoamidopropylamine oxide; sodium chloride; glycerin
OcuSoft Solution and Pads	Polyethylene glycol 80 sorbitan laureth; sodium trideceth sulfate; cocoamidopropyl hydroxysulftaine; polyethylene glycol 150 distearate; lauroamphocarboxyglycinate; sodium laureth-13 carboxylate; polyethylene glycol 15 tallow polyamine; quaternium-15
Prosthesis Lubricant/Cleaner	
Enuclene Solution	Tyloxapol 0.25%; hydroxypropyl methylcellulose 0.85%; benzalkonium chloride 0.02%

[a] Product containing thimerosal.

[b] Preservative-free product.

for long-term therapy. Hypertonic saline, however, is nontoxic to the external ocular tissues, and allergic reactions are rare.

Contraindications

Perhaps the most important contraindication to topical hyperosmotic sodium chloride is its use to clear edematous corneas with traumatized epithelium. The intact corneal epithelium exhibits only limited permeability to inorganic ions; therefore, an absent or compromised corneal epithelium will promote increased corneal penetration of the hyperosmotic and thereby reduce the osmotic effect. Consequently, the management of corneal edema associated with traumatized epithelium requires the use of organic hyperosmotic agents that are available only by prescription.[35] Patients whose history or physical appearance suggests a damaged corneal epithelium should be referred for immediate professional eye care.

Loose Foreign Substances in the Eye

Etiology/Signs and Symptoms of Loose Foreign Substances in the Eye

Despite the protective effect of the lids, foreign substances often contact the ocular surface. The immediate response of the eye is watering. If the substance causes only minor irritation and does not abrade the eye surface, self-treatment is appropriate.

Treatment of Loose Foreign Substances in the Eye

Treatment Outcomes

The goal in treating loose foreign substances in the eye is to remove the irritant by irrigating the eye.

General Treatment Approach

If reflex tearing does not remove the foreign substance, the eye may need to be flushed. Lint, dust, and similar materials can usually be removed by rinsing the eye with sterile saline or specific eyewash preparations (irrigants).

Pharmacologic Therapy (Ocular Irrigants)

Indications/Mechanism of Action

Ocular irrigants are used to cleanse ocular tissues while maintaining their moisture; these solutions must be physiologically balanced with respect to pH and osmolality. Because the tissues with which they come in contact obtain nutrients elsewhere, the role of irrigants is primarily to clear away unwanted materials or debris from the ocular surface. Patients should use ocular irrigants only on a short-term basis. All the ophthalmic irrigating solutions are available without a prescription and, therefore, can be used by patients and practitioners alike. (See Table 22–6 for examples of these products.)

In the ophthalmic practitioner's office, irrigating solutions come in handy after certain clinical procedures, and they are often used to wash away mucous or purulent exudates from the eye. They are also administered in the hospital to clean out eyes between changes of ocular dressings.

Dosage/Administration Guidelines

See Table 22–7 for instructions on how to use ophthalmic irrigants.

Contraindications/Precautions/Warnings

Ocular irrigants should not be used for open wounds in or near the eyes. These agents should also not be applied with contact lenses in place because the solutions tend to cause contact lens irritation by reducing the mucin component of the tear film. In the case of rigid gas–permeable lenses, the solutions reduce the hydrophilicity of the lens surface.[36] Furthermore, absorption of the preservatives BAK or phenylmercuric acetate by soft lenses can have a deleterious effect on the corneal epithelium. Although irrigating solutions may be used to wash out the eyes after contact lens wear, they have no particular value as contact lens wetting, cleansing, or cushioning solutions.

In cases in which the patient experiences continuous eye pain, changes in vision, or continued redness or irritation of the eye, or in which the ocular condition persists or worsens, evaluation by an eye practitioner should similarly be strongly encouraged. Commercial irrigating products that use an eyecup should generally be avoided because of difficulties in cleaning the eyecup, with the resultant risk of bacterial or fungal contamination.

Table 22–7

Administration Guidelines for Ophthalmic Irrigants

1. If provided, discard the eyecup that comes with the irrigant. Preventing viral, fungal, or bacterial contamination of the cup is very difficult.
2. Bend over a sink or bathtub, and slightly tilt one ear downward.
3. Hold the bottle near the corner of the eye that is next to the nose, being careful not to touch the eye.
4. Squeeze the bottle, and allow the irrigant to flow across the entire eye surface.
5. If necessary, adjust the angle of the head during instillation of the irrigant to ensure that the entire eye surface is flushed.
6. Blot excessive solution from around the eye.
7. If both eyes are affected, repeat the procedure for the other eye.

Minor Eye Irritation

Etiology/Signs and Symptoms of Minor Eye Irritation

Nonallergenic, minor eye irritation can be caused by loose foreign substance in the eye; contact lens wear; or exposure of the eye to wind, sun, smog, chemical fumes, or chlorine. Snow skiing without protective eye goggles may often be the cause of such sun exposure. Redness of the eye is the common sign of minor irritation.

Treatment of Minor Eye Irritation

Minor irritation often responds well to artificial tear solutions or nonmedicated ointments. (For a discussion of these ophthalmic agents, see the section "Treatment of Dry Eye.")

Zinc sulfate, a mild astringent, may be recommended for temporary relief of minor ocular irritation. The dosage is generally one to two drops up to four times daily.

The homeopathic product known as Similasan eye drops #1 is marketed to relieve dryness and redness caused by smog, contact lenses, and other causes. The active homeopathic ingredients are belladonna, *Euphrasia*, and mercurius sublimatus. (See Chapter 46, "Homeopathic Remedies," for further discussion of these types of products.) Controlled clinical trials have not demonstrated the efficacy of this formulation.

Prevention of Ophthalmic Disorders in Artificial Eyes

Aside from the obvious aesthetic benefits, clearing dried mucus or fluid secretions from the surfaces of artifical eyes removes a potential medium for bacterial growth. A sterile isotonic buffered solution containing 0.25% tyloxapol and 0.02% BAK is available especially for cleaning and lubricating ophthalmic prostheses.

Tyloxapol is a detergent surfactant that liquefies solid matter on the prosthesis, and BAK aids tyloxapol in wetting the artificial eye. The solution is used in the same matter as ordinary artificial tears. With the artificial eye in place, one or two drops of solution should be applied three or four times daily. In addition, the solution can be used as a cleaner to remove oily or mucus deposits; in this case, the artificial eye is then rubbed between the fingers and rinsed with tap water before reinsertion.

Macular Degeneration

Age-related macular degeneration is the leading cause of blindness in the United States. It takes two forms: hemorrhagic (wet or bleeding) and atrophic (dry). Currently, there are no proven therapies for the atrophic form. Side effects and the number of people eligible for therapy limit treatment of the hemorrhagic form. Animal models have shown that oxidative mechanisms play a role in developing both forms of this disorder. Numerous human studies have indicated a general inverse association with antioxidant level.[37]

Beta carotene (a specific vitamin A group), ascorbic acid (vitamin C), and tocopherol (vitamin E), as well as the trace elements zinc and selenium, have been implicated as helpful in reducing progression of the disorder.[37] The efficacy of these products is unknown.[38] All studies to this point have been limited, and definitive clinical trials are only now under way. The possible association of antioxidants to aid this disorder has led to the development of numerous nonprescription ophthalmic preparations containing these vitamins. Because other treatment options are limited and side effects are rare, optometrists and ophthalmologists will frequently recommend these products to their patients diagnosed with age-related macular degeneration.

Given the lack of other effective treatments, patients will ask pharmacists for product selection recommendations. These products are generally taken once or twice a day and are usually well tolerated, with gastrointestinal side effects rarely reported. (See Chapter 19, "Nutritional Deficiencies," for discussion of these effects.) Pharmacists should make sure that ophthalmic vitamin products are not taken in conjunction with other multivitamin supplements, which could lead to possible hypervitaminosis.

Contact Dermatitis

Etiology/Signs and Symptoms of Contact Dermatitis

Contact dermatitis of the eyelid can be either a reaction to an allergen or an irritant. A change in cosmetics or soap or an exposure to some foreign substance is usually the cause. The equal involvement of each eyelid suggests allergy because both eyes are often exposed. Swelling, scaling, or redness of the eyelid along with profuse itching are common with contact dermatitis.

Treatment of Contact Dermatitis

Questioning the patient about use of new products (e.g., eyeliner and eye shadow) quickly identifies the offending substance. Discontinuing use of the suspected products is the best treatment. If swelling of the eyelid is marked, nonprescription oral antihistamines along with cold compresses applied three to four times a day will help reduce the inflammation and itching.

Lice Infestation of the Eyelid

Etiology/Signs and Symptoms of Lice Infestation of the Eyelid

Infestation of the eyelids with the organisms *Phthirus pubis* (crab louse) or *Pediculus humanus capitis* (head louse) may cause symptoms similar to blepharitis (i.e., red, scaly, thickened eyelids). These organisms are also responsible for sexually transmitted lice infestation. Children are rarely affected by the crab louse but are commonly affected by the head louse.

Treatment of Lice Infestation of the Eyelid

A bland (nonmedicated) ophthalmic ointment (e.g., petrolatum) used for 10 days is the recommended self-treatment. The ointment suffocates the louse and deprives its eggs of adequate oxygen to hatch. Pharmacists should carefully instruct patients about the need to take hygienic measures, such as washing clothing and bedding that may contain unhatched eggs.

Blepharitis

Etiology/Signs and Symptoms of Blepharitis

Blepharitis is an extremely common inflammatory condition of the eyelid margins. The most common causative factors are *Staphylococcus epidermidis, Staphylococcus aureus,* seborrheic dermatitis, or a combination of these factors.[39] Red, scaly, thickened eyelids—often with loss of the eyelashes—are typical signs of blepharitis. Itching and burning are the most common accompanying complaints. All forms of blepharitis tend to be chronic, and individuals are often aware of their diagnosis.

Treatment of Blepharitis

Treatment Outcomes

The goals in treating blepharitis are to (1) control the disorder with good eyelid hygiene and (2) provide symptomatic relief.

Case Study 22–2

Patient Complaint/History

Craig, a 37-year-old male, presents to the pharmacist after being told by his eye practitioner to treat a "scabies" infestation of his eyelids by scrubbing the eyelids and then applying an ointment to them. The patient complains of itching and burning of his eyelids. When questioned about the presence of other symptoms, the patient admits that he also has itching of the scalp and genitals. Physical observation reveals reddened eyelid margins.

To treat the scabies infestation, Craig's eye practitioner prescribed doxycycline 250 mg qid po for 30 days. The patient selected the following nonprescription products for additional treatment of his condition: Lacrilube Ophthalmic Ointment, Eye-Scrub solution, and 1% Nix cream rinse. (See Chapter 31, "Insect Bites and Stings and Pediculosis," for discussion of pediculicides.)

Clinical Considerations/Strategies

The reader can use the following considerations/strategies to determine whether treatment of this disorder with nonprescription products is warranted:

- Determine whether the patient has had this disorder before. If so, find out whether he used the described nonprescription medication regimen to treat the previous occurrences.
- Assess the appropriateness of the patient-selected ophthalmic products.
- Assess the need to treat the disorder with the prescribed and patient-selected products.
- Assess the appropriateness of the patient-selected nonophthalmic products.
- Assess the need for additional nonophthalmic products.

Patient Counseling/Education

The reader can use the following strategies to develop a patient education/counseling plan that will help ensure optimal therapeutic outcomes:

- Explain the potential toxicity of nonophthalmic products when used on or around the eye.
- Indicate the appropriate duration of treatment for each product.
- Explain strategies to prevent spread of the scabies infestation.
- Explain the appropriate use and possible reuse of the nonophthalmic products.
- Explain the proper application of ophthalmic ointments and the use of eyelid scrub solutions.

General Treatment Approach

Careful eyelid hygiene is the mainstay of therapy for the many forms of blepharitis. The chronic nature of blepharitis makes the use of careful lid hygiene preferable to the long-term use of topical antibiotics. Ocular lubricants can be used if eye irritation is also present. (See the section "Treatment of Dry Eye.")

The patient can implement good lid hygiene by using hot compresses for 15 to 20 minutes, two to four times daily. Each application of a compress should be followed by lid scrubs using a mild detergent cleanser compatible with ocular tissues.

Pharmacologic Therapy (Lid Scrubs)

Lid scrub procedures are usually effective and well tolerated. Table 22–8 gives instructions on how to perform lid scrubs. This procedure can also be used for hygienic eyelid cleansing in people who wear contact lenses. Although baby shampoo is often used for lid scrubs, recent experience has shown other commercially available cleansers to be as effective with potentially less ocular stinging, burning, and toxicity.[40]

Commercial lid scrub products are specifically intended for the removal of oils, debris, or desquamated skin associated with the inflamed eyelid. (See Table 22–6 for examples of these products.) Some commercial products are packaged with gauze pads, which provide an abrasive action to augment the cleansing properties of the detergent solution.

Eyelid scrubs using commercially available detergents are most effective in patients with noninfectious blepharitis. If

Table 22–8

Administration Guidelines for Eyelid Scrubs

1. Wash hands thoroughly.
2. Apply three to four drops of baby shampoo or eyelid cleanser to cotton-tipped applicator or gauze pad.
3. Close one eye, and clean the upper eyelid and eyelashes using side-to-side strokes, being careful not to touch eyeball with applicator or fingers.
4. Open eye, look up, and clean lower eyelid and eyelashes using side-to-side strokes.
5. Repeat the procedures on the other eye using a clean applicator or gauze pad.
6. Rinse eyelids and eyelashes with clean, warm water.

the patient's signs or symptoms fail to improve, the patient should be referred for professional ocular examinations and treatment with appropriate antibacterial agents.

Hordeolum/Chalazion

Etiology/Signs and Symptoms of Hordeolum/Chalazion

An internal hordeolum is an inflammation of the meibomian gland, whereas an external hordeolum is an inflammation of the glands of Zeis and Moll. (See Figure 22–1.) A palpable, tender nodule is always present. Swelling of the eyelid, almost to the point of closure, can occur with a severe internal hordeolum. The cause is invariably one of the staphylococcal species associated with blepharitis.

A chalazion, which is a sterile granuloma, is very similar in appearance to an internal hordeolum. However, a chalazion is not tender to gentle touching, whereas a hordeolum is typically quite tender.

Treatment of Hordeolum/Chalazion

A hordeolum typically responds well to hot compresses applied three to four times daily for 5 to 10 minutes at each session. Clearing usually occurs within 1 week. An external hordeolum may be treated with a topical antibiotic, however an internal hordeolum does not respond well to such treat-

Table 22–9

Differentiation of Ophthalmic Disorders That Require Medical Referral

Disorder	Signs/Symptoms	Potential Complications	Treatment Approach
Blunt trauma	Ruptured blood vessels, bleeding into eyelid tissue space, swelling, ocular discomfort	Internal eye bleeding, secondary glaucoma, detached retina	Medical referral
Foreign particles trapped/embedded in the eye	Reddened eyes, profuse tearing, ocular discomfort	Corneal abrasions/scarring, chronic red eye, interocular penetration from metal striking metal at high speeds	Medical referral for removal of particles
Ocular abrasions	Partial/total loss of corneal epithelium, blurred vision, profuse tearing, difficulty opening the eye	Risk of bacterial/fungal infection if eye exposed to organic material	Medical referral
Infections of eyelid/eye surface	Red, thickened lids; scaling	Scarring of lids, dry eye	Medical referral
Eye exposure to chemical splash, solid chemical, or chemical fumes	Reddened eyes, watering, difficulty opening eye	Scarring of eyelids and eye surface, loss of vision	To prevent/reduce scarring of eyelids from chemical burns, flush eye immediately for at least 10 minutes with preferably sterile saline/water. If neither is available, flush with tap water. (This treatment may not prevent/reduce scarring of ocular surface.) After flushing eye, arrange immediate transportation to an emergency facility. Make no recommendation for acid–base balance
Thermal injury to eye (welder's arc)	Reddened eyes, pain, sensitivity to light	Corneal scarring, secondary infection	Medical referral for definitive care, including possible eye patching
Bacterial conjunctivitis	Reddened eyes with purulent (mucous) discharge, ocular discomfort, eyelids stuck together on awakening	Typically self-limiting in 2 weeks	Medical referral for treatment with topical antibiotics if patient desires to clear infection more quickly
Chlamydial conjunctivitis	Watery or mucus discharge, ocular discomfort, low-grade fever, possible blurred vision	Scarring	If infection with *Chlamydia* sp. is known or suspected, or if symptoms are too vague to rule in viral or allergic conjunctivitis, medical referral is mandatory

ment and is best treated with a course of oral prescription antibiotics. Surgical drainage may be required in recalcitrant cases.

Hot compresses applied the same as for treatment of hordeola are usually sufficient to drain a chalazion. If either disorder does not drain within 1 week or has been present chronically, medical referral is appropriate. Periodic use of lid scrubs may reduce the recurrences of chalazion and hordeolum. (See Table 22–8.)

Patient Assessment of Ophthalmic Disorders

For patients who have not seen an eye practitioner, the pharmacist must determine whether the ophthalmic disorder is self-treatable or requires medical referral. The pharmacist must also take great care in assessing a patient with a new, acute problem. Ocular inflammation and irritation can be caused by many conditions, some of which can be treated safely and effectively with nonprescription ophthalmic products. These products are used primarily to relieve minor symptoms of burning, stinging, itching, and watering. The FDA has suggested that self-treatment may be indicated for tear insufficiency, corneal edema, and external inflammation or irritation.[41] Self-treatment may also be effective in managing hordeolum (stye), blepharitis, and allergic and viral conjunctivitis.[42]

Exclusions to self-treatment include blunt trauma to the eye, trapped/embedded foreign objects in the eye, and thermal/chemical burns of the eyelid and eye surface. Medical referral is also appropriate for ocular abrasions and bacterial and chlamydial conjunctivitis. Table 22–9 describes the major features of these disorders.

Asking the patient the following questions will help elicit the information needed to accurately assess the disorder and to recommend the appropriate treatment approach.

Q~ Is this an acute or chronic problem? Have you sought professional care for this problem? What is the current recommended treatment?

A~ If the disorder is chronic with a well-established diagnosis, recommend the appropriate nonprescription product for the disorder and counsel the patient on product use. Be sure to advise the patient not to instill nonprescription medications immediately after instilling the prescription medication.

Q~ Is your vision blurred?

A~ Blurred vision may accompany both minor and severe ophthalmic disorders. *Identify which self-treatable and non–self-treatable disorders are associated with blurring. (See Table 22–9 and the sections describing signs and symptoms of self-treatable disorders.)* Significant blurring of vision may indicate internal eye damage. Refer such patients immediately to an eye practitioner.

Q~ Do you have other eye symptoms (double vision, flashing lights, floating spots)?

A~ Refer patients with these symptoms to an eye practitioner.

Q~ Do your eyes hurt? Is the pain sharp or dull? Is it constant or intermittent?

A~ Because pain may occur in minor and serious disorders, it is not a good clue as to the severity of the problem. The pharmacist should try to determine whether eye irritation or pain is present. If this determination cannot be made, refer the patient to an eye practitioner.

Q~ Have you recently been in an accident or injured your eye or head in any way?

A~ Refer all cases of eye trauma to an eye practitioner.

Q~ Have your eyes been exposed to chemicals?

A~ If yes and the patient has not flushed the eye for 10 minutes with an ocular irrigant, administer this procedure; then refer the patient immediately to an emergency facility.

Q~ Do you wear contact lenses? Are the eye surfaces red?

A~ Contact lenses are often a source of infectious organisms. *Identify other ophthalmic disorders that can cause acute reddening of the eyes. (See Table 22–9 and the sections describing signs and symptoms of self-treatable disorders.)* Refer patients with acute reddening of the eyes to an eye practitioner.

Q~ Does your problem seem to be on the lids or on the eye? If on the eyelid, is there swelling with or without a nodule? Are the eyelids red?

A~ *Identify the disorders that cause swelling of the eyelids or are associated with a nodule. Identify the most likely causes of red eyelids. (See Table 22–9 and the sections describing signs and symptoms of self-treatable disorders.)* Determine the appropriate self-treatment for each.

Q~ Do your eyelids itch?

A~ *Identify the self-treatable eyelid disorders associated with itching. (See Table 22–9 and the sections describing signs and symptoms of self-treatable disorders.) Determine the appropriate self-treatment for each.*

Q~ Is your eye surface red? Is there a discharge from the eye? Is it watery? Have you recently had a head cold, sinus problem, or been exposed to "pink eye"?

A~ *Identify the self-treatable disorder these symptoms most likely indicate. (See Table 22–9 and the sections describing signs and symptoms of self-treatable disorders.) Determine the appropriate self-treatment.*

Q~ Is your eye surface red? Is there a mucus discharge from your eye?

A~ *Identify the non–self-treatable disorder these symptoms most likely indicate. (See Table 22–9.)*

Q~ Do you have allergies? If so, to what are you allergic? Do your eyes itch? Have you used a new product or been exposed to an irritative agent?

A~ If the patient's response indicates a history of allergic rhinitis or a known exposure to environmental or pharmacologic agents, recommend avoiding the allergen or irritant and then recommend the appropriate treatment. (Nonprescription ophthalmic products or contact lens care products may be causing the symptoms.) *Identify the appropriate self-treatment measures for allergic conjunctivitis and contact dermatitis.*

Q~ Do your eyes burn or sting? Do they have a gritty sensation? Do they water excessively?

A~ *Identify the self-treatable condition these symptoms most likely indicate. (See the sections describing signs and symptoms of self-treatable disorders.)* Ask whether the patient is exposed to environmental conditions that can cause tear evaporation.

Q~ Are you taking any prescription or nonprescription medications? Do you have other medical conditions?

A~ *Identify the medications that can interact with nonprescription ophthalmic products. Identify the medical conditions that contraindicate the use of these products. (See the sections that discuss adverse effects and contraindications for the various products.)*

Patient Counseling for Ophthalmic Disorders

Before counseling a patient, the pharmacist should carefully consider the nature and extent of ocular involvement. It is important for patients with acute ocular disease to receive a prompt definitive diagnosis, including baseline visual acuity, before the pharmacist considers the appropriateness of nonprescription therapy. Some acute conditions, which may or may not involve ocular pain or blurred vision, can be appropriately treated with nonprescription agents, but a recent diagnosis from the ophthalmic practitioner can give the pharmacist additional reassurance and confidence in recommending such treatment. Although the cost-effectiveness of ophthalmic care can be greatly improved through the use of nonprescription agents, severe visual impairment, including blindness, can be a serious clinical and medicolegal complication if the pharmacist delays referral for definitive diagnosis and treatment. After careful consideration of the history, the pharmacist should always counsel patients on the indications for and limitations of self-treatment. The algorithms in Figures 22–2 and 22–3 can assist the pharmacist in recommending the appropriate treatment for disorders of the eye surface and eyelid, respectively.

Numerous nonprescription ophthalmic products for treating minor ocular irritations are commercially available for self-administration by the patient under minimal or no supervision. Such products are also adequate for treating certain clinical conditions that have been diagnosed by health practitioners. First-line therapy should always include counseling on nonpharmacologic treatment. These treatments are frequently sufficient in and of themselves to relieve the ocular symptoms or are necessary as an adjunct to the ophthalmic drug therapy. Proper drug instillation technique is critical if the target tissue (the eye) is to receive the maximum benefit from the medication. Ophthalmic solutions and ointments, as well as eyelid scrubs, are often misused. By carefully instructing patients in the proper self-administration procedures, the pharmacist can help ensure maximum safety and effectiveness of these agents. Appropriate patient education and counseling must accompany dispensation of any ophthalmic product.

Although drug side effects and interactions are rare with topically applied ophthalmic products, the potential for such effects does exist. Therefore, the pharmacist should advise the patient of possible adverse effects, including the clinical signs of drug toxicity or allergy.

The pharmacist must actively assist patients in selecting the appropriate product that will enhance adherence, minimize or avoid side effects, and reduce the attendant costs of therapy. The other major considerations in making therapeutic recommendations are whether the person has sensitivity to one of the product constituents, whether the product can be used with contact lenses on the eyes, and whether the product has the potential to wash out prescription ophthalmic drugs that the person may be using. Outside of ophthalmic antihistamines and decongestants, little product-to-product comparative research has been done for nonprescription ophthalmic preparations. The pharmacist must, therefore, make therapy recommendations based on the patient's diagnosis and the products the patient is currently using. The box "Patient Education for Ophthalmic Disorders" lists specific information to provide patients.

Evaluation of Patient Outcomes for Ophthalmic Disorders

Patients who self-treat allergic conjunctivitis, loose foreign substances in the eye, or minor eye irritation should be advised to see an eye practitioner if the symptoms persist after 72 hours of treatment. Those who are self-treating viral conjunctivitis should seek medical care if vision loss occurs or symptoms persist after 3 weeks. Dry eye is often a chronic

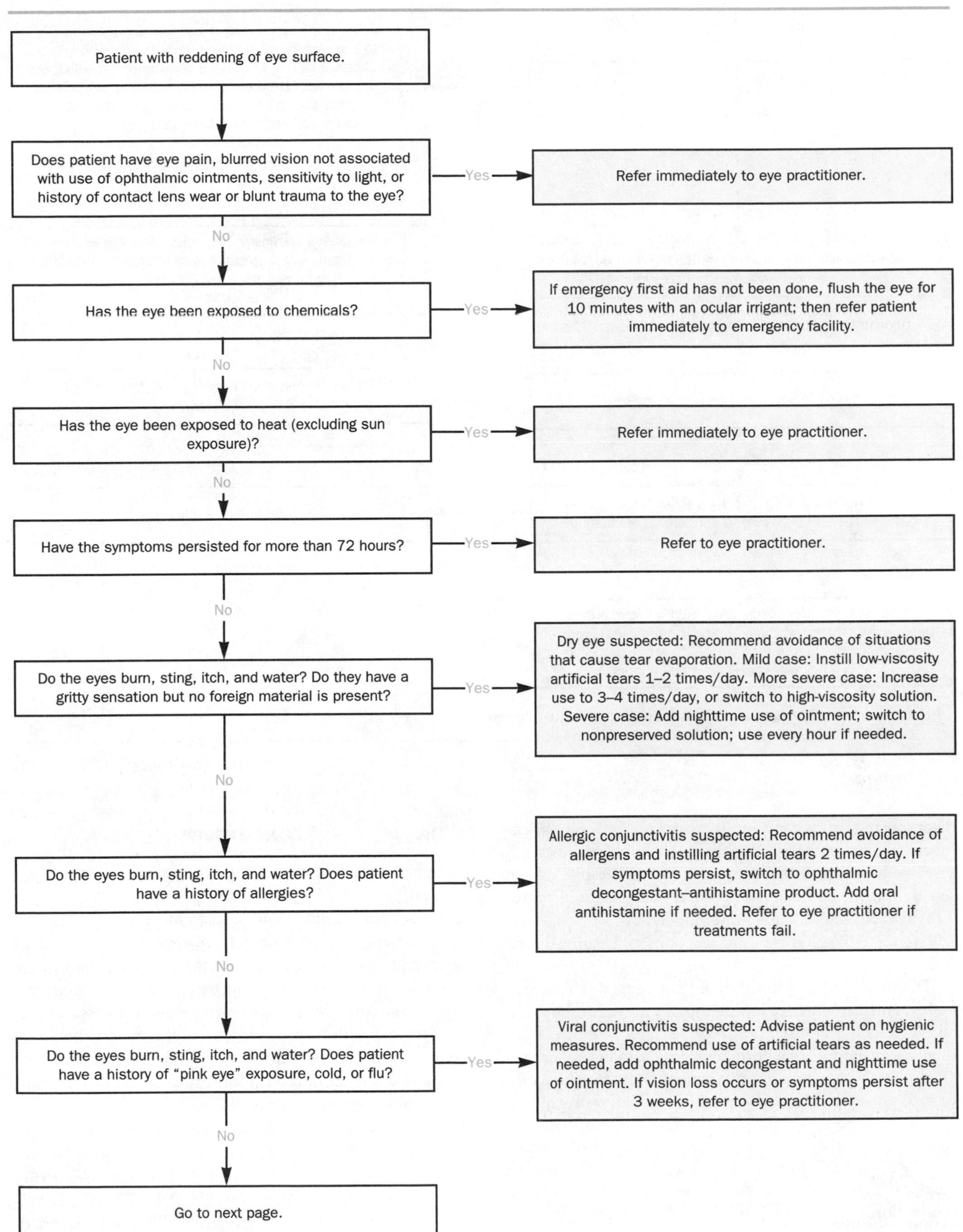

Figure 22–2 Self-care of eye surface disorders.

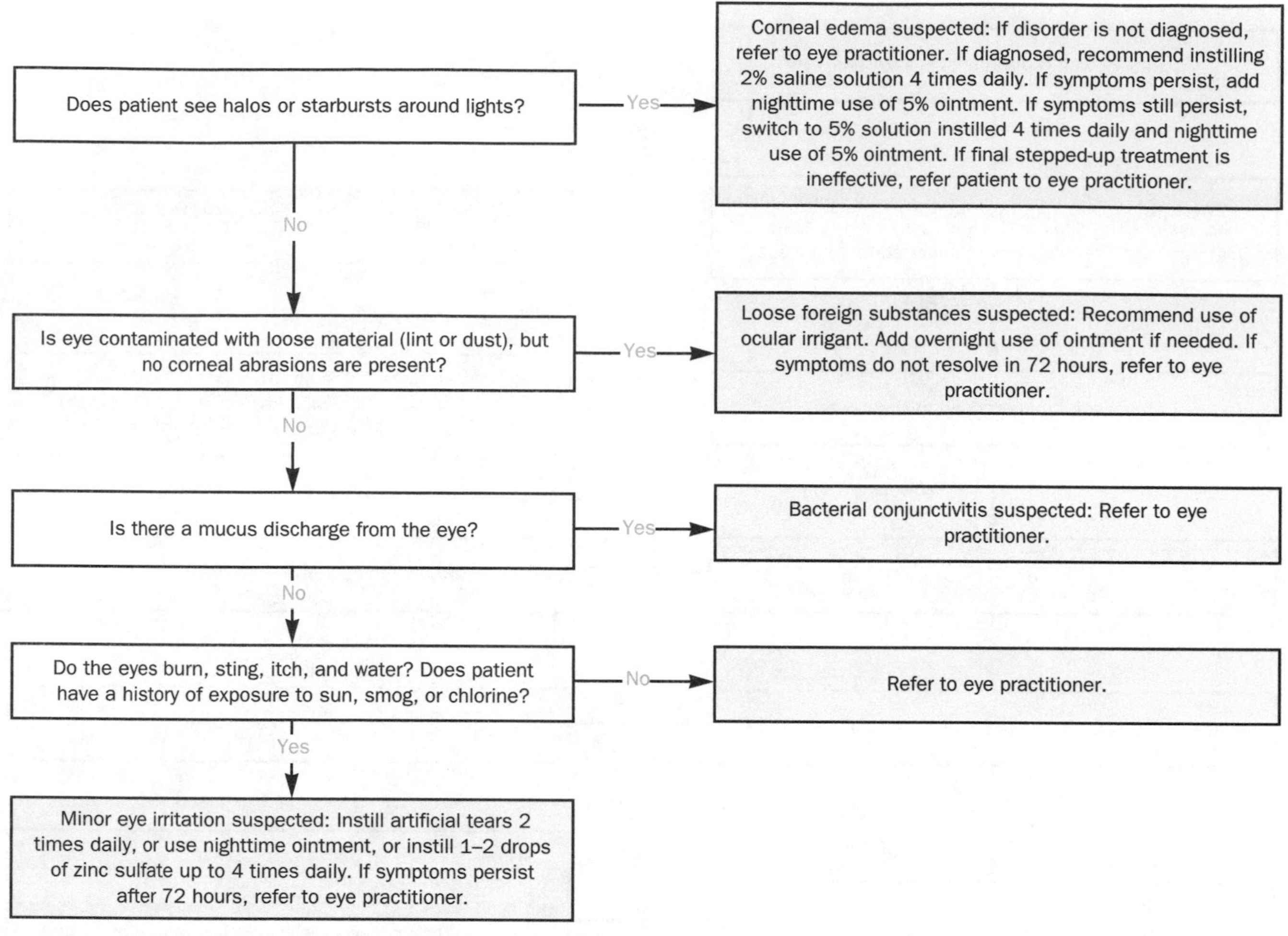

Figure 22–2 Self-care of eye surface disorders (continued).

disorder, requiring continuous treatment with ophthalmic lubricants. Patients with this disorder should be advised to seek medical care if the symptoms worsen despite diligent self-treatment. Patients with corneal edema should consult an eye practitioner if the symptoms persist or worsen despite adherence to the physician's instructions for treating the disorder.

The treatment period for eyelid disorders differs considerably. Patients with lice infestation of the eyelids should see an eye practitioner if symptoms persist after 10 days of treatment. If the nodule of a hordeolum/chalazion is not drained after 1 week of treatment, the patient should seek medical care. Symptoms of contact dermatitis should resolve quickly once the offending substance is removed. If symptoms persist, the patient should see an eye practitioner. Blepharitis usually requires chronic treatment. Patients with diagnosed blepharitis should self-treat the disorder daily as described in the section "Treatment of Blepharitis"; however, if symptoms worsen, the patient should seek medical care.

CONCLUSIONS

The pharmacist is strategically positioned in the community to treat patients with ophthalmic pathology or to recommend self-management with one or more nonprescription drugs. Several such pharmaceuticals are available to manage the symptoms of minor acute or chronic conditions of the eye and eyelid. By understanding the pathophysiology of certain ocular conditions and knowing how to assess patients who present with such conditions, a pharmacist should be able to optimize the safe, appropriate, effective, and economical use of nonprescription drugs to manage various conditions of the eye and eyelid.

Nonprescription ophthalmic products should be used only in cases of minor pain or discomfort. If doubt exists concerning the nature of the problem, the pharmacist should refer the patient for professional care. Nonprescription ocular medications should not be recommended to patients who have demonstrated an allergy to any of the active ingredients,

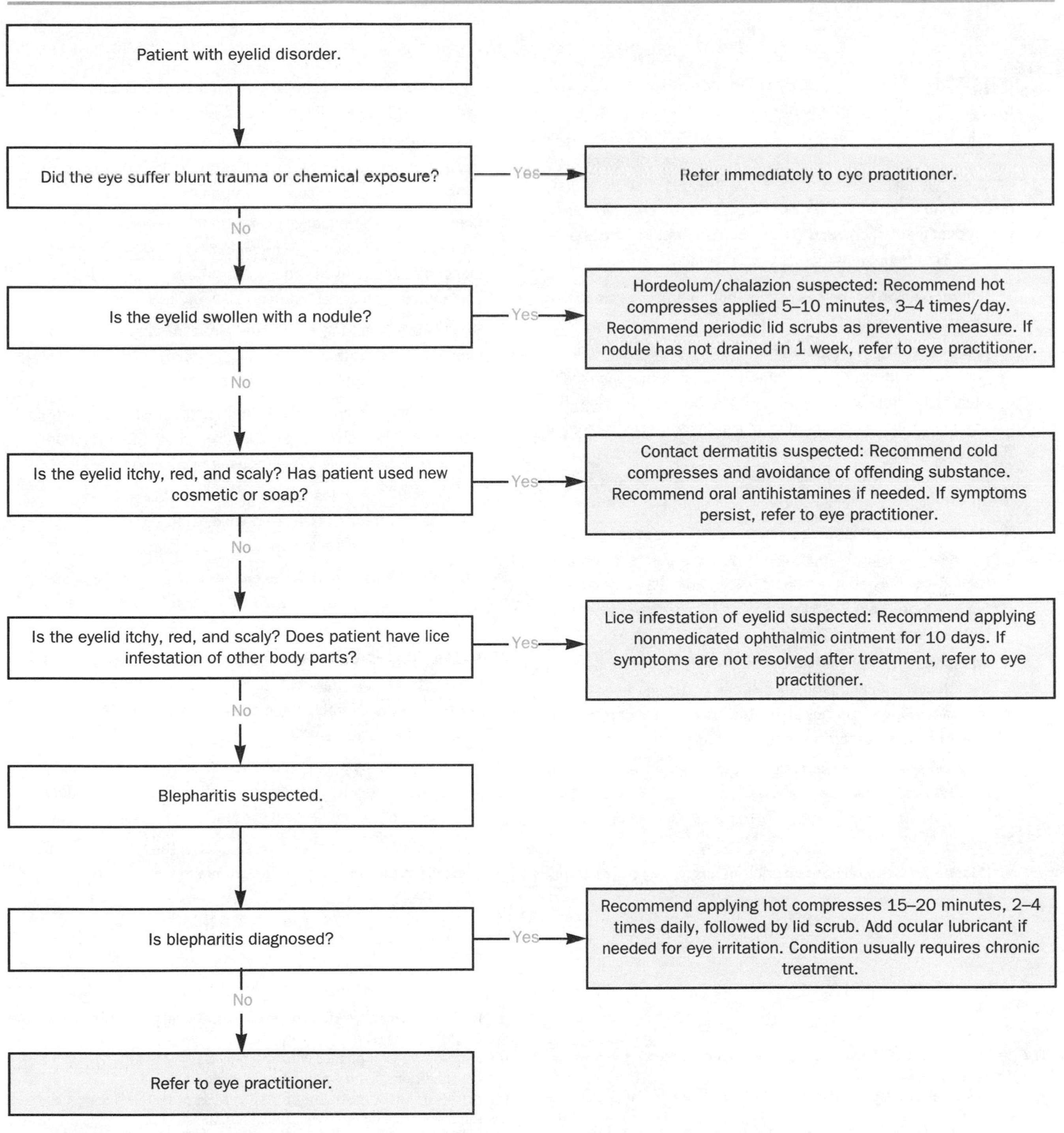

Figure 22–3 Self-care of eyelid disorders.

preservatives, or other excipients in the product. Patients who are already using a prescription ophthalmic product should use nonprescription products only after consulting with an ophthalmic practitioner or pharmacist. Patients with a history of narrow anterior chamber angles or narrow-angle glaucoma should not use topical ocular decongestants because of the risk of angle-closure glaucoma. Drug application should be conservative in patients with hyperemic conjunctiva because of the potential for increased systemic drug absorption and the risk of adverse effects. The lowest concentration and conservative dosage frequencies should be used, and overdosage should be avoided. Ophthalmic products are frequently misused; therefore, counseling on appropriate application of products is crucial.

Patient Education for Ophthalmic Disorders

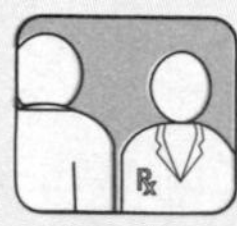

The objectives of self-treatment are (1) to relieve the symptoms of minor ophthalmic disorders, using the appropriate nonprescription products or nondrug measures, and (2) to use nonprescription products as adjunct treatment of ophthalmic disorders diagnosed by an eye practitioner. For most patients, carefully following product instructions and the self-care measures listed below will help ensure optimal therapeutic outcomes.

- If **blunt trauma to the eye** occurs, obtain an eye examination as soon as possible.
- If you have **dry eye syndrome** and the first ophthalmic lubricants used to treat it are not effective, ask the pharmacist about the following treatment options: increasing the dosage, switching to a product of increased viscosity, and/or switching to a nonpreserved product. (See Table 22–1 for examples of dry eye products. See Tables 22–2 and 22–3 for guidelines on instilling eye drops and ointment.)
- When treating **allergic conjunctivitis**, do not exceed recommended dosages of ophthalmic decongestants or antihistamine–decongestant products. (See Table 22–4 for product listings. See Table 22–5 for dosages.) Do not use these medications longer than 72 hours.
- When treating **viral conjunctivitis**, wash hands after touching the infected eye and properly dispose of tissues used to blot the infected eye. Do not share towels or other objects that might come in contact with the infected eye.
- If **eye exposure to chemicals** occurs, irrigate the eye for 10 minutes and seek immediate eye care. (See Table 22–6 for examples of eye irrigants. See Table 22–7 for usage guidelines.)
- If **loose foreign substances** such as lint, dust, or pollen enter the eye, flush the substance from the eye using an eye irrigant. (See Tables 22–6 and 22–7.)
- If a **foreign substance becomes imbedded in the eye** or trapped under the eyelid, see an eye practitioner. Failure to remove the substance could cause an eye infection.
- Consult an eye practitioner before treating **corneal edema**. If hyperosmotic solutions are recommended, follow the recommended dosages even though the product may sting. (See Table 22–6 for product listings.)
- Be aware that taking ophthalmic vitamin supplements for **macular degeneration** along with general multivitamins may result in gastrointestinal upset or toxicity.
- For treatment of **chronic blepharitis**, maintain lid hygiene with the regular use of lid scrubs. (See Table 22–6 for product listings. See Table 22–8 for usage guidelines.)
- Do not treat **lice infestations of the eyelids** with pediculicides (lice products); use a nonmedicated ointment for 10 days instead. (See Table 22–3 for usage guidelines.)
- If **contact dermatitis of the eyelid** occurs, identify the cause of the reaction and try to avoid future contact with the substance.
- To clear a **hordeolum or chalazion,** apply hot compresses three to four times daily for 5 to 10 minutes at each session. Consult an eye practitioner if the disorder persists after 1 week of treatment.
- Discard or replace eye drop bottles 30 days after the sterility safety seal is opened. The manufacturer's expiration date does not apply once the seal is broken.

If the disorder persists or worsens after the recommended length of therapy, consult an eye practitioner.

References

1. Schein OD, Munoz B, Tielsch JM, et al. Prevalence of dry eye among the elderly. *Am J Ophthalmol.* 1997;124:723–8.
2. Warwick R. In: *Anatomy of the Eye and Orbit.* 7th ed. Philadelphia: WB Saunders; 1975:195–219.
3. Milder B. The lacrimal apparatus. In: Moses RA, Hart WM, eds. *Adler's Physiology of the Eye.* 8th ed. St Louis: CV Mosby; 1987:15–35.
4. Mishima S, Gasset A, Klyce SO, et al. Determination of tear volume and tear flow. *Invest Ophthalmol.* 1966;3:264–76.
5. Jordan A, Baum J. Basic tear flow. Does it exist? *Ophthalmology.* 1980;9: 920–30.
6. Harris LS, Galin MA. Dose response analysis of pilocarpine-induced ocular hypotension. *Arch Ophthalmol.* 1970;1:605–8.
7. Pfister RR, Burstein N. The effects of ophthalmic drugs, vehicles, and preservatives on corneal epithelium; a scanning electron microscope study. *Invest Ophthalmol.* 1976;15:246–59.
8. Norn MS. Desiccation of the precorneal film: I. Corneal wetting time. *Acta Ophthalmol.* 1969;47:865–80.
9. Lopez-Bernal D, Ubels JL. Quantitative evaluation of the corneal epithelial barrier effect: effect of artificial tears and preservatives. *Curr Eye Res.* 1991;7:645–66.
10. Swanson M. Compliance with and typical usage of artificial tears in dry eye conditions. *J Am Optom Assoc.* 1998;69:649–55.
11. Berdy GJ, Abelson MB, Smith LM, et al. Preservative free artificial tear solutions. *Arch Ophthalmol.* 1992;110:528–32.
12. Jaanus SD. Lubricants and other preparations for ocular surface disease. In: Bartlett JD, Jaanus SD, eds. *Clinical Ocular Pharmacology.* Boston: Butterworth-Heinemann; 1995:355–67.
13. Schilling H, Koch JM, Waubke TN, et al. Treatment of dry eye with vitamin A acid: an impression cytology controlled study. *Fortschr Ophthalmol.* 1989;5:530–4.
14. Mullen W, Sheppard W, Leibowitz J. Ophthalmic preservatives and vehicles. *Surv Ophthalmol.* 1973;17:469–83.
15. Sabiston DW. The dry eye. *Trans Ophthalmol Soc N Z.* 1969;21:96–100.
16. Linn ML, Jones LT. Rate of lacrimal excretion of ophthalmic vehicles. *Am J Ophthalmol.* 1968;65:76–8.
17. Burstein NL. Ophthalmic drug formulations. In: Bartlett JD, Jaanus SD, eds. *Clinical Ocular Pharmacology.* Boston: Butterworth-Heinemann; 1995:21–45.

18. Burstein NL. Preservative cytotoxic threshold for benzalkonium chloride and chlorhexidine digluconate in cat and rabbit corneas. *Invest Ophthalmol Vis Sci.* 1980;19:308–13.
19. Wilson WS, Duncan AJ, Jay JL. Effect of benzalkonium chloride on the stability of the precorneal tear film in rabbit and man. *Br J Ophthalmol.* 1975;59:667–9.
20. Mondino BJ, Salamon SM, Zaidman GW. Allergic and toxic reactions in soft contact lens wearers. *Surv Ophthalmol.* 1982;26:337–44.
21. Miller J, Wolf EM. Antazoline phosphate and naphazoline hydrochloride, singly and in combination for the treatment of allergic conjunctivitis—a controlled double-blind clinical trial. *Ann Allergy.* 1975;35: 81–6.
22. Soparkar CN, Wilhelmus KR, Koch DD, et al. Acute and chronic conjunctivitis due to over the counter ophthalmic decongestants. *Arch Ophthalmol.* 1997;115:34–8.
23. Jaanus SD, Pagano VT, Bartlett JD. Drugs affecting the autonomic nervous system. In: Bartlett JD, Jaanus SD, eds. *Clinical Ocular Pharmacology.* Boston: Butterworth-Heinemann; 1989:69–148.
24. Abelson MB, Yamamoto GK, Allansmith MR. Effects of ocular decongestants. *Arch Ophthalmol.* 1980;98:856–8.
25. Jaanus SD, Hegeman SL, Swanson MW. Antiallergy drugs and decongestants. In: Bartlett JD, Jaanus SD, eds. *Clinical Ocular Pharmacology.* Boston: Butterworth-Heineman Publishers; 1995:337–53.
26. Krupin T, Silverstein B, Faitt M, et al. The effect of H1 blocking antihistamines on intraocular pressure in rabbits. *Ophthalmology.* 1980;87: 1167–72.
27. Abelson MB, Allansmith MR, Freidlaender MH. Effects of topically applied ocular decongestant and antihistamine. *Am J Ophthalmol.* 1980;90:254–7.
28. Petrusewicz J, Kalizan R. Blood platelet adrenoreceptor: aggregatory and antiaggregatory activity of imidazole drugs. *Pharmacology.* 1986;33: 249–55.
29. Pahissa A, Guardia J, Botil JM, et al. Antazoline induced allergic pneumonitis. *Br Med J.* 1979;2:1328.
30. Bengtsson U, Larsson O, Lindstedt G, et al. Antazoline induced immune hemolytic anemia, hemoglobulinuria, and acute renal failure. *Acta Med Scand.* 1975;198:223–7.
31. Neilsen JL, Dahl R, Kissmeyer-Neilsen F. Immune thrombocytopenia due to antazoline. *Allergy.* 1981;36:517–9.
32. Ogbuihi S, Audick W, Bohn G. Sudden infant death-fatal intoxication with pheniramine. *Z Rechtsmed.* 1990;103:221–5.
33. Berdy GJ, Abelson MB, George MA, et al. Allergic conjunctivitis—a survey of new antihistamines. *J Ocul Pharmacol.* 1991;7:313–24.
34. Gelmi C, Occuzzi R. Mydriatic effect of ocular decongestants studied by pupillography. *Ophthalmologica.* 1994;208:243–6.
35. Lamberts DW. Topical hyperosmotic agents and secretory stimulants. *Int Ophthalmol Clin.* 1980;20:163–9.
36. Hales RH. Contact lens solutions. In: *Contact Lenses: A Clinical Approach to Fitting.* Baltimore: Williams & Wilkins; 1978:32–50.
37. Christen WG. Antioxidant vitamins and age-related eye disease. *Proc Assoc Amer Phys.* 1999;111:16–21.
38. Sperduto RD, Ferris FL, Kurinij N. Do we have a nutritional treatment for age-related cataract or macular degeneration? *Arch Ophthalmol.* 1990;108:1403–5.
39. Jones DB, Liesegang TJ, Robinson NM. Laboratory diagnosis of ocular infections. Paper presented at: Annual Meeting of the American Society for Microbiology; May 26–30, 1981; Washington, DC.
40. Polack FM, Goodman DF. Experience with a new detergent lid scrub in the management of chronic blepharitis. *Arch Ophthalmol.* 1988;106: 719–20.
41. Ophthalmic drug products for over-the-counter human use; final monograph. *Federal Register.* 1988;53(43):6997–8.
42. Ophthalmic drug products for over-the-counter human use; establishment of a monograph; proposed rulemaking. *Federal Register.* 1980;45(89):30002–50.

CHAPTER 23

Prevention of Contact Lens–Related Disorders

Janet P. Engle

Chapter 23 at a Glance

Annual sales of contact lens care products exceed $400 million in pharmacies and $900 million overall; these sales are growing faster than any other category of nonprescription items. With the introduction of soft contact lenses in the 1970s, the greatly enhanced comfort of lenses has led to a significant expansion of the contact lens market. Similarly, developments with rigid gas–permeable (RGP) hard lenses provide the comfort of soft lenses and the enhanced optical qualities of hard lenses. Extended-wear lenses, toric lenses for astigmatism, tinted lenses, bifocal contact lenses, and disposable lenses have also greatly expanded the potential patient population.

Although much of the motivation to wear contacts may be cosmetic, properly fitted lenses can provide significant vi-

Editor's Note: This chapter is based, in part, on the 11th edition chapter titled "Contact Lens Products," which was written by Janet P. Engle.

sion advantages over spectacles. Of the 32 million Americans currently wearing contact lenses, nearly 90% use the lenses to correct the vision of an otherwise healthy eye. Contact lenses reduce size distortion and prismatic effects and improve peripheral vision. Elimination of spectacle fogging, dirt accumulation, and frame distraction may also be a significant advantage to many users. Most soft contact lens wearers say their lenses are more comfortable than eyeglasses.

However, it has been well established that contacts, even when expertly fitted, somewhat alter ocular tissues and change the corneal metabolism. These effects make it imperative that both the user and the health care professional understand the proper care, maintenance, and safe use of these products. Failure to do so can greatly increase the chance of corneal infection, corneal ulcers, and other ocular conditions that may result in permanent eye damage. Fortunately, however, most side effects of contact lens use are reversible if attended to promptly.

More than 200 nonprescription contact lens care products are available, and consumers are likely to be overwhelmed by the variety. Except for the prescriber, pharmacists are the most qualified to counsel contact lens wearers as to which products to choose.[1] Product selection depends on the products' compatibility with each other as well as with the specific contact lens. Therefore the pharmacist's responsibility is to understand this area of professional practice and provide effective, up-to-date information when consulting with the contact lens wearer.

Table 23–1

Comparisons of Contact Lens Characteristics

	Conventional Hard Lenses	Soft Lenses	Rigid Gas–Permeable Lenses
Lens Characteristics			
Rigidity	+++	0	+++
Durability	+++	+	++
Oxygen transmission	0	+	+++
Chemical adsorption	0	+++	0
Optical Quality			
Visual acuity	+++	+	+++
Correction of astigmatism	Yes	Toric	Yes
Photophobia	+++	+	++
Spectacle blur	+++	0	++
Convenience			
Comfort	+	+++	++
Adaptation period	Weeks	Days	Days
Extended wear	No	Yes	Yes
Intermittent wear	No	Yes	No

Key: + indicates the degree to which the characteristic is present. 0 means the characteristic is not present.

Characteristics of Contact Lenses

Contact lenses are often broadly classified into three distinct groups based on their chemical makeup and physical properties. (See Table 23–1.) Lenses that are relatively inflexible, do not appreciably absorb water (less than 10%), and retain their shape when removed from the eye are commonly called rigid lenses. Rigid lenses made of polymethylmethacrylate (PMMA) are not permeable to oxygen and are often called hard lenses. Rigid lenses made of less inflexible polymers are permeable to oxygen and are called rigid gas–permeable, or RGP lenses. Hard lenses are seldom prescribed initially but may be replaced for individuals who successfully wore them before the advent of RGP lenses. Contact lenses that are moderately to highly flexible, absorb a high percentage of water (greater than 10%), and conform to the shape of a supporting structure are commonly called soft lenses. Although the overwhelming majority of contact lenses fall into these three categories, a few do not. Those few may be called flexible nonhydrogel lenses.

Subgroups of contact lenses are extended-wear lenses and disposable lenses. Extended-wear lenses can be either soft or, occasionally, RGP lenses that are designed to be worn for an extended time before removal. Disposable lenses are designed to be worn for 1 to 14 days and then thrown away.

Contact lenses are manufactured from polymers that vary widely in their chemical and physical properties. Each material has physical and surface characteristics that correlate to the specific problems the patient may encounter.[2]

Physical characteristics of contact lenses include dimensional stability, physical breakage, and polymer stability. Generally, hard lenses are dimensionally stable and tend to hold their parameters with little change. Soft lenses, however, are much less stable physically; water content, to a large extent, dictates their physical strength. RGP lenses generally have a high degree of dimensional stability. As they dehydrate, however, curvature of the plastic surfaces may alter slightly.

The characteristics of the different contact lenses account for most of the problems that patients encounter. Unfortunately, many patients do not know which type of lens they are wearing. This underscores the importance of the pharmacist establishing an excellent relationship with contact lens practitioners in the area.

To maintain a healthy cornea, an adequate amount of oxygen is needed. The more oxygen that passes through the contact lens, the more adequately corneal metabolism can be maintained. Oxygen permeability describes the ability of a specific material to permit the passage of oxygen. Oxygen permeability is expressed as the *Dk* value of the material, where *D* is the diffusion coefficient, and *k* is the solubility coefficient. The higher the *Dk* value, the higher the oxygen permeability. The *Dk/L* value, in which *L* corresponds to the thickness of the material, is a measure of oxygen transmissibility (i.e., the amount of oxygen that can be transmitted through a contact lens of specific thickness) and is thus the value to which most practitioners and manufacturers refer. Because the lens thickness varies depending on the power of the lens, many manufacturers report the *Dk/L* value for a lens with a –3.00D prescription. For example, a lens that corrects a large myopia (minus lens) will be thinner in the center than a lens that corrects hyperopia (plus lens), which will be thicker in the center than on the periphery.

The minimal oxygen transmission values needed to prevent corneal edema in most patients have been extensively debated. For a daily-wear soft lens, the *Dk/L* value ([cm mL O_2]/[sec mL mm Hg]) should be at least 24.1×10^{-9}; for extended-wear soft lenses, the *Dk/L* value should be 34.3×10^{-9}. This limits overnight corneal swelling to approximately 8% and provides for adequate daytime deswelling to occur.[3] Paradoxically, RGP lenses now have a greater oxygen capability than do soft lenses but, owing to a "tear fluid–pumping" mechanism where oxygen-saturated tears help oxygenate the cornea, do not require the oxygen transmissibility to be as high.

Oxygen transmission primarily depends on the water content of the soft lens. The higher the water content, the more oxygen is transmitted through the lens. However, as water content increases, durability decreases, and the lens must be made thicker, which hinders oxygen permeability. Thus, a thick lens with a high water content may transmit the same amount of oxygen as a thin lens with a lower water content.[4] Another problem is that, as water content increases, the lenses tend to attract tear deposits such as lipids, proteins, and polysaccharides. Further, and especially if large pores or many pores are present, lenses with a high water content tend to be more susceptible to the growth of bacteria and fungi on the surface than lenses with a lower water content.[5]

Types of Contact Lenses

The majority of contact lens–wearing patients (82%) are fitted with soft (hydrophilic) lenses.[6] Rigid (primarily RGP) lenses are prescribed for 18% of patients. Extended-wear lenses (soft or RGP) are worn by 15% of patients wearing contact lenses. Approximately 87% of patients wearing contact lenses wear some type of disposable or planned replacement lenses.[7]

Hard Lenses

Hard contact lenses were the first lenses to be used in the United States. Hard lenses are polymerized products of esters of acrylic acid or methacrylic acid. The most common plastic found in hard lenses is PMMA, which is known commercially as Lucite or Plexiglas.

PMMA is not significantly permeable to oxygen; therefore, for the cornea to remain healthy, the lens must be able to slide and rock over the corneal surface in response to a blink so that oxygenation can occur. As the hard lens moves, a layer of tears forms under it and is continually recirculated by the sliding and rocking motion of the tear fluid–pumping phenomenon. To allow this movement over the eye, hard lenses are made relatively small in diameter (8.0 to 9.5 mm) and thus may pop out of the wearer's eye.

Contact lenses made of PMMA are hydrophobic, and PMMA is now rarely used for new contact lens fittings because of its negligible permeability to oxygen. However, PMMA possesses many characteristics that make it ideal for a corrective lens in contact with the ocular surface.

Advantages

Hard lenses offer the following distinct advantages to the wearer: (1) The lenses are very light because of a specific gravity of 1.18 to 1.20. (2) Their refractive index, 1.49 to 1.50, is similar to that of glass spectacle lenses. (3) The lenses allow a light transmission of 90% to 92%. (4) The lenses are not affected by weak alkalis or weak acids. (5) The plastic does not cause sensitivity reactions when placed on the cornea.

Disadvantages

In rigid lenses, a small colored dot marker or an etch mark on one lens identifies it as being for the right eye. This marker, located at the outer periphery of the lens, is not perceived by the wearer when the lens is on the cornea.

One phenomenon associated primarily with hard lenses is spectacle blur. A hard lens, while in place on the cornea, alters the surface topography of the eye and creates hypoxic edema. As a result, the patient may not see well with glasses immediately after removing the lens. Generally, spectacle blur abates in 20 to 30 minutes. The hardness of these lenses is less than that of glass but is more than that of RGP or soft lenses. Thus, reasonable care must be exercised with hard lenses to avoid scratching or chipping them. Inadequate care or neglect of hard lenses may lead to corneal problems or wearer discomfort, but the lens will still maintain its optical qualities.

Rigid Gas-Permeable Lenses

The new generation of RGP lenses combines the optical qualities of PMMA and the oxygen permeability of soft lenses. Generally, RGP lenses can deliver two to three times more oxygen to the cornea than soft lenses of the same thickness. Although, to maintain rigidity (important for correcting astigmatism and the lens fit), RGP lenses are generally thicker than soft lenses, most recent RGP lenses still transmit much more oxygen to the cornea than do soft lenses while covering only the central 75% of the cornea. RGP lenses, unlike soft lenses, also exchange up to 20% of the postlens tear volume per blink.

RGP lenses have been investigated for extended-wear use, and some have been approved for 1 to 7 days of extended wear. The use of extended-wear lenses is somewhat controversial as these lenses have been implicated in causing corneal ulcers (eruptions on the corneal surface), which in rare instances can lead to partial or complete blindness.

RGP lenses are available in several materials. One type of RGP lens is composed of silicone acrylates that combine silicone with methyl methacrylate and methacrylic acid and/or hydroxyethyl methacrylate (HEMA) in varying amounts. This material is relatively stable and fairly inflexible. Examples of this type of lens include Polycon II and Paraperm O_2.

Fluorine may also be a component of RGP lenses. This may be in the form of fluorosilicone acrylate or fluoropolymer lenses. An example of this type of lens is the Boston Equalens.

Alkyl styrene copolymers, another type of RGP lens, are moderately oxygen permeable and lighter than other RGP lens materials. They also have low density and a relatively high refractive index. Although these lenses are seldom prescribed, Novalens is an example.

Of the many RGP materials available, the silicone acrylates and the fluorosilicone acrylates are the most commonly used.[8]

Advantages

Advantages of RGP lenses vary depending on the type of materials used. Fluorinated lenses offer the advantages of increased oxygen transmissibility and reduced liphophilicity problems. These lenses also have less surface reactivity, thereby decreasing tear deposits. Alkylstyrene copolymers have the advantage of being lighter than other RGP lens materials.

Disadvantages

Disadvantages of RGP lenses also vary depending on the type of materials used. Silicone acrylate lenses have less surface wettability than PMMA because silicone has relatively higher hydrophobicity. Silicone acrylates also tend to have a negative surface charge, which can attract lysozymes and other positively charged deposits. Fluorinated lenses have the disadvantage of greater mass, which can affect RGP lens fit. These lenses also tend not to be highly wettable. Alkyl styrene copolymer lenses are brittle, have poor wettability, and lack surface stability.[9]

Soft Lenses

The main chemical difference between the hydrophobic rigid lens and the hydrophilic soft lens is that the soft lens contains hydroxyl or hydroxyl and lactam groups, which allow it to absorb and hold water. Table 23–2 classifies the different types of soft contact lenses into four groups according to water content and ionic charge based on 1986 Food and Drug Administration (FDA) recommendations. Soft lenses are composed of hydrophilic groups, including hydroxyl, amide, lactam, and carboxyl, with small amounts of cross-linking agents that form a hydrophilic gel (hydrogel) network. The degree of cross-linking determines lens hydrophilicity and water content. Greater cross-linking means fewer hydrophilic groups are available to interact with water, which in turn produces a less flexible, less hydrated lens than those originally available.

Table 23–2

Soft Contact Lens Classification

Soft Contact Lens Classification
Group I: Low Water, Nonionic
Polymacon
Hefilcon A and B
Tefilcon
Tetrafilcon A
Group II: High Water, Nonionic
Lidofilicon A and B
Surfilcon
Netrafilcon A
Group III: Low Water, Ionic
Bufilcon A (45%)
Etafilcon (43%)
Phemfilcon A (38%)
Group IV: High Water, Ionic
Bufilcon A (55%)
Perfilcon
Phemfilcon A (55%)
Etafilcon A (58%)

Ionic lenses have a negative surface charge, which tends to attract more protein deposits than nonionic lenses; soaking ionic lenses in sorbate-preserved saline yellows the lenses prematurely. Nonionic lenses are electrically neutral and tend to be less reactive with the tear film, resulting in a more deposit-resistant lens. High-water lenses (greater than 50%), which tend to attract tear film deposits into their matrix, usually cannot withstand daily heat disinfection. If soaked in enzymes for a prolonged period, these lenses may also cause sensitivity reactions.

The water content of soft lenses has gradually increased since they were introduced. Increasing the water content improves the oxygen permeability of a material. However, permeability also depends on lens thickness. Highly hydrated lenses are more comfortable but are also more fragile. Because these lenses must therefore be thicker to offset their fragility, the two factors often cancel each other out regarding oxygen transmissibility. Lowering the water content produces a more durable and longer-lasting lens. The water content of a HEMA-type (2-hydroxyethyl methacrylate) material can vary between 5% and 90%, but a theoretical ideal value might be 75% to 78%, which matches the hydration of the corneal stroma. However, reducing the percentage of water in a soft HEMA lens also reduces the thickness of the hydrated lens, thereby improving the wearer's comfort. Thus, the optimum water content actually appears to be between 55% and 65%, given the thicknesses at which these materials can be reliably worn. Many lens wearers find they cannot tolerate lenses with a thickness above 0.4 mm because of lid discomfort. For those who cannot tolerate regular soft lenses, several ultrathin soft lenses are available with a thickness as low as 0.04 mm.

Soft lenses in the nonhydrated (dry) state are rigid and extremely brittle and should not be handled by the wearer. When hydrated, the lenses expand as water is absorbed into the gel matrix. These lenses are most comfortable when they are larger than the diameter of the cornea, have thin edges, and undergo just enough movement on the eye to ensure lubrication of the ocular surface under the lens.

Types

The increased oxygen permeability and reduced eyelid interaction of soft contact lenses enable certain lenses to be broken in more quickly and worn continuously. Table 23–3 lists examples of some of the soft contact lenses approved for wear in the United States.

Extended-Wear Lenses Soft extended-wear lenses were originally intended to be worn for weeks. However, as with RGP extended-wear lenses, problems with contamination, infection, and ulceration suggest that they should not be worn for more than 7 days.[10] Some evidence strongly supports removing them overnight, at least once per week, to reduce the risk of ulcerative keratitis.[11,12] At this time, there is a trend towards lens care practitioners discouraging overnight wear of contact lenses because of the potential for adverse effects.

Disposable and Planned Replacement Lenses Disposable lenses represent the fastest-growing segment of the soft lens market. Depending on the lens, there are several approved wearing schedules. Some lenses are worn for 1 day and then discarded; others are worn daily for up to 2 weeks and then discarded; still others can be worn as extended-wear lenses for up to 2 weeks, with the patient wearing them for 6 nights and then removing them for 1 night. Planned replacement lenses are discarded and replaced usually after 1 to 3 months of wear, depending on how quickly the lenses build up deposits and on how well the patient complies with lens care. Planned replacement lenses and disposable lenses other than the daily disposables are cared for similarly to other soft contact lenses. In most patients, an enzymatic cleaner is generally not necessary when using disposable lenses that will be discarded after a few weeks of wear.

Daily disposable lenses have the following advantage: (1) Each lens is sterile prior to removal from its package for immediate insertion into the eye. (2) No cleaning regimen is necessary since the lens is just thrown out after wear. (3) Deposit formation is minimal. (4) Lens-related problems such as giant papillary conjunctivitis or allergic reactions to lens care solutions occur less often. However, at a cost of up to $2 per day for daily disposable lenses to correct both eyes, they are not yet affordable for some patients.

Specialty Lenses Some soft contacts are classified as specialty lenses. These include toric, bifocal, and tinted lenses. Toric soft lenses have been developed specifically to correct astigmatic (improper focusing attributed to an irregularly shaped cornea) visual conditions. Traditional soft lenses do not correct astigmatism because they conform to the corneal surface rather than retain their original shape, as do rigid lenses. Toric soft lenses are fabricated with both spherical and cylindrical optical corrections and remain on axis because of design features such as weighting on the bottom edge of the lens. Spherical soft lenses can be fitted to eyes with an upper limit of astigmatism of about 1.00 diopters (a

Table 23–3

Examples of Soft Contact Lenses

Trade Name (Manufacturer)	Water/Saline Content (%)	Group Classification[a]
Daily Wear Soft Lenses		
Cibasoft (CIBA Vision)	37.5	I
Durasoft 2 (Wesley-Jessen)	38.0	III
Satureyes (Metro)	55.0	II
Soflens (Bausch & Lomb Optics)	38.6	I
Hydrasoft Standard (Coopervision)	55.0	IV
Extended Wear Soft Lenses		
Cibathin (CIBA Vision)	37.5	I
DuraSoft 3 (Wesley-Jessen)	55.0	IV
Permaflex Natural (Coopervision)	74.0	II
Permalens (Coopervision)	71.0	IV
Disposable Soft Lenses		
1 Day Acuvue (Vistakon)	58.0	IV
New Vues (CIBA Vision)	55.0	II
SeeQuence (Bausch & Lomb Optics)	38.0	I
Soft Toric Lenses		
Optima Toric (Bausch & Lomb Optics)	45.0	I
Eclipse (Sunsoft)	55.0	IV
Soft Bifocal Lenses		
Hydrocurve II (Wesley-Jessen)	45.0	III
PA1 (Bausch & Lomb Optics)	38.6	I

[a] See Table 23–2 for group classifications.

unit of refracting power used as a quantitative measure of the abnormal refraction of light at surfaces such as the cornea). However, this figure highly depends on the criticality and motivation of the patient.

Bifocal lenses, which can be weighted in a fashion similar to that of toric lenses, are prescribed to correct presbyopia (ocular changes caused by age).

Tinted lenses are available to facilitate handling and for cosmetic purposes (to change eye color) as well as for corrective uses. Three types of tinted lenses are available: translucent lenses, opaque lenses, and lenses that absorb ultraviolet radiation. Translucent lenses can be tinted in varying degrees, from light/number 1 intensity to facilitate handling and increase the visibility of the lens, to medium/number 2 and dark/number 3 intensities to enhance eye color. Translucent lenses work best on light eye colors. Opaque lenses cover the iris and hide its natural color; they can completely change the apparent eye color, even in individuals with dark brown eyes. These lenses may also be used as a prosthetic to mask corneal scarring or to cover an amblyopic (lazy) eye. Finally some lenses have material incorporated into them that absorbs ultraviolet radiation. To help protect from the harmful effects of ultraviolet radiation, these lenses are used in cases of aphakia patients (patients in whom the crystalline lens of the eye is removed because of an opacified lens or cataract and an intraocular lens is not implanted).

Advantages

Soft lenses are easier to remove and are considerably more comfortable than rigid lenses. This effect is most apparent during the initial break-in period. Photophobia is not likely to occur with soft lenses, and glare is significantly reduced. As with rigid lenses, however, flare around the periphery may be noticed at night, particularly in individuals who have large pupils. This flare is caused by refractive light entering the eye through the edge margin of the contact lens.

Soft lens wearers can change more easily from their lenses to eyeglasses after a period of wear. The typical soft lens wearer does not usually experience the spectacle blur common among hard lens wearers and even occasionally experienced among RGP wearers.

Soft lenses are less likely than rigid lenses to trap dust particles, eyelashes, or other foreign material under the lens. They are also less likely to become dislodged or fall out. Therefore, soft lenses are often better suited for occasional wear and sports, including contact sports.

Disadvantages

Although many people prefer the comfort of soft lenses, not all soft lens wearers can achieve excellent visual acuity. The hydration of the lens may change either in or out of the eye, particularly with extreme temperatures and low relative humidity. This change can decrease the quality of the visual image. Because a soft lens conforms in large part to the corneal shape, it is difficult to project the degree of vision improvement before the lens is actually placed on the eye. Further, because soft lenses cannot be as precisely tailored to the specific requirements of an individual cornea, the fitting process is less exact than it is with rigid lenses. As a result, the overall quality of vision with soft contact lenses does not usually equal that of a properly fitted pair of rigid lenses. Fortunately, these differences are often small and should not concern many wearers.

Unlike rigid lenses, soft lenses can absorb chemical compounds from topically administered ophthalmic products.[13] As previously discussed, ocular irritation may result, and the lens may be damaged. With the exception of specially formulated rewetting solutions, no solution should be instilled into the eye with the soft lens in place. If a drug solution is instilled into the eye prior to lens insertion, the wearer must wait to insert a lens until the solution has cleared from the precorneal (conjunctival) pocket—about 5 minutes. A nonprescription ophthalmic product not specifically designed for use with contact lenses should not be used when lenses are in the eye. When topical ophthalmic ointments, gels, or suspensions are being used, the lenses should not be worn at all.

Unlike rigid lenses, soft lenses cannot be easily marked to identify which is for the left and right eyes. A soft lens wearer who is uncertain of the identity of the lenses may have to see the vision specialist.

Soft lenses generally cost more than hard lenses. Although the initial cost of acquiring soft lenses has decreased, the overall cost is greater because they must be replaced more often because of changes in the refractory requirements of the eye. Soft lenses are also more costly because they are less durable than hard ones and require more cleaning and disinfecting products.

The care given to contact lenses varies considerably with each wearer. Soft lenses rapidly degenerate to useless pieces of plastic if they are neglected. When used with a fastidious care and cleaning program, however, daily wear soft lenses can have an average life of 12 to 18 months compared with 18 to 36 months for similarly used RGP lenses.

Use of Contact Lenses

In a few cases, use of contact lenses is contraindicated. Most people though can wear one or more types of contact lenses without problems if certain precautions are taken.

Indications for Contact Lenses

Some patients wear contact lenses because eyeglasses cannot provide satisfactory vision. Others wear them for cosmetic reasons or because they find eyeglasses a hindrance during sports or other life activities. However, most patients with vision problems can use either eyeglasses or contact lenses for purely visual reasons.

Therapeutic Necessity

The decision to wear contact lenses rather than eyeglasses is sometimes based on therapeutic necessity. For example, with keratoconus, a gradual protrusion of the central cornea, satisfactory vision is usually unattainable with ordinary eyeglasses but can be obtained with rigid contact lenses.[14] Other examples of therapeutic necessity are lenses used as collagen shields and soft contact lenses saturated with antibiotic agents.

Aphakic individuals characteristically see better with contact lenses than with spectacles. Extended-wear contacts are particularly beneficial for such patients because their poor vision makes it difficult for them to insert and remove lenses.

Visual aberrations caused by corneal scarring are also often better corrected with rigid contact lenses. Whereas eyeglasses simply correct refractive error by changing the focus of light incident on the cornea, the proximity of the rigid contact lens actually masks irregularities in the corneal topography. Prosthetic lenses may also make corneal scarring cosmetically unnoticeable.

Refractive Exam

Other indications for the use of contacts include refractive errors such as myopia (nearsightedness), hyperopia (farsightedness), astigmatism, and presbyopia.

Astigmatism occurs when an unequal curvature of the refractive surfaces of the eye results in a fuzzy image. RGP lenses, hard lenses, and toric soft lenses, to a lesser extent, can be used to correct an astigmatism.

Presbyopia (old vision) is a condition caused by aging, in which the crystalline lens cannot properly focus on near objects. More than 50% of visually corrected patients are presbyopic. Contact lenses have not been overly successful for these patients. Because vision correction is needed for both near and far, two optical corrections are required in each bifocal contact lens. For most bifocal contact lenses to be successful, the patient should be highly motivated and should engage in an occupation or sports activities with rigorous visual demands.[15,16]

To correct presbyopia with spectacles, bifocal or trifocal lenses (often called multifocal lenses) are needed. If properly selected and indoctrinated, patients trying bifocal contacts can be successful 60% to 70% of the time. Monovision is one method of presbyopic contact lens correction that has been successful in some cases: The dominant eye is fitted with a lens for far vision; the other eye is fitted with a lens that corrects for close-up objects and reading. In most individuals, the eyes adjust in a relatively short time; reading is done with the nondominant eye, and distant objects are noted with the dominant one.

Other Benefits

Perhaps the main reason for choosing contact lenses is the perceived improvement in personal appearance. Other strongly influencing factors include (1) no obstruction of vision from eyeglass frames, (2) greater clarity in peripheral vision, (3) no fogging of lenses caused by sudden temperature changes, and (4) more freedom of motion during vigorous activity (e.g., sports). A number of factors, such as increased sensitivity to light and improved quality of the retinal image, contribute to the subjective perception of vision improvement by the contact lens wearer. With eyeglasses, the myopic individual sees a smaller-than-normal image and the hyperopic individual sees a larger-than-normal image. With contacts, both myopic and hyperopic individuals see objects in nearly their true sizes; for highly myopic persons, the image size increase with contact lenses is significant and decidedly beneficial.

Contraindications for Contact Lenses

Some individuals who require vision correction cannot or should not wear contact lenses. Contraindications are often based on lifestyle as well as on medical history.

Occupational Hazards

Occupational conditions that may prohibit the wearing of contact lenses include exposure to wind, glare, molten metals, irritants, dust and particulate matter, tobacco smoke, chemicals, and chemical fumes.[17] Certain chemical fumes have been suggested as being particularly hazardous because of the potential concentration of irritants under a hard lens or inside a soft lens. The lens theoretically prolongs contact of such substances with the cornea and can lead to corneal toxicity. However, these theoretical occupational contraindications have not been proven.

Medical Conditions

Contact lenses should not be used for cosmetic reasons if a patient has active pathologic intraocular or corneal conditions. Medical reasons that contraindicate contact lens wear include (1) chronic conjunctivitis; (2) blepharitis; (3) recurrent viral, bacterial, or fungal infections; and (4) poor blink rate or incomplete blink. Insufficient tear production, a deficiency or excess of mucin, excessive lipid production, or excessively dry environments may also preclude successful contact lens use.

Diabetic patients are often advised against extended-wear contact lenses because of retarded healing processes and the tendency toward prolonged corneal abrasion with such use. This precaution is probably unnecessary for daily wear of lenses unless problems occur.

Chronic common colds or allergic conditions such as hay fever and asthma may also make lens wear extremely uncomfortable or impossible.

In women, the corneal topography may be altered by pregnancy or the use of oral contraceptives. The fluid-retaining properties of estrogen may lead to edema of the cornea and eyelids as well as to decreased tear production. Dry spots on the cornea, often found in postmenopausal women, may also preclude successful contact lens wear. These spots, possibly caused by the absence of the precorneal film, are often identified with lacrimal insufficiency.

Contact lenses can be used with care by elderly persons; care is needed because of possible lacrimal insufficiency and loose lid tissues, which create a sagging conjunctival cul-de-sac and therefore make lens retention difficult. Contact lenses should be used with caution by patients with severe arthritis. Individuals with arthritis may lack the dexterity needed to insert lenses.

Lens wearers moving from a low to a high altitude may encounter hypoxia (low oxygen content of the cornea) or metabolic deficiency, resulting in irritation and corneal abrasions.

During the period needed for adapting to rigid contact lenses, the eyelids may become hyperemic (congested with excess blood); this condition may lead to blepharitis (inflammation of the eyelids), especially in the upper lid. Short pseudoblinks, by new wearers of hard lenses, may irritate the conjunctiva of the upper eyelid. Chin elevation and squinting may result from the patient's efforts to minimize the irritation.

Precautions for Contact Lenses

Contact lenses generally can match or exceed the vision obtained with spectacles. However, depending on the type of lens, vision may become worse in certain situations.[18] Some patients wearing lenses with high water content may experience hazy vision around the edges of objects. In some cases, patients wearing hard lenses experience nighttime ghosting, which occurs when the patient's pupil dilates enough to see the edges of the lens. This can sometimes be corrected with larger-diameter lenses. Other patients complain of spiderweb vision, usually at night; this can be due to crazing, the development of fine cracks, usually in RGP lenses.

Potential Transmission of Viral Infections

The human immunodeficiency virus (HIV) has been isolated from the tears of infected individuals as well as from the contact lenses worn by infected individuals. This seemingly becomes an issue in the case of trial contact lenses, which may be reused by different patients in the lens-fitter's office. Generally, these lenses are not dispensed to a patient except as loaner lenses (i.e., to a patient waiting for new replacement lenses). Even in this scenario, after the lenses have been used in any patient, they are disinfected with heat or chemicals before being dispensed to another patient. Studies have shown that heat and the routinely available hydrogen peroxide products are effective in inactivating the HIV virus. The FDA also requires that all contact lens regimens kill herpes simplex, another enveloped virus. No reported cases of HIV transmission via a contact lens fitting have been reported.[19]

Adverse Effects of Drugs

Many undesired effects have been reported when a patient who wears contact lenses ingests or applies certain drugs or encounters certain drugs. (See Table 23–4.) The pharmacist must understand these drug-induced problems to counsel patients effectively.

Topical Drugs In general, patients should be counseled not to place any ophthalmic solution, suspension, gel, or ointment into the eye when contact lenses are in place. The only exceptions to this rule are products specifically formulated to be used with contact lenses, such as rewetting drops, or those products that an eye care practitioner has specifically recommended for use with contact lenses.

Topical administration of ophthalmic drugs may have physiologic consequences or may modify pharmacologic responses to drugs. The use of solutions that may be considered benign, such as artificial tears, may reduce tear breakup time and alter the distribution of the mucoid, aqueous, and lipid components of tears, perhaps causing initial discomfort upon instillation of the drops.[13] The pharmacologic effect of a topically administered drug while soft lenses are in place may be exaggerated: The soft lens may absorb the drug and either release it over time, thus creating a sustained-release

Table 23–4

Drug–Contact Lens Interactions

Changes in Tear Film and/or Production	
Tear Volume Decreased	
Anticholinergic agents	Timolol (topical)
Antihistamines	Tricyclic antidepressants
Diuretics	
Tear Volume Increased	
Cholinergic agents	Reserpine
Changes in Lens Color (Primarily Soft Lenses)	
Diagnostic dyes (i.e., fluorescein)	Phenolphthalein
Epinephrine (topical)	Phenylephrine
Fluorescein (topical)	Rifampin
Nicotine	Sulfasalazine
Nitrofurantoin	Tetracycline
Phenazopyridine	Tetrahydrozoline (topical)
Phenothiazines	
Changes in Tonicity	
Pilocarpine (8%)	Sodium sulfacetamide (10%)
Lid/Corneal Edema	
Chlorthalidone	Oral contraceptives
Clomiphene	Primidone
Ocular Inflammation/Irritation	
Gold salts	Salicylates
Isotretinoin	Diclofenac (topical ophthalmic)
Changes in Refractivity (Induction of Myopia)	
Acetazolamide	Sulfamethoxazole
Sulfadiazine	Sulfisoxazole
Sulfamethizole	
Miscellaneous Agents/Effects	
Digoxin (increased glare)	
Ribavirin (cloudy lenses)	
Topical ciprofloxacin/Prednisolone acetate (precipitate)	
Hypnotics/Sedatives/Muscle relaxants (decreased blink rate)	

Adapted with permission from Engle JP. Contact lens care. *Am Druggist.* 1990;201:54–65.

dosage form, or bind it tightly so that none of it is released into the eye. Further, the presence of any kind of contact lens may increase the amount of time the medication is in contact with the eye. Finally, some increased drug absorption may occur secondary to a compromised corneal epithelium that is present during contact lens wear.[13]

In certain cases, patients will be treated with topical ophthalmic medications while wearing contact lenses. For example, such medications are used in conjunction with disposable soft contact lenses as an alternative to bandage contact lenses in the treatment of persistent epithelial corneal defects. Yet some case reports of an opaque precipitate have been noted in patients using SeeQuence disposable contact lenses when treated with topical ciprofloxacin and topical prednisolone acetate concurrently.[20] When studied in the laboratory, neither drug alone produced precipitates in the contact lens; white crystalline deposits were noted only when the two topical agents were used in combination. Another study noted that the combination of topical gentamicin and methylprednisolone produced precipitates.[21] Thus, if a patient who wears contact lenses is treated with a topical antibiotic and steroid combination, the eye care practitioner must carefully monitor for deposits in the lenses. If deposits are noted, the lenses should be removed and replaced with a new pair.

Additionally, the preservatives, vehicles, tonicity factors, and pH of the solution instilled into the eye could alter the lenses. For instance, instilling of hypertonic solutions such as sodium sulfacetamide 10% or pilocarpine 8% may cause soft lens dehydration and lens disfigurement. Topical medications with an acidic pH promote lens dehydration and steepening; alkaline medications promote hydration and flattening.[22] Topical suspensions may lead to lens intolerance because particulate matter builds up and causes discomfort. Gel and oil formulations may alter the surface relationship between the contact lens and the cornea.[13] Finally, the active ingredient of certain topical products may discolor lenses. For example, exposure to light and air causes epinephrine to form adrenochrome deposits, which range in color from pink to brown.

Airborne Drugs Some drugs present in indoor air may damage lenses. For example, some nurses who care for patients receiving ribavirin have reportedly experienced cloudy lenses after repeated exposure to the drug.[23,24] Similarly, contact lens wearers exposed to a large amount of cigarette smoke may discover a brown discoloration and nicotine deposits on their lenses. This is especially true for those who smoke and have nicotine-stained fingers.[25]

Systemic Medications Some systemic medications are secreted into tears and may interact with (primarily soft) contact lenses through this mechanism. For example, rifampin will stain the lenses and tears orange. Drugs such as gold salts are secreted into the tears and may cause ocular irritation. Others drugs may affect tear production, the refractive properties of the eye, the shape of the cornea, or the actual lens.[26] (See Table 23–4.)

Use of Cosmetics

Patients who wear contact lenses should choose—and use—cosmetics with care.[27] Individuals should insert lenses before applying makeup and should avoid touching the lens with eyeliner or mascara. Cosmetics, moisturizers, and makeup removers with an aqueous base should be used because oil-based products may cause blurred vision and irritation if they are deposited on the lens. Cream eye shadows are preferable to powder shadows. Water-resistant as opposed to waterproof mascara (which requires an oil-based remover) should be applied only to the very tips of the lashes. Eyeliners should never be applied inside the eyelid margin as the liner can clog glands in the eyelid and contaminate the contact lens. Any aerosol products, in particular, must be used with caution: Irritation may occur if some of the spray particles are trapped in the tear layer beneath the lens, and some sprays may actually damage the lens. One way to avoid a problem is to insert the lenses, go to another room, cover the eyes with a cloth, use the spray, and then leave the area with the eyes still closed.

Nail polish, hand creams, and perfumes should also be applied only after the lenses have been inserted. Nail polish and remover can destroy a lens. Men often contaminate their lenses with hair preparations and spray deodorants; they should take special care to clean their hands thoroughly before handling their contacts. Soaps containing cold cream or deodorants should be avoided because they can leave a film on the fingers after rinsing. This residue readily transfers to a lens and can cause blurred vision. Moreover, if a lens comes in contact with residual petrolatum-based lotion on the patient's fingers, the lens's surface can be modified. This modification cannot be detected by inspection; it will be noted, however, once the lens is worn. Approximately 20 to 30 minutes after insertion of the lens, the surface-wetting properties of the lens are disrupted.[28]

Corneal Hypoxia and Edema

An adequate supply of oxygen exists only if the cornea is continuously bathed with oxygenated tears.[29] During blinking, metabolic byproducts from the surface epithelium are flushed from under the contact lenses, and oxygen is brought in as the lenses move toward and away from the cornea. Even when properly fitted, however, both rigid and soft lenses can produce a progressive hypoxia of the cornea while the lenses are in place, especially in persons who have low blink frequency or incomplete blinks.

One major effect of this hypoxia is edema of the corneal tissues. It has been demonstrated that corneal thickness is increased to a greater extent by hard (PMMA) lenses. After approximately 16 hours of continuous wear, hard and, to a lesser extent, soft lenses cause the glycogen content of the cornea to fall to a level that is accompanied by significant edema. Symptoms associated with corneal edema include photophobia, rainbows around a light, sensations of hotness, grittiness and itchiness, fogging of vision, and blurred vision. Although it is not usually necessary, a patient experiencing corneal edema from overuse of contact lenses can be treated with one to two drops of sodium chloride (2% or 5%) every 3 to 4 hours after the lenses have been removed. (See Chapter 22, "Ophthalmic Disorders.") The patient should be counseled that transient stinging or burning may occur upon instilling the drops. Further, the patient should be counseled not to overuse the lenses.

Another effect of corneal hypoxia is neovascularization. The development of new vessels is potentially irreversible. Routine follow-up visits to the lens care specialist are important to monitor this effect of contact lens wear.

Corneal Abrasions

Corneal abrasions are surface defects in the epithelial layer of the cornea. Causes of these abrasions range from poorly fitted lenses or simple overwear to scratches caused by the entrapment of foreign bodies under the lens. The cornea is sensitive to abrasion, so blepharospasm (reflex lid closure), tearing, and rubbing the affected eye are immediate. However, rubbing the eye must be avoided because it can cause more extensive damage while the lens remains in the eye.

Fortunately, the pain associated with corneal abrasion is usually of greater magnitude than the damage. The epithelium regenerates quickly: Most minor epithelial defects (i.e., those 22 mm in diameter or less) generally heal within 12 to 24 hours. The lens should be left out for 2 to 7 days. The wearer may then proceed using a modified break-in schedule suggested by the vision specialist.

More extensive abrasions require the attention of an eye care specialist.

Symptoms of Lens Problems

Lens wearers may initially encounter various problems in adapting to lenses, particularly RGP ones; even longtime wearers occasionally experience difficulty. Many of these problems arise from different causative factors, and identifying and solving a specific problem may require a trained vision specialist. The following list provides a perspective for counseling a lens wearer who seeks advice. Most of this information is particularly applicable to rigid lens wear.

- *Deep aching of eye:* This pain persists even after the lens is removed, and it may be caused by poorly fitted lenses. The eye care practitioner must be consulted.
- *Blurred vision:* This effect may be produced by improper refractive power, lenses switched right for left, lenses placed on the eye inside out, tear film buildup, cosmetic film buildup, corneal edema, or use of oral contraceptives.
- *Excessive tearing:* Tearing is normal when lenses are first worn; however, poorly fitted lenses or chipped, rough edges on the lenses may also cause tearing.
- *Fogging:* Misty or smoky vision can be caused by corneal edema, overwearing of contact lenses, coatings or deposits on lens surfaces, or poor wetting of the lens while on the eye.
- *Flare:* Point sources of light having a sunburst or streaming quality can be caused by inadequate optic zone size or decentration of a poorly fitting lens.
- *Itching:* This symptom may be caused by allergic conjunctivitis and may be treated with short-term use of topical steroids.
- *Lens falling out of eye:* Poorly fitted lenses could be the cause. However, even properly fitted rigid lenses may occasionally slide off the cornea or be blinked out of the eye.
- *Inability to wear lenses in the morning:* This problem may be caused by corneal edema or mild conjunctivitis. Most likely, however, the patient's eyes dry out overnight because of incomplete eyelid closure.
- *Pain after removal of lens:* This effect is usually caused by corneal abrasion. The presence of the lens anesthetizes the cornea because of hypoxia; sensation returns after 4 to 6 hours and pain develops.
- *Sudden pain in the eye:* A foreign body or chipped or folded lens may be the problem.
- *Squinting:* This effect is caused by excessive lens movement or a poorly fitted lens. The wearer squints to center the optical portion of the lens over the pupil.

Lens Care Products and Procedures

Lens care products include surface-active cleaners, enzymatic cleaners, disinfecting solutions, wetting and rewetting solutions, and multipurpose solutions that combine several steps into one. Each type of contact lens has specific care procedures.

Formulation Considerations

The manufacturing and the marketing of contact lenses are regulated by the ophthalmic devices division of the FDA. Even though contact lens solutions are not considered drug products, formulation considerations still apply. Contact lens wearers should use only lens care products that have been approved by the FDA for use with their specific contact lens.

The basic considerations for a well-formulated contact lens solution include pH, viscosity, isotonicity with tears, stability, sterility, and provision for maintenance of sterility (bactericidal action). The pH range of comfort is not well defined because while normal tear pH is 7.4, tear pH varies among individuals. It is best to have a weakly buffered solution that can readily adjust to any tear pH, given that highly buffered solutions can cause significant discomfort, even ocular damage, when instilled. However, as with therapeutic ophthalmic solutions, stability of the solution components takes precedence over comfort. For this reason, many contact lens solutions are formulated with pH values above or below 7.4. These systems are weakly buffered and are usually well tolerated by the eye.

Routine daily use of any contact lens solution allows the potential for bacterial contamination. Depending on specific lens care procedures, a single container may last for a month or more. The solution must therefore contain a bactericidal agent that is both effective over the long term and nonirritating with daily use in the eye. Few preservatives fulfill these criteria. Commonly used agents are benzalkonium chloride, thimerosal, and sorbic acid products, all of which can cause irritation, depending on concentration and patient sensitivity.

Solutions from different manufacturers should not be mixed because a precipitate may result. For instance, a product containing alkaline borate buffers forms a gummy, gel-like precipitate on lenses if mixed with a wetting solution containing polyvinyl alcohol. Further, solutions containing cationic preservative, such as chlorhexidine, polyquaternium-1 (Polyquad), or polyaminopropyl biguanide (Dymed), should not be mixed with solutions containing an anionic preservative such as sorbic acid because this, too, will cause a precipitate.[30]

Preservatives Several preservatives are used in contact lens products. Older types of preservatives used include benzalkonium chloride, thimerosal, sorbic acid, chlorhexidine, EDTA. (For a detailed discussion of these preservatives, see Chapter 22, "Ophthalmic Disorders.") Several newer preservatives (polyquaternium-1 and polyaminopropyl biguanide) have been introduced in recent years. These preservatives are thought to cause less adverse effects than some of the older preservatives.

Polyquaternium-1 Polyquaternium-1 is a quaternary ammonium preservative shown to be effective against certain bacteria, fungi, and yeast. Few toxicity or sensitivity problems have been noted with this preservative thus far. When first introduced to the market, formulations containing Polyquad were not compatible with lenses that had a high water content since the methacrylic acid component of the lens had the ability to adsorb the preservative in toxic levels. However, recent formulations do not seem to have this problem.

Polyaminopropyl Biguanide Polyaminopropyl biguanide is a cationic polymeric biguanide effective against certain bacteria and yeast although its activity against *Acanthamoeba* and fungi does not appear to be optimal. *Acanthamoeba*, of which there are 15 species, is an opportunistic protozoan. Usually nonpathogenic, *Acanthamoeba* has been isolated from airborne dust, soils, surface water, tap water, and even distilled water. In unfavorable environments, it forms a very resistant cyst that can survive many antimicrobial agents, even though its vegetative form (trophozoite) may be susceptible. Viable cysts have been found in swimming pools and hot tubs that are adequately chlorinated to kill trophozoites. *Acanthamoeba* infection was very rare until contact lenses become popular. Some solutions were formerly preserved with chlorhexidine, and there were reports of contamination of the solution with *Serratia marcescens*, which is able to feed on the high molecular weight wetting agents. However, no significant adverse effects to polyaminopropyl biguanide have been reported in lens wearers. One manufacturer of RGP solutions uses higher concentrations of this preservative than are found in soft lens solutions; this is necessary because the RGP solutions contain high molecular weight wetting agents, which decrease the effectiveness of the preservative. The higher concentrations do not seem to cause toxicity to the wearer because RGP lenses do not adsorb the preservatives to the degree that soft lenses do.

Care of Hard Lenses

Lens care products help minimize the stress on the eye from hard contacts. These products aid the wearer, providing comfort and safety.

Hard lens care involves three important steps: cleaning, soaking, and wetting. (See Figure 23–1.) For optimal lens care, all three steps should be performed each time the lenses are removed from the eye.

Cleaning Solutions

Normal tears are composed of secretions from many specialized glands lining the lacrimal apparatus, conjunctiva, and lids. Many components are somewhat hydrophobic and tend

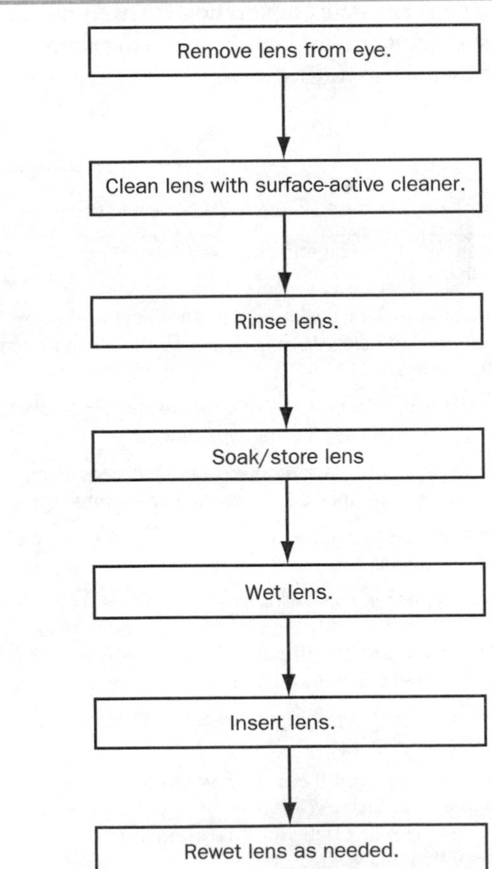

Figure 23–1 Self-care of hard lenses.

to adhere to the surface of a hard lens during normal daily wear. This residue, primarily proteinaceous debris and oils, acts as a growth medium for bacteria. If it is not routinely removed by daily cleaning, the residue may harden to form coatings or tenacious deposits that create an irregular surface on the lens. This residue will eventually irritate the eyelids and corneal epithelium, and it may progress to infection or other pathology. Decreased visual acuity and lens wear time are likely consequences of a cloudy lens or allergenic reactions to the residue.

Typical cleaning solutions contain nonionic or amphoteric surfactants that emulsify oils and aid in solubilizing other debris. Proteins and lipids are soluble in highly alkaline media, but high pH can cause lens decomposition. Weak alkaline solutions may dislodge deposits from the lens in conjunction with the surface tension-lowering properties of the surfactants. Homemade cleaning solutions such as baking soda mixed with distilled water or cleaning solution may scratch lenses and may not rinse off easily.[31] Use of household cleansers should be strongly discouraged to prevent lens damage and ocular irritation. Tables 23–5 and 23–6 provide instructions for properly cleaning hard lenses.

Soaking Solutions

A soaking solution is used to store hard contact lenses whenever they are removed from the eyes. The solution maintains the lens in a constant state of hydration for maximum comfort and visual acuity. It also aids in removing deposits that accumulate on the lens during wear.

Table 23–5

General Cleaning Procedures for All Lens Types

- Wash hands with noncosmetic soap and rinse thoroughly before handling lenses.
- Clean contact lenses only with agents specifically made for that purpose. Homemade cleansers can scratch the lenses or cause eye irritation or injury.
- Care for each type of lens only with commercially manufactured products made specifically for that type of lens.
- Do not mix contact lens care products from different manufacturers unless a lens care specialist says they are compatible.
- When handling lenses over a sink, cover or close the drain to prevent loss of a lens.
- During cleaning, check lenses for scratches, chips, or tears, and the presence of foreign particles, warpage, or discoloration. Also, check that lenses are clean and thoroughly rinsed of cleaner. These factors could cause eye discomfort.
- When cleaning a lens, rub it in a back-and-forth rather than a circular direction.
- Clean the second lens as thoroughly as the first to prevent "left lens syndrome," in which the left lens has more deposits than the right lens because the right lens is often removed first and cleaned more thoroughly.
- Discard cleansers and other lens care products if the labeled expiration date has passed.

Table 23–6

Specific Cleaning Procedures for Hard Lenses

- Apply appropriate cleaning solution to both surfaces of the lenses; rub the lens between thumb and forefinger or between forefinger and palm of opposite hand for approximately 20 seconds.
- Do not wipe lenses dry with tissue as that may scratch lenses.
- Avoid overvigorous cleaning of lenses as that may cause scratches or warpage.
- Always clean hard lenses before storing them.

A rigid lens absorbs between 1% and 3% moisture by weight. Upon exposure to air, the lens dehydrates; it subsequently rehydrates when it comes in contact with a soaking solution or the lacrimal fluid. Placing a dehydrated lens into the eye causes discomfort as the lens absorbs tears from the precorneal area. In addition, a dehydrated lens is flatter than a hydrated lens; this factor causes problems with both comfort and visual acuity.

If lenses are allowed to dry out during overnight storage, accumulated deposits are more difficult to remove by normal cleaning. Storage in a soaking solution reduces the likelihood of deposits forming.

To maintain sterility, storage solutions use essentially the same preservatives as wetting solutions. The main difference is that the concentration can be somewhat higher in a soaking solution because the solution is rinsed from the lens before insertion. However, preservative levels are carefully selected because higher levels do not necessarily give increased effectiveness and may lead to impaired wetting or corneal irritation because of the adsorption of preservatives onto the lens.

Wetting Solutions

An ideal wetting solution performs the following functions: (1) converting the hydrophobic lens surface to a hydrophilic surface by means of a uniform film that does not easily wash away; (2) increasing comfort by providing cushioning and lubrication between the corneal surface and the inner surface of the lens, and between the lens and the inner surface of the eyelid; (3) placing a viscous coating on the lens to protect it from oil on the fingers during insertion; and (4) stabilizing the lens on the fingertip to ease insertion, particularly for individuals with poor manual dexterity or unsteady hands.

If the lens is thoroughly cleaned before insertion, lacrimal fluid can adequately wet the lens. Indeed, the wetting action of popular wetting solutions is sometimes not significantly better than that of saline. Further, patients whose tears are capable of wetting a lens almost immediately upon insertion often do not use these solutions.

The basic wetting solution comprises components from the following main categories: (1) cushioning agents (e.g., viscosity-inducing additives such as methylcellulose or hydroxypropyl methylcellulose); (2) wetting agents (e.g., polyvinyl alcohol or other surfactants); (3) preservatives (e.g., benzalkonium chloride, thimerosal, polyquaternium-1, sorbic acid, and polyaminopropyl biguanide); and (4) buffering agents and salts added to adjust the pH and tonicity.

The cushioning effect of a wetting solution is achieved by hydrophilic polymers that lubricate the interface between the lens and the surfaces of the cornea and eyelid. Cellulose gum derivatives are often used. Although compounds such as methylcellulose possess a degree of surfactant activity, they do not promote uniform wetting of a rigid lens. For this reason, polyvinyl alcohol is also often used to decrease surface tension.

The concentration of the cushioning polymer in wetting solutions affects both eye comfort and the quality of vision immediately following insertion. In some individuals, a concentration that is too low causes discomfort after only a short time. In other wearers, a high polymer concentration results in blurred vision because the viscous solution mixes poorly with tears. Overspill of solution onto the lids and eyelashes causes crusting as the solution dries; this crusty residue can be a source of foreign material falling into the eye. Saliva should never be used to wet contact lenses because it can lead to infection by *Acanthamoeba, P. aeruginosa,* or other pathogens.

Multipurpose Products

Initially, manufacturers recommended three different solutions for the cleaning, soaking, and wetting of hard contact lenses. However, there has been a trend toward using combination solutions for these functions: Some single solutions claim to be effective for all three procedures.

The major problem with an all-purpose solution is that ingredients required in its formulation perform different and somewhat incompatible functions. For example, high concentrations of benzalkonium chloride are necessary to kill bacteria in soaking solutions; however, these same concentrations can cause ocular irritation when placed directly on the eye with a contact lens. If lenses are stored overnight in a solution containing a high concentration of polymers for cushioning and wetting, the lenses may become gummy and cause discomfort. Similarly, if lenses are stored overnight in a cleaning solution containing an anionic surfactant, the detergent may eventually build up on the lens and cause irritation.

No single agent that will optimally perform all three basic functions currently exists. The present all-purpose solutions are compromises. They are marginally effective but cannot be expected to perform as well as separate solutions.

Rewetting Solutions

Rewetting solutions are intended to clean and rewet the contact lens while the lens is in the eye. These solutions depend on the use of surfactants to loosen deposits; removal is assisted by the natural cleaning action of blinking. An agent used to promote this action is polyoxyl 40 stearate. Although these products function well to recondition the lens, the cornea benefits more if the lens is actually removed, cleaned, and rewetted. Removing the lens for even a brief time allows the cornea to be resurfaced with a new proteinaceous or mucinaceous layer.

Other Products

Other ophthalmic products are available to the hard lens wearer for occasional use. Some, such as artificial tears and ocular decongestants, are not recommended for use with the lenses in place. Because of their emollient and lubricating effect, artificial tears can be used to soothe the eye. Ocular decongestants reduce mild conjunctival hyperemia associated with prolonged lens wear. However, these topical decongestants can induce conjunctival hypoxia, which may harm the patient.[32] Thus, routine use of these products should be avoided. If symptoms requiring their use persist, a visit to a vision specialist is advised.

Product Selection Guidelines

The variety of lens care solutions available to hard lens wearers poses a selection problem. (See Table 23–7 for examples of these products.) The availability of single- and multipurpose products within the same product line can further frustrate and confuse some wearers. Thus, product selection is an area in which pharmacists can perform a much-needed role as a consultant. Unfortunately, information at hand is not always sufficient to provide a complete foundation for patient consultation. One factor that could help determine which products to recommend is the adequacy of the labeling. Product labeling is often incomplete or limited to general information. The specific agents and concentrations of preservatives are usually adequately listed, but concentrations of cushioning and lubricating polymers are often absent. Other ingredients are often listed simply as cleaning agents or buffers, making alternate selections a random process. A surfactant cleaner, a soaking solution, a wetting solution, and a rewetting solution should be recommended.

Insertion and Removal

See Tables 23–8 and 23–9 for instructions on inserting and removing hard lenses.

Care of Rigid Gas-Permeable Lenses

The diversity and variation in materials used in RGP lenses preclude generalizations. Lens wearers should be advised by their eye practitioners about the products and regimens recommended for their particular lenses. The labeling on contact lens products also indicates the lenses for which they are approved.

Procedures

The care of an RGP lens is similar to that of a hard contact lens. (See Figure 23–2.) Unlike hard lenses, however, RGP lenses should be cleaned in the palm of the hand, not between fingertips, to reduce the risk of chipping an edge.[33] (See Tables 23–5 and 23–10 for the proper cleaning procedures.)

Table 23–7

Selected Hard Contact Lens Products

Trade Name	Primary Ingredients
Cleaning Solutions	
LC-65 Daily Contact Lens Cleaner	Cocoamphocarboxyglycinate; sodium lauryl sulfate; hexylene glycol; NaCl; sodium phosphate; EDTA
Opti-Clean Daily Cleaner[a]	Nylon 11; polysorbate 21; hydroxyethyl cellulose; thimerosal 0.004%; EDTA 0.1%; boric acid; sodium borate; NaCl
Opti-Clean II Daily Cleaner for Sensitive Eyes	Nylon 11; polysorbate 21; hydroxyethyl cellulose; polyquaternium-1; EDTA; boric acid; sodium borate; NaCl
Opti-Free Daily Cleaner	Nylon 11; polysorbate 21; hydroxyethyl cellulose; polyquaternium-1, 0.001%; EDTA; boric acid; sodium borate; NaCl; hydrochloric acid and/or sodium hydroxide
Cleaning/Soaking Solutions	
Clean-N-Soak[a]	Surfactant cleaning agent; phenylmercuric nitrate 0.004%
MiraFlow Extra Strength[b]	Isopropyl alcohol 20%; poloxamer 407; amphoteric
Wetting Solutions	
Adapt	Hydroxyethyl cellulose; poloxamer; povidone; thimerosal 0.004%; EDTA; sodium phosphate; NaCl
Liquifilm	Hydroxypropyl methylcellulose; polyvinyl alcohol; benzalkonium chloride 0.004%; EDTA; NaCl; KCl
Wetting/Soaking Solutions	
Soac-Lens[a]	Hydroxyethyl cellulose; polyvinyl alcohol; thimerosal 0.004%; EDTA 0.1%; NaCl; sodium phosphate
Rewetting/Lubricating Solutions	
Adapettes Sensitive Eyes	Sorbic acid 0.2%; EDTA 0.1%; boric acid; sodium borate; NaCl
Bausch & Lomb Global Lens Lubricant[a]	Polyoxyethylene; povidone; thimerosal 0.004%; EDTA 0.1%
Clerz 2	Hydroxyethyl cellulose; sorbic acid 0.1%; EDTA 0.1%; NaCl; KCl; sodium borate; boric acid
Lens Fresh	Hydroxyethyl cellulose; sorbic acid 0.1%; EDTA 0.2%; NaCl; boric acid; sodium borate
Multipurpose Solutions	
Bausch & Lomb Global Wetting & Soaking Solution	Hydroxyethyl cellulose; polyvinyl alcohol; cationic cellulose derivatives; poloxamer 407; chlorhexidine gluconate 0.006%; EDTA 0.05%
Total All-in-One Contact Lens	Polyvinyl alcohol; benzalkonium chloride; EDTA

[a] Product containing thimerosal or phenylmercuric nitrate.

[b] Preservative-free product.

Some RGP lenses have a high silicone content and thus have decreased surface wettability. As previously noted, the lens surface tends to have a negative charge, which promotes the binding of positively charged tear constituents. Cleaners designed for conventional hard or RGP lenses may not effectively remove the more tenacious deposits. Other cleaners formulated for this type of lens (i.e., Boston Advance Cleaner) contain silica gel, which acts to mechanically break the adhesive bonds that have formed between the lens and the deposits.

Because high-silicone lenses have decreased surface wettability, conditioning solutions are generally used instead of soaking solutions to aid the formation of a cushioning tear layer. A conditioning solution is essentially a specially formulated wetting solution. The conditioner system enhances wettability of the lens, increases comfort, and disinfects the lens. The lenses must be soaked at least 4 hours in this solution before they are reinserted into the eyes. It is important to counsel the patient that the Boston Advance Conditioning solution must be discarded 90 days after opening. There is a space on the label to record the date that the product is opened.

Reconditioning/rewetting drops may also be used while the lens is on the eye to rewet the lens as necessary. Boston Rewetting Drops must be discarded 60 days after opening. Heat disinfection cannot be used with RGP lenses.

Table 23–8

Insertion of Hard and Rigid Gas–Permeable Lenses

- After washing hands, remove one lens from the lens storage case, rinse it with fresh conditioning/soaking solution, and inspect it for cleanliness and signs of damage (cracks or chips).
- If a wetting or conditioning solution is being used, place a few drops on the lens.
- Place the lens on the top of the index finger as shown in drawing A.
- Place the middle finger of the same hand on the lower lid and pull it down as shown in drawing B.
- With the other hand, use a finger to lift the upper lid and then place the lens on the eye as shown in drawing C.
- Release the lids and blink.
- Check vision immediately to see if the lens is in the proper position.
- If vision is blurred, blink three to four blinks. If vision is still blurred, the lens may be off center, on the wrong eye, or dirty.
- Instill one to three drops of rewetting or reconditioning drops into the eye.
- If vision is not improved, remove the lens, place several drops of wetting/conditioning solution onto both surfaces, and reinsert.
- Repeat all steps with the other lens.

A

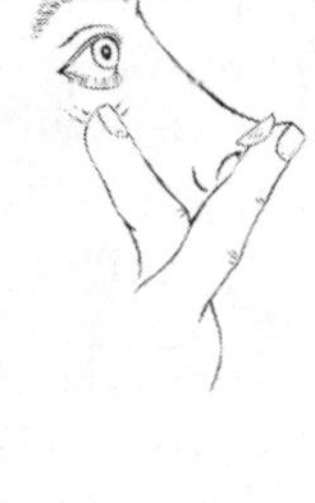

B

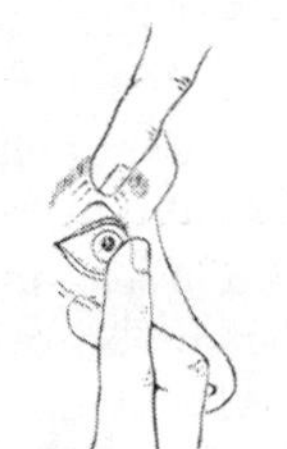

C

Table 23–9

Removal of Hard and Rigid Gas–Permeable Lenses

- Before removing the lens, fill the storage cases with soaking/conditioning solution.
- Remove the top from the cleaning solution.
- Place a hand (or a towel) under the eye.
- Use one of the following methods to remove the lens from the eye.

Two-Finger Method of Removing Lenses

- Place the tip of the forefinger of one hand on the middle of the upper eyelid by the lashes as shown in drawing A.
- Place the forefinger of the other hand on the middle lower lid margin as shown in drawing A.
- Push the lids inward and then together as shown in drawing B. The lens should pop out.
- If the lens only becomes decentered onto the white part of the eye, recenter the lens and try again.

Temporal Pull/Blink Method of Removing Lenses

- Place an index finger on the temporal edge of the lower and upper lids. Initially, widen the eyelids a little as shown in drawing C.
- Stretch the skin outward and slightly upward without allowing the lid to slide over the lens. Blink briskly as shown in drawing D. The lens will pop out because of the pressure of the eyelids at the top and bottom of the lens. Blinking facilitates removal after the lids have been tightened around the lens.

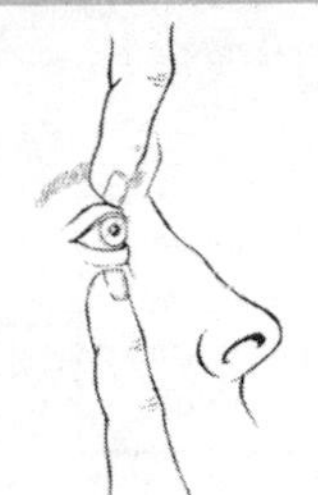

A

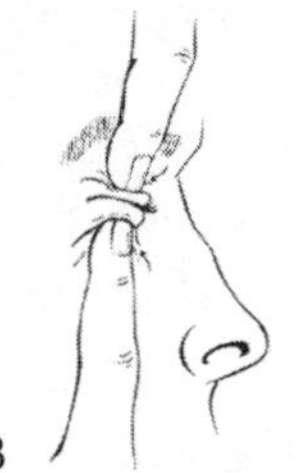

B

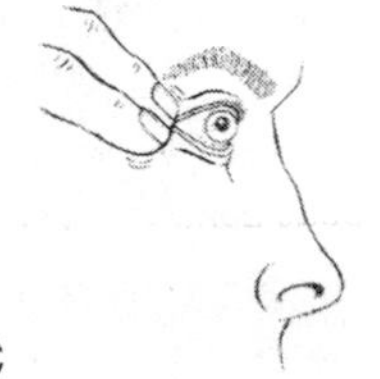

C

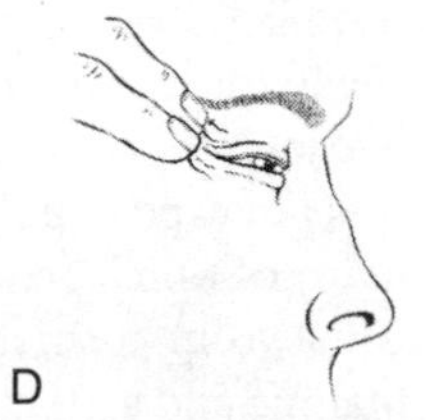

D

As the silicone content of RGP lenses increases, so does the amount of protein adherence. Silicone acrylate lenses have an active surface that promotes the binding of tear constituents. Protein deposits on the lens will decrease the oxygen permeability, and the patient may experience discomfort.[34] Lenses of this type should be cleaned with an enzymatic product once weekly. Failure to comply with this cleaning step may result in the need for professional polishing or replacement of the lens.

Products containing chlorhexidine gluconate should not be used with silicone or styrene lenses because this agent will make the lens surface more difficult to wet and may also cause surface clouding. Fluorosilicone acrylate lenses should not be disinfected with hydrogen peroxide or cleaned more than one time with MiraFlow. Cracking, changes in parameters, and brittleness have been noted when this type of lens is cleaned repeatedly with MiraFlow.

Product Selection Guidelines

The appropriate lens care regimen for RGP lenses must be compatible with the particular lens. Lens wearers should be advised against substituting other products for those specifically recommended by their eye practitioner. Patients wearing RGP lenses should be advised to purchase a surface-active cleaning product, an enzymatic product, and a conditioning or soaking solution, depending on the type of lens worn. A rewetting or reconditioning product should also be recommended. Table 23–11 lists examples of products for RGP lenses.

Insertion and Removal

Wearers of RGP lenses should be counseled to follow the insertion and removal procedures for hard lenses. (See Tables 23–8 and 23–9).

Care of Soft Lenses

Conventional hard lens solutions should never be used with soft lenses because absorption of the ingredients can damage the lenses. Because soft lenses contain a high percentage of water, they are most prone to bacterial contamination. Lens

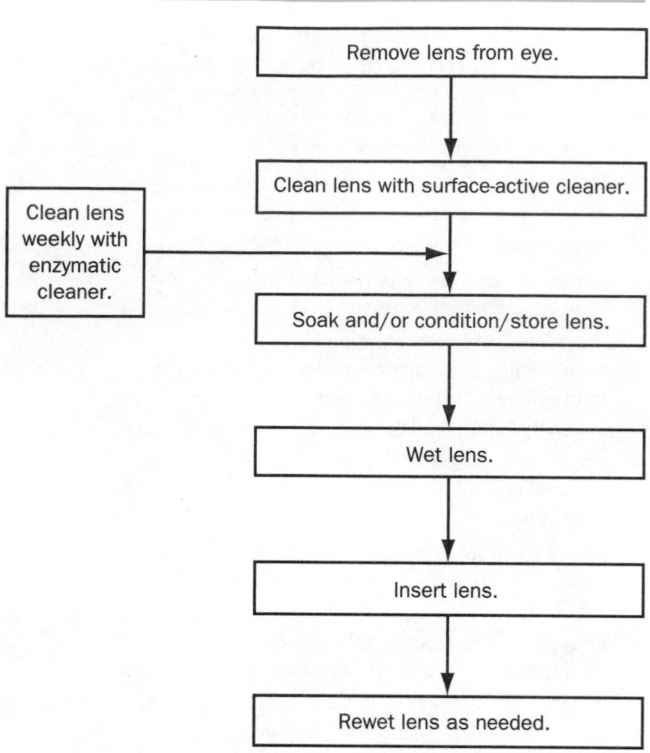

Figure 23–2 Self-care of rigid gas–permeable lenses.

disinfection is crucial to prevent ocular infection and damage to the lens material by bacteria and fungi. Wearers of soft hydrophilic contact lenses should also be particularly cautious in exposing their lenses to chemicals. These chemicals, many of which penetrate and bind with the lens material, can come from cosmetics, environmental pollutants, and ophthalmic and systemic products.

The basic care regimen for soft lenses is different from that for hard lenses. (See Figure 23–3.) All steps must be completed to avoid ocular complications. The only exception is with daily-wear disposable soft lenses. Because these lenses are disposed of within 2 weeks, enzymatic cleaners are usually not necessary. Disposable lenses should, however, be cleaned and disinfected after each wearing until disposal. Products such as Opti-One are multipurpose solutions (for cleaning and disinfecting) formulated specifically for contact lenses that have a replacement schedule of 2 weeks or less.

Cleaning Products

A troublesome aspect of soft lens wear is the accumulation of deposits on the lens.[35] The nature of these deposits varies, but generally they consist of proteins and lipids from the wearer's lacrimal secretions. Deposits are a greater problem with the more highly hydrated lenses, but the rate at which these deposits accumulate depends on the lens and the tears. Some wearers experience little difficulty and wear soft lenses for long periods without significant buildup; others may show deposits in as little as 2 or 3 days. Whatever the cause or accumulation rate, the result is an uncomfortable lens of poor optical quality.

Soft contact lenses require two cleaning steps to rid them of debris. (See Tables 23–5 and 23–12.) Cleaning with a surface-active cleaner must be done daily or, in the case of extended-wear lenses, each time they are removed from the eyes. Cleaning with an enzymatic cleaner should be done weekly or biweekly and can be done more often if necessary.

Soft lens cleaning solutions generally contain a nonionic detergent, a wetting agent, a chelating agent, buffers, preservatives, and, in some cases, polymeric cleaning beads.

Although the surface-active cleaners generally are quite effective in removing lipid deposits, they less successfully remove tenacious protein debris. Enzymatic cleaners are an additional cleaning aid that can help solve this problem. These enzymes hydrolyze polypeptide bonds of protein and dissolve the protein deposits. For the enzyme solution to work properly, however, the lens must be cleaned with a surface-active cleaner first; enzymes are ineffective on debris that covers or is mixed with protein.

With most enzymatic products, the lens then must be disinfected as a separate step to complete the cleaning procedure. Some enzymatic regimens however were developed to be used simultaneously with thermal or chemical disinfection. Products that combine enzymatic cleaning and disinfecting steps tend to increase compliance since they decrease the number of lens care steps a patient must perform. Table 23–13 lists characteristics of various enzymatic products, including whether they can be used concurrently with a disinfecting process.

Table 23–10

Specific Cleaning Procedures for Rigid Gas–Permeable Lenses

- Use the cleansing, soaking, and conditioning products recommended by your eye practitioner to clean your lenses.
- At least once a day apply appropriate cleaning solution to both surfaces of the lenses; rub the lens between forefinger and palm of opposite hand to avoid chipping an edge, which may occur if lenses are cleaned between the fingers.
- When cleaning the lens, do not apply too much pressure. If debris is still on the lens, soak a cotton swab in the surfactant cleaner, and use the swab to clean the lens.
- For RGP lenses with high silicone content only, use a silica gel cleaner (i.e., Boston Advance) if other cleaners do not remove deposits.
- Clean silicone acrylate RGP lenses once a week with an enzymatic cleaner to avoid the need for professional polishing or replacement of lenses.
- If unsure of lens type, ask the eye practitioner about proper cleaning procedures.
- After cleaning RGP lenses, soak them in a soaking or a conditioning solution recommended by the eye practitioner for the specified amount of time. Rewet lenses before inserting them in the eyes.

Table 23–11

Selected Products for Rigid Gas–Permeable Lenses

Trade Name	Primary Ingredients
Cleaning Solutions	
Bausch & Lomb Global Concentrated Cleaner[a]	Silica gel; sulfate surfactant; alkyl ether sulfate; titanium dioxide; NaCl
Boston Advance Cleaner[a]	Silica gel; alkyl ether sulfate; ethoxylated alkyl phenol; triquaternary cocoa-based phospholipid
Boston Cleaner[a]	Silica gel; alkyl ether sulfate; titanium dioxide; NaCl
Opti-Clean II Daily Cleaner for Sensitive Eyes[b]	Cleaning agent; polysorbate 21; hydroxyethyl cellulose; thimerosal 0.004%; EDTA 0.1%; boric acid; sodium borate; NaCl; sodium hydroxide
Opti-Free Daily Cleaner	Nylon 11; polysorbate 21; hydroxyethyl cellulose; polyquaternium-1; EDTA; boric acid; sodium borate; hydrochloric acid and/or sodium hydroxide
Resolve/GP Daily Cleaner[a]	Cocoamphocarboxyglycinate; surfactants; sodium lauryl sulfate; fatty acid amide; hexylene glycol; alkyl ether sulfate
Enzymatic Cleaning Tablets	
ComfortCare GP Dual Action Daily Enzymatic Cleaner	Subtilisin; poloxamer 338; povidone; potassium carbonate; citric acid; sodium benzoate
Opti-Zyme Weekly Enzymatic Cleaner[a]	Pancreatin
Pro Free/GP Weekly Enzymatic Cleaner	Papain; EDTA; NaCl; sodium carbonate; sodium borate
Wetting/Soaking/Disinfecting Solutions	
Bausch & Lomb Global Wetting & Soaking Solution	Hydroxyethyl cellulose; polyvinyl alcohol; cationic cellulose derivatives; poloxamer 407; chlorhexidine gluconate 0.006%; EDTA 0.05%
Boston Advance Comfort Formula Conditioning Solution	Cellulosic viscosifier; polyvinyl alcohol; cationic cellulose derivative polymer; derivatized polyethylene glycol; chlorhexidine gluconate 0.003%; polyaminopropyl biguanide 0.0005%; EDTA 0.05%
Boston Conditioning Solution	Hydroxyethyl cellulose; polyvinyl alcohol; cationic cellulose derivatives; poloxamer 407; chlorhexidine gluconate 0.006%; EDTA 0.05%
ComfortCare GP Wetting & Soaking Solution	Polyvinyl alcohol; povidone; chlorhexidine gluconate; EDTA; octylphenoxy (oxyethylene) ethanol; propylene glycol; NaCl
Wet-N-Soak Plus	Polyvinyl alcohol; benzalkonium chloride 0.003%; EDTA
Rewetting/Lubricating Solutions	
Boston Rewetting Drops	Hydroxyethyl cellulose; polyvinyl alcohol; cationic cellulose derivatives; poloxamer 407; chlorhexidine gluconate 0.006%; EDTA 0.05%
ComfortCare GP Comfort Drops	Hydroxyethyl cellulose; potassium sorbate 0.13%; EDTA 0.1%; oxtylphenoxy (oxyethylene) ethanol; NaCl
Wet-N-Soak	Hydroxyethyl cellulose; WSCP 0.006%; borate
Multipurpose Solutions	
Boston Simplicity	Betaine surfactant; PEO sorbitan monolaurate; cellulosic viscosifier; silicone glycol polymer; derivatized polyethylene glycol; chlorhexidine gluconate 0.003%; polyaminopropyl biguanide 0.0005%; EDTA 0.05%

[a] Preservative-free product.
[b] Product containing thimerosal.

Disinfecting Methods

The FDA recommends disinfecting soft contact lenses before each reinsertion. Disinfection occurs after cleaning the lens. Two methods of disinfection are currently approved: thermal and chemical. Studies have shown that microorganisms do not actually enter the matrix of soft lenses but that surface contamination could lead to ocular infection.[36] Both disinfecting methods are reliable for most ocular pathogens. Chemical disinfection with hydrogen peroxide has increased in popularity with certain types of lenses over thermal and earlier chemical disinfectants because of decreased ocular allergenicity and toxicity.

Thermal Disinfection Table 23–14 describes the basic and alternative method of thermal disinfection. Originally, lenses were disinfected by raising the temperature to the boiling point for about 20 minutes. Units that use a lower temperature (about 176°F [80°C]) for a longer time are now avail-

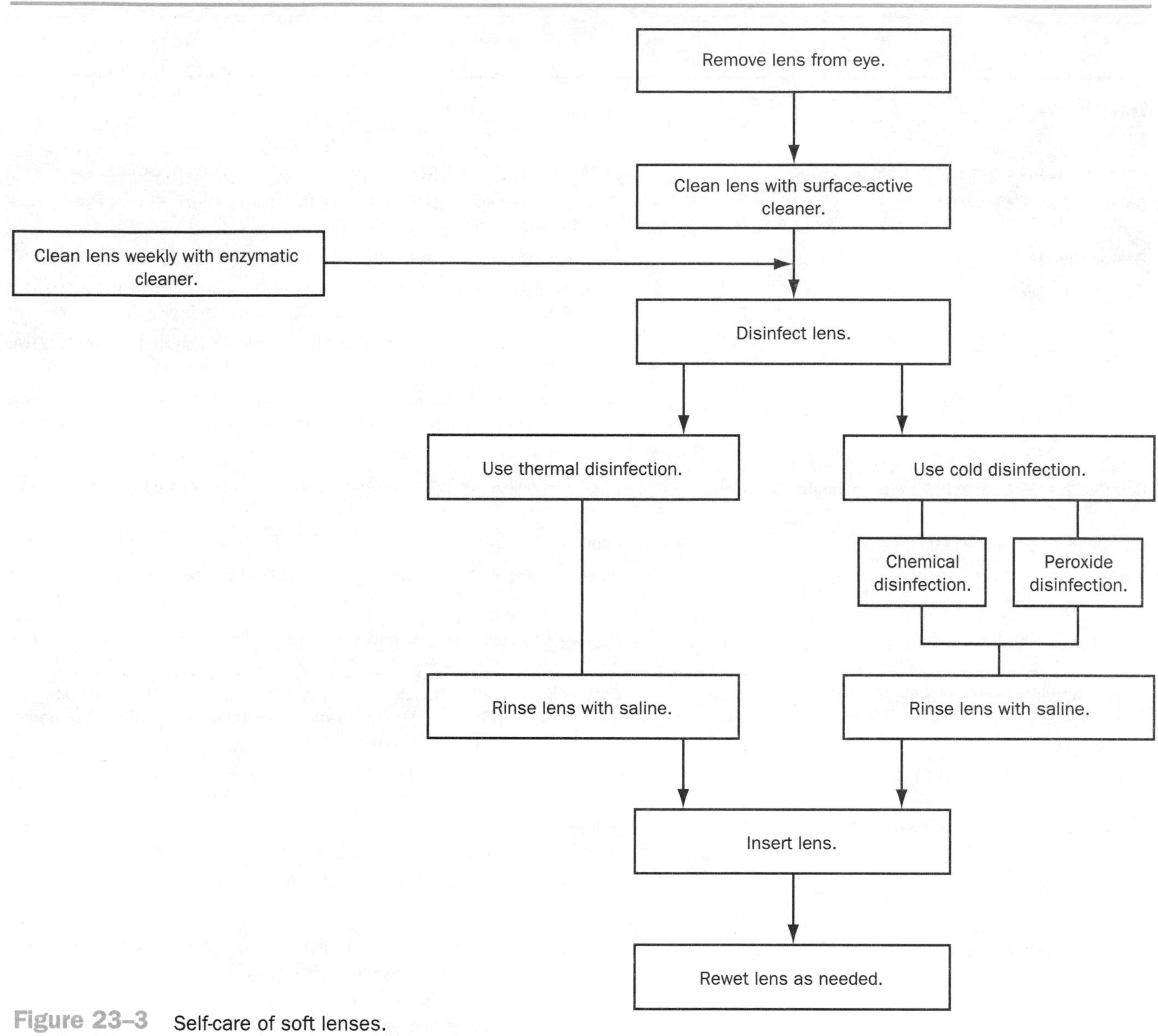

Figure 23–3 Self-care of soft lenses.

able. The FDA requirement is at least 176°F (80°C) for a minimum of 10 minutes. This process is as effective as boiling for most organisms, and it prolongs lens life. The procedure is usually done at night.

Advantages Thermal disinfection has several advantages: (1) It can be done with a preservative-free solution and is therefore less likely to cause eye irritation. (2) It kills microbial contamination better than any other method. (3) It is the only approved contact lens disinfecting method known to be effective against cysts of *Acanthamoeba.* (4) It is generally more effective against chemically resistant microorganisms such as fungi and bacillus species. (5) It kills organisms on and surrounding the contact lens case, further preventing potential contaminants from entering the lenses.

Disadvantages Thermal disinfection also has several drawbacks: (1) Lenses with a high water content cannot withstand daily heating. (2) Some individuals find the method cumbersome and less convenient than chemical disinfection. (3) There is a high initial cost for equipment, although long-term costs of chemical disinfectant solutions may offset this. (4) The user must take care to remove proteinaceous and other debris by cleaning the lenses first. (5) Lens cases used with thermal units, and the units themselves, must be routinely inspected for damage, cracks, or leaks and replaced at the earliest sign of a problem.

Table 23–12

Specific Cleaning Procedures for Soft Lenses

- Clean regular soft lenses daily with a surface-active cleaner. Clean extended-wear and disposable soft lenses with a surface-active cleaner after each wearing.
- Place several drops of a cleaning product on the lens; gently rub the lens between the thumb and forefinger or between the fingertip of the forefinger and the palm of the opposite hand for 20 to 30 seconds.
- Avoid cutting the lens with a fingernail or scratching the lens surface with grit or dirt on the hands.
- Rinse lenses with a sterile isotonic buffered solution. Never use tap water: It is not isotonic and contains harmful microorganisms.
- Clean lenses at least weekly with enzymatic cleaners, either as a step separate from disinfection or as part of the disinfecting process.
- When combining enzyme cleaning and disinfecting of the lenses as one step, see Table 23–13 for the appropriate combinations of products.
- When using enzymatic cleaners as a step separate from disinfection, clean lenses according to the following instructions weekly, biweekly, or more often, if needed:
  —Place enzyme tablet (papain, pancreatin, or subtilisin) in solution recommended by the product manufacturer; allow lens with high-water content to soak for 15 minutes; allow lenses with low-water content to soak overnight
  —Thoroughly rinse lenses with saline solution to prevent eye irritation.
- Disinfect lenses to complete the cleaning procedure, using either thermal or chemical disinfection. (See Table 23–14.) Make sure lenses are cleaned thoroughly before disinfecting them.
- Discard any enzyme cleaner that is discolored.

Chemical Disinfection In chemical disinfection, the lenses are stored for a prescribed period of time in a solution containing bactericidal agents that are compatible with soft lens materials. There are two basic chemical disinfection methods available in the United States. The first method is based on the original chemical disinfecting solutions, which consisted of antimicrobial preservatives of sufficient concentration in storage solutions primarily composed of saline. These initial disinfecting solutions contained chlorhexidine and thimerosal, both of which induce sensitivity reactions in many soft lens wearers. These solutions no longer contain thimerosal, but several still contain chlorhexidine. Patients are less sensitive to chlorhexidine and apparently can tolerate it better than thimerosal. To avoid sensitivity reactions, solutions with several new disinfecting preservatives are currently being marketed for soft contact lens care. These preservatives are sorbic acid, polyquaternium-1, TrisChem, and polyaminopropyl biguanide, which are touted to be much less toxic or allergenic than their predecessors. However, these agents may also be less effective, especially against fungi and protozoans.

The second chemical method uses hydrogen peroxide as the antimicrobial agent. (See Table 23–14.) Soft lenses are placed in purified hydrogen peroxide and are disinfected by the liberation of oxygen from peroxide. Household hydrogen peroxide solution should not be used because its pH is too low and it may discolor lenses.[37] Following disinfection, the peroxide is neutralized to trace levels by soaking the lenses in a neutralizing solution or by the catalytic action of a platinum disc.

Most hydrogen peroxide systems that require two steps for disinfection and neutralization (Consept 1, MiraSept Step

Table 23–13

Enzymatic Cleaners

Trade Name	Active Ingredient	Product Odor	Separate Disinfection Step	Concurrent Use with Thermal Disinfection	Concurrent Use with Chemical Preservative Disinfection	Concurrent Use with Hydrogen Peroxide Disinfection
Allergan Complete Weekly Enzymatic	Papain	Yes	Yes	No	No	No
Opti-Free SupraClens	Pancreatin	No	No	No	Yes with Opti-One or Opti-Free Express	No
ReNu Effervescent	Subtilisin	No	Yes	No	No	No
ReNu 1 Step	Subtilisin	No	No	No	Yes with ReNu Multipurpose Solution	No
ReNu Thermal	Subtilisin	No	No	Yes	No	No
Ultrazyme/Unizyme	Subtilisin	No	No	No	No	Yes with Ultra-Care or Oxysept

Table 23–14

Guidelines for Disinfecting Rigid Gas–Permeable and Soft Lenses

Conventional Thermal Disinfection

- Do not use thermal disinfection for RGP lenses, tinted lenses, or soft lenses with water content greater than 50%.
- Place cleaned lenses into separate compartments of storage case filled with saline solution.
- Place case in heat disinfecting unit.
- Turn on unit and heat lenses and solution for at least 10 minutes.
- Rinse lenses with saline.

Alternative Thermal Disinfection

- When heat disinfecting unit is not available, place tightly closed lens case containing lenses and saline solution in a pot of boiling water for at least 10 minutes (15 minutes if at an altitude above 7000 ft). Do not allow water to boil away.
- Remove pot from heat; allow to cool for 30 minutes.
- Rinse lenses with saline.
- Resume use of heat disinfecting unit as soon as possible.

Chemical Preservative Disinfection

- Store lenses for prescribed period of time (usually a minimum of 4 hours) in a preservative disinfecting solution appropriate for the lenses.
- If lenses are stored longer than 3 days in the disinfectant, clean and disinfect them again for 4 hours before inserting them.
- If using Quick CARE, rub the hypertonic starting solution onto the lens to clean and disinfect; rinse lenses thoroughly with saline; soak in finishing solution for 5 minutes.
- Rinse lenses thoroughly with saline to remove disinfecting solution.

Chemical Disinfection with Hydrogen Peroxide

- Using the cup provided with the hydrogen peroxide product, place lenses in a commercial purified hydrogen peroxide for the length of time specified by the manufacturer. Do not use lens cups or cases that came with other products.
- Do not soak lenses in peroxide solution longer than recommended; otherwise, neutralization of the peroxide will take longer. To neutralize hydrogen peroxide, remove lenses and soak them in a solution containing catalase, sodium pyruvate, or sodium thiosulfate for the length of time specified by the manufacturer.
- Do not mix neutralizers from different peroxide systems because ingredients may interact and form a precipitate. Lenses may be ruined.
- To disinfect and neutralize in one step, place platinum catalytic disc in lens case and leave the disc there until time to replace it; add hydrogen peroxide; insert lenses and leave for at least 6 hours.
- Never place neutralizing solution in lens case with a catalytic disc. An unwanted chemical reaction may occur, or a gummy residue may form on the disc.
- Make sure hydrogen peroxide is completely neutralized before inserting lenses in the eyes.
- Rinse lenses thoroughly with saline.

Combination Enzyme Cleaning and Disinfection

- When combining enzyme cleaning and disinfecting of the lenses as one step, select products compatible with your disinfecting system. (See Table 23–13.)
- Add appropriate solution (saline or disinfecting preservative) to separate compartments of storage case of disinfecting system.
- Add lenses to separate compartments.
- Add appropriate enzymatic cleaner to each compartment.
- Follow directions above for appropriate disinfecting system.
- Rinse lenses thoroughly with saline to remove residual disinfecting or neutralizing solutions.

1, Oxysept 1, and Ultra-Care) work in only 20 to 30 minutes. The neutralizing solutions for these systems contain catalase (Oxysept 2 and Ultra-Care), sodium pyruvate (MiraSept Step 2), or sodium thiosulfate (Consept 2). For most patients, one of these systems is appropriate. The patient may use these products in the morning just before inserting the lenses; the neutralizing step is easy; and if the neutralizing agent contains a preservative, there is less chance that the resultant solution will become contaminated. Mirasept neutralizing solution, however, is good for only 4 months after being opened.

One potential disadvantage of hydrogen peroxide disinfection is that patients may insert the lens directly from the peroxide solution without neutralization. A peroxide-soaked lens placed on the eye will cause great pain, photophobia, redness, and, perhaps, corneal epithelial damage. If this occurs, the patient should immediately remove the lens from the eye and flush the eye with sterile saline solution. The pain should subside within a few hours. If it does not, the patient should consult an eye or vision care specialist. If the patient has any doubt as to whether the peroxide was neutralized, the entire disinfection cycle should be started over again to avoid the risk of inserting a peroxide-soaked lens without a neutralizing step.

Three hydrogen peroxide products help the patient avoid the possibility of forgetting to do the neutralization step: AO Sept, Pure Eyes, and Ultra-Care.

Patients who use the AO Sept platinum disc for neutralization should replace the disc after 100 uses or 3 months, whichever comes first. Failure to comply with these instructions may result in disc failure, and the patient may sustain a peroxide burn on the cornea. Although the catalytic disc systems only require one step, that step takes 6 hours for disinfection and neutralization, which decreases the flexibility of the system and rules out morning use. Suboptimal disinfection is another concern with AO Sept. The catalytic disc will neutralize the surrounding peroxide quickly, and there may not be adequate time for disinfection. Once the catalytic disc neutralizes the peroxide, a nonpreserved solution remains. If the lenses are left in the case for several days, bacterial contamination may occur. Patients should not store their lenses in neutralized AO Sept for more than 24 hours unless they disinfect the lenses again prior to insertion. Another option for patients using a catalytic disc system is Pure Eyes. This system contains a new storage case and catalytic disc with every bottle of solution, allowing the patient to throw out the old case and disc each time they buy a new bottle of Pure Eyes.

With Ultra-Care, the user adds a delayed-release neutralizing tablet at the beginning of the 2-hour disinfecting cycle. Disinfection and neutralization then occur at the appropriate time intervals. This tablet contains catalase and cyanocobalamin; the latter ingredient turns the solution pink, thus reminding the user that the tablet has been added. Exposure of the lenses to the disinfecting effects of hydrogen peroxide for 2 hours allows optimal activity against *Acanthamoeba*. Patients using Ultra-Care should know the following:

- This product requires a minimum of 2 hours to complete disinfection and neutralization of the peroxide.
- The neutralizing tablet should not be crushed or used if there are cracks in the coating; the tablet will start neutralizing the peroxide before adequate disinfection occurs.
- MiraFlow or Pliagel, which are used for surface-active cleaning, can leave a film on the lenses and lens cup if not carefully rinsed off the lens. This may result in foaming and overflow of the peroxide–neutralizer solution.[38] If this occurs, lenses should be rinsed more carefully or another surface-active cleaner should be used.
- Before lenses are removed from the eye, the lens container should be filled with fresh Ultra-Care disinfection solution, the cap tightened, and the cup turned upside down so that the solution bathes the upper portion of the cup and the top. The cup is left in this position until the patient is ready to disinfect the lenses.
- Ultra-Care should not be used with Illusions opaquely tinted soft contact lenses. Lens damage may result.
- If the lenses are not going to be worn for awhile, they can be stored unopened in the neutralized solution; however, they should be disinfected once weekly and just before wear.

Multipurpose Products

In many patients, separate solutions for surface-active cleaning, protein removal, and disinfection of soft contact lenses are recommended. However, there has been a trend toward using multipurpose solutions for these functions. Some of the cold disinfection systems are considered multipurpose solutions. Examples include ReNu MultiPlus MultiPurpose Solution, ReNu Multipurpose Disinfecting Solution, Opti-Free Express, SOLO-care, Complete and Consept. All of these solutions are indicated for surface-active cleaning of the lens as well as disinfection. ReNu MultiPlus MultiPurpose Solution also performs protein removal as well.

These products are useful for patients with planned replacement lenses as these lenses are usually discarded before a significant amount of protein or lipid builds up on the lens. Patients who wear traditional soft contact lenses usually benefit from using separate solutions for cleaning, protein removal, and disinfection rather than from using multipurpose solutions.

Saline Solutions

The hydrophilic soft contact lens must be maintained in a constant state of hydration. Furthermore, the hydrated lens must be isotonic with tears because changes in tonicity can alter the conformation and optical properties of the lens. Isotonic normal saline is the basic solution used for rinsing, thermally disinfecting, and storing soft contact lenses.

Prepared saline is available in either preserved or preservative-free forms. Because thimerosal and chlorhexidine can cause sensitivity reactions or irritation in a great many patients, sorbic acid–preserved products are commonly promoted for sensitive eyes and appear to be acceptable to most wearers. Salines preserved with Polyquad and Dymed are also available for patients who are sensitive to other preservatives.

Several preservative-free salines are also available. Preservative-free buffered saline is available in unit-of-use containers (which should be used and discarded once opened) and

Case Study 23–1

Patient Complaint/History

Jessica, who is 34 years old, presents to the pharmacy with complaints of eye discomfort associated with soft contact lenses. Questioning the patient reveals that she began wearing soft contact lenses, and this particular pair of lenses, 2 months ago; she is unsure of the brand name of the lenses. Jessica did not experience discomfort when she first began wearing the lenses; however, over the past 2 to 3 weeks she has noticed discomfort and some irritation that occurs only when she wears the lenses. She does not complain of other symptoms such as discharge from the eye. Her last visit to the lens prescriber was 2 months ago when she received the soft lenses.

The patient's lens care regimen includes cleaning the lenses with Bausch & Lomb Global Sensitive Eyes Daily Cleaner each time she removes them. She then soaks the lenses in Ultra-Care with a neutralization tablet (hydrogen peroxide disinfection system) for 2 hours. Further, she always uses fresh solutions and cleans her storage container once a week according to the manufacturer's recommendations. Although Jessica does wear a water-resistant mascara (but no eyeliner), she inserts her lenses before she applies any cosmetics. She also washes her hands with a noncosmetic soap before inserting the lenses.

Questions about the patient's medical history reveal no history of ocular problems, no known allergies, no current use of prescription medications (including oral contraceptives), and no past or present history of pregnancy; her family history is noncontributory. Her use of nonprescription medications includes acetaminophen for occasional headaches. The patient does not smoke; she drinks five to six beers a week.

Clinical Considerations/Strategies

Readers can use the following considerations/strategies to determine the best recommendation for this patient and to select the appropriate contact lens products:

- Assess the contact lens care regimen. Call the lens prescriber to determine the appropriate care regimen and to discuss suggested changes in the care regimen.
- Assess the patient's history of lens wear along with symptomatology and allergy history.

Patient Education/Counseling

Readers can use the following strategies to develop a patient education/counseling plan that will help ensure optimal therapeutic outcomes:

- Describe a lens care regimen that is optimal for compliance and ease of use.
- Justify changes in the care regimen.
- Explain proper use of new product(s) added to the regimen.
- Educate the patient about contact lens wear and symptoms of lens problems.

in multiuse bottles (which must be discarded 14 days after opening) Nonpreserved salines are also available as aerosol sprays.

Patients using nonpreserved saline should be counseled that only aerosolized and unit-of-use saline solutions can be used to rinse lenses just before insertion into the eye. Multipurpose nonpreserved saline (e.g., Unisol 4) should never be used to rinse lenses just before insertion unless the bottle is new and has not been opened. Once these products have been opened, they should only be used if a disinfection step will be performed prior to insertion.

Patients should avoid using other forms of saline such as intravenous normal saline or saline squirts because these products are usually too acidic for use with soft contact lenses.

Some persons prepare their own preservative-free saline using salt tablets and USP purified water. Using salt tablets is inexpensive, but the clear superiority of commercial salines argues strongly against it. The use of homemade saline from salt tablets and the application of improper lens care are the greatest predisposing factors to *Acanthamoeba* keratitis and to many anterior eye infections contracted by hydrophilic lens wearers.[39] The FDA no longer condones the use of salt tablets, and neither should a concerned pharmacist.

When contact lens patients started using homemade salt tablet solutions, there was a resurgence of *Acanthamoeba* infections. Most victims of *Acanthamoeba* keratitis have used improper lens hygiene, gone swimming without removing their contact lenses, used nonsterile saline solution made from salt tablets and distilled water, or used tap water in the maintenance of their soft contact lenses. Because they are very resistant, *Acanthamoeba* cysts often can survive attempts to eradicate them antimicrobially from the eye. Multiple antibiotic regimens have been applied with variable or poor therapeutic response. Many cases of *Acanthamoeba keratitis* are severe enough to require keratoplasty, a partial or complete cornea transplant, in an attempt to save the eye. Unfortunately, the persistent presence of cysts gives this eye infection a poor prognosis, which, in many cases, ultimately leads to enucleation—the partial or total removal of the affected eye.

Rewetting Solutions

Accessory solutions for use with soft lenses permit lubricating and rewetting (and, in some cases, cleaning) of the lens in the eye. These solutions typically contain a low concentration of a nonionic surfactant to promote cleaning and a polymer to lubricate the lens surface, along with buffering agents. These solutions are particularly useful to patients with highly hydrated lenses, such as the extended-wear type. Exposing lenses to wind and high temperature causes some dehydration, even of the lens in the eye. The resulting discomfort is sometimes relieved by one or two drops of rewetting solution. To minimize contamination, the tip of the applicator bottle should not touch the eye, eyelid, or any other surface. The pharmacist should be aware of the preservative content of these products. Some are available without thimerosal and may be less sensitizing to patients with preservative allergies.

Product Selection Guidelines

Many problems associated with soft lens wear arise from the way people handle their lenses; unsatisfactory results may stem from improper procedures rather than from inadequate products.[40] Table 23–15 lists examples of products designed specifically for soft contact lenses. In one investigation, only 26% of contact lens wearers fully complied with care instructions, and the occurrence of signs and symptoms of potential wearing problems was directly correlated with noncompliance. Specific questions about the care and maintenance regimen used by a wearer can often bring these problems to light.

Surface-Active Cleaners Some surface-active cleaners have a lower viscosity and may be easier to rinse off the lens (e.g., Bausch & Lomb Global Sensitive Eyes Daily Cleaner). These products are good choices for patients who have difficulty completely rinsing the cleaner off their lens.

In addition to surfactants, some products (e.g., Opti-Clean II) contain mild abrasives that aid in the removal of lens deposits. Patients who have difficulty removing deposits from their lenses will benefit from this type of cleaner. These products should be shaken before use. Some patients may have difficulty rinsing these cleaners off their lenses. Care should be taken to be sure that no residue from the cleaning solution remains on the lens prior to insertion. Finally, one surfactant cleaner (MiraFlow) contains isopropyl alcohol. This product is useful for patients who discover heavy lipid deposits on their lenses.

Enzymatic Cleaners Enzymatic cleaners can be recommended based on the disinfection system the patient uses. If the patient uses thermal disinfection, ReNu Thermal is a good choice because it eliminates the need to perform the enzymatic cleaning and disinfection steps separately. Ultrazyme and Unizyme are choices for the patient using a hydrogen peroxide cleaning system. These products can be placed in the peroxide solution, thus cleaning and disinfecting at the same time. If the patient uses Opti-Free disinfecting solution, Supra-Clens or Opti-Free Enzymatic Cleaner would be a good choice as it can be placed directly in the Opti-Free solution during the disinfection cycle. If the patient uses another chemical disinfection system, the comparisons between products become very idiosyncratic unless the patient is allergic to one of the components.

Disinfecting Methods When counseling a patient about the best disinfecting method to use, the pharmacist should ask what type of lenses the patient wears. If the patient wears low-water lenses, heat disinfection or Ultra-Care (2-hour exposure to hydrogen peroxide) is best because they are the only methods that eradicate *Acanthamoeba*. If a patient wears high-water lenses or is not sure what type of lenses he or she has, a hydrogen peroxide system or a second-generation chemical system (i.e., Opti-Free or ReNu) can be recommended.

When choosing a chemical disinfection product, several factors can be considered. If the patient has a history of sensitivity reactions to lens solutions or is unsure if sensitivity exists, it is best to recommend a product containing one of the nonsensitizing preservatives. A recommendation can be made based on the brand and type of enzymatic cleaner the patient is using. For example, if the patient is using Supra-Clens Enzymatic cleaner, then Opti-Free or Opti-Free Express should be recommended as the disinfecting agent. If the patient is using ReNu 1 Step Enzymatic Cleaner, then the best recommendation is ReNu Multipurpose Disinfecting Solution. If a patient has no preference for a particular enzymatic product, then any of the chemical disinfection solutions that can be used concurrently with an enzymatic product are appropriate.

Soft lens wearers may freely switch from thermal to chemical disinfecting methods, but the switch from chemical to thermal may present problems. If lenses that have been chemically disinfected are not completely free from all traces of the chemicals, they can be damaged by heating. Prolonged soaking in several changes of saline is recommended to clean the lenses before using a heating unit.

Product Incompatibility Several incompatibilities may occur when mixing soft lens products. Most manufacturers test for compatibility within their own product lines; however, compatibility with other manufacturers' products is usually not determined. Generally, chemical disinfecting solutions should not be interchanged or used concurrently. If a patient mixes a disinfecting solution containing chlorhexidine and thimerosal (i.e., Flex-care) with a product containing a quaternary ammonium compound (i.e., Allergan Hydrocare), a toxic keratopathy known as mixed solution syndrome may occur. Patients should be counseled not to switch from a chlorhexidine-containing chemical disinfection system to a hydrogen peroxide system unless they procure new lenses. A fine black precipitate may form on the

Table 23–15

Selected Products for Soft Lenses

Trade Name	Primary Ingredients
Surface-Active Cleaning Solutions	
Bausch & Lomb Global Daily Cleaner[a]	Tyloxapol; hydroxyethyl cellulose; polyvinyl alcohol; thimerosal 0.004%; EDTA 0.2%; sodium phosphate; NaCl
Bausch & Lomb Global Sensitive Eyes Daily Cleaner	Hydroxypropyl methylcellulose; sorbic acid 0.25%; EDTA 0.5%; NaCl; borate buffer; poloxamine
LC-65 Daily Contact Lens Cleaner[a]	Sodium lauryl sulfate; cocoamphocarboxyglycinate; thimerosal 0.001%; EDTA; hexylene glycol; NaCl; sodium phosphate; EDTA
MiraFlow Extra Strength	Isopropyl alcohol 20%; poloxamer 407; amphoteric 10
Opti-Clean Daily Cleaner[a]	Nylon 11; polysorbate 21; hydroxyethyl cellulose; thimerosal 0.004%; EDTA 0.1%; boric acid; sodium borate; NaCl
Opti-Clean II Daily Cleaner for Sensitive Eyes	Nylon 11; polysorbate 21; hydroxyethyl cellulose; polyquaternium-1; EDTA; boric acid; sodium borate; NaCl
Opti-Free Daily Cleaner	Nylon 11; polysorbate 21; hydroxyethyl cellulose; polyquaternium-1, 0.001%; EDTA; boric acid; sodium borate; hydrochloric acid and/or sodium hydroxide
Pliagel	Sorbic acid 0.25%; EDTA 0.5%; poloxamer 407; KCl; NaCl
Pure Eyes 1	Pluronic surfactant; sodium perborate (releasing up to 0.006% of hydrogen peroxide); boric acid; sodium borate; phosphoric acid
Enzymatic Cleaning Products	
Allergan Complete Weekly Enzymatic Cleaner Tablet	Subtilisin A
Opti-Free Enzymatic Cleaner for Sensitive Eyes Tablet	Pancreatin; povidone; citric acid; sodium bicarbonate; polyethylene glycol; dehydrated alcohol
Opti-Free SupraClens Daily Protein Remover Solution[b]	Highly purified porcine pancreatin enzymes; polyethylene glycol; sodium borate
Opti-Zyme Enzymatic Cleaner Tablet	Pancreatin
ReNu 1 Step Enzymatic Cleaner Tablet	Subtilisin; sodium carbonate; NaCl; boric acid
ReNu Effervescent Enzymatic Tablet	Subtilisin; PEG; sodium carbonate; NaCl; tartaric acid
ReNu Thermal Enzymatic Tablet	Subtilisin; PEG; sodium carbonate; NaCl; boric acid
Ultrazyme Enzymatic Cleaner Tablet	Subtilisin A; effervescing agents; buffers
Unizyme Tablet	Subtilisin
Chemical Preservative Disinfecting Solutions	
Bausch & Lomb Global Disinfecting Solution[a]	Chlorhexidine gluconate 0.005%; thimerosal 0.001%; EDTA 0.1%; NaCl; sodium borate; boric acid
Flex-Care for Sensitive Eyes	Chlorhexidine gluconate 0.005%; EDTA 0.1%; NaCl; sodium borate; boric acid
Opti-Free Rinsing, Disinfecting & Storage Solution	Polyquaternium-1, 0.001%; EDTA 0.05%; citrate buffer; NaCl
Hydrogen Peroxide Disinfecting Solutions and Rinsing/Neutralizing Products	
AO SEPT	Disinfecting solution: Hydrogen peroxide 3%; NaCl 0.85%; phosphate buffers; phosphoric acid Neutralizer: Platinum disc
Soft Mate Consept	Consept 1 (disinfecting solution): Hydrogen peroxide 3%; sodium stannate; sodium nitrate; phosphate buffers; polyoxyl 40 stearate Consept 2 (rinse/neutralizer): Sodium thiosulfate 0.5%; chlorhexidine gluconate 0.001%; borate buffers
MiraSept	MiraSept Step 1 (disinfecting solution): Hydrogen peroxide 3%; sodium stannate; sodium nitrate MiraSept Step 2 (rinse/neutralizer): Sorbic acid; EDTA; boric acid; sodium borate; sodium pyruvate
Oxysept	Oxysept 1 (disinfecting solution): Hydrogen peroxide 3%; sodium stannate; sodium nitrate; phosphate buffers Oxysept 2 (neutralizer): Catalase tablet; buffering agents; tableting agents

Table 23–15

Selected Products for Soft Lenses (continued)

Trade Name	Primary Ingredients
Pure Eyes 2	Hydrogen peroxide 3%; NaCl 0.85%; phosphate buffers; phosphoric acid; packaged with plastic lens case with built-in neutralizing disc
Quick CARE System	Starting step: Polyoxypropylene; polyoxyethylene block copolymer, isopropanol, disodium lauroamphodiacetate, NaCl Finishing step: Sodium perborate (releases up to 0.006% hydrogen peroxide); sodium borate; boric acid; phosphoric acid
Ultra-Care	Disinfecting solution: Hydrogen peroxide 3%; sodium stannate; sodium nitrate; phosphates Neutralizer: Catalase tablet; cyanocobalamin (color indicator)
Preserved Saline Solutions	
Bausch & Lomb Global Preserved Saline[a]	Thimerosal 0.001%; EDTA; NaCl; boric acid
Bausch & Lomb Global Sensitive Eyes Saline	Sorbic acid 0.1%; NaCl; borate buffer; EDTA
Bausch & Lomb Global Sensitive Eyes Saline Plus	Polyaminopropyl biguanide; NaCl; KCl
Bausch & Lomb Global Sensitive Eyes Saline/ Cleaning Solution	Sorbic acid; NaCl; borate buffer; surfactant
ReNu Saline	Polyaminopropyl biguanide; EDTA: NaCl; boric acid
SoftWear Saline	Sodium perborate (releases up to 0.006% hydrogen peroxide); NaCl; sodium borate; boric acid; phosphoric acid
Preservative-Free Saline Products	
Bausch & Lomb Global Sensitive Eyes Saline Aerosol	NaCl; boric acid; sodium borate
Ciba Vision Saline Solution	NaCl; boric acid
Lens Plus Sterile Saline Solution	NaCl; boric acid
Unisol 4 Saline Solution	NaCl; sodium borate; boric acid
Rewetting/Lubricating Solutions	
Bausch & Lomb Global Sensitive Eyes Plus Lubricating Drops	Hydroxypropyl methylcellulose; sorbic acid; EDTA; poloxamine; NaCl
Bausch & Lomb Global Sensitive Eyes Rewetting Drops	Sorbic acid 0.1%; EDTA; borate buffer
Ciba Vision Lens Drops	Hydroxyethyl cellulose 0.7%; poloxamer 407; sorbic acid 0.15%; EDTA 0.2%; NaCl; borate buffer; carbamide
Clerz 2	Hydroxyethyl cellulose; sorbic acid 0.1%; EDTA 0.1%; NaCl; KCl; sodium borate
Lens Fresh	Hydroxyethyl cellulose; sorbic acid 0.1%; EDTA 0.2%; NaCl; boric acid; sodium borate
Lens Plus[b]	NaCl; boric acid
Opti-Free Rewetting Drops	Polyquaternium-1, 0.001%; citric acid; sodium citrate; NaCl
Opti-Soak Soothing Drops	Hydroxypropyl methylcellulose; Dextran; polyquaternium-1, 0.001%; EDTA; NaCl; KCl
Opti-Tears Soothing Drops	Hydroxypropyl methylcellulose; Dextran 70; polyquaternium-1, 0.001%; EDTA 0.1%; NaCl; KCl; sodium hydroxide and/or hydrochloric acid
ReNu Rewetting Drops	Sorbic acid 0.15%; EDTA; borate buffer; poloxamine; NaCl
Multipurpose Solutions	
Complete Multi-Purpose Solution	Tyloxapol; hydroxypropyl methylcellulose; polyhexamethylene biguanide 0.0001%; EDTA; NaCl; tromethamine
Opti-Free Express Multipurpose Solution	Polyquaternium-1, 0.001%; EDTA; sodium citrate; NaCl; citric acid
Opti-One Multi-Purpose Solution	Polyquaternium-1, 0.0011%; EDTA 0.05%; sodium citrate; NaCl; citric acid; sodium hydroxide and/or hydrochloric acid
ReNu Multi-Purpose Solution	Polyaminopropyl biguanide; EDTA; NaCl; sodium borate; boric acid; poloxamine
ReNu MultiPlus Solution	Polyaminopropyl biguanide; EDTA; NaCl; sodium borate; boric acid; poloxamine
SOLO-care Multi-Purpose Solution	Polyhexanide 0.0001%; disodium edetate dihydrate 0.025%; NaCl; polyoxyethylene polypropylene; block copolymer; dibasic sodium phosphate; monobasic sodium phosphate

[a] Product containing thimerosal.

[b] Preservative-free product.

lenses if chlorhexidine is still present in the lens matrix. Other chemical disinfection system residue on soft lenses may cause the lens to turn pink, yellow, brown, black, or purple if the lens is exposed to a hydrogen peroxide system. Barnes Hind Daily Cleaner should not be mixed with a cleaner containing poloxamer 407 (i.e., Mirasoft) because cloudy precipitates may form on the lens.[30]

Insertion and Removal

See Table 23–16 for instructions on inserting and removing soft lenses.

Lens Storage Case

Choice of a lens storage case is important. The case should have left and right clearly identified on the caps and in the lens wells. The lens wells should have ridges or flutes so that the RGP lens does not adhere to the case, an occurrence that is common in smooth cases and can cause warpage of the lens or inversion upon removal.

As important as lens care is the proper care and cleaning of the contact lens storage case. A storage case should be able to hold at least 2.5 mL of the storage solution.[41] This minimizes the chance that the soaking solution will be overwhelmed by an inoculum of bacteria. The lens case should be cleaned thoroughly on a routine basis and replaced at least every 3 months.[42] Routine cleaning entails air drying the case between periods of use and scrubbing it weekly. Air drying should be done daily as it discourages biofilm formation. Some manufacturers recommend cleaning the case twice weekly using a few drops of lens cleaner and hot water.[43] If the case can routinely withstand boiling (such as those cases made of polycarbonate or noryl plastic), it can be boiled in a pot of water for 10 minutes weekly.[44] Examine for cracks and replace periodically. Lens cases can be contaminated with a biofilm that will attract pathogens and increase the risk of infection.

Table 23–16

Insertion and Removal of Soft Lenses

Insertion

- Wash the hands with noncosmetic soap and rinse thoroughly; dry the hands with a lint-free towel.
- Remove the lens for the right eye from its storage container.
- Rinse the lens with saline solution to dilute any preservatives left from disinfection.
- Place the lens on the top of a finger and examine it to be sure it is not inside out. This can be done by using the "taco test." Gently fold the lens at the apex (not the edges) between the thumb and forefinger. The edges should look like a taco shell with the edges pointed inward. If the edges roll out, the lens is inverted and must be reversed.
- Examine the lens for cleanliness. If necessary, clean it and rinse again with saline.
- Insert the lens on the right eye using the same procedure as for hard and RGP lenses. (See Table 23–8.)
- Repeat the process for the left eye.

Removal

- Before removing the lenses, wash hands with a noncosmetic soap; rinse the hands thoroughly and dry them with a lint-free towel.
- Using the right middle finger, pull down the lower lid of the right eye. Touch the right index finger to the lens and slide the lens off the cornea as shown in drawing A.
- Using the index finger and thumb, grasp the lens and remove it as shown in drawing B.
- Repeat the procedure for the left eye.

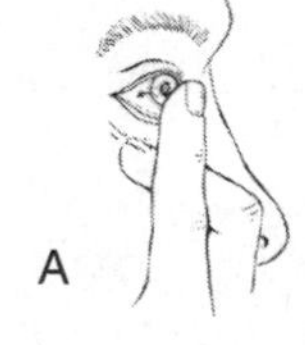

A

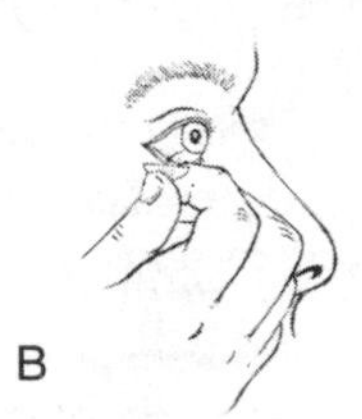

B

Patient Assessment of Contact Lens-Related Problems

Although contact lenses are usually safe, lens wearers can experience a variety of problems. During the patient interview, the pharmacist should first determine what type of eye problems exist and how long the patient has been experiencing them. Asking the patient whether a history of eye problems exists and what medications are currently being taken will give a general sense of the etiology and urgency of the current eye problem. The answers will also help the pharmacist determine whether the problem is related to noncompliance with care regimens or to drug–lens interactions. Many lens care–related problems are minor and can be easily solved by the knowledgeable pharmacist. When lens care is appropriate but the lenses are old or, in the case of hard lenses, chipped or scratched, the patient should see an eye care practitioner for replacement lenses. Other situations that require referral are suspected vision changes, deep aching of the eyes, an eye examination occurred longer than 1 year ago, and a suspected interaction between the lenses and oral contraceptives or other systemic medications.

Finding out which type of contact lenses a patient is wearing and for how long is crucial in assessing problems related to improper lens care or deteriorated lenses. Each type of lens has unique physical characteristics that in turn dictate which methods and products for cleaning and disinfecting lenses are appropriate. Patients should be asked to describe how they care for their lenses, which lens care products they use, and whether they have recently changed products. Asking the patient the following questions will elicit the information needed to recommend either changes in lens care regimens or referral to an eye practitioner.

Case Study 23–2

Patient Complaint/History

Jack, a 42 year-old man who began wearing soft contact lenses 3 weeks ago, comes to the pharmacy seeking information about the proper care of his lenses. He had worn hard contact lenses for the prior 17 years. He says that his lens prescriber told him to clean the soft lenses with Opti-Clean II each time he removes them; however, he cannot remember the rest of the care regimen. He also says that his lenses will be replaced every 3 months.

Questioning the patient reveals that he is wearing soft contact lenses (brand unknown) and that his lenses don't seem to be as "clear" as when he first got them. He reports occasional blurry vision but denies any discharge from the eye.

Jack's lens care regimen includes cleaning the lenses with Opti-Clean II each time he removes them and then soaking them in aerosolized saline. He has used the same saline solution for the past week and has not added fresh saline solution. He also has not cleaned his storage container since purchasing it.

Although questions about the patient's medical history reveal no history of prior ocular problems, a history of sensitivity to thimerosal is revealed; his family history is noncontributory. Jack does not take any medications. He does not smoke and is only a social drinker.

Clinical Considerations/Strategies

Readers can use the following considerations/strategies to determine the best recommendation for this patient and to select the appropriate contact lens products:

- Assess the contact lens care regimen. Call the lens prescriber to determine an appropriate care regimen and to discuss suggested changes in the regimen.
- Assess the patient's history of lens wear along with symptomatology, allergy history, and medication history.

Patient Education/Counseling

Readers can use the following strategies to develop a patient education/counseling plan that will help ensure optimal therapeutic outcomes:

- Describe a lens care regimen that is optimal for compliance and ease of use.
- Justify changes in the care regimen.
- Explain proper use of new product(s) added to the regimen.
- Reinforce proper principles of lens care.
- Educate the patient about contact lens wear and symptoms of lens problems.

General Assessment of Contact Lens Wearers

Q~ What types of lenses do you wear? Hard, soft, or rigid gas-permeable? Are your lenses disposable or for extended wear? How do you take care of your lenses? Have you recently changed brands of any of your solutions?

A~ Determine whether the patient is complying with the prescribed lens care regimen and is using compatible solutions. If the patient is unsure how to care for the lenses, explain the care regimen and recommend products for the patient's type of lenses.

Q~ How long have you been wearing lenses? When did you start wearing this pair, in particular? When did the problems start?

A~ If the problem is associated with an old pair of lenses, refer the patient to an eye care practitioner.

Q~ What types of problems are you having with your lenses? Are they related to eye irritation or changes in vision? When did the problems start?

A~ *Identify potential problems for lens wearers. (See the section "Precautions for Contact Lenses.") Identify symptoms of lens problems and their possible causes. (See the section "Symptoms of Lens Problems.")* Determine whether the patient's problem is acute or chronic. If vision changes have occurred, refer the patient to an eye care practitioner.

Q~ How many hours per day do you wear your lenses before problems start? Do you remove your lenses during the day?

A~ Determine whether overwear and/or corneal edema are possible causes of the problem.

Q~ When did you last see your optometrist or ophthalmologist?

A~ If the last eye examination was longer than 1 year ago, refer the patient to an eye care practitioner to determine whether a serious problem exists or whether the patient's lenses are wearing out.

Q~ How often do you change your storage solutions?

A~ If the solutions are being used too long, advise the patient how often to exchange the solutions and not to use solutions past the manufacturer's expiration date.

Q~ How often do you clean or replace your storage case? Does it need to be replaced?

A~ *Identify the proper care procedures for storage cases. (See the section "Lens Storage Case.")* If the storage case is not being cleaned or has been used too long, advise the patient that bacterial contamination of the container could cause eye infections.

Q~ Have you become pregnant or begun using oral contraceptives since you were prescribed lenses?

A~ If yes, advise the patient that changes in estrogen levels might be affecting the way a lens fits. Refer the patient to an eye care practitioner.

Q~ What nonprescription and prescription medications are you now taking?

A~ *Identify medications that can interact with contact lenses. (See Table 23–4.)* Advise the patient that only nonprescription ophthalmic products specifically designed for use with contact lenses should be used when lenses are in the eye. If the patient is taking a systemic medication known to interact with contact lenses, refer the patient to an eye care practitioner.

Q~ Do you have allergies?

A~ If yes, advise the patient that allergies may affect the ability to wear contact lenses.

Assessment of Hard Lens Wearers

Q~ Do you soak your lenses when they are not in use?

A~ If no, advise the patient that lenses should not be stored dry.

Q~ How often do you clean your hard lenses? How often do you clean them?

A~ *Identify proper care procedures for hard lenses. (See Figure 23–1 and Tables 23–5 and 23–6.)* If the cleaning procedure is incorrect or not frequent enough, instruct the patient on proper lens care.

Q~ What lens care products do you use? Do you use a multipurpose solution, which may not provide optimal lens care?

A~ If the lens care products are inappropriate, recommend the appropriate products and advise the patient not to use multipurpose solutions.

Q~ Do you inspect your lenses regularly for chips and scratches?

A~ If no, advise the patient that chips and scratches can cause corneal abrasions and ocular discomfort.

Assessment of Rigid Gas-Permeable Lens Wearers

Q~ What brand of RGP lenses do you wear?

A~ Base care recommendations on the brand of lens the patient wears.

Q~ Do you routinely use enzymatic cleaners? How often? What do you use to dissolve the enzymatic tablet?

A~ *Identify proper care procedures for RGP lenses. (See Figure 23–2 and Tables 23–5 and 23–10.)* If the cleaning procedure is incorrect or not frequent enough, explain proper care procedures for the lenses.

Q~ Do you clean your lenses immediately after removing them from the eye?

A~ If no, advise the patient that lens deposits may be more difficult to remove if cleaning the lenses is delayed.

Q~ Do you routinely use a soaking/conditioning solution formulated for your type of RGP lenses?

A~ *Identify the benefits of soaking the lenses. (See the section "Care of Rigid Gas-Permeable Lenses.")* If this procedure is not being implemented, advise the patient of its benefits.

Assessment of Soft Lens Wearers

Q~ What type of soft lenses do you wear (i.e., brand, high- or low-water content, ionic or nonionic)?

A~ Base care recommendations on the characteristics of the lens the patient wears.

Q~ Do you clean your lenses before disinfecting? What method of disinfection do you use? How often do you disinfect your lenses? Do you routinely use enzymatic cleaners? How often? How do you dilute the enzymatic tablet?

A~ *Identify proper cleaning and disinfecting procedures for soft lenses. (See Figure 23–3 and Tables 23–5, 23–12, and 23–14.)* If the patient's response indicates improper lens care, explain the prescribed lens care regimen.

Q~ Do you use commercial saline solutions or do you mix your own? How often do you replace your solution?

A~ If the patient uses homemade solutions or does not replace the solution often enough, explain that these practices can cause an eye infection.

Q~ Do you apply any cosmetics to the eye area? How do you apply these products?

A~ If eye cosmetics are used, explain how to apply them and which cosmetics to avoid.

Q~ Are your lenses extended-wear lenses? If so, how long do you wear them?

A~ Advise patients with extended-wear lenses that adverse effects can occur if the lenses are worn for long periods of time.

Patient Education for Preventing Contact Lens–Related Disorders

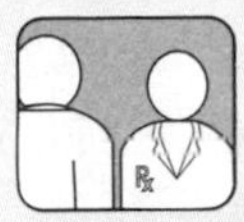

The objective of contact lens care is to prevent lens-related problems such as abrasions or infections of the cornea. For most patients, following the prescribed lens care regimen, product instructions, and the self-care measures listed below will help ensure trouble-free use of contact lenses.

General Instructions for All Contact Lens Types

- Wash hands with noncosmetic soap and rinse thoroughly before touching contact lenses.
- Avoid wearing oily cosmetics while wearing lenses. Bath oils or soaps with a bath oil or cream base may leave an oil film on the hands that will be transferred to the lenses.
- To avoid mixing up the lenses, always work with the same lens first. Check hard lenses for a dot in the lens periphery to avoid confusing lenses.
- If the lenses are not comfortable after insertion or if vision is blurred, check to see if they are on the wrong eyes or inside out.
- To avoid damaging lenses, apply aerosol cosmetics and deodorants either before lens insertion or with eyes closed until the air is clear of spray particles.
- Except for prescription extended-wear lenses do not wear lenses while sleeping.
- To avoid excessive dryness of the eyes, do not wear lenses while sitting under a hair dryer, overhead fans, and air ducts.
- When lenses are worn outside on windy days, protect the eyes from soot and other particles that may become trapped under the lens and scratch the cornea.
- Use eye protection in industry, sports, or any other occupation or hobby that has the potential for eye damage.
- Store contact lenses in a proper lens case when not in use.
- Never reuse contact lens solutions.
- Replace soaking solutions in lens cases after each use.
- Never store lenses in tap water.
- Do not wear contact lenses in swimming pools, hot tubs, ocean waters, or other natural bodies of water without external eye protection such as goggles.
- To prevent contamination, do not touch dropper tips or the tips of lens care product containers.
- While wearing lenses, apply to the eyes only ophthalmic solutions specifically formulated for contact lens use.
- Never use saliva to wet contact lenses. This practice can result in eye infections.

⚠ Do not insert lenses in red or irritated eyes. If the eyes become irritated while lenses are being worn, remove the lenses until the irritation subsides. Should irritation or redness not subside, consult an eye care practitioner.

⚠ If an eye infection is suspected, see an eye practitioner immediately.

Instructions for Hard Lenses

- Do not store lenses dry.
- Clean lenses every time they are removed from the eyes. See Tables 23–5 and 23–6 for cleaning procedures.
- Be aware that multipurpose solutions may not provide optimal lens care.
- Inspect lenses regularly for chips and scratches.
- Do not rub eyes while lenses are in place.
- Do not rinse contact lenses with very hot or very cold water because temperature extremes may warp the lenses.
- Do not get oils or lanolin on the lens.

Instructions for Rigid Gas-Permeable Lenses

- See Tables 23–5 and 23–10 for guidelines on cleaning RGP lenses.
- Do not use tap water to rinse off a cleaner or to rewet lenses. If tap water is used, disinfect lenses before inserting them in the eyes.[45]
- Do not disinfect these lenses with thermal disinfecting systems.
- See Table 23–14 for guidelines on using other types of disinfecting systems.

Instructions for Soft Lenses

- See Tables 23–5 and 23–12 for guidelines on cleaning these lenses.
- Handle soft lenses carefully because they are very fragile and can easily be torn.
- Remove these lenses before instilling any ophthalmic preparation not specifically intended for concurrent use with soft contact lenses. Wait at least 20 to 30 minutes before reinserting the lenses unless directed otherwise by an eye practitioner.
- Do not wear lenses when a topical ophthalmic ointment is being used.
- Do not wear soft contact lenses in the presence of irritating fumes or chemicals.
- Wear disposable soft contact lenses under the supervision of an eye practitioner and strictly follow manufacturer's guidelines for wear.

(continued)

Patient Education for Preventing Contact Lens–Related Disorders (continued)

Instructions for Extended-Wear Lenses (Rigid Gas-Permeable or Soft)

- Do not wear extended-wear soft lenses continuously for more than 7 days without completely cleaning and disinfecting the lenses.
- For female patients, remove mascara before sleeping because mascara can flake off during sleep and become trapped underneath the lens.[46]
- If lenses appear to be lost upon awakening, check eyes to see if the lenses were displaced. Soft lenses can fold over on themselves and get lodged underneath the top or bottom eyelid.

⚠ Each morning, check eyes carefully for unusual, persistent redness, discharge, or pain. If redness does not abate within 45 minutes or discharge or pain is present, remove the lens and call the lens care practitioner.

⚠ Check vision after inserting lenses. (Some hazy vision is normal upon awakening because of corneal hypoxia, which develops overnight.) Apply a few drops of rewetting solution to improve hydration of the lens and help resolve hypoxia. If the problem is not resolved, remove lenses, clean them, and reinsert. If vision is not improved within an hour, remove lenses and call the lens care practitioner.

Patient Counseling for Contact Lens Care

Following the prescribed lens care program is the best strategy for avoiding lens wear–related problems. The pharmacist should explain the care regimen for the patient's particular lens type and stress that the patient should use only the products recommended for their lenses. Instructions on avoiding practices or situations that can cause eye irritation or lens damage are also important in educating the patient about successful wearing of contact lenses. The patient should also be advised of signs and symptoms that indicate medical care is needed. The box "Patient Education for Preventing Contact Lens–Related Disorders" lists specific information to provide patients.

References

1. MacKeen DL. Contact lens solutions. *Am Pharm.* 1986;26:691–6.
2. Feldman GL. Contact lens materials. *Int Ophthalmol Clin.* 1981;21:155–62.
3. Holden BA, Mertz GW. Critical oxygen levels to avoid corneal edema for daily and extended wear contact lenses. *Invest Ophthalmol Vis Sci.* 1984;25:1161–7.
4. Hayworth NA, Asbell PA. Therapeutic contact lenses. *CLAO J.* 1990;16:137–42.
5. Yamaguchi T et al. Fungus growth on soft contact lenses with different water contents. *CLAO J.* 1984;10:166–71.
6. Barr JT. The 1998 annual report on contact lenses. *Contact Lens Spectrum* 1999;14(1):25–8.
7. Capaldi-O'Brien P, Barr JT. Disposable and planned replacement lens update. *Contact Lens Spectrum* 1998;13(7):23–7.
8. Callender MG. Contact lenses and care systems. *Pharm Pract.* 1990;6:26–45.
9. Lembach RG. Rigid gas permeable contact lenses. *CLAO J.* 1990;16:129–34.
10. Weinstock FJ, Zucker JL. Extended-wear cosmetic contact lenses. *Int Ophthalmol Clin.* 1991;31:25–33.
11. Schein OD et al. The relative risk of ulcerative keratitis among users of daily-wear and extended-wear soft contact lenses. *N Engl J Med.* 1989;321:773–8.
12. Kershner RM. Infectious corneal ulcerations with over-extended wear of disposable contact lenses. *JAMA.* 1989;261:3549–50.
13. Krezanoski JZ. Topical medications. *Int Ophthalmol Clin.* 1981;21:173–6.
14. Lembach RG. Keratoconus. *Int Ophthalmol Clin.* 1991;31:71–82.
15. Stein HA. Contact lenses in the management of presbyopia. *Int Ophthamol Clin.* 1991;31:61–70.
16. Stein HA. The management of presbyopia with contact lenses: a review. *CLAO J.* 1990;16:33–8.
17. Freeman MI. Patient selection. *Int Ophthalmol Clin.* 1991;31:1–12.
18. Kastl PR. Is the quality of vision with contact lenses adequate? Not in all instances. *Cornea.* 1990;9(suppl 1):S20–2.
19. Pepose JS. Contact lens disinfection to prevent transmission of viral disease. *CLAO J.* 1988;14:165–8.
20. Macsai MS et al. Deposition of ciprofloxacin, prednisolone phosphate, and prednisolone acetate in SeeQuence disposable contact lenses. *CLAO J.* 1993;19:166–8.
21. Lee BL et al. The solubility of antibiotic and corticosteroid combinations. *Am J Ophthalmol.*1992;114:212–5.
22. Plotnik RD, Mannis MJ, Schwab IR. Therapeutic contact lenses. *Int Ophthalmol Clin.* 1991;31:35–52.
23. Diamond SA, Dupuis LL. Contact lens damage due to ribavirin exposure. *DICP Ann Pharmacother.* 198;23:428–9.
24. Rodriguez WJ et al. Environmental exposure of primary care personnel to ribavirin aerosol when supervising treatment of infants with respiratory syncytial virus infections. *Antimicrob Agents Chemother.* 1987;31:1143–6.
25. Broich J, Weiss L, Rapp J. Isolation and identification of biologically active contaminants from soft contact lenses. *Invest Ophthalmol Vis Sci.* 1980;19:1328–35.
26. Miller D. Systemic medications. *Int Ophthalmol Clin.* 1981;21:177–83.
27. Koetting RA. Cosmetics. *Int Ophthalmol Clin.* 1981;21:185–93.
28. Mandell RB, Respicio SG. Efficacy of contaminant removal by RGP lens cleaners. *Contact Lens Spectrum.* 1988;3:57–60.
29. White PF, Miller D. Corneal edema. *Int Ophthalmol Clin.* 1981;21:3–12.
30. Rakow PL. Mixing contact lens solutions. *J Ophthalmic Nurs Technol.* 1989;8(2):67–8.
31. Diefenbach CB, Seibert CK, Davis LJ. Analysis of two home remedy contact lens cleaners. *J Am Optom Assoc.* 1988;59(7):518–21.
32. Butrus SI, Abelson MB. Contact lenses and the allergic patient. *Int Ophthalmol Clin.* 1986;26:73–81.
33. Terry R, Schnider C, Holden BA. Rigid gas permeable lenses and patient management. *CLAO J.* 1989;14:305–9.
34. Mobley CL. Letter. *Contact Lens Forum.* 1989;14(suppl 4):13–4.
35. Stenson S. Soft contact lens deposits. *JAMA.* 1987;257:2823.
36. Tripathi BJ, Tripathi RC, Rhee JM. Adherence of bacteria to soft contact lenses. In: Dabezies OH, ed. *Contact Lenses, The CLAO Guide to Basic Science and Clinical Practice.* 2nd ed. Boston: Little, Brown and Co; 1992:42.1–42.17.
37. Harris MG. Practical considerations in the use of hydrogen peroxide disinfection systems. *CLAO J.* 1990;16(suppl 1):S53–S60.
38. Wittman G. Personal communication of data on file at company. Irvine, CA: Allergan, Inc; January 17, 1995.

39. Fiscella RG. New eye infection: difficult to detect, easier to prevent. *US Pharm.* 1989;14:75–81.
40. Lowther G, Shannon BJ, Weisbarth R, eds. The importance of compliance. In: *The Pharmacist's Guide to Contact Lenses and Lens Care.* Atlanta: CIBA Vision; 1988:23–5.
41. Krezanoski JZ, Dabezies OH. Hard lens hygiene. In: Dabezies OH, ed. *Contact Lenses, The CLAO Guide to Basic Science and Clinical Practice.* 2nd ed. Boston: Little, Brown and Co; 1992:31.1–31.17.
42. Driebe WT. Contact lens cleaning and disinfection. In: Kastl PR, ed. *Contact Lenses, The CLAO Guide to Basic Science and Clinical Practice.* 3rd ed. Dubuque, IA: Kendall/Hunt Publishing; 1995;II:237–62.
43. *Boston Equalens Patient Care Guide.* Polymer Technology Corporation; 1987.
44. Callender MG. Contact lens care systems: part 1. hard and gas permeable lenses. *Pharm Pract.* 1990;6:26–31.
45. Campbell RC, Caroline PJ. RGPs and tap water. *Contact Lens Forum.* 1990;15:64.
46. Key JE, Bennett ES. Rigid gas-permeable extended wear contact lenses. In: Kastl PR, ed. *Contact Lenses, The CLAO Guide to Basic Science and Clinical Practice.* 3rd ed. Dubuque, IA: Kendall/Hunt Publishing;1995;II:51–74.

CHAPTER 24

Otic Disorders

Linda Krypel

Chapter 24 at a Glance

Ear complaints are common and vary from simple complaints of excessive earwax (cerumen) or itching to painful ear infections. A survey indicated that patients with ear disorders seek medical care 87% of the time.[1] Cerumen impaction can affect up to 6% of the general population and is one of the most frequent otologic problems encountered by physicians.[2] Ear disorders affect all ages, with the young and the elderly being most prone.

Self-treatment with nonprescription medications and alternative remedies should be restricted to external ear disorders, which include disorders of the auricle and the external auditory canal (EAC). Excessive cerumen and water-clogged ears are self-treatable EAC disorders for which the Food and Drug Administration (FDA) has approved nonprescription otic medications. Other self-treatable disorders of the auricle include allergic and contact dermatitis, seborrhea, psoriasis, and boils. Nonprescription medications used to treat these

Editor's Note: This chapter is based, in part, on the 11th edition chapter titled "Otic Products," which was written by Keith O. Miller.

disorders when they appear on other parts of the body are also appropriate for treating the auricle.

Diseases in the head and neck can cause referred pain, which the patient often perceives as pain from the ear. The pharmacist's greatest challenge in self-care of otic disorders is differentiating whether an otic disorder is causing the symptoms and, if so, whether the disorder is self-treatable. For that reason, patient assessment of self-treatable disorders is covered in one section: "Patient Assessment of Otic Disorders." This section also highlights symptoms of otic disorders that are not amenable to self-treatment. Collective discussions of patient counseling and evaluation of patient outcomes for the various self-treatable disorders are also presented at the end of the chapter.

Anatomy and Physiology of the Ear

The external ear consists of the auricle (also called the pinna) and the EAC. (See Figure 24–1.) The external ear is closed by the tympanic membrane, which is part of the middle ear.[3] The auricle is composed of a thin layer of highly vascular skin that is tightly bound to cartilage. Adipose or subcutaneous tissue, which would insulate blood vessels, is absent except in the lobe. The lobe has fewer blood vessels and is composed primarily of fatty tissue. The triangular piece of cartilage in front of the ear canal adjacent to the cheek (not shown in Figure 24–1) is called the tragus.

The EAC consists of an outer cartilaginous portion, which composes one-third to one-half its length, plus an inner body or osseous portion.[3] The canal forms a blind cul-de-sac. Children have a shorter, straighter, and flatter EAC than that of adults, whose canals tend to lengthen and form an "S" shape.[3,4] At the same time, an adult's eustachian tube (part of the inner ear) lengthens downward as it enters the nasal cavity. This shape helps promote drainage and inhibits aspiration of throat and nasal contents into the middle ear through the eustachian tube, explaining why children suffer from more middle ear infections than do adults.[4]

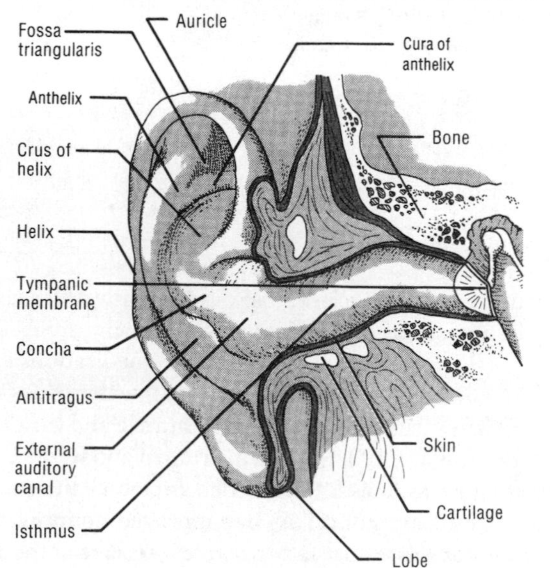

Figure 24–1 Anatomy of the auricle and external ear.

The skin that covers the auricle is especially susceptible to bleeding when scratched because of the lack of flexibility usually afforded by a subcutaneous layer of fat and the profuse blood supply to the area.[3] The skin is highly enervated, causing a disproportionate otalgia (ear pain) when inflammation is present. Skin farther into the EAC is thicker and contains apocrine and exocrine glands as well as hair follicles.[5] The skin in the canal is continuous with the outer layer of the tympanic membrane.

Oily secretions from the exocrine glands mix with the milky, fatty fluid from the apocrine glands to form cerumen, which appears on the skin's surface of the outer half of the EAC. Cerumen lubricates the canal, traps dust and foreign materials, and provides a waxy, waterproof barrier to the entry of pathogens.[6,7] It also contains various antimicrobial substances, such as lysozymes, and exhibits an acidic pH, which aids in the inhibition of bacterial and fungal growth.[5,6,7]

The canal skin is shed continuously and mixes with cerumen. This debris-laden cerumen migrates outward when jaw movements, such as chewing and talking, take place in a self-cleaning process.[6] Cerumen may appear dry and flaky or oily and pastelike. Color varies from light gray to orange or brown and may darken on exposure to air.[8]

The normal tympanic membrane or eardrum is smooth, translucent, and pearl-gray. It is concave and oval with an average thickness of 0.074 mm and is composed of three layers. The continuous skin layer of the EAC forms the outer tympanic membrane layer. The middle layer is fibrous tissue, and the internal layer is a mucous membrane continuous with the lining of the middle ear.[3] The tympanic membrane transmits sound waves and acts as a protective barrier to the middle ear.[9]

The natural defenses of the ear canal include the skin layer with its protective coating of cerumen, an acidic pH, and hairs that line the outer half of the canal. Together they protect against injury from foreign material and infection. An understanding of the normal role and function of cerumen is important for the pharmacist to assist in educating patients.

Pathophysiology of Otic Disorders

Because the EAC forms a blind cul-de-sac, it is especially susceptible to collecting moisture. A dark, warm, moist environment is ideal for bacterial growth. In the preinflammatory stage, the lipid layer covering the skin is removed by moisture, local trauma, or both. Local trauma from fingernails, cotton-tipped swabs, or other items inserted into the canal can abrade the skin and allow pathogens to enter. Because a normal, healthy ear canal is impervious to potentially pathogenic organisms, skin integrity generally must be interrupted before an organism can produce an infection. Trauma to the ear from thermal injuries, sports injuries, ear piercing, and poorly fitting or improperly cleaned ear molds or hearing aids can contribute to the breakdown of the EAC's natural defenses.[9] Dermatologic skin disorders, such as contact dermatitis, seborrhea, psoriasis, and malignancies, also compromise these defenses.[6,7,10]

Viral illnesses, such as colds and upper respiratory infections, can contribute to the breakdown of natural defenses of the middle and inner ear, especially in children, who are very susceptible to inner ear infections following such illnesses. Because a child's eustachian tube is shorter and angled flatter than an adult's, nasopharynx secretions can easily be aspirated and accumulate in the middle ear, leading to bacteria proliferation. Holding back or trying to stifle a sneeze can force secretions into the middle ear and thus should be strongly discouraged, even in adults.

Excessive/Impacted Cerumen

Cerumen has been referred to as " . . . an under-valued defense system."[11] Widespread misinformation has often led the public to believe that cerumen production is a pathologic condition that must be continually removed. Rather, improper attempts to remove cerumen can actually damage the EAC.[12]

Epidemiology/Etiology of Excessive/Impacted Cerumen

Individuals with abnormally narrow or misshapen EACs and/or excessive hair growth in the canal are predisposed to impacted cerumen. These physiologic anomalies disrupt the normal migration of cerumen to the outer EAC. Individuals who have overactive ceruminous glands or who wear hearing aids, ear plugs to prevent water from entering the ear, and sound attenuators often suffer from impacted cerumen. Devices in the ear can inhibit the migration of cerumen and cause wax buildup.[9,13]

The elderly often experience impacted cerumen resulting from atrophy of ceruminous glands.[8] This population secretes drier cerumen, which is more difficult to expel from the ear.

Signs and Symptoms of Excessive/Impacted Cerumen

The most common symptoms of impacted cerumen are a sense of fullness or pressure in the ear and a gradual hearing loss. A dull pain is sometimes associated with this disorder.

Case Study 24–1

Patient Complaint/History

Margo is a 72-year-old woman who complains of a slight hearing loss in her left ear. She is not experiencing pain, dizziness, or other symptoms. She has no family history of hearing loss nor has she been hospitalized recently. Margo explains that she has always had too much earwax but " . . . a good squirt with an ear syringe usually takes care of it." Flushing the ear has failed to dislodge anything this time. Margo asks whether you have anything to help dissolve earwax. She admits that she was tempted to use a cotton swab or toothpick to poke the wax out even though her doctor told her not to ever use them in her ear.

Margo is being treated for high blood pressure and takes atenolol 50 mg every morning and acetaminophen 1000 mg as needed for mild osteoarthritis of her knees. She also takes a vitamin/mineral supplement daily and extra calcium (1000 mg calcium carbonate) daily.

Clinical Considerations/Strategies

Readers can use the following considerations/strategies to determine whether treatment of the patient's condition with nonprescription medications is warranted:

- Assess whether the current condition warrants medical referral or a regimen with one or more nonprescription medications or devices.
- Select an appropriate treatment regimen to relieve excessive accumulation of cerumen in the ear.

Patient Counseling/Education

Readers can use the following strategies to develop a patient counseling/education plan that will help ensure optimal therapeutic outcomes:

- Provide proper patient counseling regarding the use of selected products, including technique, dose, frequency of administration, and duration of therapy.
- Explain the proper otic irrigation technique and the dangers of using too much force. (See the section "Treatment of Excessive/Impacted Cerumen.")
- Recommend a course of action to take if current symptoms persist and/or worsen or if new symptoms develop.
- Remind the patient of the techniques for proper ear hygiene once the current condition resolves and of the potential consequences of inappropriate ear hygiene such as cerumen impaction or infection.

Complications of Excessive/Impacted Cerumen

Attempting to remove cerumen by means of cotton-tipped applicators, bobby pins, toothpicks, fingernails, or other such objects can force the cerumen into the inner half of the EAC where it becomes hardened and compacted over time.[14] Hearing loss can occur along with vertigo (a sensation of spinning or whirling) or pain.[8,13] The delicate skin of the auditory canal can also be scratched or damaged, providing an entry for water and pathogens.[12] Hardened cerumen generally does not cling to cotton-tipped applicators and using them may serve only to remove the protective waxy layer and force the cerumen plug further into the canal.[9] Cerumen whose migration to the outer EAC is blocked by devices will also harden and become compacted.

Treatment of Excessive/Impacted Cerumen

Treatment Outcomes

Softening cerumen with safe and effective agents and using proper methods to remove it from the ear are the primary goals for self-treatment of excessive/impacted cerumen. These measures in turn will restore temporary hearing loss and eliminate other symptoms.

General Treatment Approach

Carbamide peroxide 6.5% in anhydrous glycerin is a proven safe and effective agent for softening cerumen.[15] After the cerumen is softened, the ear is gently irrigated, using an otic bulb syringe filled with warm water. Cotton-tipped swabs or other foreign objects should not be used to remove cerumen. The algorithm in Figure 24–2 outlines the appropriate self-treatment of excessive/impacted cerumen.)

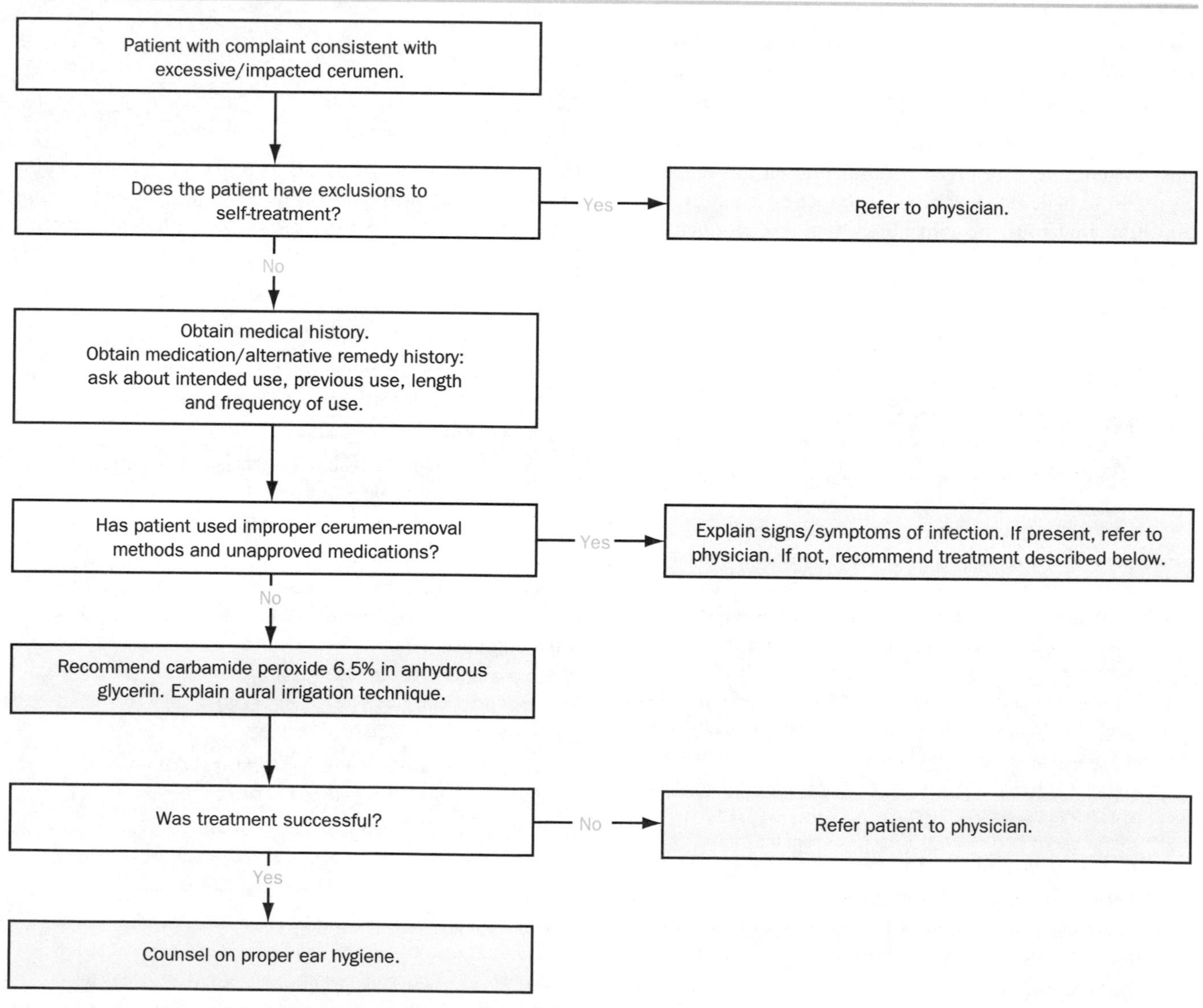

Figure 24–2 Self-care of excessive/impacted cerumen.

Bleeding or discharge from the ear and the presence of pain preclude irrigation of the ear. Presence of a ruptured tympanic membrane, ear surgery in the past 6 weeks, or signs of infection or trauma also exclude self-treatment. Further, the pharmacist should not recommend self-treatment if the patient appears incapable of following proper procedures.

Nonpharmacologic Therapy

Earwax should be removed only when it has migrated to the outermost portion of the EAC. The only recommended nonpharmacologic method of removing cerumen is to use a wet, wrung-out washcloth draped over a finger. This method of removing cerumen is not effective once cerumen becomes impacted. However, making this procedure part of daily aural hygiene can prevent impacted cerumen if physiologic abnormalities or physical devices are not the cause of the impaction.

Pharmacologic Therapy

Carbamide peroxide 6.5% in anhydrous glycerin is currently the only FDA-approved nonprescription cerumen-softening agent. Other agents such as mineral oil, olive oil (sweet oil), glycerin, and dilute hydrogen peroxide have been used by physicians and patients as inexpensive home remedies to soften cerumen. No data support these remedies as being more effective than carbamide peroxide in anhydrous glycerin. Docusate sodium has even been used in attempts to soften cerumen because of its emulsifying properties.

Carbamide Peroxide

Carbamide peroxide 6.5% in anhydrous glycerin is approved as safe and effective in softening, loosening, and removing excessive earwax in adults and in children ages 12 years and older.[15] (See Table 24–1 for instructions on the proper instillation of ear drops.) Carbamide peroxide is prepared from hydrogen peroxide and urea. When carbamide peroxide is exposed to moisture, nascent oxygen is released slowly and acts as a weak antibacterial. The effervescence that occurs during this process along with urea's effect on tissue debridement helps to mechanically break down and loosen cerumen that has been softened by anhydrous glycerin.

Any cerumen remaining after treatment may be removed with gentle, warm water irrigation using a rubber otic bulb syringe. (See Table 24–2.) Improper use of an otic syringe or using an oral jet irrigator to remove cerumen can leave excess moisture in the canal or further compress cerumen. These actions can also cause otitis externa, perforated tympanic

Table 24–1

Guidelines for Administering Ear Drops

1. Wash your hands with soap and warm water; then dry them thoroughly.
2. Carefully wash and dry the outside of the ear, taking care not to get water in the ear canal.
3. Warm ear drops to body temperature by holding the container in the palm of your hand for a few minutes. Do not warm the container in hot water. Hot ear drops can cause ear pain, nausea, and dizziness.
4. If the label indicates, shake the container.
5. Tilt your head (or have the patient tilt his or her head) to the side as shown in drawing A. Or lie down with the affected ear up as shown in drawing B. Use gentle restraint, if necessary, for an infant or a young child.
6. Open the container carefully. Position the dropper tip near, but not inside, the ear canal opening. Do not allow the dropper to touch the ear, because it could become contaminated or injure the ear. Ear drops must be kept clean.
7. Pull your ear (or the patient's ear) backward and upward to open the ear canal as shown in drawing A. If the patient is a child younger than 3 years old, pull the ear backward and downward as shown in drawing B.
8. Place the proper dose or number of drops into the ear canal. Replace the cap on the container.
9. Gently press the small, flat skin flap over the ear canal opening to force out air bubbles and to push the drops down the ear canal.
10. Stay (or keep the patient) in the same position for the length of time indicated in the product instructions. If the patient is a child who cannot stay still, the doctor may tell you to place a clean piece of cotton gently into the child's ear to prevent the medication from draining out. Use a piece large enough to remove easily, and do not leave it in the ear longer than an hour.
11. Repeat the procedure for the other ear, if needed.
12. Gently wipe excess medication off the outside of the ear, using caution to avoid getting moisture in the ear canal.
13. Wash your hands.

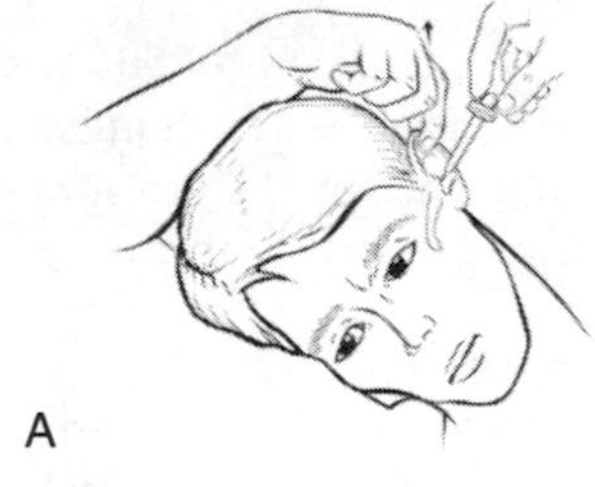
A

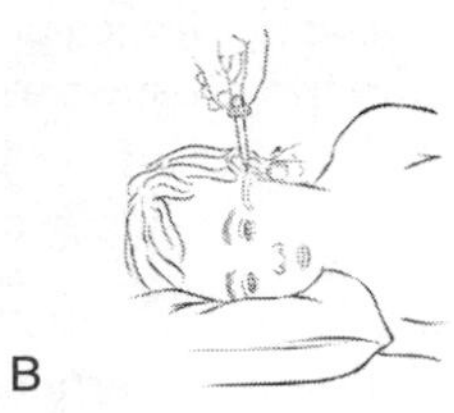
B

Source: *APhA Special Report: Medication Administration Problem Solving in Ambulatory Care.* Washington DC: American Pharmaceutical Association; 1994:9.

Table 24–2

Guidelines for Removing Excessive/Impacted Cerumen

1. Place 5 to 10 drops of the cerumen-softening solution into the ear canal, and allow it to remain for at least 15 minutes. (See Table 24–1.)
2. Prepare a warm (not hot) solution of plain water or other solution as directed by your doctor. Eight ounces of solution should be sufficient to clean out the ear canal.
3. To catch the returning solution, hold a container under the ear being cleaned. An emesis basin is ideal because it fits the contour of the neck. Tilt the head down slightly on the side where the ear is being cleaned.
4. Gently pull the ear lobe down and back to expose the ear canal.
5. Place the open end of the syringe into the ear canal with the tip pointed slightly upward toward the side of the ear canal as shown in drawing A. Do not aim the syringe into the back of the ear canal. Make sure the syringe does not obstruct the outflow of solution.
6. Squeeze the bulb gently—not forcefully— to introduce the solution into the ear canal and to avoid rupturing the ear drum. (Note: Only health professionals trained in aural hygiene should use forced water sprays [e.g., Water Pik] to remove cerumen.)
7. Do not let the returning solution contact the eyes.
8. If pain or dizziness occurs, remove the syringe and do not resume irrigation until a doctor is consulted.
9. Rinse the syringe thoroughly before and after each use, and let it dry.
10. Store the syringe in a cool, dry place (preferably, in its original container) away from hot surfaces and sharp instruments.
11. Do this procedure twice daily for no longer than 4 consecutive days.

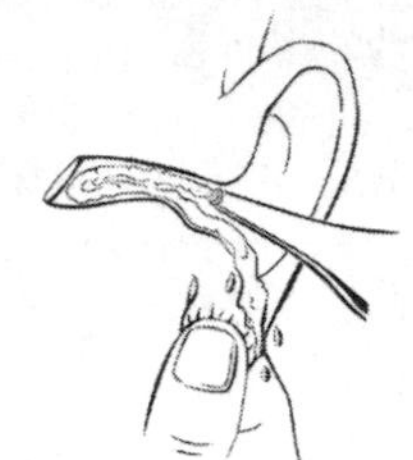

Source: Reprinted with permission from *Ohio Pharmacist*. 1996;14(5):10.

membrane, pain, vertigo, otitis media, tinnitus (ringing, hissing, or buzzing noises in the ear), and cough.[13,16,17]

Carbamide peroxide solutions may be used twice daily for up to 4 days. If symptoms persist after 4 days, the patient should see a physician for evaluation.[18]

Glycerin

Glycerin has emollient and humectant properties and is widely used as a solvent and vehicle. It is safe and nonsensitizing when applied to abraded skin. It can be used to soften earwax.

Hydrogen Peroxide

Hydrogen peroxide releases nascent oxygen when exposed to moisture that acts as a weak antibacterial.[19] A 1:1 solution of warm water and 3% hydrogen peroxide can be used to flush the ear canal when softening or removing earwax. This solution, however, is not an effective ear-drying agent. Overuse of 1:1 aqueous hydrogen peroxide solutions may predispose to infection from tissue maceration because of excessive water left in the canal.

Olive Oil (Sweet Oil)

Olive oil is used as an emollient and is helpful for softening earwax.[20] It may be instilled into the ear canal to alleviate itching.

Product Selection Guidelines

Although overall costs of FDA-approved and nonapproved agents are low, docusate sodium is more expensive, has poor results, and causes superficial erythema in some cases.[21] Table 24–3 lists examples of cerumen-softening and other otic products.

Alternative Remedies

Although major herbal references do not list herbal remedies for otic disorders,[22–25] other alternative (folk) remedies remain popular in many regions. One of the more interesting—and dangerous—is the use of ear candles to remove cerumen. A hollow candle is burned with one end inserted in the ear canal. The intent is to create negative pressure and draw cerumen from the ear. Studies have shown this method does not aid in removing cerumen but has caused serious ear injuries. Candle wax was deposited in the ear canal in some patients, and severe blockages and burns occurred. A survey of 122 otolaryngologists identified 21 ear injuries resulting from the use of ear candles.[26]

Water-Clogged Ears

Water-clogged ears is a separate disorder from swimmer's ear (external otitis). No nonprescription products have FDA approval for preventing or treating external otitis. Manufacturers have argued that removing moisture from water-clogged ears with an approved agent may prevent tissue maceration, which can lead to inflammation and infection of the external EAC (commonly referred to as swimmer's ear). The FDA prohibits this extrapolation, and, thus, manufacturers may no longer label their products as preventing

Table 24–3

Selected Products for Otic Disorders

Trade Name	Primary Ingredients
Cerumen-Softening Agents	
Bausch & Lomb Global Earwax Removal System	Carbamide peroxide 6.5%; anhydrous glycerin base; packaged with syringe
Debrox Drops	Carbamide peroxide 6.5%; glycerin
E.R.O. Drops	Carbamide peroxide 6.5%; anhydrous glycerin
E.R.O. Earwax Removal System	Carbamide peroxide 6.5%; anhydrous glycerin; packaged with syringe
Murine Earwax Removal System	Carbamide peroxide 6.5%; glycerin; alcohol 6.3%; packaged with syringe
Ear-Drying Agents	
AURO-DRI Drops	Isopropyl alcohol 95%; glycerin 5%
Ear-Dry Drops	Isopropyl alcohol 95%; anhydrous glycerin 5%
Miscellaneous Otic Products	
Aurocaine 2 Drops	Boric acid 2.75%; isopropyl alcohol
Earsol-HC Drops	Alcohol; hydrocortisone 1%

swimmer's ear. Most available nonprescription products for water-clogged ears have been reformulated to contain only FDA-approved ingredients.

Epidemiology/Etiology of Water-Clogged Ears

Some patients are more prone to retaining water because of the shape of their ear canals or the presence of excessive cerumen,[5] which can swell, trapping water. Excessive moisture in the ears can result from hot, humid climates, sweating, swimming, bathing, or improper use of aqueous solutions to cleanse the ear. Thus, simple attempts to remove water by mechanical manipulation may be insufficient.

Signs and Symptoms of Water-Clogged Ears

A feeling of wetness or fullness in the ear, accompanied by gradual hearing loss, can occur after exposure to any of the etiologic factors. The trapped moisture can compromise the natural defenses of the EAC, causing tissue maceration, which in turn can lead to itching, pain, inflammation, or infection.[10]

Treatment of Water-Clogged Ears

Treatment Outcomes

Using a safe and effective agent to dry already water-clogged ears is one objective of self-treatment. Another is to prevent recurrences in persons who are prone to retaining moisture in the ears.

General Treatment Approach

Before recommending an agent to treat water-clogged ears, the pharmacist should determine whether a patient has a ruptured tympanic membrane or a tympanostomy tube. Ear-drying agents are very painful if instilled in either of these situations. Further, if signs of infection or trauma are present or if the patient has had ear surgery in the past 6 weeks, medical referral is the appropriate recommendation. All nonprescription otic preparations may be contraindicated in individuals who are susceptible to local irritation and hypersensitivity. The algorithm in Figure 24–3 outlines the appropriate treatment of water-clogged ears.

The pharmacist should recommend either a product containing 95% isopropyl alcohol in 5% anhydrous glycerin or an extemporaneously compounded 50 : 50 mixture of 95% isopropyl alcohol and 5% acetic acid.

Nonpharmacologic Therapy

Tilting the affected ear downward and gently manipulating the auricle can expel excessive water from the ear. This procedure should be followed after swimming or bathing, or during periods of excessive sweating, especially by persons who are prone to developing this disorder. Using a blow-dryer on a low setting immediately after swimming or bathing may help dry the ear canal.

Pharmacologic Therapy

FDA has approved only 95% isopropyl alcohol in 5% anhydrous glycerin as a safe and effective "ear-drying aid."[27] (See Table 24–3 for examples of products containing these agents.) In addition, the American Academy of Otolaryngology recommends a 50 : 50 mixture of acetic acid 5% (white household vinegar) and 95% isopropyl alcohol to help dry water-clogged ears.[28]

Isopropyl Alcohol in Anhydrous Glycerin

Alcohol is highly miscible with water and acts as a drying agent. Alcohol in concentrations greater than 70% are also effective skin disinfectants. Glycerin has been used in pharmaceutical preparations for its solvent, emollient, or hygroscopic properties. It is safe and nonsensitizing when applied to open wounds or abraded skin. Combined with alcohol, glycerin provides a product that reduces moisture in the ear without overdrying.

Ear-drying agents, which are recommended for use in adults and children ages 12 years and older, may be used whenever ears are exposed to water. Table 24–1 presents guidelines for administering these agents. Medical referral is

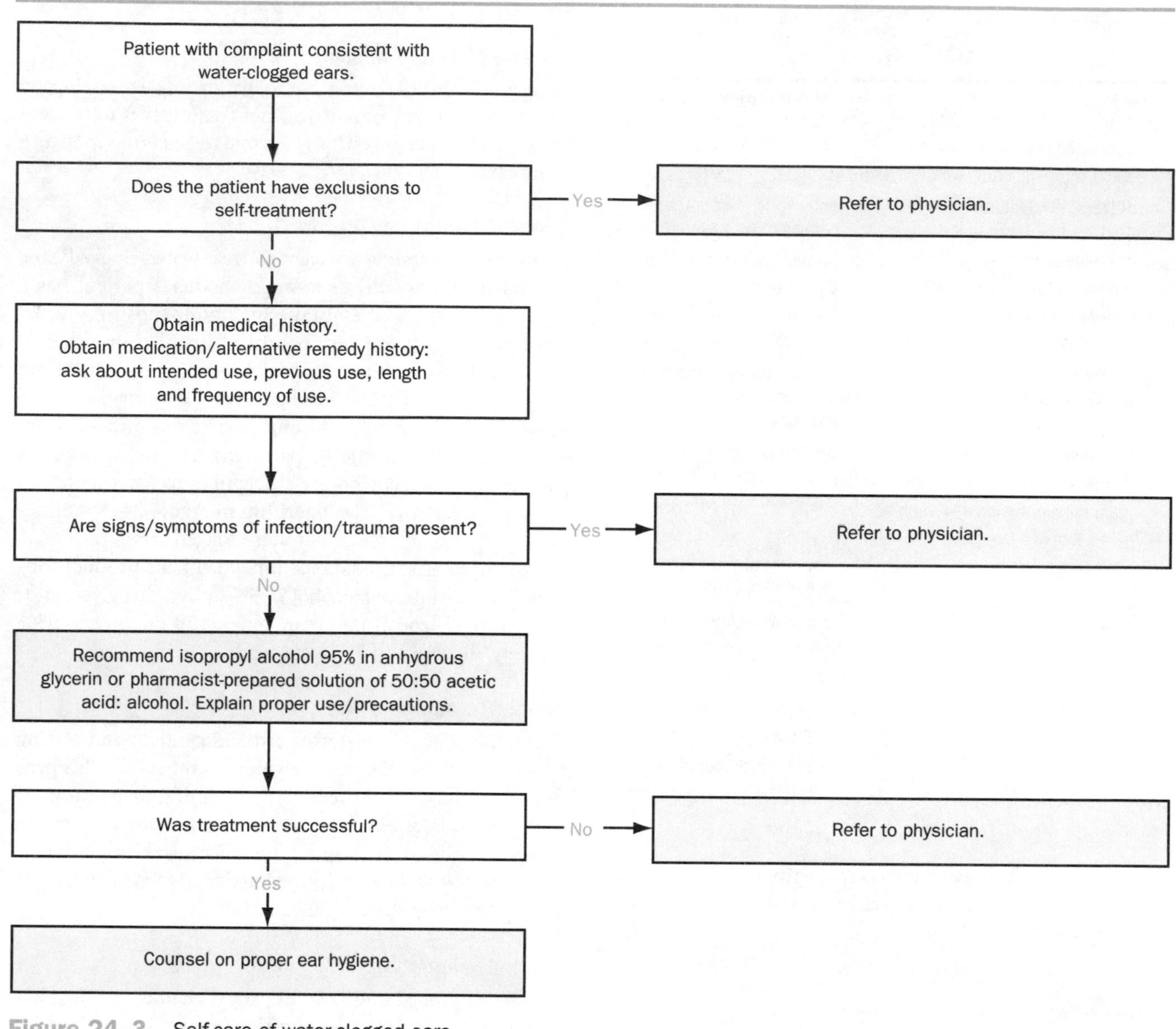

Figure 24–3 Self-care of water-clogged ears.

necessary if symptoms persist after several days of simultaneous use of ear-drying agents and prevention of exposure of ears to water. Symptoms of infection also require medical referral.

Acetic Acid

The acetic acid in the 50:50 mixture of acetic acid 5% and 95% isopropyl alcohol has bactericidal and antifungal properties. Species of *Pseudomonas, Candida, and Aspergillus* are particularly sensitive to this agent. As discussed previously, alcohol has anti-infective properties as well, is highly miscible with water, and helps to remove water from the ear. Care must be taken to advise patients against using cider vinegar instead of white vinegar. Cider vinegar is produced from fruit and contains impurities that could hinder antibacterial activity.

A 50:50 mixture of these two agents provides a 2.5% acetic acid solution. Concentrations of acetic acid between 2% and 3% may lower the pH of the ear canal below the optimal pH of 6.5 to 7.5 needed for bacterial growth.[29] This solution is well-tolerated, is nonsensitizing, and does not induce resistant organisms.[30] It may sting or burn slightly, especially if the skin is abraded. The pharmacist can best provide an accurately compounded solution in a proper dropper bottle.

Boric Acid

Boric acid is added to some commercially prepared ear products to increase product acidity. It is also a very weak germicide. Solutions containing boric acid should be applied only to unbroken skin because it may be toxic if absorbed through broken skin or if accidentally swallowed. As little as 5 g of boric acid powder ingested orally can cause serious poison-

Case Study 24–2

Patient Complaint/History

David is a 15-year-old member of the high school swim team. He has experienced a feeling of wetness and fullness in the ears each morning after swimming for the previous 2 weeks. When questioned about self-treatment of the disorder, David explains that he has been using some 3% hydrogen peroxide daily after swimming in an attempt to dry his ears. The last few days his symptoms have been getting worse. His right ear started itching and is now painful when he talks or chews food; on inspection you notice that his EAC appears swollen. David mentions that he had some drainage from his ear last night. He admits to using a pencil to scratch his ear during school a few days ago in an attempt to stop the itching.

David is currently in good health and does not take any prescription drugs, but he does occasionally use nonprescription pain relievers such as ibuprofen for muscle aches. He has never used tobacco nor does he drink alcohol during swim season.

Clinical Considerations/Strategies

Readers can use the following considerations/strategies to determine whether treatment of the patient's condition with nonprescription medications is warranted:

- Assess the patient's use of 3% hydrogen peroxide as an ear-drying agent.
- Assess the patient's use of a pencil to scratch the ear canal and advise of the dangers associated with this practice.
- Assess whether the current condition warrants medical referral or a regimen of one or more nonprescription medications.

Patient Counseling/Education

Readers can use the following strategies to develop a patient counseling/education plan that will help ensure optimal therapeutic outcomes:

- Educate the patient regarding proper otic hygiene to prevent the reoccurrence of this complaint.
- Explain the proper use of nonprescription medications used to prevent water-clogged ears.

ings.[19] Children are particularly vulnerable to the risk of accidental ingestion.

Dermatologic Disorders of the Ear

Self-treatable dermatologic disorders of the external ear include contact dermatitis, seborrhea, psoriasis, and boils.

Contact Dermatitis

Contact dermatitis is categorized as either allergic contact dermatitis or irritant contact dermatitis. The external ear is susceptible to both types of this dermatitis.

Etiology/Signs and Symptoms of Contact Dermatitis

Topical neomycin, nickel in earrings, poison ivy, and the chemicals used to process the rubber or plastic of hearing aid molds or earphones typically cause allergic reactions of the external ear.[6,7] Allergic dermatitis is associated with various skin manifestations, including maculopapular rash and formation of vesicles. The rash in turn causes pruritus, erythema, and edema. Soaps and detergents are mild irritants, which generally require repeated or extended contact to cause a significant inflammatory response. However, such substances have been shown to cause reactions similar to allergic contact dermatitis.[6,7]

Treatment of Contact Dermatitis

Ear dermatitis frequently is treated with an astringent such as 1:40 aluminum acetate solution. Solutions of aluminum acetate have antipruritic, anti-inflammatory, and limited antibacterial properties. They are useful for treating itchy, weeping, swollen conditions of the external ear when diluted to concentrations of 1:10 to 1:40.[19,30] Astringents precipitate proteins and dry the affected area by reducing the secretory function of skin glands.[19] The dilute solution has an acidic pH that inhibits bacterial and fungal growth. A wet compress of diluted aluminum acetate solution applied several times a day is useful for acute dermatitis.

Seborrhea and Psoriasis

Seborrhea and psoriasis are chronic dermatologic disorders usually associated with the scalp, face, and trunk. Seborrhea can usually be managed with nonprescription medications. Psoriasis that involves mild inflammation is sometimes responsive to nonprescription medications. However, a physician should make the initial diagnosis of psoriasis.

Etiology/Signs and Symptoms of Seborrhea and Psoriasis

See Chapter 28, "Scaly Dermatoses," for a detailed discussion of the etiology of these disorders.

Pruritus with visible drying and flaking of the skin is the most common manifestation of seborrhea. Skin fissures may develop, compromising the skin's protective barrier and possibly leading to acute bacterial external otitis.[7,9] Psoriasis of the scalp can extend to the external ear. Psoriasis exhibits as thickened, erythematous, silvery scaling lesions that occur most frequently on the knees, elbows, torso, and scalp. Cold weather and stress appear to aggravate psoriasis.[31]

Treatment of Seborrhea and Psoriasis

Treating the scalp with antiseborrheic shampoos often relieves the symptoms of this disorder.[9] Medicated shampoos can be used to treat mild cases of psoriasis of the scalp. Topical hydrocortisone is also useful in treating these disorders.

A Word about Fluid Monitors

In 1997, a medical device that detects the presence of fluid in the middle ear was approved for marketing and for use by patients aged 6 months to adult.[32] It is marketed as an aid to monitoring fluid resolution in the middle ear following middle ear infections. The device uses sonar-like technology to detect the presence of fluid by measuring reflected sound. An acoustic transducer emits a soft, complex series of sound waves into the ear canal. In a normal ear, the tympanic membrane is flexible and vibrates when sound waves reach it. When fluid is in the middle ear, the tympanic membrane is not as mobile and reflects sound waves differently from that of the normal ear. The intensity of the reflected sound is measured by the device, using a microphone and microprocessor.

Three color levels are coded according to the probability of fluid being present. Green (level 1) indicates fluid is unlikely, yellow (level 2) indicates that fluid is possible, and red (levels 3–5) indicates fluid is likely. The higher the red level number, the higher the probability of middle ear fluid. Given a red reading, users are urged to contact a physician who can then determine whether an infection is present or treatment is necessary.[33]

The device is expensive, which limits its usefulness for the general public. Users of the device should be reminded that the presence of fluid in the middle ear does not always indicate an infection. The device will not work if a tympanostomy tube, a ruptured eardrum, or impacted cerumen is present. Normal amounts of cerumen in the canal do not appear to affect the results. Cautions with use of the device include not reusing the disposable tips and not forcing the tip far into the ear.

Table 24–4

Differentiation of Common Otic Disorders

Disorder	Etiology	Pain
Ruptured tympanic membrane	Otitis media or trauma to ear such as sharp blows, diving into water, forceful irrigation of ear	Brief, severe
External otitis (swimmer's ear)	Local trauma to EAC caused by excessive moisture or abrasions; subsequent fungal/bacterial infections	Acute onset, varies from mild to severe, increases with movement of tragus/auricle
Otitis media	Bacterial infection of middle ear, usually following upper respiratory tract infections	Sharp, steady, frequently unilateral; does not increase with movement of tragus/auricle
Foreign object in ear	Insects, insertion of objects by children, hearing aids, sound attenuators	Dull to severe pain with sense of fullness/pressure while chewing
Trauma to ear	Burns from curling iron, frostbite, hematomas/injuries from contact sports or ill-fitting helmets, ear piercing, improper cerumen removal techniques, abrasions of EAC, rapid changes in air pressure (barotrauma)	Varies from sharp and steady to brief and severe
Tinnitus	Hearing disorders, blockage of EAC, exposure to high noise levels, acoustic trauma, systemic diseases, drug toxicities (salicylate, quinidine, aminoglycosides, and other antibiotics)	Possible
Excessive/impacted cerumen	Overactive ceruminous glands; obstructed migration of cerumen	Rare, dull pain if present
Water-clogged ears	Excessive moisture in EAC	None
Boils	Localized staphylococcal infections of hair follicles	Often

(See Chapter 28, "Scaly Dermatoses," for discussion of these agents.)

Boils

Boils (furuncles) are usually localized infections of the hair follicles. Boils on the auricle are self-treatable; those that appear in the EAC require medical referral.

Etiology/Signs and Symptoms of Boils

In a high percentage of cases in young adults, no specific causative or predisposing factor for boils can be established. Poor body hygiene may contribute to their development. The etiologic organism is usually a *Staphylococcus* species.[6]

A boil often involves the anterior portion of the EAC. It usually begins as a red papule and develops into a round or conical superficial pustule with a core of pus and erythema around the base. The lesion gradually enlarges, becomes firm, and then generally softens and opens within 2 weeks, discharging the purulent contents. Because the skin is very taut, even minimal swelling may cause severe pain.

Treatment of Boils

Boils are usually self-limiting; however, they may be severe, autoinoculable, and multiple. Warm compresses followed by topical antibiotics are often recommended. Antibiotics do not readily penetrate boils; therefore, incision and drainage by a physician may be required. Multiple boils, boils that do not respond rapidly to topical treatment, or boils in the EAC should be referred to a physician.[6,7]

Patient Assessment of Otic Disorders

The most common complaints of ear disorders are otalgia, pruritus (itching), and hearing loss. Common symptoms of non–self-treatable disorders include lymphadenopathy (enlarged lymph nodes), discharge, fever, and malaise. Dizziness, tinnitus, and vertigo are less common symptoms. Infections of the EAC (external otitis) and middle ear (otitis media), which require medical referral, are often the cause of a patient's complaints. Because use of home remedies and nonprescription medications may delay the patient from seeking medical care in such cases, the pharmacist plays a key role in helping patients understand when self-treatment is appropriate and when referral is warranted. Patients who recently have had ear surgery or a ruptured eardrum should always be referred to a physician.[15,34] Further, if discharge, pain, or dizziness are present or an infection is suspected, medical referral is the appropriate recommendation.[15,34]

Evaluating the characteristics of particular symptoms, such as pain and hearing loss, and the specific combination of symptoms is the key to assessing otic disorders. To that end, the following discussion of common otic symptoms describes their possible causes. Further, Table 24–4 compares the signs and symptoms and other features of common otic disorders.

Itching	Loss of Hearing	Discharge	Other Features
No	Abrupt	If associated with otitis media	May be associated with otitis media (see below)
Yes	Seldom	Occasionally, clear discharge changing to seropurulent	Swollen ear canal, stuffiness, discharge, swollen lymph nodes, fever, usually occurring in summer or in warm, humid climates
No	Sometimes decreased	Possible exudate through perforated eardrum	Perforated or bulging eardrum, lymph nodes sometimes swollen, fever, dizziness, usually occurring in winter
Yes	Yes	Possible exudate from secondary bacterial infection	If obstruction not removed promptly, acute otitis externa and tinnitus may develop
Rare	Varies from abrupt to seldom	Seldom	Untreated hematomas may cause swelling/scarring; ear piercing may cause metal sensitivities, keloids, perichondritis, toxic shock syndrome, hepatitis B
No	Yes	No	Continuous or intermittent alien noises in ear such as ringing, roaring, or humming
No	Often	None	Sense of fullness or pressure in the ears
No	Often	None	Sense of fullness or wetness
No	Rare	Rare, except on rupture	Round or conical, superficial pustules with cores of pus

Etiology of Common Otic Symptoms

Etiology of Otalgia

Otalgia can be intrinsic (directly related to the ear) or extrinsic (not associated with the ear).[9,12,35,36] Many disorders such as trauma, foreign objects, perichondritis (inflammation of the connective tissue around the ear cartilage), and infection of the EAC or middle ear can be intrinsic.[36,37] The skin covering the ear is stretched tightly over the auricle and canal. Thus, even minor swelling can cause severe pain disproportionate to the visible swelling. The following disorders can cause referred, or extrinsic, otic pain: ill-fitting dentures or tooth problems, temporomandibular joint dysfunction, nasopharyngeal infections, tumors, cysts, migraines, neuralgias, and cervical arthritis.

Excessive/impacted cerumen, a foreign object or water in the ear, or tooth and jaw disorders may manifest as a dull pain or sense of fullness in the ear. Excessive moisture can cause cerumen to swell, leading to tissue maceration that in turn can cause itching and pain. Brief, severe pain followed by abrupt hearing loss characterizes a ruptured eardrum. Rapid barometric pressure changes, such as those caused by riding in airplanes or a fast-moving elevator, can create a negative pressure in the ear, causing severe pain and possibly vertigo. A sharp, steady pain characterizes otitis media, whereas pain from external otitis has an acute onset and increases with movement of the auricle or tragus. Contrary to folklore, no evidence exists that wind in the ear will cause pain, unless a preexisting pathology is present.

Warmed olive oil, which may seem soothing, has been used inappropriately by patients to treat ear pain. If pain is due to an infection, using this method may delay proper treatment. Improperly heated oil can also cause burns.

Pain intensity alone cannot be relied on to determine whether a disorder is serious. Malignancies may cause little pain, whereas external otitis may be very painful. Unless the pharmacist can determine that the cause of pain is a self-limiting (e.g., boil, minor cut, scrape) or self-treatable (excessive/impacted cerumen or water-clogged ears) disorder, the patient should be referred to a physician.

Etiology of Otic Pruritus

Contact dermatitis, seborrhea, and psoriasis can cause itching of the ear; this symptom is often associated with allergic rhinitis. Itching may signal the onset of external otitis caused by either bacteria or fungi (otomycosis). Itching is the chief complaint of chronic external otitis.[5] Further, lack of normal sebum production, often seen in the elderly, can result in excessively dry ear canals and can cause itching.[8,38]

Patients will usually attempt to stop the itch by rubbing the ear, instilling remedies such as alcohol, olive oil (sweet oil), or mineral oil, or pulling on the auricle or tragus. Although 1 to 2 drops of mineral oil applied in the ear at bedtime may be helpful in treating excessively dry ears, overuse of alcohol may dry the ear canal excessively and can aggravate itching. Occasionally, physicians may need to prescribe cortisone ear drops to control the itching.

Some patients may use more forceful methods to alleviate itching, such as scratching the EAC with objects. These objects can abrade the EAC, providing an entry for pathogens. The resultant inflammation results in more itching and pain, and a scratch-itch-scratch cycle develops. Improper use of an otic bulb syringe or overusing aqueous solutions may leave excess moisture in the canal that in turn can cause tissue maceration and itching, and lead to the same cycle.

Etiology of Hearing Loss

Foreign objects, water trapped in the canal, infections of the external or middle ear, and neoplasms can all cause hearing loss. Occlusion of the canal impairs the transmission of sound waves to the tympanic membrane. Congestion associated with an upper respiratory tract infection can cause loss of hearing. Decreased hearing may be associated with otitis media, a common sequela of upper respiratory tract infections. Abrupt loss of hearing associated with brief but severe pain can result from perforation of the tympanic membrane. Sharp blows to the head with a cupped hand, water sports such as diving, and forceful irrigation of the ear canal can lead to perforation. A slower onset of hearing loss can be due to excessive or impacted cerumen and is not associated with severe pain. A gradual hearing loss is common in noise-induced hearing loss and Meniere's disease.[39] Medications associated with hearing loss include many antimicrobials, salicylates and nonsteroidal anti-inflammatory drugs (NSAIDs), loop diuretics, antineoplastic agents, and other miscellaneous drugs.[40]

Sustained hearing loss in infants and children can slow the development of speech. Hearing loss in the elderly can be mistaken for early dementia. If hearing loss is not attributable to either water in the ear or excessive cerumen, a physician should be consulted. Table 24–5 provides a 5-minute hearing test that can be self-administered by the patient to facilitate hearing loss assessment.

Etiology of Dizziness

Vertigo, which is often imprecisely referred to as dizziness, is a whirling or spinning sensation caused by lesions within the labyrinth of the inner ear. Lesions elsewhere in the ear may cause a variety of symptoms such as dizziness, lightheadedness, pressure, or ataxia (incoordination).[41] The most frequent cause of dizziness in children is otitis media.[41] Changes in pressure (rapid barometric changes) on the tympanic membrane, migraine, ototoxic drugs (e.g., aminoglycosides, vancomycin, macrolides), postural hypotension, cardiac disease, and tumors are some other causes of dizziness. Using hot or cold water to irrigate the ear can cause severe dizziness.[13,14,16,21] Because of its potential seriousness, all complaints of dizziness (not associated with motion sickness) should be referred to a physician for evaluation.

Table 24–5

Five-Minute Hearing Test

	Almost Always	Half the Time	Occasionally	Never
1. I have a problem hearing over the telephone.				
2. I have trouble following the conversation when two or more people are talking at the same time.				
3. People complain that I turn the television volume too high.				
4. I have to strain to understand conversations.				
5. I miss hearing some common sounds like the phone or doorbell ringing.				
6. I have trouble hearing conversations in a noisy background such as a party.				
7. I get confused about where sounds come from.				
8. I misunderstand some words in a sentence and need to ask people to repeat themselves.				
9. I especially have trouble understanding the speech of women and children.				
10. I have worked in noisy environments (on assembly lines, with jackhammers, around jet engines, etc.).				
11. Many people I talk to seem to mumble (or do not speak clearly).				
12. People get annoyed because I misunderstand what they say.				
13. I misunderstand what others are saying and make inappropriate responses.				
14. I avoid social activities because I cannot hear well and feel I will reply improperly.				
To be answered by a family member or friend:				
15. Do you think this person has a hearing loss?				

Mark the column that best describes the frequency with which you experience each situation or feeling. To calculate your score, give yourself 3 points for every time you checked "almost always," 2 for every "half the time," 1 for every "occasionally," and 0 for every "never." If you have a blood relative who has a hearing loss, add another 3 points. Total your points.

Scoring:

0 to 5: Your hearing is fine. No action is required.

6 to 9: Suggest you see an ear, nose, and throat (ENT) physician.

10 and above: Strongly recommend you see an ENT physician.

Source: Reprinted with permission from the American Academy of Otolaryngology—Head and Neck Surgery, Inc., Alexandria, VA.

Etiology of Tinnitus

Tinnitus is defined as a continuous or intermittent alien noise in the ear, which is subjective and audible only to the patient. The noise is described as sounding like steam escaping from a small pipe, ringing, roaring, or humming.[39] Patients' reactions to tinnitus are varied: Some complain of only minor distraction, while others develop severe mental depression.

Blockage of the auditory canal can cause tinnitus and is easily remedied. Exposure to high noise levels, acoustic trauma, systemic disease, or drug toxicity can also cause tinnitus. Salicylates, quinidine, aminoglycosides, and other antibiotics have been frequently linked with tinnitus. Discontinuing the offending drug often brings relief.[42] Patients who experience tinnitus should receive a medical examination and evaluation. This symptom may be the first and only sign of a hearing disorder. Nonprescription medications are not effective and thus are not recommended for treating tinnitus.

Assessment of Common Otic Symptoms

Asking the patient the following questions will help elicit the information needed to accurately assess an otic disorder and to recommend the appropriate treatment approach. The questions are grouped under the three most common symptoms.

Assessment of Otalgia

Q~ Describe the pain. How long has it been occurring?

A~ *Identify the otic disorders associated with pain and the type of pain characteristic of each disorder. (See the sec-*

tion "Etiology of Otalgia" and Table 24–4.) Use the patient's description to determine the likely cause of the pain. If the pain has been present for longer than 24 hours, refer the patient to a physician.

Q~ Do you have a fever or discharge from the ear?

A~ *Identify the disorders with which these symptoms occur. (See Table 24–4.)* Refer patients with these symptoms to a physician.

Q~ Have you recently had a cold or the flu?

A~ *Identify the otic disorder often associated with these respiratory tract infections. (See Table 24–4.)* Refer any patient whose ear pain is associated with one of these respiratory disorders to a physician.

Q~ Have you attempted to remove the wax from your ears recently? If so, describe the method used.

A~ *Identify the proper method for removing cerumen. (See the section "Treatment of Excessive/Impacted Cerumen" and Table 24–2.)* If the patient used an improper method to dry the EAC, explain the signs and symptoms of an infection, and advise the patient to see a physician if they occur. If a proper method was used unsuccessfully, refer the patient for treatment of possible impacted or hardened cerumen.

Q~ Have you been swimming recently, or do you routinely have problems with water remaining in your ears after bathing? Have you tried to remove the water? If so, describe the method used.

A~ *Identify the role excessive ear moisture can play in causing otic pain. (See the section "Signs and Symptoms of Water-Clogged Ears".)* If assessment of the pain and other symptoms indicates self-treatment, recommend an appropriate product. If the patient used an improper method, explain the signs and symptoms of an infection and advise the patient to see a physician if they occur. (See Table 24–4.)

Q~ Have you recently been in an airplane or fast-moving elevator in which the air pressure changed suddenly?

A~ Refer patients with ear pain related to air pressure changes to a physician.

Q~ Have you recently had any ear surgery, or have you ever had a ruptured eardrum?

A~ Refer patients with underlying otic pathology to a physician.

Q~ Have you experienced recent trauma to the ear?

A~ Refer patients with ear trauma to a physician to prevent perichondritis or permanent disfigurement such as cauliflower ear.

Q~ Do you wear dentures or a hearing aid?

A~ If the patient wears either and referred pain seems likely, refer the patient to a dentist or physician for evaluation of the devices.

Q~ Have you taken any medications to treat the pain?

A~ If yes, advise the patient that aspirin, acetaminophen, or NSAIDs can mask a fever and do not treat the cause of ear pain.

Assessment of Otic Pruritus

Q~ When did your ears first start to itch?

A~ *Identify the otic disorders with which itching is associated. (See the section "Etiology of Otic Pruritus" and Table 24–4.)*

Q~ What have you done to relieve the itching? Have you used any objects such as cotton-tipped swabs to relieve the itching? Have you attempted to remove the wax from your ears recently? If so, describe the method used. Did these measures help or make the itching worse?

A~ If the patient has used improper methods to relieve itching or to remove cerumen, explain the signs and symptoms of an infection. Advise the patient to see a physician if they occur.

Q~ Do you have a problem with seborrhea or psoriasis or other dermatologic conditions?

A~ Determine whether the itching is related to one of these disorders. If so, recommend the appropriate self-treatment. (See Chapter 27, "Atopic Dermatitis, Contact Dermatitis, and Dry Skin," and Chapter 28, "Scaly Dermatoses.")

Q~ Have you been swimming recently, or do you routinely have problems with water remaining in your ears after bathing? Have you tried to remove the water? If so, describe the method used.

A~ *Identify the proper and improper methods of removing excessive water from the ear. (See the section "Water-Clogged Ears.")* If the patient's method of removal was improper, explain the signs and symptoms of an infection. (See Table 24–4.) Advise the patient to see a physician if they occur.

Assessment of Hearing Loss

Q~ When did you notice that your hearing is not as good as it used to be?

A~ *Identify the possible causes of hearing loss. (See the section "Etiology of Hearing Loss" and Table 24–4.)* If the hearing loss has lasted for longer than 1 week, refer the patient to a physician.

Q~ Do you have an upper respiratory tract infection such as a cold?

A~ Inform the patient that congestion from the cold can affect hearing. Advise the patient holding back or stifling sneezes can force secretions into the middle ear and allow otitis media to develop.

Q~ Are you taking any prescription, nonprescription, or alternative medications? Have you discontinued any medications recently?

A~ *Identify medications that can induce hearing loss or tinnitus. (See the sections "Etiology of Hearing Loss" and "Etiology of Tinnitus.")* If prescribed medications are being taken, advise the patient to see a physician. If nonprescription analgesics are being taken, advise the patient to discontinue use and return in 1 week for reassessment.

Q~ Would you be interested in taking a self-scored, 5-minute hearing test for your own information?

A~ Advise the patient that a written hearing test can help to determine the extent of hearing loss. (See Table 24–5.)

Patient Education for Self-Treatable Otic Disorders

Excessive/Impacted Cerumen

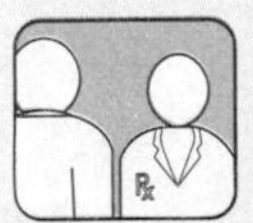

The objective of self-treatment is to soften and remove excessive or impacted cerumen (earwax) that is already present or to prevent the disorder from recurring in susceptible patients. For most patients, carefully following product instructions and the self-care measures listed below will help ensure optimal therapeutic outcomes.

Nondrug Measures for Excessive or Impacted Cerumen

- Use a washcloth draped over a finger to remove earwax from the outer canal.
- Do not insert objects in the ear to remove earwax. Such attempts may injure the ear canal or have a negative effect on the earwax.
- Never use the hollow candle method to remove earwax; it can cause serious ear injury.

Nonprescription Medications for Excessive or Impacted Cerumen

- See Tables 24–1 and 24–2 for guidelines on using carbamide peroxide to remove excessive or impacted earwax.
- Do not let the medication contact the eyes.
- Do not use this medication if you have a fever, ear drainage, pain more severe than a dull pain, dizziness, or a ruptured eardrum, or if you had ear surgery within the past 6 weeks.
- Do not use this medication to treat inflamed ear tissue, swimmer's ear, or itching of the ear canal.

⚠ Prolonged contact between carbamide peroxide solution and skin of the ear canal can cause dermatitis. Discontinue treatment if irritation or a rash appears.

⚠ Monitor your hearing and symptoms of infection such as pain and itching. If severe pain occurs or your hearing worsens, see a physician immediately. Severe pain may indicate a ruptured eardrum.

Water-Clogged Ears

The objective of self-treatment is to remove water from ears already clogged with water or to prevent the disorder in persons who are susceptible to excessive moisture in the ears. For most patients, carefully following product instructions and the self-care measures listed below will help ensure optimal therapeutic outcomes.

Nondrug Measures for Water-Clogged Ears

- Tilt the affected ear down, and gently manipulate it to help drain water from the ear.
- Immediately after swimming or bathing, use a blow-dryer on a low setting to help dry the ear canal.

Nonprescription Medications for Water-Clogged Ears

- Use a product that reduces moisture content in the ear without overdrying. Isopropyl alcohol 95% in anhydrous glycerin 5% or a solution of one part isopropyl alcohol to one part white vinegar is acceptable.
- Do not use the medications if you have a ruptured eardrum or tympanostomy tubes.
- Place 5 to 10 drops of the solution in the ear canal, and allow the solution to remain for 1 to 2 minutes.
- See Table 24–1 for instructions on instilling the medication.
- Do not let the medication contact the eyes.

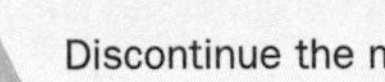

⚠ Discontinue the medication if stinging or burning occurs.

⚠ If pain, fever, or discharge develops, see a physician immediately.

Dermatologic Disorders of the Ear

The objective of self-treatment is to relieve the symptoms. For most patients, carefully following product instructions and the self-care measures listed below will help ensure optimal therapeutic outcomes.

(continued)

Patient Education for Self-Treatable Otic Disorders (continued)

Contact Dermatitis

- Avoid substances known to cause allergic or irritant reactions.
- Apply a wet compress of diluted (1:10 to 1:40) aluminum acetate solution several times a day to relieve itching and weeping of affected areas.
- If needed, apply hydrocortisone to relieve inflammation.

Seborrhea and Psoriasis

- Treat the scalp and the external ear with the appropriate medicated shampoo.

Boils

- Do not self-treat multiple boils or a boil in the ear canal.
- Apply warm compresses to a boil located on the outside of the ear; then apply topical antibiotics.

If the boil does not respond to the topical treatment within 4 days, see a physician.

Patient Counseling for Otic Disorders

Patients who self-treat otic disorders must understand how easily the EAC can be injured. The pharmacist should discourage common harmful practices of relieving itching of the ear and then should instruct patients on the proper methods of removing excessive cerumen and moisture from the ears. Patients who are susceptible to these disorders should be advised to incorporate the removal methods as part of their aural hygiene. The pharmacist should explain the proper use and possible adverse effects of all recommended medications. The box "Patient Education for Self-Treatable Otic Disorders" lists specific information to provide patients.

Evaluation of Patient Outcomes for Otic Disorder

If the symptoms of excessive/impacted cerumen or water-clogged ears persist or worsen after 4 days of proper treatment, the patient should consult a physician. The patient should also consult a physician if ear pain or discharge develops during treatment.

If the symptoms of any self-treatable dermatologic disorder of the ear persist after 4 days of proper treatment, the patient should consult a physician.

CONCLUSIONS

Ear disorders affect all ages. Visible signs are not always consistent with the degree of severity or pain experienced. Disorders of the external ear include disorders of the auricle and the EAC. Nonprescription medicines are restricted to minor, self-limiting disorders affecting these areas. Nonprescription medicines should not be used to treat middle ear disorders.

Taking a proper history and assessing the patient's complaint are important for the pharmacist to be able to judge whether self-treatment or referral to a physician is indicated. Using products inappropriately—or when non–self-treatable conditions exist—can delay the institution of proper medical care. Educating patients about proper ear hygiene is important in preventing further problems or complaints. Patients should be reminded that earwax is important for the normal function and protection of the EAC. Attempts to remove earwax with anything besides a washcloth-draped finger should be strongly discouraged. Using objects, such as cotton-tipped swabs or sharp objects, may scratch or damage the delicate skin and may cause infections. The warning, "Never clean the ear with anything smaller than the elbow" is frequently given as advice by physicians to help patients remember proper ear care.

Patients should always use products proven to be safe and effective. Appropriate directions for use are important for the patient to understand. If symptoms do not resolve with proper treatment after 4 days, or if symptoms worsen, the patient should be encouraged to contact a physician.

References

1. Dorgan CA, ed. Medical attention for acute conditions: 1991. In: *Statistical Record of Health and Medicine.* Detroit: Gale Research Inc; 1995:43.
2. Jabor MA. Cerumen impaction. *J La State Med Soc.* 1997;149(10):358–62.
3. Alvord LS, Farmer BL. Anatomy and orientation of the human external ear. *J Am Acad Audiol.* 1997;8(6):883–9.
4. Hoppe MW, Kolling WM. Ear infections and their treatment in pediatrics. *Drug Topics.* August 17, 1998:93–7.
5. Balkany TJ, Ress BD. Infections of the external ear. In: Cummings CW, Fredrickson JM, Harker LA, et al., eds. *Otolaryngology, Head and Neck Surgery.* 3rd ed. St. Louis: Mosby; 1998:2979–80.
6. Hirsch BE. Diseases of the external ear. In: Bluestone CD, Stool SE, Kenna MA, eds. *Pediatric Otolaryngology.* 3rd ed. Philadelphia: WB Saunders Co; 1996:378–9, 382, 384.
7. Roland PS, Marple BF. Disorders of the external auditory canal. *J Am Acad Audiol.* 1997;8:367–78.

8. Roeser RJ, Ballachanda BB. Physiology, pathophysiology, and anthropology/epidemiology of human ear canal secretions. *J Am Acad Audiol.* 1997;8(6):391–8.
9. Amundson LH. Disorders of the external ear. *Primary Care.* 1990;17(2):215–7, 220–1.
10. Austin DF. Diseases of the external ear. In: Ballenger JJ, Snow JB Jr, eds. *Otorhinolaryngology, Head and Neck Surgery.* 15th ed. Media, PA: Williams & Wilkens; 1996:974–5, 981.
11. Pray WS. Earwax: an under-valued defense system. *US Pharmacist.* April 1992:20–4.
12. Dolitsky JN. Otalgia. In: Bluestone CD, Stool SE, Kenna MA, eds. *Pediatric Otolaryngology.* 3rd ed. Philadelphia: WB Saunders Co; 1996: 235–41.
13. Sharp JF, Wilson JA, Ross L, et al. Earwax removal: a survey of current practice. *BMJ.* 1990;301:1251–3.
14. Warwick-Brown NP. Cotton-tipped "buds" as a source of otological trauma. *Practitioner.* 1986; 230: 301.
15. *Federal Register.* 1986;51:28656–61.
16. Grossan M. Cerumen removal-current challenges. *Ear Nose Throat J.* 1998;77(7):541–6.
17. Wilson PL, Roeser RJ. Cerumen management: professional issues and techniques. *J Am Acad Audiol.* 1997;8(6):428.
18. *Physicians' Desk Reference for Nonprescription Drugs.* 13th ed. Montvale, NJ: Medical Economics Data; 1992:677–8.
19. Gennaro AR, Chase GD, Marderosian AD, et al., eds. *Remington: The Science and Practice of Pharmacy.* 19th ed. Easton, PA: Mack Pub Co; 1995:871, 1147, 1151, 1267, 1400, 1407.
20. Gennaro AR, Chase GD, Marderosian AD, et al., eds. *Remington: The Science and Practice of Pharmacy.* 18th ed. Easton, PA: Mack Pub Co; 1990:1309.
21. Spiro SR. A cost-effectiveness analysis of earwax softeners. *Nurse Pract.* 1997;22(8):28–31, 166.
22. Blumenthal M, Busse WR, Goldberg A, et al. *The Complete German Commission E Monographs: Therapeutic Guide to Herbal Medicines.* Boston: Integrative Medicine Communications; 1998.
23. *PDR for Herbal Medications.* Montvale, NJ: Medical Economics Co; 1998:626–7, 1098–9.
24. Tyler VE. *The Honest Herbal.* 3rd ed. New York: Pharmaceutical Products Press; 1993.
25. Tyler VE. *Herbs of Choice: The Therapeutic Use of Phytomedicinals.* New York: Pharmaceutical Products Press; 1994.
26. Seely DR, Quigley SM, Langman AW. Ear candles—efficacy and safety. *Laryngoscope.* 1996;106: 1226–9.
27. "Ear drying aids" monograph status proposed by FDA. *FDC Reports—The Tan Sheet.* 1999:7(34):4.
28. *Swimmer's Ear: Itchy Ears and Fungus* [pamphlet]. Alexandria, VA: American Academy Otolaryngology—Head and Neck Surgery Inc; 1993.
29. Aminifarshidmehr N. The management of chronic suppurative otitis media with acid media solution. *Am J Otol.* 1996;17(1):24–5.
30. *AMA Drug Evaluations Annual.* Chicago: American Medical Association; 1995:1291, 1630, 1631.
31. Nowakowski PA, Rumsfield JA, West DP. Common skin disorders: acne and psoriasis. In: DiPiro JT, Talbert RL, Yee GC, et al., eds. *Pharmacotherapy: A Pathophysiologic Approach.* 3rd ed. Stamford, CT: Appleton & Lange; 1997:1824.
32. *FDA Consumer.* 1997;31(7):37.
33. *How EarCheck Works.* Woburn, MA: MDI Instruments Inc; 1999.
34. *Federal Register.* 1982;47:30014, 30018.
35. Bluestone CD, Klein JO. Methods of examination: clinical examination. In: Bluestone CD, Stool SE, Kenna MA, eds. *Pediatric Otolaryngology.* 3rd ed. Philadelphia: WB Saunders Co; 1996:150–9.
36. Hathaway H. Diagnosing referred otalgia: the ten Ts. *J Craniomandibular Prac.* 1992; 10(4):333–4.
37. Lau D, Watson D. Referred otalgia: an unusual presentation of a laryngeal foreign body. *Hosp Med.* 1998;59(2):161.
38. Oliveira RJ. The active ear canal. *J Am Acad Audiol.* 1997;8(6):409–10.
39. Snow JB, Martin JB. Disturbances of smell, taste, and hearing. In: Wilson JD, Braunwald E, Isselbacher KJ, et al., eds. *Harrison's Principles of Internal Medicine.* 12th ed. New York: McGraw-Hill; 1991:156.
40. Lesar TS. Drug-induced ear and eye toxicity. In: DiPiro JT, Talbert RL, Yee GC, et al., eds. *Pharmacotherapy: A Pathophysiologic Approach.* 3rd ed. Stamford, CT: Appleton & Lange; 1997:1763–70.
41. Busis SN. Vertigo. In: Bluestone CD, Stool SE, Kenna MA, eds. *Pediatric Otolaryngology.* 3rd ed. Philadelphia: WB Saunders Co; 1996:285.
42. Black FO, Lilly DJ. Tinnitus in children. In: Bluestone CD, Stool SE, Kenna MA, eds. *Pediatric Otolaryngology.* 3rd ed. Philadelphia: WB Saunders Co; 1996:304–5, 308.

CHAPTER 25

Prevention of Hygiene-Related Oral Disorders

Chapter 25 at a Glance

Dental diseases are among the most prevalent chronic diseases in our society. Pertinent supporting statistics include the following:

- Among all Americans, 50% need dental treatment.
- Only 42% of adults ages 65 years and older visit a dentist during a year.
- Of all 12- to 17-year-olds, 68% have experienced tooth decay.
- The average adult has 21.5 decayed or filled tooth surfaces.
- Each year, dental conditions cause 7.05 million days of work loss.
- Nearly 80% of all Americans have some degree of periodontal disease.
- Nearly 44% of Americans ages 75 years and above have lost all their natural teeth but that percentage is declining. The increasing number of elderly with natural teeth has many dental implications.[1]

Improper oral hygiene is a direct cause of dental caries, gingivitis, halitosis, and some cases of denture-related discomfort. Nonprescription products are widely available in the pharmacy for prevention of oral disease. An analysis of 1997 retail sales for four categories of oral health care products (toothpaste, dental accessories, mouthrinses [mouthwashes], and denture products) indicated overall sales at approximately $3.5 billion. Drugstore sales for these categories totaled about $1 billion (29%) and accounted for 20% of all sales in the toothpaste category, 25% of the mouthrinse category, and the highest market share (34%) in the dental accessories category.

Editor's Note: This chapter is based, in part, on the 11th edition chapter titled "Oral Health Products," which was written by Arlene A. Flynn.

Anatomy and Physiology of the Oral Cavity

The teeth and supporting structures are necessary for normal mastication and articulation and for aesthetic appearance. The primary dentition first appears at approximately age 6 months when the mandibular (lower jaw) central incisors erupt; it is usually complete with the eruption of the upper second molars at approximately age 24 months. There are 20 deciduous teeth, 10 in each arch. Generally, the permanent dentition first appears when the mandibular first molar erupts behind the deciduous second molar at approximately age 6 years, and it continues in a regular pattern, usually replacing shedding deciduous teeth. The last permanent teeth to erupt are the third molars (wisdom teeth), which may appear between ages 17 and 21 years.

Anatomically, the teeth are grossly viewed as having two parts, the roots and the crown. (See Figure 25–1.) The roots are normally below the gingival (gum) line or margin and are essential in supporting and attaching the tooth to the surrounding tissues. The crown is above the gingival margin and is responsible for mastication. Each tooth has four basic components: enamel, dentin, pulp, and cementum.

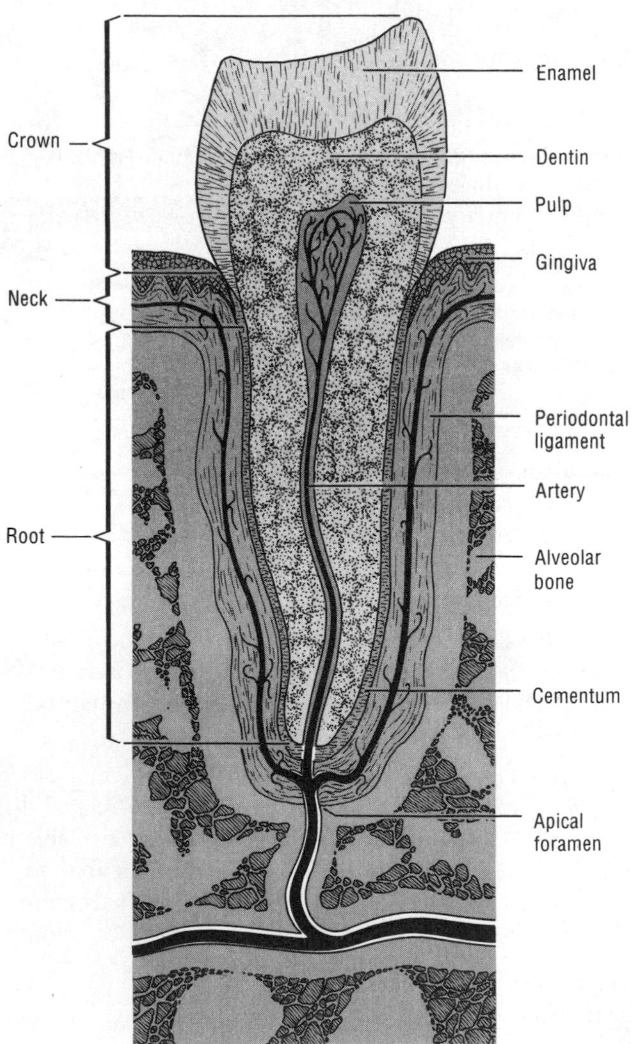

Figure 25–1 Anatomy of the tooth.

Enamel is composed of very hard, crystalline calcium salts (hydroxyapatite). It protects the underlying tooth structure and covers the crown of the tooth to the cementoenamel junction, thus enabling the crown to withstand the wear of mastication. Dentin, which is softer, lies beneath the enamel and makes up the largest part of the tooth structure. Its tubules transport nutrients from the dental pulp. Dentin protects the dental pulp from mechanical, thermal, and chemical irritation.

The pulp occupies the pulp chamber and is continuous with the tissues surrounding the tooth by means of the apical foramen, which is an opening at the apex of the root. The pulp consists primarily of vascular and neural tissues. The only type of nerve endings in the pulp is free nerve endings; thus, any type of stimulus to the pulp is interpreted as pain.

The periodontium comprises the tissues that support the teeth, including the cementum, the periodontal ligament, the encompassing alveolar bone, and the gingiva. The bone-like cementum is softer than dentin and covers the root of the tooth, extending apically from the cementoenamel junction. Its major function is to attach the tooth to the periodontal ligament by periodontal fibers. The periodontal ligament is connective tissue that attaches the tooth to the surrounding alveolar bone and gingival tissue. The four functions of the periodontal ligament are supportive, formative, sensory, and nutritive. The alveolar bone forms the sockets of the teeth. Alveolar bone is thin and spongy, and it attaches to the principal fibers of the periodontal ligament, as well as to the gingiva. The gingiva is the soft tissue surrounding the teeth. It is normally pink and keratinized, and it is attached to the cementum by the gingival group of periodontal ligament fibers.

The mucosa covering the pharyngeal region, soft palate, floor of the mouth, vestibule (between the alveolar ridge and cheek), and cheeks is normally more pinkish red than the gingiva. This coloration is because the outer surface of the mucosa, which is stratified squamous epithelium, does not have a keratinized stratum corneum outer layer as do the gingiva and hard palate.

The tongue functions in mastication, swallowing, taste, and speech. Its dorsal or upper surface is usually irregular and rough in appearance. Taste buds are usually small, oval-shaped organs of flat epithelial cells surrounding a small opening (taste pore).

The major salivary glands are the parotid, submandibular, and sublingual glands. They are responsible for secreting saliva, which is an alkaline, slightly viscous, clear secretion that contains enzymes (lysozymes and ptyalin), albumin, epithelial mucin (a mucopolysaccharide), immunoglobulin, leukocytes, and minerals. Normal salivary gland function promotes good oral health in several ways. Saliva components clear carbohydrates and microorganisms from the oral cavity. Saliva also buffers the decline in pH that is caused by the acid formed by carbohydrate fermentation. Its mineral components have a protective role in the demineralization and remineralization process of tooth enamel.

Caries

Since the 1970s, the incidence of dental caries has declined significantly in school-aged children in this country, and the proportion of caries-free children has increased. The percentage of 12- to 17-year-old children in the United States who are free of caries has increased threefold, from 10.4% in the early 1970s to 32.7% in the late 1980s. Similar declines are reported in younger children. The 1988–1991 survey of the National Health and Nutrition Examination III reported that 50% of 5- to 9-year-olds and 83% of 2- to 4-year-old children were free of caries in the primary dentition.[2] Nevertheless, dental caries remains a public health problem, and the importance of prevention should not be ignored.

The percentage of the U.S. population ages 65 years and older is increasing, and this increase is predicted to continue well into the 21st century. Projections for the year 2030 suggest that 20% of the population will be older than age 65 years and that 3%, or about 8.8 million people, will be older than age 85 years.[3] Edentulism (toothlessness) is decreasing; more than half of older Americans have retained natural dentition. This statistic has many dental implications. Root caries, an age-related problem that affects the root surfaces of adult teeth exposed by gingival recession, is becoming more prevalent as adults retain greater numbers of teeth later in life.[2]

Epidemiology of Caries

Patients with poor oral hygiene are at greatest risk for developing caries. Some patients at increased risk for caries are those with orthodontic appliances, xerostomia (dry mouth), and gum tissue recession that exposes root surfaces to caries, as well as patients undergoing head and neck radiation therapy.

Evidence also supports the association of smokeless tobacco with increased dental caries (because these products contain sugar that is kept in contact with the teeth) and with cervical erosion of the teeth.[4] The use of tobacco (both smoked and smokeless) has been linked to the formation of dental caries and to discoloration of teeth. Because alcohol consumption can cause xerostomia, individuals who consume alcohol may have a higher risk of caries.

Etiology/Pathophysiology of Caries

Dental caries is a destructive microbial disease that affects the calcified tissues of the teeth. Certain plaque bacteria generate acid from dietary carbohydrates; the acid demineralizes tooth enamel, leading to the formation of carious lesions (pits or perforations) that will eventually destroy the tooth if untreated. Dental caries formation requires growth and attachment of cariogenic microorganisms (e.g., *Streptococcus mutans*, *Lactobacillus casei*, and *Actinomyces viscosus*) to exposed surfaces. *S. mutans* is the primary organism to initiate carious process. Lactobacilli continue the process after entering established pits and fissures in biting surfaces of teeth, whereas *A. viscosus* is associated with root caries. These organisms are spread by saliva—from mother to infant—by sharing a spoon, by kissing, by blowing on food, and by other shared activities. Most children are infected by age 2 years, and 83% are infected by age 4 years.[5] If oral hygiene is neglected, dental plaque containing these organisms remains on the tooth surfaces and in time attracts more bacteria, thereby promoting decay.

The carious process is characterized by alternating periods of destruction and repair. Demineralization is caused by organic acids, such as lactic and formic acids, which are produced (usually anaerobically) by microbial metabolism of low–molecular-weight carbohydrates (sugars) that readily diffuse into plaque. The resulting reduction of pH on the tooth surface causes demineralization of dental enamel. Repeated and frequent sugar intake will keep plaque pH low and prolong demineralization. A carious lesion starts slowly on the enamel surface and initially produces no clinical symptoms. Once the demineralization progresses through the enamel to the softer dentin, the destruction is much more rapid and becomes clinically evident as a carious lesion.

At this point, the patient can become aware of the process by visualization or by symptoms of sensitivity to stimuli, such as heat, cold, or chewing. If untreated, the carious lesion can result in damage to the dental pulp itself (with continuous pain as a common symptom) and, eventually, in necrosis of vital pulp tissue. Because an opening exists between the pulp and surrounding supporting tissues through the apical foramen, the infectious process can progress apically and can result in bone loss, abscesses, cellulitis, or osteomyelitis. Saliva, rich in calcium and phosphate ions, has a role in remineralizing early carious lesions. Fluoride ion in the mouth also promotes remineralization and thus retards enamel dissolution.

Plaque is commonly recognized as the source of microbes that cause caries and periodontal disease; thus, plaque buildup is related to the incidence of oral disease.[6] Plaque begins with the formation of acquired pellicle on a clean tooth surface. Pellicle appears to be a thin, acellular, glycoprotein–mucoprotein coating that adheres to the enamel within minutes after a tooth is cleaned. Its source is thought to be saliva. The pellicle seems to serve as an attachment for cariogenic bacteria that produce, along with acids, long-chain polymers such as dextrans and levans that adhere to the pellicle and tooth surface. The resulting sticky adherent mass is soft and readily disrupted by toothbrushing or flossing.

After meals, food residue may be incorporated into plaque by bacterial degradation. Left undisturbed, plaque thickens and bacteria proliferate. Plaque growth begins in protected cracks and fissures and along the gingival margin.[7] If not removed within 24 hours, dental plaque (especially in areas opposite the salivary glands) begins to calcify by calcium salt precipitation from the saliva; then it forms calculus, or tartar. This hardened, adherent deposit is removable only by professional dental cleaning.[7]

Calculus is generally considered to be a substrate on which additional plaque can develop, and it is not regarded as the primary causative oral accumulation in periodontal disease.[7] However, most periodontists agree that supragingival (above) and subgingival (below the gingival margin) calculus can promote the progression of periodontal disease by accumulating new bacterial plaque in contact with sensitive tissue sites and by interfering with local self-cleaning efforts to remove plaque. Subgingival calculus may also intensify the inflammatory process. Thorough removal of subgingival calculus in periodontal therapy is an important step in delaying the reestablishment of periodontal pathogens and the resolution of inflammation.[8,9]

Prevention of Caries

The key to preventing caries is controlling dental plaque. Because a combination of diet (carbohydrate substrate), oral bacteria, and host resistance is involved in developing caries, prevention should be aimed at modifying these factors.[7] Frequency of refined carbohydrate intake should be reduced; plaque, which supports cariogenic bacterial growth, should be removed; and host resistance should be increased through appropriate exposure to fluoride ion. The declining prevalence of dental caries in children may be attributed to a combination of these interventions (e.g., increased exposure to fluoride in drinking water, dentifrices, and mouthrinses; changed patterns of diet; and improved oral hygiene).[10]

Dietary Measures

Cariogenic foods should be avoided in favor of less cariogenic foods. A food is considered highly cariogenic if it contains more than 15% sugar, clings to the teeth, and remains in the mouth after it is eaten. Conversely, foods are less cariogenic if they have a high water content (e.g., fresh fruit), stimulate the flow of saliva (fibrous foods that require lots of chewing), or are high in protein (e.g., dairy products). Both the water content of fresh fruit and the flow of saliva tend to wash the sugar away and to neutralize the acid it creates. Milk protein also raises pH and tends to block binding of bacteria.

Although sucrose is the most cariogenic sugar, other types of fermentable carbohydrates, such as fructose and lactose, also are cariogenic.[10] Oral hygiene products such as mouthrinses and dentifrices may contain a low concentration of saccharin, which is a potent noncariogenic sugar substitute that appears to present no caries hazard.[7] The Food and Drug Administration (FDA) limit on saccharin is 1.0 g per day for adults; ingestion from normal use of both mouthrinse and dentifrice would result in a total saccharin exposure of only about 20 to 40 mg per day.[7]

Other sugar substitutes such as sorbitol, xylitol, and aspartame are currently used to sweeten numerous products. Claims for the noncariogenicity of sorbitol need substantiation through further clinical trials.[1] Xylitol has been shown to be noncariogenic, and aspartame appears to be so. Some clinical trials have reported that xylitol-containing chewing gum is cariostatic and others have shown that xylitol activity may aid in remineralization.[1,11]

In 1996, FDA approved health-claim labeling of foods that contain sugar alcohol. The approved sugar alcohols are xylitol, sorbitol, mannitol, maltitol, isomalt, lactisol, hydrogenated starch hydrolysates, hydrogenated glucose syrups, erythritol, or a combination of these. Products may claim that they reduce the risk of dental caries, that the sugar alcohol in the food does not promote tooth decay, or both.[12]

Plaque Removal

Mechanical methods (i.e., brushing with a dentifrice and flossing) of plaque removal are used most often. Chemical management of plaque (e.g., using specific products to prevent plaque accumulation or to aid in its removal) is a recent innovation in oral hygiene. The best way to ensure healthy teeth and gingival tissues is to mechanically remove plaque buildup by brushing at least twice daily and by flossing at least once a day. Toothbrushing removes plaque from the lingual (tongue) side, buccal (cheek) side, and occlusal (biting) surfaces of the teeth. Plaque found on interproximal (between the teeth) surfaces can be removed efficiently only with dental floss and other interdental cleaning aids (e.g., interproximal brush, dental tape, or tapered picks). Effective plaque removal will help prevent both dental caries and periodontal disease by removing disease-causing bacteria and by preventing their growth.

Chemical management of plaque and calculus can enhance mechanical removal either by acting directly on the plaque bacteria or by disrupting components of plaque to aid its removal during routine oral hygiene. The use of chemical agents in plaque control may be particularly appropriate for selected patients who may be either unable to brush and floss effectively or inhibited from doing so. Physically or mentally handicapped individuals (who may not be able to master the manual techniques necessary) and orthodontia patients or those with fixed prostheses may benefit from adding antiplaque agents to their oral hygiene regimen.

Desirable characteristics for antiplaque agents include the following:

- Selective antibacterial activity, interference with the rate of accumulation, or metabolism of supragingival plaque.

- Substantivity (sustained retention of the agent in the mouth).
- Compatibility with dentifrice ingredients.
- Lack of undesirable side effects for the user.
- Noninterference with the natural ecology of the normal oral microflora.[13,14]

Dentifrices

Dentifrices are used with a toothbrush for cleaning accessible tooth surfaces. Use of a dentifrice enhances removal of dental plaque and stain, resulting in a decreased incidence of dental caries and gum disease, reduced mouth odors, and enhanced personal appearance.[7]

Dentifrices are available as powders, pastes, or gels. (See Table 25–1 for examples of commercially available products.) The powder forms commonly contain abrasive and flavoring agents and sometimes a surfactant (foaming agent). Dentifrice powders are either moistened to form a slurry and applied with a dry brush or used dry with a brush moistened in water. The powder is more abrasive when used dry. In the final rule for anticaries drug products, monograph status is approved for powdered dentifrice containing sodium fluoride with a sodium bicarbonate abrasive.[15] The gels and pastes commonly contain an abrasive, a surfactant, a humectant (moistening agent), a binder/thickener, a sweetener, flavoring agents, and, commonly, a therapeutic agent such as fluoride for anticaries activity.

Abrasive Ingredients Dentifrice abrasives are pharmacologically inactive and insoluble compounds. Common abrasives include silicates, dicalcium phosphate, alumina trihydrate, calcium pyrophosphate, calcium carbonate, and sodium metaphosphate.[7] Although dentifrices vary in their degree of abrasiveness, abrasion is an essential property for removing stained pellicle from teeth.[1,7] The ideal abrasive would maximally aid in cleaning and minimally cause damage to tooth surfaces. Unfortunately, because of the variance in patient brushing techniques and oral conditions, the ideal dentifrice abrasive does not exist.

Low-abrasive dentifrices, which make up most dentifrice formulations currently marketed in the United States,[7] usually have a low concentration (10% to 25%) of silica abrasives, whereas high-abrasive dentifrices typically have higher concentrations (40% to 50%) of the inorganic calcium or aluminum salts listed above. Baking soda, a mild abrasive, is found in a number of dentifrices. Although safe to use, toothpastes with baking soda have not been shown to be better at cleaning teeth than are toothpastes without this substance. Baking soda is water soluble, and, even at higher concentrations, its polishing action is limited.[16,17]

Cosmetic dentifrices make no therapeutic claims and are usually chosen by patients because of taste, whitening ability, or antistain properties. Some dentifrices claiming to remove stubborn coffee or tobacco stains may contain higher concentrations of abrasives. High-abrasive formulations are not advised for long-term use or for use by patients with exposed root surfaces. Plain baking soda, which is a mild abrasive, or toothpastes containing baking soda have limited polishing and stain-removal capacity. Other products may contain a pigment (e.g., titanium dioxide) that produces a temporary brightening effect. Rembrandt Whitening Toothpaste contains a chemical complex of aluminum oxide, a citrate salt, and papain. Whitening dentifrices containing oxygenating agents depend on debriding action to remove stained pellicle. Numerous products offer a combination of baking soda and peroxide with fluoride. Whitening dentifrices should not be confused with the tooth-bleaching products discussed in the box "A Word about Tooth-Bleaching Products."

Popular gel dentifrices are flavored and disperse rapidly in the mouth. Manufacturers of gel dentifrices have advertised that children brush longer and more thoroughly because of the gel's consistency, translucence, dispersibility, and flavor. This claim has not been substantiated, but many dentifrices marketed for children are of the gel type. The children's products usually have fruit flavors rather than the breath-freshening minty or cinnamon flavors that adults prefer.

Chemotherapeutic Ingredients The most common therapeutic agent added to dentifrice is fluoride for its anticaries activity. Other therapeutic ingredients include potassium nitrate to treat hypersensitive dentin; triclosan, an antibacterial ingredient, which was recently added for its antigingivitis properties; and a stabilized stannous fluoride for its antigingivitis and anticaries properties. Other agents with antiplaque potential for inclusion in dentifrices include plant extracts (sanguinarine), metal salts (zinc and stannous), and essential oils (thymol and eucalyptol).[13,14,18] Hydrogen peroxide and sodium bicarbonate have also been added for plaque reduction.

Combinations of ingredients (e.g., triclosan and zinc citrate) have been shown to reduce plaque accumulation significantly and to be more effective at lower concentrations than are higher concentrations of either agent alone.[13,18] Few clinical data support inclusion of enzymes (e.g., dextranases and oxidases) for antiplaque purposes, and quaternary ammonium compounds are incompatible with most conventional toothpaste ingredients.[18]

Fluoride Fluoride dentifrices are indicated for both preventing and treating carious lesions. Use of fluoride-containing dentifrices is the one method of caries prevention common to all countries that show a reduction in caries.[19] ADA accepts as safe and effective the fluoride-containing toothpaste and fluoride-containing gel dentifrice formulations with compatible abrasive systems. FDA promulgated a final rule for nonprescription anticaries drug products in 1995 and determined that 0.22% sodium fluoride, 0.76% sodium monofluorophosphate, and 0.4% stannous fluoride dentifrices containing 850 ppm to 1150 ppm of theoretical

Table 25–1

Selected Dentifrices

Trade Name	Primary Ingredient
Fluoride Toothpastes	
Aim Extra Strength Gel	Hydrated silica; sodium monofluorophosphate 1.2%
Aim Regular Strength Gel	Hydrated silica; sodium monofluorophosphate 0.8% (fluoride 0.14%)
Aquafresh Extra Fresh Toothpaste	Calcium carbonate; hydrated silica; sodium monofluorophosphate
Close-Up Classic Red Gel	Hydrated silica; sodium monofluorophosphate 0.8% (fluoride 0.14%)
Colgate Toothpaste[a]	Dicalcium phosphate dihydrate; sodium monofluorophosphate 0.76%
Colgate Junior Gel[a]	Hydrated silica; sodium monofluorophosphate 0.243%
Crest Cavity Protection Gel	Hydrated silica; sodium fluoride 0.243%
Pepsodent Original Toothpaste	Hydrated silica; sodium monofluorophosphate 0.8% (fluoride 0.14%)
Tartar-Control Toothpastes	
Aquafresh Tartar Control Toothpaste	Hydrated silica; sodium fluoride; tetrapotassium pyrophosphate; tetrasodium pyrophosphate
Close-Up Tarter Control Gel	Hydrated silica; sodium monofluorophosphate 0.79% (fluoride 0.15%)
Colgate Baking Soda & Peroxide Tartar Control Toothpaste[a]	Hydrated silica; sodium bicarbonate; sodium monofluorophosphate 0.76%
Crest Tartar Protection Gel/Toothpaste	Silica; sodium fluoride 0.243%; tetrapotassium pyrophosphate; disodium pyrophosphate; tetrasodium pyrophosphate
Mentadent Gum Care Gel/Toothpaste	Hydrated silica; sodium bicarbonate; sodium fluoride 0.24% (fluoride 0.15%); zinc citrate trihydrate 1.8%
Pepsodent Tartar Control Toothpaste	Hydrated silica; sodium monofluorophosphate 0.8% (fluoride 0.14%); zinc citrate trihydrate
Viadent Fluoride Gel/Toothpaste	Hydrated silica; sodium monofluorophosphate 0.8%; zinc chloride; sanguinaria extract
Antiplaque/Antigingivitis Toothpastes	
Colgate Total Toothpaste	Hydrated silica; sodium bicarbonate; sodium fluoride 0.243%; triclosan 0.3%
Crest Baking Soda Tartar Gel/Toothpaste	Hydrated silica; sodium bicarbonate; sodium fluoride 0.243%; tetrasodium pyrophosphate; disodium pyrophosphate; tetrapotassium pyrophosphate
Crest Gum Care Gel/Toothpaste	Hydrated silica; stannous fluoride 0.454%
Whitening Toothpastes	
Aquafresh Whitening Gel/Toothpaste	Hydrated silica; sodium fluoride; titanium dioxide
Colgate Baking Soda Peroxide Whitening Toothpaste	Hydrated silica; sodium bicarbonate; aluminum oxide; sodium monofluorophosphate 0.76%; titanium dioxide
Colgate Platinum Whitening Toothpaste	Silica; aluminum oxide; sodium monofluorophosphate 0.76%; titanium dioxide
Mentadent Advanced Whitening Gel/Toothpaste	Hydrated silica; sodium bicarbonate; sodium fluoride 0.15%; titanium dioxide
Pearl Drops Whitening Extra Strength Toothpaste[a,b]	Hydrated silica; calcium pyrophosphate; dicalcium phosphate; sodium monofluorophosphate; titanium dioxide
Rembrandt Whitening Natural Toothpaste[b]	Dicalcium phosphate; silica; sodium monofluorophosphate; papain
Ultra Brite Toothpaste[a]	Hydrated silica; alumina; sodium monofluorophosphate 0.76%; titanium dioxide

[a] Sucrose-free product.

[b] Dye-free product.

total fluorine in a compatible base will meet monograph conditions. (See Table 25–2.) Although previously recognized as safe, clinical data submitted in the final rulemaking process established efficacy for enhanced anticaries benefit from a 1500 ppm theoretical total fluorine concentration of sodium monofluorophosphate.

Because of concerns about dental fluorosis in children, FDA required that dentifrice products with sodium

A Word about Tooth-Bleaching Products

Some home bleaching products include an acidic rinse in addition to the oxygenating whitening agent. The potential exists for damage to enamel, dentin, and some restorative materials. Concern also exists for possible pulp damage with the long-term use of whitening agents over a period of several weeks.[20] Patients should be strongly discouraged from attempting tooth bleaching without a dentist's direct supervision because serious adverse effects (i.e., loss of surface enamel) resulting from misuse or overuse of such products have been reported.[21]

Tooth whiteners, which claim to bleach teeth, contain oxidizing ingredients such as hydrogen peroxide, carbamide peroxide, or perhydrol urea in gel or liquid form. These products were previously marketed as cosmetics but are now considered drugs by FDA. The drug classification makes the products subject to rigorous new drug application requirements that will document their safety and effectiveness. Safety concerns related to long-term exposure of oral tissue to oxidizing agents include (1) the possibility of soft tissue damage or delayed wound healing, (2) the potential for damage to tooth pulp, and (3) the potential for mutating or enhancing the carcinogenic effects of other agents (e.g., tobacco).[22]

The American Dental Association (ADA) approved safety and efficacy guidelines for peroxide-containing oral hygiene products for dentist-prescribed/home use as tooth whitening agents, and ADA has accepted professional products intended for office use.[20,23] However, ADA accepts none of the available nonprescription products for unsupervised consumer use as a tooth-whitening agent.[23]

Early reports of dentist-supervised home bleaching of natural teeth began with the use of nonprescription oral antiseptic products containing 10% topical carbamide peroxide (e.g., Gly-Oxide, Proxigel). Patients were instructed to expose extrinsically stained teeth to the peroxide gel by using custom-made mouth trays coated with a thin gel film. Anecdotal reports emerged about successful tooth bleaching. One double-blind study reported effective whitening with minimal and reversible adverse effects (e.g., unpleasant taste, mucosal irritation, and tooth sensitivity) during treatment.[22]

monofluorophosphate containing 1500 ppm of theoretical total fluorine carry the following label: "Keep out of the reach of children under 6 years of age."[15] Aim Extra Strength toothpaste is an extra-strength monofluorophosphate fluoride product that is accepted by ADA; data support clinical and statistical superiority of its regular-strength counterpart.[24]

A possibility of staining exists with stannous fluoride. About 10% to 20% of patients may experience slight, but noticeable, tooth discoloration after 2 to 3 months of continuous use. The discoloration is not permanent and may be readily removed at the next professional dental cleaning.

Table 25–2

FDA-Approved Active Ingredients for Anticaries Dentifrices

Ingredient	Concentration (ppm)	Dosage Form
Sodium fluoride	850 to 1150	Dentifrice paste
	850 to 1150	Dentifrice powder
Sodium monofluorophosphate	850 to 1150 1500	Dentifrice paste Dentifrice paste
Stannous fluoride	850 to 1150	Dentifrice paste

Source: Reference 15.

This product is for use by adults and children ages 12 years and older.

Triclosan Colgate Total contains triclosan, an antibacterial agent and promoter of substantivity, which has antigingivitis and antiplaque activity. The product also contains fluoride for caries protection and a copolymer delivery system for the triclosan. This product was the first toothpaste approved by FDA in the antiplaque/antigingivitis category. It is also the only toothpaste currently accepted by ADA for this indication. Approval was based on clinical data for safety and efficacy. The product is not intended for use in children younger than 6 years.

An improved and stabilized stannous fluoride dentifrice, Crest Gum Care is marketed as an antigingivitis and anticaries product. The levels of bioavailable stannous fluoride for antimicrobial action exceed those required for anticaries action (through mineral reactivity). Clinical studies have demonstrated that it affects bacterial flora and metabolic processes that result in clinically reducing gingivitis.[25,26]

Zinc Chloride, Zinc Citrate, and Soluble Pyrophosphates A number of fluoride dentifrices contain anticalculus or tartar-control compounds. Although plaque, not supragingival calculus, is the primary etiologic factor in marginal periodontal disease, reducing calculus formation is still a goal of oral hygiene.[7,28] The ingredients incorporated to prevent or retard new calculus formation are zinc chloride, zinc citrate, and soluble pyrophosphates, which act to inhibit crystal growth. Placebo-controlled clinical studies have reported efficacy;

A Word about the American Dental Association Seal of Acceptance

The ADA's seal of acceptance program has been the consumer's guide to dental product safety and efficacy. ADA evaluates the safety and efficacy of dental products used by dental professionals and the public through the Seal of Acceptance's evaluation program of its Council on Scientific Affairs. Manufacturers voluntarily submit their products for detailed analysis of safety and efficacy. Moreover, product labels and promotional material must comply with ADA standards. Only claims that can be supported by appropriate clinical studies and scientific data are allowed to appear in conjunction with the seal. Dental products are evaluated on the basis of data regarding their safety and effectiveness for their intended use. Products that carry ADA seals or statements have scientifically earned their recognition. Once a product has earned the ADA seal, it may display that seal for 3 years, provided it continues to meet all the requirements.[23] The ADA's on-line home page www.ada.org provides searchable access to a current listing of dental consumer products that have been awarded the ADA Seal of Acceptance.

The ADA Council on Scientific Affairs holds that "because plaque is the etiologic agent for gingivitis and other oral diseases, the only accepted chemotherapeutic products that will be allowed to make plaque control or plaque modification claims will be those that can also demonstrate a significant effect against gingivitis. If a product can only demonstrate a significant plaque reduction without a concomitant significant reduction in gingivitis, it will not be eligible for Acceptance."[27] The council has developed stringent guidelines for acceptance of these products. They have approved two statements to be used for products classified under these guidelines—one for both gingivitis and plaque reduction and one for gingivitis reduction only.

> [Product Name] has been shown to help prevent and reduce [whichever is appropriate] gingivitis [and supragingival plaque accumulation] when used as directed in a conscientiously applied program of oral hygiene and regular professional care. Its effect on periodontitis has not been determined.[27]

Manufacturers of dentifrices or mouthrinses with therapeutic potential for gingivitis and supragingival dental plaque control may voluntarily submit data to ADA for evaluation.

findings have shown significant reduction in calculus occurrence and severity.[28,29]

ADA regards inhibition of supragingival calculus as a nontherapeutic use and, therefore, does not evaluate anticalculus claims. However, all advertising claims made for accepted products are reviewed for accuracy. ADA has directed that the following additional statement appear on all package and container labeling for accepted fluoride dentifrice products with calculus-control activity: "[Product name] has been shown to reduce the formation of tartar above the gumline, but has not been shown to have a therapeutic effect on periodontal diseases."[30]

Use of tartar-control toothpastes has been related to a type of contact dermatitis in the perioral region.[31] Adding pyrophosphate compounds to these products increases alkalinity and requires increased concentrations of other components, such as flavorings and surfactants for solubilizing. It is hypothesized that the pyrophosphates, either alone or in combination with the higher concentrations of inactive ingredients, are implicated as the cause of irritant contact dermatitis. Patients experiencing such a reaction should be advised to discontinue the tartar-control dentifrice and should switch to a non–tartar-control fluoride product. The skin eruption has been shown to resolve by decreasing or eliminating exposure.[31]

Sanguinarine, Sodium Bicarbonate, and Hydrogen Peroxide In a review of clinical studies on sanguinarine-containing dentifrices, only one in five trials reported a significant antiplaque effect.[32] The Plaque Subcommittee of the FDA Dental Products Panel requested more studies to prove antiplaque claims for sodium bicarbonate, hydrogen peroxide, and sanguinarine before a final monograph expected in 2000. All three ingredients are considered safe. Hydrogen peroxide used at the low concentrations in toothpaste and not swallowed appears to be safe.

Administration Guidelines Table 25–3 describes the proper method for brushing teeth using a fluoride dentifrice. Children are usually unable to brush by themselves until they are ages 4 or 5 years, and they may require supervision until age 8 or 9 years to clean effectively. FDA recommends that parents instruct children ages 6 to 12 years about good brushing and rinsing habits to minimize swallowing of fluoride.[15] Parents should apply the toothpaste (only a pea-sized amount) to a child-size toothbrush and should brush the teeth of preschoolers until the children can manage it properly themselves. Children should be taught to rinse thoroughly and expectorate after brushing.[33] Only regular-strength fluoride toothpaste is recommended for use in children from age 2 years up to age 6 years. Use in children younger than age 2 years should be under direction of the dentist or pediatrician.

All fluoride dentifrice products must contain the following warning on the labeling: "Warning: Keep out of the reach of children under 6 years of age. If you accidentally swallow more than used for brushing, seek professional assistance or contact a Poison Control Center immediately."

Table 25–3

Guidelines for Brushing Teeth

- Brush teeth after each meal, or at least twice a day.
- If using a toothpaste, apply a small amount of paste to the toothbrush.
- If using a powder, apply the powder to a wet toothbrush, completely covering all bristles.
- Use a gentle scrubbing motion with the bristle tips at a 45-degree angle against the gumline so that the tips of the brush do the cleaning.
- Do not use excessive force because such force may result in bristle damage, cervical abrasion, irritation of delicate gingival tissue, and gingival recession with associated hypersensitivity.
- Brush for at least 30 seconds, cleaning all tooth surfaces systematically.
- Gently brush the upper surface of the tongue to reduce debris, plaque, and bacteria that can cause oral hygiene problems. If using a powder, reapply powder as before and brush again. (Two applications of powder are needed to deliver an amount of sodium fluoride comparable to one application of a paste formulation.)
- Rinse the mouth, and spit out all the water.

Product Selection Guidelines Unless advised otherwise by their dentists, patients—especially those with periodontal disease, significant gum recession, and exposed root surfaces—should choose the least abrasive dentifrice that effectively removes stained pellicle. Although dentifrice abrasives do not pose a risk to dental enamel, toothbrushing action and excessive abrasiveness, which may lead to tooth hypersensitivity, can damage the softer material of exposed root surfaces (cementum) and dentin.[7]

Children younger than 6 years should not use a fluoride dentifrice. Extra-strength fluoride dentifrices, however, may be beneficial to patients who have a greater tendency to develop cavities or who reside in an area with nonfluoridated water.

Plaque Removal Devices

Toothbrushes, dental floss, specialty aids (e.g., interproximal dental brushes), and oral irrigating devices are the primary devices used in facilitating plaque removal.

Toothbrushes The toothbrush is the most universally accepted device available for removing dental plaque and for maintaining good oral hygiene. Toothbrush sales at retail are estimated in the $500-million range.

The proper frequency and method of brushing will vary from patient to patient, depending on individual factors. Thoroughness of plaque removal without gingival trauma is more important than the method used. Table 25–3 describes the proper method of brushing teeth.

Types of Toothbrushes Manual toothbrushes vary in size, shape, texture, and design, with new product designs proliferating rapidly. These toothbrushes have either nylon or natural bristles. The firmness of the bristles is usually rated as soft, medium, or firm.

Electric toothbrushes, which are available from numerous manufacturers, use essentially three brush-head motions to clean (i.e., back and forth, up and down, and a combination pattern).

Best results can be expected if a patient uses a brush carrying ADA's seal of acceptance and follows the specific directions of a dental professional. ADA's criteria for acceptance are based on safety and efficacy concerns. Advertising may mention plaque reduction but may not claim to improve any existing oral disease.[1] Comparative studies to date have yielded mixed results and modest differences. Variations in study design and specific patient factors or situations have influenced interpretation. Positive results (i.e., significant reductions in dental plaque accumulation) depend to some extent on proper use of the device, implying a need for patient education.[34]

Replacement of Toothbrushes There is no definite answer as to how often a patient should buy a new toothbrush, although 3 months has been suggested as a guide for toothbrush life expectancy. Marketing data suggest that consumers on average replace their toothbrushes only 1.7 times per year.[35] Two major reasons exist for replacing toothbrushes frequently: wear and bacterial accumulation. Different methods of brushing cause bristles to wear differently. Worn, bent, or matted bristles do not remove plaque effectively. Thus, patients should replace toothbrushes at the first sign of bristle wear rather than after a set period of use. Ideally, they should rotate two or three toothbrushes to allow each to dry completely between use, thereby decreasing bristle wear and matting.

Toothbrushes have been found to be a receptacle for bacteria. One study has reported that it takes just 17 to 35 days to accumulate a heavy buildup of bacteria on a toothbrush.[36] Patients with infectious diseases of the oral tissues (e.g., gingival or periodontal disease) should change brushes every 2 weeks, and it is advisable to replace a toothbrush following a respiratory infection to prevent reinfection.[36] Patients should be advised to rinse their toothbrushes thoroughly after each use to dislodge food debris and dilute sugar residue, both of which may serve as media for bacterial growth.

Product Selection Guidelines Dentists recommend toothbrushes according to the individual patient's manual dexterity, oral anatomy, and periodontal health. The toothbrush should be of a size and shape to allow the patient to reach every tooth in the mouth. Many dentists and dental hygienists prefer soft, rounded, multitufted, nylon bristle brushes. This preference is because nylon bristles are more durable and easier to clean than are natural bristles and because soft, rounded bristle tips are more effective in removing plaque below the gingival margin and on proximal tooth surfaces. Unfortunately, toothbrush firmness is not standardized;

toothbrushes designated as soft, medium, or hard may not be comparable across manufacturers. Innovations in head shapes and bristle configurations continue to be introduced in an attempt to improve cleaning contact with tooth and gumline surfaces.[37]

The handle size and shape of a toothbrush should allow the individual to maneuver the brush easily while maintaining a firm grasp. Many modifications have been introduced that may improve contact between the bristles and some less-accessible tooth surfaces, such as angle bends or flexible areas in the handle.

Standard electric toothbrushes mimic the motion of hand brushing. Although they have not consistently proven superior to properly manipulated manual toothbrushes, electric toothbrushes may benefit patients who are handicapped, who lack manual dexterity, who require someone else to clean their teeth, or who wear orthodontic appliances. These devices may also be useful for young children when parents do the brushing and for patients who may be motivated by the novelty of a powered toothbrush to increase the frequency and efficiency of their oral hygiene.[38,39] It has been suggested that "level of instruction, motivation, cost, ease of use, and maintenance will determine long-term acceptance by patients."[37]

Soft bristles are recommended for children's toothbrushes. A child's toothbrush is smaller than an adult's and is available in a baby (for children up to age 6 or 7 years) and a junior (ages 7 years to teens) size. Toothbrush size and shape should be individualized according to the size of the child's mouth. Children can usually remove plaque more easily with a brush that has short and narrow bristles.

Dental Floss Plaque accumulation in the interdental spaces contributes to proximal caries and periodontal pocketing. Interdental plaque removal has been reported to reduce gingival inflammation and prevent periodontal disease and dental caries.[39] Dental flossing is the most widely recommended method of removing dental plaque from proximal tooth surfaces that are not adequately cleaned by toothbrushing alone.[39] Besides removing plaque and debris interproximally, proper flossing also polishes the tooth surfaces, massages interdental papillae, and reduces gingival inflammation. Proper flossing technique requires some finger dexterity and practice. If done improperly, flossing can injure gingival tissue and cause cervical wear on proximal root surfaces.[1] Table 25–4 describes the proper use of dental floss.

Types of Dental Floss Most floss is a multifilament nylon yarn that is available in waxed or unwaxed form and in varying widths, from thin thread to thick tape. Many brands feature product lines of flosses that are impregnated or coated with additives, such as baking soda and fluoride. Also, several manufacturers are marketing floss made of materials with superior antishredding properties (e.g., Colgate Total, Glide, Reach Floss Easy Slide). ADA has recognized nearly 100 brands of dental floss and tape as safe and effective.[23]

Table 25–4

Guidelines for Using Dental Floss

- Pull out approximately 18 inches of floss, and wrap most of it around the middle finger.
- Wrap the remaining floss around the same finger of the opposite hand. About an inch of floss should be held between the thumbs and forefingers.
- Do not snap the floss between the teeth; instead use a gentle, sawing motion to guide the floss to the gumline.
- When the gumline is reached, curve the floss into a C-shape against one tooth, and gently slide the floss into the space between the gum and tooth until you feel resistance.
- Hold the floss tightly against the tooth, and gently scrape the side of the tooth while moving the floss away from the gums.
- Curve the floss around the adjoining tooth, and repeat the procedure.

Product Selection Guidelines Because no particular product has proven superior, patient factors (e.g., tightness of tooth contacts, tooth roughness, manual dexterity, and personal preference) should be considered in product selection.[40] Similarly, clinical studies show no difference between waxed and unwaxed floss in terms of removing plaque and preventing gingivitis.[41,42] Concern about a residual wax film deposited on tooth surfaces when using waxed floss is not supported by available evidence.[43]

Waxed floss may pass interproximally between tight-fitting teeth without shredding easier than unwaxed floss can. If contacts at the crowns of teeth are too tight to force floss interdentally, floss threaders can be used to pass floss between the teeth and around fixed bridges. Floss threaders, which are available in reusable and disposable forms, are usually thin plastic loops or soft plastic, needle-like appliances. Floss holders have one or two forks rigid enough to keep floss taut and a mounting mechanism that allows quick rethreading of floss.[40] Floss threaders should be used cautiously so as not to physically traumatize the gingiva. Floss holders may promote compliance among some people and are recommended for patients who lack manual dexterity and for caregivers who assist handicapped or hospitalized patients.

Specialty Aids Cleaning devices that adapt to irregular tooth surfaces better than dental floss are recommended for interproximal cleaning of teeth with large interdental spaces, such as is found in patients with periodontal disease.[40] The Flossbrush is such a device; it features woven dental floss with a time-release fluoride system that is molded into a plastic handle for interdental cleaning. The most common aids are tapered triangular wooden toothpicks (Stim-U-Dent), holders for round toothpicks (Perio-aid), miniature bottle brushes (Py-Co-Prox or Proxabrush), rubber stimulator tips, denture brushes, and denture clasp brushes.

Conflicting findings are reported for plaque-removal efficacy among these interproximal cleaning devices. Differences in methodology and patient populations prevent generalizations, while individual patient motivation and dexterity may influence results.[44] The dental professional considers the patient's oral anatomy, the presence of periodontal disease, the size of the interproximal spaces, and the patient's dexterity when recommending an interdental cleaning aid.

Oral Irrigating Devices Oral irrigators work by directing a high-pressure stream of water through a nozzle to the tooth surfaces. Studies have shown that these devices can remove only a minimal amount of plaque from tooth surfaces.[39,45] Thus, oral irrigators cannot be viewed as substitutes for a toothbrush, dental floss, or other plaque-removal devices but should be considered as adjuncts in maintaining oral hygiene.[39] ADA views these devices as potentially useful for "removing loose debris from those areas that cannot be cleaned with the toothbrush such as around orthodontic bands and fixed bridges."[39] Several brands on the market carry the ADA seal.[23]

A multicenter study of periodontitis patients receiving supportive periodontal treatment (maintenance phase) determined that adjunctive daily water irrigation provided meaningful clinical outcomes.[46] Oral irrigators have also been valuable as vehicles for administering chemotherapeutic agents that inhibit microbial growth in inaccessible regions of the mouth.[47]

Yet ADA cautions that patients with advanced periodontal disease should use these devices only under professional supervision because it is possible for transient bacteremia to occur after manipulative procedures with the oral irrigator.[39] Oral irrigation devices should also be considered contraindicated in patients predisposed to bacterial endocarditis.

Plaque Disclosing Agents Disclosing agents are used at home by the patient for self-evaluation of plaque removal and in the dental office when the dentist is instructing the patient in proper cleaning technique. Disclosing agents contain a vegetable dye (e.g., erythrosin or FD&C Red No. 3) that stains dental plaque so that the patient can easily see it. This visualization enables patients to evaluate their oral hygiene efforts and to detect areas they missed (e.g., where more thorough brushing and flossing is indicated). The dye stains plaque but not tooth enamel, gingiva, or restorations, and it is easily rinsed away because it is soluble in water. (See the "Color Plates," photograph 1.)

Disclosing agents are available for home use as either a solution or a chewable tablet. These agents are not intended for daily or continuous long-term use; they should be used intermittently as a plaque indicator to monitor cleaning technique. Chewable tablets (e.g., Red-Cote Dental Disclosing Tablets) may be preferred for normal home use because they are individually wrapped in unit-of-use doses, thereby eliminating any problems with spilling that might occur with the liquids. The patient should be instructed to rinse the mouth first with water. The tablet is chewed, swished around the mouth for 30 seconds, and then expectorated—never swallowed. After the patient rinses with water and expectorates again, red areas remain to indicate areas of plaque accumulation. The dark red color should be removed by thorough brushing and flossing. Solutions may be preferred in some cases because another person can apply the agent with a cotton-tipped applicator to a handicapped patient's or child's dentition, and the solution can be diluted with water.

Because disclosing tablets are sweet, usually containing mannitol or sorbitol, and are brightly colored, the tablets may be mistaken for candy.[48] Thus, these products should be kept out of the reach of children, and use by children should be supervised. Patients should not swallow disclosing products and should always rinse the mouth with water and then expectorate the water.

Antiplaque Products

In 1990, FDA issued a call for data on oral health care products that make antiplaque and related claims.[49] This call was the initial step in developing the final segment of the rulemaking for over-the-counter (OTC) oral health care drug products, which will address antiplaque and related claims. Because plaque reduction or removal is intended to prevent disease (i.e., gingivitis, caries, and periodontal disease), FDA considers claims of removing or reducing plaque to be drug claims.[49] At the time of this publication, no final rule has been issued. However, the Plaque Subcommittee of the FDA Dental Products Panel is engaged in continuing discussions to develop guidelines for determining the safety and effectiveness of antiplaque products. That panel will advise the FDA Commissioner on the promulgation of a monograph establishing conditions under which oral antiseptic drugs for antiplaque and antiplaque-related use are generally recognized as safe and effective.[50]

Two classes of oral health care products have made antiplaque claims. These classes include (1) those products that rely on the mechanical action of abrasives to remove plaque and (2) those that claim to reduce or remove plaque by chemical or antimicrobial activity. These products are available in multiple forms (e.g., dentifrices and mouthrinses). ADA has adopted Acceptance Program Guidelines for Adjunctive Dental Therapies for the Reduction of Plaque and Gingivitis. The guidelines apply to the design of clinical trials that will evaluate the safety and effectiveness of products intended to mechanically remove dental plaque and reduce gingivitis. Separate guidelines evaluate products that contain chemotherapeutic agents for control of gingivitis.

Mouthrinses and Gels A mouthrinse with plaque or calculus control properties is indicated as an adjunct to proper flossing and toothbrushing with a fluoride toothpaste. In some cases, further research is necessary to determine how efficacious the antiplaque activity is.

Mouthrinse and dentifrice formulations are very similar. Like dentifrices, mouthrinses may be cosmetic or therapeutic. Both may contain surfactant(s), humectant(s), flavor, coloring, water, and therapeutic ingredient(s). Table 25–5 lists examples of commercially available products.

Cosmetic Mouthrinses A mouthrinse approximates a diluted liquid dentifrice that contains alcohol but no abrasive. Alcohol adds bite and freshness, enhances flavor, solubilizes other ingredients, and contributes to the cleansing action and antibacterial activity. Flavor contributes to pleasant taste and breath freshening. Surfactants are foaming agents that aid in removal of debris. Other active ingredients may include astringents, demulcents (soothing agents), antibacterial agents, and fluoride.[7]

Cosmetic mouthrinses freshen the breath and clean some debris from the mouth. Mouthrinses can be classified by appearance, alcohol content, and active ingredients. In general, mouthrinses are minty (green or blue) or spicy (red), medicinal or alcoholic, and they contain various miscellaneous ingredients such as (1) glycerin, a topical protectant that tastes sweet and is soothing to oral mucosa; (2) benzoic acid, an antimicrobial agent; and (3) zinc chloride/citrate, an astringent that neutralizes odoriferous sulfur compounds produced in the oral cavity. The most popular cosmetic mouthrinses are phenolic (medicinal) and mint flavored. To have some degree of oral malodor (e.g., morning breath) is normal in a healthy individual. This malodor is because reduced activity of tongue, cheeks, and salivary flow enhance bacterial activity and production of odoriferous sulfur compounds.[7] Thus, products that are intended to eliminate or suppress mouth odor of local origin in healthy people with healthy mouths are considered by the FDA Advisory Review Panel on Over-the-Counter Oral Health Care Products to be cosmetics unless they contain antimicrobial or other therapeutic agents.[51] ADA's acceptance program does not evaluate mouthrinses labeled and advertised only as cosmetic agents.

An important consideration is the potential for breath-freshening mouthrinses to disguise and delay treatment of pathologic conditions that may contribute to lingering oral malodor (e.g., periodontal disease, purulent oral infections, and respiratory infections). ADA suggests that "if marked breath odor persists after proper toothbrushing, the cause should be investigated" and not masked with mouthrinse.[39]

Therapeutic Mouthrinses Over the past decade, nonprescription mouthrinses promoted for antiplaque or tartar-control activity have proliferated. Ingredients added to mouthrinses for plaque control include (1) plant extracts (sanguinarine); (2) aromatic oils (thymol, eucalyptol, menthol, and methyl salicylate), which are antibacterial and have some local anesthetic activity; and (3) agents with antimicrobial activity (e.g., quaternary ammonium compounds). Of the latter, cetylpyridinium chloride is a cationic surfactant that is capable of bactericidal activity although it does not penetrate plaque well; domiphen bromide is a bactericidal agent similar to cetylpyridinium. Another ingredient, phenol, is a local anesthetic, antiseptic, and bactericidal agent that penetrates plaque better than either cetylpyridinium or domiphen does.

Listerine, containing the active ingredients thymol, eucalyptol, methyl salicylate and menthol, was the first mouthrinse to be accepted by ADA as a nonprescription antiplaque/antigingivitis mouthrinse. The phenol oils (active ingredients) control plaque by destroying bacterial cell walls, inhibiting bacterial enzymes, and extracting bacterial lipopolysaccharides.[52] ADA has since accepted Cool Mint and FreshBurst Listerine and more than 100 similarly formulated private-label antiseptic mouthrinses in the antiplaque/antigingivitis category of accepted therapeutic products.[23]

The quaternary ammonium and sanguinarine compounds have some merit, but studies of their efficacy in plaque and gingivitis reduction are mixed.[52] Although sanguinarine has shown effectiveness against plaque-forming bacteria in vitro, widely divergent findings that range from significant reduction of plaque and gingivitis to negligible or no effect have been reported in numerous short-term and several long-term clinical studies.[32]

Clinical trials with mouthrinses containing cetylpyridinium chloride alone or in combination with domiphen bromide have reported reductions in plaque accumulation.[53] On the basis of available data, the potential for oral toxicity with these agents is low, and the potential for a gingival health benefit exists.[7,14,54] However, studies consistent with ADA guidelines have not been evaluated, and further study is needed to substantiate antigingivitis efficacy. At least one study[54] has reported no difference in plaque control and gin-

Table 25–5

Selected Mouthrinses and Gels

Trade Name	Primary Ingredients
Cepacol Mouthwash/Gargle[a]	Alcohol 14%; cetylpyridinium chloride 0.05%
Listerine	Alcohol 26.9%; eucalyptol 0.092%; thymol 0.064%; methyl salicylate 0.06%; menthol 0.042%
Mentadent Cool Mint Mouthwash	Alcohol 10%; methyl salicylate
Plax Advanced Formula	Alcohol 8.7%; sodium lauryl sulfate; tetrasodium pyrophosphate
Scope Baking Soda	SD alcohol 38F 9.9%; cetylpyridinium chloride; domiphen bromide; sodium bicarbonate
Scope Cool Peppermint	SD alcohol 38F 14%; cetylpyridinium chloride; domiphen bromide
Targon Smokers' Mouthwash[a]	SDA alcohol 38B 15.6%
Viadent Oral Rinse	Alcohol 10%; zinc chloride 0.2%; sanguinaria extract

[a] Sucrose-free product.

gival health between a cetylpyridinium rinse and a placebo when the former was used as a prebrushing rinse. It was suggested that the order of rinsing and brushing may be relevant: Reduced activity may have been influenced by the interaction of the cationic surfactant with anionic detergents in the toothpaste. Rinsing after brushing or at a time separate from brushing may be indicated. Cepacol, Scope, Clear Choice, and Oral-B Anti-Plaque Rinse are examples of products in this category. Because cetylpyridinium is chemically related to chlorhexidine, it too may stain teeth but to a much lesser degree.[54] Staining is usually associated with overuse.

Another approach to plaque control does not rely on antimicrobial activity but is based on principles of surfactant action to loosen plaque. Plax, intended for use as a prebrushing rinse, has been reformulated. The new product, Advanced Formula Plax, contains an enhanced level of detergent (sodium lauryl sulfate) and the addition of detergent builders, tetrasodium pyrophosphate and sodium benzoate. Approximately 1 to 2 tablespoons of the product is vigorously swished between the teeth and then spit out. Patients should refrain from eating, drinking, or smoking for 30 minutes after use.

Findings reported in clinical trials with the original formula of Plax were contradictory. Although there were early reports of efficacy for plaque removal in short-term clinical trials,[55,56] a number of studies[57–59] reported results comparable to those of placebo. A more recent clinical evaluation[60] indicated the new formula significantly reduced subjects' plaque levels when compared with placebo.

Mouthrinses claiming anticalculus or tartar-control activity contain the same active ingredients as anticalculus dentifrices. Although ADA regards inhibition of supragingival calculus as a nontherapeutic use and does not evaluate mouthrinse anticalculus claims, FDA included these mouthrinses in the aforementioned 1990 call for data on ingredients contained in products bearing antiplaque and antiplaque-related claims. FDA will eventually rule on safety and effectiveness for this indication.[49]

Anticavity fluoride treatment mouthrinses and gels are therapeutic topical applications of fluoride for prevention of dental caries. These agents are discussed in the section "Use of Fluoride."

Usage Guidelines Plaque or calculus control mouthrinses are intended for use twice daily after brushing, with the exception of Advanced Formula Plax, which should be used before brushing. In general, an amount equal to 1 to 2 tablespoons of rinse should be swished vigorously in the mouth and between the teeth for about 30 seconds and then expectorated; the rinses should not be swallowed. Patients should be advised to refrain from smoking, eating, or drinking for 30 minutes following use. Children younger than 12 years should be instructed to develop good rinsing habits (to minimize swallowing) until they are capable of using mouthrinses without supervision.

Adverse Effects Mouthrinses and gels are generally safe when used as directed, but occasional adverse reactions (e.g., burning sensation, irritation) have been reported. Overuse should be discouraged. Consultation with a health professional is indicated if irritation occurs and persists after the patient discontinues use of the product.

Contraindications/Precautions/Warnings Unsupervised use is contraindicated in patients with mouth irritation or ulceration. These products should be kept out of the reach of children. In case of accidental ingestion, the caregiver should seek professional assistance or contact a poison control center.[53]

The alcohol content in mouthrinses ranges from zero to 27%; most popular adult mouthrinses contain between 14% and 27%.[61] This issue has drawn attention for two reasons. Ingestion of alcohol-containing products poses a danger for children, who may be attracted by bright colors and pleasant flavors, and concern exists for a potential association between the use of mouthrinses containing alcohol and an increased risk of oral cancer.

Toxicity data concerning children's ingestion of an alcohol-containing mouthrinse demonstrate that the amount of alcohol in available mouthrinse preparations is sufficient to cause serious illness and injury to children.[61] Acute alcoholic intoxication and death resulting from high-dose ingestion is possible. For a child weighing 26 pounds, 5 to 10 ounces of a mouthrinse containing alcohol can be lethal.[1] Responding to concern over the potential danger to children, the Consumer Products Safety Commission issued a final rule in January 1995[61] that required child-resistant packaging for mouthrinses with 3 g or more of absolute alcohol per package—the amount that is present in a small quantity (approximately 2.6 ounces) of mouthrinse with 5% alcohol. "For the purposes of this final rule, the term *mouthwash* includes liquid products that are variously called mouthwashes, mouthrinses, oral antiseptics, gargles, fluoride rinses, anti-plaque rinses, and breath fresheners. It does not include throat sprays or aerosol breath fresheners."[61] These products should be kept out of the reach of children and should not be administered to children younger than 12 years. Labeling includes a warning not to swallow but to seek professional assistance or to contact a poison control center immediately in case of accidental ingestion.

The Dental Products Panel considered the use of alcohol in oral health care products in 1994 and again in 1996. The FDA Plaque Subcommittee has recommended that the alcohol content of mouthrinse products be clearly stated on the principal display panel.[62] Following review of information submitted in response to their call for more data to investigate a possible connection between the use of alcohol-containing mouthrinses and oral cancer, the subcommittee withdrew its call for more follow-up studies in 1996.[63] Alcohol-free formulations in the various mouthrinse categories are available. (See Table 25–5.)

Plaque Control Chewing Gum Recent additions to the plaque control market include baking soda chewing gum (e.g., Arm & Hammer Dental Care Chewing Gum, Trident

Advantage) for plaque reduction. Gum chewing contributes to increased saliva flow that apparently produces a beneficial buffering effect against acids in the oral cavity.[64] Thus, especially for patients with a dry mouth condition, these products may have some value as an adjunct to their oral hygiene. In addition, the chewing gums are sugar free and are sweetened with sugar alcohols (e.g., xylitol, sorbitol) that do not promote caries and may reduce the risk.[65]

The patient is directed to chew two pieces of gum daily after eating. These products are not regulated for their antiplaque claims by FDA and should not substitute for a regular program of brushing, flossing, and rinsing to remove plaque.

Special Population Considerations for Plaque Removal At birth, the 20 primary teeth that will erupt are present but not visible. It is important to start oral hygiene early in life. Thus, the pharmacist should recommend removal of plaque and milk residue by wiping the baby's gums with a wet gauze pad after each feeding. The deciduous teeth will usually start to erupt at about age 6 months and can decay at any time. "Baby bottle caries" results when an infant is allowed to nurse continuously from a bottle of juice, milk, or sugar water. The prolonged contact of teeth with the cariogenic liquid promotes caries. When the teeth have erupted, a soft child-size toothbrush can be used for cleaning. Parents must do the brushing and should take care to use only a very small amount of fluoride toothpaste or none at all. Children at this age will swallow the toothpaste, which will contribute to overall systemic fluoride ingestion. Therefore, younger children need to be taught the proper brushing technique or supervised while brushing.

In patients with fixed orthodontia, very careful attention to oral hygiene to prevent gingivitis and caries is required. Patients with these appliances need a combination of toothbrush types to clean all surfaces effectively. Use of powered dentifrices or oral irrigating devices may help to remove plaque and debris around orthodontic bands. It may be advisable for orthodontic patients to use a nonprescription fluoride mouthrinse while undergoing treatment.

Patients with removable orthodontic appliances should consult their orthodontist about using a denture cleanser. Some dental practitioners have recommended a denture cleanser in addition to brushing to remove plaque, tartar, odor-causing bacteria, and stain that accumulates on orthodontic appliances.[66]

In geriatric patients with natural dentition, topical fluoride application in the form of dentifrice, rinse, or gel is indicated to prevent coronal and root caries. Pharmacists should continue to recommend fluoride anticaries products to their older patients. When a pharmacist counsels geriatric patients on oral health care, it becomes very important to consider medication profiles. Because the elderly are more likely to be taking multiple medications, the likelihood increases for drug-induced or disease-related changes in oral physiology.

Use of Fluoride

Fluoride is thought to help prevent dental caries through a combination of effects. Incorporated into developing teeth, fluoride systemically reduces the solubility of dental enamel by enhancing the development of a fluoridated hydroxyapatite (which is more resistant to demineralizing acids) at the enamel surface. The topical effect facilitates remineralization of early carious lesions during repeated cycles of demineralization and remineralization. Some evidence exists that fluoride interferes with the bacterial cariogenic process. Fluoride that is chemically bound to organic constituents of plaque may interfere with plaque adherence and may inhibit glycolysis, the process by which sugar is metabolized to produce acid.[1]

Fluoridated Water Supplies

Fluoridation of the public water supply is an effective and economically sound public health measure that has played a major role in decreasing the incidence of caries. More than half of the U.S. population resides in communities in which the public water supply contains either naturally occurring or added fluoride at optimal levels for decay prevention (e.g., 1 ppm or 1 mg/L).[67] Besides reducing dental caries in children, fluoridation has benefits that extend through adulthood, resulting in (1) fewer decayed, missing, or filled teeth; (2) greater tooth retention; and (3) a lower incidence of root caries. Systemic fluoride supplementation in children is based on the preventive mechanism of fluoride when incorporated into developing enamel. Current concepts of the action of fluoride relative to its presence in saliva and plaque provide a rationale for its topical application to prevent caries in all age groups. It must be noted, however, that any decision to supplement fluoride intake must take into account the concentration of fluoride present in the drinking water.[1,39]

Fluoride Rinses and Gels

Mouthrinses and gels that contain sodium fluoride are therapeutic topical applications of fluoride for prevention of dental caries. (See Table 25–6 for examples of commercially available products.) Fluoride mouthrinsing enables patients to apply fluoride interproximally. Studies of fluoride mouthrinsing have given consistently positive results. Studies in which subjects used 0.05% sodium fluoride rinse once daily have demonstrated a significant reduction (by 17% to 47%) in caries incidence, especially among children living in areas with nonfluoridated water.[33]

Examples of patients who may benefit from fluoride rinsing are those with orthodontic appliances, those with decreased salivary flow for whatever reason, those at risk for developing root caries, and anyone with difficulty maintaining good oral hygiene. Orthodontic patients are at risk of developing decalcified areas while under treatment, and their ability to clean interdental spaces thoroughly may be inhibited.[33]

Because fluoride rinses and gels provide a therapeutic fluoride treatment, package directions should be followed

Table 25–6

Selected Topical Fluoride Products

Trade Name	Primary Ingredients
Fluoride Foam	Fluoride 1.23% (from sodium fluoride and hydrogen fluoride)
Fluorigard Anti-Cavity Rinse[a]	Sodium fluoride 0.05%
Reach Act Adult Anti-Cavity Rinse[b]	Sodium fluoride 0.05%; cetylpyridinium chloride
Reach Act for Kids Rinse[b]	Sodium fluoride 0.05%; cetylpyridinium chloride
Rembrandt Age Defying Adult Formula Mouthwash[b]	Sodium fluoride 0.05%

[a] Dye-free product.

[b] Alcohol-free product.

Table 25–7

Guidelines for Using Topical Fluoride Treatments

- Use topical fluoride treatments no more than once a day.
- Brush teeth with a fluoride dentifrice before using a fluoride treatment.
- If using a fluoride rinse, measure the recommended dose (most commonly 10 mL), and vigorously swish it between the teeth for 1 minute.
- If using a fluoride gel, brush the gel on the teeth. Allow the gel to remain for 1 minute.
- After 1 minute, spit out the fluoride product. Do not swallow it.
- Do not eat or drink for 30 minutes after the treatment.
- Supervise children as necessary until they can use the product without supervision.
- Instruct children younger than 12 years in good rinsing habits to minimize swallowing of the product.
- Consult a dentist or doctor before using fluoride products in children younger than 6 years.

Source: Reference 2.

closely. To maximize the safe and effective use of these products, FDA requires labeling to instruct consumers to read the directions. Table 25–7 describes the proper method of applying fluoride rinses and gels. When recommending a nonprescription fluoride mouthrinse, the pharmacist should stress that children younger than 12 years should be supervised as necessary until they are capable of using the product correctly. Further, children younger than 6 years should use these products only as directed by a dentist or physician. Some concern has been raised about whether unsupervised home use of the fluoride gels is justified.[33]

Fluoride Dentifrices

Fluoride dentifrices provide a means of increasing contact of fluoride with the tooth surfaces, where fluoride exerts its greatest protection.[68] Brushing with a fluoride dentifrice provides anticaries protection; however, the fluoride does not reach the surfaces between teeth adequately. Thus, the high-risk patients mentioned above may especially benefit from multiple sources of fluoride application. Fluoride-containing dental products are thought to be of greatest benefit when used in areas with a nonfluoridated public water supply. However, they can help reduce the caries incidence even in patients residing in communities with a fluoridated water supply.[39] FDA proposed that the following statement be applied to fluoride-containing dental care products: "The combined daily use of a fluoride treatment ('rinse' or 'gel') and a fluoride toothpaste can aid in reducing the incidence of dental cavities."[69]

Patients who form heavy calculus between dental visits may consider using a fluoride dentifrice with added tartar-control ingredients instead of a plain fluoride dentifrice. A patient's appearance may benefit from a lessening of visible supragingival calculus buildup, and reports indicate that professional dental cleaning may be easier because the calculus that does form is less adherent.[30]

Dental Fluorosis

Fluoride dentifrices contribute to the total amount of fluoride ingested by children. Other sources are dietary products, recommended systemic supplements, and any other topical fluoride preparations. When chronic fluoride ingestion from all sources is considered, children who live in a community with an optimally fluoridated water supply may exceed optimal daily amounts. This excess places them at risk for mild forms of dental fluorosis, a mottled appearance of surface enamel. Although a mild degree of fluorosis is an aesthetic concern, more severe cases can result in pitting and surface defects.[70] (See the "Color Plates," photograph 2.)

Related to this concern, FDA considered comments regarding formulation of a reduced-strength fluoride dentifrice during the anticaries final rule process. It was determined that mild dental fluorosis does not compromise oral health or tooth function as do dental caries. Therefore, the risk of dental caries from inadequate fluoride protection is a greater health hazard than the cosmetic detriment of fluorosis. The increased incidence of mild fluorosis appears to be caused by a combination of factors.

In 1994, ADA revised its recommendations for fluoride supplement dosing in children. The new schedule slightly lowers the dose amounts, recommends beginning treatment not earlier than age 6 months, and extends the age limit from 13 to 16 years. Evaluation of current studies reporting on the intake of fluoride among children prompted the revision.[71]

Studies of dentifrice ingestion by children show great variation in the amount of dentifrice retained and consistently show that younger children are more likely than older ones to swallow some dentifrice.[33] Limiting ingestion of fluoride dentifrice is advised as discussed in the section "Administration Guidelines" under "Dentifrices."

Fluoride rinsing presents a similar problem for children (ages 3 to 5 years) who may swallow significant amounts of rinse each time they swish. A usual dose of 0.05% rinse contains 2 mg of fluoride ion and may contribute to mild fluorosis in the presence of a fluoridated public water supply. Alcohol content of most nonprescription fluoride rinses ranges from 6% to 8% and may pose a hazard for very young children. Alcohol-free formulations are now available. Fluoride rinses should be used only by children ages 6 years and older who have mastered the swallowing reflex. These products should be kept out of the reach of children, and children younger than 12 years should be supervised when rinsing. High-dose ingestion requires prompt medical assistance. Toxicity is related to fluoride content and alcohol content. Parents should be able to identify the product and to estimate the amount ingested.[68]

Patient Assessment of Caries

When asked to recommend plaque-control products, the pharmacist should determine what dental care measures the patient is taking, whether these measures meet recommended oral hygiene standards, and how often the patient sees a dentist. The patient's concern about caries should alert the pharmacist to ask whether the patient has a history of caries and whether the patient suspects a new carious lesion has developed. Asking the patient the following questions will help elicit the information needed to determine the patient's level of oral hygiene and to recommend any additional needed preventive measures.

Q~ Are you having symptoms of a toothache?

A~ If yes, refer the patient to a dentist for evaluation of possible advanced caries or other dental problem.

Q~ Are you using any plaque-control measures? How do you brush your teeth and how often? Do you use dental floss and how often? Do you use supplemental fluoride in any form?

A~ Evaluate whether the patient's plaque-control measures meet recommended standards for oral hygiene. If not, advise the patient of which measures to add and recommend the appropriate products.

Q~ Do you smoke or use any tobacco (including smokeless tobacco) product? Do you drink alcohol?

A~ If yes, advise the patient these substances are risk factors for caries.

Q~ Do you see a dentist regularly? Has a dentist treated you for dental caries in the past?

A~ If the patient is not seeing a dentist regularly, stress the importance of dental cleanings in controlling caries. Stress to patients who have already experienced tooth decay the importance of implementing the dentist's preventive measures. Advise the patient of dietary measures that also aid in preventing caries.

Patient Education for Prevention of Caries, Gingivitis, and Halitosis

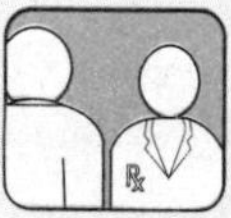

The primary objective of self-care is the removal of plaque to prevent caries, gingivitis, and halitosis. For most patients, carefully following product instructions and the self-care measures listed below will help ensure good oral hygiene.

Lifestyle Measures and Other Considerations

- Avoid cariogenic foods such as foods that contain more than 15% sugar, that cling to the teeth, and that remain in the mouth after they are eaten.
- Eat low-cariogenic foods such as foods that have a high water content (e.g., fresh fruit), that stimulate the flow of saliva (e.g., fibrous foods that require lots of chewing), or that are high in protein (e.g., dairy products).
- To help prevent mouth odor, drink at least eight 8-ounce glasses of water a day. Also, if you wear dentures, do not wear them while sleeping.
- Note that use of alcohol and tobacco can cause caries, gingivitis, and halitosis.
- Note that hormonal changes during pregnancy increase the risk of gingivitis.
- Consider incorporating gum massage as an antigingivitis measure, using such devices as soft brushes, special rubber cup massagers, a Stim-U-Dent, or toothpicks.

Plaque Removal

Brushing Teeth

- Mechanically remove plaque buildup by brushing teeth at least twice daily with a fluoride dentifrice. (See Table 25–3 for proper brushing technique.)
- Use a brush with soft nylon bristles.
- Replace the brush when the bristles show signs of wear.
- For children younger than 2 years, clean the teeth with a soft cloth, and massage the gums.
- For preschool children, apply a pea-sized amount of toothpaste to a child-size toothbrush, and brush the child's teeth until the child can brush properly.

- Use only regular-strength fluoride toothpaste for children from ages 2 years to 6 years. Consult a dentist before using fluoride toothpastes in children younger than 2 years.
- Teach children how to rinse the mouth and to spit out the toothpaste to avoid swallowing fluoride.
- Note that tartar-control toothpastes have been related to a type of contact dermatitis in the perioral region. Discontinue the tartar-control dentifrice, and switch to a non–tartar-control fluoride toothpaste if you experience itching or irritation of the mouth after brushing.
- If you are prone to developing caries or gingivitis, consider using a toothpaste classified as having antiplaque/antigingivitis activity. Such toothpastes contain triclosan (Colgate Total) or stannous fluoride.

Flossing Teeth

- Floss your teeth at least once a day. (See Table 25–4 for proper flossing technique.)
- Use a waxed floss if you have tight contacts between teeth.

Using Plaque-Disclosing Products

- For maximum plaque removal, use a plaque-disclosing product to see whether toothbrushing and flossing have removed all the plaque.
- Rinse the mouth with water.
- Chew a disclosing tablet, or apply a solution to the teeth with a cotton-tipped applicator.
- Swish the product around the mouth for 30 seconds, and then spit out the product.
- Rinse the mouth with water, and spit out the solution.
- Look for red areas on the teeth that indicate areas of plaque accumulation. If teeth are red, brush and floss again.

Using Mouthrinses and Gels

- To freshen breath, use a mouthrinse that contains zinc chloride (Viadent) and zinc citrate. These ingredients eliminate odoriferous sulfur compounds.
- If you are prone to developing caries or gingivitis, consider using a mouthrinse classified as having antiplaque/antigingivitis activity. Such mouthwashes contain thymol, eucalyptol, methyl salicylate, and menthol.
- To use plaque-softening mouthrinses (Advanced Formula Plax) effectively, use them before brushing. Vigorously swish 1 to 2 tablespoons of rinse in the mouth and between the teeth for about 30 seconds, and spit out the rinse. Do not smoke, eat, or drink for 30 minutes following use.
- Note that overuse of mouthrinses containing cetylpyridinium can stain teeth.

Using Topical Fluoride Treatments

- If your drinking water is not fluoridated or if you are prone to developing caries, consider using topical fluoride treatments. (See Table 25–7 for proper use of these products.)
- Supervise children younger than 12 years until they are capable of using the product correctly.
- Consult a dentist or physician before using these products in children younger than 6 years.

See a dentist if any of the following occur:
—You develop symptoms of a toothache.
—Your teeth develop a mottled appearance (a sign of fluorosis).
—Your gums bleed, swell, or become red.
—Mouth odor persists despite regular use of a fluoride toothpaste, or the cause of the odor cannot be identified.

Patient Counseling for Caries

The pharmacist should tailor to the patient's level of knowledge all explanations of the purpose of various oral hygiene products and the methods for using them. Patients with a history of caries should be encouraged to brush after meals and to check with a dentist about using topical fluoride products. The pharmacist should explain the precautions for these products as well as the possible adverse effects of some therapeutic ingredients in other products. Patients should be advised of signs and symptoms that indicate a dental evaluation is necessary. The box "Patient Education for Prevention of Caries, Gingivitis, and Halitosis" lists specific information to provide patients about plaque-induced oral disorders.

Because dental disease is the most frequently encountered health problem in the United States, and because pharmacists see many people with dental problems, today's pharmacist needs a well-developed knowledge of oral health care products and their use. Useful resources, references, and information related to ongoing FDA and ADA evaluations of nonprescription dental products are easily available on the Internet. Sites maintained by government agencies, industry, and professional associations provide valuable professional

Table 25–8

Internet Oral Health Care Resources for the Pharmacist

Agency/Organization	Web Site	Available Resources/Services
American Dental Association	www.ada.org	Patient education, product news, research, publications, references, accepted products
Federal Register	www.access.gpo.gov	OTC Advisory Committee actions and recommendations; proposed and final rules, etc.
National Institute of Dental and Craniofacial Research	www.nidr.nih.gov (site maintained by National Institutes of Health)	Health care and patient information, *NIDCR Research Digest*, and links to oral health resources
Academy of General Dentistry	www.agd.org	Reliable source for consumer dental health information
American Dental Hygienists' Association	www.adha.org	Consumer oral health information and related links
American Association of Public Health Dentistry	www.pitt.edu/~aaphd	Databases and links to Internet resources on oral health
National Oral Health Information Clearinghouse	www.aerie.com/nohicweb	Information for special care populations; Oral Health Database; resource links
Combined Health Information Database (CHID)	www.chid.nih.gov	Database produced by health-related agencies of the federal government; health information and health education resources
Various manufacturers of oral health care products	Search for home pages on the Internet	Product information and links to related dental sites

and patient education material. Table 25–8 lists some of these organizations.

Gingivitis

Periodontal disease, the prevalence and severity of which is related primarily to oral health care, remains the principal cause of tooth loss in adults older than 45 years.[2] Yet controlling buildup of plaque and calculus can prevent or control this common and significant public health problem. All forms of periodontal disease are associated with oral hygiene status, not with age. However, as lifespans increase and as people retain more teeth later in life, both the number of teeth at risk and the time for risk of periodontal disease increases.[1]

Gingivitis, a reversible and the mildest form of periodontal disease, affects nearly everyone. Gingivitis may progress to more severe periodontal diseases, such as acute necrotizing ulcerative gingivitis and periodontitis. The latter can cause significant, irreversible alveolar bone loss.

Acute necrotizing ulcerative gingivitis, also referred to as Vincent's stomatitis and trench mouth, is an acute bacterial infection characterized by necrosis and ulceration of the gingival surface with underlying inflammation. The disease may involve a single tooth, a group of teeth, or the entire oral cavity. Localized symptoms often include severe pain, bleeding gingival tissue, halitosis, foul taste, and increased salivation. Lymphadenopathy, fever, and malaise may accompany the localized symptoms.

Trench mouth is seen most frequently in the United States in teenagers and young adults. Predisposing factors include anxiety, emotional stress, smoking, malnutrition, and poor oral hygiene. Factors resulting in decreased host resistance that alter the host–bacteria relationship have been implicated.[72] Professional dental treatment is indicated and consists of local debridement and systemic drug therapy coupled with elimination of predisposing factors.

Periodontitis and gingivitis can be distinguished in the following way. Whereas gingivitis is the inflammation of the gingiva without loss or migration of epithelial attachment to the tooth, periodontitis occurs when the periodontal ligament attachment and alveolar bone support of the tooth have been compromised or lost.[73] This process involves apical migration of the epithelial attachment from the enamel to the root surface. (See the "Color Plates," photographs 3 and 4.)

Most adults with periodontitis have moderately progressing disease, and perhaps 10% have rapidly progressing disease. Patients have a good prognosis if an initial comprehensive course of therapy is successful. Unfortunately, in some cases, alveolar bone loss is irreversible. Prospects for disease control are not good if plaque and calculus control is poor or if resolution of inflammation is inadequate despite comprehensive treatment.[73]

Pharmacists can assist patients in preventing gingivitis and the more advanced periodontal diseases when they counsel patients on the selection of oral hygiene products and encourage patients to practice good oral hygiene.

Epidemiology of Gingivitis

Because caries and gingivitis can result from buildup of plaque, the epidemiology of caries can be extended to that of gingivitis. (See the section "Epidemiology of Caries.") In addition, hormonal changes influence gingivitis, thereby accounting for its increased frequency during puberty and pregnancy.

Pregnant patients are more susceptible to both dental caries and gingivitis.[74] An inflammatory condition so common that it is called pregnancy gingivitis is characterized by red, swollen gingival tissue that bleeds easily. This gingivitis is caused by local factors, as it is in any patient. Pregnancy modifies the host's response, however, making gingival tissue more sensitive to bacterial dental plaque. Hormone level or increased production of prostaglandins has been implicated in the heightened inflammatory response.[1] Pregnancy gingivitis can be prevented or resolved with thorough plaque control. The severity of the inflammatory response and the resulting gingivitis will decrease postpartum and will return to prepregnancy levels after approximately 1 year.

Pathophysiology/Signs and Symptoms of Gingivitis

The basic pathologic process of gingivitis is an inflammatory reaction caused by bacterial plaque. If dental plaque is not controlled, specific bacteria (first gram-positive cocci such as *S. sanguis* and *S. mitis* and later *Actinomyces* spp. and gram-negative organisms) colonize the gum tissue to produce the following symptoms: swelling, redness, changes in gum form and position, and bleeding (when gums are brushed or probed). Pink-tinted toothbrush bristles should be a sign to patients of possible gingivitis.

The marginal gingiva (the border of the gingiva surrounding the neck of the tooth) is held firmly to the tooth by a network of collagen fibers. Microorganisms present in the plaque in the gingival sulcus (the space between the gingiva and the tooth) are capable of producing harmful products, such as acids, toxins, and enzymes, that damage cellular and intercellular tissue. Dilatation and proliferation of gingival capillaries, increased flow of gingival fluid, and increased blood flow with resultant erythema of the gingiva are found in early stages. The gingiva may also enlarge, change contour, and appear puffy or swollen as a result of the inflammation. (See the "Color Plates," photograph 3.) In the early stage of gingivitis, the inflammatory process is reversible with effective oral hygiene.

In time and with neglect, the condition becomes chronic as capillaries become engorged, as venous return is slowed, and as localized anoxemia gives a bluish hue to areas of the reddened gingiva. Chronic gingivitis may be localized to the area around one or several teeth, or it may be generalized, involving the gingiva around all the teeth. The inflammation may involve just the marginal gingiva, or it may be more diffuse and may involve all the gingival tissue surrounding the tooth. Changes in gingival color, size, and shape, as well as ease of gingival bleeding, are common indications of chronic gingivitis that both the patient and the pharmacist can recognize. The flat knife-edge appearance of healthy gingiva is replaced by a ragged or rounded edge. The presence of red cells in extravascular tissue and the breakdown of hemoglobin also deepen the color of gingival tissue. Progression of these conditions is usually slow and insidious—and often painless.

Left untreated, chronic gingivitis may advance to the inflammatory condition of chronic destructive periodontal disease, or periodontitis. (See the "Color Plates," photograph 4.) Bacterial species that predominate in periodontitis but are not present in healthy periodontium have been found in low proportions in gingivitis. Progression of gingivitis may parallel the increasing proportions of bacterial species implicated in the genesis of periodontitis.

Etiology of Gingivitis

Gingivitis results from the accumulation of supragingival bacterial plaque.[75] If the accumulation of this plaque is not controlled, it proliferates and invades subgingival spaces. At the same time, as specific types of bacteria are associated with plaque at different stages of accumulation, the composition of the bacterial flora changes to a more complex mix of organisms.[76] The transition from supragingival to subgingival plaque accumulation is significant because the patient cannot remove the subgingival plaque adequately by mechanical means. Thus, the accumulation of supragingival plaque over time can eventually result in gingivitis. Although not all gingivitis progresses to periodontitis, the progression from supragingival plaque to gingivitis to periodontitis is relatively common, so that controlling gingivitis is a reasonable approach to limiting periodontitis.[1]

Gingivitis also may manifest as a result of (1) blood dyscrasias such as leukemia, (2) mucocutaneous diseases such as lichen planus, and (3) viral infections such as acute herpetic gingivostomatitis. And most important, disturbances of the immune system (as occur in AIDS) can lead to a severe form of this disease.[77]

Other possible etiologies include medications such as nifedipine, cyclosporine, and phenytoin. Anticholinergics and antidepressants may cause gingivitis by reducing flow of saliva. The use of tobacco (both smokeless and smoked) has also been linked to periodontal disease.

Prevention of Gingivitis

Because prevention of gingivitis and caries depends on calculus prevention and plaque control, the same measures described in the section "Prevention of Caries" pertains to gingivitis. The active antigingivitis ingredients in dentifrices, mouthrinses, and other plaque removal and antiplaque products are triclosan (an antibacterial ingredient recently introduced for its antigingivitis properties) and a stabilized stannous fluoride added for its antigingivitis and anticaries properties. Stannous fluoride inhibits the types of bacteria that infect supragingival spaces.[78] Triclosan is both an antiplaque and an anti-inflammatory agent; it inhibits production of prostaglandins by several means.[79]

Brushing and flossing can cure early gingivitis that arises from irritating food debris and plaque. Adequate removal and control of supragingival plaque is the single most important factor in reversing gingivitis and in preventing and controlling periodontal disease. Gum massage is also recommended, using such devices as soft brushes, special rubber cup massagers, a Stim-U-Dent, or toothpicks. Pharmacists should immediately refer for dental care any patient who describes bleeding during brushing or shows signs of early gingivitis.

Patient Assessment of Gingivitis

Before recommending oral hygiene products, the pharmacist should evaluate the patient's oral hygiene regimen. At a minimum, the pharmacist should find out whether the patient has a history of gingivitis, whether signs and symptoms of gingivitis are currently present, and what preventive measures the patient has tried or is using. Checking the patient's medical and medication history will identify asymptomatic patients who are at risk for gingivitis.

The pharmacist will quite often be alerted to pregnancy gingivitis during counseling on prescription prenatal vitamins. Besides monitoring the pregnant patient's medications for safety, the pharmacist has an opportunity to advise a dental checkup and careful attention to brushing and flossing to avoid oral health complications.

In addition to the questions in the section "Patient Assessment of Caries," the pharmacist should ask the following questions to determine whether gingivitis or the risk of the disorder is present and to recommend measures to prevent plaque buildup.

Q~ Do you have a history of gingivitis?

A~ *Identify predisposing factors for gingivitis. (See the sections "Epidemiology of Caries" and "Epidemiology of Gingivitis.")* Suspect that patients with a history of gingivitis have poor oral hygiene practices or predisposing factors for gingivitis.

Q~ Are you having any symptoms of gingivitis, such as bleeding during brushing of teeth? If so, how long has it been occurring?

A~ Refer any patient with symptoms of gingivitis to a dentist. Advise the patient that delayed treatment could result in a more serious disorder such as periodontitis.

Q~ (If female) Are you pregnant?

A~ If yes, advise the patient that hormonal changes increase the risk of gingivitis.

Patient Counseling for Gingivitis

Because gingivitis is usually not associated with pain, patients are unlikely to seek a pharmacist's advice for this problem alone. More likely patients will be asking for oral hygiene information and product recommendations. The pharmacist may have to suggest oral hygiene methods and to alert the patient to the possible adverse effects of certain products. The box "Patient Education for Prevention of Caries, Gingivitis, and Halitosis" lists specific information to provide patients.

The pharmacist should also use this opportunity to warn patients with suspected gingivitis (bleeding, swollen gums) that this disease is a serious problem that warrants professional attention. The pharmacist should stress, especially to pregnant patients, that adherence to an oral hygiene program is vital to preventing gingivitis.

Halitosis

Halitosis, an offensive odor emanating from the oral cavity, may be symptomatic of oral pathology. However, in 90% of cases, poor oral hygiene is the cause.

Pathophysiology of Halitosis

Most foul breath odors occur because of a breakdown of sulfur-containing proteins into volatile sulfur compounds by gram-negative bacteria in an alkaline environment. Some degree of oral malodor (e.g., morning breath) is normal in a healthy individual.[7]

Etiology of Halitosis

Common oral causes related to poor oral hygiene include odoriferous decaying food particles, cellular and nutritional debris, plaque-coated tongue, caries, bleeding gums, and periodontal disease. Xerostomia and stomatitis can also cause mouth odor. Other oral disorders, such as postsurgical states, purulent infections, and extraction wounds, can contribute to halitosis. Medications that have anticholinergic properties can result in dry mouth, which can lead to halitosis. Garlic can also cause halitosis but by a different mechanism. The use of tobacco (both smoked and smokeless) is another etiologic factor. Mouth odor in denture wearers is usually related to keeping dentures in the mouth at night or not cleaning them properly.

Pulmonary diseases that cause halitosis include purulent lung infections, tuberculosis, bronchiectasis, sinusitis, tonsillitis, and rhinitis. Renal failure, carcinoma, and hepatic failure can also cause mouth odor. Other non-oral causes include the elimination of chemical substances from the blood through the lungs on exhalation. Examples include alcoholic breath or acetone breath in patients with severe hyperglycemic diabetes.

Prevention of Halitosis

Prevention of halitosis relies on the removal of plaque and the prevention of calculus formation as described in the section "Prevention of Caries." In addition to brushing the teeth and tongue and to flossing regularly, drinking at least eight 8-ounce glasses of water a day will help to prevent mouth odor.

Any patient who complains of severe or lingering halitosis without a readily identifiable cause (e.g., smoking) should be advised to see a dentist for a thorough evaluation. Masking foul taste and odor with cosmetic mouthrinses may delay necessary dental or medical assessment and any needed treatment.

Patient Assessment of Halitosis

When assessing a patient for halitosis, the pharmacist should evaluate the patient's dental hygiene. Ideally, the pharmacist would obtain a medication and medical history to determine whether the halitosis might arise from one of the illnesses discussed in the section "Etiology of Halitosis." (See also the section "Xerostomia" in Chapter 26, "Oral Pain and Discomfort.")

Asking the patient the questions in the sections "Patient Assessment of Caries" and "Patient Assessment of Gingivitis" will help to determine whether the patient's oral hygiene is adequate and whether the risk for periodontal disease exists. The following questions will help elicit the information needed to recommend the appropriate treatment approach and to determine whether the halitosis is related to other causes.

Q~ Does your mouth feel abnormally dry?

A~ If yes, evaluate the patient further for xerostomia. (See the section "Xerostomia" in Chapter 26, "Oral Pain and Discomfort.")

Q~ Have you recently had dental surgery or a tooth extraction?

A~ If yes, refer the patient to a dentist or endodontist for reevaluation of the dental procedures.

Q~ Do you have any soreness, swelling, redness, or pus-filled sores in your mouth?

A~ If yes, refer the patient to a dentist for evaluation of possible gingivitis, inflammation, or infection.

Q~ Do you wear dentures? If so, do you remove your dentures at night? How do you clean them?

A~ Advise patients that sleeping with the dentures in can cause mouth odor. If needed, advise the patient on proper cleaning of dentures. (See the section "Prevention of Hygiene-Related Denture Problems.")

Q~ Do you have conditions such as lung infection or inflammation, tuberculosis, sinusitis, tonsillitis, and rhinitis?

A~ Advise the patient that these conditions can cause mouth odor and that resolution of the condition may eliminate the mouth odor.

Patient Counseling for Halitosis

For patients with mouth odor related to poor dental hygiene, the pharmacist should recommend the appropriate products and should explain their use. Nondrug measures should also be explained. The pharmacist should stress to patients whose mouth odor is related to medical conditions that proper oral hygiene is still necessary to prevent tooth and gum problems. The box "Patient Education for Prevention of Caries, Gingivitis, and Halitosis" lists specific information to provide patients.

Hygiene-Related Denture Problems

Pain along the gingival ridge under a denture prosthesis suggests conditions such as denture stomatitis (an inflammation of the oral tissue in contact with a removable denture), inflammatory papillary hyperplasia, and chronic candidiasis. Denture stomatitis, which results from poor cleaning of dentures, can lead to chronic candidiasis.

Etiology/Pathophysiology of Hygiene-Related Denture Problems

Dentures accumulate plaque, stain, and calculus by a process very similar to the process occurring on natural teeth.[80] The denture plaque mass in contact with oral tissues produces predictable toxic results. Poor denture hygiene contributes to fungal and bacterial growth and so not only affects the patient aesthetically (unpleasant odors and staining) but also seriously affects the patient's oral health (inflammation and mucosal disease) and ability to wear the dentures successfully.[81]

Chronic atrophic candidiasis, sometimes referred to as denture stomatitis or denture sore mouth, is common in patients with full or partial dentures. This condition may be attributed to infection with *Candida albicans*, which can be found resident on the denture base.[66] Symptomatically, the inflamed denture-bearing area may appear granular or erythematous and edematous with soreness or a burning sensation.[81] (See the "Color Plates," photograph 5.) Inflammation secondary to *Candida* organisms is generalized to the entire denture-bearing tissue area, whereas inflammation secondary to the trauma of ill-fitting dentures is usually localized to the specific area of the trauma. It appears that the candidal organisms either adhere to the denture material or reside in pores of the denture material and can reinfect the mouth.[66] Failure to remove the denture at bedtime and to clean it regularly worsens this condition. Angular cheilitis is commonly associated with chronic atrophic candidiasis and other forms of oral candidiasis.[81]

Prevention of Hygiene-Related Denture Problems

Removing plaque from dentures helps prevent gum infections, staining of dentures, and mouth odor. Specialty brushes and aids are available to remove plaque from hard-to-clean areas (e.g., spaces around a fixed bridge, implants, or orthodontic bands) and dentures. Dentures should be cleaned thoroughly at least once daily to remove unsightly stain, debris, and potentially harmful plaque. Abrasive and chemical cleansers formulated specifically for dentures are available. (See Table 25–9 for examples of these products.) A combination regimen of brushing dentures with an abrasive cleaner and soaking them in a chemical cleanser is recommended.[82]

Abrasive Denture Cleansers

Denture (paste or powder) cleansers containing mild abrasives (e.g., calcium carbonate) must be applied properly with specialty brushes adapted to the denture's contour to remove stains, plaque, and calculus. Overly vigorous scrubbing can abrade the acrylic materials of dentures and can bend the metal clasps. To prevent irritation of oral tissues, the patient should rinse the abrasive cleaner thoroughly from the denture.

The brushing routine can be followed by soaking the denture in an alkaline peroxide cleansing solution to help remove remaining plaque and bacteria. Plaque removal is then enhanced by brushing the denture after it has soaked; instructions for doing so are included on some products.[83]

Chemical Denture Cleansers

The other method of cleaning is to use a soaking solution containing one of the three chemical cleansers: alkaline hypochlorite, alkaline peroxide, or dilute acids.

Alkaline peroxide cleaners are the most commonly used chemical denture cleansers. These powders or tablets become alkaline solutions of hydrogen peroxide when dissolved. The ingredients are alkaline detergents and perborates, the latter of which cause oxygen release for a mechanical cleaning effect. These products are most effective on new plaque and stains that are soaked for 4 to 8 hours. The alkaline peroxides have few serious disadvantages and do not damage the surface of acrylic resins.[83]

Alkaline hypochlorites (bleach) remove stains, dissolve mucin, and are both bactericidal and fungicidal. Denture plaque consists of cells embedded in a matrix that serves as a surface on which calculus may develop. Hypochlorite cleansers act directly on the organic plaque matrix to dissolve its structure, but they cannot dissolve calculus once formed.[83] The most serious disadvantage of hypochlorite is that it corrodes metal denture components such as the framework and clasps of removable partial dentures, solder joints, and possibly the pins holding the teeth.[66] The addition of anticorrosive phosphate compounds has greatly reduced this effect, but these products should be used for 15-minute soaks to limit exposure[83] and should not be used more often than once a week.

Acid-containing soaking solutions can also be corrosive to metals, and short soaking times in these solutions are recommended. A sonic or ultrasonic cleaning device when used with a commercially prepared solution is easier to use and cleans more effectively than soaking alone. However, some hand brushing may still be required.

Table 25–9

Selected Denture Cleansers

Trade Name	Primary Ingredients
Ban-A-Stain Liquid	Phosphoric acid 25%
Dentu-Cream Paste	Dicalcium phosphate dihydrate; calcium carbonate; aluminum silicate
Efferdent Antibacterial Tablets	Sodium carbonate; sodium bicarbonate; potassium monopersulfate; sodium perborate
Efferdent Plus Tablets	Sodium bicarbonate; sodium perborate; potassium monopersulfate; detergents
Efferdent 2 Layer Tablets	Sodium bicarbonate; sodium carbonate; potassium monopersulfate; detergents

Precautions

All denture-cleansing products should be completely rinsed off the denture before insertion. Abrasive cleansers coming in contact with oral or other mucous membranes may cause tissue irritation. Chemical cleansers may cause tissue irritation or possibly severe chemical burns.[83] All denture cleansers should be kept out of the reach of children because of the potential for eye or skin irritation or for toxicity from accidental ingestion.[83] A dentist should evaluate stains that are resistant to proper denture brushing and soaking in available solutions.[83]

Unapproved Denture Cleaners

Only products specifically formulated for denture cleansing should be used. Household cleansers (used for soaking) are not appropriate and may either be ineffective or damage denture material. The use of whitening toothpastes meant for natural dentition should be discouraged because their abrasivity is too high for them to be used safely on denture material.

Patients should not soak or clean dentures in hot water or hot soaking solutions because distortion or warping may occur.

Product Selection Guidelines

Geriatric or handicapped patients may prefer an alkaline peroxide soak solution for daily, overnight cleaning. Alkaline peroxide cleansers do not corrode metal components of dentures as do alkaline hypochlorite and acid cleansers.

Patient Assessment of Hygiene-Related Denture Problems

Before recommending any type of oral hygiene product, the pharmacist should determine what denture care measures the patient is taking and whether those measures are adequate. At a minimum, the pharmacist should find out whether the patient suffers from denture stomatitis or from inflammation secondary to ill-fitting dentures.

Asking the patient the following questions will help elicit the information needed to accurately assess the disorder and to recommend the appropriate treatment approach.

Q~ Do you have a bad taste in your mouth? How do you clean your dentures? How often?

A~ Evaluate the effectiveness of the patient's denture hygiene measures. If inadequate, suspect the problem is related to hygiene. Recommend the appropriate hygiene measures.

Q~ Are your dentures loose? Do you have sore spots?

A~ If yes to these questions, suspect that ill-fitting dentures are the cause of the problem. Refer the patient to a dentist for evaluation of the dentures and their fit.

Q~ Is the entire area under the denture painful?

A~ If yes, suspect denture stomatitis caused by poor hygiene. Refer the patient to a dentist for evaluation of the disorder. Recommend appropriate denture hygiene measures to prevent recurrences.

Q~ How long have you worn dentures? Did you have problems with mouth irritation or infection before you needed dentures?

A~ If denture wear began recently, suspect that fit is the problem. Refer the patient to a dentist for evaluation of the dentures. If the patient had mouth irritation or infection before wearing dentures, suspect an underlying pathology. Refer the patient to a dentist or physician.

Patient Counseling for Hygiene-Related Denture Problems

Denture wearers may tend to blame any oral discomfort on the appliances, rather than on their hygiene regimen. The pharmacist should stress that diligent plaque removal from dentures is the key to preventing denture stomatitis. The methods of cleaning dentures, including their advantages and disadvantages, should be explained. Using the patient's preferences, the pharmacist should recommend a denture cleanser and should reinforce the methods of use. The box "Patient Education for Hygiene-Related Denture Problems" lists specific information to provide patients.

Patient Education for Hygiene-Related Denture Problems

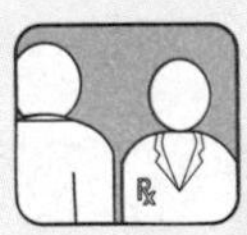

The objective of self-care is to prevent bacterial or fungal infections of the mouth by removing plaque from the dentures. For most patients, carefully following product instructions and the self-care measures listed below will help ensure good denture hygiene.

- Clean dentures thoroughly at least once daily to remove unsightly stain, debris, and potentially harmful plaque.
- Preferably, brush dentures with an abrasive cleaner, and then soak them in a chemical cleanser. This combination regimen is more effective in removing plaque and bacteria.
- Apply the abrasive cleaner to the denture, using a brush designed to adapt to the denture's contour.
- Do not scrub the denture surface vigorously; such action can abrade the acrylic materials and bend the metal clasps.
- To prevent irritation of oral tissues, rinse the abrasive cleaner thoroughly from the denture.
- After brushing the dentures, soak them in an alkaline peroxide cleansing solution for 4 to 8 hours. Rinse the dentures thoroughly to avoid chemical burns of the mouth.
- If possible, brush the dentures again, and rinse them thoroughly.
- Note that alkaline peroxide cleansers cannot damage the denture as can alkaline hypochlorite or dilute acid (phosphoric acid) cleansers.
- If using an alkaline peroxide or acid cleanser, soak the dentures for only 15 minutes to avoid corrosion of metal denture components.
- Keep all denture cleansers out of the reach of children. These agents can cause eye or skin irritation or toxicity if accidentally ingested.
- Do not use household cleansers or whitening toothpastes to clean dentures. These agents may damage denture material.
- Do not soak or clean dentures in hot water or hot soaking solutions. Distortion or warping of the denture may occur.
- Do not sleep with your dentures in. Decreased levels of saliva during sleep may contribute to plaque buildup on the denture.

⚠ If the mouth becomes sore or shows sign of infection, see a dentist.

CONCLUSIONS

For prevention of caries, plaque removal products, products containing anticaries ingredients, and products with antigingivitis/antiplaque ingredients are indicated. Preventive measures aimed at the oral plaque diseases (dental caries, gingivitis, periodontal disease) are largely under the patient's control. Meeting dental health care needs of the public is a responsibility shared by the patient, dentist, dental hygienist, and pharmacist. Given that the pharmacy is the source for nonprescription products intended to prevent oral plaque–related diseases, the pharmacist has an opportunity to educate the patient about consumer advertising, clinical data, FDA regulations, and ADA acceptance guidelines. Pharmacists can also offer their patients assessment, including disease states and medication profile, triage, referral to a dental professional if necessary, or proper instruction on self-care with nonprescription products proven to be safe and efficacious. With open lines of communication to dental practitioners, pharmacists can better serve their patients as oral health consultants and members of the dental health care team.

References

1. Harris NO, Garcia-Godoy F. *Primary Preventive Dentistry.* 5th ed. Stamford, Conn: Appleton & Lange; 1999:64–9,88–9,110,115–6,145, 177,206,361,381,426,435,564–5.
2. Gluck GM, Morganstein WM, eds. *Jong's Community Dental Health.* 4th ed. St. Louis: Mosby-Year Book Inc; 1998:127–33.
3. Niessen LC, Williams GC. Aging in America: Implications for dentistry. *Pharm Times.* 1988;54:36–40.
4. Glover ED, Edmundson EW, Edwards SW, et al. Implications of smokeless tobacco use among athletes. *Physician and Sportsmedicine.* 1986;14: 95–104.
5. Smith RW, Staff of the Columbia School of Dental and Oral Surgery. *Columbia University Guide to Family Dental Care.* WW Norton & Co: New York; 1997:87–8.
6. McHugh WD. Role of supragingival plaque in oral disease initiation and progression. In: Loe H, Kleinman DV, eds. *Dental Plaque Control Measures and Oral Hygiene Practices.* Oxford, England: IRL Press; 1986: 1–12.
7. Pader M. *Oral Hygiene Products and Practice.* New York: Marcel Dekker, Inc; 1988:45–59,89,101,226–8,333–8,426–53,489–504.
8. Greenwell H, Bissada NF, Wittwer JW. Periodontics in general practice: Professional plaque control. *J Am Dent Assoc.* 1990;121:642–6.
9. Low SB, Ciancio SG. Reviewing nonsurgical periodontal therapy. *J Am Dent Assoc.* 1990;121:467–70.
10. Kidd EAM, Joyston-Bechal S. *Essentials of Dental Caries.* Bristol, England: IOP Publishing Ltd; 1987:3–15,82.
11. Bar A. Caries prevention with xylitol. *World Rev Nutr Diet.* 1988;55: 1–27.
12. *Federal Register.* 1996 August 23;61:43433–47.
13. Marsh PD. Dentifrices containing new agents for the control of plaque and gingivitis: microbiological aspects. *J Clin Periodontol.* 1991;18: 462–7.
14. Hogg SD. Chemical control of plaque. *Dent Update.* 1990;17:330,332–4.
15. *Federal Register.* 1995 October 6; 60:52474,52479–82,52508.
16. Sears C. Baking soda toothpastes. *Am Health.* 1994;13:19.
17. A guide to good dental care. *Consumer Rep.* 1992;57:602–4.
18. van der Ouderaa F, Cummins D. Anti-plaque dentifrices: Current status and prospects. *Int Dent J.* 1991;41:117–23.
19. Glass RL. Fluoride dentifrices: The basis for the decline in caries prevalence. *J R Soc Med.* 1986;79(suppl 14):15–7.
20. American Dental Association. *ADA Statement on the Safety of Hydrogen-Peroxide-Containing Dental Products Intended for Home Use.* Chicago: American Dental Association; 1997.
21. Cubbon T, Ore D. Hard tissue and home tooth whiteners. *CDS Rev.* 1991;84:32–5.
22. Howard WR. Patient-applied tooth whiteners: Are they safe, effective with supervision? *J Am Dent Assoc.* 1992;123:57–60.
23. Council on Scientific Affairs. *Products of Excellence ADA Seal Program.* Chicago: American Dental Association; 1998.
24. Council on Dental Therapeutics. Council on Dental Therapeutics accepts Extra-Strength Aim. *J Am Dent Assoc.* 1988;117:785.
25. Mandel ID. The new toothpastes. *Texas Dent J.* 1998; December:8–13.
26. White DJ. A "return" to stannous fluoride dentifrices. *J Clin Dent* (special issue). 1995;6:29–36.
27. Council on Scientific Affairs. *Guidelines for Acceptance of Chemotherapeutic Products for the Control of Gingivitis.* Chicago: American Dental Association; 1997.
28. Lobene RR, Soparkar PM, Newman MB, et al. Reduced formation of supragingival calculus with the use of fluoride–zinc chloride dentifrice. *J Am Dent Assoc.* 1987;114:350.
29. Zacherl WA, Pfeiffer HJ, Swancar JR. The effect of soluble pyrophosphates on dental calculus in adults. *J Am Dent Assoc.* 1985;110:737–8.
30. Naleway CA, Whall CW Jr. What benefits do tartar control dentifrices provide your patrons? *Pharm Times.* 1987;53:32–7.
31. Beacham BE, Kurgansky D, Gould WM. Circumoral dermatitis and cheilitis caused by tartar control dentifrices. *J Am Acad Dermatol.* 1990;22:1029–32.
32. Balanyk TE. Sanguinarine: comparisons of antiplaque/antigingivitis reports. *Clin Prev Dent.* 1990;12:18–25.
33. Ripa LW. A critique of topical fluoride methods (dentifrices, mouthrinses, operator- and self-applied gels) in an era of decreased caries and increased fluorosis prevalence. *J Public Health Dent.* 1991;51: 23–41.
34. Mueller LJ et al. Rotary electric toothbrushing: Clinical effects on the presence of gingivitis and supragingival dental plaque. *Dent Hyg.* 1987;613:546–50.
35. Lazarus G. Colgate's smile still bright in toothbrush sales. *Chicago Tribune.* March 27, 1995;4:2.
36. Toothbrush may be link to sore throat, infections. *Med World News.* 1986 March 10;27:68.
37. Mandel ID. The plaque fighters: Choosing a weapon. *J Am Dent Assoc.* 1993;124:71–4.
38. Bratel J, Berggren U, Hirsch JM. Electric or manual toothbrush? *Clin Prev Dent.* 1988;10:23–6.
39. Council on Dental Therapeutics. *Accepted Dental Therapeutics.* 40th ed. Chicago: American Dental Association; 1984:64–5,79,321–4,386–8, 395–420.
40. Carranza FA Jr. *Glickman's Clinical Periodontology.* 7th ed. Philadelphia: WB Saunders Co; 1990:706.
41. Lamberts DM, Wunderlich RC, Caffesse RG. The effect of waxed and unwaxed dental floss on gingival health: Part I. Plaque removal and gingival response. *J Periodontol.* 1982;53:393–9.
42. Hill HC, Levi PA, Glickman I. The effects of waxed and unwaxed dental floss on interdental plaque accumulation and interdental gingival health. *J Periodontol.* 1973;44:411–3.
43. Perry DA, Pattison G. An investigation of wax residue on tooth surfaces after the use of waxed dental floss. *Dent Hyg.* 1986;60:16–9.
44. Kiger RD, Nylund K, Feller RP. A comparison of proximal plaque removal using floss and interdental brushes. *J Clin Periodontol.* 1991;18: 681–4.
45. Frandsen A. Mechanical oral hygiene practices. In: Loe H, Kleinman DV, eds. *Dental Plaque Control Measures and Oral Hygiene Practices.* Oxford, England: IRL Press; 1986:100.
46. Newman MG, Cattabriga M, Etienne D, et al. Effectiveness of adjunctive irrigation in early periodontitis—multi-center evaluation. *J Periodontol.* 1994;65:224–9.
47. Greenstein G. Effects of subgingival irrigation on periodontal status. *J Periodontol.* 1987;58:827–36.
48. Controlling plaque limits periodontal disease. *US Pharm.* 1987;12:70–6.
49. *Federal Register.* 1990 September 19;55:38560–2.
50. *Federal Register.* 1994 February 9;59:6084.
51. *Federal Register.* 1982 May 25;47:22809,22842–4.

52. Mandel ID. Antimicrobial mouthrinses—overview and update. *J Am Dent Assoc.* 1994;125:S2–S10.
53. Gossel TA. Counseling the consumer on antiplaque mouthrinses. *US Pharm.* 1988;13:46–8,51.
54. Moran J, Addy M. The effects of a cetylpyridinium chloride prebrushing rinse as an adjunct to oral hygiene and gingival health. *J Periodontol.* 1991;62:562–4.
55. Bailey L. The effect of a detergent-based pre-brushing dental rinse on plaque accumulation. *J Clin Dent.* 1990;II:6–10.
56. Emling RC, Yankell SL. An analysis of the clinical plaque removal efficacy of a pre-brushing dental rinse in a three center study design. *J Clin Dent.* 1990;II:11–6.
57. Grossman E. Effectiveness of a prebrushing mouthrinse under single-trial and home-use conditions. *Clin Prev Dent.* 1988;10:3–6.
58. Beiswanger BB, Mallatt ME, Mau MS, et al. The relative plaque removal effect of a prebrushing mouthrinse. *J Am Dent Assoc.* 1990;120:190–2.
59. Freitas BL, Collaert B, Attstrom R. Effect of the pre-brushing rinse, Plax, on dental plaque formation. *J Clin Periodontol.* 1991;18:713–5.
60. Schiff TS, Border LC. The effect of a new experimental prebrushing dental rinse on plaque removal. *J Clin Dent.* 1994;4:107–10.
61. *Federal Register.* 1995 January;60:4536–41.
62. *NDMA Executive Newsletter.* 1994;43:2.
63. *NDMA Executive Newsletter.* 1996;12:1.
64. Consensus: Oral health effects of products that increase salivary flow rate. *J Am Dent Assoc.* 1988;116:757.
65. NIH consensus development conference: Health implications of smokeless tobacco use. *Am Pharm.* 1986;26:18–20.
66. Abelson DC. Denture plaque and denture cleansers: Review of the literature. *Gerodontics.* 1985;1:202–6.
67. Fluoride: still a good public health value. *Pharm Times.* 1990;56:105–7,111.
68. Adair SM. Risks and benefits of fluoride mouthrinsing. *Pediatrician.* 1989;16:161–9.
69. *Federal Register.* 1985 September 30;50:39859,39872.
70. Baker KA, Levy SM. Review of systemic fluoride supplementation and consideration of the pharmacist's role. *Drug Intell Clin Pharm.* 1986;20:935–42.
71. Jakush J. New fluoride schedule adopted. *ADA News.* 1994 May 16:12,14.
72. Pinkham JR. *Pediatric Dentistry: Infancy through Adolescence.* Philadelphia: WB Saunders Co; 1988:507–8.
73. Genco RJ, Goldman HM, Cohen DW, eds. *Contemporary Periodontics.* St. Louis: CV Mosby; 1990:63–81,348–59.
74. Klatell J, Kaplan A, Williams G Jr. *Family Guide to Dental Health.* New York: Macmillan; 1991:37,83.
75. Barrington EP, Nevins M. Diagnosing periodontal diseases. *J Am Dent Assoc.* 1990;121:460–4.
76. Loe H. The specific etiology of periodontal disease and its application to prevention. In: Carranza FA Jr, Kenney EB, eds. *Prevention of Periodontal Disease.* Chicago: Quintessence Pub Co; 1981.
77. Eisen DE, Lynch DP. *The Mouth; Diagnosis and Treatment.* Mosby: St. Louis; 1998.
78. Mengel R, Wissing E, Smitz-Habben A, Flores-de-Jacoby L. Comparative study of plaque and gingivitis prevention by AmF/SnF2 and NaF. A clinical and microbiological 9-month study. *J Clin Periodont.* 1996;23:372–8.
79. Modeer T, Bengtsson A, Rolla G. Triclosan reduces prostaglandin biosynthesis in human gingival fibroblasts challenged with interleukin-1 in vitro. *J Clin Periodont.* 1996;10:927–33.
80. Gossel TA. Counseling patients on denture cleansing products. *US Pharm.* 1988;13:56–8,61–2,76.
81. Budtz-Jorgensen E, Bertraum U. Denture stomatitis: I. The etiology in relation to trauma and infection. *Acta Odontol Scand.* 1970;28:71–92.
82. Zacharczenko N. Dentures and denture care. *Pharm Times.* 1991;57:42.
83. Council on Dental Materials, Instruments, and Equipment. Denture cleansers. *J Am Dent Assoc.* 1983;106:77–9.

CHAPTER 26

Oral Pain and Discomfort

Chapter 26 at a Glance

Editor's Note: This chapter is based, in part, on the 11th edition chapter titled "Oral Health Products," which was written by Arlene A. Flynn.

Everyone has experienced oral pain and discomfort. Pain can accompany many common oral problems. Different features of pain indicate different underlying problems. Tooth pain that is triggered or worsened by stimuli such as heat, cold, or pressure on biting will often indicate a pulpal response to deep carious lesions or a cracked or broken tooth. Continuous tooth pain may indicate a pulpal infection and necrosis, an abscess, or a serious periodontal disease. Fever, malaise, and swelling may indicate an oral abscess; a patient who exhibits such symptoms should be referred to a dentist for immediate professional care.

Similarly, pain in the mucosa of the oral cavity and lips can be traced to a spectrum of causes, ranging from mouth injury to recurrent aphthous stomatitis (canker sores) and herpes simplex labialis (cold sores). Some of these problems are self-limiting and may be treated with nonprescription palliatives. By distinguishing the patient's self-treatable problems from those potentially requiring professional care, the pharmacist plays an important advisory role in oral health care.

Orofacial Pain

Self-treatable orofacial pain includes tooth hypersensitivity and teething pain. Resolution of pain associated with toothache and ill-fitting dentures requires professional dental care. Although denture adhesives are available as nonprescription products, their use can delay treatment and can worsen the condition. Ill-fitting dentures and loose, misfitting, or broken removable dental prostheses (partial or full dentures) can also contribute to accelerated bone loss, ulceration, irritation, tumorous growths, and compromised oral function. Refitting, relining, or repairing dentures to ensure proper functioning requires professional dental treatment.

Toothache and Tooth Hypersensitivity

Varying degrees of pulp injury cause toothache. The mildest form is called hypersensitivity. Tooth hypersensitivity (as distinguished from toothache) affects approximately 40 million adults at some time, and about one-fourth of these adults experience a chronic condition.[1]

Etiology/Pathophysiology of Toothache and Tooth Hypersensitivity

Hypersensitive teeth result from exposed areas of the root at the cementoenamel junction. (See the section "Anatomy and Physiology of the Oral Cavity" in Chapter 25, "Prevention of Hygiene-Related Oral Disorders," for a discussion of tooth anatomy.) Exposed dentin allows stimuli (heat, cold, percussion, acid) to reach the nerve fibers within the pulp. These irritations do not damage the pulp. But pain may be intense and may condition patients to limit oral hygiene, which, in turn, contributes to plaque accumulation and the progression of oral plaque diseases.[2] Causes of dentinal hypersensitivity may relate to a postsurgical condition, braces, gum recession, trauma, or excessive brushing with an abrasive dentifrice or hard-bristle brush.

The next levels of injury involve further exposure or loss of dentin. If left untreated, dental caries will progress to destroy the barrier of enamel and dentin, allowing bacteria to reach the pulp. The inflammatory response to bacteria in the pulp (called pulpitis) will stimulate free nerve endings, resulting in pulpalgia, or common toothache.

Patients with poor oral hygiene practices or systemic illness may be prone to dental decay and toothaches. Although toothache usually indicates dental pathology involving the tooth substance, dental pulp, or supporting periodontium, pain may also be referred to the teeth from the sinuses, eyes, or ears. Often acute sinusitis is precipitated by cold viruses, and the toothache is resolved soon after recovery from the cold by drainage of the sinuses. Other nondental causes of toothache include facial neuralgia, vitamin deficiencies, herpes zoster (facial shingles), and cluster headaches.

Signs and Symptoms of Toothache and Tooth Hypersensitivity

Whereas the pain of tooth hypersensitivity tends to be short and stabbing, the pain of pulpitis is lasting and throbbing. Pulpitis can be either reversible (after removing decay and filling the tooth) or irreversible (requiring root canal therapy). Pain that is intermittent often indicates viable pulp with reversible damage. But pain that is continuous and throbbing usually indicates irreversible pulp damage.

Sensitivity to hot and cold is normal in the weeks following the filling of a tooth. It also occurs as a result of clenching teeth and from gumline grooves formed by abrasive or inappropriate toothbrushing technique. This problem reverses after cessation of these activities. If a cold drink relieves the pain of a tooth that is sensitive to heat only, that tooth's nerve probably has been damaged.

When dental nerves become inflamed, quite often the ligament that attaches the root to its bony socket becomes inflamed. This situation results in chewing (biting) sensitivity. If the sensitivity on tapping the tooth is not mild but rather a sharp, acute ache, then a serious condition (infection of the nerve and inflammation of the ligament at the root) is indicated. Even if the pain later disappears, the nerve is further degenerating and an abscess or granuloma may be forming.

Treatment of Toothache and Tooth Hypersensitivity

Effective nonprescription oral products are available for treating tooth hypersensitivity. Self-treatment of toothache, however, is limited to use of oral and topical analgesics for temporary pain relief until the source of the problem is corrected.

Treatment Outcomes

The goals of self-treating tooth hypersensitivity are to (1) repair the damaged tooth surface using the appropriate toothpastes and (2) stop abrasive toothbrushing practices.

General Treatment Approach

The patient with a toothache should be advised to seek professional dental assistance. The presence of swelling or fever usually indicates the need for antibiotic therapy.

If the patient wears a removable prosthesis that attaches to the painful tooth, removing the appliance may help temporarily. Nonprescription internal analgesics such as ibuprofen, aspirin, or acetaminophen may be taken for short-term pain relief until a dentist corrects the problem. (See Chapter 3, "Headache and Muscle and Joint Pain" for discussion of these agents.) None of these products—and particularly not aspirin—should ever be placed locally on gingival tissue or in a cavity; doing so can result in chemical burns of sensitive tissue. (See the "Color Plates," photograph 6.) For temporary relief, nonprescription topical anesthetic products containing lidocaine or benzocaine may also be used. (See the section "Topical Oral Anesthetics" under "Treatment of Recurrent Aphthous Stomatitis" for a discussion of these agents.) Patients with allergy to "caine" anesthetics should use other topical products. Such drugs are also indicated for posttreatment pain associated with tooth extractions or root canals.

The American Dental Association (ADA) has not accepted eugenol or clove oil as safe and effective nonprescription drugs for toothache. These drugs are generally ineffective in the hands of the patient and can cause damage to viable pulp and soft tissue.

In addition to toothache, exclusions to self-care with nonprescription oral products include mouth soreness associated with poor-fitting dentures; the presence of fever or swelling; loose teeth; bleeding gums in the absence of trauma; broken or knocked-out teeth; severe tooth pain triggered or worsened by hot, cold, or chewing; and trauma to the mouth with bleeding, swelling, and soreness.

Once a dentist has diagnosed tooth hypersensitivity, the patient should brush with a desensitization toothpaste. A single application of these toothpastes has no effect; for some patients, long-term use may be necessary to relieve the symptoms. Figure 26–1 outlines the self-treatment of tooth hypersensitivity.

Nonpharmacologic Therapy

Ice may provide temporary relief for toothaches, but not all toothaches respond to it. Heat from hot packs may cause the bacterial infection to spread and, therefore, is contraindicated. If the tooth is infected, hot or sweet foods will exacerbate the problem. Patients should be advised not to delay treatment of a toothache even if nondrug measures provide relief.

For diagnosed tooth hypersensitivity at or near a receding gumline, flexible gum stimulators with or without densensitizing toothpastes can help.

Pharmacologic Therapy

Patients with hypersensitive teeth may get pain relief from brushing less vigorously with a standard fluoride toothpaste and a soft-bristled brush. If these measures do not relieve the sensitivity after 5 to 7 days, special desensitizing toothpastes containing potassium nitrate, strontium chloride, or potassium chloride are available. Two well-controlled clinical studies and three supportive studies provided sufficient data to the Food and Drug Administration (FDA) to establish the effectiveness of 5% potassium nitrate for protection against painful sensitivity of the teeth caused by cold, heat, acids, sweets, or contact. As a tooth desensitizer, 5% potassium nitrate remains the only Category I agent at this time.[3] Dibasic sodium citrate in pluronic gel and 10% strontium chloride were classified as Category III pending further evidence of effectiveness. FDA has proposed a Category I classification for the combination of a Category I fluoride ingredient with a 5% potassium nitrate to be used to relieve dentinal hypersensitivity and to prevent dental caries.[4] Such a combination product would be a good recommendation. Table 26–1 lists examples of commercial products currently available.

Mechanism of Action/Indication A tooth desensitizer acts on the dentin to block the perception of stimuli that are not usually perceived by subjects with normal teeth. Because the most common cause of tooth sensitivity is exposed dentin, a desensitizing dentifrice must inhibit sensitization while being nonabrasive.

Dosage/Administration Guidelines For optimum effectiveness, patients should apply at least a 1-inch strip of dentifrice to a soft-bristle brush and use the product twice daily. Brushing thoroughly for at least 1 minute will apply the desensitizing agent to all sensitive surfaces. Onset of effect is not immediate and may take several days to 2 weeks. These dentifrices should be used until the sensitivity subsides or as long as a dentist recommends. The patient should then switch to a low-abrasion dentifrice. In about 25% of adults, hypersensitive teeth are a chronic problem and require long-term treatment.

Contraindications/Precautions/Warnings Dentifrices containing 5% potassium nitrate are not recommended for children younger than 12 years. Patients with hypersensitive teeth should be cautioned against using high-abrasion toothpastes such as cosmetic pastes that whiten or remove stains.

Product Selection Guidelines The best choice of products at present is limited to either a desensitization toothpaste containing the only Category I agent, 5% potassium nitrate, or a combination product containing this desensitizing agent and fluoride. FDA has proposed a Category I classification for this combination product. Such a product relieves dentinal hypersensitivity and prevents dental caries, making it a good recommendation.

Patient Assessment of Toothache and Tooth Hypersensitivity

Before recommending self-treatment of tooth pain, the pharmacist should find out whether a dentist has diagnosed the cause. The pharmacist should also find out whether the

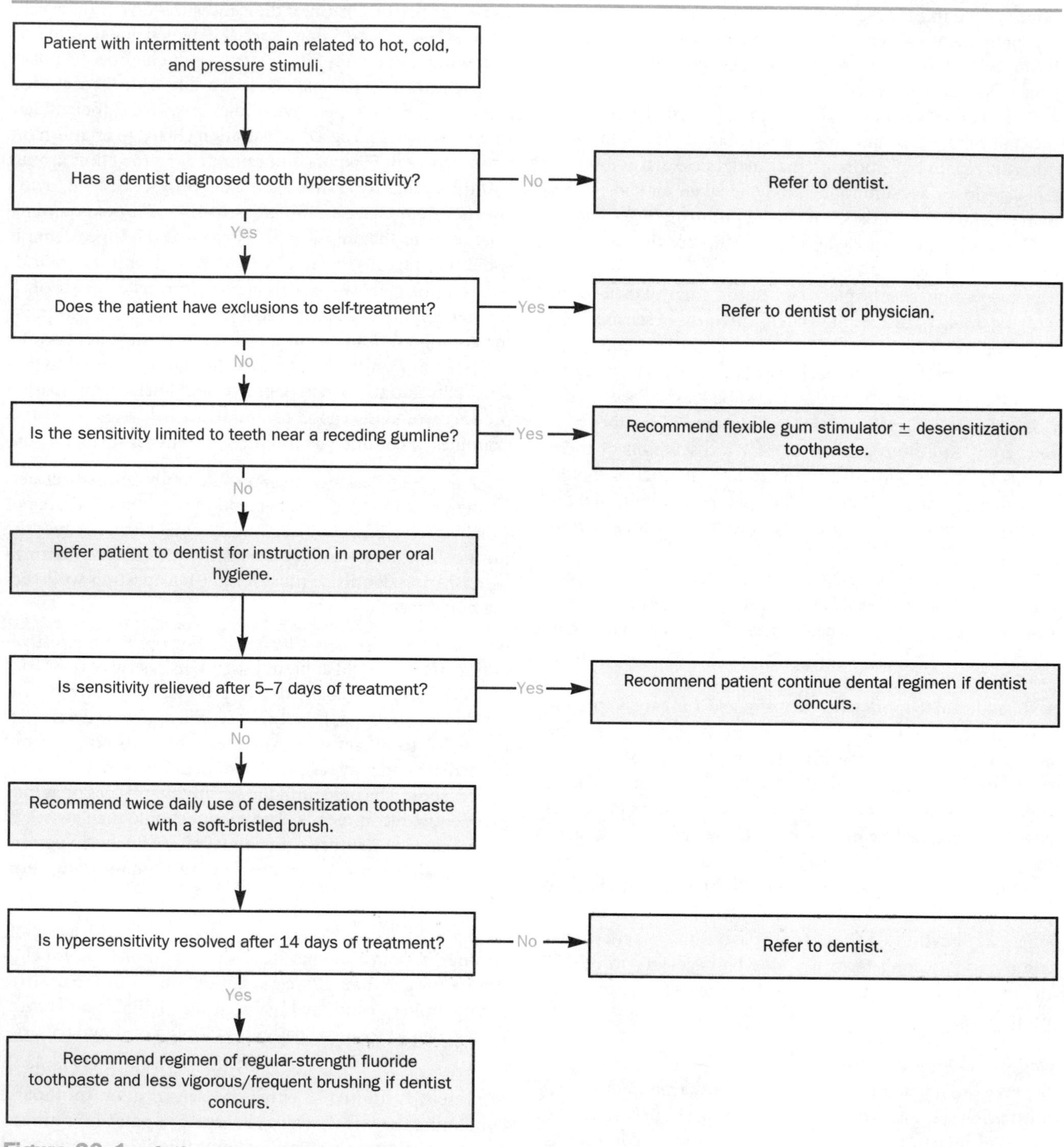

Figure 26–1 Self-care of tooth hypersensitivity.

patient has a history of dental problems (caries, abscess, periodontal, or endodontal problems) and how the patient removes plaque from the teeth. This information will help to determine whether the patient's oral hygiene is adequate. Use of plaque removal products should be evaluated for possible misuse, abuse, or inappropriate response.

Although a dentist should evaluate all cases of tooth pain, asking the patient the following questions will help elicit information to support the pharmacist's recommendation to have a dentist diagnose the disorder.

Q~ Have you consulted a dentist about the pain?

A~ If yes, find out the dentist's diagnosis and, if appropriate, recommend self-care measures and products. If no, refer the patient to a dentist.

Q~ Where is the pain? Is it severe? Is the area swollen?

Color Plates

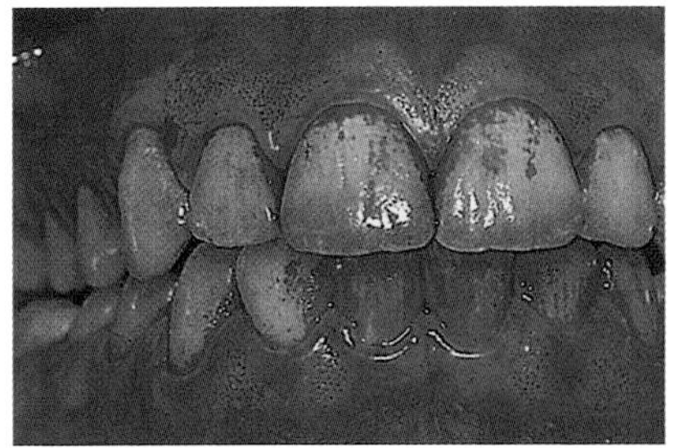
1

1 **Disclosing agents,** such as erythrosin (FD& C Red No. 3), aid patients in evaluating the effectiveness of their brushing and flossing by staining mucinous film and plaque on teeth. These agents reveal the presence and extent of deposits on teeth that otherwise appear clean. (See Chapter 25, "Prevention of Hygiene-Related Oral Disorders.")

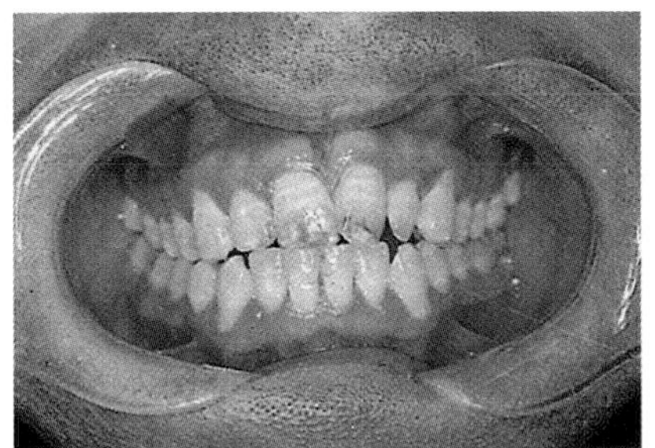
2

2 **Dental fluorosis (mottled enamel)** occurs during the time of tooth formation and is caused by the long-term ingestion of drinking water containing fluoride at concentrations greater than 1 ppm. Discoloration of the teeth varies, depending on the level of fluoride in the water, and ranges from white flecks or spots to brownish stains, small pits, or deep irregular pits that are dark brown in color. (See Chapter 25, "Prevention of Hygiene-Related Oral Disorders.")

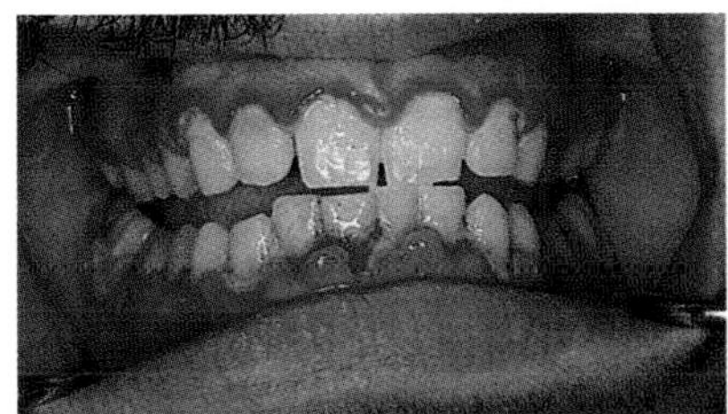
3

3 **Chronic gingivitis,** an asymptomatic inflammation of the gingivae (gums) at the necks of the teeth, is an early stage of periodontitis and is usually caused by poor oral hygiene. The gingivae are erythematous (red) and may have areas that appear swollen and glossy. In addition, mild hemorrhage may occur during teething brushing. (See Chapter 25, "Prevention of Hygiene-Related Oral Disorders.")

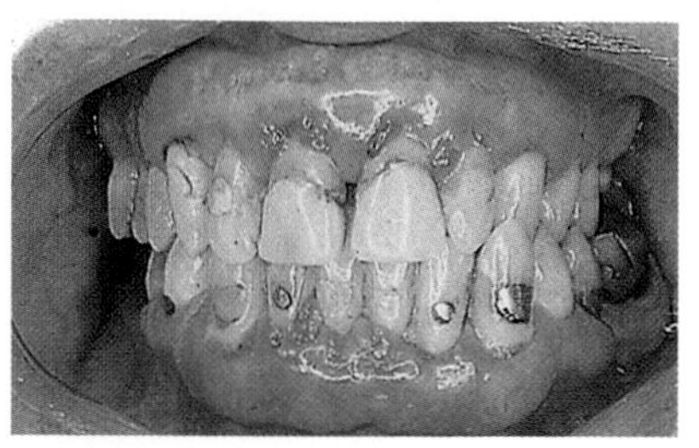
4

4 **Chronic periodontitis (pyorrhea)**, an inflammation of the tissues surrounding the teeth, including the gingivae, periodontal ligaments, alveolar bone, and the cementum (bony material covering the root of a tooth), is caused by plaque accumulation resulting from poor oral hygiene. The gingivae may be erythematous and swollen and may recede from the necks of the teeth. The condition is not painful and usually is accompanied by halitosis, loosening of the teeth, and mild hemorrhage during teeth brushing. (See Chapter 25, "Prevention of Hygiene-Related Oral Disorders.")

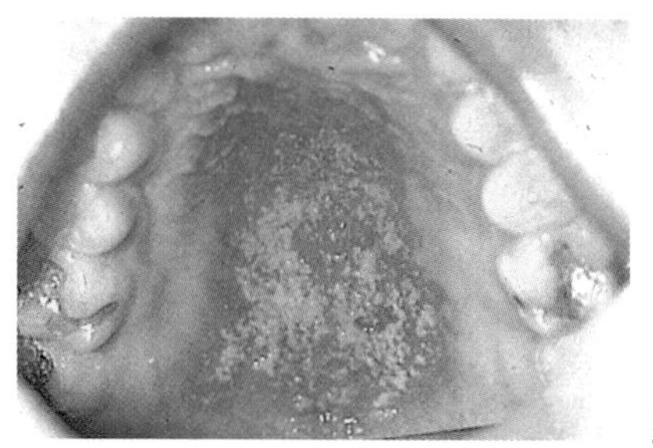
5

5 **Candidiasis (candidosis, moniliasis, thrush)**, an infection caused by overgrowth of *Candida albicans,* tends to occur in people with debilitating or chronic systemic disease or those on long-term antibiotic therapy. Candidiasis commonly presents as a whitish-gray to yellowish, soft, slightly elevated pseudomembrane-like plaque on the oral mucosa; the plaque is often described as having a milk curd appearance. If the membrane is stripped away, a raw bleeding surface remains. A dull, burning pain is often present. (See Chapter 25, "Prevention of Hygiene-Related Oral Disorders," and Chapter 26, "Oral Pain and Discomfort.")

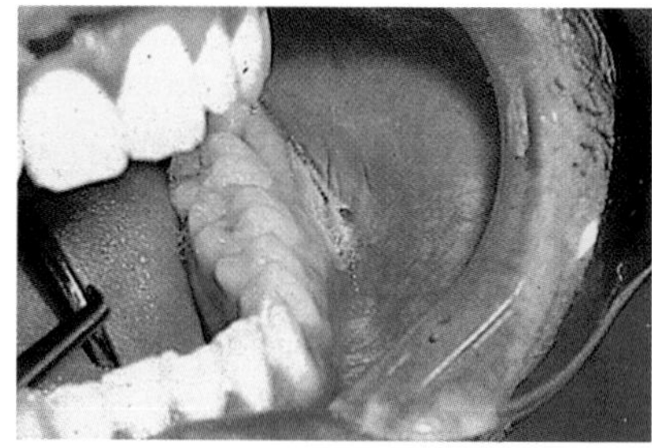
6

6 **Aspirin burn** results from the topical use of aspirin to relieve toothache. An aspirin tablet is placed against the tooth, where it is held in place by pressure from the buccal (cheek) mucosa. The mucosa becomes necrotic and is characterized by a white slough that rubs away, revealing a painful ulceration. (See Chapter 26, "Oral Pain and Discomfort.")

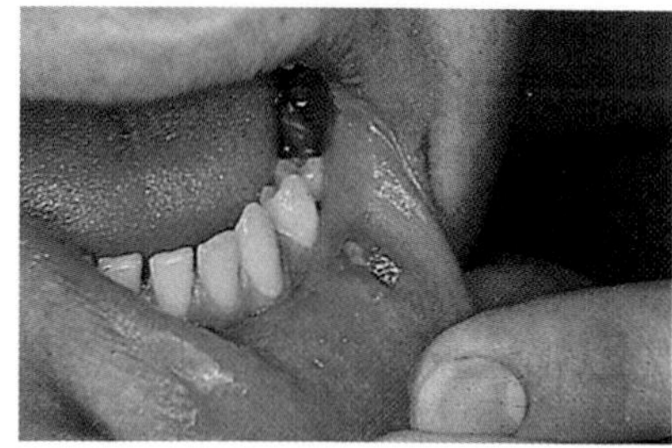
7

7 **Recurrent aphthous ulcers (canker sores)** are recurrent, painful, single or multiple ulcerations of bacterial origin. The central ulceration is sharply demarcated, often has a yellow to white surface of necrotic debris, and is surrounded by an erythematous margin. (See Chapter 26, "Oral Pain and Discomfort.")

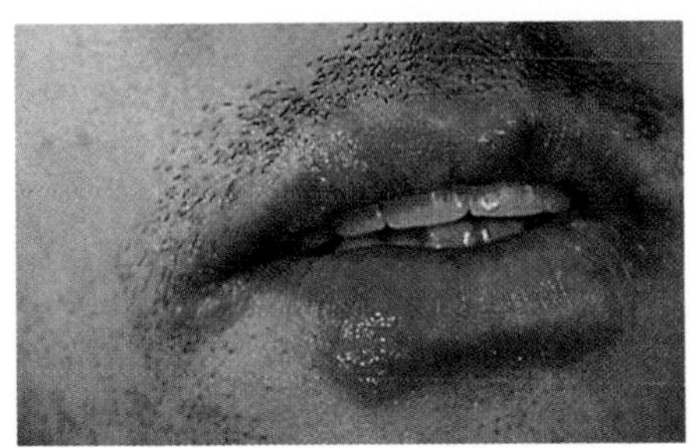
8

8 Herpes simplex lesions of the mouth and the eye usually start as a small cluster of vesicles (tiny blisters) that subsequently heal over with a serosanguinous (blood-tinged) crust. Local stinging, burning, and pain often herald the onset of lesions. Eye involvement should always be referred to an ophthalmologist. (See Chapter 26, "Oral Pain and Discomfort.")

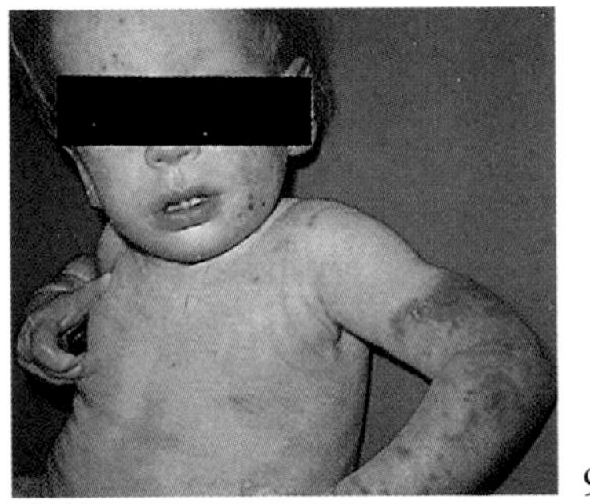
9A

9A, B, and C Atopic dermatitis (eczema) is an inflammatory condition that occurs on the extensor surface of the elbows and knees (**A**) during the first year of life and then involves predominantly the flexors (**B**). The hands, feet, and face are often involved as well (**C**). The dermatitis is characterized by erythema, scale, increased skin surface markings, and crusting; secondary infection is common. (See Chapter 27, "Atopic Dermatitis, Contact Dermatitis, and Dry Skin.")

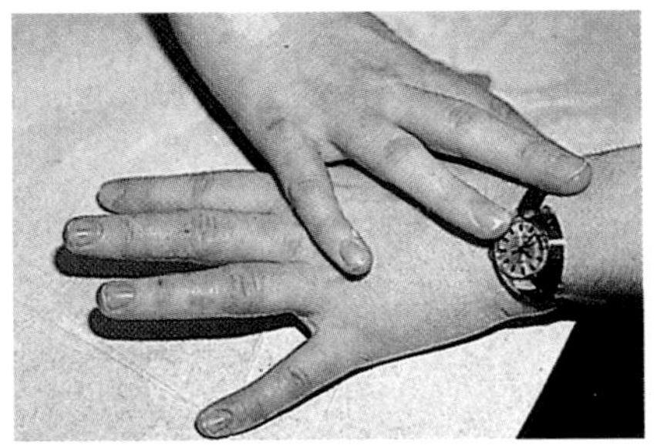
9B

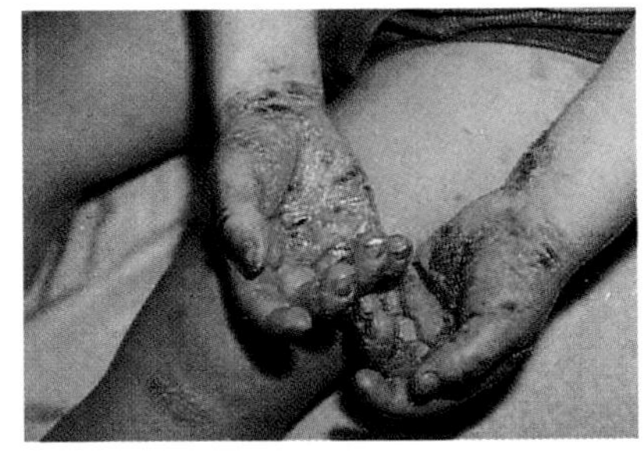
9C

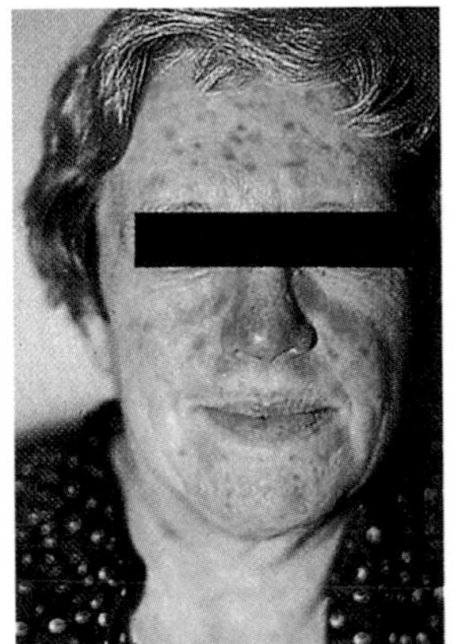
10

10 Seborrhea (seborrheic dermatitis) is a red scaling condition of the scalp, midface, and upper midchest of adults. This dermatitis is marked by characteristic greasy, yellowish scaling and is associated with erythema. (See Chapter 28, "Scaly Dermatoses.")

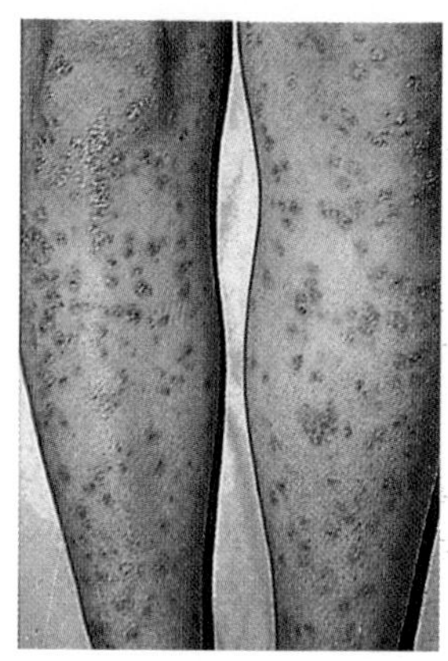

11A

11A, B, and C Psoriasis is a scaling condition in which erythematous plaques (red raised areas) are covered by a thick adherent scale. The borders of the lesions are well developed and vary from guttate (very small drop-shaped plaques) to much larger plaques: (**A**) guttate; (**B**) medium-sized plaques; (**C**) large plaques. (See Chapter 28, "Scaly Dermatoses.")

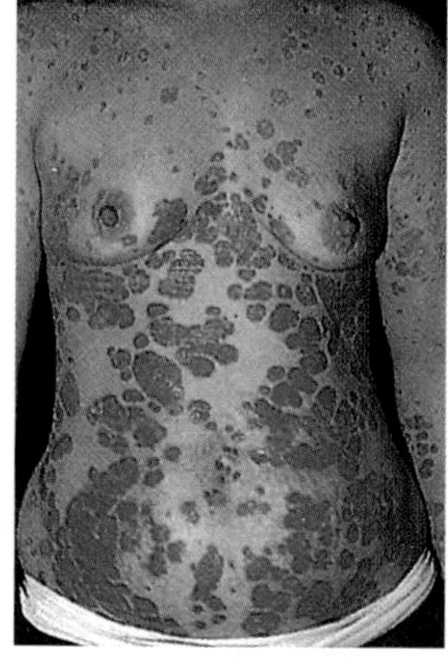

11B

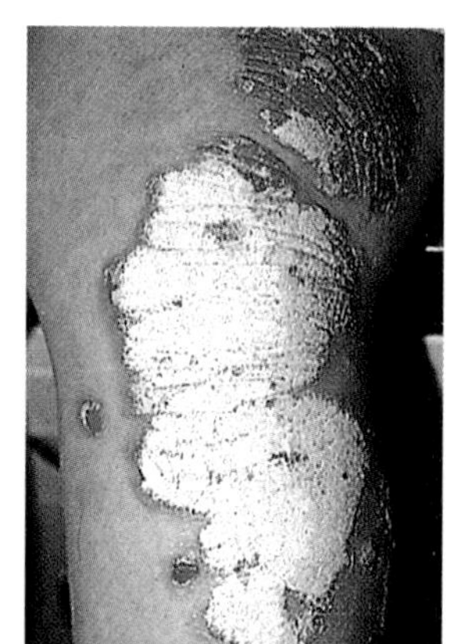

11C

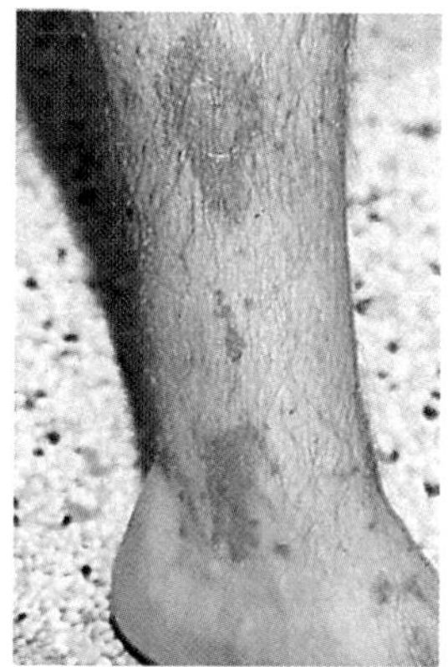

12A

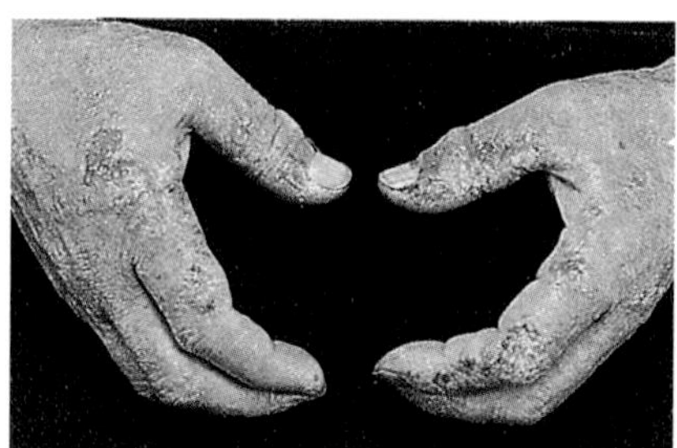

12B

12A and B Poison Ivy causes a linear erythema that can develop into large blisters (**A, B**). Similar reactions can also be caused by poison oak and poison sumac. (See Chapter 29, "Poison Ivy/Oak/Sumac Dermatitis.")

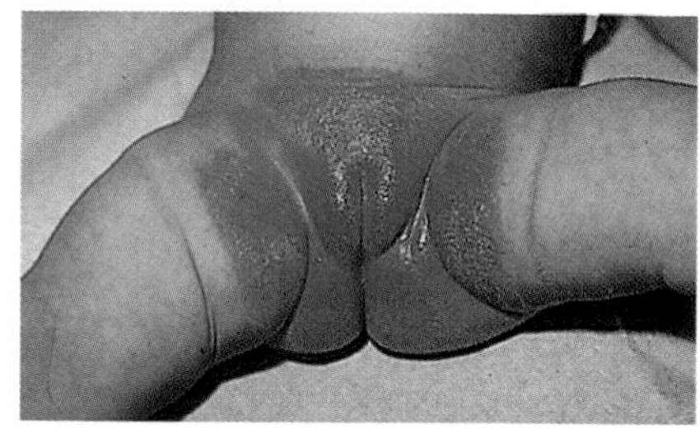

13

13 Diaper dermatitis presents as erythema of the groin (crease area around the genitals) and is common in infants. The case shown here was caused by a contact allergen. Contact irritants, such as urine and feces, and secondary bacterial and yeast infections may also cause problems in this area. (See Chapter 30, "Diaper Dermatitis and Prickly Heat.")

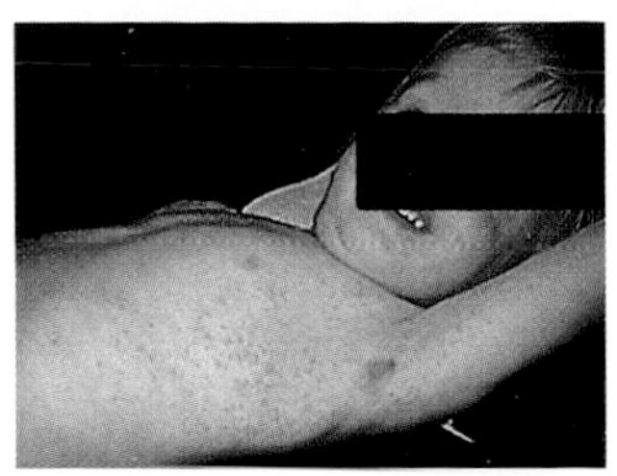
14

14 **Miliaria rubra (heat rash)** is an obstruction of sweat glands. Superficial involvement results in only tiny vesicles (blisters) appearing on the skin surface (miliaria crystallina). When deeper inflammation is present, the surrounding erythema is characteristic of miliaria rubra. (See Chapter 30, "Diaper Dermatitis and Prickly Heat.")

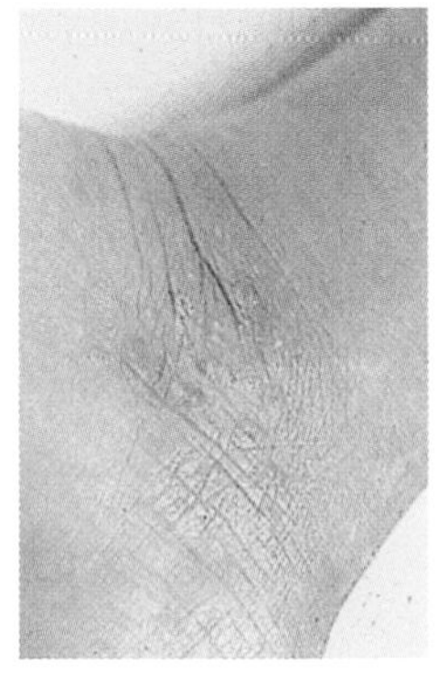
15

15 **Scabies** is caused by a small mite that burrows under the superficial skin layers. Small linear blisters that cause intense itching can be seen between the finger webs, on the inner wrists, in the axilla, around the areola (nipple) of the breast, and on the genitalia. (See Chapter 31, "Insect Bites and Stings and Pediculosis.")

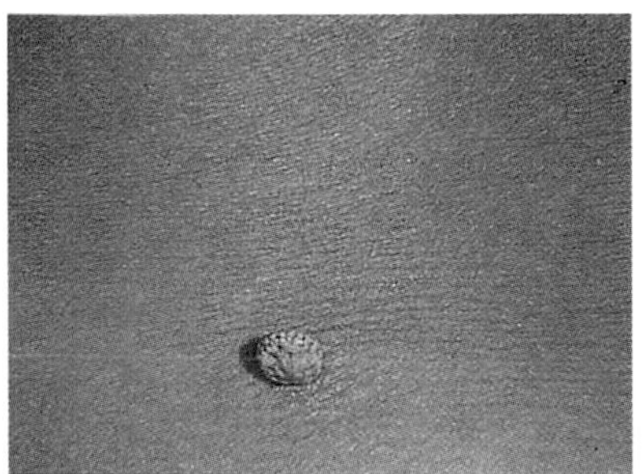
16

16 **Ticks** can attach to human skin and burrow into superficial skin layers. With careful examination, the back of the organism is usually visible on the skin surface. Ticks are vectors of several systemic diseases. (See Chapter 31, "Insect Bites and Stings and Pediculosis.")

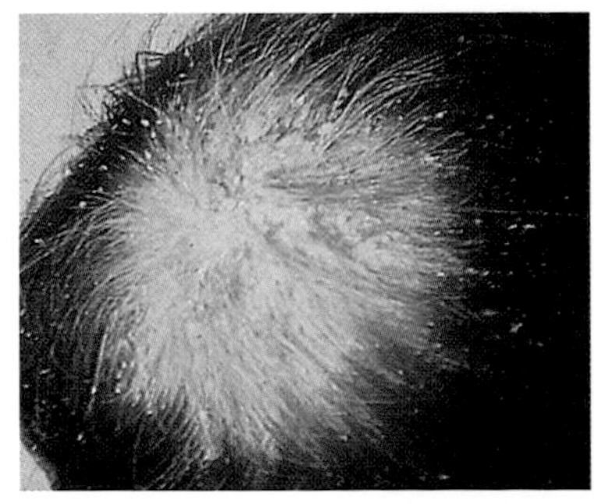
17A

17B

17 A and B **Pediculosis humanus capitis** is a louse infestation of the scalp. Examination of the scalp hair in this infestation shows tiny nits (eggs) attached to the hair shaft (**A**). The organism shown is only occasionally seen (**B**). (See Chapter 31, "Insect Bites and Stings and Pediculosis.")

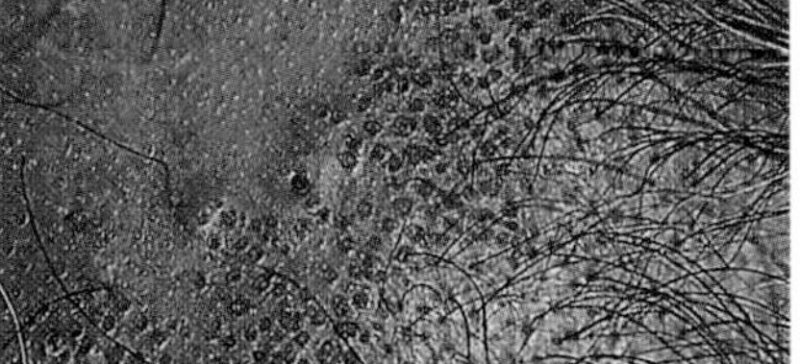
18

18 **Comedonic acne (noninflammatory)** occurs when follicles become plugged with sebum, forming a comedone on the surface. The black color is caused by oxidation of lipid and melanin, not dirt as is commonly believed. (See Chapter 32, "Acne.")

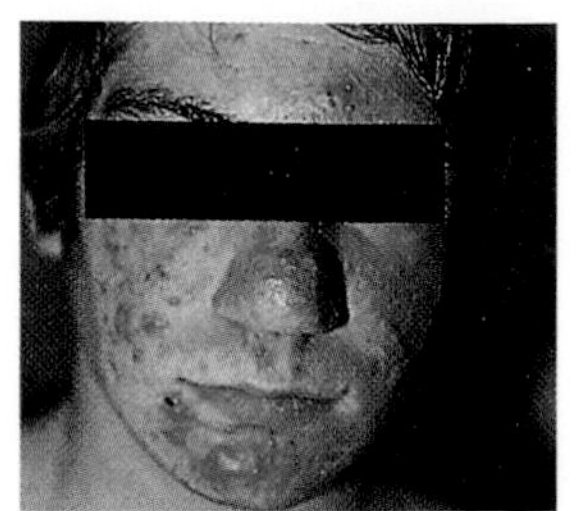

19

19 Pustular acne (inflammatory) presents as inflamed papules that are formed when superficial hair follicles become plugged and rupture at a deeper level. Superficial inflammation results in pustules; deep lesions cause large cysts to form with possible resultant scarring. (See Chapter 32, "Acne.")

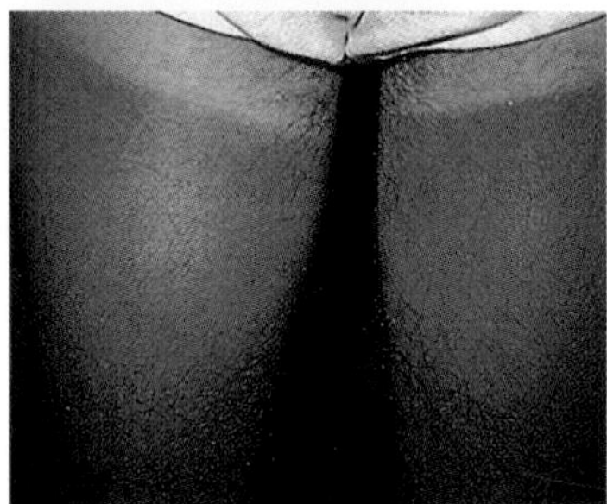

20

20 Sunburn presents as an erythema that occurs after excessive sun exposure; severe burns can result in large blister formation. Proper sunscreen application can provide photoprotection for susceptible patients. (See Chapter 33, "Prevention of Sun-Induced Skin Disorders," and Chapter 34, "Minor Burns and Sunburn.")

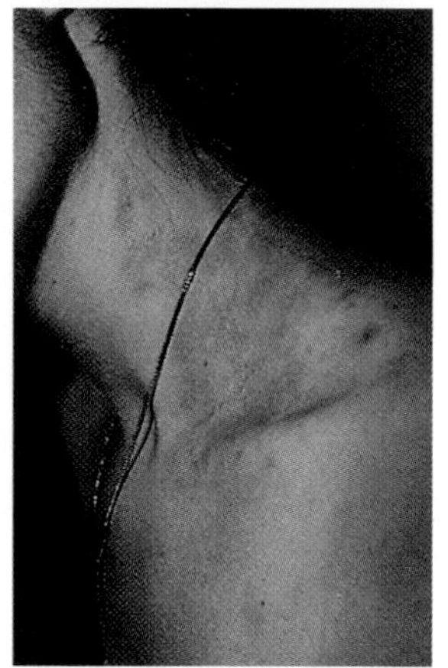

21

21 Cosmetic-induced photosensitivity can be caused by ingredients in certain topical colognes and perfumes. This immunologic reaction produces a local erythema that leaves characteristic postinflammatory pigmentation. (See Chapter 33, "Prevention of Sun-Induced Skin Disorders," and Chapter 34, "Minor Burns and Sunburn.")

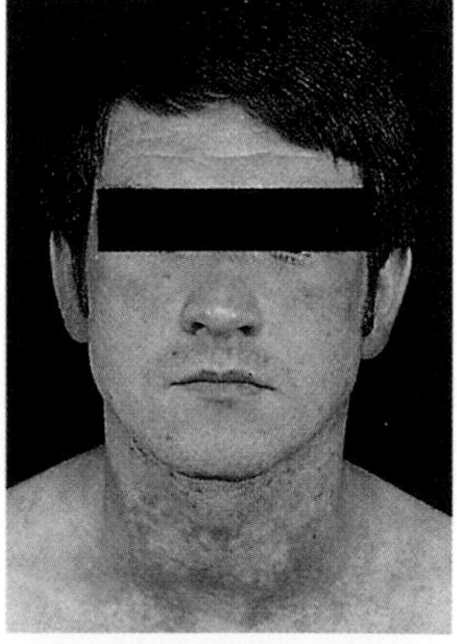

22

22 Drug-induced photosensitivity is a reaction that occurs on sun-exposed surfaces of the head, neck, and dorsum (back) of the hands. The erythema does not occur on photoprotected areas (under the nose and chin, behind the ears, and between the fingers). (See Chapter 33, "Prevention of Sun-Induced Skin Disorders," and Chapter 34, "Minor Burns and Sunburn.")

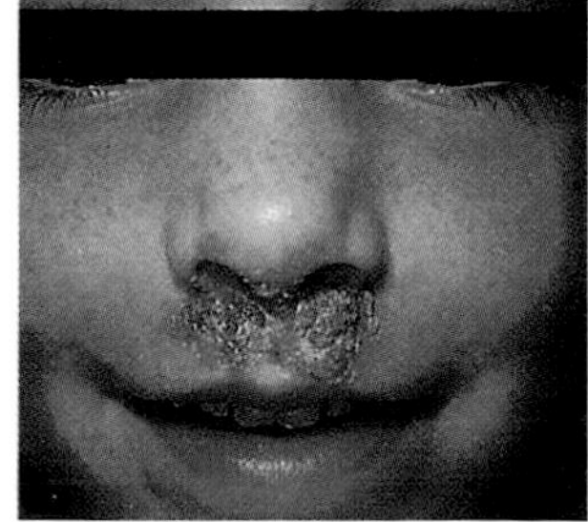

23

23 Impetigo is a bacterial infection characterized by honeycomb crusts on erythematous bases. A bullous (blistering) form can also occur. (See Chapter 35, "Minor Wounds and Skin Infections.")

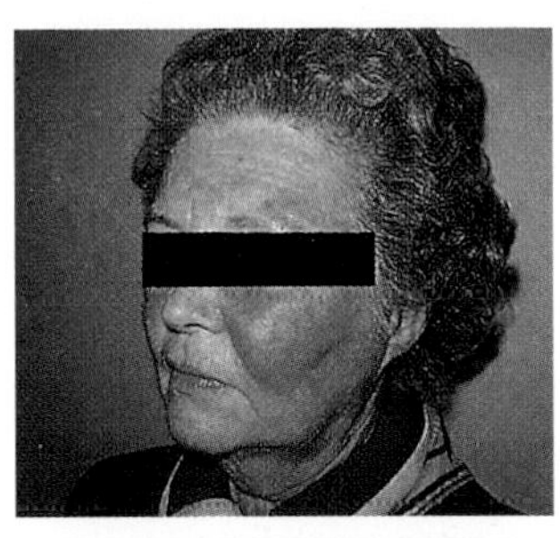

24

24 **Erysipeloid** is a streptococcal infection that often involves the face or extremities. The infected area is red and raised, with local warmth and edema. The margins of the infected area change rapidly, often forming serpiginous (irregular) patterns. (See Chapter 35, "Minor Wounds and Skin Infections.")

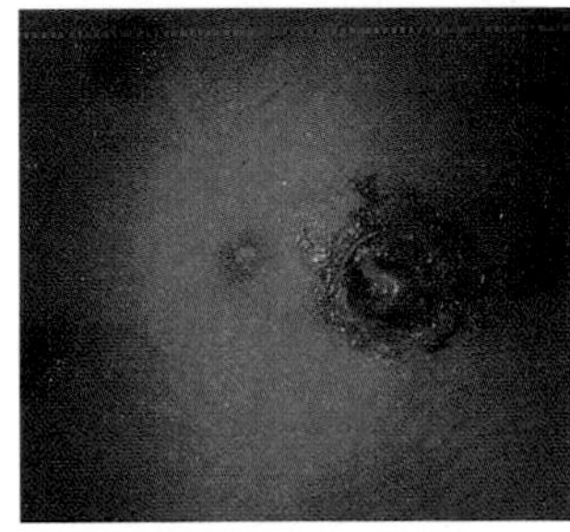

25

25 **Infections of the hair follicles** are usually caused by staphylococcal or streptococcal organisms. Superficial infections (folliculitis) can occur; deeper infections are called furuncles (small boils). Carbuncles form when adjacent hair follicles are involved. (See Chapter 35, "Minor Wounds and Skin Infections.")

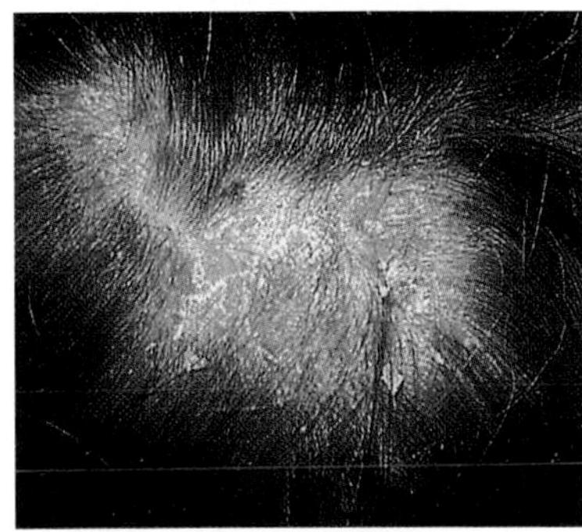

26

26 **Tinea capitis**, a fungal infection of the scalp, is marked by scale on the scalp with local breaking or loss of hair; erythema (redness) is usually not observed. (See Chapter 35, "Minor Wounds and Skin Infections.")

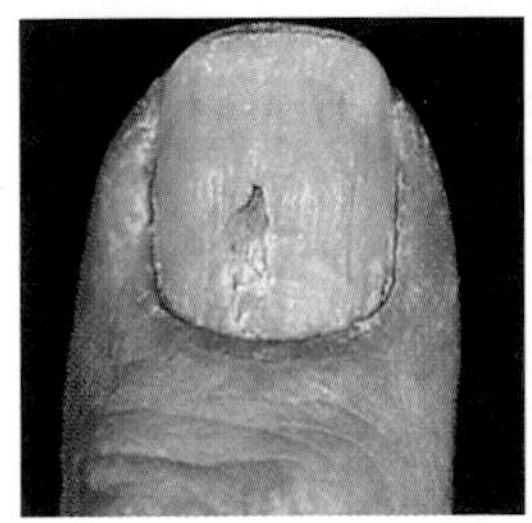

27

27 **Paronychia** is usually caused by overexposure of the nails to water, causing cuticle loss and inflammation around the nail folds. Approximately 50% of cases involve candidal infection. (See Chapter 35, "Minor Wounds and Skin Infections.")

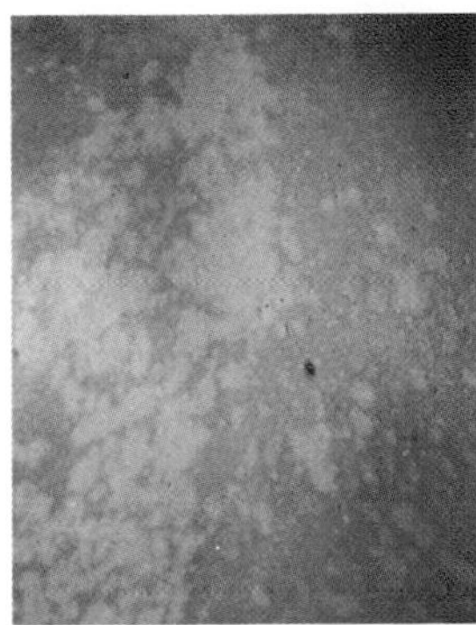

28A

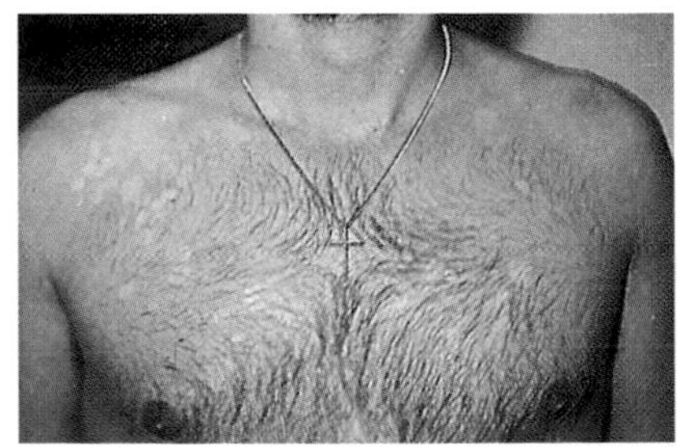

28B

28A and B **Tinea versicolor** is caused by a yeast organism that overgrows locally, resulting in hyperpigmentation or hypopigmentation (**A**). These mildly scaling eruptions characteristically occur on the chest, upper back, and arms (**B**). (See Chapter 35, "Minor Wounds and Skin Infections.")

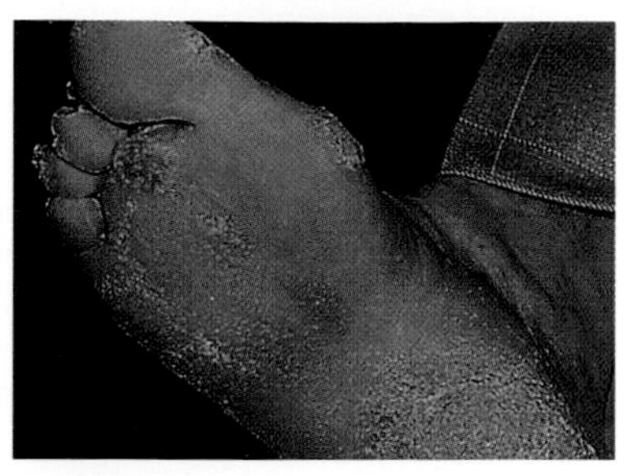
29

29 Calluses are thickened scales that often form on joints and weight-bearing areas. A callus on the plantar surface of the foot is shown here. (See Chapter 36, "Minor Foot Disorders.")

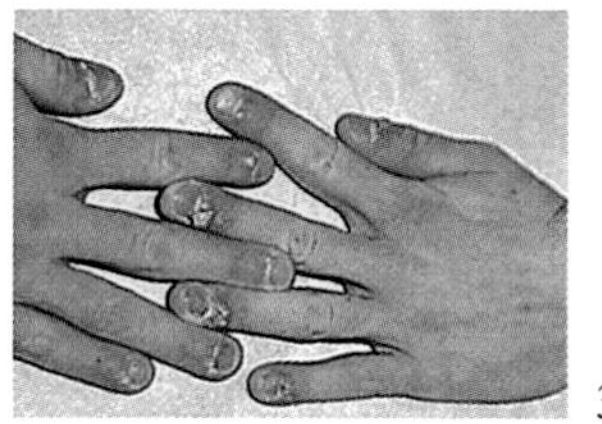
30

30 Common warts are viral-induced lesions that present as localized rough accumulations of keratin (hyperkeratosis) containing many tiny furrows. If the wart's surface is pared, small bleeding points can be seen. (See Chapter 36, "Minor Foot Disorders.")

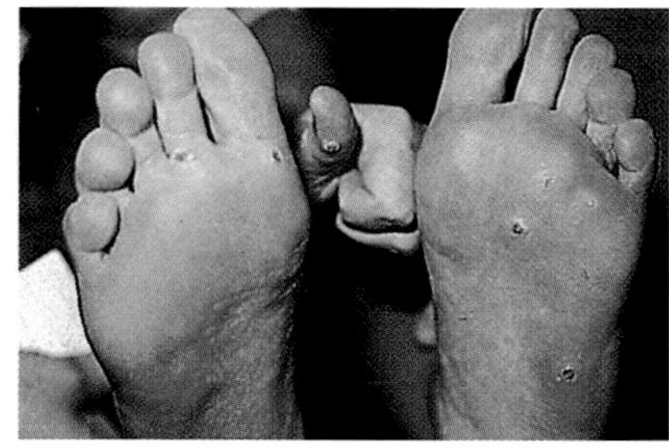
31

31 Plantar warts, caused by a viral infection, are often found on the plantar surface of the foot and present with hard localized accumulations of keratin. The punctate bleeding points seen when the lesions are pared distinguish plantar warts from calluses. (See Chapter 36, "Minor Foot Disorders.")

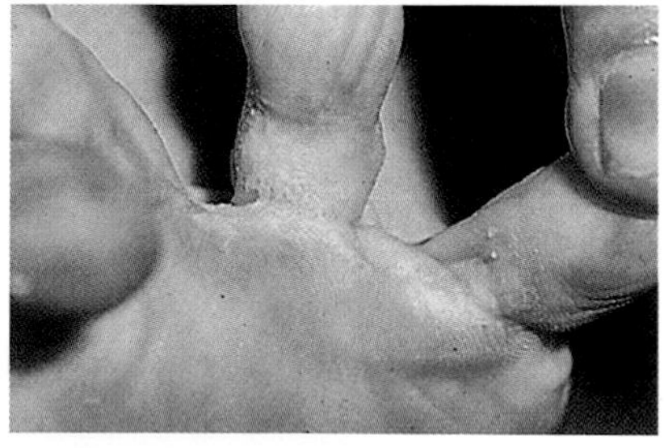
32

32 Tinea pedis infection of the toes characteristically starts between the fourth and fifth web space and spreads proximally. Scaling can progress to maceration with resultant small fissures. (See Chapter 36, "Minor Foot Disorders.")

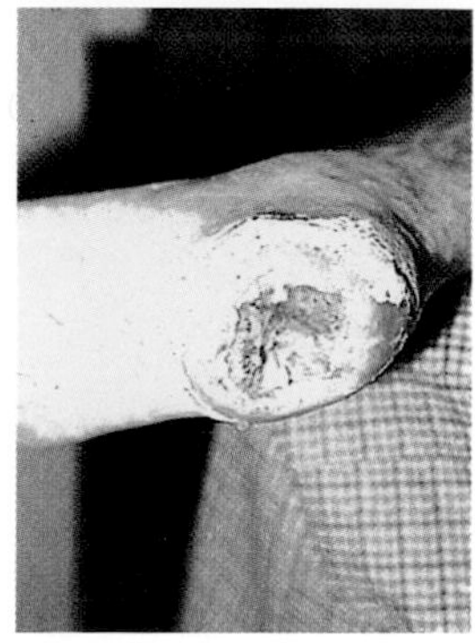
33

33 Gangrene of the foot is a serious and common complication of diabetes caused by trauma that has gone unrecognized because of neuropathy (loss of sensation) or vascular lesions. Eventually, the trauma may lead to gangrene when the necrotic (dead) skin is removed and ulceration results (as shown). (See Chapter 39, "Diabetes Mellitus.")

Table 26–1

Selected Desensitization Toothpastes

Trade Name	Primary Ingredients
Aquafresh Sensitive Toothpaste	Hydrated silica; potassium nitrate; sodium fluoride
Crest Sensitivity Protection Toothpaste[a]	Hydrated silica; potassium nitrate 5%; sodium fluoride 0.15%
Orajel Gold Sensitive Teeth Gel	Hydrated silica; potassium nitrate 5%; sodium monofluorophosphate 0.2%
Sensodyne Baking Soda Toothpaste[a,b]	Silica; sodium bicarbonate; potassium nitrate; sodium fluoride
Sensodyne Cool Gel[b]	Silica; sodium fluoride; potassium nitrate

[a] Dye-free product.
[b] Sucrose-free product.

A~ Advise the patient that these symptoms could indicate toothache or other serious oral pathology.

Q~ Is the pain continuous and throbbing, or does it come and go? Is the pain triggered or made worse by hot or cold food or drink or by chewing?

A~ *Distinguish the symptoms of tooth hypersensitivity from those of pulpitis. (See the section "Etiology/Pathophysiology of Toothache and Tooth Hypersensitivity.")* Advise the patient that even the intermittent pain associated with tooth hypersensitivity should be diagnosed by a dentist.

Q~ Do you feel ill? Do you have a fever? Do you have a cold or a sinus or ear infection?

A~ If yes to any of the questions, suspect referred pain from nondental causes. Ask whether the patient has had past episodes of toothache in conjunction with either cold or a sinus or ear infection.

Q~ Is the pain associated with braces?

A~ Advise patients with braces that the pain could be related to the devices and that an orthodontist should evaluate the disorder.

Q~ Does the pain occur after brushing the teeth?

A~ If yes, suspect the patient has been brushing excessively with a hard-bristle brush, an abrasive dentifrice, or both. Advise the patient of proper brushing methods. Offer to recommend products for hypersensitive teeth once a dentist has diagnosed the disorder.

Patient Counseling for Toothache and Tooth Hypersensitivity

Patients should be counseled that because a differential diagnosis of toothache is needed to rule out other conditions that produce this pain, the problem can be serious and it warrants the attention of a physician or dentist. The pharmacist may recommend a nonprescription analgesic to relieve toothache pain during the interval preceding the patient's dental appointment.

Subsequent to a definite diagnosis of tooth hypersensitivity, the pharmacist should explain the proper use of desensitization toothpastes and the safe methods of toothbrushing. The pharmacist should also explain precautions for using the toothpastes. The box "Patient Education for Tooth Hypersensitivity" lists specific information to provide patients.

Evaluation of Patient Outcomes for Toothache and Tooth Hypersensitivity

The patient with hypersensitive teeth should return for evaluation after 14 days of treatment with desensitization toothpastes. If the pain is resolved, the patient should continue treatment as recommended by a dentist. The patient should be advised to continue the recommended hygienic measures. If the pain persists or worsens or if new symptoms develop, the patient should see a dentist for further evaluation.

Teething Discomfort

Not all babies suffer discomfort during teething. For those who do, nonprescription products can provide symptomatic relief.

Etiology of Teething Discomfort

Teething is the eruption of the deciduous teeth through the gingival tissues. Usually this physiologic process is uneventful. However, it can cause sleep disturbances or irritability in some infants.

Signs and Symptoms of Teething Discomfort

Teething is not associated with pain, vomiting, diarrhea, nasal congestion, malaise, fever or rashes, but these symptoms may be a sign of ear or stomach infection. Irritation, reddening, or slight swelling of the gums may precede or accompany the other symptoms (sleep disturbances or irritability).

Bluish and soft, round swellings (called eruption cysts) sometimes form over emerging incisors and molars. Eruption cysts are not the result of infection and will disappear if

Case Study 26–1

Patient Complaint/History

Theodora, a 25-year-old woman who is the head of a household with two children and geriatric parents, had previously reported tooth pain in two quadrants. She correlated this pain with drinking coffee in the morning and brushing her teeth. At the pharmacist's suggestion, she went to her dentist and was diagnosed as having hypersensitive teeth. Her dentist gave her a sample of a dentifrice for hypersensitive teeth and advised her to use a nonprescription fluoride rinse. Although the patient did not like the taste of the dentifrice, she used up the sample; however, she is still experiencing pain.

Theodora, who is at the pharmacy today to pick up her mother's prescription, mentions her disappointment with the dentifrice provided by her dentist. She also has some questions she forgot to ask the dentist: Can the whole family use this new toothpaste? Can she use the same fluoride rinse that her children use? Currently, the children (6 and 10 years old) use a fluoride rinse before breakfast each day.

Clinical Considerations/Strategies

Readers can use the following considerations/strategies to determine whether treatment of the patient's condition with nonprescription medications is warranted:

- Determine which ingredients are appropriate for treating hypersensitive teeth.
- Recommend alternative products for relief of the symptoms.

Patient Education/Counseling

Readers can use the following strategies to develop a patient education/counseling plan that will help ensure optimal therapeutic outcomes:

- Address the patient's concerns about the apparent failure of the desensitization dentifrice that was recommended by the dentist.
- Explain proper use of the nonprescription medication regimen that was recommended to provide symptomatic relief for hypersensitivity and for prevention of caries.
- Include consideration of prevention of caries in other family members.

Patient Education for Tooth Hypersensitivity

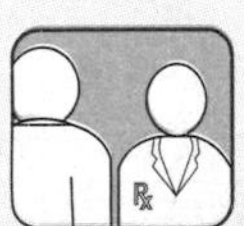

The objectives for self-care of diagnosed tooth hypersensitivity are to (1) repair the damaged tooth surface using the appropriate toothpastes and (2) stop abrasive toothbrushing practices. For most patients, carefully following product instructions, the dentist's recommendations, and the self-care measures listed below will help ensure optimal therapeutic outcomes:

- Use flexible gum stimulators with or without a desensitization toothpaste for sensitive teeth at or near a receding gumline.
- If recommended, try less vigorous brushing for generalized sensitivity, using a regular-fluoride toothpaste or a soft-bristled brush.
- If a desensitization toothpaste is needed, apply a 1-inch strip of toothpaste to a soft-bristled brush. Brush for at least 1 minute twice daily.
- Note that relief of the sensitivity may take several days to 2 weeks.
- Use the toothpaste as long as the dentist recommends; then switch to a low-abrasion dentifrice.
- Note that some cases of hypersensitive teeth require long-term treatment.
- Do not use desensitization toothpastes in children younger than 12 years.
- Do not use high-abrasion toothpastes such as cosmetic pastes that whiten or remove stains.

See a dentist if the pain worsens during treatment or if new symptoms develop.

left alone. In addition, three bumps (called mamelons) may develop on the biting surfaces of emerging incisors. The mamelons will wear away within 6 months. If the underside of the tongue becomes irritated, a dentist may try to smooth the edges of the mamelons to prevent further irritation.

Treatment of Teething Discomfort

Treatment Outcomes

The goal of self-care of teething discomfort is to relieve gum pain and irritation, thereby reducing the child's irritability and sleep disturbances.

General Treatment Approach

Parents should be cautioned to exercise restraint in treating a child's teething discomfort. Eruption cysts are a part of the physiologic process and should be left alone to resolve spontaneously. If cut or punctured, the cysts will leave scars that may delay the tooth's eruption. Parents should also exercise restraint in the use of nonprescription teething products.

Various nondrug measures are recommended for alleviating teething discomfort. Parents should try all measures to determine which are helpful. If additional treatment is needed, topical analgesics that are approved specifically for teething discomfort can be used.

Nonpharmacologic Therapy

If the baby cooperates, massaging the gum around the erupting tooth may provide relief. Babies may be made more comfortable by giving them a frozen pacifier (teething ring), a cold wet cloth, or food such as dry toast to chew on.

Pharmacologic Therapy

Pharmacologic management of teething discomfort is limited to topical analgesics that are approved for use in infants and to pediatric doses of systemic analgesics.

Topical Oral Analgesics FDA's review of nonprescription drug products for relief of oral discomfort has included benzocaine 5% to 20% and phenol 5% preparations as Category I topical anesthetic/analgesics for teething pain. Teething products are available as liquids and gels. Table 26–2 lists examples of commercially available products.

Indications Teething products are labeled "For the temporary relief of sore gums due to teething in infants and children 4 months of age and older."[3]

Dosage/Administration Guidelines Products containing benzocaine in solution or suspension should be rubbed onto the gums not more than four times daily. Concentrations of benzocaine in commercial teething products range from 7.5% to 10%. Teething preparations containing phenol or phenolate sodium equivalent to 0.5% phenol in aqueous solution or suspension may be applied to the affected area up to six times daily. Gels are easier to apply without dripping. The use of an alcohol-free product, one that FDA accepts, is preferred.

Contraindications/Precautions/Warnings In the highest (20%) concentration, benzocaine is too potent for infants and can even cause death from drug overdose. The risk of hypersensitivity to caine-type anesthetics also exists.

Teething products must carry a warning that fever and nasal congestion are not symptoms of teething and may indicate the presence of an infection.

Systemic Analgesics Pediatric doses of systemic nonprescription analgesics (e.g., acetaminophen) may be used to relieve teething discomfort. (See Chapter 3, "Headache and Muscle and Joint Pain," for appropriate doses.)

Product Selection Guidelines Although benzocaine is known to cause hypersensitivity, most commercial teething products contain this agent in a 7.5% concentration. As the trade name indicates, a product containing 10% benzocaine (Oragel Baby Nighttime) might be preferable for nighttime use to help babies sleep.

For ease of application, gels are the best choice; unlike liquids, they do not drip when applied. ADA recommends using an alcohol-free product. Parents should be advised to check the ingredients of teething products for alcohol.

Alternative Remedies

Chamomile has been used to treat teething discomfort. (See Chapter 45, "Herbal Remedies," for discussion of these types of products.)

Table 26–2

Selected Teething Products

Trade Name	Primary Ingredients
Anbesol Grape Baby Gel	Benzocaine 7.5%
Anbesol Original Baby Gel	Benzocaine 7.5%
Numzit Teething Gel	Benzocaine 7.5%
Orabase Baby Gel[a]	Benzocaine 7.5%
Orajel Baby Gel/Liquid[a]	Benzocaine 7.5%
Orajel Baby Nighttime Gel[a]	Benzocaine 10%

[a] Alcohol-free product.

Patient Assessment of Teething Discomfort

In most cases, the pharmacist has to base an assessment of teething discomfort on the parent's description of the child's symptoms. If the child cooperates, visual inspection of the gums may confirm that the child is teething. Still, the pharmacist must distinguish the signs and symptoms of teething from those of an infection.

Asking the parent the following questions will help elicit the information needed to accurately assess the disorder and to recommend the appropriate treatment approach.

Q~ What are the baby's symptoms?

A~ *Identify typical signs and symptoms of teething discomfort. (See the section "Signs and Symptoms of Teething Discomfort.")* If possible, look at the baby's gums. Determine whether the signs and the described symptoms are typical of teething discomfort.

Q~ Has the baby had vomiting, diarrhea, fever, or rashes recently?

A~ If yes, advise the parent that these are not typical symptoms for teething discomfort. Recommend that a pediatrician evaluate the baby.

Q~ Has the baby had a cold or nasal congestion recently?

A~ If yes, suspect an ear infection. Advise the parent to take the child to a pediatrician to rule out an infection.

Patient Counseling for Teething Discomfort

The pharmacist should be prepared to suggest both pharmacologic and nonpharmacologic remedies for teething discomfort. Parents should be urged to contact a physician when symptoms uncharacteristic of teething discomfort are present. The box "Patient Education for Teething Discomfort" lists specific information to provide parents.

Evaluation of Patient Outcomes for Teething Discomfort

The pharmacist should ask the parent to call after 3 to 5 days of treatment. If neither nonpharmacologic therapy nor nonprescription medications are relieving the symptoms, the parent should be advised to take the baby to a physician or pediatrician. Further, if symptoms uncharacteristic of teething discomfort have developed, the baby should be evaluated by a physician or pediatrician.

Fractured Dentition and Restorations

Teeth, fillings, or crowns may crack, break, or be knocked out. These problems may occur as a result of trauma (an accident or fight), chewing on a hard object, or the abrasive action of a filling. They may also appear for no apparent reason.

Pain may be associated with sudden exposure of or damage to nerves in a fractured tooth. Irritation or injury of gums and mucosa can also cause pain. Complications include malocclusion, rapid carious breakdown, compromised mastication, and infection. Loose, displaced, or broken fillings, crowns, or bridges may cause loss of normal function, tooth breakdown, or malocclusion. Only a dentist can evaluate and treat these conditions adequately. As with other disorders involving tooth pain, the pharmacist should advise the patient to see a dentist without delay.

Oral Mucosal Lesions

Two of the most common oral problems for which patients seek treatment advice are recurrent aphthous stomatitis (canker sores) and herpes simplex labialis (cold sores/fever blisters). Both disorders respond to symptomatic self-treatment, and the conditions should be self-limiting unless a secondary infectious process occurs. Patients frequently seek a pharmacist's recommendations for nonprescription products to relieve symptoms of these disorders. This interaction provides an excellent opportunity for the pharmacist to intervene on the patient's behalf. However, although many

Patient Education for Teething Discomfort

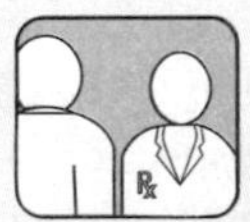

The objective of self-care of teething discomfort is to relieve gum pain and irritation, thereby reducing the child's irritability and sleep disturbances. For most patients, the parent's careful following of product instructions and the self-care measures listed below will help ensure optimal therapeutic outcomes.

Nondrug Measures

- To reduce irritation of the underside of the tongue, have a dentist smooth the edges of the erupting teeth.
- Do not cut or puncture gum cysts. Doing so will leave scars that may delay the tooth's eruption.
- If possible, massage the gum around the erupting tooth to provide relief.
- Give the baby a frozen pacifier (teething ring), a cold wet cloth, or food such as dry toast to chew on.

Nonprescription Medications

Topical Analgesics

- Rub commercial teething products containing benzocaine onto the gums not more than four times daily.
- Note that although benzocaine in concentrations of 5% to 20% was approved for teething preparations, the 20% concentration is too potent for infants and can even cause death from drug overdose.
- Rub teething products containing 0.5% phenol onto the gums not more than six times daily.
- Preferably, use alcohol-free products that carry the American Dental Association (ADA) acceptance seal.
- Note that benzocaine can cause hypersensitivity. If redness or irritation of the gum increases after use of this medication, stop using it.

Systemic Analgesics

- If desired, use pediatric formulations of oral nonprescription analgesics such as acetaminophen to relieve teething discomfort.
- Read the label carefully, and do not exceed recommended doses or frequency of use.

⚠ If the baby is vomiting or has diarrhea, a fever, nasal congestion, malaise, pain, or other symptoms not typical of teething discomfort, take the baby to a physician or pediatrician.

nonprescription products are available for symptomatic treatment of cold sores and canker sores, none has been shown conclusively to decrease the recurrence rate of lesions or to be curative.

Recurrent Aphthous Stomatitis

The minor clinical form of canker sores, also referred to as recurrent aphthous ulcers or recurrent aphthous stomatitis (RAS), is self-treatable. As Table 26–3 shows, 85% of cases of canker sores are of this form.

Epidemiology/Etiology of Recurrent Aphthous Stomatitis

RAS affects approximately 20% of Americans. The incidence is slightly higher in stressed populations and in women.[5] The disease usually begins in childhood or early adolescence. After age 50 years, RAS declines in frequency and severity.

The cause of recurrent aphthous ulcers is unknown; however, evidence suggests that they may result from a hypersensitivity to bacteria found in the mouth. Precipitating or contributing factors may include food allergy, nutritional deficiency (possibly related to iron, B_{12}, or folate deficiency), genetic predisposition, stress, and hormonal changes. Trauma (e.g., chemical irritation, biting the inside of cheeks or lips, or injury caused by toothbrushing or braces) has also been implicated.[6]

Patients with inflammatory bowel disease,[7] systemic lupus erythematosus,[8] or Behçet's disease[9] manifest ulcerations that are clinically similar to RAS lesions, prompting some investigators to believe systemic diseases can cause RAS. Cell-mediated immunity may also play a role. Recent studies suggest that recurrent aphthous ulcers are caused by a dysfunction of the immune system and may be initiated by a trigger event such as a minor trauma.[6]

Recurrent aphthous ulcers are neither viral in origin nor contagious.

Signs and Symptoms of Recurrent Aphthous Stomatitis

Recurrent aphthous lesions appear as an epithelial ulceration on nonkeratinized mucosal surfaces of movable mouth parts, such as the tongue, the floor of the mouth, the soft palate, or the inside lining of the lips and cheeks. Rarely, ulcerations affect keratinized tissue such as gingiva. Most recurrent aphthous ulcerations persist for 7 to 14 days and heal spontaneously without scarring.[6] The ulcers usually range from 0.5 to 3.0 cm in diameter; however, larger lesions can develop in clusters. Individual ulcers are usually (1) round or oval, (2) flat or crater-like in appearance, and (3) gray to grayish yellow with an erythematous halo of inflamed tissue surrounding the ulcer. (See the "Color Plates," photograph 7.)

Table 26–3

Differentiation of Aphthous Ulcers (Canker Sores) and Herpes Simplex Labialis (Cold Sores)

	Major Aphthae	Herpetiform Aphthae	Herpetiform Aphthous Stomatitis (Minor Aphthae)	Herpes Simplex Labialis (Cold Sores)
Manifestation	Gray/grayish yellow round/oval ulcers, either flat or crater-like with erythematous halo of inflamed tissue around ulcer	Similar to canker sores	Similar to canker sores	Begins as small, red papules of fluid-containing vesicles; lesions may coalesce; crusted mature lesions have erythematous base
Number of lesions	1–10	1–5	5–100	1 to multiple
Incidence (%)	85	10	5	—
Pain	None–moderate	Moderate–severe	Mild–moderate	None–moderate
Size of ulcers	<1 cm	1–3 cm	1–4 mm	1–3 mm
Duration (days)	7–14	30–60	7–14	10–14
Scarring	Rare	Common	None	Rare
Location	Buccal and labial mucosa, lateral tongue, floor of mouth	Palate, oropharynx and lips	All sites	Labial—usually at junction of mucous membrane and skin of lips or nose
Comments	Resembles viral infections; induced by trauma, hematologic abnormalities	Common in HIV, may be initial manifestation of GI disease	Not caused by herpesvirus infection	Induced by HSV-1

Key: HIV = Human immunodeficiency virus; GI = gastrointestinal; HSV = herpes simplex virus 1.

Source: Adapted from reference 10.

Some patients may experience a painful sensation before the lesion actually appears. Patients may develop single or multiple lesions. The lesions can be very painful—with the pain increasing on eating and drinking—and may inhibit normal eating, drinking, swallowing, and talking, as well as routine oral hygiene. Although many patients have recurrent episodes of oral lesions with periods of remission, some patients may chronically experience one or more lesions in the mouth for very long periods. Usually no fever or lymphadenopathy accompanies RAS; however, such symptoms may arise if a secondary bacterial infection is present.

Treatment of Recurrent Aphthous Stomatitis

Recurrent aphthous ulcerations cannot be cured; however, nonprescription medications can provide symptomatic relief.

Treatment Outcomes

The goals in treating RAS are to (1) control discomfort, thus allowing healing so that the patient can eat, drink, and perform routine oral hygiene; and (2) prevent complications such as secondary infection.

General Treatment Approach

Treatment should focus on protecting the ulcerations from irritating stimuli and on reducing the duration and severity of pain and irritation. Figure 26–2 outlines the self-care of RAS.

Exclusions to self-care include any underlying condition that could manifest RAS, lesions that do not resolve by 14 days, discomfort that is not relieved by self-treatment, lesions that recur with increased frequency, and symptoms of systemic illness such as fever or malaise.

Nonpharmacologic Therapy

If a nutritional deficiency (e.g., iron, folate, vitamin B_{12}) is suspected as a contributing factor, the patient can increase consumption of foods high in these nutrients or can take nutritional supplements. Spicy foods should be avoided until ulcerations improve.

Ice applied directly to the lesions can give temporary relief. However, hot packs may cause the spread of infection (if present) and should not be used.

Pharmacologic Therapy

Several types of nonprescription medications provide symptomatic relief of RAS: oral debriding and cleansing agents, topical oral anesthetics, topical oral protectants, oral rinses, and systemic analgesics. Table 26–4 lists commercial products containing these agents. Cauterizing lesions with silver nitrate is not effective. Further, this agent may stain teeth and damage healthy tissue.

Oral Debriding and Wound-Cleansing Agents Products that release nascent oxygen can be used as debriding and cleansing agents to exert temporary relief of RAS discomfort. After a thorough review process, FDA has determined that four active ingredients are generally recognized as safe and effective for use as nonprescription debriding agents or oral wound cleansers for oral health care. This proposed ruling applies to carbamide peroxide 10% to 15% in anhydrous glycerin, hydrogen peroxide 3%, sodium perborate monohydrate (1.2 g), and sodium bicarbonate.[11] The FDA has determined that no ingredient is generally recognized as safe and effective for use as a nonprescription healing agent for oral wounds.[12]

Mechanism of Action Peroxides and perborates release molecular oxygen. Hydrogen peroxide and carbamide peroxide do so immediately on contact with tissue enzymes (catalase and peroxidase), but tissue and bacterial exposure to the oxygen is very brief.[13] The foaming of the liberated oxygen exerts a mechanical action, which loosens particulate matter and cleanses debris from wounds. The efficacy of oxidizing products in killing anaerobic bacteria when treating infections and periodontitis is equivocal and has not been established.[13]

Dosage/Administration Guidelines For direct application, drops of carbamide peroxide or hydrogen peroxide are placed on the affected area and allowed to remain in place for 1 minute. As a rinse, carbamide peroxide drops are placed on the tongue, mixed with saliva, and swished in the mouth for 1 minute. A 3% aqueous solution of hydrogen peroxide should be mixed with an equal amount of water before rinsing the mouth. Some products (e.g., Peroxyl Rinse and Perimed) are a 1.5% solution of hydrogen peroxide and should be used full strength. Sodium perborate monohydrate powder (1.2 g) should be dissolved in 1 ounce of water and used immediately.

Such products can be used up to four times daily (after meals) but should be used for no longer than 7 days. In all cases, it is important to follow package directions carefully. The solution should be spit out, not swallowed.

Contraindications/Precautions/Warnings Prolonged rinsing with oxidizing products could lead to soft-tissue irritation, transient tooth sensitivity from decalcification of enamel, cellular changes, and overgrowth of undesirable organisms that will possibly lead to black hairy tongue.[14–16]

Labeling of these products includes the following warning:

> Do not use this product more than 7 days unless directed by a dentist or doctor. See your doctor or dentist promptly if sore mouth symptoms do not improve in 7 days; if irritation, pain, or redness persists or worsens; or if swelling, rash, or fever develops.[3]

Topical Oral Anesthetics FDA has classified topical oral anesthetic/analgesic products containing benzocaine 5% to 20%, butacaine sulfate 0.05% to 0.1%, dyclonine 0.05% to 0.1%, hexylresorcinol 0.05% to 0.1%, menthol 0.04% to 2.0%, phenol 0.5% to 1.5%, phenolate sodium 0.5% to 1.5%, benzyl alcohol 0.05% to 0.1%, and salicylic alcohol 1% to 6% as safe and effective for temporary relief of pain associated with RAS.[3]

Benzocaine and butacaine are the most commonly used

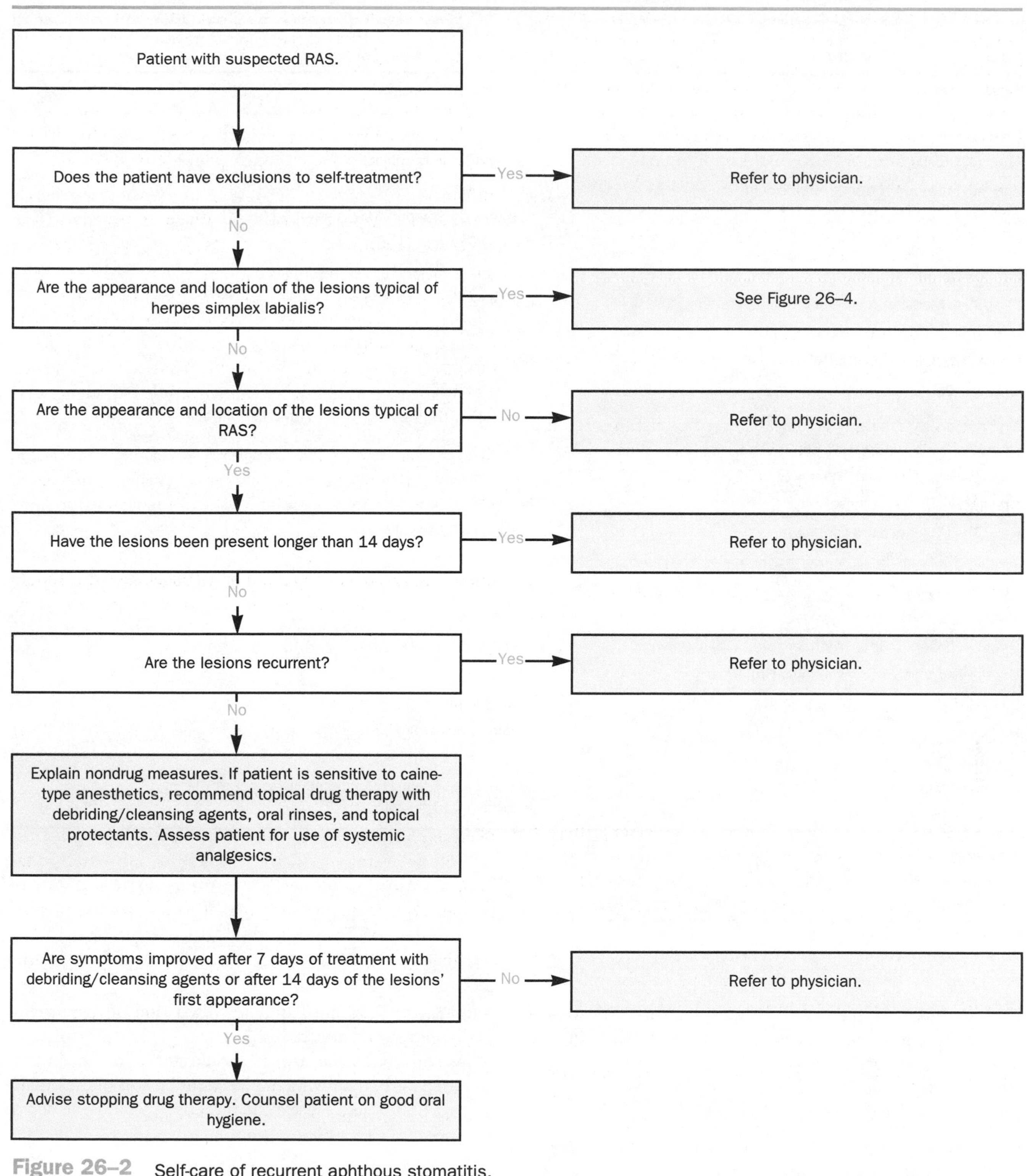

Figure 26–2 Self-care of recurrent aphthous stomatitis.

local anesthetics in nonprescription products. However, benzocaine is a known sensitizer (allergen) and should not be used by patients with a history of hypersensitivity to other benzocaine-containing products.

The patient should avoid using potentially inflammatory products containing ketone or alcohol counterirritants (e.g., menthol, phenol, camphor, and eugenol) as anesthetic, counterirritant, or antiseptic treatments for RAS. These agents may cause tissue irritation and damage or systemic toxicity, especially if overused.[17]

Table 26–4

Selected Products for Recurrent Aphthous Stomatitis and Herpes Simplex Labialis

Trade Name	Primary Ingredients
Topical Anesthetics	
Anbesol Gel/Liquid	Benzocaine 6.3%; phenol 0.5%
Anbesol Maximum Strength Gel/Liquid	Benzocaine 20%
Blistex Lip Medex Ointment	Camphor 1%; menthol 1%; phenol 0.5%
Campho-Phenique Gel[a]	Camphor 10.8%; phenol 4.7%
Carmex Lip Balm Ointment[a–c]	Menthol; camphor; salicylic acid; phenol
ChapStick Medicated Lip Balm Stick/Ointment	Camphor 1%; menthol 0.6%; phenol 0.5%
Kank-A Professional Strength Liquid	Benzocaine 20%
Numzident Adult Strength Gel	Benzocaine 10%
Orabase Gel	Benzocaine 15%
Orabase Lip Cream[a]	Benzocaine 5%; menthol 0.5%; camphor; phenol
Orabase-B with Benzocaine Paste[a]	Benzocaine 20%
Orajel Mouth-Aid Liquid/Gel	Benzocaine 20%
Orajel Regular Strength Gel	Benzocaine 10%
Red Cross Canker Sore Ointment	Benzocaine 20%; phenol
Debriding/Cleansing Agents (Not for use on cold sores)	
Cankaid Liquid	Carbamide peroxide 10%
Gly-Oxide Liquid	Carbamide peroxide 10%
Orajel Perioseptic Spot Treatment Oral Cleanser Liquid	Carbamide peroxide 15%
Orajel Perioseptic Super Cleaning Oral Rinse	Hydrogen peroxide 1.5%
Peroxyl Hygienic Dental Rinse Liquid/Gel	Hydrogen peroxide 1.5%
Proxigel[b,c]	Menthol; carbamide peroxide 10%
Oral Skin Protectants	
Orabase Plain	Pectin; gelatin; carboxmethylcellulose; polyethylene; mineral oil; tragacanth

[a] Alcohol-free product.
[b] Dye-free product.
[c] Sucrose-free product.

Topical Oral Protectants Coating the ulcers with topical oral protectants (e.g., Orabase or denture adhesives) can be effective in protecting ulcerations, decreasing friction, and affording temporary symptomatic relief.[13] These products can be applied as needed. (See Table 26–4.)

Oral Rinses Saline rinses (1 to 3 teaspoons of table salt in 4 to 8 ounces of warm tap water) may soothe ulcers and can be used before topical application of a medication. Similarly, a paste of baking soda applied to the lesions for a few minutes may soothe irritation. Zinc in astringent mouthrinses is of equivocal value in promoting healing.

Systemic Analgesics Systemic nonprescription analgesics (e.g., aspirin, ibuprofen, and acetaminophen) afford additional relief of mouth discomfort. (See Chapter 3, "Headache and Muscle and Joint Pain," for discussion of these agents and their recommended dosages.)

As with toothache, aspirin should not be retained in the mouth before swallowing or placed in the area of the oral lesions. The acid can cause a chemical burn with tissue necrosis. (See the "Color Plates," photograph 6.)

Product Selection Guidelines All four currently available oral debriding agents/wound cleansers—carbamide peroxide 10% to 15% in anhydrous glycerin, hydrogen peroxide 3%, sodium perborate monohydrate (1.2 g), and sodium bicarbonate—are Category I agents. Sodium bicarbonate rinses or pastes can be made at home, making this agent the least expensive choice for wound cleansing. This agent also temporarily soothes discomfort.

Patients with known hypersensitivity to caine-type anesthetics should use a product containing one or more of the other Category I agents: butacaine sulfate 0.05% to 0.1%, dyclonine 0.05% to 0.1%, hexylresorcinol 0.05% to 0.1%, menthol 0.04% to 2.0%, phenol 0.5% to 1.5%, phenolate sodium 0.5% to 1.5%, benzyl alcohol 0.05% to 0.1%, and salicylic alcohol 1% to 6%. As with benzocaine, patients with known sensitivity to aspirin should avoid salicylic alcohol. Only products containing menthol, phenol, and/or camphor in the concentrations approved as Category I should be used for RAS. Higher concentrations are potentially inflammatory.

Patient Assessment of Recurrent Aphthous Stomatitis

The pharmacist should find out whether the patient has a history of RAS. If possible, the lesions should be inspected to determine whether their appearance and location are characteristic of RAS. The patient's medical history will help in ruling out underlying pathology that can cause lesions that resemble RAS. Finally, the pharmacist should ask about previous self-treatments and their effectiveness.

Asking the patient the following questions will help elicit the information needed to accurately assess the disorder and to recommend the appropriate treatment approach.

Q~ How long have you had this problem?

A~ *Identify the normal healing time for RAS. (See the section "Signs and Symptoms of Recurrent Aphthous Stomatitis.")* Determine whether the patient's ulcerations are chronic or recurrent according to the longevity of the problem. Refer patients with chronic or recurrent cases to a physician.

Q~ Are the lesions visible? What is their color? Are they crusted or erythematous? Where in the mouth do they occur?

A~ *Distinguish the ulcerations of RAS from those of herpes simplex labialis and more severe aphthous lesions. (See Table 26–3.)* Determine whether the signs and symptoms are characteristic of RAS or herpes simplex labialis. Recommend appropriate treatment.

Q~ Do you have discomfort? Is the discomfort continuous? Is it localized? Does talking, eating, or drinking aggravate it? Do you have a discharge from the lesion? Can you associate the appearance of the lesion(s) with any event?

A~ Evaluate the patient's answers to determine whether the symptoms are characteristic of RAS or indicate underlying abnormalities, infection, trauma, or other causes. Refer patients with any disorder other than minor RAS lesions to a physician.

Q~ Do your gums bleed when you brush your teeth? Do you have a bad taste in your mouth? Do you have bad breath or loose teeth?

A~ If yes to any of these questions, suspect poor oral hygiene or infection as the cause of the symptoms. Refer the patient to a dentist or physician for evaluation of the lesions. Offer to discuss oral hygiene measures and products with the patient if the dentist confirms poor hygiene as the problem.

Q~ Do you wear dentures? Are they loose? Do your dentures cause sore spots, or are the lesions in contact with dentures?

A~ If yes to any of these questions, refer the patient to the dentist for evaluation of possible ill-fitting dentures.

Q~ What nonprescription medications have you used in the past? Do you have any drug-related allergies?

A~ Recommend alternative treatments for patients with allergy to aspirin or caine-type anesthetics.

Patient Education for Recurrent Aphthous Stomatitis

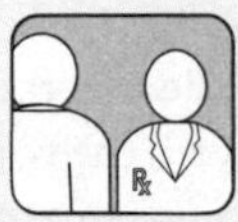

The primary objective of self-treatment is to relieve pain and irritation so that the lesions can heal and the patient can eat, drink, and perform routine oral hygiene. The secondary objective is to prevent complications such as secondary infection. For most patients, carefully following product instructions and the self-care measures listed below will help ensure optimal therapeutic outcomes.

Nondrug Measures

- If a deficiency of iron, folate, or vitamin B_{12} is suspected as a contributing factor, increase consumption of foods high in these nutrients, or take nutritional supplements.
- Avoid spicy foods until the lesions heal.
- If desired, apply ice directly to the lesions.
- Do not use hot packs. If infection is present, heat may spread the infection.
- Apply a paste of baking soda directly to the lesions to soothe the discomfort.

(continued)

Patient Education for Recurrent Aphthous Stomatitis (continued)

Nonprescription Medications

- If longer lasting relief is desired, ask your pharmacist to recommend one or more of the following types of nonprescription medications: debriding and cleansing agents, topical oral anesthetics, topical oral protectants, oral rinses, and systemic analgesics.
- Do not cauterize lesions with silver nitrate. This treatment is not effective and may stain teeth and damage healthy tissue.

Debriding and Cleansing Agents

- Use a product containing either 10% to 15% carbamide peroxide, 3% hydrogen peroxide, or perborates after meals up to four times daily.
- Do not use these medications longer than 7 days. Chronic use can cause tissue irritation, decalcification of enamel, and black hairy tongue.
- Do not swallow these medications.

Topical Oral Anesthetics

- Ask your pharmacist to recommend a product containing one of the following medications: benzocaine 5% to 20%, benzyl alcohol 0.05% to 0.1%, butacaine sulfate 0.05% to 0.1%, dyclonine 0.05% to 0.1%, hexylresorcinol 0.05% to 0.1%, or salicylic alcohol 1% to 6%.
- Do not use benzocaine if you have a history of hypersensitivity to other benzocaine-containing products.
- Avoid potentially inflammatory products containing substantial amounts of menthol, phenol, camphor, or eugenol. These agents may cause tissue irritation and damage or systemic toxicity.

Topical Oral Protectants

- Use topical oral protectants (e.g., Orabase Plain or denture adhesives) to coat and protect the lesions. These agents will also provide temporary relief of discomfort.
- Apply these products as needed.

Oral Rinses

- Rinse the mouth with Listerine to hasten healing of the lesions.
- Rinse the mouth with a saline solution to soothe the discomfort or to prepare the lesion for application of a topical medication. For saline solution, add 1 to 3 teaspoons of table salt to 4 to 8 ounces of warm tap water.

Systemic Analgesics

- If desired, take an oral analgesic (e.g., aspirin, ibuprofen, or acetaminophen) for additional relief of mouth discomfort.
- Do not hold aspirin in the mouth or place it on oral lesions. The acid can cause a chemical burn with tissue necrosis.

See a physician if any of the following occur:

—Symptoms do not improve after 7 days of treatment with debriding/wound-cleansing agents.
—The lesions do not heal in 14 days.
—Symptoms worsen during self-treatment.
—Symptoms of systemic infection such as fever, rash, or swelling develop.

Patient Counseling for Recurrent Aphthous Stomatitis

The pharmacist should explain all drug and nondrug measures for treating RAS. The patient should be warned about ineffective or harmful therapies. Possible adverse effects, contraindications, and precautions should be explained for all nonprescription agents. In addition, the pharmacist must alert patients to the conditions that warrant dental or medical evaluation. The box "Patient Education for Recurrent Aphthous Stomatitis" lists specific information to provide patients.

Evaluation of Patient Outcomes for Recurrent Aphthous Stomatitis

The patient should return for reevaluation after 7 days of treatment with debriding and cleansing agents. If the symptoms have improved, the patient should discontinue treatment but continue hygienic measures. Symptoms that persist or that worsened during treatment require medical evaluation.

The patient should return for reevaluation after 14 days of treatment with the other discussed agents. If the ulcerations have disappeared or if symptoms have improved, the patient should discontinue treatments and continue hygienic measures. Persistent or worsening symptoms should be evaluated by a physician.

Minor Oral Mucosal Injury or Irritation

Minor wounds or inflammation resulting from minor dental procedures, accidental injury (e.g., biting the cheek or suffering abrasion from sharp, crisp foods), or other irritations of the mouth or gums may be treated with various nonprescription medications.

Treatment of Minor Oral Mucosal Injury or Irritation

Treatment of mouth injury and irritation is very similar to that of RAS. However, RAS warrants separate discussion because of its specific etiology and some specific treatment considerations.

Treatment Outcomes

The goals of treating minor mucosal injury and irritation are to (1) control discomfort and pain, (2) aid healing with the appropriate use of drug and nondrug measures, and (3) prevent secondary bacterial infection.

General Treatment Approach

Treatment should focus first on relieving discomfort. Local anesthetics, oral analgesics, and saline rinses are safe and effective choices. Application of ice is another method of relieving discomfort. Once discomfort is taken care of, patients should focus on healing the affected area. Homemade sodium bicarbonate rinses and oral debriding/cleansing agents can help achieve this objective. Finally, concomitant use of oral protectants can relieve discomfort and can aid healing by protecting the area from further irritation. (See the algorithm in Figure 26–3.)

Oral mucosal irritation or injuries that are not amenable to self-care include mouth soreness associated with orthodontic appliances or ill-fitting dentures; loose teeth; bleeding gums in the absence of trauma; broken or knocked-out teeth; toothache; severe tooth pain triggered or worsened by hot, cold, or chewing; and trauma to the mouth with bleeding, swelling, and soreness. The presence of fever indicates a systemic disorder and rules out self-treatment.

Nonpharmacologic Therapy

Sodium bicarbonate ($^1/_2$ to 1 teaspoon in 4 ounces of water) solutions can act as oral debriding/wound cleanser agents. The solution is swished in the mouth over the affected area for at least 1 minute and then spit out. Sodium bicarbonate's mucolytic action is related to its alkalinity. Saline rinses can cleanse and soothe the affected area. The patient should add 1 teaspoon to 3 teaspoons of salt to 4 to 8 ounces of warm tap water.

When tissues of the lips and cheeks are bruised, direct application of ice may reduce the swelling. Ice should not be applied longer than 20 minutes in a given hour. Longer than that time may cause tissue damage.

Pharmacologic Therapy

As with RAS, topical analgesics/anesthetics, astringents, oral protectants, and oral debriding/wound-cleansing agents are the mainstay of pharmacologic therapy.

Topical analgesics/anesthetics are applied for pain relief. Astringents cause tissues to contract or to arrest secretions by causing proteins to coagulate on a cell surface.[3] Oral mucosal protectants are pharmacologically inert substances that coat and protect the area. Debriding agents/oral wound cleansers may be used to (1) aid in the removal of debris or phlegm, mucus, or other secretions associated with sore mouth; (2) cleanse minor wounds or minor gum inflammation; and (3) cleanse recurrent aphthous ulcers.[11] (See the section "Treatment of Recurrent Aphthous Stomatitis" for discussion of these agents.)

Dentists may suggest that their patients use oxidizing mouthrinses or drops as an adjunctive treatment of specific conditions or as a postoperative aid to cleaning and relieving discomfort.

The review of oral antiseptic products found insufficient data to support efficacy for oral antiseptic use (i.e., to decrease the chance of infection in minor oral irritation).[18]

Patients who dislike complicated regimens may wish to use a combination preparation. (See Table 26–4.) These preparations may contain (1) a single anesthetic/analgesic with either a single astringent, an oral mucosal protectant, or a denture adhesive; or (2) benzocaine combined with menthol or phenol preparations.

Patient Assessment of Minor Oral Mucosal Injury or Irritation

The cause and nature of the injury or irritation are the primary considerations in patient assessment. If the disorder is self-treatable, the pharmacist should find out whether the patient has had previous episodes, how they were treated, and whether the patient has known contraindications to the nonprescription medications used to treat these disorders.

Asking patients the following questions will help elicit the information needed to accurately assess the disorder and to recommend the appropriate treatment approach.

Q~ How and when did your injury occur? Do you have pain? Are your lips (cheeks) bruised?

A~ Refer to a dentist those patients with trauma other than irritation from biting the cheek or eating sharp foods. If pain is severe, is related to teeth, or is associated with fever, swelling, or bleeding of the mouth or gums, refer the patient to a physician or dentist.

Q~ Do you wear dentures or braces? Do you have a bad taste in your mouth? How do you clean your dentures or teeth? How often? Do you have sore spots, or is the entire mouth sore?

A~ Refer patients with dentures or braces to a dentist or orthodontist. Ill-fitting devices can cause localized pain. If oral hygiene is poor, refer the patient to a dentist for evaluation of gingivitis and caries. (See Chapter 25, "Prevention of Hygiene-Related Oral Disorders.")

Q~ Have you ever self-treated an oral mucosal injury before? If so, how? Are you hypersensitive to analgesics or anesthetics?

A~ Tailor product recommendations to patient factors (e.g., medication hypersensitivity) as well as to patient preferences. Also consider previously successful treatments when selecting products.

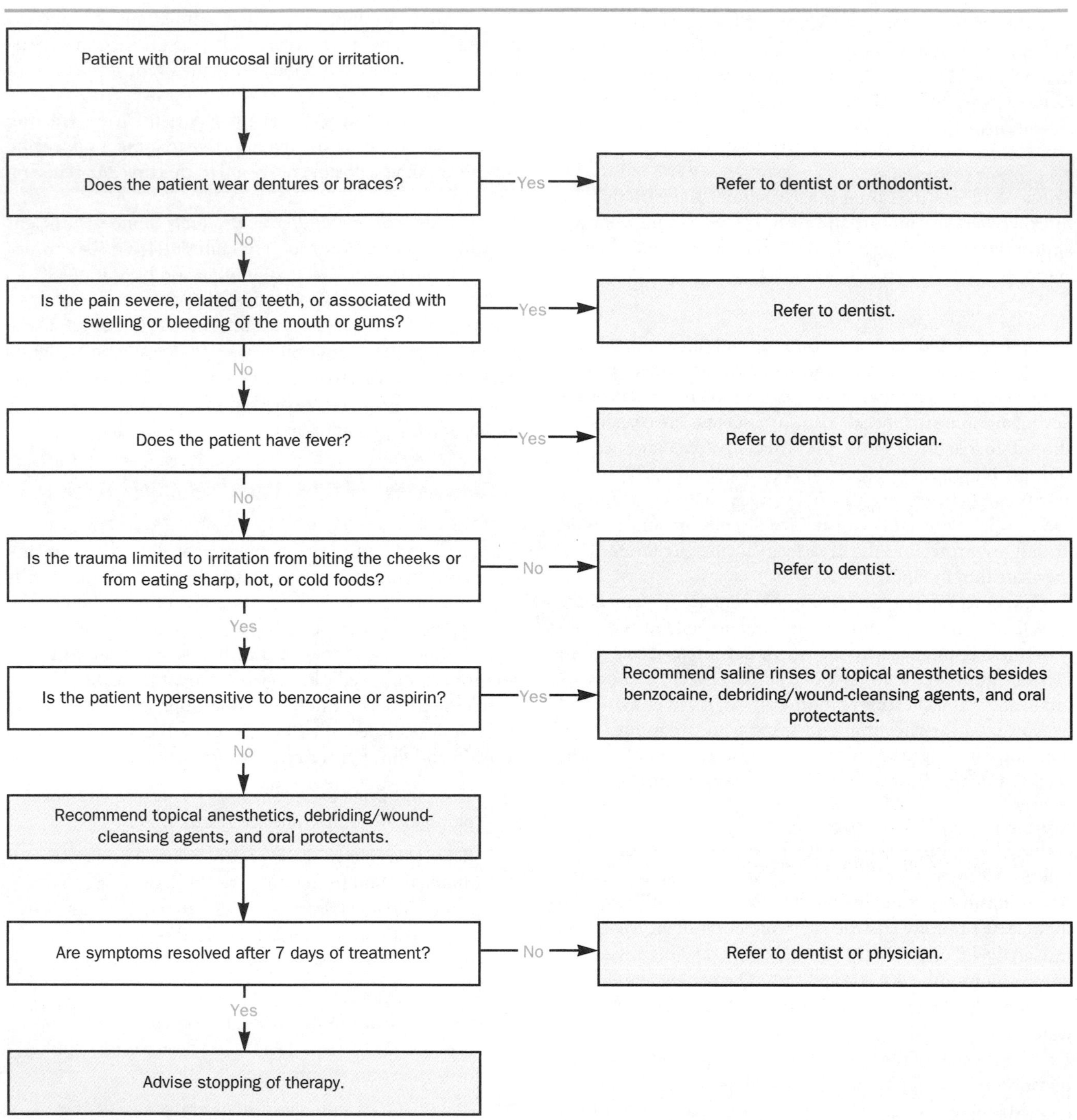

Figure 26–3 Self-care of minor oral mucosal injury or irritation.

Patient Counseling for Minor Oral Mucosal Injury or Irritation

Once the problem is assessed as minor irritation or injury of the mouth, the pharmacist should explain (1) the steps in the treatment regimen, (2) the purpose of each agent, and (3) the length of time the products can be used safely. Signs and symptoms that indicate infection should also be explained. The box "Patient Education for Minor Oral Mucosal Injury or Irritation" lists specific information to provide patients.

Evaluation of Patient Outcomes for Minor Oral Mucosal Injury or Irritation

The patient should return for reevaluation after 7 days of treatment with oral mucosal healing agents. If the symptoms are resolved, no further treatment is needed. If symptoms

Patient Education for Minor Oral Mucosal Injury or Irritation

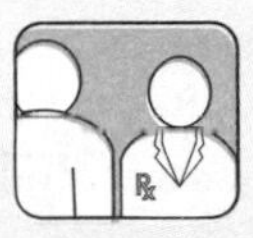

The objectives of self-treatment are to (1) control discomfort and pain, (2) aid healing with the appropriate use of drug and nondrug measures, and (3) prevent secondary bacterial infection. For most patients, carefully following product instructions and the self-care measures listed below will help ensure optimal therapeutic outcomes.

Nondrug Measures

- Rinse with a sodium bicarbonate solution to debride (remove injured tissue) and cleanse the affected area. Add $^1/_2$ to 1 teaspoon to 4 ounces of water. Swish the solution in the mouth over the affected area for 1 minute, and then spit out the solution.
- Use saline rinses to cleanse and soothe the affected area. Add 1 to 3 teaspoons of salt to 4 to 8 ounces of warm tap water.
- For bruised lips or cheeks, apply ice to reduce swelling. Do not apply ice longer than 20 minutes in a given hour.

Nonprescription Medications

- If longer-lasting relief is desired, ask your pharmacist to recommend one or more of the following types of nonprescription medications: debriding and cleansing agents, topical oral anesthetics, topical oral protectants, and systemic analgesics.

Debriding and Cleansing Agents

- Use a product containing either carbamide peroxide 10% to 15%, hydrogen peroxide 3%, or perborates after meals up to four times daily.
- Do not use these medications longer than 7 days. Chronic use can cause tissue irritation, decalcification of enamel, and black hairy tongue.
- Do not swallow these medications.

Topical Oral Anesthetics

- Ask your pharmacist to recommend a product containing one of the following medications: benzocaine 5% to 20%, benzyl alcohol 0.05% to 0.1%, butacaine sulfate 0.05% to 0.1%, dyclonine 0.05% to 0.1%, hexylresorcinol 0.05% to 0.1%, or salicylic alcohol 1% to 6%.
- Do not use benzocaine if you have a history of hypersensitivity to other benzocaine-containing products.
- Avoid potentially inflammatory products containing substantial amounts of menthol, phenol, camphor, or eugenol. These agents may cause tissue irritation and damage or systemic toxicity.

Topical Oral Protectants

- Use topical oral protectants (e.g., Orabase Plain) or denture adhesives to coat and protect the lesions.
- Apply these products as needed.

Systemic Analgesics

- If desired, take an oral analgesic (e.g., aspirin, ibuprofen, or acetaminophen) for additional relief of mouth discomfort.
- Do not hold aspirin in the mouth or place it on oral lesions. The acid can cause a chemical burn and tissue necrosis.

See a physician if any of the following occur:
—Symptoms persist after 7 days of treatment.
—Symptoms worsen during self-treatment.
—Symptoms of systemic infection such as fever, rash, or fever develop.

persist or worsen or if swelling, rash, or fever develops, the patient should see a dentist or physician for evaluation.

Herpes Simplex Labialis

Because herpes simplex labialis (cold sores) are viral disorders, any person who comes in contact with the virus has the potential to become infected. Once the virus has infected a host, it can go through periods of dormancy and reactivation.

Epidemiology of Herpes Simplex Labialis

Among the triggers of viral reactivation is ultraviolet radiation (sun tanners should use caution), stress, fatigue, chilling, and windburn. Other possible triggers include fever, any kind of injury, menstruation, dental work, infectious diseases (cold and flu), other factors that depresses the immune system.[19]

Pathophysiology of Herpes Simplex Labialis

Herpes simplex virus 1 (HSV-1) is contagious and is thought to be transmittable by direct contact. Fluid from herpes vesicles contains live virus and may serve to transmit the virus from patient to patient.[13] Herpes simplex virus 2 (HSV-2), which causes genital lesions, is sexually transmitted. However, it has been demonstrated in herpes lesions of the lip and can be caused by oral–genital contact or by hand-to-mouth transfer.

Herpes simplex labialis (HSV-1) infects through a break in the skin or through intact mucous membranes. Invasion of sensory neurons follows, and then the virus migrates to sensory ganglia where it may remain dormant. Because the virus is viable for several hours on surfaces, contaminated objects may also be a source of infection. Once infected, an individual may have recurrent lesions throughout life. Herpes simplex labialis is self-limiting and heals without scarring, usually within 10 to 14 days. The recurrence rate and extent of lesions vary greatly from patient to patient. Some patients may experience several large lesions every few weeks; other patients may have only a single small lesion at infrequent intervals.

Etiology of Herpes Simplex Labialis

Cold sores or fever blisters are lesions generally caused by HSV-1. They are referred to as herpes simplex labialis because they commonly occur on the lip or on areas bordering the lips; the usual site is at the junction of mucous membrane and skin of the lips or nose. The lesions are recurrent, painful, and cosmetically objectionable. About half of all patients who have sustained a primary (initial) HSV-1 infection will experience recurrent local lesions after some unpredictable latent interval; the lesions often arise in the same location repeatedly. After the primary infection, the virus apparently remains in host cells. The primary infection is reported most often in childhood. Patients may relate a history of primary herpetic stomatitis (viral-induced inflammation of the mouth), which usually manifests itself by vesicles (blisters) in the mouth. However, most primary oral infections of herpes virus seem to be subclinical, and most patients are unaware of their previous primary exposure.

Any of the human herpesviruses (cytomegalovirus, Epstein-Barr virus, and others—not just HSV-1 and 2) can cause oral lesions. Most people are sufficiently protected by their immune systems from manifesting symptoms. But in a setting of immunosuppression, repeated reactivation of latent infection becomes possible.

Signs and Symptoms of Herpes Simplex Labialis

The lesions are often preceded by a prodrome in which the patient notices burning, itching, tingling, or numbness in the area of the forthcoming lesion. The lesion first becomes visible as small, red papules of fluid-containing vesicles 1 mm to 3 mm in diameter. Often, many lesions coalesce to form a larger area of involvement. An erythematous, inflamed border around the fluid-filled vesicles may be present. A mature lesion often has a crust over the top of many coalesced, burst vesicles; its base is erythematous. The presence of pustules or pus under the crust of a herpes virus lesion may indicate a secondary bacterial infection and should be evaluated promptly and treated with an appropriate antibiotic. (See the "Color Plates," photograph 8.)

A related disease, acute herpetic gingivostomatitis, is mainly seen in children but can occur in adults, especially adults who are immunocompromised. Although they commonly occur on the lip, on areas bordering the lips, or on the gums, the oral lesions of this disease can develop anywhere on the oral mucosal surface, whereby they can resemble RAS lesions. Acute gingivostomatitis caused by herpesvirus can be distinguished from RAS by the fact that the infected gums are very red, are covered by a pseudomembrane, or are studded with ulcerations.

The appearance of herpes simplex labialis and RAS should easily be distinguished from the candidal plaque. In the mouth, candidiasis is often referred to as thrush, and white plaques with a milk curd appearance characterize it. Such plaques, which are attached to the oral mucosa, can usually be detached easily, displaying erythematous, bleeding, sore areas beneath. (See the "Color Plates, photograph 6.)

Treatment of Herpes Simplex Labialis

Although the etiology of herpes simplex labialis and RAS differs, treatment of these disorders is similar. Of the products listed in Table 26–4, debriding and cleansing agents are not used to treat herpes simplex labialis.

Treatment Outcomes

The goals of treating herpes simplex labialis are to (1) relieve the discomfort of the lesions, (2) prevent secondary bacterial infection, and (3) prevent autoinoculation or spread of the virus to others.

General Treatment Approach

Cleansing the affected area and using topical skin protectants can protect the lesions from infection. Skin protectants can also relieve dryness and keep lesions soft. Topical local anesthetics in bland, emollient vehicles aid in relieving the discomfort of burning, itching, and pain. If evidence of secondary bacterial infection is seen, topical application of a thin layer of triple-antibiotic ointment (e.g., Mycitracin or Neosporin) three to four times daily is recommended, along with systemic antibiotics if indicated. Systemic nonprescription analgesics may provide additional pain relief. (See Figure 26–4.)

Exclusions to self-treatment include lesions that have persisted longer than 14 days, outbreaks that are occurring with increased frequency, patients who are immunocompromised, and symptoms (e.g., fever, swollen glands, rash) that indicate an infection.

Nonpharmacologic Therapy

Lesions should be kept clean by gently washing with mild soap solutions. Hand washing is important in preventing lesion contamination and in minimizing autoinoculation of herpesvirus. The lesion should be kept moist to prevent drying and fissuring. Cracking of the lesions may render them more susceptible to secondary bacterial infection, may delay healing, and usually will increase discomfort.

Factors that delay healing (e.g., stress, local trauma, wind, sunlight, and fatigue) should be avoided. Patients who identify sun exposure as a precipitating event should be advised to use a lip and face sunscreen product routinely.

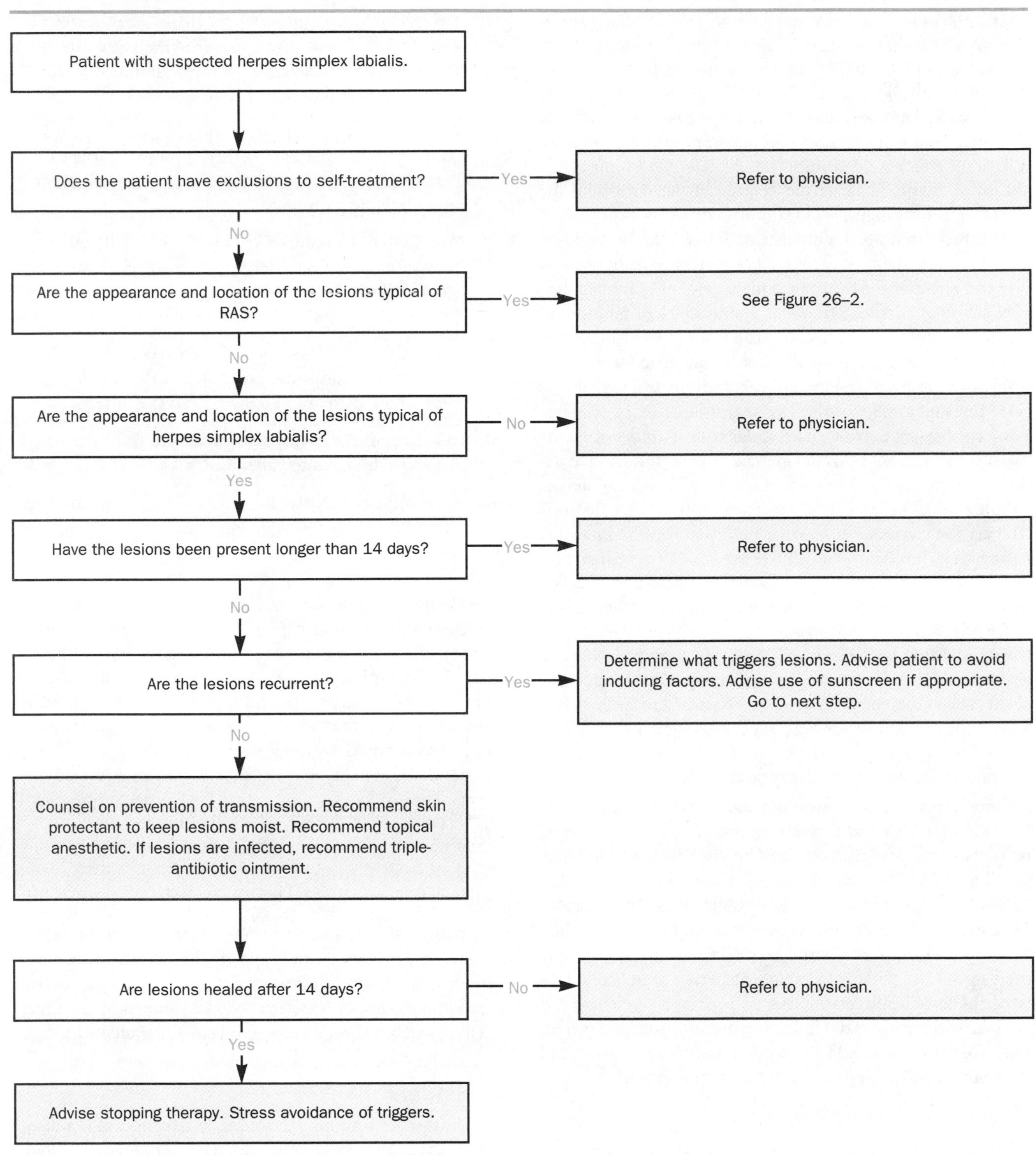

Figure 26–4 Self-care of herpes simplex labialis.

Pharmacologic Therapy

FDA has proposed the use of topically applied nonprescription skin protectants or externally applied analgesic/anesthetic drug products as the only currently effective nonprescription treatment for relieving the discomfort of herpes simplex labialis.[20]

FDA's review of over-the-counter (OTC) products for herpes simplex labialis classified external analgesics, alcohols, ketones, and amine- and caine-type local anesthetics as Category I.[21] A partial listing of Category I ingredients includes benzocaine 5% to 20%, dibucaine 0.25% to 1%, dyclonine hydrochloride 0.5% to 1%, benzyl alcohol 10% to 33%, camphor 0.1% to 3%, and menthol 0.1% to 1%.[22] These ingredients offer analgesic, anesthetic, and antipruritic effects in relieving the pain and itching of herpes simplex labialis.

Higher concentrations of certain ingredients (i.e., camphor greater than 3% and menthol greater than 1%) that stimulate cutaneous sensory receptors and produce a counterirritant effect are contraindicated.[23] Herpes simplex labialis is not considered a steroid-responsive dermatosis, so the use of topical steroids is contraindicated.[13]

Products that are highly astringent should be avoided. Tannic acid and zinc sulfate are not generally recognized as safe and effective for the topical management of herpes simplex labialis.[23] Because frequent applications of tannic acid to the lip and oral cavity could cause a patient to ingest it when eating or drinking, FDA was concerned about the drug's potential for oral mucosal absorption and toxicity.

Numerous orally administered products (e.g., preparations containing *Lactobacillus acidophilus, L. bulgaricus*, the essential amino acid L-lysine, citrus bioflavonoids, or pyridoxine) have also been proposed for the treatment of herpes simplex labialis. However, evidence conclusively demonstrating their efficacy is lacking. FDA determined in a final ruling that "no orally administered active ingredient has been found to be generally recognized as safe and effective for OTC use to treat or relieve the symptoms or discomfort of fever blisters and cold sores."[20]

Lesions that are secondarily infected with bacteria can also be coated three times a day with a triple-antibiotic ointment. (See Chapter 35, "Minor Wounds and Skin Infections," for more information about these agents.)

Patient Assessment of Herpes Simplex Labialis

Although many of the same nonprescription medications are indicated for RAS and for herpes simplex labialis, the pharmacist still needs to differentiate the disorders. Because herpes simplex lesions are contagious, additional measures are necessary to prevent transmission of the virus. The pharmacist should obtain the patient's medical and medication history to determine whether an underlying pathology predisposes the patient to recurrent herpes simplex labialis or could complicate treatment.

Asking the patient the following questions will help elicit the information needed to accurately assess the disorder and to recommend the appropriate treatment approach.

Q~ How long have you had this problem?

A~ Refer patients who have had herpes simplex labialis longer than 14 days to a physician.

Q~ Are the lesions visible? What color are they? Are they crusted or erythematous? Where in the mouth do they occur? On the skin bordering lips or nose?

A~ *Identify the characteristic signs of RAS and herpes simplex labialis. (See Table 26–3.)* Determine whether the patient's lesions are characteristic of herpes simplex labialis.

Q~ Do you have discomfort? Is the discomfort continuous? Does talking, eating, or drinking aggravate it? Do you have a discharge from the lesion? Do you have other symptoms?

A~ Recommend products or methods to relieve the discomfort. Refer patients with symptoms atypical of herpes simplex labialis to a physician for evaluation of underlying pathology.

Q~ Are the lesions recurrent? Do they occur in certain situations, such as after sun exposure or during stressful periods?

A~ *Identify known triggers of herpes simplex labialis. (See the section "Epidemiology of Herpes Simplex Labialis.")* If the lesions are associated with known triggers, advise the patient to avoid such situations.

Q~ What products have you used in the past? Do you have any drug-related allergies?

A~ Determine if the patient has any allergy to aspirin or caine-type anesthetics.

Patient Counseling for Herpes Simplex Labialis

The pharmacist should stress that herpes simplex lesions are contagious and should explain measures to prevent transmission of the virus. Patients should be advised that the disorder is self-limiting and that pharmacologic therapy can only keep the lesions moist and supple, remove the itch and pain, and protect the lesions from secondary bacterial infection. The pharmacist should explain the action of each recommended product, its proper use, and possible adverse effects. The box "Patient Education for Herpes Simplex Labialis" lists specific information to provide patients.

Evaluation of Patient Outcomes for Herpes Simplex Labialis

The patient should return for reevaluation after 14 days. If the symptoms have resolved, no further treatment is necessary. But if the condition worsens (pain and itching persist, redness increases, or signs of secondary infection are apparent), the patient should see a physician for evaluation.

Xerostomia

Xerostomia, commonly referred to as dry mouth, is a disorder in which salivary flow is limited or completely arrested.

Epidemiology/Etiology of Xerostomia

Epidemiologic factors for dry mouth correlate with its causes. Individuals having the diseases, taking the medications, or exhibiting lifestyle practices discussed below are most prone to this disorder. About 20% of the elderly are affected with dry mouth. Chronic diseases and polypharmacy are probably responsible for the high incidence of dry mouth in this population.

Patient Education for Herpes Simplex Labialis

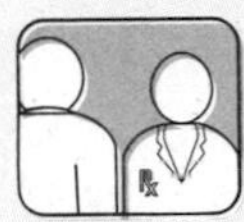

The objectives of self-treatment are to (1) relieve pain and irritation while the sores are healing, (2) prevent secondary infection, and (3) prevent spread of the lesions. For most patients, carefully following product instructions and the self-care measures listed below will help ensure optimal therapeutic outcomes.

Nondrug Measures

- Keep lesions clean by gently washing them with mild soap solutions.
- Wash hands frequently to prevent contaminating the lesions and to avoid spreading the virus.
- Avoid factors believed to delay healing such as stress, injury to the lesions, wind, sunlight, and fatigue.
- If outbreaks are related to sun exposure, use a lip and face sunscreen routinely.

Nonprescription Medications

- Use skin protectants such as allantoin, petrolatum, and cocoa butter to keep lesions moist and to prevent cracking of the lesions. (See Chapter 34, "Minor Burns and Sunburn," for discussion of these agents.) These measures help prevent secondary bacterial infection.
- Use topical anesthetics such as benzocaine or dibucaine to relieve burning, itching, and pain. Do not use benzocaine if you have a history of hypersensitivity to other benzocaine-containing products.
- If using products containing camphor and menthol, make sure that the concentration of camphor does not exceed 3% and that the concentration of menthol does not exceed 1%.
- Do not apply hydrocortisone to the lesions.
- If evidence of secondary bacterial infection is seen, apply a thin layer of triple-antibiotic ointment (e.g., Mycitracin or Neosporin) three to four times daily.
- If desired, take oral nonprescription analgesics (e.g., aspirin, ibuprofen, or acetaminophen) for additional pain relief.
- Do not hold aspirin in the mouth or place it on oral lesions. The acid can cause a chemical burn and tissue necrosis.

See a physician if any of the following occur:

—The lesions do not heal in 14 days.
—Self-treatment measures do not relieve the discomfort.
—Symptoms of systemic illness such as fever, malaise, rash, or swollen lymph glands occur.

The usual causes of xerostomia are disease (e.g., Sjögren's syndrome, diabetes, and depression), drugs with anticholinergic activity, or drugs that cause depletion of salivary flow volume (e.g., antihypertensives, antihistamines, antipsychotics, stimulants, tricyclic antidepressants, tranquilizers, and diuretics). Radiation therapy of the head and neck can cause atrophy of the salivary glands. Nonpharmacologic causes include use of alcohol, tobacco, caffeine, and breathing through the mouth.

Older patients are more likely to be taking multiple medications for chronic diseases. However, if xerostomia is drug-induced and the medication can be changed, the condition may be reversed.

Signs and Symptoms of Xerostomia

Xerostomia can result in difficulty in talking and swallowing, stomatitis and burning tongue, and halitosis. Food cannot be tasted when not moistened; thus xerostomia can cause loss of appetite and eventually decline of nutritional status.[24]

Complications of Xerostomia

Depending on the status of dentition, this disorder also can increase the incidence of caries, gingivitis, and more severe periodontal disease or can reduce denture-wearing time. Further, reduced flow of saliva can disturb the balance of microflora in the oral cavity and can predispose it to candidiasis. The absence of lubrication and buffering can lead to tooth erosion, decalcification, and decay.[24]

Treatment of Xerostomia

Dry mouth should never be discounted as inconsequential. Failure to treat it can result in serious complications for some patients.

Treatment Outcomes

The goals in treating dry mouth are to (1) relieve discomfort and (2) reduce the risk of dental decay.

General Treatment Approach

The patient should discontinue using substances that dry the mouth or erode tooth enamel. The commercially available artificial saliva products can be used as needed to relieve soft-tissue discomfort as outlined in Figure 26–5. These products are more effective and longer lasting than simple rinses and lozenges.

Exclusions to self-care include complications of dry mouth as described previously, as well as the presence of the following disorders: mouth soreness associated with poor-fitting dentures; fever or swelling; loose teeth; bleeding gums in the absence of trauma; broken or knocked-out teeth; severe tooth pain triggered or worsened by hot, cold, or chewing; and trauma to the mouth with bleeding, swelling, and soreness.

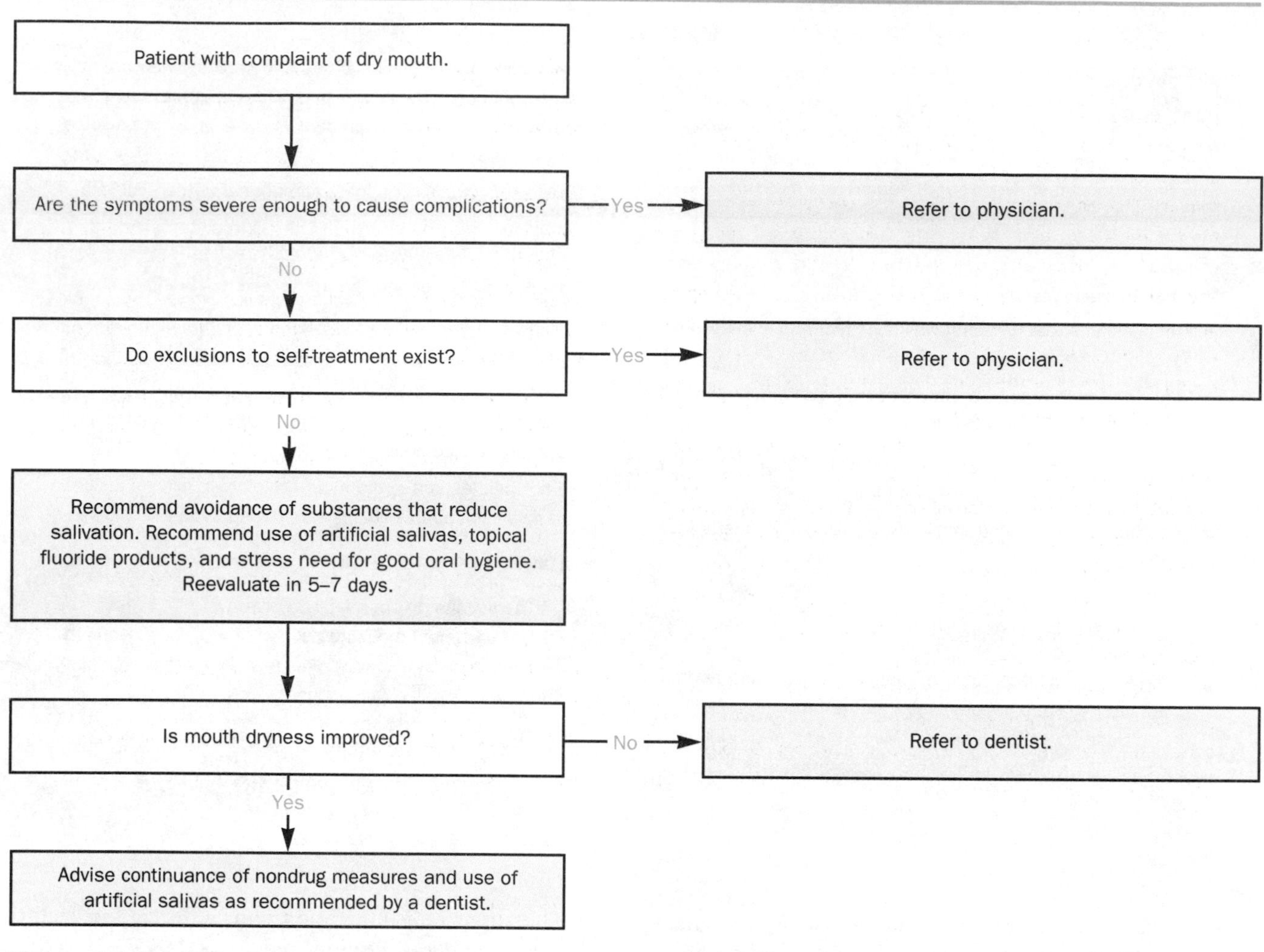

Figure 26–5 Self-care of xerostomia.

Table 26–5

Selected Artifical Saliva Products

Trade Name	Primary Ingredients
Glandosane Mouth Moisturizer Aerosol Spray	Sodium carboxymethylcellulose 0.51 g; sorbitol 1.52 g; sodium chloride 0.043 g; potassium chloride 0.061 g; calcium chloride dihydrate 0.007 g; magnesium chloride hexahydrarte 0.003 g; dipotassium hydrogen phosphate 0.017 g
Optimoist Liquid	Hydroxyethyl cellulose; sodium benzoate; citric acid; malic acid; sodium phosphate monobasic; calcium chloride; sodium monofluorophosphate; xyitol; polysorbate 20; sodium hydroxide
Oralbalance Moisturizing Gel	Hydroxyethyl cellulose; glycerate polyhydrate; glucose oxidase; lactoperoxidase; lysozyme; lactoferrin; xylitol
Salivart Synthetic Saliva Solution[a]	Sodium carboxymethylcellulose 1%; sorbitol; sodium chloride; potassium chloride; calcium chloride; magnesium chloride; potassium phosphate

[a] Preservative-free product.

Case Study 26–2

Patient Complaint/History

Colin, a 54-year-old man, picks out several nonprescription products and brings them to the pharmacy counter. He asks which product should be used to treat a crusted erythematous sore that is visible on the skin bordering his upper lip. He reveals that several days ago, after sensations of tingling and burning occurred at the lesion site, a cluster of small blisters appeared. The sore has since enlarged and formed a crust; it now hampers speaking and eating. Other symptoms include itching and pain at the site. Colin expresses concern for his overall health because he was told this type of lesion indicates an infection with the virus that causes chickenpox.

During conversation with the patient, the pharmacist determines that the lesions are recurrent. Colin acknowledges that this outbreak is the third such episode this year: one episode occurred on a 10-day winter vacation in the Caribbean; two other episodes occurred this past summer. He is very interested in preventing future occurrences and asks about preventive medications, specifically pyridoxine (vitamin B_6), which he heard can minimize or prevent these outbreaks.

The nonprescription drugs brought to the counter for the pharmacist's evaluation and recommendation include a hydrocortisone 1% topical cream, Blistex Lip Ointment, Orabase Lip Healer cream, Vaseline petroleum jelly, and pyridoxine 50 mg tablets. Colin mentions that he is allergic to aspirin.

Clinical Considerations/Strategies

Readers can use the following considerations/strategies to determine whether treatment of the patient's condition with nonprescription medications is warranted:

- Assess the patient's complaint.
- Assess individually the appropriateness of the four topical products (creams/ointments) and the pyridoxine for treating the lesion.
- Determine which ingredients in these products will have little positive effect on the symptom complex or in preventing secondary complications.
- Assess the specific value, or lack of value, that topical steroids have in treating herpes simplex labialis.
- Assess the specific value, or lack of value, that orally administered pyridoxine has in treating the symptoms.
- Propose a nonprescription topical medication regimen that is based on patient-specific factors and that focuses on products containing emollients and local analgesics/anesthetics.
- Define the role of oral nonprescription analgesics (acetaminophen, ibuprofen, naproxen, ketoprofen) in managing pain associated with herpes simplex lesions.

Patient Education/Counseling

Readers can use the following strategies to develop a patient education/counseling plan that will help ensure optimal therapeutic outcomes:

- Explain the etiology of the lesion as well as the tendency for recurrence, predisposing factors, and preventive measures.
- Define reasonable therapeutic goals in treating the lesion.
- Emphasize the importance of keeping the lesion and hands clean.
- Support the logic for changes in the nonprescription medication regimen selected by the patient. Provide the patient with appropriate information regarding product use (e.g., dose, frequency of administration, and duration of therapy).
- Define techniques and procedures for using the nonprescription medication regimen that was recommended by the pharmacist to provide symptomatic relief and prevent complications.

Nonpharmacologic Therapy

The patient should avoid substances that reduce salivation. Tobacco (smoked and smokeless) and products that contain alcohol (including mouthrinses), antihistamines, or central nervous system stimulants (pseudoephedrine and phenylpropanolamine) are common causes of impaired salivation.

To prevent tooth decay, the patient should limit intake of sugary and acidic foods. The sugar promotes bacterial growth, and the acid creates caries and increases tooth erosion. Similarly, the patient should avoid sucking on hard candy or lozenges sweetened with sugar because of the cariogenic potential. Chewing gum sweetened with sugar alcohols (e.g., xylitol), however, may be of benefit. Chewing gum increases salivary flow, and xylitol has been shown to have noncariogenic activity.[14,25] Finally, the use of very soft toothbrushes will help prevent decay by minimizing tissue abrasion.

Pharmacologic Therapy

Artificial saliva products are the primary products for relieving the discomfort of dry mouth. Topical fluoride products help reduce the risk of caries.

Artificial Saliva Products Artificial salivas are of value and can be used on an as-needed basis in patients with little or no flow of saliva. An ADA-accepted artificial saliva is Salivart Synthetic Saliva.[26] (See Table 26–5 for other examples of commercially available products.)

Artificial salivas are designed to mimic natural saliva both chemically and physically. Because they do not stimulate natural salivary gland production, however, they must be considered as replacement therapy, not as a cure for xerostomia. Artificial saliva closely resembles natural saliva and is formulated with the following properties:

- Viscosity. Carboxymethylcellulose and glycerin are used to mimic natural saliva viscosity.
- Mineral content. All products contain calcium and phosphate ions, and some also contain fluoride. With normal use, no product has demonstrated the ability to remineralize enamel. Therefore, ADA does not recognize any such claims made by the manufacturers.
- Preservatives. Salivart does not contain preservatives because it is packaged as a sterile aerosol. Other products do contain preservatives, such as methyl- or propylparaben, which may cause hypersensitivity reactions in certain patients.
- Palatability. Flavorings (e.g., mint or lemon) and sweeteners (e.g., sorbitol and xylitol) are commonly used.

Patients on low-sodium diets should avoid artificial salivas that contain sodium.

Topical Fluoride Products Xerostomic patients with a history of susceptibility to caries should use a professionally designed topical fluoride program in addition to artificial saliva products. Chapter 25, "Prevention of Hygiene-Related Oral Disorders," discusses the use of topical fluoride products and other oral hygiene measures.

Patient Assessment of Xerostomia

The pharmacist should inquire about the patient's history of xerostomia, oral hygiene practices, and regularity of dental visits. The pharmacist should then evaluate the patient's symptoms to determine whether the symptoms have progressed to the point that complications are likely. A review of the patient's medical and medication history will rule in or out the presence of diseases and/or use of medications known to reduce salivation. Further, the pharmacist should find out whether lifestyle or other practices could be contributing to dry mouth.

Asking the patient the following questions will help elicit the information needed to accurately assess the disorder and to recommend the appropriate treatment approach.

Q~ What symptoms are you having?

A~ Identify signs and symptoms characteristic of dry mouth. (See the section "Signs and Symptoms of Xerostomia.") Determine whether the patient's symptoms indicate dry mouth.

Q~ What drugs (prescription and nonprescription) are you taking? How long have you been taking them?

A~ Identify drugs known to reduce salivation. (See the section "Epidemiology/Etiology of Xerostomia.") Refer patients taking any of these medications to a physician for possible adjustments in medications.

Q~ Do you use alcohol or tobacco? Do you consume foods or drinks that contain caffeine?

A~ Advise patients who smoke, drink alcohol, or drink caffeinated beverages that these substances contribute to dry mouth.

Q~ Are you losing weight? Are you having difficulty eating? Do you have any mouth inflammation or soreness?

A~ Refer patients with severe symptoms such as these to a physician.

Q~ Do you have toothaches or other denture or dental pains? How frequently do you visit your dentist? Are you using fluoride treatments?

A~ Evaluate the risk for tooth decay on the basis of the patient's oral hygiene practices.

Patient Counseling for Xerostomia

Patients need to know which appropriate drug and nondrug measures will keep the oral cavity moist and can be taken to treat dry mouth. The pharmacist should warn these patients of the increased risk for tooth decay. They should be encouraged to practice good oral hygiene measures and to see their dentists regularly. Finally, the pharmacist must alert patients to signs and symptoms that indicate complications from dry mouth. The box "Patient Education for Xerostomia" lists specific information to provide patients.

Evaluation of Patient Outcomes for Xerostomia

The patient with xerostomia should return for evaluation after 5 to 7 days of self-treatment. If the mouth dryness is improved, the patient should continue using artificial salivas as recommended by a dentist. The patient should also be advised to continue the nondrug measures. If the dryness becomes worse or symptoms of complications develop, the patient should see a dentist for further evaluation.

CONCLUSIONS

For treatment of minor oral problems, the goal of therapy is to minimize discomfort, to allow healing, and, in the case of herpes simplex labialis, to prevent spread of the virus. Given that the pharmacy is the source for nonprescription products for symptomatic treatment of minor oral problems, the pharmacist has an opportunity to interpret consumer advertising, clinical data, FDA's regulations, and ADA's acceptance guidelines for the patient. These services are important components for educating and counseling patients about oral problems and for monitoring their oral health care needs. Pharmacists can also offer patients assessment services such as an evaluation of disease states and medication profiles,

Patient Education for Xerostomia

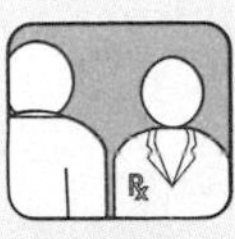

The objectives of self-treatment are to (1) relieve the discomfort of dry mouth and (2) reduce the risk of dental decay. For most patients, carefully following product instructions and the self-care measures listed below will help ensure optimal therapeutic outcomes.

Nondrug Measures

- To prevent reduced levels of saliva, avoid use of cigarettes and smokeless tobacco.
- Do not use products that contain alcohol (including mouthrinses), antihistamines (allergy medications, decongestants) and the drugs pseudoephedrine and phenylpropanolamine. These substances reduce saliva levels.
- Avoid foods or drinks that contain caffeine.
- To prevent tooth decay, limit consumption of sugary and acidic foods. Do not suck on hard candy or lozenges sweetened with sugar.
- If desired, chew gum sweetened with sugar alcohols such as xylitol to help increase flow of saliva.
- To help prevent tooth decay, use a very soft toothbrush to reduce abrasion of the teeth.

Nonprescription Medications

- Use artificial saliva products to relieve the discomfort of dry mouth.
- If you are on a low-sodium diet, avoid artificial salivas that contain sodium.
- Use topical fluoride products to help reduce the risk of tooth decay. Also, brush your teeth at least twice daily using a regular toothpaste with fluoride, floss at least once daily, and see your dentist regularly.

If your symptoms do not improve or if they worsen, see a dentist.

triage, referral to a dental professional if necessary, or proper instruction on self-care with nonprescription products that have proven to be safe and efficacious. By establishing open lines of communication with dental practitioners, pharmacists can better serve their patients as oral health consultants and as members of the oral health care team.

References

1. Kanapka JA. Over-the-counter dentifrices in the treatment of tooth hypersensitivity. *Dent Clin North Am.* 1990;34:545–60.
2. Gossel TA. Hypersensitive teeth: OTCs take the pain away. *US Pharm.* 1991;16:23–32.
3. *Federal Register.* 1991 September 24;56 : 48308–10,48315–6,48325, 48335–46.
4. *Federal Register.* 1992 May 11;57:20115.
5. Pray WS. Oral mucosal lesions. *US Pharm.* 1990;15:21–2,24–5,66.
6. Antoon JW, Miller RL. Aphthous ulcers—a review of the literature on etiology, pathogenesis, diagnosis, and treatment. *J Am Dent Assoc.* 1980;101:603–8.
7. Rehberger A, Puspok A, Stallmeister T, et al. Crohn's disease masquerading as aphthous ulcers. *Eur J Dermatol.* 1998;8:274–6.
8. Bonaccorso A, Tripi TR. Oral lesions in systemic lupus erythematosus. I. The etiopathogenic aspects of lupus erythematosus. *Minerva Stomatol.* 1998;47:27–31.
9. Krause I, Rosen Y, Kaplan I, et al. Recurrent aphthous stomatitis in Behçet's disease: Clinical features and correlation with systemic disease expression and severity. *J Oral Pathol Med.* 1999;28:193–6.
10. Eisen DE, Lynch DP. *The Mouth; Diagnosis and Treatment.* Mosby: St. Louis; 1998.
11. *Federal Register.* 1988 January 27;53:2453,2456.
12. *Federal Register.* 1986 July 18;51:26113.
13. Council on Dental Therapeutics. *Accepted Dental Therapeutics.* 40th ed. Chicago: American Dental Association; 1984 : 64–5,79,321–4,386–8, 395–420.
14. Harris NO, Garcia-Godoy F. *Primary Preventive Dentistry.* 5th ed. Stamford, CT: Appleton & Lange; 1999:64–9,88–9,110,115–6,145,177, 206,361,381,426,435,564–5.
15. American Dental Association. *ADA Statement on the Safety of Hydrogen-Peroxide-Containing Dental Products Intended for Home Use.* Chicago: American Dental Association; 1997.
16. Gossel TA. Debriding agents and oral wound cleansers. *US Pharm.* 1990;15:28–36.
17. *Federal Register.* 1982 May 25;47:22809,22842–4.
18. *Federal Register.* 1994 February 9;59:6084.
19. Scully C. Orofacial herpes simplex infections: Current concepts in the epidemiology, pathogenesis, and treatment, and the disorders in which the virus may be implicated. *Oral Surg Oral Med Oral Path.* 1989;68: 701–10.
20. *Federal Register.* 1992 June 30;57:29173.
21. *Federal Register.* 1990 January 31;55:3372,3379.
22. Council on Dental Materials, Instruments, and Equipment. Denture cleansers. *J Am Dent Assoc.* 1983;106:77–9.
23. *Federal Register.* 1993 May 10;58:27638.
24. Klatell J, Kaplan A, Williams G Jr. *The Mount Sinai Medical Center Guide to Dental Health.* New York: Macmillan Publishing; 1991: 269,273–4.
25. *Federal Register.* 1996 August 23;61:43433–47.
26. Council on Scientific Affairs. *Products of Excellence ADA Seal Program.* Chicago: American Dental Association; 1998.

SECTION VIII

DERMATOLOGIC DISORDERS

CHAPTER 27

Atopic Dermatitis, Contact Dermatitis, and Dry Skin

Nina H. Han and Dennis P. West

Chapter 27 at a Glance

Skin disorders are common, with an estimated 5% of people suffering from a chronic skin, hair, or nail condition and many others experiencing acute or seasonal disorders. A majority of people ages 65 and older have two or

Editor's Note: This chapter is based, in part, on the 11th edition chapter titled "Dermatologic Products," which was written by Dennis P. West and Phillip A. Nowakowski.

more skin conditions such as seborrheic dermatitis, fungal infections, and neoplastic growths.[1]

Pharmacists play a key role in providing services to manage skin disorders in the community. In a study of some 300 consumers who purchased nonprescription skin products, 42% bought products that were recommended by pharmacists while 18% were recommended by physician recommendation. The most frequently described skin disorders included dermatitis, dry skin, acne, and tinea.[2]

Dermatitis is a nonspecific term that describes a vast number of dermatologic conditions that are inflammatory and generally characterized by erythema (redness). The terms *eczema* and *dermatitis* are often used interchangeably to describe a group of inflammatory skin disorders of unknown etiology. When the cause of a particular skin condition is elucidated, the disorder is given a specific name. Known causes of dermatitis include allergens, irritants, and infections. However, several distinct forms of dermatitis exist for which the causes remain unclear.

This chapter discusses the most common forms of dermatitis—atopic dermatitis and contact dermatitis (irritant or allergic)—and dry skin, another common dermatologic complaint. Almost everyone has experienced dry or chapped skin (xerosis). In some people, it is a seasonal occurrence, while it is a chronic condition in others. Although dry skin is often not serious, it may be annoying and uncomfortable because of the attendant pruritus and, in some cases, pain and inflammation. In addition, dry skin is more prone to bacterial invasion than is normal skin.

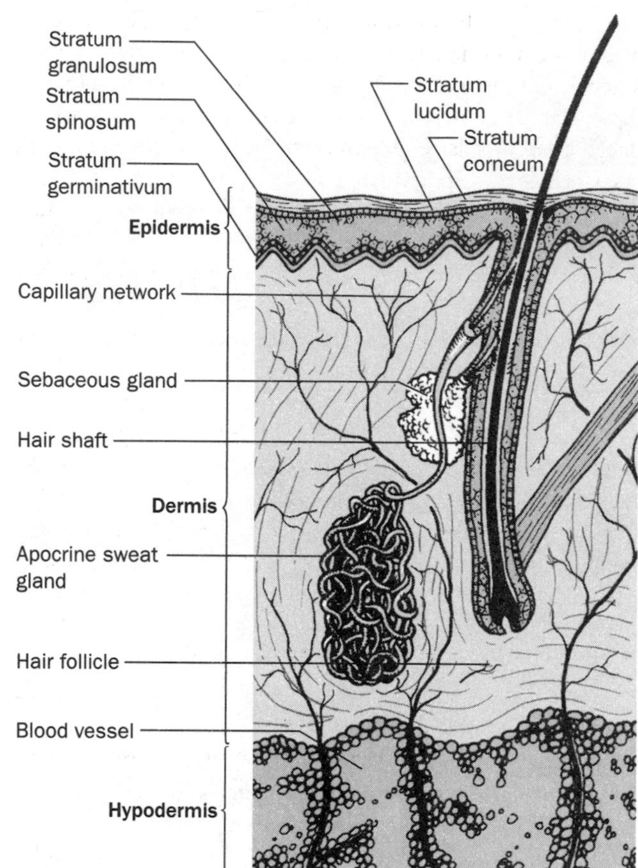

Figure 27–1 Cross section of human skin.

Anatomy and Physiology of the Skin

The skin is the largest organ of the body; it is involved in numerous physical and biochemical processes.[3] Skin thickness is variable but it averages about 1 to 2 mm, with the thickest skin on the palms of the hand and soles of the feet, and the thinnest skin on the eyelids and scrotum. These thinner areas are more permeable and allow substances to be absorbed through the skin more easily than thicker skin areas do. Although it is exposed to a wide variety of chemical and environmental insults, skin demonstrates remarkable resiliency and recuperative ability.

Skin Regions

Human skin is composed of three functionally distinct regions: epidermis, dermis, and hypodermis. Figure 27–1 shows these three regions and their components.

Epidermis

The epidermis is the outermost layer and consists of compact, avascular stratified squamous epithelial cells. There are five distinct layers. Innermost, in close association with the dermis, is the basal cell layer (stratum germinativum). This layer consists of columnar/cuboidal epithelial cells, or keratinocytes, which divide and move upward. As keratinocytes migrate to the skin surface, they change from living cells to dead, thick-walled, flat, nonnucleated cells that contain keratin (a fibrous, insoluble protein). The basal cell region is predominately involved in the mitotic processes of epidermal regeneration and repair.

Above the basal cell layer is the prickle cell unit (stratum spinosum), which is thicker in the palms and soles than in other anatomic skin sites. This layer is composed of prickle cells or polygonal epithelial cells that are produced by cellular division. The stratum spinosum contains keratinocytes, the pigment-forming melanocytes that contain melanin precursors and melanin granules.

Above the prickle cells is the granular region (stratum granulosum), which is several thicknesses of flattened polygonal cells. These cells are rich in granules of keratohyalin.

A translucent, thin area (stratum lucidum), which is present in the palms and soles, lies between the stratum granulosum and the stratum corneum. The stratum lucidum is a narrow band of flattened, closely packed cells believed to be derived from keratohyalin.

The outermost layer, the stratum corneum, is composed of flat, scaly, dead (keratinized) tissue. The stratum corneum is the layer normally exposed to the environment. The stratum corneum is highly lipophilic and, thus, is likely to store fat-soluble materials rather than allow them to pass into the systemic circulation. Its outermost cells are flat (squamous) plates that are constantly shed (desquamated) and are replaced by new cells generated by the mitotic processes of the basal cell layer. Specifically, newer cells push older ones closer to the surface. In the process, the older cells are flattened, lose water, become more compact, and gradually lose their nuclei before taking their place on the skin surface, where they are shed. Because the keratinized, or "horny," layer of the stratum corneum is constantly being shed and regenerated, the epidermis is maintained at a uniform thickness. The complete cycle, from basal cell formation to shedding is 28 to 45 days. This cycle length is important because some topically applied medications may not be effective until the complete cycle is over.

Flexibility of the stratum corneum depends on its water content, which is normally between 10% and 20% by weight. Many factors, including humidity, temperature, surfactants, and physical or chemical trauma, influence the water content of the stratum corneum.[4] Keratin can absorb many times its weight in water, and thus retains water to maintain the skin's flexibility and integrity. Intracellular spaces of the stratum corneum contain a complex mixture of hygroscopic substances (e.g., free amino acids, pyrrolidine carboxylic acid, urea, uric acid, ammonia, creatinine, sodium, calcium, potassium, magnesium, phosphate, chloride, lactate, citrate, formate, sugars, organic acids, and peptides) called the natural moisturizing factor, which holds water and allows absorption of water-soluble drugs. When the skin's water content drops below 10%, chapping occurs and the stratum corneum becomes brittle and cracks easily. This chapping allows irritants and bacteria to penetrate more easily, causing inflammation and possibly infection.

Dermis

About 40 times thicker than the epidermis, the dermis supports the epidermis physically and separates it from the lower fatty layer. The dermis consists mainly of elastic and connective tissue (collagen and elastin) embedded in a mucopolysaccharide substance. Fibroblasts and mast cells are found throughout. A network of nerves and blood supply is found in the dermis. This network is composed of the neurovascular supply to dermal appendages (hair follicles, sebaceous glands, and sweat glands). Because this layer of skin contains nerve fibers, it is responsible for cutaneous sensations. The sensation of itching arises in the upper portion, that of stinging arises in the middle portion, and that of pain arises in the portion closest to the layer of subcutaneous fat. The main regions of the dermis are the papillary and reticular layers. The papillary layer, which is adjacent to the epidermis, is rich in blood vessels and is thought to assist in bringing nutrients to the avascular epidermis. Below the papillae, the reticular layer contains coarser tissue that connects the dermis with the hypodermis.

Hypodermis

The hypodermis, or subcutaneous tissue, is the innermost area of the skin. It is composed of loose connective tissue and adipose tissue firmly anchored to the dermis. Subcutaneous tissue is of varying thickness and provides necessary pliability for human skin. This layer also includes a fatty component that facilitates thermal control, holds a food reserve, and provides cushioning or padding.

Skin Functions

Normal skin and its appendages (hair and nails) have many functions, the most important being to serve as a protective barrier between the body and the environment. The ability of the skin to protect the body from harmful external agents such as pathogenic organisms and chemicals[5] depends on age, immunologic status, underlying disease states of the individual, use of certain oral or topical medications, and preservation of an intact stratum corneum.[6]

The acid mantle has been postulated to be a protective mechanism because infected areas of skin typically have higher pH values than areas of normal skin. Several fatty acids (e.g., propionic, caproic, and caprylic) found in sweat and sebum help inhibit microbial and fungal growth. Therefore, the importance of the acid mantle concept lies not only in the inherent pH of the acid mantle but also in the specific compounds responsible for the acidity.

Another protective mechanism is the buffer capacity of skin surface secretion. When pH is altered, the skin tends to readjust to a normal pH. Moreover, normal skin flora acts as a defense mechanism by controlling the growth of potential pathogenic organisms and their possible invasion of the skin and body.

The skin also contributes to sensory experiences and is involved in temperature control, pigment development, and synthesis of some vitamins. It is also important in hydroregulation because it controls moisture loss from the body and moisture penetration into the body.

Skin hydration is important to the health and normal function of the skin. If the stratum corneum becomes dehydrated, it loses elasticity and its permeation characteristics become altered. The stratum corneum can be hydrated by water transfer from lower regions of the skin and by water accumulation (perspiration) induced by occlusive coverings such as impervious bandages or oleaginous pharmaceutical vehicles (e.g., petrolatum). Generally, such moisture accumulation seems to "open" the compactness of the stratum corneum for renewed suppleness and for more-effective penetration by some drug molecules. Aging skin becomes more fragile, requiring a longer recovery time after injury. Excessive or aggressive bathing insults aging skin more than younger skin.

Percutaneous Absorption of Drugs

A drug must be released from its vehicle if it is to exert an effect at the desired site of activity (the skin surface, the epidermis, or the dermis). Release occurs at the interface between the skin surface and the applied layer of product. The physical–chemical relationship between the drug and the vehicle determines the rate and amount of drug released. Considerations such as the drug's solubility in the vehicle, its diffusion coefficient in the vehicle, and its partition coefficient into the sebum and stratum corneum are significant to its efficacy.[7] Molecular weight, molecular size, and melting point of a compound are factors that influence percutaneous absorption. A drug with a strong affinity for the vehicle has a lower rate and extent of percutaneous absorption than does a drug with weaker affinity for its vehicle. Thus, a drug with a proper balance of polar and hydrocarbon moieties (i.e., a partition coefficient) penetrates the stratum corneum more readily than one that is either highly polar or highly lipoidal.

Other factors influencing drug release include degree of hydration of the stratum corneum, p*Ka* of the drug, pH of the drug vehicle and the skin surface, drug concentration, thickness of the applied layer, and temperature. As temperature increases at the site of application, blood flow in the area also increases, as does the rate of percutaneous absorption. These factors apply to drug release from all topical forms (e.g., powders, ointments, pastes, emulsified creams or lotions, gels, suspensions, and solutions).

Oily hydrocarbon bases such as petrolatum are transiently occlusive, promote hydration, and generally increase molecular transport. Hydrous emulsion bases are less occlusive. Water-soluble bases (polyethylene glycols) are minimally occlusive, may attract water from the stratum corneum, and may decrease drug transport. Powders with hydrophilic ingredients presumably decrease hydration because they promote evaporation from the skin by absorbing available water.

Substances are transported from the skin surface to the general circulation through percutaneous absorption. The routes of such transport have not been proven, but it is presumed that they involve passage through skin between the keratinized units of the stratum corneum and through skin appendages (e.g., hair follicles, sweat glands, and sebaceous glands). The major mechanism of drug absorption is by passive diffusion through the stratum corneum, followed by transport through the deeper epidermal regions and then the dermis.

Drug movement into and through the skin meets with varying degrees of enhancement or inhibition depending on the physical–chemical properties of a drug, the sebum, and area of skin. The stratum corneum provides the greatest resistance and is often a rate-limiting barrier to percutaneous absorption. Because it is nonliving tissue, the stratum corneum may be viewed as having the general characteristics of an artificial and semipermeable membrane. Molecular passage through the stratum corneum occurs mostly by passive diffusion. Once a molecule has crossed this layer, there is much less resistance to its transport through the rest of the epidermis and into the dermis.

When the stratum corneum is hydrated, drug diffusion is generally accelerated. Hydration swells the stratum corneum, loosening its normally tight, densely packed arrangement, thus making diffusion easier. Occlusion also increases hydration of the stratum corneum, which enhances the transfer of most drugs. The increased amount of water present in the skin under such conditions probably further enhances the transfer of polar molecules.

Wounds, burns, chafed areas, and dermatitis can alter the integrity of the stratum corneum and can result in artificial shunts of the percutaneous absorption process. Inflammation can also enhance percutaneous absorption of topically applied medications, which may result in dangerous systemic drug levels. Therefore, caution should be used in applying topical medication to compromised skin, particularly if large surface areas are involved.

Atopic Dermatitis

Epidemiology of Atopic Dermatitis

Atopic dermatitis occurs primarily in infants, children, and young adults. It is considered the most common dermatologic condition seen in children, with more than 10% of children affected by age 6 months. In adults, it is often associated with other skin conditions, such as dry skin, hand dermatitis, and contact dermatitis. Areas commonly affected (e.g., the face, the flexural areas on the inside of the knees and elbows, and the collar area of the neck) depend on the patient's age.

Etiology/Pathophysiology of Atopic Dermatitis

The word "atopy" literally means uncommon or "not in the right place." Atopic dermatitis is diagnosed according to clinical criteria. No established laboratory tests exist, although many patients have shown an elevated immunoglobulin E (IgE) level and peripheral blood eosinophilia. Atopic dermatitis may be accompanied by allergic respiratory disease, but often is the initial clinical manifestation of an allergic disease.

Common exacerbating factors include soaps, detergents, chemicals, temperature changes, mold, dust, pollens, and emotional changes. Patients with atopic dermatitis are generally very sensitive to irritants; thus, it is important for patients affected to minimize exposure to irritants and allergens.[8]

Atopic dermatitis is not contagious and is thought to be genetically linked. If one parent has the condition, the child has a greater than 25% chance of developing it. If both parents have atopic dermatitis, the child has a greater than 50% chance of developing it. Although the etiology of the condition is unknown, patients and immediate family members often have associated asthma, hay fever, or chronic allergic rhinitis.[9]

Signs and Symptoms of Atopic Dermatitis

Although atopic dermatitis is often first manifested in infancy, it is rarely present at birth. If it does develop early in life, it typically occurs within the first year (often beginning at ages 2 to 3 months) in approximately 80% of the cases. It initially appears as redness and chapping of the infant's cheeks, which may continue to affect the face, neck, and trunk. At times, this dermatitis may progress to become more generalized with crusting developing on the forehead and cheeks.[10] Crusting (or scabs) is dried exudate containing proteinaceous and cellular debris from erosion or ulceration of primary skin lesions. Remission usually occurs between ages 2 and 4 years, with recurrences often diminishing in intensity or even disappearing as the child approaches adulthood.[4]

A classic case of infantile or childhood atopic dermatitis involves the cheeks and extensor surfaces of the forearms and legs. (See the "Color Plates," photographs 9 A, B, and C.) Later manifestations of atopic dermatitis typically present on flexor surfaces. Lesions are typically symmetric in atopic dermatitis patients.

The primary symptom of atopic dermatitis is severely intense pruritic papules (solid, circumscribed, elevated lesions less than 1 cm in diameter) and vesicles (sharply circumscribed, elevated lesions containing fluid). The pruritis is often intermittent, leading to vigorous itch–scratch cycles.[9] The skin may show inflammation and may produce scales; infection may result.[10]

The itching can be exacerbated by environmental and psychologic factors. Affected skin can progress to erythematous, excoriated, and scaling lesions. After repeated scratching and itching, the skin becomes thick, or lichenified (increased epidermal markings). This lichenification is often considered characteristic and sometimes diagnostic of atopic dermatitis.[10]

Complications of Atopic Dermatitis

Secondary or associated cutaneous infections can be common, difficult to prevent, and typically aggravate the condition. Patients should be counseled to seek medical attention promptly when signs of bacterial or viral skin infection such as pustules (circumscribed, elevated lesions less than 1 cm in diameter containing pus), vesicles (especially exudate or pus-filled), crusting (dried exudate), and herpes simplex (fever blisters or cold sores) are noticed.[11]

Special Considerations for Atopic Dermatitis

Atopic dermatitis may be exacerbated by various factors such as irritants, allergens, extremes of temperature and humidity, dry skin, emotional stress, and cutaneous infections. The patient should be encouraged to identify the role of these factors (if any) so that they may be minimized or avoided.

Irritants (e.g., solvents, industrial chemicals, fragrances, soaps, fumes, tobacco smoke, paints, bleach, wool, and astringents) may cause burning, itching, or redness of the skin.[11] Patients with atopic dermatitis may be especially sensitive to low concentrations of irritants that would not generally cause a reaction on normal skin.

Allergens—typically, plant or animal proteins from food, pollens, or pets—may aggravate atopic dermatitis. However, the role of food allergies in exacerbating atopic dermatitis is unclear. It is claimed that up to 20% of children with atopic dermatitis are affected by allergic reactions to foods through either ingestion or skin contact,[11] and specific hypersensitivities to milk products and eggs have been identified. Dietary management needed to achieve strict avoidance often poses overwhelming compliance problems. Moreover, while dietary restriction may show some improvement in the condition initially, complete resolution is unlikely to occur. Thus, it is probably best to reserve dietary management for patients who have severe symptoms and are unresponsive to other treatments.[4,12]

Patients with atopic dermatitis are often intolerant of sudden and extreme changes in temperature and humidity. High humidity may enhance perspiration, which may lead to increased itching. Low humidity, often found in heated buildings during the winter, dries the skin and increases itching. Use of humidifiers in dry environments will provide some benefit. Similar to asthma, emotional stress is an exacerbating factor in some patients. A calm environment and biofeedback techniques may prove beneficial for some of these patients.

Treatment Overview of Atopic Dermatitis

Treatment Outcomes

The goals in treating atopic dermatitis are to (1) maintain skin hydration, (2) relieve or minimize symptoms of itching and weeping, and (3) avoid or minimize factors that trigger or aggravate the disorder.

General Treatment Approach

Regardless of a patient's age, the stratum corneum in patients with atopic dermatitis contains less moisture than normal skin. Enhancing skin hydration can be achieved through nonpharmacologic measures, as well as through the use of emollients and moisturizers. Hydrocortisone can help relieve itching and the weeping of vesicles. The most-effective measure is avoiding factors known to trigger the allergic reaction. The algorithm in Figure 27–2 outlines the self-treatment of this disorder.

If the condition is severe or involves a large area of the body or if the patient is age 2 years or younger, a physician should be consulted. There is a general understanding that topical medications should not be used on children age 2 years or younger except under the advice and supervision of a physician. Part of the rationale is that infants have immature hepatic enzyme systems, as well as higher body surface area-to-weight ratios than do older individuals. Therefore, infants are at increased risk for systemic effects from topically applied drugs.

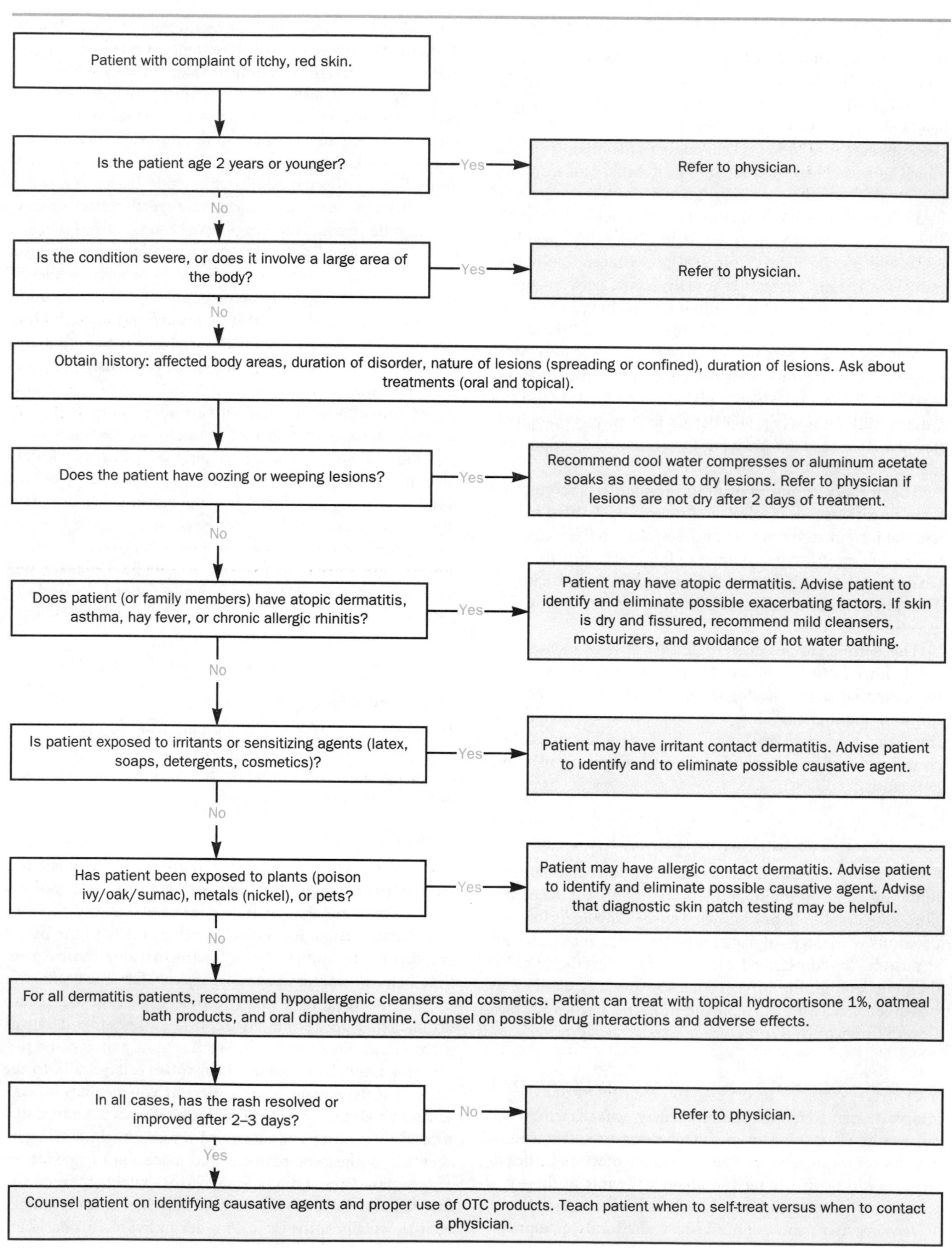

Figure 27–2 Self-care of dermatitis.

Nonpharmacologic Therapy

Excessive bathing with soap and water—with its concomitant frequent warming (vasodilatation from hot water) and cooling (evaporation from skin surface)—may actually increase dryness and aggravate the dermatitis. Bathing can also contribute to the disease by developing microfissures and cracks in the skin that can serve as a portal of entry for irritants and allergens. Therefore, the first step is to ensure that bathing is not too frequent, preferably every other day, and to substitute sponge baths with tepid water for full-body bathing several days per week. Because of the significant drying effect of most soaps, mild non-soap cleansers (e.g., Cetaphil, Oilatum AD) are recommended and better tolerated.

Treatment of acute weeping or oozing lesions is directed toward drying the lesions. Wet compresses using tap water should be applied for 20 minutes, four to six times daily. Bathing with tepid water containing colloidal oatmeal may be soothing.

For itching, simply telling a patient not to scratch is generally ineffective. Therefore, adjunctive measures may be used to minimize scratching and the damage it produces. Fingernails should be kept short, smooth, and clean. Because scratching may increase at night, even while the patient is sleeping, wearing cotton gloves or socks on the hands at night may lessen scratching.

Recommendations can be made regarding avoidance of environmental trigger factors. The patient should avoid occlusive, tight clothing. If possible, patients should remain in moderate temperature settings and in low humidity conditions.

Pharmacologic Therapy

Treatment of chronic lesions focuses on measures to maintain skin hydration and to decrease itching. Colloidal oatmeal that contains natural oils may be used for bathing, or a water-miscible bath oil may be added to the water near the end of the bath. The skin should be gently patted dry because vigorous rubbing produces irritation. An emollient should be applied while the skin is still damp. Although ointments with a petrolatum or water-in-oil base maintain hydration best, sweating after the application of heavy ointments may add to the propensity for itching. Oil-in-water preparations are often more cosmetically acceptable, but they may need to be applied more frequently. If applied correctly, they should have a good emollient effect and not produce dryness.

Hydrocortisone in an oil-in-water base may also be used to dry weeping lesions and is indicated to relieve itching. In some patients, itching may disrupt sleep. (See the section "Treatment of Atopic Dermatitis, Contact Dermatitis, and Dry Skin" for further discussion of these agents.)

Antihistamines are of limited value in decreasing the itching, but those with a significant sedative effect (e.g., diphenhydramine) may be used to promote sleep. (See Chapter 9, "Disorders Related to Cold and Allergy," for discussion of these agents.) A major limitation with the use of classic antihistamines is the undesired drowsiness or residual sedation or "hangover" effect that may be experienced the following morning.[12]

Contact Dermatitis

Contact dermatitis, one of the most common ailments directed to pharmacists for consultation, refers to a rash that results from an allergen or irritant in contact with susceptible skin. It is further categorized into either irritant or allergic contact dermatitis,[13] with irritants accounting for 70% to 80% of all cases. Although the cause of each type is different, the signs, symptoms, and treatment of both are similar. As with other forms of dermatitis, itching is the primary symptom.[14] Skin diseases make up approximately one-half of all occupational hazards, with a large majority of that percentage of patients being diagnosed with contact dermatitis.[15]

Epidemiology of Contact Dermatitis

The true incidence of contact dermatitis is difficult to determine because most patients do not seek medical advice. Children younger than 8 years and elderly patients seem to be more susceptible to irritant dermatitis, with reactions being less acute and slower in onset in older patient groups. Hand dermatitis is more common among women, but again, this correlation may result from women being more prone than men to perform "wet work" (i.e., dishpan hands) or from women being more likely to seek treatment.[16]

Etiology/Pathophysiology of Contact Dermatitis

Irritant contact dermatitis is a nonallergenic and nonimmunologic reaction caused by exposure to irritating substances. Irritant contact dermatitis is often occupation-related and thus most commonly seen in people in the food, plastics, oil, agriculture, or construction industries. Inflammation may be produced by exposure to many substances if concentration and duration of contact are sufficient. A primary or strong irritant, such as a strong acid or alkali, generally elicits a response on first exposure. The injury it causes to the skin may not be limited to erythema and vesiculation but may result in ulceration and tissue necrosis. Mild irritants (e.g., soaps, detergents, sunscreens, and cosmetics) generally require repeated or extended contact to cause a significant inflammatory response. A secondary irritant is nonirritating to the skin when applied alone, but it may cause irritation in combination with an agent that enhances its absorption, such as a surfactant or keratolytic. Previously damaged or compromised skin is more easily irritated than undamaged skin.[17,18]

Acute irritation is more likely if the area is under occlusion, which minimizes evaporation and causes the skin to become more permeable to chemicals. Gloves, clothing, and diapers often increase susceptibility and should be changed often. Combinations of various irritants can also influence potential response. The absorption of an irritant substance may depend on the vehicle, which can itself affect the reaction.[16]

Other agents that may act as sensitizers include iodine-containing products, sulfonamides, mercury-containing antiseptics, and ethylenediamine. Health care and laboratory workers may be sensitized to latex as well as formaldehyde. Many topical skin preparations used for medicinal effect, including some used for itching and skin rashes, may also be a source of allergens. Local anesthetics containing esters such as benzocaine have been used topically for pruritus, local pain, and sunburn and can sensitize individuals. Benzocaine can cross-react with related chemicals such as hair dyes and with sunscreens containing aminobenzoic acid (PABA) to produce allergic contact dermatitis. Topical products containing pramoxine may sometimes be recommended as an alternative to benzocaine. Cross sensitivity probably does not occur among topical anesthetics of different types. Topical antihistamines such as diphenhydramine may also cause sensitization. Once a patient has become sensitized by topical diphenhydramine, oral administration of the agent may also produce dermatitis.[19]

Allergic contact dermatitis is immunologically mediated and is manifested as a delayed hypersensitivity reaction to contact allergens. It involves contact of the skin with an allergenic material functioning as a hapten, which becomes attached to protein carriers on specific cells in the epidermis. An initial sensitizing exposure is necessary for the reaction to occur. On subsequent contact with the allergen, reactive skin areas typically present an eczematous clinical picture, typically appearing within minutes to hours after exposure. Although it may often diminish substantially with old age, susceptibility to allergic contact dermatitis may last virtually a lifetime.[18]

An example of a contact allergen is urushiol from the *Toxicodendron* genus of plants (e.g., poison ivy, oak, and sumac). (For additional information, see Chapter 29, "Poison Ivy/Oak/Sumac Dermatitis.")

A number of metals (e.g., cobalt, chromium, and nickel) may cause allergic contact dermatitis. This sensitivity is important to keep in mind because nickel, often with cobalt as a contaminant, is widely used in costume jewelry, watches, and blue jean studs. Chromium is present in cement and may pose an occupational hazard to construction workers and masons.[18] Rubber has often been implicated as an allergenic substance. However, it is not the rubber or latex itself that typically causes the reaction, but rather the chemical accelerators and antioxidants used in processing the rubber.

Signs and Symptoms of Contact Dermatitis

Hands are most often involved in adults, particularly the dorsal surface or back of the hands. Eruptions can occur on the upper back, thighs, axillary areas, feet, and face. Lesions are often asymmetric in distribution and sharply demarcated (well-defined), reflecting where contact with the substance occurred. Mild irritants often produce erythematous, vesicular, and oozing lesions. The chronic phase is likely to be dry, thickened, and fissured skin. Irritants cause inelasticity and stiff-feeling skin, dryness, and pruritus. Allergic contact dermatitis is similar to an irritant eruption in symptomatology.

Clinically, reactions may be acute, chronic, delayed, or cumulative. Strong irritants cause the acute reactions, which results in an immediate erythematous, edematous reaction with vesicles. Chronic reactions are seen commonly in hairdressers and those involved in wet work, with erythematous, chapped skin developing after months of exposure. Some chemicals can produce a delayed reaction, with the appearance of inflammation 8 to 24 hours or longer postexposure. A cumulative reaction, the most common type of irritant dermatitis, is a reaction that persists as a result of consistent exposure.

Treatment Overview of Contact Dermatitis

Treatment Outcomes

The goals of treating contact dermatitis are to (1) relieve the discomfort and (2) prevent or minimize exposure to irritant or allergenic substances by identifying and avoiding offending substances.

General Treatment Approach

Choice of treatment for contact dermatitis depends on the severity of the condition. Decreasing exposure to irritants such as detergents, soaps, and solvents are good preventive measures. Patients who have experienced topical allergic reactions should avoid contact with known allergens. Many allergens are occult in nature and may require diagnostic patch testing. Regardless, because there is a potential that the allergen may never be identified, patients should be treated.

Mild-to-moderate dermatitis is usually amenable to treatment with nonprescription agents. Astringents such as aluminum acetate can dry lesions, whereas calamine lotion, colloidal oatmeal, or hydrocortisone can relieve itching. Hydrocortisone also reduces erythema. The algorithm in Figure 27–2 outlines the use of such agents.

If the condition does not begin to improve in several days or if it worsens, the patient should consult a physician.[4,20] Similarly, a patient with a severe reaction or involvement of large areas of the body should also be referred to a physician. Patients age 2 years or younger require medical referral.

Nonpharmacologic Therapy

In addition to well-known irritants (e.g., detergents, soaps, and solvents) the patient should avoid any substance that has caused adverse skin reactions. The patient should also avoid

Case Study 27-1

Patient Complaint/History

Sam, a 20-year-old healthy college student, presents to the pharmacist with a complaint of irritated hands. He requests assistance in choosing a product to treat his condition. The patient is working this summer as a construction laborer; his main tasks are mixing and transporting brick mortar. He does not wear gloves while working. After performing these tasks for 3 to 4 weeks, he noticed his hands had become progressively irritated.

Physical observation reveals that the patient's hands appear dry with minimal fissuring at the flexors; no vesicles, weeping, or infection is apparent; and the forearms are uninvolved. Sam says that his hands itch periodically and feel tight—as though the skin would crack with any movement.

Clinical Considerations/Strategies

Readers can use the following considerations/strategies to determine whether treatment of the patient's condition with nonprescription medications is warranted:

- Determine what additional information is needed from the patient before therapy can be recommended.
- Determine what nondrug measures may be helpful.
- Recommend a nonprescription product to relieve the dryness and itching.

Patient Education/Counseling

Readers can use the following strategies to develop a patient education/counseling plan that will help ensure optimal therapeutic outcomes:

- Explain the therapeutic goals for the recommended product.
- Explain the adverse effects, if any, of the recommended therapy.

occlusion of the skin, which can make it more permeable to chemicals, and should frequently change gloves (especially latex gloves used for cleaning chores) and clothing. In infant patients, diapers should be changed frequently.

Patients with allergic contact dermatitis may react to preservatives, fragrances, hair care products, nail polish, hair dyes, and deodorants. These patients should use hypoallergenic cosmetics and soapless cleansers.

Pharmacologic Therapy

The involved area should usually be washed gently, but well, to remove traces of the offending agent. If the area is oozing, compresses of cool tap water or of aluminum acetate should be applied for 20 minutes, four to six times daily. These compresses may be recommended to aid in drying the lesions. Applying calamine lotion between compress applications and using colloidal oatmeal baths may be soothing and may help relieve itching. Topical hydrocortisone cream may be added to the regimen to reduce inflammation and itching. At times, oral antihistamines, such as diphenhydramine taken at bedtime, can be recommended. (See the section "Treatment of Atopic Dermatitis, Contact Dermatitis, and Dry Skin" for further discussion of such agents.)

The duration of therapy is often relatively short because the condition usually improves upon withdrawal of the allergen or irritant, typically within hours. However, a patient may be sensitive to or irritated by more than one drug or chemical. Therefore, before recommending any product for treating contact dermatitis, the pharmacist should first encourage the patient to try to identify the possible offending substance(s).

Dry Skin

Dry skin can be related to occupational or environmental factors. Occupational dry skin involves mostly hands or other body parts directly involved in the occupation. Environmental dry skin is heavily associated with the patient's taking long, hot showers or not consuming enough water.

The prevention and care of dry skin may become a major focus for the pharmacist as the elderly population continues to increase. There is a heightened awareness among those caring for elderly people that prophylactic dry skin care can reduce morbidity by minimizing the risk of skin breakdown and thus can ultimately reduce the cost of dermatologic health care.[21,22]

Epidemiology of Dry Skin

Dry skin is more common in elderly people. With advancing age, the epidermis changes because of abnormal maturation or adhesion of the keratinocytes, resulting in a superficial, irregular layer of corneocytes. This condition may be described as a thinning of the entire epidermis, which produces a roughened skin surface. The skin's hygroscopic substances also decrease in quantity with advancing age. Hormonal changes that accompany aging result in lowered sebum output and, therefore, lowered skin lubrication.[23]

Other epidemiologic factors correlate with etiologic factors of dry skin. (See the section "Etiology/Pathophysiology of Dry Skin.") For example, individuals who live or work in arid, windy, or cold environments have an increased risk for dry skin.

Etiology/Pathophysiology of Dry Skin

Conditions of dry skin can result from various etiologies. Dry skin can be caused by disruption of keratinization and impairment of water binding properties.[24] Dry skin is especially prevalent during the winter months and is often referred to as "winter itch." It may occur secondary to prolonged detergent use, malnutrition, or physical damage to the stratum corneum. It may also signal a systemic disorder such as hypothyroidism or dehydration.

It is a common misconception that dry skin is caused by a lack of natural skin oils. On the contrary, dry skin is caused by a lack of water retention in the stratum corneum. The pathophysiology of dry skin, therefore, can be described by examining the factors involved in skin hydration. One factor is frequent or prolonged bathing or showering with hot water, as well as excessive use of soap, both of which increase dryness of the skin. Soap removes the skin's natural oils, and the short duration of contact with water is usually insufficient to hydrate dry skin. The second factor is environmental conditions, such as low humidity. Dry air allows the outer skin layer to lose moisture, become less flexible, and crack when flexed, which leads to an increased rate of moisture loss. High wind velocity also causes skin moisture loss. A third factor is physical damage to the stratum corneum, which dramatically increases transepidermal water loss. However, after the insult is removed, partial recovery occurs within 1 or 2 days with the formation of a temporary barrier consisting of incompletely keratinized cells. This newly formed barrier provides approximately 50% of normal barrier function and moisture retention with the barrier effect being restored in 2 to 3 weeks if the dry skin is not severe.

Signs and Symptoms of Dry Skin

Xerosis is characterized by one or more of the following signs and symptoms: roughness, scaling, loss of flexibility, fissures, inflammation, and pruritus.

Two dermatologic conditions difficult to differentiate from simple dry skin are asteatotic eczema and ichthyosis vulgaris. Asteatotic eczema is characterized by dry, fissured skin, inflammation, and pruritus. Sebaceous secretions are scanty or absent. The condition is more common during dry winter weather and in elderly individuals as an extension of the dry skin condition.

Ichthyosis vulgaris affects 0.3% to 1.0% of the population and is usually identified in the first few months of life. It is a genetic disorder (autosomal dominant) that should be suspected when a patient complains of a familial tendency to excessive dryness and chapping. Patients may have an associated history of atopic disease. Symptoms of ichthyosis include dryness and roughness of the skin, accompanied by small, fine, white scales. The condition tends to appear on the extensor aspects of the arms and legs. Dryness of the cheeks, heels, and palms may also be noted. In severe forms of the disease, a classic fish scale appearance of the stratum corneum is noted. Extreme cases have been described as "alligator," "porcupine," or "lizard" skin.[17,25] Ichthyosis vulgaris may be placed at most severe end on a continuum of dermatitis conditions, with common dry skin at the least severe end.

Treatment Overview of Dry Skin

Treatment Outcomes

The goal in treating dry skin is to restore skin hydration and barrier function.

General Treatment Approach

The key to preventing dry skin is to maintain skin hydration. The same nondrug measures that maintain hydration (avoiding drying hygiene practices and consuming adequate fluids) can be used to restore dehydrated skin. Nonprescription products such as bath oils, emollients/moisturizers, humectants, and keratolytic agents also aid in restoring and maintaining barrier function. If needed, topical hydrocortisone can be used to reduce pruritus and erythema.

Ichthyosis vulgaris and related ichthyoses respond minimally to topical corticosteroid therapy although short-term use of topical corticosteroids may reduce symptoms of erythema and pruritus.[25] Such patients should consult a physician. Blanching erythema (i.e., skin that loses the "red" appearance when mechanical pressure is applied by the finger) generally indicates a steroid-responsive disorder, whereas nonblanching erythema (i.e., redness caused by vessel wall breakdown and leakage into the skin) is usually not responsive to topical steroids. Although topical hydrocortisone is generally safe in full-term infants when used for a short duration of treatment (less than 15 days), these products should not be used in children younger than 2 years.

Nonpharmacologic Therapy

Nondrug measures to restore and maintain hydration include reducing full-body bathing to every other day or less often. The patient should avoid long, hot showers. Taking sponge baths or quick showers will also reduce loss of hydration. In fact, the patient should use warm rather than hot water for all types of bathing. Patients should also maintain internal hydration by drinking plenty of water—between 3 and 4 liters per day—and should not drink sodas, coffee, or teas as a substitution.

Pharmacologic Therapy

Products such as colloidal oatmeal, oilated oatmeal, or bath oil added near the end of the bath may be used to enhance skin hydration. The patient should apply oil-based emollients immediately after bathing while the skin is damp and should reapply them frequently. More severe cases of dry skin may require a urea-containing or lactic acid–containing product to enhance hydration. The patient may apply topical hydrocortisone ointment on a short-term basis (no longer than 7 days) to reduce inflammation and itching. If resolution does not occur within 1 or 2 weeks, a physician should be consulted.[4]

Dry skin is more prone to itching, inflammation, and development of secondary infections. Most moisturizers are mixtures of oils and water. Moisturizers that contain 12% ammonium lactate have improved the appearance of skin covered with cracks and fissures.[26] α-Hydroxy acids (AHAs) and related compounds have been shown to normalize keratinization and to result in more normal stratum corneum.[24] Indications for using AHA products include treatment of xerosis (dry skin), melasma, acne, and photoaging. The recent emergence of such products allows the pharmacist to choose from a vast array of nonprescription products. (See the following section for discussion of these agents.)

Treatment of Atopic Dermatitis, Contact Dermatitis, and Dry Skin

Nonprescription products for dermatitis and dry skin that restore skin hydration include bath products, emollients, hydrating agents, and keratin-softening agents. (See Table 27–1 for examples of commercially available products.) Astringents, antipruritics, protectants, and hydrocortisone are

Table 27–1

Selected Dry Skin Products

Trade Name	Primary Ingredients
Alpha Keri Moisture Rich Cleansing Bar	Mineral oil; lanolin oil; glycerin
Aveeno Bath Treatment Moisturizing Formula Powder[a]	Mineral oil; colloidal oatmeal 43%
Aveeno Bath Treatment Soothing Formula Powder[a]	Colloidal oatmeal 100%
Aveeno Moisturizing Cream/Lotion[a]	Petrolatum; dimethicone; isopropyl palmitate; cetyl alcohol; colloidal oatmeal 1%; glycerin
Carmol 10 Lotion	Urea 10%
Carmol 20 Cream	Urea 20%
Cetaphil Gentle Cleanser Liquid[a]	Cetyl alcohol
Complex 15 Therapeutic Moisturizing Cream/Lotion[a]	Glycerin; lecithin
Corn Huskers Lotion	Glycerin
Curél Nutrient Rich Severe Dry Skin Lotion	Petrolatum; dimethicone; isopropyl palmitate; glycerin
Jergens Advanced Therapy Dry Skin Care Lotion	Dimethicone; lanolin; cetearyl alcohol; isopropyl myristate; glycerin
Jergens Advanced Therapy Dual Healing Cream	Mineral oil; dimethicone; petrolatum; cetyl dimethicone; isopropyl palmitate; glycerin
Jergens Advanced Therapy Ultra Healing Lotion	Petrolatum; mineral oil; dimethicone; cetearyl alcohol; cetyl alcohol; glycerin; allantoin
Keri Original Formula Therapeutic Dry Skin Lotion	Mineral oil; lanolin oil; glyceryl stearate; propylene glycol
Keri Silky Smooth Lotion	Petrolatum; dimethicone; cetyl alcohol; glycerin
Lubriderm Bath and Shower Oil	Mineral oil
Moisturel Cream/Lotion[a]	Petrolatum; dimethicone; cetyl alcohol; glycerin
Neutrogena Body Oil	Isopropyl myristate; sesame oil
Neutrogena Norwegian Formula Cream	Glycerin 41%
Pacquin Medicated Hand and Body Cream	Dimethicone 1%; cetyl alcohol; glycerin 12%
Pacquin Plus Dry Skin Hand and Body Cream	Lanolin anhydrous 0.5%; cetyl alcohol; glycerin 12%
Sardo Bath Oil	Mineral oil; isopropyl palmitate
Sardoettes Wipe	Mineral oil; isopropyl palmitate
Vaseline Dermatology Formula Lotion	White petrolatum 5%; mineral oil 4%; dimethicone 1%; glyceryl stearate; cetyl alcohol; glycerin

[a] Fragrance-free product.

Table 27–2

Selected Dermatitis Products

Trade Name	Primary Ingredients
Bactine Hydrocortisone 1% Cream	Hydrocortisone 1%; hydrocortisone alcohol; aluminum sulfate; calcium acetate
Cortaid Maximum Strength Ointment/Cream	Hydrocortisone 1%
Cortaid Sensitive Skin Cream	Hydrocortisone 0.5%
Cortizone-10 Ointment	Hydrocortisone 1%
Cortizone-10 Cream	Hydrocortisone 1%; aluminum sulfate; calcium acetate
Cortizone-5 Ointment	Hydrocortisone 0.5%
Cortizone-5 Cream	Hydrocortisone 0.5%; aluminum sulfate; calcium acetate
Kericort 10 Maximum Strength Cream	Hydrocortisone 1%; stearyl alcohol

used to relieve weeping and/or itching of lesions and to protect the affected area. Table 27–2 lists examples of commercial products for these agents.

Keratolytics (salicylic acid and sulfur) are usually avoided in dermatitis unless extensive lichenification (thickening/hardening of skin into an irregular plaque due to excessive rubbing/scratching) has occurred. These agents and those that reduce the mitotic rate of the epidermis, such as tars, should be used cautiously because of their irritant potential. (See Chapter 28, "Scaly Dermatoses," for discussion of such agents

Bath Products

Bath Oils

Bath oils generally consist of a mineral or vegetable oil, plus a surfactant. Mineral oil products are adsorbed better than vegetable oil products. Adsorption onto and absorption into the skin increase as temperature and oil concentration increase. Bath oils are minimally effective in improving a dry skin condition because they are greatly diluted in water. Their major effect is the slip or lubricity they impart to the skin, which may be important to the patient. This effect may be maximized by adding the oil near the end of the bath and by patting the skin dry rather than rubbing it. When applied as wet compresses, however, bath oils (1 teaspoon in one-fourth cup of warm water) help lubricate dry skin and may allow a decrease in the frequency of full-body bathing.[4,27]

Bath oils make the tub and floor slippery, creating a *safety hazard* especially for elderly patients or children. They also make cleansing the skin with soaps more difficult. There is no clear superiority of one type of bath oil product over another; however, patients with dermatologic disorders should generally avoid products with fragrance.

Oatmeal Products

Colloidal oatmeal bath products contain starch, protein, and a small amount of oil. They are less effective than bath oils; however, oilated oatmeal products combine the effect of oatmeal and a bath oil. Colloidal oatmeal is claimed to be soothing and antipruritic, and it does have a lubricating effect. The pharmacist should inform patients that colloidal oatmeal products, if used on a regular basis, may clog waste pipes.

Cleansers

Typical bath soaps generally contain salts of long-chain fatty acids (commonly oleic, palmitic, or stearic acid) and alkali metals (e.g., sodium and potassium). Combined with water, such products act as surfactants that will remove many substances from the skin, including the lipids that normally keep the skin soft and pliable. Some authorities recommend special soaps that contain extra oils to minimize the drying effect of washing. However, these soaps usually lather and clean poorly. Unscented Dove is one example of a nonsoap cleansing agent with minimal drying effect to skin.[4,23]

Glycerin soaps, which are transparent and more water soluble, have a higher oil content than standard toilet soaps because of the addition of castor oil. They are closer to a neutral pH and are, therefore, regarded as less drying than soaps, which are alkaline. Although little objective proof exists to prove their superiority, the glycerin soaps are advertised for and well accepted by people with skin conditions.

The pharmacist should recommend mild cleansers such as Cetaphil or Oilatum AD if soap is to be avoided. Most of these products consist primarily of surfactants and may contain an oil. On application, they foam mildly, and on gentle wiping, they leave a thin layer of lipid material on the skin, which helps to retain water in the stratum corneum.

Emollients/Moisturizers

Some of the most commonly used emollients include petrolatum and mineral oil. Petrolatum is one of the most occlusive and best emollients if applied correctly. The Food and Drug Administration (FDA) has given this agent a Category I (safe and effective) status as a skin protectant. Mineral oil and silicones are not as effective as complete barriers.

Attempts have been made to formulate products that try to function like sebum. Because sebum and skin surface lipids contain a relatively high concentration of fatty acid glycerides, vegetable and animal oils such as avocado, cucumber, mink, peanut, safflower, sesame, turtle, and shark liver are included in dry skin products, presumably because of their unsaturated fatty acid content. However, although use of such oils contributes to skin flexibility and lubricity, their occlusive effect is less than that of petrolatum.

Mechanism of Action

Emollients are occlusive agents and moisturizers that are used to prevent or relieve the signs and symptoms of dry skin. Such products act primarily by leaving an oily film on the skin surface through which moisture cannot readily escape.

Cosmetically, emollients make the skin feel soft and smooth by helping to reestablish the integrity of the stratum corneum. Lipid components make the scales on the skin translucent and flatten them against the underlying skin. This flattening eliminates air between the scales and the skin surface, which is partly responsible for a dry, scaly appearance.[21]

Dosage/Administration Guidelines

Some clinicians believe that minimizing transepidermal water loss is not enough to maintain adequate hydration. Therefore, a patient may be advised to hydrate the skin by soaking the affected area in water for 5 to 10 minutes, patting it dry, and applying an occlusive agent while the skin is still damp. In this way, moisture is retained more adequately in the skin. In addition, drinking plenty of water should again be stressed.

Frequency of application depends on the severity of the dry skin condition, as well as on the hydration efficiency of the occlusive agent. For dry hands, the patient may need to apply the occlusive agent after each hand washing, as well as at numerous other times during the day. However, care should be exercised to avoid excessive hydration, which may lead to tissue maceration.

Dosage Forms

Emollient products are available in a wide variety of formulations. Ointments containing petrolatum typically feel very greasy and generally lack consumer appeal because of their texture, difficulty of spreading and removing, and staining properties. Pharmacists can play a key role in stressing correct application of emollient ointments. To avoid any greasy feel, patients should be advised to apply a small amount and to massage it into the skin very well.

Ointments are inappropriate for an oozing dermatitis. Lotions and creams are either water-in-oil or oil-in-water emulsions. The higher the lipid content, the greater is the occlusive effect. In most cases, patients prefer the less effective but more-aesthetic oil-in-water emulsions for their cosmetic acceptability. Such agents help alleviate the pruritus associated with dry skin by virtue of their cooling effect as water evaporates from the skin surface. Moreover, enough oil exists in most oil-in-water emulsions to form a continuous occlusive film.[4,21]

Adverse Effects

Lanolin, a natural product derived from sheep wool, is found in many nonprescription moisturizing products. Rarely, patients develop an allergic reaction to this substance, presumably because its wool wax fraction is recognized as antigenic. Patients with a previous history of allergic reactions to lanolin should generally avoid lanolin-containing products. However, refined lanolin-containing products are generally less likely to be sensitizing and may even be tolerated by those with a history of allergic contact reactions to unrefined lanolin.

Precautions/Warnings

In addition, although most commercial formulations generally are bland, contact with the eye or with broken or abraded skin should be avoided because formulation ingredients may cause irritation. This irritation is especially true with emulsion systems because the surfactants in them denature protein and may thus produce further irritation.

Petrolatum should not be applied over puncture wounds, infections, or lacerations because its high occlusive ability may lead to maceration and further inflammation. Applying petrolatum to intertriginous areas, mucous membranes, and acne-prone areas should be minimized and used with caution. Similar precautions should be taken with dimethicone.

Humectants

Humectants or hydrating agents are hygroscopic materials that may be added to an emollient base. Commonly used hydrating agents are glycerin, propylene glycol, and phospholipids.

Humectants draw water into the stratum corneum to hydrate the skin. Water may come from the dermis or from the atmosphere. However, high relative humidity (80% or greater) is necessary for the latter to occur. Humectants are distinct from emollients, which serve to retain water already present.

Because of glycerin's hygroscopic properties, high concentrations may actually increase water loss by drawing water from the skin rather than from the atmosphere. However, humectants such as glycerin help decrease water loss by keeping water in close contact with skin and by accelerating moisture diffusion from the dermis to the epidermis. In addition, glycerin provides lubrication to the skin surface.

Propylene glycol is a viscous, colorless, odorless solvent with hygroscopic properties. It is less viscous than glycerin and is included in many skin care formulations for its humectant action. However, it can cause skin irritation, usually on a concentration-dependent basis.

Phospholipid products contain lecithin, which is a water-binding compound normally present in the skin. Each phospholipid molecule can complex with up to 15 molecules of water. Hydrolysis yields fatty acids, which help retain water.

Keratin-Softening Agents

Chemically altering the keratin layer softens skin and cosmetically improves its appearance. This treatment approach does not need a substantial addition of water, but all the attendant dry skin symptoms may not be alleviated unless water is added to the keratin layer. Agents used as keratin softeners in nonprescription dry skin products are urea, lactic acid, and allantoin.

Urea

Urea (carbamide) in concentrations of 10% to 30% is mildly keratolytic and increases water uptake in the stratum corneum, giving it a high water-binding capacity. Urea has a direct effect on stratum corneum elasticity because of its ability to bind to skin protein. It accelerates fibrin digestion at about 15% and is proteolytic at 40%. It is considered safe and has been recommended for use on crusted necrotic tissue. Concentrations of 10% have been used on simple dry skin; 20% to 30% formulations have been used for treating more-resistant dry skin conditions. Formulations containing urea may be better to help remove scales and crusts, while urea in emollient ointments (e.g., urea in Aquaphor) may be better at rehydration of the skin. However, urea preparations can cause stinging, burning, and irritation, particularly on broken skin.

Lactic Acid/α-Hydroxy Acid

Lactic acid is an AHA that has been useful in concentrations of 2% to 5% for treating dry skin conditions. Lactic acid increases the hydration of human skin and may act as a modulator of epidermal keratinization rather than as a keratolytic agent. Lactic acid may be added to urea preparations for both its stabilizing and its hydrating effects.

Other AHAs, found in many fruits, are used for a number of common skin conditions such as dry skin, acne, melasma, and photoaging. Such acids include malic acid (in apples), citric acid (in oranges and lemons), tartaric acid (in grapes), and glycolic and gluconic acids (in sugar cane).[28] (See Chapter 37, "Skin Hyperpigmentation and Photoaging" for examples of commercially available products.)

Allantoin

Allantoin and allantoin complexes are claimed to soften keratin by disrupting its structure. Allantoin is a product of purine metabolism and is considered to be a relatively safe compound. However, it is less effective than urea. FDA classifies allantoin as a Category I skin protectant for adults, children, and infants when applied in concentrations of 0.5% to 2.0%.[17]

Astringents

Astringents retard oozing, discharge, or bleeding of dermatitis when applied to the unhealthy skin or mucous membranes. They work by coagulating protein. When applied as a wet dressing or compress, they cool and dry the skin through evaporation. They vasoconstrict and reduce blood flow in inflamed tissue, and they cleanse the skin of exudates, crust, and debris. Because they generally have a low cell penetrability, their activity is limited to the cell surface and interstitial spaces. The protein precipitate that forms may serve as a protective coat, allowing new tissues to grow underneath.[17]

FDA has identified two astringent solutions as Category 1: aluminum acetate (Burow's solution) and witch hazel (hamamelis water). Aluminum acetate solution (USP) contains approximately 5% aluminum acetate. The solution must be diluted 1 : 10 to 1 : 40 with water before use. It is commercially available in tablet or powder form. Witch hazel is no longer listed in the official compendia, but it has been used for centuries as an astringent solution. A natural product prepared from the twigs of *Hamamelis virginiana*, it contains tannins, trace amounts of volatile oils (which give it a characteristic pleasant odor), and 14% to 15% alcohol, all of which contribute to its astringent activity. The product may be applied as often as necessary in the treatment of minor skin irritations. Numerous other ingredients, including alum and zinc oxide, have been promoted as astringents. However, data are lacking to demonstrate their safety and effectiveness as astringents.[29]

The patient may soak the affected area in the astringent solution two to four times daily for 15 to 30 minutes. Alternatively, the patient may loosely apply a compress of washcloths or small towels soaked in the solution and then wrung gently so they are wet but not dripping. The dressings should be rewetted and applied every few minutes for 20 to 30 minutes, four to six times daily. Isotonic saline solution, tap water, or diluted white vinegar (one-fourth cup per pint of water) may also be used in this fashion.[4,17]

Topical Hydrocortisone

Hydrocortisone is currently the only corticosteroid available without a prescription for the topical treatment of dermatitis. Though its exact mechanism is unknown, it relieves the redness, heat, pain, swelling, and itch associated with various dermatoses, possibly because of a vasoconstrictive effect. FDA monograph indications for its use include temporary relief of itching associated with minor skin irritations, inflammation, and rashes caused by dermatitis, seborrheic dermatitis, insect bites, poison ivy, poison oak, poison sumac, soaps, detergents, cosmetics, and jewelry.

When hydrocortisone was initially switched from prescription to nonprescription status in 1980, the concentrations available were 0.25% and 0.5%. However, the efficacy of hydrocortisone preparations of less than 0.5% concentration has not been established. Concentrations of 0.5% to 1% are regarded as appropriate for treating localized dermatitis. In August 1991, FDA approved the nonprescription marketing of hydrocortisone in strengths up to 1%.[30]

Hydrocortisone should be applied sparingly to the affected area three or four times a day. An ointment formulation is best for chronic, non-oozing dermatoses.

Before recommending a hydrocortisone-containing product, be certain that the area of application is not infected. Signs of bacterial or fungal infection can include erythema, warmth, exudate, and crusting or scaling. Topical hydrocortisone may mask the symptoms of dermatologic infections and may allow the infection to progress.

Topical hydrocortisone will rarely produce systemic complications because systemic absorption is relatively minimal. Approximately 1% of hydrocortisone solution applied to normal skin on the forearm is absorbed systemically. Absorption increases in the presence of skin inflammation or with the use of occlusive dressings. Certain local adverse effects such as skin atrophy may arise with prolonged use because collagen production is inhibited, which thereby weakens the skin's "infrastructure." In practice, however, clinically detectable atrophy rarely occurs with hydrocortisone in the concentrations available without a prescription; it is more common with the more potent products available by prescription only. Because response to topical corticosteroids decreases with continued use, intermittent courses of therapy are advised.[4]

Antipruritics

The itching associated with dermatitis may be mediated through several different mechanisms, which may explain how three major classes of pharmacologic agents—local anesthetics, antihistamines, and corticosteroids (discussed previously)—are useful as antipruritics. Cooling the area through application of a soothing, bland lotion may reduce the extent of the pruritus, but this action is only transitory in its effect.

The itching sensation is mediated by the same nerve fibers that carry pain impulses. Local anesthetics block conduction along axonal membranes, thereby relieving itching as well as pain. However, because local anesthetics may cause systemic side effects, they should not be used in large quantities or over long periods of time, particularly if the skin is raw or blistered. Nonprescription topical anesthetics that appear to be safe and effective are dyclonine, pramoxine, lidocaine, and benzocaine. Benzocaine (5%–20%) may be applied to the affected area three or four times daily. However, these agents may have a sensitizing effect in a small number of people.

Itching may be mediated by various endogenous substances, including histamine. Accordingly, topical antihistamines such as diphenhydramine, tripelennamine, and pyrilamine are effective in alleviating this symptom. Their activity stems from an ability to compete with histamine at H_1-receptor sites and to exert a topical anesthetic effect. Local anesthesia may be the more important mechanism of action because the cause of itching in many conditions (e.g., atopic dermatitis) has not been established and may not be related to histamine release at all. Antihistamines are considered safe and effective for use as nonprescription external analgesics. However, because of their significant sensitizing potential, FDA does not recommend the topical use of such agents for more than 7 consecutive days except under the advice and supervision of a physician.[18,31]

Oral antihistamines have been used to treat the itching of dermatologic disorders with variable results. Some researchers claim that the antipruritic effect is a result of the sedative side effect; others claim the efficacy is caused by antihistaminic activity, although with a delay in onset of several days. If histamine is involved, it has already reached and stimulated the receptor sites to produce itching, and a finite time is required for the antihistamine to displace it. In either case, central nervous system depression may be a problem, as may the anticholinergic side effects in patients with conditions such as prostatic hypertrophy or glaucoma.[12,15]

Protectants

Skin protectants are substances that protect injured or exposed skin surfaces from harmful or annoying stimuli. Zinc oxide (1%–25%) is one of the most widely used and clinically accepted skin protectants, and it is claimed to be mildly astringent and antiseptic. It may be applied as a paste (Lassar's), an ointment, or a lotion (calamine). Patients should be cautioned that covering the lesions or applying a product with an occlusive barrier may increase the degree of tissue maceration and may prevent heat loss, resulting in discomfort. Any powder-based aqueous product that dries weeping through water adsorption or astringency should be used with caution. Such agents have a tendency to crust, and removing the crusts may cause bleeding and infections.[17,18]

Product Selection Guidelines

When deciding on which product to recommend for dermatitis or dry skin, the pharmacist must evaluate the active ingredients and the vehicle. Primary active ingredients contained in nonprescription skin products are water and oil. However, a wide variety of secondary ingredients are added to enhance product elegance and stability, and many of them have the potential for producing contact dermatitis through either an irritant or a sensitizing effect. The agents may include the following:

- Emulsifiers: cholesterol, magnesium aluminum silicate, polyoxyethylene lauryl ether (Brij), polyoxyethylene monostearate (Myrj), polyoxyethylene sorbitan monolaurate (Tween), propylene glycol monostearate, sodium borate plus fatty acid, sodium lauryl sulfate, sorbitan monopalmitate (Span), or triethanolamine plus fatty acid.
- Emulsion stabilizers (thickening agents): carbomer, cetyl alcohol, glyceryl monostearate, methylcellulose, spermaceti, or stearyl alcohol.
- Preservatives: cresol or the parabens.

The type of vehicle (e.g., ointment, cream, lotion, gel, solution, or aerosol) may have a significant effect on dermatitis. The following guidelines may be used to choose an appropriate vehicle:

- "If it's wet, dry it." If a drying effect is desired, the pharmacist may recommend solutions, gels, and occasionally creams. However, components of these systems may quickly diffuse into the underlying tissue and possibly cause irritation.
- If slight lubrication is needed, creams and lotions should be preferred.
- "If it's dry, wet it." If the lesion is very dry and fissured, ointments are the vehicle of choice. However, avoid use in intertriginous areas because of their maceration potential. Also, in an acute process, ointments may cause further irritation because of their occlusive effect.

Table 27–3

Amount of Topical Medication Needed for Three Times Daily Application for 1 Week

Part of the Body	Cream/ Ointment (g)	Lotion/Solution/ Gel (mL)
Face	5–10	100–120
Both hands	25–50	200–240
Scalp	50–100	200–240
Both arms of both legs	100–200	240–360
Trunk	200	360–480
Groin and genitalia	15–25	120–180

Source: Adapted from reference 32.

- The pharmacist may recommend aerosols, gels, or lotions when the dermatitis affects a hair-covered area of the body.

Numerous cosmetic dry skin formulations are commercially available and may contain natural oils, vitamins, or fragrances that have a psychologic appeal. However, the fragrances and dyes found in many formulations may be irritating or allergenic to sensitive, dry skin and should be avoided. Efficacy of any skin care product may need to be sacrificed or compromised somewhat to achieve patient acceptance. The pharmacist should recommend the most efficacious product that the patient will accept.

Topical nonprescription products come in varying package sizes and strengths. Table 27–3 lists the amount of drug needed to cover a given area of the body three times daily over a 1-week period. By being aware of such details, the pharmacist can serve the patient economically as well as therapeutically.

Patient Assessment for Atopic Dermatitis, Contact Dermatitis, and Dry Skin

Initially, the signs and symptoms are similar for most forms of dermatitis. These signs may include pruritus (itching), erythema (redness), and edema (swelling). Edema may be accompanied by fluid-filled vesicles, which often break and cause weeping or oozing from the skin. Evaporation of water from the exudate results in crusting and scaling. Over time, the weeping may diminish, giving way to a dry, scaly condition. Lesions may also be patchy in distribution.[17] During an acute phase of dermatitis, it is common to observe vesicles on an erythematous base in the lesional area.[17]

The dermatitis is further characterized as weeping or oozing. If the dermatitis is chronic and if the weeping present in the acute phase has subsided, the skin will become dry and scaly, and fissures may appear. If itching results in excessive scratching, the epidermis may appear thickened and ridged (lichenification). Infections may occur as sequelae to pruritus-induced scratching. Pigment production may be altered, and hyperpigmentation or hypopigmentation may become evident.[4]

Because atopic dermatitis is primarily a disease of the young, patient age is important in assessment. The pharmacist should determine whether the patient (or patient's family) has a history of atopic disorders. Inquiries should be made regarding onset and duration of the eruption, anatomic location, and distribution of the lesions.

When recommending the use of an appropriate nonprescription product or when referring the patient to a physician, the pharmacist must consider the cosmetic, psychologic, and work- or recreation-related aspects of a dermatologic disorder in addition to the underlying pathology.

Thorough questioning of the patient's total environment (e.g., home, work, recreation, laundry products, cosmetics, wearing of unwashed new clothes, and medication use) is important to identify the offending substance. Removal of the causative agent will usually result in improvement. Because no well-defined types of lesions are associated with many types of contact dermatitis, assessment is often through exclusion by asking questions about the patient's environment and practices. Except for the obvious exposure like poison ivy, the cause of allergic contact reactions may often be elusive.

An accurate assessment is made on the basis of the character, configuration, and location of the rash and itching. (See Table 27–4.) Diagnostic skin patch testing may be useful in assessing some allergic contact reactions.[33] Accurate assessment may be difficult, however, if the contact dermatitis is superimposed over another dermatologic condition. Moreover, skin that is in a reactive state may be more easily reactive to other irritating or allergenic substances, making assessment and treatment even more complicated.[34] For example, a minor cutaneous bacterial infection may produce a rash and may be treated with a topical antibiotic containing neomycin. Because such agents are commonly sensitizing, the neomycin may produce allergic contact dermatitis at the treatment site. Thus, while the infection itself may heal, the allergic contact dermatitis produced by the neomycin persists. Not recognizing that the initial infection has resolved, the patient may continue to use the offending neomycin-containing product, thus setting up a reaction cycle.[17,20]

Dry skin is typically visible to the eye, with roughness and scaling. Pharmacists can question the patient about their bathing habits, the soaps and detergents used, and any other medical condition that may predispose them to excessive dryness. Patients should note that changes in climate can also affect their skin, such as winter air resulting in drying even though it may be raining.

Asking the patient the following questions will help elicit the information needed to accurately assess the disorder and to recommend the appropriate treatment approach.

Table 27–4

Characteristics of Selected Forms of Dermatitis and Dry Skin

Condition	Symptoms	Location	Signs
Atopic dermatitis	Itching, scratching	2 months: chest face	Red, raised vesicles; dry skin; oozing
		2 years: scalp, neck, and extensor surface of extremities	Less acute lesions; edema; erythema
		2–4 years: neck, wrist, elbow, knee	Dry, thickened plaques; hyperpigmentation
		12–20 years: flexors, hands	
Contact dermatitis (irritant and allergic)	Acute: itching	Irritant: contact areas	Irritant (mild, acute): red, oozing blisters
	Chronic: stiffness, dry	Allergic: exposed contact areas (transferable by touch)	Irritant (mild, chronic): dry, thick, fissured skin Irritant (severe): blisters, ulcers Allergic: unusual pattern of lesions; sharp margins with angles and straight lines
Hand dermatitis	Itching, dry	Sides of fingers, occasionally	Red, dry, chapped, fissured skin
Dry skin (chapped)	Often none; moderate-to-severe itching	Lower legs, backs of hands, forearms, occasionally entire body	Dry, fine scale; patches, diffuse or round; if severe, fissures

Source: Adapted from Ricciatti-Sibbald DJ. In: Clark C, ed. *Self-Medication: A Reference from Health Professionals.* 4th ed. Ottawa: Canadian Pharmaceutical Association; 1992:65.

Q~ What is your age? How long have you had this condition? When did it first appear?

A~ Suspect atopic dermatitis if the disorder first appeared at a young age. If the patient is an adult, ask if the recurrences have become less frequent.

Q~ What skin areas—including mucous membranes, hair, and nails—are involved?

A~ *Identify the body areas that these three disorders typically affect. (See Table 27–4.)* Using a visual inspection or the patient's description of affected areas, determine which disorder(s) could be present.

Q~ Do you or any family members have allergies, asthma, or hay fever?

A~ If yes, suspect atopic dermatitis.

Q~ Do you notice a seasonal change in the disorder?

A~ Suspect dry skin if symptoms worsen in the winter.

Q~ What is your occupation?

A~ Suspect dry skin if the occupation requires working in dry or windy environments. Suspect contact dermatitis if the patient is exposed to chemicals or other irritants in the workplace.

Q~ Is there anything such as work activities, hobbies, house cleaning, cleansers or cosmetics, medications, or jewelry that seems to make the disorder worse?

A~ Suspect contact dermatitis if worsening of symptoms is related to jewelry, glues or solvents used in hobbies, or medications known to be sensitizers. Consider contact dermatitis and dry skin if household cleansers and body soaps worsen the disorder.

Q~ How often do you bathe or shower? How long do you typically stay in the tub or shower? Do you use hot or warm water for bathing or showering?

A~ Suspect dry skin if the patient takes frequent or long showers using hot water.

Patient Counseling for Atopic Dermatitis, Contact Dermatitis, and Dry Skin

Patients with atopic dermatitis should be educated on achieving control of their disease with proper education on the chronic nature of the disease, exacerbating factors, and appropriate treatment options.

For patients with contact dermatitis, the pharmacist should stress that avoiding substances known to induce irritant or allergic skin reactions is the best "treatment." Appropriate treatment options for the discomfort of skin reactions should also be explained.

Patients with dry skin should be informed that they have more control over mild-to-moderate forms of this disorder than most other types of dermatologic disorders. The pharmacist should also explain factors that cause dry skin and the

Patient Education for Atopic Dermatitis, Contact Dermatitis, and Dry Skin

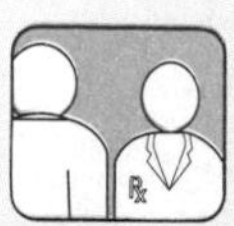

The primary objectives of self-treating atopic and contact dermatitis are to (1) relieve symptoms of itching and weeping and (2) avoid or minimize exposure to factors that trigger or aggravate the disorders. The primary objectives in self-treating dry skin, restoring skin moisture and the skin's barrier function, can also help relieve the discomfort of atopic and contact dermatitis. For most patients, carefully following product instructions and the self-care measures listed below will help ensure optimal therapeutic outcomes.

Atopic Dermatitis

Nondrug Measures

- Avoid factors that trigger allergic reactions. Do not wear occlusive, tight clothing. Remain in moderate temperature settings and in low humidity conditions.
- Bathe or shower preferably every other day. Take short showers or baths, using warm water and a nonsoap cleanser such as Cetaphil or Oilatum AD.
- If possible, substitute sponge baths with tepid water for full-body bathing.
- To dry weeping lesions, apply wet tap water compresses for 20 minutes, four to six times daily.
- To prevent injury to the affected area caused by scratching, keep your fingernails short, smooth, and clean. At night, wear cotton gloves or socks on your hands to lessen scratching.

Nonprescription Medications

- To decrease itching, bathe in tepid water that contains colloidal oatmeal, or add a water-miscible bath oil to the water near the end of the bath.
- Gently pat your skin dry, and apply an emollient while your skin is still damp.
- Use hydrocortisone to dry weeping lesions and to relieve itching. Do not use this medication for longer than 7 days.
- If itching keeps you awake at night, take an antihistamine such as diphenhydramine, with a sedative effect, to help you sleep. Be aware that such medications can cause drowsiness the next morning.

If the atopic dermatitis does not improve or worsens after 2 to 3 days of treatment, consult a physician.

Contact Dermatitis

Nondrug Measures

- Decrease exposure to common skin irritants such as detergents, soaps, and solvents.
- Avoid occlusion of the skin, which can make it more permeable to chemicals, by changing gloves (especially latex gloves used for cleaning chores), diapers, and clothing more frequently.
- If you have experienced topical allergic reactions, avoid contact with known allergens.
- To avoid potential allergic reactions, use hypoallergenic cosmetics and soapless cleansers.
- Wash the affected area gently to remove traces of the offending agent.

Nonprescription Medications

- To dry up lesions, apply compresses of cool tap water or aluminum acetate for 20 minutes, four to six times daily.
- Apply calamine lotion between compress applications, and take colloidal oatmeal baths to soothe and help relieve itching.
- Use hydrocortisone to relieve itching and/or inflammation.
- If itching keeps you awake at night, take an antihistamine, such as diphenhydramine, with a sedative effect, to help you sleep. Be aware that such medications can cause drowsiness the next morning.

If the contact dermatitis does not begin to improve in 2 to 3 days or if it worsens, consult a physician.

Dry Skin

Nondrug Measures

- Reduce full-body bathing to every other day or less often.
- Do not take long, hot showers.
- If possible, take sponge baths or quick showers, using warm water.
- Drink up to 3 to 4 liters of water per day. Do not substitute sodas, coffee, or teas for water.

Nonprescription Medications

- Add products such as colloidal oatmeal, oilated oatmeal, or bath oil near the end of your bath to enhance skin hydration.
- Apply an oil-based emollient immediately after bathing while your skin is damp. Reapply the emollient frequently.
- For more severe cases of dry skin, use a product that contains urea or lactic acid.
- Apply topical hydrocortisone ointment to reduce inflammation and itching. Do not use this medication for longer than 7 days.

If skin dryness is not resolved within 7 days, consult a physician.

appropriate measures for restoring barrier function. The box "Patient Education for Atopic Dermatitis, Contact Dermatitis, and Dry Skin" lists specific information to provide patients.

Evaluation of Patient Outcomes for Atopic Dermatitis, Contact Dermatitis, and Dry Skin

The pharmacist should reevaluate a patient with atopic or contact dermatitis within 2 to 3 days of the patient's initial visit. A patient with dry skin should be reevaluated in 7 days.

Visual assessment is the best method of determining treatment response. Therefore, a scheduled pharmacy visit is the preferred method of follow-up. If the symptoms have not improved or have worsened, the patient should see a physician.

CONCLUSIONS

Many individuals suffer from atopic and contact dermatitis and dry skin. The pharmacist performs a valuable service by educating patients about the disorder in question and by recommending the most effective nonprescription therapy or, if applicable, referral for medical treatment. Nonprescription products are effective in the short-term treatment of the itching and inflammation, which are often associated with these disorders. Long-term treatment should include avoidance of factors or practices that cause these disorders.

References

1. Kligman AM, Koblenzer C. Demographics and psychological implications for the aging population. *Dermatol Clin.* 1997;15:549–53.
2. Yeatman JM, Kilkenny MF, Stewart K, et al. Advice about management of skin conditions in the community: who are the providers? *Australas J of Dermatol.* 1996;37:S46–7.
3. Odland GF. Structure of the skin. In: Goldsmith LA, ed. *Physiology, Biochemistry, and Molecular Biology of the Skin.* New York: Oxford University Press; 1991:3–62.
4. Ricciatti-Sibbald DJ. Dermatitis. In: Clark C, ed. *Self-Medication: A Reference for Health Professionals.* 4th ed. Ottawa: Canadian Pharmaceutical Association; 1992:65.
5. Guy RH, Hadgraft J. In: Bronaugh RL, Maibach HI, eds. *Percutaneous Absorption.* 3rd ed. New York: Marcel Dekker; 1999:13–26.
6. Roth RR, James WD. Microbiology of the skin: resident flora, ecology, infection. *J Am Acad Dermatol.* 1989;20:367–90.
7. Cascella PJ, Powers JE. *US Pharm.* 1988;13:26.
8. Leung DY, Hanifin JM, Charlesworth EN, et al. Disease management of atopic dermatitis: a practice parameter. Joint Task Force on Practice Parameters, representing the American Academy of Allergy, Asthma and Immunology, the American College of Allergy, Asthma and Immunology, and the Joint Council of Allergy, Asthma and Immunology, Work Group on Atopic Dermatitis. *Ann Allergy Asthma Immunol.* 1997;79:197–209.
9. Holden CA, Parish WE. In: Champion RH, Burton JL, Burns DA, et. al, eds. *Textbook of Dermatology.* 6th ed. Oxford, England: Blackwell Scientific Publications; 1998:681–708.
10. Vickers CHF. Eczematous diseases. In: Orkin M, Maibach III, eds. *Dermatology.* 1st ed. Norwalk, CT: Appleton & Lange; 1991:466–70.
11. Pearce M. Atopic dermatitis. *Pharm Times.* 1990:88–92.
12. David TJ, Devlin J, Ewing CI. Atopic and seborrheic dermatitis: practical management. *Pediatrician.* 1991;18:211–7.
13. Burns DA, Rycroft RJG. In: Champion RH, Burton JL, Breathnach SM, eds. *Textbook of Dermatology.* 6th ed. Oxford, England: Blackwell Scientific Publications; 1998:821–60.
14. Belsito D. In: Freedberg IM, et al, eds. *Dermatology in General Medicine.* 5th ed. New York: McGraw-Hill; 1999:1447–61.
15. Andersen KE, Maibach HI. Contact dermatitis. In: Orkin M, Maibach HI, eds. *Dermatology.* 1st ed. Norwalk, CT: Appleton & Lange; 1991:405–13.
16. Denig NI, Hoke AW, Maibach HI. Irritant contact dermatitis: clues to causes, clinical characteristics, and control. *Postgrad Med.* 1998;103:199–200, 207–8, 212–3.
17. Robinson JR. Dermatitis, dry skin, dandruff, seborrheic dermatitis, and psoriasis products. In: Feldmann EG, Blockstein WL, eds. *Handbook of Nonprescription Drugs.* 9th ed. Washington, DC: American Pharmaceutical Association; 1990:811–40.
18. Keefner KR, DeSimone EM. Contact dermatitis: skin reactions to irritants. *US Pharm.* 1991;16 (skin care suppl):36–9.
19. Fisher AA. Allergic contact dermatitis associated with OTC topical anesthetics and antihistamines. *Pharm Times.* 1991;57:65–8.
20. Gossel TA. Therapeutic relief of contact dermatitis. *US Pharm.* 1990;15:12–6.
21. Lazar AP, Lazar P. Dry skin, water, and lubrication. *Dermatol Clin.* 1991;9:45–51.
22. Hamacher DP. Facial moisturizers. *NARD.* 1991;113:63.
23. Fitzpatrick JE. Common inflammatory skin diseases of the elderly. *Geriatrics.* 1989;44:40–6.
24. Kempers S, Katz HI, Wildnauer R, et al. An evaluation of the effect of an alpha-hydroxy acid-blend skin cream in the cosmetic improvement of symptoms of moderate to severe xerosis, epidermolytic hyperkeratosis, and ichthyosis. *Cutis.* 1998;61:347–50.
25. Shwayder T, Ott F. All about ichthyosis. *Pediatr Clin North Am.* 1991;38:835–57.
26. Roenigk HH Jr. Treatment of the aging face. *Dermatol Clin.* 1995;13:245–61.
27. Gossel TA. Dry skin. *US Pharm.* 1990;15:20–4.
28. Jackson EM. AHA-type products proliferate in 1993. *Cosmet Dermatol.* 1993;6:22–4.
29. *Federal Register.* 1982;47:39444–8.
30. *Federal Register.* 1991;56:43025–6.
31. *Federal Register.* 1979;44:69768–866.
32. Bingham EA. Topical dermatologic therapy. In: Rook A, Parish LC, Beare JM, eds. *Practical Management of the Dermatologic Patient.* Philadelphia: JB Lippincott; 1986:227–8.
33. Wahlberg JE. Patch testing. In: Rycroft RJG, Menne T, Frosch PJ, eds. *Textbook of Contact Dermatitis.* 2nd ed. Berlin: Springer-Verlag; 1995:241–68.
34. Angelini G. Topical drugs. In: Rycroft RJG, Menne T, Frosch PJ, eds. *Textbook of Contact Dermatitis.* 2nd ed. Berlin: Springer-Verlag; 1995:477–503.

CHAPTER 28

Scaly Dermatoses

Nina H. Han and Dennis P. West

Chapter 28 at a Glance

Dandruff, seborrheic dermatitis (seborrhea), and psoriasis are chronic, scaly dermatoses. They may be placed on a spectrum ranging from dandruff (a minor problem that is primarily cosmetic) to psoriasis (a clinical condition that can have significant physical, psychologic, and economic consequences).

Nonprescription products are appropriate treatment for all degrees of dandruff. Many cases of seborrheic dermatitis will respond to the same pharmacologic therapy used to treat dandruff. Psoriasis that involves mild inflammation may be responsive to nonprescription treatment. However, initial diagnosis of psoriasis and management of acute flare-ups require the attention of a physician.[1]

Editor's Note: This chapter is based, in part, on the 11th edition chapter titled "Dermatologic Products," which was written by Dennis P. West and Phillip A. Nowakowksi.

Dandruff

Dandruff is a chronic, noninflammatory scalp condition that results in excessive scaling of scalp epidermis. Dandruff is clinically visible in approximately 20% of the population. Scalp scaling has a high public profile; although it is commonly associated with significant distress, the medical profession has a tendency to dismiss this problem as rather trivial.[2] Severity of dandruff declines in the summer and is not proved to be aggravated by emotional states. Authorities disagree over whether inadequate shampooing exacerbates dandruff; however, agreement exists that a consistent washing routine is important in managing the condition.[1,2]

Epidemiology of Dandruff

Dandruff generally appears at puberty, reaches a peak in early adulthood, levels off in middle age, and declines in advancing years (occurring only rarely after 75 years of age).

Etiology/Pathophysiology of Dandruff

Dandruff is technically a physiologic event and condition much like the growth of hair and nails, except that the end product is visible on the scalp and has a substantial cosmetic and social stigma associated with its presence. It correlates with the proliferative activity of the epidermis.

Dandruff is characterized by accelerated epidermal cell turnover, an irregular keratin breakup pattern, and the shedding of cells in large scales. It is normal for epidermal cells on the scalp to continually slough off just as they do elsewhere. The turnover rate of epidermal cells is greater on the scalp than on other parts of the body. In patients with dandruff, however, the turnover rate of epidermal cells on the scalp is about twice that of normal scalp.[3] This rate assists in distinguishing dandruff from seborrhea and psoriasis: Psoriasis has a higher turnover rate than seborrhea, which has a higher rate than dandruff.

Dandruff scales often appear around a hair shaft because of the epithelial growth at the base of the hair. This phenomenon does not occur on the normal scalp because the horny substance breaks up in a much more uniform fashion. The horny layer of the scalp normally consists of 25 to 35 fully keratinized, closely coherent cells per square millimeter arranged in an orderly fashion. However, in dandruff, the intact horny layer has fewer than 10 normal cells per square millimeter, and nonkeratinized cells are common. With dandruff, crevices occur deep in the stratum corneum, resulting in cracking, which generates relatively large scales. If the large scales are broken down to smaller units, the dandruff becomes less visible.

As the rate of keratin cell turnover increases, so too does the number of incompletely keratinized cells, a situation characterized by the retention of nuclei in keratin layer cells. Incompletely keratinized cells in dandruff appear in clusters, possibly as a result of tiny inflammatory foci that are incited when capillaries discharge a load of inflammatory cells into the epidermis, causing accelerated epidermal growth in a small area. These microfoci are found on all scalps but are increased proportionately in dandruff.[3]

The specific cause of accelerated cell growth seen in dandruff is unknown. Debate continues as to whether dandruff is a result of elevated microorganism levels—particularly of *Pityrosporum ovale* (a yeast-like fungus that is normal flora of the scalp).[4]

Signs and Symptoms of Dandruff

Dandruff is diffuse rather than patchy and is not inflammatory. Dandruff alone typically does not cause pruritus. Scaling, the only visible manifestation of dandruff, is the result of an increased rate of horny substance production on the scalp and the sloughing of large scales. Unlike seborrheic dermatitis, which can result in scaling with erythema or inflammation, dandruff lesions are noninflammatory, diffuse scalings.

Treatment Overview of Dandruff

Treatment Outcomes

The goal of treating dandruff is to reduce the epidermal turnover rate of the skin of the scalp, thereby minimizing the likelihood of visible scaling. The patient needs to understand that the disorder can be controlled but that no direct cure for dandruff exists.

General Treatment Approach

Dandruff is more of a cosmetic than a medical problem, and treatment is fairly straightforward. Washing the hair and scalp with a nonmedicated shampoo every other day or daily is often sufficient to control dandruff. If it is not, the pharmacist may recommend medicated nonprescription antidandruff products. With medicated shampoos, contact time improves effectiveness. The pharmacist should counsel the patient to allow medicated shampoo to remain on the hair for several minutes before rinsing and repeating. Thorough rinsing is important in the use of all shampoo products.

A cytostatic agent (e.g., pyrithione zinc, selenium sulfide, or coal tar) is recommended. Such agents reduce scaling by decreasing the epidermal turnover rate. However, the coal tar–containing shampoos may tend to discolor light hair as well as clothing and jewelry and, thus, may not appeal to some patients. A keratolytic shampoo containing salicylic acid or sulfur may also be used. (See the section "Treatment of Scaly Dermatoses.") If dandruff proves resistant to these agents, the patient should be referred to a physician for treatment.[1,5] Scalp conditions in children younger than 2 years should be referred to a physician for evaluation.

Seborrhea

Seborrheic dermatitis describes a group of eruptions that occur predominantly in the areas of greatest sebaceous gland activity (e.g., the scalp, face, and trunk).

Epidemiology of Seborrhea

Seborrheic dermatitis affects approximately 12 million Americans and occurs mostly in otherwise healthy middle-aged and elderly people, particularly men. It is also commonly found in people with parkinsonism, zinc deficiency, endocrine states associated with obesity, and human immunodeficiency virus infection. Quadriplegics and patients who have experienced a cerebrovascular accident or a myocardial infarct also seem prone to seborrheic dermatitis. Because nonprescription therapy is effective in a significant percentage of cases, the pharmacist can play a key role in managing seborrheic dermatitis.[6]

Etiology/Pathophysiology of Seborrhea

Seborrheic dermatitis is marked by accelerated epidermal proliferation and sebaceous gland activity.[7] The cause is unknown, although it appears to be a genetic predisposition. Proposed etiologic factors have included vitamin B complex deficiency, food allergies, autoimmunity, climate changes, and low relative humidity. Emotional and physical stress serve as aggravating factors. The characteristic accelerated cell turnover and enhanced sebaceous gland activity give rise to the prominent scale displayed in the condition. However, no clear-cut quantitative relationship exists between the degree of sebaceous gland activity and susceptibility to seborrhea.

It is commonly believed that seborrheic dermatitis is an extension of dandruff, and the controversy regarding involvement of *P. ovale* extends to seborrhea. Some researchers, however, dispute the link with dandruff, offering evidence that seborrhea is a separate condition. Incompletely keratinized cells commonly make up 15% to 25% of the corneocyte count in seborrheic dermatitis but rarely exceed 5% in dandruff.[6]

Signs and Symptoms of Seborrhea

The distinctive characteristics of the disorder are its common occurrence in hairy areas (especially the scalp); the appearance of dull, yellowish red lesions, which are well demarcated; and the associated presence of oily-appearing, yellowish scales. Pruritus is common.[8] The most common form, seborrhea of the scalp, is characterized by greasy scales on the scalp that often extend to the middle third of the face with subsequent eye involvement. (See the "Color Plates," photograph 10.) Lesions can occur on the face, particularly around the nasal area, with ear involvement also being common. Other areas affected can include the groin, axillae, sternum, and the back.

If the lesion is located in the groin, tinea cruris (jock itch) must be considered, especially during warm weather. Scalp lesions must be evaluated for the possibility of tinea capitis (ringworm of the scalp).[3] Signs and symptoms of bacterial or fungal infection can include erythema, warmth, exudate, and crusting or scaling. At times, concomitant bacterial or fungal infections can be present, which can make treatment difficult.[9] Many patients with severe acne also have seborrheic dermatitis.[2]

When seborrhea of the scalp occurs in newborns and infants, it is referred to as "cradle cap" and is treated primarily by gentle massaging with baby oil, followed by a nonmedicated shampoo to remove scales. Pruritus does not typically accompany cradle cap, and the condition often clears spontaneously by ages 8 to 12 months.[1,6,10]

Treatment Overview of Seborrhea

Treatment Outcomes

The goals of treating seborrhea are to reduce inflammation and reduce the epidermal turnover rate of the skin of the scalp, thereby minimizing or eliminating visible erythema and scaling.

General Treatment Approach

The treatment of seborrheic dermatitis is similar to that of dandruff. It generally responds to shampoos containing pyrithione zinc, selenium sulfide, sulfur, ketoconazole, salicylic acid, or coal tar. However, a minority of patients may complain that selenium sulfide makes the scalp more oily and that it may have exacerbated the seborrheic condition.

A primary difference between the treatment of dandruff and that of seborrheic dermatitis is the use of topical corticosteroids. Such products are not indicated for dandruff but may be used to manage seborrheic dermatitis whenever erythema is persistent after therapy with medicated shampoos. Hydrocortisone lotions for scalp dermatitis are available without a prescription. The pharmacist should advise the patient to apply the hydrocortisone product two to three times a day until symptoms subside and then intermittently to control acute exacerbations. The patient should also be instructed in the proper technique of application. The hair should be parted and the product applied directly to the scalp and massaged in thoroughly. The patient should repeat this process until desired coverage of the affected area is achieved. The absorption of medication into the scalp is enhanced if the lotion is applied after shampooing; skin hydration promotes drug absorption. Shampooing removes natural body oils, which allows better medication penetration.

The pharmacist should encourage the patient to minimize prolonged and continued use of hydrocortisone in treating seborrheic dermatitis because a rebound flare may occur when prolonged therapy is discontinued. If the condition worsens or symptoms persist longer than 7 days, a physician should be consulted. At this point, a more potent topical steroid may be indicated.[3]

If the seborrheic dermatitis spreads to the ear canal, eyelashes, or eyelids, a physician should be consulted for appropriate therapy. This therapy may include the use of prescription otic and ophthalmic agents, along with systemic antibiotics in some cases.[2]

Nonprescription products used to treat seborrheic dermatitis are to be avoided for children younger than 2 years, except under the advice and supervision of a physician.[11] (See the section "Treatment of Scaly Dermatoses.")

Psoriasis

Psoriasis is estimated to afflict 1% to 3% of the U.S. population. Lesions are often localized but may become generalized over much of the body surface and may result in disability.[12] Remissions and exacerbations are unpredictable. Approximately 30% of people with psoriasis find that lesion involvement may clear spontaneously. In fact, psoriasis may be so mild that many people do not even know they have it. However, unrelenting generalized psoriasis may cause enough psychologic distress to affect lifestyle and career choice adversely. With an associated psoriatic arthritis, psoriasis may

Case Study 28–1

Patient Complaint/History

Joel, a 24-year-old man, comes to the pharmacy complaining of excessive dandruff with itchy, flaky scalp. He states that the shampoos he has used have not been successful. While you are questioning him, you notice that he has some yellow, oily scales around his nose and mouth.

Clinical Considerations/Strategies

Readers can use the following considerations/strategies to determine whether treatment of this condition with nonprescription products is warranted:

- Assess the possible etiologies of the patient's dermatitis.
- Determine which nonprescription medications would manage the "dandruff."
- Further assess the oily, yellow scales around the patient's nose.
- Determine which nonprescription products would manage the possible seborrheic dermatitis.

Patient Education/Counseling

Readers can use the following strategies to develop a patient education/counseling plan that will help ensure optimal therapeutic outcomes:

- Explain how to use the recommended therapy.
- Stress the amount of contact required for effective treatment.

result in disability and deformity.[13] Treatment of severe psoriasis can also produce a significant physical and economic burden.[1,14]

Epidemiology of Psoriasis

The incidence of psoriasis is distributed almost equally among men and women. Psoriasis is common to all races and geographic regions, but the incidence is lower in people living in countries close to the equator and among African Americans, Native Americans, and Asians.[14]

There appear to be two subgroups with respect to age of onset, with the most common being the second decade of life and the other being the fourth to fifth decades. Some researchers subdivide psoriasis on the basis of age into Type I and Type II. Type I patients typically present at the early age, have a strong family history, and have a higher frequency of histocompatibility locus antigen (HLA) antigens, whereas Type II would be those developing psoriasis in the later decades of life.

Etiology/Pathophysiology of Psoriasis

Accelerated epidermal proliferation leading to excessive scaling is one hallmark of psoriasis. Normal epidermal cell turnover is 25 to 30 days, whereas in a psoriatic plaque, it is 3 to 4 days. The duration of psoriasis is variable, and lesions may last a lifetime or may disappear quickly. When lesions disappear, they may leave the skin either hypopigmented or hyperpigmented. The disease course is marked by spontaneous exacerbations and remissions, and it tends to be chronic and relapsing.

Although it is not contagious, patients seem to have an inherited predisposition to psoriasis, given that about 30% of psoriatic patients show an associated family history. Evidence supports an autosomal dominant mode of inheritance, and genetic markers as determined by the major HLA system have been identified. Mononuclear cells and polymorphonuclear (PMN) leukocytes can be found in the dermis and also tend to infiltrate the epidermis. Extracts of psoriatic scale contain factors that can induce directed migration (chemotaxis) of inflammatory cells. The presence of inflammatory cells in psoriatic skin may induce epidermal proliferation and has led to various theories about the possible role of the immune system in the pathogenesis of psoriasis.[3]

Environmental factors are not to be underestimated. Controlled exposure to sunlight usually improves the condition. Some observers believe that emotional stress, smoking, and higher alcohol intake often affect psoriasis adversely. Medications such as lithium carbonate increase the total mass of circulating PMN leukocytes and are, therefore, associated with an induction or exacerbation of psoriatic symptoms. Other associated medications include antimalarial agents and β-blockers. Abrupt withdrawal of corticosteroids in psoriatic patients may precipitate a rebound flare.[1,14]

Psoriasis assumes several pathologic forms, the most common being psoriasis vulgaris, a chronic, plaque-type psoriasis occurring in about 80% of cases. The plaques may be any size and may be quite extensive.[1] Guttate psoriasis is less common and is characterized by many small, teardrop-shaped lesions that are distributed more or less evenly over the body. These lesions may later coalesce to form large characteristic plaques. (See the "Color Plates," photographs 11A, B, and C.)

Signs and Symptoms of Psoriasis

Psoriasis is a papulosquamous erythematous skin disease marked by the presence of silvery scales. These scales cover flat-topped lesions, which are pink or dull red. Edges of the lesions are sharply delineated, and individual diameters may vary from a few millimeters to 20 cm or more. When psoriatic scales are removed, small bleeding points (Auspitz's sign) often appear. Untreated psoriatic skin represents an altered barrier that allows greater permeability for some substances. For example, psoriatic skin may lose water 8 to 10 times faster than normal skin. In fact, when large areas of the body surface are involved, transepidermal water loss may be as much as 2 to 3 L daily in addition to normal perspiration loss. Evaporation of this volume of water requires more than 1000 calories. For this reason, psoriatic patients may show increased metabolic rates manifested as tissue catabolism, and muscle wasting may occur.[3]

Psoriatic lesions tend to appear on the scalp, elbows, knees, fingernails, and lower back and in the genitoanal region. Lesions may develop at sites of trauma (Koebner's phenomenon), such as vaccination or skin tests, scratch marks, or surgical incisions. In fact, the response to skin trauma is so predictable that it can be used in the assessment of up to 40% of patients afflicted. Itching is a significant manifestation of the disease in 30% to 70% of cases, and the name *psoriasis* originates from the Greek word for *itch*.[14]

Besides skin, tissues known to be clinically involved are the nails and synovium. In many patients with coexisting joint disease and psoriasis, the arthritic component is not easily distinguishable from rheumatoid arthritis. About 7% of psoriatic patients, however, have psoriatic arthritis, which is recognized as a distinct clinical entity. Nail involvement includes onycholysis (separation of the nail from the nail bed), pitting, and yellow discoloration. Unlike rheumatoid arthritis, psoriatic arthritis is often asymmetric in its joint involvement. Usually, the rheumatoid factor is absent, and prognosis is better than it is with rheumatoid arthritis.

Treatment Overview of Psoriasis

Treatment Outcomes

The goals in treating psoriasis are to control or eliminate the signs and symptoms (scales, itching, and inflammation) and to prevent or minimize the likelihood of flares.

General Treatment Approach

The Food and Drug Administration (FDA) recommends that only mild cases of psoriasis be self-treated. Individuals with moderate-to-severe cases, involving more than 10% of body surface, should be under a physician's care.[3] Severe, generalized psoriasis sometimes necessitates day care or hospitalization. Recalcitrant cases or cases in children younger than 2 years should be referred to a physician for evaluation.

Pruritic dry skin is common in psoriasis, and emollients and lubricating bath products often provide relief for these symptoms. (See Chapter 27, "Atopic Dermatitis, Contact Dermatitis, and Dry Skin," for discussion of these products.) Gentle rubbing with a soft cloth following the bath helps to mechanically remove scales. Depending on the anatomic site, self-treatment may progress to the use of topical hydrocortisone, coal tar products, and/or keratolytic agents such as salicylic acid.[1] The patient should avoid vigorous rubbing, which can aggravate the lesions.

Acute localized flares, characterized by bright red lesions, call for soothing local therapy with emollients and hydrocortisone. The patient must avoid tars, salicylic acid, and aggressive ultraviolet (UV) radiation therapy at this stage because of potential exacerbating effects. After the flare has subsided and the usual thick-scaled plaques appear, the patient may use therapy with agents such as keratolytics. Many patients respond well to simple measures, whereas others are refractory even to aggressive treatments.[3]

In the case of psoriatic arthritis, the psoriatic lesions may be treated topically, but the joint involvement is usually treated with nonsteroidal anti-inflammatory drugs (NSAIDs) or with prescription agents such as methotrexate.[1,14] (See Chapter 3, "Headache and Muscle and Joint Pain," for discussion of NSAIDs.) No reliably effective nonprescription treatment is available for nail psoriasis.

Previous guidelines for nonprescription therapy with a medicated shampoo for dandruff and seborrhea are applicable to treating scalp psoriasis with tar-based as well as salicylic acid–based products. Again, sufficient contact time is the key to successful therapy, the goal of which is scale removal. In addition, although 1% hydrocortisone products for facial lesions, scalp itching, and mild lesional skin involvement may be used, widespread involvement dictates that the patient be treated by a physician. If a nonprescription product is used, the pharmacist should counsel the patient to consult a physician if the condition does not improve in 1 to 2 weeks or if it worsens.

Because intertriginous areas (e.g., armpits and genitoanal region) are sensitive to irritants such as coal tar and salicylic acid, such agents should be used with extreme caution, if at all, to treat psoriasis in these areas. Instead, hydrocortisone cream may be applied sparingly two or three times a day and should be used less often as improvement occurs.

Salicylic acid products may be more cosmetically acceptable than coal tar products to some patients and may encourage compliance. Such products are most useful if thick scales are present. Soaking the affected area in warm (not hot) water for 10 to 20 minutes before applying a salicylic acid product enhances keratolytic activity.

Coal tar products may be applied to the body, arms, and legs at bedtime. Because coal tar stains most materials, the patient should be advised to use appropriate bed linen and clothing during applications. The overnight application is followed by a bath in the morning to remove residual coal tar and to loosen psoriatic scales. Topical 1% hydrocortisone ointment for the body may be applied sparingly to lesions and massaged into the skin thoroughly but gently. (See the section "Treatment of Scaly Dermatoses.")

Psoriasis cannot be cured, but signs and symptoms can usually be controlled adequately with appropriate patient education and treatment. The patient should be reassured that, in most cases, control is possible. Such reassurance increases compliance with burdensome and prolonged treatment regimens. Also, if the pharmacist can help the patient gain some understanding and acceptance of the condition, that knowledge may reduce the patient's emotional stress and psychogenic exacerbations. Prevention of flares, which can be achieved by minimizing identified precipitating factors such as emotional stress, skin irritation, and physical trauma, should be emphasized.

Treatment of Scaly Dermatoses

Cytostatic agents and keratolytic agents, usually in the form of medicated shampoos, are used to reduce epidermal turnover rate. Ketoconazole, an antifungal agent, is used in self-treatment of seborrhea. Hydrocortisone controls the inflammation associated with seborrhea and psoriasis. Table 28–1 summarizes the concentrations and indications of these agents, whereas the algorithm in Figure 28–1 outlines self-treatment with these agents.

Patients should shampoo with a nonmedicated, nonresidue shampoo to remove scalp and hair dirt, oil, and scale before using a medicated shampoo. Many shampoos leave a residue on the hair shaft and scalp that may aggravate scaly dermatoses of the scalp. Nonresidue shampoos (e.g., Prell, Breck, and Johnson's Baby Shampoo) do not interfere with these scalp conditions but rather leave the scalp clean and receptive to optimal effects from medicated shampoos. A nonresidue shampoo application and rinse may be followed by a pyrithione zinc shampoo worked into the scalp for at least 2 minutes and then rinsed out thoroughly. The patient can use this treatment as often as daily until symptoms are relieved, then use it two to three times weekly or as needed.[1]

Table 28–1

Concentrations of Approved Nonprescription Ingredients for Products Used to Treat Dandruff, Seborrheic Dermatitis, and Psoriasis

	Concentration (%)		
Ingredient	**Dandruff**	**Seborrheic Dermatitis**	**Psoriasis**
Coal tar	0.5–5	0.5–5	0.5–5
Ketoconazole	1	1	—
Pyrithione zinc (brief exposure)	0.3–2	0.95–2	—
Pyrithione zinc (residual)	0.1–0.25	0.1–0.25	—
Salicylic acid	1.8–3	1.8–3	1.8–3
Selenium sulfide	1	1	—
Sulfur	2–5	—	—

Source: Reference 11.

Cytostatic Agents

Although their mechanism of action is not completely understood, cytostatic agents are known to decrease the rate of epidermal cell replication. This action increases the time required for epidermal cell turnover, which, in turn, allows the possibility of normalizing epidermal differentiation, resulting in a dramatic decline in visible scales. Thus, cytostatic agents represent a direct approach to controlling dandruff and seborrheic dermatitis. (See Table 28–2 for examples of commercially available products.)

Pyrithione Zinc

Pyrithione zinc's action is likely caused by a nonspecific toxicity for epidermal cells. The pyrithione moiety is apparently the active part of the molecule. Product effectiveness is influenced by several factors. First, pyrithione zinc is strongly bound to both hair and the external skin layers, and the extent of binding correlates with clinical performance. Second, the drug minimally penetrates into the dermal region. Third, its absorption increases with contact time, temperature, concentration, and frequency of application. Some researchers consider pyrithione zinc to be slower acting than selenium sulfide.[3]

For pyrithione zinc products that are intended to be applied and washed off within minutes, FDA allows concentrations of 0.3% to 2% for treating dandruff and 0.95% to 2% for treating seborrheic dermatitis. Concentrations for products intended to be applied and then left on the skin or scalp are 0.1% to 0.25% for treating both dandruff and seborrheic dermatitis.[15] Shampoos and soaps are currently available in 1% and 2% concentrations.

Long-term use of 1% to 2% pyrithione zinc rinse-away products has rarely been associated with toxicity. Nevertheless, patients should be cautioned against using this agent on broken or abraded skin because rare cases of contact dermatitis have been reported.

Ketoconazole

Ketoconazole, a synthetic azole antifungal agent, is available as a nonprescription shampoo formulation. Nizoral AD (ketoconazole 1%) is active against most pathogenic fungi but is indicated specifically for *P. ovale*. Thus, it is used to treat seborrheic dermatitis of the scalp. Although it has been suggested that *P. ovale* may be associated with the development of dandruff, a definite causal relationship has not yet been established. Regardless, some studies have demonstrated efficacy in dandruff conditions. In addition to ketoconazole shampoo, other antifungals such as clotrimazole and miconazole (cream or solution) have been used to treat seborrheic dermatitis of areas other than the scalp.

As with other medicated shampoos, contact time cannot be stressed enough. The scalp and hair should be wet; then the shampoo should be massaged well into the scalp and left on for 1 to 3 minutes. The scalp and hair should be thoroughly rinsed and the process repeated. The patient should

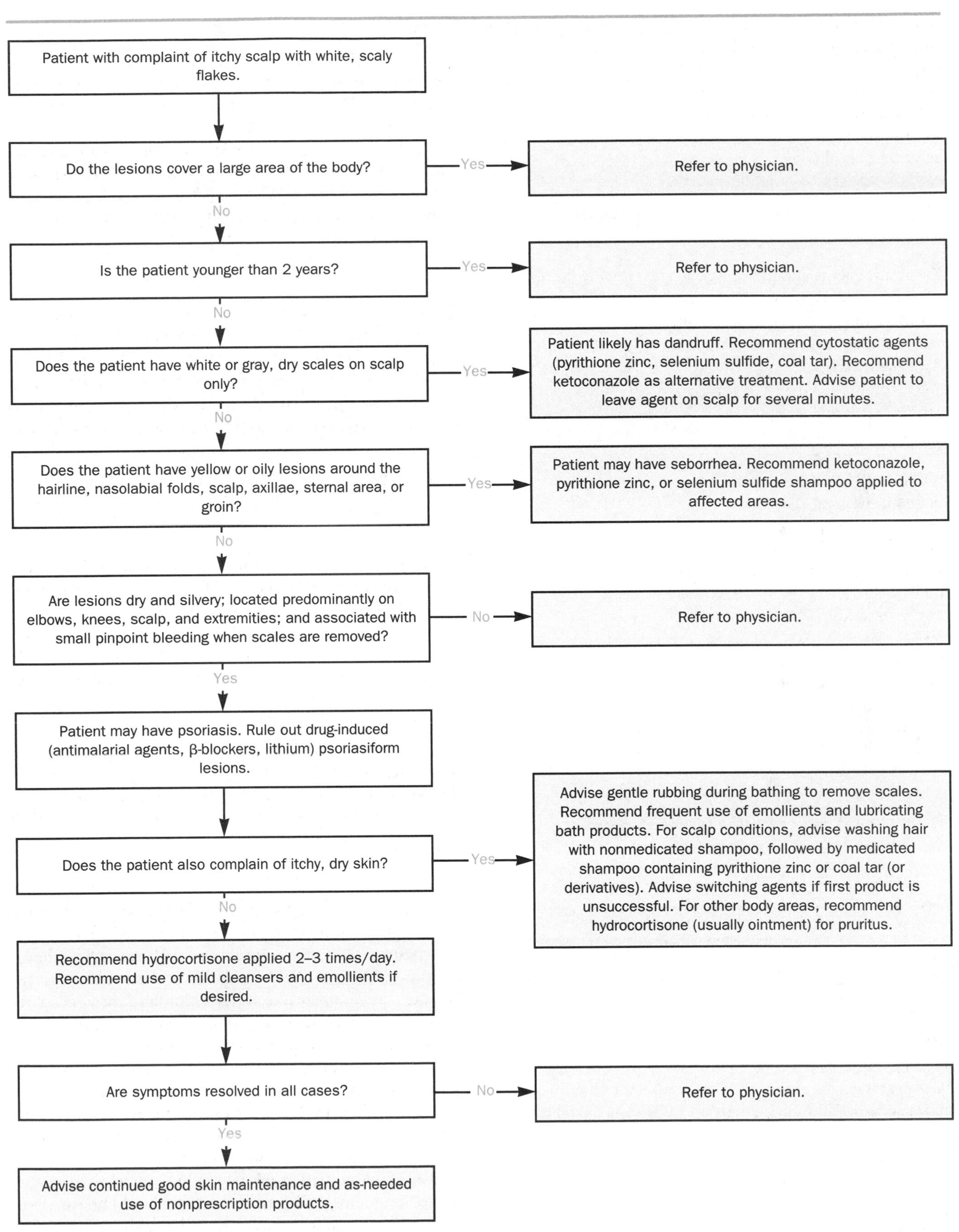

Figure 28–1 Self-care of scaly dermatoses.

Table 28–2

Selected Cytostatic Products for Scaly Dermatoses

Trade Name	Primary Ingredients
Balnetar Bath Oil	Coal tar 2.5%
Denorex Dandruff for Dry Scalp Shampoo and Conditioner	Coal tar extract 2% (equivalent to 0.5% coal tar)
Denorex Medicated Shampoo and Conditioner	Coal tar solution 9% (equivalent to 1.8% coal tar)
Denorex Extra Strength Medicated Shampoo and Conditioner	Coal tar solution 12.5% (equivalent to 2.5% coal tar)
DHS Tar Shampoo	Coal tar 0.5%
DHS Tar Gel Shampoo	Coal tar 0.5%
DHS Zinc Shampoo	Pyrithione zinc 2%
Head & Shoulders Dandruff 2-in-1 Shampoo	Pyrithione zinc 1%
Head & Shoulders Dandruff Shampoo	Pyrithione zinc 1%
Head & Shoulders Dry Scalp Shampoo	Pyrithione zinc 1%
Head & Shoulders Intensive Treatment Shampoo	Selenium sulfide 1%
Ionil T Shampoo	Coal tar solution 5% (equivalent to 1% coal tar)
Ionil T Plus Shampoo	Coal tar 2%
MG217 for Psoriasis Lotion	Coal tar solution 5%
MG217 for Psoriasis Ointment	Coal tar solution 10%
MG217 for Psoriasis Shampoo	Coal tar solution 15%
Neutrogena T/Derm Body Oil	Tar 5% (equivalent to 1.2% coal tar)
Neutrogena T/Gel Extra Strength Therapeutic Shampoo	Tar 4% (equivalent to 1% coal tar)
Neutrogena T/Gel Shampoo or Conditioner	Tar 2% (equivalent to 0.5% coal tar)
Oxipor VHC Lotion	Coal tar solution 25% (equivalent to 5% coal tar)
Pantene Pro-V Anti-Dandruff Shampoo	Pyrithione zinc 1%
Pert Plus Dandruff Shampoo	Pyrithione zinc 1%
Polytar Shampoo	Tar 4.5% (equivalent to 0.5% coal tar)
Polytar Cleansing Bar	Tar 2.5% (equivalent to 0.5% coal tar)
Sebulon Shampoo	Pyrithione zinc 2%
Selsun Blue 2-in-1 Treatment Shampoo	Selenium sulfide 1%
Selsun Blue Balanced Treatment Shampoo	Selenium sulfide 1%
Tarsum Shampoo/Gel Shampoo	Coal tar solution 10%
Tegrin Cleansing Bar/Cream	Coal tar solution 5% (equivalent to 0.8% coal tar)
Tegrin Shampoo	Coal tar solution 7% (equivalent to 1.1% coal tar)
X-Seb Plus Shampoo	Pyrithione zinc 1%
X-Seb T Plus Shampoo	Coal tar solution 10% (crude coal tar 2%)
ZNP Cleansing Bar	Pyrithione zinc 2%

use ketoconazole shampoo twice a week for 4 weeks, with at least 3 days in between each treatment.

Adverse effects are minimal, but reports of hair loss, irritation, abnormal hair texture, and dry skin have been reported.

Selenium Sulfide

Selenium sulfide is thought to have a direct antimitotic effect on epidermal cells. Like pyrithione zinc, it is more effective with longer contact time and thus should be applied in a similar manner. The product must be rinsed from the hair thoroughly or discoloration may result, especially in blond, gray, or dyed hair. Frequent use of selenium sulfide tends to leave a residual odor and an oily scalp.

Selenium sulfide has been approved in a 1% concentration as an active ingredient in nonprescription products to treat dandruff and seborrhea.[15] A higher concentration is available by prescription for use in resistant cases.

Cytostatic toxicity from selenium sulfide is minimal, but the product can cause irritation of scalp and adjacent skin areas and should be avoided if such irritation occurs. Contact with the eyes should be avoided because of the potential for irritation. If such contact does occur, the patient should flush the eyes with copious amounts of water. Selenium sulfide is toxic if ingested. Because of the risk of systemic toxicity, it should be applied only to intact skin.[2]

Coal Tar

Coal tar products have long been popular for treating dandruff, seborrheic dermatitis, and psoriasis. Many nonprescription products are available. Crude coal tar, which consists of a heterogeneous mixture of thousands of hydrocarbon compounds, is produced by the destructive distillation of bituminous coal. Its composition varies, depending on the source of the coal and the process used. Crude coal tar is considered the most active, whereas the refined tars and the coal tar solution (liquor carbonis detergens, or LCD) are less active.[1]

Although its mechanism of action is not known, coal tar has been attributed with antiseptic, antipruritic, keratoplastic, antiparasitic, antifungal, antibacterial, antimitotic, vasoconstrictive, and photosensitizing capabilities.

Crude coal tar 1% to 5% and UV radiation therapy have been used to treat psoriasis since 1925 in a method known as the Goeckerman treatment. A therapeutic benefit of both the tar alone and the irradiation alone has been demonstrated, but the combination is more effective than either agent by itself. Remissions lasting up to 12 months have been reported after 2 to 4 weeks of therapy. The coal tar is removed from the skin before irradiation takes place; otherwise, the UV radiation will not reach the skin.

For many years, the therapeutic response to this form of therapy was believed to be caused by phototoxicity, but this theory has been challenged. Now it is thought that the beneficial effect of coal tar may lie in its ability to cross-link with DNA. Coal tar in combination with UV radiation may also increase prostaglandin synthesis in the skin, which may contribute to its beneficial effect. Combinations of 1% crude coal tar with long-wave UV (UVB) radiation and 6% crude coal tar with UVB radiation have been shown to be equally effective. Hence, only modest levels of coal tar are needed.[3]

Coal tar is available in creams, ointments, pastes, lotions, bath oils, shampoos, soaps, and gels. This variety of products has partly resulted from an attempt to develop a cosmetically acceptable product, one that masks the odor, color, and staining properties of crude coal tar that most patients find aesthetically unappealing. LCD is a 20% tincture of coal tar that has been useful in developing acceptable tar products. It is used in concentrations of 3% to 15%.

Tar gels represent a special product form that appears to deliver the beneficial elements of crude coal tar in a form both convenient to apply and cosmetically acceptable. These gels are nongreasy, nonstaining, and nearly colorless. The pharmacist should caution the patient, however, that many of these gels may have a drying effect on the skin, necessitating the use of an emollient.

Certain side effects are associated with the use of coal tar, including folliculitis (particularly of the axilla and groin); stains to the skin and hair (particularly blond, gray, and dyed hair); photosensitization; and dermatitis caused by irritation.[2] Certain patients may even show a worsening of the condition being treated when they are exposed to coal tar products. This situation is of particular concern in the acute phase of psoriasis, when topical corticosteroids are recommended to reduce inflammation before coal tar preparations are used.[1]

Because of the relatively short contact time, and thus the low lifetime exposure, FDA considers the benefits of coal tar to outweigh the risks for use in shampoo formulations. Thus, coal tar is available in concentrations of 0.5% to 5% for the self-treatment of scalp conditions such as dandruff, seborrheic dermatitis, and psoriasis.[15]

Keratolytic Agents

The keratolytic agents salicylic acid and sulfur are used in dandruff and seborrheic dermatitis products to loosen and lyse keratin aggregates, thereby facilitating their removal from the scalp in smaller particles. These agents act by dissolving the "cement" that holds epidermal cells together. Vehicle composition, contact time, and concentration are important factors in the success of a keratolytic agent. The keratolytic concentrations in nonprescription scalp products are not sufficient to impair the normal skin barrier but do affect the abnormal, incompletely keratinized stratum corneum. (See Table 28–3 for examples of commercially available products.)

Keratolytic agents may produce several adverse effects, and the patient should be counseled accordingly. These agents have a primary, concentration-dependent irritant effect, particularly on mucous membranes and on the conjunctiva of the eye. They also have the potential of acting on

Table 28–3

Selected Keratolytic Products for Scaly Dermatoses

Trade Name	Primary Ingredients
MG217 Sal-Acid for Psoriasis Ointment/Solution	Salicylic acid 3%
Neutrogena Healthy Scalp Anti-Dandruff Shampoo	Salicylic acid 1.8%
Neutrogena T/Sal Maximum Strength Therapeutic Shampoo	Salicylic acid 3%
Scalpicin Maximum Strength Foam/Solution	Salicylic acid 3%
Sebucare Lotion	Salicylic acid 1.8%
Sebulex Conditioning Shampoo with Protein	Salicylic acid 2%; sulfur 2%
Sulfoam Medicated Antidandruff Shampoo	Sulfur 2%
Sulray Cleansing Bar	Sulfur 5%
Sulray Dandruff Shampoo	Sulfur 2%

hair and skin keratin. Thus, hair appearance may be altered as a result of extended use. The directions and precautions for the use of keratolytic shampoos are similar to those for shampoos containing cytostatic agents.

Salicylic Acid

Salicylic acid decreases skin pH, causing increased hydration of keratin and, thus, facilitating its loosening and removal. Because contact time is minimal for a shampoo, absorption of the agent by the skin should be minimized.

Topical salicylic acid is useful for psoriasis when thick scales are present. A patient should soak the psoriatic lesion(s) in warm water for 10 to 20 minutes before applying the preparation, which may then be covered by an occlusive dressing. However, the patient should avoid application over extensive areas because of the potential for percutaneous absorption and systemic toxicity. Initially, the patient should use lower concentrations to minimize the possibility of causing irritation and worsening the condition.[3]

Salicylic acid has been approved in concentrations of 1.8% to 3% for the self-treatment of dandruff, seborrheic dermatitis, and psoriasis.[15] At these concentrations, the keratolytic effect typically takes 7 to 10 days. In higher concentrations for other uses, the keratolytic effect may be evident in 2 to 3 days.

Sulfur

Sulfur is believed to cause increased sloughing of cells and to reduce corneocyte counts. Sulfur has been approved in concentrations of 2% to 5% for the self-treatment of dandruff only. Although it is approved as a single-entity active ingredient, sulfur is often combined with salicylic acid. For the control of dandruff, the sulfur–salicylic acid combination is useful if both ingredients are present within the approved concentrations.[15] Although not an official indication, this combination has been commonly used for the self-treatment of seborrheic dermatitis.[6]

Topical Hydrocortisone

Topical hydrocortisone 1% is available without a prescription and has been promoted for the temporary relief of itching caused by body and scalp dermatoses. Hydrocortisone is generally efficacious as an antipruritic agent when used in concentrations of at least 1%. It is not indicated, nor is evidence available that it is effective, in treating dandruff. However, it may be useful for seborrhea accompanied by inflammation that is unresponsive to medicated shampoos.[6]

Nonprescription hydrocortisone products can play a role in managing mild psoriasis. A problem with topical corticosteroids is that a rebound flare may occur when topical therapy is discontinued. Relapse occurs more quickly after use of topical corticosteroids than after use of tar therapy. Nevertheless, corticosteroids are more appealing to the patient on cosmetic grounds, which are a consideration in long-term therapy.[14]

Topical corticosteroids have several effects (e.g., anti-inflammatory, antimitotic/antisynthetic, antipruritic, vasoconstrictive, and immunosuppressive) on cellular activity. Efficacy may be enhanced by an occlusive dressing. However, continued use of topical corticosteroids beyond 2 or 3 weeks may render the drug less effective. If the patient does not respond adequately to hydrocortisone, physician referral is appropriate because the use of more potent corticosteroids may be in order. Selection of the proper prescription corticosteroid may be complex because of the common assumption that potency and adverse effects are linked directly to halogenation.[16,17]

Adverse effects associated with the use of topical corticosteroids include local atrophy after prolonged use as well as the aggravation of certain cutaneous infections. The possibility of systemic sequelae exists and is enhanced by the use of the more potent compounds, by occlusive dressings, or by application to large areas of the body. Because children have a greater surface area-to-body mass ratio, they are at greater risk for developing systemic complications. In general, however, the concentrations of hydrocortisone available in nonprescription preparations are highly unlikely to cause systemic sequelae.[16,17]

The patient should be instructed to apply the hydrocortisone as a thin film two to four times a day at the onset of therapy and intermittently thereafter to control exacerbations. The medication should be thoroughly, but gently, massaged into the skin. Continued use of hydrocortisone should be discouraged because topical corticosteroids may become less effective with prolonged use and may cause adverse local effects.

Systemic use of corticosteroids is contraindicated in all but the most severe forms of psoriasis. This restriction relates to undesirable side effects that accompany systemic use of corticosteroids and to rebound flare that may occur after discontinuance.[14] Intralesional injections of corticosteroids have a limited use in treating isolated lesions and nail psoriasis.[1]

Other Agents

Detergents are not generally considered to be active ingredients in antidandruff products. However, for mild forms of dandruff, frequent and vigorous washing with a nonmedicated shampoo may help control excess scaling. Massaging the scalp produces a dispersion of scales into smaller, less-visible subunits. Detergents may contribute to this effect by virtue of their surfactant activity. Detergents found in shampoos include sodium lauryl sulfate, polyoxyethylene ethers, triethanolamine, and quaternary ammonium compounds such as benzalkonium chloride, benzethonium chloride, and isoquinolinium bromides.[3]

Although ordinary vitamin D is of no known value in treating psoriasis, topical calcipotriene (a synthetic vitamin D_3 analog) is available by prescription. This product is useful for treating localized lesions and can be combined with other forms of treatment.[18,19]

Patient Assessment of Scaly Dermatoses

Differentiation of the scaly dermatoses involves several factors. The appearance of the scales in the early stages of a disorder is not always definitive. In these cases, the presence and nature of other symptoms or the location of the dermatitis provide additional important clues to its assessment. Factors that precipitate or exacerbate the disorder are also helpful in defining the disorder. Table 28–4 describes the distinguishing features of these three dermatoses.

Asking the patient the following questions will help elicit the information needed to accurately assess the disorder and to recommend the appropriate treatment.

Case Study 28–2

Patient Complaint/History

Ileana, a 50-year-old woman, presents to the pharmacy complaining of new "scales" around her knees and legs. The patient admits to "picking" at her lesions and noticing some little bleeding marks.

The patient's profile reveals that Ileana began taking a β-blocker 4 months ago for recently diagnosed hypertension.

Clinical Considerations/Strategies

Readers can use the following considerations/strategies to determine whether treatment of this condition with nonprescription products is warranted:

- Determine which questions to ask about the characteristics of the scales.
- Determine what disorder the bleeding marks indicated.
- Determine what disorder the prescription medication could induce.
- Determine which nonprescription medications would manage the disorder.

Patient Education/Counseling

Readers can use the following strategies to develop a patient education/counseling plan that will help ensure optimal therapeutic outcomes:

- Explain how to use the recommended therapy.
- Advise the patient of signs and symptoms that indicate medical attention is needed.

Table 28–4

Distinguishing Features of Dandruff, Seborrhea, and Psoriasis

	Dandruff	Seborrhea	Psoriasis
Location	Scalp	Adults and children: head and trunk; Children only: back, intertriginous areas	Scalp, elbows, knees, trunk, and lower extremities
Exacerbating factors	Generally a stable condition, exacerbated by inadequate washing, dry climate	Exacerbated by many external factors, notably stress and low relative humidity	Exacerbated by medical irritation, stress, climate, drugs, infection, and endocrine factors
Appearance	Thin, white, or grayish flakes; even distribution on scalp	Patchy lesions with margins; mild inflammation; oily, yellowish scales	Usually symmetrical, red, patchy plaques with sharp border; silvery white scale; small bleeding points when removed. Difficult to distinguish from seborrhea in early stages or in intertriginous zones
Inflammation	Absent	Present	Present
Epidermal hyperplasia	Absent	Present	Present
Epidermal kinetics	Turnover rate is 2 times faster than normal	Turnover rates is about 5–6 times faster than normal	Turnover rate is about 5–6 times faster than normal
Percentage of incompletely keratinized cells	Rarely exceeds 5% of total corneocyte count	Commonly makes up 15%–25% of corneocyte count	Commonly makes up 40%–60% of corneocyte count

Source: Reference 1 and the following:

McGinley KJ, Marples RR, Plewig G, et al. A method for visualizing and quantitating the desquamating portion of the human stratum corneum. *J Invest Dermatol*. 1969;53:107.

Kligman AM, et al. *J Soc Cosmet Chem*. 1974;25:73.

Q~ What skin areas, including mucous membranes, hair, and nails, are involved?

A~ If only the scalp is involved, suspect dandruff or seborrhea as a more likely cause than psoriasis. Suspect seborrhea as a more likely cause than psoriasis if scales appear on the scalp and on the eyes or eyebrows. Suspect psoriasis if silver or white scales are present on the elbows, knees, extremities, and nails. If the lesions involve fine, white scales that also appear in intertriginous areas, consider a fungal infection as a more likely cause than psoriasis.

Q~ Describe the appearance of the affected area.

A~ Suspect dandruff if evenly distributed white or grayish scales occur primarily on the scalp without the presence of pruritus or erythema. Suspect seborrhea if patchy areas of dull, yellowish red lesions, often associated with oily-appearing yellowish scales, appear primarily in hairy areas, hairline areas, and nasolabial folds. Suspect psoriasis if bright red plaques associated with dry, silvery scales are present and if small pinpoint bleeding areas occur when scales are removed.

Q~ How does the affected area feel (e.g., painful, itchy)? Is it dry or oozing?

A~ Suspect seborrhea or psoriasis as a more likely cause than dandruff if pruritus is present. Consider bacterial infection if an exudate is present.

Q~ Have you had this disorder before? Does it seem to come and go?

A~ Suspect dandruff if the disorder is stable, and other characteristics are typical of dandruff.

Q~ Are there activities or situations that seem to make the disorder better or worse?

A~ Suspect psoriasis if emotional stress exacerbates the condition.

Q~ Do other family members have a similar disorder?

A~ If yes, suspect psoriasis but also consider seborrhea.

Q~ Do you notice a seasonal change in the disorder?

A~ Consider psoriasis if sun exposure during warm seasons improves the disorder.

Q~ Do you have swelling or pain in any joints?

A~ If yes, suspect psoriasis (psoriatic arthritis).

Q~ Have you consulted a physician about the disorder? If so, what was your diagnosis and what treatment was recommended? Have current or previous treatments been effective?

A~ Consider the patient's satisfaction or dissatisfaction with previous treatments when recommending nonprescription products.

Q~ Are you currently using any prescription or nonprescription medications? If so, what are they?

A~ *Identify medications that can exacerbate psoriasis. (See the section "Etiology/Pathophysiology of Psoriasis.") Identify medications that can interact with nonprescription agents used to treat scaly dermatoses. (See the section "Treatment of Scaly Dermatoses.")* On the basis of the patient's disorder and medication use, explain possible drug therapy problems. Base treatment recommendations on the patient's medication use.

Patient Education for Scaly Dermatoses

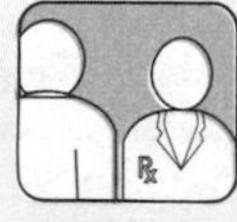

The primary objective for self-treating dandruff, seborrhea, and psoriasis is to reduce the turnover rate of skin cells, which is responsible for the scaly lesions. Controlling inflammation and itching of the affected areas is another treatment objective for seborrhea and psoriasis. Although these disorders cannot be cured, most patients who carefully follow product instructions and the self-care measures listed below will be able to effectively control the disorders.

Dandruff

- Use a medicated shampoo containing ketoconazole, pyrithione zinc, selenium sulfide, or coal tar. If these agents are ineffective, use a medicated shampoo containing sulfur or salicylic acid.
- Note that coal tar can stain light hair, and can cause folliculitis (inflammation of hair follicles), dermatitis, and photosensitization (sensitivity of the skin to sunlight).
- Shampoo the hair with the medicated shampoo, and leave it on the hair for several minutes. Rinse the hair thoroughly and repeat.

Seborrhea

- Use a medicated shampoo containing ketoconazole, pyrithione zinc, or selenium sulfide as described above. Note that selenium sulfide may increase scalp oiliness or worsen seborrhea in some individuals.
- If redness persists after therapy with medicated shampoos, apply hydrocortisone two to three times a day until symptoms

subside and then intermittently to control acute exacerbations. Do not use this agent longer than 7 days. Prolonged use can cause rebound flare-ups when the hydrocortisone is discontinued.

- After shampooing, part the hair, apply the product directly to the scalp, and massage it in thoroughly. Repeat this process until the affected area is covered.

Psoriasis

- For itchy, dry skin use emollients and lubricating bath products. (See Chapter 27, "Atopic Dermatitis, Contact Dermatitis, and Dry Skin.") Remove scales by gently rubbing them with a soft cloth following the bath. Do not rub vigorously.
- For scalp psoriasis, use medicated shampoos containing coal tar or salicylic acid as described above.
- For daytime treatment of itchiness, apply hydrocortisone 1% cream three to four times daily. Reduce frequency of application as the condition improves. Do not use this agent longer than 7 days.
- To help loosen and remove scales during the day, soak the affected body area in warm (not hot) water for 10 to 20 minutes. Then apply a salicylic acid product. Do not apply salicylic acid to extensive areas of the body. The agent may be absorbed into the blood stream.
- For more effective removal of scales, apply coal tar products to the body, arms, and legs at bedtime. Note that this agent stains bed linen and clothing. Bathe in the morning to remove residual coal tar and also to loosen psoriatic scales. If preferred, apply salicylic acid at bedtime as described above.
- For psoriasis of the armpits, genital areas, and anus, use hydrocortisone instead of coal tar or salicylic acid.
- When bright red lesions are present, use only emollients and hydrocortisone until the flare-up has subsided. Resume therapy with coal tar and salicylic acid when the thick-scaled plaques appear.
- Prevent flare-ups by minimizing factors such as emotional stress, skin irritation, and physical trauma that you know will exacerbate the disorder.
- Consult a physician before treating psoriasis with UV radiation therapy (sun exposure).
- Take a nonsteroidal anti-inflammatory drug (e.g., aspirin, ibuprofen, naproxen, or ketoprofen) for swelling of joints associated with psoriatic arthritis. (See Chapter 3, "Headache and Muscle and Joint Pain.")

⚠ Consult a physician if the condition does not improve or if it worsens after 1 to 2 weeks of treatment with nonprescription medications.

Patient Counseling for Scaly Dermatoses

Patients need to know that scaly dermatoses are rarely cured by pharmacotherapy; rather, nonprescription agents help to control the signs and symptoms of the disorders. The pharmacist should also explain that fluctuation in severity of seborrhea and psoriasis may be related to emotional, physical, or environmental factors. The patient should be advised to avoid exacerbating factors if possible.

Explanations of the proper use of cytostatic and keratolytic agents should include information about the length of time to leave the agent on the affected area. The pharmacist should also explain possible adverse effects and drug interactions with recommended agents. Finally, the pharmacist should advise the patient what signs and symptoms indicate medical attention is needed. The box "Patient Education for Scaly Dermatoses" lists specific information to provide patients.

Evaluation of Patient Outcomes for Scaly Dermatoses

Follow up on the patient's progress should occur after 1 week of self-treatment. A scheduled visit to the pharmacy is preferable if the lesions are on a part of the body that can be inspected. If the symptoms persist or have worsened after 1 week of treatment, the patient should consult a physician. If the disorder has not worsened, the pharmacist should ask the patient to return after a second week of treatment. If the symptoms persist or have worsened after this period, the patient should consult a physician.

CONCLUSIONS

Mild-to-moderate scaly dermatoses can often be effectively managed with topical nonprescription products. Products should be selected on the basis of the patient's history and prior response to treatment, as well as on the basis of a careful evaluation of the risks and benefits of using the nonprescription products.

References

1. Wright DE. Psoriasis, seborrheic dermatitis, and dandruff. In: Clark C, ed. *Self-Medication: A Reference for Health Professionals*. 3rd ed. Ottawa: Canadian Pharmaceutical Association; 1988:87–98.
2. Hay RJ, Graham-Brown RAC. Dandruff and seborrheic dermatitis: causes and management. *Clin and Exp Dermatol*. 1997;22:3–6.
3. Robinson JR. Dermatitis, dry skin, dandruff, seborrheic dermatitis, and psoriasis products. In: *Handbook of Nonprescription Drugs*. 9th ed. Washington, DC: American Pharmaceutical Association; 1990:811–40.
4. Dolnick E. A flaky concern. *Hippocrates*. 1989;3:28–30.

5. Cauwenbergh G, De Doncker P, Schrooten P, et al. Treatment of dandruff with a 2% ketoconazole scalp gel: a double-blind placebo-controlled study. *Int J Dermatol.* 1986;25:541.
6. Gossel TA, Slattery CD. Self-treatment of seborrhea. *US Pharm.* 1991;16:24–34.
7. Burton JL, Holden CA. In: Champion RH, Burton JL, Ebling FJG, eds. *Textbook of Dermatology.* 5th ed. Oxford, England: Blackwell Scientific Publications; 1998:638–43.
8. Plewig G, Jansen T. Seborrheic dermatitis. In: Freedberg IM, Eisen AZ, Wolff K, et al., eds. *Fitzpatrick's Dermatology in General Medicine.* 5th ed. New York: McGraw-Hill; 1999:1482–3.
9. Pandya AG. Seborrheic dermatitis or tinea capitis: don't be fooled. *Int J Dermatol.* 1998;37:827–8.
10. David TJ, Devlin J, Ewing CI. Atopic and seborrheic dermatitis: practical management. *Pediatrician.* 1991;18:211–7.
11. *Federal Register.* 1982;47:54646–84.
12. Christophers E, Mrowietz U. Psoriasis. In: Freedberg IM, Eisen AZ, Wolff K, et al., eds. *Fitzpatrick's Dermatology in General Medicine.* 5th ed. New York: McGraw-Hill; 1999:495–521.
13. Sege-Peterson K, Winchester RJ. Psoriatic arthritis. In: Freedberg IM, Eisen AZ, Wolff K, et al., eds. *Fitzpatrick's Dermatology in General Medicine.* 5th ed. New York: McGraw-Hill; 1999:522–33.
14. Pray WS. Psoriasis: it can be dangerous. *US Pharm.* 1991;16(skin care suppl):28–34.
15. *Federal Register.* 1991;56:63554–69.
16. Vonderweidt J. Sorting out topical corticosteroids. *US Pharm.* 1988;13:54–65.
17. Trozak DJ. Topical corticosteroid therapy in psoriasis vulgaris. *Cutis.* 1990;46:341–50.
18. Araujo OE, Flowers FP, Brown K. Vitamin D therapy in psoriasis. *DICP.* 1991;25:835–9.
19. McQueen KD. Is vitamin D effective in treating psoriasis? *DICP.* 1991;25:753–4.

CHAPTER 29

Poison Ivy/Oak/Sumac Dermatitis

Kenneth R. Keefner

Chapter 29 at a Glance

Poison ivy/oak/sumac dermatitis, which has been referred to as *Rhus* dermatitis, is the principal cause of allergic contact dermatitis (ACD) in the United States and exceeds the incidence of all other causes of ACD combined. No other plant in the United States can compare with the *Toxicodendron* genus in the magnitude of disease caused.[1] Several million cases of poison ivy are reported each year in the United States, and they account for the largest number of worker's compensation claims. These plants are the primary cause of injuries in the field for U.S. Forestry Service personnel.[2]

Epidemiology of Poison Ivy/Oak/Sumac Dermatitis

The incidence of poison ivy/oak/sumac dermatitis in the average patient begins as early as age 3 years. It continues to rise through early adulthood and begins to decline only during the mid-30s. After this period, its incidence peaks once again and continues to climb throughout the fifth decade of life. Primarily because of diminished exposure after age 65 years, the incidence of this dermatitis again declines and remains low throughout the remainder of the human life cycle.

As much as 80% of the U.S. population is estimated to be sensitive to poison ivy's urushiol, the oleoresin that causes the dermatitis, while only 50% of the population will show a dermatologic reaction to urushiol. Ordinary patch testing is not used to confirm poison ivy sensitivity. Many researchers believe that patch testing will act as a sensitizing process for the patient who is not already sensitive to urushiol.

Newborn infants are not sensitive to poison ivy, although experimental results show that 70% to 85% of infants and children may be easily sensitized to poison ivy or urushiol through a single exposure to the plant or its constituents. Although newborn infants are not born sensitive to urushiol, they may be sensitized with as little as one application in a localized area, and by age 3 years they demonstrate peak reactivity to urushiol exposure. Elderly patients, in contrast, appear to have a declining sensitivity with age, because of reduced response, but have a prolonged duration of symptoms. Itching in elderly patients has been observed to be greater than in younger adults. Presentation of symptoms in

Editor's Note: This chapter is based, in part, on the 11th edition chapter titled "Poison Ivy, Oak, and Sumac Products," which was written by Henry Wormser.

the elderly may be explained in part by a general decline in immune competence that occurs with age and by a reduced ability to be sensitized to a new antigen.[3] The peak ages at which adults show their greatest reactivity and sensitivity to urushiol are between ages 25 and 50 years. Several reports exist of dark-skinned people being less susceptible to urushiol than are other individuals.[4]

The primary incidences of poison ivy rash occur through outdoor recreation and exercise. Of equal importance are various occupations linked with *Toxicodendron* exposure in the daily work environments, as shown in Table 29–1.

Table 29–1

Occupations at Risk for Developing Poison Ivy/Oak/Sumac Dermatitis

- Civil engineers
- Construction workers
- Farm and agricultural workers
- Fire fighters
- Forestry personnel and conservationists
- Gardeners and grounds keepers
- Geologists
- Highway and road construction crews
- Land surveyors
- Loggers
- Park maintenance personnel
- Police officers
- Power utilities and maintenance personnel
- Truck and traffic drivers

Adapted from: Reference 5; used with permission.

In the past, poison ivy/oak/sumac dermatitis has been the major cause of occupational skin diseases. It accounts for 8% to 11% of occupational injuries caused by an occupational plant dermatitis.[6,7,8] Dermatitis caused by this family of plants provides an excellent opportunity for pharmacists to apply the tenets of good pharmaceutical care while directing the care and treatment of patients afflicted with this uncomfortable rash.

Etiology of Poison Ivy/Oak/Sumac Dermatitis

In the United States, five species of *Toxicodendron* plants are primarily responsible for the dermatoses associated with exposure to plants. (See Table 29–2.) All of these species are part of the family of plants known as the Anacardiaceae. Many of these plants were previously considered to belong to the genus *Rhus,* but the term *Toxicodendron* is now the accepted genus for this group of antigenic plants. This genus will be used throughout the chapter to refer to these plants. The change in genus and the difficulty in classifying these plants is the result of the variability in the morphology of the plants. Botanists claim that such variability is based on the effects associated with geographic location, soil, water, and climatic conditions. The plants were reclassified into the genus *Toxicodendron*, but terms such as *Rhus radicans*, *Rhus rash*, and *Rhus dermatitis* are still used when referring to such plants and their dermatologic effects, especially in early literature and reference works.

Species of poison ivy and oak are the primary causes of rashes induced by *Toxicodendron* plants. Although all five species are common to the United States, they are somewhat indigenous to specific regions of the country. These species

Table 29–2

Toxicodendron Plants Indigenous to North America

Plant (Genus, Species)	Other Common Names	Common Geographic Location
Poison Ivy		
T. radicans	Poison vine, markweed, three-leaved ivy, and poor man's liquid amber	Several subspecies exist throughout North America, ranging throughout the United States (Central, Midwest, Southcentral, Southeastern, lower Mississippi Valley regions); states (specifically SE Arizona, SW and E Texas, Great Lake states, and Oklahoma); Canada (Ontario, Nova Scotia); and Mexico.
T. rydbergii		The most northerly species exists in southern Canada, United States, Texas, and Arizona
Poison Sumac		
T. vernix	Poison elder, poison ash	Species commonly exists from Quebec to Florida in primarily the eastern third of the U.S. coast.
Western Poison Oak		
T. diversilobum		Species exists from Baja, California, to British Columbia, Canada, but less so in the northern ranges.
Eastern Poison Oak		
T. toxicarium		Species exists widely in the southeastern United States.

Adapted from: Reference 9; used with permission.

are most easily identified as having three leaves emanating from a central stem with the middle leaflet appearing at the terminal end of the stem. The plants flower in the spring and produce small, waxy, white five-petaled flowers. In the late fall, the plants develop berries that are greenish white, pale yellow, or tan. In the fall, the leaves turn brilliant red or orange. A saying taught to youngsters to help identify the plant and to avoid exposure to urushiol is "Leaves of three; Let it be!" In general, this statement is true, but other members of the genus differ in the number of leaflets attached to the central stalk, and in the berry and leaf morphology.

Poison Ivy

The most common *Toxicodendron* plant found throughout the United States is poison ivy (*T. radicans* and *T. rydbergii*). It is quite common throughout the central and northeastern United States and Canada. Poison ivy has been described as a scrambling shrub or a climbing hairy vine that commonly grows up poles, trees, and building walls. It also grows along roads, hiking trails, streams, dry rocky canyons, or embankment slopes. *T. radicans* is composed of nine subspecies that can exist as a shrub or may become a climbing vine, while *T. rydbergii* is a dwarf shrub that has large, broad, spoon-shaped leaves with a hairy underside. (See Figure 29–1.) *T. rydbergii* is the principal variety of poison ivy that grows in the northern United States and southern Canada. *T. radicans* grows over much of the United States and is a climbing vine with aerial rootlets.

Poison Oak

Poison oak has two species indigenous to the United States: *T. diversilobum*, which inhabits the West Coast, and *T. toxicarium*, which inhabits the East Coast. Both species possess leaves similar to oak trees, with most having an unlobed leaf edge and commonly displaying three leaflets per stem. (See Figure 29–2.) The leaves and berries of eastern poison oak (*T. toxicarium*) are covered with fine hairs. The plant ordinarily exists as a nonclimbing shrub. Western poison oak (*T. diversilobum*) differs by usually possessing between 3 and 11 leaflets per stem, and it bears fruit covered with numerous fine hairs. Its leaves are quite similar to California live oak. Poison oak exists as a shrub capable of climbing to distances as high as 131 feet (40 m). Poison oak grows along streams, in thickets, on wooded slopes, and in dry woodlands. As a rule, poison oak grows well at altitudes below 4000 to 5000 feet.

Poison Sumac

Poison sumac (*T. vernix*) grows in remote areas of the eastern third of the United States in peat bogs and swampy areas. Although highly antigenic, its remoteness from human contact limits the incidence of human dermatoses manifested. It appears as a shrub or small tree and attains a height of roughly 9.8 feet (3 m) and may resemble, to some extent, either elder or ash trees. Hence, it has been given the name "poison elder or poison ash." Its leaves are pinnate and may

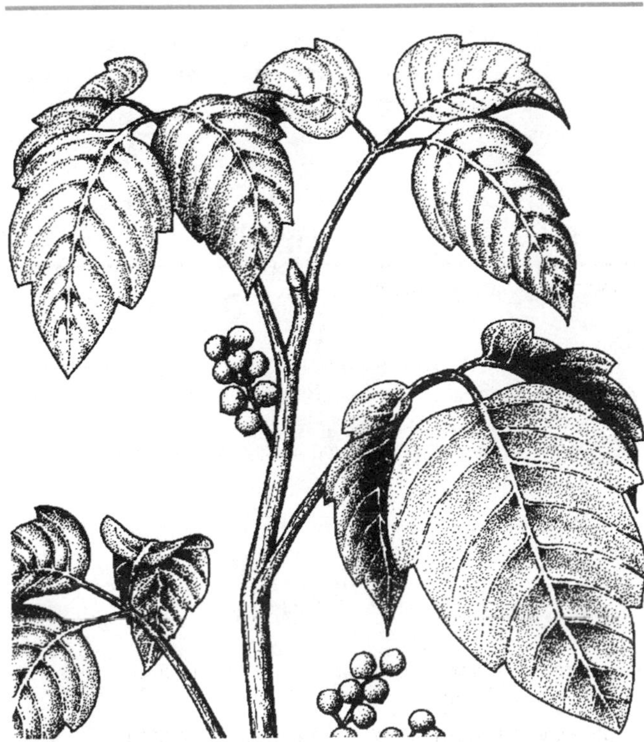

Figure 29–1 Poison ivy.

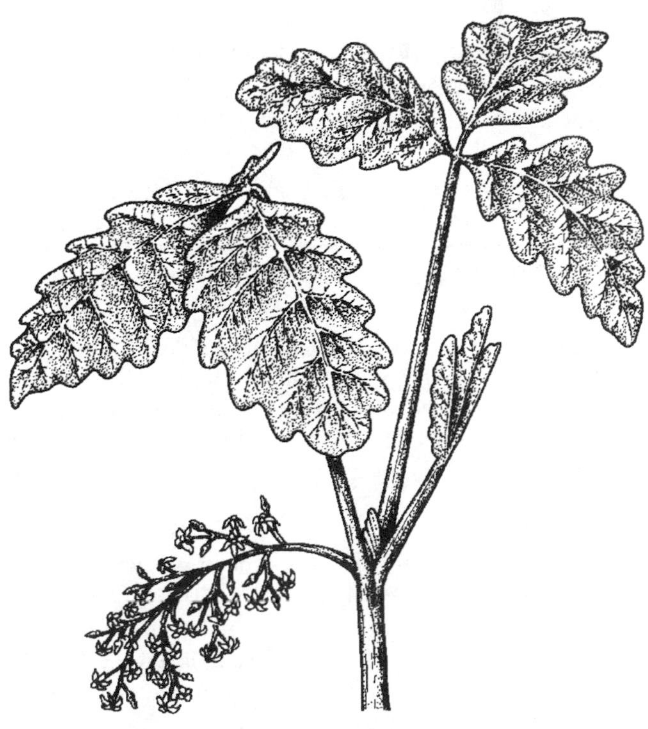

Figure 29–2 Poison oak.

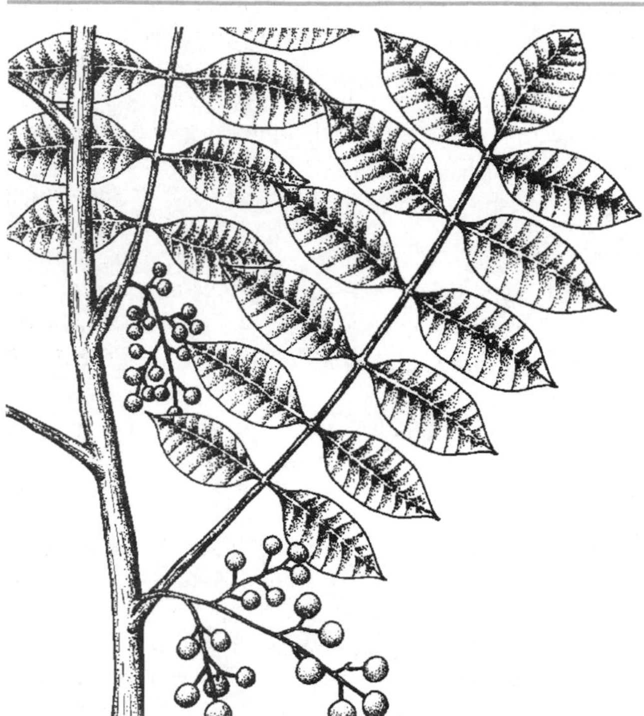

Figure 29–3 Poison sumac.

be almost 16 inches (40 cm) in length; they are odd-numbered, ranging between 7 and 13 leaflets. The edges of the leaves are smooth and come to a tip. (See Figure 29–3.)

Other Causative Plants

In addition to the genus *Toxicodendron*, several other plants are known to have cross-sensitivity with these urushiols, causing a poison ivy-like dermatitis in individuals who have been previously sensitized to urushiol. Although the plants enumerated in this discussion are not all-inclusive, several deserve specific mention. The cashew nut tree (*Anacardium occidentale* L.) bears an edible nut—the shells of which contain oils that share a cross-sensitivity to urushiol and that produce a similar rash. The peel of the mango fruit (*Magnifera indica* L., Indian mango, king of the fruits, apples of the tropics)[10] contains an antigenic substance that has been responsible for facial, oral, and lip dermatitis and cheilosis associated with exposure to only the peel of the fruit. The mango allergen is found in the stems, leaves, and peel, but not in the edible fruit of the mango itself. Even poison ivy-sensitive patients can freely eat the fruit after it has been peeled. Such rashes are commonly encountered in Malaysia and Hawaii when urushiol-sensitive visitors to these locations are exposed to the peels of fresh mangoes.

People throughout the world have enjoyed the fine lacquered wood boxes and other items finished by using the dark resinous liquid obtained from the Japanese lacquer tree (*T. vernicifluum*). This lacquer has been used as an ingredient in the finish used to manufacture varnished boxes, rifle stocks, floors, bar rails, tea pots, canes, and toilet seats. Urushiol-sensitive individuals who are exposed and reexposed to such lacquered products may continue to have recurrent episodes of ACD.[11] The fruit of the ginkgo tree (*Ginkgo biloba* L.) contains a cross-sensitive resin that leads to rashes on the lower extremities (caused by walking through an area with fallen fruit) and to dermatitis of the mucous membranes, cheilitis, stomatitis, proctitis, or rectal itching associated with consumption of the fruit.

Pathophysiology of Poison Ivy/Oak/Sumac Dermatitis

The allergenic substance responsible for the dermatologic conditions caused by this genus of plant is known as urushiol. Urushiol has been identified as several chemically similar catechols (3-*n*-alk-(en)-*Y* chols) that vary in concentration according to the species of plant.[12] Urushiol is quite sensitive to oxidation by ambient air. It changes in appearance from clear fluid to a black inky lacquer that becomes tarry and may harden on the damaged portion of the plant in a matter of minutes. This oddity has been used as a visual identifier to confirm the existence of poison ivy, oak, or sumac in the surrounding foliage.[13,14]

The release of urushiol from the plant can occur only through damage to some portion of the plant itself, either through direct damage by an individual who bruises the plant by lying, sitting, kneeling, or stepping on it or by contact after damage resulting from natural causes (e.g., wind, rain, insects, or animals eating or damaging the plant). The antigenic urushiol is contained and carried only within resin canals of the plant that do not communicate to the surface of the plant. It has been reported that as little as 2 to 2.5 mcg or less of urushiol is enough to stimulate the typical dermal rash in sensitive patients.[15,16] In patients who are tolerant or show subclinical reactions to the same level of urushiol, as much as 5, 10, or 50 mcg may be necessary to elicit an allergic response. Therefore, one should note that as long as the plant remains intact and undamaged, no urushiol is released to the plant's outer surface and, hence, no exposure to urushiol can occur.

Apparently, all subsurface parts of the poison ivy plant contain the resin. Researchers have identified urushiol in the roots, stems, leaves, berries, and flowers of the plant. Even dead and dried plants or its dried parts (e.g., leaves, stems, and roots) retain resin that is capable of creating a rash in sensitive patients.[17] Researchers believe that the resin enters the superficial layers of the human dermis in 10 minutes or less, where it attaches to tissue proteins to produce a hapten. Urushiol is not a volatile substance, but it has been implicated in producing dermatitis when the plant was burned. The mechanism for this occurrence is that urushiol is contained in the particulate material in the smoke emanating from burned plants. The urushiol carried by particulates is capable of affecting body surface areas ordinarily viewed as protected (e.g., genitals, buttocks, anus, and lungs). This source of exposure is a primary cause of poison ivy and oak occupational illnesses that occur in personnel who fight forest fires, especially in California and other states along the West Coast.

Patients sometimes present with poison ivy dermatitis in midwinter or off-season periods. When assessing patients who have a documented history of urushiol dermatitis but are unable to accurately identify the source of urushiol exposure, the pharmacist must ask about their recent use of contaminated fomites (inanimate objects). It is well recognized that urushiol can remain active for long periods of time on inanimate objects and that it continues to be active within dead and dried parts of the plant. For example, it has been reported that the urushiol contained in dried plants stored at a herbarium—for more than 100 years—still retains its ability to incite a dermal rash.[18] The dried, dormant remnants of plants in the field can retain antigenicity, especially if the plant has been kept in a dry location that is relatively free from ambient moisture. The oleoresin is inactivated when it is exposed to wet environmental conditions. A fomite may easily become contaminated with the oleoresin, and fomite is a common source of oddly timed dermatitis. It is not unusual for fomites to become contaminated in one growing season; the contaminating urushiol retains its antigenicity throughout the winter and causes rashes with each use of the fomite in succeeding seasons. Urushiol-contaminated shoes, boots, clothing, garden and work tools, golf clubs, baseball bats, fishing rods, and other recreational equipment or the fur of domestic pets have all been implicated as sources of nonseasonal poison ivy rash, as well as of recurrent seasonal rashes.

The reaction to poison ivy is described as a Type IV delayed hypersensitivity reaction, or ACD. In general, this reaction requires an initial exposure to the antigenic substance (the *Toxicodendron* plant oleoresin, or urushiol). This initial exposure causes a dermal sensitization to the offending allergen to develop. Most clinicians think that the initial exposure is not ordinarily associated with dermal symptoms, although some reports suggest that the initial exposure in very sensitive patients may not only sensitize the patient to urushiol, but also lead to a resulting dermatitis as much as 2 to 10 days later.[17] The first sensitizing dose may not produce a rash until as long as 3 weeks after the initial exposure.[1] Other reports suggest that numerous, recurrent exposures may be needed to develop the dermatitis clinically in highly resistant or tolerant patients. Individuals who are exposed to the urushiol oleoresin succumb to a vesiculopapular rash that itches intensely at the resin contact site on the skin. In people previously sensitized, the rash and related symptoms may appear at any time between 2 and 48 hours after the second exposure.

The allergic response appears to be a two-step process: initial sensitization (step one), followed by a delayed hypersensitivity reaction (step two) in the dermal layers of the skin. Some clinicians think the urushiol rapidly enters the skin and attaches to protein molecules found on the surface of Langerhans cells (specialized white blood cells) in the epidermis and to macrophages in the dermis. The Langerhans cells communicate the antigen information to lymphocytes (inducer cells); these cells, in turn, proliferate into circulating T-effector and T-memory lymphocytes. This process allows the immune lymphocytes to become sensitized to future entry of urushiol into the skin layers. With succeeding urushiol exposure, the patient has a delayed hypersensitive reaction that allows T cells to invade the skin area containing the newly deposited urushiol. Symptoms of pruritus, erythema, vesiculation, and local edema are the result of this cytotoxic immune response, which is typical of *Toxicodendron* rashes.[19,20]

Signs and Symptoms of Poison Ivy/Oak/Sumac Dermatitis

After exposure to urushiol has taken place, the dermal process begins to develop erythematous itchy patches on the affected, exposed areas of the body. The intensity and magnitude of the rash may continue to increase for several days and will depend on the sensitivity of the specific body area exposed, the amount of urushiol on the skin surface, the amount of urushiol that entered the dermis, the duration of the exposure, the rapidity with which the area was cleaned after exposure, and the individual's sensitivity and genetic makeup.

The initial dermal reaction to urushiol is an intense itching of the skin's surface areas exposed to the antigen. This itching is followed by erythema and finally the formation of vesicles (blisters) or bullae, depending on an individual's sensitivity. (See the "Color Plates," photographs 12A and B.) Patients scratch the area and may spread the urushiol to other unexposed skin surfaces. As the dermatitis progresses, vesicles or bullae form and may be easily broken open, releasing their fluid. Vesicular fluid does not contain any antigenic material to further spread the dermatitis. Patients may continue to scratch for several days after exposure and may excoriate the surface dermal layer, leading to open lesions and the potential for secondary wound infections. Oozing and weeping of the vesicular fluid continues to occur for several days, until the affected area develops crusts and begins to dry.

Poison ivy rash usually occurs on skin unprotected by clothing. Poison ivy rashes on the East Coast generally occur in the spring and summer, while in the southwestern United States poison oak rashes may appear anytime, because outdoor living is common throughout the year.[10] Rashes commonly occur on exposed or unprotected skin surfaces such as the hands and fingers, forearms, ankles, calves of the legs, and areas with thin skin, especially around the eyes, face, and neck. A common patient description that highly suggests poison ivy or oak exposure is streaks of vesicles that correspond to the points of urushiol contact from the damaged plant. In fact, specks of black oxidized urushiol may form on the skin and clothing after contamination.[1] Lesions may develop on skin that is ordinarily considered protected (e.g., the genitals, anus, buttocks, or other covered body surfaces) and occurs primarily through contact with urushiol-contaminated fingers and hands. Unwashed, contaminated hands and fingernails are the principal sources of rash on protected areas of the body. Numerous reports describe the dermatitis on the face and around the eyes, lips, underarms, buttocks and anus, as well as on the genitalia of the affected patient and his or her sexually intimate partner.

Mild Dermatitis

Mild dermatitis characteristically consists of localized patches of pruritus and erythema followed by the appearance of vesicles and papules, often in a linear streaking arrangement where the damaged plants have deposited the urushiol. The urushiol from the plants may cause marked swelling of the eyelids without associated swelling of other parts of the face,[10] and is caused by rubbing the eyelids with urushiol-contaminated fingers and hands. Clinically, the dermatitis is localized in distinct patches on the unprotected lower and upper extremities where initial, direct plant contact has occurred.

Moderate Dermatitis

Signs and symptoms of moderate dermatitis include the appearance of bullae and edematous swellings of various body parts, in addition to the pruritus, erythema, papules, and vesicles of mild dermatitis.

Severe Dermatitis

Severe dermatitis is distinguished by extensive involvement and edema of the extremities and the face. Often the eyelids are swollen closed. Extreme itching, irritation, and formation of severe vesicles, blisters, and bullae may also be present. Further, daily activities may be hampered in some patients. If the dermatitis or edema from the allergic reaction affects large areas of the face, the eyes, or the genitalia, such patients should be referred at once to a physician for systemic or parenteral therapy.

Dark-skinned patients may experience a permanent discoloration in areas of dermatitis where severe inflammatory changes and blistering have taken place.[1]

Complications of Poison Ivy/ Oak/Sumac Dermatitis

On rare occasions, various other diseases have been associated with exposure to *Toxicodendron* plants and the development of ACD. Such diseases have included eosinophilia (ordinarily seen with exposure to poison ivy), secondary mania,[21] erythema multiforme,[22] acute respiratory distress syndrome (caused by inhaling urushiol particles carried in smoke),[23] renal failure,[24] dyshydrosis of the hands and feet,[17] and urethritis.[25]

Treatment of Poison Ivy/ Oak/Sumac Dermatitis

Treatment Outcomes

Therapy is indicated primarily to relieve symptoms associated with the ACD and to avoid secondary infections of excoriated portions of the skin caused by excessive scratching.[1] Customarily, the first several days following the initial appearance of the dermatitis are usually the most uncomfortable for the patient. Treated or untreated poison ivy dermatitis will naturally resolve in approximately 10 to 21 days as a result of the patient's own immune system or through use of adjuvant topical, symptomatic treatment. Patients will seek the pharmacist's counsel principally because of the intensity of itching, burning, and pain associated with a mild localized rash, or because of the widespread nature of the dermatitis and the magnitude of symptoms.

The goals of self-treating this dermatitis are to (1) protect the area affected during the acute phase of developing the rash, (2) prevent itching and excessive scratching that may lead to open lesions and potential secondary skin infections, and (3) prevent the accumulation of debris and resulting complications that arise from the vesicle fluids oozing, crusting, and scaling, thereby preventing spread of the dermatitis to the surrounding area of inflammation.

General Treatment Approach

The aggressiveness and type of treatment depends on the severity of the allergic reaction: mild, moderate-to-severe, or severe. (See the algorithm in Figure 29–4 for a summary of appropriate treatments.) If, at the time of presentation, the patient exhibits mild dermatitis (only localized patches of rash with intense pruritus and erythema), the pharmacist may initially recommend treatment that includes the topical application of an antipruritic (shake) lotion containing calamine, menthol, phenol, camphor, and antipruritic agents, or the application of a hydrocortisone cream or ointment. As long as the rash does not begin to weep and remains dry, the patient may use shake lotions and ointments. When a rash is present, the patient should avoid further exposure to *Toxicodendron* plants or to plants with cross-sensitivity to prevent exacerbating the dermatitis.

If the rash spreads to larger areas but does not affect the eyes or genitals and does not cover the body (moderate-to-severe reaction), the patient may use astringent compresses and baths to treat the rash.

Patients with one or more of the following symptoms or factors should seek medical attention:

- Extreme itching; irritation; and severe vesicle and bullae formation are present.
- The rash is widespread and/or the body or the extremities are swollen.
- The eyes are affected (e.g., the eyes are swollen or the eyelids cannot be opened).

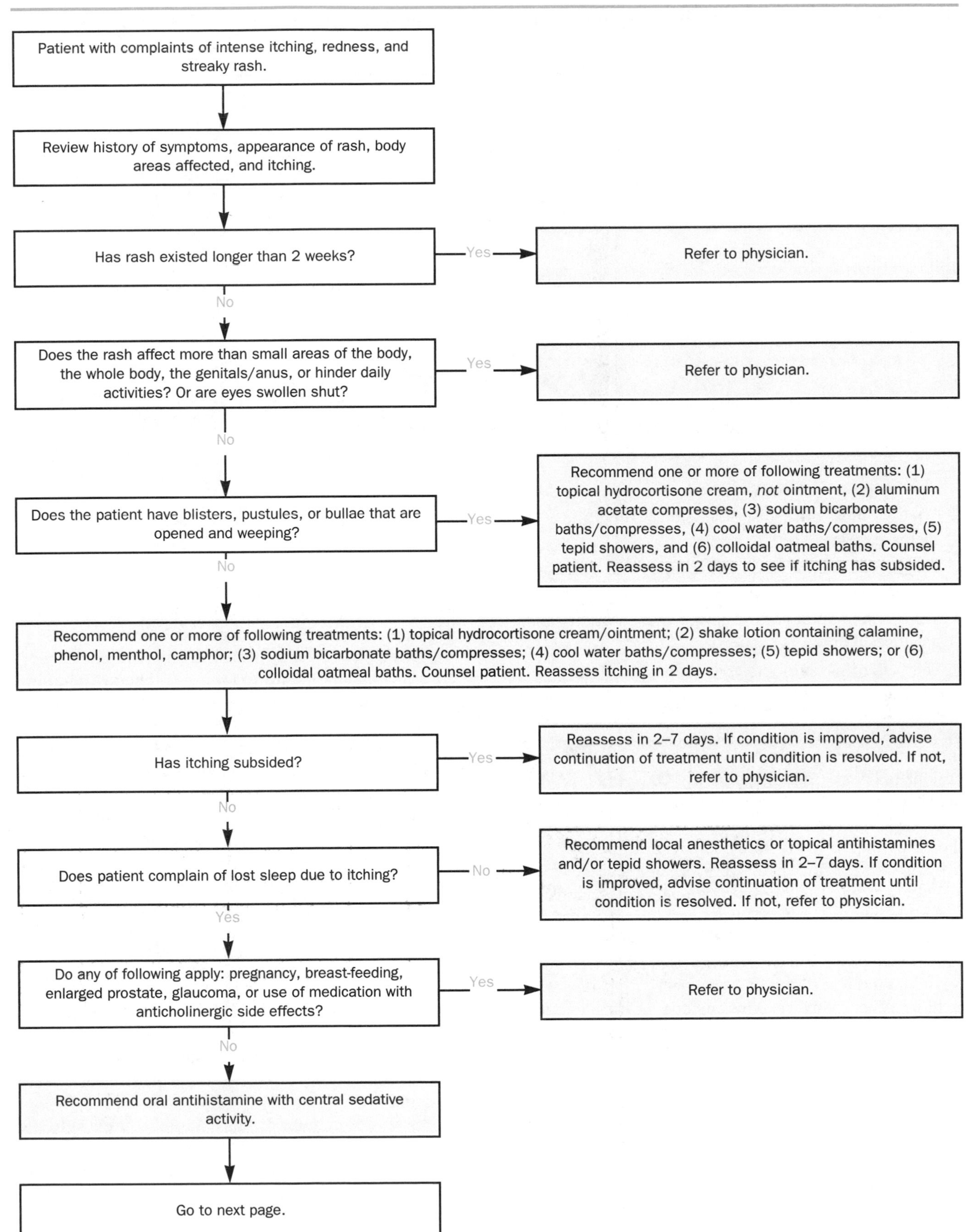

Figure 29–4 Self-care of poison ivy/oak/sumac dermatitis.

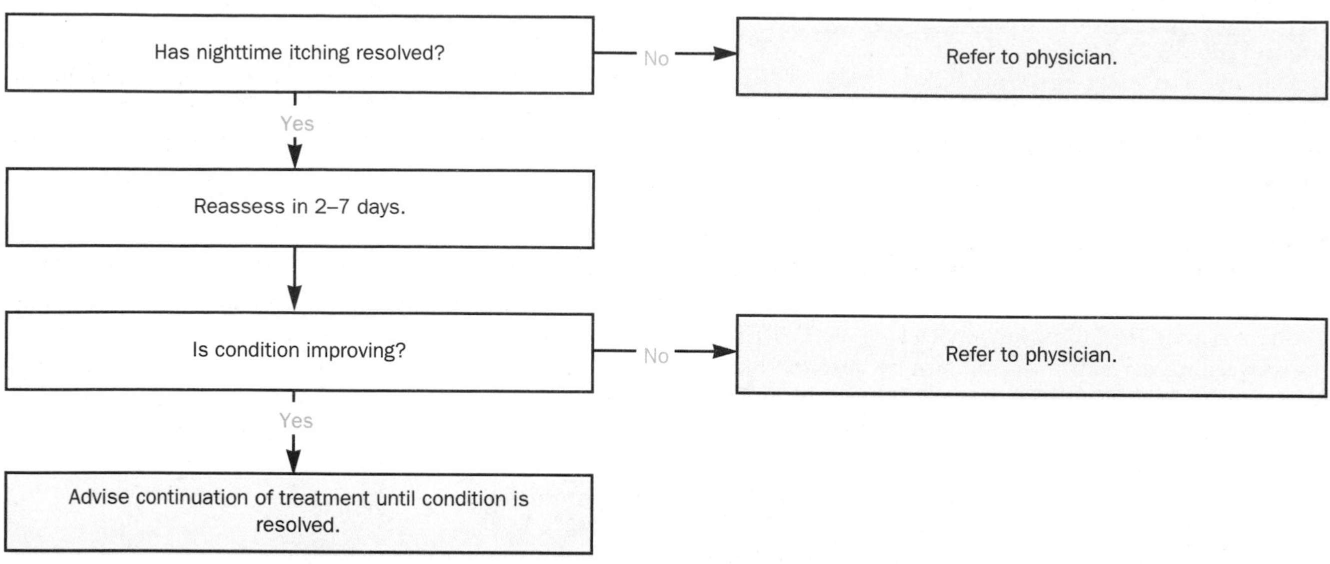

Figure 29–4 Self-care of poison ivy/oak/sumac dermatitis (continued).

- Extensive areas of edema, dermatitis, itching, and erythema are present on the face.
- The genitalia are affected or are uncomfortable from itching, redness, swelling, or irritation.
- Mucous membranes of the mouth, eyes, nose, or anus are affected or display urticaria.
- The patient has a low tolerance for pain, itching, or symptom discomfort.[26]

Measures for Mild Dermatitis

Initial treatment recommendations may consist of several options to relieve pruritic symptoms. One option is the use of a shake lotion consisting of calamine lotion with the addition of phenol (1%) and/or menthol (0.25%). The lotion should be shaken well before being applied topically to the itchy or erythematous areas every 4 hours as needed for the relief of pruritus. The lotion leaves a light flesh-colored film in the application area and may be cosmetically distasteful to the patient, especially when applied to the face. Instead, the patient may prefer using a topically applied hydrocortisone cream or ointment to the affected area. Hydrocortisone may be more esthetically acceptable and does not bring attention to the affected areas, especially when a cream base is used.

Alternatively, patients may use sodium bicarbonate either as a paste or as a cool compress. For paste application, the patient should add cool tap water to sodium bicarbonate powder in sufficient quantity to prepare a paste for direct application to the vesicles to relieve itching and irritation. In addition, one or two cupfuls of sodium bicarbonate powder may be added to a warm bath. The patient should be told to soak the affected areas for 15 to 30 minutes and then apply the paste. The patient should be told to dry off by patting rather than wiping so a film of baking soda will remain on the skin. For very localized dermatitis, baking soda compresses may be applied for 15 to 30 minutes and may be repeated as often as necessary. Patients should be warned not to use baking soda near the eyes and to consult a physician if relief is not obtained within 7 days of treatment. Baking soda should not be applied to patients younger than 2 years.

Applying topical ointments and creams containing anesthetics (benzocaine); antihistamines (diphenhydramine), which are used for their antipruritic qualities; or antibiotics (neomycin), which are used for secondary infections of the blisters, has been questioned in the past and should be avoided, because these agents are known sensitizers and are capable of producing a drug-induced dermatitis along with the existing poison ivy contact dermatitis. Conversely, there may be instances when the recommended topical treatments are not effective. When traditional treatments have failed, pramoxine or benzocaine may be used on a trial basis if the patient is monitored closely for untoward dermatologic reactions.

Measures for Moderate-to-Severe Dermatitis

Treatment of numerous large, coalesced bullae should be referred to a physician who may open and drain them under sterile conditions. A safe initial recommendation is for the patient to apply a cool water compress to the affected area for as long and as often as needed. The patient should apply cool compresses of aluminum acetate solution (Burow's) to the edematous areas as an astringent to reduce weeping and irritation. Mild edema or swelling of the eyelids should be treated with only cold water dressings.

The patient may prepare a 1:40 ratio strength dilution of Burow's solution from prepackaged tablets or powder by adding one tablet or package to 1 pint of cool tap water. The patient should then soak clean white compresses in the solution and apply the compress to the affected areas for 30 minutes, four times a day or as often as needed. The patient should discard any remaining solution and prepare a fresh solution for each application. Burow's solution provides an astringent action on the papulovesicular lesions of the dermatitis that dries the weeping vesicles.[27,28] In addition, Burow's solution is useful in softening and removing crusting and in preparing the skin for the application of a hydrocortisone cream or ointment.

Shake lotions are not recommended for treating large areas of weeping dermatitis on the face because the lotions have a tendency to cake and to generate debris that can make the skin uncomfortable and stiff. An application of Burow's compresses may help the patient and should be followed with a cream or lotion application that will provide an emollient effect and may be better tolerated.

The pharmacist may recommend colloidal oatmeal baths to cleanse and soothe the lesions, as well as to reduce the itch. Patients should use one packet (30 g) of the colloidal oatmeal in a tub full of water. The pharmacist should tell the patient to turn the water on high, to choose a comfortably warm water temperature, and then to sprinkle the oatmeal into the running bath water to allow for good mixing of the milled oatmeal. Stirring the bath water occasionally will help to avoid having lumps develop. The pharmacist should caution the patient to take extreme care in entering and exiting the tub. Colloidal oatmeal becomes extremely slippery when used in bath water. The patient should use a rubber mat in the tub and should have a dry rug or towel on the floor to avoid falling. Holding a grab rail/bar or other such convenience securely will provide additional safety for entering and exiting the tub. The patient should soak for 15 or 20 minutes at least twice each day. The oatmeal bath water should be drizzled over areas that can't be soaked while sitting in the tub. After bathing in the colloidal oatmeal, patients should pat themselves dry rather than wiping, because it is advantageous to leave a film of colloidal oatmeal on the skin.

Although topical antihistamines have no role in treating poison ivy rash, the pharmacist may recommend oral antihistamines to provide rest at night from the intolerable pruritus that accompanies many cases of dermatitis. Diphenhydramine is an antihistamine that possesses a therapeutic sedative effect and is commonly used in numerous nonprescription drug products for its sedative action.

Measures for Severe Dermatitis

Symptomatic topical treatment of severe dermatitis remains quite similar to that used in moderately severe cases, except that the physician will likely prescribe a potent anti-inflammatory glucocorticoid systemically as well as topically. The pharmacist should ensure a good treatment outcome by recommending a systemic glucocorticoid that consists of a tapering dosage of not fewer than 12 days to as long as 21 days of therapy. On average, about 1 mg/kg body weight per day (approximately 40 to 100 mg) of prednisone is used when initiating therapy and is tapered over the next 2 to 3 weeks. The use of prepackaged dosage packs of glucocorticoid (tapered over 6 days) in numerous instances has led to the use of a second or third dose pack, or may even lead to rebound dermatologic symptoms if this shorter therapy period is selected.[29]

Nonpharmacologic Therapy

Nonpharmacologic treatment of the allergic reaction is limited primarily to showers. However, hypersensitive patients who suspect poison ivy exposure can take measures to prevent or lessen the severity of the dermatitis. All individuals should avoid contact with *Toxicodendron* plants and, if exposed, should take the steps discussed next to remove oleoresin from the skin.

Hygienic Measures

The primary nondrug measure to relieve symptoms of *Toxicodendron* dermatitis is to take very cold or tepid soapless showers to temporarily relieve the pruritus. A tepid shower is approximately 90°F or cooler. The pharmacist should recommend that a patient be cautious about taking a hot shower (temperatures greater than 105°F), because it may cause scalding or thermal skin injuries (second degree burns).[30–32] The pharmacist may recommend that patients bathe or shower using bland face soap to maintain cleanliness; they should never use harsh soaps. Furthermore, when a rash is present, affected areas should not be vigorously scrubbed. Men should be encouraged to shave, because shaving cleanses the facial area of caked and crusted fluid from pustules or bullae. If the dermatitis is allowed to become crusted and hardened in the hairs and stubble of the beard, shaving will become very uncomfortable for the patient. Along with applying topical treatment, all patients, both adults and children, should be advised to trim their fingernails to help reduce the degree of scratching injury.

Preventive/Protective Measures

For any individual who is sensitive to urushiol from *Toxicodendron* plants, the best preventive measure against exposure is total avoidance of the plants. (See Table 29–3.) Any recreational or work-related outdoor activity should include a brief survey of the surrounding vegetation to determine the potential risk of exposure. The individual should avoid frequenting areas that have indigenous poison ivy or poison oak plants. In addition, a proactive educational process that includes descriptive and photographic representations of the plants should help patients identify the plants that naturally occur in the areas in which they live. From the description of the *Toxicodendron* genus and from observations of other experts in this field,[15,33] readers will know that the plants vary in morphology according to geographic location, soil, and climate.

Use of Protective Clothing Individuals should wear additional protective clothing that can be removed and immedi-

Table 29–3

Preventive and Protective Measures for Poison Ivy/Oak/Sumac Dermatitis

Preventive Measures

- Learn the physical characteristics and usual habitat of *Toxicodendron* plants.
- Eradicate *Toxicodendron* plants near your residence either by mechanically removing the plant and its roots or by applying a herbicide recommended by the state Farm Bureau or the USDA Extension Services.
- Apply bentoquatam on exposed areas of body to reduce the risk of contamination before visiting an outdoor site. Repeat application every 4 hours until your potential exposure has ended. This application should be followed by flushing the area with water to remove bentoquatam and any urushiol deposited on the skin surface.
- Survey the area of an outdoor visit, identify surrounding plants, and assess potential risk for exposure to *Toxicodendron* plants.
- Take the protective measures listed below for suspected exposure.

Protective Measures

- Remove all clothing worn during exposure.
- Wash the suspected area with soap and water as soon as possible.
- If thorough washing is not possible, rinse with water as soon as possible.
- At earliest convenience, take a complete shower instead of a bath, using soap and water. Avoid bathing right after exposure, because bathing will allow the oleoresin to remain in the tub and potentially affect other unaffected areas.
- Meticulously clean under the fingernails to avoid transferring trapped urushiol to clean skin surfaces.
- Wash all clothing exposed to urushiol separate from other clothes in a washing machine using ordinary detergent. If clothes are dry cleaned to remove urushiol, warn cleaning personnel of the possible contamination. Put contaminated clothing in a plastic bag for transport.
- Thoroughly wash with soap and water, or with water alone, any shoes, gloves, jackets, or other protective garments; sports equipment; garden and work tools; and any equipment that is capable of carrying urushiol, as soon after use as possible. Wear vinyl gloves for washing contaminated objects. Allow this clothing and equipment to dry and then store them for the next use.
- Cleanse the fur of pets after known or suspected exposures to poison ivy plants.

ately washed after exposure. They should use ordinary laundry detergent to wash clothes contaminated with urushiol separate from noncontaminated clothing.

Removal of Urushiol from Skin To reduce the spread of poison ivy rash, the individual should immediately wash the area that was exposed to the poison ivy plants. Even though urushiol is a water-insoluble compound, clinicians have shown that immediate and early washing of urushiol-exposed areas with soap and water may avoid or reduce the severity of the rash. Researchers have shown[4] that washing the contaminated area must take place within 10 minutes of exposure to significantly reduce the risk of dermatitis. Studies have also revealed that, for up to 30 minutes after exposure, washing will remove unreacted oleoresin. Therefore, washing after the initial 10-minute period is still useful in removing any oleoresin that remains on the skin's surface and that has not entered the dermal layers. Once urushiol has entered the skin and attached to tissue proteins it can no longer be removed.

"In the field" washing is without a doubt difficult, but simply using large volumes of water will rinse away much of the surface oleoresin. Previously, physicians and many home remedies recommended vigorous scrubbing of contaminated skin surfaces with a harsh soap (such as Fels Naphtha, or homemade lye soap). Instead, today's recommendation is to use a mild face soap and water to wash all body areas thought to have been exposed to urushiol. In lieu of this approach, copious amounts of plain water may be sufficiently helpful to reduce the chance of dermatitis. In addition, it is crucial to impress on the at-risk patient that good hand washing, including meticulous cleansing under the fingernails, is needed to avoid contaminating other clean skin surfaces with urushiol that has been trapped under the fingernails.

Other cleansers and organic solvents have been used to rinse off skin surface urushiol, including isopropyl alcohol. However, general thought holds that although the urushiol is soluble in alcohol, its use should be followed immediately by a mild soap and water wash to remove any remaining surface oleoresin. Alcohol may serve to dissolve and transport the surface oleoresin to clean skin surfaces and may thus generate additional areas of dermatitis. Alcohol may also remove natural protective oils from the skin and can be a source of irritation.

One product used as a cleanser is Technu Outdoor Skin Cleanser, whose constituents include mineral spirits, water, a soap, and a surface active agent. The cleanser was originally developed as an agent to wash away radioactive matter from the skin surface of exposed individuals. This product is recommended for use after exposure and should be rubbed into the affected area as soon after exposure as possible. The patient should use the liquid to cleanse the contaminated area for a minimum of 2 minutes. No water is required for the initial cleansing application, but the cleanser may be wiped away with a cloth or rinsed with cool water. The manufacturer recommends using the product before eating, smoking, or using the bathroom in an effort to minimize the spreading of urushiol to uncontaminated skin.

Use of Barrier Products Several studies have evaluated the use of barrier creams and lotions as agents to prevent urushiol from entering the skin. The most recent comprehensive study[34] identified three products that had notable protective qualities when used in subjects who were experimentally challenged with *Toxicodendron* extract. The three products (Hydropel, Hollister Moisture Barrier, and Stokogard Outdoor Cream) reduced dermatitis severity by 48%, 52%, and 59%, respectively. At the present time, Stokogard is in extremely short supply and is available from only one midwestern supplier. The manufacture of additional product is not planned. The active ingredient was a dimer of linoleic acid, whose presumed mechanism of action was probably the obstruction of urushiol penetration into the skin. Disadvantages of this product included its tacky, greasy nature and an unpleasant fishy odor.[33] The remaining two products (Hydropel and Hollister Moisture Barrier Cream) do not claim protection from poison ivy dermatitis, but instead claim prevention from irritant contact dermatitis or diaper rash.

The first barrier product that has gained Food and Drug Administration (FDA) approval on the basis of a New Drug Application to provide protection against exposure to poison ivy, oak, and sumac has been IvyBlock Lotion. This product's active ingredient is an organoclay known as quaternium-18 bentonite (bentoquatam),[35,36] which is manufactured by reacting bentonite clay with quaternium-18 (a dimethyl dihydrogenated tallow quaternary ammonium compound). The product contains 5% bentoquatam in a lotion containing alcohol. Bentoquatam is a nonsensitizing and nonirritating organoclay that appears to possess little antigenicity or toxicities when it is applied topically. The mechanism by which this ingredient works is not presently known, but it is thought to physically block urushiol from being absorbed into the skin. It is effective in protecting patients from exposure to the urushiol common to all *Toxicodendron* plants, as well as urushiol that adheres to smoke particles from burned plants.

This barrier lotion claims protection when it is topically applied at least 15 minutes before *Toxicodendron* exposure. It should be reapplied once every 4 hours or as needed after the initial application to maintain effective protection. The lotion should be shaken vigorously before applying to skin that is likely to be exposed to poison ivy, oak, or sumac. The individual must generously apply the lotion to clean dry skin, leaving a smooth wet film of lotion where it is applied. One may determine skin coverage by looking for the faint white coating that appears when the lotion has dried. After the period of exposure has ended, the patient may remove the lotion by washing with soap and water.[37] This product is flammable, and patients should be cautioned not to use the lotion around the eyes and not to apply it if the patient already has a poison ivy rash. Its use is not recommended in children younger than 6 years.

Eradication of* Toxicodendron *Plants The eradication of *Toxicodendron* plants has been both suggested and recommended in situations where extremely sensitive individuals are affected by close proximity to the plant and its oleoresin. Two methods of eradication have been recommended: either mechanically removing (hand grubbing of plants and the root system) or applying an appropriate herbicide. When considering the use of herbicides, patients should contact their state's Farm Bureau or U.S. Department of Agriculture (USDA) Extension Service to determine the recommended choice of herbicide and the prescribed methods of application for the species of *Toxicodendron* plant that is indigenous to the area.

Hyposensitization History and scientific literature are replete with folklore and stories of Native American Indians who ate poison ivy to desensitize themselves from poison ivy dermatitis. Beginning in the early 1940s, numerous oral and injectable forms of poison ivy extract products were available for use. Their purpose was to desensitize patients to urushiol. From the numerous studies published since these products were introduced, clinicians have learned that such desensitization methods are incapable of adequately desensitizing the patient to poison ivy. Although hyposensitization was possible, it can be maintained only with consistent maintenance doses of injectable extracts. Any protection provided through hyposensitization was lost within 3 months of discontinuing maintenance doses. Several hundred milligrams of urushiol were required to provide clinical hyposensitization. Injectable products could be given only in small doses because of the development of poison ivy symptoms and the side effects associated with administering higher doses. Physicians have long doubted the potency of such commercial products. However, some clinicians prepared their own injectables, which then led to overall claims that were confusing and were not convincing in support of the hyposensitization process.

The FDA's Advisory Panel on the review of allergenic extracts recommended an efficacy review of numerous allergenic extract products. In the proposed rulemaking that was reported in the *Federal Register*[38] of January 23, 1985, FDA recommended that licenses for the manufacture of all injectable *Toxicodendron* oleoresins (poison ivy or poison oak) extracts be suspended. The *Federal Register*[39] of November 16, 1994, suspended licenses for the manufacture of all injectable *Toxicodendron* oleoresin (poison ivy or poison oak) extracts effective December 16, 1994. Since these FDA actions, the manufacturers of the *Toxicodendron* oleoresin extracts have removed their products from the marketplace. No products currently exist that can be recommended as hyposensitization programs for human use.[40]

Pharmacologic Therapy

The agents used for topical relief of symptoms come from several different therapeutic classes. Because treatment is primarily aimed at relieving itching, patients should use topical hydrocortisone, topical antihistamines, and other antipruritic agents. Patients can use astringents to promote drying of the moist, wet, oozing lesions and to provide a protective covering for the inflamed, tender skin beneath the lesional areas. Combination products that contain one or more of these ingredients are available for use. Many dosage forms exist that may be used on the dermatitis, according to the skin condition and patient-specific preferences. In addition, antiseptics can be included in the formulation to theoretically provide antimicrobial protection.

Topical Anesthetics

Two local anesthetic agents appear in most nonprescription drug products that relieve itching: benzocaine and pramoxine. Benzocaine is available in concentrations as high as 20%. Pramoxine is ordinarily used in a concentration of 1%. Anesthetic agents affect the impulses carried by the sensory neurons emanating in the areas affected by the dermatitis. By relieving the itch, anesthetic agents indirectly protect the inflamed tissues from further scratching injury and may reduce the risk of a secondary infection. The dosage forms in which anesthetic agents are available include creams, ointments, sprays, and gels. In many instances, these agents are formulated in combination with other antipruritic agents such as camphor and menthol. The pharmacist should reserve these topical anesthetic ingredients for treatment only after other forms of antipruritic therapy have failed to relieve the itching. These agents should be applied no more than three to four times daily. As previously mentioned, benzocaine may be the source of a secondary dermatitis and increased itching, because it has known sensitizing capabilities. (See Chapter 34, "Minor Burns and Sunburn," for additional information about local anesthetics.) If the patient experiences additional itching, redness, or worsening of the dermatitis or urticaria after applying the anesthetic, the pharmacist should advise the patient to wash off the local anesthetic product with mild soap and water and not to apply any more product to the area.

Hydrocortisone

Hydrocortisone is the most effective form of topical therapy for treating the symptoms of mild to moderately severe poison ivy dermatitis that does not involve extensive areas of the skin and edema. Hydrocortisone is a nonsynthetic, low-potency, naturally occurring corticosteroid that is capable of relieving pruritus and reducing inflammation associated with dermatitis. The FDA's Advisory Panel and dermatologists feel that it is safe to apply to all parts of the body, except the eyes and eyelids. It may be applied to large areas of dermatitis, including areas that contain open lesions. It is free of systemic side effects such as adrenal suppression that may result from the absorption of more potent topically or systemically administered anti-inflammatory steroids. Hydrocortisone may be applied up to three or four times a day and is available in concentrations from 0.25% to 1%. Topical hydrocortisone should not be used for children younger than 2 years, except on a physician's advice.[41] Pharmacists should advise patients that hydrocortisone dosage forms should not be used if the dermatitis persists for longer than 7 days, or if symptoms clear and then reappear in a few days, unless patients have consulted with a physician. (See Chapter 28, "Scaly Dermatoses," for additional information about this agent.)

Other Topical Antipruritics

Several long-standing external analgesics have been used for their local antipruritic and anesthetic properties and are incorporated into nonprescription products to relieve the pruritus of poison ivy or poison oak. Phenol, camphor, and menthol appear in numerous products at various low concentrations. (See Chapter 5, "Musculoskeletal Injuries and Disorders," for additional information about these agents.) Using such products on open lesions and tender, inflamed tissues may cause local burning and irritation at the application site. Menthol is capable of depressing the skin's receptors, which will contribute to its topical analgesic effectiveness.

Astringents

Astringents are pharmacologic entities that are known protein precipitants used to stop or reduce the oozing of capillaries or the fluid release from blisters or inflamed tissues. Such substances promote drying of wet dermatitis and, in turn, promote reduced inflammation and healing. The ingredients approved by the FDA's Advisory Panel[42] include aluminum acetate (Burow's solution), zinc oxide, zinc acetate, sodium bicarbonate, calamine, and witch hazel (hamamelis water). They are often used as soaks or in wet compresses that are applied to the area several times a day. This type of application aids in cleansing and in removing crusting or surface debris that arises from the natural progression of poison ivy or poison oak dermatitis. Therapy may be continued for approximately 5 to 7 days, when the dermatitis is moist and oozing.

After the use of astringents, patients may notice drying, tightening, and contracting of the skin. As a note of caution, prolonged use of calamine lotion and of zinc oxide lotion or paste may lead to a buildup of debris and caked material on the skin, which will lead to further irritation and discomfort. Regular cleansing of the affected area to avoid buildup is recommended. The pharmacist may recommend the use of colloidal oatmeal baths to help provide skin hydration, to aid in cleansing or removing skin debris, and to allay the drying and tightening symptoms noted after frequent use. Also available is an oleated form of colloidal oatmeal, which contains mineral oil to provide an emollient action on the skin.

Antihistamines

Antihistamines are used to treat poison ivy in two ways: the first is for their topical anesthetic activity, and the second is for their central sedative action. Although antihistamines are blockers of the histamine$_1$ (H_1) receptor, such receptors do not play a significant role in Type IV cell-mediated responses. Other antihistamines have been included in topical formulations for a similar anesthetic action. Topical antihistamines can act as dermatologic sensitizers, which are responsible for causing secondary inflammatory dermatologic conditions. Just as with the local anesthetics, if the patient experiences additional itching or redness, worsening of the dermatitis or urticaria after applying a topical antihistamine, the patient should be advised to wash off the local antihistamine product with mild soap and water and not to apply any more. (See Chapter 31, "Insect Bites and Stings and Pediculosis," for additional information about these agents.)

When administered orally to provide relief from poison ivy or poison oak pruritus during the night, sedating antihistamines give the patient a restful night's sleep. Diphenhydramine is an example of an antihistamine that is used both orally and topically for such purposes. When recommending oral antihistamine administration, the pharmacist must remember that several patient populations and disease states have a potential for adverse reactions related to the antihistamine's anticholinergic side effects. These populations include individuals who are predisposed to urinary hesitancy or retention, bronchial asthma, glaucoma, hyperthyroidism, cardiovascular disease, or hypertension; pregnant patients; nursing mothers; and patients who are already taking medications that possess anticholinergic activity. The usual recommended adult dosage is 25 to 50 mg at bedtime. Children over 10 kg body weight are usually dosed between 12.5 and 25 mg, or approximately 5 mg/kg. (See Chapter 9, "Disorders Related to Cold and Allergy," for additional information about systemic antihistamines.)

Unapproved Agents

Formerly, some nonprescription products used zirconium for its drying and astringent action on poison ivy/oak rashes and on other forms of weeping dermatitis. Reports have appeared in the literature showing that zirconium caused lesions known as zirconium granulomas on the skin where it was applied. The granulomas were superimposed on the existing dermatitis and thus complicated the existing condition.[43–45] Products that contain zirconium are no longer available on the market, although some brand names once used to connote zirconium content still remain in use today. Again, such products do not contain zirconium, but they may contain other approved nonprescription ingredients.

Product Selection Guidelines

Numerous dosage forms are available for nonprescription recommendation by the pharmacist. The choice of dosage form will depend on several factors, especially the severity of the dermatitis and the presence of vesicles (dry or weeping). Ointments will hold moisture within the skin and act as a reservoir for the active ingredient, holding it on the affected site. Ointments are effective agents when they are applied before the lesions open and begin oozing fluid. Ointments

Case Study 29–1

Patient Complaint/History

Lonnie is a 37-year-old man who works for a local roofing company as a sales associate. The patient has just recently purchased some lakefront property on which he intends to build a cabin for use by friends and family. He and his wife have spent the past several weeks cutting down saplings so that they can move into a temporary mobile home until their permanent home is established. On Tuesday morning, after the Sunday when they burned some of the brush and saplings, Lonnie presents at the pharmacy complaining of intense itching and reddening of the inner aspects of his thighs, along with swelling of his penis and scrotum. He was awakened several times during the night because his thighs and groin itched. After taking a shower this morning, the itching and rash felt somewhat better, but then he noted what looked like blisters forming on his thighs. Lonnie finds it very difficult to arrange an appointment with his physician because of his own busy schedule, so he has not called his physician.

The patient's past medical history includes treatment for mild hypertension and hypercholesterolemia. Presently, he takes hydrochlorothiazide and Pravachol.

Clinical Considerations/Strategies

Readers can use the following considerations/strategies to determine whether treatment of the patient's condition with nonprescription medications is warranted:

- Assess the possible etiology of the patient's dermatitis.
- Discuss with the patient your hypothesis on the etiology of the symptoms.
- Assess the severity of the patient's symptoms.
- Determine which nonprescription medications are most likely to produce a significant degree of symptomatic relief.
- Determine possible drug–drug interactions.

Patient Education/Counseling

Readers can use the following strategies to develop a patient education/counseling plan that will help ensure optimal therapeutic outcomes:

- Explain how the condition will most likely progress and when resolution of the symptoms is most likely to occur.
- Explain possible complications and what to do if they occur.
- Explain the importance of nonprescription drug therapy and when and how to use the recommended therapy.

should not be applied to open lesions for several reasons. Ointment removal from an open lesion is more difficult when it is applied to the skin surface. Ointments may potentially trap bacteria beneath the oleaginous film, which may lead to secondary infections.

Applying a cream base does allow vesicle fluid to flow freely from the blisters and does not trap bacteria, because creams are quickly absorbed into the skin. Gels offer ease of application and a rapid absorption of active ingredients into the skin. Some gels may contain alcohol or similar organic solvents that may cause irritation or burning when applied to open lesions.

Spray products provide the easiest form of drug application. They allow even distribution to relatively larger areas and are convenient to use, but they are somewhat more expensive. One advantage of a spray product is that touching the area of dermatitis is not necessary and this advantage may curtail additional scratching. Aerosol sprays may contain propellants that may cause additional inflammation. Table 29–4 lists examples of products that contain primarily colloidal oatmeal, astringents, or bentoquatam. (See Chapter 31, "Insect Bites and Stings and Pediculosis," for examples of products that contain local anesthetics, hydrocortisone, or topical antihistamines.)

Table 29–4

Selected Products for Treating Poison Ivy/Oak/Sumac Dermatitis

Trade Name	Primary Ingredients
Aveeno Bath Treatment Moisturizing Formula Powder	Colloidal oatmeal 43%
Aveeno Bath Treatment Soothing Formula Powder	Colloidal oatmeal 100%
Bluboro Powder	Aluminum sulfate 53.9%
Domeboro Powder	Aluminum sulfate 1191 mg
Ivarest 8-Hour Medicated Cream	Diphenhydramine HCl 2%; calamine 14%
Ivy Dry Cream	Benzyl alcohol 10 mg/g; camphor 6 mg/g; menthol 4 mg/g; zinc acetate 20 mg/g
Ivy Dry Liquid	Isopropyl alcohol 12.5%; zinc acetate 20 mg/mL
Ivy Super Dry Liquid	Benzyl alcohol 0.1 mg/g; camphor 4 mg/g; menthol 2 mg/g; isopropyl alcohol 35%; zinc acetate 20 mg/mL
IvyBlock Lotion	Benzyl alcohol; SDA alcohol 40 25%; bentoquatam (quaternium-18 bentonite 5%

Alternative Remedies

Jewel weed (*Impatiens biflora, Impatiens pallida*) is a well-known natural product and folk remedy used by Native Americans to treat a vast array of dermal conditions, including the prevention of poison ivy/oak/sumac dermatitis. The juice of the stems is applied to the area where urushiol contact occurred to prevent the ensuing rash. In a recent double-blind study,[46] fresh juice from the stems of *Impatiens pallida* was applied to the skin where freshly crushed poison ivy (*T. radicans*) was applied for 15 minutes. Three treatment approaches were tried: (1) application of jewel weed juice, (2) application of saline solution, and (3) no treatment. The study's conclusions revealed that jewel weed juice applied directly after fresh poison ivy exposure did not reduce or prevent poison ivy dermatitis in humans. A second study[47] concluded that boiled jewel weed extract was not an effective treatment for preventing poison ivy/oak dermatitis.

Patient Assessment of Poison Ivy/Oak/Sumac Dermatitis

Assessment of a suspected plant-induced dermatitis is based on characteristic symptoms, history of sensitivity, and activities that indicate exposure to causative plants. Determining the type and success of previous treatments of such rashes will aid in recommending the appropriate nonprescription medications. Asking the patient the following questions will help elicit the information needed to accurately assess the disorder and to recommend the appropriate treatment approach.

Q~ Describe your symptoms, the appearance of the rash, and the specific body parts and areas affected. When did your rash, redness, itching, or other symptoms first appear?

A~ *Identify the characteristic symptoms of poison ivy/oak/sumac dermatitis and the time frame in which they are usually manifested. (See the sections "Pathophysiology of Poison Ivy/Oak/Sumac Dermatitis" and "Signs and Symptoms of Poison Ivy/Oak/Sumac Dermatitis.")* Consider urushiol-induced dermatitis if the patient's symptoms are characteristic. Suspect causes other than urushiol for rashes of longer than 2 weeks duration.

Q~ Have you recently visited or worked outdoors in the past several days or weeks?

A~ If yes, determine whether the time of year coincides with the growing season of *Toxicodendron* plants. Consider possible exposure to such plants if the season is appropriate and if the outdoor activity was short. If outdoor activity was prolonged, consider that the dermatitis is chronic in nature or is related to a more serious disease.

Q~ Have you used any sporting equipment or any work tools, shoes, or clothing that have not been laundered or cleaned since they were last used or worn?

A~ If recent outdoor activity has been ruled out or if it is not the growing season for *Toxicodendron* plants, consider exposure to dead plants, inanimate objects such as gardening tools or sports equipment, and fur of domestic pets as possible sources of exposure to urushiol.

Q~ Have you had similar symptoms in the past 1 to 5 years? Have you ever had a poison ivy/oak/sumac rash?

A~ If yes, determine whether the present symptoms are similar to other *Toxicodendron*-induced rashes and suspect that the patient is sensitive and reactive to urushiol. If the dermatitis occurred more than 5 years ago, consider other causes of the dermatitis. To determine whether the patient has a prior history of dermatologic problems or symptoms, ask whether the patient has previously seen a physician for this or similar conditions.

Q~ What has worked best for you in treating the rash and symptoms in the past? What have you used to treat your present condition?

A~ Evaluate the appropriateness of present treatments. Drawing on the success of previous treatments, evaluate whether other untried therapies will offer any relief to the patient or whether the patient should be referred to a physician.

Q~ Have you had any allergic symptoms or difficulties with antihistamines, anesthetics, or other topical nonprescription or prescription medications? What products or ingredients are you allergic or sensitive to?

A~ Avoid further aggravation of the patient's dermatitis and associated symptoms by basing product recommendations on any preexisting allergies. Minimize potential drug interactions by evaluating the patient's current medication use.

Patient Counseling for Poison Ivy/Oak/Sumac Dermatitis

When approached by a patient with a plant-induced dermatitis, the pharmacist should take the opportunity to explain preventive and protective measures, as well as treatment measures. If the patient cannot identify *Toxicodendron* plants, the pharmacist should show them illustrations of the plants, if possible, or refer patients to an appropriate reference. The pharmacist should also explain the purpose and appropriate use of nonprescription agents, their possible adverse effects, and signs and symptoms that indicate medical referral is appropriate. The box "Patient Education for Poison Ivy/Oak/Sumac Dermatitis" lists specific information to provide patients.

Evaluation of Patient Outcomes for Poison Ivy/Oak/Sumac Dermatitis

After recommending treatment for a poison ivy rash, the pharmacist may chose to follow up with the patient after several days of treatment, or instead may encourage the patient to call for additional advice if the itching has not subsided significantly within 5 to 7 days. If, at follow-up, the rash has significantly increased in size, affects the eyes or genitals, or covers extensive areas of the face, the pharmacist must reassess the patient for further therapy or physician referral. Overall, complete remission of the dermatitis may take up to 3 weeks. However, the patient should see slow but steady reduction in itching, weeping, and dermatitis after 5 to 7 days of therapy.

CONCLUSIONS

Members of the plant genus *Toxicodendron* can be found throughout the United States and North America. As much as 70% to 80% of people in the United States are sensitive to urushiol, although only 50% of all Americans will have a dermatologic response. Exposure to urushiol oleoresin, which is responsible for poison ivy dermatitis, can occur only through contact with fresh or dried plants that have been damaged. Urushiol oleoresin that is deposited on inanimate objects can remain antigenically active for many months or years.

Patients who are sensitive to poison ivy urushiol may take precautions to eliminate unnecessary exposure by avoiding geographic areas endemic with *Toxicodendron* plants, by wearing protective clothing, and by applying liberal and timely applications of bentoquatam barrier lotion every 4 hours until the exposure period is over. Once exposure to urushiol has taken place, the patient can take protective measures that include bathing with mild soap and water, or using large volumes of cool water immediately after or within 10 minutes of exposure to reduce the risk of dermatitis. Dermatitis appearance may begin as localized streaks of highly pruritic rash proceeding to larger areas on exposed extremities. The rash may affect eyelids, face, and, in some cases, areas ordinarily considered protected. The pharmacist should refer patients to a physician if the rash causes edema of the eyelids, closes the eyelids, affects the external genitalia or anus, or produces massive areas of body rash or edema.

Treatment of localized, pruritic streaky rash consists of a topical application of hydrocortisone cream or ointment, sodium bicarbonate paste, compresses, or baths. Weeping of vesicles or bullae, which is caused by the patient's scratching, may be treated with aluminum acetate compresses as an astringent to soothe and dry the weeping. Colloidal oatmeal baths may be used to treat the pruritic rash, to soothe, and to provide an emollient action on dry skin. For pruritus that has not been resolved with the use of hydrocortisone products,

Patient Education for Poison Ivy/Oak/Sumac Dermatitis

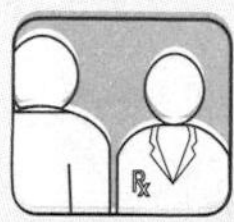

The objectives of self-treatment are to (1) reduce or prevent itching and excessive scratching that may lead to secondary skin infections, (2) protect the affected area, and (3) prevent the accumulation of skin debris and oozing, crusting, and scaling of vesicle fluids, which could spread the infection to the area surrounding the inflammation. For most patients, carefully following product instructions and the self-care measures listed below will help ensure optimal therapeutic outcomes.

Nondrug Measures

- Take the preventive measures outlined in Table 29–3 to prevent poison ivy/oak/sumac dermatitis.
- If exposure is suspected and if preventive measures were not taken, implement the protective measures outlined in Table 29–3.
- Take tepid, soapless showers to relieve the itching of this dermatitis.
- When cleansing the affected areas, do not use harsh cleansers or scrub vigorously.

Nonprescription Medications

- Note that the dermatitis will dissipate with or without treatment in 14 to 21 days.
- If treatment is desired, consult a pharmacist about the use of one or more of the following nonprescription medications to relieve the intense itching, inflammation, weeping, and crusting that may accompany this dermatitis.
- If desired, use sodium bicarbonate paste or compresses as follows to relieve itching:
  —Apply paste directly to the rash to reduce itching.
  —Use clean white cloths to apply cool water compresses and apply for 20 to 30 minutes as often as needed or desired. Use a fresh solution with each new application.
- If desired, apply topical hydrocortisone cream or ointment as follows to reduce the itching and to dissipate the dermal inflammation and erythema:
  —Apply sparingly to affected areas four times a day.
  —Avoid direct application around the eyes or eyelids.
  —Note that ointment dosage forms appear to maintain hydrocortisone application for longer periods of time than cream forms.
- To avoid potential dermal infections, do not apply ointments to open or excoriated pustules or lesions.
- Use aluminum acetate (Burow's solution) compresses as follows to dry open and weeping pustules or lesions:
  —Mix a prepackaged tablet or packet of aluminum acetate with a pint of cool tap water and use it to wet cloth compresses for application to rash areas.
  —Apply compresses for 30 minutes at least four times a day or as needed.
  —Prepare fresh Burow's solution for each application period.
- Use colloidal oatmeal baths or soaks as follows to soothe and cleanse areas of rash as well as to reduce pruritus:
  —Sprinkle 30-gram packets or a cup full of milled oatmeal into fast-running bath water and mix water periodically to avoid lumping of the oatmeal.
  —Take a 15- to 20-minute soak in the oatmeal bath at least twice a day. Pat skin dry rather than wiping it.
  —Be cautious on entry and exit from the bathtub because oatmeal baths are quite slippery.
- If you are not sensitive to local anesthetics (e.g., benzocaine) or topical antihistamines (e.g., diphenhydramine), use these agents as follows to provide relief of itching:
  —Apply agents sparingly to the affected area three or four times a day.
  —Avoid prolonged use beyond 7 days unless directed by your physician.
  —Note that antihistamines and anesthetic agents are sensitizing agents and may cause additional dermatitis and inflammation in areas where they are applied.
- For nighttime relief of itching and restful sleep, take oral antihistamines such as diphenhydramine as follows for their sedating effect:
  —Adult doses of diphenhydramine range from 25 to 50 mg and may be taken just before bedtime.
  —Pediatric doses of diphenhydramine for children weighing more than 10 kg range from 12.5 to 25 mg, or 5 mg/kg of body weight.
  —Caution should be exercised in recommending oral antihistamines to some patients on the basis of (1) their disease state, (2) medications they presently take, or (3) existing physiologic conditions.

Contact a physician for systemic and topical treatment in the following situations:
—Symptoms become worse.
—The rash becomes more widespread on the body.
—The rash covers large areas of the face or causes swelling of the eyelids.
—The rash involves the genitalia.

the patient may topically apply a local anesthetic or antihistamine agents for additional anesthetic activity. The pharmacist should advise caution when recommending these agents because they are sensitizing substances and are capable of producing additional dermatitis and itching. In an effort to provide a restful night's sleep, pharmacists could recommend oral antihistaminic agents, which possess a central sedating effect and are used before bedtime. Pharmacists should use caution when recommending anticholinergic antihistamines for patients who are already taking medications with anticholinergic side effects, for nursing mothers, or for patients with preexisting physiologic conditions.

Resolution of poison ivy /oak/sumac dermatitis will occur in approximately 10 to 21 days with or without topical therapy. Nonprescription medication recommendations will, in part, serve to relieve the intense itching, inflammation, weeping, and crusting that may accompany this dermatitis.

References

1. Dannaker C, Maibach HI. Allergic contact dermatitis due to plants. In: Lovell CR, ed. *Plants and the Skin.* London: Blackwell Scientific Publications; 1993:105–20.
2. Klingman DL, Davis DE, Knake ED, et al. *Poison Ivy, Poison Oak, Poison Sumac.* Washington, DC: Extension Service, U.S. Dept of Agriculture; 1983.
3. Lejman E, Stoudemayer T, Grove G, et al. Age differences in poison ivy dermatitis. *Contact Dermatitis.* 1984;11:163–7.
4. Fisher AA. Poison ivy/oak dermatitis. Part 1: prevention—soap and water, topical barriers, hyposensitization. *Cutis.* 1996;57:384–6.
5. Gellin GA, Wolf CR, Milby TH. Poison ivy, poison oak, and poison sumac: common causes of occupational dermatitis. *Arch Environ Health.* 1971;22:280–6.
6. Bureau of Labor Statistics, U.S. Department of Labor. Number of nonfatal occupational injuries, and illnesses involving days away from work by source of injury or illness and selected natures of injuries or illness, 1993. Available at: http://stats.bls.gov/case/ostb0025.pdf. Accessed March 26, 1999.
7. Bureau of Labor Statistics, U.S. Department of Labor. Incidence for nonfatal occupational injuries and illnesses involving days away from work per 10,000 full-time workers by source of injury or illness and selected natures of injuries or illness, 1996. Available at: http://stats.bls.gov/case/ostb0570.pdf. Accessed March 21, 1999.
8. Bureau of Labor Statistics, U.S. Department of Labor. Incidence for nonfatal occupational injuries and illnesses involving days away from work per 10,000 full-time workers by source of injury or illness and selected events or exposures leading to injuries or illness, 1995. Available at: http://stats.bls.gov/case/ostb0403.pdf. Accessed March 21, 1999.
9. Botanical Dermatology Database. Anacardiaceae. Available at: http://www.uwcm.ac.uk/uwcm/dm/BoDD/BotDermFolder/BotDermA/ANAC.html. Accessed February 8, 1999.
10. Reitschel RL, Fowler JF, eds. *Fisher's Contact Dermatitis: Toxicodendron Plants and Spices.* 4th ed. Baltimore: Williams & Wilkins; 1995:461–74.
11. Kawai K, Nakagawa M, Kawai K, et al. Heat treatment of Japanese lacquerware renders it hypoallergenic. *Contact Dermatitis.* 1992;27:244–9.
12. Johnson RA, Baer H, Kirkpatrick CH, et al. Comparison of the contact allergenicity of the four pentadecylcatechols derived from poison ivy urushiol in human subjects. *J Allergy Clin Immunol.* 1972;49:27–35.
13. ElSohly MA, Adawadkar PD, Ma CY, et al. Separation and characterization of poison ivy and poison oak urushiol components. *J Nat Products.* 1982;45:532–8.
14. Guin JD. The black spot test for recognizing poison ivy and related species. *J Am Acad Dermatol.* 1980;2:332–3.
15. Epstein WL, Epstein JH. In: Auerbach PL, ed. *Wilderness Medicine Management of Wilderness and Environmental Emergencies: Plant Induced Dermatitis.* 3rd ed. St. Louis: Mosby-Year Book; 1995:843–61.
16. Epstein WL, Baer H, Dawson CR, et al. Poison oak hyposensitization: evaluation of purified urushiol. *Arch Dermatol.* 1974;109:356–60.
17. Klingman AM. Poison ivy (Rhus) dermatitis: an experimental study. *AMA Archives Dermatol.* 1958;77:149–80.
18. Gillis WT. The systematics and ecology of poison ivy and the poison oaks. *Rhodora.* 1971;73:72–159, 161–237, 370–443, 465–540.
19. Gayer KD, Burnett JW. Toxicodendron dermatitis. *Cutis.* 1988;42:99–100.
20. Epstein WL. Plant-induced dermatitis. *Ann Emerg Med.* 1987;16:950–5.
21. D'Mello DA, MacAuley L. Poison ivy dermatitis and secondary mania. *J Nerv Ment Dis.* 1994;182:116–7.
22. Cohen LM, Cohen JL. Erythema multiforme associated with contact dermatitis to poison ivy: three cases and a review of the literature. *Cutis.* 1998;63:139–42.
23. Gealt L, Osterhoudt KC. Adult respiratory distress syndrome after smoke inhalation from burning poison ivy. *JAMA.* 1995;274:358–9.
24. Devich KB, Lee JC, Epstein WL, et al. Renal lesions accompanying poison oak dermatitis. *Clin Nephrol.* 1975;3:106–13.
25. Watts WJ. Poison oak urethritis. *N Engl J Med.* 1989;321:194.
26. Guin JD, Klingman AM, Maibach HI. Treating poison ivy, oak, and sumac. *Patient Care.* 1989;23(11):227–37.
27. Williford PM, Sheretz EF. Poison ivy dermatitis: nuances in treatment. *Arch Fam Med.* 1994;3:184–8.
28. McGuffey EC. What methods are effective to prevent or treat poison ivy/oak/sumac? *Am Pharm.* 1993;33:18.
29. Ives TJ, Tepper RS. Failure of a tapering dose of oral methylprednisolone to treat reactions to poison ivy. *JAMA.* 1991;266:1362.
30. Drake DC. Pruritus of poison oak dermatitis—other views [letter]. *West J Med.* 1984;141:111.
31. Tomovitch TA, Stegman SJ, Glogau R. Pruritus of poison oak dermatitis—other views. [letter] *West J Med.* 1984;141:111.
32. Gross DA. Pruritus of poison oak dermatitis—other views [letter]. *West J Med.* 1984;141:111–2.
33. Epstein WL. Occupational poison ivy and oak dermatitis. *Dermatol Clin.* 1994;12:511–6.
34. Grevelink SA, Murrell DF, Olsen EA. Effectiveness of various barrier preparations in preventing and/or ameliorating experimentally produced *Toxicodendron* dermatitis. *J Am Acad Dermatol.* 1992;27(2 Pt 1):182–8.
35. Epstein WL. Topical prevention of poison ivy/oak dermatitis. *Arch Dermatol.* 1989;125:499–501.
36. Marks JG Jr, Fowler JG Jr, Sheretz EF, et al. Prevention of poison ivy and poison oak allergic contact dermatitis by quaternium-18 bentonite. *J Am Acad Dermatol.* 1995;33(2 Pt 1):212–6.
37. EnviroDerm Pharmaceuticals, Inc. IvyBlock Lotion product information. 1998.
38. Biological products; allergenic extracts; implementation of efficacy review. *Federal Register.* 1985;50:3082–288.
39. Biological products; allergenic extracts classified in category IIIB; final order; revocation of licenses. *Federal Register.* 1994;59:59228–37.
40. Scott PM. Personal communication. Bayer Allergy Products, Miles, Inc., Spokane, WA, confirmed the fact that Bayer Allergy Products will no longer manufacture the oral poison/oak extract capsule for hyposensitization use. March 1999.
41. Hydrocortisone marketing status as an external analgesic drug product for over-the-counter human use; notice of enforcement policy. *Federal Register.* 1991;56:43025–6.
42. Skin protectant drug products for over-the-counter use; proposed rule making for poison ivy, poison oak, poison sumac and insect bites drug products. *Federal Register.* 1989;54:40808–27.
43. Epstein WL, Allen JR. Granulomatous hypersensitivity after use of zirconium-containing poison oak lotions. *JAMA.* 1964;190:162–4.
44. LoPresti PJ, Hambrick GW. Zirconium granuloma following treatment of Rhus dermatitis. *Arch Dermat.* 1965;92:188–91.
45. Bale GR. Granulomas from topical zirconium in poison ivy dermatitis. *Arch Dermat.* 1965;91:145–8.
46. Zink BJ, Otten EJ, Rosenthal M, et al. The effect of jewel weed in preventing poison ivy dermatitis. *J Wilderness Med.* 1991;2:178–82.
47. Long D, Ballentine NH, Marks JG Jr. Treatment of poison ivy/oak allergenic contact dermatitis with an extract of jewelweed. *Am J Contact Dermat.* 1997;8:150–3.

CHAPTER 30

Diaper Dermatitis and Prickly Heat

Victor A. Padrón

Chapter 30 at a Glance

Diaper dermatitis (also called diaper rash) is the general name for a group of acute dermatitis lesions of the skin characterized as an inflammatory condition in the region of the perineum, buttocks, lower abdomen, and inner thighs. (In Europe diaper rash is called nappy rash because the diaper is called a napkin or nappy.) Although most often seen in infants, diaper rash can appear in adults.

Prickly heat (also known as miliaria or miliaria rubra) is a transient inflammation of the skin that appears as a very fine, usually red, rash. It can appear in the diaper area or on other parts of the body such as the chest and axilla regions.

Neither dermatitis produces serious illness in most circumstances. These conditions can cause discomfort, irritation, or itching and, in infants and adults, can result in fussiness, agitation, and easy irritability. Most infants, however, may have no behavioral symptoms and may experience no apparent discomfort.

Editor's Note: This chapter is based, in part, on the 11th edition chapter titled "Diaper Rash, Prickly Heat, and Adult Incontinence Products," which was written by Gary H. Smith, Victor A. Elsberry, and Martin D. Higbee.

Diaper Dermatitis

Epidemiology of Diaper Dermatitis

The vast majority of cases of diaper rash appear in infants who are still in diapers. Infants younger than 20 months are the most-affected population. A report from the mid-1980s indicated that roughly two-thirds of infants had experienced some symptoms of diaper dermatitis, with one-fourth to one-third progressing to moderate or severe forms of the disease.[1] By 1995, the number of infants with diaper dermatitis had not improved. It still stood at about two-thirds of all infants; however, the number that had moderate-to-severe diaper rash had dropped to 2%.[2] The disposable diaper has been available since the 1960s, and the decline in moderate-to-severe diaper rash is suspected to be a result of the rise in affordability and widespread acceptability, use, and advertising of disposable diapers since 1985.

Breast-fed infants have less diaper rash than do bottle-fed infants. Studies[3,4] have shown that starting a child on solid food early has no effect on the incidence of diaper rash in infants. The feces of breast-fed infants is less copious, less alkaline, and less caustic to the skin. Foods that increase the urinary and fecal pH, such as high-protein diets, may contribute to diaper rash.[5]

Diaper rash can also be a manifestation of other diseases such as Kawaski's syndrome, granuloma gluteale infantum, and cytomegalovirus.[6–9] Infants born to compromised mothers, such as those who are human immunodeficiency virus (HIV) positive or those with genital herpes or other chronic, congenital, or sexually transmitted diseases, should be considered at increased risk of unusual manifestations of diaper rash. Infants with yeast infection (*Candida albicans*) should be checked for oral candidiasis (oral thrush).

Because of the aging of the general population and the rise of incontinence causing the elderly to use adult diapers, the incidence of reported diaper dermatitis (incontinence dermatitis) in the elderly, especially in nursing home patients, is expected to increase.

Etiology of Diaper Dermatitis

According to the Food and Drug Administration (FDA) review panel, diaper rash is believed to be caused by one or more of the following factors: moisture, occlusion, chafing, continued contact with urine or feces or both, or mechanical or chemical irritation.[10] The presence of gastrointestinal (GI) enzymes and bile salts in infant feces and the changes in skin pH are also possible factors in diaper rash.[11] It was previously believed that urine was the chief culprit in diaper rash, probably because of the ammonia smell associated with diapers, especially if left unchanged for a time or left to percolate in diaper pails. Ammonia is a known skin irritant and caustic that can rapidly produce a serious chemical burn. Fecal contamination was implicated because urea-splitting bacteria from the colon were believed responsible for diaper rash by converting urea from urine into ammonia. The resulting ammonia raised the pH of the skin, making it more susceptible to damage or infection. Others felt that mechanical irritation of the skin was the initial insult that broke down the epidermis, allowing other irritants to assault the skin.

Taken all together the most likely scenario for developing diaper rash is some combination of all of these factors. Occlusion, moisture, bacteria, a shift away from the normal acidic skin pH (pH 4 to 5.5) to a more alkaline pH, mechanical chafing and friction (as the infant becomes more active and more mobile), and proteolytic enzymes and bile salts from the GI tract all combine in additive or synergistic ways to cause diaper rash.

Tight-fitting, stiff, or rough diapers and the use of occlusive plastic or rubberized covers or pants over the diaper contribute to occlusion of the skin. Infrequent changing of the diaper contributes to increased skin moisture. Skin left in contact with wetness for long periods becomes waterlogged or hyperhydrated, which plugs sweat glands and makes skin more susceptible to irritation and the absorption of chemicals.[12] The typical infant begins to urinate within 24 hours after birth. Urination occurs in infants up to 20 times a day up to approximately age 2 months, falling to about 8 times a day until age 8 years. Defecation occurs from 3 to 6 times a day up to about age 8 months. Then, as the infant's autonomic and muscular control develops, it gradually declines to 1 to 3 times a day.[13] In the first months of life, it is common for infants to need an average of six diaper changes per day.

Reusable cloth diapers can also contribute to diaper rash and skin irritation through inadequate washing. A contributing factor can be the use of harsh chemicals to clean the diapers, which in turn may leave chemical residues on the diaper that then come in contact with the skin. One study concluded that infants who wear cloth diapers have a slight, but not statistically increased, incidence of diaper rash. If cloth diapers are used, a professional diaper service is preferred over home laundering. Cloth diapers are generally perceived to be more environmentally friendly because they can be reused, can be used for other children, and can be converted to dust cloths and rags when no longer needed as diapers. Disposable diapers deposit raw feces and urine into landfills, and it has been shown that disposable diapers are not significantly biodegraded in landfills. Discussions of the advantages of cloth diapers usually fail to consider the amount of water consumed to wash them, and the tons of detergents, bleach, and softener used to process them for reuse. The actual costs to the environment, taking all factors into account, give the edge to the disposable diaper.[13–15]

Medications can affect the motility and flora of the GI tract and the autonomic control of urination and defecation. They can also be irritating on elimination from the body. Antibiotics can produce diarrhea secondary to changes in GI flora that can lead to diaper dermatitis. The type, frequency, and route of administration of the medication can influence the development of diaper rash.

Pathophysiology/Signs and Symptoms of Diaper Dermatitis

In infants, the skin of the perineal region is relatively thin, being about one-half to one-third the thickness of adult skin. Because the area is typically enclosed by a diaper and has little exposure to the air, air currents, or sunlight, it tends to hold moisture and wetness, predisposing it to irritation and infection. It is also a less-effective barrier to the absorption of drugs and toxins. Adult skin, being thicker, is less susceptible to this irritation and to the absorption of drugs and chemicals.[1,16]

Diaper rash usually presents as red to bright red (erythematous), sometimes shiny, wet-looking patches or lesions on the skin. (See the "Color Plates," photograph 13.) They may appear maroon or purplish on darker skin. More severe diaper rash may progress to maceration, papule formation, the presence of vesicles or bullae, oozing, erosion of the skin, and ulceration.

Generally, diaper rash occurs in the skin spaces and creases covered by the diaper, but severe cases can spread outside the diaper area, moving up the abdomen or onto the upper buttocks and lower back. If the infant lies primarily on his or her abdomen, the rash may appear more forward of the perineum. If the infant lies primarily on his or her back, the rash may appear posterior to the perineum.

A disconcerting feature of diaper rash is that it can occur in a matter of a few hours and can take days to resolve. The onset of clearly observable diaper rash can occur in the time between two diaper changes. Most likely, the process of skin breakdown is not initially pronounced or observable, and the breakdown goes from mild to moderate in a matter of hours. The entire process from normal to noticeably inflamed skin takes longer than the time between diaper changes. It may be worth noting that populations that do not use diapers do not experience diaper rash. No diaper rash is found in cultures in which infants are essentially naked, wear loin cloths that leave the genitals uncovered, or wear clothing with slits.[2]

Complications of Diaper Dermatitis

Diaper rash can predispose the skin to secondary infection. Opportunistic infection by normal skin flora, such as streptococci or staphylococci, or by fungi have been known to occur. There is at least one report of herpes simplex diaper rash.[3] The change in skin pH tends to foster the overgrowth of normal and abnormal organisms (e.g., yeasts). The longer diaper rash goes untreated, the more likely the disease is to progress to ulceration of the skin and secondary infection. Severe diaper rash can cause maceration, ulceration, and infection of the penis or vulva, which can progress to urinary tract infection. Untreated or infected diaper rash has caused adhesions and scarring of the genitals, necessitating cosmetic or reconstructive surgery.

In addition to secondary infection, diaper rash can coexist with other skin conditions such as psoriasis and seborrhea. If skin conditions are seen on other parts of the body, they may also coexist with diaper rash or may be misdiagnosed as diaper rash.

Treatment of Diaper Dermatitis

Treatment Outcomes

Once diaper rash has been determined, the overall goals of treatment are to (1) rid the patient of the rash, (2) relieve the symptoms, and (3) prevent recurrences.

Case Study 30-1

Patient Complaint/History

An underweight (5th percentile for age) infant about 4 months old presents with diarrhea and diaper rash. The mother requests a product to treat the diarrhea. Visual inspection of the infant's diaper area reveals dusky to maroon skin that covers the entire diaper area without break. Peeling is present in some skin creases. The child is not fussy or irritable. When asked about presence of fever, the mother replies the baby's temperature is not that high, only 99.5°F.

Questioning about the diarrhea reveals that the present episode began this morning but that the infant had diarrhea a month ago. The diaper area skin began to turn reddish 3 days ago, but there is no history of previous diaper rash. The mother changes the diapers about six times during the day and twice in the night. Although other children are in the house, none has diarrhea or diaper rash.

When asked about the child's weight and feeding, the mother explains the infant was born prematurely. Because of the low birth weight, the baby was last seen by a physician about a week after being born. She is not sure whether the infant has lost any weight, and the child is still being breast-fed. Questioning about the mother's diet within the past 24 hours reveals no dietary changes.

The infant's medication history shows no prescription or nonprescription medications. In response to questions about family history of allergies, the mother states that only she has allergies (seafood).

Clinical Considerations/Strategies

Readers can use the following considerations/strategies to determine whether treatment of the disorder with nonprescription medications is warranted:

- On the basis of its manifestation, determine whether the diaper rash is self-treatable.
- Determine the appropriate treatment approach when diarrhea coexists with diaper rash, especially in an underweight infant.
- Evaluate the significance of the child's temperature.
- Evaluate the need for physician supervision of this child's health.

Patient Education/Counseling

Readers can use the following strategies to develop a patient education/counseling plan that will help ensure optimal therapeutic outcomes:

- Advise the mother that diarrhea can cause diaper rash and that a physician must determine the cause of the diarrhea.
- Explain that the rash has spread beyond the diaper area and may indicate a disorder more serious than diaper rash.
- Explain the need for close physician supervision of a low-birth-weight infant.
- Stress that the infant should be taken to a physician immediately for evaluation.

General Treatment Approach

The general approach to diaper rash is the use of nondrug therapy or a combination of drug and nondrug therapy as outlined in Figure 30–1.

The best treatment for diaper rash is prevention. The ideal nonpharmacologic therapy would be to change the diaper each time the child defecates or urinates. This treatment is very impractical because it would require a 24-hour vigil and a way to know immediately when the infant defecated or urinated. It is difficult enough for modern parents to make six or more diaper changes in a typical day. Hence, nonpharmacologic therapy encompasses both prevention and treatment of diaper rash.

Therefore, the steps in nonpharmacologic therapy are to

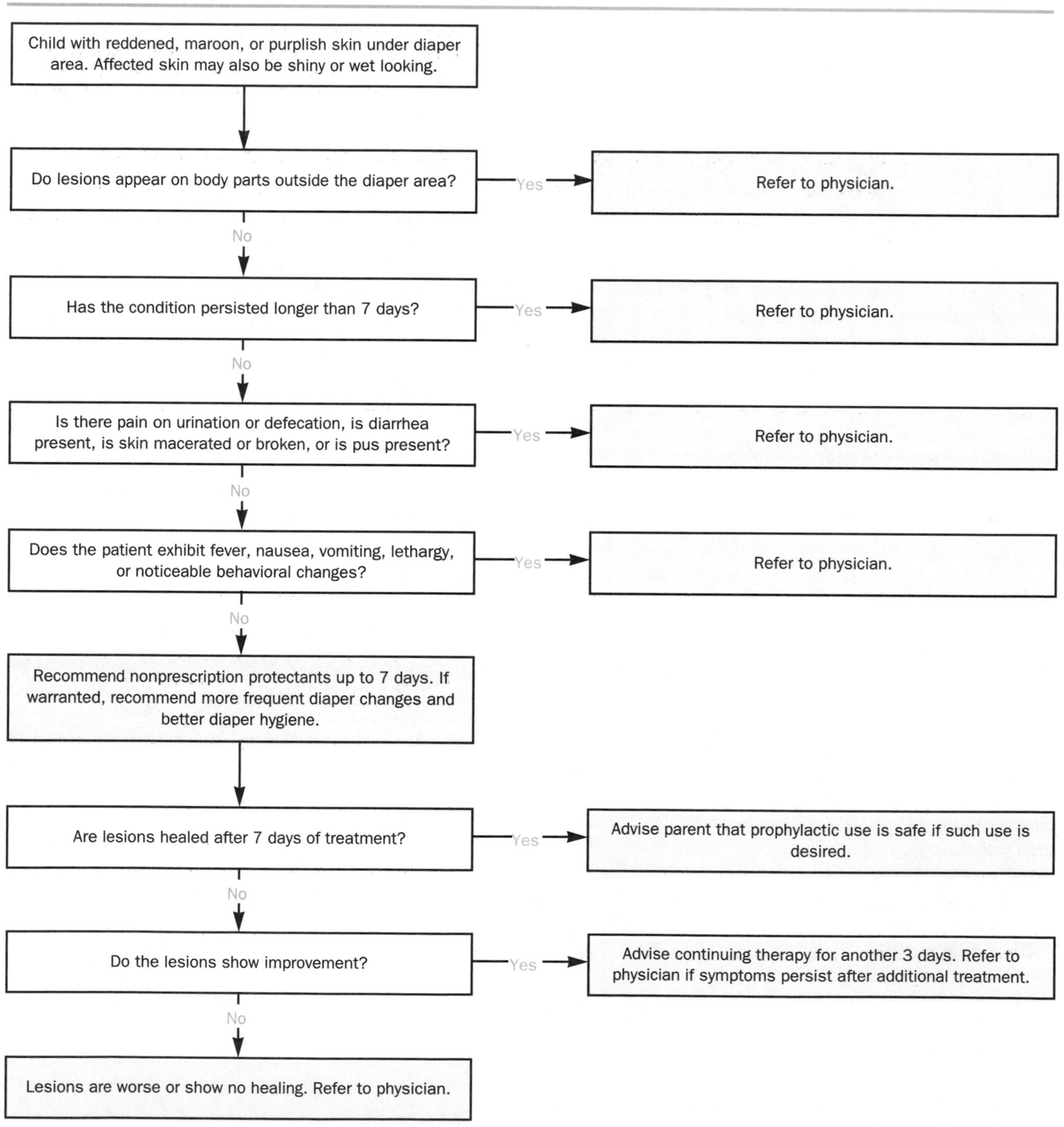

Figure 30–1 Self-care of diaper dermatitis.

(1) reduce occlusion (2) separate feces from urine, (3) reduce contact time of urine and skin, (4) reduce mechanical irritation and trauma to the inguinal and perineal skin, (5) protect the skin from further irritation, (6) encourage healing, and (7) discourage the onset of secondary infection.

The steps in pharmacologic therapy are to (1) dry the skin, (2) protect the skin from further contact with urine and feces, (3) encourage healing, (4) soothe any discomfort caused by the lesion(s), and (5) discourage the onset of secondary infection.

Treatment should be limited to diaper rash that is uncomplicated and mild to moderate in presentation. The patient should be referred to a physician when the diaper rash manifests one or more of the following:

- Has been present longer than 7 days.
- Has not improved in 7 days despite appropriate self-care.
- Is complicated by secondary infection.
- Is part of or a result of another disease state.
- Has spread outside the diaper region of the body.
- Has broken the skin or caused ulceration or peeling.
- Has an onion-skin-like appearance or has bullae formation.
- Oozes blood or pus.
- Is associated with constitutional symptoms, such as fever, diarrhea, nausea, vomiting, rash, or skin lesions on other parts of the body.
- Is associated with significant behavioral changes in the patient.
- Appears chronic or recurs frequently.
- Is associated with urinary tract infection or when disfigurement of the penis or vulva is possible.
- Is associated with comorbid conditions, such as HIV, transplantation or immune suppressive therapy, history of dermal hepatic infections, and so forth.

Nonpharmacologic Therapy

Treatment of mild-to-moderate diaper rash should be initiated with nondrug therapy. If the child achieves adequate improvement with nondrug methods, exposure to drugs can be reduced, and the drugs can be held in reserve. Increasing the frequency of diaper changes to six a day may be a good starting place. If feasible, more than six changes a day combined with careful diaper change procedures may ameliorate mild symptoms of redness. During each and every diaper change, careful flushing of the skin with plain water followed by gentle nonfriction drying is to be encouraged.[17] The apparently unsoiled part of the diaper should not be used to clean or wipe the infant because this action can spread fecal bacteria.

Anecdotally, both professional and nonprofessional caregivers have suggested using a shower sprayer on a low power setting to rinse the child because a sprayer head is maneuverable and can flush skinfolds and natural skin creases without directly touching the area. Another method is holding the infant in a sitting position in a basin of lukewarm water and gently washing the area; however, this action may spread fecal contamination to other parts of the body. Holding the child over a basin or sink as the infant is washed is better, but holding a wiggling wet infant may not be as simple as it sounds. Some caregivers will let the child air dry and run naked for a spell, but there is the risky possibility that the infant has more urine or bowel contents ready to evacuate.

Other caregivers have ventured to use a hair dryer set to its lowest temperature and lowest speed to help dry the child more thoroughly and more quickly. Obviously, the child must be securely held during these kinds of procedures, and care must be taken not to burn or scald the infant with a high heat setting or by placing the hair dryer too close to the skin. None of these procedures has been subjected to scientific analysis for reliability, safety, or clinical value.

The use of detergents or ordinary lye-based soaps to launder diapers may be irritating and may further aggravate diaper rash or cause contact dermatitis.[18] Starched or very stiff diapers should be avoided in diaper rash because they can also irritate the skin. The use of commercial baby wipes is controversial. Some are chemically bland for use on diaper rash, but the friction of their use may be irritating. Commercial baby wipes should be considered for use with great caution. Some wipes contain alcohol, perfumes, soap, and other ingredients that can cause contact dermatitis, or actually burn or sting the infant, leading to pain, further irritation, and a screaming infant.[18,19]

The controversy over the use of disposable versus cloth diapers continues. The trend, however, is toward the use of disposable diapers and is probably driven by convenience to the caregiver, by advertising, and by a quelling of environmental issues with the advent of biodegradable disposable diapers. As the technology of disposable diapers has improved, the disposable diaper has become a critical component of nondrug therapy for diaper rash. Disposable diapers are now available in various absorbencies to match the waste output of the infant. Some disposable diapers are available that contain absorptive gel beads that pull the moisture away from direct contact with the skin to reduce maceration and the mixing of urine with feces. Newer still is a disposable diaper that has the protectant already in the diaper. These innovations in the technology would seem to favor the disposable diaper. This conclusion is supported by acceptable studies[19–22] that compare cloth and disposable diapers as well as low- versus high-absorbency disposable diapers.

If cloth diapers are used, the following guidelines should be observed:

- Wash with mild detergent.
- Avoid harsh detergents and water softeners.
- If bleach or other bactericidal agents are used, conduct additional rinses to remove chlorine or chemical residues.

Case Study 30–2

Patient Complaint/History

A frustrated mother calls you at the pharmacy during a down time and tells you the following story. Her 5-month-old child has diaper rash. The child has had the rash intermittently over a period of 6 weeks. She started out using the standard therapy of a zinc oxide ointment product, and for several days the diaper rash got better. She increased the frequency of diaper changes, even resorting to changing the diaper during the night. After 3 days of improvement, she opened the diaper one morning and found that full-blown diaper rash had returned.

Again, she went through a week of therapy, alternating zinc oxide and A&D ointment. This time she resorted to prophylactic corn starch when the lesions appeared to be close to resolution. She had no problem for 4 days; then it came back again. This time she took the child to her doctor who diagnosed diaper rash and gave her a prescription steroid cream to help heal the lesions. She tried the product for a week and got some decline in the rash, but it never really went away.

The mother informed her doctor by telephone of the status of the rash. He then recommended that she bathe the child daily in colloidal oatmeal, continue the prescription ointment, and use Tucks disposable wipes to clean the child during diaper changes. The doctor also had her seat the child for 15 minutes in a solution of aluminum acetate each evening before bedtime. She changed to a so-called "rash prevention" diaper. She followed this regimen over a 2-week period, and the skin seemed to return to normal. The child had not complained.

An additional 5 days went by, and again one morning she had the surprise of a bright, wet-looking bottom on the child at the morning diaper change. Again she called the doctor who told her the child had the "most stubborn case of diaper rash I have ever seen." He made another appointment for her for the following week.

The mother and her doctor tried everything they could think of to give this child lasting relief, but the mother thought she would call her pharmacist for other recommendations. When asked about cultures and blood tests, she replied that the physician did culture the diaper rash area and took a blood sample.

Questioning about the use of other medications and the history of fever reveals that the child is taking only the medications mentioned and occasionally has a high temperature that never exceeds 100°F. When asked about the child's diet, the mother replies she is breast-feeding and has had no difficulty in feeding the child. Questions about her health reveals that she had a candidal infection over a month ago but the infant is not showing signs of thrush (white patches in the throat).

Clinical Considerations/Strategies

Readers can use the following considerations/strategies to determine whether treatment of the disorder with nonprescription medications is warranted:

- Evaluate the diaper hygiene in this infant.
- Evaluate the significance of the child's temperature.
- Evaluate the appropriateness of the self-treatments if the disorder was uncomplicated diaper rash.
- Determine possible causes of this rash other than the common causes of poor diaper hygiene, diet, or medication use.
- Determine the appropriate treatment approach for recalcitrant rashes.

Patient Education/Counseling

Readers can use the following strategies to develop a patient education/counseling plan that will help ensure optimal therapeutic outcomes:

- Advise the mother that the steps she has taken should have cleared up an uncomplicated diaper rash.
- Advise her to take the child back to the physician for further evaluation but to continue the present treatments until she sees the physician.

Another suggestion from caregivers is to place a cup of vinegar in the final rinse water of a half-full wash load to lower the pH of the diapers. Exposing the diapers to ultraviolet (UV) radiation by hanging them to dry in the sun has a bactericidal effect, and the heat of ironing diapers can further kill bacteria, fungi, and yeasts. A commercial diaper service may be a more convenient way to accomplish this preventive measure because reputable diaper services sterilize diapers, press them, and return them neatly folded.

Pharmacologic Therapy

The FDA's review panel did not address or classify ingredients for use in diaper rash drug products. In 1990, FDA issued proposed rules for four types of products: antimicrobials, external analgesics, skin protectants, and antifungals. Subsequently in 1993, FDA ruled that antifungal and external analgesic ingredients are not permitted and that an approved new drug application would be required for such ingredients. Since 1993, labeling claims for antifungal or external analgesics for diaper rash are considered misbranding and subject to FDA enforcement action. Meanwhile, FDA has not issued final rules for the skin protectant or the antimicrobial monographs.

Skin Protectants

The skin protectants are a group of products that serve as a physical barrier between the skin and outside irritants. By preventing further insult or aggravation, they protect surfaces that are healing. Protectants serve as a lubricant in ar-

Table 30–1

Skin Protectants Approved to Treat Diaper Rash

Agent	Concentration (%)
Allantoin	0.5–2
Calamine	1–25
Cod liver oil (in combination)	5–13.5
Dimethicone	1–3
Kaolin	4–20
Lanolin (in combination)	15.5
Mineral oil	50–100
Petrolatum	30–100
Talc	45–100
Topical cornstarch	10–98
White petrolatum	30–100
Zinc oxide	1–25
Zinc oxide ointment	25–40

Source: Reference 10.

eas of the skin in which skin-to-skin or skin-to-diaper friction could aggravate diaper rash or could predispose to diaper rash. Protectants absorb moisture or prevent moisture, including urine and feces, from coming into direct contact with the skin. The protective effects of these products allow the body's normal healing processes to work. In 1990, FDA proposed the 12 ingredients listed in Table 30–1—all skin protectants—for treating diaper rash.[10]

It is common for two or more of the proposed ingredients to be combined in commercial products for treating diaper rash. Proposed ingredients for diaper rash have been combined with ingredients that are not protectants, which has produced combinations of dubious usefulness. Also, products that contain a proposed ingredient may be combined with an ingredient that is unsafe for treating diaper rash. A benzocaine ointment product contains a protectant base and petrolatum; however, the benzocaine is not useful or approved for diaper rash and can lead to sensitization when applied to macerated skin. Products that are intended for use as first aid and that contain one or more antibacterials may have a protectant as their vehicle, but they are not suitable for use on diaper rash. Because a product has an acceptable diaper rash ingredient in the formulation does not make it satisfactory for use on diaper rash. The other ingredient(s) may be unsuitable or even toxic when applied to skin impaired by diaper rash. Hence, pharmacists should recommend only those products that are labeled for diaper rash or that contain only one or more of the 12 proposed ingredients.

Zinc oxide is a mild astringent with minor antiseptic properties, but it is an excellent protectant. Zinc oxide is typically formulated as a powder or ointment dosage form. The ointment is acceptable in concentrations of 1% to 40%. Other dosage forms are acceptable only up to 25%. Zinc oxide paste USP is a preparation containing 25% zinc oxide, 25% corn starch, and 50% white petrolatum; it is a seminal example of the protectant group of products. The major drawback to the zinc oxide products is that they are tacky to the touch at higher concentrations and removal from the skin requires wiping with mineral oil. Zinc oxide preparations are often combined with other ingredients that may or may not have FDA recommendation. Ingredients such as vitamins A and D, peruvian balsam, silicone, aluminum acetate, aluminum hydroxide, microporous cellulose, colloidal oatmeal, glycerin, sodium bicarbonate, or aloe vera may be found in combination with zinc oxide. Use of plain zinc oxide paste avoids irritation and possible allergic response from additive ingredients. A 40% zinc oxide product has been compared to soap and talcum powder for treatment of diaper rash; zinc oxide ointment was found to be superior.[23] Few useful comparative studies of the protectants are available. Existing comparisons are complicated by added ingredients, poor study design, and an inability to rule out the benefits of the bases used versus the added ingredients.

Calamine, a mixture of zinc and ferrous oxides, has absorption properties and is available in numerous dosage forms. Allantoin is rarely seen as a single-entity product. It is a purine that complexes with and renders harmless many sensitizing agents on the skin. Mineral oil coats the skin with a water-impenetrable film that must be washed off with each diaper change to avoid buildup in pores and subsequent folliculitis. Lanolin is proposed for use only in combination with other ingredients. By itself, lanolin is very tacky and difficult to remove by washing. Some people are allergic to lanolin, and it should not appear in products at more than 20% concentration, whereby it may become irritating.[10]

Petrolatum is a yellow oleaginous hydrocarbon that, when decolorized, becomes white petrolatum. In either form, it is an excellent protectant and a ubiquitous ointment base. Kaolin is a clay-like material of hydrated aluminum silicate. It is mined from the earth and then highly purified. This protectant absorbs moisture and perspiration. Cod liver oil is a protectant oil that is rich in vitamin A. (In alternative medicine, vitamin A is thought to be a wound-healing agent.) Dimethicone is a silicone-based oil that repels water and that soothes and counteracts inflammation.

Talc and topical corn starch are almost exclusively used as loose powders and have a long history of use in diaper rash and prickly heat. Talc is a finely milled form of hydrous magnesium silicate, and it is more a lubricant than an absorbent. It reduces friction between folds of skin and between body parts, such as the thighs, buttocks, and inguinal area. It adheres well to the skin, but it should never be applied to broken or oozing skin because it can cake on the edges of wounds and can lead to infection or retard healing.

Talc carries an FDA warning against inhalation of the powder because of a history of injury and fatality from improper use of the powder in infants.[10] Corn starch carries the same FDA warning against inhalation as does talc. The warning states: "Do not use on broken skin. Keep powder away from child's face to avoid inhalation, which can cause breathing problems." Powders should be carefully applied close to the body at the place of application.

Corn starch, which is literally derived from the grain heads of corn plants, is effective as an absorbent. The use of corn starch in diaper rash has been controversial because yeasts are known to thrive on cornstarch, metabolizing it to ethanol. No controlled studies show a cause-and-effect relationship between the use of corn starch on diaper rash and the onset of yeast infections. Corn starch and talc are often combined with other ingredients (e.g., magnesium stearate) to increase adhesion of the products to the skin. Calcium carbonate, zinc stearate, and microporous cellulose may be added to increase absorption of moisture.

Because the skin protectants are remarkably safe, their use either as treatment or as prophylaxis is acceptable. An infant with no diaper rash symptoms should not be exposed to diaper rash products needlessly. If the infant has diaper rash, or if the infant has recently had a bout of diaper rash, then prophylaxis with these products is reasonable. If diaper rash is anticipated, as when an infant has a history of diarrhea or diaper rash or both when being treated with an antibiotic, prophylaxis may be warranted. If prophylaxis is used for some length of time, it should be discontinued periodically to determine whether further use is still necessary.[10]

Contraindicated Agents

Patients with secondary infections (viral, bacterial, or fungal) should not be treated with nonprescription products. The general public is not considered adequately educated or trained to diagnose and treat infectious diseases in infants in the inguinal area. Topical nonprescription antibiotic and antifungal agents are, therefore, not appropriate to use in diaper rash. External analgesics are not recommended because they can alter sensory perception in a population that cannot communicate changes in sensory perception.[10] They may excoriate macerated skin, be painful, retard healing, and further complicate diaper rash.

Hydrocortisone, although indicated for minor skin irritation, should not be used in diaper rash without a physician's supervision. In infants, this contraindication is especially true for a number of reasons. Hydrocortisone may suppress local immune response, an action that may be undesirable if even the threat of secondary infection exists. Second, the diaper area is a significant portion of the infant's body surface area. Hydrocortisone absorption into the skin is enhanced under occlusive conditions. When applied to macerated skin or a large surface area, absorption of hydrocortisone may lead to therapeutic blood levels that interfere with the pituitary–adrenal axis of the infant. It may also cause local skin atrophy. Nonprescription hydrocortisone is labeled not to be used in patients younger than 2 years.[2,8,9] (See Chapter 27, "Atopic Dermatitis, Contact Dermatitis, and Dry Skin," for further discussion of this agent.)

Product Selection Guidelines

Caregivers for diaper rash patients should be informed that drug therapy is only an adjunct to good diaper hygiene and diaper changing practices. When there is diaper rash, the pharmacist should inform caregivers about their choices be-

Table 30–2

Selected Products for Diaper Dermatitis and Prickly Heat

Trade Name	Primary Ingredients
A + D Ointment with Zinc Oxide	Zinc oxide 10%; dimethicone 1%
A + D Original Ointment	Petrolatum 80.5%; lanolin 15.5%
Aveeno Bath Treatment Moisturizing Formula Powder	Colloidal oatmeal 43%; mineral oil
Aveeno Bath Treatment Soothing Formula Powder	Colloidal oatmeal 100%
Desitin Ointment	Zinc oxide 40%; cod liver oil; petrolatum; lanolin; talc
Desitin Cornstarch Baby Powder	Zinc oxide 10%; corn starch 88.2%
Desitin Creamy Ointment	Zinc oxide 10%; dimethicone; petrolatum; mineral oil
Diaparene Cornstarch Baby Powder	Corn starch 88%
Johnson's Baby Cream	Dimethicone 2%; lanolin; mineral oil
Johnson's Baby Powder	Talc
Johnson's Baby Powder Cornstarch	Corn starch 95%
Johnson's Medicated Baby Powder	Zinc oxide; corn starch
Johnson's Diaper Rash Ointment	Petrolatum; zinc oxide; benzethonium chloride (antimicrobials not recommended for diaper rash)
Mexsana Medicated Powder	Zinc oxide 10.8%; corn starch; kaolin; benzethonium chloride (antimicrobials not recommended for diaper rash)
Vaseline Pure Petroleum Jelly	White petrolatum 100%

tween solid and powdered protectants. (See Table 30–2 for examples of commercially available products.) Caregivers may be more comfortable with a semisolid product if the patient does not find the hands-on application painful or uncomfortable or if there is anxiety about the inhalation warning on the powders. Semisolid products can be applied with disposable tongue depressors or washable rubber spatulas. Caregivers can also apply the products while wearing rubber gloves if they desire. If the powders are chosen, it is important to describe to the caregiver how to apply the products to avoid inhalation pneumonitis. The pharmacist should point out expiration dates on both types of products. It is important to distinguish between acute and prophylactic use of the products to outline therapeutic end points. Fortunately, the products in this category are relatively inexpensive, and socioeconomic status tends not to be a major issue in treating diaper rash. Infant caregivers may need to be reassured that, at one time or another, the overwhelming majority of infants have an episode of diaper rash and that this pathology is not a social stigma.

Pharmacists should advise caregivers of agents to be avoided (i.e., alcohol wipes) and of product ingredients that may be useless or even harmful. Although the products in this therapeutic category generally have a wide margin of safety, the pharmacist should not recommend them indiscriminately.

Patient Assessment of Diaper Dermatitis

When a parent or guardian consults a pharmacist about a suspected diaper rash, the pharmacist should find out whether factors conducive to diaper dermatitis are present. Specifically, the parent should be asked what type of diaper is being used and how frequently diapers are changed. Drawing on that response, the pharmacist must consider whether increasing the frequency of diaper changes would reduce the diaper rash problem.

If cloth diapers are used, the pharmacist should find out how they are laundered and should determine whether the laundering method is adequate to remove chemical residues or fecal bacteria. The pharmacist should also ask how the infant is cleaned during diaper changes. The parent's response may indicate a cleaning method that does not remove all fecal bacteria or the use of commercial wipes that may cause skin irritation. To find out whether occlusion of the diaper area is a problem, the pharmacist should find out whether plastic pants are being used with the diaper or whether high absorbency diapers are being used.

Asking the parent or caregiver the following questions will help elicit the information needed to accurately assess the disorder and to recommend the appropriate treatment approach.

Q~ What does the "rash" look like?

A~ *Identify the typical symptoms of diaper rash. (See the section "Pathophysiology/Signs and Symptoms of Diaper Dermatitis.")* If the infant's diaper area has an onion-skin-like appearance, suspect chronic contact dermatitis. (See Chapter 27, "Atopic Dermatitis, Contact Dermatitis, and Dry Skin," for discussion of this disorder.) If raised lesions with well-demarcated borders are present, suspect early bullae formation. If the lesions are donut-shaped, tiny white scales, suspect yeast infection. (See Chapter 35, "Minor Wounds and Skin Infections.") Refer these infections to a physician.

Q~ Does the diaper rash have regular or irregular borders?

A~ Refer to a physician any rash with unusual or irregular lesions that look like patterned warts or that have what looks like white or silvery patches in the skin folds. These manifestations could suggest hepatic infection, candidal dermatitis, or candidiasis superimposed over diaper rash.

Q~ Does the infant have a fever?

A~ If yes, consider systemic infection or infectious diarrhea that can be an underlying cause of diaper rash. Refer either case to a physician for resolution. Often, eliminating the diarrhea will make a major contribution to clearing up the diaper rash.

Q~ Has the infant had fungal (yeast) infections on the skin, the genitals, or the mouth? Does the mother have a history of vaginal candidal infections?

A~ In either of these situations, suspect a candidal superinfection in the diaper region. Refer such cases to a physician.

Q~ Has the infant recently been weaned? Has any other change of diet occurred on or near the onset of the diaper rash?

A~ If weaning occurred recently, consider a diaper rash caused by changes in the pH of the skin, feces, or urine brought about by changes in the pH of the diet. If diaper rash does not quite fit the normal description, consider some form of deficiency in the diet that may manifest as diaper rash (e.g., *Acrodermatitis enteropathica* or a zinc deficiency.)[2]

Q~ Does your family have a history of allergic disorders, or is the child using any medication?

A~ Consider allergic contact dermatitis or atopic dermatitis in the diaper region if an allergic history exists. Consider diaper dermatitis related to drug-induced diarrhea if the child is taking medications, especially antibiotics.

Q~ Is the skin in the diaper area broken? Is the infant acutely distressed, or does he or she cry violently following or during urination or defecation?

A~ If the skin is broken, caution the parent that secondary

bacterial infection could occur. If urination or defecation is causing distress, suspect severe diaper rash. In either situation, refer the patient to a physician to prevent further complications, such as adhesions and scarring of the genitals or infection of the penis or vulva that could progress to urinary tract infection.

Q~ Have you seen major changes in the infant's behavior with the onset of the diaper rash? Is the infant lethargic or less alert than previously?

A~ If yes, refer the infant to a physician for evaluation of early signs of a serious systemic problem that has manifested initially as a diaper rash.

Q~ Is there a history of repeat or multiple infections in the infant?

A~ If yes, refer the infant to a physician. Refer the following infants for immediate medical attention: infants who present with diaper rash accompanied by failure to thrive; bleeding lesions; fever of unknown origin; chronic otitis media; swollen lymph nodes; swollen lips, hands or feet; peeling skin; abdominal enlargement; or other unusual signs or symptoms.

Q~ How long has the child had the rash? What have you done to treat it?

A~ Refer to a physician those infants whose rash has been present a week or more without treatment or whose rash has been present a week or longer and reasonable nonprescription therapy has not resulted in improvement or elimination.

Patient Education for Diaper Dermatitis

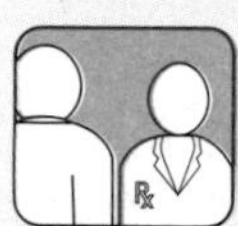

The objectives of self-treatment are to (1) eliminate the rash, (2) relieve the symptoms, and (3) prevent recurrent rashes. For most patients, carefully following product instructions and the self-care measures listed below will help ensure optimal therapeutic outcomes.

Nondrug Measures

- Change diapers frequently, at least six times a day, to prevent prolonged exposure of the infant's skin to moisture and feces.
- To prevent occlusion of skin in the diaper area, avoid putting rubber pants over cloth diapers or using highly absorbent disposable diapers. Tightly covering the skin causes it to break down.
- During every diaper change, flush the infant's skin with plain water and gently pat it dry.
- Do not wipe the infant with any part of the diaper. Even areas that appear unsoiled may be contaminated with fecal bacteria.
- To prevent irritating the infant's skin, do not use detergent or ordinary lye-based soaps to launder diapers; starched or very stiff diapers; and commercial baby wipes that contain alcohol, perfumes, and soap, which may burn or sting the skin.

Nonprescription Medications

- To treat diaper rash, use a product containing one or more of the skin protectants listed in Table 30–1. The product can be used even after the rash clears to prevent recurrences, but use should be stopped for a short time to see whether the rash returns.
- Do not use products that contain ingredients listed in Table 30–1 combined with benzocaine or an antibacterial such as benzethonium chloride. Benzocaine can cause an allergic reaction; antibacterials are not suitable for use on diaper rash.
- Do not use hydrocortisone or external analgesics such as phenol, menthol, methyl salicylate, or capsaicin to treat diaper rash. These medications are inappropriate for use on infant skin.
- Sprinkle or gently rub powders onto the skin, using a sufficient amount to cover the affected area. Keep powder away from the child's face to avoid inhalation that can cause breathing problems.
- Apply sufficient cream or ointment by hand or with a disposable or washable spatula to cover the affected area.
- If using mineral oil, wash it off at every diaper change to avoid clogging skin pores, which may lead to folliculitis, an inflammation of hair follicles.
- Do not apply products containing talc to broken or oozing skin because it can cake on the edges of wounds and lead to infection or can retard healing.
- Discard products that are discolored or whose expiration date has passed.

Consult a physician if any of the following occur:

—The rash does not improve after 7 days of treatment, or the symptoms worsen despite therapy.
—Symptoms such as fever, nausea, vomiting, or diarrhea occur.
—The affected skin ruptures or pus forms.
—The diaper rash causes pain on urination or defecation.
—The infant cries incessantly.
—Concurrent dermatitis appears on other parts of the body.
—The rash spreads outside the diaper area.
—The infant develops a fever or becomes lethargic.
—The rash recurs repeatedly.

Patient Counseling for Diaper Dermatitis

The pharmacist should review proper cleaning of the diaper area with the parents or guardian. The caregivers should be cautioned to avoid occlusion of the area and to prevent prolonged contact of urine or feces with the infant's skin. The pharmacist should explain the proper methods of applying nonprescription skin protectants and should warn the caregivers of signs and symptoms that indicate the dermatitis has worsened and needs medical attention. The box "Patient Education for Diaper Dermatitis" lists specific information to provide patients.

Evaluation of Patient Outcomes for Diaper Dermatitis

Treatment of diaper dermatitis should be relatively short—approximately a week. If 7 days have elapsed and the condition is improved but not healed, therapy should be continued beyond the seventh day until healing has occurred. If the condition has not improved or has worsened at the seventh day, a physician should be consulted. At each diaper change, the parent should inspect the lesions for signs of improvement. At the end of therapy, the skin should have returned to normal.

Prickly Heat

Epidemiology of Prickly Heat

Prickly heat has a more even age distribution than does diaper rash in that it can occur at any age in anyone who has active sweat glands. It is probably significantly underreported because it is less troublesome than diaper rash is and clears up very rapidly if left alone and/or if its cause is removed. Prickly heat occurs in infants and the elderly, and in any age group in between. Because the elderly are less tolerant to heat, sweat less, are less physically active, and spend more time indoors and in controlled environments than do younger people, they may have less opportunity to develop prickly heat.

Etiology of Prickly Heat

Prickly heat results from blocked or plugged sweat glands. Prickly heat can arise from quite normal skin with little or no anatomic prodrome. The condition is most often associated with very hot, humid weather or can occur during illnesses that cause significant or profuse sweating. It can also result from inability of the skin to "breathe" (interact with air) because of wearing excessive clothing, wearing very tight clothing, wearing occlusive clothing such as leather and polyester, or wearing athletic protective or safety garments and devices.

Pathophysiology/Signs and Symptoms of Prickly Heat

In prickly heat, the pores that house the sweat glands are obstructed. The inability of sweat to be secreted and to escape the pore causes dilation and rupture of the epidermal sweat pores. This situation causes an acute inflammation of the dermis that may manifest as stinging, burning, or itching. The pinpoint-sized lesions are raised and red or maroon, forming erythematous papules. (See the "Color Plates," photograph 14.) Common sites for prickly heat dermatitis include the axilla (arm pits), chest, upper back, back of the neck, abdomen, and inguinal area. The lesions usually follow the pattern of the occlusion and, in uncomplicated cases, do not extend beyond the occlusion area. Lesions can occur on the body wherever occlusion occurs. If the lesions are not tended to in a reasonable length of time, they can evolve into the same kinds of complications seen in diaper rash (e.g., infection, pustule formation, generalized dermatitis).

Treatment of Prickly Heat

Treatment Outcomes

The lesions of prickly heat will resolve without pharmacologic treatment if the cause is removed; therefore, eliminating the cause is the overall goal.

General Treatment Approach

The steps in nonpharmacologic therapy of prickly heat include (1) reducing occlusion of the skin, (2) protecting the skin from further irritation, (3) promoting healing of the skin, and (4) discouraging the onset of secondary bacterial infection.

Some of the steps in pharmacologic therapy have the same goal as the nondrug measures but involve the use of nonprescription products. These products help to (1) keep the skin dry, (2) promote healing, (3) soothe any discomfort caused by the lesion(s), and (4) discourage the onset of secondary infection. The algorithm in Figure 30–2 outlines the self-treatment of prickly heat.

Nonpharmacologic Therapy

Nondrug therapy for prickly heat consists of decreasing sweating. Letting the patient rest, cool off, or enter a cool environment is a start. If the sweating is caused by a fever, the use of internal antipyretics is appropriate, if not contraindicated. The wearing of loose, light-colored, and light-weight clothing is palliative in prickly heat and is also good prevention if it allows air flow to the skin. In infants, frequent diaper changes and the sparing use of soap or chemical irritants can reduce the discomfort of existing prickly heat. Bathing or soaking in bath products such as colloidal oatmeal can be soothing and can make the skin more comfortable. Pharmacists should warn patients not to apply oleaginous or oily substances to prickly heat lesions because these substances plug up the pores that need to be patent.

Pharmacologic Therapy

Nonprescription treatment of prickly heat should be limited to mild-to-moderate, uncomplicated cases. The contraindication for using hydrocortisone to treat diaper rash in infants also applies to its use in prickly heat. However, in the adult, hydrocortisone may be useful if the surface area involved is equal to or less than approximately 10% of the body surface area. Prickly heat should not be occluded during therapy.

Case Study 30–3

Patient Complaint/History

Dewey, who appears to be in his late teens or early 20s, approaches the pharmacist for advice about a rash on his upper chest, upper back, and inner surface of the upper arm. He describes the rash as tiny little red "bumps" that were "itchy." He says he observed them when he woke up this morning. He speculates that some insect must have bitten him. He reports that the rash felt better after a hot shower and the bumps "don't itch much now." He wants to know what the disorder is and what medicine he should use for it. He has not tried to treat it.

Visual inspection of the rash reveals a fine red rash that has discrete lesions without a red or raised base. The distribution is over the areas the patient described and is without any coalescence, signs of skin breakage, or indications of infection.

When asked about insect infestation of his residence, the patient reports no suspected infestation until now. Questioning about his allergy history reveals no known allergies. When asked about recent activities that could have caused sweating, the patient replies he danced for about 7 hours at a party the previous night and then went to bed in his clothes: a western shirt of silk material with a leather yoke, jeans, boots, and a leather rodeo belt. The patient reports that the shirt was still "pretty yucky" when he awoke this morning. He denies having symptoms such as headache, fever, nausea, vomiting; he experienced only a "little sour stomach from eating junk food and drinking beer."

Clinical Considerations/Strategies

Readers can use the following considerations/strategies to determine whether treatment of the disorder with nonprescription medications is warranted:

- Determine possible causes of the rash.
- Drawing on the patient's reaction to the symptoms, determine the severity of the disorder.
- On the basis of its manifestation, determine whether the prickly heat is self-treatable.
- Determine the appropriate treatment approach.

Patient Education/Counseling

Readers can use the following strategies to develop a patient education/counseling plan that will help ensure optimal therapeutic outcomes:

- Explain the factors that caused the disorder.
- Explain how to treat the disorder and prevent recurrences.
- Explain the signs and symptoms that indicate medical attention is needed.

Prickly heat can be ameliorated in less time resulting in less total drug exposure than in diaper rash. Because prickly heat rapidly clears without drug therapy, the only real use for hydrocortisone would be to relieve itching. For prickly heat, washing the skin with bland soap and soaking in colloidal oatmeal may be all that is needed with infants. (See Chapter 27, "Atopic Dermatitis, Contact Dermatitis, and Dry Skin," for discussion of colloidal oatmeal products.)

Oral antihistamines might be both safer and more economical than hydrocortisone application in older children and adults. (See Chapter 9, "Disorders Related to Cold and Allergy," for discussion of oral antihistamines.) Topical antihistamines carry the risk of sensitization, and their effectiveness is doubtful. (See Chapter 31, "Insect Bites and Stings and Pediculosis," for discussion of topical antihistamines.)

Petrolatum and oils are not desirable in prickly heat because they trap moisture beneath it and keep the area hydrated. In prickly heat, the patient should keep the skin dry and moisture dissipated. To absorb moisture and help prevent wetness, powders are more appropriate. However, prolonged use or overuse of powders can lead to clogged pores and can precipitate prickly heat. If applied to the chest or neck, as in the case of prickly heat, corn starch or talc powder should be placed in the hand and manually applied to the skin with light friction. Pharmacists should be very careful not to recommend any product for infants that has an ingredient (e.g., phenols or boric acid) that could be toxic if easily absorbed through thin, compromised skin.

For prickly heat, the choice of a drug product should be limited to one product that relieves burning and itching and that does not block skin exposure to the air. The patient should avoid oleaginous products. A powder may be acceptable to help dry the skin, or a water-washable antipruritic product may be used. (See Table 30–2 for examples of commercially available products.)

Bathing or showering with a mild soap or soaking in a tub of colloidal oatmeal may be adequate to reduce or to stop burning or itching.

Patient Assessment of Prickly Heat

Patient assessment for prickly heat involves identifying the site of the lesions and having patients reconstruct their activities and attire over the past 24 hours. If the patient is an infant, the pharmacist should ask whether the infant sleeps in a warm or humid environment and whether additional clothing or occlusive coverings are used at night or when the infant is asleep.

Patient Counseling for Prickly Heat

The pharmacist should stress to the patient that prickly heat is easily prevented by removing factors that clog skin pores.

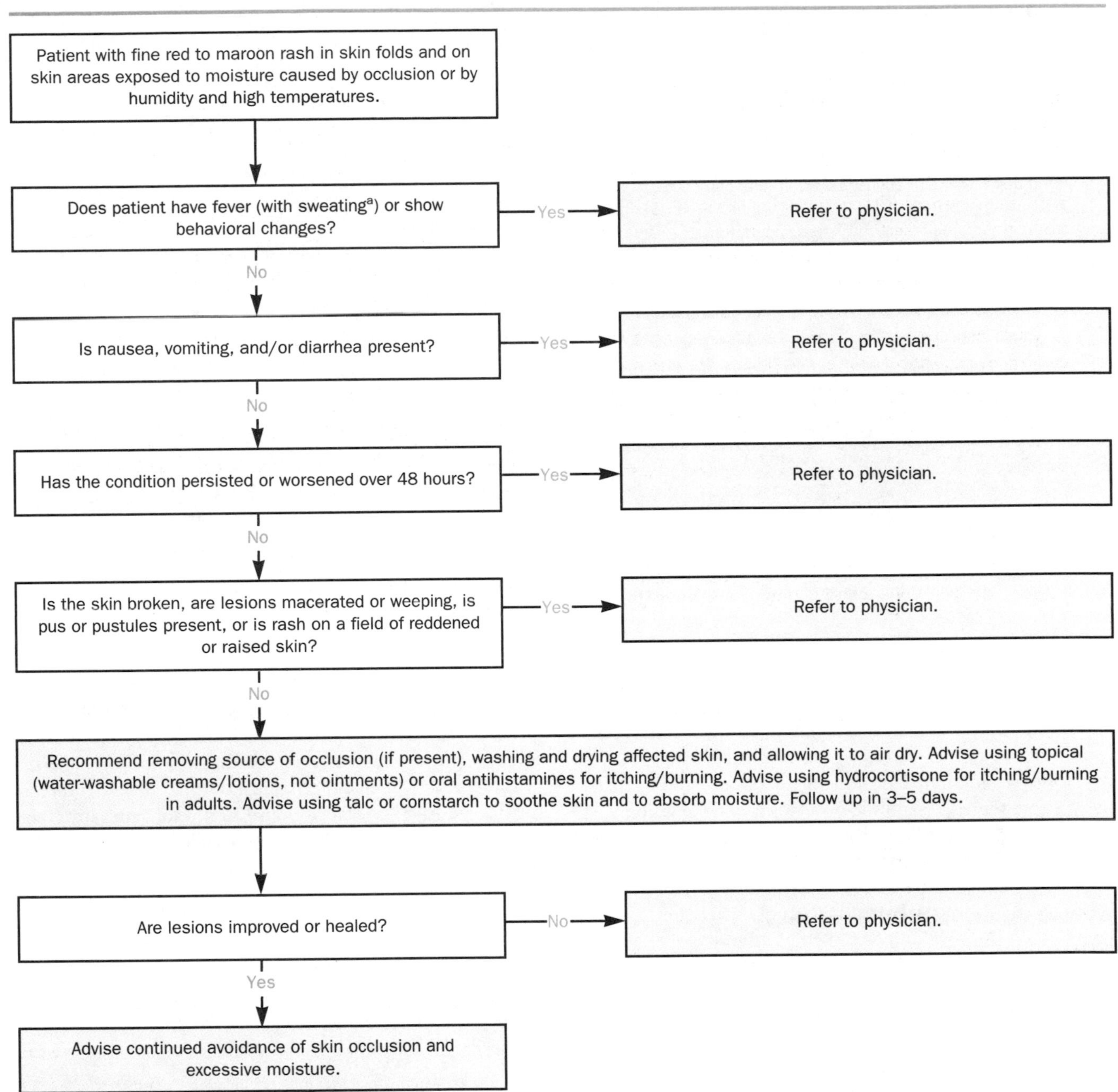

[a] High fever without sweating, high pulse rate, possible increased respiration, or hot flushed dry skin (patient seems to be "burning up") may indicate hyperpyrexia ("heat stroke" or "sunstroke"). Refer the patient immediately to a physician and/or transport patient to an emergency facility. Slow or weak pulse, lethargy, cold pale clammy skin, absence of fever, or disorientation may indicate heat exhaustion. Move patient to a cool environment, and have the patient recline and take regular sips of water or slightly salty liquids or electrolyte solutions every few minutes.

Figure 30–2 Self-care of prickly heat.

Appropriate nondrug and drug measures for healing a prickly heat rash should be explained. The pharmacist should explain that skin protectants can exacerbate the disorder. The box "Patient Education for Prickly Heat" lists specific information to provide patients.

Evaluation of Patient Outcomes for Prickly Heat

Treatment of prickly heat should be relatively short—approximately a week. This disorder may take less time to heal.

Patient Education for Prickly Heat

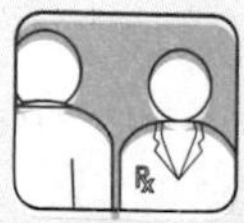

The objectives of self-treatment are (1) to relieve the discomfort of prickly heat and (2) to eliminate its cause. For most patients, carefully following product instructions and the self-care measures listed below will help ensure optimal therapeutic outcomes.

Nondrug Measures

- To prevent clogging skin pores, avoid excessive sweating by resting, cooling off, or going to a cool environment.
- Wear loose, light-colored, and light-weight clothing to allow air flow to the skin.
- Decrease the discomfort of prickly heat in infants by changing diapers frequently and by using soaps or possible chemical irritants (e.g., baby wipes) sparingly.

Nonprescription Medications

- Unless a pharmacist or physician advises otherwise, use internal analgesics (e.g., aspirin, acetaminophen, ibuprofen, ketoprofen, or naproxen) to reduce a fever and the sweating it can cause.
- Do not apply oleaginous or oily substances to prickly heat lesions because they clog skin pores.
- Use powdered skin protectants to absorb moisture and help prevent wetness. (See Table 30–2.) Place corn starch or talc powder in the hand, and apply to the skin with light friction. Note that prolonged use or overuse of powders can lead to clogged pores and can precipitate prickly heat.
- Do not use hydrocortisone on infants. However, it may be used to relieve itching in adult cases of prickly heat if no more than 10% of the body surface area is involved.
- For older children and adults, consider using oral antihistamines for relief of itching. Note that topical antihistamines can cause allergic reactions.
- To soothe discomfort in infants, wash the skin with bland soap or soak the skin in colloidal oatmeal.

If the condition has not improved or has worsened after 7 days of treatment, consult a physician.

If the condition is improved after 7 days of treatment, therapy should be continued until healing has occurred. If the condition has not improved or has worsened at the seventh day, a physician should be consulted. Monitoring of treatment success involves simple observation of the lesions. At the end of therapy, the skin should have returned to normal.

CONCLUSIONS

Diaper rash and prickly heat are two dermatologic conditions that are caused by a combination of environmental factors, the most important of which are moisture and occlusion. The pharmacist should be prepared to help the patient distinguish between ordinary diaper rash or prickly heat and complicated cases that warrant referral to a physician. Fortunately, most diaper rash and prickly heat cases are mild and heal readily when the causes are removed. Both respond well to nonprescription products that are intended to treat them, and both are amenable to some fairly simple prophylactic measures. Prevention is still the best method to deal with the heat, humidity, and occlusion problems at the core of these pathologies.

In the case of diaper rash, prompt and regular changing of the diaper may bring a patient's risk of exposure to this disease to a minimum. As many as 20% of infants do not experience diaper rash at all. In the case of prickly heat, care should be taken to ensure that the skin always "breathes" and that clothing and equipment do not block sweat glands.

The drug treatments for these diseases consist of skin protectants primarily as powders and ointments that dry the skin, provide a physical barrier to further moisture, and lubricate the skin against mechanical trauma. By recommending preventive measures and rational therapy, the pharmacist can prevent medical complications, and reduce parent and caregiver anxieties.

References

1. Weston WL. *Practical Pediatric Dermatology*. 2nd ed. Boston: Little, Brown; 1985:1–2.
2. Hansen RC, Bernice R, Krafchik MB, et al. Diaper dermatitis. *Supplement to Contemporary Pediatrics*. Montvale, NJ: Medical Economics Company; 1998:8.
3. Jordan WE, Lawson KD, Berg RW, et al. Diaper dermatitis: frequency and severity among a general infant population. *Pediatr Dermatol*. 1986: 3:198–207.
4. Forsyth JS, Ogston SA, Clark A, et al. Relation between early introduction of solid food to infants and their weight and illnesses during the first two years of life. *Br Med J*. 1993;306(6892):1572–6.
5. Brown CP, Wilson FH. Diaper region irritations: pertinent facts and methods of prevention. *Clin Pediatr*. 1964;3:409–13.
6. Hara M, Watanabe M, Tagami H, et al. Jacquet erosive diaper dermatitis in a young girl with urinary incontinence. *Pediatr Dermatol*. 1991: 8:160–1.
7. Thiboutot DM, Beckford A, Mart CR, et al. Cytomegalovirus diaper dermatitis. *Arch Dermatol*. 1991;127:396–8.
8. Bluestein J, Furner BB, Phillips E. Granuloma gluteale infantus: case report and review of the literature. *Pediatr Dermatol*. 1990;7:196–8.
9. Friter BS, Luck AW. The perineal eruption of Kawasaki syndrome. *Arch Dermatol*. 1988;124:1805–10.
10. *Federal Register*. 1990;55:25246,25234,25204,25240.
11. Longhi F, Carlucci G, Bellucci R, et al. Diaper dermatitis: a study of contributing factors. *Contact Dermatitis*. 1992;26:248–52.

12. Berg RW. Etiologic factors in diaper dermatitis: a model for development of improved diapers. *Pediatrician.* 1987;14(suppl 1):27–33.
13. Sutton MB, Weitzman M, Howland J. Baby bottoms and environmental conundrums: disposable diapers and the pediatrician. *Pediatrics.* 1991;88:386–9.
14. Seitz ML. Disposable diapers vs the environment [letter; comment]. *Pediatrics.* 1992;89:523.
15. Scott N. Diaper debate continues [letter; comment]. *Pediatrics.* 1992;90:654–5.
16. Gowdy JM, Ulsamer AG. Hexachlorophene lesions in newborn infants. *Am J Dis Child.* 1976;130:247–50.
17. *Federal Register.* 1982;47:39415,39464.
18. Gallichio V. Nappy rash. *Aust Fam Physician.* 1988;17:971–2.
19. Sires UI, Mallory SB. Diaper dermatitis. *Postgrad Med.* 1995;98:79–82,84,86.
20. Austin AP, Milligan MC, Pennington K, et al. A survey of factors associated with diaper dermatitis in thirty-six pediatric practices. *J Pediatr Health Care.* 1988;2:295–9.
21. Campbell RL. Clinical tests with improved disposable diapers. *Pediatrician.* 1987;14(suppl 1):34–8.
22. Lane AT, Rehder PA, Helm K. Evaluations of diapers containing absorbent gelling material with conventional disposable diapers in newborn infants. *Am J Dis Child.* 1990;144:315–8.
23. Research report. New York: Leeming/Pacquin Pharmaceutical Co; 1974.

CHAPTER 31

Insect Bites and Stings and Pediculosis

Farid Sadik

Chapter 31 at a Glance

Insect bites and stings are common occurrences. The reaction to these injuries is usually local in nature and confined to a limited area of the vicinity of the site injury. However,

Editor's Note: This chapter is based, in part, on the 11th edition chapter titled "Insect Sting and Bite Products," which was written by Farid Sadik.

for a group of sensitive individuals, stings from some insects can produce allergic reactions that range from a mild reaction to potentially life-threatening anaphylaxis. Many of the deaths that occur as a result of anaphylaxis could be prevented if adequate precautions and treatment were initiated. Thousands of people are admitted annually to hospitals because of the allergic reactions precipitated by insect stings.

Most encounters with biting and stinging insects are brief. Pediculosis, or lice infestation, and scabies, however, are parasitic infections. The arachnids that cause these disorders will stay on the host until eradicated. Pediculosis is a common disorder, especially among children. In addition to being an annoying pest, lice can transmit diseases such as typhus.

Although the public usually refers to all biting and stinging invertebrate animals as "insects," such animals are members of the phylum Arthropoda, which includes insects, arachnids, and crustaceans. While this chapter covers only the stings of insects, it covers the bites of both insects and arachnids (ticks, mites, spiders, and lice). Because few patients will be familiar with the term "arthropod," the chapter uses the term "insect" to cover general statements about these invertebrates

Insect Bites

Epidemiology of Insect Bites

Individuals who enjoy outdoor activities, those whose occupation requires them to remain outdoors, and those who spend time in their backyard are at risk for insect bites and stings. Practically all victims of insect bites experience local reactions at the site of the injury. The exact number of people who experience systemic allergic reactions to the salivary secretions of biting insects is unknown.

Etiology of Insect Bites

Bites from insects such as mosquitoes, fleas, and bedbugs and from the arachnids ticks and chiggers are nonvenomous in nature. These insects usually attack and pierce the skin of the victim by inserting their biting organs to feed by sucking blood from their hosts. To keep the victim's blood flowing, an anticoagulant saliva, which consists of antigenic substances, is introduced into the pierced skin.

Mosquitoes

Mosquitoes are found in abundance worldwide, particularly in a humid, warm climate. Because mosquito larvae can live only in water, these insects always live and breed near wet areas. The adult mosquitoes become active in the evening.

Fleas

Fleas are tiny (1.5 to 4 mm long), bloodsucking, wingless, laterally compressed insects with strongly developed posterior legs used for leaping. Fleas act as parasites on various avian and mammalian hosts. Body warmth and exhaled carbon dioxide are believed to attract fleas to the host. Fleas are found throughout the world (including arctic regions), but they breed best in warm areas with relatively high humidity. They may survive and multiply without food for several weeks. However, females need a blood meal to deposit eggs. Places that have been vacant for weeks may be heavily infested, partly because of the hatching of eggs, which are usually deposited in floor crevices or on rugs, particularly those on which pets have been sleeping. Humans are often bitten by fleas after moving into a vacant, infested habitat or when living with infested pets. Fleas are not only annoying but also responsible for transmitting diseases, such as bubonic plague and endemic typhus.

Sarcoptes scabiei

Scabies, commonly called "the itch," is a contagious parasitic skin infection caused by *Sarcoptes scabiei,* a very small and rarely seen arachnid mite. It burrows beneath the stratum corneum but neither bites nor stings. This mite is transmitted from an infected individual to others through physical contact.

Bedbugs

Bedbugs have a short head and a broad, flat body (4 to 5 mm long and 3 mm wide). Bedbugs usually hide and deposit their eggs in crevices of walls, floors, picture frames, bedding, and other furniture. They normally hide during the day, become active at night, and bite their sleeping victims. People may also be bitten in subdued light by day while sitting in theaters or other public places.

Ticks

Ticks feed on the blood of humans and of both wild and domesticated animals. Certain species of ticks can transmit systemic disease such as Lyme disease. This disease was first recognized in 1975 when a number of juvenile rheumatoid arthritis cases occurred in Lyme, Connecticut. It was described and named by Dr. Allen Steere in 1977.[2] Five years later, Dr. Willy Burgdorf recognized that Lyme disease is a systemic infection caused by a spirochete found in deer ticks (*Ixodes dammini*) and is transmitted into the victim following tick bites. The spirochetes, which were named *Borrelia burgdorferi,* appear as irregular coils that range from 10 to 30 micrometers in length and 0.18 to 0.25 micrometers in diameter. The deer tick is very small compared with dog ticks; it is about one-eighth of an inch in diameter and, thus, is difficult to find as a parasite on animals. (See Figure 31–1 for the life cycle of the deer tick.) The tick inserts its mouthpiece into its prey to suck blood. During the feeding process, *B. burgdorferi* are released at the bite site and spread throughout the body through circulation to initiate the infection.

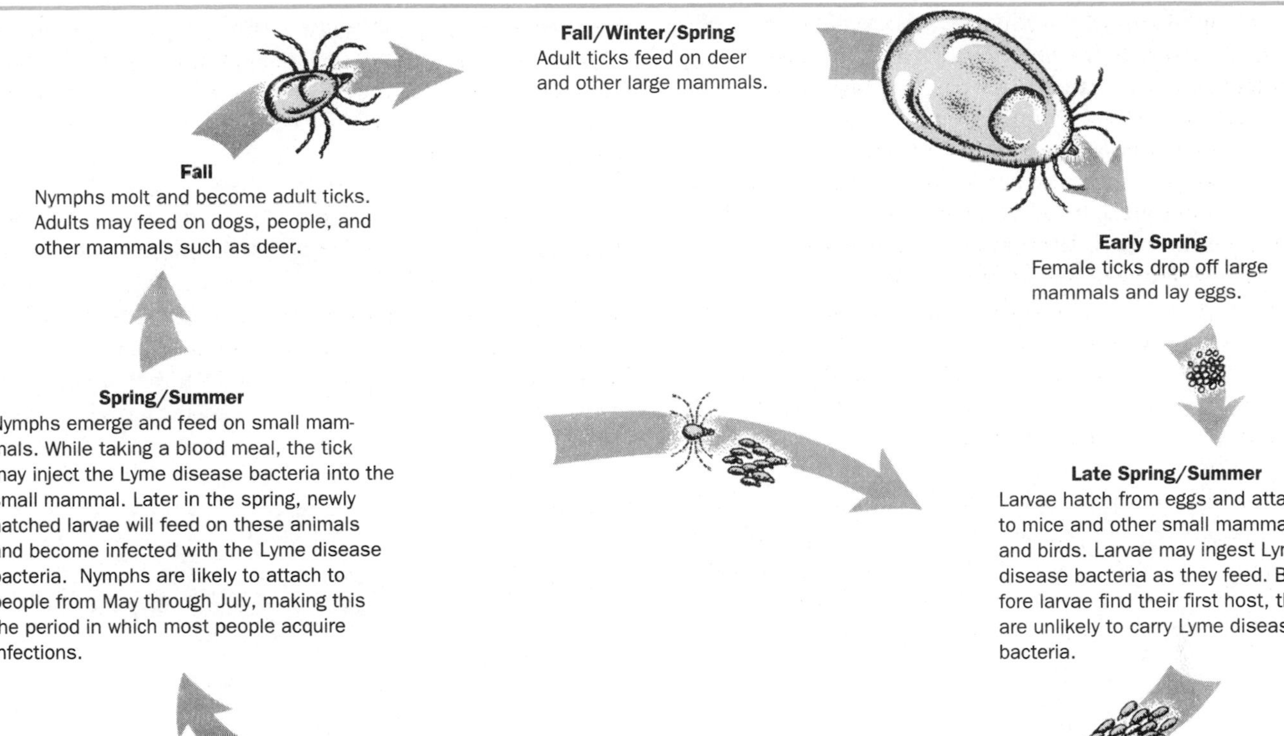

Figure 31–1 Life cycle of the deer tick (*Ixodes dammini*). Reprinted from: *Lyme Disease in Wisconsin: An Update.* Madison, WI: Wisconsin Department of Natural Resources and Department of Health and Social Services; 1989; used with permission.

Chiggers

Chiggers, or redbugs, are very annoying pests that live in shrubbery, trees, and grass. Only the chigger larvae bite. The larvae insert their mouthpart into the skin and secrete a digestive fluid that causes cellular disintegration of the affected area and intense itching.

Spiders

Spiders, including black widows, are found throughout the country, especially in the warmer regions. This spider's bite may not be noticed initially, but the victim may develop symptoms to the bite within a short time. Bites from the brown recluse spider are also initially painless but later may cause local and/or systemic reactions.

Pathophysiology/Signs and Symptoms of Insect Bites

As the following discussions show, each biting arthropod has distinctive biting organs and salivary secretions. These factors produce characteristic signs and symptoms for each type of bite.

Mosquitoes

When a mosquito alights on the skin, it cuts through the skin with its mandibles and maxillae. A fine, hollow-like, flexible structure (proboscis) is introduced into the cut and probes the tissue for a blood vessel. Blood is sucked directly from a capillary lumen or from previously lacerated capillaries with extravasated blood. During feeding, the mosquito injects into the wound a salivary secretion containing an anticoagulant and antigenic components that cause the characteristic sign of a welt and the symptom of itching. The bites usually occur on exposed parts of the body (face, neck, forearms, and legs), but mosquitoes can also bite through thin clothing.

Fleas

Flea bites are usually multiple and grouped. Most people are bitten by fleas about the legs and ankles. Each lesion, which is characterized by an erythematous region around the puncture, causes intense itching.

Sarcoptes scabiei

The impregnated female *S. scabiei* is responsible for scabies. She burrows into the stratum corneum with her jaws and her first two pairs of legs, forming tunnels up to 1 cm long in which she lays eggs and excretes fecal matter. In a few days, the hatched larvae form their own burrows and develop into adults. The adult mites copulate, and the impregnated females burrow into the stratum corneum to start a new life cycle. The most common infestation sites are the interdigital spaces of the fingers, the flexor surface of the wrists, the external male genitalia, the buttocks, and the anterior axillary fold. (See the "Color Plates," photograph 15.) Scabies is characterized by secondary inflammation and intense itching.

No effective nonprescription product is available to treat scabies.

Bedbugs

A bedbug's mouthparts consist of two pairs of stylets used to pierce the skin. The outer part has barbs that saw the skin, and the inner part is used to suck blood and to allow salivary secretions to flow into the wound. A bedbug can engorge itself with blood within 3 to 5 minutes and then typically seeks its hiding place. Depending on the sensitivity of the bitten individual, the reaction may range from irritation at the site of the bite to a small dermal hemorrhage.

Ticks

During feeding, the tick's mouthparts are introduced into the skin, enabling it to hold firmly. If the tick is removed, the mouthparts are torn from the tick and remain embedded, causing intense itching and nodules, which may need to be surgically excised. (See the "Color Plates," photograph 16.) If the tick is left attached to the skin, it becomes fully engorged with blood and remains for as long as 10 days before it drops off. Ticks should be removed intact from the skin by using fine tweezers. If fingers are used, they should be protected by using gloves and washed afterward. Fingernail polish or mineral oil may be applied on the tick to facilitate its removal.

The local reaction to tick bites consists of itching papules that disappear within 1 week.

Most of the acute stages of Lyme disease are heralded by a skin rash and flulike symptoms. The rash appears first as a papule at the bite site and may become an enlarged circle with a clear center referred to as a "bull's eye" or erythema migrans. The infection then gradually spreads to various parts of the body. The lesions are usually tender and urticarial in nature. They appear 3 to 30 days after the bite and disappear spontaneously within 3 to 4 weeks, but when they are treated with antibiotics, remission occurs within several days. The flu-like symptoms include fever, muscle and joint pain, and, in severe cases, conjunctivitis. If left untreated, neurologic symptoms (e.g., aseptic meningitis, headache, stiff neck, partial paralysis, and paresthesias [a sensation of pricking, tingling, or creeping of the skin]); cardiac symptoms (e.g., tachycardia); and musculoskeletal symptoms may develop and last up to several months. The final and most durable symptoms are arthritis and the appearance of red discoloration of the skin of the hands, wrists, feet, or ankles.

Lyme disease can be diagnosed by studying the medical history of the patient and by conducting laboratory examinations, such as enzyme-linked immunosorbent assays, immunoblotting technique, and indirect fluorescent antibody. Early diagnosis and prompt treatment of Lyme disease can prevent the development of neurologic, cardiac, and rheumatologic manifestations. The disease is treated with antibiotics such as tetracycline, doxycycline, amoxicillin, and cephalosporins.

Chiggers

Only the chigger larvae, which are nearly microscopic, attack the host by attaching to the skin and sucking blood. Once in contact with the skin, the larvae insert their mouthparts into the skin and secrete a digestive fluid that causes cellular disintegration of the affected area, a red papule, and intense itching. Chiggers do not burrow in the skin; however, the injected fluid causes the skin to harden and a tiny tube is formed. The chigger lies in this tube and continues to feed until engorged, after which it drops off and changes into an adult.

Spiders

Even though spider bites are seldom fatal, infants, the elderly, and individuals with allergies are at risk. The reaction to black widow bites includes delayed intense pain, stiffness and joint pain, abdominal disturbances, fever, chills, and dyspnea. In addition to the aforementioned symptoms, brown recluse spiders may cause a spreading, ulcerated wound at the site of the bites.

Complications of Insect Bites

Secondary bacterial infection of insect bites can occur if the skin of the affected area is scratched. This method of relieving itching should be discouraged because it can abrade the skin, allowing contamination of the injury with infectious organisms.

Treatment of Insect Bites

Nonprescription external analgesics are labeled for use in treating insect bites. However, these agents are not effective for scabies.

Treatment Outcomes

The goals of self-treating insect bites are (1) to relieve the symptoms and (2) to prevent secondary bacterial infections.

General Treatment Approach

Application of an ice pack may provide sufficient relief of the pain and irritation of bites from mosquitoes, chiggers, bedbugs, or fleas. If not, applying an external analgesic to the site should relieve these symptoms. A skin protectant may help prevent secondary bacterial infection of injuries. Patients should be advised to avoid scratching the bite. Trimming children's fingernails short and filing them smooth may prevent further injury from scratching. Measures to prevent future insect bites, especially those from ticks and spiders, is important patient information.

Self-treatment of insect bites with a nonprescription product is appropriate if the reaction is confined to the site and if the patient is older than 2 years. Because of possible systemic effects, a physician should evaluate and treat bites from ticks and spiders. The algorithm in Figure 31–2 outlines the treatment of insect bites.

Nonpharmacologic Therapy

Nondrug measures include the two methods of preventing insect bites: avoiding insects and using repellents.

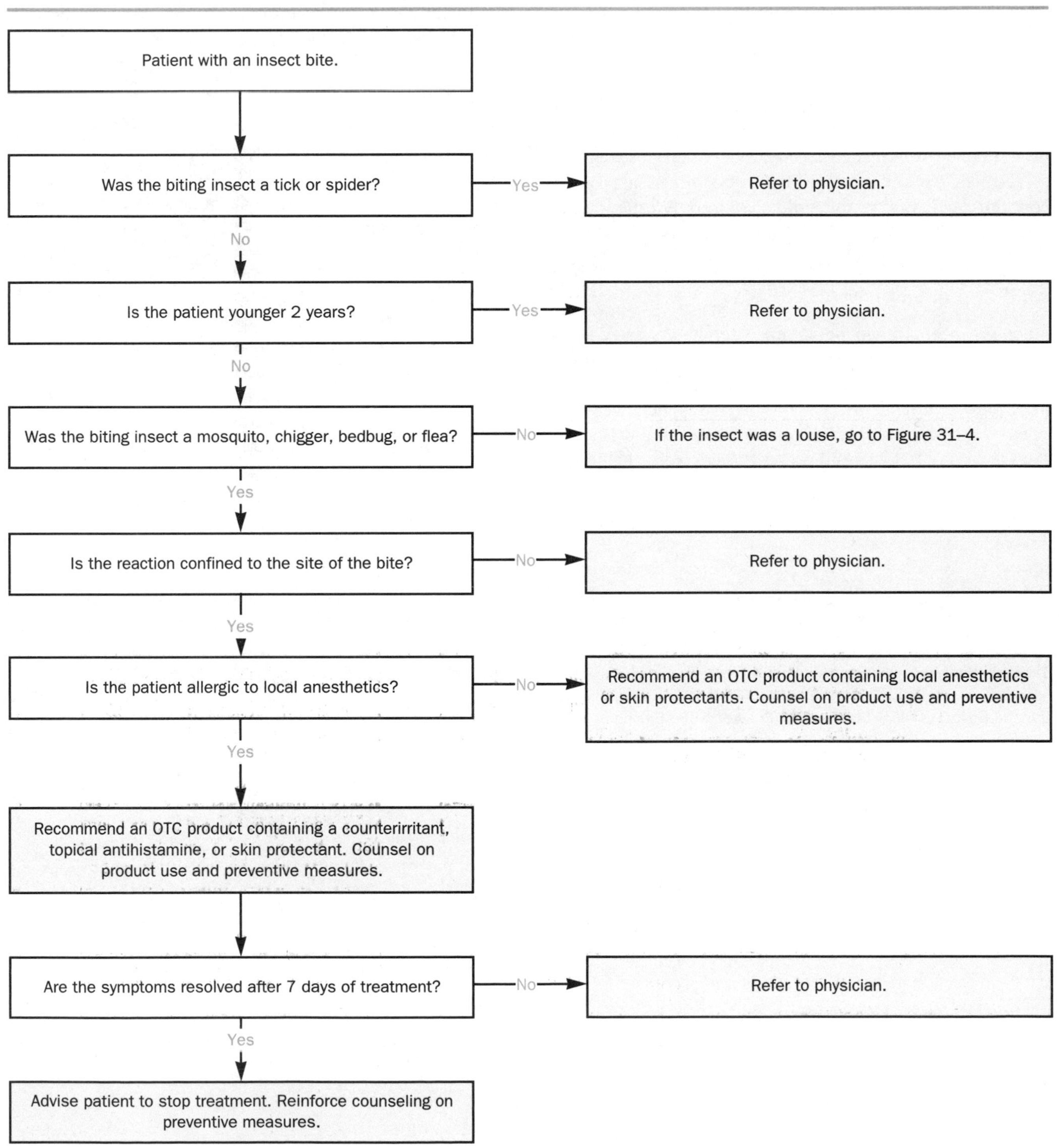

Figure 31–2 Self-care of insect bites.

Avoidance of Insects

Measures to avoid insect bites include covering the skin as much as possible with clothing and socks; cuffing clothing around the ankles, wrists, and neck; avoiding swamps and dense woods and brush that harbor ticks and chiggers; and keeping pets free of pests. To prevent transmission of scabies, people should avoid sharing articles such as combs, brushes, towels, caps, hats, and clothes.

Use of Insect Repellents

Applying insect repellents is useful in preventing insect bites, but they are not effective in repelling stinging insects. An insect repellent should have an inoffensive odor, protect for several hours, be effective against as many insects as possible, be relatively safe, withstand all weather conditions, and have an aesthetic feel and appearance. Most commercial products contain *n,n*-diethyl-*m*-toluamide, commonly called DEET. (See Table 31–1 for examples of these products.)

n,n-diethyl-m-toluamide The best all-purpose repellent is *n,n*-diethyl-*m*-toluamide.

Mechanism of Action/Indication Repellents are used to protect the skin against insect bites. Even though the exact mechanism of action is not fully known, DEET, like other repellents, does not kill insects. The volatile repellent, when applied to skin or clothing, has vapors that tend to discourage the approach of insects and prevents them from alighting.

Dosage/Administration Guidelines Repellents, which are available in the form of sprays, solutions, and creams, are applied to the skin as needed. The use of insect repellents on children younger than 2 years should be discouraged.

Adverse Effects Repellents may be toxic if taken internally. People who are sensitive to these chemicals may develop skin reactions (e.g., itching, burning, and swelling or smarting) when applied to broken skin or mucous membranes.

Contraindications/Precautions/Warnings Repellents should not be applied on the skin of people who are sensitive to such chemicals. These agents should be applied carefully around the eyes because they may burn. Use of these chemicals should be discontinued if irritation or burning develop.

Other Insect Repellents Other insect repellents include ethohexadiol, dimethyl phthalate, dimethyl ethyl hexanediol carbate, and butopyronoxyl. Most commercial repellents, however, contain DEET. A few products contain citronella, an oil extracted from a fragrant grass of southern Asia.

Pharmacologic Therapy

External analgesics such as local anesthetics, counterirritants, topical antihistamines, and hydrocortisone are approved for treating the pain and itching of insect bites. These agents are not approved for use in children younger than 2 years.

Calamine, zinc oxide, and titanium dioxide are useful in preventing secondary bacterial infections. These agents, however, are not approved for treating the symptoms of insect bites. First-aid antiseptics and antibiotics can also help

Table 31–1

Selected Insect Repellents

Trade Name	Primary Ingredients
Banana Boat Bite Block Sunblock for Children SPF 15 Lotion	*n,n*-diethyl-*m*-toluamide 9%; octyl methoxycinnamate; oxybenzone
Banana Boat Bite Block Sunblock SPF 15 Lotion	*n,n*-diethyl-*m*-toluamide 19%; octyl methoxycinnamate; oxybenzone
Coppertone Bug & Sun Adult Formula SPF 15 Lotion	*n,n*-diethyl-*m*-toluamide 9.5%
Coppertone Bug & Sun Kids Formula SPF 30 Lotion	*n,n*-diethyl-*m*-toluamide 9.5%
Cutter Backwoods Aerosol Spray	*n,n*-diethyl-*m*-toluamide 21.85%
Cutter Outdoorsman Lotion/Stick	*n,n*-diethyl-*m*-toluamide 28.5%
Cutter Pleasant Protection Pump Spray/Aerosol Spray	*n,n*-diethyl-*m*-toluamide 6.65%
Natrapel Lotion/Pump Spray	Citronella 10%
Off! Deep Woods Aerosol Spray	*n,n*-diethyl-*m*-toluamide 23.75%
Off! Deep Woods Aerosol Spray for Sportsmen	*n,n*-diethyl-*m*-toluamide 28.5%
Off! Skintastic for Kids Pump Spray	*n,n*-diethyl-*m*-toluamide 4.75%
Off! Skintastic Lotion with Sunscreen	*n,n*-diethyl-*m*-toluamide 9.5%; octocrylene; octyl methoxycinnamate; benzophenone-3
Repel 100 Pump Spray	*n,n*-diethyl-*m*-toluamide 100%
Repel Classic Sportsmen Formula Aerosol Spray	*n,n*-diethyl-*m*-toluamide 38%
Repel Sportsmen IPF 20 Formula Lotion	*n,n*-diethyl-*m*-toluamide 19%
Repel Sportsmen IPF 29 Formula Aerosol Spray	*n,n*-diethyl-*m*-toluamide 27.55%

prevent secondary infections. (See Chapter 35, "Minor Wounds and Skin Infections.")

Local Anesthetics

Local anesthetics such as benzocaine are used widely in topical preparations for the relief of itching and irritation caused by insect bites. Other local anesthetics include pramoxine, benzyl alcohol, lidocaine, dibucaine, and phenol.

Mechanism of Action Local anesthetics cause a reversible blockade of conduction of nerve impulses at the site of the application, thereby producing a loss of sensation. Phenol exerts topical anesthetic action by depressing cutaneous sensory receptors.

Indications Local anesthetics carry the following labeling as recommended by the Food and Drug Administration (FDA) panel: "For temporary relief of pain and itching due to minor burns, sunburns, minor cuts, abrasions, insect bites, and minor skin irritation."

Dosage/Administration Guidelines Topical preparations containing local anesthetics are used as antipruritics and are applied in the form of cream, ointment, aerosol, or lotion. Table 31–2 lists dosages for these and other external analgesics.

Table 31–2

Dosage Guidelines for External Analgesics Used to Treat Insect Bites and Stings[a]

Agent	Concentration (%)	Frequency/Duration of Use
Local Anesthetics[a]		External analgesics are applied up to 3–4 times daily for no longer than 7 days.
Pramoxine	0.5–1	
Benzocaine	5–20	
Benzyl alcohol	5–20	
Lidocaine	2–5	
Dibucaine	0.5–1.5	
Phenol	0.25–1	
Topical Antihistamines[b]		
Diphenhydramine	0.5–2	
Counterirritants[a]		
Camphor	0.1–3	
Menthol	0.1–1	
Corticosteroids[a]		
Hydrocortisone	0.25–1	

[a] These agents should not be used in children younger than 2 years.

[b] These agents should not be used in children younger than 12 years.

Adverse Effects Even though local anesthetics, including benzocaine, are relatively nontoxic when applied topically, sensitization may occur. Adverse effects of pramoxine are not common and exhibit less cross-sensitivity than do other local anesthetics. Adverse reactions with benzyl alcohol are also rare. Phenol is caustic when applied in undiluted form to the skin. Aqueous solutions of greater than 2% are irritating and may cause sloughing and necrosis. The concentration of phenol in nonprescription products, however, ranges from 0.5% to 1.5%.

Precautions/Warnings Local anesthetics should not be used longer than 7 days. Some individual agents have specific precautions or warnings.

Benzocaine Preparations containing benzocaine should not be applied to the skin of individuals with confirmed or suspected hypersensitivity to benzocaine or other ester-type local anesthetics.

Dibucaine Although in the same class as benzocaine, dibucaine products carry specific additional labeling: "Warning: Do not use in large quantities, particularly over raw surfaces or blistered areas." Convulsions, myocardial depression, and death have been reported from systemic absorption.

Phenol Nonprescription products that contain phenol should include the following specific warning: "Do not apply this product to extensive areas of the body or under compresses or bandages."

Topical Antihistamines

Diphenhydramine hydrochloride in concentrations of 0.5% to 2% is the agent used in most products that contain a topical antihistamine.

Mechanism of Action Topical antihistamines exert an anesthetic effect by depressing cutaneous receptors, thereby relieving pain and itching.

Indications Topical antihistamines carry the following labeling as recommended by the FDA panel: "For temporary relief of pain and itching due to minor burns, sunburns, minor cuts, abrasions, insect bites, and minor skin irritation."

Dosage/Administration Guidelines Table 31–2 lists dosing information for topical diphenhydramine.

Adverse Effects Although some absorption occurs through the skin, these ingredients are not absorbed in sufficient quantities to cause systemic side effects even when applied to damaged skin. However, antihistamines are capable of acting as haptens, producing hypersensitivity reactions. Continued use of these agents for 3 to 4 weeks increases the possibility of allergic contact dermatitis. In addition, their continued antipruritic action over a period of time is questionable.

Precautions/Warnings Topical antihistamines should not be used longer than 7 days except under the advice of a physician.

Counterirritants

Counterirritants reduce pain and itching by stimulating cutaneous sensory receptors to provide a feeling of warmth, coolness, or milder pain, which obscures the more severe pain of the injury. The activity of these agents depends on the concentration. In low concentrations, they may depress the cutaneous receptors, resulting in an anesthetic effect. At higher concentrations, they stimulate these receptors. Low concentrations of the counterirritants camphor and menthol are used in some external analgesic products. Chapter 5, "Musculoskeletal Injuries and Disorders," discusses these agents in more detail. A brief discussion of their use follows; their recommended dosages are listed in Table 31–2.

Camphor At concentrations of 0.1% to 3%, camphor depresses cutaneous receptors, thereby relieving itching and irritation. However, camphor-containing products can be very dangerous if ingested. Patients should be warned to keep these (and all drugs) out of the reach of children. Should a child ingest this agent, the parent should contact a physician or a poison control center immediately.

Menthol In concentrations of less than 1%, menthol depresses cutaneous receptors and exerts an analgesic effect. Menthol is considered a safe and effective antipruritic when applied to the affected area in concentrations of 0.1% to 1%.

Hydrocortisone

FDA has approved topical preparations containing hydrocortisone in concentrations up to 1% for nonprescription use.

Mechanism of Action Topically applied, hydrocortisone is an anti-inflammatory agent capable of preventing or suppressing the development of edema, capillary dilation, swelling, and tenderness that accompanies inflammation. Reduction in inflammation results in relief of pain and itching.

Pharmacokinetics Topical absorption of hydrocortisone is increased following the use of occlusive dressings. Following application, a minimal amount of hydrocortisone may enter circulation; however, this penetration increases if the skin is broken or inflamed.

Indications Hydrocortisone topical preparations are indicated for temporary relief of minor skin irritations, itching, and rashes caused by dermatitis, insect bites, poison ivy/oak/sumac dermatitis, soaps, cosmetics, and jewelry.

Dosage/Administration Guidelines Table 31–2 lists dosing information for hydrocortisone.

Adverse Effects Prolonged administration of hydrocortisone may cause atrophy of the epidermis, acneiform eruptions, irritation, folliculitis, and tightening and cracking of the skin.

Contraindications Patients who suffer from scabies, fungal or bacterial infections, and moniliasis should be warned against using topical hydrocortisone. Not only may the underlying conditions be worsened but hydrocortisone may also mask these disorders, thereby making accurate diagnosis difficult.

Skin Protectants

Medications such as zinc oxide, calamine, and titanium dioxide are applied to insect bites mainly in the form of lotions, ointments, and creams. These agents act as astringents and tend to relieve inflammation and irritation. They also exert mild antiseptic, and antibacterial actions. Thus, they are capable of preventing secondary bacterial infections. Zinc oxide and calamine tend to absorb fluids from weeping lesions.

FDA considers preparations containing zinc oxide and calamine to be safe and effective in nonprescription drugs containing 1% to 25%. Titanium dioxide has action similar to that of zinc oxide. However, FDA has not determined the safety and effectiveness of this ingredient. These preparations should be applied to the affected area as needed. They have minimal adverse effects and are recommended for adults, children, and infants.

Product Selection Guidelines

Sensitization can occur with local anesthetics. If such agents are preferred, pramoxine and benzyl alcohol are less likely to cause adverse effects. Dibucaine and phenol have the most potential for adverse effects, especially if systemic absorption occurs from improper application.

Adverse effects and systemic absorption are generally not a concern with short-term use of the topical antihistamine diphenhydramine hydrochloride. Prolonged use of this agent can, however, cause hypersensitivity reactions. Similarly, short-term use of hydrocortisone usually does not cause adverse effects or systemic absorption. However, patients with scabies, bacterial infections, or fungal infections, especially moniliasis, should not use this agent. Hydrocortisone can worsen or mask these disorders, making accurate diagnosis difficult. Camphor-containing products can be very dangerous if ingested, making them an inappropriate choice for use in children.

Topical diphenhydramine's side-effect profile makes it the safest external analgesic to recommend; however, patients must understand that external analgesics should not be used longer than 7 days.

The patient's preference of dosage forms should also guide product recommendations. Creams, lotions, and sprays are the most commonly used dosage forms. If cost is a consideration, generic external analgesic preparations are probably effective even though no clinical studies have evaluated these preparations for insect bites. Table 31–3 lists examples of commercially available products.

Patient Assessment of Insect Bites

The pharmacist should first find out what type of insect inflicted the injury. A physician should evaluate bites from ticks and spiders because of the serious diseases or adverse ef-

Table 31–3

Selected External Analgesic Products for Insect Bites and Stings

Trade Name	Primary Ingredients
Local Anesthetics	
Bactine Antiseptic/Anesthetic First-Aid Spray	Lidocaine HCl 2.5%; benzalkonium chloride 0.13%
Bicozene External Analgesic Creme	Benzocaine 6%; resorcinol 1.67%
Caladryl Lotion/Cream	Pramoxine HCl 1%; calamine 8%
Chigger-Tox Liquid	Benzocaine 2.1%
Chiggerex Ointment	Benzocaine 2%
Itch-X Gel/Pump Spray	Benzyl alcohol 10%; pramoxine HCl 1%
Lanacane Aerosol Spray	Benzocaine 20%
Lanacane Creme	Benzocaine 6%
Lanacane Maximum Strength Cream	Benzocaine 20%
Nupercainal Ointment	Dibucaine 1%
Rhuli Bite-Aid Stick	Benzocaine 10%; benzyl alcohol 10%
Solarcaine Medicated First Aid Aerosol Spray	Benzocaine 20%
Unguentine Plus Cream	Lidocaine HCl 2%; phenol 0.5%
Topical Antihistamines	
Benadryl Itch Relief Extra Strength Stick	Diphenhydramine HCl 2%
Benadryl Itch Stopping Extra Strength Cream/Spray	Diphenhydramine HCl 2%
Benadryl Itch Stopping Regular Strength Cream/Spray	Diphenhydramine HCl 1%
Bio-Sentry Anti-Itch Pump Spray	Diphenhydramine HCl 2%
Counterirritants	
Gold Bond Medicated Powder, Extra Strength	Menthol 0.8%
Gold Bond Medicated Powder, Regular Strength	Menthol 0.15%
Sarna Lotion	Camphor 0.5%; menthol 0.5%
Corticosteroids	
Bactine Hydrocortisone 1% Cream	Hydrocortisone 1%
Cortaid FastStick	Hydrocortisone 1%
Cortaid Intensive Therapy Cream	Hydrocortisone 1%
Cortaid Maximum Strength Ointment/Cream	Hydrocortisone 1%
Cortaid Sensitive Skin Cream	Hydrocortisone 0.5%
Kericort 10 Maximum Strength Cream	Hydrocortisone 1%
Lanacort 10 Cream/Ointment	Hydrocortisone 1%
Combination Products	
Aveeno Anti-Itch Cream/Lotion	Pramoxine HCl 1%; camphor 0.3%; calamine 3%
Benadryl Itch Stopping Extra Strength Gel	Diphenhydramine HCl 2%; camphor
Benadryl Itch Stopping Original Strength Gel	Diphenhydramine HCl 1%; camphor
Rhuli Gel	Benzyl alcohol 2%; menthol 0.3%; camphor 0.3%
Rhuli Spray	Benzocaine 5%; camphor 0.7%; benzyl alcohol
Sting Kill Stick	Benzocaine 20%; menthol 1%
Sting-Eze Drops	Diphenhydramine HCl; camphor; phenol; benzocaine

fects associated with these bites. For other insect bites, the pharmacist should evaluate the seriousness of the reaction before recommending a nonprescription product or nondrug measure. If a nonallergic reaction is present, the pharmacist should recommend the appropriate external analgesic for symptomatic relief. The pharmacist should explain to the patient the proper use of the selected product, as well as its possible adverse effects. If the patient is a child, recommendation of a skin protectant to prevent secondary bacterial infection is appropriate.

Asking the patient or caregiver the following questions will help elicit the information needed to accurately assess the cause and seriousness of the injury and to recommend the appropriate treatment approach.

Q~ Do you know what type of insect bit you?

A~ Refer tick and spider bites to a physician. If the cause of the bite is unknown, refer the patient to a physician.

Q~ Have you previously had severe reactions to insect bites? Is the reaction limited to the site of the bite?

A~ Refer a patient who has had severe reactions to insect bites to a physician. If the patient has no history of severe reactions and if the present symptoms do not indicate an allergic reaction, recommend the appropriate treatment.

Q~ What, if anything, have you used to treat the bite?

A~ Determine whether the self-treatment was appropriate. If not, recommend appropriate therapy. If the self-treatment was appropriate but ineffective, recommend an alternative treatment.

Q~ Have you ever had adverse reactions to topically applied products?

A~ Tailor product recommendations to the patient's history with these products.

Patient Counseling for Insect Bites

Counseling for insect bites includes an explanation of how to treat the injury as well as how to prevent future occurrences. The pharmacist should explain nondrug measures and/or the proper use of recommended nonprescription products. The explanation should include potential adverse effects of these agents plus the signs and symptoms that indicate the injury needs medical attention. The box "Patient Education for Insect Bites" lists specific information to provide patients.

Evaluation of Patient Outcomes for Insect Bites

Follow up of the pharmacist–patient interaction should occur after 7 days of self-treatment. Either a telephone call or scheduled visit to the pharmacy is an appropriate method of follow-up. The patient should be advised to seek medical attention if the symptoms worsen during treatment. Medical attention is also necessary if the symptoms persist after 7 days of treatment.

Insect Stings

Epidemiology of Insect Stings

As with insect bites, persons who work or spend time outdoors are at risk for insect stings. An estimated 0.5% of the population may show signs of allergic reactions to insect stings. About 40 deaths caused by anaphylaxis are reported annually in the United States.[1]

Etiology of Insect Stings

Venomous insects such as bees, wasps, hornets, yellow jackets, and fire ants belong to the order Hymenoptera. They attack their victims to defend themselves or to kill other insects. The injected venom contains a number of allergenic proteins as well as several pharmacologically active molecules. These contents vary among different families within the Hymenoptera order. Therefore, venoms are discussed here in general terms.

Wild Honeybees, Wasps, Hornets, and Yellow Jackets

Wild honeybees are most commonly found in the western and midwestern United States, and they usually nest in hollow tree trunks. Paper wasps, hornets, and yellow jackets are more commonly found in the south, central, and southwestern United States. Paper wasps tend to nest in high places, under eaves of houses, or on branches of high trees, whereas hornets prefer to nest in hollow spaces, especially hollow trees. Yellow jackets, considered the most common stinging culprits, usually nest in low places, such as burrows in the ground, cracks in walks, or small shrubs.

Fire Ants

Fire ants, which were imported from South America early in the 20th century, are now found in the southern and western United States, live in underground colonies, and form large raised mounds. Fire ants are considered a health hazard because of the severity of reactions to their bite.

Pathophysiology of Insect Stings

Although they are small, many insects have a venom as potent as that of snakes. However, whereas death from a snakebite is usually caused by toxicity of the venom and occurs within 3 hours to several days, death from an insect sting is usually related to allergic hypersensitivity, which could lead to an anaphylactic reaction within 5 to 30 minutes after the sting. Simultaneous, multiple stings of 500 or more may cause death from toxicity. In the United States, more people die of insect stings than of the bites of all poisonous animals combined.

Stinging insects inject the venom into their victims through a piercing organ (stinger), a modified ovipositor delicately attached to the rear of the female's abdomen.

Patient Education for Insect Bites

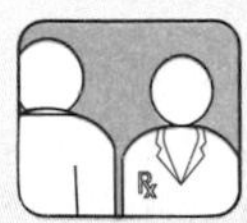

The objectives of self-treatment are to (1) relieve the pain and itching of insect bites and (2) prevent scratching (especially among children), which may lead to secondary bacterial infection. A secondary objective is to prevent future insect bites. For most patients, carefully following product instructions and the self-care measures listed below will help ensure optimal therapeutic outcomes.

Nondrug Measures

- Apply ice promptly to the site of the bite to help reduce itching, swelling, and pain.
- Avoid scratching the affected area. Also, keep fingernails trimmed short and filed smooth to minimize possible damage to the affected area if scratching occurs.
- Do not wear rough and irritating clothing, especially wool, over an area that has been irritated by insect bites.

Preventive Measures

- Cover the skin as much as possible with clothing and socks. Use cuffed clothing around the ankles, wrists, and neck.
- Avoid swamps, dense woods, and dense brush, which harbor mosquitoes, ticks, and chiggers.
- Keep pets free of pests.
- To prevent transmission of scabies, do not share articles such as combs, brushes, towels, caps, hats, and clothes.
- If desired, apply an insect repellent as needed to repel biting insects. Be aware that repellents do not deter stinging insects.

Nonprescription Medications

External Analgesics

- Use an external analgesic to relieve the pain and itching of insect bites. Choice of medications include local anesthetics, topical antihistamines, counterirritants, and hydrocortisone.
- See Table 31–2 for dosage guidelines. Do not apply these agents to children younger than 2 years. Also, do not use these agents longer than 7 days.
- Note that local anesthetics can cause sensitization. If such agents are preferred, pramoxine and benzyl alcohol are less likely to cause adverse effects.
- Do not use dibucaine in large quantities, particularly over raw surfaces or blistered areas. Such use could cause convulsions, myocardial depression, and death.
- Do not apply phenol to extensive areas of the body or under compresses or bandages. Such application increases systemic absorption of the medication.
- Do not use topical diphenhydramine hydrochloride longer than the recommended 7 days. Prolonged use can cause hypersensitivity reactions.
- Do not use hydrocortisone if you have scabies, bacterial infections, or fungal infections, especially moniliasis. Hydrocortisone can worsen these disorders.
- Do not allow children to ingest camphor-containing products. This medication is toxic when ingested.

Skin Protectants

- If needed to prevent secondary bacterial infection, use a skin protectant such as zinc oxide or calamine.
- Apply the protectant to the affected area as needed.
- Note that protectants can be applied to the skin of children younger than 2 years.
- Note that some insect bite products contain external analgesics and skin protectants.

⚠ Seek medical attention if the condition worsens during treatment or symptoms persist after 7 days of topical treatment.

(Males do not have an ovipositor and, consequently, are stingless.) The stinger consists of two lancets made of highly chitinous material and separated by the poison canal. The venom flows through the canal from the venom sac attached to the stinger's dorsal section. The tip of the stinger, which is directed posteriorly, has sharp barbs, and the base enlarges into a bulb-like structure. Most species of bees and wasps have two types of venom glands under the last abdominal segment. The larger gland secretes an acidic toxin directly into the venom sac; the small one at the base of the sac secretes a less-potent alkaline toxin. The injected venom is usually a mixture of the two toxins.

When the honeybee stings, it attaches firmly to the skin with tiny, sharp claws at the tip of each foot, arches its abdomen and immediately jabs the barbed stinger into the skin. The barbs firmly embed the stinger, and when the honeybee pulls away or is brushed off, the entire stinging apparatus (stinger, appendages, venom sac, and glands) is detached from the bee's abdomen. The disemboweled bee later dies. The abandoned stinger, driven deeper into the skin by rhythmic contractions of the venom sac's smooth muscle wall, continues to inject venom.

The stinging mechanism of wasps, hornets, and yellow jackets resembles that of the honeybee except that the stingers are not barbed. Their stingers can be withdrawn easily after the venom is injected, enabling these insects to survive and sting repeatedly.

The major antigenic proteins found in the venom are the enzymes hyaluronidase and phospholipase A. Hyaluronidase breaks down hyaluronic acid, which is the binding agent in connective tissue. By altering tissue structure, hyaluronidase acts as a spreading factor, allowing for enhanced penetration of venom substances. Phospholipase A attacks phospholipids in cell membranes. It also contracts smooth muscle, causes hypotension, increases vascular permeability, and destroys mast cells. Other venom components include histamine, meletin, apamin, and mast cell degranulating peptide. Of the components, only meletin is antigenic, and not all people make antibodies against it. Although these mediators do not directly contribute to insect sting anaphylaxis, they do affect the rate at which venom antigens become available to the systemic circulation following a sting. These molecules have direct and indirect effects on mast-cell mediator release, vascular permeability, and smooth muscle contractions.

Some ants only bite; others bite and sting simultaneously. Stinging ants (fire ants; *Solenopsis invecta*) use their mandibles to cling to the skin of their prey; then they bend their abdomen, sting the flesh, and empty the contents of their poison vesicle into the wound. Because these ants use their mandibles, it is often believed that the bite causes the reactions. Their sting causes intense itching, burning (hence the name), vesiculations, necrosis, and anaphylactic reaction in hypersensitive persons. It appears that very limited or no cross-sensitivity exists between the venom of fire ants and that of bees, wasps, hornets, and yellow jackets.

The intensity of the allergic reactions to venomous insect stings varies significantly. The thrust of the stinger into the flesh and the subsequent injection of venom causes a sharp pain. The reaction that follows depends on the person's sensitivity to the venom. To develop sensitivity, a person should have been previously exposed to the venom. The first sting is considered the sensitizing one. Systemic and local allergic manifestations usually occur in people who have been stung previously.

The venom may trigger a mild reaction or may precipitate anaphylaxis, a rapid allergic reaction that may affect more than one part of the body and, if severe, may result in death. Following the initial sting, the antibody immunoglobulin E (IgE) is formed and binds to receptors on the mast cells and basophils. Each subsequent sting produces more antibodies and intensifies the allergic manifestations. When the allergen (venom) reaches the IgE on the mast cells, a reaction takes place, causing the degranulation of the mast cells and the release of chemical mediators such as histamine, prostaglandins, and leukotrienes. These inflammatory mediators are potent vasodilators and bronchoconstrictors. The vasodilation results in a rapid fall in blood pressure as well as an increase in the permeability of the blood vessels, thus causing seepage of fluid into the surrounding tissue and subsequent swelling (angioedema.) The severity of the anaphylactic reactions depends largely on the amounts of chemical mediators produced. The skin, respiratory, cardiovascular, and gastrointestinal systems are most commonly involved during anaphylaxis.

Signs and Symptoms of Reactions to Insect Stings

Most people experience no allergic reactions to insect stings. However, many may complain of pain, itching, and irritation at the site of the sting but may have no systemic effect. People who are allergic to insect stings may experience hives, itching, swelling, and burning sensations of the skin. The vasodilation and loss of fluid from blood vessels can cause a fall in blood pressure, and the person may experience lightheadedness or even loss of consciousness. Obstruction of the nose and throat may occur, resulting in hoarseness and a choking sensation. Likewise, the bronchial tree may become constricted, causing chest tightness, dyspnea , and wheezing. Nausea, vomiting, abdominal cramps, and diarrhea are common. In women, uterine contractions may occur, resulting in pelvic cramps.

Treatment of Insect Stings

Although labeling of nonprescription products for insect-related injuries mentions only "insect bites" as an indication, FDA had intended the term to cover stings as well.

Treatment Outcomes

The goal of self-treating insect stings is to relieve the itching and pain of cutaneous nonallergic reactions. Allergic reactions require evaluation and treatment by a physician.

General Treatment Approach

Removal of the stinger and application of an ice pack are the first steps in treating insect stings. Applying a local anesthetic, skin protectant, antiseptic, or counterirritant to the sting site is appropriate if the reaction is confined to the site, if the patient has never been stung before or never had a previous severe reaction to a sting, if the patient has no personal or family history of allergic reactions such as hay fever, and if the patient is older than 2 years.

Nonprescription systemic antihistamines can also be taken to alleviate itching. The algorithm in Figure 31–3 outlines the treatment of insect stings.

Avoiding future insect stings can prevent a person from developing allergic reactions to stings. If symptoms of an allergic reaction develop, emergency treatment should be administered, and the patient should seek medical attention. Patients with severe allergic reactions might want to consider prophylactic treatment such as hyposensitization therapy. Such patients should be advised to wear a bracelet or carry a card identifying the nature of the allergy.

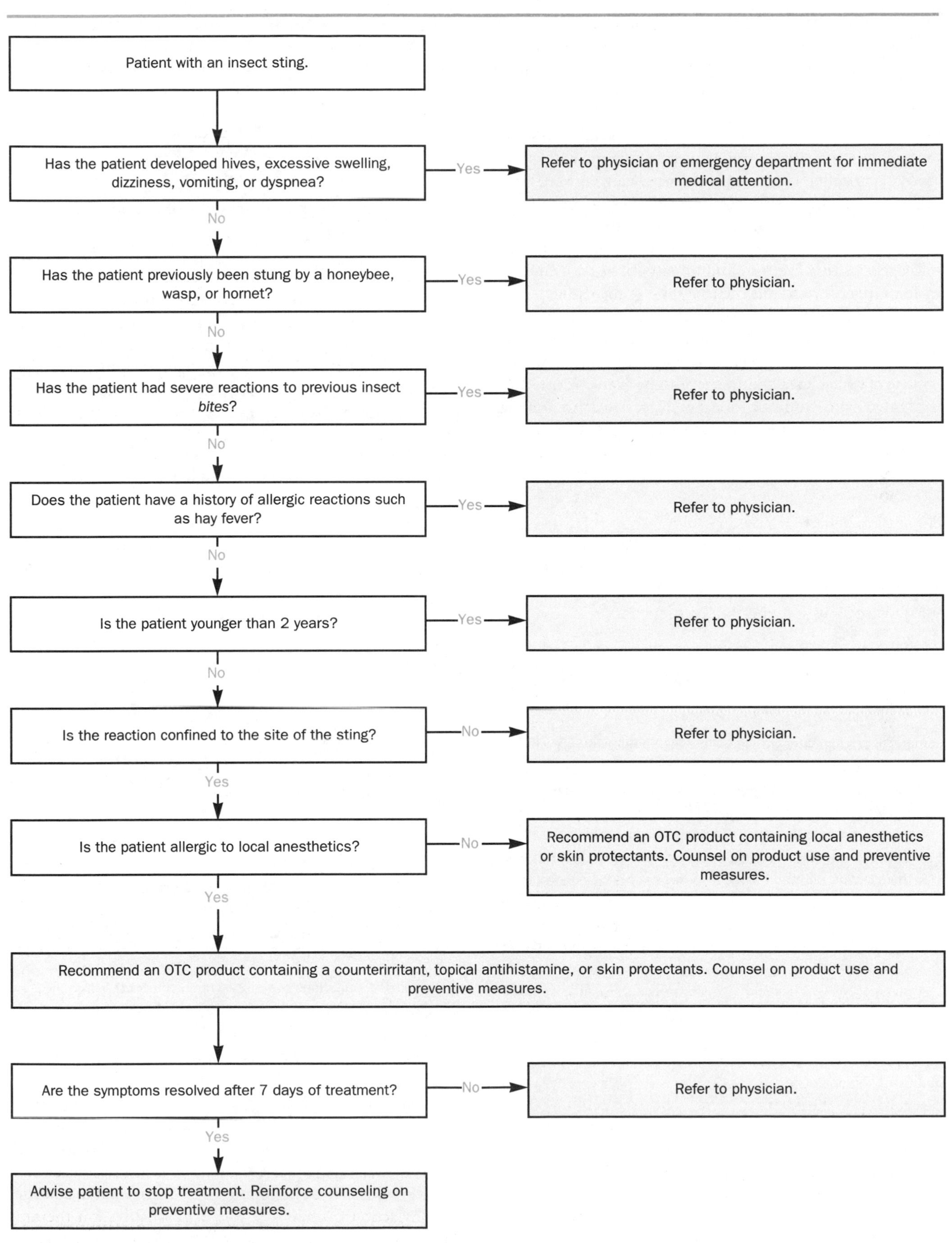

Figure 31–3 Self-care of insect stings.

Nonpharmacologic Therapy

Prompt application of ice packs to the sting site helps to slow absorption and reduce itching, swelling, and pain. Removal of the honeybee's stinger and venom sac, which usually are left in the skin, is another measure that should be offered or explained, particularly to patients who are allergic to insect venom. The patient should remove the stinger before all venom is injected; it takes approximately 2 to 3 minutes to empty all the contents from the honeybee's venom sac. The patient should not squeeze the sac because rubbing, scratching, or grasping it releases more venom. Scraping the stinger with tweezers or a fingernail minimizes the venom flow. After the stinger is removed, an antiseptic should be applied.

To avoid stinging insects, the patient should adhere to the following measures: avoid wearing perfume, scented lotions, and brightly colored clothes; control odors in picnic and garbage areas; change children's clothing if it becomes contaminated with summer foods such as fruits; wear shoes when outdoors; and destroy nests of stinging insects near homes.

Pharmacologic Therapy

The section "Pharmacologic Therapy" under "Treatment of Insect Bites" discusses the following external analgesics approved for treatment of insect bites and, by inference, insect stings: local anesthetics, topical antihistamines, counterirritants, hydrocortisone, and skin protectants.

Product labels for systemic antihistamines do not include treatment of itching associated with insect stings as an indication. One of the most commonly used antihistamines in systemic antihistamines is diphenhydramine hydrochloride. Chapter 9, "Disorders Related to Cold and Allergy," discusses systemic antihistamines in detail.

Emergency Treatment of Allergic Reactions

The initial drug of choice for combating anaphylactic reactions precipitated by insect stings is epinephrine. Antihistamines are often used in conjunction with epinephrine hydrochloride and are given either orally or parenterally to relieve itching. The latter agents act too slowly in counteracting the effects of histamine and other chemical mediators to be beneficial in life-threatening anaphylactic reactions.

Epinephrine is an α_1, β_1, and β_2 agonist. Activation of α_1 receptors, which control blood vessels in the internal organ, mucosa surface, and skin, results in a systemic increase in blood pressure. Because β receptors control the bronchial tree, activation of these receptors results in bronchial dilation, thereby relieving chest tightness, dyspnea, and wheezing. Patients who are allergic to insect stings should carry an injectable form of epinephrine with them to use only when stung. Epinephrine is not used as a maintenance therapy. A product such as EpiPen Auto-Injector, which contains a 0.3 mg subcutaneous dose of 1:1000 epinephrine in a 2 mL disposable prefilled injector, is easier and faster to use than

Case Study 31–1

Patient Complaint/History

Bill, a 20-year-old man, was walking barefooted on the lawn of his backyard when he was stung by a wasp. Within minutes, he experienced difficulty in breathing, nausea, and dizziness. He was rushed to the emergency room where he was given intramuscular injection of 0.25 to 0.3 mg of epinephrine hydrochloride (1:1000) and a capsule containing 50 mg of diphenhydramine. Even though his condition stabilized, he was kept in the hospital for observation for 5 hours and then was released. The next day, Bill revealed to his pharmacist that he suffers from hay fever and that his mother is an asthmatic. He also revealed that he had been stung previously by bees on several occasions but that his previous reaction was milder than the recent one. Bill never consulted a physician or a pharmacist, and, evidently, he did not realize the seriousness of his condition.

Clinical Considerations/Strategies

Readers can use the following considerations/strategies to determine whether treatment of the patient's condition with nonprescription medications is warranted:

- Assess the patient's reaction to the bee sting.
- Assess the appropriateness of trying to self-treat this type of reaction.

Patient Education/Counseling

Readers can use the following strategies to develop a patient education/counseling plan that will ensure optimal therapeutic outcomes:

- Assess the patient's understanding of his progressively severe hypersensitivity reaction to bee stings.
- Advise the patient about the pathogenesis of anaphylactic reactions.
- Explain the limitations of nonprescription products in treating anaphylactic reactions and the need to minimize the risk of bee stings.
- Explain the importance of always having immediate access to an epinephrine-containing injection 1:1000 epinephrine in a disposable, prefilled injection.
- Explain the importance of informing family, friends, and coworkers about the severity of the hypersensitivity and the need for immediate medical intervention following a bee sting.

epinephrine in ampules, which must be withdrawn and injected with a syringe.

Prophylactic Treatment of Insect Stings

Hymenoptera venom is used prophylactically to treat patients who have had reactions to stings. Venom immunotherapy is accomplished by subcutaneous injection of small amounts of venom at regularly scheduled intervals. The dose of the venom is gradually increased over many weeks until a predetermined maintenance dose is reached. For patients who have had mild-to-moderate reactions to insect venoms, 2 to 3 years of immunotherapy are sufficient. Longer periods are necessary for those who have experienced severe symptoms and who continue to show positive skin-test sensitivity.[3]

Patient Assessment of Insect Stings

The critical determination in assessing a patient with an insect sting is whether the patient is allergic to the venom. Patients experiencing allergic reactions should be immediately referred for medical attention. Asking the patient the following questions will help elicit the information needed to determine whether an allergic reaction is likely and to recommend the appropriate treatment approach.

Q~ Have you been stung previously by a honeybee, wasp, or hornet?

A~ If no, suspect that the reaction is nonallergic in nature. If yes, refer the patient to a physician. The previous sting may have sensitized the patient.

Q~ Is the reaction limited to the site of the sting?

A~ If the reaction is confined locally, suspect that the reaction is nonallergenic in nature. If not, refer the patient to a physician.

Q~ Are you experiencing hives, excessive swelling, dizziness, vomiting, or difficulty in breathing?

A~ If yes, refer the patient to a physician, preferably an allergist, who may initiate immunotherapy or prescribe an insect sting emergency kit. If no, suspect a local reaction that is nonallergenic in nature.

Q~ Have you previously had severe reactions to insect stings?

A~ If yes, refer the patient to a physician for evaluation and treatment of a possible anaphylactic reaction that could intensify and become fatal. If no, suspect a local reaction that is nonallergenic in nature.

Q~ Have you ever consulted a physician after experiencing a sensitivity reaction?

A~ If no, urge the patient to seek medical advice. The next insect sting could prove fatal.

Q~ Do you have a personal or family history of allergic reactions such as hay fever?

A~ If yes, advise the patient that heredity plays an important role in allergic disorders and that he or she is an excellent candidate for developing allergic reactions to insect stings.

Patient Counseling for Insect Stings

The pharmacist should advise the patient that local reactions to insect stings (e.g., itching, pain, and irritation) are usually transient and are experienced by the vast majority of the population. The pharmacist should also explain that severe reactions to insect stings can occur if sensitization to the insect venom develops. The symptoms of allergic reactions should also be explained. The pharmacist should stress the importance of consulting a physician if such symptoms occur. Encounters with patients who have a known hypersensitivity to insect stings are opportunities to educate the patients about (1) anaphylaxis, (2) the importance of prompt medical attention following insect stings, (3) the limitations of nonprescription drugs in treating their condition, and (4) the importance of avoiding stinging insects.

For nonallergic reactions to stings, the pharmacist should recommend one or more topical products to manage the immediate symptoms and should explain techniques and procedures for properly applying the products. Possible adverse effects and any contraindications to use should also be explained. The box "Patient Education for Insect Stings" lists specific information to provide patients.

Evaluation of Patient Outcomes for Insect Stings

Follow-up for nonallergic reactions to insect stings should occur 7 days after the pharmacist–patient interaction. Either a telephone call or scheduled visit to the pharmacy is an appropriate method of follow-up. The patient should be advised to seek medical attention if the symptoms worsen during the treatment period or persist after 7 days of treatment.

Follow-up for patients with allergic reactions should occur the same day if possible. In addition to expressing concern for the patient's welfare, the pharmacist should ask about the emergency treatment and find out whether the patient needs a supply of epinephrine for future emergencies.

Pediculosis

Pediculosis is lice infestation. Lice are wingless parasites with well-developed legs. They do not jump like fleas, nor do they fly.

Patient Education for Insect Stings

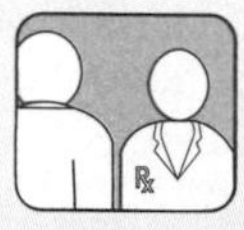

The objectives of self-treatment are to (1) relieve the pain and itching of insect stings and (2) monitor any reaction to the sting to determine whether an allergic reaction is developing. A secondary objective is to prevent future insect stings. For most patients, carefully following product instructions and the self-care measures listed below will help ensure optimal therapeutic outcomes.

Nondrug Measures

- For honeybee stings, remove the honeybee stinger by scraping it with tweezers. This action reduces the amount of injected venom. Do not squeeze, rub, scratch, or grasp the stinger. These actions will actually release more venom.
- Apply ice promptly to the sting site to help slow absorption of the venom. This action will reduce itching, swelling, and pain.

Preventive Measures

- Avoid scratching the affected area. Also, keep fingernails trimmed short and filed smooth to minimize possible damage to the affected area if scratching occurs.
- Avoid wearing brightly colored clothing as well as scented lotions or perfume that attract stinging insects.
- If you are hypersensitive to stings, wear a bracelet or carry a card showing the nature of the allergy.

Treatment of Allergic Reactions

- To prevent an allergic reaction, administer 0.25 to 0.3 mg of epinephrine hydrochloride 1:1000 subcutaneously immediately following a sting. Repeat the dose every 20 minutes, but do not administer the medication longer than 24 hours.
- If desired, take an oral antihistamine in conjunction with epinephrine hydrochloride to relieve itching.

Nonprescription Medications for Nonallergic Reactions

- Apply a topical nonprescription external analgesic such as a local anesthetic, topical antihistamine, counterirritant, or hydrocortisone to the affected site to relieve pain and itching.
- See the box "Patient Education for Insect Bites" for specific information about these agents. See Table 31–2 for recommended dosages.

⚠ Seek medical attention if symptoms (hives, excessive swelling, dizziness, vomiting, or difficulty in breathing) of an allergic reaction develop.

⚠ Seek medical attention if the pain and itching worsen during treatment or they do not improve after 7 days of topical treatment.

Epidemiology/Etiology of Pediculosis

In addition to being irritating pests, lice may act as vectors of epidemic diseases such as typhus. Lice infestations in the United States are common. Three types of lice that infest humans are head lice (*Pediculus humanus capitis*), body lice (*P. humanus corporis*), and pubic lice (*Phthirus pubis*). Epidemiologic variables correlate with the type of lice infestation.

Head Lice

Head lice are the most common lice infestation, affecting more than 10 million Americans annually. Most cases involve children 1 to 12 years of age. Outbreaks of lice infestation are common in crowded places such as schools, day care centers, and nursing homes. Outbreaks usually peak after the opening of schools each year between the months of August and November. The National Pediculosis Association recommends school-wide screenings after school opens, before Christmas, and before school is dismissed for the summer.

Body Lice

Body lice live, hide, and lay their eggs in clothing, particularly in the seams and folds of underclothing, which they periodically leave to invade the host's body to feed. Infestations occur in individuals who do not change clothing frequently, such as homeless people and soldiers in extended military campaigns. These insects are larger than head lice and twice as long, and the female body louse lays more eggs (as many as 300).

Pubic Lice

Pubic lice, commonly called crab lice because of their crab-like appearance, may be encountered in all people, even those with high standards of hygiene. An infestation of pubic lice is identified by the presence of the parasite and its nits. The lice are usually found in the pubic area, but may infest armpits and occasionally eyelashes, mustaches, beards, and eyebrows. They may be transmitted through sexual contact, toilet seats, shared undergarments, or sheets. A female adult pubic louse deposits 50 eggs during her lifetime.

Pathophysiology of Pediculosis

Head lice usually infest the head and live on the scalp (See the "Color Plates," photographs 17A and B.) The female deposits 10 to 150 eggs (nits), which become glued to the hair and hatch in 5 to 10 days. The nit is about 5 mm in diameter and has yellowish or grayish-white color. Once hatched, the louse must begin the feeding process within 24 hours or it dies. The nymph (newly hatched, immature louse) resembles an adult and matures within 8 to 9 days.

The lifespan of an adult is about 1 month. The nymph is active and tends to move about the head, whereas the adults are less active.

Signs and Symptoms of Pediculosis

The bite of a louse causes an immediate wheal to develop around the bite. A local papule appears within 24 hours. Itching and subsequent scratching result in excoriation or secondary pyogenic infection.

Treatment of Pediculosis

If used properly, nonprescription pediculicide agents are very effective in ridding a patient of lice. These products cannot prevent a lice infestation, however. Awareness of the problem and appropriate actions by health officials, school authorities, and parents are essential in stopping the spread of lice.

Treatment Outcomes

The goal of treating pediculosis is to rid the infested patient of lice by killing the adult and nymph lice and by removing nits (lice eggs) from the patient's hair.

General Treatment Approach

To rid the patient of lice, a pediculicide is applied to the infested body area for the designated amount of time. The hair is then combed with a lice/nit comb to remove loosened nits from the hair shaft. Combing will also remove dead lice. Once rid of lice, patients should be instructed on how to avoid future infestations. The algorithm in Figure 31–4 outlines the treatment of lice infestations.

Nonpharmacologic Therapy

To prevent future lice infestations, the patient should avoid direct physical contact with an infested individual and should never share articles such as combs, brushes, towels, caps, and hats.

Pharmacologic Therapy

Two nonprescription pediculicide agents are available for treating pediculosis: pyrethrins and permethrin.

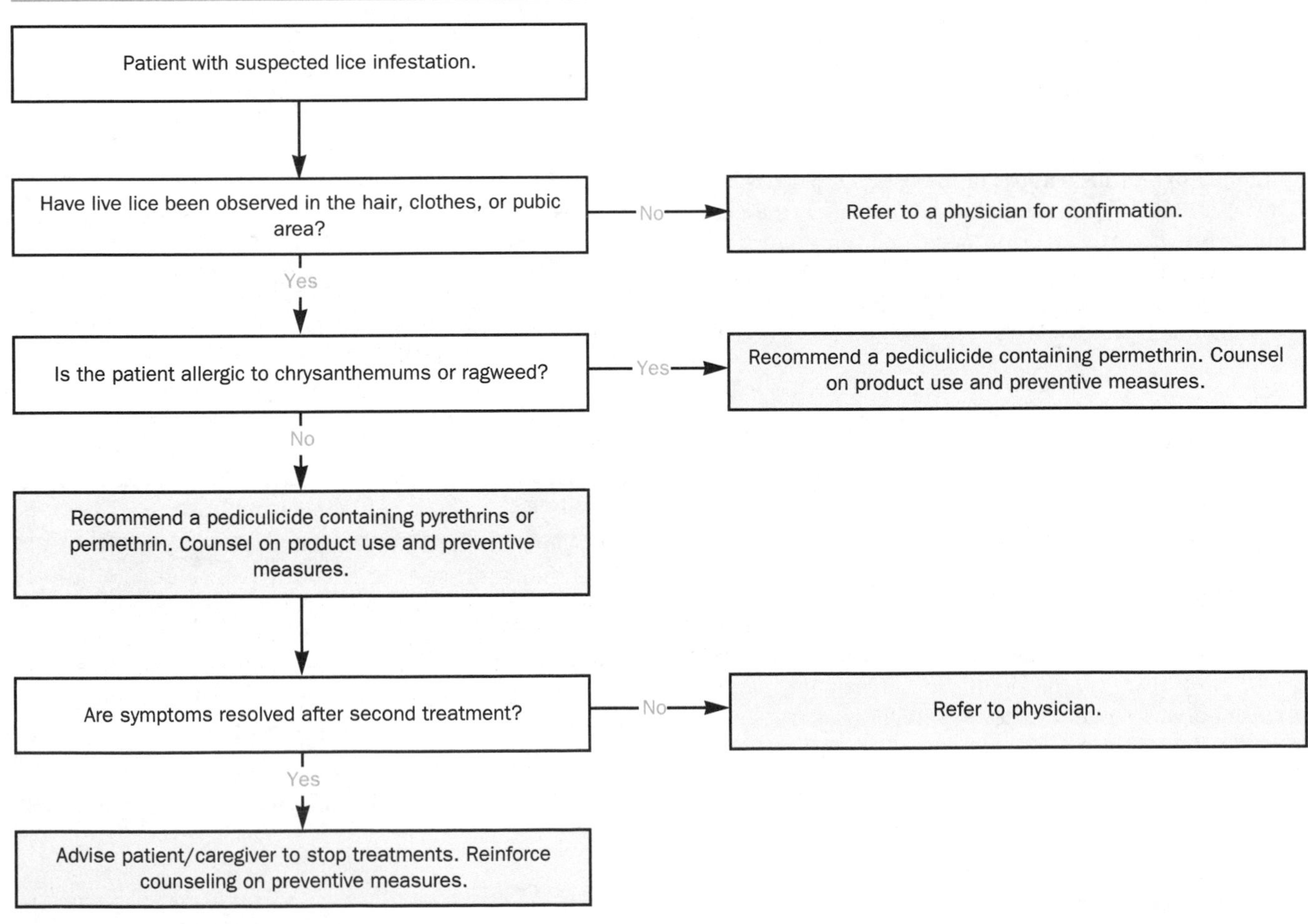

Figure 31–4 Self-care of pediculosis.

Pyrethrins

Pyrethrins are obtained from chrysanthemum flowers and occur as a viscous, brown, liquid oleoresin.

Mechanism of Action Following penetration of the chitinous exoskeleton of insects, pyrethrins block nerve impulse transmission causing the insect's paralysis and death.[4]

Pharmacokinetics When applied topically, pyrethrins are absorbed through the skin. Ingested pyrethrins are inactivated by the gastric fluid.

Indications Pyrethrins are approved for treating head and pubic lice.

Dosage/Administration Guidelines Pyrethrins in concentrations ranging from 0.17% to 0. 33% are generally used in combination with 2% to 4 % piperonyl butoxide. This combination is considered to be an effective pediculicide when applied topically in the form of solution, shampoos, or gels. The medication is applied to the affected area and then repeated in 7 to 10 days to kill lice larvae. The drug should not be applied more than twice in 24 hours.

Adverse Effects When applied according to directions, pyrethrins have a low order of toxicity. Most of the adverse reactions are cutaneous and include irritation, erythema, itching, and swelling. Contact with mucous membranes should be avoided.

Contraindications/Precautions/Warnings Individuals who are allergic to pyrethrins or to chrysanthemums should not use this agent. Ragweed-sensitive individuals should not use unrefined pyrethrins because of the risk of cross-sensitivity. This agent should not be applied to the patient's eyelashes and eyebrows. Instead a nonmedicated ointment such as petrolatum can be applied to these areas to smother the lice. (See discussion of lice infestation of the eyelid in Chapter 22, "Ophthalmic Disorders.")

Special Population Considerations Pyrethrin-containing preparations may be used on infants, young children, and pregnant or lactating women.

Permethrin

In 1991, FDA approved reclassifying of permethrin cream rinse from a prescription to a nonprescription medication for treating head lice. Although permethrin is effective, lice may develop resistance to it.[5] Permethrin is more effective than pyrethrin and piperonyl butoxide when used in a single application. However, no significant difference exists in effectiveness when used for a second application.[6,7]

Mechanism of Action Permethrin is a synthetic pyrethroid that acts on the nerve cell membrane of lice. It disrupts the sodium channel, delaying repolarization and causing paralysis of the parasite.

Pharmacokinetics When permethrin is applied to the skin, it is estimated that less than 2% is absorbed, after which the agent is metabolized.

Indication Permethrin is indicated for treating head lice only.

Dosage/Administration Guidelines The 1% cream rinse should be applied in sufficient quantities to cover or saturate the hair and scalp. It should be left on the hair for 10 minutes before rinsing.

Adverse Effects The main adverse effects include transient pruritus, burning, stinging and irritation to the scalp. Two cases of respiratory difficulty have been reported as well as two cases of minor musculoskeletal injury.[4]

Contraindications/Precautions/Warnings The drug is contraindicated in patients who are sensitive to pyrethrins or chrysanthemums. Permethrin should not be used on infants younger than 2 years.

Therapeutic Comparison

Pyrethrins in combination with piperonyl butoxide have comparable efficiency to benzene hexachloride shampoo, a prescription pediculicide. The cure rate is as high as 95% with pyrethrins and 87.9% with benzene hexachloride. Additionally, pyrethrins are less toxic. Permethrin has been shown to be as effective as pyrethrins and benzene hexachloride in treating head lice.

Product Selection Guidelines

Pyrethrins may be recommended for treating pubic lice. For treatment of head or body lice, the choice between pyrethrins and permethrin is based on patient sensitivity to chrysanthemums or ragweed. Permethrin is the appropriate agent for patients with such sensitivities. This agent is also the best choice for patients who prefer a single-application product. Table 31–4 lists examples of products containing these agents.

Table 31–4

Selected Pediculicides

Trade Name	Primary Ingredients
A-200 Lice Killing Shampoo	Piperonyl butoxide 4%; pyrethrins 0.33%
End-Lice Liquid	Piperonyl butoxide 4%; pyrethrins 0.33%
InnoGel Plus Gel	Piperonyl butoxide 4%; pyrethrins 0.33%
Licide Shampoo	Piperonyl butoxide 4%; pyrethrins 0.33%
Licide Blue Gel	Pyrethrins 0.2%
Nix Cream Rinse	Permethrin 1%
Pronto Lice Killing Shampoo	Piperonyl butoxide 4%; pyrethrins 0.33%
R&C Shampoo/Conditioner	Piperonyl butoxide 3%; pyrethrins 0.33%
RID Lice Killing Shampoo	Piperonyl butoxide 4%; pyrethrins 0.33%

Case Study 31–2

Patient Complaint/History

Sharon, a healthy 8-year-old girl, complained to her mother of itching on her scalp. The itching, which provokes scratching, interferes with her sleep and studies. This symptom began 2 weeks after she spent a night with a friend. Her mother asked the pharmacist about this problem.

Clinical Considerations/Strategies

Readers can use the following considerations/strategies to determine whether treatment of the patient's condition with nonprescription medication is warranted:

- Advise the mother on how to identify the type of problem.
- Advise the patient of the contagious nature of lice infestations.
- Evaluate the clinical appropriateness of using permethrin and pyrethrins in combination with piperonyl butoxide.

Patient Education/Counseling

Readers can use the following strategies to develop a patient education/counseling plan that will ensure optimal therapeutic outcomes:

- Recommend procedures for proper application of the topical products.
- Counsel the mother on how to prevent reinfestation.

Patient Education for Lice Infestation

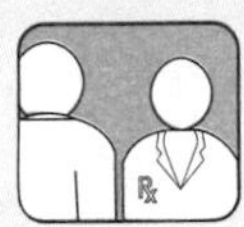

The objective of self-treatment is to rid the body of lice. A secondary objective is to implement measures to prevent future infestations. For most patients, carefully following product instructions and the self-care measures listed below will help ensure optimal therapeutic outcomes.

Nondrug Measures

- Use hot water to wash hairbrushes, combs, and toys of infested patients for 10 minutes.
- Use hot water to wash the clothes, bedding, and towels of infested patients. Dry the items on the hottest dryer setting the fabric permits.
- Either discard objects or clothing that cannot be washed, or seal them in plastic bags for the length of the louse's life cycle when it is unable to feed on a host (2 weeks).

Preventive Measures

- Avoid direct physical contact with an infested patient.
- Do not share articles such as combs, brushes, towels, caps, and hats.

Nonprescription Medications

- Note that when a member of a family becomes infested with lice, all members of the family should be treated.
- If using a shampoo, apply it to the wet hair and scalp. Allow it to remain for 10 minutes.
- Work the shampoo into a lather and then rinse thoroughly.
- If using a cream rinse, shampoo the hair, apply the rinse to the wet hair and scalp, and allow it to remain for 10 minutes.
- Dry the hair. Then use a fine-toothed comb to remove dead lice and eggs.
- Note that the pediculicide can cause temporary irritation, erythema, itching, and swelling of the scalp.
- Avoid contact of the pediculicide with mucous membranes.
- To ensure all lice are killed, repeat the entire process in 7 to 10 days.

Seek medical attention if symptoms of a lice infestation persist after the second treatment.

Patient Assessment of Pediculosis

In some cases of pediculosis, visual inspection of the scalp will verify the presence or absence of head lice or nits. Similarly, body lice can be determined by identifying adult lice and nits in the seams of clothing. If a patient does not want such inspection or if lice has not been confirmed by another health care professional, the pharmacist should not recommend a pediculicide. When the disorder is confirmed, the pharmacist should recommend the appropriate pediculicide according to the patient's allergic history to chrysanthemums or ragweed.

Patient Counseling for Pediculosis

Many individuals still associate pediculosis with poor hygiene. For that reason, patients and caregivers are often reluctant to seek counseling for using pediculicides. Pharmacists must not appear judgmental or repulsed when providing such information. In fact, pharmacists are in an ideal setting to aid community-wide education about lice infestations.

Patients with confirmed lice infestations should be counseled on which product is best for their clinical situation and on how to use the product properly. Preventive measures should also be discussed. The box "Patient Education for Lice Infestation" lists specific information to provide patients.

Evaluation of Patient Outcomes for Pediculosis

Follow-up of lice infestations should occur 10 days after the initial pharmacist–patient encounter. Either a telephone call or scheduled visit to the pharmacy is an appropriate follow-up method. The pharmacist should advise the patient to seek medical attention if symptoms of lice infestation persist after a second application of a pediculicide.

CONCLUSIONS

Stings of honeybees, yellow jackets, hornets, wasps, and fire ants can cause pain, discomfort, illness, and severe local and systemic reactions. In people who are not hypersensitive, insect stings and bites cause local irritation, inflammation, swelling, and itching that provoke rubbing and scratching. In hypersensitive people, anaphylactic reactions may pose serious emergency problems.

People sensitized to insect venom may react violently when stung. They need immediate, active treatment such as the administration of epinephrine hydrochloride. Partial desensitization may be accomplished by insect venom immunotherapy. The pharmacist can play a significant role by advising hypersensitive individuals about emergency procedures for insect stings. The pharmacist should also advise and educate patients about treating and preventing lice infestation, tick-induced disease, and other insect bites.

Nonprescription products are of minimal value to hypersensitive patients. Immunotherapy is an option for the hypersensitive patient and must be accomplished under a physician's supervision.

The temporary relief of itching and the pain that follows insect bites may be achieved by topically applied preparations that should not be used for prolonged periods. Topical nonprescription preparations that contain local anesthetics, antihistamines, hydrocortisone, or counterirritants are considered safe and effective when used properly for adults and children 2 years of age and older. Preparations of zinc oxide and calamine may be applied to adults, children, and infants to prevent secondary bacterial infections.

Treating allergic reactions to insect stings is usually of short duration, lasting from hours to a few days. Once the emergency situation disappears, no further active treatment is required.

For most patients or caregivers, the social embarrassment of pediculosis is a major concern. They may not be aware of the risk of contracting typhus from lice. Available nonprescripition pediculicides contain either pyrethrins or permethrin. Both agents are effective in treating lice infestations.

Prevention of insect stings and bites, including bites from lice, is the best "treatment" for these disorders. Pharmacists should include prevention of future stings and bites in their counseling of patients who seek products to treat such injuries. School officials, health officials, and health care professionals should work together to educate the public about pediculosis and the methods of preventing it.

References

1. Valentine MD. Anaphylaxis and stinging insect hypersensitivity. *JAMA.* 1992;268:2830–3.
2. Steere AC. Lyme disease. *N Engl J Med.* 1989;321:586–96.
3. Reisman RE. Duration of venom immunotherapy: relationship to the severity of symptoms of initial insect sting anaphylaxis. *J Allergy Clin Immunol.* 1993;92:831–6.
4. DeSimone ED II, McCracker G. September lice alert. *US Pharmacist.* 1994;9:32–40.
5. Dawes M, Hicks NR, Fleminger M, et al. Treatment of head lice. *Br Med J.* 1999;318:385.
6. Carson DS, Tribble PW, Weart CW. Pyrethrins combined with piperonyl butoxide (RID) vs 1% permethrin (NIX) in the treatment of head lice. *Am J Dis Child.* 1998;142:768–9.
7. DiNapoli JB, Austin RD, Englender SJ, et al. Eradication of head lice with a single treatment. *Am J Public Health.* 1998;78:978–80.

CHAPTER 32

Acne

Joye Ann Billow

Chapter 32 at a Glance

Acne vulgaris, the most common adolescent skin disorder, is often linked to the onset of puberty. Although not a physical threat, acne may have a significant negative psychosocial effect on an adolescent during a time when physiologic changes necessitate emotional and social adjustments. Acne may precipitate problems of low self-esteem, social phobias, and depression and may even trigger obsessive–compulsive disorders or psychosis. However, medical treatment may manage acne symptoms and thus alleviate these psychosocial conditions.[1,2]

More than an estimated 60% of U.S. teenagers use nonprescription products to treat acne, and more than 65% of reported sales of acne remedies occur in pharmacies.[3] Thus, the pharmacist can be instrumental in assisting teenagers to make informed choices about a treatment that may greatly affect their cosmetic and psychosocial well-being. This contact also represents a tremendous opportunity for pharmacists to introduce a new group of consumers to the value of pharmaceutical care.

Editor's Note: This chapter is based, in part, on the 11th edition chapter titled "Acne Products," which was written by Joye Ann Billow.

Epidemiology of Acne

The incidence of acne is nearly universal; approximately 85% of all people between the ages of 12 and 24 years will develop it to some degree.[4] Acne typically develops in males ages 16 to 18 years and in females ages 15 to 17 years. Acne lesions may precede other signs of puberty and may be diagnosed as early as age 7 years. Papular lesions generally appear during the mid-teen years, and nodular lesions appear in the late teens. In males, acne generally clears by the mid-20s. However, in females it may persist through the third and fourth decades (in each case, among approximately 30% of women) and may worsen during menopause.[5] It may be exacerbated by cosmetics (acne cosmetica) at any age.[6] Acne may disappear spontaneously in adults for reasons that are not readily apparent.

Anatomy and Physiology of Skin

Acne vulgaris has its origin in the pilosebaceous units in the dermis. (See Figure 32–1A.) These units, consisting of a hair follicle and the associated sebaceous glands, are connected to the skin surface by a duct (the infundibulum) through which the hair shaft passes. Epithelial tissue (an ex-

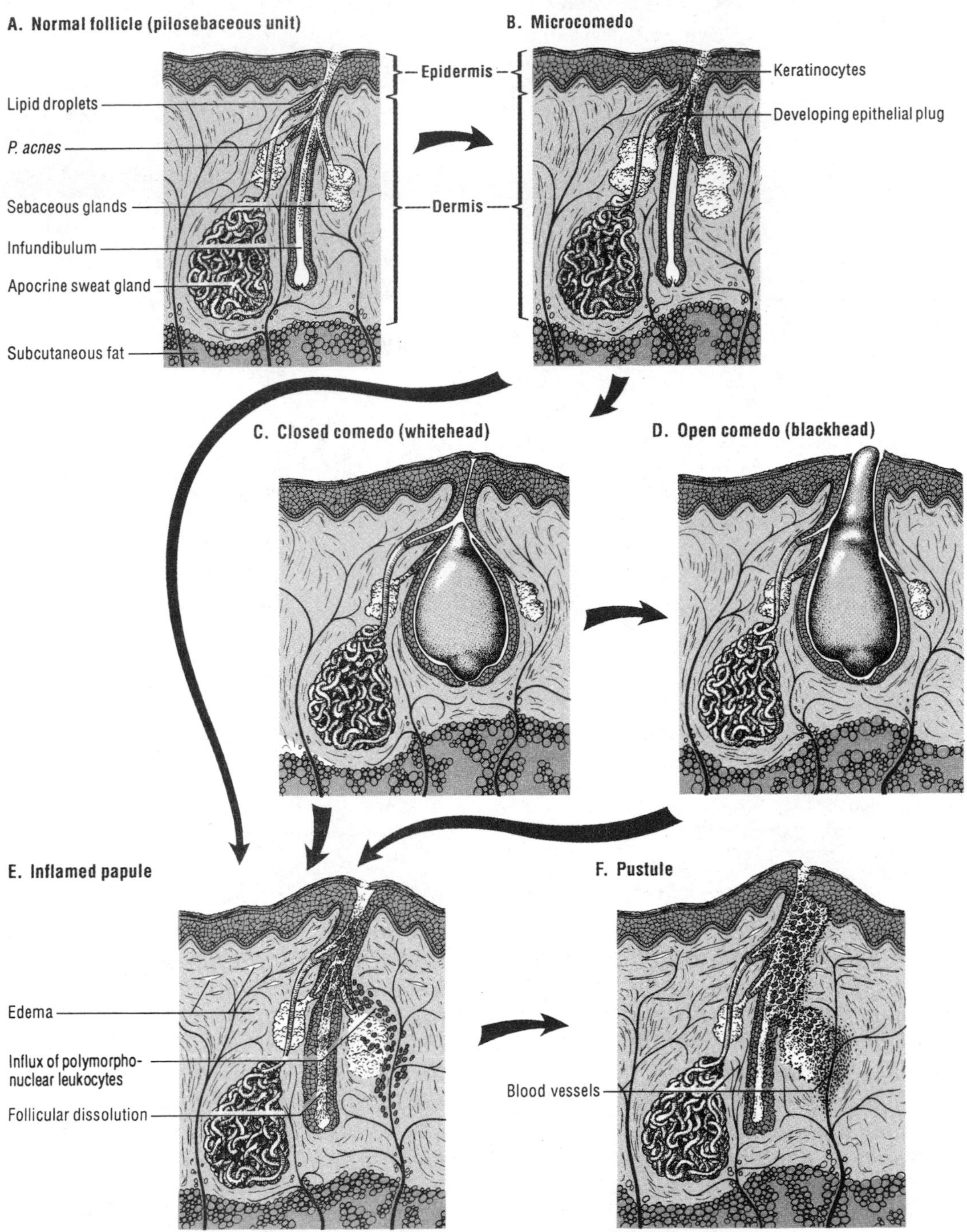

Figure 32–1 Pathogenesis of acne. Adapted with permission from Fulton JE, Bradley S. *Cutis.* 1976;7:560.

tension of the epidermis) forms the lining of the infundibulum. The sebaceous glands produce sebum, which passes to the skin surface through the infundibulum and then spreads over the skin to retard water loss and to maintain hydration of the skin and hair. Because the sebaceous glands are more common on the face, back, and chest, acne tends to occur most often in those areas.

Etiology of Acne

The production of androgenic hormones increases as a male or female approaches puberty. Although the precise cause of acne is not known, processes linked to this increase are closely related to acne development. Specifically, androgenic hormones stimulate the sebaceous glands with the resultant appearance of acne usually being noticed at the actual onset of puberty.[7] Four processes linked to the pubertal increase in androgens are closely related to acne development: (1) an abnormal keratinization of cells in the infundibulum, (2) an increase in sebum productions, (3) an accelerated growth of *Propionibacterium acnes*, and (4) the occurrence of inflammation.[5,7] These four processes are discussed in detail in the next section.

Pathophysiology of Acne

The abnormal keratinization of the cells shed in the infundibulum produces greater than normal cohesiveness and results in obstruction of the follicle rather than the normal removal of cells to the skin surface. The trapped, keratinized cells plug and distend the follicle to form a microcomedo, the initial pathologic lesion of acne. (See Figure 32–1B.) As more cells and sebum accumulate, the microcomedo enlarges and becomes visible as a closed comedo, or whitehead, and is visible as a small, pale nodule just beneath the skin surface. This lesion is the precursor to developing other acne lesions.

The hair in the follicle may play a significant role in comedo development. If it is thin and small, the hair may become entrapped in the plug. The heavier hair of the scalp and beard push the developing plug to the surface, preventing comedo formation.

An open comedo or blackhead occurs when sufficient material accumulates behind the plug, and the orifice of the follicular canal becomes distended, allowing the plug to protrude. The tip of the plug of the open comedo may darken because of melanin (not dirt or oxidized fat).

The increase in circulating androgens stimulates production of sebum, which is prevented from reaching the skin surface by the obstructing keratinized cells. At the same time, *P. acnes* (an anaerobic rod and the main microorganism found in the sebaceous duct) undergoes accelerated growth. *P. acnes* is a major contributor to causing inflammatory acne lesions through lipase production and the breakdown of sebum to free fatty acids. Its colony counts are higher in patients with acne than in those without acne. The resultant inflammation causes localized tissue destruction.[5,7]

Inflammatory acne begins with closed comedones that distend the follicle, causing the cellular lining of the walls to spread and become thin. Primary inflammation of the follicle wall develops with the disruption of the epithelial lining and lymphocyte infiltration. A severe inflammatory reaction results if the follicle wall ruptures spontaneously or is ruptured by picking, squeezing, or attempted expression with a comedo extractor, or if the contents are discharged into the surrounding tissue. The results may be abscesses, which may cause scars or pits after healing. The pustules or purulent nodules of inflammatory acne are more likely to cause permanent scarring than those of noninflammatory acne.

Signs and Symptoms of Acne

Acne involves the oil glands and hair follicles of the skin, primarily on the face and trunk. The disease is characterized by whiteheads, blackheads, acne pimples, and acne blemishes.[8] Whiteheads and blackheads are noninflammatory lesions also known as closed and open comedones. (See Figure 32–1C and D.) Noninflammatory acne is characterized by the presence of closed or open comedones. (See the "Color Plates," photograph 18.)

Inflammatory acne is characterized by pimples (i.e., small, prominent, inflamed elevations of the skin), which may rupture to form a papule. (See Figure 32–1E.) Papules are inflammatory lesions appearing as raised, reddened areas on the skin, which may enlarge to form pustules. Pustules also appear as raised, reddened areas filled with pus. (See Figure 32–1F and the "Color Plates," photograph 19.) More extensive penetration into surrounding and underlying tissue produces necrotic, purulent nodular lesions, previously designated as cysts, and may lead to pitting and scarring if left untreated.

The typical acne patient presents with a combination of lesions: comedones (open and closed), papules, and pustules. The lesions are typically found on the face, chest, and back where sebaceous glands are common, but they may also appear on other body surfaces.[5,7,9]

A Word about Rosacea

Rosacea (acne rosacea, or "adult acne") is a generalized disorder of the blood vessels. It can be differentiated from acne vulgaris in various ways. Onset is not typically linked to endocrine changes associated with surges in androgen levels, which occur from adolescence to the early or mid-20s. The condition may occur in early adulthood or at any time later. Symptoms may be progressive and may consist of sensitivity to the touch, reddening of the face, enlarged blood vessels, and formation of solid red papules or pustules. Factors that may aggravate symptoms include alcohol ingestion, overexposure to sunlight, spicy foods, smoking, hot drinks, temperature extremes, friction, irritating cosmetics, and systemic corticosteroid use. Symptoms tend to diminish and to flare in a somewhat cyclic pattern. Lesions tend to be localized to the central portion of the face (e.g., center of forehead, nose, and chin). Comedones are not typically present.

As with acne vulgaris, there is no cure for rosacea. Medical referral is required, and treatment is directed toward relieving symptoms. If untreated, symptoms may progressively worsen. Oral antibiotics (e.g., erythromycin, tetracycline), topical metronidazole gel (0.75%), or oral isotretinoin may be required to treat the lesions.[10]

Classification System for Acne

Various systems have been used to classify the severity of acne vulgaris. Table 32–1 presents a synthesized classification system that is based on the older Pillsbury scheme. The synthesized system indicates the severity level of the acne from the mildest form (consisting primarily of comedones often localized on one portion of the face) through the most severe form (consisting of necrotic, purulent nodules, often called cystic acne, nodulocystic acne, or acne conglobata in which moderate to severe scarring is likely).[7,11–13]

Acne classification was addressed by the Consensus Conference on Acne Classification convened by the American Academy of Dermatology in 1990. The consensus panel concluded that a strictly quantitative classification of acne cannot be established and that "acne grading can best be accomplished by the use of a pattern-diagnosis system, which would include a global (total) evaluation of lesions and their complications such as drainage, hemorrhage, and pain."[13] The division of acne into inflammatory and noninflammatory types has not changed. However, the opinion is that noninflammatory acne, presenting as comedones only, can rarely be classified as severe even if the comedones are present in large numbers. A recent reexamination of acne classification requires the presence of a microcomedo as the initial pathologic condition.

Special Considerations for Acne

Several factors are known to exacerbate existing acne or cause periodic flare-ups of acne in some patients. Other factors widely assumed to cause acne have not been proven as etiologic factors.

Substantiated Exacerbating Factors for Acne

The patient may have control over some exacerbating factors, such as environmental, physical, and emotional issues or cosmetic use. One predisposing factor, heredity, cannot be controlled. The chances of offspring developing acne are higher when both parents have had acne than when only one parent has the disorder.[14]

Environmental and Physical Factors

Hydration decreases the size of the pilosebaceous duct orifice; therefore, exposure to high-humidity environments or other situations that induce frequent and prolonged sweating can exacerbate acne by reducing the orifice and preventing the loosening of comedones. Tight-fitting clothes that restrict air movement and prevent evaporation of skin moisture also increase skin hydration.

Acne symptoms may increase because of local irritation or friction. Occlusive clothing, headbands, helmets, or other friction-producing devices can aggravate acne (acne mechanica). Even resting the chin or cheek on the hand often or for long periods creates localized conditions conducive to lesion formation in acne-prone individuals.

Exposure to dirt, vaporized cooking oils, or certain industrial chemicals, such as coal tar and petroleum derivatives, may cause occupational acne.[15]

Cosmetic Use

Acne cosmetica is a low-grade, mild form of acne on the face, cheek, and chin. The lesions are typically closed, noninflammatory comedones and cannot easily be distinguished from similar lesions of acne vulgaris. Acne cosmetica is more common in women because they are more likely to use cosmetics. Some products may contain oils that are comedogenic (e.g., lanolin, mineral oil, or cocoa butter). Oil-based cosmetics, including shampoos, may be occlusive and plug the follicles, thus exacerbating or even initiating acne.

Pomade acne, most often seen in African Americans and manifested by comedones along the hairline on the forehead and temples, is caused by the long-term use of hair dressing that contains occlusive or liquid petrolatum.

Emotional Factors

Severe or prolonged periods of stress or other emotional extremes may exacerbate acne; however, they do not cause

Table 32–1

Assessment of Acne Severity

Grade of Acne	Qualitative Description	Quantitative Description
I	Comedonal acne	Comedones only, <10 on face, none on trunk, no scars; noninflammatory lesions only
II	Papular acne	10–25 papules on face and trunk, mild scarring; inflammatory lesions <5 mm in diameter
III[a]	Pustular acne	More than 25 pustules, moderate scarring; size similar to papules but with visible, purulent core
IV[a]	Severe/persistent pustulocystic acne	Nodules or cysts, extensive scarring; inflammatory lesions >5 mm in diameter
—	Recalcitrant severe cystic acne	Extensive nodules/cysts

[a] Some overlap with previous grade of acne.

Case Study 32–1

Patient Complaint/History

Claudia, a 34-year-old female, presents to the pharmacist with a skin disorder that resembles noninflammatory acne. Her cheeks are red and rough; lesions that are typical of closed comedones are also present. The patient says the condition has worsened in the past year. She wants to treat the disorder with a nonprescription acne product and asks the pharmacist to recommend a product.

Next Claudia reveals that she rarely had acne blemishes as a teenager and, up until a year ago, did not regard herself as having had acne. She mentions that the condition seems to worsen before her menstrual period and that she often has eye irritation. Physical observation reveals a few small telangiectasias (spider veins) on the patient's cheeks.

Claudia's current medications include the following: Lo/Ovral-28 one tablet q am for 21 days, one inert tablet for 7 days; Tavist-D one tablet q 12 h prn.

Clinical Considerations/Strategies

Readers can use the following considerations/strategies to determine whether treatment of the patient's condition with nonprescription medications is warranted:

- Determine whether the lesions are actually acne vulgaris.
- Assess whether the condition may be a side effect induced by current medications.
- Attempt to determine the presence of exacerbating factors.
- Evaluate the patient to determine whether a relationship may exist between the facial lesions, ocular irritation, and telangiectasias.
- Assess the feasibility and appropriateness of a medical referral.
- Assess the potential of any nonprescription acne product to produce positive results.
- Determine the ingredient(s) in nonprescription acne products that would most likely produce a positive outcome.
- Determine the most appropriate dosage form for this patient.

Patient Education/Counseling

Readers can use the following strategies to develop a patient education/counseling plan that will help ensure optimal therapeutic outcomes:

- Explain the etiology and pathogenesis of the probable condition.
- Explain nondrug measures for acne management.
- Explain optimal use of nonprescription acne products, the warnings/precautions pertinent to these products, and the adverse effects associated with them.
- Explain the risk related to overexposure to UVA and UVB radiation, especially in the presence of photosensitizing chemicals.
- Encourage the patient to seek the advice of a dermatologist to confirm the assessment.

acne. How these factors increase acne severity is not known.

Hormonal Factors

Many women with acne experience a premenstrual flare-up of symptoms. Hormonal changes associated with ovulation and pregnancy are also related to flare-ups. Oral contraceptives containing androgenic progestins with higher androgen activity are implicated in the production of acne, as are certain cyclic progestins used in menopausal hormone replacement therapy. Although progestins with high androgenic activity have been implicated in acne production, some contraceptives with low androgenic progestins and some estrogens in higher dosage ranges have paradoxically been approved for acne treatment in women.[16]

Medication Use

Although medications can exacerbate preexisting acne vulgaris, medication-induced acne (acne medicamentosa) is not a true acne. Corticosteroids, both systemic and topical, may induce hypertrophic changes by sensitizing the follicle and producing steroid acne. Table 32–2 lists other drugs known to precipitate acneiform eruptions.[17,18]

Unsubstantiated Etiologic Factors

Little evidence supports a direct relationship between diet and acne. Several studies have demonstrated that chocolate does not affect acne even though some clinicians and patients remain unconvinced. Other clinicians think that dietary restrictions are unwarranted because no convincing evidence has been presented to implicate nuts, fats, colas, or carbohydrates. However, an indirect relationship has been proposed between acne and a diet high in fat and refined carbohydrates and low in fiber, suggesting that dietary habits may be a risk factor in acne.[19] People should avoid any particular food that seems to exacerbate their acne.

There is no evidence that sexual activity causes or exacerbates acne. Because acne usually begins at puberty and sexual activity may begin in the same time frame, some people have interpreted the two events as having a cause and effect relationship.

Treatment of Acne

Acne symptoms can be controlled to varying degrees because in most cases the disorder is self-limiting. Available therapeutic regimens and patient compliance will reduce symp-

Table 32–2

Medications That Can Induce Acne

Androgens	Haloperidol
Azathioprine	Halothane
Bromides	Iodides
Contraceptives, oral with a high progestin level	Isoniazid
Corticosteroids, systemic and topical	Lithium
Dantrolene	Phenytoin and other hydantoins
Ethionamide	Rifampin
	Thyroid preparations
	Trimethadione

Source: References 17 and 18.

toms and minimize permanent scarring. Because acne persists for long periods, often from adolescence to the early 20s or beyond, treatment must be long-term, continuous, and consistent.

Treatment Outcomes

The primary goal in self-treating acne is consistent, long-term use of methods to unblock pilosebaceous ducts and to keep the orifice open. Avoiding factors that exacerbate acne, such as physical irritation of the skin and oil-based cosmetics and cleansers, is another important goal in acne treatment. These two goals should aid in achieving the desired outcome: relieving the patient's physical and social discomfort.

General Treatment Approach

Self-treatment of acne is most effective in patients mature enough to understand that treatment will be long-term and that symptoms can be controlled but not cured. The treatment algorithm in Figure 32–2 outlines this approach to self-care by patients who have acne but have none of the exclusions to self-treatment.

Treatment of noninflammatory comedonal acne usually consists of using pharmacologic agents along with nonpharmacologic measures, such as cleansing the skin, to unblock pilosebaceous ducts and to keep them open. Irritants, such as nonprescription acne medications, also aid in unblocking the ducts. To improve the chances of a positive outcome for noninflammatory acne, the patient should avoid physical, environmental, and emotional factors that can exacerbate acne.

Treatment of inflammatory acne typically requires both nonprescription and prescription medication, such as oral and topical antibiotics and retinoids, as well as possible excision and drainage of inflammatory lesions. The effectiveness of oral antibiotics (e.g., erythromycin, clindamycin, minocycline, meclocycline, tetracycline, or doxycycline) and topical antibiotics (e.g., tetracycline, erythromycin, or clindamycin) in treating inflammatory acne is due to their ability to suppress the bacterial population of the sebaceous duct and to reduce lipase activity. Notwithstanding, these patients also benefit from properly cleansing the skin and from avoiding exacerbating factors.

Self-treatment is appropriate for only patients with grade I acne (i.e., noninflammatory acne of mild-to-moderate severity). This grade of acne presents with open or closed comedones. Situations in which physician referral is required include inflammatory acne consisting of observed papules, pustules, and nodules that are extensive. Also, if acne is associated with the use of a drug with comedogenic (e.g., androgenic) activity, the patient should contact a physician. If acne lesions persist beyond the mid-20s or develop in the mid-20s or later, the symptoms may signal rosacea rather than acne vulgaris. These conditions need to be medically differentiated because the approach for treating rosacea, although similar to that for treating acne vulgaris, also has unique elements.[10]

A physician must direct suppressing or altering hormonal activity, correcting disfiguring effects, and using prescription drugs to treat acne. Further, the patient should not add nonprescription medications to prescribed regimens unless the prescriber recommends them.

Nonpharmacologic Therapy

Numerous products, medicated and nonmedicated, are available for cleansing the skin. Acne patients often need guidance in selecting the appropriate products for their special skin care needs. Information about avoiding situations that can worsen acne is also important.

Cleansing the Skin

Removing excess sebum from the skin in a program of daily washing produces a mild drying of the skin and, perhaps, mild erythema. The affected areas should be thoroughly but gently washed at least twice daily (more frequently if skin is oily) with warm water, medicated or unmedicated soap, and a soft washcloth; then patted dry. Washing should not be excessively vigorous; it should cause barely noticeable peeling that can loosen comedones. Washing intensity and frequency should be reduced and a less drying soap should be considered if tautness occurs.

Facial soaps that do not contain moisturizing oils are usually satisfactory. Soaps that contain antibacterial agents have no clinical value. Salicylic acid, sulfur, and a combination of sulfur and resorcinol or resorcinol monoacetate are safe and effective for self-treating acne, but their effectiveness as soaps is questionable because little, if any, residue is left on the skin after washing.[20]

Soap substitutes that contain surfactants have been suggested for acne because they are less drying to the skin. Because a mild degree of drying is desirable, a facial soap should be tried first. Some cleansing preparations contain pumice, polyethylene, or aluminum oxide particles to add abrasive action. Used gently, abrasive agents may be helpful in treat-

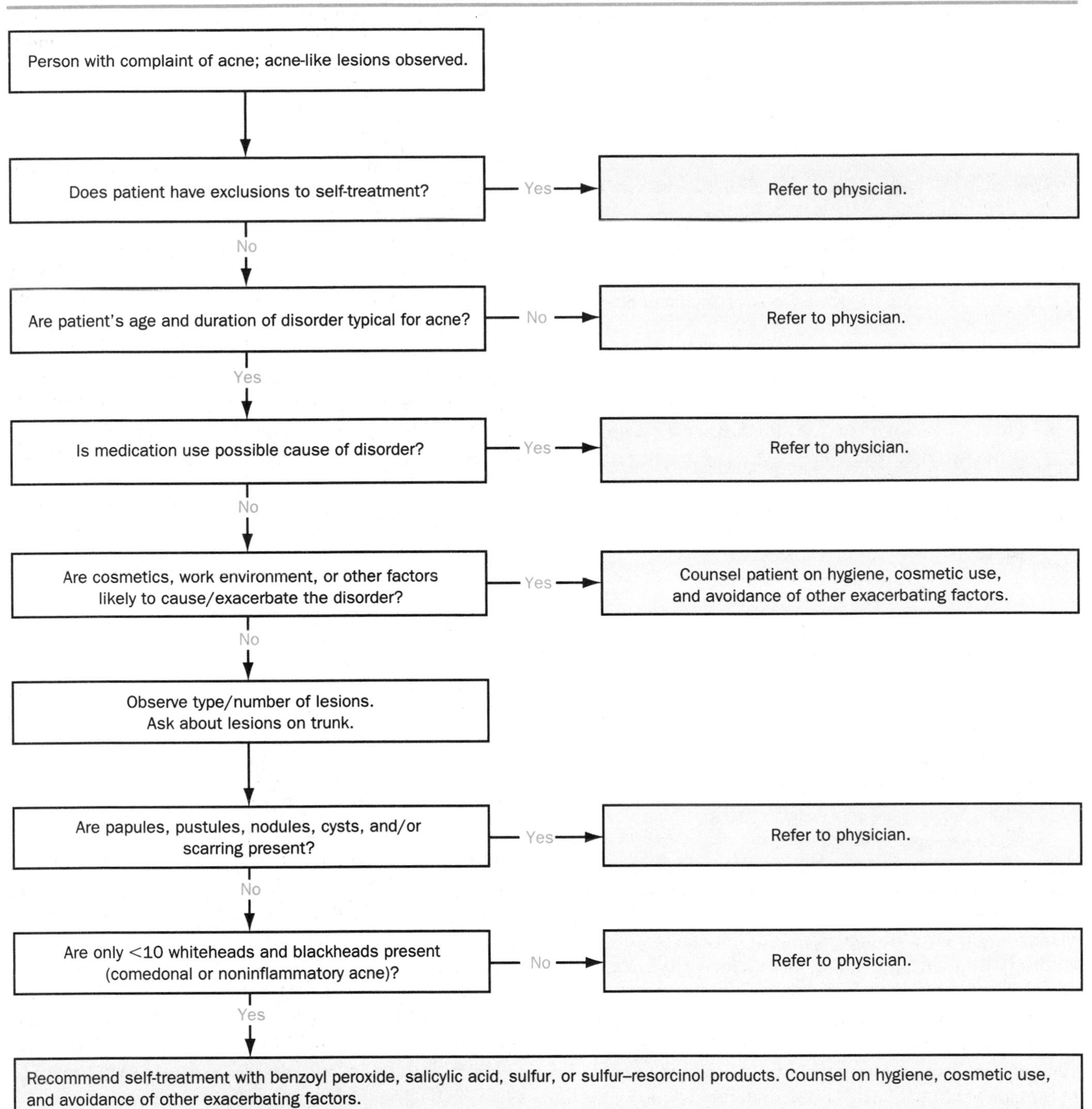

Figure 32–2 Self-care of acne.

ing noninflammatory acne. They should be avoided in inflammatory acne because of increased irritation. If it is inconvenient to wash during the day, the patient can use cleansing pads that contain alcohol, acetone, and a surfactant while at school or work.

Minimizing Exacerbating Factors

Minimizing exacerbating factors conducive to developing acne can help prevent the condition. If acne lesions are present where clothes, headbands, helmets, or other devices cause friction, preventing friction-induced irritation should be discussed with the patient. Irritation also occurs as a result of routinely resting the face or chin on the hand; if problematic, this habit should be avoided or minimized.

The patient should use water-based cosmetic products and frequently wash oily hair with a water-based shampoo.

If exposure to environmental factors (e.g., dirt, dust, oil, or chemical irritants) exacerbates the acne, the patient should be counseled on how to minimize or avoid such exposures.

To prevent infection, the patient should not pick or squeeze the lesions. Open comedones may be regarded as unsightly by the patient, but a trained professional can easily express them, using a clean comedo extractor.

Pharmacologic Therapy

Benzoyl peroxide is the most effective and widely used nonprescription medication currently available for treatment of comedonal acne. Although proposed and initially classified as a Category I (generally recognized as safe and effective by the Food and Drug Administration [FDA]) ingredient, it was temporarily reclassified to Category III (i.e., more data needed to determine safety) because of concern over its tumorigenic potential. (See the section "Safety and Effectiveness" under "Benzoyl Peroxide" for further discussion of safety issues involving this agent.)

Category I topical anti-acne ingredients include 0.5% to 2% salicylic acid, 3% to 8% sulfur, and a combination of 3% to 8% sulfur with either 2% resorcinol or 3% resorcinol monoacetate.[8]

Benzoyl Peroxide

Benzoyl peroxide is commonly available in concentrations of 2.5%, 5%, and 10% in such diverse dosage forms as lotions, gels, creams, cleansers, masks, and soaps. Benzoyl peroxide products in concentrations of 4%, 5.5%, and 20% are also available.

Mechanism of Action Benzoyl peroxide causes irritation and desquamation that prevents closure of the pilosebaceous orifice. Its irritant effect causes an increased turnover rate of the epithelial cells lining the follicular duct, which then increases sloughing and promotes resolution of the comedones. Its oxidizing potential may contribute to bacteriostatic and bactericidal activity, thus suppressing the local population of *P. acnes* and reducing the formation of irritating free fatty acids. It also exhibits irritant, drying, and sensitizing effects.

Case Study 32–2

Patient Complaint/History

Jason, a 20-year-old male, approaches the pharmacy counter and asks to speak with the pharmacist. The young man has typical symptoms of moderate acne. His facial lesions consist of numerous noninflammatory comedones on the cheeks, nose, and forehead, plus several inflammatory pustules on the chin. Jason is planning a trip during spring break to Florida in 2 weeks. He asks for help in selecting a nonprescription acne product to clear the flare-up on his chin.

Jason reveals that he is taking an oral antibiotic to treat the acne and that the prescribing dermatologist suggested supplementation with nonprescription products. The dermatologist left the choice of product up to the patient, who indicates he has never used nonprescription acne products. Pharmacy records show that the patient has been compliant in taking tetracycline 250 mg one capsule daily; he is not currently taking other medications.

Clinical Considerations/Strategies

Readers can use the following considerations/strategies to determine whether treatment of the patient's condition with nonprescription medications is warranted:

- Assess the presence of external exacerbating factors that can be controlled by the patient.
- Assess the potential value of a supplemental nonprescription acne product.
- Determine the ingredient(s) in nonprescription acne products that would produce a positive outcome and that would be tolerated if used properly.
- Determine the most appropriate dosage form and strength for this patient.
- Assess nonpharmacologic measures that should be added to the treatment regimen.
- Assess the use of adjunctive nonprescription acne preparations that may be appropriate for the upcoming vacation environment.

Patient Education/Counseling

Readers can use the following strategies to develop a patient education/counseling plan that will help ensure optimal therapeutic outcomes:

- Explain the pathogenesis, as well as etiologic and confounding factors of acne.
- Explain the importance of proper hygiene of affected areas.
- Explain the importance of nonpharmacologic measures, and identify exacerbating situations to avoid or minimize.
- Explain the value and proper use of nonprescription drug therapy.
- Support/justify the use of recommended supplementary nonprescription product(s).
- Explain optimal use of nonprescription acne products, the warnings/precautions pertinent to these products, and the adverse effects associated with them.
- Encourage the patient to comply with the suggested pharmacologic and nonpharmacologic measures.
- Emphasize the long-term nature of the treatment.

Therapeutic Comparison of Dosage Forms Clinical response to all concentrations is similar in reducing the number of inflammatory lesions. However, the different formulations are not equivalent. The drying effect of the alcohol gel base enhances benzoyl peroxide's effectiveness; therefore, this form is superior to a lotion of the same concentration. Some products, mainly gels, are available by prescription only. Although washes and cleansers containing benzoyl peroxide are widely used as acne treatment adjuncts, they have little or no comedolytic effect.[21]

Dosage/Administration Guidelines See Table 32–3 for instructions on the proper use of topical nonprescription benzoyl peroxide products.

Adverse Effects Excessive dryness, marked peeling, some skin sloughing, erythema, or edema indicates that lower concentrations should be used for shorter periods of time. Use of the drug may cause transient stinging and burning, but patients should not be alarmed unless it persists or becomes worse.

Precautions/Warnings Benzoyl peroxide may bleach hair and clothing. Care must be taken to avoid exposing these items to the product.

Other sources of irritation, such as sunlamps and excessive exposure to the sun, should also be avoided.

The drug should not be used concurrently with other topical products unless a physician or pharmacist recommends concomitant use.

Safety and Effectiveness Safety studies are ongoing to determine whether benzoyl peroxide enhances the ability of ultraviolet radiation to produce skin cancer. Meanwhile, the product remains on the market, but a rule proposed by the FDA requires additional warning statements and directions on the label.[22] The FDA has delayed final action on this medication, pending further study[8,23,24] because of reports that benzoyl peroxide is a tumor promoter and progressor but is neither an initiator nor a complete carcinogen.[25,26] Thus, while studies are being conducted and analyzed, the FDA is unable to state that this ingredient is unsafe for use. The FDA acknowledges that this research, as well as a final determination on benzoyl peroxide's safety, may take a number of years.[27–29]

A recent interim 52-week study by the Nonprescription Drug Manufacturers Association (NDMA), filed March 1, 1999, with FDA, concluded that benzoyl peroxide "is not carcinogenic in the skin or in 'select internal organs' of mice and rats." A second 52-week study sponsored by NDMA indicates that the medication "does not enhance photocarcinogenesis in mice."[30] At press time, FDA had not revised its 1991 final monograph for acne products.

Salicylic Acid

A mild comedolytic agent, salicylic acid is available in various nonprescription acne products in concentrations of 0.5% to 2%.

Table 32–3

Administration Guidelines for Benzoyl Peroxide

Using a nonmedicated soap, gently cleanse the affected area plus any area likely to be affected; then pat dry.

- Smooth a small quantity of the preparation over the area once or twice daily.
- To determine sensitivity to the product, limit initial applications to one or two small areas at the 2.5% or 5% concentration.
- Leave initial application on the skin for only 15 minutes; then wash off.
- If no discomfort occurs, increase the time benzoyl peroxide is left on the skin in 15-minute increments as tolerance allows.
- Once the product is tolerated for 2 hours, leave it on overnight. The once-a-day application may be all that is needed. If desired, apply a morning dose if tolerable.
- For fair-skinned individuals, initiate therapy with the 2.5%, 4%, or 5% strength and apply only once daily during the first few weeks of therapy.
- Because it is highly irritating, use benzoyl peroxide with great care near the eyes, mouth, lips, and nose, as well as near cuts, scrapes, and other abrasions.
- Do not use this product concurrently with other topical products unless a physician or pharmacist recommends such use.
- If excessive dryness, marked peeling, some skin sloughing, erythema, or edema occur, use lower concentrations for shorter periods of time.
- If needed, apply cool compresses to relieve the discomfort of inflamed skin.
- Be aware that the product can bleach hair and clothing.
- Do not be alarmed if transient stinging and burning occur unless the symptoms persist or become worse. If excessive stinging and burning occur after application, remove the preparation with soap and water; then wait until the next day to reapply.
- Avoid exposure to other sources of irritation, such as sunlamps or excessive time in the sun. Use a sunscreen if sun exposure is unavoidable. Apply the sunscreen after applying the benzoyl peroxide.
- Adhere to the treatment regimen for at least 4 to 6 weeks to see the full therapeutic effect.

Pharmacologically, salicylic acid acts as a surface keratolytic.[4] The keratolytic effect and possible enhanced absorption of other agents provide the rationale for the topical use of salicylic acid. However, its safety is questionable when used over large areas for prolonged periods of time.[22]

The use of salicylic acid in cleansing preparations is considered adjunctive acne treatment in reducing comedonal lesions and in improving the overall condition.[21] A recent review indicates that salicylic acid pads are safe, effective, and superior to benzoyl peroxide in preventing and clearing both the comedones and inflammatory lesions of acne.[31]

Sulfur

Sulfur has met the criteria of the FDA Advisory Review Panel for Over-the-Counter Topical Acne Products, although the claim for its antibacterial effects was disallowed.[8] Alternate forms of sulfur, such as sodium thiosulfate, zinc sulfate, and zinc sulfide, are not recognized in the monograph as safe and effective.

Sulfur, in a precipitated or colloidal form, is included in acne products as a keratolytic in concentrations of 3% to 10%. It is generally accepted as an effective agent for promoting the resolution of existing comedones, but, on continued use, it may have a comedogenic effect.

Sulfur-containing products are applied in a thin film to the affected area one to three times daily.[32] They have a noticeable color and odor, characteristics that must be considered when their selection and use are being recommended. Compliance may be enhanced by recommending fleshtone products or by suggesting usage after school and at bedtime.

Resorcinol and Resorcinol Monoacetate

Although resorcinol and resorcinol monoacetate are not considered to be efficacious as single agents in treatment of acne, they have been offered in concentrations of 1% to 2%. Doubt exists as to whether percutaneous absorption of resorcinol may precipitate systemic toxicity when these agents are applied to extensive areas of the body. The FDA advisory review panel concluded that, when used alone, these agents in lower concentrations are safe but not effective in the topical treatment of acne. Therefore, FDA placed such products in Category II (not generally recognized as safe and effective, or unacceptable indications).[12]

Sulfur–Resorcinol Combination Products

FDA includes the combination of 3% to 8% sulfur with 2% resorcinol or 3% resorcinol monoacetate in the Category I list of active ingredients for nonprescription acne products.[8] The precise mechanism by which this combination helps resolve acne lesions has not been determined. The agents function primarily as keratolytics, fostering cell turnover and desquamation.

Sulfur–resorcinol products have the characteristic color and odor noted for the sulfur-only products. Additionally, resorcinol may produce a dark brown scale on some darker-skinned individuals, who should be forewarned and reassured that the reaction is reversible when the medication is discontinued.

Therapeutic Comparison of Acne Agents

See Table 32–4 for a comparison of the therapeutic properties among the major acne products.

Product Selection Guidelines

Nonprescription medications for treating acne are applied topically, so the most important patient factor is willingness to comply with the treatment. The mental and emotional maturity to be patient with the long-term nature of the treatment is necessary for success. The cosmetic appearance of the product may influence patient compliance. In these instances, the pharmacist should recommend the most effective cosmetic formulation.

Cleansing bars, liquids, suspensions, lotions, creams, and gels are generally used for anti-acne preparations. Cleansing products alone are of little value because they leave little active ingredient residue on the skin. Lotions and creams with a low-fat content do not counteract drying (astringent effect) and peeling (keratolytic effect). They are an acceptable alternative to the more effective gels and are recommended for dry or sensitive skin and for use during dry winter weather. Generally, gels are the most effective formulations because they are astringents and remain on the skin the longest. Nonfatty gels dry slowly if formulated in a completely aqueous base. Ethyl or isopropyl alcohol added to liquid preparations and gels hastens their drying to a film. The drying effect of the volatile solvents may enhance the effectiveness of the various preparations, but the solvents' greater irritant effect may be unacceptable to the patient.[33]

Thickening agents in preparations should not dry to a sticky film. Solids in most preparations leave a film that is not

Table 32–4

Comparison of Nonprescription Topical Acne Agents

	Benzoyl Peroxide	Sulfur	Salicylic Acid	Resorcinol/Resorcinol Monoacetate
Bactericidal	Yes	—	—	—
Keratolytic	—	Yes	Yes	When combined with sulfur
Comedolytic	—	Yes	Yes	—
Dose	2.5%–10%	2%–10%	0.5%–2%	1%–3%
Administration	1–2 times daily	1–3 times daily	Used mainly as cleanser, then rinsed off	Usually combined with sulfur
Adverse Effects	Bleached hair, clothing	Color, odor	Potent keratolytic at high concentration	Systemic toxicity if applied to large areas of body; may produce reversible brown scale in darker-skinned persons

Source: Adapted from reference 32; used with permission.

noticeably visible and does not need coloring to blend in with the skin. However, some products are intended to hide blemishes by depositing an opaque film of insoluble masking agents such as zinc oxide on the skin. Those products are tinted to improve their cosmetic effect; however, they rarely produce a satisfactory color match.

In general, cream formulations should be recommended for individuals with fair complexions and gels for those with dark complexions. Table 32–5 lists examples of acne products in these and other formulations.

Alternative Remedies

Kampo formulations, or Japanese herbal medicines that are combinations of powdered extracts of crude drugs, have been studied, both in vitro and in clinical trials, as acne treatments. These products were found to have antibacterial activity against *P. acnes.*[34,35] (See Chapter 45, "Herbal Remedies," for discussion of other herbal acne remedies.)

Patient Assessment of Acne

Patient assessment begins with asking questions to define the condition. Physical assessment, which involves observing the affected area and further questioning the patient, is the next step in evaluating the disorder. This evaluation helps determine whether the condition is acne vulgaris or another dermatologic condition with similar signs and symptoms. Physical assessment also determines whether the severity of the condition precludes self-treatment. (See Table 32–1.) Before self-care is recommended, an assessment of current medication use (prescription and nonprescription) is necessary to reveal prescribed treatments for the disorder or use of medications known to cause acne. (See Table 32–2.)

Asking the patient the following questions will help elicit the information needed to accurately assess the disorder and to recommend the appropriate treatment approach.

Q~ How old are you?

A~ *Identify the typical age range for acne. (See the section "Epidemiology of Acne.")* If the patient's age is outside the range typical for acne, refer the patient to a physician, preferably a dermatologist. If the age is within the range, continue the assessment process.

Q~ How long have you had acne?

A~ If the acne has persisted beyond puberty or if onset did not coincide with puberty, refer the patient to a physician, preferably a dermatologist.

Q~ Is the acne a problem on areas other than your face (e.g., neck, shoulders, chest, or back)?

A~ *Identify the severity grades of acne. (See Table 32–1.)* The greater the area involved, the more aggressive the treatment needs to be and may dictate referral to a physician.

Q~ What type of cosmetics, including makeup, after-shave, or hair preparations, do you use? Do they seem to aggravate the acne?

A~ Determine whether the location of either the newly affected areas or exacerbated affected areas coincide with the use of these products. Determine whether the patient is receptive to using water-based cosmetic products.

Q~ How often do you shampoo your hair? What type of shampoo do you use?

A~ Determine whether the affected areas occur along the hairline or in other areas the hair contacts. Determine whether the patient is receptive to shampooing more frequently or to using water-based cosmetic products.

Q~ How often do you wash your face? How (e.g., with pads or washcloths) do you wash? What type of cleanser do you use?

A~ Determine whether the frequency of washing or the cleansing products used (e.g., alcohol-impregnated pads) may be causing excessive drying of the skin. If so, recommend less drying cleansers.

Q~ Are you routinely exposed to environmental conditions such as heat or humidity or cooking oils in the air?

A~ If yes, exposure to dirt, vaporized cooking oils, or industrial chemicals such as petroleum derivatives may be causing the acne. Discuss with the patient ways to reduce exposure to these elements.

Q~ Are you currently using any medications, either prescription or nonprescription? If so, what are they?

A~ *Identify drugs known to induce acne. (See Table 32–2.)* If the patient is taking one of those drugs, refer the patient to a physician. Note that contraceptives with low-androgenic progestins and high dosages of estrogen are approved acne treatments for women.

Q~ Have you consulted a physician about your acne? If so, what treatment was suggested? Are you currently following it?

A~ Self-care treatments should not be added to prescribed regimens unless recommended by the prescriber. Advise the patient to contact the prescriber and return to the pharmacy if the prescriber recommends adjunctive nonprescription acne products.

Q~ Have you already tried acne treatment? If so, which ones? How did you use them? For how long did you use them? How effective were they?

A~ Attempt to find out whether a product was used

Table 32–5

Selected Products for Acne

Trade Name	Primary Ingredients
Benzoyl Peroxide Products	
Clean & Clear Persa-Gel 5	Benzoyl peroxide 5%
Clean & Clear Persa-Gel 10	Benzoyl peroxide 10%
Clearasil Maximum Strength, Tinted or Vanishing Cream	Benzoyl peroxide 10%
ExACT Adult Medication Cream	Benzoyl peroxide 2.5%
ExACT, Tinted or Vanishing Cream	Benzoyl peroxide 5%
Fostex 10% Benzoyl Peroxide Vanishing Gel	Benzoyl peroxide 10%
Neutrogena Acne Mask	Benzoyl peroxide 5%
Oxy Balance Deep Action Night Formula Gel	Benzoyl peroxide 2.5%
Oxy Balance Emergency Spot Treatment Gel	Benzoyl peroxide 5%
Oxy-10 Balance Emergency Spot Treatment, Cover-Up or Invisible Formula Gel	Benzoyl peroxide 10%
Salicylic Acid Products	
Clean & Clear Invisible Blemish Treatment Gel	Salicylic acid 2%
Clean & Clear Oil Controlling Astringent Liquid	Salicylic acid 2%
Clean & Clear Oil Controlling Astringent, Sensitive Skin Liquid	Salicylic acid 0.5%
Clearasil Clearstick Regular Strength	Salicylic acid 1.25%
Clearasil Clearstick Maximum Strength or Sensitive Skin	Salicylic acid 2%
Clearasil Maximum Strength Pads	Salicylic acid 2%
ExACT Pore Treatment Gel	Salicylic acid 2%
Neutrogena Clear Pore Treatment Gel	Salicylic acid 2%
Neutrogena Multi-Vitamin Acne Treatment Cream	Salicylic acid 1.5%
Noxzema 2 in 1 Astringent Liquid	Salicylic acid 2%
Noxzema 2 in 1 Maximum Strength Pads	Salicylic acid 2%
Noxzema 2 in 1 Regular Strength Pads	Salicylic acid 0.5%
Stri-Dex Clear Gel	Salicylic acid 2%
Stri-Dex Maximum Strength, Single or Dual Textured Pads	Salicylic acid 2%
Stri-Dex Regular Strength, Dual Textured Pads	Salicylic acid 0.5%
Sulfur Products	
Fostril Lotion	Sulfur 2%
Sulmasque Mask	Sulfur 6.4%
Sulpho-Lac Cream	Sulfur 5%
Combination Products	
Clearasil Adult Care Cream	Sulfur 3% or 8%; resorcinol 2%
Pernox Lotion	Sulfur 2%; salicylic acid 1.5%
Rezamid Acne Lotion	Sulfur 5%; resorcinol 2%
Sulforcin Lotion	Sulfur 5%; resorcinol 2%

properly. Do not recommend a product that has been used unsuccessfully. If a product was used incorrectly or for too short a time, counsel the patient on its proper use. (See the box "Patient Education for Acne.") If product use was correct, recommend another product.

Q~ Do you prefer one type of acne treatment product (e.g., lotion, cream, gel, or soap) over another?

A~ To improve adherence to the regimen and the ultimate outcome, recommend a product in the preferred dosage form.

Patient Education for Acne

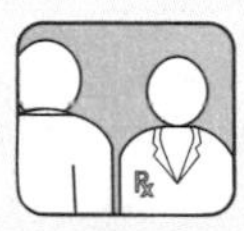

The objective of self-treatment is to control mild acne, thus preventing more serious forms from developing. Acne usually goes away on its own. Meanwhile, its symptoms can be managed with diligent and long-term treatment. The best approaches to controlling acne are using cleansers and medications to keep the skin ducts and orifices open and avoiding situations that worsen acne. For most patients, carefully following product instructions and the self-care measures listed below will help ensure optimal therapeutic outcomes.

Nondrug and Preventive Measures

- Cleanse skin thoroughly but gently at least twice daily to produce a mild drying effect that will loosen comedones. Use a soft washcloth, warm water, and facial soap without moisturizing oils.
- To prevent or minimize acne flare-ups avoid or reduce exposure to environmental factors, such as dirt, dust, petroleum products, cooking oils, or chemical irritants.
- To prevent friction or irritation of the body that may cause acne flare-ups, do not wear tight-fitting clothes, headbands, or helmets; avoid resting the chin on the hand.
- To minimize acne related to cosmetic use, do not use oil-based cosmetics and shampoos.
- To prevent excessive hydration of the skin, which can cause flare-ups, avoid areas of high humidity and do not wear tight-fitting clothes that restrict air movement.
- Try to maintain a proper diet even though a link between diet and acne is unfounded.
- Avoid stressful situations. Stress may play a role in acne flare-ups, but it does not cause acne.
- Note that sexual activity plays no role in the occurrence or worsening of acne.

Nonprescription Medications

- Keep all acne products away from eyes, eyelids, and mucous membranes.

Benzoyl Peroxide

- Benzoyl peroxide is the most effective and widely used nonprescription medication for treating acne. See Table 32–3 for administration guidelines and possible adverse effects.

Salicylic Acid, Sulfur, and Sulfur-Resorcinol Combination Products

- See Table 32–4 for administration guidelines and possible adverse effects of those agents.

Patient Counseling for Acne

Before recommending self-treatment, the pharmacist should evaluate the patient's attitude toward treatment and willingness to comply with a skin care program that involves a continued daily regimen of washing affected areas and applying or ingesting medication. The pharmacist should clearly explain the basis for the recommended treatment. Comedonal and mild papular acne can usually be successfully self-treated if the recommended measures are stringently followed. Patients with moderately severe papular, pustular, and nodular acne should be encouraged to see a physician, preferably a dermatologist, for effective treatments.

Once the decision is made on which approach to recommend, the pharmacist should explain acne as a medical condition, describe the treatment program, and correct any misconceptions the patient might have. The patient should be advised about scalp and hair care; the use of cosmetics; and, above all, the need for long-term, conscientious care. Also, the myths about acne being related to diet and sexual activity should be discounted.

The box "Patient Education for Acne" lists specific information to provide patients.

Because acne cannot be cured but only controlled, reassurance and emotional support are often necessary to reduce patient concern.

The Internet lists supplemental information about acne in lay language, including discussions of acne, nonprescription drugs used to treat it, and treatment expectations. The following selected sites provide accurate information: ACNE NET Home Page (www.derm-infonet.com/acnenet), FaceFacts (www.facefacts.com), 4Acne.Com (www.4acne.com), and articles from the *FDA Consumer* as shown on FDA home page (www.fda.gov). If not copyrighted, these materials can be printed and given to the patient during the consultation. If the material is copyrighted, the pharmacist should instead give the patient the website address.

Evaluation of Patient Outcomes for Acne

Although the patient may expect complete resolution of the acne, an improvement in the disorder is a realistic expectation. A decrease in the number, extent, and severity of the lesions indicates effective self-treatment. The pharmacist should determine whether patients whose acne shows no improvement after 6 weeks of self-treatment are following the recommended treatment regimen. If they have been compliant, medical referral is appropriate. Patients who have not diligently followed the regimen should be encouraged to do so. The pharmacist should again explain the expected results of treatment and the rigor with which treatment must be pursued to maintain the results.

CONCLUSIONS

Acne vulgaris mostly occurs in young adults from their early teens to their mid-20s and occasionally in prepubertal and older people. Acne cannot be cured; however, it may be controlled enough to improve cosmetic appearance and to prevent developing severe acne with its resultant scarring. If given empathy and reassurance, patients with acne may understand that the condition will not exist forever but that they must care for the affected areas for a long time before improvement will occur.

References

1. Koo JYM, Smith LL. Psychologic aspects of acne. *Pediatr Dermatol.* 1991;8(3):185–8.
2. Gupta MA, Johnson AM, Gupta AK. The development of an acne quality of life scale: reliability, validity, and relation to subjective acne severity in mild to moderate acne vulgaris. *Acta Derm Venereol.* 1998;78(6):451–6.
3. Gossel TA. OTC anti-acne medications. *US Pharm.* October 1990;15:24–34.
4. Somnath P. 17 million persons have acne vulgaris. *US Pharm.* April 1997;22(4):15.
5. Rothman KF, Lucky AW. Acne vulgaris. *Adv Dermatol.* 1993;8:347–75.
6. White GM. Recent findings in the epidemiologic evidence, classification, and subtypes of acne vulgaris. *J Am Acad Dermatol.* 1998;39:S34–7.
7. Hurwitz S. Acne vulgaris: pathogenesis and management. *Pediatrics Rev.* February 1994;15(2):47–52.
8. *Federal Register.* August 16, 1991;56:41018–20.
9. Kligman AM. An overview of acne. *J Invest Dermatol.* 1974;62:268–87.
10. Patient counseling. Facial skin problems may be rosacea. *Am Pharm.* January 1992;32(1):9–10.
11. Pillsbury DM. *A Manual of Dermatology.* Philadelphia: WB Saunders; 1971;173–4.
12. *Federal Register.* March 23, 1982;47:12430–77.
13. Pochi PE, Shalita AR, Strauss JS, et al. Report of the Consensus Conference on Acne Classification. *J Am Acad Dermatol.* March 1991;24(3):495–500.
14. Pochi PE. Treatment of teenage acne. *Drug Ther.* January 21, 1991;56–62.
15. Popovich NG. Acne: control is a slow process. *US Pharm (skin care supplement).* June 1991;16:20–7.
16. Brown SK, Shalita AR. Acne vulgaris. *Lancet.* 1998;351:1871–76.
17. Nguyen QH, Kim YA, Schwartz RA. Management of acne vulgaris. *Am Fam Physician.* July 1994;50(1):89–100.
18. Pochi PE. The pathogenesis and treatment of acne. *Annu Rev Med.* 1990;41:187–98.
19. Rosenberg EW, Kirk BS. Acne diet reconsidered. *Arch Dermatol.* April 1981;117:193–5.
20. *Federal Register.* January 15, 1985;50:2172–82.
21. Shalita AR. Comparison of a salicylic acid cleanser and a benzoyl peroxide wash in the treatment of acne vulgaris. *Clin Ther.* 1989;11(2):264–7.
22. *NDWA Executive Newsletter.* February 17, 1995;4–95:7.
23. Slaga TJ, Klein-Szanto AJ, Triplett LL, et al. Skin-tumor promoting activity of benzoyl peroxide, a widely used free radical-generating compound. *Science.* 1981;213:1023–5.
24. Kurokawa Y, Takamura N, Matsushima Y, et al. Studies on the promoting and complete carcinogenic activities of some oxidizing chemicals in skin carcinogenesis. *Cancer Lett.* 1984;24:299–304.
25. Schweizer J, Lochrke H, Edler L, et al. Benzoyl peroxide promotes the formation of melanotic tumors in the skin of 7,12-dimethyl benz[a]antracene-initiated syrian golden hamsters. *Carcinogenesis.* 1987;8(3):479–82.
26. Swauger JE, Dolan PM, Zweier JL, et al. Role of the benzoyloxyl radical in DNA damage mediated by benzoyl peroxide. *Chem Res Toxicol.* March–April 1991;4:223–8.
27. *Federal Register.* August 7, 1991;56:37622–35.
28. *Federal Register.* February 17, 1995;60(33):9554–65.
29. *Federal Register.* May 19, 1995;60(97):26835–8.
30. Benzoyl peroxide carcinogenicity not shown in NDMA interim study results. *FDC Reports—The Tan Sheet.* 1999;7(11):13.
31. Zander E, Weisman S. Treatment of acne vulgaris with salicylic acid pads. *Clin Ther.* 1992;14(2):247–52.
32. Koh-Knox CP, Scott SA, Popovich NG. Therapy and topical treatment of acne vulgaris. *US Pharm Health Systems Ed.* 1997;22(4):40.
33. Ives TJ. Benzoyl peroxide. *Am Pharm.* 1992;32(8):33–8.
34. Higaki S, Morimatsu S, Morohashi M, et al. Susceptibility of propionibacterium acnes, staphylococcus aureus and staphylococcus epidermidis to 10 kampo formulations. *J Int Med Res.* November–December 1997;25(6):318–24.
35. Akamatsu H, Asada Y, Horio T. Effect of keigai-rengyo-to, a Japanese kampo medicine, on neutrophil functions: a possible mechanism of action of keigyo-rengyo-to in acne. *J Int Med Res.* September–October 1997;25(5):255–65.

CHAPTER 33

Prevention of Sun-Induced Skin Disorders

Edward M. DeSimone II

Chapter 33 at a Glance

Sunbathing is one of the most popular ways to spend leisure time in the United States. The association in the 1950s of tanned skin with good health spawned a major industry that revolved around suntanning, including suntan lotions, sunless tanning products, and tanning beds and booths. During the past 25 years, however, research has generated an understanding of the effects of ultraviolet radiation (UVR) and the discovery that this type of radiation is harmful.

Whether sun exposure is recreational or occupational, sunburn can occur, the severity of which depends on an individual's natural skin type as well as on the measures used (e.g., protective clothing, sunscreens) to protect the skin. Most people consider sunburn with its accompanying swelling and tenderness, to be a minor, albeit painful, inconvenience. However, repeated exposure to UVR is cumulative and can produce serious, long-term problems such as premature aging of the skin. In addition, cumulative exposure from childhood to adulthood, even without a serious sunburn ever developing, may cause both precancerous and cancerous skin conditions. This fact is now clear: Avoiding excessive exposure to UVR will reduce the incidence of premature aging of the skin, skin cancer, and other long-term dermatologic effects.

With this new understanding of the dangers of UVR has come a multitude of sunscreen (rather than suntan) products intended not only to help darken but also to protect the skin from the harmful effects of exposure to the sun. Applied properly, these products can block most of the sun's harmful UV rays. Unfortunately, the average consumer shows a considerable lack of understanding of both the process of tanning and the necessity of using sunscreens properly. Thus, pharmacists need to educate the public on the safe and effective use of sunscreen and suntan products. To perform this function, pharmacists must be aware of the hazards of UVR as well as the criteria for selecting and properly using sunscreen products. They are encouraged to become involved in an education program to help minimize the morbidity and mortality associated with UVR exposure.

According to published data from 1995, the market for sun care products was $460 million with a market share of 44% by pharmacies.[1] The pharmacy market share was down 3.1% whereas that of mass merchandisers was up 11%. Sun-

Editor's Note: This chapter is based, in part, on the 11th edition chapter titled "Sunscreen and Suntan Products," which was written by Edward M. DeSimone II.

screen/sunblock products represented 61% of the total market; suntan products, 20%; and self-tanning products, 17%. The change in distribution of sales from pharmacies to mass merchandisers moves consumers away from pharmacists and could have a negative effect on the overall skin care health of the population.

Epidemiology of Sun-Induced Skin Disorders

The most common skin problem caused by UVR is sunburn. However, quite a few other conditions are either directly caused or are exacerbated by UVR. These conditions include both drug and nondrug photosensitivity. Photodermatoses are skin eruptions that are idiopathic (self-originated) or exacerbated (photoaggravated) by radiation of varying wavelengths, including ultraviolet A (UVA) and some visible light. Ultraviolet B (UVB), however, is most often responsible for the reactions. More than 20 known disorders are classified as photodermatoses; Table 33–1 lists the most common ones. Almost all cases of nondrug photodermatosis are manifested as one of four diseases: polymorphic light eruption (PMLE), systemic lupus erythematosus (SLE), solar urticaria, and the porphyrias.[2] PMLE appears to affect approximately 10% of the population, with a first occurrence usually before age 30 years.[3,4] It affects women more often than men. In addition to the idiopathic photodermatoses, UVR can precipitate or exacerbate many photoaggravated dermatologic conditions, including herpes simplex labialis (cold sores), SLE and associated skin lesions, and chloasma, which may affect pregnant women and women taking oral contraceptives. One of the other long-term hazards of UVR is premature photoaging of the skin. It is now believed that up to 80% of all photoaging damage occurs by age 20 years.[5]

Numerous epidemiologic studies have been conducted since the 1950s that demonstrate a strong relationship between chronic, excessive, and unprotected sun exposure and human skin cancer. Skin cancer is the most common type of cancer by far, accounting for approximately 33% of all malignancies. Chronic, unprotected sun exposure accounts for up to 90% of skin cancer. About 80% of all skin cancers occur on the most exposed areas of the body, such as the face, head, neck, and back of hands.

Table 33–1

Most Common Photodermatoses

Idiopathic Disorders	
Actinic prurigo	Polymorphic light eruption
Chronic actinic dermatitis	Solar urticaria
Photoaggravated Disorders	
Acne vulgaris	Erythema multiforme
Atopic dermatitis	Herpes simplex labialis
Atopic eczema	Lichen planus
Bullous pemphigoid	Psoriasis
Chloasma	Rosacea
Dermatomyositis	Seborrheic dermatitis
Drug photosensitivity	Systemic lupus erythematosus

Source: References 6–8.

The two most common types of nonmelanoma skin cancer (NMSC) are basal cell carcinoma and squamous cell carcinoma. Other UVR-induced disorders include premalignant actinic keratosis (which usually develops into squamous cell carcinoma if left untreated), keratoacanthoma, and malignant melanoma. During 1999, an estimated more than 1 million people were diagnosed with skin cancer in the United States.[9] The majority of these cancers break down into basal cell (800,000) and squamous cell carcinomas (200,000). The rate at which these carcinomas grow and invade tissue is relatively slow, and more than 99% are curable with early detection and treatment. By contrast, an estimated 42,000 new cases of malignant melanoma were diagnosed in 1999, representing almost 5% of all skin cancers.[10] The mortality rate from malignant melanoma is estimated to be as high as 20% to 25% among all those who develop the condition.

During the 1980s, a large number of studies linking skin cancer with UVR exposure was reported. This relationship has become accepted by most health professionals. Since 1990, however, additional studies have produced some evidence that, although the relationship does exist, the type of cancer varies significantly according to the causes and contributing factors.

For example, studies have shown conclusively that skin cancer occurs more often in Caucasians than in other ethnic groups.[6] This finding is believed to be because individuals with darker pigmentation have more melanin in the skin. Melanin functions to absorb UVR, thereby preventing the radiation from penetrating into the tissue. Accordingly, Gallagher et al.[11] reported the corroboration of other researchers in finding that individuals with blond or red hair, a history of freckling, and light skin plus a tendency to burn rather than tan are at greater risk of developing squamous cell carcinoma.

Another risk factor was found to be a history of severe sunburn. Gallagher et al.[11] reported that occupational sun exposure increased the risk of squamous cell carcinoma, but only during the 10 years before the cancer developed. Another finding of this study—that lifetime or recreational UVR exposure showed no effect—is contrary to current opinion. In a parallel study on basal cell carcinoma, however, Gallagher et al.[12] reported an elevated risk from childhood (ages 5 to 15 years) sun exposure but not from recreational exposure at other ages and no effect from occupational sun exposure. As in the study on squamous cell carcinoma, freckling was also shown as a risk factor for basal cell carcinoma. One implication from the data on sun exposure is that avoiding the sun as an adult may not alter the chances of developing basal cell carcinoma later in life. Kricker et al.[13] reported no association between basal cell carcinoma and occupational sun exposure but did find an association with recreational exposure.

These studies have raised many new questions and identified new confounding factors. Most researchers agree that follow-up corroborating studies need to be done before a definitive relationship can be made between the type of sun exposure and the type of skin cancer. However, there is no question that skin cancer is linked to sun exposure.

Another factor affecting skin cancer has been generally accepted: its relationship to latitude. It has been shown that the incidence of skin cancer increases steadily in populations closer to the equator. The quantity of harmful UVR that reaches Earth's surface increases as the angle of the sun to a reference point on Earth approaches 90° and as the distance of the sun to Earth decreases.[14] People in the southern part of the United States are at greater risk from the harmful effects of UVR than are those in northern areas. In the United States as elsewhere, a constant rate of increase in the incidence of skin cancer is found as one approaches the equator from north to south; the incidence approximately doubles for every 3°48′ reduction in latitude.[15] Also, the irradiance of UVB increases by 4% for every 1000 feet of altitude. This increase may be of particular concern to skiers and to people who live and work in higher elevations.

Etiology of Sun-Induced Skin Disorders

The various bands of UVR cause or exacerbate sun-induced skin disorders. UVR is commonly referred to as UV light. However, *light* technically refers to only the visible spectrum; thus, the correct terminology in this context is *radiation*.[16]

Bands of Ultraviolet Radiation

The UV spectrum is divided into three major bands: UVC, UVB, and UVA.

Ultraviolet C Radiation

The wavelength of UVC, also known as germicidal radiation, is within the 200 to 290 nm band. Little UVC radiation from the sun reaches the surface of Earth because it is screened out by the ozone layer of the upper atmosphere. However, UVC is emitted by some artificial sources of UVR, and most of the UVC that strikes the skin is absorbed by the dead cell layer of the stratum corneum.[16] Although UVC does not stimulate tanning, it can cause some erythema (redness) of the skin.[16]

Ultraviolet B Radiation

The wavelength of the UVB band is between 290 and 320 nm. This position is the most active UVR wavelength for producing erythema, which is why it is called sunburn radiation. The irradiance (i.e., intensity of the radiation reaching Earth's surface) of UVB is most intense from late morning to early afternoon (10 am to 3 pm).

Cutaneous UVB exposure is responsible for vitamin D_3 synthesis in the skin. Current consensus suggests that this vitamin is the only true therapeutic effect of UVB.[17] Although vitamin D deficiency does not seem to be a problem for infants in the United States who receive vitamin D–fortified milk, it may be a problem for chronic shut-ins or for elderly people who spend little time outdoors if they do not receive adequate vitamin D in their diet or as a vitamin supplement. Its therapeutic benefit notwithstanding, however, UVB is considered to be primarily responsible for inducing skin cancer, and its carcinogenic effects are believed to be augmented by UVA.[18] In addition, UVB is primarily responsible for wrinkling of the skin, epidermal hyperplasia, elastosis, and collagen damage.[19] The discovery of the effects of UVR on the immune system has led to developing the field of photoimmunology.[20]

Ultraviolet A Radiation

The wavelength of UVA radiation ranges from 320 to 400 nm. Although most concerns regarding the hazards of sun exposure to date have focused specifically on UVB, concern about the adverse effects of UVA has been slowly developing since the early 1980s.[21] It is now known that UVA radiation penetrates deeper into the skin than UVB, thereby having a greater effect on the dermis than on the epidermis. This deeper penetration can cause both histologic and vascular damage.[22,23] Evidence suggests that subsequent UVA exposure may cause further and more serious acute and chronic damage to the underlying tissue than UVB exposure. In a recent study,[24] UVA was found to cause sagging of the skin, thickening of the dermis and epidermis, and an increase in the activity of elastase. It was thought previously that only UVB produced premature aging effects on the skin. Now UVA is believed to be involved in suppression of the immune system as well as in damage to DNA.[19,25]

On the basis of research into the effects of UVA on the skin and underlying structures, the UVA band has been divided into two subsets: UVA II (320 to 340 nm) and UVA I (340 to 400 nm).[26] It has been suggested that the degree of damage caused by UVR parallels the degree of erythema across the UV spectrum.[27] That is, the damage at 290 nm is 100 times greater than that at 320 nm, the damage caused at 320 nm is believed to be 10 times higher than that at 340 nm, and the damage at 320 nm is 100 times greater than that at 400 nm. According to these data, UVA II radiation is the most damaging to the skin after UVB.[28] This situation has significant implications for sunscreen products and the type of protection they offer.

The results of this research have caused some controversy about the relative importance of UVA effects on skin as compared with those of UVB. Although approximately 20 times more UVA than UVB reaches Earth's surface at noon (30 times more in winter), erythemogenic activity is relatively weak in the UVA band, requiring up to 200 times more UVA energy than UVB energy.[29] In addition, the irradiance of UVA varies by a factor of 4 to 1 throughout the day and 3 to 1 from summer to winter; however, the significance of this variation is being debated.[29] UVA also represents the wavelength in which most photosensitizing chemicals such as 8-

methoxypsoralen, are active. This activity is true throughout the UVA band but especially above 360 nm.

Ultraviolet Radiation in Tanning Booths and Sunbeds

Since 1980, manufacturers have shifted the composition of UVR emitted by tanning booths and sunbeds from UVB to UVA. The newer types of tanning devices use UVR sources composed of more than 96% UVA and less than 4% UVB, a considerably different mix of UVR than that obtained from natural sunlight.[26] Some tanning devices in commercial use are almost exclusively UVA, although all of them contain a minimal amount of UVB necessary to stimulate tanning. The emission spectrum of tanning devices varies significantly, and the user has no way of knowing what effects to expect.[30]

It would appear that UVA, if used properly, could generate a tan without producing an erythematous sunburn. However, a concern exists about UVB contamination of UVA lamps. It is believed that even 1% UVB emission can cause a significant increase in the incidence of skin cancer. In addition, some UVA lamps produce more than five times as much UVA per unit of time than does sunlight.[28] A small but growing body of evidence suggests that the use of sunlamps and sunbeds is related to the rising incidence of malignant melanoma worldwide.[31,32] It has been speculated that the lack of sufficient corroborating data is partly because of a latent period between exposure and the development of melanoma. The effects of the transition to predominantly UVA sunlamps and sunbeds since 1980 may only just now be beginning to surface.

UVA also presents other hazards, such as deeper tissue penetration than UVB, as described earlier. UVA radiation may trigger the eruption of herpes simplex labialis. In addition, it can produce a photosensitivity reaction in patients who have ingested or applied photosensitizing agents. A recent study[33] reported a phototoxic reaction with the use of a home tanning bed. Moreover, because UVA is less likely to produce the overt burning (erythema) of UVB, patients may become complacent and forgo the use of eye goggles. This practice will produce eye burns and may increase the risk of subsequently developing cataracts. In one study[34] on eye injuries from UV tanning devices, ophthalmologists treated 152 patients over a 12-month period for various ocular injuries, primarily of the cornea and retina. Only 24% of patients wore safety goggles while using the devices. (See the box "A Word about Sun-Induced Ocular Damage.")

The Food and Drug Administration (FDA) sets standards for sunlamp products and UV lamps.[35] These regulations deal with issues such as timers, exposure time, and device labeling, as well as the use of goggles with specified transmittance limits. Despite all of FDA's precautions and warnings, however, its regulations do not include any specified limits on the amount or ratio of UVA and UVB emitted from tanning devices. Pharmacists should advise patients that the possibility of long-term hazards related to UVA has not yet been fully assessed and that there are currently no accepted health benefits from tanning devices.

Transmission/Reflection of Ultraviolet Radiation

Contrary to popular opinion, cloud cover filters very little UVR; rather, 70% to 80% of UVR will penetrate clouds. Although varying amounts of visible sunlight may not pass through cloud cover and although clouds tend to filter out the infrared radiation that contributes to the sensation of heat, this reduction in heat sensation provides a false sense of security against a burn.[39] Fresh snow will reflect 85% to 100% of the light and radiation that strikes it, creating the need for sunglasses when one is skiing on a sunny day. This

A Word about Sun-Induced Ocular Damage

Concern has been expressed regarding the relationship between UVR and eye damage such as cataracts or long-term retinal damage.[36] UVR may also cause temporary injuries such as photokeratitis (a painful type of snow blindness associated with highly reflective surfaces). Another concern involves an increase in the incidence of uveal (iris plus ciliary body) melanoma.[37] Such concerns are even more serious because of the erroneous belief that all sunglasses screen out UVR. In response, the Sunglass Association of America, working with FDA, has developed a voluntary labeling program. Abbreviated information concerning the UVR screening properties is directly attached to each pair of sunglasses, and brochures describing the appropriate use of each type of lens are available at outlets selling the sunglasses. According to its UVR filtration properties, each pair of sunglasses is placed in one of the following three categories:[38]

- Cosmetic sunglasses block at least 70% of UVB, 20% of UVA, and less than 60% of visible light. They are recommended for activities in nonharsh sunlight, such as shopping.
- General purpose sunglasses block at least 95% of UVB, at least 60% of UVA, and 60% to 92% of visible light. With shades that range from medium to dark, they are recommended for most activities in sunny environments, such as boating, driving, flying, or hiking.
- Special purpose sunglasses block at least 99% of UVB, 60% of UVA, and 20% to 97% of visible light. They are recommended for activities in very bright environments, such as ski slopes and tropical beaches.

reflected radiation is also why a skier can receive a significant sunburn, even on a cloudy day, and thus should use a sunscreen. Similarly, sand and white-painted surfaces, although not as reflective as snow, nevertheless reflect a significant amount of the radiation striking them. Therefore, a person sitting in the shade of a beach umbrella may still be bombarded by UVR reflecting off the sand. This reflection contributes to the overall radiation received, and a severe sunburn may result.

Water reflects no more than 5% of UVR and allows the remaining 95% to penetrate and burn the swimmer. Therefore, time in the water, even if the swimmer is completely submerged, should be considered as part of the total time spent in the sun. In addition, although dry clothes reflect almost all UVR, wet clothes allow transmission of approximately 50% of UVR. However, if light passes through dry clothing when held up to the light, UVR will also penetrate that clothing. Tightly woven material offers the greatest protection.

Although UVB does not penetrate window glass, UVA does.[40] Patients sensitive to UVA (e.g., those with photodermatoses or taking photosensitizing drugs) should use appropriate sunscreens even when driving with the window closed.

Pathophysiology/Signs and Symptoms of Sun-Induced Skin Disorders

Sunburn and Suntan

The degree to which a person will develop a sunburn or a tan depends on a number of factors, including (1) the type and amount of radiation received, (2) the thickness of the epidermis and stratum corneum, (3) the pigmentation of the skin, (4) the hydration of the skin, and (5) the distribution and concentration of peripheral blood vessels.[41] Most UVR that strikes the skin is absorbed by the epidermis.

A sunburn is the result of an inflammatory reaction that involves a number of mediators, including histamine, lysosomal enzymes, kinins, and at least one prostaglandin. Such mediators produce peripheral vasodilatation as the UVR penetrates the epidermis; then an inflammatory reaction involving a lymphocytic infiltrate develops. Swelling of the endothelium and leakage of red blood cells from capillaries will also occur. Although the exact mechanism is not fully understood, it is believed that UVB radiation produces erythema by first causing damage to cellular DNA. The intensity of the UVB-induced erythema peaks at 12 to 24 hours after exposure.[41]

Sunburn is, in fact, a burn. It is most often seen as a first-degree (superficial) burn, with a reaction ranging from mild erythema to tenderness, pain, and edema. Severe reactions to excessive UVR exposure can sometimes produce a second-degree burn, with the development of vesicles (blisters) or bullae (many large blisters), as well as with the constitutional symptoms of fever, chills, weakness, and shock. Shock caused by heat prostration or hyperpyrexia can lead to death. (See Chapter 34, "Minor Burns and Sunburn," for discussion of treatment of sunburn.)

A tan is produced when UVR stimulates the melanocytes in the germinating skin layer to generate more melanin and when UVR oxidizes the melanin already in the epidermis. Both processes serve as protective mechanisms by diffusing and absorbing additional UVR. Although UVB and UVA contribute to the tanning process, they induce pigmentation by different mechanisms. UVB acts by stimulating epidermal hyperplasia as well as by shifting of melanin up through the skin. UVA acts by increasing the total amount of melanin in the basal layer. Because of the location of melanin in each case, greater photoprotection from UVB-induced pigmentation is available than from UVA-induced pigmentation.[2] UVA produces a tan through two processes. The first process is known as immediate pigment darkening (IPD), which involves photooxidation of existing melanin.[42] It begins to be visible from 5 to 10 minutes after exposure and reaches its maximum effect in 60 to 90 minutes. The effects of IPD begin to fade very quickly and may be gone within 24 hours. The second process is delayed tanning, or melanogenesis, which involves an increase in the number and size of melanocytes, as well as in the number of melanosomes or pigment granules produced by melanocytes. This delayed tanning contributes to the development of a slow natural tan.

Drug Photosensitivity

Photosensitivity encompasses two types of conditions: photoallergy and phototoxicity. Drug photoallergy, a relatively uncommon immunologic response, involves an increased, chemically induced reactivity of the skin to UVR and/or visible light. UVR (primarily UVA) triggers an antigenic reaction in the skin, which is characterized by urticaria, bullae, and/or sunburn. This reaction, which is not dose related, is usually seen after at least one prior exposure to the involved chemical agent or drug.

Phototoxicity is an increased, chemically induced reactivity of the skin to UVR and/or visible light. However, this reaction is not immunologic in nature. It is often seen on first exposure to a chemical agent or drug, it is dose related, and it usually exhibits no drug cross-sensitivity. Phototoxicity is most likely to appear as an exaggerated sunburn.[3] Some of the drugs associated with phototoxicity are tetracyclines (especially demeclocycline), sulfonamides, antineoplastics (e.g., 5-fluorouracil), hypoglycemics, thiazides, phenothiazines (especially chlorpromazine), and the psoralens. Table 33–2 lists other photosensitizing drugs. This type of reaction is not limited to drugs but is also associated with plants, cosmetics, and soaps.

Photodermatoses

The most common of the idiopathic photodermatoses is PMLE. This condition usually manifests itself in a single morphologic form that includes erythema, vesicles, or

Table 33–2

Selected Groups of Medications Associated with Photosensitivity Reactions

Antidepressants
Amitriptyline
Amoxapine
Clomipramine
Desipramine
Doxepin
Imipramine
Isocarboxazid
Maprotiline
Nortriptyline
Phenelzine
Protriptyline
Trazodone
Trimipramine

Antihistamines
Astemizole
Azatadine
Brompheniramine
Buclizine
Carbinoxamine
Chlorpheniramine
Clemastine
Cyclizine
Cyproheptadine
Dexchlorpheniramine
Dimenhydrinate
Diphenhydramine
Doxylamine
Hydroxyzine
Meclizine
Methapyrilene
Methdilazine
Pheniramine
Promethazine
Pyrilamine
Terfenadine
Trimeprazine
Tripelennamine
Triprolidine

Antihypertensives
Captopril
Diltiazem
Enalapril
Hydralazine
Labetalol
Lisinopril
Methyldopa
Minoxidil
Nifedipine

Antipsychotics
Acetophenazine
Chlorpromazine
Fluphenazine
Haloperidol
Mesoridazine
Perphenazine
Prochlorperazine
Promazine
Thioridazine
Thiothixene
Trifluoperazine
Triflupromazine

Coal Tar and Derivatives
Denorex Medicated Shampoo
DHS Tar Gel Shampoo
Doak Tar Shampoo
Estar Gel
Ionil T Plus Shampoo
Neutrogena T/Derm Body Oil
Neutrogena T/Gel Extra Strength Therapeutic Shampoo
Tegrin Shampoo
Zetar Shampoo

Diuretics (Thiazides)
Bendroflumethiazide
Benzthiazide
Chlorothiazide
Chlorthalidone
Cyclothiazide
Hydrochlorothiazide
Hydroflumethiazide
Methyclothiazide
Polythiazide
Trichlormethiazide

Estrogens/Progestins

Estrogens
Chlorotrianisene
Diethylstilbestrol
Estradiol
Estrogens, conjugated
Estrogens, esterified
Estropipate
Ethinyl estradiol
Megestrol

Progestins
Medroxyprogesterone
Norethindrone
Norgestrel

Hypoglycemics
Acetohexamide
Chlorpropamide
Glipizide
Glyburide
Tolazamide
Tolbutamide

Nonsteroidal Anti-Inflammatory Drugs
Diclofenac
Diflunisal
Fenoprofen
Flurbiprofen
Ibuprofen
Indomethacin
Ketoprofen
Meclofenamate
Nabumetone
Naproxen
Piroxicam
Sulindac
Tolmetin

Psoralens
Methoxsalen
Trioxsalen

Sulfonamides
Sulfadiazine
Sulfamethizole
Sulfamethoxazole
Sulfapyridine
Sulfasalazine
Sulfinpyrazone
Sulfisoxazole

Tetracyclines
Chlortetracycline
Demeclocycline
Doxycycline
Methacycline
Minocycline
Oxytetracycline
Tetracycline

Other Agents

Anticancer Drugs
Dacarbazine
Daunorubicin
Fluorouracil
Flutamide
Methotrexate
Procarbazine
Vinblastine

Anti-Infectives (Other)
Alatrofloxacin
Ciprofloxacin
Dapsone
Enoxacin
Ethionamide
Flucytosine
Gentamicin
Griseofulvin
Levofloxacin
Lomefloxacin
Nalidixic acid
Norfloxacin
Ofloxacin
Pyrazinamide
Sulfonamides
Trimethoprim
Trovafloxacin

Antiparasitic Drugs
Bithionol
Chloroquine
Quinine
Thiabendazole

Diuretics (Other)
Acetazolamide
Amiloride
Furosemide
Metolazone
Triamterene

Table 33–2

Selected Groups of Medications Associated with Photosensitivity Reactions (continued)

Sunscreens	Menthyl anthranilate	Carbamazepine (anticonvulsant)	Lovastatin (antihyperlipidemic)
Aminobenzoic acid	Oxybenzone	Disopyramide (antiarrhythmic)	Nabilone (antiemetic)
Aminobenzoic acid esters	**Miscellaneous**	Etretinate (antipsoriatic)	Phenytoin (anticonvulsant)
Benzophenones	Amiodarone (antiarrhythmic)	Gold salts (antiarthritic)	Quinidine sulfate (antiarrhythmic)
Cinnamates	Benzocaine (local anesthetic)	Isotretinoin (antiacne)	Selegiline (antiparkinsonism)
Homosalate	Benzyl peroxide	Lamotrigine (anticonvulsant)	Tretinoin (antiacne)

Source: Albrant DH, ed. *The American Pharmaceutical Association Drug Treatment Protocols.* Washington, DC: American Pharmaceutical Association; 1999:417; *Med Lett.* 1993;37:946; *Medications That Increase Sensitivity to Light: A 1990 Listing.* FDA Pub No. 91-8280. Washington, DC: US Department of Health and Human Services, Public Health Service; 1995; and *Drug Facts and Comparisons.* St. Louis: JB Lippincott Co; 1993.

plaques on skin exposed to UVR. It is usually seen in people who can experience a burn, including people who tan well.

Another disorder that has shown an increase is a phytophotodermatitis, also known as "weed wacker dermatitis."[43] This disorder usually occurs when the sap of plants bruised by high-speed weed-cutting machines (used by many homeowners) gets on the skin and the skin is then struck by UVR. The only protection is to cover the skin with clothing before using such equipment.

Premature Aging

Premature aging is genetically determined. For example, Caucasians are more susceptible than African Americans. The condition, which is most easily characterized by wrinkling and yellowing of the skin, is called premature photoaging because the obvious physical findings are similar to those seen in natural aging. However, histologic and biochemical differences distinguish such degenerative changes from those associated with normal aging. Conclusive evidence reveals that prolonged exposure to UVR in susceptible people results in elastosis (degeneration of the skin due to a breakdown of the skin's elastic fibers). Pronounced drying, thickening, and wrinkling of the skin may also result.[7] Other physical changes include cracking, telangiectasia (spider vessels), solar keratoses (growths), and ecchymoses (subcutaneous hemorrhagic lesions).[8] (See Chapter 37, "Skin Hyperpigmentation and Photoaging," for discussion of measures for reversing photoaging.)

Skin Cancer

Of all the skin cancers, melanoma has stimulated the most interest in recent years. Melanoma exhibits a pathophysiology different from the NMSCs. Risk factors include light skin, large numbers of melanocytic nevi (moles), and excessive sun exposure.[44] One finding, also noted by Kricker et al.[13] for basal cell carcinoma, is the development of melanoma on any area of the body subjected to intense, intermittent sun exposure, such as the legs and trunk. It seems clear that an increased (but modest) risk of developing melanoma exists if frequent sunburn episodes occur.[45] One of the most common locations for oral cancer is the lips, because few melanocytes are present. Thus, lips burn rather than tan and are prone to develop cancer that has been associated with exposure to UVR.

Prevention of Sun-Induced Skin Disorders

The short-term goals in preventing sun-induced skin disorders are relatively simple: avoiding or minimizing sunburn, photosensitivity reactions, and UVR-induced or exacerbated photodermatoses. The expected long-term outcomes are prevention of skin cancer and premature aging of the skin.

UVR-induced skin disorders can be prevented in one of two ways: The individual must avoid exposure to UVR or must use sunscreen agents. The selection of a sunscreen product and the degree of protection will vary, depending on the patient's intended use for the product as well as the conditions under which the product will be used. (See the algorithm in Figure 33–1.)

The greater the risk a patient has of developing a UVR-induced skin disorder, the greater the need to avoid sun exposure. However, most people do not want to spend a warm, sunny July afternoon sitting at home or in a hotel room. People do not normally go to the beach or to the pool enthusiastically wearing lots of clothing. Therefore, the pharmacist can assist the patient in striking a balance between totally avoiding sun exposure, wearing protective clothing, and using sunscreen products. If, however, the patient suffers from a UVR-induced skin disorder, such as lupus (SLE), little choice is available. In regard to preventing sunburn, the patient's natural skin type will be the primary factor in deciding the potency of the sunscreen product to be used. The lighter the natural skin color is (and the more quickly a burn develops), the higher is the required potency of the sunscreen product.

Avoidance of Sun Exposure

Complete avoidance of UVR is often the best approach for patients with the following characteristics or history:

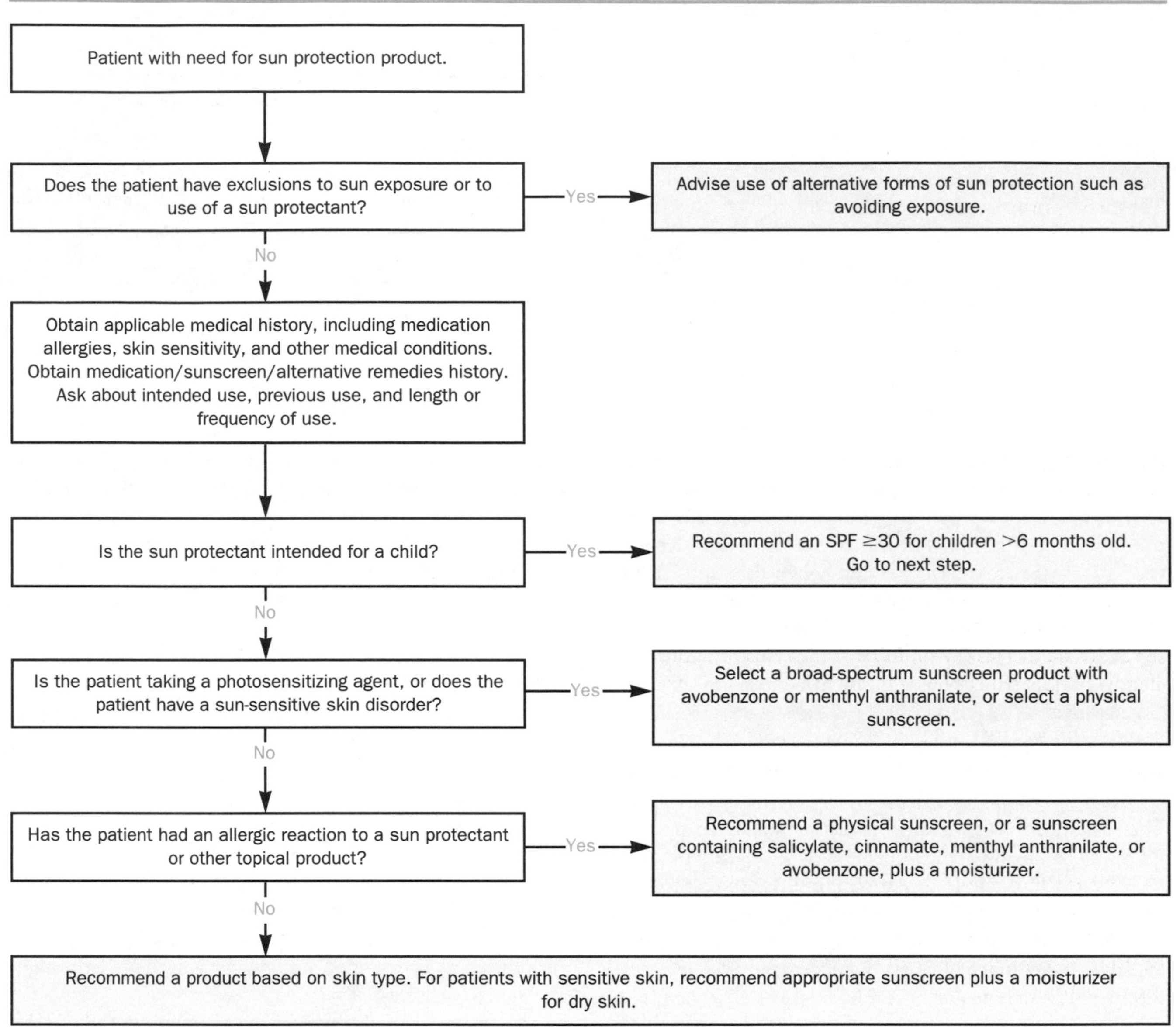

Figure 33–1 Self-care for sun protection.

- Light skin that always burns and never tans.
- A history of one or more serious sunburns.
- Blonde or red hair.
- Blue, green, or gray eyes.
- A history of freckling.
- A growth on the skin or lip caused by sun exposure.
- The existence of a UVR-induced disorder.
- Current use of a photosensitizing drug.

For people who refuse to stay indoors or who must be outdoors for extended periods, the pharmacist should recommend using protective clothing such as a hat with a brim, long pants, and a long-sleeved shirt. In situations in which the patient is unwilling to avoid the sun or to wear protective clothing, the next best choice is to use a sunscreen product.

Use of Sunscreens

The Advisory Review Panel on Topical Analgesic, Antirheumatic, Otic, Burn, and Sunburn Prevention and Treatment Drug Products issued the advance notice of proposal rulemaking (ANPR) on over-the-counter (OTC) sunscreen agents in 1978.[46] Because of the number of responses to the ANPR and significant new developments in the area of photobiology, FDA delayed issuing guidelines on sunscreen products for 15 years. In May 1993, FDA published the tentative final monograph (TFM).[47] The final monograph (FM) was published in 1999, but the mandated changes became effective May 21, 2000. However, several key issues such as UVA protection factors and professional labeling were not addressed because they are still under review.[48]

Labeled Uses

In the FM, FDA decided to limit the labeled uses of sunscreen products. Only the term *uses* and not *indications* is allowed. The two approved uses are to provide protection (minimal/moderate/high) against sunburn and tanning. The degree of protection is related to the sun protection factor (SPF) of a sunscreen.

Sunscreen Efficacy

Purchasers of sunscreens are usually familiar with SPF, one parameter for determining the effectiveness of sunscreens for UVB protection. Another parameter, minimal erythema dose (MED), is used to calculate the SPF of a sunscreen. A comparable index of protection for UVA radiation is yet to be developed.

Minimal Erythema Dose It is difficult to ascertain the efficacy of sunscreens on humans because individual responsiveness to UVR varies greatly. The standardized measure is the MED, defined as the "minimum UVR dose that produces clearly marginated erythema in the irradiated site, given as a single exposure."[41] It is a dose of radiation and not a grade of erythema. The MED is indicative not only of the amount of energy reaching the skin but also of the responsiveness of the skin to the radiation. For instance, 2 MEDs will produce a bright erythema; 4 MEDs, a painful sunburn; and 8 MEDs, a blistering burn. Different types of MEDs may also be on different parts of the body because of variations in the thickness of the stratum corneum. In addition, the MED for African Americans with heavy pigmentation has been estimated to be up to 33 times higher than that for Caucasians with light pigmentation.

Sun Protection Factor Another important measure is the SPF, derived by dividing the MED of protected skin by the MED of unprotected skin. For example, if a person requires 25 mJ/cm^2 of UVB radiation to experience 1 MED on unprotected skin and requires 250 mJ/cm^2 of radiation to produce 1 MED after applying a given sunscreen, the product would be given an SPF rating of 10. The higher the SPF, the more effective the agent is in preventing sunburn. If it normally takes 60 minutes for someone to experience 2 MEDs (a bright erythematous sunburn), a sunscreen with an SPF of 6 will allow that person to stay in the sun six times longer (or 6 hours) before receiving this same sunburn (assuming the sunscreen is reapplied at the recommended intervals). The SPF is product specific because it is calculated on the basis of the final formulation of the product and cannot be determined on the basis of the active ingredient alone.

Table 33–3 presents the newly revised product category designations with recommended SPF. The five categories of SPF have been reduced to three, whereas the associated skin type for each category has been eliminated. A separate classification has been created to show the relationship between patient skin type and sunburn/tanning history. (See Table 33–4.) However, the latter classification is not allowed on product labeling. It is to be used only as part of manufacturers' testing procedures for sunscreen products.

Table 33–3

Product Category Designations

SPF	Category Designation
2–<12	Minimal sunburn protection
12–<30	Moderate sunburn protection
30+	High sunburn protection

Source: Adapted from reference 48.

Table 33–4

Sunburn and Tanning History[a]

Skin Type	Sunburn/Tanning History
I	Always burns easily; never tans (Sensitive)
II	Always burns easily; tans minimally (Sensitive)
III	Burns moderately; tans gradually (Normal)
IV	Burns minimally; always tans well (Normal)
V	Rarely burns; tans profusely (Insensitive)
VI	Never burns; deeply pigmented (Insensitive)

[a] Used for selection of test subjects for general testing procedures and is not to be used as part of any sunscreen label.

Source: Adapted from reference 48.

Perhaps the most controversial change in the FM, as well as one that will affect the greatest number of sunscreen consumers, sets a maximum SPF of 30 for all commercial sunscreen products. Since 1978, SPFs have climbed all the way to a high of 50, triggering debate about whether products with an SPF greater than 30 offer any advantage to users. For example, a product with an SPF of 15 blocks out 93% of UVB. Raising the SPF to 30 increases UVB protection to only 96.7%, and SPF-40 blocks out 97.5%.[47] It is believed that to achieve this small gain in protection (from 30 to 40) might require up to 25% more sunscreen ingredients. This requirement could add to the problems of possible systemic effects and of local adverse effects, as well as to a significant increase in cost. A hypothetical SPF of 70 would increase UVB protection to only 98.6%.[47]

However, some researchers argue in favor of no SPF limits for medical reasons. It has been pointed out that patients with SLE and other lupus-related disorders require a minimum SPF of 40 to prevent triggering the disease.[47] Another comment to FDA stated that patients taking photosensitizing drugs require an SPF of 45 to provide adequate protection.

In response, FDA has decided that an SPF of 30 provides adequate protection for all skin types, including patients with UVR-induced disorders. When one determines protection from photosensitivity, the wavelength at which the product absorbs or reflects the UVR is more important than the SPF. For example, no evidence exists that an SPF of 40 will protect against photosensitivity if the reaction is triggered at 370 nm and if the product absorbs only up to 340 nm.

The question remains as to whether an SPF of 30 provides adequate protection for all individuals and whether the risks of higher SPF products outweigh the benefits. It is interesting to note here that in a study[49] of actinic keratoses, the use of a waterproof, ultra-high (SPF 29) sunscreen product reduced the incidence of new growth development compared with a placebo. Because actinic keratoses develop into squamous cell carcinomas, the implication is that regular sunscreen use will reduce the incidence of such cancers. The study results show a greater reduction of actinic keratoses in patients with lighter skin and in patients with a greater number of preexisting lesions at the time of the study. A protective effect even existed for individuals with naturally darker skin. FDA does acknowledge that a sunscreen with an SPF greater than 30 may be of some benefit. As a compromise for the time being, products with an SPF greater than 30 may be marketed but can have only "30 plus" or "30+" on the label. However, the FM labeling rules no longer allow use of the term *sunblock*, although it has been a common labeling claim for many years.

Measures of UVA Protection With concern growing about the long-term adverse effects of UVA, the utility of the SPF value has been questioned. SPF provides a measure of a patient's erythemogenic response to UVB when using a sunscreen. However, UVA is at least 200 times less potent than UVB in producing erythema, and its effects on the skin are somewhat different from those produced by UVB.[29] Investigations have shown that sunscreens with similar SPFs demonstrate significant differences in their abilities to protect against UVR-induced immunologic injury to the skin.[50] Data suggest that high SPF products block significant amounts of UVA. However, among products of equal SPF, UVA blockage may vary considerably. SPF is not considered to be a reliable measure of UVA protection. As a temporary measure, FDA has extended the rule from the TFM that allows a product to make a claim of UVA protection so long as the ingredients have an absorption spectrum that extends to at least 360 nm.[47]

One area of considerable discussion and debate is how best to measure UVA protection. FDA received many comments as well as several proposals in this regard. The key is to create an index of protection analogous to the SPF. FDA stated in the TFM that the various UVA protection factors being proposed by sunscreen manufacturers are not yet "meaningful."[47] Although it has issued an FM on sunscreen products, FDA did not address the issue of UVA, which will be dealt with sometime in the future.

Substantivity The efficacy of a sunscreen is also related to its substantivity—that is, its ability to remain effective during prolonged exercising, sweating, and swimming. This property can be a function of the active sunscreen, the vehicle, or both. Generally speaking, products with cream-based (water in oil) vehicles appear more resistant to removal by water than those with alcohol bases and will reduce desquamation of the skin. One should remember, however, that part of a sunscreen's effectiveness may relate to the ability of the active agent to bind with constituents of the skin. This binding characteristic may be independent of the vehicle. Oil-based products have traditionally been the most popular and are the easiest to apply. However, they tend to have lower SPF values.

The following are FM requirements for sunscreen product substantivity according to sweating, perspiring, or participating in water activities.

- The product is water resistant: retains its SPF for at least 40 minutes.
- The product is very water resistant: retains its sun protection for at least 80 minutes.

The category of *very water resistant* is intended to replace *waterproof*, which is currently in use. This terminology is one of the areas in which manufacturers do not agree with FDA and have chosen to continue to label products as waterproof since the TFM was published. However, labeling will have to change with the effective date of the FM. Related to this situation, the FM does not allow for the use of labeling that claims a specific number of hours of protection or "all-day protection." The only allowed labeling will be "Higher SPF gives more sunburn protection."

Mechanism of Action

The mechanism of action of sunscreens is related to the definitions for the two therapeutic sunscreen types.[47]

- Sunscreen active ingredient: An active ingredient absorbs at least 85% of the radiation in the UV range at wavelengths from 290 to 320 nm but may or may not allow transmission of radiation to the skin at wavelengths longer than 320 nm.
- Sunscreen opaque sunblock: An opaque sunscreen active ingredient reflects or scatters all light in the UV and visible range at wavelengths from 290 to 777 nm, and the sunscreen thereby prevents or minimizes suntan and sunburn.

Types of Sunscreens

According to the therapeutic definitions, topical sunscreens can be divided into two major subgroups: chemical and physical sunscreens. Chemical sunscreens work by absorbing and thus blocking the transmission of UVR to the epidermis. Physical sunscreens are generally opaque and act by reflecting and scattering UVR rather than absorbing it.

Chemical Sunscreens The FM lists 14 chemical agents and 2 physical agents as being safe and effective for use as sunscreens. Table 33–5 lists these agents, their UVR absorbance range, and their maximum concentrations. Because the SPF is product specific and does not depend on the sunscreen's active agent alone, the FM has eliminated a required minimum strength for sunscreens that contain a single active ingredient. (See Table 33–6 for examples of commercially available products.)

Aminobenzoic Acid and Derivatives For many years, aminobenzoic acid (formerly known as para-aminobenzoic acid, or PABA) has been used in many sunscreen products. Because of the continuing confusion about the name of this sunscreen, the FM requires that the name shall be aminobenzoic acid (not para-aminobenzoic acid), and each time this name appears on product labeling, it shall be followed by "(PABA)" so that consumers know which chemical entity they are using.

Aminobenzoic acid is an effective UVB sunscreen, especially when formulated in a hydroalcoholic base (maximum of 50% to 60% alcohol). The SPF of such formulations increases proportionally as the concentration of aminobenzoic acid increases from 2% to 5%. Evidence exists that some UVA is also blocked at the 5% or higher level.[51]

One advantage of this agent is its ability to penetrate into

Table 33–5

Sunscreens Considered to Be Safe and Effective

Sunscreen Agent	Absorbance Range (nm)	Maximum Range (nm)	Approved Maximum Concentration (%)
ABA and Derivatives			
Aminobenzoic acid (PABA)	260–313	288.5	15
Padimate O	290–315	310	8
Anthranilates			
Menthyl anthranilate	260–380[a]	340[a]	5
Benzophenones			
Dioxybenzone	260–380[b]	282[c]	3
Oxybenzone	270–350	290[d]	6
Sulisobenzone	260–375	285[e]	10
Cinnamates			
Cinoxate	270–328	310	3
Octyl methoxycinnamate	290–320	308–310	7.5
Octocrylene	250–360	303	10
Dibenzoylmethane Derivatives			
Avobenzone[f]	320–400	360	3
Salicylates			
Octyl salicylate	280–320	305	5
Homosalate	295–315	306	15
Trolamine salicylate	260–320	298	12
Miscellaneous			
Phenylbenzimidazole sulfonic acid	290–320	302	4
Titanium dioxide[g]	290–770	—	25
Zinc oxide	290–770	—	25

[a] Values are for concentrations higher than those normally found in nonprescription drugs.
[b] Values are achieved when used in combination with other sunscreen agents.
[c] Second peak occurs at 217 nm.
[d] Second peak occurs at 329 nm.
[e] Second peak occurs at 324 nm.
[f] Agent is currently marketed through a new drug application.
[g] Agent scatters, rather than absorbs, radiation in the 290 nm to 770 nm range.
Source: References 46–48; Shaath NA. Encyclopedia of UV absorbers for sunscreen products. *Cosmetic Toiletries*. 1987;102:21–36.

Table 33–6

Selected Sunscreen Products

Trade Name	SPF Value	Sunscreen Ingredients
Bain de Soleil All Day for Kids Waterproof Sunblock Lotion[a]	30	Octyl methoxycinnamate; octocrylene; oxybenzone; titanium dioxide
Bain de Soleil Le Sport Lotion	30	Octyl methoxycinnamate 7.5%; octocrylene 4%; oxybenzone 2%; titanium dioxide 2%
Bain de Soleil Orange Gelee	8·15	Octyl methoxycinnamate; octocrylene; octyl salicylate; oxybenzone
Banana Boat Faces Sensitive Skin Sunblock Lotion	15·23	Octyl methoxycinnamate; oxybenzone; octyl salicylate
Banana Boat Quik Blok Spray Lotion[b]	15·25	Octyl methoxycinnamate; octyl salicylate; homosalate; oxybenzone
Banana Boat Tan Express Lotion/Spray Lotion	4	Octyl methoxycinnamate; octyl salicylate; oxybenzone
Banana Boat Tan Express Atomic Gel	4	Phenylbenzimidazole sulfonic acid
Blistex Ultra Protection Lip Balm Stick	30	Octyl methoxycinnamate 7.4%; oxybenzone 5.2%; octyl salicylate 5%; menthyl anthranilate 4.8%; homosalate 4.5%
ChapStick Ultra Stick	30	Octocrylene 10%; octyl methoxycinnamate 7.5%; octyl salicylate 5%; oxybenzone 5%; titanium dioxide
Coppertone Kids Colorblock Purple Disappearing Sunblock Lotion[a]	30·40	Octyl methoxycinnamate; oxybenzone; octyl salicylate; homosalate
Coppertone Moisturizing Sunblock Lotion	30·45	Octyl methoxycinnamate; octyl salicylate; oxybenzone; homosalate
Coppertone Moisturizing Sunscreen Lotion	4·8·15	Octyl methoxycinnamate; oxybenzone
Coppertone Oil-Free Sunblock Lotion	8·15	Octyl methoxycinnamate; oxybenzone
Coppertone Shade Sunblock Oil-Free Gel	30	Octyl methoxycinnamate; homosalate; oxybenzone
Coppertone Sport Lotion	48	Octyl methoxycinnamate; oxybenzone; octyl salicylate; homosalate
Coppertone Water Babies UVA/UVB Sunblock Lotion[a]	30	Octyl methoxycinnamate; octyl salicylate; homosalate; oxybenzone
Hawaiian Tropic Baby Faces Sunblock Lotion[a]	35·50	Octyl methoxycinnamate; octyl salicylate; titanium dioxide
Hawaiian Tropic Herbal Tanning Lotion	4	Octyl methoxycinnamate; benzophenone-3
Hawaiian Tropic Protection Plus Lotion	15·30·45	Octyl methoxycinnamate; octyl salicylate; titanium dioxide
Hawaiian Tropic Protective Tanning Dry Oil Pump Spray	6	2-Octyl methoxycinnamate; homosalate; menthyl anthranilate
Neutrogena Oil Free Sunblock Lotion	30	Homosalate; octyl methoxycinnamate; benzophenone-3; octyl salicylate
Neutrogena Sensitive Skin Sunblocker Lotion	17	Titanium dioxide
Neutrogena Sunless Tanning Cream	8	Octyl methoxycinnamate
PreSun 15 or 30 Active Gel[b]	15·30	Benzophenone-3; octyl methoxycinnamate; octyl salicylate
PreSun 30 Ultra Gel[b]	30	Avobenzone; octyl methoxycinnamate; octyl salicylate; oxybenzone

[a] Pediatric formulation.

[b] Fragrance-free product.

the horny layer of the skin and to provide lasting protection. It has significant substantivity on sweating skin although not so much on skin that is immersed in water. The primary advantage of aminobenzoic acid derivatives over aminobenzoic acid itself is that the derivatives do not stain clothing. The only Category I derivative is padimate O.

The disadvantages of alcoholic solutions of aminobenzoic acid include contact dermatitis, photosensitivity, stinging and drying of the skin, and yellow staining of clothes on exposure to the sun.[52] Patients who have experienced a photosensitivity reaction to a sunscreen product containing aminobenzoic acid or any of its derivatives should avoid using such products.

Anthranilates The anthranilates are ortho-aminobenzoic acid derivatives. Menthyl anthranilate, the menthyl ester of anthranilic acid, is a weak UV sunscreen with maximal absorbance in the UVA range. It is usually found in combination with other sunscreen agents to provide broader UV coverage.

Benzophenones Three agents are in the benzophenone group: dioxybenzone, oxybenzone (benzophenone-3), and sulisobenzone (benzophenone-4). As a group, these agents are primarily UVB absorbers, with maximum absorbance between 282 and 290 nm. However, their absorbance extends well into the UVA range, with oxybenzone up to 350 nm and dioxybenzone up to 380 nm. Because of their extended spectrum of action, benzophenones are often found combined with other sunscreens to provide a broad spectrum of coverage.

Because of the possibility of allergic reactions to aminobenzoic acid and its derivatives and because of the wider spectrum of action of the benzophenones, more sunscreen products contain benzophenones in their formulations. Because of this formulation and the fact that oxybenzone, found in some cosmetic formulations, is a significant sensitizing agent, there has been a rise in reports of sensitivity to the benzophenones.[53]

Cinnamates Cinnamates include three sunscreens: cinoxate, octyl methoxycinnamate, and octocrylene. As shown in Table 33–5, cinoxate and octyl methoxycinnamate have similar absorbance ranges, as well as maximum absorbances. Octocrylene, however, has an absorbance range of 250 to 360 nm, well into the UVA range. Octocrylene is currently found in many more commercial sunscreen preparations than it was in the past, possibly reflecting its broader spectrum of absorbance. Unfortunately, cinnamates do not adhere well to the skin and must rely on the vehicle in a given formulation for their substantivity.

Dibenzoylmethane Derivatives Avobenzone (butyl methoxydibenzoylmethane, originally known as Parsol 1789) is the first of a new class of sunscreen agents effective throughout the entire UVA range (320 to 400 nm; full spectrum). It has a maximum absorbance at approximately 360 nm.[54] This agent entered the market through a new drug application (NDA) and was officially approved in the recently published FM. Although avobenzone absorbs UVR through all of the UVA spectrum, its absorbance falls off sharply at 370 nm. Therefore, reactions from photosensitive drugs and chemicals that are highly reactive in the 370 to 400 nm range could still occur. Avobenzone, however, offers the best protection in the UVA range when compared with the other chemical sunscreens on the market.

Salicylates Salicylic acid derivatives are weak sunscreens and must be used in high concentrations. They do not adhere well to the skin and are easily removed by perspiration or swimming.

Other Chemical Sunscreens Phenylbenzimidazole sulfonic acid does not fit into any of the above classes. It is a pure UVB sunscreen with an absorbance range of 290 to 320 nm.

Physical Sunscreens Physical sunscreens scatter rather than absorb UVR and visible radiation (290 to 777 nm). They are most often used on small and prominently exposed areas by patients who cannot limit or control their exposure to the sun (e.g., lifeguards). The nose and tops of the ears are often coated with a white or colored substance containing zinc oxide or titanium dioxide, although manufacturers have developed a way to make titanium dioxide transparent while maintaining efficacy as a sunscreen. Their disadvantages are that they can discolor clothing and may occlude the skin to produce miliaria (prickly heat) and folliculitis. Because titanium dioxide increases the effective SPF of a product and extends the spectrum of protection well into the UVA range, the number of commercial products containing this agent has increased. The FM allows for zinc oxide to be used alone or combined with any of the other sunscreen agents except avobenzone because of a lack of data on effectiveness.

Combination Products FDA has not recommended any limits on the number of sunscreen agents that may be used together in a nonprescription product. However, FDA is concerned that additional sunscreen agents must contribute to the efficacy of a product and must not be included merely for marketing promotion purposes. Therefore, the FM requires that (1) each active ingredient contribute a minimum SPF of not less than 2, and (2) the finished product must have a minimum SPF of not less than the number of sunscreen active ingredients used in the combination multiplied by 2.

Dosage/Administration Guidelines

The two major causes of poor sun protection with sunscreen use are application of inadequate amounts and infrequent reapplication. In a report[55] on sunscreen application to eight areas of the face, the degree of complete coverage ranged from 8% periorbital and 18% ears to 80% forehead and 94% cheeks. Although many sunscreen products that prevent burning of the lips (or nose) are available, the lips are often neglected. Although they differ in ingredients and in the UVA and UVB spectrum, products for the lips carry most of the same labeling, including the SPF, as do sunscreen lotions. The SPF of products for lips is usually at least 15. Studies have shown that lip protection not only helps prevent drying and burning of the lips but also helps prevent the development of cold sores or fever blisters triggered by the herpes simplex virus in patients who are susceptible to recurrent outbreaks.

Sunscreens must be liberally applied to all exposed areas of the body and reapplied as often as the label recommends for maximum effectiveness. Although these two factors drive up the cost of sunscreen use, the long-term benefits of proper sunscreen use far outweigh the costs.

The FDA standard for application of sunscreens is 2 mg/cm^2 of body surface area. This standard means that, for sufficient protection, the average adult in a bathing suit should apply nine portions of sunscreen of approximately ½ teaspoon each, or approximately 4 ½ teaspoons (22.5 mL) total. The sunscreen should be distributed as follows:[56]

- Face and neck: Apply ½ teaspoon.
- Arms and shoulders: Apply ½ teaspoon to each side.
- Torso: Apply ½ teaspoon each to front and back.
- Legs and top of feet: Apply 1 teaspoon to each side.

Because of the cost of sunscreen products and the need to apply them often and in sufficient amounts, people may use far less sunscreen than is necessary to provide adequate protection. One study[57] demonstrated that the effective SPF of commercial products was only 50% of the labeled value when subjects were allowed to apply sunscreen according to their own assessment of need.

Reapplying a sunscreen does not extend the amount of time a person can spend in the sun. Outdoor exposure to UVR should be within the limits of the SPF value of the sunscreen. Another factor to consider is the time that it takes the sunscreen to bind to the various skin constituents and to become fully effective. For most sunscreen products, the interval is 15 to 30 minutes, although at least one product claims immediate effectiveness. Because this lag time varies from product to product, the FM allows each product to include its individual lag time on the label. Sunscreens should be reapplied as often as label instructions direct. Water-resistant products are reapplied every 40 minutes, whereas very water-resistant products are reapplied every 80 minutes.

If properly applied, products with an SPF of 15 to 30 allow an individual to stay out in the sun for long periods and to slowly develop a tan over several days to weeks. It is important to remember, however, that as an individual tans, a natural protection against burning also develops. Therefore, an individual who insists on tanning should begin the summer using a product with an SPF of at least 15 to 30 (depending on skin type and tanning history) and should switch to a product with a lower SPF (e.g., 12, then 10, then 8, etc.) as the natural tan progresses. This change will allow a more rapid deepening of the tan while helping to build up natural protection in the skin. The individual can, however, continue to use the product with the higher SPF; it will simply take longer to achieve the desired tan.

Patients should be advised that, although tanning and thickening of the skin serve as protective mechanisms against future injury, peeling of the skin removes part of this protection. The amount of exposure to the sun as well as the SPF of the product being used must be reevaluated as tanning and peeling occur.

Adverse Effects

The development of a rash, vesicles (blisters), hives, or an exaggerated sunburn is most likely a sign of either a photosensitivity or allergic reaction. The FM labeling rule is very simple. Product labels must state the following: "Stop use if skin rash occurs." The patient should be referred to a physician for evaluation of the situation. The degree of the reaction will determine what type of medical intervention (if any) is necessary.

Recently, questions have arisen as to whether the substantivity of a sunscreen may affect the temperature-regulating ability of the body. One study[58] reported that exercising in hot weather after applying a sunscreen product may increase the risk of overheating. Under hot, humid conditions, sweating is increased but evaporation is poor. When the humidity is low, overheating during exercise may still occur, possibly because the oily vehicle of the sunscreen may block the pores. Therefore, sunbathers should be cautious when exercising in hot weather after applying a sunscreen product.

One study reported individuals ingesting aminobenzoic acid in doses of up to 1 g daily to prevent phototoxic reactions.[59] However, no evidence demonstrates the safety or efficacy of aminobenzoic acid when used in this manner. Moreover, oral ingestion has been associated with a lowered white blood cell count, drug fever, and organ damage, and thus should be vigorously discouraged.

Precautions/Warnings

In 1998, stories began to circulate about a 2-year-old boy who went blind after getting sunscreen in his eye. This study turned out to be one of the many myths that seem to be launched and perpetuated on the Internet. The issue was investigated and found to be without merit.[60] However, the FM does include the label warning "Keep out of eyes."

Additional Product Considerations

Sunscreens in Cosmetic Products The FM addresses a troublesome gray area that has allowed the proliferation of cosmetics claiming to offer sun protection. It stipulates that sunscreen products will be classified as drugs rather than cosmetics because consumers expect that sunscreens will protect them from some of the sun's damaging effects. However, cosmetics that contain sunscreen agents will be classified as cosmetics as long as no therapeutic claims are made, and the sunscreen is intended for a nontherapeutic, nonphysiologic purpose. In addition, if the term "sunscreen" appears on the product labeling, a statement must appear that describes the cosmetic purpose of the sunscreen (e.g., "Contains a sunscreen—to protect product color").

Suntan Products Two types of products fall under the general heading of suntan products: Those that contain a pigmenting agent and those that do not. Products that do not contain a pigmenting agent are formulated with oily vehicles (such as mineral oil) that tend to concentrate UVR onto the skin. Although they are also formulated with emollients, this type of product provides no protection whatsoever against all the short- and long-term hazards of UVR exposure. The other type of suntan product contains the pigmenting agent, dihydroxyacetone (DHA). It may be formulated with or without an oily vehicle. For years, DHA has been the major ingredient in products that claim to tan without the sun. DHA produces a reddish-brown color by binding with specific amino acids in the stratum corneum. The intensity of the tan is related to the thickness of the skin. If the product is not washed off the hands immediately after application, however, the palms may also develop this tan (turn orange). In addition, dry areas, such as elbows and kneecaps, will absorb the DHA more readily, resulting in uneven coloration. The color fades after 5 to 7 days with desquamation of the stratum corneum.

The FM issued new rules concerning suntan products.

Any product that is labeled for suntanning purposes cannot contain any sunscreen ingredients intended to provide protection from UVR. In addition, the product label must carry the following warning:

> **Warning** This product does not contain a sunscreen and does not protect against sunburn. Repeated exposure of unprotected skin while tanning may increase the risk of skin aging, skin cancer, and other harmful effects to the skin even if you do not burn.

Unapproved Suntan Agents

Oral Pigmenting Agents During the past several years, a number of products have claimed to be effective oral tanning compounds. Their active ingredients are the dyes canthaxanthin and β-carotene, which are chemically similar to one another. β-Carotene and canthaxanthin are both approved by FDA as color additives in foods and drugs, and β-carotene is also approved for use in cosmetics. Canthaxanthin is a synthetic dye that is similar to dyes found naturally in fruits, vegetables, and flowers. Both agents are used to enhance the appearance of foods such as pizza, barbecue and spaghetti sauces, soups, salad dressings, fruit drinks, baked goods, pudding, cheese, ketchup, and margarine. However, they are present in food in lower concentrations than they are in oral products that claim to produce tanning. For example, the daily dietary intakes of β-carotene and canthaxanthin as food colorants are about 0.3 mg and 5.6 mg, respectively;[61] in one brand of tanning tablet, however, the daily intakes are 12 mg and 100 mg, respectively.

The dyes alter skin tone by coloring the fat cells under the epidermal layer. Because of variations in fat cells and epidermal thickness, the extent of the tan varies from person to person. Canthaxanthin is dosed by body weight, with a 20-day schedule necessary to achieve a significant change in skin tone. This process is followed by doses of one to two capsules per day to maintain the color. The promotional literature cautions the user that if the palms turn orange, too much of the product is being consumed.

According to the 1960 Color Additive Amendment, any new use of a color additive must be submitted to FDA for approval.[62] FDA has not yet approved either β-carotene or canthaxanthin for artificial tanning. One major concern is the discoloration of the feces to brick red, which could mask gastrointestinal bleeding. A second concern is the long-term adverse effects that may be associated with the large doses recommended. Although β-carotene is used on a prescription basis to help prevent photosensitivity in patients with erythropoietic protoporphyria, no evidence documents the safety of canthaxanthin at the high doses found in oral tanning products. In fact, a case has been reported of fatal aplastic anemia associated with canthaxanthin ingestion from an oral tanning product. Reported cases of retinopathy, hepatitis, and urticaria associated with the use of oral tanning agents has prompted FDA to issue further warnings on such products.[63] In addition, Canada, which previously allowed the nonprescription sale of canthaxanthin for tanning purposes, has decided that there is insufficient evidence of its safety, and Canada no longer allows such sales.

Tan Accelerators Tan accelerators are cosmetic products that claim to stimulate a faster and deeper tan. Their major ingredient is tyrosine, an amino acid necessary to produce melanin. Product literature recommends application of these products once daily for at least 3 days before sun exposure. However, one study that tested two commercial products using indoor UVR found no evidence of benefit.[64] The TFM recognizes this fact and states that "any product containing tyrosine or its derivatives and claiming to accelerate the tanning process is an unapproved new drug."[47] These agents are not addressed in the FM.

Melanotropins and Melanin Products A hormone known as α-melanotropin or α-melanocyte-stimulating hormone (α-MSH) has been located within the human central nervous system. The role of α-MSH in humans, if any, has not yet been identified. However, this hormone is produced by the pituitary gland of numerous vertebrates and has been shown to affect skin color through its action on melanocytes. α-Melanotropin is currently under investigation to determine whether it can affect skin tanning.[65] Also, the FM states that melanin and artificial melanin ingredients are not recognized sunscreens and that any product containing these agents and making sunscreen claims must be under an NDA.

Product Selection Guidelines

Two primary factors will determine the best product for a given patient: the intended use of the product and specific patient characteristics. These factors are not mutually exclusive categories. The decision on which sunscreen product to use must be based on the information obtained from both categories.

Intended Use Some patients may wish to use sunscreens to prevent the photoaging effects of UVR or to protect themselves from skin cancer. Others may need protection from sun exposure because they are taking photosensitive drugs or they have a photodermatosis.

The higher the SPF of the sunscreen product, the greater the protection it provides against sunburn and tanning. Studies have shown that even low protective sunscreens (SPF-2) can reduce the incidence of NMSCs from 36% to 54% if properly used beginning in childhood.[66] However, some investigators and clinicians have suggested that products with an SPF of less than 6 not be recommended routinely to patients.[51] Because of the hazards associated with UVR, they recommend instead the selection of a product with an SPF of 15 or higher. Any product in the SPF range of 15 to 30+ will significantly reduce the total amount of UVB and UVA radiation received when compared with lower SPF products.

For other purposes, intervention by health professionals to recommend the use of a sunscreen product is often

Case Study 33–1

Patient Complaint/History

Regina, a 23-year-old student, asks for a recommendation for a sunscreen product because her physician told her to avoid excessive exposure to the sun. The weather is turning warmer and she enjoys sunbathing. When she is questioned, it is determined that she has recently been diagnosed with systemic lupus erythematosus (SLE). She has brown hair and brown eyes. She states that she can get a sunburn but generally tans well. A check of her medication record shows that she is currently taking a corticosteroid and an NSAID for her lupus. She is on no other medication.

Clinical Considerations/Strategies

Readers can use the following considerations/strategies to determine whether use of nonprescription sunscreens is warranted:

- Determine the clinical considerations of sun exposure in patients with lupus.
- Determine the best management of this clinical situation.
- Identify the primary indicator that the situation is being successfully managed.

Patient Education/Counseling

Readers can use the following strategies to develop a patient education/counseling plan that will help ensure optimal therapeutic outcomes:

- Identify the important points for counseling the patient about her disease.
- Identify the appropriate measures for protecting the patient from sun exposure.

needed. FDA has stated that it received no comments for professional labeling. Therefore, FDA has decided not to issue any regulations dealing with professional labeling, although it will reconsider in the future if such reconsideration becomes warranted. Generally, if a product is to be used to prevent skin cancer, reduce the chances of a photosensitivity reaction, or reduce the risk of triggering a UVR-induced or aggravated skin disorder, a 30+ SPF is best.

If the patient has a potential for a photosensitivity reaction or photodermatosis that is likely to be triggered by UVA, the sunscreen product should be broad spectrum. It should protect through as much as possible of the UVA range and still provide coverage in the UVB range.

The question remains about what constitutes a true broad-spectrum sunscreen. A number of commercial products claim to be broad spectrum; the TFM allows such claims if the product contains ingredients that absorb or reflect UVB (290 to 320 nm) *and* absorb up to 360 nm.[4] Products with equal SPFs may still differ significantly in total UVR protection, depending on the absorbances of the various sunscreens they contain. Most currently available broad-spectrum products have a minimum of two sunscreen ingredients, whereas many others incorporate three or even four sunscreens.

Although UVA II is more damaging to the skin than UVA I, the lack of a standardized UVA protection factor does not allow such considerations to be taken into account in product selection. Thus, no one generally accepted measure exists to evaluate the actual efficacy of a product that claims to provide UVA protection. The best recommendation would be to select a product that contains a combination of sunscreen agents that protect throughout the entire UVB range and across the widest possible UVA range. A product labeled as broad spectrum that contains avobenzone and has an SPF of at least 15 is an excellent choice for patients who have UVR-induced disorders or who are taking photosensitizing drugs. A very broad spectrum of coverage can be obtained by using a sunscreen product containing padimate O with one of the benzophenones, octocrylene, or menthyl anthranilate. An increasing number of products have added micronized titanium dioxide to increase the SPF and to provide a broad spectrum of coverage.

Patient Factors In cases not dealing with photosensitivity, photodermatoses, or skin cancer, product selection is much simpler. The following factors can serve as a guide in selecting products with the appropriate properties for a patient's particular situation.

Skin Type and Tanning History The most important factors in product selection are the individual's natural skin type and tanning history. A high SPF product of 30+ should be given to people who always burn easily and tan minimally at best. The average person who uses sunscreen products does so to avoid getting burned while still obtaining a tan. For that individual, a product with an SPF of 12 to 30 is recommended with the lower end for people who always tan well and the higher end for those who tan gradually. An SPF from 2 to 12 is recommended for people who are deeply pigmented or who tan profusely. A higher SPF product can always be recommended. The tanning that occurs will do so at a slower rate.

Physical Activity A second consideration is the physical conditions under which the product will be used. If the individual plans to swim, participate in vigorous activity (e.g., sand volleyball), or work outdoors, the sunscreen product must be able to adhere to the skin more substantially than if the individual just lies on the beach. The expected duration of the physical activity can also help determine which sunscreen to use. Water-resistant products are usually effective for at least 40 minutes when used under the above activities, whereas very water-resistant products are labeled as effective for at least 80 minutes.

Adverse Reactions to Sunscreen Agents If a patient has had a prior reaction to a sunscreen product, the pharmacist should try to ascertain the name of the product and the ingredients it contained. This action may be difficult because product formulations change with significant frequency. Photosensitivity and contact dermatitis are more likely to occur with aminobenzoic acid and its esters, although other sunscreens have also been reported to produce both conditions. Such sunscreens include the benzophenones, the cinnamates, homosalate, avobenzone, and menthyl anthranilate. In addition, patients who are allergy prone and have allergies to various drugs (e.g., benzocaine, thiazides, or sulfonamides) may also develop an allergic reaction to either aminobenzoic acid or its esters.

Cosmetic Considerations Some patients may avoid using sunscreens because of cosmetic concerns. For example, at least one-third of the commercial products currently available are labeled noncomedogenic, fragrance free, and hypoallergenic. Noncomedogenic products do not plug the pores and, therefore, do not exacerbate acne. This property is especially important for teenagers, who generally spend more time out of doors than other age groups and would generally prefer not to use comedogenic sunscreens. Regarding fragrance-free and hypoallergenic properties, many patients are sensitive to various ingredients, including fragrances, emulsifiers, and preservatives. In a randomized, placebo-controlled study of adverse reactions to sunscreens, 16% of subjects developed a local reaction to the topically applied product.[67] Of these subjects, 53% agreed to be patch tested and photopatch tested. None of this subset showed a sensitivity to the sunscreen agents. Instead, all the reactions were found to be caused by formulation ingredients such as fragrances and preservatives. This finding seems to reinforce the belief that, although some patients are sensitive to certain sunscreen products, most of that sensitivity may be caused by nonsunscreen ingredients. Although it may not be possible to figure out what specific ingredient a patient is sensitive to, patients who have a history of sensitivity to certain types of ingredients would do well to use a fragrance-free, hypoallergenic product.

Some patients have normally dry skin. Sunbathing can further exacerbate this problem. These patients should avoid ethyl and isopropyl alcohols, which are included in a number of commercial sunscreen products, and can dry the skin additionally.

Use in Young Children Special consideration is needed when recommending a sunscreen product for young children. The consensus is that the absorptive characteristics of human skin in children younger than 6 months are different from those of adult skin. Related to this consensus is the belief that the metabolic and excretory systems of children younger than 6 months are not fully developed to handle any sunscreen agent absorbed through the skin. Therefore, only patients older than 6 months are considered to have adult

Case Study 33–2

Patient Complaint/History

Lucas is a 61-year-old executive. He plays golf two to three times a week. He is in the pharmacy today looking at sunscreen products. He explains that he usually protects his head and neck from sun exposure by wearing a hat. However, he would like to keep a sunscreen product in his golf bag in case he forgets his hat. Physical observation of the patient reveals that he suffers from male pattern baldness and has numerous nevi. Further, the top of his head, his neck, and his arms are red and appear to have a fading sunburn. Lucas admits that he tans slowly and gets sunburned several times each year. He has had several sun-related growths removed from his arms and face, although his physician said that he did not have skin cancer. He is in fairly good health and does not take any medication.

Clinical Considerations/Strategies

Readers can use the following considerations/strategies to determine whether use of nonprescription sunscreens is warranted:

- Determine the clinical considerations of sun exposure in this case.
- Determine the best recommendation for this clinical situation.
- Identify the primary indicator that the situation is being successfully managed.

Patient Education/Counseling

Readers can use the following strategies to develop a patient education/counseling plan that will help ensure optimal therapeutic outcomes:

- Identify the important points for counseling the patient about occurrences of skin growths.
- Identify the important points for counseling the patient about preventive measures.

human skin. The FM requires that sunscreen products be labeled with the statement "children under 6 months of age: ask a doctor." Caregivers should be extremely wary regarding sun exposure in children, especially those younger than 6 months. Regular use of an SPF-15 product starting after age 6 months and continuing through age 18 years can reduce the incidence of skin cancer over a lifetime by as much as 78%.[66] Even better would be a product with an SPF of 30+. Such usage would result in a reduction in sunburn and a reduced risk of premature skin aging and other skin problems.

Patient Assessment of Sun-Induced Skin Disorders

The approach to UVR-induced skin disorders is different from that used in most self-care situations. Such disorders are addressed from a preventive rather than a treatment standpoint. In 1999, FDA issued an FM on OTC sunscreen drug products.[48] The primary indication for sunscreen products is to protect against sunburn. A voluntary labeling "sun alert" may also advise that such products "may reduce the risks of skin aging, skin cancer, and other harmful effects of the sun."

Because this type of pharmacist–patient self-care situation involves prevention rather than treatment, assessment of the patient must focus on the *intended use* of the product. Two primary situations exist in which pharmacist interventions with patients occur. The first situation involves a request by the patient for the pharmacist to recommend a sunscreen product, either to prevent a burn and/or to allow for developing a tan. The second situation is initiated by the pharmacist when a patient is placed on a drug that can produce a photosensitivity reaction. In this second scenario, no real patient assessment is needed because prevention of exposure to UVR is the standard approach.

Asking the patient the following questions will help elicit the information needed to determine the intended use of a sunscreen and to recommend the appropriate product.

[Note: The term "sun exposure" is intended to include all sources of UVR, including tanning beds and booths.]

Q~ Do you have light skin with a tendency to burn?

A~ If yes, advise the patient that a sunscreen with a high SPF is needed for protection from sun exposure. Explain that the use of other measures, such as protective clothing, will also be helpful.

Q~ Have you ever had a severe sun reaction or a severe burn?

A~ If yes, advise the patient that any exposure to UVR should probably be avoided because a high risk exists of developing a sunburn as well as the long-term risk of skin cancer. Explain that wearing protective clothing is essential.

Q~ Have you ever had a growth on your skin or lip caused by sun exposure? Observe the patient to see whether he or she has blonde or red hair; blue, green, or gray eyes; or a history of freckling.

A~ If the patient has any of these risk factors for developing skin cancer, explain that avoiding UVR and using protective clothing are required.

Q~ Do you normally spend much time outdoors because of your job, sports, or other activities? How long can you stay out in full sun before your skin starts to turn red?

A~ Determine from the patient's answers the optimal SPF required for adequate protection from UVR exposure.

Q~ Will you be using the product while swimming, skiing, participating in strenuous activities, or working?

A~ Advise a patient who will be using a sunscreen under such conditions to use a very water-resistant sunscreen. Explain that this type of product will adhere better to the skin.

Q~ Have you ever had a reaction to any sunscreen product?

A~ If yes, try to find out which sunscreen ingredients the product contained. Advise the patient that local or systemic reactions can occur to any topically applied product but that certain sunscreen ingredients are more likely than others to produce such a reaction.

Q~ Is the patient younger than 6 months?

A~ If yes, explain that sunscreens should never be used on children this young. Advise the parent to consult a physician about use of sunscreens for the child.

Patient Counseling for Sun-Induced Skin Disorders

Pharmacists can provide a great service by counseling consumers about the suntanning process and about properly selecting and using sunscreens. In one study[68] involving almost 500 subjects, a considerable amount of misinformation was found to exist concerning sunscreen use. For example, 51% of those surveyed did not know the definition of SPF or its significance; 26% were not even aware of the existence of sunscreens before the study; of the 41% who used sunscreens, one-third thought the products would promote tanning.

One simple way to find out if a patient is using a sunscreen properly is to ask how long the current bottle has lasted. When applied properly, according to the suggested dosing guidelines and in accordance with the appropriate substantivity of the product, a sunbather could easily use about 1 ounce every 80 to 90 minutes. This use would amount to several ounces a day and several bottles per week. Incredibly, many frequent sunbathers use only one bottle in

Patient Education for Protection from Sun Exposure

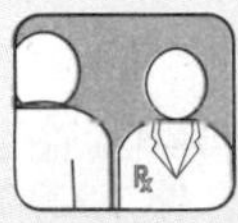

The objectives of self-care depend on a patient's specific goal or health status. Protection from sun exposure can prevent sunburn or tanning, as well as prevent photosensitivity reactions in susceptible persons or prevent exacerbation of sun-induced photodermatoses. The primary long-term benefits are to prevent skin cancer and premature aging of the skin. For most patients, carefully following product instructions and the self-care measures listed below will help ensure optimal therapeutic outcomes.

Avoiding/Minimizing Sun Exposure

- Avoid exposure to the sun and other sources of ultraviolet radiation such as tanning beds/booths and sunlamps.
- Note that the rays of the sun are the most direct and damaging between 10 am and 3 pm. Avoid sun exposure during this time of day as much as possible.
- Note also that 70% to 80% of UVR penetrates clouds. Sunburn, therefore, can occur on a cloudy or overcast day.
- Wear protective clothing such as long pants, a long-sleeved shirt, and a hat with a brim. Tightly woven fabrics that do not allow light to pass through will provide the most protection.
- Note that wet clothing and water allow significant transmission of UVR. Consider time in the water, even if the body is completely submerged, as part of the total time spent in the sun.

Use of Sunscreens

- Note that an SPF of 30+ provides the greatest protection against sunburn and other UVB-induced skin problems.
- Note that a broad-spectrum sunscreen product (such as avobenzone used in combination with padimate O and/or one of the benzophenones, octocrylene, menthyl anthranilate, or titanium dioxide) provides optimal protection against sun exposure. This type of sunscreen is especially recommended if you have a sun-induced disorder or are taking photosensitizing drugs, or if you just wish to prevent as much sun exposure as possible.
- Apply approximately 1 ounce of sunscreen to all exposed areas of the body. Avoid contact with the eyes.
- Reapply the sunscreen according to the label instructions—usually every 40 minutes for water-resistant sunscreens or 80 minutes for very water-resistant sunscreens.
- Note that altitude and latitude affect the amount of UVR an individual is exposed to. Take proper precautions, including use of a sunscreen with a high SPF, to protect skin from UVR.
- Note that snow and sand reflect ultraviolet radiation. Take proper precautions, such as wearing sunglasses and using sunscreens, to protect exposed skin.

Stop using the sunscreen if a skin rash occurs.

an entire season. This diminished usage demonstrates the importance of individuals receiving adequate counseling from pharmacists to get the protection they desire. The box "Patient Education for Protection from Sun Exposure" lists specific information to provide patients.

Evaluation of Patient Outcomes for Sun-Induced Skin Disorders

The short-term outcomes for sunscreen use are readily apparent. Within 24 hours of use, there will be no obvious sunburn, photosensitivity reaction, or eruption of photodermatosis. This success indicates that the appropriate sunscreen agents and/or SPF were used. However, the long-term effects of UVR (e.g., skin cancer and premature aging of the skin) may take from several years to 20 to 30 years to become evident. The lack of sunburn is at least one indicator that the patient is using an adequate SPF. However, this initial response still does not provide an indication of protection from the long-term effects of UVA. The best predictor of long-term protection from the damaging effects of UVR is the use of the most appropriate sunscreen product. This protection refers to using a product with an SPF according to the patient's skin type and tanning history. In addition, the product should be broad spectrum, absorbing or reflecting UVR across the entire spectrum from 290 to 400 nm. Also, patients should be asked about the quantity used and the frequency with which it is reapplied.

- A sunscreen product with an SPF of 30+ provides the greatest protection against UVR-induced skin damage.
- For optimal protection against UVR-induced skin damage, a broad-spectrum sunscreen should be selected regardless of its intended use.
- The patient should apply approximately 1 ounce of sunscreen to all exposed areas of the body.
- The sunscreen should be reapplied according to the labeled substantivity (usually either every 40 or 80 minutes).

CONCLUSIONS

Sunscreens prevent sunburn, photosensitivity reactions, and photodermatosis as well as preventing premature aging of the skin and skin cancer. Avoiding UVR and using protective clothing are important factors in reducing skin damage from UVR exposure.

The selection of a sunscreen product (SPF) should be based on the patient's skin type and tanning history. A sunscreen product with an SPF of 30+ provides the greatest protection against UVR-induced skin damage. For optimal protection against UVR-induced skin damage, patients should use a broad-spectrum sunscreen regardless of its intended use. The patient should be counseled to apply the recommended amount of sunscreen to all exposed areas of the body and to reapply it according to the labeled substantivity.

References

1. *NARD J.* 1996;118:43–4.
2. Morison WL, Hadley TP, Gilchrest BA, et al. Photobiology. *J Am Acad Dermatol.* 1991;25:327–9.
3. Bernhard JD, Pathak MA, Korheuar IE, et al. Abnormal reactions to ultraviolet radiation. In: Fitzpatrick TB, Eisen AZ, Wolff K, et al., eds. *Dermatology in General Medicine.* 3rd ed. New York: McGraw-Hill; 1987: 1480–507.
4. Taylor CR, Hawk JL. Recognizing photosensitivity. *Ann Rheum Dis.* 1994;53:705–7.
5. Leyden JJ. Clinical features of aging skin. *Br J Dermatol.* 1990;122(Suppl 35):1–3.
6. Pathak MA, Fitzpatrick TB, Parrish JA. Photosensitivity and other reactions to light. In: Fitzpatrick TB, Eisen AZ, Wolff K, et al., eds. *Dermatology in General Medicine.* 3rd ed. New York: McGraw-Hill; 1987: 254–62.
7. Guercio-Hauer C, Macfarlane DF, Deleo VA. Photodamage, photoaging, and photoprotection of the skin. *Am Fam Physician.* 1994;50: 327–32.
8. Kligman LH, Kligman AM. Photoaging. In: Fitzpatrick TB, Eisen AZ, Wolff K, et al., eds. *Dermatology in General Medicine.* 3rd ed. New York: McGraw-Hill; 1987:1470–5.
9. Skin Cancer Foundation. More than a million—basal cell carcinoma & squamous cell carcinoma. Available at: http://www.skincancer.org/morethan/index.html. Accessed 3/29/00.
10. Skin Cancer Foundation. Melanoma. Available at http://www.skincancer.org/melanoma/index.html. Accessed 3/29/00.
11. Gallagher RP, Hill GB, Bajdik CD, et al. Sunlight exposure, pigmentation factors, and risk of nonmelanocytic skin cancer: II. Squamous cell carcinoma. *Arch Dermatol.* 1995;131:164–9.
12. Gallagher RP, Hill GB, Bajdik CD, et al. Sunlight exposure, pigmentary factors, and risk of nonmelanocytic skin cancer: I. Basal cell carcinoma. *Arch Dermatol.* 1995;131:157–63.
13. Kricker A, Armstrong BK, English DR, et al. A dose-response curve for sun exposure and basal cell carcinoma. *Int J Cancer.* 1995;60:482–8.
14. Urbach F, O'Beirn S, Judge P, et al. The influence of environment and genetic factors on cancer of the skin in man. *Tenth International Cancer Congress* (Abstracts). Philadelphia: JB Lippincott; 1970:109–10.
15. Averbach H. Geographic variation in incidence of skin cancer in the United States. *Public Health Rep.* 1961;76:345–8.
16. Kochevar IE, Pathak MA, Parrish JA. Photophysics, photochemistry, and photobiology. In: Fitzpatrick TB, Eisen AZ, Wolff K, et al., eds. *Dermatology in General Medicine.* 3rd ed. New York: McGraw-Hill; 1987: 1441–51.
17. Forbes PD, Davies RE, Urbach F, et al. In: Jackson EM, ed. *Photobiology of the Skin and Eye.* New York: Marcel Dekker; 1986:67–84.
18. Willis I, Menter JM, Whyte HJ. The rapid induction of cancer in the hairless mouse utilizing the principle of photoaugmentation. *J Invest Dermatol.* 1981;76:404–8.
19. Cole CA, Van Fossen R. Testing UVA protective agents in man. In: Urbach F, ed. *Biological Responses to Ultraviolet A Radiation.* Overland Park, KS: Valdenmar; 1992:335–45.
20. Kripke ML. Ultraviolet radiation and immunology: something new under the sun—Presidential Address. *Cancer Res.* 1994;54:6102–5.
21. Kligman LH. Photodamage to dermal connective tissue by UVA. In: Urbach F, Gange RW, eds. *The Biological Effects of UV-A Radiation.* New York: Praeger; 1986:98–110.
22. Gilchrest BA, Soter NA, Hawk JL, et al. Histologic changes associated with ultraviolet A-induced erythema in normal human skin. *J Am Acad Dermatol.* 1983;9:213–9.
23. Staberg B, Worm AM, Brodthager H, et al. Direct and indirect effects of UVA on skin vessel leakiness. *J Invest Dermatol.* 1982;79:358–60.
24. Motoyoshi K, Ota Y, Takuma Y, Takenouchi M, et al. Wrinkles from UVA exposure. *Cosmetic Toiletries.* 1998;113:51–6, 58.
25. Ruenger TM, Epe B, Moeller K. Repair of ultraviolet B and singlet oxygen-induced DNA damage in xeroderma pigmentosum cells. *J Invest Dermatol.* 1995;104:68–73.
26. Mutzhas MF, Cesarini JP. Risk-benefit calculations for UV tanning devices. In: Passchier WF, Bosnjakovic BFM, eds. *Human Exposure to Ultraviolet Radiation: Risk and Regulations.* Amsterdam, The Netherlands: Elsevier Science Publishers; 1987:345–52.
27. McKinlay AF, Diffey BL. A reference action spectrum for ultraviolet induced erythema in human skin. *J Int Commission Illumination.* 1987;6: 17–22.
28. National Institutes of Health. *Consensus Development Conference Statement on Sunlight, Ultraviolet Radiation, and the Skin.* Bethesda, MD: National Institutes of Health; May 8–10, 1989.
29. Urbach F. Ultraviolet A transmission by modern sunscreens: is there a real risk? *Photodermatol Photoimmunol Photomed.* 1993;9:237–41.
30. Daxecker F, Blumthaler M, Ambach W. Ultraviolet exposure of cornea from sunbeds [letter]. *Lancet.* 1994;344:886.
31. Autier P, Dore JF, Lejeune F, et al. Cutaneous malignant melanoma and exposure to sunlamps or sunbeds: an EORTC multicenter case–control study in Belgium, France and Germany. *Int J Cancer.* 1994;58:809–13.
32. Westerdahl J, Olsson H, Masback A, et al. Use of sunbeds or sunlamps and malignant melanoma in southern Sweden. *Am J Epidemiol.* 1994;140:691–8.
33. Cohen JB, Bergstresser PR. Inadvertent phototoxicity from home tanning equipment [letter]. *Arch Dermatol.* 1994;130:804–6.
34. Injuries associated with ultraviolet tanning devices—Wisconsin. *Morbid Mortal Wkly Rep MMWR.* 1989;38:333–5.
35. Sunlamp products and ultraviolet lamps intended for use in sunlamp products. 21 CFR 1040.20 (1992):519–22.
36. Taylor HR, West SK, Rosenthal FS, et al. Effect of ultraviolet radiation on cataract formation. *N Engl J Med.* 1988;319:1429–33.
37. Horn EP, Hartge P, Shields JA, et al. Sunlight and risk of uveal melanoma. *J Natl Cancer Inst.* 1994;86:1476–8.
38. *SAA UV Labeling Policy.* Norwalk, CN: Sunglass Association of America; 1989.
39. Pathak MA, Fitzpatrick TB, Creiter F, et al. Preventive treatment of sunburn dermatoheliosis and skin cancer with sun protective agents. In: Fitzpatrick TB, Eisen AZ, Wolff K, et al., eds. *Dermatology in General Medicine.* 3rd ed. New York: McGraw-Hill; 1987:1507–77.
40. Johnson JA, Fusaro RM. Broad-spectrum protection: the roles of tinted auto windows, sunscreens, and browning agents in the diagnosis and treatment of photosensitivity. *Dermatology.* 1992;185:237–41.
41. Gange RW. Acute effects of ultraviolet radiation in the skin. In: Fitzpatrick TB, Eisen AZ, Wolff K, et al., eds. *Dermatology in General Medicine.* 3rd ed. New York: McGraw-Hill; 1987:1451–7.
42. Pathak MA. Immediate and delayed pigmentary and other cutaneous responses to solar UVA radiation (320–400 nm). In: Urbach F, Gange RW, eds. *The Biological Effects of UV-A Radiation.* New York: Praeger; 1986:156–67.
43. Reynolds NJ, Burton JL, Bradfield JW, et al. Weed wacker dermatitis [letter]. *Arch Dermatol.* 1991;127:1419–20.
44. Williams ML, Pennella R. Melanoma, melanocytic nevi, and other melanoma risk factors in children. *J Pediatr.* 1994;124:833–45.
45. Marks R, Whiteman D. Sunburn and melanoma: how strong is the evidence? *Br Med J.* 1994;308:75–6.
46. *Federal Register.* 1978;43:38206–69.
47. *Federal Register.* 1993;58:28194–302.
48. *Federal Register.* 1999;64:27666–93.
49. Naylor MF, Boyd A, Smith DW, et al. High sun protection factor sun-

screens in the suppression of actinic neoplasia. *Arch Dermatol.* 1995;131:170–5.

50. Mommaas AM, van Praag MC, Bouwes Bavinck JN, et al. Analysis of the protective effect of topical sunscreens on the UVB-radiation-induced suppression of the mixed-lymphocyte reaction. *J Invest Dermatol.* 1990;95:313–6.
51. Roelandts R, Vanhee J, Bonamie A, et al. A survey of ultraviolet absorbers in commercially available sun products. *Int J Dermatol.* 1983;22: 247–55.
52. Pathak MA. Sunscreens: topical and systemic approaches for protection of human skin against harmful effects of solar radiation. *J Am Acad Dermatol.* 1982;7:285–312.
53. Ferguson J, Collins P. Photoallergic contact dermatitis to oxybenzone. *Br J Dermatol.* 1994;131:124–9.
54. Kaidbey K, Gange RW. Comparison of methods for assessing photoprotection against ultraviolet A in vivo. *J Am Acad Dermatol.* 1987;16: 346–53.
55. Loesch H, Kaplan DL. Pitfalls in sunscreen application. *Arch Dermatol.* 1994;130:665–6.
56. Sunscreens. *Consumer Rep.* 1980;45:353–6.
57. Stenberg C, Larko O. Sunscreen application and its importance for the sun protection factor. *Arch Dermatol.* 1985;121:1400–2.
58. Wells TD, Jessup GT, Langlotz KS. Effects of sunscreen use during exercise in the heat. *Physician Sportsmed.* 1984;12:132–42.
59. Letter to the editor. *JAMA.* 1984;251:2348.
60. Anonymous. E-mail myth: sunscreen won't cause blindness. Available at: http://accessatlanta.com/living/news/1998/08/31/sunscreen.html. Accessed 3/29/00.
61. Fenner L. The tanning pill, a questionable dye job. *FDA Consumer.* 1982;16:23–4.
62. *Tanning Pills. Talk Paper.* Rockville, MD: Food and Drug Administration, US Department of Health and Human Services; July 1981.
63. Bluhm R, Branch R, Johnstone P, et al. Aplastic anemia associated with canthaxanthin ingested for "tanning" purposes. *JAMA.* 1990;264: 1141–2.
64. Jaworsky C, Ratz JL, Dijkstra JWE. Efficacy of tan accelerators. *J Am Acad Dermatol.* 1987;16:769–71.
65. Levine N, Sheftel SN, Eytan T, et al. Induction of skin tanning by subcutaneous administration of a potent synthetic melanotropin. *JAMA.* 1991;266:2730–6.
66. Stern RS, Weinstein MC, Baker SG. Risk reduction for nonmelanoma skin cancer with childhood sunscreen use. *Arch Dermatol.* 1986;122: 537–45.
67. Foley P, Nixon R, Marks R, et al. The frequency of reactions to sunscreens: results of a longitudinal population-based study on the regular use of sunscreens in Australia. *Br J Dermatol.* 1993;128:512–8.
68. Johnson EY, Lookingbill DP. Sunscreen use and sun exposure: trends in a white population. *Arch Dermatol.* 1984;120:727–31.

CHAPTER 34

Minor Burns and Sunburn

John D. Bowman and Robert H. Moore III

Chapter 34 at a Glance

Although the number of burn injuries is not known, each year approximately 2 million people are burned seriously enough to seek medical care.[1] These injuries result in more than 500,000 emergency department visits and about 70,000 hospitalizations annually. A substantially greater number of minor burns and sunburns occur and are self-treated with nonprescription products. Because deep burn injuries can lead to scarring and nonhealing wounds, it is important to accurately assess the injury and determine whether self-care or medical referral is appropriate.

Epidemiology of Minor Burns and Sunburn

In 1995, approximately 3600 deaths and 18,600 injuries were attributed to residential fires.[2] Burn deaths occur more often in individuals younger than 5 or older than 64 years. During 1991, residential fires were the second leading cause of injury deaths (after motor vehicle injuries) among children aged 1 to 9 years, and the sixth leading cause of injury deaths among those 65 years of age and older.[3] Sunburn, in comparison, occurs regardless of age.

More than 80% of minor burns occur in the home. Among household burns, 63% are on the hands and arms, and 34% are on the face and legs. Of the minor burns that occur outside the home, sunburn is the most common. The incidence and significance of sunburn has been underrated, and the injury goes unreported in most burn surveys because the public often does not consider sunburn in the same context as thermal, electrical, and chemical burns.

Anatomy and Physiology of the Skin

The skin is the largest organ of the human body, accounting for approximately 17% of the body weight of an average per-

Editor's Note: This chapter is based, in part, on the 11th edition chapter titled "Burn and Sunburn Products," which was written by Robert H. Moore III and John D. Bowman.

son. The skin performs a number of vital physiologic functions. It protects the body from injury and serves as a barrier against microorganisms. By synthesizing melanin, the skin protects underlying tissues from certain forms of irradiation. Additionally, the skin is a sense organ, receiving sensory input (especially touch and temperature) from the proximal environment. Fat deposits in the subcutaneous tissue play a role in lipid biotransformation. Cholecalciferol (vitamin D_3), which is involved in calcium regulation, is produced in the skin through exposure to ultraviolet (UV) radiation. The skin plays a major role in thermoregulation; cutaneous blood flow and perspiration are vitally important in maintaining the core body temperature at a normal level. Cutaneous blood flow and perspiration also help maintain water balance in the body. Sebaceous glands produce oil, which lubricates and prevents excessive drying of the skin.

Figure 34–1 shows a cross-section of the anatomy of the skin and the depths of injury caused by thermal burns. (See Chapter 27, "Atopic Dermatitis, Contact Dermatitis, and Dry Skin," for further discussion of skin anatomy and physiology.)

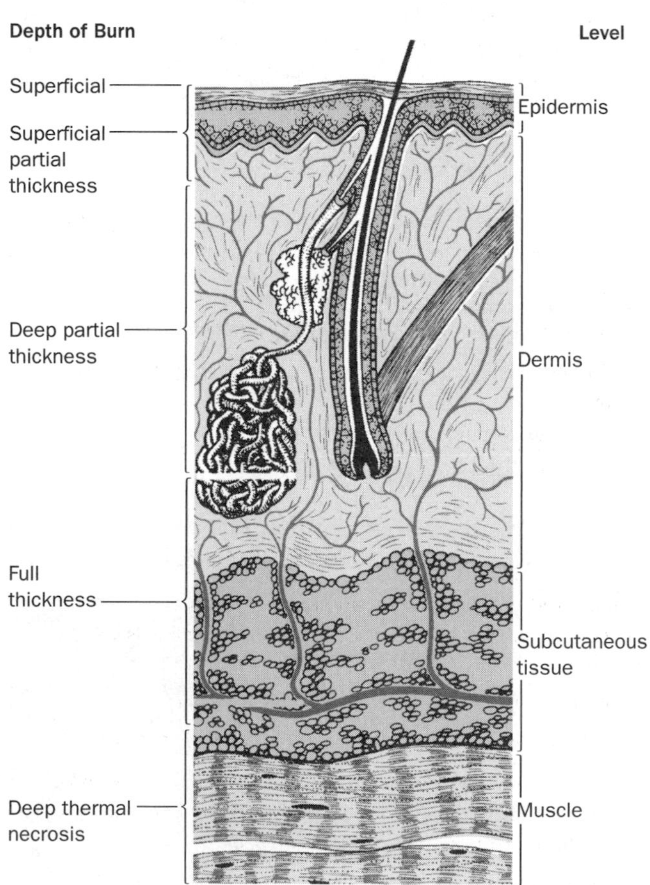

Figure 34–1 Cross-section of skin showing depth of burns.

Etiology/Types of Burns

Burns are tissue injuries caused by thermal, electrical, chemical, and UV radiation exposure. Most burns occur in the home and are usually thermal burns.

Thermal Burns

Thermal burns result from skin contact with flames, scalding liquids, or hot objects (e.g., oven broiler elements, hot pans, curling irons) or from inhaling smoke or hot vapors. The leading causes of thermal burns in children are (1) playing with fire-ignition sources, such as matches (37%); (2) faulty or misused heating devices (19%); and (3) faulty or misused electrical sources (11%). Among the elderly, the leading causes are (1) careless smoking (33%), (2) faulty or misused heating devices (19%), and (3) faulty or misused electrical sources (12%).[3] Most fire-related deaths occur during December through February. The increased occurrence of deaths during the winter months reflects the seasonal use of space heaters, portable heaters, fireplaces and chimneys, and Christmas trees.

Thermal damage to the respiratory tract from exposure to steam or hot gases can cause immediate upper airway obstruction as well as obstruction of the lower bronchioles caused by slowly developing edema. Smoke inhalation produces extensive lung damage because of toxic particles. Resultant injury to small airway alveolar capillaries can cause progressive respiratory failure. If smoke or heated gas inhalation has occurred, paramedics should quickly transport the patient to a hospital emergency room.

Electrical Burns

There are two types of electrical burns: flash electrical burns that result from a high-temperature arc of current close to the skin, and contact electrical burns that are caused by contact with a high-voltage source. Contact electrical burns generally have entry and exit sites, and tissue at every depth along its path can be injured, including bone. Electrical burns result from exposure to heat of up to 9000°F (5000°C). Most resistance to an electrical burn is at the skin, but electrical burns can cause extensive damage to underlying tissues and may be of any size and depth. Progressive necrosis and sloughing are usually greater than the initial lesion indicates. The pharmacist should refer such injuries to a physician for emergency care.

Chemical Burns

Chemical burns can result from skin contact with acids or alkalis contained in household products or from substances used in the workplace. Chemical burns can be partial or full thickness. (See the section "Classification Systems for Burns.") If not properly treated, chemical burns will occasionally extend for several hours after exposure. Thus, all efforts should be made to remove the chemical to prevent further injury, including removal of exposed clothing.

Sun Exposure

Sunburn is caused by acute overexposure of the skin to UV radiation for periods that overcome the ability of melanin, skin thickness and hydration, and vascular supply to protect the skin from injury. (See the "Color Plates," photograph 20.) Sunburn from natural sunlight is mainly caused by ultraviolet band B (UVB).[4] Tanning beds can also cause sunburn. They emit primarily an ultraviolet band A (UVA) radiation, which penetrates the skin more deeply than UVB. However, it takes an estimated 1000 times greater dose of UVA than UVB to produce erythema. (See Chapter 33, "Prevention of Sun-Induced Skin Disorders," for discussion of UV radiation bands.)

Photosensitive reactions (photoallergy and phototoxicity) to sun exposure have signs and symptoms similar to those of sunburn. Of the two types of reactions, photoallergy is relatively uncommon. It is characterized by an intensely pruritic eczematous dermatitis that may evolve into thickened leathery changes in sun-exposed skin.[5] (See the "Color Plates," photograph 21.) Products that usually cause this reaction include sulfonamides, phenothiazines, thiazide diuretics, piroxicam, and cosmetics that contain fragrances such as musk ambrette, sandalwood oil, and bergamot oil.

Phototoxicity usually appears as an exaggerated erythema, relative to the time of exposure, that quickly desquamates within several days.[6] Edema, vesicles (blisters), and bullae (large blisters), may occur. Sun-exposed skin is the only area of involvement. (See the "Color Plates," photograph 22.) This reaction occurs more often to systemic than to topical medications. Medications that usually cause phototoxic reactions include tetracycline antibiotics, furosemide, phenothiazines, fluoroquinolones, 5-fluorouracil, and amiodarone.

Chapter 33, "Prevention of Sun-Induced Skin Disorders," lists other medications that can elicit photosensitive reactions. Not every individual taking such medications will experience an adverse reaction to UV radiation, and those who do will not exhibit the same degree of symptomatic response.

Pathophysiology of Minor Burns and Sunburn

The extent of thermal injury to the skin is a function of the temperature generated and the duration of exposure. The skin can tolerate temperatures up to 104°F (40°C) for relatively long periods of time before injury. Temperatures above this produce a logarithmic increase in tissue destruction.[1] Cell damage occurs as a result of protein denaturation. This damage is reversible unless temperatures exceed 113°F (45°C). At this temperature, protein denaturation exceeds the capacity for cellular repair. The pathophysiology and manifestations of skin burns are related to the depth of the injury. For that

Case Study 34–1

Patient Complaint/History

Shawna, a fair, green-eyed, 18-year-old coed with strawberry blond hair, presents to the pharmacist with erythema on the face, arms, neck, and legs in a pattern consistent with overexposure to ultraviolet radiation. She requests advice on products to relieve the burning and stinging sensations. Because she wanted to develop a tan and eliminate facial acne before an upcoming social event, the patient used the services of a local tanning salon for less than an hour on the previous day.

Shawna's current medications include benzoyl peroxide 5% lotion at bedtime and tetracycline 250 mg one capsule daily for acne prophylaxis.

Clinical Considerations/Strategies

Readers can use the following considerations/strategies to determine whether treatment of this patient's condition with nonprescription medications is warranted:

- Assess possible causes of the erythema, including excessive UVA sunlamp exposure, drug-induced photosensitization, and contact dermatitis.
- Attempt to determine any change in soaps, cosmetics, or other topical interventions that might account for contact dermatitis.
- Assess the appropriateness of the nonprescription medication currently used to manage acne symptoms.
- Support/justify any change in the current nonprescription medication regimen.
- Consider referring the patient to her prescriber for reevaluation of the tetracycline therapy.

Patient Education/Counseling

Readers can use the following strategies to develop a patient education/counseling plan that will help ensure optimal therapeutic outcomes:

- Explain the etiology and pathogenesis of acne.
- Explain the nondrug measures for acne management.
- Explain the optimal use of nonprescription acne products, the warnings/precautions pertinent to these products, and the adverse effects associated with them.
- Explain the risk related to overexposure to UVA and UVB radiation, especially in the presence of photosensitizing chemicals.

reason, the specific pathophysiologic processes and the signs and symptoms for specific depths of burns are discussed in the section "Classification Systems for Burns."

Signs and Symptoms of Minor Burns and Sunburn

See the specific classification of burns in the section "Classification Systems for Burns."

Classification Systems for Burns

Skin burns are classified primarily according to depth of injury. This criterion is customarily used to determine whether a burn patient needs emergency medical care. A second system developed by the American Burn Association classifies burns by the severity of the injury. (See Table 34–1.) Either system can be used to assess a patient's burn; this chapter uses the depth of injury classification however.

Table 34–1

American Burn Association Injury Severity Grading System

Type of Burn	Criteria
Minor burn	15% BSA superficial and superficial partial-thickness burn in an adult 10% BSA superficial and superficial partial-thickness burn in a child 2% BSA deep partial-thickness or full-thickness burn in a child or adult not involving the eyes, ears, face, or genitalia
Moderate burn	15%–25% BSA superficial partial-thickness burn in an adult 10%–20% BSA superficial partial-thickness burn in a child 2%–10% BSA deep partial-thickness or full-thickness burn in a child or adult not involving the eyes, ears, face, or genitalia
Major burn	25% BSA superficial partial-thickness burn in an adult 20% BSA superficial partial-thickness burn in a child. All deep partial-thickness or full-thickness burns greater than 10% BSA All burns involving the eyes, ears, face, or genitalia All inhalation injuries Electrical burns Complicated burn injuries involving fractures or other major trauma All poor-risk patients (preexisting condition such as closed head injury, cerebrovascular accident, psychiatric disability, emphysema or lung disease, cancer, or diabetes)

Source: Adapted from reference 5.

Classification by Depth of Burn

The traditional classification of burns as first, second, or third degree has become obsolete, being replaced by the terms *superficial, superficial partial-thickness, deep partial-thickness,* and *full-thickness.* Although sunburn can be classified as one or more of these depths of burns, it is discussed separately to emphasize the damage that excessive sun exposure can cause.

Superficial Burns

Superficial burns usually result from a brief exposure to low heat, causing a painful area of erythema, which is similar to sunburn but is without significant damage to epithelial cells. Superficial burns involve only the epidermis. In most circumstances, no blistering occurs. Redness, warmth, and slight edema are present. The burn may be painful because the sensory nerve endings are intact. Avoidance of additional injury and symptomatic relief of pain and fever are usually the only treatment required. Sunburn is classified most often in this category. The majority of superficial burns can be managed through ambulatory care centers or through self-care.

Superficial Partial-Thickness Burns

Higher levels of heat than that involved in superficial burns will damage the outer epidermal layers and produce painful blistering, causing a superficial partial-thickness burn. If the damage does not involve the deeper proliferating area of the epidermis, rapid regeneration of a normal epidermis usually results. Superficial partial-thickness burns are often moist and weeping, and they blanch with pressure. They are painful and sensitive to temperature and air. They can occur from a splash or spill of hot liquid, a brief contact with a hot object, or a flash ignition. Healing is generally spontaneous, occurring within 2 to 3 weeks, with minimal or no scarring. However, if this type of burn occurs in a child or a patient with multiple medical problems, or covers more than 10% body surface area (BSA), fluid restoration may be required and the patient should be transported to a hospital emergency room. Lesser degrees of superficial partial-thickness burn injuries can often be managed in an ambulatory setting, and small burns (1% to 2% BSA) can usually be managed through self-care.

Deep Partial-Thickness Burns

Deep partial-thickness burns result from more extensive heat exposure than that involved in superficial partial-thickness burns. The heat damages deeper layers of the skin including the dermis, resulting in a blanched rather than moist erythematous wound. Such burns result from a spill of scalding liquid, contact with a hot object, flash ignition, and chemical contact, as well as from flame exposure. Such wounds can resurface because of surviving nests of epithelial cells that line the hair follicles and sweat glands. In this case, healing may be slow and scarring is likely to occur. In addition, these injuries are prone to infection because of the loss of barrier function and the loss of vasculature. Infection will worsen the severity of a burn injury, its depth, or both.

Deep partial-thickness burns involve the entire depth of the epidermis and may extend into the dermis. The appearance may be a patchy white to red area, and large blisters may be present. Blanching indicates loss of blood vessels to the area. Pain is usually more intense than in superficial burns because of the irritation to nerve endings, although some areas may be insensate. More of the dermis is involved than in superficial partial-thickness burns, so these burns take longer to heal (up to 6 weeks) and may cause thick scar formation (hypertrophic scarring or cheloid). Itching and hypersensation of the scar often occur when deep partial-thickness wounds are allowed to heal without skin grafting. Patients with deep partial-thickness burns should be examined in a hospital's emergency room. Such burn injuries can convert to full-thickness injuries if not properly and promptly managed.

Full-Thickness Burns

Even more extensive heat exposure than that involved in deep partial-thickness burns will cause death of the full thickness of skin in the affected area, resulting in a dry, leathery area that is painless and insensate. These full-thickness burns result from immersion in scalding liquid, flame exposure, electricity, and chemical contact and are considered serious. The body attempts to heal these wounds by sloughing off the dead layer and contracting the wound. If the wounds are not surgically managed, significant scarring may result, as well as failure to completely heal. Even deeper wounds cause necrosis of underlying structures including muscle and bone.

Full-thickness burns destroy both the dermis and epidermis and may extend into underlying tissues. Initially, the wound may appear red but will fade to white over 24 hours. Usually the burn is not edematous because the vascular supply to the area has been destroyed. Because nerve terminals are destroyed, pain will be absent or diminished in comparison with other degrees of burns. No sensation of pressure or temperature is noted in the burn wound. Healing occurs slowly over months, and grafting is often required to achieve wound closure. Scarring usually results. Hospitalization is normally required for treatment of full-thickness burns, and patients should seek emergency care as soon as possible.

Sunburn

Sunburn causes a superficial burn injury, characterized by erythema and slight dermal edema resulting from an increase in blood flow to the affected skin. The increased blood flow begins approximately 4 hours after exposure and peaks between 12 and 24 hours following exposure. Severe sunburn can lead to blistering (partial-thickness injury), fever, vomiting, delirium, and shock. If blisters occur, they will desquamate or "peel" over a period of several days. There is a slight chance of bacterial infection because of the loss of the outer skin barrier. Signs and symptoms of sunburn are seen in 4 to 24 hours following excessive exposure. (See the "Color Plates," photograph 20.) With mild exposure, erythema with subsequent scaling and exfoliation ("peeling") of the skin occurs. Pain and low-grade fever may accompany the erythema. More prolonged exposure causes pain, edema, skin tenderness, and possibly blistering. Systemic symptoms similar to those of thermal burn, such as fever, chills, weakness, and shock, may be seen in people in whom a large portion of the BSA has been affected. Following exfoliation and for several weeks thereafter, the skin will be more susceptible than normal to burning.

Classification by Severity of Injury

The American Burn Association's Injury Severity Grading System classifies burns as minor, moderate, and major.[5] Table 34–1 lists the criteria for these burn classifications, including the percentage of affected BSA, location of burn, and cause of burn. Minor burns account for about 95% of all burns treated in the United States and can often be managed in an outpatient environment if the eyes, ears, face, or perineum (genitalia) are not involved.

Complications of Minor Burns and Sunburn

A specialist should promptly examine patients who have received burns to the ear or eye, because loss of function in these structures may be devastating. Facial burns may be associated with respiratory injuries caused by inhalation. Burns that are more than superficial may result in permanent scarring that is much more consequential than scarring on less-visible body areas.

Hand burns can result in scarring and loss of range of motion, leading to major functional problems. Feet burns are often slow to heal, particularly in adults, and may become infected. Perineal burn victims are often chair-bound elderly or paraplegic patients suffering spill scalds. Such wounds are difficult to dress and readily infected by fecal organisms. Patients who are immunocompromised or otherwise at high risk of infection, such as the elderly and diabetics, can develop serious infections without specialized care of the burn injuries. All these patients should be referred to a physician.

Repeated sunburns are a risk factor for melanoma, particularly in children. Excessive unprotected exposure to the sun can also cause photoaging and ocular damage.[4] (See Chapter 33, "Prevention of Sun-Induced Skin Disorders," for further discussion of these disorders.)

Treatment of Minor Burns and Sunburn

Treatment Outcomes

The goals in treating superficial and superficial partial-thickness burns are to (1) relieve pain associated with the burn, (2) provide physical protection, and (3) provide a favorable environment for healing that minimizes the chances of infection and scarring.

Case Study 34–2

Patient Complaint/History

Wanda, a 39-year-old woman, comes to the pharmacy counter and requests help in selecting a topical product for a thermal burn. She burned her hand and forearm earlier that day when hot oil from a wok splashed onto her right hand and forearm. Because the patient does not have medical insurance, she hopes to find an aloe-containing product to relieve the pain associated with the burn.

Physical observation of the patient reveals thermal injury to the entire back of the right hand, scattered areas on the fingers of the right hand, and areas of the forearm composing about one-fourth of its dorsal surface. The burn areas are erythematous with some small elevated blisters present in some of the areas; the hand and forearm appear edematous.

Wanda is not currently taking any medications; she is allergic to codeine and penicillin however.

Clinical Considerations/Strategies

Readers can use the following considerations/strategies to determine whether treatment of the patient's condition with nonprescription medications is warranted:

- Assess the degree of severity and extent of the burn injuries.
- Using the previous assessment, make appropriate recommendations.
- Taking into consideration the patient's reluctance to seek medical attention, determine whether recommending a nonprescription topical product is appropriate.
- If deemed appropriate, recommend nonprescription products to treat the burn.
- Discuss with the patient the potential consequences of failing to obtain appropriate medical care for an acute injury of this type.
- Determine the pharmacist's duty in this situation.

General Treatment Approach

The treatment of a burn depends on its depth and severity. When a patient with burns presents for treatment, it is critical to assess the extent and depth of the injury, both initially and again in 24 to 48 hours. If appropriate and the patient has not already done so, the pharmacist should administer first aid. If the burn is self-treatable, the patient should follow the treatment approach outlined in Figure 34–2 and discussed below.

Most patients with superficial or superficial partial-thickness burns complain of pain. A number of therapeutic strategies can be used to alleviate the pain, including topical cold compresses, skin protectants, external anesthetics, topical corticosteroids, and oral nonsteroidal anti-inflammatory drugs (NSAIDs).

Superficial burns are not likely to become infected and do not pose a problem with exudates. Physical protection for comfort can be provided by a number of dressings and skin protectants that are currently marketed.

Superficial partial-thickness burns in which the epithelium is lost and the surface is weeping are prone to surface infection. Blisters should not be disturbed because blister fluid protects the skin below. Once debrided, a blistered area may become infected and should be cleansed periodically. Systemic antibiotics are not used—even for severe burns—unless symptoms warrant. For ambulatory or self-care, first-aid antiseptics or antibiotics are sufficient. Dressings and skin protectant agents should be used to protect the injured area.

Generally, if the burned area is 2% or larger and consists of superficial partial-thickness or greater injury, medical attention is needed. The inflammatory response to a burn injury evolves over the first 24 to 48 hours; thus the initial appearance of the injury often leads to an underestimation of its actual severity. As a rule, the patient should return after that period for reevaluation of the injury.

The location and type of burn are also critical in determining whether self-treatment is appropriate. Burns involving the eyes, ears, face, hands, feet, or perineum should not be self-treated. First-aid measures for chemical burns should be quickly administered; then the patient should go directly to the hospital's emergency department. Electrical burns and inhalation burns should be immediately referred for emergency care.

Other factors to assess include the presence of any underlying medical disorders or use of medication. Medication use can indicate the patient's health status. In addition, some medications can cause a photosensitivity reaction. (See the section "Sun Exposure.") Such reactions require medical referral. Patients with multiple medical disorders may need to restore body fluids, ruling out self-treatment. Immunocompromised patients or other patients at high risk for infection (the elderly or patients with diabetes) need specialized care.

First-Aid Measures

The initial treatment of superficial and superficial partial-thickness thermal burns is to cool the affected area in cool tap water (no ice) for 10 to 30 minutes. This phase of treatment does not apply when the depth or extent of the burn or both are serious because such action would delay emergency treatment. Cool immersion decreases cutaneous vasodilation and has been shown to decrease the area of redness, and thus edema, associated with tissue surrounding the burn. This treatment may help prevent blister formation. An internal analgesic drug product such as aspirin, NSAIDs, or ac-

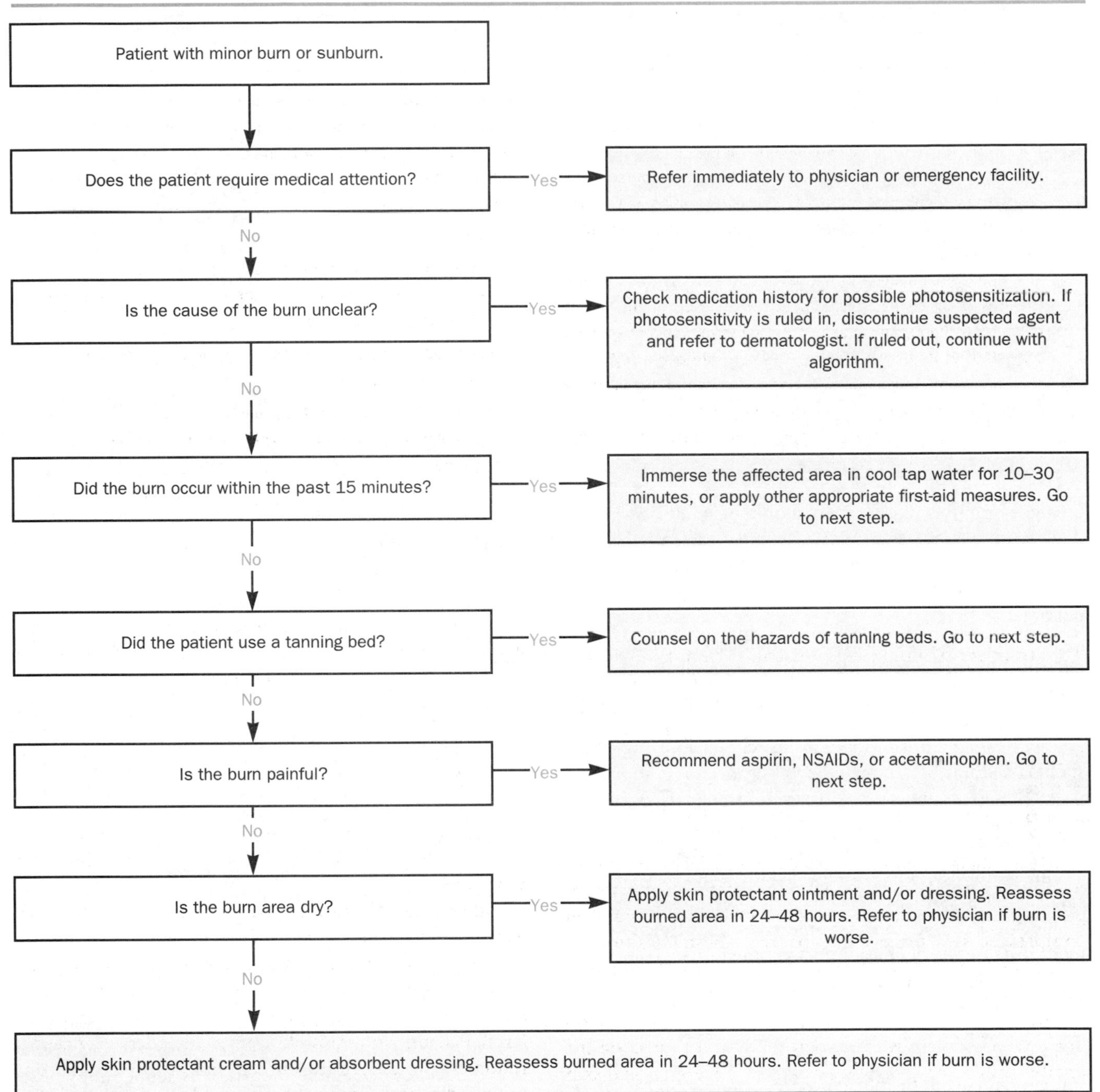

Figure 34–2 Self-care of minor burns and sunburn.

etaminophen can be given to reduce pain. Table 34–2 lists the appropriate doses.

Patients with deep partial-thickness or full-thickness injuries should be transported to an emergency center promptly. If some delay is anticipated before emergency care can be initiated, the patient should drink water, if possible, to replace vascular losses. An oral analgesic drug product such as aspirin or an NSAID can be given to reduce pain if the patient is conscious. If there is an inhalation injury, edema of the larynx or other structures may obstruct breathing.

In the case of chemical burns, the patient should immediately remove any clothing on or near the affected area. The affected area should then be washed with tap water for anywhere from 15 minutes to 2 hours until the offending agent has been removed.

If the eye is involved, the eyelid should be pulled back and the eye irrigated with tap water for at least 15 to 30 minutes. The irrigation fluid should flow from the nasal side of the eye to the outside corner to prevent washing the contaminant into the other eye. When the offending agent is identified, the

Table 34–2

Nonprescription Oral Analgesics for Minor Burn Pain in Adults

Agent	Dose (mg)	Maximum Daily Dose (mg)	Frequency of Use
Aspirin (e.g., Bayer)	325–650	4000	Every 3–4 hours, as needed
Acetaminophen (e.g., Tylenol)	325–650	4000[a]	Every 4–6 hours, as needed
	1000	4000[a]	3–4 times a day, as needed
Ibuprofen (e.g., Advil, Motrin IB, Nuprin)	200–400	1200[b]	Every 4–6 hours, as needed
Naproxen (e.g., Aleve)	200[c]	600	Every 12 hours, as needed
Ketoprofen (e.g., Orudis KT, Actron)	12.5[d]	75	Every 4–6 hours, as needed

[a] The maximum daily dose should not be exceeded. Consult physician if use extends beyond 10 consecutive days for adults or beyond 3 days in the presence of fever.

[b] The maximum daily dose should not be taken for pain that persists beyond 10 days or for fever that persists beyond 3 days unless directed by a physician.

[c] Initial dose of 400 mg may provide better relief.

[d] Initial dose of 25 mg may provide better relief.

area poison information center should be contacted immediately for treatment guidelines. In most cases of chemical burns and chemical contact with the eye, further medical attention is encouraged and should be sought as soon as possible.

No attempt should be made to counteract or neutralize a chemical burn. Such action may produce an exothermic (heat-generating) chemical reaction, which can damage the injured area more than the original offending agent. For example, treating a burn caused by an acid by applying a base such as sodium bicarbonate is inappropriate. It should be noted that for certain chemicals, even a small area of contact could produce serious or lethal injury. For example, hydrofluoric acid, an industrial chemical, has caused death within 2 or 3 hours following exposure that burns areas as small as 2.5% BSA.[7]

Electrical contact burns should receive emergency treatment because the depth of injury can be much greater than that suggested by the size of the entry or exit wounds. In an unconsciousness patient, other injuries may not be immediately apparent.

Initial treatment for minor sunburn is to get out of the sunlight and avoid further exposure. Minor sunburn can be relieved to some extent with cool compresses or a cool bath. Administering nonprescription oral analgesics (e.g., aspirin, NSAIDs, or acetaminophen) for treatment of pain is recommended. (See Table 34–2).

Heat stroke may occur with excessive exposure to sunlight in an environment that is hot or humid, or both. Because of complications from heat stroke, patients exhibiting fever, confusion, weakness, or convulsions should be referred to a physician or an appropriate medical facility immediately.

Nonpharmacologic Therapy

Preventing or reducing the number of burn injuries is an important public health measure. However, if a burn does occur, nondrug measures such as cleansing and protecting the burn are important therapeutic components.

Preventive Measures

Several public health strategies are effective in reducing burn injuries. People should install smoke alarms in all homes and periodically test them. Families should develop escape plans; remove fire-ignition sources from homes with children; and teach children not to play with matches, lighters, and the like. People should inspect electrical cords and portable heaters, clean chimneys periodically, and use fire screens in front of fireplaces. They should also use the correct fuel (not gasoline) in kerosene heaters.[2,3]

Sunburn can be prevented by avoiding overexposure to sunlight and by using appropriate sunscreen agents. (See Chapter 33, "Prevention of Sun-Induced Skin Disorders.")

Cleansing Procedures

After cool moisture is applied to a burned area to help stop the progression of the burn injury, reduce local edema, and relieve pain, the patient should gently cleanse the area with water and a bland soap, such as a baby wash or a surfactant (e.g., Shur-Clens). Alcohol-containing preparations should not be used because they cause pain to denuded skin and dehydrate the area. After the burn is cleansed, a nonadherent, hypoallergenic dressing may be applied if the area is small. A skin protectant or lubricant may be applied instead of or in addition to a dressing for small areas, particularly if the burn is extensive or in an area that cannot be dressed easily. (See Table 34–3.) If the burn is weeping, soaking it in cool tap water three to six times a day for 15 to 30 minutes will provide a soothing effect and diminish the weeping. Minor burns usually heal without additional treatment. For blistering burns in which blisters are no longer intact, cleansing once or twice daily to remove dead skin is recommended. Patients should be advised to avoid pulling at loose skin or peeling off burned skin because viable skin may be removed in the process, thereby delaying healing.

Table 34–3

Skin Protectant Ingredients Used in the Treatment of Minor Burns and Sunburn

Ingredient	Proposed Concentrations (%)
Allantoin	0.5–2
Cocoa butter	50–100
Petrolatum	30–100
Shark liver oil	3
White petrolatum	30–100

Source: Adapted from reference 8.

Protective Measures

Sterile, nonadherent gauze dressings are the most convenient way to cover a small burn on a body area that is easily bandaged, such as the arm or leg. For superficial burns, films that are self-adhesive, waterproof, and semipermeable will provide a protective barrier that is transparent and permits wound inspection without dressing changes (e.g., OpSite or Tegaderm).[9] Pressure points should be covered with self-adherent hydrocolloid dressings such as Duoderm or Comfeel.

Newer dressings have been designed to incorporate the desirable characteristics of exudate absorption with occlusiveness (e.g., DuoDerm, Vigilon, and Viasorb). Blistering burns should be dressed with these absorbent hydrocolloid dressings. If the dressing remains dry and intact, it may be left in place for 5 days. (See Chapter 35, "Minor Wounds and Skin Infections," for further discussion of wound dressings.)

Pharmacologic Therapy

Various products are useful in treating minor burns and sunburn. Some agents relieve pain, swelling, and/or inflammation. Others either protect the burn from infection or aid in healing the skin.

Skin Protectants

According to recommendations of its Advisory Review Panel on Over-the-Counter (OTC) Skin-Protectant Drug Products, the Food and Drug Administration (FDA) has recognized the agents in Table 34–3 as safe and effective for the temporary protection of minor burns and sunburn.[8]

Skin protectants benefit patients with minor burns by making the wound area less painful. They protect the burn from mechanical irritation caused by friction and rubbing, and they prevent drying of the stratum corneum. Rehydrating the stratum corneum helps relieve the symptoms of irritation and permits normal healing to continue. Skin protectants provide only symptomatic relief. The FDA has proposed revised labeling for the indications of skin protectants as follows: "For the temporary protection of minor cuts, scrapes, burns, and sunburn."[10] In selecting a skin protectant for burns, the pharmacist should choose products that prevent dryness and provide lubrication. Accordingly, the FDA has proposed that bismuth subnitrate, boric acid, sulfur, and tannic acid not be considered safe or effective when used as skin protectants. Drawing on advisory panel recommendations, the FDA has also proposed that products with labeling claims of "cures any irritation" or "prevents formation of blisters" should not be generally recognized as safe and effective and should not be included in the proposed skin protectant monograph. The FDA has not accepted claims that certain substances (e.g., allantoin, live yeast cell derivatives, or zinc acetate) contained in skin protectants are safe and effective in accelerating wound healing.

Liver oils have been used for many years as folk remedies for wound healing. Shark liver oil contains a high concentration of vitamin A and is proposed as a skin protectant. Vitamin A and D ointment has been used to treat minor skin burns and abrasions. The FDA recommends that the restriction preventing the use of skin protectants on children under 2 years of age be waived except for products containing live yeast cell derivatives, shark liver oil, and zinc acetate.

Generally, the patient with minor burns may apply a skin protectant as often as needed. If the burn has not improved in 7 days or if it worsens during or after treatment, the patient should consult a physician promptly.

Analgesics

An initial step in treating the patient with a minor burn is to recommend the short-term administration of an internal analgesic, preferably one with anti-inflammatory activity, such as the NSAIDs (aspirin, naproxen, ketoprofen, or ibuprofen).

Mechanism of Action As prostaglandin inhibitors, NSAIDs may decrease the erythema and edema in the burned area. The NSAIDs may be especially beneficial in the patient with mild sunburn, especially in the first 24 hours after overexposure to UV radiation.

For patients who cannot tolerate the NSAIDs, acetaminophen can provide pain relief. The dose of acetaminophen should not exceed 4 g per day, and prolonged use should be discussed with a pharmacist or physician. Although acetaminophen is a weak prostaglandin inhibitor and is not an anti-inflammatory agent, it may still produce beneficial analgesia. Further guidelines for the proper use of internal analgesic agents are included in Chapter 3, "Headache and Muscle and Joint Pain."

The use of various systemic NSAIDs has been shown to decrease inflammation caused by exposure to UV radiation. However, this effect has been found to last only about 24 hours,[11] possibly because the initial inflammation of sunburn is mediated by prostaglandins, whereas the later ensuing inflammation is primarily associated with leukocytes. The combined use of a topical corticosteroid and oral ibuprofen or another NSAID was found to produce more effective sunburn relief than either agent used alone.[12] Ibuprofen may decrease early inflammation by inhibiting prostaglandin formation, and the corticosteroid provides later relief by decreasing leukocyte infiltration into the area.

Dosage/Administration Guidelines See Table 34–2 for recommended dosages.

Adverse Effects Aspirin can cause hearing impairment, gastrointestinal (GI) upset, and occult bleeding when used chronically. GI distress, occult bleeding, diarrhea, vomiting, dizziness, and skin rash occur occasionally with NSAIDs.

Drug–Drug Interactions Alkalinizing agents (e.g., acetazolamide, antacids) and corticosteroids can reduce salicylate levels. Large doses of aspirin can increase oral anticoagulant effect; even small doses can increase risk of bleeding with anticoagulants. NSAIDs may inhibit the antihypertensive response to angiotensin converting enzyme (ACE) inhibitors, β blockers, diuretics, and hydralazine. NSAIDs may decrease renal lithium clearance.

Precautions/Warnings Because of the association with Reye's syndrome, the use of aspirin in children and teenagers with flu-like symptoms or chickenpox is not recommended. Aspirin and NSAIDs should be used with caution in patients with renal disease, peptic ulcer disease, bleeding tendencies, hypoprothrombinemia, or during anticoagulant therapy. Patients who develop bronchospasm to aspirin may develop a similar reaction to other NSAIDs. NSAIDs should be used cautiously in patients with congestive heart failure or cirrhosis.

Topical Anesthetics

The pain of minor burns and sunburn can be attenuated by the judicious use of topical anesthetics. Agents proposed as safe and effective in providing temporary relief of pain associated with minor burns are listed in Table 34–4.

Mechanism of Action Topical anesthetics relieve pain by inhibiting the transmission of pain signals from pain receptors. Relief is short-lived, lasting only 15 to 45 minutes.

Dosage/Administration Guidelines Benzocaine (5% to 20%) and lidocaine (0.5% to 4%) are the two amine external anesthetics most often used in nonprescription drug preparations. Dibucaine (0.25% to 1%), tetracaine (1% to 2%), butamben (1%), and pramoxine (0.5% to 1%) are also found in external anesthetic preparations. The higher concentrations of the topical anesthetics are appropriate for burns in which the skin is intact. Lower concentrations of topical anesthetics are preferred when the skin surface is not intact because absorption is enhanced, but they should be applied only to small areas to avoid systemic toxicity.

Topical anesthetics should be applied no more often than three or four times daily. Because their duration of action is short, continuous pain relief cannot be obtained with these agents. Increasing the number of applications increases the risk of a hypersensitivity reaction and, more important, the chance for systemic toxicity.

Adverse Effects Benzocaine produces a hypersensitivity reaction in about 1% of patients, a higher incidence than that seen with lidocaine. In a patch test study of 4000 patients with dermatitis, 9% were sensitive to benzocaine, and only neomycin was more sensitizing (10%).[13] In contrast, benzocaine is essentially devoid of systemic toxicity, whereas the systemic absorption of lidocaine can lead to a number of side effects. Systemic toxicities caused by lidocaine are rare, however, if the product is used on intact skin, on localized areas, and for short periods.

Table 34–4

External Analgesic Ingredients for the Treatment of Minor Burns and Sunburn

Agent	FDA-Approved Concentrations (%)
Amine and "Caine"-Type Local Anesthetics	
Benzocaine	5–20
Butamben picrate	1
Dibucaine	0.25–1
Dibucaine hydrochloride	0.25–1
Dimethisoquin hydrochloride	0.3–0.5
Dyclonine hydrochloride	0.5–1
Lidocaine	0.5–4
Lidocaine hydrochloride	0.5–4
Pramoxine hydrochloride	0.5–1
Tetracaine	1–2
Tetracaine hydrochloride	1–2
Alcohol and Ketone Counterirritants	
Benzyl alcohol	10–33
Camphor	0.1–3
Camphorated metacresol	
Camphor	3–10.8
Metacresol	1–3.6
Camphor and phenol[a]	
Camphor	3–10.8
Phenol	4.7
Juniper tar	1–5
Menthol	0.1–1
Phenol	0.5–1.5
Phenolate sodium	0.5–1.5
Resorcinol	0.5–3
Antihistamines	
Diphenhydramine hydrochloride	1–2
Tripelennamine hydrochloride	0.5–2
Hydrocortisone Preparations	
Hydrocortisone	0.25–0.5
Hydrocortisone acetate	0.25–0.5

[a] When combined in a light mineral oil, USP vehicle.

Source: Adapted from reference 10.

Topical Hydrocortisone

Although not FDA-approved for use in treating minor burns, 1% topical hydrocortisone is often used in the first-aid treatment of minor burns covering a small area.

An anti-inflammatory agent, hydrocortisone should be used with caution if the skin is broken because its use may allow infections to develop. Topical corticosteroid treatment with high-potency agents has been shown to decrease collagen synthesis and delay reepithelialization in dermal wounds, while low-potency 1% hydrocortisone ointment does not interfere with resurfacing of the skin.[14] (See Chapter 28, "Scaly Dermatoses," for additional information about this agent.)

Antimicrobials

The patient should always use topical antimicrobial therapy for major burns; most often the prescription preparations silver sulfadiazine and mafenide are used.[15] However, for minor burns, nonprescription first-aid antibiotic or antiseptic products are of limited value, especially on burns in which the skin is intact. These preparations may be used on minor burns when the skin has been broken. Drawing from data and information submitted to the rule-making panel for over-the-counter (OTC) topical antimicrobial drug products, the FDA issued an amended proposed rule for first-aid antiseptics.[16] Chapter 35, "Minor Wounds and Skin Infections," discusses preparations that may be used to help prevent infection in minor burns or sunburn. The petrolatum base present in some first-aid products, such as triple antibiotic ointment, is a skin protectant that can provide symptomatic relief.

Vitamins

Vitamin supplements are commonly used by burn centers for severe burn injuries. Although the benefits of vitamin supplementation for minor burns are not known, a frank deficiency of vitamin C (ascorbic acid) or vitamin A will impair wound healing. No evidence suggests that vitamin dosages beyond the normal daily requirements accelerates wound healing. However, vitamin C does play a key role in healing wounds because it is required for collagen synthesis. Because vitamin C is not stored in the body, it is reasonable to recommend up to 2 g of vitamin C daily from the time of injury until healing is complete.

Animal studies indicate that vitamin A enhances healing in a variety of wounds. Following serious injury, the patient may have an increased requirement for vitamin A. In addition, deficiency states are associated with increased infections. Because vitamin A is stored in large amounts in the liver, supplemental vitamin A should not be used for long periods. Minor burn injuries will probably not benefit from supplemental oral vitamin A, but topical vitamin A (fish or shark liver oil-based products) may be helpful.

Deficiency of B vitamins may retard wound healing, so B vitamins should be supplemented if nutritional status is poor. Excess vitamin E may delay wound healing and does not play a role in burn injury. Vitamin D is not significantly involved in healing wounds.

Administering zinc is not beneficial in people who are not zinc deficient. Iron deficiency anemia can decrease the oxygen supply to the healing area and should be corrected if present. Copper deficiency may impair healing and can be corrected through normal dietary intake.

Oral supplementation with vitamins E and C, as well as dietary fish oil, may reduce sunburn.[17,18] Beta-carotene supplementation does not alter sunburn reactions.[19]

In summary, burned individuals with good nutritional status may not benefit from vitamin or mineral supplementation. However, patients whose dietary intake may be suboptimal will not be harmed by, and could benefit from, temporary supplementation with standard multivitamin or mineral preparations. Assurance of adequate vitamin C intake is recommended during healing from burn injury.

The ability of topical forms of aloe vera and vitamin E to aid in the healing of minor burns and sunburn has not been substantiated, so the FDA has not approved these agents as healing aids.

Counterirritants

Although counterirritants, such as camphor, menthol, and ichthammol, are currently proposed for use in minor burn treatment, the FDA is still evaluating such agents, and they should not generally be used for burns. Such agents do reduce pain by stimulating sensory nerve fibers, but they increase blood flow to the area, causing further development of edema. They also irritate the already sensitized and damaged skin.

Miscellaneous Agents

Small studies suggest that so-called inert topical preparations may alter wound healing in either a positive or a negative manner. Topical nitrofurantoin, a liquid detergent, and some petrolatum-containing products have been shown to retard epithelial healing, while an oil-in-water cream, triple antibiotic ointment, silver sulfadiazene cream, and benzoyl peroxide lotion 10% and 20% have increased the rate of healing.[14]

Combination Products

Rarely will a product that is intended to treat minor burns contain only one ingredient. The FDA proposed that two or more of the skin-protectant ingredients listed in Table 34–3 may be combined, provided that each ingredient in the combination is within the concentration range in the proposed monograph.[8]

Additionally, the FDA recognized that skin protectants are suitable inactive vehicles for delivering active ingredients in other categories, such as topical analgesics and sunscreens. (See Chapter 5, "Musculoskeletal Injuries and Disorders," and Chapter 33, "Prevention of Sun-Induced Skin Disorders," respectively, for discussions of these active ingredients.)

Product Selection Guidelines

If a topical anesthetic or hydrocortisone is to be used, the pharmacist should recommend the most appropriate product formulation. Such products are available as ointments, creams, solutions (lotions), and sprays (aerosols).

Ointments are oleaginous-based preparations. They provide a protective film to impede the evaporation of water from the wound area, which helps keep the skin from drying. However, if the skin is broken, an ointment may not be appropriate because of its impermeability. The presence of excessive moisture trapped beneath the application may promote bacterial growth or maceration of the skin, thus delaying healing. Ointments are more appropriate for minor burns in which the skin is intact. Creams are emulsions that allow some fluid to pass through the film and that are best for broken skin. Generally, creams are easier to apply and remove than are ointments. To prevent contaminating the preparation, the patient should not apply ointments and creams directly onto the burn from the container.

Lotions spread easily and are easier to apply when the burn area is large. However, lotions that produce a powdery cover should not be used on a burn because they tend to dry the area, are difficult (and possibly painful) to remove, and provide a medium for bacterial growth under the caked particles.

Generally, aerosol and pump sprays are more costly than other topical dosage forms. Sprays offer the advantage of precluding the need to physically touch the injured area, so there is less pain associated with applying the medication. Proper application requires holding the container approximately 6 inches from the burn and spraying for 1 to 3 seconds. This method decreases the chances of chilling the area. However, sprays are not usually protective in that the aerosol is typically water- or alcohol-based and will evaporate.

Table 34–5 lists examples of products appropriate for treating minor burns and sunburn.

Alternative Remedies

Therapy for minor burns and sunburn is largely empirical, with little scientific study. The use of alternative preparations

Table 34–5

Selected Products for Minor Burns and Sunburn

Trade Name	Primary Ingredients
Skin Protectants	
A + D Ointment with Zinc Oxide	Zinc oxide 10%; cod liver oil (contains vitamins A and D)
A + D Original Ointment	Petrolatum 80.5%; lanolin 15.5%; cod liver oil (contains vitamins A and D)
Delazinc Ointment	Zinc oxide 25%; white petrolatum
Skin Protectants–Antiseptics	
Unguentine Ointment	Petrolatum; zinc oxide; phenol 1%
Vaseline First Aid Anti-Bacterial Petroleum Jelly	Petrolatum 98.3%; chloroxylenol 0.53%; phenol
Local Anesthetics	
Americaine Aerosol	Benzocaine 20%
Banana Boat Sooth-A-Caine Gel	Lidocaine
Butesin Picrate Ointment	Butamben picrate 1%
Dermoplast Aerosol	Benzocaine 20%
Gold Bond Medicated Anti-Itch Cream	Pramoxine HCl 1%
Nupercainal Cream	Dibucaine 0.5%
Solarcaine Aloe Extra Burn Relief Cream/Gel/Spray	Lidocaine 0.5%
Tronothane Hydrochloride Cream	Pramoxine HCl 1%
Xylocaine Ointment	Lidocaine 2.5%
Local Anesthetics–Antiseptics	
Bactine First Aid Liquid/Spray	Lidocaine HCl 2.5%; benzalkonium chloride 0.13%
Bicozene External Analgesic Creme	Benzocaine 6%; resorcinol 1.67%
Burntame Spray	Benzocaine 20%; 8-hydroxyquinoline
Foille Plus Aerosol	Benzocaine 20%; benzethonium chloride 0.15%
Foille Medicated First Aid Aerosol/Ointment	Benzocaine 5%; chloroxylenol
Lanacane Aerosol	Benzocaine 20%; benzethonium chloride 0.1%
Lanacane Creme	Benzocaine 6%; benzethonium chloride 0.1%
Lanacane Maximum Strength Cream	Benzocaine 20%; benzethonium chloride 0.2%
Medi-Quik First Aid Aerosol	Lidocaine 2%; benzalkonium chloride 0.13%
Solarcaine Medicated First Aid Aerosol	Benzocaine 20%; SD alcohol 40, 35%; triclosan 0.13%
Unguentine Plus Cream	Lidocaine HCl 2%; phenol 0.5%

such as herbals is also empirical, but in some societies such remedies have been used for many generations. Plants such as *Calendula*, *Aloe vera*, *Garcinia morella*, and *Datura metol* are said to have healing properties.[20] In fact, the traditional way of treating lightning burns in southern India involves smearing coconut oil on plantain (banana) leaves and dressing wounds with them. Externally applied extracts of *Picrorhiza kurrea*, *Cassia fistula*, *Emblica officinalis*, *Euphorbia thymifolia*, and *Curcuma longa* have antimicrobial effects, while *Allium sativum*, *Boerhaevia diffusa*, *Curcuma longa*, and *Ricinus communis* possess anti-inflammatory properties. (See Chapter 45, "Herbal Remedies," for further discussion of these types of remedies.)

Aloe gel has been widely used externally for its wound-healing properties, although controversy exists concerning the effectiveness of commercial preparations compared with fresh aloe gel.[21] Differences in extraction and processing techniques may be related to variable results in artificial cell culture systems for processed aloe gel. A few small clinical studies suggest the effectiveness of fresh aloe gel and some prepared products in skin ulcers, burn wounds, frostbite injuries, and psoriasis. Aloe gel's effects may result from inhibition of the pain-producing substance bradykinin. Aloe gel may also inhibit thromboxane and prostaglandins and may have antibacterial and antifungal properties. The FDA does not recognize aloe gel as safe and effective for treating any condition because of insufficient evidence. Nonetheless, aloe gel products are widely used for burns and sunburns, and freshly prepared aloe gel may be worth considering for self-care of minor burns.

Comfrey consists of the leaves or root of *Symphytum officinale* and has been used to treat various wounds.[21] However, variability in species use and inherent toxic alkaloids raise concerns about its safety. The patient should avoid internal use or any use of the plant's root. Only mature leaves should be applied externally and then only to unbroken skin for a limited time. The levels of carcinogenic pyrrolizidine alkaloids in American products are unknown.

Tea tree oil is prepared from the leaves of an Australian tree, *Melaleuca alternifolia*.[21] It has antimicrobial activity and has been used for treating cuts, abrasions, burns, insect bites, and other skin and vaginal infections.

The dried flower heads of *Arnica montana* have been prepared as hydroalcoholic extracts and creams.[21] Arnica has been shown to have antimicrobial, antiedema, and anti-inflammatory properties. The German Commission E has approved arnica for external application because of its anti-inflammatory, analgesic, and antiseptic properties.

A prospective randomized trial of honey versus silver sulfadiazine for superficial burns demonstrated that honey dressings resulted in faster healing and fewer infections than did the silver sulfadiazine dressings.[22]

A home remedy to relieve sunburn is to brew a quart of strong tea (e.g., orange pekoe or black tea) with no additives, then to chill it until cold. The patient dips washcloths in the tea, wrings them out, and gently lays the cloths over the sunburned area(s) until the cloths feel warm to the touch. Applications are repeated until the pain is relieved. This method also prevents blistering and tans the reddened areas.

Patient Assessment of Minor Burns and Sunburn

When a patient presents with a burn, the pharmacist should immediately assess the severity of the burn by determining the depth of the injury and the percentage of BSA involved. The percentage of the adult body that has been burned can be estimated by the rule of nines. (See Figure 34–3.) The total BSA is divided into 11 areas, each accounting for 9% or a multiple of 9. An easy way to estimate the percentage of burned BSA is to use the back of the hand as 1% of BSA. The rule of nines is reliable for adults but inaccurate for children and patients with small body surfaces. Table 34–6 illustrates how the BSA of the head, extremities, and other parts of the body changes with age.

In addition to the physical assessment, asking the patient the following questions will help elicit the information needed to accurately assess the disorder and to recommend the appropriate treatment approach.

Q~ Does the affected area have a leathery, white, or charred appearance?

A~ *Identify this type of burn. (See the section "Classification by Depth of Burn.")* Advise the patient that the

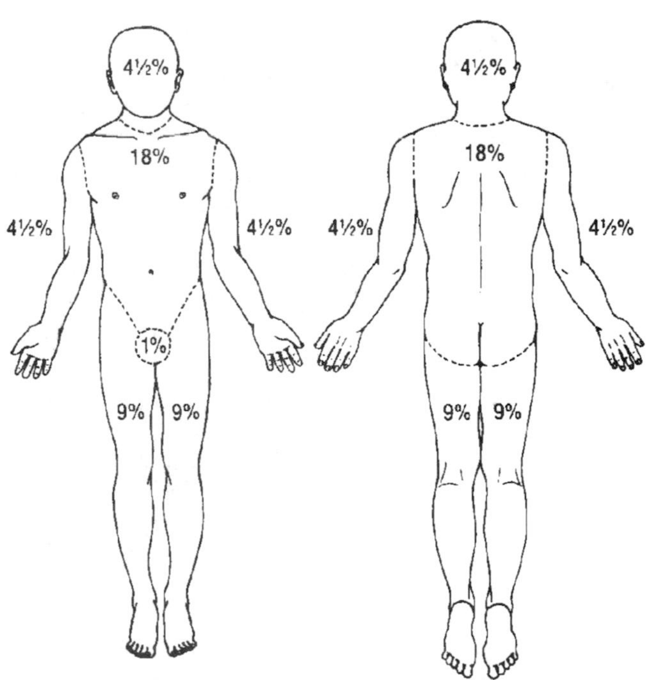

Figure 34–3 Rule-of-nine method for quickly establishing the percentage of adult body surface burned. Adapted with permission from *The Guide to Fluid Therapy*. Deerfield, IL: Baxter Laboratories; 1969:111.

Table 34–6

Age-Related Changes in Body Surface Area (%)

Surface	Age: Birth	1 year	5 years	10 years	15 years	Adult
Head	19	17	13	11	9	7
Neck	2	2	2	2	2	2
Trunk (anterior)	13	13	13	13	13	13
Trunk (posterior)	13	13	13	13	13	13
Buttocks	5	5	5	5	5	5
Perineum	1	1	1	1	1	1
Arms	8	8	8	8	8	8
Forearms	6	6	6	6	6	6
Hands	5	5	5	5	5	5
Thighs	11	13	16	17	18	19
Legs	10	10	11	12	13	14
Feet	7	7	7	7	7	7

absence of pain does not mean the burn is not severe. Arrange immediate transportation of the patient to the hospital's emergency department.

Q~ Is the wound blanched rather than erythematous, and is it moist and weeping?

A~ *Identify this type of burn.* Arrange immediate transportation of the patient for emergency treatment to prevent the burn from progressing to a full-thickness burn.

Q~ Is the burned area blistered and erythematous?

A~ *Identify this type of burn.* Assess the percentage of BSA affected. If the burn covers more than 10% BSA or the patient is a child or has multiple medical disorders, arrange transportation of the patient to the hospital for treatment of the burn and for possible fluid restoration. If the patient is an adult without multiple disorders and the affected BSA is less than 10%, recommend treatment in an ambulatory care center. If affected BSA of an adult is 1% to 2%, recommend appropriate self-treatment. (See the section "Treatment of Minor Burns and Sunburn.")

Q~ Is the burned area red and painful without blistering?

A~ *Identify this type of burn.* Recommend appropriate self-treatment for symptomatic relief of pain and swelling. Also, discuss with the patient measures to avoid further injury to the affected area.

Q~ Has the patient been sunburned?

A~ Ask the patient how soon the signs and symptoms occurred after the sun exposure. *Identify the typical time frame after sun exposure for manifestation of a sunburn.* If the time frame is characteristic of minor sunburn, recommend appropriate self-treatment. If the symptoms occurred sooner than this time frame, see the next question. If the signs and symptoms are characteristic of severe sunburn or stroke, refer the patient to a hospital.

Q~ Is the cause of the burn unclear?

A~ If the patient is unsure of the cause but has been exposed to the sun even for only minutes, do a complete drug history. *Identify the medications that can cause photosensitivity reactions.* (See the section "Sun Exposure.")

Q~ Has the patient inhaled hot vapors or smoke?

A~ If yes, call paramedics to transport the patient quickly to a hospital's emergency department. Either injury can cause extensive, progressive damage to the lungs.

Q~ Did electricity or chemicals cause the burn?

A~ If a chemical caused the burn, administer first aid. (See the section "First-Aid Measures.") Refer the patient to the emergency department. If the patient has an electrical burn, refer the patient immediately for emergency care to prevent progression of the injury.

Q~ Does the burn involve the eyes, ears, face, hands, feet, or perineum? Is the patient immunocompromised or otherwise at high risk for infection?

A~ *Identify possible complications for these situations. (See the section "Complications of Minor Burns and Sunburn.")* Refer all such burns to a physician or specialist for treatment and prevention of complications.

Patient Education for Minor Burns and Sunburn

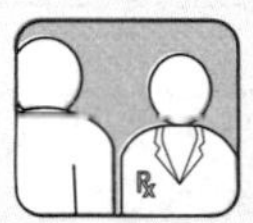

The objectives of self-treatment are to (1) relieve the pain and swelling, (2) protect the burned area from further physical injury, and (3) avoid infection and scarring of the burned area. For most patients, carefully following product instructions and the self-care measures listed below will help ensure optimal therapeutic outcomes.

Nondrug Measures

- Treat superficial burns with no blistering as follows:
  —Immerse the affected area in cool tap water for 10 to 30 minutes.
  —Cleanse the area with water and a mild soap.
  —Apply a nonadherent dressing or skin protectant to the burn.
- For small burns with minor blistering, follow the first two steps above but use a hydrocolloid dressing to protect the burn.
- If possible, avoid rupturing blisters.
- For sunburns, avoid further sun exposure and follow the appropriate procedures above based on whether blistering is present.

Nonprescription Medications

- For superficial burns (including sunburn) with unbroken skin, treat the affected area with skin protectants, topical anesthetics, or topical hydrocortisone.
- If the skin is broken, use topical antibiotics to prevent infection.
- If nutritional status is poor, take supplements for vitamins A, B, and C.
- Do not apply camphor, menthol, or ichthammol to the burn.
- For temporary relief of pain, take aspirin, acetaminophen, ibuprofen, naproxen, or ketoprofen. (See Table 34–2 for dosage guidelines.)
- Do not give aspirin to children or teenagers with flu-like symptoms or chickenpox. Reye's syndrome, a rare but potentially fatal condition, may result.
- Take aspirin with food, milk, or a full glass of water to minimize stomach upset.
- Take ibuprofen, naproxen, or ketoprofen with a small amount of food, milk, or antacid to minimize stomach upset.
- If a skin rash, weight gain, swelling, or blood in the stool occurs while taking pain relievers, report these side effects to a physician.

Report immediately to a physician any redness, pain, or swelling that extends beyond the boundaries of the original injury.

If the burn is not healed significantly in 7 days, see a physician for further treatment.

Patient Counseling for Minor Burns and Sunburn

Once a burn is assessed as self-treatable, the pharmacist should address the patient's immediate concern: relieving the pain and swelling. Some patients may not realize the potential complications of even minor burns; therefore, advice on how to protect the injury is vital in preventing possible infection and scarring. Using a 24- to 48-hour follow-up evaluation of the burn, the pharmacist should either recommend continuation of self-treatment or refer the patient for medical care. If self-treatment continues, the patient needs to know how long healing of the burn will take and the signs and symptoms that indicate worsening of the injury. The box "Patient Education for Minor Burns and Sunburn" lists specific advice for successful treatment of these injuries.

Evaluation of Patient Outcomes for Minor Burns and Sunburn

Burn wounds should be reassessed after 24 to 48 hours, because the full extent of skin damage may not be initially apparent. If the burn has progressed or worsened, the patient should seek medical attention.

If the wound has not healed significantly in 7 days, a surgeon experienced in burn wound management should examine it. Although such wounds may ultimately heal on their own, surgical excision and skin grafting may be the preferred treatment to shorten the healing process and minimize the degree of scarring. Typically, deep partial-thickness and full-thickness wounds managed surgically will heal within 2 weeks. After self-treating unsuccessfully for weeks, the patient will be distressed to learn that surgical management is needed and that healing could have been achieved much earlier.

The burn wound should exhibit decreased redness during healing. Signs of cellulitis or tissue infection, such as increasing redness, pain, and swelling that extend beyond the boundaries of the original wound, require examination by a physician.

Burned skin is more susceptible to sunburn for several weeks after initial injury, so avoiding sun exposure and using sunscreen agents during this period is recommended.

CONCLUSIONS

Minor burns and sunburn can often be treated with self-care. However, deeper burn injuries or burns affecting more than 1% to 2% of the body surface area require medical attention. Burn injuries may increase in severity over the first 24 to 48 hours, so reassessment is always necessary. Patient complaints usually focus on pain. Skin protectants and dressings should be recommended, and aspirin or NSAIDs are often helpful. The type of dressing or skin protectant used depends on whether the wound is dry or weeping. Blisters should not be ruptured. Topical hydrocortisone or anesthetics may provide additional relief in some patients, but should be used sparingly on broken skin. Counterirritants should be avoided. Vitamins, whether systemic or topical, are generally of no value unless the patient is malnourished. Photosensitization reactions can often be assessed by history and must be distinguished from ordinary sunburns.

References

1. Robson MC, Burns BF, Smith DJ. Acute management of the burned patient. *Plast Reconstr Surg.* 1992;89(6):1155–68.
2. Deaths resulting from residential fires and the prevalence of smoke alarms—United States, 1991–1995. *MMWR Morb Mortal Wkly Rep.* 1998;47(38):803–6.
3. Deaths resulting from residential fires—United States, 1991. *MMWR Morb Mortal Wkly Rep.* 1994;43(49):901–4.
4. Rapaport MJ, Rapaport V. Preventive and therapeutic approaches to short- and long-term sun damaged skin. *Clin Dermatol.* 1998;16: 429–39.
5. Edlich RF, Larkham N, O'Hanlan JT, et al. Modification of the American Burn Association injury severity grading system. *J Am Coll Emerg Phys.* 1978;7:226.
6. Bickers DR. Photosensitivity and other reactions to light. In: Fauci AS, ed. *Harrison's Principles of Internal Medicine.* 14th ed. New York: McGraw-Hill; 1998:1254–62.
7. Greco RJ. Hydrofluoric acid–induced hypocalcemia. *J Trauma.* 1988;28:1593–6.
8. Proposed rule, Part 348—External analgesic drug products for over-the-counter human use. *Federal Register.* 1983;48:5867–8.
9. Judson R. Minor burns—modern management techniques. *Aust Family Physician.* 1997;26(9):1023–6.
10. Proposed rule, Part 347—Skin protectant drug products for over-the-counter human use. *Federal Register.* 1983;48:6820–33.
11. Greenberg RA, Eaglestein WH, Turnier H, et al. Orally given indomethacin and blood flow responses to UVL. *Arch Dermatol.* 1975;111:328–30.
12. Eaglestein WH, Ginsberg LD, Mertz PM. Ultraviolet irradiation-induced inflammation: effects of steroids and nonsteroidal anti-inflammatory agents. *Arch Dermatol.* 1979;115(12):1421–3.
13. Bandmann HJ, Calnan CD, Cronin E, et al. Dermatitis from applied medicaments. *Arch Dermatol.* 1972;106(3):335–7.
14. Eaglestein WH, Mertz BA, Alvarez OM. Effect of topically applied agents on healing wounds. *Clin Dermatol.* 1984;2:112–5.
15. Kaye ET, Kaye KM. Topical antibacterial agents. *Infect Dis Clin N Am.* 1995;9(3):547–61.
16. Proposed rule—Topical antimicrobial drug products for over-the-counter human use. *Federal Register.* 1991;56(140):33644–80.
17. Fuchs J, Kern H. Modulation of UV-light-induced skin inflammation by D-alpha-tocopherol and L-ascorbic acid: a clinical study using solar simulated radiation. *Free Radical Biol Med.* 1998;25(9):1006–12.
18. Rhodes LE, Durham BH, Fraser WD, et al. Dietary fish oil reduces basal and ultraviolet B-generated PGE2 levels in skin and increases the threshold to provocation of polymorphic light eruption. *J Invest Dermatol.* 1995;105(4):532–5.
19. Garmyn M, Ribaya-Mercado JD, Russel RM, et al. Effect of beta-carotene supplementation on the human sunburn reaction. *Exper Dermatol.* 1995;4(2):104–11.
20. Sai KP, Babu M. Traditional medicine and practices in burn care: need for newer scientific perspectives. *Burns.* 1998;24:387–8.
21. Robbers JE, Tyler VE. *Tyler's Herbs of Choice.* New York: The Haworth Herbal Press; 1999:215–24.
22. Subrahmanyam M. A prospective randomised clinical and histological study of superficial burn wound healing with honey and silver sulfadiazine. *Burns.* 1998;24:157–61.

CHAPTER 35

Minor Wounds and Skin Infections

Edwina S. Chan and Raymond L. Benza

Chapter 35 at a Glance

Editor's Note: This chapter is based, in part, on the 11th edition chapter titled "First-Aid Products and Minor Wound Care," which was written by Edwina Chan and Raymond Benza. The discussion of fungal infections is based on sections of the 11th edition chapters "Dermatologic Products," written by Dennis P. West and Phillip A. Nowakowski, and "Foot Care Products," written by Nicholas G. Popovich and Gail D. Newton.

The skin is a versatile, multifunctional organ whose intricate workings depend on a delicate balance between structure and function. When a wound alters or disturbs this balance, prompt restoration is required to ensure body homeostasis. Restoration of the homeostasis is accomplished through the process of wound healing, a complex cascade of localized biochemical and cellular events regulated by the immune system and orchestrated by the skin. Although the skin is well adapted to heal minor wounds over time, proper cleansing and the use of antibiotics, antiseptics, and dressings facilitate healing and prevent scar formation.

Certain bacteria and the fungus *Candida albicans* inhabit the skin and protect it against invasion by other pathogenic microorganisms. Under certain conditions, these microorganisms can become pathogenic and can cause skin infections. Bacterial skin infection may occur secondary to a contaminated wound or may present as a primary pyodermic infection. Primary bacterial infections are discussed briefly to aid the pharmacist in differentiating them from secondary infection of an injury. Common fungal infections that may infect wounds or macerated skin are also discussed. Self-treatable viral infections, such as warts and herpes simplex labialis (cold sores) are discussed in Chapter 36, "Minor Foot Disorders," and Chapter 26, "Oral Pain and Discomfort," respectively.

Anatomy and Physiology of the Skin

The skin is composed of two anatomic layers, the epidermis and the dermis, supported by a variably thick subcutaneous layer called the hypodermis. (See Table 35–1 and Figure 27–1 in Chapter 27, "Atopic Dermatitis, Contact Dermatitis, and Dry Skin.") The epidermis, the most superficial layer of the skin, is normally in direct contact with the outside environment. Approximately 0.04 mm thick and avascular, it consists of five layers of stratified squamous epithelium (keratinocytes).[1] This stratified organization results from the upward migration of dividing cells from the stratum germinativum (basilar layer lying adjacent to the dermis) toward the stratum corneum (uppermost layer). As the cells migrate, they lose their nucleus, die, and become tightly packed and keratinized. This keratinized layer provides a tough, resistant, waterproof covering for the skin. Aside from its protective function, the epidermis serves several other functions as well, as it contains the cell types necessary for immune regulation (Langerhans' cells), skin color (melanocytes), and proprioception (Merkel's tactile cells). Skin appendages, including the sweat glands and hair follicles, are also derived from the epidermis.

The dermis is the layer directly below the epidermis. It is approximately 0.5 mm thick[1] and contains a rich vascular supply, multiple nerve endings, lymphatics, collagen proteins, and connective tissue. It also contains two main cell types: fibroblasts and macrophages.[2] The main function of fibroblasts is to produce collagen, a structural support protein necessary for scar formation. Macrophages, however, are multifunctional cells that are vital for wound repair. They serve as both immune and growth regulators, functions that are necessary for the sterilization, debridement, and eventual healing of the wound. The dermis also contains the basilar projections of epidermally derived sweat glands and hair follicles.

Table 35–1

Structure and Function of the Skin

Epidermis
Thickness of 0.04 mm
No blood supply
Composed of epithelium
Resident flora
Appendages: hair follicles, sebaceous glands, sweat glands
Five layers (two are stratum corneum and stratum germinativum or basement layer)
Dermis
Thickness of 0.5 mm
Main support structure
Contains nerve endings, lymphatics, vasculature
Normally moist
Extension of epidermal appendages
Subcutaneous Tissue (Hypodermis)
Variable thickness
Reservoir for fat storage
Temperature insulator
Shock absorber
Stores calories
Contains all structures and appendages found in dermis

Source: Reference 1; used with permission.

The subcutaneous tissue contains mostly adipocytes and is the origination site for dermal blood vessels. Its major function is to provide insulation, padding, and protection against mechanical injury. It also stores calories in the form of fat, and it provides the skin with a moderate degree of mobility, protecting it against friction and shear-related injury.[1]

The skin has five basic functions: protection, sensation, thermoregulation, immunomodulation, and production of vitamin D.[3] Its protective features are twofold: It provides the body with a barrier against physical injury from chemicals, sunlight, dehydration, and bacterial invasion, and it acts as a "shock absorber" against mechanical trauma. The skin modulates sensation through its vast network of pressure and touch receptors localized primarily in the dermis and subcutaneous layers. Its thermal regulation lies in its ability to modify fluid and electrolyte balances. Specialized cells within the epidermis act as antigen-processing sites, thus forming the basis of the skin's immunomodulation activity. In addition, vitamin D_3, which is important for calcium homeostasis, is synthesized in the epidermis by a process in which an endogenous cholesterol 7-dehydrocholesterol is photolyzed by UV radiation.

The skin has several other specialized features. Its surface is inhabited by bacteria (skin flora), including *Staphylococcus epidermidis* and *Staphylococcus aureus* as well as the fungus *C.*

albicans.[3] These skin flora serve to protect against invasion by other pathogenic bacteria. The pH of the skin is acidic (range between 4.2 and 5.6),[3] which allows it to regulate the number and activity of the skin flora. This feature is important as these normal flora can become pathogenic under certain conditions.

Wounds

The approach to wound care has dramatically changed over the past decade. Problems related to wound healing were approached empirically in the past, and solutions were usually based on anecdotal experience. Popular opinion dictated that wounds be left exposed to air to encourage drying and scab formation. Occlusive dressings were expressly avoided because it was thought that the moist, warm environment they created promoted bacterial colonization. Today, despite clear evidence to support the benefits of a moist, wound-healing environment,[4,5] clinical practice has lagged behind in instituting moist, wound-healing therapy. Traditional gauze dressings, which promote dehydration of the wound, continue to predominate over the newer, synthetic products that provide a moist environment. Thus, the goal of this discussion of wounds is to educate pharmacists and health care providers as to the principles of the moist, wound-healing method and its proper implementation through the use of selected first-aid products.

This goal will be accomplished through a review of skin anatomy and function, the physiology of wound healing, the classifications and type of wounds and superficial skin infections, the management of wounds and dermal-related infections through the use of drugs and/or dressings, and, finally, a schematic approach to triaging wounds. This discussion should enable pharmacists to communicate effectively with physicians on issues related to care of wounds and dermal infections, as well as to provide a firm foundation for effective outpatient counseling on the processes and treatments of these disorders.

Physiology of Wound Healing

Wound healing begins immediately after injury and consists of three overlapping stages: the inflammatory, proliferative, and maturation (remodeling) stages.[6] (See Figure 35–1.)

Inflammatory Phase

The inflammatory phase is the body's immediate response to injury. This phase, which lasts approximately 3 to 4 days, is responsible for preparing the wound for subsequent tissue development and consists of two primary parts: hemostasis and inflammation.

In the initial portion of the inflammatory phase, the wound becomes hypoxic and acidotic. Hemostasis is then initiated by the release of thromboplastin from injured cells. Thromboplastin, in turn, activates the body's intrinsic clotting system. The activated clotting factors, along with recruited platelets, form a clot within the first several hours. The newly formed clot stops the bleeding and allows healing to progress. The recruited platelets are crucial to the initial phases of healing because they release cytokines such as platelet-derived growth factor (PDGF) and the transforming growth factor, TGF-β. These cytokines stimulate chemotaxis of polymorphonuclear neutrophil (PMN) leukocytes, monocytes, and fibroblasts. Cytokines will also subsequently promote mitogenesis and collagen synthesis.[7]

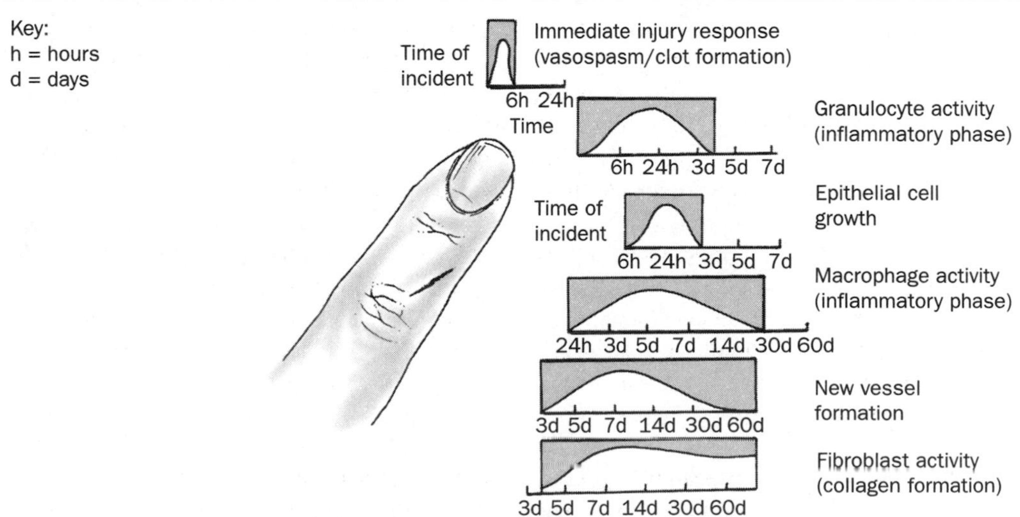

Figure 35–1 The chronology of early wound healing: activity of wound healing components. Adapted with permission from Trott A. Surface injury and wound healing. In: *Wounds and Lacerations: Emergency Care and Closure*. St. Louis: Mosby-Year Book; 1991:15.

After hemostasis is achieved, an active inflammatory phase begins, the primary function of which is to cleanse the wound. Inflammation begins with the recruitment of PMN leukocytes within the first 24 to 48 hours. PMN leukocytes, which require oxygen to function, phagocytize debris and bacteria in the wound. Yet the wound can heal in the absence of these cells. This healing is because platelets release bradykinin, histamine, and prostaglandins into the wound during this time, thereby initiating an intense vasodilatation of the vessels surrounding the wound and then flooding the wound in a type of rinsing action with water, plasma proteins, electrolytes, antibodies, and complement.[7] As a result, the wound becomes erythematous and edematous.

After the first 24 hours, blood monocytes are recruited into the wound by released chemotactic factors and become tissue macrophages. Without the macrophages, the wound would not heal. Macrophages function as phagocytes, releasing more chemotactic factors and, most important, releasing growth factors. Such growth factors stimulate epithelial mitogenesis and endothelial angiogenesis. They also induce fibroblasts to synthesize collagen,[8,9] which provides a healthy bed of granulation tissue for future epithelial cells.

The final portion of the inflammatory phase involves epithelial migration into the wound. Epithelial cells from the stratum germinativum migrate from the intact wound edges and epithelial appendages to cover the denuded area of the wound. As mentioned earlier, the successful migration and adherence of epithelial cells to the wound require a clean, healthy bed of granulation tissue. Once the epithelial cells become established on their granulation bed, they provide the initial (one-cell-thick) layer of new skin for the wound.[10] Epithelial cells can migrate under the clot and eschar (scab) in the wound, but, in doing so, they delay healing time and promote scar formation.

Proliferative Phase

The next phase of healing is the proliferative phase in which the wound is filled with new connective tissue and covered with new epithelium. This phase starts on about day 3 and continues for about 3 weeks. It involves the formation of granulation tissue, which is a collection of new connective tissue (fibroblasts and newly synthesized collagen), new capillaries, and inflammatory cells. The formation of this matrix involves several key coexisting and ongoing processes, including neoangiogenesis (capillary formation) and collagen synthesis.[4] The process of neoangiogenesis is stimulated by the acidic environment of the wound and directed by a variety of cytokines produced by stimulated macrophages, platelets, and endothelial cells, including TGF-α, TGF-β, and angiogenesis growth factor.

Collagen synthesis by fibroblasts is also directed by cytokines produced by stimulated macrophages, including PDGF, TGF-α and TGF-β, fibroblast growth factor, monocyte/macrophage-derived growth factor, and interleukin-2.[11] Collagen synthesis also requires oxygen, zinc, iron, and vitamin C. As granulation tissue is being laid down, epithelial cells, which began to migrate during the inflammatory phase, resurface the wound defect. It is important to remember that epithelial cells do not migrate across a dry or necrotic surface. The final portion of this phase involves the action of cytokine-recruited smooth muscle cells, which begin the process of wound contraction. This process involves the mobilization and pulling together of the wound edges.

Maturation Phase

The final phase of healing is known as the maturation or "remodeling" phase. The longest phase, it begins at about week 3, when the wound is completely closed by connective tissue and resurfaced by epithelial cells, and can continue for approximately 2 years after the injury. It involves a continual process of collagen synthesis and breakdown, replacing earlier, weak collagen with high–tensile-strength collagen.[10] The result is a scar with approximately 70% to 80% of the original strength of the skin it replaced.

As stated previously, all the healing phases involve and use cell-derived growth factors or cytokines. The cytokines are polypeptides that promote cellular growth, chemotaxis, proliferation, and differentiation as well as collagen synthesis, contraction, and eventual healing of the wound.[11] These features make cytokines an attractive new source of first-aid products to facilitate wound healing. One such product is topical silver nitrate impregnated with epidermal growth factor, which has been shown in animal models to shorten healing time when applied to burns.[12,13] Topical TGF-β has also been used to reverse the deleterious effects of glucocorticoids on wound tensile strength and hypocellularity.[14] The description, source, and cellular targets of these cytokines are beyond the scope of this chapter.

Factors Affecting Wound Healing

Several local and systemic factors can affect how efficiently and to what extent a wound will heal. Some of the important systemic factors[3] that can affect the healing process include the following:

- Inadequate tissue perfusion and oxygenation at the wound site.
- The patient's overall nutritional status, age, and weight.
- The presence or absence of local infection.
- Coexistence of diabetes mellitus.
- Certain medications.
- Wound characteristics.

Tissue Perfusion and Oxygenation

Adequate tissue perfusion and oxygenation promote and enhance phagocytosis and angiogenesis, which, in turn, stabilize cell structure and stimulate collagen synthesis. Lack of adequate tissue perfusion and oxygenation results in impaired collagen synthesis, decreased epithelial proliferation and migration, and reduced tissue resistance to infection.

Decreased perfusion and oxygenation can result from hypovolemia, severe anemia (hematocrit equal to 20 g/dL), peripheral vascular occlusive disease, congestive heart failure, or severe lung disease resulting in resting hypoxemia.[15]

Nutrition

Maintenance of adequate nutrition is extremely important in providing the building blocks for wound repair. Protein, carbohydrates, vitamins, and trace elements are needed for collagen production and cellular energy. Vitamins A and C are important for producing and maintaining wound integrity. Vitamin A stimulates collagen synthesis and epithelialization and can help reverse the harmful effects of steroids on wound repair (with the exception of steroid-induced failure of wound contraction).[16] Vitamin C is necessary to maintain proper cellular membrane integrity.[16] Zinc also promotes cell proliferation.[17]

Age and Weight

A patient's age and body composition are important systemic factors affecting proper wound repair. Aging can cause a delayed inflammatory response and is associated with increased capillary fragility, reduced collagen synthesis, and neovascularization.[18] Aging is also associated with slow epithelialization. Patients who are obese (more than 20% of ideal body weight) experience the same difficulties as those who are elderly.[3] They also have more problems with poor perfusion (adipose tissue lacks vascular tissue) and delayed development of tensile strength.[15]

Infection

All traumatic wounds are contaminated with bacteria to some degree; such contamination is usually restrained by phagocytic action. However, an infection will develop if the following factors are present: (1) a high level of bacterial contamination (e.g., greater than 10^5 bacteria per gram of wound tissue), (2) a compromised tissue microenvironment (e.g., eschar, necrosis), (3) systemic conditions (e.g., age, steroid therapy, malnutrition), and (4) immunoincompetence.[10,19]

The presence of localized infection in the wound delays collagen synthesis and epithelialization and prolongs the inflammatory phase, causing additional tissue destruction. Bacteria in the wound compete with fibroblasts and macrophages for the available oxygen supplies, thus impeding the roles of these cells in wound restructuring. The most common bacteria implicated in community-acquired wound infections include gram-positive *S. aureus*, *Streptococcus faecalis*, and pyogenes. Gram-negative *Escherichia coli*, *Pseudomonas aeruginosa*, and *Klebsiella* species are often associated with hospital-acquired or chronic wounds. Anaerobic organisms, such as *Bacteroides* species, are particularly infective in wounds with necrotic or poorly perfused tissue.[10]

The classic signs and symptoms of a local wound infection include erythema, edema, induration, pain, crepitation, and the presence of purulent or odorous exudate in the affected area.[15] Fever, flulike symptoms, and leukocytosis are frequently associated with systemic infections. Wound cultures should be taken to identify the infecting organisms when the classic clinical signs of infection are present. Usually, if these signs are severe, fever and systemic leukocytosis will be present.[15]

Coexisting Diabetes Mellitus

Patients who have coexisting diabetes mellitus may have particular difficulties with proper wound healing. Poorly controlled diabetes is usually associated with reduced collagen synthesis, impaired wound contraction, delayed epidermal migration, and reduced PMN leukocytes chemotaxis and phagocytosis. Strict professional attention should be given to wounds in patients with diabetes because of these inherent difficulties.[15]

Medications

Pharmacists can play a key role in identifying potential detriments to proper wound closure. Certain medications, for example, can act directly to impede healing through their interaction at various stages of the healing process. Corticosteroids (topical or systemic) reduce phagocytosis, angiogenesis, and collagen synthesis.[20] Antineoplastic drugs and radiation therapy interfere with the cellular division necessary for fibroblast function and reepithelialization.[21] Immunosuppressive agents and anticoagulants can also interfere, especially in the early inflammatory phase. Patients who are taking these medications should be carefully followed by a wound care specialist to ensure that proper healing occurs.

Wound Characteristics

Local characteristics of the wound site are factors in regulating wound healing. Local features that may impair wound closure include the presence of necrotic tissue (eschar) or foreign bodies (e.g., glass, dirt), the lack of moisture, and the presence of infection.[15] Pharmacists who are aware of and can recognize problems with such local factors can, through careful counseling, do their part to ensure proper wound healing.

Classification of Wounds

Classification of wound type is necessary for implementing proper and specific wound therapy; hence, it is imperative that pharmacists who are recommending outpatient first-aid products be aware of these classifications. Wounds can be classified according to their acuity and/or depth.

Classification by Acuity

Using the acuity classification, wounds can be either acute or chronic.

Acute Wounds

Acute wounds are usually abrasions, punctures, lacerations, or burns. Burns are discussed in Chapter 34, "Minor Burns and Sunburn."

Abrasions Abrasions usually result from a rubbing or friction injury to the epidermal portion of the skin and extend to the uppermost portion of the dermis. These wounds should be cleansed with soap and water and then covered with a sterile, semipermeable dressing that is nonadhering to the wound bed.[22]

Punctures Punctures usually result from a sharp object that has pierced the epidermis and lodged in the dermis or deeper tissues. It is important for a physician to inspect these wounds to ensure that no foreign bodies are retained and to update tetanus prophylaxis, if necessary. If no debris are present, the wounds should then be cleansed with either water or sterile saline. The wounds should be left open, elevated, and soaked with soapy water daily to allow for proper healing.[22]

Lacerations The last acute form of injury is laceration, which results from sharp objects cutting through the various layers of the skin. Lacerations should be inspected by a physician, debrided, and flushed; again, tetanus prophylaxis is important. If they are clean, the wounds can be sutured to facilitate their contracture. If they are grossly contaminated by foreign particles or inorganic matter or if they show evidence of early infection, the wounds should instead be left open and covered with a sterile, nonadhering, semipermeable dressing to facilitate healing by secondary closure,[22] as detailed in the section "Nonpharmacologic Therapy (Wound Dressings)."

Chronic Wounds

Chronic wounds include pressure ulcers, or decubiti, and arterial and venous ulcers. Among these, pressure ulcers deserve special attention because they often require intense supervision and professional aid to heal properly.

Pressure Ulcers Pressure ulcers, which are commonly encountered in bedbound or neurologically impaired, immobile patients,[23] are initiated by three forces that are usually present in such patients. These forces include pressure, shear, and friction. (See Figure 35–2). Pressure is the perpendicular force exerted on a unit of body tissue, shear refers to the forces that move fascia and skin in opposition to each other, and frictional forces are produced when two surfaces move across one another (e.g., skin and sheets).[10] Acting together, the three forces result in the avulsion of local arteries supplying blood to an area of skin (Figure 35–3). Once perfusion decreases, tissue hypoxia ensues, resulting in skin necrosis and decubiti formation.

Demographic risk factors for the development of these forces include obesity, malnutrition, incontinence, and generalized debilitation. Common areas of involvement include the bony prominences of the body, especially the sacrum, trochanters, heels, and elbows.[24]

Pressure ulcers can be further subdivided according to their depth or color. (See Table 35–2.) Because color classifications are often used by the lay public to describe these wounds, it is particularly important for the pharmacist to recognize the descriptions, to counsel patients properly, and to facilitate appropriate wound management. Red wounds usually involve a partial-thickness loss of the skin layers. (See the section "Classification by Wound Depth.") The wound base is moist, red, painful, and free of necrotic tissue;[24] the base is red and granular. Yellow wounds involve tissue loss that extends through the dermis. The wound exhibits devitalized tissue that appears yellow or grayish in the base.[25] Moisture is usually present and the wound is painless. Black wounds are usually covered by eschar, a thick, black, leatherlike crust of dead tissue,[25] which blocks visualization of the wound base.

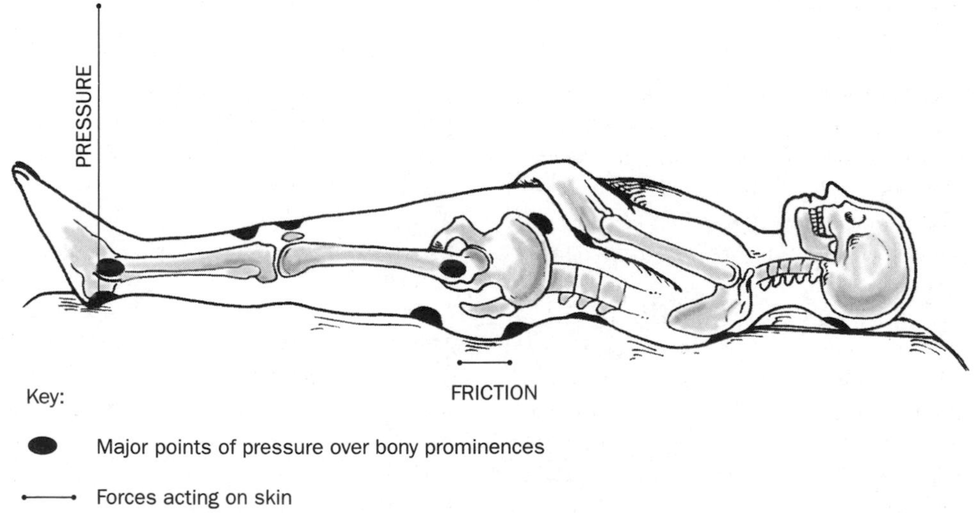

Figure 35–2 Stresses on skin.

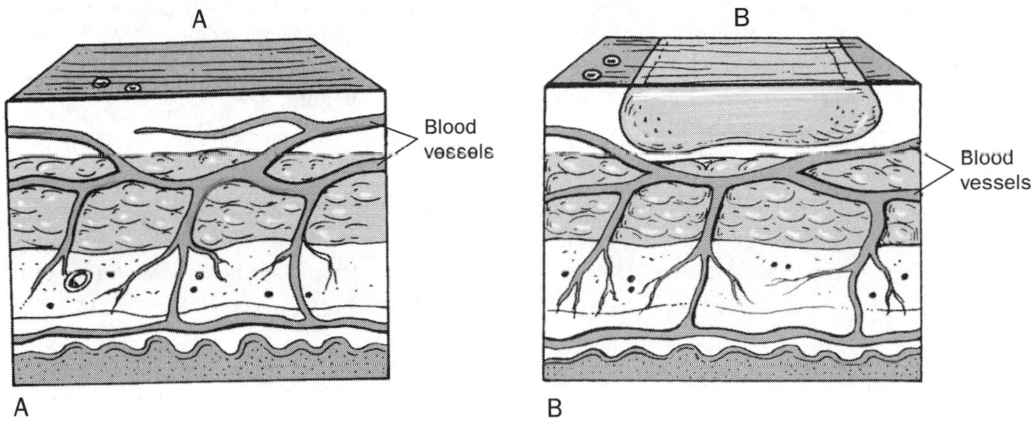

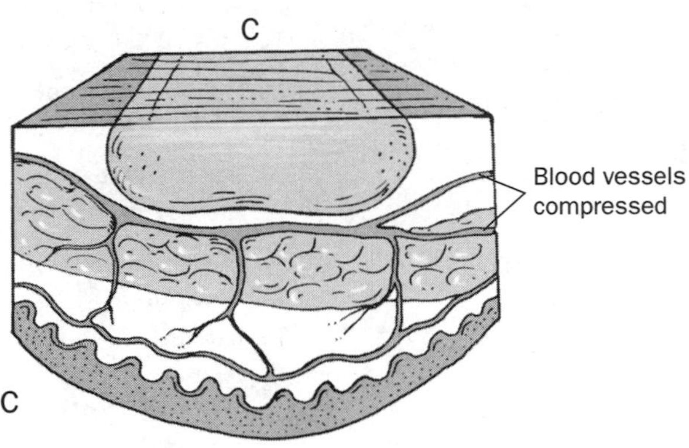

Figure 35–3 Diagrammatic representation of the decubitus ulcer developmental process. A, Normal skin is kept healthy by capillary blood supply. B, In some places of the body, large bony prominences lie close to the skin, especially at the hips, sacrum, heels, elbows, and so forth. C, When a patient is lying down, the skin is compressed between the bones and the bed, which impedes the blood supply to that area of the body. At this point, there is great risk of developing decubitus ulcers. Adapted with permission from reference 10.

Table 35–2

Decubitus Ulcer Assessment Scale

Grade of Score	Comments
0	Erythema/induration noted (potential sore)
1	Blister skin formation; erythema that does not disappear within 30 minutes after pressure is relieved
2	Superficial skin break in the dermal layers
3	Tissue necrosis involving loss of subcutaneous tissue
4	Tissue cavity formation, extending to bones

Pharmacists should counsel patients that the management of decubiti should be closely supervised by individuals trained to treat such wounds. The selection of products to assist in this treatment is based on the extent and depth of the wound, as detailed in the section "Classification by Wound Depth." Close attention should be given to alleviating the cause of these wounds, keeping in mind the forces that initiated them and the risk factors that promote these forces.

Arterial and Venous Ulcers Arterial and venous ulcers are the second form of chronic wounds. (See Table 35–3). Arterial ulcers are usually secondary to severe peripheral vascular occlusive disease. They are commonly encountered in the lower extremities and are painful. Venous ulcers are secondary to incompetent venous valves. Incompetent valves allow fibrin to leak from the blood vessels and to form obstructive rings around capillaries, causing tissue ischemia and breakdown.[26]

Classification by Wound Depth

Wound depth classification is used primarily by health care personnel and is based on the extent or number of skin layers damaged during the wound-initiating process. This classification has been divided, for simplicity's sake, into four descriptive stages. Stage I does not involve loss of any skin layers and consists primarily of reddened, unbroken skin. Stage II includes developing a blister or partial-thick-

Table 35–3

Ischemic Ulcers

	Arterial	Venous
Cause of ulcer	Arterial occlusion curtails blood flow	Incompetent perforator valves
Initiating factor	Arteriosclerosis; atherosclerosis	Deep vein thrombosis
Location	Toes, heels	Above medial malleolus
Pain	Extreme; increases with leg elevation	Medium; decreases with leg elevation
Pedal pulses	Usually absent	Usually present
Appearance	Punched-out lesion with pale or white bed	Irregular lesion with brown and blue color

Source: Reference 10; adapted with permission.

Case Study 35–1

Patient Complaint/History

A mother presents to the pharmacist with her 5-year-old son, Hyun, who injured his upper, left arm 24 hours earlier by scraping it on a tree branch. The wound, which is about 1 inch long, contains no foreign matter or necrotic tissue. However, the pinkish skin surrounding the wound indicates that the slight abrasion is inflamed. Hyun says that the wound feels warm but does not hurt.

The mother asks whether a triple-antibiotic ointment is appropriate to use on the wound. She previously scrubbed the wound with Dial soap and water, applied hydrogen peroxide with a cotton ball, and covered the wound with an adhesive bandage. She has also taken the child's temperature several times and reports that the temperature measurements were normal.

Hyun's patient profile shows no current medical problems or known drug allergies. The mother confirms that the child is not taking any medications.

Clinical Considerations/Strategies

Readers can use the following considerations/strategies to determine whether treatment of the patient's condition with nonprescription medications is warranted:

- Assess the appropriateness of the mother's cleaning of the wound. If warranted, propose an alternative cleaning procedure.
- Explain to the mother why the wound is warm and the skin surrounding it is pink.
- Respond to the mother's question about using the triple-antibiotic ointment on the wound.
- Identify symptoms that would warrant contacting the child's physician.

Patient Education/Counseling

Readers can use the following strategies to develop a patient education/counseling plan that will help ensure optimal therapeutic outcomes:

- Explain the appropriate technique and procedure for cleaning the wound and maintaining wound hygiene.
- Explain how to monitor the wound and what changes in the wound's appearance would warrant contacting the child's physician.
- Explain when and how to apply topical medications to the wound.
- Explain the appropriate type of dressing to use in covering the wound, how often to change the dressing, and when to stop using a dressing.

ness skin loss involving all the epidermis and part of the dermis. Stage III, full-thickness skin loss, includes damage to the entire epidermis, dermis, and dermal appendages. Stage IV is an extension of stage III but further involves the subcutaneous tissue and underlying muscle, tendon, and bone. Understanding these stages helps in selecting appropriate dressings for proper wound closure as discussed in the next section.

Treatment of Wounds

Treatment Outcomes

The goal in treating wounds is to promote healing by protecting the wound from infection or further trauma. Treatment should include a stepwise approach that involves cleansing the wound, selectively using antiseptics and antibiotics, and creating closure with an appropriate dressing.

General Treatment Approach

Uncontaminated wounds (e.g., minor cuts, scrapes, and burns) require only basic supportive measures, including the use of mild soap and water for proper cleansing and using a wound dressing to prevent entry of bacteria into the affected area. Topical nonprescription antibiotic and antiseptic preparations can also be useful in preventing secondary infection, but these agents should be viewed as extensions of supportive treatment. The algorithm in Figure 35–4 outlines the triage and treatment of acute wounds.

More serious or deeper tissue infection (e.g., puncture wounds, severe burns) requires physician consultation to assess the need for systemic or topical prescription antibiotics. The basic instructions for treating acute wounds may not apply to chronic wounds. For that reason, patients with chronic wounds should also seek medical advice concerning wound care. These patients should also do the following:

- Consult a physician about any slow-healing wound because the underlying defect in healing probably requires systemic treatment as well as local wound care.
- Prevent pressure ulcers by repositioning the body regularly and often and by using pressure-relieving devices.
- Watch for early signs of skin redness over bony prominences as prompt intervention can prevent skin breakdown.

Nonpharmacologic Therapy (Wound Dressings)

Traditional wound management involves leaving the wound open to air or covering it with an nonocclusive textile dressing (gauze). However, this type of management leads to several important problems. It promotes eschar formation, which impedes reepithelialization of wounds and creates unwanted scars (Figure 35–5A). It also offers excessive exudate control, which dehydrates wounds and delays healing. Removal of gauze dressings tears away not only the eschar but also the new tissue under the eschar. Finally, this treatment promotes bacterial entry into the wound, increasing the incidence of infection and delaying healing. These cumulative problems have led physicians and nurses to develop new treatment strategies on the basis of creating a moist wound environment (Figure 35–5B). Such an environment prevents eschar development, removes excess exudate without dehydration, and prevents bacterial invasion of the wound. Accordingly, it uses semipermeable dressings that promote optimal moisture, exudate removal, and gas exchange. This technique has been shown to accelerate healing and prevent scarring.[4,5,10] Additionally, it reduces pain and promotes epithelialization and the healing of chronic wounds.

Before discussing wound dressings, a brief mention should be made as to the techniques of wound closure. These techniques should be used for the more extensive wounds that fall under a physician's supervision. Closure of the wound depends on the degree of contamination and extent of the wound. Primary closure with sutures or adhesives is used only for clean, uncontaminated wounds. Secondary closure is used mainly for contaminated wounds; wounds are left open so they can be filled in by the normal healing process under the close supervision of a physician. Tertiary closure (delayed primary closure) is for contaminated and extensive wounds. With this approach, wounds are left open for several days to initiate the healing process and are then later sealed by primary closure techniques.[10]

The primary goal in wound healing is to minimize scarring, and scarring is closely related to the type of dressing used; occlusive dressings cause less scarring than do gauze dressings.[26] The timing of the dressing placement is also important; immediate occlusion leads to resurfacing of epithelium faster than delayed occlusion.[26] Turner[22] has developed a set of criteria for the optimal dressing: The ideal dressing (1) removes excess exudate, (2) maintains a moist environment, (3) is permeable to oxygen, (4) thermally insulates the wound, (5) protects the wound from infection, (6) is free of particulate or toxic contaminants, and (7) can be removed without disrupting delicate new tissue. A plethora of solutions and coverings for wounds are available today, and the range of choices may be overwhelming to an individual trying to choose an appropriate dressing. Jeter and Tintle[28] have developed a schema to assist clinicians in choosing the most appropriate dressing according to the wound's severity. (See Figure 35–6.)

Most superficial wounds (minor abrasions and lacerations) that pharmacists encounter may simply require the application of adhesive bandages such as Band-Aids. Pharmacists should consider the various features of these bandages (e.g., contour, size, padding, allergenicity, impregnation with medication) in their recommendations for patients. As discussed previously, the more extensive wounds require the pharmacist to triage the patient to a physician or a wound care specialist for further evaluation. Table 35–4 and Figure 35–6 describe and illustrate the major categories of wound care products available today and provide an overview of their indications, advantages, and disadvantages. Although none of these products meets all of Turner's criteria, many do approach his description of the optimal dressing.

Pharmacologic Therapy

First-Aid Antiseptics

Antiseptics are chemical substances designed for application to intact skin up to the edges of a wound for disinfection purposes.[29] When effective antisepsis is combined with proper wound care technique, including gentle handling of tissue, the infection rate is low—about 1.6%.[29] Ideally, antiseptics should exert a sustained effect against all microorganisms without causing tissue damage. However, even when used in therapeutic concentrations, the agents have been shown to be leukocytotoxic. Increased intensity and duration of inflammation, tissue necrosis, endothelial damage, and thrombosis have been observed in wound models treated with various antiseptics.[30] Thus, the current recommendation in

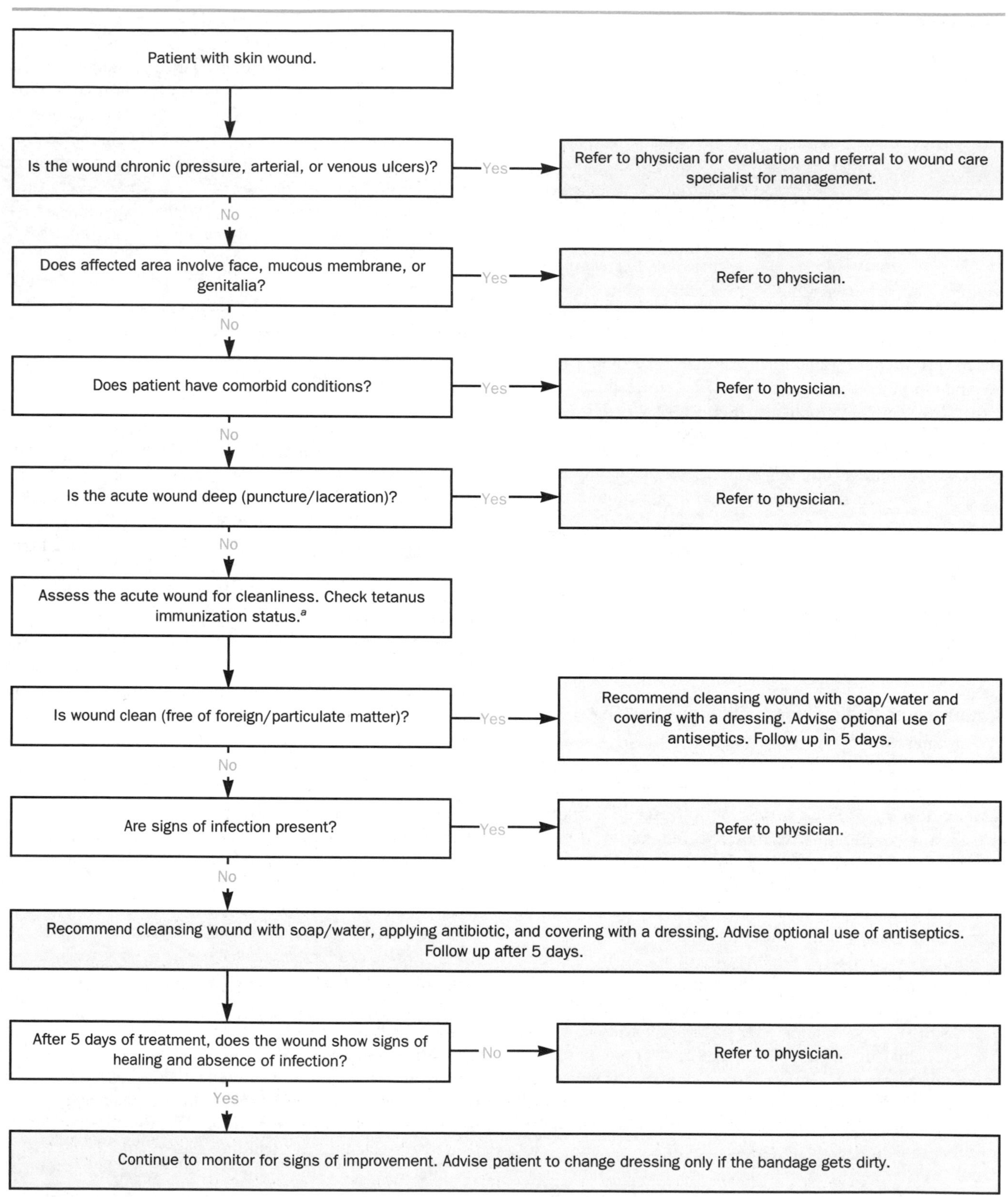

[a] If basic series has been completed, one dose is required every 10 years.[27]

Figure 35–4 Self-care of skin wounds.

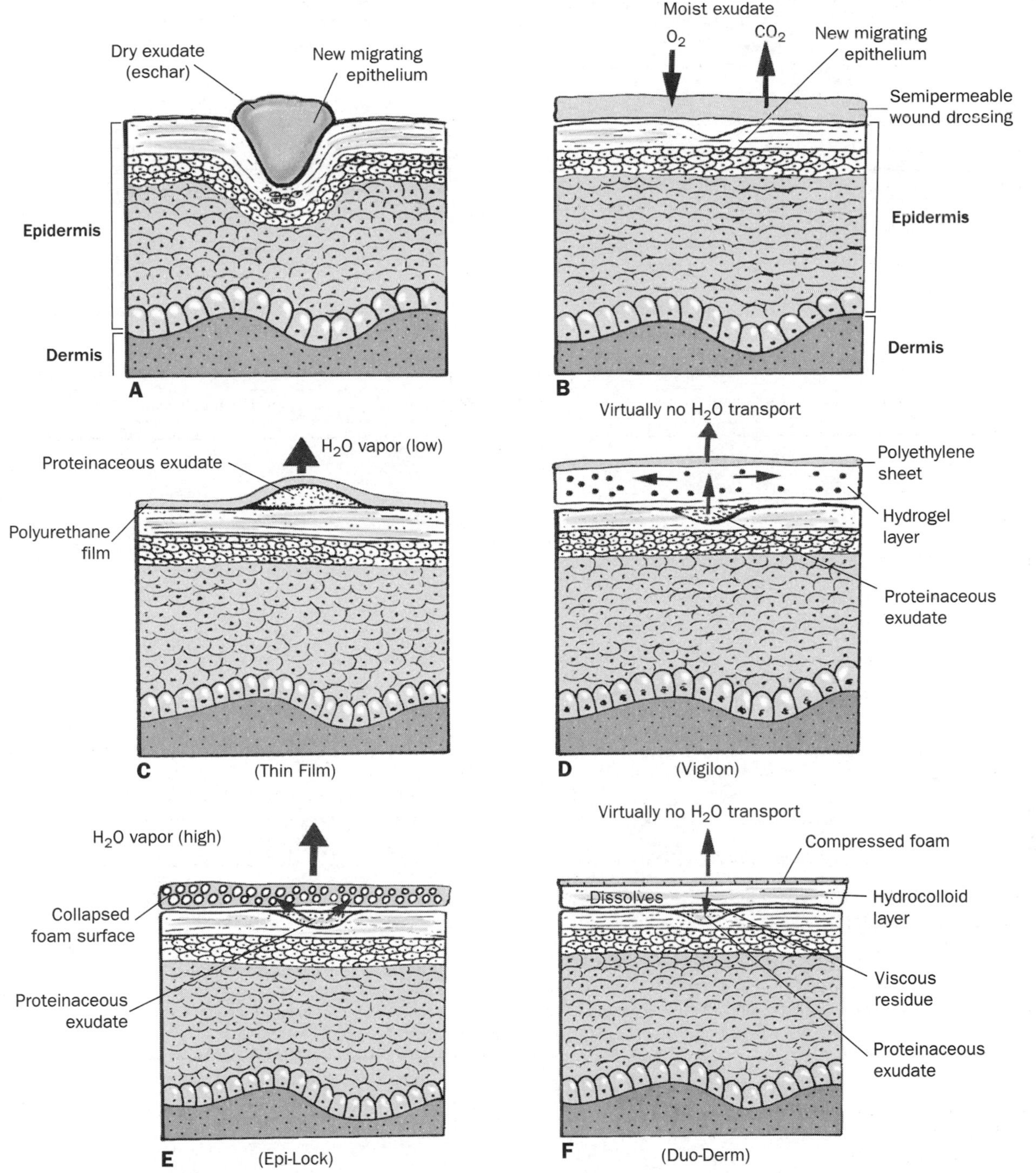

Figure 35–5 Mechanisms by which semipermeable wound dressings create a moist environment for wound healing. A, Regenerating epidermal cells are forced to "tunnel" below the dry wound eschar to attain wound closure. This tunneling delays wound closure. B, Semipermeable wound dressings prevent formation of eschar by maintaining an optimal moisture level at the wound bed. Unhindered by the presence of a dry eschar, migrating epithelial cells are able to migrate and close the wound. C, Mechanism of water vapor transmission in thin films. D, Mechanism of action of a hydrogel wound dressing (Vigilon). E, Mechanism of action of a hydrophilic polyurethane foam dressing (Epi-Lock). F, Mechanisms of action of a hydrocolloid wound dressing (DuoDerm). Adapted with permission from reference 10.

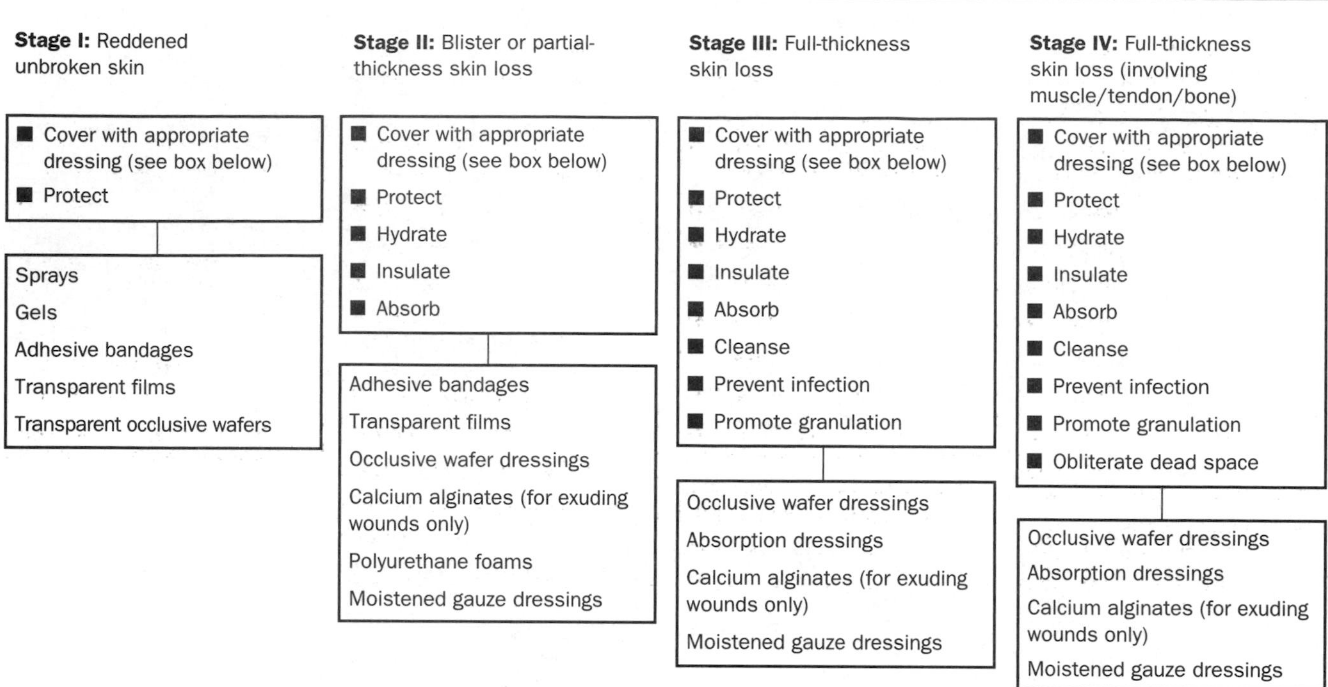

Figure 35–6 Guidelines for product selection based on wound severity. Adapted with permission from reference 28.

the literature is to avoid using antiseptics on open wounds but to use them instead for what they were originally intended: disinfection of intact skin.

Antiseptics, which are subject to the ongoing review by the Food and Drug Administration (FDA) of over-the-counter (OTC) topical antimicrobial products, encompass four groups of products that may contain the same active ingredients but are labeled and marketed for different intended uses. The first group covers products that are generally intended for use by health care professionals as patient preoperative skin preparations, personnel hand washes, and surgical hand scrubs. The second group encompasses antiseptic hand washes purchased by consumers for personal use in the home. The third group includes first-aid antiseptics to help prevent infection in minor scrapes, cuts, and burns. (See Table 35–5.) The fourth group covers hand cleansers used by food handlers to prevent disease caused by contaminated food.

FDA's proposed classification of first-aid antiseptic ingredients for safety and effectiveness was published in July 1991.[31] With a myriad antiseptic active ingredients available for use, only five of the ingredients listed in Table 35–5—alcohol (60% to 95%), isopropyl alcohol (50% to 91.3%), iodine topical solution (USP), iodine tincture (USP), and povidone–iodine complex (5% to 10%)—are recognized as safe and effective (Category I) for use both as preoperative skin preparations by health care professionals and as first-aid products. Only two of these ingredients, alcohol and povidone–iodine, are considered Category I for all antiseptic uses. (See Table 35–5). Other common agents such as hydrogen peroxide, phenolic compounds, hexylresorcinol, and quaternary ammonium compounds are considered Category I for use as first-aid products only. The following discussion of antiseptic agents is confined to their use as first-aid antiseptics. (See Table 35–6 for examples of commercially available products.)

Alcohol Alcohol has good bactericidal activity in a 20% to 70% concentration. For first-aid uses, it decreases the risk of infection in minor cuts, scrapes, and burns. Caution must be used, however, when applying it to the intact skin surrounding the wound because direct application of alcohol to the wound bed can cause tissue irritation. Alcohol usually contains denaturants that will dehydrate the skin when applied topically at high concentrations. It is also highly flammable and must be kept away from fire or flame. Alcohol wash may be used one to three times daily and may be covered with a sterile bandage after the washed area has dried.[32]

Isopropyl Alcohol Isopropyl alcohol, which has somewhat stronger bactericidal activity and lower surface tension than ethanol, is generally used for its cleansing and antiseptic effects on the skin. It can be used undiluted or as a 70% aqueous solution. Denaturants are not added because isopropyl alcohol itself is not potable. However, isopropyl alcohol has a greater potential for drying the skin (astringent action) because its lipid solvent effects are stronger than those of alcohol. Like alcohol, it is flammable and must be kept away from fire or flame.

Table 35–4

Options in Wound Management

Description (Trade Name)[a]	Use Indications	Advantages	Disadvantages
Transparent Adhesive Films			
Semiocclusive translucent dressings with partial or continuous adhesive composed of polyurethane or copolyester thin film (e.g., ACU-derm, Op-Site, Uniflex) (See Figure 35–5C)	Stages I, II, shallow Stage III Clean granular wounds Minimally exuding wounds Autolysis Can use with absorption products and alginates Can be used in conjunction with some enzymatic debriders	Semiocclusive Gas permeable Easy inspection Autolysis Protection Impermeable to fluids/bacteria Comfortable Self-adherent Reduce pain Moist environment Resist shear	For uninfected wounds only Not absorptive May cause periwound trauma on removal With continuous adhesive, may reinjure wound on removal With large amounts of exudate, maceration may occur
Nonadherent Dressings			
Nonadherent, porous dressings. Lightly coated dressings allow easy flow-through of exudate (e.g., Adaptic, Telfa)	Skin donor sites Stage II, shallow stage III Staple/suture lines Abrasions Lacerations	Readily available Less adherent than plain gauze	Need secondary dressing May have traumatic/painful dressing removal Some impregnated dressings may delay healing May require frequent dressing changes Some may cause exudate pooling
Alginates			
Hydrophilic, nonwoven dressings of calcium-sodium (percentages vary between products) alginate fibers. Alginates are processed from brown seaweed into pad or twisted fiber form. Exudate transforms fibers to gel at wound interface (e.g., Kaltostat, Sorbsan)	Light to heavy exuding wounds Stages II, III, IV Moist wound environment Autolysis Skin donor sites	Absorptive Reduce pain Nonocclusive Moist wound environment Conformable Easy, trauma-free removal Can use on infected wounds Accelerate healing time Less frequent dressing changes Potential to aid in control of minor bleeding	Require secondary dressing Characteristic odor May need wound irrigation May desiccate May promote hypergranulation
Exudate Absorbers			
Hydrophilic dressings that absorb exudate, dead dells, and bacteria (e.g., Debrisan Beads, Hydragran)	Stages II, III Exuding wounds Nontunneling deep wounds Infected wounds	Absorb exudate Moist environment Nonocclusive Reduce odor Conformable Inert Clean debris Many distributed in unit dose packs	Contraindicated with tunneling May be difficult to remove May increase wound pH May sting on application Need secondary dressing Application techniques vary
Debriding Agents			
Debriders digest necrotic tissue by differing methods (e.g., Elase, Santyl)	Stages II, III, some stage IV Dermal ulcers Second- and third-degree burns	Nonsurgical method of debridement Some will not damage healthy tissue	May require frequent dressing changes Require secondary dressing May require cross-hatching of eschar Some may damage healthy tissue Application techniques vary significantly Need moist wound environment Some require refrigeration

(continued)

Table 35–4

Options in Wound Management (continued)

Description (Trade Name)[a]	Use Indications	Advantages	Disadvantages
Gauze Dressings			
Nonocclusive fiber dressing with loose, open weave	Stages II–IV Minimal to heavy exuding wounds/topicals Infected wounds Debridement Wound rehydration	Readily available Deep wound packing May use with infected wounds/topicals Mechanical debridement Nonocclusive Conformable	Wound bed may desiccate if dressing is dry Nonselective debridement May cause bleeding/pain on removal Need secondary dressing Frequent dressing changes Some dressings may "shed"
Hydrogels/Gels			
Nonadherent, nonocclusive dressings with high moisture content that come in the form of sheets and gels (e.g., Elasto-Gel, Vigilon) (see Figure 35–5D)	Stages II, III, some approved for stage IV Granular or necrotic wound beds Autolysis Some used on partial- and full-thickness burns	Nonadherent Most are nonocclusive Trauma-free removal Varying absorption capabilities Conformable Some can be used in conjunction with topicals Thermal insulation Reduce pain Moist environment	Most require secondary dressings May macerate periwound skin Some products may dehydrate Slow to minimal absorption rate in most Most require frequent/daily dressing change
Composite/Island Dressings			
Nonadherent absorptive center barrier with adhesive at perimeter (e.g., Airstrip, Viasorb)	Stages II, III Moderate to heavy exuding wounds	Nonadherent over wound Semiocclusive Autolysis Suture/staple lines Protective Reduce pain	May cause periwound trauma on removal No secondary dressing required Impermeable to fluids/bacteria
Foams			
Semipermeable, absorptive, nonwoven, inert polyurethane foam dressings (e.g., EPIGARD, LYOfoam) (See Figure 35–5E)	Stage II, shallow stage III Minimal to moderate drainage Autolysis First- and second-degree burns Containdicated for third-degree burns	Most are nonadhesive Some can be used with infected wounds/topicals Thermal insulation Reduce pain Nonocclusive Moist environment Conformable Less frequent dressing changes Trauma-free removal Absorbent	Most require secondary dressing May require cutting May cause wound desiccation May be difficult to determine wound contact surface
Hydrocolloids			
Wafer dressings composed of hydrophilic particles in an adhesive form covered by a water-resistant film or foam (e.g., Comfeel, ULTEC) (See Figure 35–5F)	Stages I, II, and shallow stage III Clean, granular wounds Autolysis Minimal to moderate exuding Can use with absorption products and alginates	Occlusive Manage exudate by particle swelling Autolysis Long wear time Self-adherent Impermeable to fluids/bacteria Conformable Protective Thermal insulation Reduce pain Moist environment	For uninfected wounds only May cause periwound trauma on removal Difficult wound assessment Characteristic odor Impermeable to gases Some may leave residue on skin or in wound

(*continued*)

Table 35–4

Options in Wound Management (continued)

Description (Trade Name)[a]	Use Indications	Advantages	Disadvantages
Carbon-Impregnated (odor control) Dressings			
Dressings with an outer layer of carbon for odor control (e.g., LYOfam "C" Odor Absorbent Dressing)	Malodorous wounds	Control odor	Require appropriate seal or odor may escape Carbon is inactivated when it becomes wet
Biosynthetics			
Semipermeable dressings that are not designed to adhere to a clean or debrided wound and remain in place without removal through the course of reepithelialization (e.g., BioBrane II)	Partial-thickness burns Donor sites Meshed autographs	Gas permeable Adherent to wound May be used in conjunction with topical antibacterial agents Reduce pain Wound visible	Permeable to fluids/bacteria May require secondary dressing or skin staples May adhere to skin at removal Not for use on necrotic tissue

[a] The trade names listed for each type of wound dressing are given as examples of available products; however, these trade names do not constitute an all-inclusive list of available wound-dressing products.

Source: An unpublished document prepared by McIntosh A, Raher E. Silver Cross Hospital, Joliet, IL, 1991; adapted with permission.

Table 35–5

Nonprescription First-Aid Antiseptic Ingredients

Category I Antiseptic Agents	Concentration (%)
Alcohol	48–95
Benzalkonium chloride	0.1–0.13
Benzethonium chloride	0.1–0.2
Chlorhexidine gluconate	4
Hexylresorcinol	0.1
Hydrogen peroxide topical solution	3
Iodine tincture	USP
Iodine topical solution	USP
Isopropyl alcohol	50–91.3
Methylbenzethonium chloride	0.13–0.5
Phenol	0.5–1.5
Povidone–iodine complex	5–10

Table 35–6

Selected Antiseptic Products

Trade Name	Primary Ingredients
Bactine Spray	Benzalkonium chloride 0.13%; lidocaine HCl 2.5%
Betadine Skin Cleanser Liquid	Povidone–iodine 7.5%
Campho-Phenique Pain Relieving Antiseptic Gel/Liquid	Camphor 10.8%; phenol 4.7%
First Aid Cream	Cetylpyridinium chloride
S.T. 37 Solution	Hexylresorcinol 0.1%
Unguentine Ointment	Phenol 1%

Iodine Iodine's broad antimicrobial spectrum against bacteria, fungi, virus, spores, protozoa, and yeast is attributed to its ability to oxidize microbial protoplasm.[32] An iodine solution (USP) of 2% iodine and 2.5% sodium iodide is used as an antiseptic for superficial wounds. An iodine tincture (USP) of 2% iodine, 2.5% sodium iodide, and about 50% alcohol is less preferable than the aqueous solution because it is irritating to the tissue. Strong iodine solution (Lugol's) must not be used as an antiseptic.

In general, bandaging should be discouraged after iodine application to avoid tissue irritation.[32] Iodine solutions stain skin, may be irritating to tissue, and may cause allergic sensitization in some people.

Povidone–Iodine Povidone–iodine is a water-soluble complex of iodine with povidone. It contains 9% to 12% available iodine, which is what accounts for its rapid bactericidal activity. Reduced concentration of povidone–iodine at 0.001% (e.g., vaginal douches) has been shown to be less toxic to leukocytes than to bacteria, so this antiseptic not only reduces bacterial counts but also allows for normal immune responses that promote wound maturation.[33] Povidone–iodine is nonirritating to skin and mucous membranes.

When used as a wound irrigant, povidone–iodine is absorbed systemically, with the extent of iodine absorption being related to the concentration used and the frequency of application. Final serum level also depends on the patient's intrinsic renal function. When severe burns and large wounds are treated with povidone–iodine, iodine absorption through the skin and mucous membranes can result in excess systemic iodine concentrations and can cause transient thyroid dysfunction, clinical hyperthyroidism, and thyroid hyperplasia. If renal function is normal, however, the absorbed iodine is rapidly excreted, and signs of hyperthyroidism do not develop. Thus, povidone–iodine should be used with discretion when treating large wounds.[34]

Detergents formed by the combination of surfactants with povidone–iodine have been found to damage wound tissue and potentiate infection. Therefore, these combination products are not recommended for scrubbing wounds.[34]

Hydrogen Peroxide Hydrogen peroxide (topical solution, USP), an antimicrobial oxidizing agent (along with sodium and zinc peroxides), is the most widely used first-aid antiseptic. Enzymatic release of oxygen occurs when the hydrogen peroxide comes in contact with blood and tissue fluids. Mechanical release (fizzing) of the oxygen has a cleansing effect on a wound, but organic matter reduces its effectiveness. The duration of action is only as long as the period of active oxygen release. Using hydrogen peroxide on intact skin is of minimal value because the release of nascent oxygen is too slow.

Hydrogen peroxide should be used where released gas can escape; therefore, it should not be used in abscesses, nor should bandages be applied before the compound dries.

Phenolic Compounds In very dilute solutions, phenol is an antiseptic and a disinfectant. It has local anesthetic activity and is claimed to be an antipruritic in concentrations of 1:100 to 1:200 (e.g., phenolated calamine lotion). In aqueous solutions of more than 1%, however, it is a primary irritant and should not be used on the skin except as a keratolytic or peeling agent.

Camphorated Phenol Oily solutions of phenol and camphor are often used as nonprescription first-aid antiseptics. Such products contain relatively high concentrations of phenol (4%) and must be used with caution. If oleaginous phenolic solutions are applied to moist areas, the phenol is partitioned out of the vehicle into water, resulting in caustic concentrations of phenol on the skin. To avoid such damaging effects, these products should be applied only to dry skin.

Hexylresorcinol Hexylresorcinol (0.1%) is more effective than phenol as an antibacterial agent and is less toxic. It has been used in mouthwashes. FDA has judged it safe and effective (Category I) as a first-aid antiseptic.[31] But even though it is used in low concentrations, it may be irritating.

Quaternary Ammonium Compounds FDA's monograph for proposed first-aid antiseptics includes the quaternary ammonium compounds benzalkonium chloride, benzethonium chloride, and methylbenzethonium chloride. These compounds are considered Category I for use as first-aid products. Quaternary ammonium compounds are cationic surfactants that have antimicrobial effects on gram-positive and gram-negative bacteria but not on spores.[32] Gram-negative bacteria are more resistant than gram-positive ones; thus, they need a longer period of exposure. The antimicrobial activity of these compounds consists of disrupting cell membranes and denaturing the lipoproteins of microbes. Quaternary ammonium compounds are sometimes included in topical anti-infective products. In addition to their antiseptic properties, these agents are used for their cleansing properties: They emulsify sebum and have a detergent effect that assists in removing dirt, bacteria, and desquamated epithelial cells. The "quats" can be inactivated by various anionic adjuvant ingredients (e.g., soaps and viscosity-building agents).

Quaternary compounds are formulated as creams, dusting powders, and aqueous or alcoholic solutions. Stock solutions are available for dilution to proper concentration for topical use. If used undiluted, these preparations may cause serious skin irritation. They are also irritating to the eyes, so caution must be used when applying them to skin near the eyes. For use on broken or diseased skin, concentrations of 1:5000 to 1:20,000 may be used. For use on intact skin and minor abrasions, a concentration of 1:750 is recommended.

First-Aid Antibiotics

Topical nonprescription antibiotic agents (e.g., tetracyclines or the combination of bacitracin, neomycin, and polymyxin B sulfate) help prevent infection in minor cuts, wounds, scrapes, and burns.[32] When applied to dirty, contaminated wounds up to 4 hours after insult, topical antibiotic combinations have been demonstrated to reduce the likelihood of wound infection by (1) removing the cause of tissue breakdown (infection and inflammation); (2) reducing pain; (3) removing necrotic tissue, the presence of which delays healing; (4) assisting in wound closure; and (5) fostering the healing process.[35]

Topical antibiotic preparations should be applied to the infected wound bed after cleansing and before applying a sterile dressing. Special caution should be taken when applying these preparations to large areas of denuded skin, however, because the potential for systemic toxicity can increase. Prolonged use of these agents may result in secondary fungal infection.[32] If healing does not occur within 5 days, the patient should consult a physician.

Currently recognized in the FDA's most recent monograph for first-aid antibiotics,[36] which was last amended in June 1990, are six ingredients considered to be generally safe and effective for use (Category I): bacitracin, neomycin, polymyxin B sulfate, tetracycline hydrochloride, chlortetracycline hydrochloride, and combination products containing oxytetracycline hydrochloride. (See Table 35–7 for examples of commercially available products.)

Bacitracin Bacitracin is a polypeptide bactericidal antibiotic that inhibits cell wall synthesis in several gram-positive organisms.[37] The development of resistance in previously

Table 35–7

Selected Antibiotic Products

Trade Name	Primary Ingredients
Betadine Brand First Aid Antibiotics + Moisturizer Ointment	Polymyxin B sulfate 10,000 IU/g; bacitracin zinc 500 IU/g
Campho-Phenique Triple Antibiotic Ointment	Polymyxin B sulfate 10,000 IU/g; bacitracin zinc 500 IU/g; neomycin sulfate 5 mg/g (equivalent to neomycin base 3.5 mg); lidocaine HCl 40 mg
Mycitracin Ointment	Polymyxin B sulfate 10,000 IU/g; bacitracin zinc 500 IU/g; neomycin sulfate 5 mg (equivalent to neomycin base 3.5 mg)
Mycitracin Plus Ointment	Polymyxin B sulfate 10,000 IU/gram; bacitracin zinc 500 IU/g neomycin sulfate (equivalent to neomycin base 3.5 mg)
Neosporin Ointment	Polymyxin B sulfate 5000 IU/g; bacitracin zinc 400 IU/g; neomycin base 3.5 mg/g
Neosporin Plus Maximum Strength Cream/Ointment	Polymyxin B sulfate 10,000 IU/g; neomycin base 3.5 mg/g; pramoxine HCl 10 mg
Polysporin Ointment/Powder	Polymyxin B sulfate 10,000 IU/g; bacitracin zinc 500 IU/g

sensitive organisms is rare. Minimal absorption occurs with topical administration. The frequency of allergic contact dermatitis (erythema, infiltration, papules, edematous, or vesicular reaction) is approximately 2%.[38] Topical nonprescription preparations usually contain 400 to 500 U/g of ointment and are applied one to three times a day.[32]

Neomycin Neomycin is an aminoglycoside antibiotic; it exerts its bactericidal activity by irreversibly binding to the 30S ribosomal subunit to inhibit protein synthesis in gram-negative organisms and some species of *Staphylococcus*. Neomycin has been demonstrated to decrease the severity of clinical infection 48 hours after treatment in tape-stripped wounds.[35] Resistant organisms may develop. Neomycin applied topically produces a relatively high rate of hypersensitivity; reactions occur in 3.5% to 6% of patients.[27] Some patients with positive results to neomycin on skin tests will also react to bacitracin. Because the two agents are not chemically related, such responses apparently represent independent sensitization rather than cross-reactions.[27] Although neomycin is not absorbed when applied to intact skin, application to large areas of denuded skin has been known to cause systemic toxicity (ototoxicity and nephrotoxicity).[32]

Neomycin is available in cream and ointment forms, alone or in combination. It is most frequently used in combination with polymyxin and bacitracin to prevent the development of neomycin-resistant organisms. Because neomycin is a relatively common cause of allergic contact dermatitis and is not essential to topical antibacterial coverage of skin infections, it is rarely recommended by the dermatologic community. The combination of bacitracin and polymyxin B sulfate is more widely accepted for clinical use in dermatology than the triple-antibiotic combination of bacitracin, polymyxin B sulfate, and neomycin.[35]

The concentration of neomycin commonly used in nonprescription products is 3.5 mg/g. Applications are made one to three times a day.

Polymyxin B Sulfate Polymyxin B sulfate is a polypeptide antibiotic effective against several gram-negative organisms because it alters the bacterial cell wall permeability.[37] However, its effect on healing is unknown. Polymyxin B is a rare sensitizer.[38] Concentrations of 5000 U/g and 10,000 U/g are available in nonprescription combination preparations. Applications are usually made one to three times a day.

Tetracyclines Tetracycline, chlortetracycline, and oxytetracycline are broad-spectrum antibiotics that, like neomycin, exert their bacteriostatic effects by binding to the 30S ribosomal subunit to inhibit bacterial protein synthesis. Tetracycline derivatives have activity against gram-positive and most gram-negative bacteria except *Proteus* and *Pseudomonas* species. Because of the high incidence of bacterial resistance, topical tetracycline and chlortetracycline are often ineffective for treating primary bacterial infection. Toxicity is rare when applied topically; however, hypersensitivity reaction may be triggered in allergic patients even by topical application. If redness, irritation, swelling, or pain persists or increases in the applied area, use of tetracycline should be discontinued.[32] Because tetracycline products oxidize in the presence of light on human skin, they may turn the skin a reversible yellow-brown color and may stain clothing.

Currently, 3% ointments of tetracycline and chlortetracycline are available as nonprescription agents. In its first-aid monograph for nonprescription first-aid antibiotics, FDA included oxytetracycline only in combination with polymyxin B sulfate in ointment or powder form. These products are usually applied one to three times per day and may be covered with a sterile bandage afterward.

Case Study 35–2

Patient Complaint/History

Fernando, a 25-year-old male college student, presents to the pharmacist with a 2-day-old wound. The puncture wound, located on his left leg above the knee, was treated by a physician; the wound did not require stitches. The wound, however, is now oozing a yellowish liquid that has a slight odor. The patient says he is taking acetaminophen 1000 mg every 6 hours for minor pain associated with the wound; he does not have a fever.

When questioned about his care of the wound, Fernando responds that he is following the physician's instructions: cleaning the wound with antiseptic soap and water and applying Polysporin daily. Because his mother told him that covering the wound would speed up the healing, the patient is also covering the wound with gauze dressing and adhesive tape.

Fernando's patient profile shows that he has been taking Florinef Acetate (fludrocortisone acetate) 0.1 mg daily for the past 5 years. The patient appears to be thin and underweight.

Clinical Considerations/Strategies

Readers can use the following considerations/strategies to determine whether treatment of the patient's condition with nonprescription medications is warranted:

- Determine the cause of the exudate and odor.
- Determine why the wound is not healing as expected.
- Identify the most common microorganisms that infect this type of wound.
- Determine whether the patient should see his physician again.

Patient Education/Counseling

Readers can use the following strategies to develop a patient education/counseling plan that will help ensure optimal therapeutic outcomes:

- Explain the appropriate procedure for cleaning and dressing the wound.
- Explain how to monitor the wound and what changes in the wound's appearance would warrant contacting a physician.
- Explain that, even when treated superficially with topical antibiotics, some wounds become infected by nonsusceptible bacteria.

Patient Assessment of Minor Wounds

The pharmacist should assess the type, depth, location, and degree of contamination of a wound. Visual inspection of the affected area usually provides an accurate evaluation of these factors. The wound should also be assessed for signs of infection. Descriptions of primary pyodermas in the section "Bacterial Skin Infections" can help in determining whether a wound has become infected or whether a bacterial infection initiated the cutaneous disorder. Because noninfectious processes, including drug-induced eruptions, could be involved, the patient's health status and current medication use should also be determined. Antimicrobial agents should generally be recommended when secondary infection is present or might occur.

Asking the patient the following questions will help elicit the information needed to accurately assess the disorder and to recommend the appropriate treatment approach.

Q~ What type of wound is present? Is the wound acute (an abrasion, puncture, or laceration) or chronic (a pressure ulcer, arterial ulcer, or venous ulcer)?

A~ Refer patients with punctures, lacerations, or any type of chronic wound to a physician. Check abrasions for cleanliness and signs of infection.

Q~ Where is the wound located? How extensive is the area involved?

A~ Refer patients with wounds that cover a large area or that involve the face, mucous membranes, or genitalia to a physician.

Q~ Are foreign objects or dead tissue present at the wound site?

A~ If yes, advise the patient that careful removal of the object and debridement of the dead tissue by a wound care specialist may be needed.

Q~ What is the color of the wound bed? What is the condition of the wound margins and the surrounding skin?

A~ *Identify the color characteristics for wounds. (See the section "Chronic Wounds.")* Advise the patient or caregiver that treatment of wounds such as pressure ulcers require supervision by a wound care specialist. If the wound margins and surrounding skin are red and hardened, caution that an infection is likely.

Q~ Is redness, warmth, swelling, and/or pain present in the affected area?

A~ If yes, suspect early infection. Assess patient for use of first-aid antiseptics and antibiotics.

Q~ Is pus present in the area? If so, what color is it and does it have an odor?

A~ Advise the patient that the presence of pus is not unusual but that medical attention is needed if the wound develops an odor.

Q~ Do you have a fever or any flulike symptoms?

A~ If yes, suspect systemic infection. Refer patient to a physician.

Q~ Do you have diabetes or any other medical conditions?

A~ Refer patients with diabetes or other medical conditions that can delay wound healing to a wound care specialist.

Q~ What medications are you currently taking?

A~ *Identify medications that can impair wound healing. (See the section "Factors Affecting Wound Healing.")* If the patient is taking any of these medications, refer the patient to a wound care specialist.

Q~ What measures or medications have you used to self-treat the wound? Were they effective?

A~ Assess whether any previous self-treatments were appropriate. If inappropriate, counsel the patient on proper wound management. If the measures were appropriate but ineffective, determine whether the patient implemented the treatments correctly and advise accordingly.

Q~ Do you have any allergies to topical medications? Do you have any other allergies?

A~ If the patient has a history of allergic sensitization, do not recommend iodine solutions. This agent is known to cause allergic sensitization in some people.

Patient Counseling for Wounds

Table 35–4 covers the major counseling points of self-treatment of minor acute wounds. The pharmacist should ensure that the patient understands the basic steps in wound care, especially the selection of appropriate wound dressings. An explanation of basic skin physiology and the wound healing process will enhance patient compliance. The box "Patient Education for Acute Wounds" lists specific information to provide patients.

Evaluation of Patient Outcomes for Wounds

The pharmacist should check the patient's progress after 5 days whether or not nonprescription medications are being used to prevent or treat secondary bacterial infections. Visual inspection, if possible, is the best method of assessing the healing process; therefore, a scheduled visit to the pharmacy is preferable. If the wound shows no signs of healing or has worsened, the patient should see a physician for more aggressive therapy.

Bacterial Skin Infections

Bacterial skin infection may occur secondary to a contaminated wound or may present as a primary pyodermic infection. Pyoderma is a broad term that refers to cutaneous bacterial infection characterized by crusted, oozing lesions with variable amounts of purulence and tenderness.[39] If the infection is deep or extensive, systemic toxicity may occur as manifested by an elevation in temperature and leukocytosis. Pyodermic infection may be either primary (no previous dermatoses exist) or secondary (a predisposing problem pre-

Patient Education for Acute Wounds

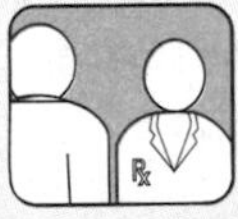

The objective of self-treatment is to promote healing by protecting the wound from infection or further trauma. For most patients, carefully following product instructions and the self-care measures listed below will help ensure optimal therapeutic outcomes.

- Position the wound above the level of the heart to slow bleeding and to relieve throbbing pain.
- If it is dirty, clean the wound with mild soap and water or with a mild wound cleanser such as normal saline solution, which is not toxic to cells. Do not use antiseptic solutions unless they are extremely dilute.
- Occlude the wound with a dressing that will keep the wound site moist. Make sure the dressing is the appropriate size and contour for the affected body part.
- Continue using a wound dressing until the wound bed has firmly closed and signs of inflammation in surrounding tissue have subsided.
- Avoid disrupting the dressing unnecessarily; change it only if it is dirty or is not intact. Frequent changes may remove resurfacing layers of epithelium and may slow the healing process.
- Use a mild analgesic to control pain.
- Observe the wound for signs of infection. Redness, swelling, and exudate are a normal part of healing; foul odor is not.

⚠ Consult a physician if infection is suspected or the wound does not show signs of healing after 5 days of self-treatment.

ceded the infection). Cultures of primary cutaneous lesions most often reveal *S. aureus* and Group A streptococci. Gram-negative *P. aeruginosa* may be present in secondary pyodermas, which are especially prevalent on warm, moist skin such as axillae, ear canals, and interdigital spaces.

Normally, the stratum corneum has only about 10% water content, which is enough to ensure elasticity but is generally below that needed to support luxuriant microbial growth.[2] However, an increase in moisture content may allow microbial growth, leading to infection. A break in the intact skin surface has a deleterious effect on the skin's defensive properties, allowing large numbers of pathogenic organisms to be introduced into the inner layers. In addition, the risk of infection may be increased by excessive scrubbing and irritation of the skin (especially with strong detergents), excessive exposure to water, prolonged occlusion, excessively elevated skin temperature, or local injury. Therefore, the presence and severity of microbial skin infection generally depend on the number of pathogenic organisms present, on the condition of the skin's defense mechanisms, and on the supportive nutrient environment for the organisms.

Types of Bacterial Skin Infections

The main pyodermic infections are impetigo, ecthyma (ulcerative impetigo), erysipeloid, folliculitis, furuncles and carbuncles, and erythrasma.[40]

Impetigo (Primary)

Impetigo is a very superficial infection of the skin caused by either *S. aureus*, Group A β-hemolytic streptococci, or a mixed infection. Impetigo is most common in preschool children and young adults. Direct contact with the infected exudate may result in transmission of the organisms. Predisposing factors include crowded living conditions, poor hygiene, and neglected minor trauma. Lesions first appear as small red spots that may evolve into characteristic vesicles filled with amber fluid. Exudate accumulates and forms yellow or brown crusts (scabs) on the skin surface, often surrounded by erythematous skin. Eruptions may be annular (circular) with clear central areas, or they may be clustered or grouped. Lesions typically last for days, accompanied by variable pruritus. Satellite lesions occur by autoinoculation. Face, arms, legs, and buttocks are common affected areas. Glomerulonephritis with certain streptococcal strains may be a complication.[40] (See the "Color Plates," photograph 23.)

Ecythma (Ulcerative Impetigo)

Ecythma refers to an ulcerative bacterial infection caused most frequently by Group A streptococci or staphylococci or both. Children, adolescents, and elderly patients are commonly affected. Ecythma is a lesion of neglect, which develops in excoriations, insect bites, minor trauma in elderly patients, soldiers, sewage workers, alcoholics, and homeless people. The lesion usually begins as an erythematous pustule that rapidly erodes and becomes crusted. These lesions extend much deeper into the dermis than those in impetigo. They have a scattered, discrete arrangement and are commonly distributed on ankles, dorsa of feet, thighs, and buttocks. Lesions are pruritic and tender; they last for weeks and often heal with a scar.[40]

Erysipeloid

Erysipeloid ("crab dermatitis") is an acute but slowly evolving cellulitis occurring at sites of inoculation, most commonly the hands. Often occupational, it is associated with handling fish, shellfish, meat, poultry, hides, and bones. Infection follows an abrasion, scratch, or puncture wound that occurs while organic material containing *Erysipelothrix rhusiopathiae*, a gram-positive rod, is being handled. The incubation period is 1 to 4 days. The highest incidence occurs in adult men during summer and early fall. Erysipeloid has a characteristic, violaceous, sharply marginated lesion composed of macules and plaques. The lesion is slightly tender and warm but not hot. Skin symptoms include itching, burning, throbbing, and pain. Occasional lymphangitis or lymphadenitis may occur. Erysipeloid is usually self-limited, subsiding in about 3 weeks. Relapse may occur. Endocarditis or septic arthritis may rarely complicate bacteremia.[40] (See the "Color Plates," photograph 24.)

Folliculitis

Folliculitis is a superficial, often bacterial inflammation of hair follicles that heals without scarring. Skin areas regularly exposed to tar, grease, mineral oil, adhesive plaster, and plastic occlusive dressings are most susceptible to folliculitis. *S. aureus* folliculitis is aggravated by shaving (e.g., beard area, axillae, legs). Skin lesions commonly last for days. They appear dirty yellow or gray with erythema. Affected areas are usually nontender or slightly tender and pruritic.[40] (See the "Color Plates," photograph 25.)

Furuncles and Carbuncles

A furuncle is an acute, deep-seated, tender, erythematous, inflammatory nodule that evolves from a staphylococcal folliculitis. A carbuncle is a conglomerate of multiple coalescing furuncles. Children, adolescents, and young adults are frequently affected, and an increased incidence is seen in boys. A chronic staphylococcal carrier state in nostrils or perineum, friction from collars or belts, obesity, and bactericidal defects (e.g., defects in cellular chemotaxis) are all predisposing factors. Chronic cases of these pyodermas should be referred to a physician for evaluation of a possible underlying disease.[40]

In these pyodermas, the lesion may start as superficial folliculitis but may develop into deep nodules. The initial erythema and swelling stage is followed by a thinning of the skin around the primary follicle, centralized pustulation, destruction of the pilosebaceous structure, discharge of the central necrotic plug, and eventual ulcer formation. The fully established furuncle is bright red, indurated, and erythematous.

These lesions commonly last for days, with associated skin symptoms of throbbing pain and, invariably, exquisite tenderness. Constitutional symptoms include low-grade fever and malaise. At times, furunculosis is complicated by bacteremia and possible hematogenous seeding of heart valves, joints, spine, long bones, and kidneys. Some patients are subject to recurrent furunculosis.[40] (See the "Color Plates," photograph 25.)

Erythrasma

Erythrasma is a chronic bacterial infection that is caused by *Corynebacterium minutissimum* and affects the intertriginous areas of the toes, groin, and axillae. Adults are generally affected, with a higher incidence in obese middle-aged blacks. Predisposing factors include diabetes and a warm, humid climate. The skin lesions are sharply marginated, brownish red, scaly eruptions that may last for months to years. Irritation may be the only skin symptom.[30]

Treatment of Bacterial Skin Infections

For the treatment of primary impetigo, a systemic or topical prescription antibiotic such as mupirocin is highly effective and preferred.[35,41] Topical nonprescription antibiotic preparations with neomycin, bacitracin, and polymyxin B sulfate seem to be most effective when lesions are superficial and are not extensive.[37] Cleaning the area with mild soap and water and gently removing loose crusts should improve response to topical therapy. Because streptococcal infection can occur in other tissues (e.g., renal, heart valve) concurrent with impetigo, most physicians treat impetigo infections with systemic as well as topical products.

For the treatment of ecthyma, folliculitis, and erysipeloid, a systemic antibiotic is usually indicated.[40] The role of topical nonprescription antibiotics in these infections is very limited; their usage is confined to very superficial infections, and their efficacy may be questionable. Furuncles and carbuncles may be resolved with incision, drainage, and the prescription of systemic antibiotics by a physician. Minor cases of erythrasma may respond to showers with povidone–iodine soap.[40] However, in most cases, systemic or topical prescription antibiotics are preferred.

Fungal Skin Infections

Fungal skin infections, often called dermatomycoses, are among the most common cutaneous disorders.[42] Characteristically, they exhibit single or multiple lesions that may produce mild scaling or deep granulomas (inflamed, nodular-sized lesions). Infections are superficial, affecting the hair, nails, and skin, and are generally caused by three genera of fungi: *Trichophyton*, *Microsporum*, and *Epidermophyton*. Species of *Candida* may also be involved.[43]

Tinea Pedis

Tinea pedis, also known as athlete's foot or ringworm of the feet, is caused by several species of fungi. (See Chapter 36, "Minor Foot Disorders," for discussion of this disorder and its treatment.)

Tinea Capitis

Transmitted by direct contact with infected people or animals, ringworm of the scalp is caused by species of *Microsporum* or *Trichophyton*. Most cases occur in children. Depending on the causative organism, the clinical presentation varies from noninflamed areas of hair loss to deep, crusted lesions that may lead to scarring and permanent hair loss. (See the "Color Plates," photograph 26.) These large lesions, similar to carbuncles in appearance, are called kerions. This fungal infection requires treatment with prescription systemic medications. Topical antifungals may be used as adjunctive treatment with a systemic agent.

Tinea Cruris

Tinea cruris (also called jock itch) is caused by *Epidermophyton floccosum*, *Trichophyton rubrum*, or *Trichophyton mentagrophytes*. It occurs on the medial and upper parts of the thighs and the pubic area and is more common in males. The lesions have well-demarcated margins that are elevated slightly and are more erythematous than the central area; small vesicles may be seen, especially at the margins. Acute lesions are bright red, and chronic cases tend to have more of a hyperpigmented appearance; fine scaling is usually present. This condition is generally bilateral with significant pruritus.

Tinea Corporis

Species of *Trichophyton* or *Microsporum* cause ringworm of the skin. A higher incidence of tinea corporis exists among persons living in humid climates. The lesions, which involve glabrous (smooth and bare) skin, begin as small, circular, erythematous, scaly, pruritic areas. They spread peripherally, and the borders may contain vesicles or pustules. Tinea corporis should be differentiated from noninfectious dermatitis; the lesions may be similar in appearance.

Tinea Unguium

Tinea unguium, also called ringworm of the nails or onychomycosis, is sometimes associated with tinea pedis. Infected nails usually look thick, yellow, and opaque. The nail may separate from the nailbed if the infection progresses. More than 18 million adult Americans (70% women) suffer from nail fungus (tinea unguium). This condition can be very embarrassing because it can cause nails to become discolored, rough, and thick.

Tinea unguium must be treated with systemic drug ther apy (e.g., terbinafine or itraconazole) or removed surgically to rid the area of the offending fungus.

Patients who wish to improve the appearance of the nail during prescription treatment can use Fungal Nail Revitalizer to reduce nail discoloration and to smooth out the thick, rough nail. This product contains calcium carbonate and urea to debride nail tissue. The patient applies the cream over the entire surface of the infected nail, scrubs this area for at least 1 minute with the provided nailbrush, and then washes and dries the nail completely. For optimum results, this procedure should be done daily for 3 weeks.

Moniliasis (Candidiasis)

Moniliasis or candidiasis, caused mainly by *C. albicans*, usually occurs in intertriginous areas such as the groin, axilla, interdigital spaces, under the breasts, and at the corners of the mouth. Involvement of the mucous membranes may be known as thrush or candidiasis, depending on the area affected. Lesions are either moist, red, and oozing or dry and scaly; they have sharp borders and are surrounded by satellite vesicles and/or pustules. Candidal paronychia is most common in people whose activities involve routine immersion of the hands in water. (See the "Color Plates," photograph 27.) Infection, malignancy, and systemic diseases such as diabetes may lower general resistance and may allow candidal infections to flourish. Certain drugs, including oral antibiotics and corticosteroids, may also contribute to candidal infection when used during prolonged periods of time.

Tinea Versicolor

Tinea versicolor is a common superficial fungal infection of the stratum corneum caused by *Pityrosporum orbiculare.* This organism is part of the normal flora in most individuals but is capable of becoming pathogenic under certain conditions. The most distinctive clinical feature of this infection is the change in pigmentation at the affected sites, ranging from white to medium brown. The shade of the macular lesions depends on the pigmentation of the individual; lesions usually occur on seborrheic areas of the body in a confetti-like configuration. (See the "Color Plates," photographs 28A and B.) Because mild scaling and pruritus are the only other sequelae, tinea versicolor is generally considered a disease of cosmetic concern.

Treatment of Fungal Skin Infections

Treatment Outcomes

The goals in treating fungal skin infections are to (1) provide symptomatic relief and (2) inhibit the growth of fungi during and after treatment.

General Treatment Approach

Nonprescription topical antifungals can be used as monotherapy to treat skin and mucous membrane fungal infections and in combination therapy with systemic agents to treat and prevent fungal infections of various tissues (skin, hair, nails, and mucous membranes). Nondrug preventive measures include keeping the skin clean and dry, avoiding the sharing of personal articles, and avoiding contact with persons who have a fungal infection. Figure 35–7 outlines the self-treatment of fungal skin infections.

Medical referral should be considered in the following situations:

- There is doubt as to the causative factor.
- Initial treatment has not been successful, or the condition is getting worse.
- Topical drug products have been applied for prolonged periods over large areas, especially on denuded skin.
- Exudate is excessive and continuous.
- Widespread infection has occurred.
- There is a predisposing illness such as diabetes, systemic infection, or an immune deficiency.
- The affected area involves the face, mucous membranes, or genitalia.
- Fever, malaise, or both will occur.
- A primary dermatitis (allergic dermatitis, psoriasis, or seborrhea) exists and becomes secondarily infected.
- Lesions are deep and extensive.
- Drainage of exudate is required to provide pain relief.

Pharmacologic Therapy

Clioquinol (3%), clotrimazole (1%), haloprogin (1%), miconazole nitrate (2%), povidone–iodine (10%), terbinafine hydrochloride (1%), tolnaftate (1%), and various undecylenates (10% to 25%) are considered safe and effective by FDA for nonprescription use in fungal skin infections.[44] Except for povidone–iodine, these agents are labeled for treatment of athlete's foot, jock itch, and body ringworm. Although considered safe and effective for treating fungal skin infections, povidone–iodine products carry no indication for these infections. In a proposed notice of rulemaking, effective February 26, 1993, FDA determined that certain topical antifungals should not be generally recognized as safe and effective for nonprescription use.[45] (See Table 35–8.) In a final rule published December 18, 1992, FDA announced that nonprescription topical antifungals were not approved for use in the treatment and/or prevention of diaper rash.[46] This final rule became effective June 18, 1993.

The active ingredients in several of these products inhibit sterol synthesis, causing cell leakage and eventually cell death. Because this product classification is so broad, the present focus is on products for use in preventing and self-treating fungal skin infections.

Clioquinol

Clioquinol, formerly called iodochlorhydroxyquin, has both antifungal and antibacterial properties. Its antibacterial properties have been used to treat cutaneous infections such as pyoderma, folliculitis, and impetigo; its antifungal prop-

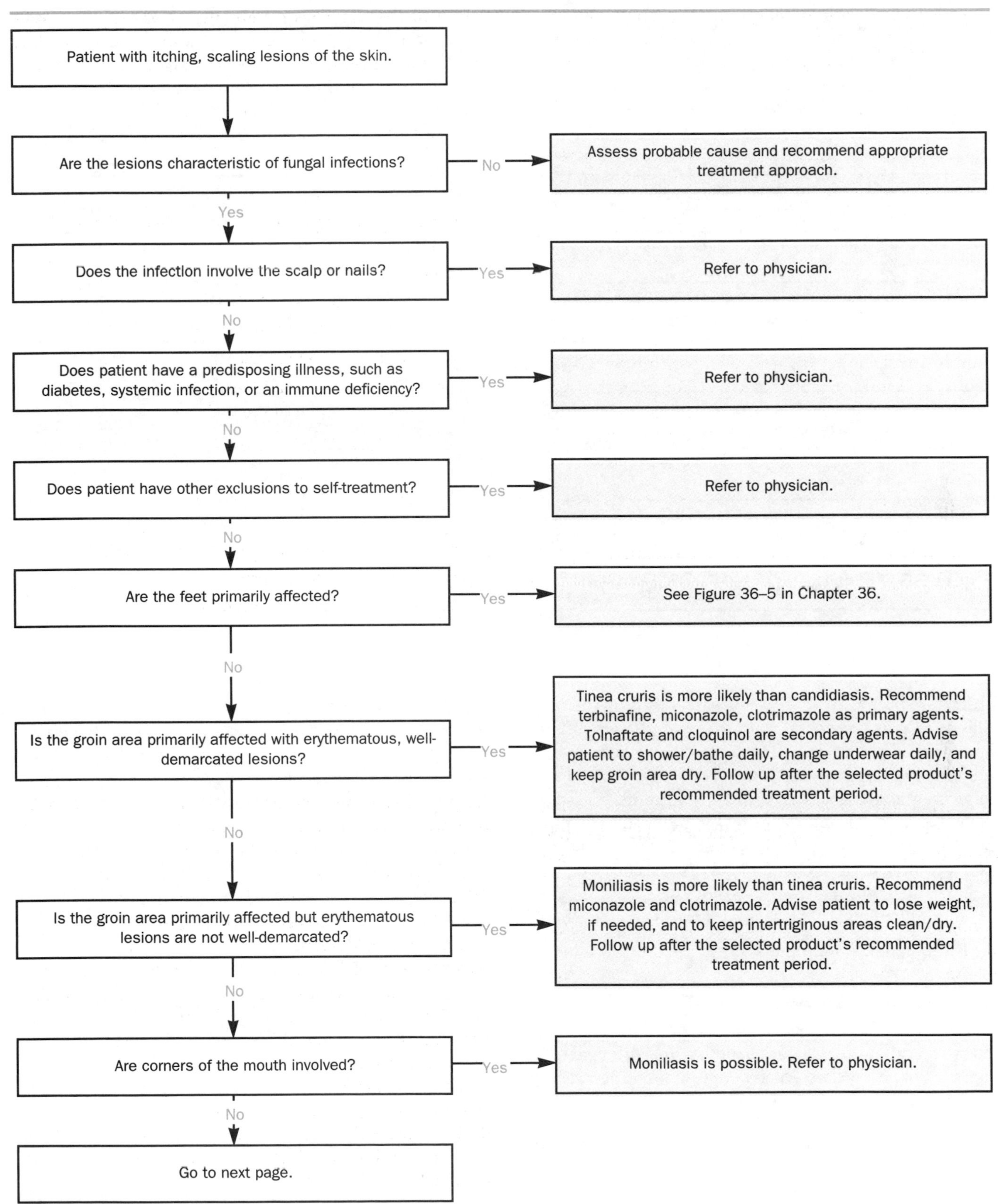

Figure 35–7 Self-care of fungal skin infections.

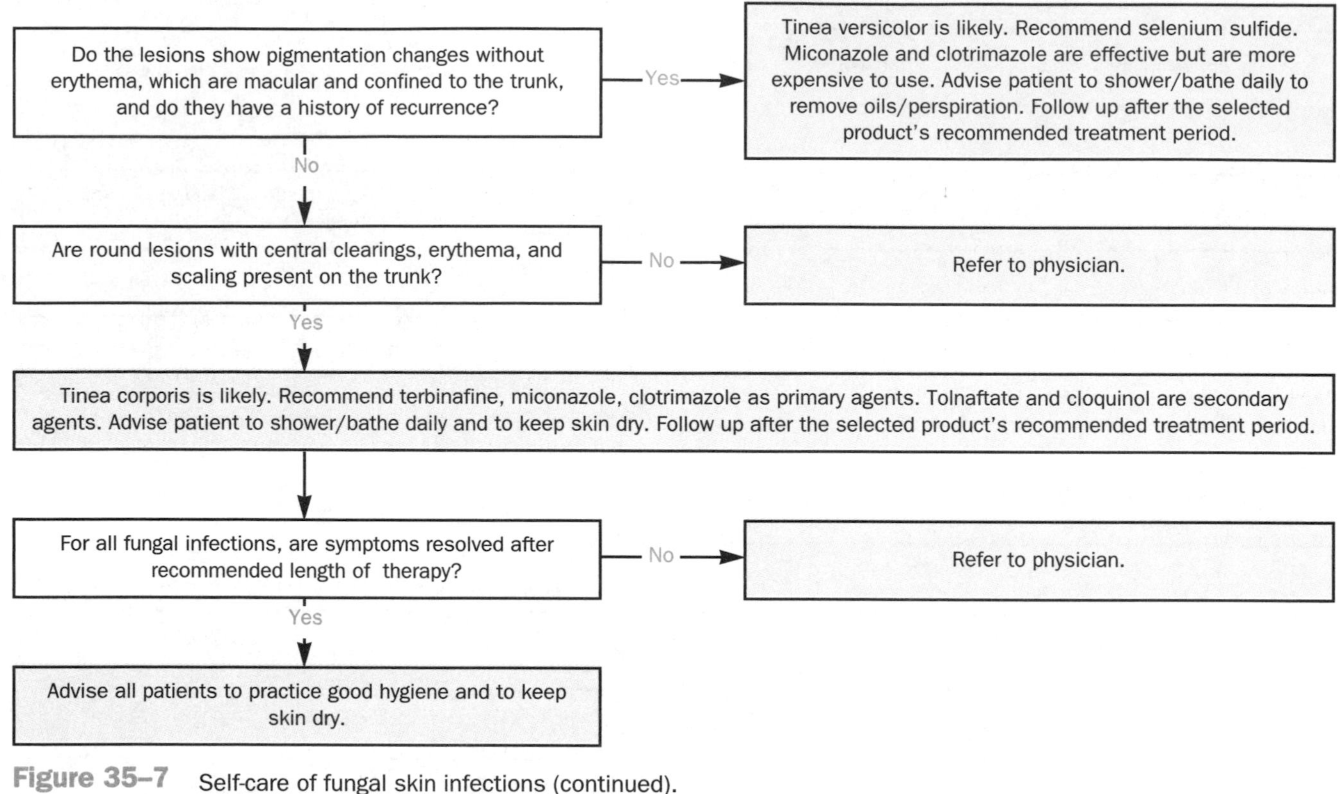

Figure 35–7 Self-care of fungal skin infections (continued).

erties have been used to treat mucocutaneous mycotic conditions such as tinea pedis, tinea cruris, and tinea corporis, and moniliasis.[47] As an irritant and a known allergen, clioquinol may cause transient stinging or pruritus as well as allergic contact dermatitis. If these symptoms persist, the patient should discontinue using the product. Several prescription product forms (lotion, cream, and ointment) contain a combination of clioquinol and hydrocortisone. FDA requires the following special warning statements: "Do not use on children under 2 years of age" and "Do not use for diaper rash."[44]

Clotrimazole and Miconazole Nitrate

Clotrimazole and miconazole nitrate are imidazole-structured topical antifungals originally approved for prescription use but now reclassified as nonprescription agents. They are active against fungi and some gram-positive bacteria.[48] Their broad spectrum includes a common dermatophyte, the organism causing tinea versicolor, and *C. albicans.*

Treatment with miconazole and clotrimazole results in a low rate of recurrent infection when therapy is continued for 2 weeks or more, depending on the clinical disorder.[49,50] However, the onset of recurrence may simply be delayed in several cases. Allergic contact sensitization is rare, and other side effects are usually self-limiting on discontinuation of the preparation.

Haloprogin

Although FDA approved haloprogin 1% for nonprescription use, no commercially available nonprescription topical antifungals contain this agent.

Terbinafine Hydrochloride

Topical terbinafine hydrochloride 1% was reclassified as a nonprescription medication in 1999 under the trade name Lamisil AT. This product is formulated as a cream. According to utilization data, the prescription version of the topical agent, Lamisil, was the number one prescription product prescribed for athlete's foot.

Terbinafine hydrochloride is indicated for interdigital tinea pedis, tinea cruris, and tinea corporis caused by *E. floccosum, T. mentagrophytes,* and *T. rubrum.* This antifungal agent inhibits squalene epoxidase, a key enzyme in fungi sterol biosynthesis. This action results in a deficiency in ergosterol and a corresponding accumulation of squalene within the fungal cell, which also causes fungal cell death. This drug is the only one available for which clinical trials demonstrated clinical and mycologic cures of athlete's foot with 1 week of treatment. Clinical data also demonstrate the following low incidences of side effects: irritation (1%), burning (0.8%), and itching/dryness (0.2%).

Oral Lamisil tablets are currently available only by prescription for the treatment of onychomycosis. However, butenafine hydrochloride (Mentax), a prescription-only

Table 35–8

Nonprescription Topical Antifungal Ingredients

Topical Nonprescription Antifungal Drug Products Generally Recognized as Safe and Effective	
Clioquinol	Povidone iodine
Clotrimazole	Terbinafine hydrochloride
Haloprogin	Tolnaftate
Miconazole nitrate	Undecylenates
Topical Nonprescription Antifungal Drug Products Not Generally Recognized as Safe and Effective[a]	
Alcloxa	Phenol
Alum, potassium	Phenolate sodium
Aluminum sulfate	Phenyl salicylate
Amyltricresols, secondary	Propionic acid
Basic fuchsin	Propylparaben
Benzethonium chloride	Resorcinol
Benzoic acid	Salicylic acid
Benzoxiquine	Sodium borate
Boric acid	Sodium caprylate
Camphor	Sodium propionate
Candicidin	Sodium propionate
Chlorothymol	Sulfur
Coal tar	Tannic acid
Dichlorophen	Thymol
Menthol	Tolindate
Methylparaben	Triacetin
Oxyquinoline	Zinc caprylate
Oxyquinoline sulfate	Zinc propionate

[a] Effective February 26, 1993.

molecule chemically related to terbinafine hydrochloride, has been shown to be effective in the topical management of onychomycosis when incorporated into a topical 20% urea cream.[51] Sixty patients ranging between ages 18 and 60 years (mean 27.4), with more than 25% involvement of the big toenail, were enrolled in the study using this topical combination. Marked improvement was observed in 73.3% of patients after 8, 16, and 24 weeks with clinically and mycological confirmed negative fungal culture. Among patients receiving the active combination dosage form, 88% were cured.

Tolnaftate

Tolnaftate is a topical antifungal agent that is effective against most superficial dermatophytes but ineffective in treating tinea versicolor and *C. albicans*. Complete clearing of cutaneous lesions may take more than a month of therapy. The mechanism of action appears to be inhibition of fungal cell wall synthesis.[52] Topically applied tolnaftate has a low incidence of toxicity; however, if local irritation occurs, treatment should be discontinued.

Undecylenic Acid

Undecylenic acid has the greatest antifungal activity of the fatty acids. Nevertheless, it is a fungistatic agent, requiring prolonged exposure at relatively high concentrations to be effective. It is used as a zinc, calcium, or copper salt in ointment, cream, powder, and aerosol forms (2% to 5% acid, 20% salt) for an additive antifungal effect.

Other Agents

Chloroxylenol In 0.5% to 3.75% concentrations, the antiseptic chloroxylenol (parachlorometaxylenol) is classified as safe to use for up to 13 weeks for treating athlete's foot, jock itch, or ringworm. However, additional safety data (for long-term, repeated use) and clinical efficacy data are needed before FDA can place chloroxylenol in Category I.[44]

Selenium Sulfide Selenium sulfide, a cytostatic agent applied as a "shampoo" lotion, is usually effective in treating tinea versicolor. The shampoo is a potential irritant if left in contact with the skin for a prolonged period of time. Contact with the eyes and sensitive skin areas, therefore, should be avoided. Although selenium sulfide is not absorbed in significant amounts when applied to the skin, it is hazardous if swallowed, producing central nervous system effects, as well as respiratory and vasomotor depression. Areas affected by tinea versicolor should be lathered with the agent for a specified period of time, usually not more than 2 to 5 minutes, and should be washed off thoroughly. This treatment should be repeated daily until a response is noted or up to 2 weeks. It should then be tapered to twice weekly and then once weekly according to response. Patients with recurrent tinea versicolor may use the product indefinitely on a weekly basis to minimize recurrent infections.

Product Selection Guidelines

Agents used for cutaneous fungal infections are found in ointments, creams, powders, and aerosols. Creams or solutions are the most-efficient and most-effective antifungal product forms for delivery of the active agent into the epidermis. Sprays and powders are less-effective products because they are often not rubbed into the skin. They are probably more useful as adjuncts to a cream or solution or as prophylactic agents in preventing new or recurrent infections. Table 35–9 lists examples of commercially available products and their dosage forms.

Patient Assessment of Fungal Skin Infections

Fungal skin infections must be differentiated from bacterial infections, as well as from noninfectious dermatitis. If possible, the pharmacist should examine the affected area to determine whether the disorder's manifestation is typical of a fungal infection. Drug-induced eruptions should also be taken into account.[53]

Table 35–9

Selected Topical Antifungal Products

Trade Name	Primary Ingredients
Aftate Aerosol Spray Liquid/Aerosol Spray Powder	Tolnaftate 1%
Cruex Aerosol Spray Powder	Total undecylenate 19% (as undecylenic acid and zinc undecylenate)
Cruex Cream	Total undecylenate 20% (as undecylenic acid and zinc undecylenate)
Cruex Prescription Strength Aerosol Spray Powder	Miconazole nitrate 2%
Cruex Prescription Strength AF Cream	Clotrimazole 1%
Cruex Squeeze Powder	Calcium undecylenate 10%
Desenex Antifungal Aerosol Spray Liquid	Tolnaftate 1%
Desenex Prescription Strength AF Aerosol Spray Powder/Aerosol Spray Liquid	Miconazole nitrate 2%
Desenex Prescription Strength AF Cream	Clotrimazole 1%
FungiCure Gel	Tolnaftate 1%
FungiCure Liquid	Undecylenic acid 10%
FungiCure Professional Formula Liquid	Undecylenic acid 12.5%
Lotrimin AF Lotion/Solution/Cream	Clotrimazole 1%
Lotrimin AF Powder/Aerosol Spray Liquid/Aerosol Spray Powder	Miconazole nitrate 2%
Micatin Jock Itch Cream/Aerosol Spray Powder	Miconazole mitrate 2%
Micatin Powder/Cream/Aerosol Spray Powder/Aerosol Spray Liquid	Miconazole nitrate 2%
Minidyne Solution	Povidone–iodine 10%
Tinactin Aerosol Spray Liquid/Aerosol Spray Powder/Cream	Tolnaftate 1%
Tinactin Jock Itch Cream	Tolnaftate 1%

Asking the patient the following questions will help elicit the information needed to accurately assess the disorder and to recommend the appropriate treatment approach.

Q~ What area of the skin is affected? How extensive is the area involved?

A~ Refer patients with fungal infections of the nails or scalp or with widespread infection to a physician.

Q~ Is there pus? Is the affected area painful?

A~ Refer patients with these symptoms to a physician

Q~ How long have you had this condition? Have you ever had it before?

A~ Refer patients with nonresponsive infections to a physician. Be aware that recurrent infections are common in some patients.

Q~ Has the disorder developed as the result of a different previous rash or skin disorder?

A~ If yes, refer the patient to a physician.

Q~ Has the disorder worsened despite treatment?

A~ If yes, refer the patient to a physician.

Q~ Do you have a fever or any flulike symptoms?

A~ Refer patients with these symptoms to a physician for evaluation of systemic infection.

Q~ Do you have diabetes? Do you have any other medical condition?

A~ Advise patients who are under the care of a physician for any medical condition to consult a physician about treating fungal infections. Diabetes and other systemic illnesses compromise the host immune system and response to these infections.

Q~ Do you have any allergies to topical medications? If so, which ones?

A~ Base product selection on the patient's allergy history.

Q~ What treatments have you tried for this disorder? Were they effective?

A~ Evaluate whether previous self-treatments were appropriate and implemented correctly. If appropriate treatments were ineffective, advise the patient on the proper usage of the agents or methods.

Patient Education for Fungal Skin Infections

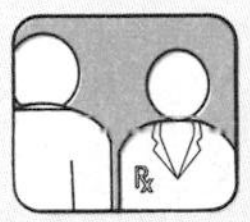

The objectives of self-treatment are to (1) relieve itching, burning, and other discomfort; (2) use antifungal medications to inhibit the growth of fungi and to cure the disorder; and (3) use antifungal medications and nondrug measures to prevent recurrent infections. For most patients, carefully following product instructions and the self-care measures listed below will help ensure optimal therapeutic outcomes.

Nondrug Measures

- To prevent spreading the infection to other parts of the body, use a separate towel to dry the affected area or dry it last.
- Do not share towels, clothing, or other personal articles with family members, especially when an infection is present.
- Launder contaminated towels and clothing in hot water to prevent spreading the infection.
- Cleanse the skin daily to remove oils and other substances that promote growth of fungi.
- If possible, do not wear occlusive clothing or shoes that cause the skin to stay wet. Wool and synthetic fabrics prevent air circulation.
- Avoid contact with people who have fungal infections.

Nonprescription Medications

- Ask a pharmacist for help in selecting an antifungal medication. These medications can contain terbinafine, clioquinol, clotrimazole, miconazole nitrate, tolnaftate, and undecylenic acid.
- Do not use clioquinol on children younger than 2 years.
- Be aware that clioquinol may cause transient stinging or pruritus, as well as allergic contact dermatitis. If these symptoms persist, stop using the product.
- When using a cream or solution dosage form, clean the affected area first; then massage the product thoroughly into the entire affected area. These dosage forms are the most efficient and effective for delivering the active ingredient into the epidermis.
- Apply the medication twice a day for the recommended length of therapy.

⚠ Contact a physician if symptoms of the infection persist after the recommended treatment period or worsen during treatment.

Patient Counseling for Fungal Skin Infections

The pharmacist should describe the proper application technique of topical antifungals to the patient to prevent overmedication or undermedication. The patient should be told what the expected duration of therapy is and how to apply the medication regularly throughout a complete course of therapy. In addition to information about product use, the pharmacist may provide information that will help control or eradicate the infection and will minimize the likelihood of recurrent infections. Such information should address proper care of the infected skin site, appropriate laundry techniques and products, minimal use of occlusive clothing, and avoidance of habits or behavior that leads to recurring infections. The patient should also be told the conditions that would indicate a need for physician-directed care (e.g., the development of a secondary bacterial infection). The box "Patient Education for Fungal Skin Infections" lists specific information to provide patients.

Evaluation of Patient Outcomes for Fungal Skin Infections

In general, the patient should see substantial improvement in 1 week; if this improvement does not occur, the patient should be referred to a physician. Recurrent skin infections may be a sign of undiagnosed diabetes, immunodeficiency, or other organic problems that require medical evaluation.

References

1. Bryant R. Wound repair: a review. *J Enterostomal Ther.* 1987;14:262–3.
2. Bauer EA, Tabas M, Goslen JB. Skin: cells, matrix, and function. In: Kelly WN, ed. *Textbook of Internal Medicine.* 1st ed. Philadelphia: JB Lippincott; 1989:971–4.
3. Norris SO. Physiology of wound healing and risk factors that impede. *AACN Clin Issues Crit Care Nurs.* 1990;1:545–52.
4. Winter GD. Formation of scab and rate of epithelialization on superficial wounds in the skin of the domestic pig. *Nature.* 1962;193:293–4.
5. Hinman CC, Maibach HI, Winter GD. Effect of air exposure and occlusion on experimental skin wound. *Nature.* 1963;200:377.
6. Cooper DM. Optimizing wound healing: a practice within nursing's domain. *Nurs Clin North Am.* 1990;25:165–80.
7. Skover GR. Cellular and biochemical dynamics of wound repair: wound environment in collagen regeneration. *Clin Podiatr Med Surg.* 1991;8:723–56.
8. Servold SA. Growth factor impact on wound healing. *Clin Podiatr Med Surg.* 1991;8:937–96.
9. Howell SM. Current and future trends in wound healing. *Emerg Med Clin North Am.* 1992;10:655–63.
10. Szycher M, Lee SJ. Modern wound dressings: a systemic approach to wounds. *J Biomater Appl.* 1992;7:142–213.
11. McGrath MH. Peptide growth factors and wound healing. *Clin Plast Surg.* 1990;17:421–32.
12. Brown GL, Nanney LB, Griffen J, et al. Enhancement of wound healing by topical treatment with epidermal growth factor. *N Engl J Med.* 1989;321:76–9.

13. Hunt TK, LaVan FB. Enhancement of wound healing by growth factors. *N Engl J Med.* 1989;321:111–42.
14. Pierce GF, Mustoe TA, Lingelbach J, et al. Transforming growth factor beta reverses glucocorticoid-induced wound healing deficits in rats: possible regulation in macrophages by platelet-derived growth factor. *Proc Natl Acad Sci USA.* 1989;86:2229–33.
15. Albritton JS. Complications of wound repair. *Clin Podiatr Med Surg.* 1991;8:773–85.
16. Reed BR, Clark R. Cutaneous tissue repair: practical implications of current knowledge. *J Am Acad Dermatol.* 1985;13:919–36.
17. Chvapil M. Zinc and other factors of the pharmacology of wound healing. In: Hunt TK, ed. *Wound Healing and Wound Infection: Theory and Surgical Practice.* New York: Appleton-Century-Crofts; 1980:143–5.
18. Tepelidis NT. Wound healing in the elderly. *Clin Podiatr Med Surg.* 1991;8:817–26.
19. Rodgers KG. The rational use of antimicrobial agents in simple wounds. *Emerg Med Clin North Am.* 1992;10:55–66.
20. Ahonen J, Jiborn H, Zederfedlt B. Hormonal influence on wound healing. In: Hunt TK, ed. *Wound Healing and Wound Infection: Theory and Surgical Practice.* New York: Appleton-Century-Crofts; 1980: 100–2.
21. Mulder GD, Daly T. In: Cloth LC, McCullough JM, Feeder J, eds. *Wound Healing Alternatives in Management.* Philadelphia: FA Davis; 1990:43–51.
22. Turner TD. Recent advances in wound management products. In: Turner TD, ed. *Advances in Wound Management.* London: John Wiley & Sons; 1986.
23. Guggisberg E, Terumalai K, Carron JM, et al. New perspectives in the treatment of decubitus ulcers. *J Palliat Care.* 1992;8:5–12.
24. Romanko KP. Pressure ulcers. *Clin Podiatr Med Surg.* 1991;8:857–68.
25. Jordon R. *Wound Management: A Treatment Plan.* Paper presented at the Kirklin Clinic: Nursing Continuing Education Seminar; July 1994.
26. Bolton L, van Rijswijk L. Wound dressings: meeting clinical and biological needs. *Dermatology.* 1991;3:146–61.
27. Hirschmann JV. Topical antibiotics in dermatology. *Arch Dermatol.* 1988;124:1697.
28. Jeter KF, Tintle TE. Wound dressings of the nineties: indications and contraindications. *Clin Podiatr Med Surg.* 1991;8:799–816.
29. McKenna PJ, Lehr GS, Leist P, et al. Antiseptic effectiveness with fibroblast preservation. *Ann Plast Surg.* 1991;27:265–8.
30. Leaper DJ. Prophylactic and therapeutic role of antibiotics in wound care. *Am J Surg.* 1994;167(suppl 1A):155–205.
31. *Federal Register.* 1991;56:33677.
32. Brown CD, Zitelli JA. A review of topical agents for wounds and methods of wounding: guidelines for wound management. *J Dermatol Surg Oncol.* 1993;19:732–7.
33. Goldenheim PD. An appraisal of povidone–iodine and wound healing. *Postgrad Med J.* 1993;69(Suppl 3):S97–105.
34. Swaim SF. Bandages and topical agents. *Vet Clin North Am.* 1990;20: 47–65.
35. Bolton L, Fattu AJ. Topical agents and wound healing. *Clin Dermatol.* 1994;22:95–120.
36. *Federal Register.* 1987;52:47312–4.
37. Sanford JP. *Guide to Antimicrobial Therapy.* Dallas: Antimicrobial Therapy; 1994.
38. Gette MT, Marks JG, Maloney ME. Frequency of post-operative allergic contact dermatitis to topical antibiotics. *Arch Dermatol.* 1992;128: 365–7.
39. Tabas M, Goslen JB, Bauer EA. Infections of skin. In: Kelly WN, ed. *Textbook of Internal Medicine.* 1st ed. Philadelphia: JB Lippincott; 1989: 1046.
40. Fitzpatrick TB et al. In: *Color Atlas and Synopsis of Clinical Dermatology: Common and Serious Diseases.* 2nd ed. New York: McGraw-Hill; 1992: 82–96.
41. Strock LL et al. Topical bactroban (mupirocin): efficacy in treating burn wounds infected with methicillin-resistant staphylococci. *J Burn Care Rehab.* 1990;11:454–9.
42. Hay RJ, Roberts SOB, MacKenzie DWR. In: Campion RH, Burton JL, Ebling FJG, eds. *Textbook of Dermatology.* 5th ed. Oxford, England: Blackwell Scientific Publications; 1992:1127–216.
43. Freeberg IM et al., eds. *Dermatology in General Medicine.* 5th ed. New York: McGraw-Hill; 1999.
44. *Federal Register.* 1989;54:51136.
45. *Federal Register.* 1992;57:38568.
46. *Federal Register.* 1992;57:60429–31.
47. Harvey SC. In: Gennaro AR, ed. *Remington's Pharmaceutical Sciences.* 18th ed. Easton, PA: Mack Publishing; 1990:1236.
48. Hildrick-Smith G. *Adv Biol Skin.* 1972;12:303.
49. Mandy SJ, Garrott TC. Miconazole treatment for severe dermatophytoses. *JAMA.* 1974;230:72–5.
50. Fulton JE Jr. Miconazole therapy for endemic fungal disease. *Arch Dermatol.* 1975;111:596–8.
51. Syed TA, Ahmadpour OA, Ahmad SA, et al. Management of toenail onychomycosis with 2% butenafine and 20% urea cream: a placebo-controlled, double-blind study. *J Dermatol.* 1998;25:648–52.
52. Barrett-Bee KJ, Lane AG, Turner RW. *J Med Vet Mycol.* 1986;24:155–60.
53. Bruinsma W, ed. *A Guide to Drug Eruptions.* 6th ed. Amsterdam: Free University Press; 1995.

CHAPTER 36

Minor Foot Disorders

Nicholas G. Popovich and Gail D. Newton

Chapter 36 at a Glance

Chapter 36 at a Glance (continued)

Annual sales of foot care products now exceed $300 million. Historically, however, Americans have seemed to use more than just these products to relieve foot disorders. For example, in 1988, a Gallup survey of family/general practitioners, dermatologists, and podiatrists identified the four most common foot disorders: corns, calluses, and plantar warts; athlete's foot; sore, aching feet; and ingrown toenails.[1] As causes of foot disorders, the survey identified harmful foot practices, such as scraping or cutting corns and calluses, opening blisters or removing the skin cover, improperly trimming toenails, and (among patients with diabetes) inappropriately using hot water to clean and bathe the feet. The survey also identified potentially harmful home remedies for foot problems, including the application of caulk plaster, WD 40 lubricant, Crisco or butter, Clorox or other bleach products, and gasoline or kerosene. Obviously, a significant need exists to educate patients about proper foot care, including self-treatment measures. Instruction in proper foot care, including the selection of proper footwear, should begin at an early age when good health habits can be nurtured. The pharmacist can serve as a valuable resource in this regard.

In some instances, foot disorders may be life-threatening to patients with diabetes, severe arthritis, and impaired circulation. Inappropriate foot care practices can be especially dangerous to such patients.[2] (See the box "A Word about Chronic Diseases and Foot Disorders.") Foot disorders may indicate serious underlying conditions. For most patients, however, such problems may cause only a substantial measure of discomfort and impaired mobility.

Editor's Note: This chapter is based, in part, on the 11th edition chapter titled "Foot Care Products," which was written by Nicholas G. Popovich and Gail D. Newton.

Epidemiology of Foot Disorders

There are three distinct groups of patients who often encounter foot problems. First are pediatric patients whose difficulty is a congenital malformation or deformity, or a specific disease that affects the foot (e.g., juvenile arthritis). These patients need special shoes and foot care provided with the oversight of an orthopedic surgeon or podiatrist. The second group comprises adolescents who experience rapid growth. Growth plates in their feet may become stressed and irritated. Athletic activity at this age can also contribute to problems, especially if associated injuries to the feet are not properly treated. Osteoarthritis, for example, can occur secondary to a foot injury. Third are geriatric patients who encounter foot problems because of aging (as the foot assumes its final shape) and disease. In particular, diabetes mellitus and arthritis can cause secondary foot problems.

An estimated 15% to 20% of the 16 million patients with diabetes will be hospitalized with a foot complication during the course of their disease.[3] Such foot problems as ulceration and infection can ultimately lead to gangrene, amputation of the foot/ankle, and even death. These are the leading causes of hospitalization for patients with diabetes.

Individuals who exercise regularly are also at risk for foot disorders. In the past two decades, society's attitude toward physical fitness and body awareness has changed dramatically. Millions of people exercise every day; jogging, running, and aerobic exercising are methods used most often to remain or get "in shape." If people do not take adequate precautions, however, problems can arise, particularly involving the feet.

Anatomy and Physiology of the Foot

At birth, an infant's foot has 35 joints, 19 muscles, more than 100 ligaments, and cartilage that will develop into 26 bones. These small components continue to develop and mature until

A Word about Chronic Diseases and Foot Disorders

Certain chronic diseases predispose certain patients to foot problems. Patients who are diabetic often have poor circulation and diminished limb sensitivity, and they are especially vulnerable to infectious foot problems. Other vulnerable patients include those with peripheral circulatory disease or arthritis. The pharmacist can identify such patients by asking about daily medication use or by reviewing the patient's drug profile. Typical drug-use patterns for high-risk patients include insulin, oral sulfonylureas, drugs for circulation (e.g., cyclandelate, isoxsuprine, papaverine, and pentoxifylline), and drugs for arthritic conditions (e.g., aspirin and nonsteroidal anti-inflammatory drugs [NSAIDs]).

Self-treatment with nonprescription products, if not properly supervised in patients with impaired circulation, may induce more inflammation, ulceration, or even gangrene, particularly in cases of vascular insufficiency in the foot. Patients with diabetes and those with peripheral circulatory impairments are particularly susceptible to gangrene. (See Chapter 39, "Diabetes Mellitus.") In addition, simple lesions may mask more serious abscesses or ulcerations. If left medically unattended, such lesions may lead to such conditions as osteomyelitis, which may require hospitalization and aggressive parenteral antibiotic therapy. If exostoses associated with corns are not excised by a physician, the corns will persist.

Diabetes Mellitus

Patients with diabetes have been known to soak their feet in water as hot as is tolerable, in Lysol solution, and in hydrogen peroxide, among others. These patients also predispose themselves to problems by walking barefoot in the home or by wearing inappropriate footwear. Because of decreased sensitivity to touch, barefoot patients may inadvertently step on objects (e.g., tacks, nails) that can lodge in the feet and may go unnoticed and lead to serious topical infections. (See Chapter 39, "Diabetes Mellitus," for further discussion of proper foot care and for potentially serious foot disorders in patients with diabetes.)

Peripheral Vascular Disease

Patients with peripheral vascular disease often have poor circulation of the feet and legs. They may complain of persistent and unusual feelings of cold, numbness, tingling, burning, or fatigue. Other symptoms may include discolored skin, dry skin, absence of hair on the feet or legs, or a cramping or tightness in the leg muscles. The most discriminating questions that a pharmacist can ask this type of patient are as follows: (1) Do you experience aching in your calves when you walk? (2) Do you have to hang your feet over the edge of the bed during sleep to relieve the soreness in your calves? A yes response to either question warrants referring the patient to a physician or podiatrist.

Coldness in only one foot may indicate a possible blockage (a clot) of circulation to the foot. Sometimes the involved foot or lower leg will appear physically larger than the other, may be red or waxy in appearance, may have no hair growth on the toes, and will exhibit thickened nails. If the patient's medication history does not indicate the use of medications intended to relieve such symptoms, the pharmacist should advise the patient with suspected circulatory problems to consult a physician or podiatrist for evaluation immediately.

A daily footbath is a simple measure that will assist these patients. After the foot is patted dry, an emollient foot cream can be applied to aid in retaining moisture and pliability. The footbath will also soften brittle toenails for clipping and filing. The feet should be kept warm and moderately exercised every day.

Arthritis

Osteoarthritis is a noninflammatory, degenerative joint disease that occurs primarily in older people. Degeneration of the articular cartilage and changes in the bone result in a loss of resilience and a decrease in the skeleton's shock absorption capability. This condition, however, is also experienced by individuals in their late teens and early twenties as a secondary complication of a previous athletic injury. This condition might be evidenced by the development of hallux limitus or rigidus of the big toe (i.e., a stiff toe or painful flexion of the big toe because of stiffness and spur formation in the metatarsophalangeal joint). Subsequently, these patients have a lot of difficulty with their shoes not fitting properly. They may also develop an osteoarthritic condition in the ankle joint. Referral to an orthopedic physician or podiatrist is appropriate.

Most patients with rheumatoid arthritis eventually have foot involvement. The major forefoot deformities in these patients is painful metatarsal heads, hallux valgus, and clawfoot. Corrective surgical procedures are often indicated to reduce pain and to improve function and mobility. Little evidence exists that conventional nonsurgical therapy (e.g., orthopedic shoes, metatarsal inserts, conventional arch supports, and metatarsal bars) is effective in such cases.

Proper foot care is especially important for arthritic patients. They should wear properly fitted shoes, pad their shoes with insoles to protect their feet from the shock of hard surfaces, and undergo regular podiatric or medical examinations.

ages 14 to 16 years for females and 15 to 21 years for males. Women will generally begin to notice changes in their feet in their 30s; men, in their 40s. After years of bearing the body's weight, the feet tend to broaden and flatten, thus stretching ligaments and causing bones to shift positions. These changes subject the feet to stress, which is compounded by prolonged standing: An estimated 40% of the U.S. population spend about 75% of their workday on their feet. Such stresses increase the potential for painful foot conditions. Thus, the simplest rule of foot care is daily inspection of the feet to note any overt signs of early problems.

Corns and Calluses

Although corns and calluses are common foot disorders, they should not be ignored. They may indicate a biomechanical problem in the feet or lead to serious complications in predisposed patients.

Etiology/Pathophysiology of Corns and Calluses

Under normal conditions, the cells in the basal cell layer undergo mitotic division at a rate that is equal to that of the continual surface cellular desquamation. Normal mitotic activity and subsequent desquamation lead to the complete replacement of the epidermis in about 1 month. During corn or callus development, however, friction and pressure increase mitotic activity of the basal cell layer,[4] leading to the migration of maturing cells through the prickle cell (stratum spinosum) and granular (stratum granulosum) skin layers. This migration produces a thicker stratum corneum as more cells reach the outer skin surface. Hardening of the skin may signal a biomechanical problem and cause abnormal weight distribution in a particular area of the foot. In this case, a podiatric examination is warranted to determine whether an imbalance is present. When friction or pressure is relieved, mitotic activity returns to normal, causing remission and disappearance of the lesion.

Signs and Symptoms of Corns and Calluses

Corns and calluses are similar in one respect: Each produces a marked hyperkeratosis of the stratum corneum. Besides this feature, however, there are marked differences.

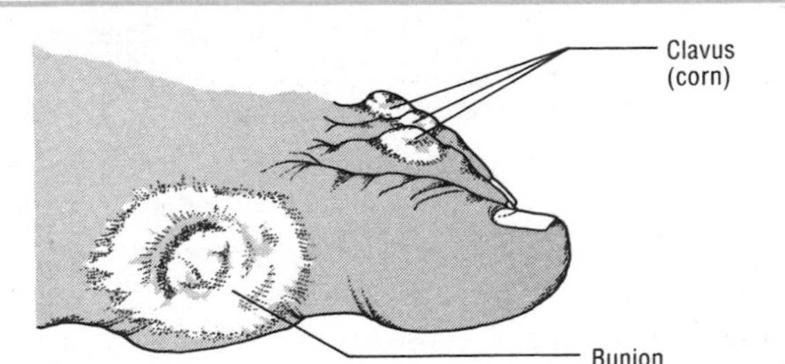

Figure 36–1 Conditions affecting the top of the foot.

Corns

A corn (clavus) is a small, raised, sharply demarcated, hyperkeratotic lesion having a central core. (See Figure 36–1). It has a yellowish gray color and ranges from a few millimeters to 1 cm or more in diameter. The base of the corn is on the skin surface; the apex of the corn points inward and presses on the nerve endings in the dermis, causing pain.

Corns may be either hard or soft. Hard corns occur on the surface of the toes and appear shiny and polished. Soft corns are whitish thickenings of the skin, usually found on the webs between the fourth and fifth toes. Accumulated perspiration macerates the epidermis and gives the corn a soft appearance. Soft corns occur because the fifth metatarsal is much shorter than the fourth, and the web between these toes is deeper and extends more proximally than the webs between the other toes.

Hard corns (usually) and soft corns (less frequently) are caused by underlying bony prominences. A bony spur, or exostosis (a bony tumor in the form of an ossified muscular attachment to the bone surface), nearly always exists between long-lasting hard and soft corns. A lesion located over non–weight-bearing bony prominences or joints—such as metatarsal heads, the bulb of the great toe, the dorsum of the fifth toe, or the tips of the middle toes—is usually a corn.[5]

Pressure from tight-fitting shoes is the most frequent cause of pain from corns. As narrow-toed or high-heeled shoes crowd toes into the narrow toe box, the most lateral toe, the fifth, sustains the most pressure and friction and is the usual site of a corn. The resultant pain may be severe and sharp (when downward pressure is applied) or dull and discomforting. Consumer research approximates that 82% of women ages 35 to 54 years suffer moderate to intense pain from corns and that 35% are consequently limited or restricted in their activities.

Calluses

A callus may be broad based or have a central core with sharply circumscribed margins and diffuse thickening of the skin. (See Figure 36–1.) It has indefinite borders and ranges from a few millimeters to several centimeters in diameter. It is usually raised and yellow, and it has a normal pattern of skin ridges on its surface. Calluses form on joints and weight-bearing areas, such as the palms of the hands, and the sides and soles of the feet. (See the "Color Plates," photograph 29.)

Friction (caused by loose-fitting shoes or tight-fitting hosiery), walking barefoot, and structural biomechanical problems contribute to the development of calluses. Structural problems include improper weight distribution, pressure, and development of bunions with age. Calluses are usually asymptomatic, causing pain only when pressure is applied. Individuals who suffer from calluses on the sole of the foot often liken their discomfort to that of walking with a pebble in the shoe.

Treatment of Corns and Calluses

Treatment Outcomes

The goals of self-treatment are to (1) remove corns and calluses and (2) prevent their recurrence.

General Treatment Approach

Effective nonprescription products are available for removing corns and calluses. However, successful treatment of corns and calluses with these products depends on eliminating the causes: pressure and friction. The algorithm in Figure 36–2 outlines self-treatment of corns and calluses.

The following circumstances indicate referral of a patient with a corn or callus to a physician for treatment.

- The patient suffers from diabetes mellitus, a peripheral circulatory disease, or another medical condition that contraindicates the use of foot care products.
- The lesion(s) is(are) hemorrhaging or oozing purulent material.
- Corns and calluses indicate an anatomic defect or fault in body weight distribution.
- Corns and calluses on the foot are extensive or painful and debilitating.
- Proper self-medication for the condition has been tried for an adequate period without success.
- The patient has a history of rheumatoid arthritis and complains of painful metatarsal heads or deviation of the great toe.
- The patient has physical or mental impairments that make following product instructions difficult.

Nonpharmacologic Therapy

Nondrug adjunctive measures include daily soaking of the affected area throughout treatment for at least 5 minutes in warm (not hot) water to remove dead tissue. Dead tissue should be removed gently rather than forcibly after normal washing to avoid further damage. A rough towel, callus file, or pumice stone effectively accomplishes this purpose. These implements for removing dead skin should be kept clean to avoid autoinoculating oneself at another body focus. Sharp knives or razor blades should not be used because they may cause bacterial contamination and infection. Petroleum jelly need not be applied to healthy skin surrounding the affected area before corrosive products are applied. However, this precaution should be suggested to patients with poor eyesight or other conditions that increase the likelihood of misapplication or accidental spillage of a salicylic acid product.

To relieve painful pressure emanating from inflamed underlying tissue and irritated or hypertrophied bones directly underneath a corn or callus, patients may use a pad such as a Dr. Scholl's with an aperture for the corn or callus. If the skin can tolerate pads, they may be used for up to 1 week or longer. To prevent the pads from adhering to hosiery, patients may wax them with paraffin or a candle and then powder them daily with a hygienic foot powder or cover them with an adhesive bandage. If, despite these measures, friction causes the pads to peel up at the edge and stick to hosiery, the pharmacist may recommend that patients cover their toes with the forefoot of an old stocking or panty hose before putting on hosiery.

Many of the disadvantages associated with older pads have been overcome with the introduction of a new cushioning material. Cushlin, a soft polymer, has been clinically proven to provide immediate, all-day relief from corns and calluses. When applied to the skin, it molds to the shape of the foot and adheres to the skin without leaving a sticky residue. Additionally, its smooth outer surface prevents snags and runs in socks and hosiery.

Pharmacists should advise patients that if at any time the pad begins to cause itching, burning, or pain, it should be removed and a physician or podiatrist should be consulted. Patients should also be advised that these pads will provide only temporary relief and will rarely cure a corn or callus.

Prevention of corns and calluses requires eliminating the pressure and friction that induces them. This prevention entails using well-fitting, nonbinding footwear that evenly distributes body weight. (See Table 36–1 for guidelines on selecting well-fitting footwear.) For anatomic foot deformities, orthopedic corrections must be made. These measures relieve pressure and friction, allowing normal mitosis of the basal cell layer to resume and the stratum corneum to normalize after total desquamation of the hyperkeratotic tissue secondary to the use of topical products.

Pharmacologic Therapy

The Food and Drug Administration (FDA) Advisory Review Panel on Over-the-Counter (OTC) Miscellaneous External Drug Products evaluated more than 20 agents for the treatment of corns and calluses. Of these agents, only salicylic acid was classified as Category I (safe and effective).[3] FDA subsequently adopted the panel's recommendation in its final monograph for nonprescription drug products that remove corns and calluses.

Salicylic Acid

Salicylic acid, the oldest of the keratolytic agents, is formulated in many strengths (0.5% to 40%), depending on its intended use and dosage form. For the self-treatment of corns and calluses, the approved concentration ranges are 12% to 40% for plaster vehicles and 12% to 17.6% in a collodion-like vehicle.[6]

Mechanism of Action Salicylic acid is thought to act on hyperplastic keratin in two ways: (1) It decreases keratinocyte adhesion, and (2) it increases water binding, which leads to a hydration of keratin. Because of the latter effect, the presence of moisture had been thought to be an important component of salicylic acid's therapeutic efficacy, and soaking the area in a warm water bath for 5 minutes before applying

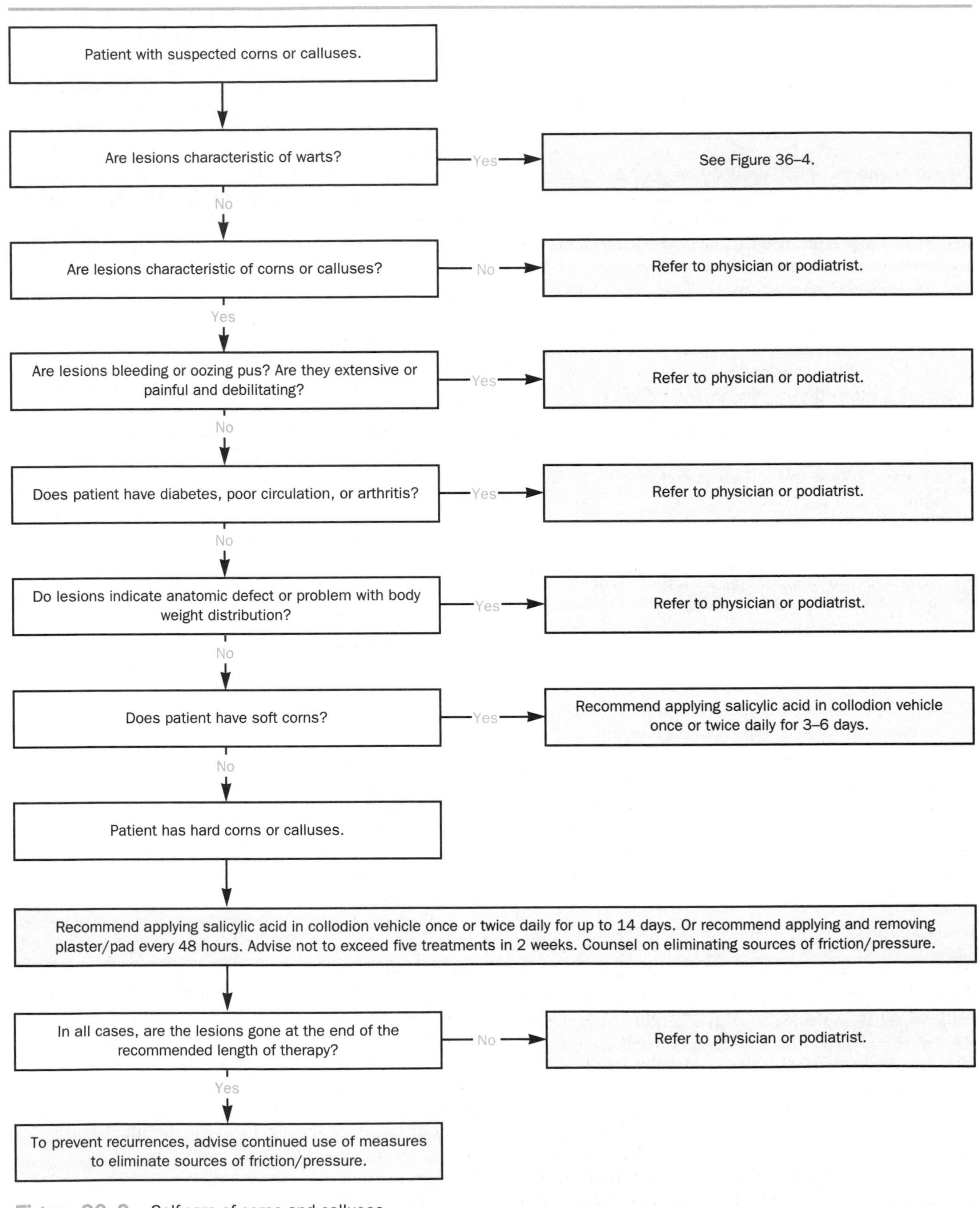

Figure 36–2 Self-care of corns and calluses.

Table 36–1

Selection of Properly Fitted Footwear

- Buy shoes in the proper size (width and length). To obtain an accurate measurement, ask a trained salesperson to measure your feet.
- Base shoe length on the longest toe of your longest foot. Make sure the toes do not bump into the front of the shoe
- For proper arch length, choose a shoe in which the metatarsal head of your foot fits the metatarsal break of the shoe.
- For proper shoe width, choose a shoe that feels comfortable at the first metatarsal joint (toes do not feel cramped in the toe box) and snug at the heel (with the shoes unlaced if a laced shoe is chosen).
- Once the shoe size is determined, choose a shoe shaped to match the shape of your foot. For example, choose a shoe shaped inward if your feet are shaped inward like a pigeon's. Choose a shoe shaped outward if your feet are shaped outward like a duck's.
- If you have abnormalities of the toes (e.g., hammer toes) or use orthotics or padding in your shoes, choose a shoe with adequate depth (vertical height) of the toe box to prevent friction of the tops of the toes.
- Make sure the heel support fits snugly and helps hold the foot straight.
- If you are physically active, make sure the shoe's midsole provides adequate cushioning and support.
- Try on both shoes at the time of purchase, preferably wearing a pair of socks or stockings of the type that will be worn normally with the new pair of shoes.
- If your feet tend to swell, select shoes at the end of the day.

Table 36–2

Selected Corn and Callus Products

Trade Name	Primary Ingredients
Dr. Scholl's Callus Remover Disk	Salicylic acid 40%
Dr. Scholl's Corn/Callus Remover Liquid	Salicylic acid 12.6%
Dr. Scholl's Cushlin Gel Callus Remover Disk	Salicylic acid 40%
Dr. Scholl's Cushlin Gel Corn Remover Disk	Salicylic acid 40%
Dr. Scholl's One Step Callus Remover Disk	Salicylic acid 40%
Dr. Scholl's One Step Corn Remover Strip	Salicylic acid 40%
Freezone Corn and Callus Remover Liquid	Salicylic acid 17.6%
Freezone One Step Callus Remover Pads	Salicylic acid 40%
Freezone One Step Corn Remover Pads	Salicylic acid 40%
Mosco Corn & Callus Remover Liquid	Salicylic acid 17.6%
OFF-Ezy Corn and Callus Remover Kit Liquid	Salicylic acid 17%

salicylic acid was recommended. However, evidence submitted to FDA indicated that presoaking produced no significant positive effects for any efficacy parameter assessed.[7] In its final rule, FDA proposed to allow the manufacturers of these products to state as an optional direction to the consumer: "May soak corn/callus (or wart) in warm water for 5 minutes to assist in removal."

Indications Products containing salicylic acid in a plaster, pad, disk, or collodion vehicle are Category I agents approved for the removal of corns and calluses.[6] FDA recognized that use of the term *plaster* includes disk and pad because these dosage forms are similar in nature. (See Table 36–2 for examples of commercially available products.)

Dosage Forms Salicylic acid is usually applied to a corn, callus, or common wart in a collodion or collodion-like vehicle. These vehicles contain pyroxylin and various combinations of volatile solvents such as ether, acetone, or alcohol, or a plasticizer, usually castor oil. Pyroxylin is a nitrocellulose derivative that remains on the skin as a water-repellent film after the volatile solvents have evaporated.

The advantages of collodions are that they form an adherent flexible or rigid film and prevent moisture evaporation. These qualities aid penetration of the active ingredient into the affected tissue and result in sustained local action of the drug. The systems are largely water insoluble, as are most of their active ingredients such as salicylic acid. They are also less apt to run onto surrounding skin than are aqueous solutions.

The liquid form is often the easiest for the patient to apply. However, this treatment mode requires patience and persistence because it takes longer to resolve the problem.

Other disadvantages of collodions are that they are extremely flammable and volatile and that, by occluding normal water transport through the skin, they may be mechanically irritating. Also, the collodion's occlusive nature allows systemic absorption of some drugs. Some patients may abuse these vehicles by sniffing their volatile aromatic solvents.

Salicylic acid may be delivered to the skin through the use of a plaster disk or pad. This delivery system provides direct and prolonged contact of the drug with the affected area. Salicylic acid plaster is a uniform solid or semisolid adhesive mixture of salicylic acid in a suitable base, spread on appropriate backing material (e.g., felt, moleskin, cotton, or plastic), which may be applied directly to the affected area. The usual concentration of salicylic acid in the base is 40%. A small piece of the 40% plaster may be cut to the size of the corn or callus and held in place by waterproof tape. More convenient, however, are corn or callus pads that have small salicylic acid disks for direct application to the skin. The patient selects the appropriately sized disk, places it directly on the affected area, and then covers it with the pad.

Table 36–3

Guidelines for Treating Corns and Calluses with Salicylic Acid Products

- Wash thoroughly and dry the affected area before applying any product.

Salicylic Acid 12% to 17.6% in Collodion-Like Vehicle

- Apply product no more than twice daily. Morning and evening are usually the most convenient times.
- Apply one drop at a time directly to the corn or callus until the affected area is well covered. Do not overuse the product.
- Allow the drops to dry and harden so that the solution does not run.
- Do not let adjacent areas of normal healthy skin come in contact with the drug. If they do, wash off the solution immediately with soap and water.
- For hard corns and calluses, the solution is applied once or twice daily for up to 14 days or, if earlier, until the corn or callus is removed.
- For soft corns between the toes, hold the toes apart until the solution has dried; then apply a dressing. Treat these corns for 3 to 6 days.
- Soak the affected foot in warm water. Then remove the macerated, soft white skin of the corn or callus by scrubbing gently with a rough towel, pumice stone, or callus file. Do not debride the healthy skin.
- After use, cap the container tightly to prevent evaporation and to prevent the active ingredients from assuming a greater concentration.
- Store the product in amber or light-resistant containers away from direct sunlight or heat

Salicylic Acid 12% to 40% Plasters/Pads

- If using plaster, trim the plaster to follow the contours of the corn or callus. Apply the plaster to the skin, and cover it with adhesive occlusive tape.
- If using disks with pads, apply the appropriately sized disk directly on the affected area, and then cover it with the pad.
- Remove the plaster/pad within 48 hours.
- Remove the dressing the next day; soak the foot and remove the macerated skin by scrubbing gently with a rough towel, pumice stone, or callus file. Do not debride the healthy skin.
- Reapply the plaster after removing the softened skin.
- Apply a maximum of five treatments over a 2-week period.

Administration Guidelines See Table 36–3 for instructions on using these dosage forms.

Adverse Effects Significant percutaneous absorption may occur when salicylic acid is applied over large body areas—for example, during therapy for extensive psoriasis on the face, trunk, or extremities. Absorbed salicylic acid is largely metabolized in the liver and excreted in the urine. Patients with impaired liver or kidney function are, therefore, predisposed to accumulation and salicylate toxicity. However, although occlusive vehicles can enhance the percutaneous absorption of salicylic acid, it is highly unlikely that salicylism will result during corn, callus, or wart therapy with recommended dosages.

Contraindications/Precautions/Warnings In years past, packaging and labeling for corn, callus, or wart removal products warned patients with diabetes or peripheral vascular disease not to use the products except under direct physician supervision. This warning was because any acute inflammation or ulcer formation caused by the topical salicylic acid could be dangerous. In its final monograph, FDA determined that the warning should be stronger and should directly caution against using the product under certain conditions rather than including an "except under" condition for use. Consequently, the revised warning is as follows:

> Do not use this product if you have irritated skin, if you have any area that is infected or reddened, if you are diabetic, or if you have poor blood circulation.[7]

Historically Used Unapproved Agents

In its final monograph, FDA classified drugs used historically for removing corns, calluses, or warts as nonmonograph ingredients.[6,8] The drugs include acetic acid, glacial acetic acid, allantoin, ascorbic acid, belladonna extract, benzocaine, calcium pantothenate, camphor, castor oil, chlorobutanol, diperodon hydrochloride, ichthammol, iodine, lactic acid, menthol, methylbenzethonium chloride, methyl salicylate, panthenol, phenoxyacetic acid, phenyl salicylate, vitamin A, and zinc chloride. Such ineffective drugs are no longer approved for self-treatment of corns, calluses, or warts and cannot be marketed for use in this regard unless they are the subject of a specifically approved application.

Patient Assessment of Corns and Calluses

For corns, calluses, and other foot disorders, the pharmacist should consider providing a private area in the pharmacy where patients can feel comfortable removing their shoe(s) to permit direct inspection of the foot by the pharmacist. Direct inspection enables the pharmacist to accurately assess the nature and extent of the problem.

Before recommending a course of action, the pharmacist must identify not only the disorder but also its possible causes. The pharmacist should determine the patient's health status and use of medications. Finally, the pharmacist should ask whether and how the patient has self-treated the disorder, as well as how successful the attempts were. This information should be recorded and regularly updated in the patient's medication profile.

Asking patients the following questions will help elicit the information needed to accurately assess the disorder and to recommend the appropriate treatment approach.

Q~ Are you the patient? If not, who is the patient?

A~ Be wary of recommending self-treatment for any patient without benefit of an interview.

Q~ What is your age?

A~ Evaluate the effect this factor might have on the feet and on the appropriateness of self-treatment. Consider also the patient's sex as a factor in developing foot problems. (See the sections "Epidemiology of Foot Disorders," "Signs and Symptoms of Corns and Calluses," and "Treatment of Corns and Calluses.")

Q~ What is your occupation?

A~ Counsel patients whose occupation requires them to stand for long periods that such action puts a lot of stress on the feet and can contribute to foot disorders.

Q~ Where is the lesion located?

A~ *Identify the typical locations of corns and calluses. (See the section "Etiology/Pathophysiology of Corns and Calluses.")* On the basis of physical inspection or the patient's description, determine whether the location of the lesions indicates corns or calluses.

Q~ How long have you had the problem?

A~ Note that long-standing problems may have caused more serious foot disorders and may require medical attention.

Q~ Did the problem begin with the use of new shoes or socks?

A~ If yes, consider that the new shoes or socks do not fit well and are causing friction or rubbing of the feet.

Q~ Is the condition painful? Is it too uncomfortable to walk?

A~ Refer patients with severe pain to a physician or podiatrist. Recommend appropriate self-treatment for minor pain of corns and calluses.

Q~ Is any bleeding or discharge present in the affected area?

A~ If yes, refer the patient to a physician or podiatrist.

Q~ Have you tried to treat the problem? If so, how?

A~ Evaluate the appropriateness of any attempts at self-treatment, as well as whether the measures were performed correctly. If the treatment was appropriate but performed incorrectly, explain the proper method.

Q~ What other medical conditions do you have?

A~ Refer patients with diabetes, peripheral vascular disease, or arthritis to a physician or podiatrist to prevent complications.

Q~ What other medications—including nonprescription medicines, dietary supplements, and home remedies—do you use?

A~ If the patient is taking another salicylate, caution that concomitant use of salicylic acid increases the risk of salicylate poisoning.

Q~ Do you have any allergies? If so, what are they?

A~ Determine whether the patient is allergic to adhesive tape, which is a component of the corn/callus pads. If so, recommend liquid forms of salicylic acid.

Q~ Does the patient have a history of other adverse reactions to medications? If so, what are they?

A~ Note that a patient who has reacted to topical vehicles or has sensitive skin may be especially sensitive to irritation.

Patient Counseling for Corns and Calluses

Remission of corns and calluses can take several days to several months. Patients suffering from corns and calluses should understand that effective treatment and maintenance depends on eliminating predisposing factors that contributed to the foot problem in the beginning. The pharmacist should counsel the patient or caregiver on how to use the medication. Because many products contain corrosive materials, they must be applied only to the corn or callus. Pharmacists should alert patients that products that contain collodions are poisonous when taken orally and that these products, as well as all other medications, should be stored out of children's reach. Collodion-containing products are volatile, have an odor similar to that of airplane glue, and may be subject to abuse by inhalation.

Nonprescription products that remove corns and calluses are not recommended for patients with diabetes or circulatory problems. Pharmacists should reinforce contraindications, warnings, and precautions with all patients to avoid the inadvertent use of such products by individuals who have such conditions.

The box "Patient Education for Corns and Calluses" lists specific information to provide patients.

Evaluation of Patient Outcomes for Corns and Calluses

The progress of patients with hard corns or calluses should be checked after 14 days of treatment. If the lesions are still present, the patient should see a podiatrist for evaluation.

Patient Education for Corns and Calluses

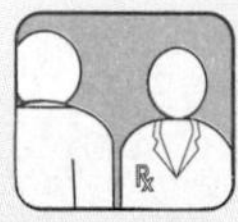

The objectives of self-treatment are to (1) remove corns or calluses and (2) prevent their recurrence. For most patients, carefully following product instructions and the self-care measures listed below will help ensure optimal therapeutic outcomes.

Nondrug Measures

- To avoid autoinoculating oneself at another body site, keep clean the implements used to remove dead skin. (See Table 36–3 for instructions on removing dead skin.)
- Do not use sharp knives or razor blades to remove dead skin of corns and calluses. Such instruments may cause bacterial contamination and infection.
- If you have trouble applying the product to only the affected area because of poor eyesight or other conditions, apply petroleum jelly to healthy skin surrounding the affected area before applying the corn and callus remover.
- For temporary relief of painful pressure from the area under a corn or callus, cover the affected area with a pad such as Cushlin that has an opening for the corn or callus. Use the pad for up to 1 week or longer unless it causes itching, burning, or pain. Consult a physician or podiatrist if these symptoms occur.

Preventive Measures

- To eliminate the pressure and friction that cause corns and calluses, wear well-fitting, nonbinding footwear that evenly distributes body weight. (See Table 36–2 for guidelines on choosing properly fitted footwear.)
- For anatomic foot deformities, consult a podiatrist about orthopedic corrections.

Nonprescription Medications

- To remove corns and calluses, use a salicylic acid product labeled for use on these types of lesions. (See Table 36–3 for instructions on using this medication.)
- Do not use this product on irritated, infected, or reddened skin.
- Do not use this product if you are diabetic or have poor blood circulation.
- Salicylic acid is poisonous: Do not allow it to come in contact with the mouth, and keep it out of the reach of children.
- Note that the medication sloughs off skin and may leave an unsightly pinkish tinge to the skin.

⚠ Stop treatment and consult a physician or podiatrist if swelling, reddening, or irritation of the skin occurs, or if pain occurs immediately when applying the product.

Warts

Warts, or verrucae, are common viral infections of the skin and mucous membranes. Treatments suggested here also apply to common warts on other self-treatable areas of the body.

Epidemiology of Warts

Approximately 9 million U.S. citizens contract warts each year. About 24% of the cases involve plantar warts. Warts are most common in children and young adults. The peak incidence of warts occurs between ages 12 and 16 years. As many as 10% of school children younger than 16 years have one or more warts.[9]

Etiology/Pathophysiology of Warts

Warts are caused by human papillomaviruses (HPVs), which contain DNA.[10] Because warts were induced when extracts from common warts and anogenital warts were injected into different sites, it was hypothesized that all warts were caused by a single agent. In the past decade, however, immunologic techniques in conjunction with DNA purification and restrictive endonuclease digestion have identified at least 50 HPV types,[11] each with its own characteristic histopathology and cytopathology.

Past studies showed that HPV-6 and HPV-11 were responsible for anogenital warts and that these strains were different from other HPVs in serologic molecular hybridization.[10,12] This finding prompted the belief that HPV type dictated the kind of wart and that these viruses were confined to specific body locations. Evidence now suggests that HPV types are not restricted to a specific site but that, for unknown reasons (perhaps epithelial cell receptor specificity), viral particles function in keratinocytes only in specific locations and will induce warts only in these locations. (See Chapter 27, "Atopic Dermatitis, Contact Dermatitis, and Dry Skin," for discussion of anatomy and physiology of the skin.)

Papillomavirus particles assemble in the nuclei of upper-layer keratinocytes and are subsequently released into the milieu within the stratum corneum. It has been demonstrated that HPVs do not bud from the cell membrane and thus lack a thermosensitive lipid envelope like that found in the herpesviruses and the human retroviruses. It is thought that the presence of a stable protein coat allows the HPV to

Case Study 36–1

Patient Complaint/History

Patrese, a 33-year-old overweight woman, presents to the pharmacy with a complaint of moderately severe pain in the fourth toe of each foot and redness of the affected toes. The pain makes walking to and from the bus stop each day difficult and interferes with her job as a retail sales clerk. She noticed a raised bump on the dorsal surface of each toe several weeks ago. The affected toes have become painful only in the last few days though.

Further questioning reveals that the pain is the most severe during the week when Patrese wears high-heeled dress shoes. To relieve the pain, she has been taking Advil 200 mg two tablets at least once a day for the past week. The analgesic helps until she walks more than a block in her high-heeled shoes. Patrese is currently taking Synthroid 0.075 mg one tablet qam and Lo-Ovral one tablet hs for 21 days, 7 days off; she is allergic to penicillins and adhesive tape.

Clinical Considerations/Strategies

Readers can use the following considerations/strategies to determine whether treatment of the patient's condition with nonprescription medications is warranted:

- Assess the patient's symptoms to determine the most likely etiology and degree of severity.
- Formulate a realistic goal for treatment of the complaint.
- Generate a list of all possible therapeutic interventions to address the patient's condition.
- Identify patient characteristics that either preclude or necessitate each therapeutic intervention.
- Create an optimal therapeutic regimen to relieve the patient's condition.
- Create a plan to monitor and document the patient's therapeutic response and progress in resolving the problem.

Patient Education/Counseling

Readers can use the following strategies to develop a patient education/counseling plan that will help ensure optimal therapeutic outcomes:

- Explain the reasons for the selected therapeutic strategy.
- Encourage the patient's adherence to the recommended pharmacologic strategy.
- Explain appropriate use of therapeutic agents as well as compliance with recommended nondrug and behavioral interventions.
- Provide the patient with alternatives in the event of a less than optimal response to recommended treatment.

remain infectious outside the host cells for substantial periods of time.

Three criteria must be met for an individual to develop a wart. First, the papillomavirus must be present. Second, an open avenue, such as an abrasion, must exist through which the virus can enter the skin. Finally, the individual's immune system must be susceptible to the virus (probably the key reason that certain individuals develop warts and others do not). Indeed, immunodeficient patients (e.g., those maintained on systemic or topical glucocorticoids), once infected, develop widespread and highly resistant warts.[13]

Warts may spread by direct person-to-person contact, by autoinoculation to another body area, or by indirect exposure through public shower floors or swimming pools. It is thought that swimming, especially in warm water with a pH greater than 5, swells and softens the horny skin layer cells on the sole of the foot. The abrasive surface of the pool and diving board also contributes to tissue debridement. Scrapings of the horny layer of plantar warts contain virus particles. Therefore, it is conceivable that the heavy traffic area of a pool can be easily contaminated by one person with a plantar wart, making inoculation in that area around the pool likely. The incubation period after inoculation is 1 to 20 months, with an average of 3 to 4 months.

Warts usually are not permanent; approximately 30% clear spontaneously in 6 months, 65% clear in 2 years, and most warts clear in 5 years.[14] The mechanism of spontaneous resolution is not fully understood.

Signs and Symptoms of Warts

Common virogenic warts are recognized by their rough, cauliflower-like appearance. They are slightly scaly, rough papules or nodules that appear alone or grouped. They can be found on any skin surface although they most often appear on the hands. (See the "Color Plates," photograph 30.) Warts begin as minute, smooth-surfaced, skin-colored lesions that enlarge over time. Repeated irritation causes them to continue enlarging. Plantar warts, hyperkeratotic lesions generally associated with pressure, are usually asymptomatic when small and may not be noticed. However, if they are large or occur on the heel or ball of the foot, they may cause severe discomfort and limitation of function.

Warts are defined according to their location. Common warts (verruca vulgaris) are usually found on the hands and fingers but may also occur on the face. Periungual and subungual warts occur around and underneath the nail beds, especially in nail biters and cuticle pickers.[10] Juvenile, or flat, warts (verruca plana) usually occur on the face, neck, and dorsa of the hands, wrists, and knees of children. Venereal warts (condyloma lata and condyloma acuminata) typically occur near the genitalia and anus; however, the penile shaft is the most common site of lesions in men. Plantar warts (verruca plantaris) are common on the soles of the feet.[8] (See the "Color Plates," photograph 31.)

Plantar warts are more common in older children and adolescents but also occur in adults. They may be confined to the weight-bearing areas of the foot (the sole of the heel, the great toe, the areas below the heads of the metatarsal bones, and the ball), or they may occur in non–weight-bearing areas of the sole of the foot. (See Figure 36–3.) Calluses are commonly found on weight-bearing areas of the foot; because of their smooth keratotic surfaces, calluses may resemble isolated plantar warts. Therefore, the distinction between a wart and a callus is sometimes unclear. However, unlike a callus, a plantar wart is tender with pressure and interrupts the footprint pattern. Optimally, a podiatrist or dermatologist will have the opportunity to assess the condition and to make a differential diagnosis. To make this assessment, the physician may shave away the outer keratinous surface to expose thrombosed capillaries in the papilloma, which appear as black dots or seeds. In instances in which the results of this procedure are inconclusive, a skin sample can be sent to a clinical laboratory to confirm or refute the presence of HPV.

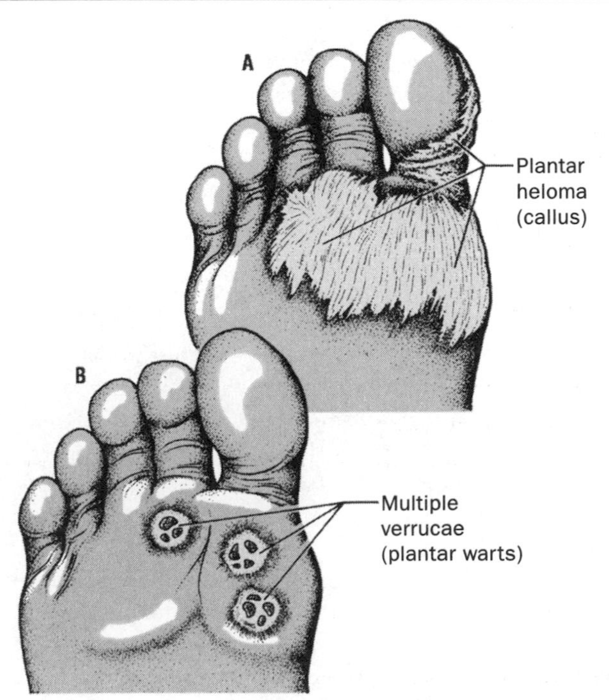

Figure 36–3A and B Conditions affecting the sole of the foot: A, plantar heloma (callus); B, multiple verrucae (plantar warts).

Plantar warts, if located on weight-bearing portions of the foot, are under constant pressure and are usually not raised above the skin surface. The wart itself is in the center of the lesion and is roughly circular, with a diameter of 0.5 to 3.0 cm. The surface is grayish and friable, and the surrounding skin is thick and heaped. Several warts may coalesce and fuse, giving the appearance of one large wart (mosaic wart).

Warts may occasionally be confused with more serious conditions, such as squamous cell carcinoma and deep fungal infections. A squamous cell carcinoma may develop rapidly, attaining a diameter of 1 cm within 2 weeks. The lesion generally appears as a small, red, conical, hard nodule that quickly ulcerates. Subungual verrucae, which occur under the nail plate, may exist in conjunction with periungual verrucae. A long-standing subungual verruca may be difficult to differentiate from a squamous cell carcinoma, especially in elderly patients.

Treatment of Warts

No specific effective medication for curing warts is available, although topical agents and procedures can sometimes help in their removal and can relieve pain.

Treatment Outcomes

The goals in treating warts are to (1) remove the wart and (2) prevent autoinoculation or transmission of the wart to other people.

General Treatment Approach

Many practitioners believe that early and vigorous treatment of warts is best. The urgency for treatment is based on considerations such as the cosmetic effect (facial warts), the number of warts present in an area, the site of the wart (weight-bearing area of the foot), and the age of the patient. Moreover, prolonged treatment with nonprescription products may increase the chance of autoinoculation. The algorithm in Figure 36–4 outlines the self-treatment of warts.

Self-treatment of warts is inappropriate in the following situations:

- The patient has extensive warts at one site or has warts on the face, around toenails or fingernails, or on or around the anus and/or genitalia.
- The patient has painful plantar warts.
- The patient has chronic, debilitating diseases, such as diabetes, or peripheral vascular disease, which contraindicate the use of foot care products.
- The patient has physical or mental impairments that make following product directions difficult.
- The patient is taking immunosuppressive medications or other medications (e.g., other salicylates) contraindicated for use of salicylic acid.

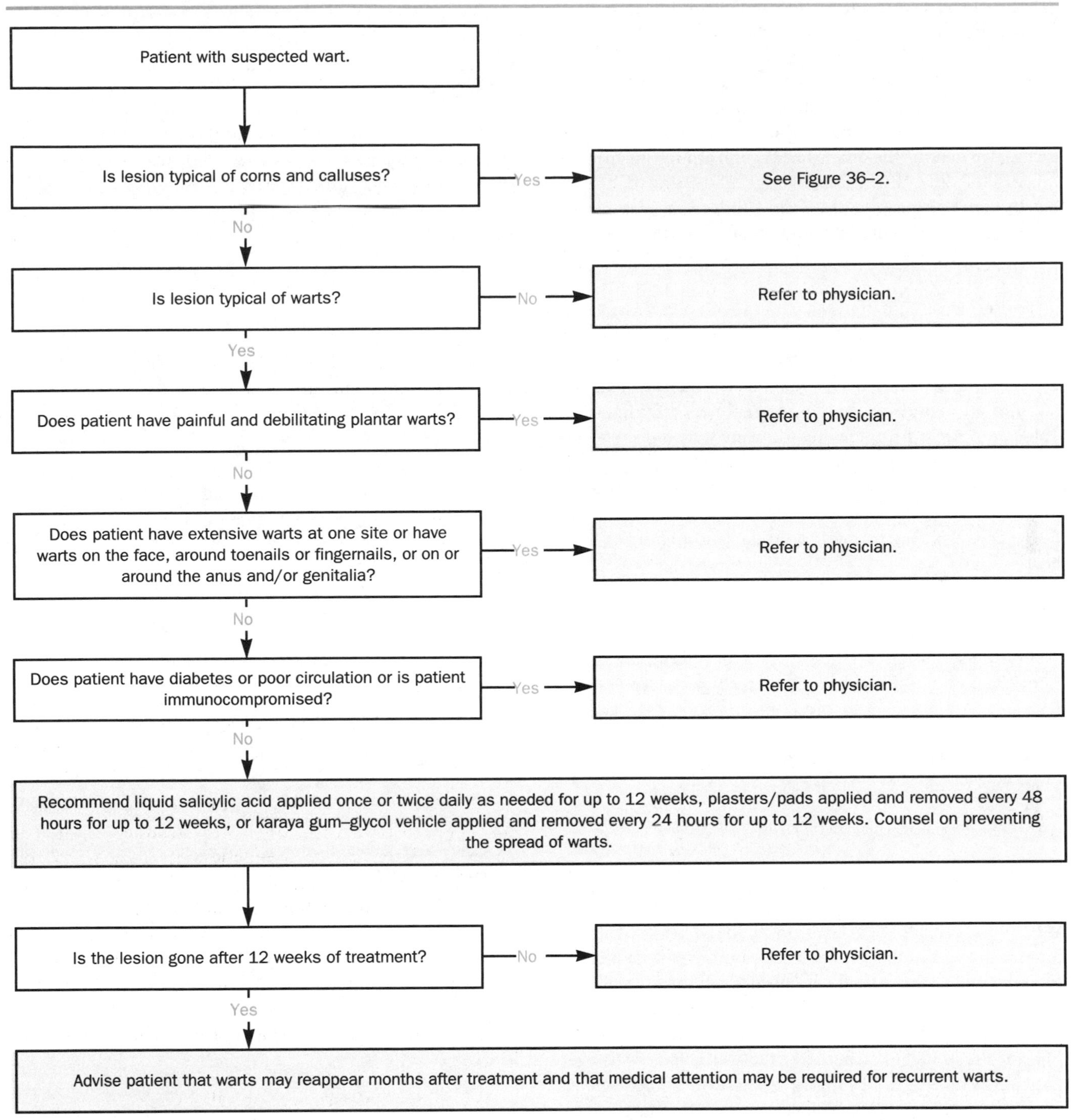

Figure 36–4 Self-care of warts.

Nonpharmacologic Therapy

To avoid the spread of warts, which are contagious, patients should wash their hands before and after treating or touching wart tissue. A specific towel should be used only for drying the affected area after cleaning. Patients should not probe, poke, or cut the wart tissue. If warts are present on the sole of the foot, patients should not walk in bare feet unless the wart is securely covered.

Pharmacologic Therapy

Salicylic Acid

Topical salicylic acid in three different vehicles has been recognized as the only drug that is safe and effective for self-treatment of common or plantar warts: salicylic acid 12% to 40% in a plaster vehicle, salicylic acid 5% to 17% in a collodion-like vehicle, and salicylic acid 15% in a karaya gum–glycol plaster vehicle.[7] (See the section "Salicylic Acid" under

"Treatment of Corns and Calluses" for a discussion of this agent's properties.) Table 36–4 lists examples of commercially available products for all three dosage forms.

FDA's Advisory Review Panel on Over-the-Counter Miscellaneous External Drug Products recommended that such products be labeled for treating only common and plantar warts.[7] It excluded the other wart types from self-therapy because of the difficulty in recognizing and treating them without the supervision of a physician.[7] Indeed, painful plantar warts—as well as multiple flat warts, facial warts, periungual warts, and venereal warts—should all be treated by a physician.[14]

For self-treatment of warts, patients will notice visible improvement within the first or second week of treatment; removal should be complete within 4 to 12 weeks of product use. Thus, selection of a convenient time to apply the product and adherence to the dosage regimen are important. Table 36–5 provides guidelines for using wart removal products.

If the wart remains after a full course of treatment, a physician should be consulted. Because of the latency factor, however, warts may reappear several months after they have been "cured."

Other Pharmacologic Therapies

Several prescription products (e.g., cantharidin, podophyllum, and podofilox) may be used to treat warts. Cryotherapy, with or without use of the prescription products, is another alternative. Detailed discussion of these treatments is outside the scope of this chapter. The reader is referred to standard pharmacy textbooks for such information.

Patient Assessment of Warts

When assessing a patient with warts, the pharmacist should inspect the lesion, if possible, to determine its suitability for self-treatment. The patient's age, health status (especially immunologic status), and use of medications for other disorders should be factored into the choice of treatment. The pharmacist should ask whether and how the patient has self-treated the disorder. The answer to these questions will help in evaluating expected compliance with self-treatment of the wart. Other important considerations before initiating treatment are the pain, the inconvenience, and the risk of scarring from the treatment. To help elicit this information, the pharmacist should ask the patient the questions in the section "Patient Assessment of Corn and Calluses," as well as the questions below.

Q~ Where is the wart located?

A~ Refer patients with warts on the face, toenails, fingernails, or genitals or with warts around the anus to a physician or dermatologist.

Table 36–4

Selected Products for Warts

Trade Name	Primary Ingredient
Clear Away OneStep Wart Remover Disk	Salicylic acid 40%
Clear Away Plantar Wart Remover Disk	Salicylic acid 40%
Compound-W OneStep Wart Remover for Kids Pad	Salicylic acid 40%
Compound-W Wart Remover Gel	Salicylic acid 17%
Compound-W Wart Remover Liquid	Salicylic acid 17%
Dr. Scholl's Wart Remover Kit Liquid	Salicylic acid 17%
DuoFilm Wart Remover Liquid	Salicylic acid 17%
DuoFilm Wart Remover Patch for Kids	Salicylic acid 40%
OFF-Ezy Wart Remover Kit Liquid	Salicylic acid 17%

Table 36–5

Guidelines for Treating Warts with Salicylic Acid Products

Wash and dry the affected area before applying the salicylic acid product.

Salicylic Acid 5% to 17% in Collodion Vehicle

- Apply the product to the wart no more often than twice daily. Morning and evening are usually the most convenient times.
- Apply the solution one drop at a time until the affected area is covered. Do not overuse the product.
- If the medication touches healthy skin, wash off the solution immediately with soap and water.
- Allow the solution to harden so that it does not run. Repeat this procedure as needed for up to 12 weeks.
- After use, cap the container tightly to prevent evaporation and to prevent the active ingredients from assuming a greater concentration.
- Store the product in amber or light-resistant containers away from direct sunlight or heat.

Salicylic Acid 12% to 40% Plaster/Pads

- If using plaster, trim the plaster to follow the contours of the wart. Apply the plaster to the skin, and cover it with adhesive occlusive tape.
- If using disks with pads, apply the appropriately sized disk directly on the affected area, and then cover it with the pad.
- Apply and remove plasters and pads every 48 hours as needed, up to 12 weeks.

Salicylic Acid 15% in Karaya Gum–Glycol Vehicle

- Apply the plaster to the wart at bedtime, and leave it on for at least 8 hours.
- Remove and discard the plaster in the morning.
- Repeat this procedure every 24 hours as needed for up to 12 weeks.

Q~ How many warts are there? How large an area is affected?

A~ Refer patients to a physician or dermatologist if they have multiple warts or warts that cover a large area.

Q~ Are you taking medications such as cancer chemotherapy, prednisone, or antirejection agents, which suppress the immune system?

A~ Refer potentially immunocompromised patients to a physician.

Patient Counseling for Warts

Patients must understand that, unlike corns and calluses, warts are contagious and can spread to other parts of the body unless proper precautions are taken. The pharmacist should point out differences in salicylic acid products used to treat warts and those used to treat corns and calluses. Pharmacists should stress the contraindications, warnings, and precautions for topical salicylic acid to prevent the wart from progressing to a more serious disorder. The box "Patient Education for Warts" lists specific information to provide patients.

Evaluation of Patient Outcomes for Warts

Because wart removal can take from 4 to 12 weeks, the pharmacist should schedule the first follow-up on the patient's progress after 4 weeks of treatment. If the wart is still present, the patient should be reminded of proper administration procedures and advised to continue the treatment. Reevaluation every 4 weeks is appropriate for persistent warts. The pharmacist should refer the patient to a physician for any warts that persist after 12 weeks of self-treatment.

Athlete's Foot

Epidemiology of Athlete's Foot

The most prevalent cutaneous fungal infection in humans is athlete's foot (dermatophytosis of the foot, or tinea pedis). Athlete's foot afflicts approximately 26.5 million people in the United States every year; of every 10 sufferers, 7 are male. It is estimated that 70% of people will be afflicted with athlete's foot in their lifetime and that approximately 45% will suffer with it episodically for more than 10 years. When exposure to infectious environments is equal, the incidence of tinea infections in women approaches that in men.

Patient Education for Warts

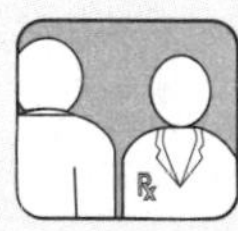

The objectives of self-treatment are to (1) remove the wart and (2) prevent the spread of warts to other parts of the body or to other people. For most patients, carefully following product instructions and the self-care measures listed below will help ensure optimal therapeutic outcomes.

Nondrug Measures

- To avoid spreading the warts, wash your hands before and after treating or touching the warts.
- Use a specific towel for drying only the affected area after cleansing. Use a separate towel to dry other parts of the body.
- Do not probe, poke, or cut the wart.
- If warts are present on the sole of the foot, do not walk in bare feet unless the wart is securely covered.

Nonprescription Medications

- Be sure to use only topical salicylic products that are labeled for use on warts. Table 36–4 lists the types of products used to treat warts. Table 36–5 gives the proper methods of applying the products.
- Treat only common or plantar warts with these agents. Ask your pharmacist or physician to identify the type of wart if you are unsure. Do not apply the medication to warts on the face, genitals, toenails, or fingernails or to warts around the anus.
- Do not use this product on irritated skin or on any area that is infected or reddened.
- Do not use this product if you are diabetic or if you have poor blood circulation.
- Salicylic acid is poisonous: Do not allow it to come in contact with the mouth, and keep it out of the reach of children.
- Note that the medication sloughs off skin and leaves an unsightly pinkish tinge to the skin.
- Expect to see visible improvement within the first or second week of treatment and complete removal of the wart within 4 to 12 weeks of product use.
- Note that warts may reappear months after the initial treatment.

⚠ Stop treatment and consult a physician or podiatrist if swelling, reddening, or irritation of the skin occurs, or if pain occurs immediately when applying the product.

⚠ If the wart remains after 12 weeks of treatment, see a physician or dermatologist.

Although there are many pathogenic fungi in the environment, the overall incidence of actual superficial fungal infections is remarkably low. Many degrees of susceptibility, from instantaneous "takes" by a single spore to severe trauma with massive exposure, produce a clinical infection. It appears, however, that trauma to the skin, especially that which produces blisters (from wearing ill-fitting footwear), may be significantly more important to the occurrence of human fungal infections than is simple exposure to the offending pathogens.

Although tinea pedis may occur at all ages, it is more common in adults, presumably because of their increased opportunities for exposure to pathogens. However, it can also occur in children. Individual susceptibility is affected by other disease processes that the patient may have. For example, dermatophytosis infections may be more severe and difficult to ameliorate in patients with diabetes mellitus, lymphoid malignancies, immunologic compromise, and Cushing's syndrome.[15]

Etiology of Athlete's Foot

Tinea pedis is an infection of relatively recent onset. It was not common until humans began wearing occlusive footwear, and it was not reported in the medical literature until 1888. Because ringworm fungi (dermatophytes) are generally the causative or initiating organisms, athlete's foot is often synonymous with a ringworm infection.[16] Tinea pedis is most commonly caused by *Trichophyton rubrum*, *Trichophyton mentagrophytes*, or *Epidermophyton floccosum*. *T. rubrum* often causes a dry, hyperkeratotic involvement of the feet; *T. mentagrophytes* often produces a blister-like or vesicular pattern; and *E. floccosum* is capable of producing both of these patterns.

In addition to specific microorganisms, other environmental factors contribute to the disease's development, such as the climatic conditions of the area and the customs of the resident population. Footwear is a key variable, as illustrated by the incidence of the disease in any population that wears occlusive footwear, especially in the summer and in tropical or subtropical climates. Nonporous shoe material increases temperature and hydration of the skin and interferes with the barrier function of the stratum corneum.

The type of dermatophytosis present varies with geographic location.[17] In Vietnam, U.S. soldiers often acquired a disabling, inflammatory *T. mentagrophytes* infection although South Vietnamese soldiers did not. In a resident population, dermatophytosis infection is often observed as chronic and noninflammatory, whereas the same infection in virgin hosts is markedly inflammatory and self-limited.[15]

Species of dermatophytes that infect humans (e.g., *T. rubrum* and *T. mentagrophytes*) are transmitted either directly by human contact or indirectly by exposure to inanimate objects. It is thought that this infection is acquired most often by walking barefoot on infected floors (e.g., hotel bathrooms, swimming pools, or locker rooms) and may be spread within families by exposure to bathroom floors, mats, or rugs. Therefore, tinea pedis is considered to be an exogenously transmitted infection in which cross-infection among susceptible individuals readily occurs.[17]

Pathophysiology of Athlete's Foot

After being inoculated into the skin under suitable conditions, the infection progresses through several stages. These stages include periods of incubation and then enlargement, followed by a refractory period and a stage of involution.

During the incubation period, the dermatophyte grows in the stratum corneum, sometimes with minimal signs of infection. After the incubation period and once the infection is established, two factors appear to play a role in determining the size and duration of the lesions. These factors are the growth rate of the organism and the epidermal turnover rate.[17] The fungal growth rate must equal or exceed the epidermal turnover rate, or the organism will quickly shed.

Dermatophytid infestations remain within the stratum corneum. This resistance to the spread of infection seems to involve both immunologic and nonimmunologic mechanisms. For example, the substance serum inhibitory factor (SIF) appears to limit the growth of dermatophytes beyond the stratum corneum. SIF is not an antibody but a dialyzable, heat-labile component of fresh sera. It appears that SIF binds to the iron that dermatophytes need for continued growth.[17]

Once into the stratum corneum, dermatophytes produce keratinases and other proteolytic enzymes. U.S. combat personnel in Vietnam demonstrated a particularly inflammatory type of *T. mentagrophytes* infection associated with elastase production.[15] This association indicated that enzymes or toxins produced by these microorganisms accounted for some of the severe clinical reactions.

Signs and Symptoms of Athlete's Foot

The clinical spectrum of athlete's foot ranges from mild itching and scaling to a severe, exudative inflammatory process characterized by fissuring and denudation. The prevalent type of athlete's foot, midway between these two extremes, is characterized by maceration, hyperkeratosis, pruritus, malodor, itching, and a stinging sensation of the feet. (See the "Color Plates," photograph 32.)

Clinically, there are four accepted variants of tinea pedis; two or more of these types may overlap. The most common is the chronic, intertriginous type,[15] characterized by fissuring, scaling, or maceration in the interdigital spaces. Typically, the infection involves the lateral toe webs, usually between the fourth and fifth or third and fourth toes. From these sites, the infection spreads to the sole or instep of the foot but rarely to the dorsum. Warmth and humidity aggravate this condition; consequently, hyperhidrosis (excessive sweating) becomes an underlying problem and must be treated along with the dermatophyte infestation.

Normal resident aerobic diphtheroids may become involved in the athlete's foot process. After initial invasion of the stratum corneum by dermatophytes, enough moisture may accumulate to trigger a bacterial overgrowth. Increased moisture and temperature then lead to the release of metabolic products, which diffuse easily through the underlying horny layer already damaged by fungal invasion. In the more severe cases, gram-negative organisms intrude and may exacerbate the condition, causing skin maceration, white hyperkeratosis, or erosions with increased patient symptomatology.

The second variant of athlete's foot is known as the chronic, papulosquamous pattern.[15] It is usually found on both feet and is characterized by mild inflammation and diffuse scaling on the soles of the feet. Tinea unguium (i.e., ringworm of the nails, or onychomycosis) of one or more toenails may also be present and may continue to fuel the infection. The toenails must first be cured with oral drug therapy, such as griseofulvin, itraconazole, ketoconazole, or terbinafine, or must be removed surgically to rid the area of the offending fungus.

The third variant of tinea pedis is the vesicular type, usually caused by *T. mentagrophytes* var. *interdigitale*.[15] Small vesicles or vesicopustules are observed near the instep and on the midanterior plantar surface. Skin scaling is seen on these areas as well as on the toe webs. This variant is symptomatic in the summer and is clinically quiescent during the cooler months.

The acute ulcerative type is the fourth variant of tinea pedis. It is often associated with macerated, denuded, weeping ulcerations of the sole of the foot. Typically, white hyperkeratosis and a pungent odor are present. This type of infection, which is complicated by an overgrowth of opportunistic, gram-negative bacteria such as *Proteus* and *Pseudomonas*, has been called dermatophytosis complex, and it may produce an extremely painful, erosive, purulent interspace that can be disabling.

Severe forms of tinea pedis may progress to disintegration and denudation of the affected skin and to profuse, serous, purulent discharge. Denudation may involve all the toe webs, the dorsal and plantar surfaces of the toes, and an area about 1 cm wide beyond the base of the toes on the plantar surface of the foot. When the disease is out of control, its progression is observed on the dorsum of the foot and the calf in the form of tiny red follicular crusts. Paradoxically, this condition may be caused by the use of reputed germicidal soaps such as pHisoHex, Dial, and Safeguard. It was hypothesized that these soaps reduce the presence of harmless saprophytes and thus promote an overgrowth of resistant pathogens (e.g., *Pseudomonas aeruginosa* and *Proteus mirabilis*) by removing their competitors.

Complications of Athlete's Foot

Secondary bacterial or other opportunistic infections can occur in patients who are already immunocompromised (e.g., diabetes mellitus, human immunodeficiency virus [HIV]) and who may already have a fungal infection.[16] Such infections are also facilitated in individuals who wear poorly ventilated shoes or whose lifestyle predisposes them to severe hyperhidrosis or profuse sweating.

Treatment of Athlete's Foot

Treatment Outcomes

The goals in treating athlete's foot are to (1) provide symptomatic relief, (2) eradicate existing infections, and (3) prevent future infections.

General Treatment Approach

Before self-medication can be effective, the type of tinea pedis and the appropriate treatment must be determined. Self-treatment of an acute, superficial tinea foot infection may be effective if certain conditions are met. In acute, inflammatory tinea pedis, characterized by reddened, oozing, and vesicular eruptions, the inflammation must be counteracted with solutions of aluminum salts before antifungal therapy can be instituted. This step is especially important if the eruptions are caused by a secondary bacterial infection.

Self-treatment is effective only if the patient understands the importance of compliance with all facets of the treatment plan. (See Figure 36–5.) Specific antifungal products must be used appropriately in conjunction with other treatment measures, including general hygienic measures and local drying. Local hygienic measures are important as a useful adjunct to specific antifungal therapy. Nonprescription topical antifungals can be used to treat and prevent athlete's foot. Nondrug preventive measures include keeping the skin clean and dry, avoiding the sharing of personal articles, and avoiding foot contact with surfaces that may harbor fungi.

If the patient has used a nonprescription antifungal product appropriately for 4 weeks without satisfactory results, a disease other than tinea pedis may be involved. Therapeutic failure may be caused by a bacterial infection, which no nonprescription antifungal product will ameliorate. Patients with such an infection, as well as with hyperhidrosis, allergic contact dermatitis, or atopic dermatitis, should consult a podiatrist or physician for treatment.

The following situations also indicate referral of a patient with suspected athlete's foot to a physician or podiatrist for treatment:

- If the toenail is involved, topical treatment is ineffective and will not allay the condition until the disease's primary focus is treated with oral itraconazole or terbinafine hydrochloride or until other preventive measures are instituted (e.g., surgical avulsion of the nail).
- If vesicular eruptions are oozing purulent material that could indicate a secondary bacterial infection, topical astringent therapy and/or antibiotic therapy may be appropriate.

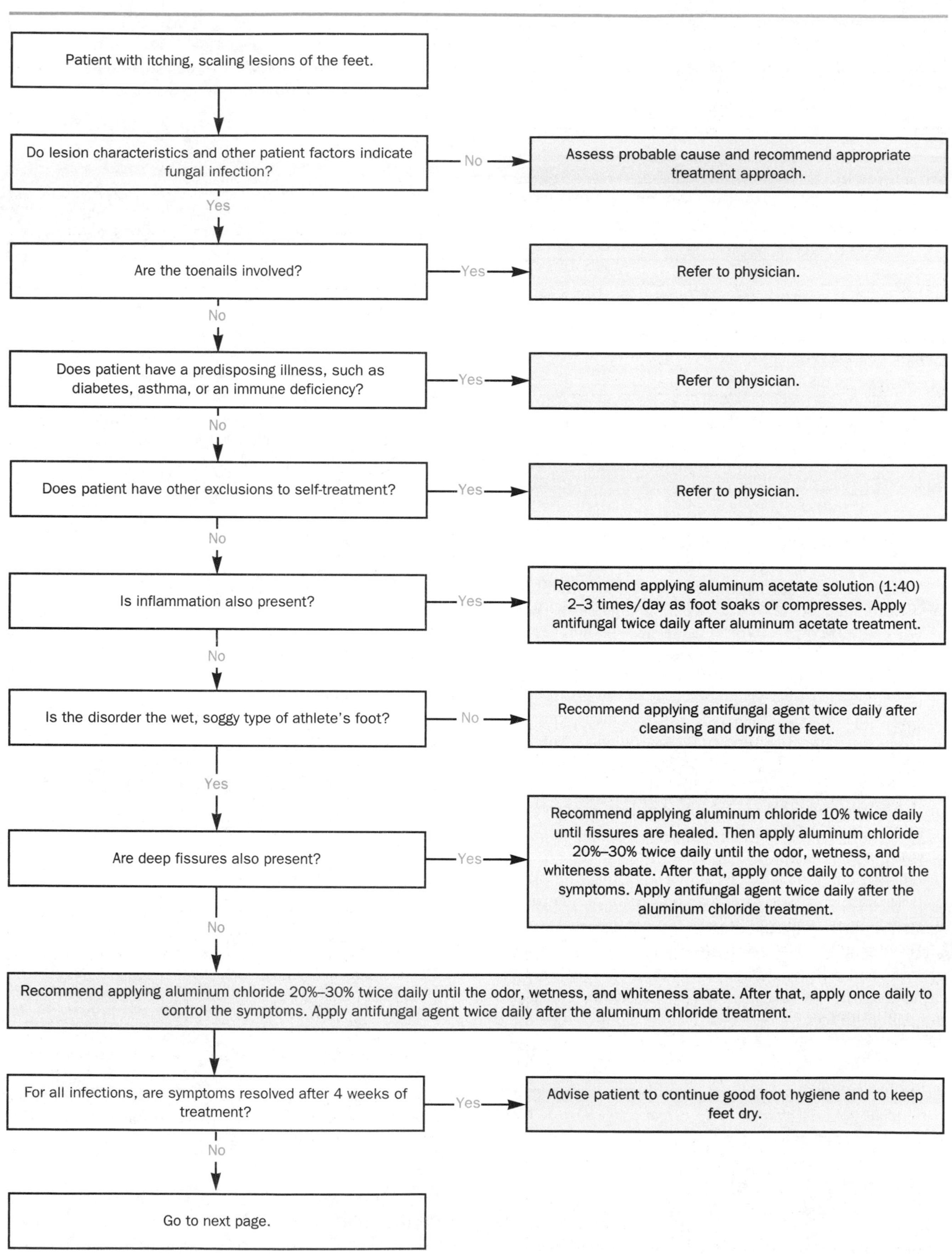

Patient with itching, scaling lesions of the feet.
Do lesion characteristics and other patient factors indicate fungal infection?
No
Assess probable cause and recommend appropriate treatment approach.
Yes
Are the toenails involved?
Yes
Refer to physician.
No
Does patient have a predisposing illness, such as diabetes, asthma, or an immune deficiency?
Yes
Refer to physician.
No
Does patient have other exclusions to self-treatment?
Yes
Refer to physician.
No
Is inflammation also present?
Yes
Recommend applying aluminum acetate solution (1:40) 2–3 times/day as foot soaks or compresses. Apply antifungal twice daily after aluminum acetate treatment.
No
Is the disorder the wet, soggy type of athlete's foot?
No
Recommend applying antifungal agent twice daily after cleansing and drying the feet.
Yes
Are deep fissures also present?
Yes
Recommend applying aluminum chloride 10% twice daily until fissures are healed. Then apply aluminum chloride 20%–30% twice daily until the odor, wetness, and whiteness abate. After that, apply once daily to control the symptoms. Apply antifungal agent twice daily after the aluminum chloride treatment.
No
Recommend applying aluminum chloride 20%–30% twice daily until the odor, wetness, and whiteness abate. After that, apply once daily to control the symptoms. Apply antifungal agent twice daily after the aluminum chloride treatment.
For all infections, are symptoms resolved after 4 weeks of treatment?
Yes
Advise patient to continue good foot hygiene and to keep feet dry.
No
Go to next page.

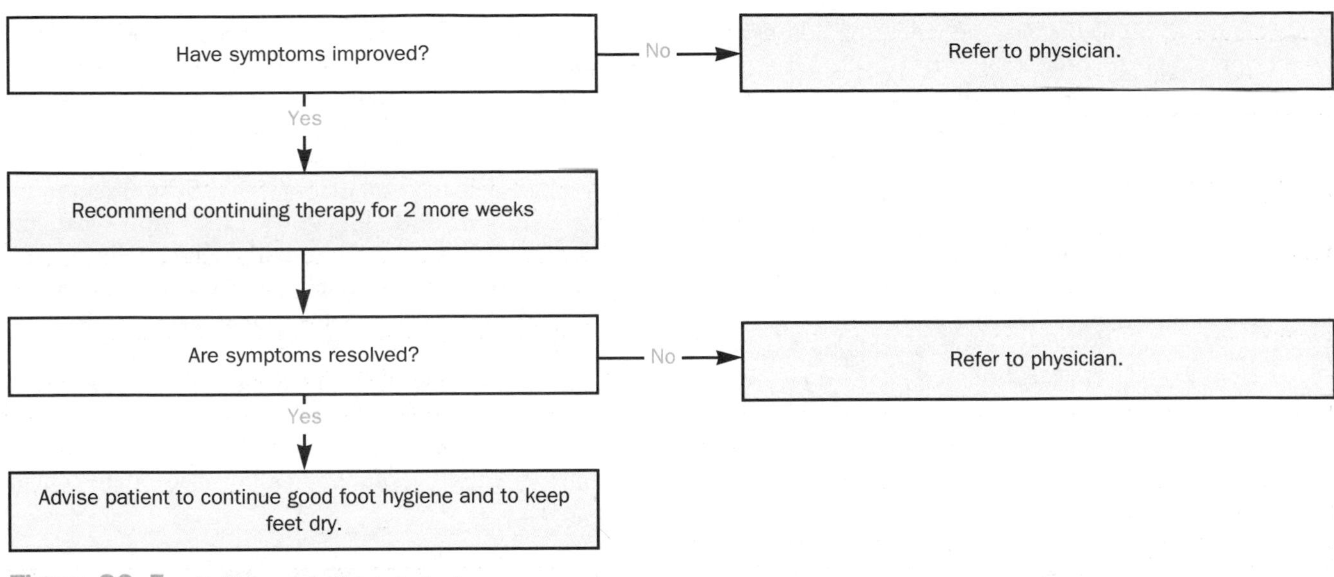

Figure 36–5 Self-care of athlete's foot.

- If the interspace between the toes is foul smelling; whitish; painful; soggy; or characterized by erosions, oozing, or serious inflammation—and especially if the condition is disabling—the patient should be referred to a physician.
- If the foot is seriously inflamed or swollen and if a major portion of it is involved, supportive therapy must be instituted before an antifungal agent may be applied.
- If the patient is a child who presents with an eczematous eruption of the feet, including that complicated by blisters and/or pyoderma, self-treatment should not be recommended.
- If the patient is under a physician's supervision for a disease such as diabetes or asthma (in which normal host defense mechanisms may be deficient), nonprescription products should not be recommended before medical consultation.

Self-treatment of athlete's foot is appropriate if the condition is not extensive, seriously inflamed, or debilitating, and if the toenails are not involved.

Nonpharmacologic Therapy

Table 36–6 provides guidelines for proper foot hygiene. The patient should follow these measures during and after treatment of the infection.

Table 36–6

Guidelines for Proper Foot Hygiene

- Cleanse the feet each day with soap and water, and thoroughly pat dry. However, do not irritate skin by scrubbing or vigorously drying the feet.
- If an infection is present, dry the feet last after bathing so that the towel does not spread the infection to other areas of the body.
- Keep feet as cool and dry as possible during the day as follows:
  —Wear shoes and light cotton socks that allow ventilation.
  —Avoid wearing fabrics such as wool and synthetic fabrics that do not allow moisture to evaporate.
  —Do not wear occlusive footwear, including canvas, leather, or rubber-soled athletic shoes, for prolonged periods.
  —Alternate shoes as often as possible so that the inside can adequately dry.
  —Dust shoes with medicated or unmedicated foot powders to help them dry.
  —Change socks daily and wash them thoroughly after use.
  —At every change of socks, dry and dust the feet with a medicated or unmedicated drying powder. Pay particular attention to the area between the toes.
  —Whenever possible, air the feet to prevent moisture buildup. Place cotton balls or Dr. Scholl's Smooth Touch Pedi-spreads between the tips of the toes to keep the web spaces open and less moist. Do not use objects such as pencil erasers because they may contain sensitizing accelerators or antioxidants.
- Wear nonocclusive protective footwear (e.g., rubber or wooden sandals) in areas of family or public use, such as home bathrooms or community showers.

Pharmacologic Therapy

Hydrocortisone, in conjunction with clioquinol (formerly iodochlorhydroxyquin), has demonstrated favorable results toward resolving uncomplicated cutaneous fungal infections (tinea cruris, tinea pedis, and moniliasis). Erythema and itching were relieved more with the combination of these two drugs than with either the drug alone or the placebo cream. However, with the availability of nonprescription topical hydrocortisone products, it is conceivable that their indiscriminate use to relieve the itching and redness of athlete's foot could complicate and delay appropriate medical care. Topical hydrocortisone by itself is contraindicated in the presence of fungal infections because it may complicate and delay healing. Nor should the pharmacist recommend the use of a nonprescription topical hydrocortisone cream in conjunction with a nonprescription antifungal product to relieve the itching associated with athlete's foot.

In its final rule for topical antifungal drug products for OTC human use,[18] FDA agreed with its Advisory Review Panel on Over-the-Counter Antimicrobial Drug Products[19] that, to best serve all consumers, a nonprescription product must provide more than temporary symptomatic relief of athlete's foot and related infections. Such products must contain a Category I antifungal ingredient capable of killing the fungus. (See Table 36–7.) The panel required each antifungal ingredient to have at least one well-designed clinical trial demonstrating its effectiveness in treating athlete's foot before being classified as Category I.[19] The advisory panel recommended treatment for a minimum of 2 to 4 weeks.[18]

Haloprogin/Povidone–Iodine

Although FDA approved haloprogin 1% for nonprescription use in treating athlete's foot, no commercially available products contain this agent. Povidone–iodine is considered safe and effective for treating fungal skin infections, but these products carry no indication for these infections.

Clioquinol

Clioquinol has demonstrated efficacy in treating athlete's foot. FDA classified it as Category I—safe and effective for topical nonprescription use in treating this condition. Evaluations of clioquinol used alone and in combination with hydrocortisone indicate the following effectiveness: clioquinol–hydrocortisone combination is greater than clioquinol alone which is greater than hydrocortisone alone and greater than placebo.

Table 36–7

FDA-Approved Topical Antifungal Drugs for Over-the-Counter Use

Drug	Concentration (%)
Haloprogin	1
Clioquinol	3
Clotrimazole	1
Miconazole nitrate	2
Terbinafine hydrochloride	1
Tolnaftate	1
Undecylenic acid and its salts	10–25
Povidone–Iodine	10

Source: Reference 18.

Clioquinol's mechanism of action is unknown. It has a low incidence of side effects; however, it may cause itching, redness, and irritation. With general, nonocclusive application, the possibility of its percutaneous absorption is low. However, if it is applied with an occlusive dressing, absorption can be rapid and extensive and may be sufficient to interfere with thyroid function tests. Thus, patients undergoing such tests must be questioned carefully to assess their prior use of iodine-containing clioquinol. Guidelines advocate that at least 3 months should elapse between the time that topical clioquinol has been discontinued and certain thyroid function determinations (e.g., protein-bound iodine, butanol-extractable iodine, radioactive iodine uptake) are performed. This drug may also stain skin, hair, and nails yellow with its application and/or inadvertent contact with fabrics.

Clotrimazole and Miconazole Nitrate

Clotrimazole and miconazole nitrate are imidazole derivatives that demonstrate fungistatic/fungicidal activity (depending on concentration) against *T. mentagrophytes, T. rubrum, E. floccosum,* and *Candida albicans.* These agents act by inhibiting the biosynthesis of ergosterol and other steroids and by damaging the fungal cell wall membrane and altering its permeability so that essential intracellular elements may be lost. These drugs have also been shown to inhibit oxidative and peroxidative enzyme activity, which results in intracellular buildup of toxic concentrations of hydrogen peroxide; this toxicity may then contribute to the degradation of subcellular organelles and to cellular necrosis. In *C. albicans,* such drugs have been shown to inhibit the transformation of blastospores into invasive mycelial form.

Both of these former prescription drugs have been reclassified as nonprescription. Both are suggested for application twice daily, once in the morning and once in the evening. Controlled studies have demonstrated their efficacy for athlete's foot, as well as for other kinds of fungal skin infections. (See Chapter 6, "Vaginal and Vulvovaginal Disorders," and Chapter 35, "Minor Wounds and Skin Infections.") Both would be expected to demonstrate efficacy comparable to that of tolnaftate (see below) for tinea pedis. In the event of treatment failure in which patient factors (e.g., noncompliance or improper foot hygiene) have been ruled out as a cause, both can be suggested as alternative treatment modalities. Rare cases of mild skin irritation, burning, and stinging have occurred with their use.

Terbinafine Hydrochloride

Topical terbinafine hydrochloride 1% was reclassified as a nonprescription medication in 1999 under the trade name Lamisil AT. This product is formulated as a cream. According to utilization data, the prescription version of the agent, Lamisil, was the number one prescription product prescribed for athlete's foot.

Terbinafine hydrochloride is indicated for interdigital tinea pedis, tinea cruris, and tinea corporis caused by *E. floc-*

cosum, T. mentagrophytes, and *T. rubrum*. This antifungal agent inhibits squalene epoxidase, a key enzyme in fungi sterol biosynthesis. This action results in a deficiency in ergosterol and a corresponding accumulation of squalene within the fungal cell, and it causes fungal cell death. This drug is the only nonprescription topical antifungal available for which clinical trials demonstrated it could cure athlete's foot with 1 week of treatment. Clinical trials to date also demonstrate a low incidence of side effects. These side effects include irritation (1%), burning (0.8%), and itching/dryness (0.2%).[20,21]

Tolnaftate

Tolnaftate has demonstrated clinical efficacy since its commercial introduction into the United States in 1965, and it has become the standard topical antifungal medication. Tolnaftate is the only nonprescription drug approved for both preventing and treating athlete's foot.[18] It acts on typical fungi responsible for tinea pedis, including *T. mentagrophytes* and *T. rubrum*. It is also effective against *E. floccosum* and species of *Microsporum*. It has no activity against *Candida* species.

Although tolnaftate's exact mechanism of action has not been reported, it is believed that tolnaftate distorts the hyphae and stunts the mycelial growth of the fungi species. Tolnaftate is effective in tinea pedis but not in onychomycosis. For treatment of onychomycosis, concomitant administration of oral griseofulvin, itraconazole, ketoconazole, or terbinafine is often necessary.

Tolnaftate is valuable primarily in the dry, scaly type of athlete's foot. Superficial fungal infection relapse has occurred after tolnaftate therapy has been discontinued. Relapse may be caused by inadequate duration of treatment, patient noncompliance with the medication, or use of tolnaftate when oral griseofulvin or ketoconazole should have been used. Because tolnaftate does not possess antibacterial properties, its value must be viewed with skepticism for use in the soggy, macerated type of athlete's foot in which bacteria are probably involved.

Tolnaftate is well tolerated when applied to intact or broken skin in either exposed or intertriginous areas, although it usually stings slightly when applied. Delayed hypersensitivity reactions to tolnaftate are extremely unlikely. As with all topical medications, however, discontinuation is warranted if irritation, sensitization, or worsening of the skin condition occurs.

Tolnaftate (1% solution, cream, gel, powder, spray powder, or spray liquid) is applied sparingly twice daily after the affected area is cleaned thoroughly. Effective therapy usually takes 2 to 4 weeks, although some individuals (patients with lesions between the toes or on pressure areas of the foot) may require treatment lasting 4 to 6 weeks. When medication is applied to pressure areas of the foot, where the horny skin layer is thicker than normal, concomitant use of a keratolytic agent (e.g., Whitfield's ointment) may be advisable. Neither keratolytic agents nor wet compresses, such as aluminum acetate solution (Burow's solution), which promote the healing of oozing lesions, interfere with the efficacy of tolnaftate. If weeping lesions are present, the inflammation should be treated before tolnaftate is applied.

As a cream, tolnaftate is formulated in a polyethylene glycol 400–propylene glycol vehicle. The 1% solution is formulated in polyethylene glycol 400 and may be more effective than the cream. The solution solidifies when exposed to cold, but, if allowed to warm, it will liquefy with no loss in potency. These vehicles are particularly advantageous in superficial antifungal therapy because they are nonocclusive, nontoxic, nonsensitizing, water miscible, anhydrous, easy to apply, and efficient in delivering the drug to the affected area.

The topical powder formulation of tolnaftate uses cornstarch–talc as the vehicle. This vehicle not only is an effective drug delivery system but also offers a therapeutic advantage because the two agents retain water. The topical aerosol formulation of tolnaftate includes talc and the propellant vehicle.

Undecylenic Acid–Zinc Undecylenate

This combination is widely used and may be effective for various mild superficial fungal infections, excluding those involving nails or hairy parts of the body. It is fungistatic and effective in mild chronic cases of tinea pedis. Compound undecylenic acid ointment (USP XXI) contains 5% undecylenic acid and 20% zinc undecylenate in an ointment base. It is believed that zinc undecylenate liberates undecylenic acid (the active antifungal entity) on contact with perspiration. In addition, zinc undecylenate has astringent properties because of the presence of the zinc ion; this astringent activity decreases the irritation and inflammation of the infection. The FDA's Advisory Review Panel on Over-the-Counter Antimicrobial Drug Products classified undecylenic acid and its derivatives (10% to 25% total undecylenate content) as Category I for treating athlete's foot.[18]

Applied to the skin as an ointment, diluted solution, or dusting powder, the combination of undecylenic acid–zinc undecylenate is relatively nonirritating, and hypersensitivity reactions are rare. The undiluted solution, however, may cause transient stinging when applied to broken skin because of its isopropyl alcohol content. Caution must be exercised to ensure that such ingredients do not come into contact with the eye or that the powder is not inhaled.

The vehicle in compound undecylenic acid ointment has a water-miscible base, making it nonocclusive, removable with water, and easy to apply. The powder uses talc as its vehicle and is absorbent. The aerosol contains menthol, which serves as a counterirritant and antipruritic. The solution contains 25% undecylenic acid in an isopropyl alcohol vehicle with either an applicator or a spray pump container. The foam dosage form contains 10% undecylenic acid.

The product is applied twice daily after the affected area is cleansed. When the solution is sprayed or applied to the affected area, the area should be allowed to air dry; otherwise, water may accumulate and further macerate the tissue. The relatively high alcohol concentration in such solutions could cause some burning; the strong odor of undecylenic acid may be objectionable to some patients, possibly promoting patient noncompliance. The usual period required for therapeutic results depends on the severity of the infection. However, if improvement does not occur in 2 to 4 weeks, the condition should be reevaluated and an alternative medication used.

Salts of Aluminum

Because they do not have any direct antifungal activity, aluminum salts were not included in the final monograph for topical antifungal drug products. However, their effectiveness as astringents and their possible use in treating athlete's foot merit their inclusion in this chapter. Historically, aluminum acetate has been the foremost astringent used for both the acute, inflammatory type and the wet, soggy type of tinea pedis. Aluminum chloride is also used to treat the wet, soggy type of infection. However, each solution has a potential for misuse (accidental childhood poisoning by ingesting the solutions or the solid tablets), and precautions must be taken to prevent this occurrence.

The action and efficacy of the aluminum salts appear to be two-pronged. First, these compounds act as astringents. Their drying ability probably involves the complexing of the astringent agent with proteins, thereby altering the proteins' ability to swell and hold water. Astringents decrease edema, exudation, and inflammation by reducing cell membrane permeability and by hardening the cement substance of the capillary epithelium. Second, aluminum salts in concentrations greater than 20% possess antibacterial activity. Aluminum chloride (20%) may exhibit that activity in two ways: by directly killing bacteria and by drying the interspaces. Solutions of 20% aluminum acetate and 20% aluminum chloride demonstrate equal in vitro antibacterial efficacy.

Aluminum acetate for use in tinea pedis is generally diluted with about 10 to 40 parts of water. Depending on the situation, the patient may immerse the whole foot in the solution for 20 minutes up to three times a day (every 6 to 8 hours) or may apply the solution to the affected area in the form of a wet dressing.

For patient convenience, aluminum acetate solution (Burow's solution) or modified Burow's solution is available for immediate use in solution or in forms (powder packets,

Case Study 36–2

Patient Complaint/History

Anwar, a 21-year-old college student, stops in to consult the pharmacist late one afternoon. He complains of a burning, itching sensation between the toes of his left foot. He says that these symptoms, which are becoming worse each day, are quite bothersome, particularly at bedtime when he is trying to fall asleep.

When questioned about the symptoms, Anwar reveals that the area between the toes is very red and seems to become worse after showering. He describes his toenails as normal in appearance; that is, the toenail beds show no apparent discoloration or brittleness. The patient mentions that he showers every day in his residence hall and at the gymnasium after his varsity baseball team's workout. He also reports that his feet sweat a lot.

The patient admits to using Lotrimin AF cream intermittently for the past week in an attempt to resolve his problem. He says that the cream seems to help a little. He asks, "Why doesn't this stuff work? It used to be a prescription drug, didn't it?"

Except for the current foot problem, Anwar is in good general health, has no known diseases or allergies, and takes nonprescription medications only on rare occasions for relief of headaches or cold symptoms.

Clinical Considerations/Strategies

Patients can use the following considerations/strategies to determine whether treatment of the patient's condition with nonprescription medications is warranted:

- Assess the patient's symptoms to determine the most likely etiology and degree of severity.
- Formulate a realistic goal for treating the patient's problem (i.e., to relieve the symptoms and resolve the problem).
- Generate a list of therapeutic drug and nondrug interventions to address the patient's condition (e.g., medical referral, nonprescription medication therapy, nondrug measures).
- Identify patient characteristics that either preclude or necessitate each therapeutic intervention.
- Create an optimal therapeutic intervention to resolve the patient's clinical condition.
- Create and agree on a plan with the patient to monitor and document progress in resolving the problem.

Patient Education/Counseling

Readers can use the following strategies to develop a patient education/counseling plan that will help ensure optimal therapeutic outcomes:

- Support/justify the selected therapeutic strategy.
- Ensure patient compliance by explaining the recommended therapeutic action plan.
- Provide the patient with alternatives in the event of a less than optimal response to the recommended treatment.

powder, and effervescent tablets) for dilution with water. These products are intended for external use only and should not be applied near the eyes. Prolonged or continuous use of aluminum acetate solution may produce tissue necrosis. In the acute inflammatory state of tinea pedis, this solution should be used for less than 1 week. The pharmacist should instruct the patient to discontinue its use if inflammatory lesions appear or worsen.

Concentrations of 20% to 30% aluminum chloride have been the most beneficial for the wet, soggy type of athlete's foot.[7] Twice-daily applications are generally used until the signs and symptoms (odor, wetness, and whiteness) abate. After that, once-daily applications control the symptoms. In hot, humid weather, the original condition may return within 7 to 10 days after the application is stopped.

Aluminum salts do not entirely cure athlete's foot but are useful when combined with other topical antifungal drugs. Application of the aluminum salt merely shifts the disease process back to the simple dry type of athlete's foot, which can then be controlled with other agents such as tolnaftate.

Because aluminum salts penetrate skin poorly, their toxicity, like that of aluminum chloride, is low. However, a few cases of irritation have been reported in patients where deep fissures were present. Thus, the use of concentrated aluminum salt solutions is contraindicated on severely eroded or deeply fissured skin. In such a case, the salts must be diluted to a lower concentration (10% aluminum chloride) for initial treatment.

Unapproved Ingredients

Historically, some organic fatty acids (e.g., caprylic acid), acetic acid (in the form of triacetin), some phenolic compounds (e.g., salicylic acid), quaternary ammonium compounds (e.g., benzethonium chloride), and quinoline derivatives (e.g., 8-hydroxyquinoline) have been used to treat athlete's foot. However, in the final monograph for topical antifungal drug products, these ingredients were not included as safe and effective for self-care purposes. The reader is referred to the 11th edition of the *Handbook of Nonprescription Drugs* for a historical perspective and detailed descriptions of these agents.

Pharmacotherapeutic Comparisons

All the topical antifungals approved for treating tinea pedis have been demonstrated to be effective. The allure of terbinafine hydrochloride is its demonstrated ability to cure athlete's foot in some patients after 1 week. However, a close analysis of the data demonstrates that the number of patients receiving resolution of the problem is low (approximately 14%) and that the effectiveness of this agent parallels that of other antifungals (e.g., clotrimazole, miconazole nitrate) recently approved for nonprescription use.

Product Ingredients and Formulations

The primary drug delivery systems used in treating tinea pedis are creams, solutions, and powders. Powders, including those in aerosol product forms, generally are indicated for adjunctive use with solutions and creams. In very mild conditions, powders may suffice as the only therapy.

Solution and cream forms should be formulated in the following manner:

- The vehicle should be nonocclusive because any moisture or sweat that is retained exacerbates the condition.
- The vehicle must be anhydrous because including water in the formulation introduces a variable that is one of the primary causes of the condition.
- The vehicle should be spreadable with minimal effort and without water.
- The vehicle must be water miscible or water washable (i.e., removable with minimal cleansing efforts) because hard scrubbing of the affected area further abrades the skin.
- The vehicle should be nonsensitizing and nontoxic when applied to intact or denuded skin because it may be absorbed into the systemic circulation.
- The vehicle should be capable of efficient drug delivery (i.e., it must not interact with the active ingredient but should allow that ingredient to penetrate to the seat of the fungal infection).

Most vehicles used to deliver topical solutions and creams are polyethylene glycol and alcohols, which meet these criteria. Polyethylene glycol bases deliver water-insoluble drugs topically and do it more efficiently than other water-soluble bases. This ability to deliver water-insoluble drugs is an added advantage because most topical antifungal drugs (e.g., tolnaftate) are largely water insoluble.

Criteria for the powder form (shaker or aerosol) are basically the same as those for creams and solutions. Certain agents in powder forms (talc and cornstarch) are therapeutic and serve as vehicles. Powders inhibit the propagation of fungi by adsorbing moisture and by preventing skin maceration. Thus, they actually alter the ecologic conditions of the fungi. The adsorbing material within the powder, rather than the intended active ingredient, may be responsible for much of the disease remission.

Many authorities consider cornstarch superior to talc for these formulations. This superiority is because cornstarch is virtually free of chemical contamination and does not tend to produce granulomatous reactions in wounds as readily as talc. Moreover, cornstarch adsorbs 25 times more moisture from moisture-saturated air than talc.

Product Selection Guidelines

Patient compliance is influenced by product selection. Therefore, the pharmacist should recommend an appropriate drug and product form that is designed to cause the least interference with daily habits and activities without sacrificing efficacy. Product selection should be geared to the individual patient. For example, elderly patients may require a preparation that is easy to use; obese patients, in whom excessive sweating may contribute to the disease, should use topical talcum powders as adjunctive therapy. Under certain patient circumstances, it may be necessary for the pharmacist to instruct the caregiver rather than the patient in the proper use of foot products.

Before recommending a nonprescription product, the pharmacist should review the patient's medical history. For example, patients with diabetes should have their blood glucose levels moderately controlled because increased glucose in perspiration may promote fungal growth. Patients with allergic dermatitides usually have a history of asthma, hay fever, or atopic dermatitis and, thus, are extremely sensitive to most oral and topical agents. By acquiring a good history, the pharmacist may be able to distinguish a tinea infection from atopic dermatitis and to avoid recommending a product that may cause skin irritation.

The pharmacist should bear in mind that prescription drugs may sometimes be more beneficial than nonprescription products. In the soggy, macerated athlete's foot complicated by bacterial infection, the broad-spectrum antifungal agents (e.g., econazole nitrate) are preferable to both tolnaftate and prescription-strength haloprogin.

The pharmacist should also bear in mind that product line extensions that have the same brand name do not necessarily have the same active ingredient(s). For example, the cream and solution formulations of Lotrimin AF contain clotrimazole 1%, whereas the topical spray and powder formulations contain miconazole nitrate 2%. In the case of the spray and powder formulations, it is prohibitively expensive for the manufacturer to pursue a new drug application that would be necessary to market these products with clotrimazole 1% as their active ingredient. It is more economically prudent to market them with an active ingredient that has already received FDA approval. Similarly, Desenex Maximum Strength Antifungal cream contains miconazole nitrate 2%, whereas the traditional Desenex Cream contains undecylenic acid and zinc undecylenate in a 25% concentration. (See Table 36–8 for examples of other commercially available products.)

Table 36–8

Selected Athlete's Foot Products

Trade Name	Primary Ingredients
Absorbine Jr. Athlete's Foot Cream/Powder	Tolnaftate 1%
Absorbine Jr. Athlete's Foot Spray Liquid Pump Spray	Tolnaftate 1%
Desenex Powder/Cream/Ointment/ Aerosol Spray Powder	Total undecylenate 25% (as undecylenic acid and zinc undecylenate)
Desenex Foot & Sneaker Deodorant Plus Powder	Calcium undecylenate 10%
Dr. Scholl's Athlete's Foot Powder/ Aerosol Spray Liquid/Aerosol Spray Powder	Tolnaftate 1%
Lotrimin AF Aerosol Spray Powder	Miconazole nitrate 2%
Odor-Eaters Antifungal Powder/ Aerosol Spray Powder	Tolnaftate 1%
Tinactin Powder/Solution/Cream	Tolnaftate 1%

Patient Assessment of Athlete's Foot

The only true determinant of a fungal foot infection is the clinical laboratory evaluation of tissue scrapings from the foot. This process involves a potassium hydroxide mount preparation of the scrapings and cuttings on a special growth medium to show the actual presence and specific identity of fungi. The procedure can be ordered and performed only at the direction of a physician, and microscopic confirmation is probably possible only in the dry, scaly type of tinea pedis. The recovery of fungi for diagnosis decreases as athlete's foot becomes progressively more severe. In typical cases of dermatophytosis complex, fungus recovery rates are only about 25% to 50%.

The pharmacist should question the patient thoroughly regarding the condition and its characteristics to determine symptoms, extent of disease, previous patient compliance with medications, and any mitigating circumstances (e.g., diabetes or obesity) that might render the patient susceptible. Patients with diabetes, for example, may present with a mixed dermatophytid and monilial infection. In general, it is appropriate to inspect the foot if privacy and sanitary conditions allow, and it is especially appropriate for patients with diabetes.

The most common complaint of patients with tinea pedis is pruritus. However, if fissures are present, particularly between the toes, painful burning and stinging may also occur. If the foot area is abraded, denuded, or inflamed, weeping or oozing may be present in addition to pain. Some patients may merely remark on the bothersome scaling of dry skin, particularly if it has progressed to the soles of the feet. Small vesicular lesions may combine to form a larger bullous eruption marked by pain and irritation. The only symptoms may be brittleness and discoloration of a hypertrophied toenail.

The pharmacist should seek to distinguish tinea pedis from diseases with similar symptoms, such as a bacterial infection, dermatitis, allergic contact dermatitis, and atopic dermatitis. For that reason, the manifestation of these disorders is briefly discussed here. In children, peridigital dermatitis or atopic dermatitis is more common than tinea pedis. Shoe dermatitis is perhaps the most common form of allergic contact dermatitis from clothing. Since 1950, the increased use of rubber and adhesives in footwear has paralleled the increase in reports of shoe dermatitis in the dermatologic and podiatric literature. Contact allergy to accelerators—the chemical compounds used to speed up the processing of rubber used in sponge-rubber insoles for tennis shoes—has also been reported.[22] In addition to accelerators, antioxidants have been implicated as major chemical allergens, and various phenolic resins used in adhesives are also troublesome. The patient is usually unaware that his or her footwear may be causing the problem.

Hyperhidrosis of interdigital spaces and of the sole of the foot is common, as is infection of the toe webs by gram-negative bacteria. In hyperhidrosis, tender vesicles cover the sole of the foot and toes and may be quite painful. The skin generally turns white, erodes, and becomes macerated. This condition is accompanied by a foul foot odor. Infection by gram-negative bacteria is characterized by a soggy wetness of the toe webs and the immediately adjacent skin; the affected tissue is damp and softened. The last toe web (adjacent to the little toe) is the most common area of primary or initial involvement because it is deeper and extends more proximally than the web between the other toes. Furthermore, abundant exocrine sweat glands, a semiocclusive anatomic setting, and the added occlusion provided by footwear enhance development of the disease at this site. The pharmacist must be careful not to confuse this condition with soft corns, which also appear between the fourth and fifth toes.

Asking the patient the following questions will help elicit the information needed to accurately assess the disorder and to recommend the appropriate treatment approach.

Q~ Where is the sore located (on or between the toes or on the sole of the foot)? Is the toenail involved?

A~ Suspect athlete's foot as the cause of the disorder if the toenail is affected. Consider atopic dermatitis, contact dermatitis, athlete's foot, and gram-negative bacterial infection as potential causes if the other mentioned areas are affected.

Q~ Is there any redness, itching, blistering, oozing, scaling, or bleeding from the lesion?

A~ If yes, consider all the disorders mentioned in the preceding question as possible causes of the foot disorder.

Q~ Do you have allergies, asthma, or skin problems?

A~ If yes, suspect atopic dermatitis as a potential cause of the foot disorder.

Q~ Is the condition painful? Is it too uncomfortable to walk?

A~ In either situation, refer the patient to a physician.

Q~ Did the problem begin with the use of new shoes, socks, or soaps?

A~ If yes, suspect contact dermatitis as a possible cause of the foot disorder.

Q~ Do your feet sweat a lot? Do you notice an odor when you take off your shoes? Do your feet sweat more when you wear socks or hosiery made of nylon or other synthetic material?

A~ If yes, consider athlete's foot, hyperhidrosis, and gram-negative bacterial infection as possible causes of the foot disorder.

Q~ Have you tried to treat this problem yourself? If so, how?

A~ Evaluate whether any attempted self-treatments were appropriate and, if so, whether they were implemented correctly. If treatments were inappropriate, recommend appropriate product and/or nondrug measures. If usage was incorrect, advise patient of the proper method. Refer the patient to a physician if product usage was correct but ineffective.

Q~ Did you see your physician about this problem? If so, what did he or she tell you to do? What have you done? Did it help?

A~ If the patient carried out the physician's instructions properly but the symptoms are not resolved, contact the physician to discuss alternative treatments. If the instructions were not carried out, advise the patient of proper technique.

Q~ Is a physician treating you for any other medical condition, such as diabetes, asthma, heart trouble, or circulatory problems?

A~ Advise patients with any condition that requires medical supervision to see their physician for evaluation of the foot disorder. Patients with diabetes and asthma may be immunocompromised. Patients with diabetes or heart or circulatory problems usually have impaired blood circulation in the feet.

Q~ What (other) prescription or nonprescription medications do you take on a routine basis?

A~ Determine whether the patient is using any topical products (e.g., salicylic acid) that, if used improperly, can predispose to fungal infections.

Patient Counseling for Athlete's Foot

Pharmacists should advise patients not to expect dramatic remission of the condition. The onset of symptomatic relief may take several days. Patients should be advised that remission depends on certain factors (e.g., the extent of the affected area and variable patient response to medication). Patients should also be told of the necessity to adhere strictly to the physician-prescribed dosage regimen or to the directions for use on the product label. Patient noncompliance contributes significantly to the failure of topical products in treating tinea pedis. Pharmacists may advise patients or caregivers to continue the medication for a few days beyond the recommended time so they can decrease the risk of relapse. Pharmacists should inform patients of the need for adjunctive protective measures that assist the topical antifungal product in eradicating the fungal infection. Finally, all topical antifungal products may induce various hypersensitivity reactions. Patients should be warned of the signs and symptoms that warrant discontinuation of the product, as well as those that indicate the disorder needs medical attention. The box "Patient Education for Athlete's Foot" lists specific information to provide patients.

Evaluation of Patient Outcomes for Athlete's Foot

The pharmacist should check on the patient's progress preferably 4 weeks after the patient's initial visit. Physical inspection of the affected area is preferable; therefore, a visit to

Patient Education for Athlete's Foot

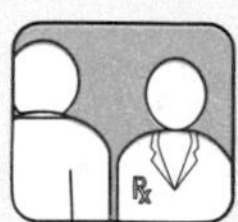

The objectives of self-treatment are to (1) relieve the discomfort of athlete's foot and (2) cure the present infection and prevent recurrences. For patients susceptible to this disorder, practicing good foot hygiene and using antifungal agents daily will help prevent future infections. For most patients, carefully following product instructions and the self-care measures listed below will help ensure optimal therapeutic outcomes.

Nondrug Measures

- Note that proper foot hygiene is required for the drug therapy to be effective. (See Table 36–6.)
- Do not share washcloths or towels with other family members.
- Wash contaminated clothing and towels in hot water.
- If needed, place odor-controlling insoles (e.g., Odor Attackers and Sneaker Snuffers) in casual or athletic shoes. These insoles also provide some support and cushioning for the feet.
- Change insoles routinely every 3–4 months or more often if the condition warrants.

Nonprescription Medications

- Ask a pharmacist for assistance in picking the appropriate antifungal agent or dosage form for your infection. Available agents include clioquinol, clotrimazole, miconazole nitrate, terbinafine, tolnaftate, and undecylenic acid–zinc undecylenate.
- Note that it usually takes 2 to 4 weeks to cure athlete's foot. Some cases may require 4 to 6 weeks of treatment.
- Apply the antifungal to clean, dry feet in the morning and the evening. Massage the medication into the feet. Note that creams and solutions are easier to work into the skin and, therefore, are probably more effective treatment forms.
- Avoid contact of the product with the eyes.
- After applying the product, wash hands thoroughly with soap and water.
- Note that topical antifungals may cause itching, redness, and irritation.
- Note that clioquinol may interfere with thyroid function tests.
- Note that tolnaftate may sting slightly.
- Note that undiluted solutions of undecylenic acid–zinc undecylenate may cause transient stinging when applied to broken skin because of its isopropyl alcohol content.
- When medication is applied to pressure areas of the foot, where the horny skin layer is thicker than normal, apply a keratolytic agent (e.g., Whitfield's ointment) to the affected area first to help the antifungal penetrate the skin.
- If oozing lesions are present, apply aluminum acetate solution (1:40) to the foot before applying the antifungal:
  - —Soak the whole foot in an aluminum acetate solution for 20 minutes up to three times a day (every 6 to 8 hours), or apply the solution to the affected area in the form of a wet dressing.
  - —Note that aluminum acetate solution (Burow's solution) or modified Burow's solution is available for immediate use in solution or in forms (powder packets, powder, and effervescent tablets) for dilution with water.
  - —Avoid contact of the eyes with the product.
  - —To avoid skin damage, use the solution less than 1 week. Discontinue use of the solution if inflammatory lesions appear or worsen.
- For the wet, soggy type of athlete's foot, apply to or soak foot in aluminum acetate solution (1:40) before applying the antifungal.
  - —Soak feet with aluminum acetate solution (1:40) twice daily until the odor, wetness, and whiteness abate. After that, soak once daily to control the symptoms.
  - —If deep fissures are present in the skin, use a more dilute solution of aluminum acetate solution for initial treatment.

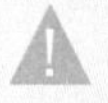 Discontinue use of the product and contact a physician if itching or swelling occurs, or if the infection worsens.

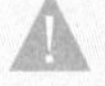 Consult a physician if the infection does not improve after 2 to 4 weeks of treatment.

the pharmacy should be scheduled. If the disorder is not resolved but shows improvement, recommend continuing treatment for 2 more weeks. If the disorder has not improved or has worsened, refer the patient to a physician for more aggressive therapy.

Bunions

Pathophysiology of Bunions

The hallux, or great toe, along with the inner side of the foot, provides the elasticity and mobility needed to walk or run. Thus, the hallux is a dynamic body part. However, this mobility causes several anatomic disorders associated with the foot, such as hallux valgus in which the great toe is angled toward the outer toes. Prolonged pressure caused by hallux valgus may result in pressure over the angulation of the metatarsophalangeal joint of the big toe, causing inflammatory swelling of the bursa and/or exostosis over that joint. (See Figure 36–6). This process may result in bunion formation as shown in Figure 36–1.

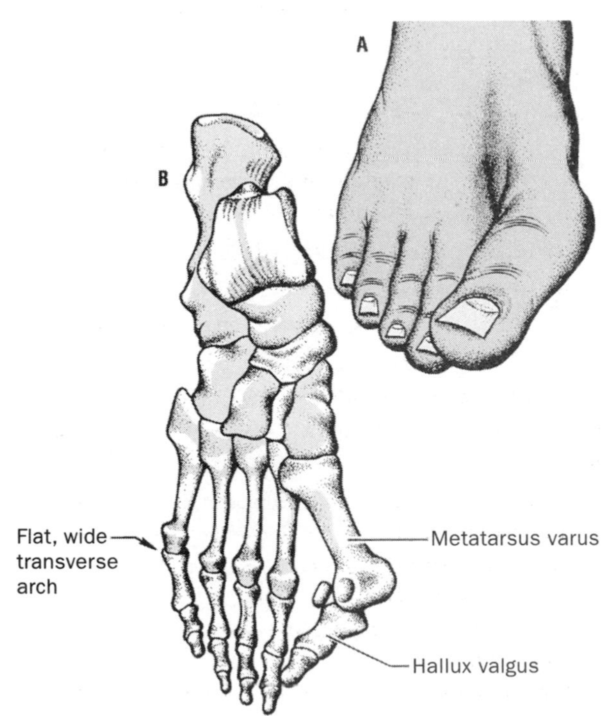

Figure 36–6 A and B Two views of hallux valgus: A, gross representation of hallux valgus; B, bone structure of hallux valgus.

Etiology of Bunions

Bunions can be caused by various conditions. Pressure may result from the manner in which a person sits, walks, or stands, but pressure from a tight-fitting shoe over a period of time generally aggravates the condition. Friction on the toes from bone malformations (wide heads or lateral bending) is also a major factor in bunion production. Some individuals have a hereditary predisposition to the development of bunions. Vigorous exercise such as running can cause bunions or exacerbate existing bunions.

Signs and Symptoms of Bunions

Bunions are usually asymptomatic but may become quite painful, swollen, and tender. The bunion itself usually is covered by an extensive keratinous overgrowth.

Treatment of Bunions

Corrective steps to alleviate bunions often depend on the degree of discomfort. In some cases, corrective surgery is necessary.

Treatment Outcomes

The goal in self-treating bunions is to decrease irritation of the affected area.

General Treatment Approach

Bunions are not amenable to topical drug therapy, nor is the routine, chronic use of oral nonprescription analgesics, particularly ibuprofen, suggested. Management of the bunion should address the cause, such as tight-fitting or high-heeled shoes, excessive pronation of the foot, or a previous injury. Thus, self-treatment includes properly fitted shoes, a wide toe box, avoidance of high-heeled shoes, and protective padding (e.g., bunion pads), as well as short-term anti-inflammatory drug therapy. Self-treatment only relieves the swelling caused by shoe friction; therefore, well-fitted shoes should be worn at all times to prevent subsequent flares of inflammation. If shoe adjustments fail to alleviate pain, referral to a properly trained health care professional is indicated.

Patients with diabetes complaining of bunions should be immediately referred to an endocrinologist and a podiatrist. The presence of a discharge or bleeding from the bunion also precludes self-treatment.

Nonpharmacologic Therapy

Selection of Footwear

See Table 36–1 for guidelines on selecting properly fitted footwear.

Bunion Pads/Cushions

Topical nonprescription padding (e.g., moleskin) can be helpful and may be all that is necessary to decrease the irritation of footwear. Eventually, padding can help decrease inflammation around the bunion area. Before the protective pad is applied, the foot should be bathed and thoroughly dried. The pad should then be cut into a shape that conforms to the bunion. If the intent is to relieve the pressure from the center of the bunion area, the pad should be cut to surround the bunion. Precut pads are available for immediate patient use. Constant skin contact with adhesive-backed pads should generally be avoided, however, unless recommended by a podiatrist or physician.

For patients who are allergic to adhesives, a nonmedicated, self-adhesive bunion cushion (i.e., Bunion Guard) is commercially available. One advantage of this product is that it protects the bunion and can be easily removed before showering. The cushion, made of a soft polymer gel, can then be reapplied for up to 3 months onto the bunion after showering. Another advantage of Bunion Guard is that it does not contain an adhesive backing that can be irritating to the patient's skin. The outer surface is smooth and not prone to snagging socks and hosiery.

Larger footwear may be necessary to compensate for the space taken up by the pad; in fact, not increasing shoe size appropriately may cause pressure in other areas. Also, protective pads should not be used on bunions when the skin is broken or blistered. Abraded skin should receive palliative treatment before pads are applied. If symptoms persist, the pharmacist should recommend that these patients consult a podiatrist or orthopedist.

Patient Assessment of Bunions

The assessment questions in the section "Patient Assessment of Corns and Calluses" are appropriate for triage of bunions. Specific information the pharmacist needs to obtain include where the lesion is located, how long it has been a problem, whether it occurs with specific footwear, and how painful it is.

Patient Counseling for Bunions

The pharmacist should stress to the patient that effective long-term "treatment" of bunions is to remove the source of irritation. Patients who do not achieve permanent relief by changing footwear should see a podiatrist or orthopedist to determine whether anatomic defects are causing bunions. The pharmacist should explain the proper short-term use of bunion pads and cushions to patients who wish to use them. The box "Patient Education for Bunions" lists specific information to provide patients.

Evaluation of Patient Outcomes for Bunions

Depending on the severity of the irritation, bunions that are not caused by biomechanical defects of the foot may take a few weeks to resolve. The pharmacist should telephone or have the patient return after 2 to 3 weeks to determine whether wearing new shoes and/or using bunion cushions or pads has eliminated the discomfort. If the patient is still experiencing discomfort, medical referral is appropriate.

Tired, Aching Feet

An estimated two-thirds of Americans suffer from tired, aching feet (the most common foot problem). In addition, 21 million adults are estimated to suffer from heel pain. People simply do not realize the daily abuse their feet must endure. With every step taken (repeated, on average, between

Patient Education for Bunions

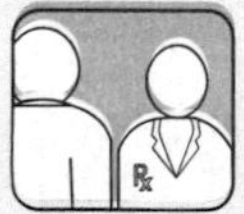

The objective of self-treatment is to decrease irritation of the bunion until the cause is corrected. For patients whose bunions are not related to anatomic defects of the foot, carefully following product instructions and the self-care measures listed below will help ensure optimal therapeutic outcomes.

- To help prevent footwear from rubbing the feet, make sure footwear fits properly. (See Table 36–1.)
- To decrease inflammation around existing bunions, apply adhesive-backed moleskin padding or a polymer gel cushion (e.g., Bunion Guard) to the bunion.
- If the skin of the bunion is broken or blistered, treat the abraded skin and wait until it heals before applying bunion pads.
- Before applying the protective pad, bathe and thoroughly dry the foot.
- Cut the pad into a shape that conforms to the bunion. Cut the pad large enough to surround the bunion.
- Note that constant exposure to the adhesive of moleskin pads may irritate the skin. If such irritation occurs, stop wearing the pads.
- If you are allergic to adhesives, use Bunion Guard. Remove the cushion before showering and reapply afterward. The cushion can be worn for up to 3 months.
- Note that larger footwear may be needed to compensate for the space taken up by the pad or cushion.

If the irritation persists after 2 to 3 weeks of implementing self-care measures, consult a podiatrist or orthopedist about the problem.

8000 to 10,000 times each day), gravity-induced pressure of up to twice the body's weight bears down on each foot, releasing powerful shocks of energy that the foot's natural padding must struggle to absorb. In an unpadded shoe, the shock as the foot strikes the ground is absorbed throughout the foot, ankle, leg, and back. This shock can fatigue muscles, resulting in tired, aching feet and/or back pain.

Etiology/Pathophysiology of Tired, Aching Feet

Aching feet can be caused by increased frequency of standing, walking (especially on hard surfaces), age-related erosion of the fat padding on the bottom of the foot, circulatory or neurologic disorders, and poorly fitting/inappropriate footwear.

The cause of heel pain is difficult to determine, which can make treatment prolonged and expensive. The two most common types of heel pain are heel spurs (i.e., bony growths on the underside of the heel bone) and plantar fasciitis. Heel spurs are the result of strained foot muscles and the wearing away of the fat tissue surrounding the heel bone. Incorrect walking or running technique, excessive running, poorly fitted shoes, being overweight or experiencing a rapid weight gain, and aging are common contributors to this condition. Heel pain can be an early sign of systemic arthritis.

Plantar fasciitis is often caused by high arches, flat feet, or repetitive foot stress during athletic activity. This disorder can be determined by the patient's description of the pain and its occurrence. Usually, the pain occurs during the day's first steps or when standing up after sitting. The sensation on the bottom of the heel is quite painful.

Treatment of Tired, Aching Feet

Treatment Outcomes

The goal in self-treating tired, aching feet is to provide additional support and shock absorbance for the feet so that foot pain/fatigue is reduced.

General Treatment Approach

The first measure to avoid tired, aching feet is to use well-fitted footwear that has sufficient padding and cushioning. (See Table 36–1.) Wearing sport-specific shoes with good arch support (e.g., running/jogging shoes) is an excellent measure for preventing heel pain.

However, active people or those who must stand for prolonged periods during the day may need to take additional measures. Some active individuals, though, prefer to wear stylish rather than orthopedic shoes. Unfortunately, many stylish shoe models are not built to provide adequate support and cushioning; however, various shoe inserts are available to enhance the comfort of most well-fitting shoes. Other self-treatment measures include replacing worn shoes or heel pads, using a night splint,[23] strapping or taping the arch, decreasing the amount of weight-bearing activity, and, if necessary, entering a weight reduction program. Anti-inflammatory treatment, including ice applications, is also appropriate. (See the section "Cryotherapy" under "Treatment of Exercise-Induced Injuries.") When self-treatment fails, referral to an appropriate health care professional for evaluation of possible bony malalignments and possible orthotic therapy is indicated.

Nonpharmacologic Therapy

Full-Shoe Inserts

Full-shoe inserts, which can provide cushioning and can absorb shock, are available in various sizes and thicknesses to accommodate most individuals. Advanced shoe inserts are now available with enhanced shock-absorbing capability. For example, Back Guard is clinically proven to decrease the incidence of lower back pain associated with shock from walking. The individual who is selecting an insert must realize that the insert should conform to the type of shoe worn. Thus, because a thick shoe insert may alter the fit of a woman's pump, a thin insole would be preferable.

Partial Insoles

Partial insoles are preferred when cushioning or support is desired in a certain portion of the shoe. For example, metatarsal arch supports, which fit into the ball-of-foot region of a woman's shoe, help lift the arch behind the toes to alleviate pain associated with the spreading of the foot, a condition that occurs with increasing age. For women who wear high-heeled shoes, inserts (i.e., Toe Squish Preventer cushions) are available to prevent the toes from becoming cramped in the pointed-toe box. A final example is the arch support insert intended to cushion and support painful longitudinal arches.

Heel Cups/Cushions

Depending on the location and extent of the pain, a heel cup or heel cushion may be indicated. For example, a heel cushion might be appropriate when the pain is confined to the bottom of the heel. The cushion can support the entire heel as it elevates the sensitive area to prevent further irritation. Alternatively, when the pain is widespread and diffuse, a heel cup might be more appropriate. Heel cups help relieve the pain caused by the breakdown of the heel's natural padding or intense athletic activity. Heel cups and cushions should be made of a lightweight, nonslip material that easily fits into any shoe, including athletic shoes.

Patient Assessment of Tired, Aching Feet

The assessment questions in the section "Patient Assessment of Corns and Calluses" are appropriate for triage of a patient who complains of tired, aching feet; bunions; and blisters. In addition, the pharmacist must determine whether the pain affects the soles of the feet, the heels, or the entire foot. The pharmacist must also evaluate lifestyle factors (e.g., occupa-

Patient Education for Tired, Aching Feet

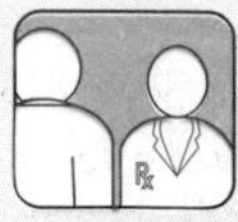

The objectives of self-treatment are to (1) reduce impact on the feet by providing additional support and shock absorbance and (2) relieve foot discomfort. For most patients, carefully following product instructions and the self-care measures listed below will help ensure optimal therapeutic outcomes.

- To reduce friction of the feet and impact on weight-bearing parts of the feet, wear well-fitted footwear that has sufficient padding and cushioning. (See Table 36–1 for guidelines on selecting footwear.)
- Consider other measures to further decrease impact on the feet, such as decreasing the length of time you stand or exercise, switching to exercises that have less effect on the feet, and, if necessary, losing weight.
- To relieve swelling or discomfort, apply an ice bag or cold wrap to the affected area. (See Table 36–10.)
- Choose a full-shoe insert when the entire foot aches. Make sure the insert conforms to the shoe. For example, choose a thin insole for a woman's pump and a thicker insole for a sneaker.
- Use partial insoles to cushion or support a certain portion of the foot, such as the ball of the foot, the arch, or the toes.
- Use a heel cushion for pain confined to the bottom of the heel.
- Use a heel cup when the pain is widespread and diffuse.

tion, daily exercise, footwear) and underlying pathology (e.g., circulatory or neurologic disorders). If underlying pathology is suspected, the pharmacist should refer middle-aged or older patients to a physician or podiatrist for initial evaluation.

Patient Counseling for Tired, Aching Feet

The pharmacist can play an integral role in counseling patients on preventing and treating foot disorders caused by friction and excessive impact. The cornerstone of preventing such disorders is selecting the appropriate footwear. If the disorder still persists, the pharmacist can help patients select in-shoe supports and can advise them of other measures to reduce weight-bearing activities. The box "Patient Education for Tired, Aching Feet" lists specific information to provide patients.

Evaluation of Patient Outcomes for Tired, Aching Feet

Resolution of pain in the soles or heels of the feet depends on the patient and the longevity of the foot problem. The pharmacist should telephone or have the patient return to the pharmacy after a few weeks to determine whether the use of new shoes and/or in-shoe supports has eliminated the discomfort. If the symptoms persist, the patient should see a podiatrist for evaluation.

Exercise-Induced Foot Injuries

The pharmacist should be aware of the problem of exercise-induced foot injuries, particularly those caused by running, jogging, or other high-impact physical activities. (See Figure 36–7.) Often, in their rush to recapture physical fitness, individuals fail to take certain precautions and dive headlong into a strenuous exercise program. Yet jogging, aerobic dance, and running are not without risk. One study documented that several exercise enthusiasts have died from heart attacks while jogging.[24] Some people, especially those older than 35 years, should consult a physician before embarking on a fitness program, and so should patients with high blood pressure or a family history of heart disease or diabetes. Ultimately, a vigorous walking program may be a more prudent form of exercise for middle-aged, unconditioned individuals than jogging or running. Walking may minimize the potential orthopedic problems described below that can result from more strenuous forms of exercise.

Types of Exercise-Induced Injuries

Patients who prefer vigorous exercise can sometimes prevent injuries by following the guidelines in Table 36–1 to make sure athletic shoes fit properly. They may also want to consider using the shoe inserts discussed previously to provide additional cushioning and/or support for their feet. Once an exercise-induced injury occurs, patients can self-treat some of the injuries with cryotherapy or compression bandages as described in the section "Treatment of Exercise-Induced Injuries." Systemic analgesics can also relieve the pain and inflammation of minor foot injuries. (See Chapter 3, "Headache and Muscle and Joint Pain," for dosing information.)

Shin Splints

The term *shin splint* is used generically to describe all the pain emanating from below the knee and above the ankle. Shin splints are an overuse phenomenon that occurs in runners or walkers who use hard surfaces. This condition may also oc-

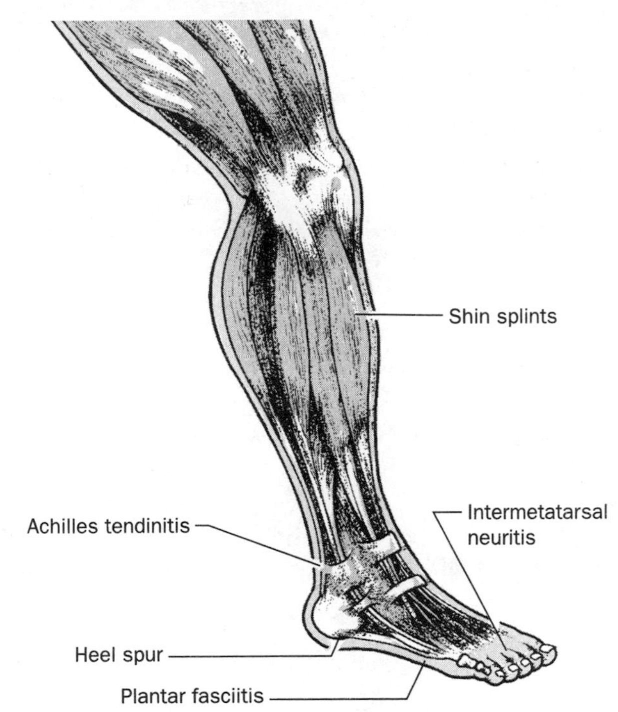

Figure 36–7 Selected foot and leg injuries associated with excessive impact shock.

cur from running on a banked track or on the sloped shoulder of a road, from wearing improper footwear, or from overstriding.

The typical complaint of a runner with shin splints is pain that's in the medial lower third of the shin and that seems to increase gradually with exercise. The patient may admit that soreness begins after running; with a continual running program, the pain will eventually occur during and after running. Complaints of pain when walking or climbing stairs may indicate a serious case of shin splints. If the discomfort is located on the anterior lateral aspect of the shin; is described as a cramping, burning tightness; and repeatedly occurs at the same distance or time during a run, then self-treatment may be ill-advised. The pharmacist should refer the runner to a physician, podiatrist, or physical therapist.

Rest and cryotherapy (e.g., an ice bag or a cold compression wrap) to the painful area are good initial treatments. Aspirin or ibuprofen can be used to relieve pain and to reduce tissue inflammation. However, the use of analgesics to suppress pain or to increase endurance during a workout is not recommended.

Stress Fracture

Stress fracture, also known as march, army, or fatigue fracture, may be encountered in runners, especially those who run repetitively on hard, inflexible surfaces. This injury usually involves the long bones of the foot or leg. It is not an overt break of the bone but rather an alteration in the architecture of the normal bone.

The onset of pain is associated with runners who drastically change aspects of their training routine (e.g., running surface, speed, or distance). Although the pain begins insidiously, the individual with a stress fracture will often complain of deep pain in the lower leg with an area of extreme tenderness. A misconception among runners is that they can "work out" the problem by continuing to jog. Runners must be instructed that pain is the body's communication mechanism to indicate that enough is enough and that something is abnormal. Treatment for stress fractures is complete rest from running, sometimes for 4 to 6 weeks, or longer if the tibia is involved.

Achilles Tendinitis

Running on hills or the beach, wearing improper footwear (e.g., running and jogging in shoes designed for racquet sports), and moving with excessive pronation (rolling in of the feet) are common causes of Achilles tendinitis. Yet this condition is not caused solely by running. It may be an early sign of arthritis or rupture of a tendon; the exact cause of the problem is difficult to distinguish. Thus, Achilles tendinitis should be referred to a physician, podiatrist, or physical therapist.

By definition, Achilles tendinitis is a painful inflammation about the Achilles tendon. However, it may not show the classic signs of inflammation, such as pain, erythema, increased skin temperature, or swelling. Typical symptoms are posterior heel pain, which is worse in the morning when getting out of bed, at the beginning of an exercise session, and when walking after prolonged sitting.

The best treatment is prevention with careful progression of training and replacement of worn footwear. Bony malalignments leading to excessive pronation should be accounted for with orthotic therapy. An orthotic device approximately positions the foot. The properties of shoe inserts (e.g., flexible or rigid) vary; the choice of insert should be based on specific treatment objectives. Shoe inserts can be custom-made or purchased off the shelf. Arch supports are intended to provide buttressing for the foot.

Symptomatic self-treatment may consist of rest, new shoes, ice applications, appropriate NSAID use, physician-prescribed temporary heel lifts, and careful calf-stretching exercises.

Blisters

Ill-fitting footwear and inappropriate hosiery can often cause or contribute to the development of blisters. When shoes are worn while running, the shoe can place excessive pressure on a specific area of the skin between the stratum corneum and stratum lucidum. Fluid quickly accumulates at this site, often on the heel, the ball of the foot, and the ends or tops of the toes. Running barefoot can also cause blisters.

Again, prevention is the key to treating blisters. Cotton or woolen socks are preferred for running. The runner can wear two pairs of socks with ordinary talcum powder sprinkled between them. Some individuals with soft skin will continue to develop blisters until their skin toughens enough to withstand friction during running. Application of compound tincture of benzoin or of a flexible collodion product (e.g., New Skin) will help toughen the skin. Applying topical antibiotics to broken skin can prevent secondary bacterial infection. (See Chapter 35, "Minor Wounds and Skin Infections," for discussion of first-aid antibiotics and antiseptics.)

Ankle Sprains

The typical mechanism of lateral ligament injury to the ankle is through rotation of the body over the fixed foot. This injury occurs most often in contact sports in which the foot remains stationary while the body is unintentionally rotated. The incidence of ankle sprains during jogging and running is low because runners usually do not take sharp diagonal cuts. However, stepping on an unnoticed stone or curb edge may also result in an ankle sprain.

The differential diagnosis of an ankle fracture from a sprained ankle is impossible without an X-ray. Rest, ice, compression, elevation (RICE) therapy is well accepted as the most appropriate immediate treatment for an ankle sprain. It remains controversial whether cold application without elevation is helpful or harmful. Regardless, treatment for a sprained ankle should be initiated as soon as possible. Sometimes an ankle sprain is perceived as a minor problem, even by trained professionals. However, the severity of ligament damage can vary widely, and an extensive ligament rupture that has been given insufficient treatment may result in a permanently unstable ankle.

Intermetatarsal Neuritis

Intermetatarsal neuritis is characterized by pain and numbness between the toes, most often within the third interspace. The cause is linked to the foot jamming forward into the shoe without enough space to accommodate the foot. Nerves become inflamed when compressed or caught in the area between the metatarsal heads and digital bases.

The solution is correct-fitting shoes with the addition of a metatarsal pad or orthotic device. Lacing of the shoe can be modified by skipping the bottom two eyelets, which will provide additional room for the ball of the foot. If the pain persists or worsens after taking these measures, the patient should consult a podiatrist. Worsening of the pain could indicate development of a neuroma.

Toenail Loss

Blisters under the toenail occur as a result of not keeping the toenails trimmed and of running in poorly fitted shoes. Long toenails catch on the sock or inside the shoe toe box, particularly when the individual is running downhill. This pressure lifts the nail and separates it from the nail bed; then blood accumulates under the nail. This condition is very painful and can result in the temporary loss of the toenail. In the latter instance, the patient should be referred to a podiatrist.

Runner's Bunion

See the section "Bunions."

Heel Pain

See the section "Tired, Aching Feet."

Treatment of Exercise-Induced Injuries

Treatment Outcomes

The best way to self-treat exercise-induced foot problems is to rest the injured foot and to institute measures that prevent further injury. If an injury is painful and/or the skin is broken, self-treatment should also include relieving the pain and/or preventing secondary bacterial infection.

General Treatment Approach

Measures to prevent exercise-induced injuries entail using proper footwear, running on the proper surface, using correct posture (i.e., running erect), and stretching muscles before exercising. Most running injuries can be successfully treated with measures for shoe modifications and in-shoe supports as discussed in the section "Treatment of Tired, Aching Feet." Measures to correct leg length discrepancies and modified training methods may also be needed.[25]

If the runner or jogger has an injured leg or foot, that activity must occasionally be interrupted to allow the injured leg or foot to rest. Relative rest (i.e., avoiding activities that produce the symptoms) is often indicated, but some runners resist this suggestion. A number of continuous days of high-intensity workouts cause accumulated fatigue and microtrauma. For this reason, the body must be allowed to recuperate after vigorous exercise. Although some runners believe that the more mileage logged per week, the better their running ability, the incidence of acquired injuries among runners increases dramatically after 25 to 30 miles per week. An increased injury rate is observed in runners who increase mileage too rapidly. A good training program entails "hard-easy" days, with extended mileage on 3 or 4 days per week and light, easy workouts on the remaining days. When an injury occurs, the pharmacist should encourage alternative exercise modes, such as swimming or bicycling (stationary or outdoor), which would allow the serious runner to maintain aerobic conditioning despite missing regular exercise.

If the injury warrants it, the pharmacist can instruct the patient on selecting and using nonprescription accessories (e.g., a compression ice wrap, ice bags, compression bandages, arch supports, or heel cushions) that will alleviate injuries or problems.

Exercise-induced injuries that are excluded from self-treatment include Achilles tendinitis, shin splints, stress fractures, and intermetatarsal neuritis. Patients with diabetes, peripheral vascular disease, or arthritis who suffer any type of foot injury should be referred to a physician or podiatrist.

Nonpharmacologic Therapy

Athletic Footwear

Shoes can be a powerful tool for manipulating human movement and can greatly influence the healing of injured tissues in both positive and negative ways. The importance of appropriate footwear has been reported by McPoil et al.[26] These authors demonstrated that a well-designed shoe, even without an orthotic, can favorably alter the center-of-pressure recordings in individuals with foot deformities. Conversely, inappropriate shoes may be problematic, as observed by Frey et al.,[27] who reported that most women surveyed indicated that they wore shoes too small for their feet and had foot pain with deformity.

A hallmark of the fitness shoe industry and the sports medicine community for decades has been that "good shoes can prevent injuries." Although shoe manufacturers modify their shoes annually with high-tech features purported to prevent injury, little or no change in the frequency and type of running injuries was reported for the period 1977 to 1987.[28]

Identifying the right shoe store and finding a knowledgeable salesperson can ease the task of selecting proper footwear. (See Table 36–1 for guidelines on choosing properly fitted footwear.) The owners or managers of independently owned and operated shoe stores are more likely to offer this kind of expertise. Although shopping at such stores may cost more, individuals with special needs should seek special service when searching for shoes. The Prescription Footwear Association in Columbia, Maryland, has a certification process for shoe sales personnel (pedorthist) and can provide a list of members.

Shoe manufacturers offer various types of shoes for different activities (e.g., running, walking, racquetball sports). Injuries and problems often develop when sport-specific shoes are used for the inappropriate activity; for example, the heel on tennis shoes is too low for jogging. Cross-training shoes are an attempt to provide features generic to many athletic activities. Pharmacists should advise individuals to use proper equipment to prevent sport-related injuries. Although the depth of the toe box in extra-depth shoes and comfort shoes is similar to that of athletic shoes,[29] only athletic shoes should be used for exercise activities.

Shoes are designed to provide stability and cushioning. Thus, as soon as a shoe becomes worn, it should be replaced. Studies on running shoes have demonstrated that the midsole of the shoe, which helps to reduce the impact on the foot by cushioning or absorbing shock, is the part of the shoe that fatigues first. Midsoles constructed of ethyl vinyl acetate or polyurethane lose 50% of their ability to attenuate force in as little as 250 to 500 miles of running.[30] Individuals with a history of stress fractures, osteoarthritis, or rigid high arches should not wait until the outer sole wears through before replacing shoes. It is wise to replace shoes early and often.

The Running Surface

The convenience, safety, and preferences of the runner often dictate the running surface (e.g., concrete sidewalk, grassy surface, or dirt shoulder of roads). Because hard surfaces have no give and provide little shock-absorbing capacity, they cause intense shock to the legs, feet, and back. Grassy surfaces, however, are often irregular, and the runner can easily incur a sprained ankle. Running on a sloping or banked surface may cause the foot to rotate excessively and may place additional stress on the tendons and ligaments of the leg and foot. Uphill running places a strain on the Achilles tendon and muscles of the lower back; downhill running places a lot of impact on the heel. The ideal running surface is relatively smooth, level, and resilient.

The ideal surface for a walker should also be relatively smooth, level, and resilient. Hard, inflexible surfaces should be avoided as much as possible. A walker who wants to increase energy expenditure may try walking on dirt or sand; such surfaces can boost energy expenditure by as much as one-third. Similarly, walking on a mild, 14-degree slope requires more muscle power than walking on a straight, flat surface. However, walkers who become overzealous on these surfaces can encounter the same problems (e.g., sprained ankle) that runners encounter.

Compression Bandages

Typically, a compression bandage (e.g., Ace) is used for an ankle sprain or knee sprain. If a compression bandage is to be used, the width of bandage needed depends on the injury site. For example, a foot or an ankle requires a 2.5- to 3-inch bandage. Table 36–9 describes the proper method of applying this type of bandage.

Cryotherapy

Applying cold compresses to an injury such as a muscle sprain anesthetizes the area and decreases the pain. Ice bags or cold wraps are useful for cold application. If an ice bag is used, the English type, which is identified by its commercial cloth material, is preferred because the patient does not have to wrap a towel around it to protect the skin. Cold packs are available as either one-use products (e.g., Faultless Instant Cold Pack) or those intended for multiple use. Table 36–10 describes the proper method of cold application to injuries.

Patient Assessment of Exercise-Induced Injuries

The pharmacist may be called on to play a triage role in treating an exercise-induced injury to the foot. Asking the patient the following questions will help elicit the information needed to accurately assess the injury and to recommend the appropriate treatment approach.

Table 36–9

Application Guidelines for Compression Bandages

- Choose the appropriate size of bandage for the injured body part. Purchase a product designed for the appropriate body part if you are unsure of the size.
- Unwind about 12 to 18 inches of bandage at a time, and allow the bandage to relax.
- If ice is also being applied to the injured area, soak the bandage in water to aid the transfer of cold. (See Table 36–10.)
- Wrap the injured area by overlapping the previous layer of bandage by about one-third to one-half its width.
- Tightly wrap the point most distal from the injury. For example, if the ankle is injured, begin wrapping just above the toes.
- Decrease the tightness of the bandage as you continue to wrap. (Follow package directions on how far to extend the bandage past the injury.) If the bandage feels tight or uncomfortable or if circulation is impaired, remove the compression bandage and rewrap it. Cold or swollen toes and fingers would indicate a bandage is too tight.
- After using the bandage, wash it in lukewarm, soapy water; do not scrub it. Rinse the bandage thoroughly and allow to air dry on a flat surface.
- Roll up the bandage to prevent wrinkles, and store it in a cool, dry place. Do not iron the bandage to remove wrinkles.

Q~ What parts of your body are affected? The toes, soles of the feet, heels, shins, or back?

A~ Try to determine the type and extent of the injury from the location of the pain or discomfort. Refer patients with suspected Achilles tendinitis, shin splints, stress fractures, and intermetatarsal neuritis to a podiatrist or physician.

Q~ Is the discomfort getting progressively worse?

A~ Advise patient to stop running to allow the injured area to heal. Suggest alternative athletic activities that reduce impact to the feet (e.g., swimming or bicycling). Find out whether the patient is wearing the appropriate type of athletic footwear and whether the shoes are properly fitted.

Q~ Has the discomfort reached a plateau level that continues to affect your running/jogging performance?

A~ If yes, a long-standing injury is indicated. Refer the patient to a podiatrist or physician.

Q~ Is the discomfort more frequent and severe while you are running? Is it present while not running?

A~ If the discomfort occurs primarily during running, suspect the patient's footwear is causing the problem. Determine whether the patient is using running shoes and, if so, whether they fit properly.

Q~ Is the discomfort causing you to compensate and to develop additional injuries?

Table 36–10

Guidelines for Applying Cold Compresses

Ice Bag Method

- Fill the ice bag one-half to two-thirds capacity with crushed or shaved ice if possible. These forms of ice will ensure greater contact with the injured body part.
- If needed, break ice into walnut-sized pieces with no jagged edges. An overfilled bag will be difficult to apply because it will not rest on the contour of the body area.
- After filling the bag, squeeze out trapped air. Then dry the outside of the bag and check for leaks.
- Bind the injured body part with a wet elastic wrap, and then apply the ice bag. The wet wrap aids transfer of cold to the injured area.
- If the ankle is being treated, keep it in a dorsiflexed position (foot toward the nose) when it is wrapped in the elastic bandage.
- Apply the ice bag to the specific body part.
- To avoid tissue damage, apply the ice bag for 10 minutes and then remove it for 10 minutes.
- Follow this procedure three to four times a day.
- Replace the ice every 2 to 4 hours.
- Continue the cryotherapy for 24 to 72 hours, depending on the severity of the injury. For ankle injuries, continue this therapy for 48 to 72 hours because maximum swelling of ankle sprains occurs within 48 hours of the injury.
- Before storing the ice bag, drain it and allow it to air dry. If possible, turn it inside out for more efficient drying. Cap the bag, and store it in a cool, dry place.

Cold Wraps

- To activate the single-use cold pack, squeeze the middle of the pack to burst the bubble. This action initiates an endothermic reaction of ammonium nitrate, water, and special additives.
- For a reusable cold wrap (cold pack or gel pack), store it in the freezer for 2 hours. Do not put the cloth cover in the freezer.
- Remove the cold wrap from the freezer, insert it in the cloth cover, and apply it to the injured body part.
- If the cold wrap is uncomfortable, remove it for a minute or two and then reapply it.
- Alternate application of the cold wrap as described above (10 minutes on; 10 minutes off) three to four times a day for 24 to 48 hours.
- After use, store the cold wrap in the freezer.
- Although some gel packs are nontoxic, keep all cold wraps out of the reach of children.

A~ If yes, refer injuries of this severity to a podiatrist.

Q~ Have attempts at self-treatment (e.g., new shoes, a change of running surface, or a change in training intensity) failed to relieve your symptoms?

A~ If yes, refer the patient to a podiatrist for evaluation of possible underlying biomechanical defects of the foot.

Patient Education for Exercise-Induced Injuries

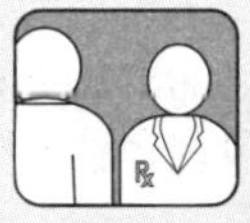

The objectives of self-treatment are to (1) rest the injured foot or limb to allow healing, (2) relieve discomfort, and (3) take measures to prevent further injury. For most patients, carefully following product instructions and the self-care measures listed below will help ensure optimal therapeutic outcomes.

- When a leg or foot injury occurs, rest the injured limb. If desired, perform other types of exercise, such as swimming or bicycling (stationary or outdoor), which do not put a great deal of force on the feet.
- Take the following actions to prevent exercise-induced injuries:
  —Stretch muscles before exercising.
  —Choose sport-specific shoes with good arch support for athletic activities.
  —Run or walk on a relatively smooth, level, and resilient surface.
  —Keep the back straight when running.

Shin Splints

- Rest the feet, and apply an ice bag or a cold wrap to the painful area. (See Table 36–10.)
- If desired, take aspirin or ibuprofen to relieve pain and to reduce tissue inflammation.
- Do not use analgesics to suppress pain or to increase your endurance during a workout.

If the discomfort becomes a cramping, burning tightness, which repeatedly occurs at the same distance or time during a run, see a physician, podiatrist, or physical therapist.

Blisters

- To prevent blisters during running, wear cotton or woolen socks. If desired, wear two pairs of socks with ordinary talcum powder sprinkled between them.
- Apply compound tincture of benzoin or a flexible collodion product (e.g., New Skin) to help toughen the skin.
- If blisters break, apply a first-aid antibiotic to the broken skin to prevent secondary bacterial infection.

Ankle Sprains

- Although maximum swelling will not occur for 48 hours, begin treatment as soon as possible.
- Stay off the injured foot, wrap a compression bandage around the ankle, apply ice, and elevate the ankle. (See Tables 36–9 and 36–10 for guidelines on applying compression bandages and ice.)

If swelling persists after 7 days, see a physician.

Toenail Blisters/Loss

- To prevent blisters under the toenail, keep toenails trimmed and run in properly fitted shoes.

If the toenail is lost, see a physician for proper treatment.

Patient Counseling for Exercise-Induced Injuries

Although a sports enthusiast is likely to resist such advice, the pharmacist should encourage the patient to rest the injured foot or limb and to allow it to heal. The pharmacist should explain measures to prevent recurrences of the patient's particular injury. When rest alone does not relieve foot discomfort, the pharmacist should explain the proper use of oral analgesics, compression bandages, and cryotherapy. At the time of purchase, the pharmacist should review with the patient the correct procedure for wrapping, which is also described on the bandage package. If there is reason to believe the patient may cause further injury through inappropriate use of a compression bandage, the pharmacist should just recommend elevating the body part and applying an ice pack or, if warranted by the severity of the injury, consulting a physician. The box "Patient Education for Exercise-Induced Injuries" lists specific information to provide patients.

Evaluation of Patient Outcomes for Exercise-Induced Injuries

The pharmacist should telephone patients with shin splints or ankle sprains 7 days after cryotherapy or other anti-inflammatory therapy is started to find out whether the symptoms are resolved. If symptoms of swelling and/or pain persist, referral to a podiatrist or physician is appropriate. Patients with blisters of the feet or under the toenail should also be reevaluated after 7 days of the recommended therapy. If signs of infection are present or if the toenail has separated from the nail bed, the patient should see a physician for further treatment.

Other Foot Disorders

Pharmacists are in a position to advise patients on self-treatment and prevention of ingrown toenails, a common foot problem. Frostbite—a less frequent but nonetheless potentially serious condition that often involves the feet—is another area in which pharmacists can educate patients and consumers about preventive measures.

Ingrown Toenails

An ingrown toenail occurs when a section of nail presses into the soft tissue of the nail groove. The nail curves into the flesh of the toe corners and becomes embedded in the surrounding soft tissue of the toe, causing pain. Swelling, inflammation, and ulceration are secondary complications that can arise from this condition.

The frequent cause of ingrown toenails is incorrect trimming of the nails. The correct method is to cut the nail straight across without tapering the corners in any way. Nails that are left sharp or jagged-edged grow outward and eventually become embedded in the soft tissue of the nail bed. This process results in microtears of the skin that, when coupled with invasion by opportunistic resident foot bacteria, can cause a superficial infection. Wearing pointed-toe or tight shoes, as well as hosiery that is too tight, has also been implicated. In such instances, direct pressure can force the lateral edge of the nail into the soft tissue, and the embedded nail may then continue to grow. Bedridden patients may develop ingrown toenails because tight bedcovers press the soft skin tissue against the nails. Nail curling, which can be hereditary or secondary to either incorrect nail trimming or a systemic, metabolic disease, can also result in ingrown toenails. Psoriatic arthritis is such a disease whereby its presence may be demonstrated in the nail.

Education is probably the best way to prevent the development of ingrown toenails. In the early stages of development, therapy is directed at providing adequate room for the nail to resume its normal position adjacent to soft tissue. This therapy is accomplished by relieving the external source of pressure and by applying medications that will harden the nail groove or help shrink the soft tissue. The patient should be referred to a podiatrist or physician if the condition is recurrent or gives rise to an oozing discharge, pain, or severe inflammation. Sometimes surgery is warranted, and even with subsequent systemic antibiotic therapy, the toe may take up to 3 to 4 weeks to heal.

Drawing on evidence currently available, FDA in its final rule for ingrown toenail relief products did not propose any OTC active ingredient for ingrown toenail relief as safe and effective and not misbranded.[31] Thus, two previously approved drugs, tannic acid and sodium sulfide,[32] were classified as Category III and were withdrawn from the market.

The pharmacist, however, must be aware of trade-name product reformulations to accommodate this rule. For example, Outgro Pain-Relieving Formula, which formerly contained tannic acid for treating ingrown toenails, now contains benzocaine 20% to relieve pain associated with ingrown toenails.

Patients with ingrown toenails often fail to realize that they may be helped by oral medication intended to allay pain and inflammation. Provided no contraindications exist for use by a particular patient, the pharmacist may recommend aspirin, ibuprofen, ketoprofen, or naproxen, which are four proven analgesics with anti-inflammatory activity. (See Chapter 3, "Headache and Muscle and Joint Pain.")

Frostbite

Frostbite is defined as the actual freezing of tissues by excessive exposure to low temperatures. To maintain normal core temperature in cold weather, the body reflexively reduces the flow of blood to the skin surface and the extremities. Therefore, frostbite usually involves areas of the body (e.g., feet, hands, earlobes, nose, and cheeks) that are the farthest from deep organs or large muscles. Minor frostbite may cause only blanching of the skin; severe frostbite may result in the loss of fingers and toes.

Predisposing factors to developing frostbite include homelessness; diabetes mellitus; alcohol ingestion; motor vehicle problems in severe, wintry weather; mental illness; and/or a previous cold injury. Additional predisposing factors to the development of frostbite include the following:

- Low temperatures (especially with high winds).
- Long periods of exposure to cold.
- Lack of proper clothing.
- Wet clothing.
- Poor nutrition, exhaustion, dehydration, and/or smoking.
- Circulatory disease.
- Immobility.
- Direct contact with metal or petroleum products at low temperatures.
- Individual susceptibility to cold.

Frostbite is not amenable to therapy with nonprescription drug products. The frostbitten part should be promptly and thoroughly rewarmed in water heated to 104°F to 108°F (45.6°C to 47.8°C). The water should *not* be hot to a normal hand at room temperature and should *not* be tested with the frozen part. The container of water should be large enough for the frozen part to move freely without bumping against the sides. Rewarming should be continued until a flush returns to the most distal tip of the thawed part. This process usually takes about 20 to 30 minutes. Dry heat (e.g., a heating pad) should be avoided because it is difficult to control the temperature and rewarm the frozen part evenly; overapplication of heat could actually burn the skin without the patient being aware. Once the injured part has been properly warmed, it should be soaked for about 20 minutes in a whirlpool bath once or twice daily until the healing process is complete.

The best treatment for frostbite is prevention; pharmacists should be able to provide a few simple rules to follow:

- Dress to maintain body warmth, taking into account the face, neck, and head as well as the extremities.
- Avoid exposure to cold during times of sickness or exhaustion.
- Do not exceed the body's tolerance to cold exposure.
- Avoid tight-fitting garments; dress with layered clothing.
- Wear clothing that allows ventilation and prevents perspiration buildup (water enhances heat loss).
- Wear insulated boots or shoes and socks (preferably wool) that fit snugly but are not tight in spots. Wear mittens instead of gloves in severe cold; the thumb should be with the rest of the fingers and not by itself.
- Never touch objects (especially cold metal or petroleum products) that facilitate heat loss.
- Think twice about traveling by automobile in inclement, wintry weather where one can be marooned (e.g., Interstate highway). This activity can be especially disastrous for a patient with poor peripheral blood circulation.

When given the opportunity, the pharmacist should seek to correct a few misconceptions. It is dangerous to rub the affected area with ice or snow even though it seems to provide warmth; this action can result in prolonged contact with the cold, and the ice crystals may lacerate cells. In addition, people should refrain from drinking alcohol for "antifreeze" purposes. Alcohol can induce a loss of body heat even though it may give the individual a feeling of warmth when ingested. Finally, frostbite victims should avoid smoking. Nicotine can induce peripheral vasoconstriction and can further reduce the blood supply to the frostbitten extremity. Thus, it would also seem prudent to forewarn patients who want to stop smoking and are taking Nicorette (i.e., nicotine polacrilex) or are using one of the topical transdermal nicotine patches (Habitrol, Nicoderm, Nicotrol, or ProStep) that they should avoid excessive exposure to the cold. (See Chapter 42, "Nicotine Addiction.")

CONCLUSIONS

The nonprescription drug of choice to treat corns, calluses, and warts is salicylic acid in a collodion-like vehicle or plaster product form, whichever is more convenient. Predisposing factors responsible for corns and calluses must be corrected. Plantar warts should be treated with a higher concentration of salicylic acid (20% to 40%); warts on thin epidermis require a lower concentration (10% to 20%). Because warts are usually self-limiting, treatment should be conservative; vigorous therapy with salicylic acid may scar tissue.

Historically, the nonprescription drug of choice to treat the dry, scaly type of athlete's foot has been tolnaftate. Other agents, such as clioquinol, clotrimazole, miconazole nitrate, and undecylenic acid and its derivatives, are also efficacious for this purpose. Topical terbinafine hydrochloride 1% was reclassified as a nonprescription medication in 1999. Some clinical trials have shown clinical and mycologic cures of athlete's foot after only 1 week of treatment with this agent. The effectiveness of topical antifungals will be limited, however, unless the patient eliminates other predisposing factors to tinea pedis. These drugs are effective in all their delivery systems, but the powder form should be reserved only for extremely mild conditions or as adjunctive therapy. Because the vehicle forms of solution and cream are spreadable, they should be used sparingly. When recommended for suspected or actual dermatophytosis of the foot, these drugs should be used twice daily (morning and night). Treatment should be continued for 2 to 4 weeks, depending on the symptoms. After that time, the patient and pharmacist should evaluate the effectiveness of the drug.

The value of any topical nonprescription product for treating the soggy, macerated type of athlete's foot is dubious. The complex nature of the topical flora (resident aerobic diphtheroids) superimposed on the fungal infection dictates rigorous therapy with broader-spectrum antifungals (e.g., ciclopirox olamine or econazole nitrate). In addition, oral therapy with either griseofulvin or ketoconazole may be indicated. Soaks and compresses of astringent agents (e.g., aluminum chloride) may be used as adjuvant therapy to dry the soggy, macerated tissue. Once this condition is converted to the dry form, the patient can appropriately use agents such as tolnaftate, clotrimazole, miconazole nitrate, and undecylenic acid derivatives.

To minimize noncompliance, the pharmacist should advise patients that alleviation of the symptoms does not occur overnight. Patients should also be cautioned that frequent recurrence of any of these problems is an indication that they should consult a podiatrist or physician.

Patients with diabetes, circulatory problems, and/or arthritis pose special challenges to the pharmacist, who plays an important role in patient education. These patients should know not to self-medicate with any topical or oral nonprescription drug without first checking with their physician, podiatrist, or pharmacist. They should understand that certain ingredients are used in such products that may threaten the delicate balance that must be maintained for their care. Misadventuring with nonprescription products could have devastating consequences and, at the least, may interfere with attaining the intended patient outcomes.

Besides understanding concepts related to good foot care for patients with the above-mentioned chronic conditions, the pharmacist must be wary about drugs that can exacerbate such conditions or can interact with other chronically used medications. Typically, patients with diabetes, for example, will have other health problems (e.g., hypertension, hyperlipidemia, or arthritis) and associated therapy regimens. Thus, the pharmacist must monitor patient progress carefully and must be attuned to patient comments that might indicate the occurrence of drug-related problems.

In an era of physical fitness and health awareness, the

pharmacist must be prepared to educate and to assist patients who develop athletic injuries. With careful questioning, the pharmacist can help the patient determine whether the problem can be addressed through self-treatment or requires the assistance of a physician, podiatrist, or physical therapist. Most running injuries can be treated with shoe modifications, in-shoe supports, modified training methods, ice applications, and stretching exercises. It is important that the pharmacist be capable of providing informed recommendations to the sports enthusiast.

References

1. Brown JA, Scholl Inc. Personal communication. Memphis, TN: 1988.
2. Plummer ES, Albert SG. Foot care assessment in patients with diabetes: A screening algorithm for patient education and referral. *Diabetes Educator.* 1995;21:47–51.
3. Frykberg RG. Diabetic foot ulcers: current concepts. *J Foot Ankle Surg.* 1998;37:440–6.
4. Stewart WD, Danto JL, Maddin S. Callus. In: *Dermatologic Diagnosis and Treatment of Cutaneous Disorders.* 4th ed. St. Louis: CV Mosby; 1978:129.
5. Gossel TA. The safe way to treat corns and calluses. *US Pharm.* 1987;12: 41–2,47–53.
6. *Federal Register.* 1990;55:33258–62.
7. *Federal Register.* 1990;55:33246–56.
8. Raskin J. Superficial fungal infections of the skin. In: Conn HF, ed. *Current Therapy 1976.* Philadelphia: WB Saunders; 1976:611–4.
9. Jarratt M. Viral infections of the skin: herpes simplex, herpes zoster, warts, and molluscum contagiosum. *Pediatr Clin North Am.* 1978;25: 339–55.
10. Reichman RC, Bonnez W. Papillomaviruses. In: Mandell GL, Douglas RG Jr, Bennett JE, eds. *Principles and Practice of Infectious Diseases.* 3rd ed. New York: Churchill Livingstone; 1990:1191–7.
11. Vance JC, Bart BJ, Hansen RC, et al. Intralesional recombinant alpha-2 interferon for the treatment of patients with condyloma acuminatum or verruca plantaris. *Arch Dermatol.* 1986;122:272–7.
12. Rock B, Shah KV, Farmer ER. A morphologic, pathologic and virologic study of anogenital warts in men. *Arch Dermatol.* 1992;127:495–500.
13. Melton JL, Rasmussen JE. Clinical manifestations of human papillomavirus infection in nongenital sites. *Dermatol Clin.* 1991;9:219–33.
14. Goldfarb MT, Gupta AK, Gupta MA, et al. Office therapy for human papillomavirus infection in nongenital sites. *Dermatol Clin.* 1991;9: 287–96.
15. Goslen JB, Kobayashi GS. Dermatophytosis. In: Fitzpatrick TB, Eisen AZ, Wolff K, et al., eds. *Dermatology in General Medicine.* 3rd ed. New York: McGraw-Hill; 1987:2193–248.
16. Hay RJ. Dermatophytosis and other special mycoses. In: Mandell GL, Douglas RG Jr, Bennett JE, eds. *Principles and Practice of Infectious Diseases.* 3rd ed. New York: Churchill Livingstone; 1990:2017–28.
17. Page JC, Abramson C, Lee WL, et al. Diagnosis and treatment of tinea pedis. *J Am Podiat Soc.* 1991;81:304–16.
18. *Federal Register.* 1993;58:49890–9.
19. *Federal Register.* 1982;47:12480–566.
20. Savin RC. Treatment of chronic tinea pedis (Athlete's Foot type) with topical terbinafine. *J Am Acad Dermatol.* 1990;23:786–9.
21. Savin RC, Zaias N. Treatment of chronic moccasin-type tinea pedis with terbinafine: a double-blind, placebo-controlled trial. *J Am Acad Dermatol.* 1990;23:804–7.
22. Jung JH, McLaughlin JL, Stannard J, et al. Isolation, via activity-directed fractionation, of mercaptobenzothiazole and dibenzothiazyl disulfide as 2 allergens responsible for tennis shoe dermatitis. *Contact Dermatitis.* 1988;19:254–9.
23. Wapner KL, Sharkey PF. The use of night splints for treatment of recalcitrant plantar fasciitis. *Foot Ankle.* 1991;12:135–7.
24. Thompson PD, Stern MP, Williams P, et al. Death during jogging or running. *JAMA.* 1979;242:1265–7.
25. Pinshaw R, Atlas V, Noakes TD. The nature and response to therapy of 196 consecutive injuries seen at a runner's clinic. *S Afr Med J.* 1984;65: 291–8.
26. McPoil TG, Adrian M, Pidcoe P. Effects of foot orthotics on center of pressure patterns in women. *Phys Ther.* 1989;69:149.
27. Frey C, Thompson F, Smith J, et al. American Orthopaedic Foot and Ankle Society women's shoe survey. *Foot Ankle.* 1993;14:79–81.
28. Noakes TD. *Lore of Running.* Cape Town, South Africa: Oxford University Press; 1985.
29. Kay RA. The extra-depth toe box: a rational approach. *Foot Ankle.* 1994;15:146–50.
30. Cook SD, Kester MA, Brunet ME. Shock absorption characteristics of running shoe. *J Am Sports Med.* 1985;13:248–53.
31. *Federal Register.* 1993;58:47602–6.
32. *Federal Register.* 1982;47:39120–5.

CHAPTER 37

Skin Hyperpigmentation and Photoaging

Nina H. Han and Dennis P. West

Chapter 37 at a Glance

Skin hyperpigmentation and photoaging are considered by many patients to be cosmetically unacceptable. Photoaging of the skin is directly related to exposure to ultraviolet (UV) radiation. Although sun exposure does not cause most cases of hyperpigmentation, such exposure during or after treatment of the pigmentation disorder will negate the therapeutic effects. Nonprescription products used to prevent sun exposure are discussed in Chapter 33, "Prevention of Sun-Induced Skin Disorders." This chapter focuses on ameliorating the effects of hyperpigmentation and photoaging once they have occurred. α-Hydroxy acids (AHAs) play a role in both disorders.

Skin Hyperpigmentation

Hyperpigmentation, or excessive color, is usually a benign phenomenon but may occasionally represent a sign of systemic disease. As a facial disorder, it can be viewed by the patient as disfigurement and may lead to a psychologic disorder. Thus, agents that can reduce pigment when applied topically are used widely around the world, especially where hyperpigmented skin is in noticeable contrast to surrounding normal skin color. Although these products serve a cosmetic function, it is important to emphasize that they are drugs and have potential toxicity and side effects.

Etiology/Pathophysiology of Skin Hyperpigmentation

Normal skin color is contributed by melanocytes, the pigment cells found in the basal layer of epidermis. Melanocytes produce melanosomes, pigment granules that contain a complex protein called melanin, a brown-black pigment. Melanocytes can be viewed as tiny one-celled glands with long projections to pass pigment particles into keratinocytes, which, in turn, synthesize keratin. As keratinocytes migrate upward, they carry pigment and deposit it on the skin surface. Melanocytes are also present in hair bulb cells, and they pass pigment granules on to the hair.

Melanin functions as an efficient sunscreen. It prevents damaging ultraviolet (UV) radiation from entering deeper regions of the skin and minimizes the risk of sunburn and deoxyribonucleic acid (DNA) damage. Solar radiation stimulates melanocytes to provide more melanin protection to minimize DNA damage, and this increase results in gradual skin darkening or a "tan." Numbers of melanocytes are the

Editor's Note: This chapter is based, in part, on the 11th edition chapter titled "Dermatologic Products," which was written by Dennis P. West and Phillip A. Nowakowski.

same in equivalent body sites in white and black skin, but the rate of production of pigment and its distribution are different. Dark skin usually has more active melanocytes than its white counterparts.[1]

Systemic as well as localized skin diseases may cause pigment cells to become overactive (resulting in a skin darkening) or to become underactive (resulting in skin lightening). Endocrine imbalances caused by Addison's disease, Cushing's disease, hyperthyroidism, pregnancy, and estrogen therapy (including oral contraceptives) are capable of altering skin pigmentation. Metabolic alterations affecting the liver and certain nutritional deficiencies can be associated with diffuse melanosis. Inflammatory dermatoses or physical trauma to the skin, such as from a thermal burn, may cause a postinflammatory hyperpigmentation that may last for a prolonged period. Also, certain drugs (e.g., chlorpromazine and hydroxychloroquine) have an affinity for melanin and may cause hyperpigmentation.

Freckles are spots of uneven skin pigmentation that first appear in childhood and are exacerbated by the sun. Melasma (also called chloasma) is a condition in which macular hyperpigmentation appears, usually on the face or neck. Melasma is often associated with pregnancy ("the mask of pregnancy") or with the ingestion of oral contraceptives, along with sun exposure. Lentigines, hyperpigmented macules that may appear at any age anywhere on the skin or mucous membranes, are caused by an increased deposition of melanin and an increased number of melanocytes. The macules are not known to be induced by UV radiation. However, solar or "senile" lentigines (age spots or liver spots) appear on the exposed surfaces, particularly in fair-skinned people, and are induced by UV radiation.

Signs and Symptoms of Skin Hyperpigmentation

Depending on the etiology of hyperpigmentation, patients can present with varying signs and symptoms. Most notably, patients complain of persistent macular discoloration on the face or other sun-exposed areas. Colors can range from brown to blue to red.[2] As noted earlier, some hyperpigmentation can occur in places of trauma or inflammation.

Treatment of Skin Hyperpigmentation

Treatment Outcomes

The goal of treating skin hyperpigmentation is to diminish the degree of pigmentation of affected areas so that the skin tone of these areas is consistent with the surrounding normal skin.

General Treatment Approach

Several types of hyperpigmentation, including freckles, melasma, and lentigines, are amenable to self-treatment with topical nonprescription skin-bleaching agents.[3] Such products diminish the hyperpigmentation by inhibiting melanin production within skin.[4] Many treatments are available for melasma, but the combination of hydroquinone with AHAs is considered to be efficacious. (See the section "Treatment of Photoaging" for further discussion of AHAs.) By using a bleaching agent, along with one that exfoliates, patients have outcomes that are acceptable with minimal adverse effects.[5,6]

To avoid negating the effects of treatment, patients must avoid even minimal exposure to sunlight and must use sunscreen agents as well as protective clothing on an indefinite, ongoing basis, even after discontinuing the bleaching agent. The algorithm in Figure 37–1 outlines the self-treatment of skin hyperpigmentation.

Diffuse pigmentation disorders and those caused by systemic factors should not be self-treated without prior evaluation by a physician. Similarly, lesions that are changing in size, shape, or color should not be self-treated, and the patient should be referred promptly to a physician. Any type of hyperpigmentation in children younger than 12 years should be evaluated by a physician.

Physician-directed management of hyperpigmentation may include topical prescription agents composed of ingredients known to cause lightening of the skin, such as tretinoin (retinoic acid), hydroquinone, and a corticosteroid. This combination of ingredients may sometimes be effective for the treatment-resistant problem of postinflammatory hyperpigmentation.

Pharmacologic Therapy

Historically, a number of topical agents have been used in skin-bleaching preparations.[7] These agents have included hydroquinone, monobenzyl and monomethyl ethers of hydroquinone, ammoniated mercury, ascorbic acid, and peroxides. However, only preparations containing hydroquinone were submitted to the Advisory Review Panel on Over-the-Counter Miscellaneous External Drug Products of the Food and Drug Administration (FDA).

Hydroquinone

FDA has recommended that only hydroquinone (*p*-dihydroxybenzene) in concentrations of 1.5% to 2.0% be available for nonprescription use.[3] (See Table 37–1 for examples of commercially available products.)[8]

Mechanism of Action Hydroquinone and its derivatives are oxidized by tyrosinase to form highly toxic free radicals that cause selective damage to the lipoprotein membranes of the melanocyte, thereby reducing conversion of tyrosine to dopa and subsequently to melanin.[9] Several studies demonstrate that topical preparations of 2% to 5% hydroquinone are effective in producing cutaneous hypopigmentation. The 2% concentration is safer and has produced results equivalent to those of higher concentrations.[8]

Monobenzone, the monobenzyl ether of hydroquinone, should never be substituted for hydroquinone. It is restricted to prescription-only use. Its action and onset time are simi-

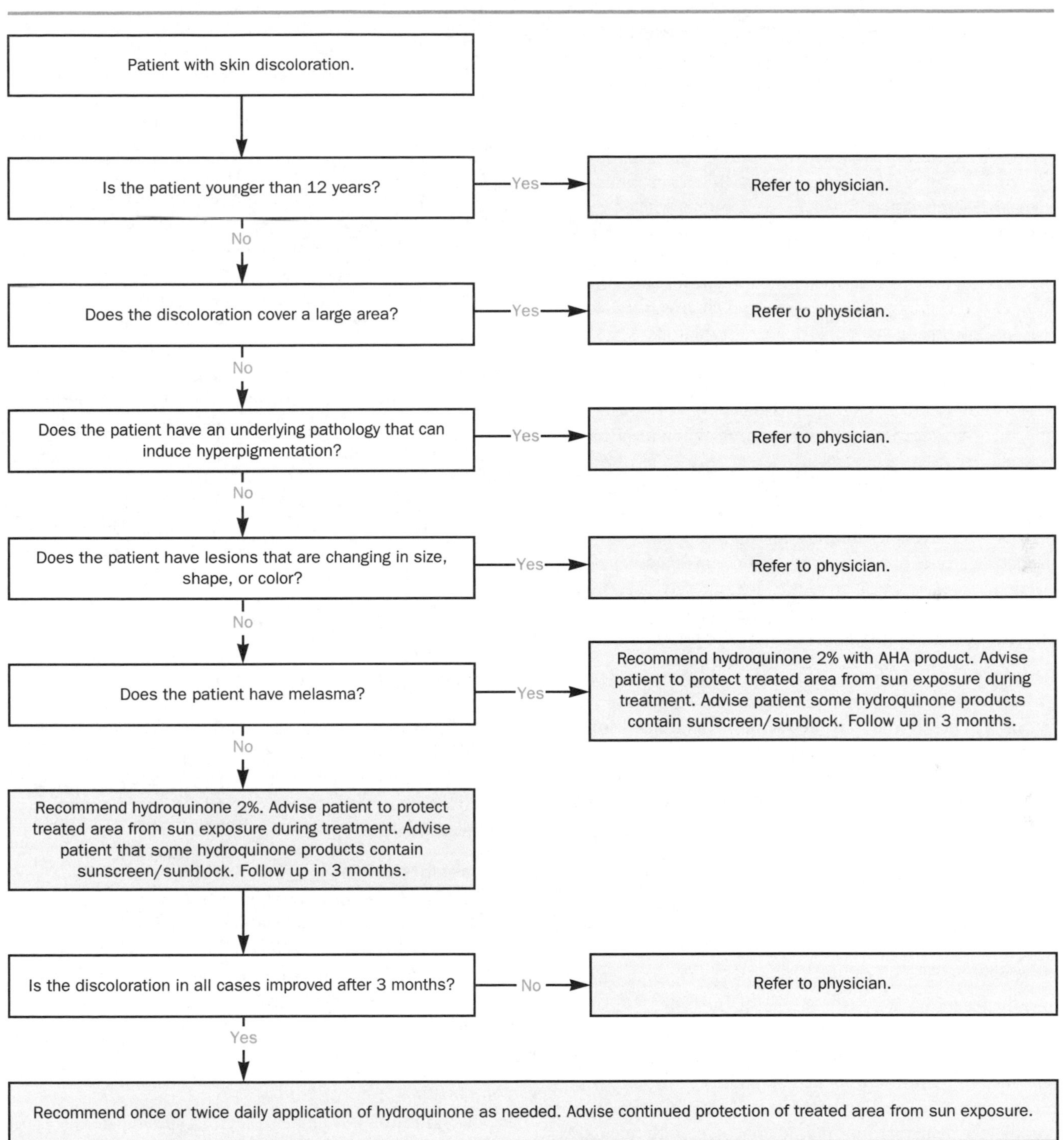

Figure 37–1 Self-care of skin hyperpigmentation.

lar to that of hydroquinone except that a complete and permanent depigmentation may occur. Its use is usually restricted to depigmenting remaining areas of normally pigmented skin in patients with extensive vitiligo (a condition resulting in patches of depigmentation, often with hyperpigmented borders).

Dosage/Administration Guidelines Hydroquinone is dosed as a thin topical application of a 2% concentration rubbed gently but well into affected areas twice daily. The agent should be applied to clean skin before the application of moisturizers or other skin-care products. It should not be applied to damaged skin or near the eyes. If no improvement

Table 37–1

Selected Skin-Bleaching Products

Trade Name	Primary Ingredients
Black & White Bleaching Cream	Hydroquinone 2%
Dr. Fred Palmer's Skin Whitener	Hydroquinone 2%
Esoterica Medicated Face Cream	Hydroquinone 2%
Esoterica Sensitive Formula	Hydroquinone 1.5%
Esoterica Sunscreen Formula	Hydroquinone 2%; octyl dimethyl PABA 3.3%; benzophenone-3, 2.5%
Nadinota Skin Cream	Hydroquinone 2%
Porcelana Skin Bleaching Cream	Hydroquinone 2%

Source: Reference 8.

is seen within 3 months, its use should be discontinued and the advice of a physician should be sought.[3] Once the desired benefit is achieved, hydroquinone can be applied as often as needed in a once- or twice-daily regimen to maintain lightening of the skin. Because of the lack of safety data, hydroquinone is not recommended for children younger than 12 years except under the supervision of a physician.

Adverse Effects Adverse effects are mild when topical hydroquinone is used in low concentrations. Tingling or burning on application and subsequent erythema and inflammation were observed in 8% of patients using a 2% concentration and in 32% of patients using a 5% concentration.[10] If desired, patients can apply the agent to a small test area and can check for signs of irritation after 24 hours. Higher concentrations frequently irritate the skin and, if used for prolonged periods, may cause side effects including epidermal thickening, pitch-black pigmentation, and colloid milium (yellowish papules associated with colloid degeneration).[11]

The effectiveness of hydroquinone varies among patients, and treatment must usually be maintained on an indefinite basis to retain lightening once it has been achieved. Results are best on lighter skin and lighter lesions. In dark skin, the response to hydroquinone depends on the amount of pigment present. Hyperpigmented areas fade more rapidly and completely than surrounding normal skin. Although treatment may not lead to complete disappearance of hypermelanosis, the results are often satisfactory enough to reduce self-consciousness. A disadvantage of treatment with hydroquinone is that it tends to overshoot the intended degree of hypopigmentation and may produce treated areas that are lighter than the surrounding normal skin color. Therefore, the patient must carefully observe the degree of lightening as the treatment progresses and must subsequently decrease applications when sufficient lightening has occurred.

When treatment is begun, melanin production may actually increase briefly. A decrease in skin color usually becomes noticeable in about 4 weeks; however, the time of onset varies from 3 weeks to 3 months. Hypopigmentation lasts for 2 to 6 months but is reversible. Although sunscreens may help, even visible light may cause some darkening. Thus, an opaque sunblock is preferable for sun protection.[12] Some nonprescription hydroquinone products are formulated with an opaque sunblock or with a sunscreen.

In some cases, lesions become slightly darker before fading. A transient inflammatory reaction may develop after the first few weeks of treatment. Occurrence of inflammation makes subsequent lightening more likely, although inflammation can occur without the development of hypopigmentation. The appearance of mild inflammation need not be considered an indication to stop therapy except in the patient whose reaction increases in intensity. In such situations, a patch can be tested for allergy to hydroquinone, although most reactions are irritant rather than allergic in nature.

Topical hydrocortisone may be used temporarily to alleviate the inflammatory reaction. Contact with the eyes should be avoided. If hydroquinone is accidentally ingested, it seldom produces serious systemic toxicity. However, oral ingestion of 5 to 15 g has produced tremor, convulsions, and hemolytic anemia.[8]

Reversible brown discoloration of nails has been reported occasionally following the application of 2% hydroquinone to the back of the hand.[13] Discoloration is probably caused by formation of oxidation products of hydroquinone. Hydroquinone is readily oxidized in the presence of light and air. Discoloration or darkening of the cream indicates product deterioration as well as a possible decline in the strength of available hydroquinone. Thus, the preferable method of packaging is in small closed dispensing containers such as squeeze tubes.

Hydroquinone Adjuvants and Combinations

Because hydroquinone is oxidized by contact with air, antioxidants such as sodium bisulfite may be added to the formulation. Hydroquinone is incompatible with alkali or ferric salts.[12] The inclusion of a sunscreen agent is rational and appropriate, provided that combination products are advertised not primarily as sunscreens but as skin-bleaching agents with added sunscreen.

Product Selection Guidelines

Product selection should be based on a suitable dosage form (i.e., cream, lotion, gel) for the patient's skin type (dry, normal, oily) and anatomic site (face, neck). For example, an emollient cream-based product may be more suitable for dry skin, whereas a gel-based preparation may be preferable for an oily skin type.

Patient Assessment of Skin Hyperpigmentation

The pharmacist should evaluate the affected areas to determine whether they are characteristic of freckles, melasma, or lentigines. The patient's medication history and health status are important factors in pinpointing possible causes of the pigmentation.

Asking the patient the following questions will help elicit the information needed to accurately assess the disorder and to determine the appropriate treatment approach.

Q~ How long has the pigmented area been present? When did it first appear?

A~ Suspect freckles if the pigmentation occurred early in life and the physical characteristics are typical of freckles. Suspect lentigines if the pigmentation occurred late in life and the physical characteristics support this assessment. Suspect melasma if the patient is female and the pigmentation first appeared during child-bearing years.

Q~ Have you suffered an injury such as a burn to that area of skin?

A~ If yes, the discoloration may be related to physical trauma. Advise the patient that the discoloration may last for a prolonged period. Refer the patient to a physician for possible management with prescription medications.

Q~ (If applicable) How long have you had that mole? Has it changed color or increased in size?

A~ Refer the patient to a physician if the described changes have occurred.

Q~ (If the patient is a woman of child-bearing age) Is there any possibility that you are pregnant?

A~ If yes, advise the patient that hormonal changes during pregnancy can cause hyperpigmentation. Recommend use of skin-bleaching product and avoidance of sun exposure during and after treatment.

Q~ Do you have any medical problems?

A~ *Identify medical problems that can cause hyperpigmentation. (See the section "Etiology/Pathophysiology Skin Hyperpigmentation.")* Refer the patient to a physician if the hyperpigmentation is related to any medical condition other than pregnancy.

Q~ Are you taking any medications, including birth control pills?

A~ *Identify medications that can induce hyperpigmentation. (See the section "Etiology/Pathophysiology of Skin Hyperpigmentation.")* Advise a patient taking birth control pills that the contraceptives can cause hyperpigmentation. Recommend use of skin-bleaching products and avoidance of sun exposure during and after treatment. If other medications are suspected as the cause, refer the patient to a physician.

Q~ Have you been using a skin hyperpigmentation product? If so, for how long?

A~ If the disorder is self-treatable and the product use has been less than 3 months, advise the patient to continue treatment until that period has elapsed. If product use has been longer than 3 months, advise discontinuation of the product, and refer the patient to a physician.

Patient Education for Skin Hyperpigmentation

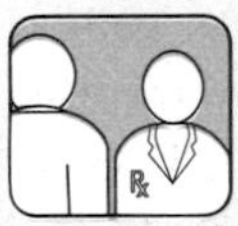

The objective of self-treatment with skin-bleaching products is to diminish the degree of pigmentation in affected areas. For most patients, carefully following the product's instructions and the self-care measures listed below will help ensure optimal therapeutic outcomes.

- Use hydroquinone to lighten only limited areas of hyperpigmented skin that are brownish discolorations.
- Do not use these products on nevi (moles) and reddish or bluish areas, such as port wine discolorations.
- Note that it may take 3 months to see noticeable results.
- Test for possible irritant reactions to the product by applying it to a small test area and by checking the area for redness, itching, or swelling after 24 hours.
- Do not apply the product near the eyes or to damaged skin.
- Apply a thin layer of the product to the affected area only.
- If moisturizers or other topical agents are being used at the same time, apply the hydroquinone first.
- If you will be outdoors for even a short time, apply an opaque sunblock or broad-spectrum (UVA and UVB) sunscreen to the affected area after applying the hydroquinone if the product does not already contain a sunscreen/sunblock in the formulation.
- Once the desired lightening of skin is reached, apply the hydroquinone once or twice daily to prevent the hyperpigmentation from recurring. Continue to protect the treated area from sun exposure.

Consult a physician

—If no improvement is seen after 3 months of using hydroquinone.

—If skin pigmentation becomes darker during treatment with hydroquinone.

Patient Counseling for Skin Hyperpigmentation

The pharmacist should explain which types of hyperpigmentation are self-treatable and stress that the therapy is short term. The avoidance of sun exposure during and after the treatment should also be stressed. To ensure a successful therapeutic outcome, the pharmacist should review the product instructions with the patient. The box "Patient Education for Skin Hyperpigmentation" lists specific information to provide patients.

Evaluation of Patient Outcomes for Skin Hyperpigmentation

The pharmacist should check on the patient's progress after 3 months of therapy. Follow-up can be achieved through a telephone call or a scheduled visit to the pharmacy. If the pigmented area shows no improvement, the patient should consult a physician. If the desired outcome has been achieved, the patient should continue applying the hydroquinone once or twice daily to maintain lightening of the skin.

Photoaging

Recent literature demonstrates that people older than 65 years represent 12% of the American population, a figure that is expected to double within the next 30 years. With the aging of the baby boomer generation, increased attention has been focused on reversing or reducing the amount of aging skin. Because members of that generation spent their formative years trying to achieve "healthy looking tans," there has been a steady increase in rates of skin cancer and prematurely aged skin.[14] Of the variety of reconstructive surgeries, skin peels, and laser treatments available, topical preparations are still most acceptable to patients. Although many products are restricted to prescriptions, many others are marketed over the counter, with AHAs being widely used to combat photoaged skin. A report in the mid-1990s indicated sales of approximately $300 million per year for AHA products.[15]

Etiology/Pathophysiology of Photoaging

Two components lead to aging skin: intrinsic and extrinsic. Clinical and histologic changes that intrinsically occur include genetically controlled skin and muscle changes, expression lines, sleep lines, and hormonal changes. The second component, extrinsic aging, relates to environmental influences such as UV radiation, smoking, wind, and chemical exposure.[16,17] Medications known to induce photosensitivity can contribute to photoaging by making the skin sensitive to UV radiation. (See Chapter 33, "Prevention of Sun-Induced Skin Disorders," for further discussion of photosensitivity.)

Prematurely aged facial skin, with creases and wrinkles, dry texture, and blotchy hyperpigmentation, is largely attributed to cumulative UV radiation, or photoaging.[18] Exposure to UVB (290 to 320 nm) light is primarily responsible for photoaging, although the longer UVA (320 to 400 nm) wavelengths also participate in damage. UVA radiation can penetrate into the deeper dermal layer and can work synergistically with UVB radiation to cause photodamage and skin cancers.[16]

Microscopically, sun-damaged skin shows dysplasia (abnormal tissue development), atypical keratinocytes, and occasional cell necrosis. Irregularity of epidermal cell alignment is also common. Deeper in the dermal layer is a loss of collagen and elastin.[14]

Signs and Symptoms of Photoaging

Clinical signs of photoaging include changes in color, surface texture, and functional capacity. (See Table 37–2.) Changes in skin may appear as a sallow yellow color, may have the appearance of discolorations, and may appear as gradual telangiectasias (visible distended capillaries). Textural changes include loss of smoothness, loss of subcutaneous tissue around the mouth, and epidermal thinning around the lip. As sebaceous glands hypertrophy, the skin begins to show coarse texture with increased pore size. In addition, fine vellus hairs can develop into unwanted terminal hairs. Other manifestations of photoaged skin can be the development of precancerous (actinic keratosis) and cancerous (basal cell and squamous cell) tumor development.[14]

Cosmetically, patients notice freckling, discolorations, "crow's feet" (small parallel lines around the eyes), and a sallow or yellowish gray coloration to the skin. Physical attractiveness, for both men and women, is correlated with occupational, educational, personal, and social rewards. Social scientists have studied behavior with physical attractiveness. Beginning in early infancy, "cute" babies are often more likely to receive attention and, thus, are likely to grow up becoming more socially adept. In a study that evaluated 24 age-related functions, the more attractive elderly patients were healthier and lived longer.[19]

Table 37–2

Classification of Photoaging

Type 1	No wrinkles; early photoaging; mild pigment changes; minimal or no makeup
Type 2	Wrinkles in motion; early-to-moderate photoaging; keratoses palpable; usually wears some foundation
Type 3	Wrinkles at rest; advanced photoaging; obvious dyschromia and keratoses; always wears heavy foundation
Type 4	Only wrinkles; severe photoaging; yellow-gray skin; cannot wear makeup because it cracks and cakes

Source: Glogau RG. Chemical peeling and aging skin. *J Geriatr Dermatol.* 1994;2:5–10.

Treatment of Photoaging

Treatment Outcomes

The goals of treating photoaging are to (1) reverse cumulative skin damage with prescription and nonprescription products and (2) protect and maintain the skin from further extrinsic damage by making lifestyle changes and, most importantly, protecting the skin from sun exposure.

General Treatment Approach

The first step in preventing and treating photoaged skin is to commit to daily sun protection. Broad-spectrum suncreens with high sun protection factor (SPF) can minimize further photodamage and promote skin repair during UV exposure.[17] (See Chapter 33, "Prevention of Sun-Induced Skin Disorders.")

Proper cleansing of the skin removes bacteria, dirt, desquamated keratinocytes, cosmetics, sebum, and perspiration. Because of marketing influence, the average American uses seven to eight times more soap than the average French citizen uses. This excessive use of soap leads to xerosis, eczematous dermatitis, and other skin conditions.[20] The use of AHAs adds moisture to the skin and repairs damaged skin by improving the skin's elasticity.

Pharmacologic Therapy

Within the vast array of available nonprescription products for skin care, the division of categories is now being questioned. For example, cosmetics and moisturizers are sold as nonprescription products, whereas antiperspirants and sunscreens are considered nonprescription drugs. Thus, although "cosmeceuticals" are a category of products recognized by pharmacists and dermatologists, no final regulatory guidance is currently available for these products from FDA. Many cosmeceutical ingredients function as active pharmaceuticals that are known to penetrate and to alter the stratum corneum.[21]

Many topical products are being used to treat aging skin. These include tretinoin (Retin-A or Renova), adapalene (Differin), vitamin C and vitamin K products, Kinerase, and AHAs and β-hydroxy acids (BHAs).

β-Hydroxy Acids

Of the BHAs, salicylic acid is the most common. Unlike the AHA products, BHAs are insoluble in water and demonstrate keratolytic effects. Although BHAs are now marketed with a cosmetic appeal, they have been used to treat skin conditions such as dermatitis and psoriasis for quite some time. Products containing BHAs as the active ingredients may be beneficial to acne-prone skin.

α-Hydroxy Acids

AHAs have generated greatly increased interest in the treatment of aging skin. The AHAs are used in various concentrations, with a wide array of available products. Most AHAs are sold as cosmeceuticals, whereas others are sold as cosmetics, and yet others are sold as pharmaceuticals through the physician. These products range in concentration from 2% to 20%, and act as a peeling agent (by aestheticians or dermatologists) from 20% to 70%.

Of the available nonprescription products, AHAs play a major role in reversing and cosmetically improving aging skin. Many types of AHAs are available, with the most common being lactic and glycolic acids. (See Table 37–3 for examples of commercially available products.) Other AHAs that are not as widely used include malic acid, citric acid, and tartaric acids.

Glycolic acid, the smallest of the AHA molecules, is colorless, odorless, water soluble, and nontoxic. Currently, FDA's advice for nonphysician-dispensed AHAs indicates use of a glycolic acid concentration between 8% to 10% with a pH from 3.5 to 4.5.[17]

Table 37–3

Selected α-Hydroxy Acid Products

Trade Name	Primary Ingredients
Aqua Glycolic Hand & Body Lotion	Mineral oil; glyceryl stearate; cetyl alcohol; glycolic acid 14%
Curél Alpha Hydroxy Moisturizing Lotion[a]	Petrolatum; dimethicone; isopropyl palmitate; glycerin; lactic acid; glycolic acid
Dermal Therapy Extra Strength Body Lotion[a]	Isopropyl myristate; cetyl alcohol; propylene glycol; urea; lactic acid
Epilyt Concentrate Lotion	Propylene glycol; glycerin; lactic acid
Nutraderm 30 Lotion	Petrolatum; dimethicone; cetaryl alcohol; cetyl alcohol; sodium PCA; glycerin; lactic acid; malic acid
Pretty Feet & Hands Replenishing Creme	Mineral oil; glyceryl stearate; cetyl alcohol
Soft Sense Alpha Hydroxy Moisturizing Lotion[a]	Petrolatum; dimethicone; isopropyl palmitate; glycerin; lactic acid
Vaseline Dual Action Alpha Hydroxy Formula Cream	Petrolatum; dimethicone; glyceryl stearate; sunflower seed oil; glycerin; lecithin; lactic acid

[a] Fragrance-free product.

Mechanism of Action Used appropriately, AHA products cause a detachment of keratinocytes; thus they result in a smoother, nonscaly skin surface with eventual normalization of keratinization. The pH of the product is important because products with a lower pH have faster results, but they may have an increased risk of irritation.

By improving the skin elasticity, AHAs have been shown to make the skin more flexible and less vulnerable to cracking and flaking. Long-term use has led to an increase in skin collagen and elastin.[5,15] Regular application of AHA results in a smoother skin texture, an evening out of fine lines, and a normalization of pigmentation.

Indications FDA-approved indications for AHA products include treatment of xerosis, solar lentigos, actinic keratoses, melasma, acne, and photoaging.[5]

Dosage/Administration Guidelines Care should be taken to apply AHAs to completely dry skin, with an estimated wait time of 10 to 15 minutes after cleansing the face. It is also helpful to apply the product slowly, starting every other night for approximately 1 week and then increasing as tolerated to a maximum of twice-daily application.

Adverse Effects Common adverse effects include sensory irritation (mild, transient stinging and burning) and dryness. Many of these effects can be ameliorated if products are applied with caution and proper counseling. Patients should also note that other topically applied products, both medications and cosmetics, may contain active ingredients (e.g., AHA, BHA, hydroquinone) that may enhance sensory irritation.

Special Population Considerations Yet another advantage of nonprescription AHAs is that they are not contraindicated in pregnancy.[17]

Product Selection Guidelines When the patient selects an AHA, the vehicle chosen depends on the skin type. Creams are appropriate for drier skin types, lotions are best for combination or normal skin, and gels or solutions are well accepted by oilier skin types. If the patient wants fast results, products with higher concentrations and a lower pH can be recommended. However, the patient should be warned that these products may also cause greater skin irritation.

N-Furfuryladenine

Kinerase (N-furfuryladenine 0.1%) is an "antiwrinkle" compound marketed as a cream or lotion to reduce wrinkles, blotchiness, and dryness. Support exists for its use as a moisturizer to improve blotchiness and skin roughness, but efficacy in reversing photodamage in comparison to available prescription products is not yet established. Kinerase may be recommended for patients with sensitive skin or for those who choose not to obtain prescription therapy for photodamaged skin.

Patient Assessment of Photoaging

If visual inspection of the patient's skin causes the pharmacist to suspect photoaging, the patient should be questioned about his or her history of sun exposure. Knowing whether the patient's current occupational or recreational habits require excessive exposure is useful not only in determining the cause of the skin disorder but also in developing a treatment plan. The patient's medication use, health status, lifestyle practices, and daily skin maintenance regimen are other important assessment criteria.

Asking the patient the following questions will help elicit the information needed to accurately assess the disorder and to recommend the appropriate treatment approach.

Q~ Have you had sunburns frequently during your life? If so, how serious were they?

A~ Suspect photoaging if the patient has a history of serious sunburns.

Q~ Does your occupation require you to work outdoors? If so, do you use sunscreens/sunblocks or clothing to protect your skin?

A~ Suspect photoaging caused by sun exposure if the patient works outdoors and uses no measures to avoid UV radiation.

Q~ Do your recreational activities involve outdoor activity? If so, do you use sunscreens/sunblocks or clothing to protect your skin?

A~ Suspect photoaging if the patient engages in frequent outdoor activities without proper sun protection.

Q~ Do you smoke cigarettes?

A~ If yes, advise the patient that smoking ages the skin even if the patient is not exposed to the sun. Ask the patient if he or she would like assistance in stopping smoking. (See Chapter 42, "Nicotine Addiction.")

Q~ What mediations, prescription and nonprescription, are you taking?

A~ *Identify medications known to induce photosensitivity reactions. (See Chapter 33, "Prevention of Sun-Induced Skin Disorders.")* If any of these medications are being taken, refer the patient to a physician for possible medication adjustments.

Patient Counseling for Photoaging

The pharmacist should advise patients that premature wrinkling, with creases, dry texture, and blotchy hyperpigmentation, is not inevitable.[18] The pharmacist should be proactive in identifying and recommending products that are appropriate for a specific patient. Patients should be encouraged to protect the skin from sun exposure and to practice good skin hygiene practices. The proper use of AHA products should be explained, including their possible irritant effects. The box "Patient Education for Photoaging" lists specific information to provide patients.

Patient Education for Photoaging

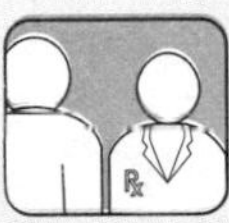

The objectives of self-treatment are to (1) reverse skin damage by using available nonprescription products and (2) protect the skin from further damage by making lifestyle changes and protecting the skin from sun exposure. For most patients, carefully following product instructions and the self-care measures listed below will help ensure optimal therapeutic outcomes.

- Protect the skin from sun exposure by covering the skin with clothing or by using a sunblock or sunscreen product.
- To prevent dry skin, cleanse the skin with a mild soap or a soap-free liquid cleanser. Do not cleanse skin more often than twice daily. After cleansing, apply a moisturizer such as an α-hydroxy acid (alpha-hydroxy acid) product.
- Note that α-hydroxy acid products contain an active ingredient and that the use of other products, including cosmetics, could result in skin irritation.
- To minimize the potential for irritation, wait 10 to 15 minutes after cleansing the face to apply an α-hydroxy acid product.
- Do not apply the product too close to the eyes or to mucous membranes.
- Begin applying this product once at bedtime, every other day for approximately 1 week. Gradually increase application to twice a day.
- Apply a sunscreen or sunblock after applying the α-hydroxy acid product.

Discontinue the α-hydroxy acid product if any irritation, such as redness or excessive dryness, occurs.

Evaluation of Patient Outcomes for Photoaging

Patients treated with nonprescription products for photoaging should set a reasonable goal. Obviously, these preparations cannot "erase wrinkles." The pharmacist should monitor the progress of the treatment and be sensitive to issues that would require additional intervention, as determined by the patient's physician.

CONCLUSIONS

Although photoaging and hyperpigmentation may be considered cosmetically unacceptable, they are usually manageable skin conditions. Patients who use the newer available products, protect their skin from sun exposure, and have reasonable expectations may be able to achieve well-maintained skin with an even tone. Pharmacists are in a key position to assess photoaging and hyperpigmentation, recommend the appropriate nonprescription products, counsel patients on the proper use of these products, and monitor patients' progress in self-treating these skin disorders.

References

1. Grimes PE, Davis LT. Cosmetics in Blacks. *Dermatol Clin.* 1991;9:53–68.
2. Nordlund JJ, Lorton CA. Disorders of pigmentation. In: Orkin M, Maibach HI, eds. *Dermatology.* 1st ed. Norwalk, CT: Appleton & Lange; 1991:261–80.
3. *Federal Register.* 1982;47:39108–17.
4. Engasser PG, Maibach HI. Cosmetics and dermatology: bleaching creams. *J Am Acad Dermatol.* 1981;5:143–7.
5. Clark CP. Alpha hydroxy acids in skin care. *Clin Plastic Surg.* 1996;23:49–56.
6. Amer M, Metwalli M. Topical hydroquinone in the treatment of some hyperpigmentary disorders. *Int J Dermatol.* 1998;37:433–53.
7. Bleehan SS, Ebling FJG, Campion RH. In: Campion RH, Burton JL, Ebling FJG, eds. *Textbook of Dermatology.* 5th ed. Oxford, England: Blackwell Scientific Publications; 1992:1561–622.
8. Fisher AA. The safety of bleaching creams containing hydroquinone. *Cutis.* 1998;61:303–4.
9. Jimbow K, Obata H, Pathak MA, et al. Mechanism of depigmentation by hydroquinone. *J Invest Dermatol.* 1974;62:436–49.
10. Arndt KA, Fitzpatrick TB. Topical use of hydroquinone as a depigmenting agent. *JAMA.* 1965;194:965–7.
11. Hoshaw RA, Zimmerman KG, Menter A. Ochronosis-like pigmentation from hydroquinone bleaching creams in American Blacks. *Arch Dermatol.* 1985;121:105–8.
12. Arndt KA. In: *Manual of Dermatologic Therapeutics.* 5th ed. Boston: Little, Brown; 1995:105–11.
13. Mann RJ, Harman RM. Nail staining due to hydroquinone skin lightening creams. *Br J Dermatol.* 1983;108:363–5.
14. Glogau RG. Physiologic and structural changes associated with aging skin. *Dermatol Clin.* 1997;15(4):555–9.
15. Stiller MJ, Bartolone J, Stern R, et al. Topical 8% glycolic acid and 8% L-lactic acid creams for the treatment of photodamaged skin. *Arch Dermatol.* 1996;132:631–6.
16. Roenigk HH. Treatment of the aging face. *Dermatol Clin.* 1995;13:245–61.
17. Gendler EC. Topical treatment of the aging face. *Dermatol Clin.* 1997;15:561–7.
18. Kligman AM. Topical treatments for photoaged skin. *Postgrad Med.* 1997;102:115–26.
19. Kligman AM, Koblenzer C. Demographics and psychological implications for the aging population. *Dermatol Clin.* 1997;15:549–53.
20. Draelos ZD. Therapeutic skin care in the mature patient. *Clin Plastic Surg.* 1997;24:369–77.
21. Draelos ZD, Jegasothy SM. Should cosmeceuticals be regulated by the FDA? *Skin & Aging.* 1999:52–4.

CHAPTER 38

Hair Loss

Nina H. Han and Dennis P. West

Chapter 38 at a Glance

Male baldness in young men is so common in the United States that some people consider it to be normal. Many women also experience thinning hair at some point in their lives. Nevertheless, hair loss is traumatic for many people and can cause depression, loss of self-confidence, and humiliation. U.S. consumers spend hundreds of millions of dollars each year on proven and unproven methods of treating hair loss.

Although only a few causes of hair loss account for the vast majority of cases, many causes and many types of baldness exist. Hair loss can be broadly categorized as nonscarring alopecia or scarring alopecia. Androgenetic alopecia (pattern hereditary hair loss), alopecia areata, anagen effluvium, telogen effluvium, cosmetic hair damage, and trichotillomania (a compulsive pulling out of one's own hair) are common forms of nonscarring alopecia. Of these disorders, the nonprescription agent minoxidil is approved to treat only androgenetic alopecia. A dermatologist must evaluate other types of nonscarring hair loss to determine their cause and proper treatment. Scarring alopecia may be related to conditions such as discoid lupus erythematosus, syphilis, sarcoid, or lichen planus.[1] These conditions must also be evaluated by a dermatologist.

Epidemiology of Hair Loss

Androgenetic alopecia is the most common form of hair loss, affecting about one-third of the U.S. male population and about one-sixth of the female population. It is characterized by progressive, patterned hair loss from the scalp. By age 30 years, about 30% of Caucasian men have androgenetic alopecia, with the incidence increasing to 50% by age 50 years. Caucasian men are four times more likely than their African American counterparts to develop premature hair loss.[2]

Alopecia areata (autoimmune hair loss) affects men and women of any race equally and occurs in 2% of the U.S. population. Most cases (60%) are in children and young adults.[3]

Telogen effluvium is a common condition internationally, but its exact prevalence has not been determined. Telogen effluvium has no racial bias and can occur at any age. Episodes are common in the first months of life. An episode can occur in either sex, but because postpartum hormonal changes are a frequent cause, the condition is believed to affect women more often than men. The chronic form of this disease has been reported mainly in women.[4]

Anatomy and Physiology of Hair Growth

A strand of hair is a cylinder of tightly keratinized cells that grows at the base of the follicle.[5] (See Figure 27–1 in Chapter 27, "Atopic Dermatitis, Contact Dermatitis, and Dry Skin.") The hair follicle, which anchors the hair strand to the skin, contains cells that produce new hairs. These germinative cells, located at the base of the follicle next to the dermal papilla, make up the follicular matrix; the matrix cells eventually keratinize to form hair.

Hair follicle activity is cyclic. In the growing phase (anagen), the follicle lengthens, the dermal papilla enlarges, and a new hair is formed. During the catagen phase—a transition phase between the growing and resting phases—cell prolifer-

Editor's Note: This chapter is based, in part, on the 11th edition chapter titled "Dermatologic Products," which was written by Dennis P. West and Phillip A. Nowakowski.

ation ceases, the hair follicle shortens, and a bulbous enlargement forms at the base of the hair. The resting phase (telogen) has an unpigmented, club-shaped root that is embedded in a shortened follicle. Telogen, or terminal, hairs are loosely held in place. Duration of the anagen phase in any individual normal scalp follicle is genetically determined and ranges from 2 to 5 years with an average duration of 1000 days.[6] The rate of human scalp hair growth averages 0.37 mm per day. The average duration of the telogen phase, however, is only 100 days, resulting in a ratio of anagen to telogen hairs of 12 : 1. Typically, 100 to 150 hairs are lost from the scalp each day as telogen hairs are shed.

The type of hair growth depends on follicle location and on the person's age and sex. Vellus hair is soft, fine, usually unpigmented, and less than 2 cm long (e.g., abdominal hair), whereas terminal hair is coarse, of greater length, and pigmented (e.g., scalp hair).

The human scalp contains approximately 100,000 to 150,000 hair follicles, which are evenly distributed.[7] These follicles have sebaceous glands whose oily secretions lubricate the scalp. Blonds apparently have greater than the usual number of follicles, and redheads, fewer. By the third decade of life, density of hair follicles usually decreases to half of that found in a newborn.[7]

Hair follicles and their sebaceous glands produce enzymes (δ-5-3β-hydroxysteroid hydrogenase [3β-HSD], 17β-HSD, and 5-α-reductase type I) that convert weak androgens (such as dehydro-3-epiandrosterone and 4-androstenedione) to testosterone and dihydrotestosterone (DHT). Testosterone and DHT stimulate production of growth factors and proteases, effect vascularization of the follicle and the composition of basement membrane proteins, and alter the amounts of cofactors required for follicle metabolism. Another enzyme (called aromatase) found in the lower portion of the outer root sheath converts androgens (4-androstenedione and testosterone) to estrogens. These enzymes are believed to maintain androgen balance in the follicle, thereby regulating the hair cycle. Androgens (testosterone and DHT) apparently bind to receptor proteins in bulbar dermal papilla cell nuclei. The complex then attaches to a DNA site that regulates the manufacture of messenger RNAs responsible for hair protein synthesis. In a scalp hair follicle, the complex down-regulates synthesis, whereas in a hair follicle on the face, the opposite occurs.[8]

Etiology/Pathophysiology of Hair Loss

Androgenetic Alopecia

In androgenetic alopecia, the hair follicle undergoes a stepwise miniaturization and change in growth dynamics. With each successive cycle, the anagen (growing) phase becomes shorter and the telogen (resting) phase becomes longer. Consequently over time, the anagen to telogen ratio decreases from 12 : 1 to 5 : 1. Because telogen hairs are more loosely anchored to follicles, their presence in increased numbers manifests eventually by an increased shedding of hairs. Also, the catagen phase (the intermediate phase between anagen regrowth and telogen shedding) increases, reducing the number of hairs. As telogen hairs are shed, they are gradually replaced by vellus-like (short and fine) hairs (mean diameter reduced from 0.08 mm to less than 0.06 mm)[9] or by anagen hairs that are too short to reach the surface. The only remaining indication of a functioning follicle is a pore.[10]

The site-specific effects on hair growth are paradoxical. Pubic, axillary, chest, and face hair follicles respond to androgens by growing into terminal hair, whereas scalp follicles respond by growing vellus hair (resembling peach fuzz). The androgen DHT, which is converted from testosterone by 5-α-reductase, is believed to be a primary repressor of hair growth by the mechanism mentioned in the previous section. This androgen also binds five times more readily than testosterone to androgen receptors. Although two forms of the 5-α-reductase are found in the scalps of bald men, the amount of DHT formed locally (in scalp hair) is small in comparison to what is available systemically (produced by the prostate gland). The relative contributions of local and systemic DHT to balding are still not known.

Increased 5-α-reductase–mediated conversion to DHT in the balding areas of women with androgenetic alopecia also supports the contention that DHT is important to this process. Women with this disease rarely lose all their hair, not simply because they have less 5-α-reductase but also because they have more aromatase that converts testosterone into estradiol.[11] In addition, women are more likely to have follicles with fewer localized androgen receptors and, therefore, are more likely to retain actively growing hair.[12]

The rate of progression and the pattern of hair loss appear to be genetically determined. Premature hair loss is not always manifested because of variability in gene expression.[13] The possibility of a different model of gene expression, such as polygenic inheritance, has not been excluded. In this model, baldness would depend on the number of baldness genes.[14]

Alopecia Areata

Alopecia areata is a disease marked by an autoimmune attack on an unidentified target. Cytotoxic T cells are believed to attack an autoantigen that is normally sequestered. Triggers that are thought to increase gene expression in alopecia areata include microtrauma, neurogenic inflammation, and microbial antigens.[15] More than one member of the patient's family may have the disease. Genetic factors may increase susceptibility to this condition.[16] Recently, the first hair-loss gene for alopecia areata was mapped. The gene was identified because it was missing from a Pakastani family that suffers from the most severe form of alopecia areata—alopecia universalis, a rare disorder that causes total body hair loss[17] This scientific development has important implications for the future (perhaps genetic) treatment of this problem.

Nonhereditary Hair Loss

Nonhereditary alopecias (such as telogen effluvium) have no characteristic pattern of hair loss, and the baldness may be asymmetrical. The cause is believed to be physiologic stress because this ailment can be a complication of or caused by the following:

- Acute illness involving fever; severe viral, fungal, or protozoan infection; major surgery; or severe trauma. The amount of time for hair loss to occur can be anywhere from a week to several months.
- Chronic illness, such as cancer (especially lymphoproliferative cancer), systemic lupus erythematosus, end-stage renal disease, or liver disease.
- Hormonal changes during and following a pregnancy (both mother and child can be affected), and endocrine disorders such as hypothyroidism and discontinuation of estrogen-containing medication.
- Dietary changes that lead to anorexia; excess dietary heavy metals, such as selenium, arsenic, and thallium; or severe nutritional deficiencies, such as low protein intake, chronic iron deficiency (runners sometimes develop anemia that leads to hair loss), or deficiencies of essential fatty acids, zinc, or biotin.
- Certain drugs, such as anticoagulants, β-blockers, angiotensin-converting enzyme inhibitors, amphetamines, retinoids (including high-dose vitamin A), propylthiouracil, and carbamazepine, may trigger hair loss.[18,19]

Antimitotic drugs, such as chemotherapy drugs used to treat cancer and antimitotics used to inhibit lactation (e.g., bromocriptine), can cause narrowing of the hair shaft, which may fracture or stop hair growth. This condition is referred to as anagen alopecia or anagen effluvium (when referring to the shedding of anagen hairs). Another disease also marked by loose anagen hairs is called "loose anagen syndrome." Loose anagen syndrome may be transmitted by autosomal dominant inheritance. This disease is predominantly found in fair-haired girls ages 2 to 9 years.[20]

Certain diseases, hair care products, and hair-grooming methods associated with scarring or burns on the scalp may result in scarring alopecia. Traction alopecia is seen primarily in children who braid their hair tightly every day. Braiding traumatizes the hair follicles, causing hairs to loosen and break. Patients who use oily moisturizers to make hair more manageable and to stop the scalp from flaking may develop folliculitis and resultant hair loss. Hot combs used to straighten hair may cause scalp inflammation and resultant scarring alopecia.[21]

Chronic papulosquamous diseases of the scalp, such as psoriasis and seborrheic dermatitis, may also lead to scarring alopecia.

Tinea capitis is another condition that may manifest as hair loss. This disease, caused by *Trichophyton tonsurans* (a fungus), must be treated with systemic antifungals such as terbinafine or griseofulvin. The illness appears as black dots where the hair breaks off at the scalp's skin surface.[21]

Psychologic stress may potentiate several types of hair loss, although the literature on this subject is still conflicting. High stress levels may depress the immune system and could lead to symptoms such as hair loss.[22]

Signs and Symptoms of Hair Loss

The scalps of patients with androgenetic alopecia show no signs of inflammation or scarring. Hair loss is gradual, and the number of hairs coming out during brushing or shampooing do not suddenly increase, in contrast to other alopecias. Typically, male androgenetic hair loss is insidious in onset and usually does not start until after puberty. Progression fluctuates considerably, with 3 to 6 months of accelerated loss followed by 6 to 18 months of no loss. Most men take 15 to 25 years to lose their hair. Male-pattern hair loss and/or gradual hair thinning usually occurs at the top rear of the head (vertex), the frontal hairline, and the occipital regions. The loss begins with a recession of the frontal hairline and continues with thinning at the vertex until all that is left is a fringe of hair at the occipital and temporal margins.

In women with androgenetic alopecia, hair loss is much more diffuse. There is a characteristic retention of the frontal hairline. Later, diffuse thinning is seen over the entire crown. Hair density remains normal but hair length does not. The woman's scalp will show a high density of hair, but the hairs will be thinner than normal, short, and tapered (rather than blunt, as seen when hair is damaged by breakage).

Androgenetic alopecia in women is a cause for suspicion of hyperandrogenism—an excess of androgen, which commonly accompanies significant acne, hirsutism (hairiness in other parts of the body), menstrual irregularities, and infertility. Androgen excess may indicate serious metabolic disturbances, such as diabetes mellitus, cardiovascular disease, and endometrial cancer.[23]

Autoimmune hair loss (alopecia areata) has three stages: sudden loss of hair in patches, enlargement of the patches, and regrowth. The cycle may take months, sometimes years, and can occur in any hair-bearing area. Axillary, pubic, and other body hairs are often not affected. However, the eyebrows and eyelashes are lost in several cases and sometimes may be the only sites affected.[24] Up to 5% of patients lose all their scalp hair (alopecia totalis), and 1% of patients lose all their body and scalp hair (alopecia universalis). Hair loss may accompany or be preceded by nail pitting or other nail abnormalities, as well as by itching, tingling, burning, or other painful sensation in the patch of hair loss.

Patients can often predict where hair loss is going to take place. A diagnostic for alopecia areata is the presence of exclamation point hairs, which are shorter than normal, have a frayed distal end, and have a narrowed root end, making them look like exclamation points when viewed under a dissecting microscope. This characteristic is often used to distinguish trichotillomania (in which hair has blunt ends) from alopecia areata. The more severe forms of alopecia areata can occur at any age but are more likely to occur when initial hair loss occurs at an early age and is very severe; they are also more likely in individuals with preexisting eczema or asthma. Patients with alopecia areata are more likely to be allergic and to have thyroid disease, vitiligo (patches of unpigmented skin), insulin-dependent diabetes, and other autoimmune diseases.[25] In addition, the incidence of alopecia areata in patients with Down's syndrome is inexplicably high.[26]

Telogen effluvium (also known as diffuse alopecia) is characterized by nonscarring, diffuse hair loss usually caused by metabolic or hormonal disturbances or by medications. The acute form is defined by shedding that lasts less than 6 months; the chronic form lasts longer than 6 months. The metabolic or physiologic disturbance usually precedes shedding by 1 to 6 months, but the identification of a specific causal event is often difficult, if not impossible. A physician will confirm a diagnosis of telogen effluvium if the hair pull test (the forced extraction of 10 to 20 hairs from the scalp) reveals that more than 25% of the hairs are in telogen phase. (Telogen hairs have a white bulb but no gelatinous hair sheath. Anagen hairs have both.)[18]

Anagen alopecia is marked by loss of primarily anagen hairs although some telogen hairs may also be removed by the gentle hair pull test. Anagen hairs stop growing or will not grow long. In other ways, the disease is very similar to telogen effluvium.

Treatment of Hair Loss

Treatment Outcomes

The goal in treating hair loss is to restore the patient's appearance by recommending (1) cosmetic camouflage and (2), where applicable, the use of topical minoxidil to regrow hair.

General Treatment Approach

At this time, the only OTC products available and approved by the Food and Drug Administration (FDA)—topical minoxidil 2% (Rogaine) and topical minoxidil 5% (Rogaine Extra Strength for Men)—are indicated for treatment of androgenetic alopecia, and specifically for loss of vertex but not frontal hair. If the patient's baldness is clearly androgenetic, treatment with 2% for women and 5% for men can be recommended. Otherwise, patients should be referred to their physician for diagnosis. The algorithm in Figure 38–1 outlines the self-treatment of hair loss.

Exclusions to self-treatment include the following signs and symptoms:

- Sudden or patchy hair loss.
- Any evidence of fever or inflammation.
- Skin lesions indicating autoimmune disease or infection.
- Scaling, sunburn, or any other damage to the scalp.
- Broken-off hair shafts, such as those produced by fungal infection or trichotillomania.
- Loss of eyebrows or eyelashes.
- Changes in nails.

Patients with hair loss who are pregnant or breast-feeding or who have discontinued oral contraceptives should consult a physician or dermatologist. Hair loss that is related to a history of endocrine dysfunction, medical treatments such as chemotherapy, medication use, and dietary deficiencies also requires medical evaluation. Patients with alopecia who have no family history of baldness or who have a positive hair-pull test are excluded from self-treatment, as are balding patients younger than 18 years.

Nonpharmacologic Therapy

Thinning hair can be camouflaged by a number of cosmetic approaches: wigs (hair pieces) and hair weaves, which are cosmetically more appealing than they were a decade ago. Hair loss that is dramatic and extensive can be emotionally very distressing. Although some people may need counseling to recover self-image and regain self-confidence, an attractive wig may ease the problem. Treatment of less-severe hair loss can be approached by using hair sprays, gels, colorants, and perms in moderation; these products can create an illusion of fullness without increasing the rate of hair loss.

Scalp massage, frequent shampooing, electrical stimulation, and Chinese herbal extracts have been proposed as treatments for hair loss; however, such remedies are considered ineffective.[27]

Acute telogen effluvium usually resolves spontaneously, and treatment is limited to comforting and reassuring the patient. Chronic telogen effluvium is slower to resolve, but the patient still needs comfort and reassurance. Where a physician has determined that the patient's hair loss is due to poor diet or iron deficiency, the patient may benefit from consulting a dietitian. Increasing protein intake, providing iron supplements, or eliminating the intake of large amounts of vitamin A may be simple solutions. Although not encouraged and of no proven value in treating telogen effluvium, the patient retains the option of treating the disease with topical minoxidil.

Hair loss that occurs as a result of trauma, such as braiding the hair (traction alopecia), using oils (inflammatory folliculitis), and compulsively pulling hair (trichotillomania), can all be readily reversed by abandoning these practices. Patients with inflammatory folliculitis may also benefit from the use of antibacterial shampoos.

Pharmacologic Therapy

Minoxidil

Both minoxidil 2% and extra-strength topical minoxidil 5%, as hydroalcoholic solutions, are the only nonprescription agents currently approved by FDA for use in regrowing hair.

Mechanism of Action Minoxidil is a potassium (K^+) channel opener and vasodilator (when used orally to control hy-

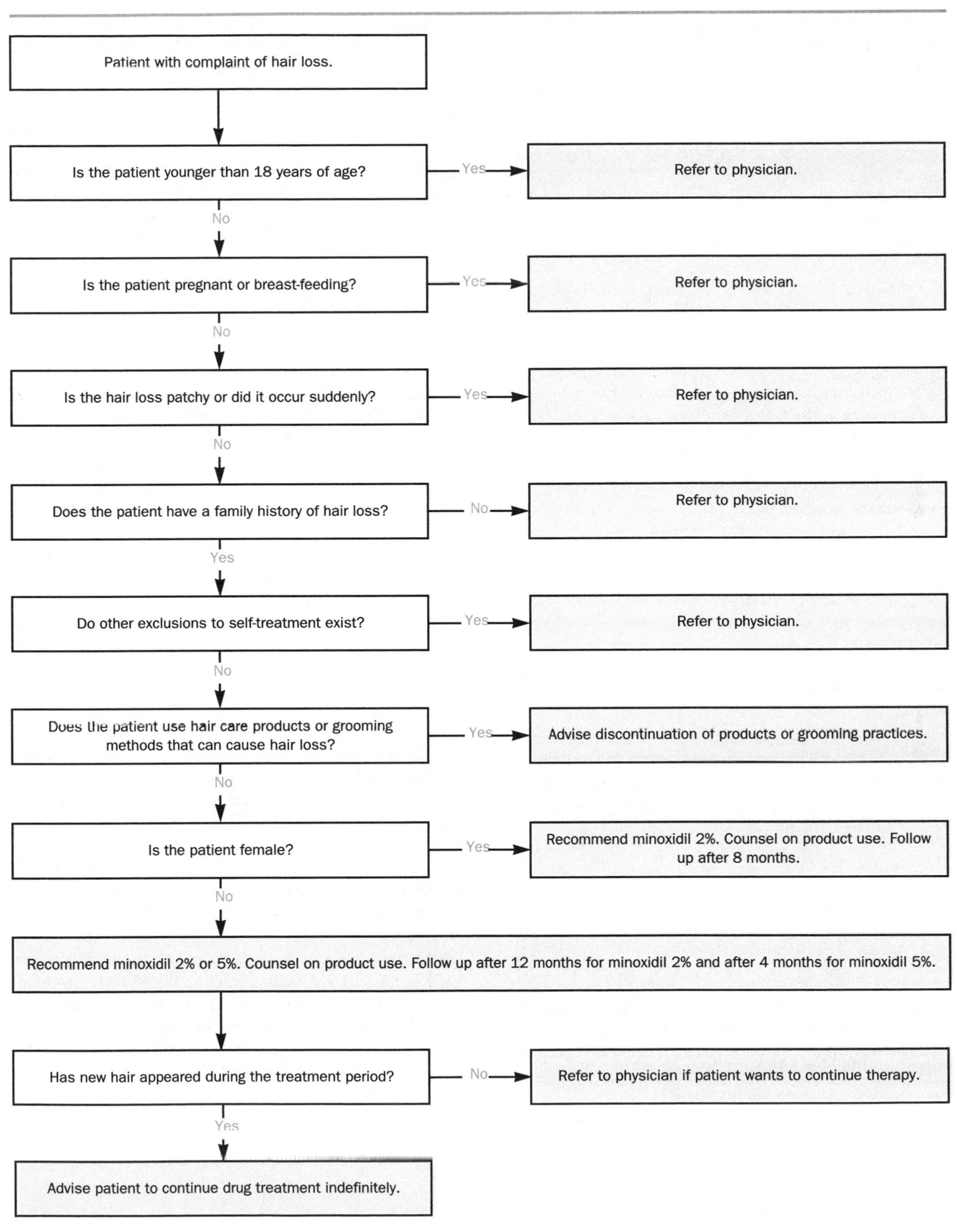

Figure 38–1 Self-care of hair loss.

pertension), but its mechanism of action as a topical medication is still unknown. According to some researchers, the drug appears to act by increasing cutaneous blood flow directly to the hair follicles, which increase in size with treatment.[28] However, others have found that cutaneous blood flow does not increase.[29] Minoxidil, which has been shown to directly stimulate follicular hypertrophy and prolong anagen phase,[30] may transform resting (telogen phase) hair follicles into active (anagen phase) hair follicles. Another study, which used a higher-than-marketed concentration of minoxidil, reported an increase in mean hair shaft diameter.[31] After up to 12 months of therapy, a subset of these same patients also revealed a reduction in the percentage of telogen hairs.

Indications Androgenetic alopecia in men and women is amenable to topical minoxidil treatment. Treatment is indicated for baldness at the crown of the head in men and for hair thinning at the frontoparietal area in women.[32] Use of the 2% product is indicated in both men and women, whereas use of the 5% product is indicated for men only.

Patients with nonpattern or sudden hair loss should first consult a physician before using minoxidil. Although topical minoxidil is not well-proven in treating alopecia areata or telogen effluvium, this medication is reported by some to be useful for selected patients. Hair often regrows spontaneously in patients with mild alopecia areata. Patients with persistent areata may respond to combination therapy in which topical minoxidil can be one of the medications used. Several combination therapies including topical minoxidil in conjunction with anthralin, topical steroids, or topical retinoids have been used, with some therapeutic advantage, for treating severe alopecia areata.[33] Topical minoxidil only slightly inhibits the amount of hair loss caused by anagen effluvium and may therefore offer less potential benefit.[34]

Dosage/Administration Guidelines Minoxidil can be applied using various methods, depending on the applicator (spray, extended spray tip, dropper, and/or rub-on assembly). Table 38–1 describes the proper application of this agent.

It may take 4 months for topical minoxidil 2% and 2 months for topical minoxidil 5% to stimulate new hair growth, which is usually colorless, soft, and very short. As treatment progresses, the hairs gradually mature and begin to look like existing hair. If hair fails to appear by 12 months for men and 8 months for women after using the 2% product, the patient should consider ending treatment. If hair fails to appear by 4 months after using the 5% product, the patient should consider ending treatment. Studies have demonstrated that once the drug is discontinued, hair density returns to pretreatment levels in a matter of months.[37]

Adverse Effects The most common side effect associated with minoxidil—local itching at the site of application (in about 7% of patients)—may be related to the hydroalcoholic vehicle. Rare side effects include acne at the site of application, increased hair loss, inflammation (soreness) of the hair roots, reddened skin, and swelling of the face.[36]

Table 38–1

Administration Guidelines for Minoxidil

- Apply minoxidil to dry scalp and hair.
- Rub about 1 mL of the product into the affected area of the scalp twice daily (morning and night).
- Wash and dry hands after applying the medication. If it gets into the eyes, mouth, or nose, rinse these areas thoroughly.
- Do not double the dose if you miss an application.
- Allow 4 hours for the drug to penetrate the scalp. Do not participate in any activity that might wash away or dilute the drug (e.g., bathing or swimming without a cap) for 4 hours after application.
- At night, apply the drug 4 hours before bedtime so that the drug does not rub off onto bed linen.
- Do not dry the scalp with a hair dryer after applying the drug. This action will reduce the drug's effectiveness.
- If applicable, apply hair grooming and styling products (e.g., sprays, mousses, and gels) or coloring agents, permanents, or relaxing agents after the minoxidil has dried. These products usually do not affect the efficacy of topical minoxidil.[35]

Source: Reference 36.

The most common side effect of long-term use is transient hypertrichosis (excessive hair growth), usually on the forehead and cheeks. Occasionally, patients may notice hypertrichosis on the chest, back, forearms and ear rims, which could indicate that the product has been applied excessively.[38] A few patients will notice increased hair loss in the first few weeks of use. Most likely, this loss represents a displacement of telogen by new anagen hairs.

Minoxidil is absorbed through the skin in relatively low concentrations, and documented systemic side effects are rare. In the unlikely event of an accidental overdose, the patient should seek emergency medical attention. Symptoms may involve low blood pressure (dizziness, confusion, fainting, lightheadedness); blurred vision or other changes in vision; headache or chest pain; irregular heart rate; sudden unexplained weight gain; swollen hands or feet; flushing of the skin; and numbness or tingling of the face, hands, or feet.[36] Although hemodynamic changes have not been detected in most controlled studies, one double-blind study reported that topical minoxidil 2% increased end-diastolic volume, cardiac output, and left ventricular mass.[39]

Drug–Drug Interactions The use of topical minoxidil is not associated with any known drug interactions. However, the concurrent use of guanethidine in patients could potentiate orthostatic hypotension, and the concurrent use of oral minoxidil could increase systemic levels of the drug, thus enhancing its effects. The application to the scalp of topical corticosteroids, such as petrolatum or tretinoin (e.g., Retin-A), with minoxidil may increase the minoxidil absorption and the risk of side effects. Scalps should not be treated with minoxidil for 24 hours before or after application of a permanent, a hair color, or a relaxant.[35]

Efficacy In a 48-week study, men displayed a mean increase in hair growth of 12.7% with minoxidil 2% and of 18.6% with extra-strength minoxidil 5%.[40] In men, minoxidil is more likely to be effective when less than one-fourth of the scalp surface has experienced hair loss or thinning. Although all of the hair usually does not grow back, even with continued treatment, progressive loss of hair is usually slowed.

Study data for men ages 18 to 49 years indicate that about one-fourth of the patients experienced moderate or better hair regrowth after using topical minoxidil.[32] One-third of the patients, however, attained only minimal hair regrowth. Minimal regrowth means that some new hairs are visible but not enough to cover thinning areas. Further, in treated areas, the hair density (i.e., how closely the hairs grow) is less than that on the untreated part of the head where significant hair loss has not occurred. With moderate regrowth, hairs may cover some or all of the thinning area and may grow more closely together. However, the hair density in the treated area will again be less than that on the rest of the head.

A minority of the patients had dense regrowth, which means that the thinning areas are almost completely covered and the hair density is equal to that on the untreated part of the head. The placebo vehicle also showed a modest response: About one-tenth of the patients had moderate or better regrowth, and about one-third had minimal regrowth.[32]

In women, topical minoxidil is more effective if less than about one-third of the scalp is thinning. Study data for women ages 18 to 45 years indicate that about one-fifth of the women experienced moderate regrowth after using topical minoxidil, whereas more than one-third experienced only minimal regrowth. In comparison, the placebo vehicle showed a 7% response rate for moderate regrowth and a 33% response rate for minimal regrowth.[32]

No studies have been done in age groups younger than 18 years or older than 65 years. No differences in side effects or other problems were demonstrated in a limited number of older patients up to age 65 years. In short, those most responsive to topical minoxidil treatment are younger patients who have limited hair loss that has existed for a relatively short period of time.[32]

Contraindications/Precautions/Warnings Patients who are allergic to minoxidil or to any component of the preparation should avoid this medication, as should patients with scalp damage from psoriasis, severe sunburn, or abrasions, which may increase minoxidil absorption. Patients should take additional precaution if corticosteroids or any agents known to increase cutaneous absorption of a drug are used concurrently with this product.

Topical minoxidil has a Pregnancy Category C rating, which means that it is not known whether the drug can harm an unborn baby. Similarly, the effect on nursing babies is not known. Therefore, pregnant women and women who are breast-feeding their babies should be advised not to use the product without first consulting a physician.

The use of the 5% product by women is contraindicated because the results with 2% and 5% are not measurably different and because the risk of facial hair growth is greater with the 5% product. Use of the product is contraindicated in patients age 18 years or younger.

The product is alcohol based and will burn or irritate eyes, mucous membranes, or abraded skin. When spraying the product, patients should take precautions to avoid inhalation and eye, nose, or mouth contact. Patients should wash and dry their hands after use, and if the product gets into the eyes, mouth, or nose, the patient should thoroughly rinse these areas. These precautions also are intended to prevent the systemic entry of minoxidil by alternative routes. Products containing minoxidil should not be used on any other part of the body.[36]

Researchers have sought a potential effect of minoxidil on systemic endocrine function but have not found one. However, measurement of plasma testosterone and excretion of urinary hydroxysteroids and ketosteroids in hypertensive patients who have been treated with oral minoxidil did not reveal any effects.[6] Further, serum cortisol, testosterone, and thyroid indexes are apparently unchanged by topical minoxidil.[41] However, unstable cardiac patients should not use the product unless supervised by a physician.

Safety and efficacy of the product in children (younger than 18 years) or in older adults (older than 65 years) have not been established, so the use of minoxidil in children and older adults must be supervised by a physician.

Product Selection Guidelines The 2% formulation should normally be recommended for use by women; however, men are usually advised to use the 5% concentration. Patient preference for method of application is another criterion in product selection. Patients with impaired vision or physical dexterity may find the rub-on method of application preferable to using sprays or droppers. (See Table 38–2 for examples of commercially available products.)

Unapproved Products

In 1980 and then again in 1989, an FDA advisory panel proposed removing from the market a number of ingredients that were known to be safe for external use but that claimed to prevent hair loss or to promote hair growth. The false claims have generally disappeared from the market, but many of these ingredients are still present in nonprescription lotions and shampoos available today. These ingredients include amino acids, aminobenzoic acid, B vitamins, hormones, jojoba oil, lanolin, polysorbates 20 and 660, sulfanilamide, tetracaine hydrochloride, urea, and wheat germ oil.[42,43]

Patient Assessment of Hair Loss

In addition to recommending treatment for hair loss, the pharmacist should first identify any possible underlying

Table 38–2

Selected Hair Regrowth Products

Trade Name	Primary Ingredients
Consort Hair Regrowth Solution Treatment for Men	Minoxidil 2%
HealthGuard Minoxidil Topical Solution for Men	Minoxidil 2%
HealthGuard Minoxidil Topical Solution for Women	Minoxidil 2%
Minoxidil Topical Solution for Men (Copley Ph'cal)	Minoxidil 2%
Minoxidil Topical Solution for Men (Alpharma)	Minoxidil 2%
Minoxidil Topical Solution for Men (Lemmon)	Minoxidil 2%
Rogaine Extra Strength Solution for Men	Minoxidil 5%
Rogaine for Men Solution	Minoxidil 2%
Rogaine for Women	Minoxidil 2%

medical cause. To assess alopecia areata or telogen effluvium, the pharmacist can direct the patient to perform a gentle hair-pull test. (See the section "Signs and Symptoms of Hair Loss.") The removal of 25% or more of the pulled hairs may indicate that the patient's hair loss is an active process (as in alopecia areata or telogen effluvium) and that the patient should be referred to a dermatologist. However, the test may be falsely negative if the patient's hair has been recently combed, brushed, or shampooed.[44] If pathology-induced and active hair loss are ruled out, the pharmacist should determine whether the balding fits the criteria for androgenetic alopecia. Asking the patient the following questions will help elicit the information needed to accurately assess the disorder and to recommend the appropriate treatment approach.

Q~ How long ago did you begin to lose your hair? What areas of the scalp are involved? How extensive are the areas involved?

A~ *Identify the characteristics of androgenetic alopecia in men and women. (See the section "Signs and Symptoms of Hair Loss.")* Suspect androgenetic alopecia if the balding has been gradual and the pattern of baldness is typical of this type of hair loss.

Q~ Have you been diagnosed with an autoimmune disorder, nutritional deficiency, or endocrine disorder?

A~ If yes, advise the patient that any of these disorders can cause hair loss and that a physician should be consulted.

Q~ Have you undergone chemotherapy or are you using a hormonal medication?

A~ Advise a patient undergoing chemotherapy that the hair loss is usually temporary. Refer patients taking a hormonal medication to a physician for evaluation of the hair loss.

Q~ (If female) Have you recently given birth?

A~ If yes, advise the patient that hormonal changes may contribute to hair loss and that this type of hair loss is usually temporary.

Q~ Have you suffered any trauma to the scalp?

A~ If yes, find out what type of injury occurred, and determine whether medical attention is needed.

Q~ Do others in your family suffer from hair loss?

A~ If yes, suspect that the patient has androgenetic alopecia.

Patient Counseling for Hair Loss

Patients should be advised that most treatment regimens for hair loss do not alter its progression, especially if the hair loss has gone on for a prolonged period of time. Some patients might instead be interested in transplantation of hair. The pharmacist should inform patients who wish to use nonprescription minoxidil that the longer the hair thinning or loss has gone on, the less likely it is that treatment will elicit a regrowth response. If the patient still wishes to use minoxidil, the pharmacist should review product instructions with the patient, making sure that the patient understands the possible adverse effects and the signs and symptoms that indicate the need for medical attention. The box "Patient Education for Hair Loss" lists specific information to provide to patients.

Evaluation of Patient Outcomes for Hair Loss

Patients should use minoxidil for the minimum recommended periods. If new hair growth does not occur after using minoxidil 2% for 12 months in men and 8 months in women, the patient should consider ending treatment. Patients using the 5% product should consider ending treatment if new hair does not appear after 4 months of using the product. If new hair does appear within the recommended periods, the pharmacist should advise the patient to continue the drug treatment indefinitely.

CONCLUSIONS

Minoxidil is suppressive, not curative. Offering cosmetic solutions may also be helpful. Patients, particularly women, are seeking treatment not only for hair loss but also for lost self-esteem resulting from the association of hair loss with illness and old age. Pharmacists and physicians should dispense medication with a measure of emotional support and should make clear the limitations of existing treatment.

Patient Education for Hair Loss

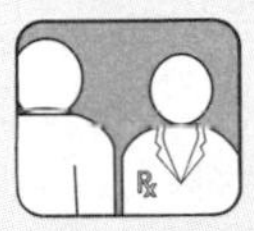

The objectives of self-treatment are to restore the appearance of the hair by (1) camouflaging thinning hair and/or (2) using minoxidil to regrow hair. For most patients, carefully following product instructions and the self-care measures listed below will help ensure optimal therapeutic outcomes.

Nondrug Measures

- If desired, use wigs to cover severe hair loss until hair is regrown.
- For less severe hair loss, use hair sprays, gels, colorants, or permanents in moderation to create the illusion of full hair. These cosmetics will not increase the rate of hair loss.
- Avoid the use of oily hair products that can cause folliculitis.
- Avoid hair styles such as tight braids that pull on the hair.

Nonprescription Medications

- Note that use of minoxidil must be continuous and indefinite to maintain regrowth. It may take up to 12 months to see results. If treatment is interrupted, regrowth will typically be lost within 4 months or less, and progression of hair loss will begin again.
- If you are pregnant, are breast-feeding, or become pregnant while using this product, consult a physician about the appropriateness of such use.
- See Table 38–1 for instructions on how to use this product.
- Do not apply the product more than twice daily. More frequent applications will not achieve better regrowth or a more rapid response.
- Do not apply the product to damaged or inflamed areas.
- Note that local itching or irritation at the site of application may occur. More rarely, allergic contact dermatitis may occur.
- Keep product containers out of the reach of children because acute ingestion of minoxidil is potentially hazardous.

⚠ If hair fails to appear within the time specified on the product, consider stopping the treatment and seeing a physician or dermatologist for further evaluation.

References

1. Sperling LC, Mezebish DS. Hair diseases. *Med Clin North Am.* 1998;82: 1155–69.
2. Sinclair R. Male pattern androgenetic alopecia. *Br Med J.* 26 Sep 1998;317:865–9.
3. Reiman P. Alopecia areata labeled autoimmune disease. *Dermatol Times.* 1999;20:43–4.
4. Camacho F. Alopecias due to telogenic effluvium. In: Camacho F, Montagna W, eds. *Trichology: Diseases of the Pilosebaceous Follicle.* Madrid, Spain: Aula Medica Group; 1997:403–11.
5. Lavker RM, Bertolino AP, Freedberg IM, et al. Biology of hair follicles. In: Freedberg IM, Eisen AZ, Wolff K, et al., eds. *Dermatology in General Medicine.* 5th ed. New York: McGraw-Hill; 1999:230–8.
6. Earhart RN, Ball J, Nuss DD, et al. Minoxidil-induced hypertrichosis: treatment with calcium thioglycolate depilatory. *South Med J.* 1977;70: 442–3.
7. Rook A, Dawber R. *Diseases of the Hair and Scalp.* Oxford, England: Blackwell Scientific Publications; 1982:9–17.
8. Sawaya ME. Biochemistry and control of hair growth. In: Arndt KA, LeBoit PE, Robinson JK, et al., eds. *Cutaneous Medicine and Surgery.* Philadelphia: WB Saunders Co; 1996:1248–9.
9. Rook A, Dawber R. *Diseases of the Hair and Scalp.* Oxford, England: Blackwell Scientific Publications; 1982:90–112.
10. Whiting D. Diagnostic and predictive value of horizontal sections of scalp biopsy specimens in male pattern androgenetic alopecia. *J Am Acad Dermatol.* 1993;28:755–63.
11. Sawaya ME, Price VH, Harris KA, et al. Human hair follicle aromatase activity in females with androgenic alopecia [abstract]. *J Invest Dermatol.* 1990;94:575.
12. Randall VA, Thornton MJ, Messenger AG. Cultured dermal papilla cells from androgen-dependent human hair follicles (such as beard) contain more androgen receptors than those from non-balding areas of the scalp. *J Endocrinol.* 1992;133:141–7.
13. Simpson NB, Barth JH. Hair patterns: hirsutes and androgenetic alopecia. In: Dawber RPR, ed. *Diseases of the Hair and Scalp.* Oxford, England: Blackwell Science; 1997:67–122.
14. Kuster W, Happle R. The inheritance of common baldness: two B or not two B? *J Am Acad Dermatol.* 1984;11:921–6.
15. Paus R, Slominski A, Czarnetski BM. Is alopecia areata an autoimmune response against melanogenesis-related proteins, exposed by abnormal MHC class I expression in the anagen hair bulb? *Yale J Biol Med.* 1993; 66:541–54.
16. Price VH, Colombe BW. Heritable factors distinguish two types of alopecia areata. *Dermatol Clin.* 1996;14:679–89.
17. Ahmad W, Faiyaz ul Haque M, Brancolini V, et al. Alopecia universalis associated with a mutation in the human hairless gene. *Science.* 1998;279:720–4.
18. Hughes ECW. Telogen effluvium. Available at: http://www.emedicine.com/derm/topic416.htm. Accessed February 4, 2000.
19. Fiedler VC. Alopecia areata and other nonscarring alopecias. In: Arndt KA, LeBoit PE, Robinson JK, et al. *Cutaneous Medicine and Surgery.* Philadelphia: WB Saunders Co; 1996:1274–8.
20. DeBerker D, Sinclair R. Defects of the hair shaft. In: Dawber RPR, ed. *Diseases of the Hair and Scalp.* Oxford, England: Blackwell Science; 1997: 296–7.
21. Talsma J. Hair disorders pose problem for African Americans. *Dermatol Times.* 1999;20:42–5.
22. Maddox J. Psychoimmunology before its time. *Nature.* 1984;309:400.
23. Mercurio MG. Androgenetic alopecia in women: Diagnosis and treatment. Available at: http://www.medscape.com/quadrant/Hospit...997/v33.n09/3309.02/hm3309.02.merc.html. Accessed February 4, 2000.
24. Messenger AG, Simpson NB. In: Dawber RPR, ed. *Diseases of the Hair and Scalp.* Oxford, England: Blackwell Science; 1997:356–7.
25. New Zealand Dermatological Society. Alopecia areata. Available at: http://www.dermnet.org.nz/dna.alopecia/alopecia.html. Accessed February 4, 2000.

26. Sinclair R, DeBerker D. Hereditary and congenital alopecia and hypertrichosis. In: Dawber RPR, ed. *Diseases of the Hair and Scalp*. Oxford, England: Blackwell Science; 1997:168–9.
27. Orentreich D, Orentreich N. Androgenetic alopecia and its treatment, a historical view. In: Inger WP, ed. *Hair Transplantation*. 3rd ed. New York: Marcel Dekker; 1995:1–33.
28. Sasson M, Shupack JL, Stiller MJ. Status of medical treatment for androgenetic alopecia. *Int J Dermatol.* 1993;32:701–6.
29. Bunker CB, Dowd PM. Alterations in scalp blood flow after the epicutaneous application of 3% minoxidil and 0.1% hexylnicotinate in alopecia. *Br J Dermatol.* 1988;117:668.
30. Kurata S, Uno H, Allenhoffmann BL. Effects of hypertrichotic agents on follicular and nonfollicular cells in vitro. *Skin Pharmacol.* 1996;9:3–8.
31. Abell E, Cary MM. The pathogenic effect of minoxidil in male pattern alopecia. *J Invest Dermatol.* 1986;86:459.
32. Minoxidil. In: *Drug Facts and Comparisons*. St. Louis: Facts and Comparisons; 1999:3239–40.
33. Fiedler VC. Alopecia areata: a review of therapy, efficacy, safety and mechanism. *Arch Dermatol.* 1992;128:1519–20.
34. Duvic M, Lemak NA, Valero V, et al. A randomized trial of minoxidil in chemotherapy-induced alopecia. *J Am Acad Dermatol.* 1996;35:74–8.
35. *Rogaine Product Information*. Kalamazoo, MI: Pharmacia & Upjohn, Inc; 1996.
36. US Pharmacopeia. Minoxidil. *The Complete Drug Reference*. 19th ed. Yonkers, NY: Consumer Reports; 1999:1148.
37. Olsen EA, Weiner MS. Topical minoxidil in male pattern baldness: effects of discontinuation of treatment. *J Am Acad Dermatol.* 1987;17:97–101.
38. Gonzalez M, Landa N, Gardeazabal J, et al. Generalized hypertrichosis after treatment with topical minoxidil. *Clin Exp Dermatol.* 1994;19:157–8.
39. Leenen FH, Smith DL, Unger WP. Topical minoxidil: cardiac effects in bald man. *Br J Clin Pharmacol.* 1988;26:481–5.
40. Propecia and Rogaine Extra Strength for alopecia. *Med Lett.* 1998;40:25–7.
41. Weiss VC, West D, Fu TS, et al. Alopecia areata treated with topical minoxidil. *Arch Dermatol.* 1984;120:457–63.
42. Hecht A. Hair grower and hair loss prevention drugs. *FDA Consumer.* 1985;19:1–3.
43. Hanover L. Hair replacement. *FDA Consumer.* 1997;31:7–10.
44. Kligman AM. Pathologic dynamics of human hair loss. *Arch Dermatol.* 1961;83:175–98.

Section IX

Other Medical Disorders

CHAPTER 39

Diabetes Mellitus

Condit F. Steil, John R. White Jr., and R. Keith Campbell

Chapter 39 at a Glance

Diabetes mellitus is a chronic syndrome characterized by abnormally high blood glucose levels and by defects in insulin production or utilization. Four types are recognized, but Type 1 (5% to 10%) and Type 2 (85% to 90%) account for the majority of cases. Table 39–1 lists distinguishing features of these two types of diabetes. The third category, gestational onset diabetes, develops in 2% to 5% of all pregnancies but usually disappears when a pregnancy is over. Gestational diabetes first becomes apparent after 24 to 28 weeks of pregnancy. The real concern with women who develop gestational diabetes is that approximately 40% will develop Type 2 diabetes. The fourth category (about 1% to 2% of all cases) includes all other factors that may induce diabetes. Because of the breadth of this category, only the inducing factors will be mentioned. These factors include malnutrition, surgery, drugs, infections, and other illnesses. Other factors include genetic defects, such as maturity-onset diabetes in youth (MODY) types 1 to 3, which are classed as

Editor's Note: This chapter is based, in part, on the 11th edition chapter titled "Diabetes Care Products and Monitoring Devices," which was written by Condit F. Steil, R. Keith Campbell, and John R. White Jr.

Table 39–1

Differentiation of Type 1 and Type 2 Diabetes Mellitus

	Type 1 (IDDM)	Type 2 (NIDDM)
Age of onset	Usually, but not always, during childhood or adolescence	Frequently >35 years
Type of onset	Abrupt	Usually gradually
Prevalence	0.5%	2%–4%
Incidence	<10%	>75%
Family history of diabetes	Frequently negative	Commonly present
Primary cause	Pancreatic β-cell deficiency	End organ (insulin receptors) unresponsiveness to insulin action
Nutritional status at time of onset	Usually thin with weight loss	Usually obese
Postglucose plasma or serum insulin,[a] mcU/mL	Absent or minimal	Normal or elevated
Symptoms	Polydipsia, polyphagia, and polyuria	Maybe none
Hepatomegaly	Rather common	Uncommon
Stability of blood glucose levels	Fluctuates widely in response to small changes in insulin dose, exercise, and infection	Fluctuations are less marked
Possible etiologic factors:		
Inheritance	Associated with specific HLA tissue types, but only 40%–50% concordance in twins	95%–100% concordance in twins, but not associated with specific HLA tissue types
Autoimmune disease	50%–80% circulating islet cell antibodies	Negative; <10% circulating islet cell antibodies
Viral infections	Coxsackie, mumps, influenza	No evidence
Proneness to ketosis	Frequent, especially if treatment program is insufficient in food and/or insulin	Uncommon except in the presence of unusual stress or moderate-to-severe sepsis
Insulin defect	Defect in secretion; secretion is impaired early in disease; secretion may be totally absent late in disease	Insulin deficiency present in some patients; others are insulin resistant
		Insulin deficiency—in most patients, insulin secretion fails to keep pace with inordinate demands caused by obesity; this defect may appear initially as a failure to respond to glucose alone, suggesting an impairment in the glucoreceptor of the pancreatic β-cell
		Insulin resistance—in some patients a defect in tissue responsiveness to insulin and evidence of hyperinsulinemia is seen; in such patients, insulin resistance may be mediated by a decreased number of insulin receptors in target cells
		Increased hepatic glucose production in response to altered cellular glucose uptake
Plasma insulin (endogenous)	Negligible to zero	Plasma insulin response may be either adequate but delayed, so that postprandial hypoglycemia may be present at diagnosis, or diminished but not absent
Vascular complications of diabetes and degenerative changes	Infrequent until diabetes has been present for ≈5 years	Frequent
Usual cause of death	Degenerative complications in target organs (e.g., renal failure caused by diabetic nephropathy)	Accelerated atherosclerosis (e.g., myocardial infarct); to lesser extent, microangiopathic changes in target tissues (e.g., renal failure)
Diet	Mandatory in all patients	If diet is used fully, hypoglycemic therapy may not be needed
Insulin	Necessary for all patients	Necessary for 20%–30% of patients
Oral agents	Rarely efficacious	Often efficacious

[a] Normal response is between 50 and 135 mcU/mL at 60 minutes and less than 100 mcU/mL at 120 minutes after 100 g of oral glucose.

genetic defects of β-cell function. Leprechaunism, Rabson-Mendenhall syndrome, type A insulin resistance, and lipoatrophic diabetes are classified as genetic defects of insulin action.

In all instances, self-care is integral to the treatment (and prevention) of this disease. Pharmacists can assist patients with diabetes by assessing their ability for self-care, teaching them how to care for themselves, monitoring self-care measures, and reinforcing patients' understanding of this information. The pharmacist can be part of the network of health care providers engaged in coordinating the patients' health care and can be their resource of information on drugs, devices, and monitoring systems used in treatment.

Type 1 Diabetes Mellitus

Patients with Type 1 diabetes mellitus have a pancreatic disability that causes them to chronically need exogenous insulin, the hormone that facilitates glucose metabolism. To survive, these patients must receive daily and lifelong insulin to control their blood glucose levels within normal limits. Thus, Type 1 diabetes mellitus is also called insulin-dependent diabetes mellitus (IDDM) and is sometimes called juvenile diabetes because it most often develops in children and young adults.

Epidemiology of Type 1 Diabetes Mellitus

More than a million people (including 123,000 under the age of 20 years) in the United States have Type 1 diabetes mellitus. Each year, 11,000 to 12,000 children are diagnosed with the disease. Risk factors for Type 1 diabetes include race and ethnicity. A family history (i.e., a first-degree relative with diabetes) of the disorder is also a risk factor. The low concordance rates of Type 1 diabetes among identical twins indicate that genetic risk factors are necessary but not sufficient. The human leukocyte antigen (HLA) region of chromosome 6 appears to be involved, but other chromosomes are implicated as well.

The risk factors that appear to accelerate the autoimmune process that stops insulin synthesis are cold environment, high growth rate, infections, and stressful life events. Risk factors that may initiate the autoimmune process are cow's milk proteins, nitrosamines, or early fetal events such as blood group incompatibility or viral infection.

Cardiovascular risks include hypertension (greater than 130/85 mm Hg) and high-density lipoprotein (HDL) cholesterol less than 45 mg/dL and/or triglyceride greater than 200 mg/dL.[1]

Physiology of Glycoprotein Metabolism

Together with glucagon, somatostatin, growth hormone, cortisol, epinephrine, and other hormones, endogenous insulin maintains blood glucose levels between 50 and 150 mg/100 mL (mg%) at all times—a level needed for systems to function normally. Insulin and glucagon, the major hormones that control glucose metabolism, are made and stored by the β- and α-cells of the pancreas, respectively. The pancreatic β-cells release insulin in response to elevated plasma glucose, and the liver rapidly clears the hormone from the system. Insulin has several functions: It stimulates glucose storage in muscle and liver cells as glycogen, increases synthesis of fatty acids and triglycerides, decreases hepatic glucose output, stimulates lipolysis and production of ketone bodies, and enhances incorporation of amino acids into proteins.

Glucagon acts as insulin's antagonist. Low blood glucose or high amino acid levels trigger glucagon secretion, which causes glycogenolysis (the breakdown of glycogen into glucose) in the liver and a rise in blood glucose. If both blood amino acids and glucose are high, the effect of glucose is dominant and causes glucagon, and consequently glucose, levels to fall.

Etiology of Type 1 Diabetes Mellitus

Diabetes mellitus is not a single disease but rather a syndrome composed of several specific diseases, all of which are characterized by hyperglycemia and a tendency to develop macrovascular or microvascular disease and neuropathy. Type 1 diabetes is characterized by an absence of functioning, insulin-secreting pancreatic islet cells.

Factors associated with the development of diabetes include heredity, obesity, age, stress, hormonal imbalance, vasculitis of the vessels supplying the β-cells of the pancreas, and viruses affecting the autoimmune responses of the body.[2] Extrinsic or environmental factors may include viruses such as mumps or Coxsackie B4, destructive cytotoxins and antibodies released by sensitized lymphocytes, or autodigestion in the course of an inflammatory disorder involving the adjacent exocrine pancreas. Specific HLA genes may increase susceptibility to a diabetogenic virus, or certain immune-response genes may predispose patients to autoimmune destruction of their own islet cells. Protective genes apparently also exist that prevent expression of the defective immune-response genes. Hence, not everyone with the Type 1 defects will develop the disease. Although genetics is a strong causal component, only a small percentage of defective genes is expressed. If both parents have Type 1 diabetes, only 20% of their children can be expected to develop the disease. This expectation contrasts with Type 2 diabetes. (See the section "Etiology of Type 2 Diabetes Mellitus.")

Pathophysiology of Type 1 Diabetes Mellitus

In Type 1 diabetes, a meal or a snack brings about hyperglycemia because insulin production is grossly lacking or totally absent. In addition, amino acids are converted into glucose by gluconeogenesis, and liver glycogen is converted into glucose by glycogenolysis. However, without insulin, the dependent tissues cannot use this glucose, and hyperglycemia becomes even more pronounced. These metabolic changes cause a rapid onset of symptoms. Specifically, the unused glucose produces an increased osmotic load in the kidney, which results in the production and excretion of large amounts of urine (polyuria), a loss of fluid, and dehydration. This osmotic diuresis may initially cause dry mouth and can progress to significant hypovolemia, electrolyte loss, and cellular dehydration. A compensatory increase in thirst (polydipsia) occurs. Because tissue cells cannot use the circulating blood glucose as a result of a lack of insulin, the nervous system signals the person to eat (polyphagia). Then eating promotes the further rise in blood glucose level.

Insulin is an inhibitor of the enzyme lipoprotein lipase, which mobilizes body fat (lipolysis). Also, circulating cholesterol indices tend to be elevated. In time, this fat metabolism and lack of carbohydrate use will cause a weight loss in Type 1 diabetes. The free fatty acids are further broken down for energy and produce acidic ketone bodies, which in the absence of insulin can eventually induce metabolic acidosis. Fully developed progression of this syndrome can induce a systemic ketoacidosis with deep and labored breathing and air hunger, or Kussmaul's respiration. This situation is an emergency that can lead to coma and death if not treated. Early detection with urine ketone testing often can limit the reaction to a milder form. Figure 39–1 shows the clinical manifestations of a patient with untreated Type 1 diabetes.[2,3]

Chronic hyperglycemia (blood glucose levels greater than 150 mg/dL) and complications in diabetes affect all major physiologic systems. A number of events, which induce changes in the blood vessels and neurologic function, have

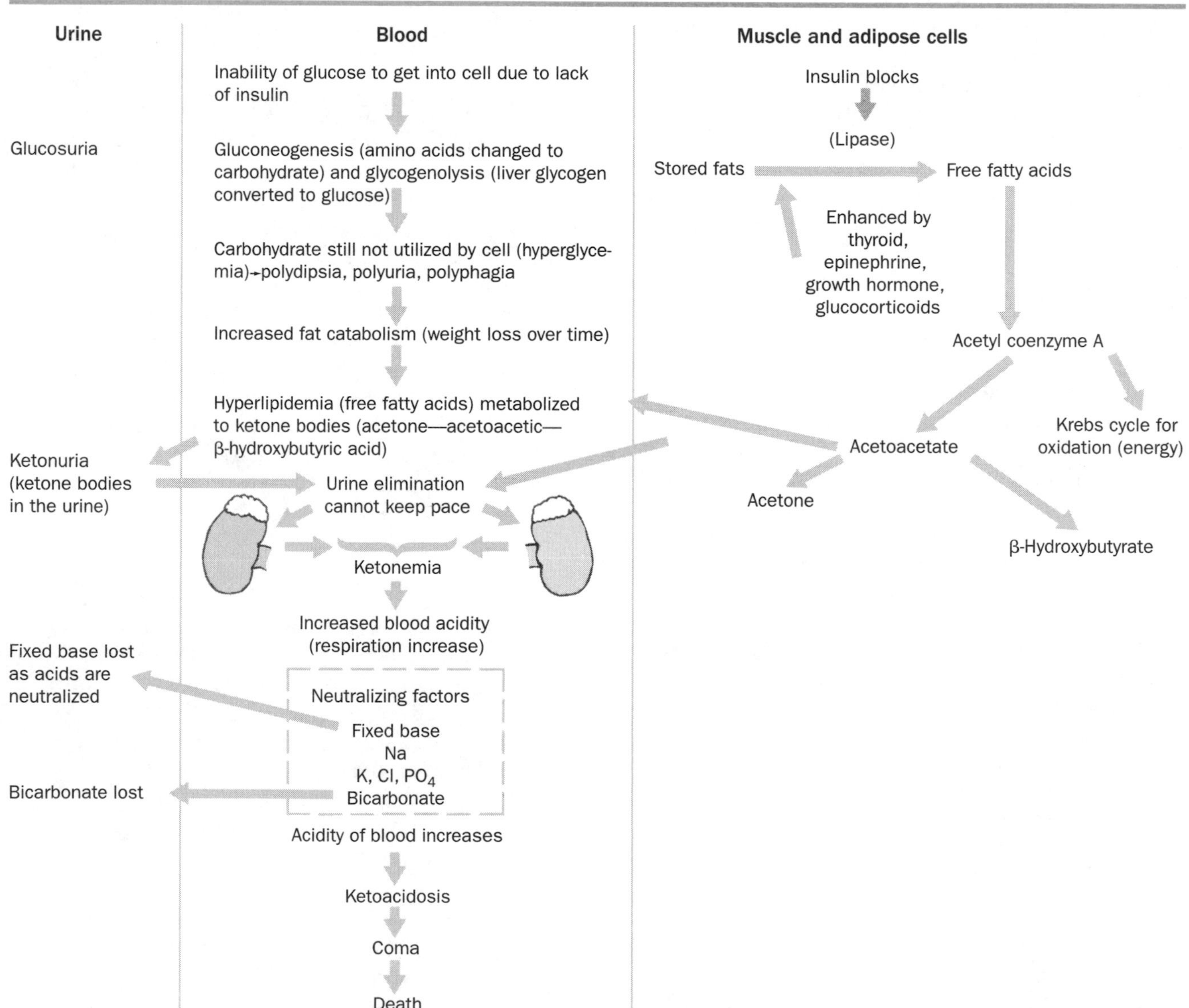

Figure 39–1 Clinical manifestations of Type 1 insulin-dependent diabetes mellitus.

been suggested as possible contributors to the following complications:

- Thickening of the capillary basement membrane.
- Osmotic damage to the lens of the eye and certain neurons, caused by increasing sorbitol levels produced by polyol pathway metabolism of glucose.
- Increased plasma viscosity.
- Decreased red blood cell flexibility.
- Faulty lipid metabolism that leads to higher fat levels and possibly to the onset of atherosclerosis.
- Abnormally high levels of glycosylated hemoglobin and advanced glycosylation end products.
- Impaired phagocytosis and subsequent inability to fight infection.
- Increased neonatal morbidity and mortality.[4]

Highly reactive glycosylated proteins form when glucose is consistently elevated. Advanced glycosylation end products form when these proteins interact and then covalently bind to amino groups on other proteins, thus accumulating and thickening the basement membrane.[5] Another such event occurs when elevated serum glucose levels generate high concentrations in non–insulin-dependent tissues, such as the lens of the eye and some neurons. The enzymes normally involved in the polyol pathway metabolize the excess glucose, increasing sorbitol and fructose concentrations in the lens and nerves, which may cause osmotic injury. When acutely elevated blood glucose levels are normalized, previously severe neuropathy symptoms may resolve.[6]

Other abnormalities of glycoprotein metabolism have been identified in both Type 1 and Type 2 patients and, in some cases, are used clinically. For instance, increase in a minor hemoglobin component, hemoglobin A_{1c}, reflects mean blood glucose concentration over the previous 2- to 3-month period and is used to assess chronic control of hyperglycemia. Hemoglobin A_{1c} is a reliable predictor for progression of diabetes complications.

Atherosclerotic lesions in people with diabetes appear similar to those in people without diabetes, but they tend to develop earlier, occur more often, and are more severe.[7] Hyperglycemia causes damage to the intimal cells of the arteries, and this damage is probably the initial lesion in atherosclerosis. Lower-than-normal levels of plasma HDL cholesterol and elevated levels of low-density lipoprotein (LDL) cholesterol may contribute to cholesterol deposition and plaque formation.[7] Patients may suffer from occlusive vascular changes in the lower extremities as a result of both atherosclerosis and damage to smaller arteries (microangiopathies). Peripheral lesions, alone or in combination with hemorheologic (blood flow) factors, may cause increased intermittent claudication (limping) and may contribute to the development of gangrene. Cardiomyopathy, cardiovascular neuropathy, and silent myocardial infarct may also occur in these patients.[7]

Hyperglycemia may impair the phagocytic activity of the body's white blood cells, which often makes the cure of bacterial infections difficult in patients with diabetes.[8]

Signs and Symptoms of Type 1 Diabetes Mellitus

Patients may be asymptomatic early in the course of the disease but typically are thirsty, have dry mouth, have increased urination, especially at night (nocturia), and have increased appetite. Some people may experience nausea or vomiting and extreme tiredness. Symptoms of long-term diabetes complications may appear well before elevated blood glucose is detected. These symptoms include numbness or pain in legs and hands, muscle weakness, vaginal itching, impotence (in men), and cessation of menses in women. Other symptoms could include frequent bladder, vaginal, and skin infections; blurred vision; depression; confusion; ear noise or buzzing; and bleeding gums.

Nonspecific symptoms for diabetes, which increase in number or become progressively more severe, may be indicators. For example, the patient may lose weight in the absence of any dietary restriction. Women may have recurrent monilial infections of the vulva and anus, signaling an increase of their blood glucose levels. Patients may have wounds, minor cuts, and scratches that take up to twice as long to heal and are more likely to become infected. Patients who wear glasses may notice they need stronger lenses more frequently.

Complications of Type 1 Diabetes Mellitus

Complications of Type 1 diabetes are categorized as microvascular, macrovascular, and neuropathic (peripheral and autonomic). Microvascular complications include retinopathy and nephropathy. Macrovascular complications pertain to atherosclerosis and to arteriosclerosis. These cardiovascular complications increase the potential for myocardial infarction and other cardiac events. Peripheral neuropathy involves degeneration of nerves in peripheral tissues (e.g., feet or hands). Autonomic neuropathy involves degeneration of nerves of the autonomic nervous system, resulting in gastroparesis, constipation, and other gastrointestinal and cardiovascular symptoms. Peripheral neuropathy and angiopathy change the character and function of the small blood vessels and thereby accelerate the potential for significant foot problems. (Data indicate that an angiotensin-converting enzyme [ACE] inhibitor, captopril, limits the progression of diabetic nephropathy.[9] Other ACE inhibitors have similar action.)

Diabetes is the leading cause of new blindness (12,000 to 24,000 new cases annually) in individuals between ages 20 and 74 years and, since 1995, has been the seventh leading cause listed on death certificates in the United States. More than half of all heart attacks are related to diabetes, with death rates from heart disease in people with diabetes about two to four times higher than in adults without diabetes. Atherosclerosis contributes to this increase in cardiovascular mortality and morbidity that occurs in people with diabetes. Less clear is to what degree atherosclerosis contributes to the development of microvascular disease.[8] Diabetic kidney disease is a leading cause of end-stage renal disease (about 40% of new cases). More than 67,000 amputations are performed annually secondary to diabetes-related complications in the foot and leg such as gangrene. (See the "Color Plates," photograph 33.) This statistic represents more than half of all amputations performed in the United States annually.[10,11] Neurologic complications, both autonomic and peripheral, also occur frequently.

People with diabetes have altered immune systems and are more susceptible to infectious diseases, such as influenza and pneumonia, than the general population. The most easily infected part of the body is the skin. In people with diabetes with related vascular and neurologic complications, infections may not be promptly detected and may require more time for healing.

Because glucose levels in saliva are increased in patients with hyperglycemia, they have a higher incidence of dental caries and gum disease. Occult abscesses of the teeth are common in hyperglycemic patients; stress caused by this complication may contribute to poor blood glucose control. Uncontrolled diabetes seems to predispose patients to the various stages of periodontal disease.

Some cases of blindness caused by diabetes can be prevented or slowed if retinopathy is detected early and the retina is photocoagulated with laser therapy, and if glaucoma is detected and treated early. Drugs with parasympatholytic effects, including anticholinergics, antihistamines, and ganglionic blockers, can alter the pupil and ciliary muscles and can result in blurred vision.

In addition, diabetic women who receive no prenatal care are likely to have at least twice the number of congenitally malformed babies as those who do receive prenatal care. Further, the rate of death among newborns of diabetic women (3% to 5%) is at least twice that of nondiabetic women.

Table 39–2 describes potential complications of diabetes and their treatment. Patients can prevent some of these com-

Table 39–2

Potential Complications of Diabetes Mellitus and Their Treatment

Body Location	Description	Treatment
Eyes	Retinopathy, cataract formation, glaucoma, and periodic visual disturbances caused by microvascular disease and other metabolic complications such as increased sorbitol; leading cause of new blindness	Strict control of blood glucose to avoid need for treatment (e.g., laser photocoagulation, vitrectomy)
Mouth	Gingivitis, increased incidence of dental caries and periodontal disease	Strict control of blood glucose and daily hygiene; see dentist regularly
Reproductive system (pregnancy)	Increased incidence of large babies, stillbirths, miscarriages, neonatal deaths, and congenital defects caused by metabolic abnormalities	Strict control of blood glucose before and during pregnancy
Nervous system	Motor, sensory, and autonomic neuropathy leading to impotence, neurogenic bladder, paresthesias, gangrene, altered gastrointestinal motility, and cardiovascular problems	Strict control of blood glucose, daily foot care, surgery, and antidepressants and phenothiazines when indicated
Vascular system	Large vessel disease resulting in atherosclerosis and microvascular disease leading to retinopathy, nephropathy, and decreased peripheral perfusion	Strict control of blood glucose
Skin	Numerous infections and specific lesions such as skin spots, diabetic bullae, lipodystrophies, and necrobiosis lipoidica diabeticorum caused by small vessel disease, increased lipids in blood, and pruritus	Strict control of blood glucose, daily hygiene
Kidneys	Diabetic glomerulosclerosis causing nephropathy	Strict control of blood glucose; eventually, diet low in proteins. Prednisone, dialysis, and renal transplantation if necessary. ACE inhibitors to limit progression.
Reticuloendothelial system (infections)	Cystitis, tuberculosis, skin infections, difficulty in overcoming infections, and moniliasis in diabetic women	Strict control of blood glucose and aggressive anti-infective therapy when indicated

Source: Pharmaceutical services for patients with diabetes. *Am Pharm* (module 4). 1986;NS26 : 8.

plications by instituting special care procedures. (See Table 39–3.)

Treatment of Type 1 Diabetes Mellitus

Successful management of Type 1 diabetes requires the combined efforts of the physician, pharmacist, nurse, dietitian, patient, patient's family, significant others, and other caregivers. Psychologic as well as clinical support is often needed to ensure adherence to the prescribed care plan.

Table 39–3

Preventive Measures for Diabetes Complications

Skin Care

- Bathe daily with mild soaps and dry skin thoroughly.
- Inspect skin daily—head to toe—for signs of potential infection.
- Cleanse minor cuts and scratches promptly with soap and water.
- See a physician immediately for a serious cut, burn, or skin puncture.
- When needed, use nonprescription topical preparations that the pharmacist and local physician consider appropriate.
- Learn the proper use and limitations for topical products.

Dental Care

- Have teeth checked at least twice each year.
- Brush and floss teeth at least twice daily, and massage gums with a brush, a Water Pik, or fingers.
- Consult a dentist at the first sign of abnormal conditions of the gums.
- Use appropriate dental care products.[12]

Eye Care

- Get an annual dilated eye exam.
- Do not use any topical ophthalmic preparations unless such products are recommended or prescribed by a physician, ophthalmologist, or optometrist.
- See a physician immediately if changes in vision or eye irritation occur.

Foot Care

- Inspect feet daily for any change, and clean them daily.
- Probe areas of the foot with a small metal filament to assess tactile sensation.
- Wear properly fitting, comfortable shoes; use caution when "breaking in" new shoes.
- Change shoes and socks a couple of times a day.
- Do not wear tight clothing, and do not cross legs when seated.
- Trim nails, preferably straight across, and file them with an emery board to the contour of the toe.
- Do not walk barefooted.
- Inspect shoes for foreign objects before inserting feet.

Treatment Outcomes

The basic objectives in the treatment of diabetes, in order of importance, are to do the following:

- Relieve and prevent diabetes-related symptoms.
- Prevent hypoglycemic and hyperglycemic reactions.
- Maintain blood glucose levels (between 80 and 150 mg/dL) and hemoglobin A_{1c} (less than 7%; take action if greater than 8%) to prevent or slow progression of chronic complications.
- Achieve and/or maintain optimal weight.
- Promote normal growth and development in children.
- Eliminate or minimize all other cardiovascular risk factors.
- Have patients become their own primary health caregiver through intensive education.

Strict adherence to a comprehensive diabetes care plan is vital to meeting these objectives. The care plan should include the following seven steps:

- Assessment of the patient's knowledge, understanding, and current care.
- Nutrition planning and instruction.
- Physical activity recommendations.
- Self-monitoring of glucose and ketone levels.
- Drug therapy.
- Patient education.
- Follow-up care to alter or adjust the plan as needed to achieve better control.

General Treatment Approach

Patients with Type 1 diabetes must inject themselves with insulin each day. The algorithm in Figure 39–2 outlines pharmacologic treatment with this agent.

Strict adherence to a dietary plan and participation in moderate exercise are also important in controlling blood glucose levels. Insulin therapy attempts to balance the effects of diet and exercise. The complications of hyperglycemia are largely preventable once this balance is achieved. To achieve the balance, patients must monitor their blood glucose levels. Not only does self-monitoring of blood glucose serve a clinical purpose, but also it gives the patient a sense of control over the disorder.

Nonpharmacologic Therapy

Nutrition and physical activity can play a crucial role in controlling blood glucose levels. A proper dietary plan for Type 1 diabetes allows a healthy daily nutritional intake. A good exercise plan includes moderate daily aerobic exercise.

Nutrition Plan

Current American Diabetes Association guidelines for nutrition control represent a change to a more individualized ap-

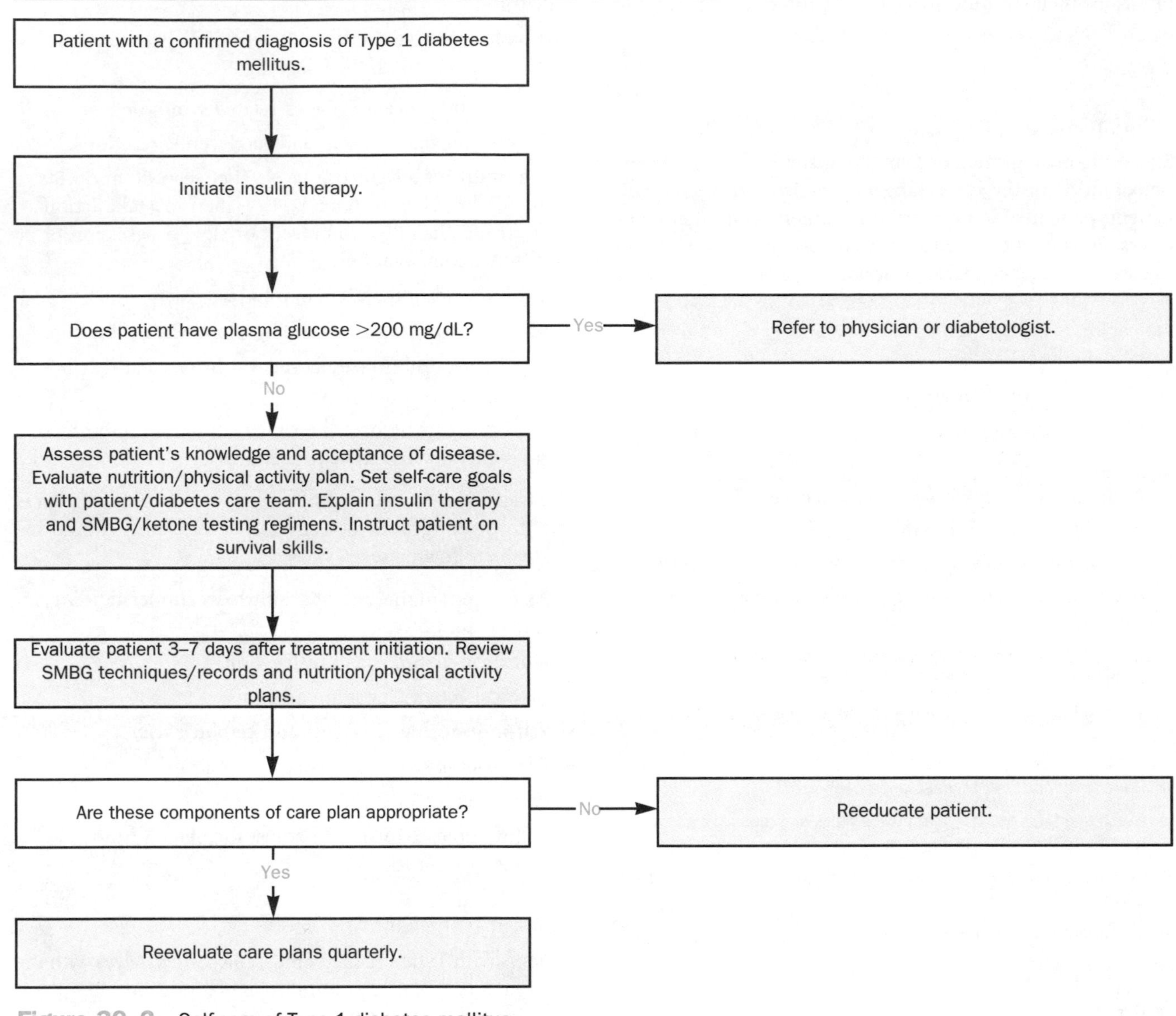

Figure 39–2 Self-care of Type 1 diabetes mellitus.

proach from previous recommendations. Limited data indicate some trends for recommending specific protein intake levels, but 10% to 20% of total calories is the generally accepted recommendation for everyone. Protein intake is less in patients with reduced renal function. Less than 10% of the total daily intake should come from saturated fats and up to 10% should come from polyunsaturated fats. For individuals with near normal weight and lipid levels, 30% or less calories should come from fat and 45% to 60% from carbohydrates. If obesity or high-lipid intake is present, the recommendation is to decrease dietary lipid or fat. Diabetes patients were taught for several years to avoid simple sugars, but little evidence shows that the assumed rapid rise in blood glucose actually occurs from sugar consumption. The message is clear to shift the concern to the total amount of carbohydrates. Sodium intake should be limited when hypertension is a risk. Pharmacists should encourage patients to keep a diet and physical activity log to link the effects of food, physical activity, and medication on blood glucose.[12,13] Patients should also be aware of the effects that sweeteners, alcohol, and caffeine can have on glycemic control.

Use of Sweeteners Non-nutritive (noncaloric) and nutritive (caloric) alternative sweetening agents are available. Non-nutritive sweeteners include saccharin or cyclamates, and nutritive sweeteners include aspartame, fructose, sorbitol, and mannitol. Saccharin is 400 times as sweet as sucrose and is a common substitute in food products. The use of sorbitol and fructose is troublesome because of their caloric content and the osmotic and laxative action of sorbitol. Fructose naturally occurs in fruits, honey, and other sources and may be used as a sweetener. All patients should contact their physician or dietitian before using a substitute sweetener. Pharmacists can support and reinforce all phases of nutrition therapy by encouraging patients to follow their meal plan and to avoid fad diets or prolonged fasting. Moreover, patients need instruction in reading food product labels and in interpreting the nutritional value of the product.

Use of Alcohol Patients with diabetes must know that alcohol (1) is considered a fat (9 calories/g) in the nutrition plan; (2) alters insulin response; (3) changes manufacture, storage, and release of glycogen; (4) impairs judgment and coordination; and (5) has chronic nerve toxicity.

Acute alcohol consumption can induce a hypoglycemic reaction, especially when consumed on an empty stomach. If the patient is going to drink alcohol, he or she should be advised to do the following:

- For men, drink no more than 2 drinks daily (4 ounces of wine, 1.5 ounces of distilled beverages, or 12 ounces of beer is considered one drink). For women, drink no more than 1 drink daily.
- Eat something first and space drinks.
- Refrain from drinking if overweight or if diabetes is uncontrolled.
- Avoid sugar-containing mixes.
- Include drinks in the caloric intake calculation.
- Refrain from drinking if neuropathy from diabetes is present, because alcohol intake can induce nerve damage.

Use of Caffeine People with diabetes may respond differently to intake of caffeine. Caffeine intake may need to be considered in patients who tend toward hyperglycemic episodes at specific times of the day. If consumed in large amounts, the caffeine in coffee, tea, soft drinks, and other products may increase liver glycogen breakdown and thus raise blood glucose levels.[14]

Physical Activity Plan

Physicians are referring patients for individual counseling about physical activity to physical therapists and exercise physiologists who are specially trained as diabetes educators. The term *physical activity* rather than *exercise* is used because many elderly individuals may feel they cannot exercise. The coordination of the physical activity and nutrition plans with the medication regimen can improve control and adherence to the care plan over the long term. Fewer episodes of hypoglycemia are reported. Physical therapists can optimize activity according to the patient's individual lifestyle and diagnosis.

Patients are encouraged to exercise the large muscle groups and to participate in aerobic activities (e.g., swimming, running, and biking). Activities that excessively strain the body, such as weight lifting, are discouraged because of the risk of optic capillary damage. Daily aerobic exercise helps lower blood glucose levels by increasing glucose penetration and metabolism in muscle cells without the assistance of insulin. Effects of physical activity on blood glucose vary. Hyperglycemia results if insulin is inadequate when the patient begins the activity, or hypoglycemia may occur if the patient's blood glucose concentration is normal or low just before physical activity. Consistent physical activity is a key component. Table 39–4 provides guidelines for the conscientious exerciser. Patients should include their activity in the aforementioned daily log.

Pharmacologic Therapy (Insulin)

Insulin is the primary medication used to treat diabetes. This agent is classified by its time–action profile and its species source.

Insulins may be divided into four groups, according to promptness of action, duration (e.g., rapid acting, short acting, intermediate acting, or long acting), and intensity of action following subcutaneous (SC) injection. Lispro (Humalog), the most rapid-acting insulin analogue available, differs from insulin by a switch in the lysine and proline residues at the insulin molecule's B-28 and B-29 amino acid sites. Short-acting insulin is regular insulin. To sustain its action, insulin can be bound to zinc and protein molecules or to zinc alone. Neutral protamine Hagedorn (NPH, which is

Table 39–4

Guidelines for Diabetic Patients Who Exercise Conscientiously

- Test blood glucose concentrations before, during, and after exercise.
- Prepare for moderate exercise (e.g., bicycling or jogging for 30–45 minutes) by decreasing the preceding dose of regular insulin by 30%–50%. If glucose concentration is normal or low before exercise, you should supplement the diet with a snack containing 10–15 g of carbohydrate.
- Avoid increased absorption of regular insulin from exercise by injecting into the abdomen or exercising 30 minutes to 1 hour following injection.
- Do not exercise if the glucose concentration exceeds 240–300 mg/dL, which indicates severe insulin deficiency and predisposes patients to hyperglycemia secondary to exercise.
- Avoid jarring exercise or exercise that involves moving the head below the waist if severe proliferative retinopathy or retinal hemorrhage is present.
- Exercise with caution if you have low glycogen stores (e.g., alcoholics, fasting individuals, and patients on diets that are extremely hypocaloric [$<$800 cal] and low in carbohydrates [$<$10 g per day]). These situations create a predisposition to the hypoglycemic effects of exercise.
- Watch for postexercise hypoglycemia (which can occur 8–15 hours following exercise). If exercise occurs during the day, increase carbohydrate intake and test blood glucose concentration during the night to detect nocturnal hypoglycemia. Patients taking insulin are more susceptible to hypoglycemia than those taking sulfonylureas. Patients with Type 2 diabetes treated with diet are unlikely to develop hypoglycemia.

Source: *Applied Therapeutics: The Clinical Use of Drugs*. Vancouver, WA: Applied Therapeutics, Inc; 1992:1697.

the classic isophane insulin) and lente insulin suspensions are intermediate-acting insulins; ultralente is long acting. (Note: The term *isophane* means that the ratio of insulin to protamine is equal; isophane insulin is made by adding equal amounts of insulin and protamine, all of which become complexed.)

In NPH, both zinc and protamine retard dissolution and absorption from the site of injection, whereas, in lente insulin, high levels of zinc slow dissolution and absorption. Mixtures of lente and ultralente insulins have two basic crystal types and are intermediate to long acting. Fixed-dose mixtures of human insulin at a ratio of 70% NPH to 30% regular and a ratio of 50% NPH to 50% regular are also available. Information concerning the time–action profiles of these insulins is contained in Table 39–5. Many factors, such as injection site, species source, and ambient temperature, affect the time–action profiles of insulins; thus, the values listed in the table have some degree of variability.[15,16]

Both the source from which insulin is derived and its antigenicity can influence the product's effect on blood glucose control, resistance, and sensitivity to its actions.[15,16] Currently, commercially available animal-derived insulin is from pork. Biosynthetic human insulin is now available from two manufacturers in the United States: Eli Lilly and Novo-Nordisk. (See Table 39–6 for examples of these insulin preparations.) Each species source of insulin has a distinct time–action profile. Human insulin acts faster and has a shorter duration of action than pork insulin. Patients who switch from one species to another require medical supervision.

In 1990, the Food and Drug Administration (FDA) decertified U-40 insulin. Unfortunately, this is the insulin that is usually available in several non–English-speaking countries. Thus, patients traveling abroad need to carry extra insulin and corresponding insulin syringes to prevent problems or errors.[15] Regular U-500 insulin is available from Eli Lilly as a prescription-only product for insulin-resistant patients who use more than 100 to 200 U per injection.

Two new prescription insulin analogues became available in early 2000: Humalog Mix 75/25 and glargine. Humalog Mix 75/25, which is available as a prefilled insulin pen, is the first premixed insulin to contain a rapid-acting insulin. This insulin contains 75% insulin lispro protamine suspension and 25% insulin lispro injection. This formulation provides the rapid onset of lispro along with the longer duration of action of a lispro protamine suspension. The lispro protamine suspension is similar to an NPH formulation. The presence of lispro in this combination product may provide a more prompt onset than that of 70/30 insulins, which contain regular insulin. Binding lispro with protamine prevents the reaction between lispro and regular insulin that occurs if lispro is mixed with NPH insulin. Preventing this reaction retains the rapid effect of the lispro, allowing patients to inject Humalog Mix 75/25 15 minutes before eating, rather than the 30 to 45 minutes recommended for 70/30 insulins.

Glargine (Lantus) is a clear, long-acting insulin in which the amino acids in the insulin have been reconfigured. This genetically engineered insulin retains the properties and actions of insulin, but provides a predictably long-acting effect, allowing additional flexibility for basal dosing throughout the day. For stability, the product is manufactured as an acidic suspension. However, the low pH induces a higher incidence of pain/stinging and skin reactions at injection sites than do the other currently marketed neutral pH insulin preparations.

With the exception of the U-500 preparation and the insulin analogues, insulin is a nonprescription drug. Although physicians prescribe insulin, pharmacists are often the health care professionals who are consulted about insulin and the problems related to its use. Thus, pharmacists should be knowledgeable about insulin products and pharmacotherapy.

Mechanism of Action

Insulin, which is produced in the β-cells of the pancreas, stimulates glucose storage in muscles and the liver as glycogen; stimulates fatty acid and triglyceride synthesis; decreases hepatic glucose output, lipolysis, and ketone production; and enhances amino acid incorporation into proteins.[17]

Indications

Insulin is indicated for the treatment of all types of diabetes mellitus.

Dosage Guidelines

Insulin treatment is usually initiated for Type 1 diabetes with a dose of 0.5 to 0.8 U per kg split into at least two doses daily. The doses are adjusted pending the patient's response. Gen-

Table 39–5

Time–Action Profile of Nonprescription Insulins

Type	Insulin Preparation	Onset (hours)	Peak Activity (hours)	Duration of Action (hours)
Rapid acting	Lispro	0.25–0.5	1–2	3–5
Short acting	Regular	0.5–1.0	3–4	6–8
Intermediate acting	NPH	1.0–1.5	6–12	18–24
	Lente	1.0–2.5	8–14	18–24
Long acting	Ultralente	4.0–8.0	12–30	up to 36
	Glargine	1.0–2.0	6–10	20–24

Table 39–6

Selected Insulin Preparations in U-100 Concentration

Trade Name	Source[a]	Onset of Action (hours)	Peak Action (hours)	Duration of Action (hours)
Short-Acting Regular Insulins				
Humulin R	Human	0.5–1	2–4	6–8
Novolin R	Human	0.5	2.5–5	8
Novolin R PenFill	Human	0.5	2.5–5	8
Novolin R Prefilled	Human	0.5	2.5–8	8
Regular Iletin II	Pork	0.5–1	1–3	5–7
Velosulin BR	Human buffered, semi-synthetic	0.5	1–3	8
Intermediate-Acting Lente Insulin[b]				
Humulin L	Human	1–3	6–12	18–24
Iletin II Lente	Pork	2–4	8–10	18–24
Lente	Pork	2.5	7–15	22
Novolin L	Human	2.5	7–15	22
Intermediate-Acting NPH Insulin[c]				
Humulin N	Human	1–2	8–12	18–24
Iletin II NPH	Pork	1–3	8–10	18–24
Novolin N	Human	1.5	4–12	24
Novolin N PenFill	Human	1.5	4–12	24
Novolin N PreFilled	Human	1.5	4–12	24
NPH	Pork	1.5	4–12	24
Long-Acting Ultralente Insulin[b]				
Humulin U	Human	4–6	8–20	24–28
Insulin Mixtures[c,d]				
Humulin 50/50	Human	0.5–1	2–12	up to 24
Humulin 70/30	Human	0.5–1	2–12	up to 24
Novolin 70/30	Human	0.5	2–12	24
Novolin 70/30 PenFill	Human	0.5	2–12	24
Novolin 70/30 PreFilled	Human	0.5	2–12	24

[a] Human insulin is produced through recombinant DNA technology.

[b] These insulins are zinc suspensions.

[c] These insulins are isophane suspensions.

[d] The 50/50 insulin mixtures contain 50% NPH and 50% regular insulin; 70/30 mixtures contain 70% NPH and 30% regular insulin.

erally, people who require insulin at diagnosis are younger than 30 years, lean, prone to developing ketoacidosis, and markedly hyperglycemic even in the fasting state.

Patients who are receiving parenteral nutrition, who require large-calorie supplements to meet increased energy needs, or who have drug-induced diabetes may require insulin exogenously on a short-term or intermittent basis to maintain normal glucose levels. By combining the appropriate modification of diet, exercise, and variable mixtures of short- and longer-acting insulins with self-monitoring, these patients can achieve acceptable control of blood glucose. Normalization of blood glucose usually requires intensified insulin regimens that involve multiple daily injections or insulin pumps.

Single-injection regimens are not advocated for people who have been newly diagnosed with Type 1 disease and do not give consistent glycemic control in most patients. Near-euglycemic blood glucose levels can be achieved by using multiple daily injections or an insulin infusion pump. Although they must monitor their blood glucose multiple—

usually four—times daily, intensively managed patients are able to maintain their usual activities and may actually increase their lifestyle flexibility by being able to more promptly adjust insulin doses to accommodate changes that occur in their activities.

The goal of intensive therapy is to mimic the insulin secretion of a functioning pancreas. Figure 39–3 depicts the glucose surges from three daily meals and the resultant insulin release from a pancreas responding to the glucose. Patients willing to use multiple injections have the option of combining insulins, depending on the individual's response pattern. Numerous regimens can be devised to fit the patient's lifestyle or other needs. (See Figure 39–3.) For example, regular insulin can be injected before meals, and an intermediate-acting insulin can be injected at bedtime to cover blood glucose levels during the sleeping hours. Another alternative would be to inject long-acting (ultralente) and regular insulin before breakfast, regular insulin before lunch, and regular and ultralente again before dinner.

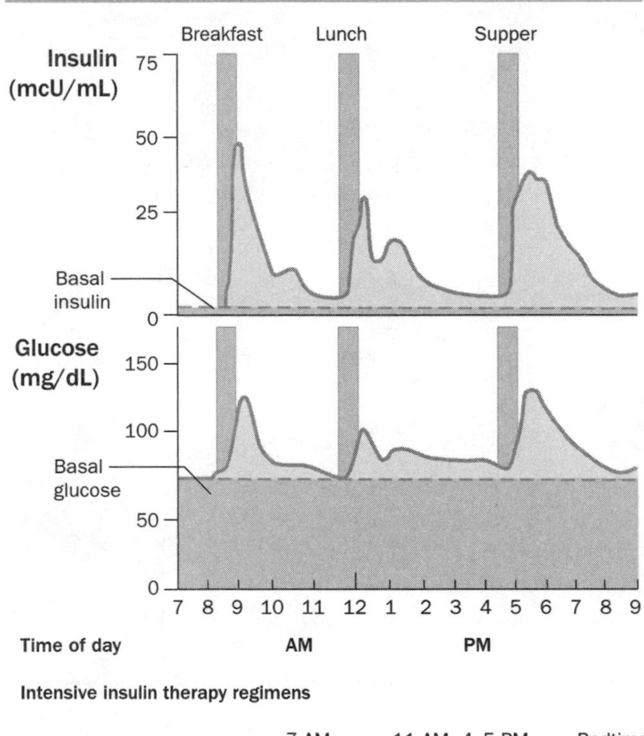

Intensive insulin therapy regimens

	7 AM	11 AM	4–5 PM	Bedtime
1. 2 doses, intermediate	x		x	
2. 2 doses, regular and intermediate	Reg. & intermed.		Reg. & Intermed.	
3. 3 doses, regular or regular and intermediate	Reg. & intermed.	Reg.	Reg. & Intermed.	
4. 4 doses, regular and long acting	Reg.	Reg.	Reg.	Long acting
5. 3 doses, regular and intermediate, regular only, intermediate only	Reg. & intermed.		Reg.	Intermed.

Figure 39–3 Relationship between insulin and glucose. Adapted with permission from *US Pharm*. 1988; 13[suppl 11]:41.

Administration Guidelines

Unless a patient is too young to inject insulin or has physical impairments that preclude self-injection, he or she should know how to mix the insulin properly with the syringe and then inject the dose properly. (See Table 39–7.)

Because the route and/or site of administration can affect the clinical use of insulin, patients should know the absorption rates of insulin for different injection routes and sites. They should also know of the various devices available for injecting or infusing insulin.

Injection Routes/Absorption Rates Regular intramuscular (IM) insulin injections absorb faster with a greater initial drop in plasma glucose levels than do injections by the SC route. Regular intravenous (IV) injections produce the most rapid rise of insulin in the least time. Insulin suspensions (e.g., NPH, lente, and ultralente) are never administered IM or IV.

The site of the injection is one of many factors that can influence the rate at which insulin is absorbed. Injection sites, in decreasing order of absorption rate, include the abdomen, upper arms (deltoid region), thighs, and hips. (See Figure 39–4.) Because of variance from one site to another, some clinicians have recommended using all areas of one site (e.g., left thigh) before switching sites. Still others have advocated using only the abdomen to eliminate the concern of dose-to-dose variance. Massaging or exercising the injection area, which will increase the rate of absorption from the injection, can affect the patient's glycemic control. Fibrosis and atrophy can be prevented by not injecting into the same site in less than 10-day intervals. Deep IM injections will produce a much more rapid onset of action because the absorption rate from the injection site is increased. Fever, exercise, extremely hot weather, or a sauna or Jacuzzi can increase peripheral blood flow, which also speeds insulin absorption. Conversely, cold packs, cold extremities, or a hypothermal blanket may slow the onset of action because the absorption rate is decreased.

Insulin absorption can be affected by exercise. Leg exercise accelerates absorption from leg but not from the arm or abdomen, and thus arm and abdominal injections reduce exercise-induced hypoglycemia. A patient whose day includes a hard game of tennis should inject that day's insulin into the abdomen rather than into the arm or leg. Also, if more than 60 U of insulin is injected at one site, absorption may be erratic. Patients receiving large doses of insulin should perhaps split the doses and inject in two different sites. These patients should be monitored closely.

Insulin is to be injected deep into SC tissue. (See Figure 39–5.) The technique for injection may need to be altered with each individual, depending on the amount of SC fat present. (See Table 39–7 for a description of proper injection

Table 39–7

Guidelines for Administering Insulin Doses

Preparation of Insulin Dose

- Inspect vials for signs of contamination or degradation.
- Wash hands with soap and water.
- Make sure the proper insulin is used—that is, the correct insulin in the correct strength from the source normally used.
- Swirl vials gently to suspend insulin before filling the syringe. All insulins, except regular insulin, are suspensions and must be evenly distributed before use.
- Gently roll the vial between the palms of the hands, or repeatedly invert it until the suspension is evenly distributed. Do not shake the bottle. If vial contains air bubbles, wait until they subside before filling the syringe.
- Wipe off the top of the vial with an alcohol swab or a cotton ball moistened with alcohol, and be sure that no cotton or cloth fibers remain on the rubber stopper.
- Remove a clean syringe from storage. Touch only the hub of the plunger and the barrel of the syringe; avoid touching the hub of the needle.
- Inject into the regular insulin vial an amount of air equivalent to the needed insulin dose.
- Inject into the intermediate-acting insulin vial an amount of air equivalent to the needed insulin dose.
- Invert the vial and syringe, and withdraw the appropriate number of units of insulin from the regular insulin vial.
- Repeat the above step with the vial of intermediate-acting insulin.
- When the correct number of units of insulin (without air bubbles) has been measured, withdraw the needle.
- Holding the syringe with the needle upright, draw an air bubble into the syringe, invert the syringe, and roll the bubble through to mix.
- Invert the syringe so the needle is upright, and tap the barrel of the syringe briskly two or three times to remove any tiny air bubbles that may have clung to the barrel.
- Expel the air bubble and recap the needle, or lay the syringe on a flat surface such as a table or shelf with the needle over the edge to avoid contamination.
- Check the administration site, and administer the insulin to the patient.

Injection of Insulin Dose

- After properly preparing the insulin dose, check the record to confirm where the insulin was injected previously. Injection sites should be rotated or alternated. (See Figure 39–4.)
- Clean the injection site with an alcohol swab or a cotton ball moistened with alcohol. Some data suggest this step may not be necessary.
- Pinch a fold of skin with one hand. With the other hand, hold the syringe like a pencil, place the needle on the skin with the beveled edge up, and push the needle quickly through the fold of skin at a 45° to 90° angle. (See Figure 39–5.) With different size needles, proper needle length enables a "straight in" (90°) approach for the injection. Before injecting the insulin, draw back slightly on the plunger (aspirate) to be sure a blood vessel has not been penetrated. If blood appears in the syringe barrel, withdraw the needle and discard. Prepare another syringe and repeat the injection in another spot on the body. Some clinicians do not recommend aspiration.
- Inject the insulin by pressing the plunger in as far as it will go.
- Withdraw the needle quickly, and press on the injection site with the swab or cotton ball moistened with alcohol.
- When injection is completed, dispose of the syringe and needle properly.
- Record the injection site.

technique.) The purpose of pinching the skin is to lift the fat off the muscle and thus avoid IM or IV injection, which may result in a more rapid onset of action and in hypoglycemia. Properly injected insulin leaves only the needle puncture dot to show the injection site. If insulin leaks through the puncture in the skin, a longer needle should be used and inserted at a right angle (90°) to the skin.

Syringes and Other Injection Devices Pharmacists should ensure that the patient is purchasing the proper type of equipment. The problems with administering the wrong insulin (source or type) have been discussed previously. Because insulin is administered in units rather than milliliters, syringes are calibrated in units. The calibration of the syringe should correspond to the concentration of the insulin used (e.g., U-100 syringes with U-100 insulin).

Types of Syringes Two types of syringes are available: glass (reusable) and plastic (disposable). Almost all patients use plastic insulin syringes even though plastic syringes are more expensive. Disposable syringes and needles ensure sterility and offer ease of penetration because needles are finer (28, 29, and 30 gauge), sharper, and silicone-coated for ease of insertion, yet they have a wide bore and a 25% smaller bevel angle. The smaller (28- or 29-gauge) needles cause less pain and have virtually no "dead space"—that is, the measurable space in the needle and at the hub of the needle and syringe, which contains drug that is not injected. Dead space is a potential

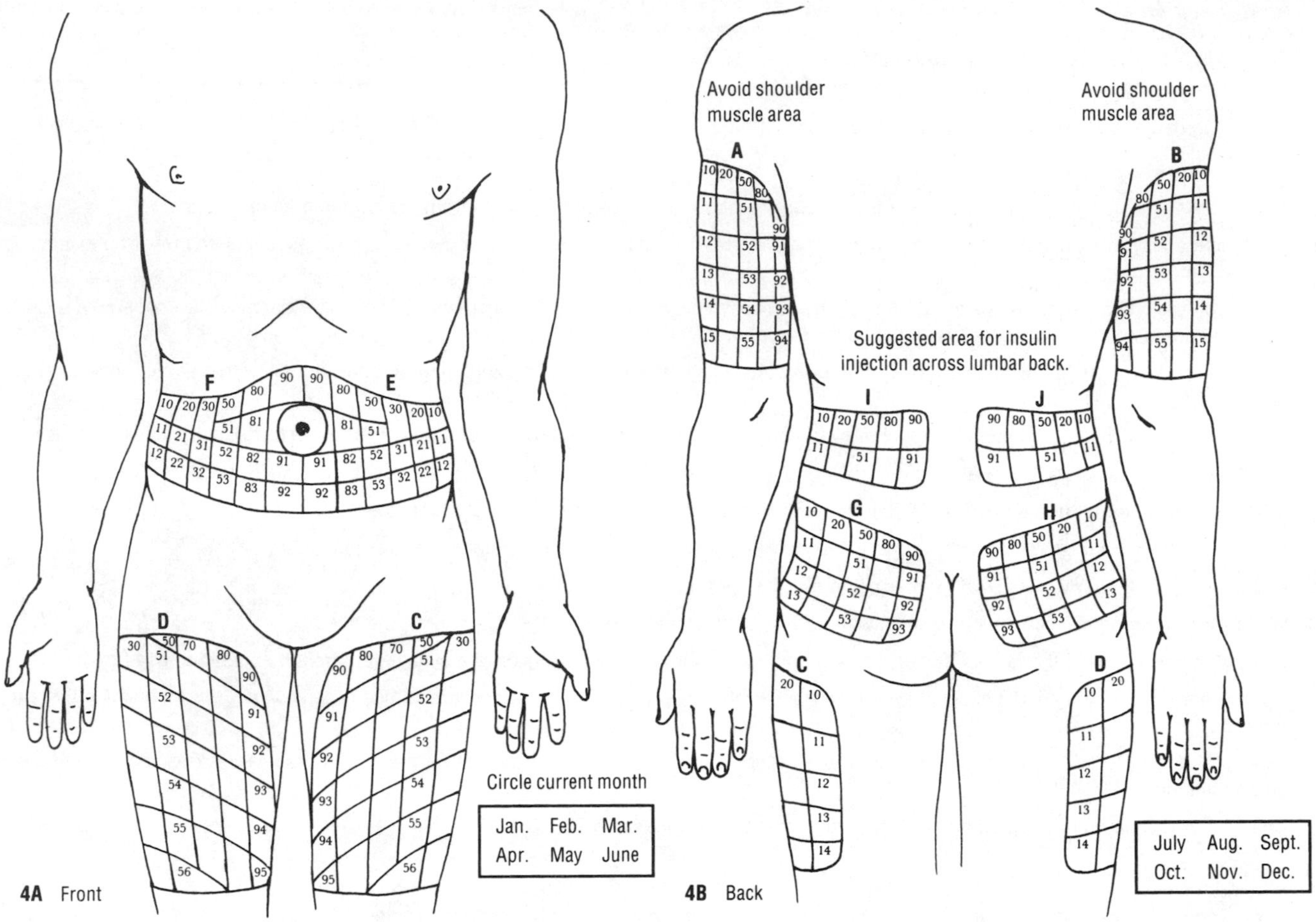

Avoid shoulder muscle area
Avoid shoulder muscle area
A
B
Suggested area for insulin injection across lumbar back.
F
E
I
J
G
H
D
C
C
D
Circle current month
Jan. Feb. Mar.
Apr. May June
July Aug. Sept.
Oct. Nov. Dec.
4A Front
4B Back

Figure 39–4 Body map of subcutaneous injection sites. This body map, which is for both hospital and home use, is designed to record insulin injection sites systematically. The numbers printed in the squares are mainly for hospital recording of insulin injection sites on each patient's chart; the numbers may be used at home, but a simpler method of recording would be to write the date of each injection in the corresponding square on the map at the time of injection. With continued use, this diagram will facilitate the rotation of insulin injection sites over the entire body and thereby avoid injection too often in a single location. Adapted with permission from *The Body Map*. Birmingham, AL: Baptist Hospitals Foundation.

source of error when two different fluids are drawn, measured, and mixed in the same syringe. Needles are available in 5/16- to 5/8-inch lengths; the longer needle is used when patients are obese and when back leakage of insulin is a problem.

Low-dose syringes are disposable U-100 syringes with the capacity of 0.3 mL (30 U) and 0.5 mL (50 U). These syringes may be used with U-100 insulin only. The low-dose syringes have a smaller-caliber barrel so that 30 U to 50 U of U-100 insulin can be measured more accurately in 1-U increments. The 1.0 mL disposable U-100 syringes, conversely, are graduated in 2-U increments and are used to inject 52 U to 100 U of U-100 insulin. The 1.0 mL syringes resemble the tuberculin syringes but should not be interchanged with them because of differences in labeling.

Several researchers have reported the reuse of insulin syringes. One study revealed that plastic disposable syringes can be reused for at least 3 days with safety and patient satisfaction. Another study indicated that patients reused sy-

Dermis
Epidermis
Subcutaneous tissue
Muscle

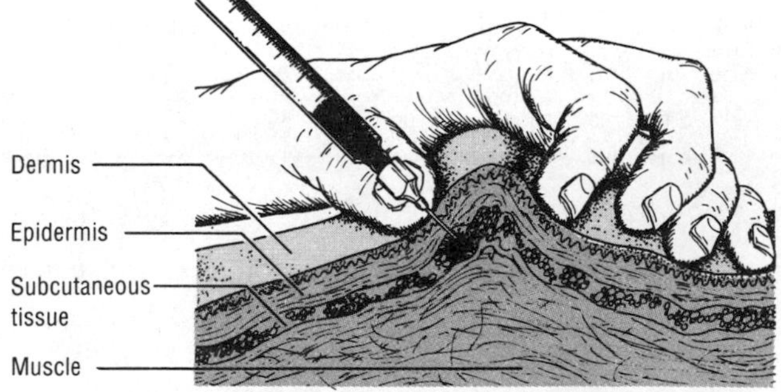

Figure 39–5 Correct method of subcutaneous insulin injection. Several techniques are good; the one illustrated serves well because the needle penetrates the skin at its thinnest area (dimple) and must enter the SC space. The needle angle should be 45° to 90° angle. With different size needles, proper needle length enables a "straight in" (90°) approach for the injection.

ringes for an average of 4 days and that dullness of the needle was a major reason for changing to a new syringe.[14] Patients have been reported to place transparent tape over the barrel of the syringe to keep the numbers from rubbing off, to refrigerate their syringes between uses, and to wipe their needles with alcohol before reusing. No reports are available of increased infection rate at the injection site in these patients, but no large, long-term, well-controlled prospective studies have been done. In general, reuse of disposable plastic syringes is not recommended, although patients who have been following this practice without problems for several years should not be discouraged. Patients who are not at increased risk for developing infection and who can safely recap the syringe may reuse syringes.[18,19] Syringes that are to be reused over a few days may be stored at room temperature. Any patient who reuses a syringe and needle must pay close attention to aseptic technique to avoid touch contamination. The needles should probably not be cleaned with alcohol because it removes the silicone coating.

Injection Devices/Aids Several different types of insulin injection devices or automatic injectors are designed for patients who have an aversion to self-injection. Such products include insertion aids, insulin pens, jet injectors, and infusers. An insertion aid is usually a jacket that fits over a filled syringe, is spring-loaded, and guides the needle into the skin. The needle may or may not be visible to the patient, depending on the design of the automatic injector. Some injectors adjust the depth and angle of skin penetration; the size of the injector will vary depending on type. The syringe may be prefilled and carried until ready to use. Insulin pens, which look like writing pens, use disposable or single-use cartridges filled with 150 U or 300 U of human insulin (regular, NPH, a 30:70 mix, or a 25:75 lispro/NPH mix). These devices can deliver preset or dial-in doses, depending on the type, and require only one hand for injection.

Jet injectors force a tiny liquid stream of insulin suspension through the skin under pressure without using a needle. The injected insulin disperses into a very thin spray as it enters the SC tissue. Patients who are first-time users may have to adjust the insulin dose because the increased tissue contact may cause faster insulin absorption. Patients who do not have enough fat tissue may actually inject insulin into muscle tissue with a jet injector. Jet injector devices cause less lipoatrophy and inflammation than the syringe and needle and also facilitate reaching and rotating the injection sites. As with any device, however, improper use can result in dose errors. For example, the jet injector must be held firmly against the skin to deliver the exact dose.

For patients who use the syringe and needle for injection but dislike sticking themselves, a small flexible catheter (the Button Infuser) can be inserted SC, usually in the abdomen, and anchored at the site. The patient can give multiple doses of insulin by simply attaching a syringe to a portal and injecting and then removing it from the SC catheter portal, which is "plugged" until the next dose is administered. The catheter can remain in place for 24 hours to 72 hours, and the patient may inject insulin several times a day through the catheter. The patient must be instructed on how to prepare the site before insertion and on how to prevent infection of the site while the catheter is in place.

Several other adapter and injector devices are being tested, including a new needle design called the sprinkler needle. This needle has a sealed end hole and 14 small holes in the side walls to sprinkle insulin into the SC tissue instead of releasing the dose as a single bolus. This device is supposed to speed the absorption of the short-acting insulin, thereby allowing patients to inject themselves immediately rather than 30 minutes before eating.

Various products are available for the visually impaired, including "drawing aids" that hold the syringe and vial, guide the needle into the vial, and help draw up the insulin. These injection aids can also be used with magnifiers, which enlarge the calibrations on an insulin syringe to twice their normal size. The syringe usually is inserted or loaded into the magnifier, or it has the magnifier attached to the side of the syringe. "Dose gauges" are available that allow doses to be dialed in or that have audible dose selectors. Some of the gauges come in Braille with raised numbers. Other dose gauges have prefilled syringes that are disposable after multiple-dose use.

Table 39–8 describes the features of selected commercially available syringes and injection aids.

Pump Infusers Intensified insulin therapy to achieve tight control of blood glucose requires either multiple daily injections, as previously discussed, or continuous insulin pump infusion (usually 0.5 U to 1.0 U per hour) plus injection of a bolus of insulin before meals and snacks. The use of portable, battery-driven, open-loop, continuous infusion pumps to administer insulin to some Type 1 and 2 patients has gained support. These pumps are referred to as open-loop devices because blood glucose level does not automatically signal the device to regulate insulin (i.e., pumps do not function like artificial pancreases). The patient must self-monitor blood glucose at least four times a day and must determine how much insulin should be injected and when. Some pumps can be programmed to change basal rates automatically at different times of the day. Patients can thereby tailor insulin therapy to their lifestyle, thereby preventing early morning rise in blood glucose and maintaining levels that approximate euglycemia.

Three pumps (MiniMed models 506/7C and 508, and H-Tron plus) are available to administer SC insulin. These devices, which are about the size of a credit card and half an inch thick, are basically microcomputers that use rechargeable batteries. They sound an alarm when the battery is running low, the infusion line is occluded, or the insulin reservoir is almost empty. These pumps use a syringe filled with diluted regular insulin and a motorized device that is programmed to push the plunger of the syringe a set distance forward. Insulin goes through a plastic tube (infusion line) attached to a 27-gauge needle or flexible cannula, which is inserted SC and taped in place. The infusion line can be dis-

Table 39–8

Selected Insulin Delivery Devices and Related Products

Trade Name	Product Features
Insulin Syringes	
B-D Micro-Fine IV Syringe	28-gauge, ½-inch needle; available in 0.3, 0.5, or 1 mL sizes; single-scale, single-unit markings for precise dosage measurement
B-D Ultra-Fine Syringe	29-gauge, ½-inch needle; available in 0.3, 0.5, or 1 mL sizes; single-scale, single-unit markings for precise dosage measurement
B-D Ultra-Fine II Short Needle Syringe	30-gauge; 5⁄16-inch needle; available in 0.3, 0.5, or 1 mL sizes; single-scale, single-unit markings for precise dosage measurement
Monoject Ultra Comfort Syringes	28- and 29-gauge needles; available in 0.3, 0.5, or 1 mL sizes; permanently attached, advanced laser-weld needle
NovoFine 30 Needle	30-gauge, ⅓-inch needles; designed for use with Novo Nordisk insulin delivery devices
Sure-Dose Plus Syringe	29-gauge, ½-inch needles; available in 0.25, 0.5, or 1 mL sizes; latex-free composition
Sure-Dose Syringe	28-gauge, ½-inch needles; available in 0.5 and 1 mL sizes; latex-free composition
Abbott Insulin Syringe	29-gauge needle; available in ¼-inch size; only insulin syringe available with 0.5-unit scale markings; latex-free composition
Insulin Pens	
B-D Pen	Pen-shaped device that uses 1.5 mL insulin cartridges and delivers 1 unit to 30 units in 1-unit increments
B-D Ultra-Fine Original Pen Needles	29-gauge, ½-inch disposable pen needles for use with B-D pens, Novolin Prefilled and NovolinPen, and NovoPen 1.5; Novo function check cannot be performed with these needles
B-D Ultra-Fine II Pen Needles	30-gauge, 5⁄16-inch disposable pen needles for use with B-D pens, Novolin Prefilled and NovolinPen, and NovoPen 1.5; Novo function check cannot be performed with these needles
B-D Ultra-Fine III Pen Needles	31-gauge, 5⁄16-inch disposable pen needles for use with B-D pens, Novolin Prefilled and NovolinPen, and NovoPen 1.5; Novo function check cannot be performed with these needles
NovolinPen	Pen-shaped device that uses 1.5 mL insulin cartridges and delivers 1 unit to 36 units in 1-unit increments
Novolin Prefilled	Pen-shaped device that is prefilled with 1.5 mL insulin cartridges and delivers up to 58 units in 2-unit increments
NovoPen 1.5	Pen-shaped device that uses 1.5 mL Novolin human insulin cartridges and delivers 1 unit to 40 units in 1-unit increments
NovoPen 3	Pen-shaped device that uses 3.0 mL Novolin human insulin cartridges and delivers 2 units to 70 units in 1-unit increments
Insulin Injection Aids	
B-D Inject-Ease	Syringe injector for use with 0.3, 0.5, or 1 mL regular or short needles. Syringe is injected by positioning device over the injection site, pressing activation button to insert needle, and then pushing in syringe plunger
B-D Magni-Guide	Device that magnifies scale calibrations on syringes two times; also designed to help guide syringe needle into insulin vial

connected from the syringe when the patient is swimming, showering, or involved in intimate activities or when the infusion line is occluded. (Buffered insulin such as Velosulin appears to be less likely to precipitate in the insulin pump and block insulin flow, although many patients use regular insulin or lispro with no reported problems.) Most patients should change the infusion line and cannula sites every 2 days to prevent soreness and infection. When empty, the syringe or reservoir is replaced. Some pumps have "runaway" alarms that sound if a runaway, or high dose, should occur. Most manufacturers say that runaways are so unlikely that such an alarm is not necessary.

The pump is programmed to deliver a continuous basal amount of SC insulin throughout a 24-hour period and to handle fluctuations in blood glucose when the patient is not eating. Guidelines for adjusting doses to account for eating, exercising, and adjusting to the results of blood glucose tests are established when the patient begins using the pump.

A number of auxiliary pump devices are also available, including infusion tubing (12 to 42 inches), batteries and battery rechargers, syringes or reservoirs that fit specific pumps, tape, tape adhesive remover, surgical soap, skin conditioner, diluting fluid for insulin, blood testing supplies, and logbooks. Some problems with pump use include the following:

Case Study 39–1

Patient Complaint/History

Emily, a 16-year-old student, was diagnosed with Type 1 diabetes approximately 16 months ago. She has been using a multiple-injection regimen that includes lispro insulin with each meal and two injections of NPH (in the morning and at bedtime). Emily came to the pharmacy today to get more supplies and to ask if she could use a pen injector or would be a candidate for a pump that she heard about in a support group last week. Her current blood glucose monitor results are obtained from her monitor's memory and reveal the following:

	Blood Glucose Levels (mg/dL)			
	6:15 am	Noon	4 pm	10 pm
Week 1	142	162	118	191
Week 2	149	151	119	199
Week 3	145	139	126	179
Week 4 (current)	122	130	131	201

Although Emily's activities have not changed significantly in the past few weeks, the patient says she has been feeling sluggish. Further, her medications have not changed in the past month. The patient asks whether the insulin timing could be a problem, because she is having a high blood glucose level in the evening.

Clinical Considerations/Strategies

Readers can use the following considerations/strategies to determine the appropriate treatment approach for this patient's situation:

- Assess the patient's nutrition and physical activity plan and recent history. What does her evening meal consist of?
- Assess the patient's injection technique.
- Assess the patient's adherence to the treatment plan (e.g., blood glucose monitoring, insulin administration, nutrition, and physical activity).
- Assess the patient's current practices for storing her insulin.

Patient Education/Counseling

Readers can use the following strategies to develop a patient education/counseling plan that will help ensure optimal therapeutic outcomes:

- Discuss with the patient the proper storage technique for insulin vials. Develop a plan for instructing her on the proper storage and use of insulin.
- Develop an individualized care plan to teach, monitor, and support the patient in controlling her diabetes.

- Some patients can go into a ketotic phase within a matter of hours should the flow of insulin be interrupted.
- Many patients do not experience the normal symptoms of hypoglycemia.
- Injection sites must be carefully monitored to prevent infections, variability in insulin absorption, and local skin reactions.

Blood glucose self-monitoring is essential for pump users, and many studies have shown that various metabolic parameters can be normalized using insulin pumps. Success in the use of insulin devices is directly correlated with patients who are highly motivated, who can participate well with a multiple daily dose regimen, and who are educable, responsible at keeping records, and willing and able to follow specific procedures and to perform and log blood tests daily. Not all patients are candidates for insulin pump therapy, however.

Insulin Mixtures As the purity of insulins has improved, the problem of stability in mixing insulins has decreased. Regular insulin may be mixed with NPH insulin in any proportion desired;[20] the resultant combination is stable for approximately 1 month at room temperature. (The manufacturers' literature actually recommends that insulin vials not be used longer than 1 month past the initial puncture of the stopper.) Lispro insulin can be mixed with NPH or lente insulin; this mixture should be injected immediately. However, lente insulin binds with regular or lispro insulin, thus decreasing the action of the regular insulin. This reaction occurs within minutes and continues for up to 24 hours. Patients mixing regular and lente insulin should either inject the mixture immediately or allow it to stand 24 hours before injection. Lente and ultralente insulins may be combined with one another in any ratio desired at any time. These mixtures are stable in any proportion for 18 months if refrigerated; however, sterility is not guaranteed. Home infusion therapy pharmacists are advised to review their policy manuals for appropriate prefilling plans. Patients should be given the smallest possible number of prefilled syringes at any one time. Novo-Nordisk's Velosulin should not be mixed with any lente preparation because of its different buffers.

Patients using infusion pumps may use either normal saline or Lilly's Insulin Dilution Fluid to dilute the insulin in the pump. Regular insulin may be mixed in any proportion with normal saline for use in the pump, but the combination should be used within 2 to 3 hours after mixing because changes in the pH and dilution of the buffer may adversely affect stability. Conversely, regular insulin may be mixed with Lilly's Insulin Dilution Fluid in any proportion, and it will be stable indefinitely. Because regular insulin may crystallize in the tubing of insulin pumps, Velosulin has added phosphate buffer to help limit or prevent this reaction.

Adverse Effects

Excessive doses of insulin can cause hypoglycemia; however, this effect can result from missed or erratic meals, insufficient amount of food, and strenuous exercise. In contrast, an insufficient or missed dose can cause hyperglycemia. (These complications are discussed in the section "Special Treatment Considerations.")

Some patients may experience redness or discomfort at injection sites. The problem may be related to insulin sensitivity or to poor injection technique.

Patients with sensitivity to insulin usually develop redness at an injection site. When a patient first begins taking animal-source insulin, such a reaction may be common and may occur over several weeks before gradually subsiding. The reactions may be treated with diphenhydramine hydrochloride (Benadryl) or hydroxyzine. The long-term solution may be changing to human insulin. Newly diagnosed patients requiring insulin are now started routinely on human insulin, and hypersensitivity reactions are very rare. Rare instances of protamine allergy have also been reported.

Newer methods of purifying insulin now ensure that all commercially available insulins are highly purified. The common pancreas contaminants (proinsulin, arginine insulin, esterified insulin, and glucagon) have been decreased, resulting in fewer insulin-sensitivity reactions. All insulin preparations available in the United States contain between 0 and 10 ppm of proinsulin. Increased insulin product purity is less antigenic and allows use of lower insulin doses. Insulin made by recombinant DNA technology is even purer.[16]

Insulin resistance, a condition in which the patient requires more than 200 U a day of insulin for more than 2 days in the absence of ketoacidosis or acute infection, occurs in about 0.001% of diabetic patients. These patients almost invariably have high titers of insulin-neutralizing immunoglobulin G antibodies and should be switched to human insulin. If this switch does not resolve the problem, glucocorticoids are indicated.

Pharmacists should stress to patients the importance of rotating/alternating injection sites to limit local irritation, tissue reactions, and lipodystrophy. Using injection devices may help the pain and inconvenience of multiple injections. To prevent skin damage, patients must learn the proper technique of using these devices.

Interactions

No insulin–drug, insulin–food (or herb) interactions have been reported.

Contraindications/Precautions/Warnings

Patients who are allergic to pork insulin should receive human insulin or at least should not receive pork insulin unless they have been successfully desensitized. Patients who have had systemic allergic reactions (e.g., hives, angioedema, or anaphylaxis) should be skin tested with each new preparation before starting therapy with that preparation.

β-Blockers may increase the chance of developing high or low blood glucose levels but can also mask blood glucose symptoms such as fast heartbeat. Topical or injected corticosteroids may increase blood glucose. Thus insulin doses may need to be increased during and for several weeks after the period of corticosteroid treatment. Pentamidine may cause the pancreas to release (if it can release) insulin too rapidly. Consequently, pentamidine and insulin doses may have to be adjusted to control blood glucose. Table 39–9 lists other medications that can alter blood glucose levels.

Contamination of Insulin

All insulins are produced at a near-neutral pH of 7.4. Regular insulin is a clear solution. If it looks cloudy or has become tinted, it may be contaminated and should not be dispensed

Table 39–9

Drugs that May Cause Hypoglycemia or Hyperglycemia

Hypoglycemia	Hyperglycemia
Acetaminophen	Acetazolamide
Alcohol (acute)	Alcohol (chronic)
Amitriptyline	Amiodarone
Anabolic steroids	Antimicrobial (pentamidine, rifampin, sulfasalazine, nalidixic acid)
β-Blockers	Asparaginase
Biguanides	β-Agonists
Chloroquine	Caffeine
Clofibrate	Calcium channel blockers
Disopyramide	Chlorpromazine
Fenfluramine	Chlorthalidone
Fluphenazine	Corticosteroids
Guanethidine	Cyclosporine
Haloperidol	Diazoxide
Imipramine	Encainide
Insulin	Estrogens
Lithium	Ethacrynic acid
Monoamine oxidase inhibitors	Fentanyl/furosemide
Norfloxacin	Indapamide
Pentamidine	Interferon α
Perphenazine/amitriptyline	Lactulose
Phenobarbital	Niacin and nicotinic acid
Prazosin	Oral contraceptives
Propoxyphene	Phenytoin
Quinine	Probenecid
Salicylates in large doses	Sugars (dextrose, fructose, mannitol, sorbitol, sucrose)
Sulfonamide antibiotics	Sympathomimetic amines
Sulfonylurea agents	Thiazide diuretics
Tetrahydrocannabinol	Thyroid preparations
	Tricyclic antidepressants

or used. All other available insulins are cloudy suspensions that will settle out after standing. If the insulin suspension rapidly settles out, it has been altered and should not be used. Similarly, if it clumps or discolors, a crystal-like glaze or frost forms on the sides of the vial, or a white flocculation develops in any of the insulins, the insulin may be contaminated and should not be dispensed or used.

Storage of Insulin

Insulin is a heat-labile protein, so all preparations must be stored carefully to maintain potency and maximum stability. Patients should be instructed repeatedly to inspect their insulin for visible changes in appearance. Color changes may be associated with protein denaturation and should be interpreted as evidence of potency loss. Regular insulin's potency may decline by as much as 1.5% per month if the insulin is stored at room temperature (59°F to 85°F [15°C to 29°C]). The rate of potency loss increases as the temperature increases. Many insulins have been shown to be physically and chemically stable in unrefrigerated areas for long periods in a controlled laboratory setting; thus, patients may keep vials of insulin currently in use at room temperature. However, the insulin should be used within 1 month and should be stored away from heaters, radiators, or sunny windows. At 100°F (38°C), all insulins lose a significant amount of potency within 1 month, as can be evidenced by clumping, precipitation, or discoloration of the insulin.

The pharmacist should advise patients to keep any extra bottles of insulin in the refrigerator (at 36°F to 46°F [2°C to 8°C]) but not in the freezer. The refrigerator door is a good location for storage to keep the insulin from being shifted to the back of the refrigerator, where it might freeze. Freezing insulin does not necessarily affect potency, but it may cause aggregation, precipitation, and clumping, which can alter the insulin action.[20] When patients are traveling for prolonged periods in warm climates, they can ensure the stability and potency of their insulin by storing it in an insulated container with ice, "blue ice," or some other form of cooling agent or in an insulated carrying case or by packing it between several layers of clothing in a suitcase. Insulin should never be stored in the glove compartment or trunk of an automobile or in uninsulated backpacks or cycle bags. Insulin should be carried with the patient when traveling by air or commercial carrier because of variance in storage conditions.

Special Treatment Considerations

Hyperglycemia

Hyperglycemia can occur if an insulin dose is missed or if the dose is insufficient to meet the body's needs. The symptoms of this adverse effect—frequent urination, dehydration, thirst, increased appetite—usually occur at blood glucose levels higher than 150 mg/dL. If ketones have developed, the patient's breath will also have a fruity odor. Untreated hyperglycemia could progress to diabetic ketoacidosis, then coma and death. Self-monitoring of blood glucose allows the patient to detect upswings in glucose levels and to adjust the insulin therapy accordingly.

Hypoglycemia

Hypoglycemia manifests as sweating, tachycardia, palpitations, confusion, and tiredness. Factors predisposing the patient to hypoglycemia include insufficient food intake (e.g., skipping meals, vomiting, diarrhea), excessive sweating, drug interactions, inaccurate measurement of insulin dose, concomitant intake of hypoglycemic drugs, very tight glycemic control, and termination of diabetogenic conditions (e.g., stopping use of drugs such as prednisone). And several factors (including overdosing insulin) can induce low blood glucose.

Morning hyperglycemia may be a result of an asymptomatic nocturnal hypoglycemia (Somogyi reaction) in patients who are otherwise well controlled on intensive insulin regimens. These patients may describe symptoms of confusion without any other signs or symptoms of hypoglycemia, and appropriate therapy may not be administered. A reflex response to the hypoglycemia causes the body to secrete epinephrine, which induces the liver to release glucose—thus, the morning hyperglycemia. Another reaction that can present with a similar morning hyperglycemia is termed the "dawn reaction."[21] Cortisol and epinephrine are released during the night in preparation for the day ahead. In response, glucose rises in the early morning hours, and insulin is released from the functioning pancreas. In people with diabetes, the insulin release may not occur, resulting again in morning hyperglycemia. Notably, the first situation is caused by too much and the second by too little insulin. Patients with morning hyperglycemia must monitor their blood glucose levels between 2:00 am and 3:00 am to determine if the glucose is low (Somogyi phenomenon) or normal/high (dawn reaction).[21] They should record the results along with any changes in their diet and activities, and they should be assisted in interpreting the results and in making adjustments in their therapy.

All manifestations of hypoglycemia are relieved rapidly by glucose. Because of the potential danger of insulin reactions progressing to hypoglycemic coma, people with diabetes should always carry packets or cubes of table sugar, a candy roll, or glucose tablets or gel. They should eat 3 teaspoons (15 g) or two cubes of sugar, five to six Lifesavers, or three glucose tablets at the onset of mild hypoglycemic symptoms (e.g., sweating, hunger, weakness, nausea, dizziness, and mood changes). (See Table 39–10 for examples of blood glucose–elevating products.) Alternatively, they may drink at least one-half cup of orange juice, one-third cup of apple juice, or 6 to 12 ounces of any sugar-containing carbonated beverage. If the glucose concentration is still below 60 mg/dL at 15 minutes, the treatment may be repeated and the carbohydrate dose increased to 15 g. Candy that contains chocolate is usually not recommended because of a slightly slower carbohydrate absorption rate, the fat content, and the accompanying potential to overshoot or overconsume a

Table 39–10

Selected Blood Glucose–Elevating Products

Trade Name	Product Features
B-D Glucose	Orange-flavored, chewable tablet containing 5 g of glucose and 19 cal
BEX4 Glucose	Grape-, lemon-, orange-, or raspberry-flavored chewable tablet containing 4 g of glucose and 15 cal
Glutose Gel	Lemon-flavored gel containing 15 g of glucose and 60 cal in the single-dose tube, and 45 g and 180 cal in the triple-dose tube
Glutose Tablets	Lemon-flavored chewable tablet containing 5 g of glucose and 20 cal
Insta-Glucose	Cherry-flavored gel in a single-dose tube containing 25 g of glucose and 96 cal
Monojel Glucose	Orange-flavored gel in an individual foil packet containing 10 g of glucose and 46 cal

proper dose. A snack consisting of 1 to 2 cups of milk, a piece of fruit, or cheese and soda crackers is generally enough to treat mild hypoglycemia if mealtime is not imminent.[22] Blood glucose should be monitored frequently to ensure adequate levels and to prevent recurrent hypoglycemia.

If symptoms are intermediate (e.g., with presenting confusion, disorientation, poor coordination, headache, and double vision), more glucose may be required. A glucagon emergency kit containing an ampule of glucagon (1 mg), a syringe of diluent, and clearly illustrated directions should be provided to every Type 1 patient in case of severe hypoglycemia-associated unconsciousness. Family members and other patient caregivers and co-workers should be taught to mix and administer glucagon by injection. Glucagon should be reconstituted with the accompanying solvent. The usual dose for adults and children weighing more than 20 kg is 1 mg; for children weighing less than 20 kg, the usual dose is 0.5 mg. Normally, the patient will regain consciousness within 5 to 10 minutes and be able to swallow some sweetened water. If no response is seen after 5 to 10 minutes, a second injection may be given. If the response is still insufficient after the second dose, the patient should be taken to an emergency room or to a physician immediately. Glucagon injection may cause nausea and vomiting up to 2 to 4 hours after injection, so care should be taken to prevent aspiration of gastric contents. One should also note that following the patient's response a regimen of food intake for the next 24 hours is needed to replenish the lost glycogen from the liver.[22] If response does occur, the physician should be informed of the episode. If a hypoglycemic person is mistakenly thought to be hyperglycemic and given insulin, severe hypoglycemia and subsequent brain damage may result. When in doubt about whether a patient is hypoglycemic or hyperglycemic, sugar should be given initially until the condition can be accurately evaluated.

Self-Monitoring of Glucose and Ketone Levels

Maintenance of blood glucose control is impossible without measurement, and self-monitoring of blood glucose (SMBG) is the gold standard and most accurate method for day-to-day assessment of glycemic control. SMBG gives the patient information needed to make immediate and accurate therapy changes, which will thereby improve the overall control of blood glucose. However, testing improves glucose control only with proper use and application.[23] Thus, the patient must be trained in the technique and given specific guidelines for therapy alterations.

As an alternative, urine glucose testing gives the patient an idea of what the blood glucose level has been in the past several hours and not what it is currently. Therefore, insulin doses should never be adjusted on the basis of urine glucose testing.

Testing for urine ketones is advised for all patients who use insulin. Additionally, all pregnant patients generally should test for urinary ketones each morning to assess the adequacy of the evening nutrition. The urine should be tested whenever blood glucose levels are greater than 240 mg/dL and during periods of illness or stress. The ketone test helps screen for the level of fat breakdown in the patient. Ketones in the urine, combined with elevated blood glucose, are the first indicators of diabetes ketoacidosis. The presence of ketones on two or more consecutive urine tests should be reported to the physician.

Cost of SMBG may be a factor for some patients, but most insurance companies and managed care organizations, under the provisions of major medical plans, will reimburse patients for all or part of the cost of SMBG, including the cost of a meter. This shift has moved rapidly since 1997 when Congress passed legislation that mandates all Medicare recipients with diabetes access to SMBG.

Although few patients with diabetes are not candidates for self-monitoring, the following patients should be strongly encouraged to self-test their blood glucose:

- Patients with an abnormal or unstable renal threshold.
- Patients with renal failure.
- Patients whose glycemic control is unstable and insulin dependent.
- Patients with impaired color vision.
- Patients who have difficulty recognizing true hypoglycemia.
- Patients who are pregnant.
- Patients who are using drug therapy or nondrug therapy for diabetes control.
- Patients who prefer to self-test their blood glucose.

A major factor to consider when recommending a method of SMBG is the type of diabetes. Patients who are brittle, or whose blood glucose level is very volatile or difficult to control, obviously need to test more often than stable Type 2 patients.

The patient's willingness to learn and perform the tasks associated with using strips and a glucose meter is also a factor in selecting home blood glucose tests. Often the health care provider's most important role is to encourage patients to alter their behavior, perhaps by performing SMBG.

Manual dexterity plays a role in product selection; urine testing and several SMBG systems cannot be manipulated by patients with trembling hands. Patients with poor vision, which is common in people with diabetes, may be unable to see the drops or the readout screens on some blood glucose meters. Problems can occur in performing the tests and in interpreting the color changes on the blood or urine glucose monitoring strips. Few visually impaired patients are able to match the strips accurately to the corresponding color chart, especially if lighting is poor; those who perform the color match by using single-source direct lighting (e.g., a table lamp) are more accurate. Special kits are available for the visually impaired patient, who may also be able to use blood glucose meters that have audio components. (See Table 39–11 for examples of commercially available monitors.)

Ketosis-prone patients are advised to test their blood for glucose; those who show elevated levels should also test their urine for ketones. All patients should periodically test their urine for protein as an indication of nephropathy. Protein in the urine can be easily determined by using an array of products.

Proper education in the methods for self-monitoring, the differences between individual meters, the importance of multiple daily tests, and the interpretation and application of test results will encourage more patients to perform SMBG consistently. Pharmacists can become distributors of the blood testing devices and can acquire the training needed to ensure that patients using such devices are themselves properly trained. Return demonstration by the patient is necessary to ensure patient understanding and to correct any errors as they are observed. The pharmacist should then document the sale and training on the profile and should correspond with the patient's primary physician regarding the training session.

Table 39–11

Selected Blood Glucose Monitors

Trade Name	Test Time (seconds)	Product Features
Accu-Check Advantage	40	Self-cleaning; no wiping of test strips; 100-test memory capacity; calibration with code chip
Accu-Check Complete	40	Self-cleaning; no wiping of test strips; 1000-test memory capacity; calibration with code chip
Accu-Check Easy	15–60	No wiping of test strips; 350-test memory capacity; calibration with code chip
Accu-Check III	120	Wiping of test strips; 20-test memory capacity; calibration with code strip; provides 7-day test average and maximum/minimum values; allows visual reading of test strips as backup measure
Accu-Check Instant	12	No wiping of test strips; 9-test memory capacity; push-button calibration; allows visual reading of test strips as backup measure
Accu-Check Instant DM	12	No wiping of test strips; 500-test memory capacity; calibration with code strip; allows visual reading of test strips as backup measure; offers graphic display of 48-hour and 7-day glucose levels
Diascan Partner	90	Wiping of test strips required; 10-test memory capacity; voice instructions for test procedure; announcement of error codes
Duet Glucose Control System	Glucose: 8 Fructosamine: 240	No wiping of test strips; 150-test memory capacity for glucose; 50-test memory capacity for fructosamine; calibration with glucose test strip; fructosamine test measures glucose control over the previous 2–3 weeks; extra-large capacity
ExacTech RSG Sensor	30	No wiping of test strips; no calibration of meter; credit-card size
Fast Take	15	Self-cleaning; no wiping of test strips; 150-test memory capacity; single-button calibration; requires very small (12.5 mL) blood sample
One Touch Basic	45	No wiping of test strips; one-test memory capacity; single-button calibration; prompts in English or Spanish; alerts user to clean monitor
One Touch Profile	45	No wiping of test strips; 250-test memory capacity; single-button calibration; prompts in any one of 19 languages; alerts user to clean meter; diabetes management software available
Precision QID	20	No wiping of test strips; 125-test memory capacity; single-button calibration; diabetes management software available
SureStep	15–30	No wiping of test strips; 150-test memory capacity; single-button calibration; test-strip confirmation that blood sample is sufficient

The patient should be encouraged to keep accurate records of the tests and to return with his or her logbook, which should also contain records of body weight, activities, diet, and medication use, so that the pharmacist can determine how well the diabetes is being controlled. The record can be quickly updated with each patient's visit. This patient data form of documentation can be invaluable to assess the outcome of pharmacist-based patient teaching.

Blood Glucose Tests Blood glucose tests are of two types: a test that uses only reagent strips and one that uses both reagent strips and a blood glucose meter.

Blood Glucose Tests Using Reagent Strips Reagent strips, which are impregnated with glucose oxidase, can be read visually to obtain a *range* of the blood glucose level. The patient places a drop of blood on the strip and waits 30 to 60 seconds before wiping or washing the blood off. Then, after another minute, the patient compares the color on the strip with the colors on a color chart. Accuracy can be achieved only when the blood is properly placed and when the correct amount of time has transpired. No known medications cause false readings.

To ensure accuracy, test strips should be stored at room temperature. Also, bottle caps should be replaced immediately and tightly after a strip is removed because most strips will react to moisture.

Blood Glucose Tests Using Glucose Meters A glucose meter used in conjunction with reagent strips gives the specific blood glucose level rather than a range. Two types of meters measure blood glucose, although both kinds are based on (oxidation) glucose oxidase or hexokinase activity. One type uses a photometric measurement based on a dye-related reaction. As in the reagent-strip method, the patient places a drop of blood on a reagent strip and blots it; the strip is then inserted into a meter, where it is read photometrically or colorimetrically. The other type of meter measures blood glucose through an electronic charge produced by a chemical reaction.

All meters are calibrated and will generally analyze the blood glucose level according to programmed data. All meters provide a digital readout of the blood glucose level as well as a visual indicator. Some have audio components or memories for later recall of recent blood glucose levels, and they can print out retained data. Many pharmacies have software from the manufacturer on their computers to allow downloading of data from a meter; the program can then plot glucose-level curves to reflect the patient's glucose pattern.

Patients who are selecting a meter can make comparisons according to size, wipe or nonwipe method, timing devices, calibration, accuracy, ease of use, memory/data management and printout features, battery types, need for cleaning, accessories required, audio capabilities, teaching materials or training available, and price. (See Table 39–11.) Other variables to assess include the precision of the product; the effect(s), if any, of temperature on accuracy; the effect on the test result of holding the meter at an angle; manufacturer support; and any specific idiosyncrasies of the particular device. FDA has set specific allowable variances for the meters. However, even when blood glucose monitoring equipment is used properly, calibrated frequently, and interpreted correctly, accuracy can vary by 5%. Finally, the blood glucose monitoring method recommended to the patient must be flexible and capable of being easily incorporated into the patient's lifestyle or daily routine. Patients should be allowed to try several meters before selecting one for home use.[24]

Lancets and Other Test Accessories In addition to these test devices, patients need blood lancets and lancet holders, alcohol swabs or cotton balls and alcohol, and other accessories. Several lancing devices are available for patient use, so pharmacists are advised to stock various brands to meet individual patient preferences. These devices allow for a finger stick with less associated pain. The patient should be instructed to use the sides of the finger, where fewer nerve endings are found than in the middle and thus less pain. Just before sticking the finger, the patient should wash his or her hands, preferably with warm water to increase blood supply. If washing is not possible, alcohol swabs can be used for cleansing. The patient should ensure however that the alcohol has evaporated before sticking the finger because alcohol can alter the test results.

Urine Glucose Tests Although blood glucose testing is strongly preferred, urine glucose testing is recommended for patients who cannot or will not monitor their own blood glucose. This group may include individuals who refuse to lance themselves, cannot be taught the proper technique, or are otherwise unreliable.

Copper reduction tests and glucose oxidase tests (also called dip-and-read tests) are used to measure glucose in urine. In the qualitative copper reduction tests, cupric sulfate (blue) in the presence of glucose yields cuprous oxide (green to orange). However, interpretation of test results is complicated by a "pass-through phenomenon"; that is, when urine glucose is more than 2%, the color reaction may change from green to orange very quickly and then fade back to brown. Because such a reaction may be erroneously interpreted as less than 2%, the patient must watch the reaction develop. Moreover, copper reduction tests detect not only glucose but also the presence of other reducing substances in the urine. Finally, care must be exercised when using test materials. The tablets and solutions are very caustic, so handling or splashing should be avoided. Also, because the tablets can be quite dangerous if accidentally ingested, they must be kept out of the reach of children.

A second qualitative method is based on the glucose oxidase–mediated conversion of glucose to gluconic acid and hydrogen peroxide (H_2O_2). In the presence of *o*-toluidine, a color change occurs. The glucose oxidase test is more convenient and less expensive than the copper reduction test, but the test strips can be affected by humidity and are not as easily read.

Patients may be taking drugs that can interfere with urine

Case Study 39–2

Patient Complaint/History

Peter Blue Cloud, a 52-year-old man, calls the pharmacy seeking help with his blood glucose meter. Six months earlier, he was diagnosed as having Type 2 diabetes for which glyburide was prescribed. Four months after the diagnosis, the physician decided that the patient needed insulin injections to control his diabetes. Currently, the patient uses Novolin 70/30 insulin 32 U every morning and 12 U every afternoon. His profile also shows that he purchased his One Touch Profile blood glucose meter and 100 test strips about 5 weeks ago. At the time of the purchase, he was instructed on the proper use of the meter.

The patient, who has been testing his blood glucose three or four times a day, asks, "What could be causing the meter to go bad so quickly?" He notes that 4 days ago, while he was out of town, he bought a new set of test strips. He goes on to explain that the results of the tests performed the past couple of days have appeared erratic and have not reflected how he feels. The patient now wants to purchase the type of strips he originally used. He also wants advice on choosing an appropriate cough and cold medication. His cold symptoms, which he describes as a runny nose and raspy cough associated with some chills, began a couple of days ago.

Based on the information provided, the pharmacist asks the patient to bring in his meter and the new test strips for evaluation.

Clinical Considerations/Strategies

Readers can use the following considerations/strategies to determine the appropriate treatment approach for this patient's situation:

- Assess the patient's current knowledge about and technique for self-monitoring of blood glucose levels.
- Assess the patient's ability to obtain an adequate blood sample for his particular meter.
- Assess the patient's ability to program his meter properly for different test strip lots.
- Assess the patient's interpretation of his blood glucose levels as they relate to control of his diabetes.
- Assess the patient's cold symptoms, and recommend a product for symptomatic relief that will not significantly interfere with his glycemic control.

Patient Education/Counseling

Readers can use the following strategies to develop a patient education/counseling plan that will help ensure optimal therapeutic outcomes:

- Describe components of a follow-up education plan that will ensure that diabetic patients understand and adhere to their treatment regimen.
- Develop a plan for continually assessing and reviewing the patient's technique in using his meter.

glucose testing methods, and they should be instructed to test their urine by both methods. If the test results differ, a drug is likely to be interfering with the test results.

Disadvantages of urine glucose tests compared with blood glucose tests include (1) the inability to detect hypoglycemia; (2) many possible drug interferences; (3) patient variance with reference to renal threshold for glucose; (4) lack of correlation between urine and blood glucose levels; (5) for some patients, difficulty in reading and performing tests; (6) more privacy required than in blood testing; and (7) inability to measure hyperglycemia.

Before purchasing a test kit, patients must consider the accuracy, sensitivity, range, ease of testing and timing, cost, availability of products, and advantages or disadvantages of multitest versus individual test kits. And as with the SMBG tests, patients must be specifically trained to use the products selected, and the pharmacist should have the patient demonstrate his or her technique to ensure accuracy and proficiency.

Urinary Ketone Tests Because ketones in the blood overflow into the urine, urinary ketone levels can be tested to detect whether metabolic changes causing ketoacidosis are occurring. The ketone bodies produced are acetone, acetoacetic acid, and β-hydroxybutyric acid. The basis for the test is that sodium nitroprusside alkali turns lavender in the presence of acetone or acetoacetic acid.

Acetest reagent tablets are specific for acetoacetic acid and acetone and will detect 10 mg of acetoacetic acid (but not β-hydroxybutyric acid) in 100 mL of serum, plasma, or whole blood. Ketostix, Chemstrip K, and other tests will detect 5 to 10 mg of acetoacetic acid in 100 mL of urine. These tests are easier to perform than Acetest, and no dropper is required. However, the improved Ketostix tests only for acetoacetic acid and thus shows a false negative result if the predominant ketobody is acetone or β-hydroxybutyric acid.

All diabetes patients, particularly those with Type 1 diabetes and pregnant women with diabetes, should test for ketones when blood glucose is 240 mg/dL or greater, and all patients should be counseled on the proper way to test for ketones in the urine. Pregnant women are commonly instructed to test for ketones each morning and sometimes more often to assess their nutritional status.

Identification Tags

All persons with diabetes should wear easily seen identification bracelets, necklaces, or tags that indicate the person has diabetes and takes medication. Patients should also carry identification cards that list the person's name, address, and telephone number; the amount and type of medication used; and the name and telephone number of the patient's physician. This identification may be lifesaving if hypoglycemia or ketoacidosis occurs. If a patient becomes unconscious through an accident or a hypoglycemic or hyperglycemic coma, medications that must be taken regularly may be missed. Because a hypoglycemic (insulin) reaction may be confused with drunkenness, hypoglycemic patients have been jailed rather than given medical care.

Travel Supplies and Preparations

The pharmacist should always counsel the traveling patient with diabetes to take enough of the following supplies for the entire trip plus 1 week:

- An extra vial of insulin.
- Extra supply of syringes because access may be limited; refrain from prefilling syringes on a trip because of potential for leakage.
- Identification cards and an identification bracelet, necklace, or tag.
- If traveling abroad, the names of English-speaking physicians in each city and some cards with several key phrases to access care in the language of the country being visited ("I have diabetes"; "Please get me a doctor").
- A summary of the patient's current medical regimen.

Patients who are traveling should control their diets carefully, allow time for physical activity, and carry candy or sugar to combat possible hypoglycemic attacks. Patients who are changing time zones should also recognize that changes of 2 hours or more require adjustments of the insulin dose. The diabetic traveler (heading west) may use the following formula to make a one-time/one-day adjustment:

New NPH/lente dose = usual NPH/lente dose × (1 + number of time zones crossed/24)

If the traveler is headed east, the formula is

New NPH/lente dose = usual NPH/lente dose × (1 − number of time zones crossed/24)

Patients using a mixture of insulins or intensive therapy may not be able to use these formulas and so should monitor their blood glucose more often to ensure control. Because patients will probably need to monitor their blood glucose more often, because of changes in diet, activity, and meal schedules, they should also take extra batteries and strips for the glucose meter, a bottle of strips that can be read visually, alcohol wipes, cotton balls, and lancets. Even if patients do not usually monitor their urine for ketones, it is advisable to do so while traveling.

Alternative Remedies

One in three Americans have sought treatment for medical conditions from alternative sources, most commonly in the

Table 39–12

Purported Herbal Remedies for Diabetes Mellitus

Product	Comments
Aloe vera	Animal and human studies show patients have a mild reduction in mean glucose levels, although not adequate to warrant clinical use.
Bitter melon	Hypoglycemic properties have been reported in several journals; the aqueous extract lowered blood glucose by 25%. Lack of standard dosed product makes recommendation difficult.
Capsaicin (cayenne pepper)	Product has beneficial effects on decreasing neuropathic pain peripherally or radiculopathy.
Dandelion root	Product contains inulin, which may have a mild but not significant effect on blood glucose.
Eucalyptus	Product has mild hypoglycemic effects in mice but is not recommended for human use.
Garlic	Active product, allylpropyl-disulphide (APDS), lowers glucose by competing with insulin in activating sites in liver. Product has limited benefit and lack of standard dose limits for use clinically.
Ginkgo biloba	Claims made that this product produces claudication; clinical trials are lacking.
Ginseng	Siberian ginseng water extract has some hypoglycemic activity in mice. A useful product with standard potency does not exist.
Licorice	Product has potential to reduce hyperphagia and polydipsia but is not useful for diabetes.
Onions	Graded doses of onion extracts can reduce blood glucose. Alicin and APDS content are active compounds but are not useful for glucose lowering in patients.
Pectin (apples)	Like guar gum, product contains high amount of fiber. Regular intake is associated with lowered total cholesterol.
Periwinkle	Conflicting reports suggest lowering blood glucose in cats, but no substantial effect is seen.
Yellow root (golden seal)	Although long-term use by Native Americans, no standardized treatment has been proven effective.
Yohimbine	Product may possibly be effective in treating psychogenic erectile dysfunction.

form of natural products, and have spent more than $14 billion annually for these remedies. Such products are marketed to patients through mail order, health food sources, and some pharmacies. The real concern is for the patient who substitutes the natural product for the oral medication or insulin in the belief that the natural product controls diabetes. The belief is that a natural product *must* be safe, because it is naturally occurring. The problem for diabetes care is that scientific support for natural product efficacy is lacking. (Very little incentive exists to conduct studies because these substances are not patentable medications.) Table 39–12 lists several of the better known products and their therapeutic claims. The following guidelines are appropriate for counseling people with diabetes who plan to use natural products:

- Research scientific proof of use of the products.
- Make sure the ingredients and the dose of each ingredient are listed.
- Know the age and sex of the patient and whether female patients are attempting to become pregnant.
- Know all the prescription and nonprescription medications the patient is taking.
- If the patient decides to take an herbal or natural remedy, advise the patient to stop the product if any adverse reaction occurs.
- Encourage patients to read the labels and to purchase standardized products.
- Encourage patients to let you and other caregivers know which products they are using.

This final point is especially important. Health care providers should not alienate patients from the system of health care because the patient chooses to use natural products. An information gap develops once the patient is not willing to tell the health care provider about using natural products.[25]

Patient Assessment of Type 1 Diabetes Mellitus

If the patient describes classic symptoms of diabetes, the pharmacist should ask whether a physician has made this diagnosis. If not, screening for diabetes is appropriate. The American Diabetes Association recommends that all individuals receive a laboratory-based glucose test by age 45 years and, if normal, repeat the test every 3 years.[26] Individuals with risk factors for diabetes should be considered for testing more frequently and at an earlier age. (See the section "Etiology of Type 1 Diabetes Mellitus.") Screening can start with the diabetes survey developed by the American Diabetes Association. (See Table 39–13.) Adding up the point values of the questions gives a person's relative risk for developing diabetes. Individuals with a high risk for the disease can then be tested by capillary blood glucose (fingerstick). Test results should be compared with the diagnostic criteria in Table 39–14. Testing itself requires literature, documentation forms, alcohol swabs, lancets, blood test strips, and a glucose meter. The pharmacist should review his or her state's specific laboratory guidelines, application of the federal Clinical Laboratory Improvements Act of 1988, and the blood and body fluid precautions issued by the Occupational Safety and Health Administration (OSHA) before performing any screening or other lab tests. Any facility that routinely has the potential for exposure to blood and body fluids must comply with OSHA guidelines.

Before recommending an insulin preparation for diagnosed diabetes, the pharmacist should determine the medications the patient is taking, any known drug allergies (particularly to porcine insulin), any concurrent diseases or infections, and the present extent of antidiabetes therapy. The pharmacist should carefully address the patient's attitude toward the disease and the impact of diabetes care on the patient's lifestyle. The assessment should provide the pharmacist with information about the patient's knowledge of the disorder and should allow for developing a diabetes education and care plan tailored to the patient's needs. At all times during the interview, the pharmacist should be prepared to answer the patient's questions concerning diabetes and to recommend proper screening steps. Asking the patient the following questions will help elicit the information needed to accurately assess the disorder and to determine the appropriate treatment approach.

Q~ Is there a history of diabetes in your family?

A~ If a first-degree relative has the disease, encourage the patient to be screened for diabetes.

Q~ What symptoms are you having? Have you been tested for diabetes? If so, what were the results?

A~ *Identify the classic symptoms of diabetes as well as the common complications of this disorder. (See the sections "Signs and Symptoms of Type 1 Diabetes Mellitus" and "Complications of Type 1 Diabetes Mellitus.")* If the patient has classic symptoms of diabetes but has not been tested for this disorder, either refer the patient to a physician for evaluation or screen the patient for diabetes if the pharmacy is certified to test blood glucose levels.

Q~ Have you seen a dietitian? If so, what were the dietitian's recommendations?

A~ Find out the patient's recommended daily caloric intake and how much of that is carbohydrates. Make sure the patient is neither losing nor gaining weight. Calculate optimal dietary intake using the ideal body weight of the patient or the grams of carbohydrate allowed in the patient's diet. (See the section "Nonpharmacologic Therapy" under "Treatment of Type 1 Diabetes Mellitus.")

Table 39–13

Diabetes Screening Questionnaire

Could you have diabetes and NOT know it?	Point Values[a]
1. My weight is equal to or above that listed in the chart below.[b]	Yes 5
2. I am under 65 years of age, and I get little or no exercise during a usual day.	Yes 5
3. I am between 45 and 65 years of age.	Yes 5
4. I am 65 years old or older.	Yes 9
5. I am a woman who has had a baby weighing more than 9 pounds.	Yes 1
6. I have a sister or brother with diabetes.	Yes 1
7. I have a parent with diabetes.	Yes 1
	Total

Women		Men	
Height (inches) (w/o shoes)	Weight (pounds)[b] (w/o clothing)	Height (inches) (w/o shoes)	Weight (pounds)[b] (w/o clothing)
57	127	61	146
58	131	62	151
59	134	63	155
60	138	64	158
61	142	65	163
62	146	66	168
63	151	67	174
64	157	68	179
65	162	69	184
66	167	70	190
67	172	71	196
68	176	72	202
69	181	73	208
70	186	74	214
		75	220

[a] A score of 3–5 indicates a low risk for diabetes; a score greater than 5 indicates a high risk for diabetes. Anyone scoring more than 5 points should see a physician promptly for evaluation.

[b] Chart lists weight 20% heavier than those recommended for men or women with medium frames.

Source: *Diabetes Alert*. Alexandria, VA: American Diabetes Association; 1995; adapted with permission.

Table 39–14

Diagnostic Criteria of Diabetes Mellitus in Nonpregnant Adults[a]

Disorder	Plasma Glucose (mg/dL)	Presence of Symptoms	Comments
Casual	≥200	+	Symptoms include polyuria, polydipsia, and unexplained weight loss. Casual is defined as any time of day without regard to time since last meal.
Fasting	≥126	—	Fasting is defined as no caloric intake for at least 8 hours.
2-Hour glucose during an OGTT	≥200	—	The test should be performed as described by World Health Organization, using a load of ≈75 g anhydrous glucose dissolved in water.

Key: OGTT = oral glucose tolerance test.

[a] These criteria should be confirmed by repeating any of the tests on a separate day, if hyperglycemia with acute metabolic compensation is equivocal.

Source: Reference 26.

Q~ When did you last review your care plan with your physician, pharmacist, nurse, dietitian, or physical therapist?

A~ If the patient's blood glucose level is under tight control, recommend that the patient's care plan be reassessed quarterly. Otherwise, recommend that the patient return for reassessment every 3 to 7 days until tight control has been established.

Q~ What prescription medications are you taking? How do you use them? Please include all medications, even for problems other than diabetes.

A~ *Identify the prescription medications that can alter glycemic control. (See Table 39-9.)* If the patient is taking any of these medications, advise the patient to return to his or her doctor for a different prescription.

Q~ Do you take any nonprescription medications?

A~ *Identify the nonprescription medications that can alter glycemic control. (See Table 39–9.)* If the patient is taking any of these medications, recommend alternative products that do not affect glycemic control. Also, advise the patient to check the sugar content of the nonprescription medications before purchasing or using them.

Q~ Are you allergic to any medications, especially sulfa drugs or pork insulins?

A~ If the patient is unaware of such allergies, advise the patient to get skin tested before using any of these medications. If the patient is allergic to pork insulin, recommend that the patient switch to human insulin.

Q~ If you use insulin, what brand do you use? How do you inject it? What injection sites do you use and how do you rotate them? Will you demonstrate your injecting technique?

A~ *Identify the four basic types of insulin and the various mixed insulin formulations.(See the section "Pharmacologic Therapy" under "Treatment of Type 1 Diabetes Mellitus.")* Evaluate the patient's injection technique and tracking system. If needed, demonstrate the proper technique and counsel the patient on keeping records of injections. (See the section "Administration Guidelines" under "Treatment of Type 1 Diabetes Mellitus.")

Q~ How do you store your insulin at home and when you travel?

A~ *Identify the proper storage conditions and time frame for insulin. (See the section "Storage of Insulin" under "Treatment of Type 1 Diabetes Mellitus.")* If needed, counsel the patient on these measures.

Q~ Do you test your blood for glucose? If so, what monitoring system do you use? How often do you test? How do you record the results? Will you show me your testing technique?

A~ If needed, demonstrate proper test techniques and logging procedures, and show the patient the least painful way to obtain a blood sample. Be sure your pharmacy meets the criteria discussed previously for diabetes screening before observing the patient's fingerstick and blood testing technique.

Q~ Do you test your urine for glucose? For ketones? Please describe your testing procedures. How do you use the test results to control your diabetes?

A~ *Identify the tests used to test glucose and ketone levels. Identify medications that could interfere with test results. (See the section "Self-Monitoring of Glucose and Ketone Levels.")* Show the patient how to avoid false-negative results when glucose is more than 2%. Advise the patient to see a doctor immediately if ketone levels are high.

Q~ Describe your diet plan. Do you have trouble following the plan? Are you currently using or have you ever used a "fad" diet? If so, describe the diet plan.

A~ Be prepared to recommend a diet plan that meets the needs, wants, and lifestyle of the patient, yet does not exceed the patient's caloric needs. Be able to calculate the patient's ideal weight and describe the point system or carbohydrate counting methods of dietary control to the patient. (See the section "Dietary Plan" under "Treatment of Type 1 Diabetes Mellitus.")

Q~ What exercise guidelines do you follow? Describe your routine exercise habits.

A~ Advise the patient to do aerobic exercise and caution against heavy lifting. Encourage the patient to monitor blood glucose before exercise and, if hypoglycemic, to eat a snack.

Q~ Do you consume alcoholic beverages? What have you been told about alcohol's effect on your diabetes?

A~ *Identify the possible effects of alcohol consumption on persons with diabetes. (See the section "Use of Alcohol" under "Treatment of Type 1 Diabetes Mellitus.")* Advise the patient of these effects; encourage the patient to limit alcohol consumption to a few drinks a week.

Q~ When did you last see an eye practitioner?

A~ *Identify the effects of chronic hyperglycemia on the eyes. (See the section "Complications of Type 1 Diabetes Mellitus.")* Advise the patient to have an annual eye exam. Counsel the patient on preventive measures. (See Table 39–3.)

Q~ When did you last see a dentist? How often do you see a dentist? Describe how you care for your teeth.

A~ *Identify the effects of hyperglycemia on teeth and gums. (See the section "Complications of Type 1 Diabetes Mellitus.")* Advise the patient to see a dentist twice a year. Counsel the patient on preventive measures. (See Table 39–3.)

Q~ Have you ever seen a podiatrist (foot specialist)? If so, how long ago and how often? Describe how you care for your feet.

A~ *Identify the effects of hyperglycemia on feet and the basics of foot care. (See the section "Complications of Type 1 Diabetes Mellitus.")* Advise the patient to see a podiatrist annually and on an as-needed basis for persistent foot problems. Counsel the patient on preventive measures. (See Table 39–3.)

Q~ What identification do you carry to show that you have diabetes?

A~ Offer the patient a choice of identification tags, and be able to advise the patient about Medic Alert identification systems.

Q~ How do you feel about having diabetes? How does your family feel about this? Does your family understand the factors that affect control of your diabetes?

A~ Find out who the members of the patient's support system are and whether they would receive training in diabetes care. Be prepared to instruct the caregivers. Find out whether the patient is depressed, and, if so, recommend the services of a counselor, psychologist, or psychiatrist.

Q~ Are you a member of the American Diabetes Association?

A~ If no, encourage the patient to join and to take advantage of the association's support and education services.

Patient Counseling for Type 1 Diabetes Mellitus

Even though a patient may seek assistance only in purchasing diabetes care products, the pharmacist should also try to determine whether the patient is adhering to the diabetes care plan. The pharmacist should stress the importance of adhering to the insulin regimen and to the diet and exercise plans. A review of techniques for administering insulin or for testing glucose and ketone levels may be necessary. If the patient wishes to switch diabetes care products (e.g., glucose meters, injection devices), the pharmacist should find out the reason for switching products and should recommend a product that best fits the patient's needs. Patients should be instructed on the correct use of any diabetes care products they purchase. The pharmacist should be familiar enough with new products to answer the patient's inquiries about them. The box "Patient Education for Diabetes Mellitus" lists specific information to provide patients.

Evaluation of Patient Outcomes for Type 1 Diabetes Mellitus

Desirable therapeutic outcomes are improved glycemic control, lower hemoglobin A_{1c}, improved lipid profile, normalized blood pressure, and, if applicable, reduced obesity. Other positive benefits are improved quality of life, improved foot care and oral hygiene, and reduced absences from work and school.[26] If the patient is not achieving such outcomes, adherence to the care plan should be assessed. Patients who are not following the plan should be reeducated about the need for and the benefits of the care plan. If compliance is not the problem, the patient should be referred to a physician.

Type 2 Diabetes Mellitus

The majority of people with diabetes mellitus and virtually all undiagnosed cases are of Type 2 diabetes mellitus. The metabolic defect here is not absence of insulin but resistance to the action of insulin. Hence, Type 2 is also known as non–insulin-dependent diabetes mellitus (NIDDM). And because the disease often occurs in adults older than 40 years, Type 2 is known as adult-onset diabetes mellitus.

Epidemiology of Type 2 Diabetes Mellitus

About 90% of the 10.3 million diagnosed and 5.4 million undiagnosed (mild or no symptoms) people with diabetes mellitus are Type 2.[27] Recent data from the U.S. Centers for Disease Control and Prevention indicate that Type 2 diabetes mellitus is especially prevalent in certain minority populations, including Hispanic Americans (1.9 times as likely to have diabetes as non-Hispanic whites), African Americans (1.7 times as likely), American Indians and Alaska Natives (2.8 times on average, but prevalence ranges from 5% to 50% between tribes), and Asian Americans and Pacific Islanders.[10,27]

Approximately 10% of patients with Type 2 diabetes are nonobese; the other 90% are obese. Nonobese Type 2 diabetes often occurs in patients during youth and is inherited in an autosomal dominant pattern. Obese Type 2 diabetes is more common in adults older than 40 years. The critical factor linking Type 2 diabetes and cardiovascular disease is the association with intra-abdominal fat. Thus, patients with Type 2 diabetes are not simply more than 20% over their

Patient Education for Diabetes Mellitus

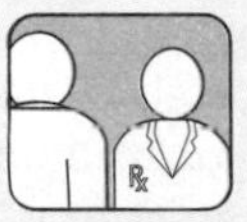

The primary objective of self-treatment is to maintain glycemic control. Achieving this objective will, in turn, ensure success with these secondary objectives: (1) prevent or reverse diabetic complications, (2) maintain normal daily activities with maximum lifestyle flexibility, (3) avoid weight gain by following a well-planned diet and exercise routine, (4) avoid infection, and (5) achieve a sense of well-being. For most patients, carefully following product instructions, the pharmacist's instructions on proper use of insulins, and the self-care measures listed below will help ensure optimal therapeutic outcomes.

Nondrug Measures

- If newly diagnosed with diabetes, meet with your doctor, nurse, dietitian, or pharmacist to develop a diet plan and exercise program that suits your lifestyle. Follow the care plan carefully.
- If you have diabetes complications, consult specialists who are specially trained to care for people with diabetes. Practice the preventive measures listed in Table 39–3 daily.
- If you exercise regularly, follow the guidelines in Table 39–4.
- Monitor your blood glucose several times a day. If your values indicate a problem, see your doctor for adjustments to your therapy.

Nonprescription Medications

- If applicable, follow your prescribed insulin regimen carefully.
- Inject your insulin at the proper sites and rotate your injection sites. (See Figure 39–4.)
- Follow the guidelines in Table 39–7 for preparing and injecting insulin doses.
- Consider using a programmable infuser pump if you have a multiple insulin-injection regimen.
- Read the labels of nonprescription medications to make sure they do not contain sugar or alcohol.
- If you have cuts and bruises that are not healing or are infected, consult with your physician.
- Sympathomimetic bronchodilators, such as ephedrine or pseudoephedrine, may raise blood glucose levels. Have your doctor prescribe an alternative medication or recommend safe dosages for these medications if you need to take them.

⚠ If you experience symptoms of hypoglycemia (sweating, tachycardia, palpitations, confusion, tiredness, etc.) or hyperglycemia (frequent urination, dehydration, thirst, increased appetite, etc.) with your prescribed insulin regimen, see a physician for reassessment of the regimen.

⚠ If your blood glucose is greater than 250 mg/dL and your urinary ketones are moderate to high, call your doctor or go to an emergency facility.

ideal body weight, but the obesity is characteristically abdominal.

Other risk factors for Type 2 diabetes include age (older than 45 years), gestational diabetes, and delivery of an infant weighing 9 pounds or more. A previous diagnosis of impaired glucose tolerance is also an indicator. In 1997, a panel of the American Diabetes Association recognized two conditions as risk factors: impaired glucose tolerance (IGT) and impaired fasting glucose (IFT). IGT occurs with a plasma glucose of greater than 140 mg/dL but less than 200 mg/dL. IFT was coined to describe a fasting glucose of greater than 110 mg/dL but less than 126 mg/dL. With both of these groups, the patients are not considered to have diabetes, but they do have an impairment in energy regulation.

Etiology of Type 2 Diabetes Mellitus

In Type 2 diabetes, the pancreas is producing insulin, but the body has developed insulin resistance, causing hyperinsulinemia. Insulin resistance corresponds to a decrease in the number of insulin receptors.[28,29] These processes are usually reversible if body weight is reduced to the ideal body weight. A defect in postreceptor binding appears to be another cause of insulin resistance. In some Type 2 patients, a decreased number of insulin receptors and a postreceptor defect may exist in combination.[30]

Reaven[31] proposed in 1988 that insulin resistance leading to hyperinsulinemia (increased serum levels of insulin) contributes directly to the development of hypertension and the appearance of factors (increased LDL and triglycerides as well as decreased HDL) leading to cardiovascular disease and atherosclerosis. The symptom cluster has been called metabolic syndrome X by Reaven and seems to parallel the development of full-blown Type 2 hyperinsulinemia and to be responsible for the increased mortality and morbidity from cardiovascular disease in these patients.

Heredity is a major cause of Type 2 diabetes mellitus. In identical twin studies, if one twin has Type 2 diabetes, nearly a 100% chance exists that both twins will have the disease. Although Type 1 diabetes also has a strong genetic component (see "Etiology of Type 1 Diabetes Mellitus"), the genes for Type 1 and Type 2 are on entirely different chromosomes.

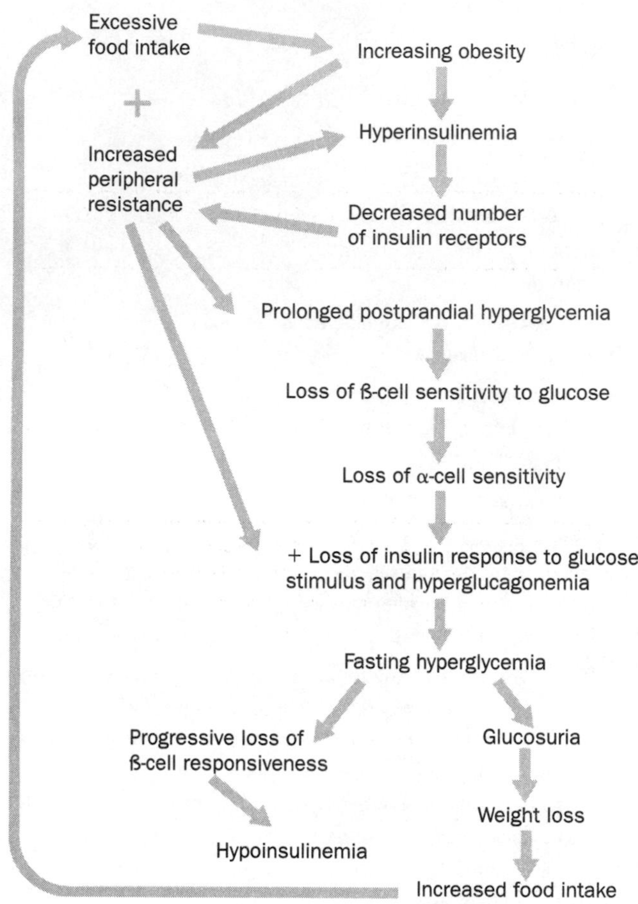

Figure 39–6 Clinical manifestation of Type 2 non–insulin-dependent diabetes mellitus.

Pathophysiology of Type 2 Diabetes Mellitus

In contrast to Type 1 diabetes, Type 2 diabetes is often not accompanied by any symptoms, at least early in the disease progression. Figure 39–6 provides a flow diagram of the pathogenesis of Type 2 diabetes. The American Diabetes Association panel that reclassified diabetes indicates that Type 2 can vary between a disorder largely caused by insulin resistance with relative insulin deficiency to one that originates from a secretory defect with some insulin resistance. Increased obesity in Type 2 patients may cause hyperinsulinemia, resulting in a down regulation or loss of insulin-receptor sensitivity to glucose, which leads to the clinical finding of hyperglycemia. (See the section "Physiology of Glycoprotein Metabolism" for a discussion of insulin's role in preventing hyperglycemia.)

Nonobese Type 2 patients may have low, normal, or high blood insulin levels, whereas obese Type 2 patients, who are in the majority, usually have normal or elevated blood insulin levels. Glucose is transported into muscle and fat cells so these patients are not usually ketosis prone and seldom develop ketoacidosis except during periods of significant stress. Because of their high blood glucose levels, they may be prone to a syndrome termed hyperglycemic, hyperosmolar, nonketotic coma. Although the acute management of this syndrome is similar to that of ketoacidosis in Type 1 patients, diagnosis is troublesome because of nonspecific symptoms in the elderly individual.

Other physiologic changes of chronic hyperglycemia that occur in Type 1 are also found in Type 2 diabetes mellitus but usually take longer to develop. (See the section "Pathophysiology of Type 1 Diabetes Mellitus.")

Signs and Symptoms of Type 2 Diabetes Mellitus

Symptoms of Type 2 diabetes are the same as those for Type 1 except that in Type 2 diabetes they can appear singly and develop at a slower pace. Patients may notice yeast infections, tingling sensations in hands or feet, or more frequent urination—especially at night. (See the section "Signs and Symptoms of Type 1 Diabetes Mellitus.")

Complications of Type 2 Diabetes Mellitus

Type 1 and Type 2 diabetes mellitus share complications of hyperinsulinemia—namely retinopathy, neuropathy, renal failure, and lower extremity disease. (See the section "Complications of Type 1 Diabetes Mellitus.") Type 2 diabetes patients rarely suffer diabetic ketoacidosis though.

Treatment of Type 2 Diabetes Mellitus

Treatment Outcomes

The primary goal of Type 2 diabetes patients is weight loss, but now meeting blood pressure, blood lipid, and blood glucose goals is emphasized as well.[12] The goals in the section "Treatment Outcomes" under "Treatment of Type 1 Diabetes Mellitus" also pertain to Type 2 diabetes.

General Treatment Approach

Early stages of Type 2 diabetes can frequently be controlled by diet and exercise alone. But as the disease develops, pharmacologic interventions will be necessary. Insulin and insulin analogues, and five different types of oral agents (sulfonylureas, meglitinides, biguanides, thiazolidinediones, and α-glucosidase inhibitors) are now available for clinical use.[32–34] Figure 39–7 outlines a potential treatment plan for the use of these agents for diabetes control. The oral agents mentioned above and in the figure are tried before, or in conjunction with, insulin treatment for patients with Type 2 (but not Type 1) diabetes.

Nonpharmacologic Therapy

The diet plan and exercise program for Type 2 and Type 1 diabetes are much the same. However, most (90%) people with Type 2 diabetes have the additional goal of reducing calories and losing weight. From this standpoint, exercise is a particularly important part of a Type 2 patient's management program. Exercise also increases the sensitivity of cell receptors to insulin and hence reduces (at least temporarily) insulin resis-

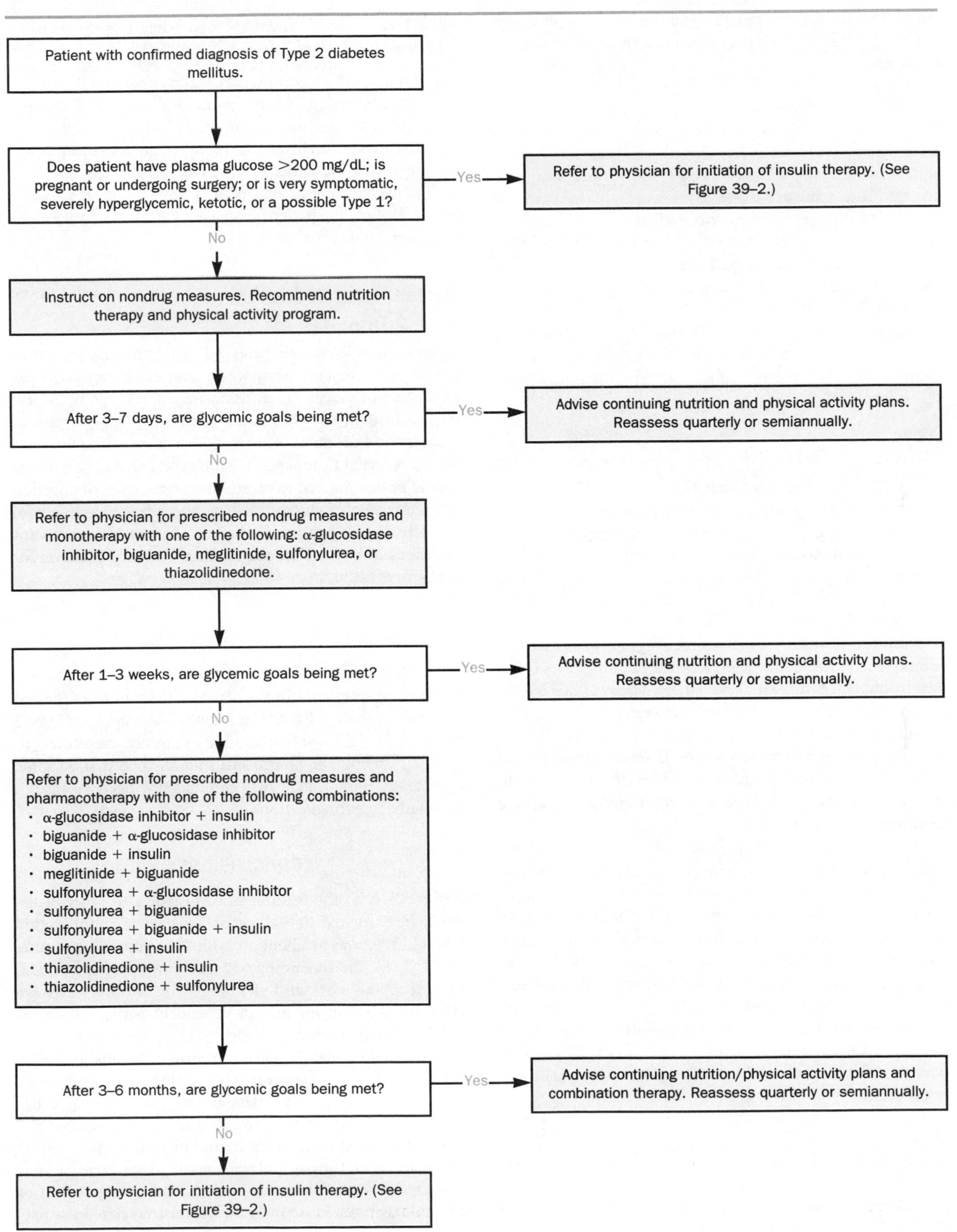

Figure 39–7 Self-care of Type 2 diabetes mellitus.

tance. Also, unlike people with Type 1 diabetes, patients with Type 2 diabetes do not need to eat extra calories before exercising unless their blood glucose levels drop below normal.

Pharmacologic Therapy

Among Type 2 patients, insulin is indicated for those who do not respond to nutrition and physical activity therapy alone or to therapy with oral agents, or for those who have fasting plasma glucose concentrations of greater than 200 mg/dL. Insulin therapy is also necessary for some Type 2 patients who are subject to situational stresses such as infection, pregnancy, or surgery. Type 2 patients must receive intensive education concerning nutrition and physical activity when they start on insulin because increased hunger and a resultant weight gain can be major problems for them. (See the section "Pharmacologic Therapy" under "Treatment of Type 1 Diabetes Mellitus" for specific information about insulin therapy.)

Patient Assessment of Type 2 Diabetes Mellitus

If the patient describes classic symptoms of diabetes, the pharmacist should find out whether the patient has been diagnosed as diabetic. If not, the patient should be screened for diabetes. (The section "Patient Assessment of Type 1 Diabetes Mellitus" describes the procedures and regulations for diabetes screening.)

Despite the results of the screening, an obese patient should be counseled on weight loss. (See Chapter 21, "Overweight and Obesity.") An obese patient who tests positive for diabetes must understand the link between obesity and Type 2 diabetes, as well as the importance of weight loss in controlling and possibly reversing the disease. Knowing that weight loss and physical exercise may obviate the need for insulin injections or oral diabetic medications may motivate the patient to lose weight.

Because obesity is linked to several serious diseases, the pharmacist should find out whether the patient has diseases other than diabetes and what medications the patient might be taking. If diabetes is confirmed, the pharmacist should carefully assess the patient's attitude toward having the disease and the impact of diabetes care on the patient's lifestyle. Asking the patient the questions below and those in the section "Patient Assessment of Type 1 Diabetes Mellitus" should provide the pharmacist with information about the patient's knowledge of the disorder. The pharmacist can then develop a diabetes education and care plan tailored to the patient's needs.

Q~ If you were diagnosed as having Type 2 diabetes, what care plan did your health care provider recommend?

A~ Determine whether the patient is taking insulin or oral diabetes medications. Also, find out whether weight loss and exercise are components of the plan.

Q~ Have you seen a dietitian? If so, what were the dietitian's recommendations?

A~ Find out the recommended daily caloric intake and the percentage of carbohydrates allowed. Calculate optimal dietary intake from the ideal body weight of the patient or from the grams of carbohydrate allowed in the patient's diet. If the patient is obese, make sure the patient is on a low-calorie diet that will allow the patient to lose weight slowly (roughly 1 or 2 pounds a month).

Patient Counseling for Type 2 Diabetes Mellitus

Patients with Type 2 diabetes will need encouragement as well as counseling on losing weight and exercising. If the patient was not successful at losing weight and has been prescribed insulin, the pharmacist should explain the various diabetes care products and should teach the patient how to use the selected products. As with Type 1 diabetes, patients should be encouraged to return for reevaluation of injection technique, use of glucose meters, and adherence to a prescribed self-care routine. For specific recommendations for Type 2 diabetes mellitus, see the box "Patient Education for Diabetes Mellitus."

Evaluation of Patient Outcomes for Type 2 Diabetes Mellitus

The patient outcomes in the section "Evaluation of Patient Outcomes for Type 1 Diabetes Mellitus" also apply to Type 2 diabetes. Weight control should be closely monitored in Type 2 patients. The pharmacist should stress that, in some cases, controlling weight may eliminate the need for insulin or oral diabetes medications.

CONCLUSIONS

Diabetes is a costly disorder in comparison to other disorders. The estimated annual cost of diabetes care in the United States in 1992 was $132 billion, with $85 billion representing direct costs. The remaining $47 billion were indirect costs, including lost work and sick days.[10] Economic costs are about 13% higher for insulin-dependent patients than for non–insulin-dependent patients.[17]

Nevertheless, diabetes care is improving because of earlier detection and tighter control of blood glucose levels. Rates of identification for diabetes patients may have increased because of the enhanced screening, the introduction of lowered acceptable blood glucose levels, and the recognition of IFG and IGT as prediabetes phenomena. Options for tight diabetes management have been enhanced by expansion of available diabetes care products, well-characterized use patterns for insulin preparations, and more and better insulin delivery products and monitoring devices.

Diabetes care requires a big investment of patient and caregiver time, effort, and change in behavior. Patients require a significant level of counseling and education to develop good coping and self-management skills and to acquire significant assistance in changing their care behavior. Patient education is a team effort to ensure the patient is able to control his or her disease. The pharmacist plays a special role in patient diabetes control with regard to mixing, storing, and injecting insulin and to monitoring the person's entire drug regimen. In addition, the pharmacist is often called on to reinforce the education and training provided by the physician, nurse, dietitian, and physical therapist. Some practice locations may not have the various practitioners listed, so the pharmacist may become the primary diabetes educator. To keep their knowledge current, concerned pharmacists should join their local diabetes associations and should consult the recent diabetes literature.

References

1. Report of the expert committee on the diagnosis and classification of diabetes mellitus. *Diabetes Care.* 2000;23(suppl 1).
2. Kahn CR. Banting Lecture. Insulin action, diabetogenesis, and the cause of type II disease. *Diabetes.* 1994;43:1066–84.
3. White JR Jr. The pharmacologic management of hyperglycemia in patients with NIDDM in the era of new oral agents and insulin analogues. *Diabetes Spectrum.* 1996;9:227–34.
4. Pharmaceutical services for patients with diabetes. *Am Pharm* (module 4). 1986;26:7.
5. Brownlee M. Glycation products and the pathogenesis of diabetic complications. *Diabetes Care.* 1992;15:1835–43.
6. Sano T, Kawamura T, Matsumae H, et al. Effects of long-term enalapril treatment on persistent micro-albuminuria in well-controlled hypertensive and normotensive NIDDM patients. *Diabetes Care.* 1994;17:420–4.
7. Nathan DM. Long-term complications of diabetes mellitus. *N Engl J Med.* 1993;328:1676–85.
8. Vlassara H. *Ann Med.* 1998;28:419–26.
9. Lewis EJ, Hunsicker LG, Bain RP, et al. The effect of angiotensin-converting-enzyme inhibition on diabetic nephropathy. The Collaborative Study Group. *N Engl J Med.* 1993;328:1456–62.
10. *ADA Vital Statistics.* Washington, DC: American Diabetes Association; 1993.
11. Diabetes Care Group, National Institute of Diabetes and Digestive and Kidney Disease. *Diabetes in America.* 2nd ed. NIH Pub No. 95–1468. Bethesda, MD: US Department of Health and Human Services; 1995.
12. Funnell MM, Hunt C, Kulkarni K, et al., eds. *A Core Curriculum for Diabetes Education.* 3rd ed. Chicago: American Association of Diabetes Educators; 1998.
13. Franz MJ, Horton SE Sr, Bantle JP, et al. Nutrition principles for the management of diabetes and related complications. *Diabetes Care.* 1994;17:490–518.
14. Vinik AI, Holland MT, Le Beau JM, et al. Diabetic neuropathies. *Diabetes Care.* 1992;15:1926–75.
15. White JR Jr, Campbell RK. Pharmacologic therapies in the management of diabetes mellitus. In Haire-Joshu D, ed. *Management of Diabetes Mellitus.* 2nd ed. St. Louis: Mosby Year Book; 1996:202–33.
16. Ahrens ER, Gossain W, Rovner DR. Human insulin. Its development and clinical use. *Postgrad Med.* 1986;60:181–4, 187.
17. Jacober S. *Diabetes Spectrum.* 1994;7:298–322.
18. Sands ML, Shetterly SM, Franklin GM, et al. Incidence of distal symmetric (sensory) neuropathy in NIDDM. The San Luis Valley Diabetes Study. *Diabetes Care.* 1997;20:322–9.
19. Walker EA. Quality assurance of blood glucose monitoring. The balance of feasibility and standards. *Nurs Clin North Am.* 1993;28:61–70.
20. White J, Campbell RK. Mixing insulin. *Hosp Pharm.* 1991;26:12.
21. Cryer PE. Banting Lecture. Hypoglycemia: the limiting factor in the management of IDDM. *Diabetes.* 1994;43:1378–89.
22. Stephenson JM, Schernthaner G. Dawn phenomenon and Somogyi effect in IDDM. *Diabetes Care.* 1989;12:245–51.
23. Diabetes care. *Clin Pract Rev.* 1991;14(suppl 2).
24. National Steering Committee for Quality Assurance in Capillary Blood Glucose Monitoring. Proposed strategies for reducing user error in capillary blood glucose monitoring. *Diabetes Care.* 1993;16:493–8.
25. Gori M, Campbell RK. Natural products and diabetes treatment. *Diabetes Educ.* 1998;24:201–8.
26. Standards of medical care for patients with diabetes mellitus. *Diabetes Care.* 1999;22:S32–41.
27. *National Diabetes Fact Sheet: National Estimates and General Information on Diabetes in the United States.* Atlanta: US Department of Health and Human Services, Centers for Disease Control and Prevention; 1997.
28. Taylor SI, Accili D, Imai Y. Insulin resistance or insulin deficiency. Which is the primary cause of NIDDM? *Diabetes.* 1994;43:735–40.
29. Leslie RD, Elliott RB. Early environmental events and cause of IDDM. Evidence and implications. *Diabetes.* 1994;43:843–50.
30. Elbein SC, Hoffman MD, Bragg KL, et al. The genetics of NIDDM. An update. *Diabetes Care.* 1994;17:1523–33.
31. Reaven, GM. Role of insulin resistance in human disease. Banting Lecture 1988. *Diabetes.* 1988;37:1595–607.
32. Lebovitz HE, ed. *Therapy for Diabetes Mellitus and Related Disorders.* 2nd ed. Alexandria, VA. American Diabetes Association; 1994.
33. White JR Jr. Oral agent/insulin therapy in patients with Type II diabetes. *Clinic Diabetes.* 1997;15:102–12.
34. Feinglos MN, Bethel MA. Oral agent therapy in the treatment of type 2 diabetes. *Diabetes Care.* 1999;22:C61–4.

CHAPTER 40

Insomnia

M. Lynn Crismon and Donna M. Jermain

Chapter 40 at a Glance

Insomnia is one of the most common patient complaints for which patients may seek a nonprescription sleep aid, ranking third behind headache and the common cold. Insomnia is not a disease; rather, it is a symptom or patient complaint for which there are no precise criteria or definitions. Patients may complain of difficulty falling asleep (sleep latency insomnia), frequent nocturnal awakening, early morning awakening, or poor quality of sleep. Because there is no ideal duration of sleep, patients who complain of a sleep disturbance may actually sleep for a similar length of time as individuals who feel that they sleep well. However, these patients usually report that it takes them more than 30 minutes to fall asleep and that their sleep duration is less than 6 to 7 hours nightly.[1] Moreover, their perceived sleep pattern and quality of daytime functioning may be more important to them than their duration of sleep. Thus, patients with insomnia are those who feel that they sleep poorly at night and that this adversely affects their daytime functioning.

Patients with other sleep disorders, such as sleep apnea, narcolepsy, nocturnal myoclonus, and restless legs syndrome, may also seek a nonprescription sleep aid from the pharmacist. Because these disorders can have significant clinical effects, patients with such complaints should see a physician.

Editor's Note: This chapter is based, in part, on the 11th edition chapter titled "Sleep Aid and Stimulant Products," which was written by M. Lynn Crismon and Donna M. Jermain.

Epidemiology of Insomnia

Annually, approximately one-third of all Americans report at least occasional difficulty sleeping, and at least 10% of the U.S. population experiences insomnia that is severe or chronic. More than 2.5% of adult Americans use a prescription hypnotic medication, and more than 3% buy a nonprescription sleep product.[1–4] Among insomniacs, 29% report having used nonprescription medications, and 28% report having used alcohol to treat their sleep disturbance.[2]

The prevalence of sleep complaints is increased among elderly patients, and it is estimated that approximately 35% of all hypnotic prescriptions are written for patients ages 65 years or older.[1] This population also has an increased incidence of sleep apnea, nocturnal myoclonus, and restless legs syndrome.[2] Significant morbidity is associated with obstructive sleep apnea, which has been linked with 38,000 cardiovascular deaths annually.[2] For these reasons, complaints of insomnia in elderly patients should be carefully evaluated.

Despite these figures, it is estimated that only a small percentage of patients with a sleep disorder actually verbalize their complaints to a physician.[4] This lack of complaint, combined with the frequent misuse of hypnotics and the availability of nonprescription agents, makes insomnia a disorder of significant concern for the pharmacist.

Physiology of Sleep

Physiologically, sleep can be categorized into different stages by using the sleeping electroencephalogram (EEG) in conjunction with electro-oculography and electromyography. Stage 1 sleep is a transitional stage, which occurs as the patient falls asleep; the EEG resembles the waking state more than sleep. Stage 2 sleep, which takes up approximately 50% of sleep time, is light sleep. Stages 3 and 4, collectively known as deep sleep or delta sleep, are characterized by the patterns of delta waves, or slow-frequency waves, on the EEG. Rapid eye movement (REM) sleep is neither light nor deep, and the EEG is characterized by an increase in high-frequency waves. REM sleep is characterized by the body being more physiologically active than it is during other sleep stages while skeletal muscles are actively inhibited. The eyes move rapidly from side to side; the blood pressure, heart rate, temperature, respiration, and metabolism are increased.[2,5]

Upon falling asleep, an individual progresses through the four stages of sleep and reaches the first REM period in about 70 to 90 minutes. This time, from falling asleep to the first REM period, is referred to as the REM latency. The first REM period is of short duration, usually 5 to 7 minutes. The sleep cycle then repeats about every 90 minutes, with each progressive REM period becoming longer and the time in deep sleep becoming shorter.[2,5] Although the effects of medication on the sleep stages are thought to be important, their relative importance in the different stages of sleep is unclear. However, prolonged suppression of REM may result in psychologic and behavioral changes.

Sleep physiology changes with increasing age. Among elderly people, less time is spent in stage 4 and REM sleep, the total duration of sleep becomes shorter, sleep becomes more shallow and disrupted, the number of nocturnal awakenings increases, and sleep latency usually remains normal.

Etiology of Insomnia

Insomnia can be classified as transient, short term, or chronic according to the duration of sleep disturbance.[2,4] Transient insomnia is often self-limiting, lasting less than 1 week. Short-term insomnia usually lasts from 1 to 3 weeks.[2,6] Unless it is managed appropriately, short-term insomnia may progress to chronic insomnia. Chronic, or long-term, insomnia lasts from greater than 3 weeks to years and is often the result of medical problems, psychologic dysfunction, or substance abuse.[4,7]

Difficulty falling asleep is often associated with acute life stresses, anxiety, and poor sleep habits. The severity of stressful situations can affect the length of insomnia. Travel, hospitalization, or anticipation of an important or stressful event can cause transient insomnia. However, if more severe stresses are present (e.g., the death of a loved one, the loss of a job, or divorce), transient insomnia may become short-term insomnia.

Some individuals are extremely sensitive to the stimulant effects of caffeine and nicotine. Drinking caffeinated beverages in the late afternoon or evening hours may cause insomnia. Alcohol, if taken in excess—especially in the evening—or on a chronic basis, can cause sleep disturbance. Alcohol will often assist the individual in falling asleep but will then result in frequent awakening and restless sleep throughout the night. Late night exercise and late evening meals can also interfere with sleep. Sleep difficulties may also result from environmental distractions, such as noise.

As shown in Table 40–1, a number of general medical disorders, including psychiatric disorders, are associated with chronic insomnia. An estimated 60% of cases of chronic insomnia are secondary to psychiatric disorders, with depression being the most common.[3,4] Insomnia concomitant with frequent nighttime awakening may be associated with various general medical (e.g., gastroesophageal reflux) and psychiatric (e.g., anxiety) conditions, as well as with environmental influences. Early morning awakening is often associated with depressive disorders. Nonprescription hypnotics are generally not helpful in these patients, and physician referral is indicated.

Individuals with psychophysiologic insomnia are thought to develop faulty sleep habits during transient or short-term insomnia that progress to a long-term sleep problem. For example, elderly people often take daytime naps, which may contribute to nocturnal sleep disturbance. Thus, it is critical to

Table 40–1

Etiology of Chronic (Long-Term) Insomnia

Medical Problems	Psychiatric Problems (30% to 70% of Cases)
Pain	Anxiety disorders
Angina pectoris	Bipolar disorder
Arthritis	Dementia
Cancer	Depression
Chronic pain syndromes	Posttraumatic stress disorder
Cluster headaches	Schizophrenia
Gastroesophageal reflux disorder	Substance abuse
Migraine	**Sleep Disorders**
Peptic ulcer	Delayed sleep phase syndrome (e.g., as in night-shift workers)
Postoperative pain	Drug-related insomnia
Respiratory Difficulty	Nocturnal myoclonus
Asthma	Psychophysiologic insomnia
Bronchitis	Restless legs syndrome
Chronic obstructive pulmonary disease	Sleep apnea
Congestive heart failure	
Other Medical Problems	
Constipation	
Epilepsy	
Hyperthyroidism	
Nocturia	
Parkinson's disease	
Renal insufficiency	
Tachyarrhythmias	

Table 40–2

Drugs That May Exacerbate Insomnia

Drugs That May Cause Insomnia	Drugs That May Produce Withdrawal Insomnia
Alcohol	Alcohol
Antidepressants Bupropion Monoamine oxidase inhibitors Serotonin-specific reuptake inhibitors Tricyclic antidepressants Venlafaxine	Antihistamines Barbiturates Benzodiazepines
Antihypertensives β-Blockers (especially propranolol) Clonidine Diuretics (at bedtime) Methyldopa Reserpine	Hypnotics (miscellaneous) Bromides Chloral hydrate Ethchlorvynol Glutethimide Monoamine oxidase inhibitors Tricyclic antidepressants
Hypnotic use (chronic) Nicotine Sympathomimetic amines Amphetamines Appetite suppressants β-Adrenergic agonists Caffeine Decongestants (e.g., phenylpropanolamine, phenylephrine)	Miscellaneous Amphetamines Cocaine Marijuana Opiates Phencyclidine
Miscellaneous Anabolic steroids Antineoplastics Corticosteroids Histamine$_2$-receptor antagonists Levodopa Methysergide Oral contraceptives Phenytoin Quinidine Theophylline Thyroid preparations	

identify the problem that is responsible for long-term insomnia if the sleep disturbance is to be appropriately managed.[3,6]

Sleep apnea can also cause chronic insomnia. Patients with this disorder complain of daytime fatigue and sedation. Sleep apnea affects the quality of sleep of both the patient and family members because of the patient's gasping and snoring during sleep. Sleep apnea appears to be more common in men, and the stereotypical patient is the middle-aged, overweight, hypertensive man. Although it is usually caused by some form of airway obstruction, sleep apnea may be produced through central nervous system (CNS) mechanisms.

Finally, medications—prescription and nonprescription—can cause withdrawal insomnia. (See Table 40–2.)

Signs and Symptoms of Insomnia

Patients with insomnia may have any number of complaints, such as difficulty falling asleep, frequent awakening, early morning awakening and inability to fall back to sleep, disturbed quality of sleep with unusual or troublesome dreams, or just poor sleep in general. Their actual duration of sleep as determined by sleep lab studies may or may not be different from that in individuals who report normal sleep.

Sleep-deprived individuals are highly symptomatic, and their quality of life is negatively affected. Some impairment in daytime functioning is necessary for a diagnosis of insomnia, and a majority of untreated patients with insomnia report "being easily upset, irritated or annoyed, blue, down in the dumps or depressed, or too tired to do things, and having more general trouble remembering things."[8] If left untreated, insomnia is associated with an increase in accidents and a rise in morbidity and mortality rates from general medical and psychiatric disorders.

Treatment of Insomnia

Treatment Outcomes

The optimal goal of treatment is a patient who reports normal sleep, awakes feeling rested, and reports no difficulty with daytime fatigue or drowsiness.

General Treatment Approach

For patients with transient or short-term insomnia—assuming there are no underlying problems—reestablishing the normal sleep cycle with a nonprescription diphenhydramine sleep aid should assist in normalizing sleep patterns. One approach is for the patient to take the medication for 2 to 3 nights, skip a night to reevaluate the quality of sleep, and then take the medication for 2 to 3 additional nights if insomnia persists. Patients complaining of continuing insomnia after 7 to 10 days of using a nonprescription sleep aid and practicing good sleep hygiene should be referred to a physician for a more thorough evaluation regarding the etiology of the sleep disturbance.[2,4] The algorithm in Figure 40–1 outlines the assessment and self-treatment of transient and short-term insomnia.

Exclusions to self-treatment include patients with frequent nocturnal awakening or early morning awakening, patients with chronic insomnia (lasting longer than 3 weeks), and patients with sleep disturbance secondary to psychiatric or general medical disorders.

Nonpharmacologic Therapy

The sleep hygiene measures in Table 40–3 should be recommended for all patients with insomnia. In many patients with sleep disturbances, these measures should be recommended before initiating pharmacotherapy.

Pharmacologic Therapy

When the Food and Drug Administration (FDA) issued its final monograph on over-the-counter sleep aids in 1989, the antihistamine diphenhydramine (hydrogen chloride or citrate) was the only agent on the list.[9,10] Although the safety and efficacy of another antihistamine, doxylamine, has not been fully established, FDA has allowed it to remain on the market.[10] No published studies supporting the efficacy of

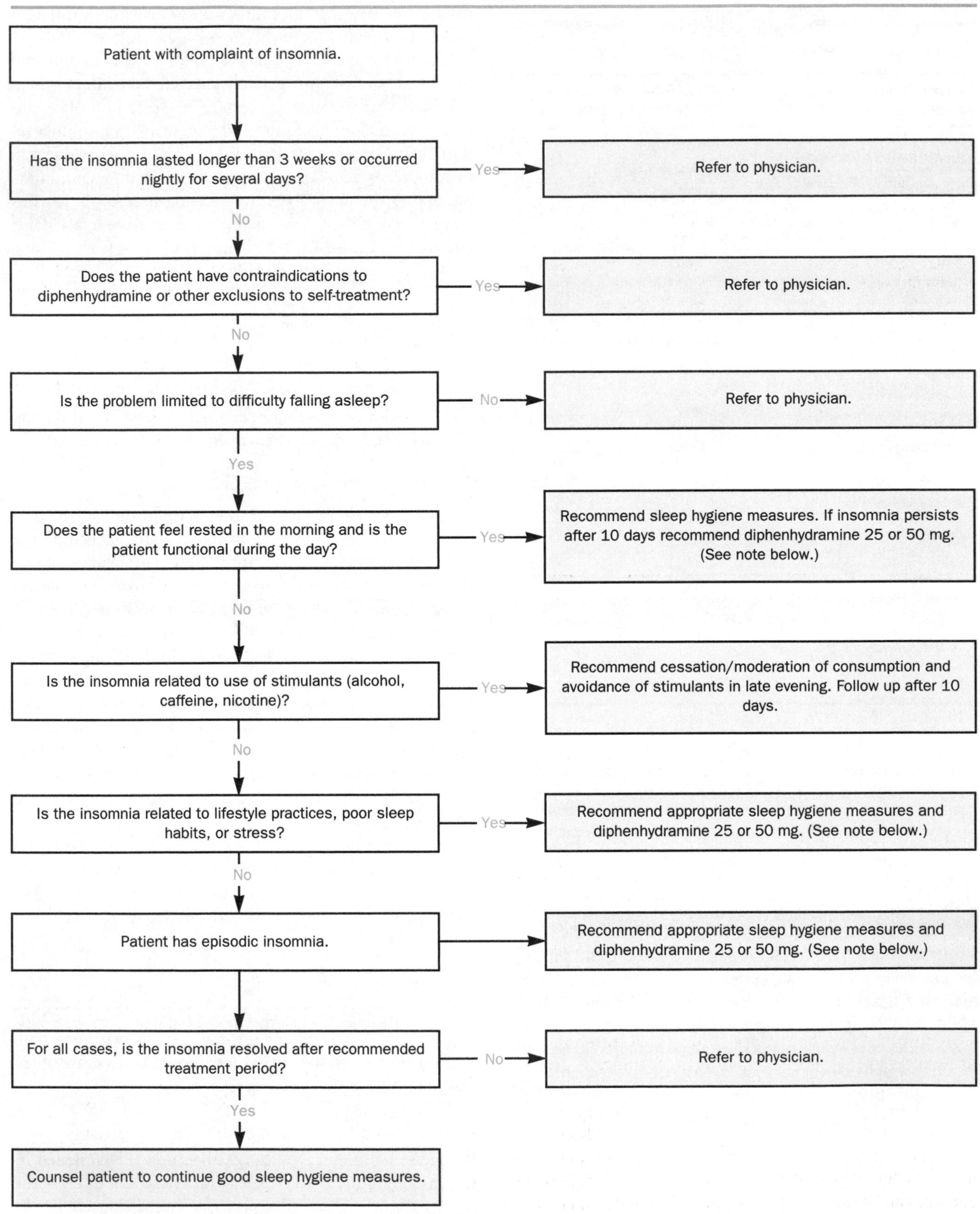

Note: Advise patient to try diphenhydramine for 2 to 3 nights and then skip a night to reevaluate the quality of sleep. If insomnia persists, advise patient to take the medication for 2 to 3 additional nights but not to take the sleep aid longer than 7 to 10 days.

Figure 40–1 Self-care of transient and short-term insomnia.

Table 40–3

Principles of Good Sleep Hygiene

- Follow a regular sleep pattern: Go to bed and arise at about the same time daily.
- Make the bedroom comfortable for sleeping. Avoid temperature extremes, noise, and light.
- Make sure the bed is comfortable.
- Engage in relaxing activities before bedtime.
- Exercise regularly but not late in the evening.
- Use the bedroom for sleep and sexual activities only, and not as an office, game room, or so forth.
- If tense, practice relaxation exercises.
- If hungry, eat a light snack, but avoid eating meals or large snacks immediately before bedtime.
- Eliminate daytime naps.
- Avoid using caffeine after noon.
- Avoid using alcohol or nicotine later in the evening.
- If unable to fall asleep, do not become anxious. Leave the bedroom and participate in relaxing activities for 20 to 30 minutes.

doxylamine as a hypnotic are currently available. Products containing pyrilamine maleate, potassium or sodium bromide, and scopolamine hydrobromide have been removed from the market.[6]

Antihistamines

Mechanism of Action Both diphenhydramine and doxylamine are members of the ethanolamine group of antihistamines. Ethanolamines are thought to affect sleep through their affinity for blocking histamine$_1$ and muscarinic receptors.[10]

Pharmacokinetics Selected clinical and pharmacokinetic properties of diphenhydramine and doxylamine are summarized in Table 40–4. Both drugs are well absorbed from the gastrointestinal tract and have short to intermediate half-lives. Diphenhydramine is metabolized in the liver through two successive *N*-demethylations, and its apparent half-life may be prolonged by a factor of approximately 1.5 in patients with hepatic cirrhosis.[11,12] A positive relationship exists between diphenhydramine plasma concentrations and drowsiness and cognitive impairment. Significant drowsiness has been shown to last from 3 to 6 hours after a single 50 mg dose of diphenhydramine, whereas impairment in performance on psychomotor tests lasts from 2 to 4 hours.[13,14] How these effects can be extrapolated to nightly dosing of diphenhydramine is unclear. However, it may indicate that patients can be assured that their ability to perform tasks requiring mental alertness and cognitive ability will not be impaired for any longer than they feel drowsy.

Patient ethnicity may account for differences in drug effect. One study indicates that Asians have lower diphenhydramine peak plasma concentrations, more rapid clearance, and less subjective sedation than do Caucasians.[11] Thus, Asians may require as much as 1.7 times more diphenhydramine than Caucasians need to experience the same level of sedation.

Indications With respect to insomnia, the primary indication for diphenhydramine is the symptomatic management of transient and short-term sleep difficulty, particularly in individuals who complain of occasional problems falling asleep.

Dosage Guidelines Although the usual optimal diphenhydramine dose is 50 mg nightly, some individuals benefit from a 25 mg dose. In children between ages 2 and 12 years, a dosage of 1 mg/kg, not to exceed 50 mg, has been reported.[10]

Tolerance to the hypnotic effects of diphenhydramine has been poorly studied but appears to result with repeated use. With the possible exception of Asians, adult patients should be advised not to exceed 50 mg nightly, because higher doses cause increased adverse effects with no additional efficacy. All patients should limit their use of diphenhydramine to no longer than 7 to 10 consecutive nights.

Overdosage Antihistamine dosage excess can result in anticholinergic toxicity,[15] which may occur as a result of drug interactions, purposeful ingestion of a large amount, or individual sensitivity. Anticholinergic toxicity is particularly common in children, in whom the symptoms are usually more severe. CNS anticholinergic toxicity is one of the primary presenting features of antihistamine excess. Patients may be anxious, excited, delirious, hallucinating, or stuporous; in more severe cases, coma or seizures may occur. Other physical signs may include dilated pupils, flushed skin, hot and dry mucous membranes, and elevated body temperature. Tachycardia and moderate QTc prolongation on the electrocardiogram are common. In severe cases, rhabdomyolysis, dysrhythmias, cardiovascular collapse, and death may occur.[16]

Table 40–4

Selected Pharmacokinetic and Clinical Properties of Nonprescription Hypnotics

	Diphenhydramine	Doxylamine
Time to maximum plasma concentration	1–4 hours	2–3 hours
Maximum sedation	1–3 hours	NA[a]
Protein binding	80%–85%	NA
Elimination half-life	2.4–9.3 hours	10 hours
Duration of sedation	3–6 hours	NA
Bioavailability	26%–61%	NA

NA = not available.

Source: References 10, 11, 13, and 14.

The primary treatment of anticholinergic toxicity includes emesis with syrup of ipecac to decrease drug absorption if ingestion is acute. If the patient is stuporous or comatose, gastric lavage and activated charcoal may be used. Activated charcoal should be followed by 240 mL of a magnesium sulfate solution to hasten gastrointestinal elimination. (See Chapter 17, "Poisoning.") Patients should receive general supportive care (e.g., hydration, antipyretics, or a cooling blanket) if needed, plus maintenance of vital signs including ventilatory support.[17] Seizures should be treated with standard anticonvulsants such as diazepam. Despite the potential pharmacologic rationale, physostigmine is not recommended as first-line therapy in anticholinergic toxicity because of its narrow therapeutic index and its short duration of action.

Adverse Effects Sedation, the intended effect when diphenhydramine is used as a hypnotic, may be associated with next morning hangover in susceptible individuals. Other primary side effects of diphenhydramine and doxylamine are anticholinergic in nature.[10] Commonly occurring adverse effects include dry mouth and throat, constipation, blurred vision, urinary retention, and tinnitus. Elderly patients, patients with comorbid general medical disorders, and patients taking multiple medications are particular susceptible to developing adverse effects.

Drug–Drug Interactions The primary drug interactions with diphenhydramine are additive sedation or anticholinergic effects when it is used in combination with other medications having these properties.[1,10] In patients on multiple medications and particularly in elderly patients, these potential interactions should be carefully monitored.

Contraindications Older male patients with prostatic hypertrophy and difficulty urinating should not use diphenhydramine. Because anticholinergics may increase intraocular pressure, narrow- (closed-) angle glaucoma is another contraindication. Patients with cardiovascular disease (e.g., angina or rhythm disturbance) may be particularly susceptible to the anticholinergic adverse effects of ethanolamine sleep aids and, therefore, should not use these agents.[10] Anticholinergics tend to decrease cognition and increase confusion in patients with dementia; diphenhydramine is contraindicated in these patients as well.

Precautions/Warnings Patients should be cautioned not to drive an automobile or operate machinery until their response to the drug is known. They should be warned of the additive CNS depressant effects of alcohol and should be encouraged not to drink alcoholic beverages while taking these drugs. Some patients may develop excitation from diphenhydramine and other highly anticholinergic antihistamines.[10] This effect occurs more often in children, elderly patients, and patients with organic mental disorders. Symptoms include nervousness, restlessness, agitation, tremors, insomnia, delirium, and, in rare cases, seizures. Elderly patients who are older than 80 years, or who have acute physical disorders or dementia, seem particularly susceptible to developing delirium from even modest doses of diphenhydramine.[18]

Special Population Considerations The safety of antihistamines during pregnancy has not been clearly established.[10] Therefore, the benefit-to-risk ratio of using these drugs during pregnancy should be carefully evaluated. Doxylamine was formerly marketed as a prescription combination product for treating morning sickness during pregnancy. However, the manufacturer voluntarily removed this combination from the market in 1976, following allegations of teratogenicity. Although it is not possible to prove conclusively that doxylamine is not teratogenic, epidemiologic studies indicate that the possibility of such a relationship is remote.[10] Nevertheless, rather than recommending a nonprescription product, pharmacists should advise pregnant women to consult their physician regarding any sleep disturbance.

There appears to be an increased risk of CNS side effects from antihistamine use in neonates. For this reason and because such drugs may inhibit lactation, pharmacists should recommend that nursing mothers not use antihistamines for sleep.

Combination Products

A combination product containing diphenhydramine and acetaminophen (e.g., Excedrin PM) is marketed.[10] No published studies are available to establish whether this product is of additive benefit in inducing sleep in patients who complain of insomnia caused by pain.

Product Selection Guidelines

Because no published efficacy and safety studies are available that document the value of doxylamine as a hypnotic, only diphenhydramine should be recommended to patients for such use at the present time. Nonprescription diphenhydramine is available as capsules, gelcaps, tablets, chewable tablets, solution, and elixir, thus allowing various forms for different patient preferences.[10] (See Table 40–5 for examples of commercially available products.)

Alternative Remedies

Melatonin

Melatonin is an endogenous hormone produced by the pineal gland. Melatonin has multiple functions in the body, many of which are poorly understood. Although it is primarily secreted at night, its physiologic effects on sleep are largely unknown.[19,20] Its secretion appears to be in some fashion related to the neuroendocrine–gonadal axis.[19] Known actions of melatonin include shifting circadian rhythms, decreasing body temperature, and decreasing alertness. Melatonin shifts circadian rhythm in a fashion that is nearly opposite to that of light exposure.[19] It delays the circadian rhythm when administered in the morning and advances it when administered in the evening. It appears to have no anxiolytic or amnestic properties.[19]

Wide variation in study methodology, including dose,

Table 40–5

Selected Sleep Aid Products

Trade Name	Primary Ingredients
Single-Entity Antihistamine Products	
Compoz Gelcaps/Tablets	Diphenhydramine HCl 50 mg
Nervine Nighttime Sleep-Aid Caplets[a]	Diphenhydramine HCl 25 mg
Nytol Caplets[a,b]	Diphenhydramine HCl 25 mg
Nytol Maximum Strength Softgels[a]	Diphenhydramine HCl 50 mg
Sominex Maximum Strength Caplets[a]	Diphenhydramine HCl 50 mg
Sominex Original Tablets[a]	Diphenhydramine HCl 25 mg
Unisom Nighttime Sleep Aid Tablets[a]	Doxylamine succinate 25 mg
Unisom Sleepgels	Diphenhydramine HCl 50 mg
Antihistamine–Analgesic Combination Products	
Alka-Seltzer PM Effervescent Tablets[c]	Diphenhydramine citrate 38 mg; aspirin 325 mg
Anacin P.M. Aspirin Free Caplets[a]	Diphenhydramine HCl 25 mg; acetaminophen 500 mg
Bayer PM Extra Strength Caplets	Diphenhydramine HCl 25 mg; aspirin 500 mg
Doan's P.M. Extra Strength Caplets	Diphenhydramine HCl 25 mg; magnesium salicylate tetrahydrate 580 mg
Excedrin PM Geltabs/Caplets/Tablets[a]	Diphenhydramine citrate 38 mg; acetaminophen 500 mg
NiteGel Liquidcaps[a]	Doxylamine succinate 6.25 mg; acetaminophen 250 mg
Sominex Pain Relief Formula Tablets[a]	Diphenhydramine HCl 25 mg; acetaminophen 500 mg
Tylenol PM Extra Strength Geltabs/Gelcaps/Caplets[a]	Diphenhydramine HCl 25 mg
Unisom Pain Relief Tablets[a]	Diphenhydramine HCl 50 mg; acetaminophen 650 mg
Melatonin Products	
Melatonex Timed-Release Tablets[a,d]	Melatonin 3 mg; pyridoxine HCl 10 mg
Nature's Vision Melatonin Liquid	Melatonin 1 mg
WorldWide Laboratories Melatonin Sustained-Release Tablets	Melatonin 1.5 mg
WorldWide Laboratories Melatonin Tablets	Melatonin 300 mcg

[a] Aspirin-free product.
[b] Dye-free product.
[c] Product containing phenylalanine.
[d] Sodium-free product.

time of administration, study population, and assessment parameters, has made it difficult to evaluate the efficacy of melatonin in insomnia. Studies with low or physiologic doses administered 1 to 2 hours before bedtime have been the most encouraging.[21] Melatonin 0.3 or 1 mg decreased both sleep latency and REM latency when compared with placebo in normal volunteers. The effects on time to fall asleep were most pronounced in patients who had longer sleep latencies (i.e., longer than 20 minutes). No residual effects on alertness were noted the next morning.[20,21] A recent study in patients with sleep maintenance insomnia showed a decreased time to fall asleep with melatonin 0.5 mg but no effect on nocturnal awakening, total sleep time, or subjective quality of sleep.[22] Studies with higher melatonin doses and studies in patients with chronic insomnia have been less positive.[21]

Melatonin has been purported to be effective in treating symptoms of jet lag. In studies of subjects traveling intercontinentally across several time zones, melatonin 5 mg daily for 4 to 5 days, beginning on the day of arrival, was shown by retrospective self-report to decrease jet lag and sleep disturbance.[23,24] In one of these studies, melatonin 0.5 mg was almost as effective as 5 mg daily.[24] However, subjects starting melatonin 3 days before the flight actually did worse than the placebo group.[23]

Some experts recommend caution with the use of melatonin.[21,25] Optimal dose and time of administration have not been determined. Similarly, potential drug interactions, side effects, and toxicity, particularly with long-term use, are largely unknown. Reports consistent with cognitive impairment and worsening of sleep apnea parameters have occurred with high-dose melatonin (greater than 5 mg daily).[21] Until more information is available, melatonin should not be recommended in pregnant women or nursing mothers.[26] Contaminants in commercial preparations of melatonin have also been reported.[27]

If the patient insists on taking a "natural product," only physiologic doses of melatonin 0.1 to 1 mg taken 1 to 2 hours before bedtime should be recommended.[19,21] Patients should be cautioned not to drive or operate machinery after administration. The pharmacist who considers recommending melatonin should be aware that FDA has not reviewed data on its efficacy and safety in treating insomnia.[26] The patient should also be counseled regarding our limited knowledge of melatonin's efficacy and safety, particularly if the product is taken on a chronic basis.

L-Tryptophan

The efficacy of L-tryptophan, an amino acid precursor of serotonin, in treating insomnia has not been clearly established. Some studies have demonstrated hypnotic efficacy; others have not.[1,28] More than 1500 cases of eosinophilia-myalgia syndrome (EMS), including at least 27 deaths, were reported in patients taking contaminated L-tryptophan before FDA, in 1990, recalled all products containing L-tryptophan except protein supplements, infant formulas, and parenteral and enteral nutritional products.[1,29]

The symptoms of EMS develop over several weeks. Primary symptoms are fatigue and myalgia, which may be severe and incapacitating. Other symptoms may include shortness of breath, cough, skin rash, arthralgia, muscle weakness, and peripheral edema. In a few severe cases, congestive heart failure, dysrhythmias, pneumonia, vasculitis, ascending polyneuropathy (similar to Guillain–Barré syndrome), and scleroderma-like skin changes have been reported. Clinical symptoms are accompanied by eosinophilia, often with more than 1000 cells per cubic millimeter. The natural course of EMS is unpredictable. Although some patients' symptoms will remit when L-tryptophan is discontinued, others will develop into some of the more severe symptoms described above.[1]

In addition to EMS, L-tryptophan has been associated with causing "serotonin storm" when used in combination with serotonin reuptake inhibitors or monoamine oxidase inhibitors. Symptoms of this drug interaction may include agitation, restlessness, confusion, aggressiveness, tremor, hyperthermia, hyperreflexia, myoclonus, diarrhea, or cramping.[1] L-tryptophan should not be initiated in combination with one of these agents in outpatients. Given its questionable efficacy and known adverse effects, pharmacists should be reluctant to recommend L-tryptophan as a sleep aid.

Alcohol

Ethanol is a CNS depressant that has been used for both its sedative and disinhibiting properties for centuries. However, alcohol does not have the positive effects on sleep that many people believe it to have. After an occasional evening consumption of one or two drinks, alcohol is effective in decreasing sleep latency. However, with heavy or continuous consumption, alcohol disrupts the sleep cycle. Although sleep latency decreases, the patient usually begins to experience restless sleep and often awakens within 2 to 4 hours. The total duration of sleep also decreases. Moreover, after alcohol is discontinued, rebound insomnia is likely to occur.[30] Chronic alcoholics usually have marked disorganization of their sleep cycle, with shortened REM periods and delta sleep. Approximately 10% to 15% of patients with chronic insomnia have problems with substance abuse, especially alcohol abuse.[7] Patients who abuse alcohol frequently abuse other CNS depressants, including benzodiazepines.

Alcohol is present in some nonprescription combination cold products, such as Nyquil, which contains 25% alcohol by volume. Products of this type are marketed and sometimes recommended by physicians and pharmacists to induce sleep. Data are limited, however, regarding the efficacy and safety of these products as hypnotics. They contain multiple ingredients, which increases the risk of side effects and interactions with other drugs. At least four cases of liver injury, possibly caused by the alcohol–acetaminophen combination, have been reported with Nyquil.[31]

Alcohol has negative effects on patients with sleep apnea. As little as 3 ounces (two shots) of 80-proof ethanol may increase the frequency and severity of apneic episodes, even in patients with mild apnea.[32] Furthermore, alcohol has been reported to cause apnea in normal individuals.[33]

Valerian

Valerian is an herbal remedy, most commonly coming from the plant, *Valeriana officinalis* L. (For further discussion of this substance, see Chapter 45, "Herbal Remedies.")

Pharmacotherapeutic Comparisons

Most published clinical trials indicate that diphenhydramine is effective in decreasing time to fall asleep (sleep latency) and in improving the reported quality of sleep for individuals with occasional sleep difficulty.[1,10] In general, diphenhydramine is not as efficacious as benzodiazepine hypnotics.[34] However, patients who have never been treated with hypnotics tend to respond better to diphenhydramine than those who have been previously treated.[35] The efficacy and dose-response relationship with melatonin are unclear. The best evidence for effectiveness is in patients who have mild-to-moderate difficulty falling asleep.[19,21]

Pharmacoeconomics

Insomnia has a significant economic impact, accounting for approximately $100 billion annually in direct and indirect costs.[26] Its occurrence is associated with an increased rate of traffic accidents, depression, alcohol abuse, and mortality. These findings make a compelling case for identifying and treating underlying causes of chronic insomnia.

The pharmacoeconomic effects of hypnotic treatment of insomnia are unknown. However, epidemiologic data indicate that patients with insomnia experience a decrease in fatigue-related sequelae after hypnotic treatment.[4]

Case Study 40–1

Patient Complaint/History

Jamal, a 28-year-old accountant, presents to the pharmacist with a complaint of difficulty sleeping for the past 2 nights. The patient, who is averaging only 5 hours of sleep instead of his usual 8, relates that once he falls asleep, he does not awake until the alarm goes off. He requests something to help him fall asleep.

During further conversation, the patient reveals that he is giving a very important business presentation in 4 days; he seems to be "stressed out" about the presentation. He goes on to say that over the past week he has increased his caffeine consumption from the usual one cup of coffee with breakfast and lunch to two cups of coffee with each meal, as well as an occasional cup between meals. Jamal has no known allergies and occasionally takes ibuprofen for muscle aches. He does not smoke and drinks only an occasional beer.

Clinical Considerations/Strategies

Readers can use the following considerations/strategies to determine whether treatment with nonprescription agents is warranted:

- Identify patient factors that may be causing the sleep problems.
- Identify principles of good sleep hygiene that may resolve the sleep problems.
- Determine whether the patient has previously used any nonprescription sleep aid products.
- Assess the value of therapy with a nonprescription sleep aid: List the advantages and disadvantages of such therapy.
- Identify key points about the nonprescription products (e.g., adverse effects, onset of action, duration of use) to discuss with the patient.

Patient Education/Counseling

Readers can use the following strategies to develop a patient education/counseling plan that will help ensure optimal therapeutic outcomes:

- Explain the importance of good sleep hygiene.
- Explain the advantages and disadvantages of any nonprescription medication used to treat the sleep problem.

Patient Assessment of Insomnia

In making an assessment of whether to recommend a nonprescription sleep product, the pharmacist should determine whether use of such products is appropriate, what nonmedication interventions should be recommended, and whether to refer the patient to a physician. Identifying acute precipitators of insomnia, poor sleep hygiene practices, or underlying medical disorders may assist the pharmacist in making a recommendation.

Asking the patient the following questions will help elicit the information needed to accurately assess the type and/or cause of insomnia and to recommend the appropriate treatment approach. The pharmacist should evaluate the patient carefully before deciding whether to recommend a nonprescription product.

Q~ Please describe the difficulty you have with sleep.

A~ Use the patient's response to establish the general nature of the patient's concern and to decide which of the following close-ended questions need to be explored.

Q~ How long have you had trouble sleeping?

A~ Refer patients with chronic insomnia to a physician. Use the following questions to explore the causes of transient and short-term insomnia.

Q~ How severe is your sleep disturbance?

A~ Refer patients with a nightly sleep disturbance, particularly if it has lasted longer than a few days, to a physician for evaluation of a psychiatric or general medical disorder.

Q~ Do you have difficulty falling asleep?

A~ If yes, suspect that acute life stresses, anxiety, or poor sleep habits are causing the insomnia. Because antihistamines tend to be most effective in decreasing the time to fall asleep, consider patients with this type of insomnia as good candidates for use of a nonprescription sleep aid. If lifestyle problems (e.g., irregular bedtimes, excessive noise or light in the bedroom) are interfering with sleep, the pharmacist can recommend specific measures of sleep hygiene that may be appropriate.

Q~ How often do you take naps?

A~ Advise patients who take daytime naps that this practice can perpetuate a transient insomnia. Encourage them to resist the temptation to take naps to make up for lost nighttime sleep.

Q~ What do you think is causing your sleep problem? What activities normally occur before you go to bed?

A~ If patients describe environmental distractions or lifestyle practices such as late night exercise or late evening meals, suspect these activities as the cause of the insomnia. If patients describe medical problems (e.g., gastroesophageal reflux, angina, depression), medical referral is appropriate.

Q~ How often and at what times during the day do you drink coffee or other caffeinated beverages? Alcoholic beverages?

A~ Suspect caffeine as the cause of insomnia if caffeinated beverages are consumed in the late afternoon or evening hours. Suspect alcohol as the cause if consumption of alcoholic beverages is excessive or chronic. If alcohol is being used as a sleep aid, explain that although it often helps someone fall asleep, it also causes frequent awakening and restless sleep throughout the night.

Q~ Do you smoke?

A~ If yes, suspect that the patient may be susceptible to the stimulant effects of nicotine.

Q~ Has there been increased stress in your life lately?

A~ If yes, consider the patient a good candidate for use of nonprescription sleep aids.

Q~ Do you wake up frequently in the night or too early in the morning?

A~ If environmental factors can be ruled out, refer patients who awake frequently at night for evaluation of potential medical and psychiatric disorders. Suspect depressive disorders in patients who awake early in the morning. Refer these patients for medical evaluation as well.

Q~ Do you feel rested when you awake in the morning?

A~ Consider the sleep complaint as clinically significant if the patient does not feel rested.

Q~ Do you have trouble functioning or staying alert during the day?

A~ Consider daytime drowsiness or difficulty staying awake as signs that the sleep disorder is clinically significant.

Q~ Do you have any health problems or physical complaints?

A~ *Identify medical disorders known to cause or worsen insomnia. (See Table 40–3.)* Refer patients with any of these disorders to a physician. Strongly suspect medical disorders as the cause of sleep disturbances in elderly patients.

Q~ Have you felt depressed or disinterested in your usual activities?

A~ If yes, refer the patient to a physician or mental health professional for further evaluation.

Q~ Have you been feeling anxious or unusually nervous?

A~ Insomnia, particularly difficulty falling asleep or frequent awakening, is commonly associated with an anxiety disorder. Refer patients with such symptoms to a physician or mental health professional for further evaluation.

Q~ What prescription and nonprescription medications do you take?

A~ *Identify medications known to cause insomnia. (See Table 40–2.)* If the patient is taking any of these medications, call the patient's physician and discuss any suspected drug-induced sleep disturbances. Also, screen for potential drug interactions before recommending a nonprescription product.

Q~ Have you ever been told that you snore loudly or are a restless sleeper?

A~ If yes, suspect sleep apnea. Refer the patient to a physician for further evaluation.

Q~ What methods or medications have you used to treat insomnia thus far? How long did you use them? Were they effective?

A~ Base treatment recommendations on the patient's success or lack of success with previous treatments. Do not recommend nonprescription sleep aids for patients who have had a poor response with prescription hypnotics or who have been taking these agents chronically. Also, do not recommend nonprescription sleep aids if the patient has been taking such products for longer than 10 days.

Patient Counseling for Insomnia

The pharmacist should encourage all patients with sleep disorders to practice good sleep hygiene measures. Depending on the precipitating factors, the pharmacist should stress the measures that will be most effective. For some patients, these measures alone will resolve the problem. If use of a nonprescription sleep aid is appropriate, the pharmacist should review the dosage guidelines with the patient and emphasize the recommended duration of therapy. The pharmacist should explain potential adverse side effects, drug interactions, and any precautions or warnings, as well as the signs and symptoms that indicate that the disorder requires medical attention. The box "Patient Education for Insomnia" lists specific information to provide patients.

Evaluation of Patient Outcomes for Insomnia

Successful outcomes include decreased time to fall asleep, improved sleep quality, and decreased daytime fatigue and

Patient Education for Insomnia

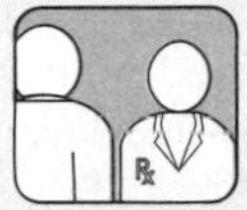

The objectives of self-treatment are to (1) improve duration and perceived quality of sleep, (2) decrease daytime fatigue and drowsiness, (3) improve daytime functioning, and (4) minimize adverse effects from treatment. For most patients, carefully following product instructions and the self-care measures listed below will help ensure optimal therapeutic outcomes.

Nondrug Measures

- See Table 40–3 for nondrug measures to prevent insomnia.
- Note that principles of good sleep hygiene may be more effective than medications in maintaining quality sleep.

Nonprescription Medications/Dietary Supplements

- Do not drive or operate machinery after taking sleep aids, including melatonin.

Diphenhydramine

- Establish a consistent bedtime, and take diphenhydramine 30 to 60 minutes before you want to go to sleep. Do not take more than 50 mg of diphenhydramine each night.
- After 2 to 3 nights of improved sleep, skip taking the medication for one night to see if the insomnia is relieved.
- Do not take the medication for longer than 10 days. Longer use will cause tolerance to the medication's sleep-inducing effects but not necessarily to its side effects.
- Note that diphenhydramine can cause morning grogginess or excess sedation, dry mouth, blurred vision, constipation, and urinary retention (particularly in older men).
- Do not take diphenhydramine with alcohol; alcohol can increase the effects of the medication on the central nervous system. Alcohol also disrupts the sleep cycle.
- Do not take diphenhydramine with prescription sleep aids in an attempt to further improve sleep.
- Consult your pharmacist or physician before taking diphenhydramine with other medications.

Melatonin

- If melatonin is being used, take it 1 to 2 hours before the established bedtime.
- Do not take more than 1 mg of melatonin each night.

If insomnia worsens or continues beyond 3 weeks, consult a physician.

drowsiness. The pharmacist should ask the patient to call if sleep has not improved within 10 days.

CONCLUSIONS

Sedating antihistamines, such as diphenhydramine, are effective in treating occasional transient or short-term insomnia, particularly if the sleep disturbance is primarily related to difficulty falling asleep. Because little published information is available regarding the hypnotic effects of doxylamine, only diphenhydramine should be recommended as a hypnotic at the present time. Before recommending a nonprescription agent, however, the pharmacist should question the patient carefully regarding the characteristics and possible etiologies of the sleep disturbance. A patient who appears to have long-term insomnia or sleep disturbance caused by an underlying disorder should be referred to a physician for further evaluation. The pharmacist should question the patient regarding medical disorders or concomitant medications that may interact with diphenhydramine, then should counsel the patient regarding diphenhydramine's side effects and particularly the additive effects of alcohol. The pharmacist should advise the patient that nonprescription hypnotics are intended for short-term use and that a physician should be consulted if sleep problems persist beyond 7 to 10 nights. Regardless of whether a nonprescription product is recommended, the pharmacist should emphasize the importance of maintaining healthy sleep habits to ensure a good night's sleep.

References

1. Eggert AE, Crismon ML. Dealing with insomnia, the evaluation and treatment of sleep disorders. *Am Druggist.* 1992;205:83–96.
2. Farney RJ, Walker JM. Office management of common sleep-wake disorders. *Med Clin North Am.* 1995;79:391–414.
3. Pagel JF. Treatment of insomnia. *Am Fam Physician.* 1994;49:1417–21.
4. Costa E, Silva JA, Chase M, et al. Special report from a symposium held by the World Health Organization and the World Federation of Sleep Research Societies: an overview of insomnias and related disorders—recognition, epidemiology, and rational management. *Sleep.* 1996;19:412–6.
5. Bixler EO, Vela-Bueno A. Normal sleep: patterns and mechanisms. *Semin Neurol.* 1987;7:227.
6. Becker PM, Jamieson AO, Bown WD. Insomnia, use of a 'decision tree' to assess and treat. *Postgrad Med.* 1993;93:66–85.
7. Lechky O. Questions about sleep should be routine part of patient visits, physician says. *Can Med Assoc J.* 1993;149:1296–8.
8. Balter MB, Uhlenhuth EH. The beneficial and adverse effects of hypnotics. *J Clin Psychiatry.* 1991;52(suppl 7):16–23.
9. FDA announces standards for nonprescription sleep-aid products and expectorants. *Clin Pharm.* 1989;8:388.

10. Antihistamine drugs. In: McEvoy GK, ed. *AHFS Drug Information 99.* Bethesda, Md: American Society of Hospital Pharmacists; 1999:27–31.
11. Spector R, Choudhury AK, Chiang C, et al. Diphenhydramine in Orientals and Caucasians. *Clin Pharmacol Ther.* 1980;28:229–34.
12. Meredith CG, Christian CD, Johnson RF, et al. Diphenhydramine disposition in chronic liver disease. *Clin Pharmacol Ther.* 1984;35:474–9.
13. Gengo F, Gabos C, Miller JK. The pharmacodynamics of diphenhydramine-induced drowsiness and changes in mental performance. *Clin Pharmacol Ther.* 1989;45:15–21.
14. Carruthers SG, Shoeman DW, Hignite CE, et al. Correlation between plasma diphenhydramine level and sedative and antihistamine effects. *Clin Pharmacol Ther.* 1978;23:375–82.
15. Koppel C, Ibe K, Tenczer J. Clinical symptomatology of diphenhydramine overdose: an evaluation of 136 cases in 1982 to 1985. *Clin Toxicol.* 1987;25:53–70.
16. Zareba W, Moss AJ, Rosero SZ, et al. Electrocardiographic findings in patients with diphenhydramine overdose. *Am J Cardiol.* 1997;80:1168–73.
17. Nash W. Treating diphenhydramine overdose. *Nursing.* 1994;24:33.
18. Tejera CA, Saravay SM, Goldman E, et al. Diphenhydramine-induced delirium in elderly hospitalized patients with mild dementia. *Psychosomatics.* 1994;35:399–402.
19. Sack RL, Hughes RJ, Edgar DM, et al. Sleep-promoting effects of melatonin: at what dose, in whom, under what conditions, and by what mechanisms? *Sleep.* 1997;20:908–15.
20. Zhdanova IV, Wurtman RJ, Lynch HJ, et al. Sleep-inducing effects of low doses of melatonin ingested in the evening. *Clin Pharmacol Ther.* 1995;57:552–8.
21. Mendelson WB. A critical evaluation of the hypnotic efficacy of melatonin. *Sleep.* 1997;20:916–9.
22. Hughes RJ, Sack RL, Lewy AJ. The role of melatonin and circadian phase in age-related sleep-maintenance insomnia: assessment in a clinical trial of melatonin replacement. *Sleep.* 1998;21:52–68.
23. Petrie K, Dawson AG, Thompson L, et al. A double-blind trial of melatonin as a treatment for jet lag in international cabin crew. *Biol Psychiatry.* 1993;33:526–30.
24. Suhner A, Schlagenhauf P, Johnson R, et al. Comparative study to determine the optimal melatonin dosage form for the alleviation of jet lag. *Chronobiol Int.* 1998;15:655–66.
25. Butler RN. A wake-up call for caution. If insomnia is the patient's problem, is over-the-counter melatonin the cure? *Geriatrics.* 1996;51:14–5.
26. Wagner J, Wagner ML, Hening WA. Beyond benzodiazepines: alternative pharmacologic agents for the treatment of insomnia. *Ann Pharmacother.* 1998;32:680–91.
27. Williamson BL, Tomlinson AJ, Gleich GJ. Contaminants in commercial preparations of melatonin. *Mayo Clin Proc.* 1997;72:1094.
28. Schneider-Helmert D, Spinweber CL. Evaluation of L-tryptophan for treatment of insomnia: a review. *Psychopharmacol.* 1986;89:1–7.
29. Kamb ML, Murphy JJ, Jones JL, et al. Eosinophilia-myalgia syndrome in L-tryptophan exposed patients. *JAMA.* 1992;267:77–82.
30. Roth T, Roehrs T, Zorick F, Conway W. Pharmacological effects of sedative-hypnotics, narcotic analgesics, and alcohol during sleep. *Med Clin North Am.* 1985;69:1281–8.
31. Foust RT, Reddy R, Jeffers LJ, et al. Nyquil-associated liver injury. *Am J Gastroenterol.* 1989;84:422–5.
32. Scrima L, Broudy M, Nay KN, Cohn MA. Increased severity of obstructive sleep apnea after bedtime alcohol ingestion: diagnostic potential and proposed mechanism of action. *Sleep.* 1982;5:318.
33. Taasan VC, Block AJ, Boysen PG, Wynne JW. Alcohol increases sleep apnea and oxygen desaturation in asymptomatic men. *Am J Med.* 1981;71:240.
34. Roehrs T, Zwyghuizen-Doorenbos A, Roth T. Sedative effects and plasma concentrations following single doses of triazolam, diphenhydramine, ethanol, and placebo. *Sleep.* 1993;16:301–5.
35. Kudo Y, Kurihara M. Clinical evaluation of diphenhydramine hydrochloride for the treatment of insomnia in psychiatric patients: a double-blind study. *J Clin Pharmacol.* 1990;30:1041–8.

CHAPTER 41

Drowsiness

M. Lynn Crismon and Donna M. Jermain

Chapter 41 at a Glance

Daytime drowsiness is a common side effect of insomnia and other sleep disorders. (See Chapter 40, "Insomnia.") The classification of insomnia as the third most-common patient complaint indicates that daytime drowsiness can also be considered a significant problem.

Caffeine-containing products are the only nonprescription stimulants available in the United States to treat drowsiness. Nearly 80% of the U.S. adult population consumes caffeine daily (usually in foods and beverages), thus making it one of the most popular drugs.[1] Many children also consume caffeine. For example, mean caffeine intake in children ages 6 to 11 months is 4.2 mg per day; in children ages 6 to 17 years, it increases to 43 mg per day.[2] In adults, mean caffeine intake is 186 mg per day (approximately two cups of coffee daily or the equivalent). Daily caffeine intake correlates with age.

Etiology of Drowsiness

Many individuals suffer from daytime drowsiness simply because they do not get enough sleep. Drowsiness is also one of the symptoms of sleep disorders, including insomnia, narcolepsy, nocturnal myoclonus, and restless legs syndrome. Other medical conditions can also cause daytime drowsiness by disrupting sleep. (See Table 40–1 in Chapter 40, "Insomnia.") As Table 40–1 shows, psychiatric problems often cause insomnia. Drowsiness is a common adverse effect of medications, including such medications as anticholinergics, antihistamines, benzodiazepines, antidepressants, and β-blockers. Poor sleep hygiene can also cause insomnia and resultant daytime drowsiness.

Paradoxically, consumption of dietary caffeine can cause daytime drowsiness by impairing sleep. Caffeine is a common ingredient in coffee, tea, soft drinks, and chocolate products.[1] (See Table 41–1.) It is also present in many prescription and nonprescription drugs, including headache and cold remedies, menstrual pain relief products, diet aids, and stimulant preparations.

Treatment of Drowsiness

Treatment Outcomes

The goal in treating daytime drowsiness is to identify and eliminate the cause of this symptom.

General Treatment Approach

The patient should be questioned extensively to determine the cause of the drowsiness. (See the section "Patient Assessment of Drowsiness.") If self-treatment is appropriate, the pharmacist should recommend good sleep hygiene measures as the preferred method of treating daytime drowsiness. If a patient insists on using caffeine products, the recommended dosages, potential adverse effects, and signs and symptoms of toxicity should be thoroughly explained. The algorithm in Figure 41–1 outlines this approach to self-treatment.

Editor's Note: This chapter is based, in part, on the 11th edition chapter titled "Sleep Aid and Stimulant Products," which was written by M. Lynn Crismon and Donna M. Jermain.

Table 41–1

Approximate Caffeine Content of Selected Beverages and Foods

Beverage or Food	Caffeine Content (mg)
Coffee (5 ounces)	
Brewed, automatic drip	60–180
Brewed, percolator	40–170
Instant	30–120
Decaffeinated, instant	1–5
Decaffeinated, brewed	2–5
Tea (5 ounces)	
Brewed, imported brands	25–110
Brewed, US brands	20–90
Instant	25–50
Iced (12 ounces)	67–76
Soft Drinks (12 ounces)	
Mountain Dew	54
Coca-Cola	45.6
Diet Coke	45.6
Dr. Pepper	39.6
Sugar-Free Dr. Pepper	39.6
Big Red	38.4
Sugar-Free Big Red	38.4
Pepsi-Cola	38.4
Diet Pepsi	36
7-Up	0
Sunkist Orange	0
Ginger ale	0
Chocolate Foods	
Chocolate cake (1/16 of a 9-inch cake)	13.8
Chocolate ice cream (2/3 cup)	4.5
Chocolate pudding, instant (1/2 cup)	5.5
Chocolate milk beverage (8 ounces)	2–7
Chocolate-flavored syrup (1 ounce)	4
Milk chocolate (1 ounce)	1–15
Dark chocolate, semisweet (1 ounce)	5–35
Baker's chocolate (1 ounce)	26
Cocoa beverage (5 ounces)	2–20

Sources: *JAMA*. August 1984;252:802–6; Lecos C. The latest caffeine scorecard. *FDA Consumer*. March 1984;18:14–6; *Hosp Pharm*. April 1984;19:257–67.

Nonpharmacologic Therapy

Good sleep hygiene principles should be discussed to address any underlying problem that may result in poor sleep and thus daytime sleepiness. (See Table 40–3 in Chapter 40, "Insomnia.")

Pharmacologic Therapy (Caffeine)

Caffeine is the only nonprescription stimulant approved by the Food and Drug Administration (FDA). Caffeine concentrations vary among the products; generally, stimulants contain the highest concentrations, averaging 100 to 200 mg per tablet. Table 41–2 lists examples of commercial products.

Pharmacologic Effects

Caffeine's pharmacologic action affects primarily the central nervous system (CNS) and the cardiovascular system. Its CNS effects temporarily counteract drowsiness.

Central Nervous System Effects In terms of CNS stimulation, caffeine is the most potent methylxanthine, even at low plasma concentrations. As caffeine plasma concentrations increase, the cortex, then the medulla, and finally the spinal cord are stimulated. (See Figure 41–2.) Caffeine doses of 50 to 200 mg can increase alertness and can decrease fatigue and drowsiness. At higher doses (200 to 500 mg), caffeine may produce tremulousness, nervousness, headache, and irritability. High plasma concentrations may also cause excitement, tinnitus, insomnia, and restlessness.

Caffeine's effect on sleep may be dose dependent, but it varies greatly among individuals. Caffeine appears to increase stage 2 sleep and decrease delta sleep. (See the section "Physiology of Sleep" in Chapter 40, "Insomnia.") Thus, it may increase awakenings and arousability although tolerance may develop to these effects.

Caffeine has varying effects on mood. Aggressive behavior has been reported to decrease with caffeine reduction. Caffeine may exacerbate anxiety, thus potentially worsening symptoms in patients with anxiety or panic disorder.[3] Depression has been reported in people consuming large amounts of caffeine (five cups of coffee a day or more).[3] However, it is difficult to know whether depressed patients self-medicate with caffeine or whether caffeine produces depression. Increased caffeine intake has been linked to a worsening in the behavioral symptoms of moderate-to-severe premenstrual syndrome.[4]

Cardiovascular Effects Pharmacologic effects of caffeine on the cardiovascular system have long been debated. Caffeine stimulates heart muscle; however, this action is often opposed by simultaneous medullary vagal stimulation. The resultant heart rate changes are variable. As the caffeine dose is increased, the myocardium stimulation overcomes the vagal effect and increased cardiac activity is noted.

Blood Pressure Caffeine causes systemic release of norepinephrine, epinephrine, and renin, producing alterations in blood pressure.[1] However, recent studies suggest that caffeine does not produce persistent increases in blood pressure because tolerance quickly develops.[5] Even in individuals who do not regularly consume caffeine, the increased blood pressure resulting from caffeine ingestion rapidly returns to normal. Thus, hypertensive patients can continue to consume moderate amounts of caffeine.

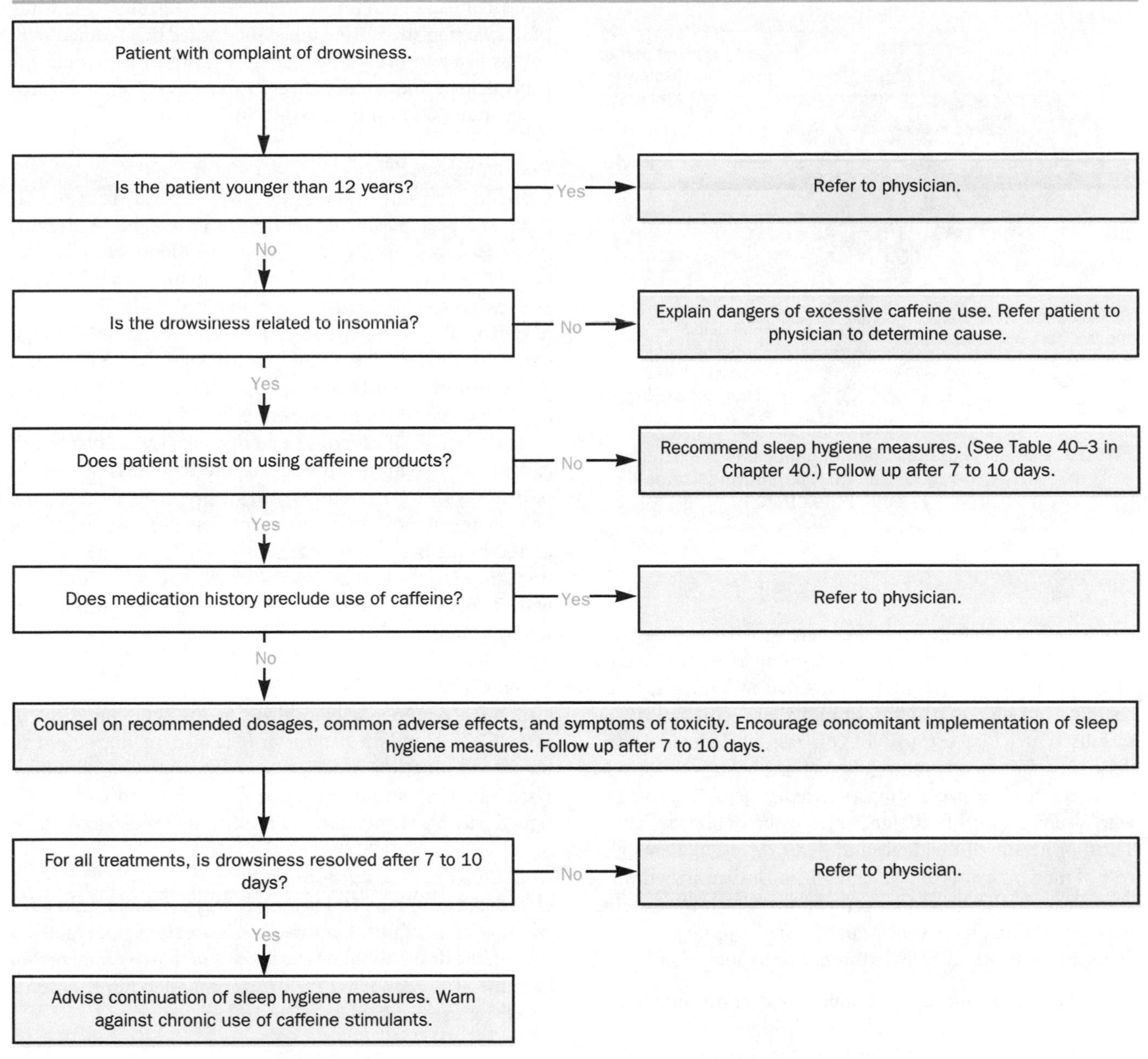

Figure 41–1 Self-care of drowsiness.

Table 41–2

Selected Stimulant Products

Trade Name	Primary Ingredients
Enerjets Lozenges[a]	Caffeine 75 mg
High Gear Gum[b]	Caffeine 25 mg
NoDoz Maximum Strength Alertness Aid Caplets[a]	Caffeine 200 mg
Vivarin Tablets/Caplets	Caffeine 200 mg

[a] Sodium-free product.

[b] Phenylalanine-containing product.

Coronary Heart Disease Several reports have suggested that heavy caffeine consumption is associated with coronary heart disease.[1,6] One prospective study involving 1130 male medical students followed for 19 to 35 years noted a positive dose–response relationship between caffeine consumption and coronary heart disease.[6] However, another 2-year prospective study involving 45,589 men with no history of cardiovascular disease found no association between coffee consumption and the risk of coronary heart disease or stroke.[7]

Cardiac Rate/Rhythm The effect of caffeine on cardiac rate and rhythm and on the possible development of arrhythmias has been studied. In 34 normal adults, high caffeine doses (1 mg/kg every 0.5 caffeine half-life) were not associated with

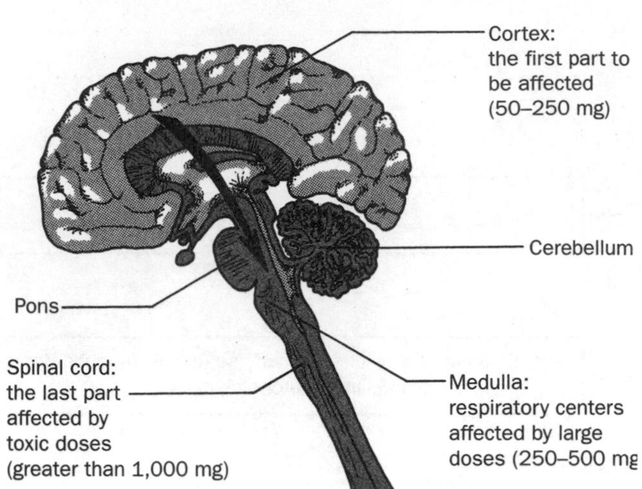

Figure 41–2 Sites of action of caffeine in the central nervous system. (The arrow indicates the progression of the effect.)

any significant change in cardiac rate or rhythm.[8] Caffeine intake of 300 to 450 mg per day did not increase the severity or frequency of arrhythmias in normal individuals, in ischemic heart disease patients, or in patients with preexisting serious ventricular ectopy.[9] In contrast, an increased incidence of spontaneous ventricular ectopic beats was noted in patients who had preexisting ventricular ectopic beats and who received 1 mg of caffeine per kilogram of body weight.[10] Thus, in healthy individuals and heart disease patients, the role of moderate amounts of caffeine in cardiac arrhythmias is unclear. In very high concentrations, however, caffeine may cause sinus tachycardia, paroxysmal supraventricular tachycardia, ventricular arrhythmias, or hypotension.[1,11]

Cholesterol Concentration Caffeine may contribute to adverse changes in lipid metabolism.[1] Some epidemiologic studies suggest a link between coffee consumption and increased concentrations of total and low-density lipoprotein cholesterol.

Miscellaneous Pharmacologic Effects Caffeine affects the respiratory, endocrine, gastrointestinal (GI), and renal systems. Caffeine is a bronchodilator, but it is only about 40% as potent as theophylline[1] and may increase the respiratory rate. Endocrine effects include increases in renin, cortisol, free fatty acids, blood glucose concentrations, and the metabolic rate. Effects on the GI system include increases in gastric acid and pepsin secretion. Caffeine may either decrease or have no effect on lower esophageal sphincter pressure, and it relaxes smooth muscle in the biliary and GI tracts. It reduces mesenteric and liver blood flow, the latter by up to 19%. Finally, caffeine has a mild diuretic effect by increasing the glomerular filtration rate and inhibiting sodium tubular reabsorption.

Caffeine has been linked to decreased fertility. One study of 104 women attempting pregnancy noted that women were half as likely to become pregnant if more caffeine than the equivalent of one cup of coffee per day was consumed.[12] Another study found similar results in 6303 women.[13]

Pharmacokinetics

Caffeine is rapidly and completely absorbed from the GI tract, and peak plasma concentrations occur 30 to 60 minutes after ingestion. Caffeine crosses the blood–brain barrier rapidly and has a volume of distribution of 0.5 to 0.8 L/kg of body weight. It is extensively metabolized in the liver by the microsomal cytochrome P-450 system, primarily through oxidative demethylation and hydroxylation. CYPIA2 is a major pathway. Furthermore, no significant first-pass effect exists. Paraxanthine, theobromine, and theophylline are active metabolites of caffeine. In adults, the average half-life of caffeine is 4 to 6 hours. In smokers, the half-life is shorter. In patients with liver cirrhosis and in pregnant women, the half-life is extended. In neonates, the half-life may be as long as 100 hours because neonates primarily eliminate caffeine unchanged by the kidneys until they are 3 months of age. The half-life of caffeine in elderly patients is not significantly different from that in younger adults.

Indications

Caffeine is commercially available as the sole ingredient in most CNS stimulant products. It is also an ingredient in many combination products such as headache remedies. Used as a CNS stimulant, caffeine is marketed to help fatigued patients stay awake and to restore mental alertness.

Dosage/Administration Guidelines

Oral doses of 100 to 200 mg are needed to achieve mild CNS stimulation in adults. If a timed-release caffeine preparation is used, the dose should not be taken less than 6 hours before bedtime. The manufacturer's recommended adult dose of timed-release products is 200 to 250 mg.

Adverse Effects

The primary adverse events associated with caffeine are CNS stimulant effects and GI irritation. Adverse CNS effects are more pronounced in children. Caffeine also can adversely affect the cardiovascular and renal systems. (See Table 41–3 for specific adverse effects related to caffeine.) Further, prolonged consumption of caffeine can result in dependence, whereas excessive consumption can result in toxicity.

Dependence/Withdrawal Prolonged caffeine consumption can cause physical dependence; withdrawal symptoms can occur following abrupt cessation.[1] The most common withdrawal symptoms are fatigue and headache. Table 41–3 lists other possible symptoms. Withdrawal symptoms generally occur 12 to 24 hours after cessation of caffeine ingestion, peak in 20 to 48 hours, and may persist for a week. A throbbing headache, the typical symptom, results from rebound

Table 41–3

Adverse Effects Associated with Caffeine Use or Overuse

Adverse Effects Associated with Recommended Dosages	Symptoms of Caffeine Withdrawal[a]
Central Nervous System	Fatigue (most common)
Insomnia	Headache (most common)
Nervousness	Anxiety
Restlessness	Nausea
Excitement	Vomiting
Tinnitus	Impaired psychomotor function
Muscular tremor	Irritability
Headache	Restlessness
Lightheadedness	Lethargy
Mild delirium	Yawning
Gastrointestinal Effects	Rhinorrhea
Nausea	**Symptoms of Caffeine Toxicity (Caffeinism)[b]**
Vomiting	Nervousness
Diarrhea	Restlessness
Stomach pain	Insomnia
Other Effects	Excitement
Extrasystoles	Diuresis Facial flushing
Palpitations	Muscle twitching
Tachycardia	Gastrointestinal disturbance
Diuresis	Tachycardia or cardiac arrhythmia
	"Rambling" flow of thought and speech
	Psychomotor agitation
	Periods of inexhaustibility

[a] Withdrawal symptoms occur after abrupt cessation, usually within 12 to 24 hours. Symptoms peak in 20 to 48 hours and may persist for a week.

[b] Diagnostic criteria of caffeinism include recent consumption of more than 250 mg of caffeine and the presence of at least five of the symptoms associated with caffeine toxicity.

Source: References 14 and 15.

vasodilatation that occurs following abrupt withdrawal. Some suggest there is a distinct clinical withdrawal syndrome consisting of headache, lethargy, and depression.[14]

Investigators have suggested that overuse of caffeine meets criteria for drug dependence. Caffeine is a reinforcer: It produces withdrawal symptoms, tolerance, and intoxication. Further research will determine whether caffeine is added to the list of agents producing drug dependence. Caffeine withdrawal is included as a research proposal in the appendixes of the *Diagnostic and Statistical Manual of Mental Disorders*, 4th edition.[15]

Toxicity Caffeinism, the ingestion of single caffeine doses greater than 250 mg can produce symptoms mimicking anxiety. The diagnostic criteria for caffeinism include recent caffeine consumption of more than 250 mg and at least five of the symptoms of caffeine toxicity listed in Table 41–3.[15] Five caffeine overdose deaths have been reported in patients who ingested caffeine-containing nonprescription products.[16] Four of the five cases were completed suicides, and the fifth was an accidental death secondary to drug abuse. The lethal dose in adults is 150 to 200 mg/kg of body weight.[17]

The primary management of caffeine toxicity includes general supportive care. For an acute ingestion, emesis should be initiated immediately with syrup of ipecac unless the patient is obtunded, comatose, or convulsing. A cathartic (e.g., magnesium sulfate, magnesium citrate, sodium sulfate, or sorbitol) should be given with or without activated charcoal. If the patient is stuporous or comatose, gastric lavage and activated charcoal should be used. Patients should receive general supportive care (e.g., hydration, antipyretics, and maintenance of vital signs, including ventilatory support and electrocardiogram monitoring). Antacids (e.g., aluminum hydroxide gel) can be used for GI irritation. Seizures should be treated with intravenous diazepam and, if they recur, with phenytoin or phenobarbital. For extremely high caffeine serum concentrations, exchange transfusion or hemoperfusion may be considered.

Drug–Drug Interactions/Laboratory Test Interferences

Drug interactions between caffeine and other agents may be clinically significant.[1,18–23] Patients using nonprescription stimulants should be warned about possible interactions with prescription or nonprescription drugs they are taking. (See Table 41–4.) Although the clinical significance of caffeine's effect on iron absorption is unclear, patients taking iron supplements should be instructed to take iron 1 hour before or 2 hours after caffeine consumption. Concomitant use of caffeine and diazepam produces antagonizing effects. For example, caffeine antagonizes diazepam-induced impairment of psychomotor performance and sedation, but does not antagonize diazepam-induced impairment of delayed recognition memory performance or immediate recall.[21] Alternatively, diazepam antagonizes caffeine-induced restlessness, alertness, arousal, and tension. Caffeine inhibits metabolism through CYPIA2, and therefore may increase the effects of drugs metabolized by this hepatic isoenzyme. Comprehensive drug interaction references should be consulted regarding current information on potential caffeine–drug interactions.

Table 41–4

Caffeine–Drug Interactions

Drug	Effect
Cimetidine, ciprofloxacin, disulfiram, enoxacin, fluvoxamine, mexiletine, norfloxacin, oral contraceptives containing estrogen	Inhibited caffeine metabolism, resulting in increased caffeine effects
Olanzapine, tertiary amine tricyclic antidepressants, fluvoxamine, clozapine, phenytoin, theophylline	Inhibited metabolism of the drugs, resulting in increased drug effects and increased risk of side effects or potential toxicity
Iron	Decreased iron absorption
Alcohol, aspirin, corticosteroids, nonsteroidal anti-inflammatory drugs	Increased gastrointestinal distress
Phenylpropanolamine	Increased blood pressure
Monoamine oxidase	Increased chance of life-threatening cardiac complications
Antiarrhythmic agents	Impaired action of antiarrhythmic agents
Diazepam	Antagonized diazepam-induced effects—specifically, impairment of psychomotor performance and sedation. Antagonized caffeine-induced effects, such as restlessness, alertness, arousal, and tension

Sources: References 1, 18–23.

Caffeine may cause false-positive diagnostic tests for both pheochromocytoma and neuroblastoma because it causes elevations in urine concentrations of vanillylmandelic acid, catecholamines, and 5-hydroxyindoleacetic acid. Also, serum uric acid concentrations may be falsely elevated.

Contraindications/Precautions/Warnings

Caffeine is contraindicated in patients with known hypersensitivity to the drug. It should be used cautiously in patients who have or have had peptic ulcer disease, and in patients with symptomatic cardiac arrhythmias and palpitations. Also, high-dose caffeine intake may result in hyperglycemia. Lower doses should be used in patients with renal dysfunction. Caffeine has been shown to worsen mental status in some patients with psychiatric disorders, and it should be used cautiously in this population.

Special Population/Therapeutic Considerations

Geriatric Considerations In elderly patients, caffeine consumption may be a factor in subjective insomnia. Caffeine has been studied for preventing postprandial hypotension. However, in the best-designed study, caffeine was not found to be efficacious. Caffeine has also been studied as a potential risk factor for developing osteoporosis. The studies suggest that if calcium intake/balance is maintained, caffeine does not pose a risk for osteoporosis.

Use during Pregnancy/Lactation The safety of caffeine during pregnancy is a significant issue because caffeine is often consumed by pregnant women and freely crosses the placenta. Caffeine also passes into breast milk.

Teratogenic Effects On the basis of the teratogenic effects of caffeine in rodents, FDA issued a warning in 1980 advising pregnant women to limit or avoid caffeine consumption.[24] However, no consistent teratogenic effects have been reported in animal studies that used massive caffeine doses.[25]

Possible teratogenic mechanisms are uncertain, but three hypotheses are proposed. First, caffeine may interfere with fetal cell growth by increasing cyclic adenosine monophosphate (cAMP).[26] Second, because it structurally resembles adenine and guanine, caffeine may directly alter nucleic acids, resulting in chromosome abnormalities. Third, caffeine may restrict uteroplacental circulation through vasoconstriction, resulting in fetal hypoxia.

Data on caffeine's teratogenic effect in humans are limited to a few studies, most of which rely on questionnaires or interviews,[27] but these limited data suggest that caffeine's teratogenic potential appears to be dose related.[25] One epidemiologic study found an increased risk for late first- and second-trimester spontaneous abortions in women consuming at least 151 mg of caffeine daily.[26] However, the study noted that larger amounts of caffeine were consumed by mothers who smoked and used alcohol relatively heavily; both practices are known to increase the risk for spontaneous abortion.[28,29]

Caffeine intake of more than 300 mg per day is associated

with intrauterine growth retardation and infants of low birth weight.[27,30] These findings are not surprising because caffeine at doses of 200 mg significantly decreases placental blood flow through vasoconstriction within the placental villi,[30] and any decrease in uteroplacental circulation is significantly correlated with decreased fetal growth. Increased fetal breathing activity was noted in mothers consuming two cups of regular or decaffeinated coffee;[31] similar results were found in mothers consuming more than 500 mg of caffeine per day.[32] Consumption of six or more cups of coffee daily during pregnancy has been associated with spontaneous abortion, stillbirth, low birth weight, breech presentation, and decreased activity and muscle tone of neonates.[25] Cleft palate and interventricular septal defect have been noted in infants of mothers consuming eight or more cups of coffee per day.[25,33] Furthermore, three cases of arrhythmias have occurred in infants whose mothers ingested large amounts of caffeine.[34] Although anecdotal case reports suggest adverse fetal effects in mothers ingesting caffeine, case–control studies involving infants with congenital malformations suggest no relationship.[35–37] In a prospective study of 286 mothers, caffeine intake was not associated with an increased incidence of breech birth, miscarriage, premature birth, or caesarian section deliveries.[38] Nor was a relationship noted between caffeine intake and low birth weight in several large prospective and retrospective studies.[39,40] Overall, information is incomplete and the data are conflicting, but no direct correlation can be made between caffeine consumption and birth defects.[27] However, it is prudent to recommend limiting caffeine intake to 300 mg per day or less because decreases in birth weight are reported to occur when daily intake exceeds this amount.[27,30]

Concentration in Breast Milk Caffeine passes into breast milk; however, the caffeine concentration in breast milk is only 1% of the mother's plasma concentration.[27] Peak caffeine concentrations in breast milk occur within 1 hour of consumption, but infant caffeine plasma concentrations are not correlated with the levels in breast milk. No adverse effects have been reported in infants of nursing mothers consuming 200 to 336 mg per day of caffeine, although wakefulness and irritability have been noted in infants of nursing mothers consuming 600 mg per day. To avoid high maternal plasma and milk concentrations, mothers should ingest caffeine, whether from medicinal or food sources, only immediately after nursing. To avoid the potential for caffeine accumulation in the infant, mothers should consume caffeine in moderation, especially when nursing infants younger than 4 months.

Usage Considerations in Neonates Liver metabolic pathways, including the cytochrome P–450 system, are immature in the neonate. Thus, newborns metabolize caffeine very slowly and may accumulate toxic caffeine concentrations. The rate of caffeine elimination increases as the liver's metabolic function matures. Caffeine clearance and half-life are correlated directly with gestational age.[41] If caffeine is used therapeutically in neonates (e.g., for treating neonatal apnea), dosing intervals should be 24 hours in infants younger than 1 month, 12 hours in infants ages 1 to 2 months, 8 hours in infants ages 2 to 4 months, and 6 hours for infants age 4 months or older.[41]

Malignancy Clinical studies proposing an association between caffeine intake and increased risk of breast cancer provide conflicting and nonconclusive results.[42–44] The causal relationship between caffeine ingestion and bladder and pancreatic cancers has been evaluated. A case–control study of 75 patients with bladder cancer and 142 control patients found no association between caffeine intake and the risk of bladder cancer.[45] Earlier studies suggest that the relative risk of developing pancreatic cancer is 2.7 (95% confidence intervals = 1.6, 4.7) in people consuming three or more cups of coffee per day;[46] however, later studies do not support this conclusion.[47–49] Thus, no conclusive data exist to suggest that caffeine ingestion is associated with any malignancy.

Benign Breast Disease Because results from various studies have been inconsistent, the possibility of a relationship between benign breast disease and caffeine is controversial.[43] Case–control studies suggest no such association.[50,51] Fibrocystic breast disease, however, may be associated with caffeine consumption.[50] Some investigators have noted the complete resolution of benign breast nodules, tenderness, pain, and nipple discharge once women with fibrocystic disease eliminated caffeine from their diet.[52]

Alternative Remedies

Herbal products with caffeine include cola nut, guarana, and mate. Guarana has a very high concentration of caffeine (3% to 5%).[53] Coffee beans, by contrast, contain 1% to 2%, and mate dried leaf contains 0.56% caffeine.[54] Damiana may also contain caffeine.[55] Caffeine content may vary significantly among herbal preparations. (See Chapter 45, "Herbal Remedies," for further discussion of this substance.)

Patient Assessment of Drowsiness

When assessing a patient with a complaint of daytime drowsiness, the pharmacist should determine the etiology of the patient's fatigue. Evaluating the patient's medical or psychiatric problems, current medication use, dietary caffeine consumption, sleep patterns, and lifestyle will help in determining the underlying cause. Given the paucity of data supporting the efficacy of caffeine, the side effects associated with recommended doses, and the effects of excessive doses of caffeine, pharmacists should usually recommend improved sleep hygiene and lifestyle modifications, when appropriate, or physician referral, rather than a caffeine-containing product.

Asking patients the following questions will help elicit the information needed to accurately assess the etiology of drowsiness and to recommend the appropriate treatment approach.

Case Study 41–1

Patient Complaint/History

Heung, a 25-year-old college student, presents to the pharmacist with a complaint of not being able to stay awake at night. Indicating the box of NoDoz in her hand, she asks if the medication will help her stay up at night. During further discussion, she reveals that she has several finals to take during the next week.

The patient reveals that she was diagnosed as mildly hypertensive last year and has been taking Dyazide daily for the past year; she has a history of mitral valve prolapse. In addition to ibuprofen for occasional headaches, she takes the oral contraceptive Tri-Levlen 21, one tablet daily, for 21 days, 7 days off. The patient, who is allergic to penicillin, reports that she drinks alcohol in moderation during social events and does not smoke.

When asked about her diet and caffeine consumption, Heung admits to drinking, on average, two cups of coffee with breakfast, two diet colas during the afternoon, and one glass of tea with dinner. She also eats a chocolate candy bar every afternoon.

Clinical Considerations/Strategies

Readers can use the following considerations/strategies to determine whether treatment with nonprescription agents is warranted:

- Assess the appropriateness of the patient using NoDoz to help stay awake.
- Assess the potential for drug–drug, drug–disease, and drug–dietary interactions if the patient were to take the NoDoz.
- Determine whether the patient has used nonprescription stimulant products before.
- Propose a response to the patient's original question: Will NoDoz help her stay awake at night?

Patient Education/Counseling

Readers can use the following strategies to develop a patient education/counseling plan that will help ensure optimal therapeutic outcomes:

- Explain the importance of the drug–drug, drug–disease, and drug–dietary interactions that might occur if NoDoz is taken.
- Explain symptoms of excessive caffeine consumption and what to do about them.

Q~ Why do you want to use a stimulant product?

A~ If the intent is to use a stimulant to stay awake while driving or studying, advise the patient that there is little information supporting the use of caffeine products for alertness. Further, advise the patient that such a product is not a substitute for adequate sleep and rest. Encourage improved sleep habits.

Q~ How long do you intend to use this product?

A~ If long-term use is intended, explore other methods of combating drowsiness. The effects of long-term use have not been adequately studied.

Q~ Do you regularly consume coffee, tea, cola, or other caffeinated beverages?

A~ Advise the patient that caffeine-containing medications should not be taken concomitantly with caffeine-containing beverages because such combination may increase the risk of side effects, including caffeinism. Also, evaluate whether drowsiness may be a symptom of caffeine-induced insomnia.

Q~ What other medications, prescription and nonprescription, do you take?

A~ *Identify medications known to interact with caffeine. (See Table 41–4.)* If the patient is taking any of these medications, discourage the use of nonprescription stimulant products. *Identify medications for which drowsiness or disturbed sleep is a side effect. (See the section "Etiology of Drowsiness.")* If such medications are being used, refer the patient to a physician for possible medication adjustments.

Q~ Are you under a physician's care? What types of medical problems do you have?

A~ *Identify disorders known to cause drowsiness. (See the section "Etiology of Drowsiness.")* If the patient has transient or short-term insomnia or has poor sleep practices, recommend the appropriate self-treatment of insomnia. (See Chapter 40, "Insomnia.") If more serious pathology is present, refer the patient to a physician.

Q~ Do you have anxiety, irritability, or any other nervous condition?

A~ If yes, suspect an underlying psychiatric condition. Refer the patient to a physician, preferably a mental health specialist.

Q~ Do you have problems sleeping?

A~ If yes, assess the patient's sleep disorder. (See Chapter 40, "Insomnia.") Consider discussing good principles of sleep hygiene with the patient. (See Table 40–3 in Chapter 40.)

Q~ Are you pregnant or breast-feeding?

A~ If yes, refer the patient to a physician.

Q~ Do you smoke cigarettes or chew tobacco?

A~ If yes, suspect that nicotine stimulation may be disrupting sleep and causing the drowsiness. Consider the additive effects of nicotine when taken in conjunction with other stimulant medications

Q~ Do you drink alcohol? If so, how much and how often?

A~ If yes, advise the patient that alcohol may be disrupting sleep, resulting in daytime drowsiness.

Patient Counseling for Drowsiness

As with insomnia, a disorder often associated with daytime drowsiness, counseling on the treatment of drowsiness should focus on practicing good sleep hygiene and eliminating factors that may be causing insomnia. If the patient insists on a caffeine product, the pharmacist should review dosage guidelines with the patient and emphasize the adverse effects that can occur with overuse of caffeine.

Pharmacists should be aware of the various prescription and nonprescription products containing caffeine. Dietary caffeine consumption may be substantial; thus, patients should be advised of the additive effects of dietary and medicinal caffeine. This advice is particularly important for elderly patients, who may be more sensitive to the stimulant effects of caffeine and may present with nervousness, anxiety, insomnia, and irritability. Elderly patients who are receiving other CNS stimulants should not take caffeine products. Agents such as theophylline, decongestants, amantadine, tricyclic antidepressants, and appetite suppressants added to caffeine may produce disorientation, delirium, and a host of other adverse effects.

Patients need to be advised of the possible drug interactions, as outlined in Table 41–4, that may occur with caffeine. The combination of caffeine and alcohol ingestion needs to be addressed. Caffeine does not antagonize the effect of alcohol, improve a person's driving ability, or lessen any of the detrimental effects of alcohol. Contrary to folklore, caffeine will not "sober up" a person intoxicated on alcohol.

The box "Patient Education for Drowsiness" lists specific information to provide to patients.

Evaluation of Patient Outcomes for Drowsiness

The pharmacist should check on the patient's progress after 7 to 10 days of the initial visit. A telephone call or scheduled visit to the pharmacy will encourage the patient to adhere to recommended strategies. If the drowsiness persists or recurs despite adherence to these strategies, the patient should consult a physician. If the drowsiness is resolved, the pharmacist should reinforce the need to continue good sleep hygiene practices.

Patient Education for Drowsiness

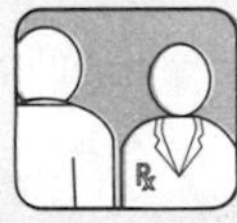

The objective of self-treatment is to maintain wakefulness. For most patients, improved sleep hygiene will help ensure optimal therapeutic outcomes. If the patient insists on taking a caffeine-containing product, the recommendations under "Nonprescription Medications" should be followed carefully.

Nondrug Measures

- Practice good principles of sleep hygiene. (See Table 40–3 in Chapter 40, "Insomnia.") A person who rests well at night should maintain wakefulness during the day.

Nonprescription Medications

- Do not exceed the recommended dose of 100 to 200 mg every 3 to 4 hours. Note that high doses of caffeine may cause multiple side effects. (See Table 41–3.)
- Do not use caffeine tablets in combination with coffee or other caffeinated products.
- If you are taking iron supplements, take iron 1 hour before or 2 hours after taking the caffeine stimulant.
- If you are taking any of the medications listed in Table 41–4, consult a physician before using caffeine stimulants.
- If you have osteoporosis, peptic ulcer disease, symptomatic cardiac arrhythmias and palpitations, or psychiatric disorders, consult a physician before using caffeine stimulants.

If drowsiness persists or recurs, consult a physician.

Seek medical attention immediately if symptoms of caffeine toxicity occur. (See Table 41–3.)

CONCLUSIONS

Caffeine is present in many foods, beverages, and drug products. Moderate use is generally considered safe, and no conclusive data exist linking regular caffeine use with various cardiovascular diseases, teratogenic effects, or cancer. However, pregnant or nursing patients and patients with cardiac dysfunction should consume caffeine in moderation, if at all.

Patients should be advised of several issues related to the use of nonprescription stimulants containing caffeine. First, caffeine toxicity may occur if higher-than-recommended doses are ingested. Second, stimulant products will not reverse alcohol impairment. Third, stimulant use should be discontinued if rapid pulse, dizziness, or heart palpitations occur. Finally, stimulant products are not intended as a substitute for normal sleep. If fatigue persists or recurs, the patient should consult a physician.

References

1. Benowitz NL. Clinical pharmacology of caffeine. *Annu Rev Med.* 1990;41:277–88.
2. Graham DM. Caffeine: its identity, dietary sources, intake, and biological effects. *Nutr Rev.* 1978;36:97–102.
3. Clementz GL, Dailey JW. Psychotropic effects of caffeine. *Am Fam Physician.* 1988;37:167–72.
4. Rossignol AM, Bonnlander H. Caffeine-containing beverages, total fluid consumption, and premenstrual syndrome. *Am J Public Health.* 1990;80:1106–10.
5. Myers MG. Effects of caffeine on blood pressure. *Arch Intern Med.* 1988;148:1189–93.
6. LaCroix AZ, Mead LA, Liang KY, et al. Coffee consumption and the incidence of coronary heart disease. *N Engl J Med.* 1986;315:977–82.
7. Grobbee DE, Rimm EB, Giovannucci E, et al. Coffee, caffeine, and cardiovascular disease in men. *N Engl J Med.* 1990;323:1026–3.
8. Newcombe PF, Rentor KW, Rautaharju PM, et al. High-dose caffeine and cardiac rate and rhythm in normal subjects. *Chest.* 1988;94:90–4.
9. Myers MG. Caffeine and cardiac arrhythmias. *Ann Intern Med.* 1991;114:147–50.
10. Sutherland DJ, McPherson DD, Renton KU, et al. The effect of caffeine on cardiac rate, rhythm, and ventricular repolarization. *Chest.* 1985;87:319–24.
11. Pentel P. Toxicity of over-the-counter stimulants. *JAMA.* 1984;252:1898–903.
12. Christianson RE, Oechsli FW, van den Berg BJ. Caffeinated beverages and decreased fertility. *Lancet.* 1989;1:378.
13. Wilcox A, Weinberg C, Baird D. Caffeinated beverages and decreased fertility. *Lancet.* 1988;2:1453–6.
14. Strain EC, Mumford GK, Silverman K, Griffiths RR. Caffeine dependence syndrome. *JAMA.* 1994;272:1043–8.
15. Organic mental syndromes and disorders. In: Frances A, Pincus HA, First MD, et al., ed. *Diagnostic and Statistical Manual of Mental Disorders.* 4th ed. Washington, DC: American Psychiatric Association; 1994: 708–9.
16. Garriott JC, Simmons LM, Poklis A, Mackrell MA. Five cases of fatal overdose from caffeine-containing "look-alike" drugs. *J Anal Toxicol.* 1985;9:141–3.
17. *Poisindex.* Vol 72. Englewood, CO: Micromedex; 1992.
18. Fazio A. Caffeine, oral contraceptives, and over-the-counter drugs. *Arch Intern Med.* 1989;149:1217–8.
19. Healy DP, Polk RE, Kanawafi L, et al. Interaction between oral ciprofloxacin and caffeine in normal volunteers. *Antimicrob Agents Chemother.* 1989;33:474–8.
20. Harder S, Fuhr U, Staib AH, et al. Ciprofloxacin–caffeine: a drug interaction established using in vivo and in vitro investigations. *Am J Med.* 1989;87(5A):89S–91S.
21. Roache JD, Griffiths RR. Interactions of diazepam and caffeine: behavioral and subjective dose effects in humans. *Pharmacol Biochem Behav.* 1987;26:801–12.
22. Ghoneim MM, Hinrichs IV, Chiang CK, Loke WH. Pharmacokinetic and pharmacodynamic interactions between caffeine and diazepam. *J Clin Psychopharmacol.* 1986;6:75–80.
23. Jefferson JW. Drug interactions—friend or foe. *J Clin Psychiatry.* 1998;59(suppl 4):37–47.
24. Caffeine and pregnancy. *FDA Drug Bull.* 1980;10:19–20.
25. Al-Hachim GM. Teratogenicity of caffeine; a review. *Eur J Obstet Gynecol Reprod Biol.* 1989;31:237–47.
26. Srisuphan W, Bracken MB. Caffeine consumption during pregnancy and association with late spontaneous abortion. *Am J Obstet Gynecol.* 1986;154:14–20.
27. Berger A. Effects of caffeine consumption on pregnancy outcome—a review. *J Reprod Med.* 1988;33:945–56.
28. Harlap S, Shiono PH. Alcohol, smoking, and incidence of spontaneous abortions in the first and second trimester. *Lancet.* 1980;2:173–6.
29. Kline J, Shrout P, Stein M, et al. Drinking during pregnancy and spontaneous abortion. *Lancet.* 1980;2:176–80.
30. Fenster L, Eskenazi B, Windham GC, Swan SH. Caffeine consumption during pregnancy and fetal growth. *Am J Public Health.* 1991;81:458–61.
31. Salvador HS, Koos BJ. Effects of regular and decaffeinated coffee on fetal breathing and heart rate. *Am J Obstet Gynecol.* 1989;160(pt 1):1043–7.
32. McGowan J, Devoe LD, Searle N, Altman R. The effects of long- and short-term maternal caffeine ingestion on human fetal breathing and body movements in term gestations. *Am J Obstet Gynecol.* 1987;157:726–9.
33. Jacobson MF, Goldman AS, Syme RH. Coffee and birth defects. *Lancet.* 1981;1:1415–6.
34. Oei SG, Vosters RPL, van der Hagen NLJ. Fetal arrhythmia caused by excessive intake of caffeine by pregnant women. *Br Med J.* 1989;298:568.
35. Coffee consumption during pregnancy. *N Engl J Med.* 1982;306:1548.
36. Rosenberg L, Mitchell AA, Shapiro S, Slone D. Selected birth defects in relation to caffeine-containing beverages. *JAMA.* 1982;247:1429–32.
37. Kurppa K, Holmberg PC, Kuosma E, Saxen L. Coffee consumption during pregnancy and selected congenital malformations: a nationwide case–control study. *Am J Public Health.* 1983;73:1397–9.
38. Watkinson B, Fried PA. Maternal caffeine use before, during, and after pregnancy and effects upon offspring. *Neurobehav Toxicol Teratol.* 1985;7:9–17.
39. Brooke OG, Anderson HR, Bland JM, et al. Effects on birth weight of smoking, alcohol, caffeine, socioeconomic factors, and psychosocial stress. *Br Med J.* 1989;298:795–801.
40. Linn S, Schoenbaum SC, Monson RR, et al. No association between coffee consumption and adverse outcomes of pregnancy. *N Engl J Med.* 1982;306:141–5.
41. Pons G, Carrier O, Richard MO, et al. Developmental changes of caffeine elimination in infancy. *Dev Pharmacol Ther.* 1988;11:258–64.
42. Wolfrom D, Welsch CW. Caffeine and the development of normal, benign and carcinomatous human breast tissues: a relationship? *J Med.* 1990;21:225–50.
43. Lubin F, Ron E. Consumption of methylxanthine-containing beverages and the risk of breast cancer. *Cancer Lett.* 1990;53:81–90.
44. Lubin F, Ron E, Wax Y, Modar B. Coffee and methylxanthines and breast cancer: a case–control study. *J Natl Cancer Inst.* 1984;74:569–73.
45. Najem GR, Louria DB, Seebode JJ, et al. Life-time occupation, smoking, caffeine, saccharine, hair dyes, and bladder carcinogenesis. *Int J Epidemiol.* 1982;11:212–7.
46. MacMahon B, Yen S, Trichopoulos D, et al. Coffee and cancer of the pancreas. *N Engl J Med.* 1981;304:630–3.
47. Hsieh CC, MacMahon B, Yen S. More on coffee and pancreatic cancer. *N Engl J Med.* 1987;316:484.
48. Hsieh CC, MacMahon B, Yen S, et al. Coffee and pancreatic cancer. *N Engl J Med.* 1986;315:587–8.

49. Hiatt RA, Klatsky AL, Armstrong MA. Pancreatic cancer, blood glucose, and beverage consumption. *Int J Cancer*. 1988;41:794–7.
50. Boyle CA, Berkowitz GS, LiVolsi VA, et al. Caffeine consumption and fibrocystic breast disease: a case–control epidemiologic study. *J Natl Cancer Inst*. 1984;72:1015–9.
51. Lubin F, Ron E, Wax Y, et al. A case–control study of caffeine and methylxanthines in benign breast disease. *JAMA*. 1985;253:2388–92.
52. Minton JP, Foecking MK, Webster DJ, Matthews RH. Response of fibrocystic disease to caffeine withdrawal and correlation of cyclic nucleotides with breast disease. *Am J Obstet Gynecol*. 1979;135:157–8.
53. Guarana [monograph]. In: DerMarderosian A, ed. *The Review of Natural Products*. St. Louis: Wolters Kluwer, Inc; May 1991.
54. Mate [monograph.] In: DerMarderosian A, ed. *The Review of Natural Products*. St. Louis: Wolters Kluwer, Inc; February 1997.
55. Damiana [monograph]. In: DerMarderosian A, ed. *The Review of Natural Products*. St. Louis: Wolters Kluwer, Inc; July 1996.

CHAPTER 42

Nicotine Addiction

Jack E. Fincham

Chapter 42 at a Glance

Cigarette smoking is the most prevalent, modifiable risk factor for increased morbidity and mortality in the United States and perhaps in the world.[1] Despite more than 30 years of accumulated, substantial evidence that describes the negative health effects of cigarette smoking in U.S. society, smoking remains a highly promoted addiction. During the past 40 years, the percentage of smokers has decreased, but an estimated 48 million U.S. adults continue to smoke.[2] Progress has been made in reducing smoking, but much work remains to be accomplished. For example, the estimated number of cigarettes sold in the United States in 1994 was equal to those sold in 1960: 480 billion.[3]

The direct and indirect costs associated with cigarette consumption exceeded $100 billion per year. Smokers use the health care system at least 50% more often than do nonsmokers.[4–6] However, health insurance coverage for the treatment of nicotine addiction has been sporadic. In 1990, only seven states had third-party payers of medical care that offer to reimburse for such treatment.[7] Although the percentage remains small, 19 states did pay for smoking cessation therapies through state Medicaid programs during 1999.

The barrage of tobacco advertisements (e.g., print, audio, video, billboards, clothing) that bombard the American public further compounds the problem of smoking. Widespread advertisements entice nonsmokers to become smokers and encourage current smokers to continue. Cigarette smoking remains a heavily promoted behavior. Many of the unwitting targets for this advertising blitz are the youth of our society.[8] Children who use alcohol, cigarettes, and smokeless tobacco are more likely also to use other substances of abuse.[9]

Studies have shown that 60% to 70% of current smokers would like to stop smoking and that 70% to 90% would consider stopping.[10] Further, receiving advice on smoking cessation in lay terms from a health professional would increase the number of individuals who stop smoking by 5% to 10%.[10] Although numerous other studies have indicated the importance of health professionals as smoking cessation counselors, many patients have noted that no health professional counseled them to stop smoking.[11]

Epidemiology of Nicotine Addiction

Anyone who smokes cigarettes or uses smokeless tobacco has the potential to become addicted to nicotine. Approximately 25% of U.S. adults smoke even though the percentage of

Editor's Note: This chapter is based, in part, on the 11th edition chapter titled "Smoking Cessation Products," which was written by Jack E. Fincham.

work sites that restrict or prohibit smoking has risen more than 50%. Many individuals still begin smoking and remain smokers for a long time.[12] Increases in the number of adolescent smokers are disturbing. An estimated 36.5% of high school students smoke, and the prevalence of smoking among high school seniors is increasing. Further, studies have indicated that 25% of children who are of elementary school age have smoked, and 12% have used smokeless tobacco. The prevalence of smoking in teens and children and the lack of continuing decreases in the percentage of adult smokers are major causes of concern.[2]

Etiology/Pathophysiology of Nicotine Addiction

Nicotine, the chief active component of tobacco, acts as an agonist to nicotinic receptors in the peripheral and central nervous systems, thereby producing both stimulant and depressant phases of action on all autonomic ganglia. The physiologic response to a nicotine dose delivered through a cigarette is almost immediate. Within seconds of inhaling the smoke, nicotine enters the pulmonary venous circulation system and is taken to the heart where it is subsequently carried through the internal carotid and anterior cerebral vessels to the brain. Tobacco use is a form of addiction that has effects comparable to opioid or narcotic addiction. These effects include euphoria during use and withdrawal symptoms after cessation of product use.[13] Tolerance to the effects of nicotine use may be caused by desensitization of nicotinic receptors at both the central and peripheral synapses.[14]

Signs and Symptoms of Nicotine Addiction

Symptoms of nicotine addiction have been referred to in terms that are normally reserved for illicit drugs: irritability, impatience, anxiety, confusion, impaired concentration, or restlessness.[15]

Complications of Nicotine Addiction

Cigarette smoking has a pervasive negative effect on countless health and disease states. It is the chief avoidable cause of death in the United States. Further, more adverse effects are being identified. A discussion of the more common complications follows.

Active and Passive Smoking Mortality

The number of smokers who die each year from tobacco-related sequelae that lead to cardiovascular disease, pulmonary disease, and cancer is increasing. In the United States, smok-

Case Study 42–1

Patient Complaint/History

Sigmund, a 55-year-old man, calls the pharmacy to complain of a "racing heart beat." He reports this effect first occurred when he began using nicotine polacrilex gum (40 4-mg dosing pieces a day) 10 days earlier and has continued that amount throughout the therapy. The patient also has been using nicotine transdermal systems for 2 weeks. He complains of a sore throat that occurs after he drinks his customary six cups of coffee in the morning. When questioned about the presence of other symptoms, the patient reports he has not suffered any withdrawal symptoms to date. He wants to stay off the cigarettes—he previously smoked two packs per day; however, the racing heart beat is frightening to him.

A review of Sigmund's patient profile reveals the following prescription medications: Theo-Dur 450 mg, one tablet three times a day for asthma (#90 filled monthly); amoxicillin 500 mg, one capsule three times a day for 10 days (filled 3 days earlier); Beconase AQ nasal spray 25 g, 2 sprays in each nostril twice a day (filled monthly); and Claritin-D, one tablet twice a day for 10 days (#20 filled 3 days earlier).

Clinical Considerations/Strategies

Readers can use the following considerations/strategies to determine whether treatment of the patient's condition with nonprescription drugs is warranted:

- Assess the probable cause of the patient's symptoms.
- Contact the patient's primary physician to explain the symptoms as described by the patient.
- Work with the physician and the patient to determine a potential revision in the theophylline dosage.
- Encourage the patient to come to the pharmacy for the counseling suggested below.

Patient Education/Counseling

Readers can use the following strategies to develop a patient education/counseling plan that will help ensure optimal therapeutic outcomes:

- Advise the patient to use only one type of nonprescription nicotine replacement therapy, never both.
- Review with the patient the proper dosing technique for administration of the nicotine polacrilex gum therapy.
- Suggest a dosage regimen and caution the patient about concurrent consumption of acidic beverages.
- Develop a pharmaceutical care plan for the patient's smoking cessation program.

ing-related deaths are in excess of 500,000 people each year, accounting for 16% of all deaths. The health risks of smoking are directly proportional to the number of cigarettes smoked per day, the number of years of cigarette smoking, and the amount of smoke inhaled. Smokers' risk for sudden cardiac death is two to four times greater than that of nonsmokers.[16] Unfortunately, such risks are not confined only to smokers. Nonsmokers are affected by second-hand smoke (sidestream smoke); they, in effect, become passive smokers when exposed to cigarette smoke. Studies have indicated the association between cardiovascular mortality and passive smoking.[17] A recent report by the U.S. Environmental Protection Agency (EPA) estimated that second-hand cigarette smoke kills 53,000 nonsmokers per year. EPA also reported that cigarette smoke is a major cause of indoor air pollution.[18] The current public debate concerning passive smoking will only intensify in coming years as more links are identified between passive smoking and various diseases.

Cardiovascular Morbidity

Nicotine affects the cardiovascular system by (1) increasing the blood pressure; (2) stimulating the heart rate; (3) inducing electrocardiographic changes (nonspecific ST and T wave changes, an increased conduction velocity, or a propensity to arrhythmias); (4) exacerbating angina in coronary patients; and (5) diminishing left ventricular performance in coronary patients.[19]

Cancer

In 1964, the U.S. surgeon general based his initial warning of the health risks of smoking on the correlation between cigarette smoking and lung cancer. Since that time, many types of cancer have been linked to smoking, including bladder, breast, cervical, esophageal, kidney, laryngeal, lip, liver, lung, nasal, oral, pancreatic, pharyngeal, prostatic, skin, gastric, tongue, and tracheal.[20,21] These cancers have been shown to occur in active smokers. Several cancers (breast, cervical, lung) have been shown to also occur in passive smokers. In men, the leading cause of smoking-related cancer mortality is lung cancer.[20] For the past 40 years, the leading cause of smoking-related cancer mortality in women has been breast cancer; however, by the early 1990s, smoking-related lung cancer had overtaken breast cancer as the leading cause of cancer in women. Cigarette smoke contains 43 carcinogenic compounds including tars; gases (e.g., carbon monoxide, hydrogen cyanide, nitrous oxide); and volatile chemicals (e.g., dioxin, formaldehyde, acrolein, benzene).

Respiratory Complications

The respiratory effects of smoking were among the first to be quantified. As early as the 1970s, smoking's negative effects on chronic obstructive pulmonary disease (COPD) were reported. At present, cigarette smoking is the chief avoidable cause of COPD.[22] In fact, 80% to 90% of COPD is caused by cigarette smoking. Smokers have a higher prevalence of cough and a greater production of phlegm in comparison with nonsmokers. Further, cigarette smoking is the major cause of COPD deaths in the United States. Rates of COPD mortality are greater in male smokers than in female smokers, reflecting men's greater consumption of cigarettes.

Lung diseases that result from smoking or conditions affected by smoking include allergies, asthma, bronchitis, emphysema, persistent cough, and pneumonia. In the large airways, smoking increases mucus secretion, cough, and sputum production. In the smaller airways, it produces inflammation, ulceration, and squamous metaplasia (abnormal replacement of squamous cells by cells of another type). These effects lead to fibrosis and airway narrowing.[22]

The most common symptoms related to passive smoking are eye irritation, headaches, cough, nasal irritation, wheezing, sore throat, and hoarseness.[23] Perhaps the most profound effects are on the lungs and respiratory system. When compared with children of nonsmokers, children of smokers have higher rates of respiratory tract infections, pneumonia, wheezing, sore throats, asthma, bronchitis, and otitis media.

Effects on Pregnancy

Smoking during pregnancy is harmful to the health of both the mother and fetus. The adverse effects of smoking on pregnancy include miscarriages, full-term babies with low birth-weights, perinatal deaths, birth defects, and preterm births. The occurrence of sudden infant death syndrome (SIDS) has also been causally linked to parental smoking behavior.[24]

Other Complications

Other disease states that are influenced by smoking[25–33] include allergies, Alzheimer's disease, cataracts, depression, diabetes, gastrointestinal disease (ulcers), Graves' ophthalmopathy, periodontal disease, and peripheral vascular disease. Table 42–1 summarizes nicotine's effect on these conditions. Some of these relationships are presently unconfirmed; for example, the data that link the occurrence of Alzheimer's disease to smoking need further clarification and amplification. Other relationships, however, are firmly established (e.g., allergies, angina, cardiovascular disease, congestive heart failure, hypertension, impotence, peripheral vascular disease). Still other relationships (e.g., ulcers, other gastrointestinal diseases) are influenced by factors such as alcohol consumption, eating habits, and duration of both the medical condition and smoking. Finally, diabetes is influenced by many factors: stress, diet, alcohol consumption, and smoking. Because nicotine can stimulate carbohydrate metabolism, diabetes is much harder to control in the smoker.

Nicotine–Drug Interactions

It may be difficult to distinguish the effect of smoking on disease states from its effect on the drugs used to treat the disease. Because of these dual effects, patients must be made

Table 42–1

Selected Disease States Adversely Affected by Smoking

Disease State	Effect of Smoking
Allergies[a]	Exacerbated allergic symptoms
Angina pectoris[a]	Increased angina symptomatology; more frequent attacks
Cataracts	Increased incidence of cataracts and lens opacities in moderate to heavy smoking (posterior subcapsular)
Chronic obstructive pulmonary disease[a]	Increased incidence of bronchitis, emphysema, asthma, and other respiratory disorders; limited daily activities; decreased tolerance for exercise; decreased quality of life
Depression	Common factors (stress, anxiety, etc.) predispose individuals to both smoking and depressive symptomatology
Diabetes mellitus	Impaired glycemic control; increased gluconeogenesis
Graves' disease	Greatly increased risk for Graves' ophthalmopathy
Hypertension[a]	Elevated blood pressure (in smokers)
Gastrointestinal disease, infections, etc.	Increased incidence of peptic ulcer disease; delayed ulcer healing; increased susceptibility to *Helicobacter pylori* infection
Periodontal disease	Negative impact on oral health
Peripheral vascular disease	Increased incidence of deep vein thrombosis; intermittent claudication

[a] Active and passive (i.e., those exposed to secondhand or sidestream smoke) smokers experience these effects.

Table 42–2

Nicotine–Drug Interactions

Drug Class	Effect
Analgesics	Decreased efficacy of acetaminophen and nonsteroidal anti-inflammatory drugs, resulting in the need for larger doses to achieve the desired effect
Anticoagulants (heparin, sodium warfarin)	Increased platelet activity, resulting in diminished efficacy of the anticoagulants
Cardiovascular agents (beta blockers, calcium channel blockers, furosemide and other loop-type diuretics, thiazide diuretics)	Decreased activity of the drugs, making the underlying conditions more difficult to treat
Estrogens (estrogen replacements for postmenopausal women, oral contraceptives containing estrogens)	Increased risk in female smokers for thromboembolic disorders (e.g., stroke, myocardial infarct, deep vein thrombosis)
Histamine$_2$-receptor antagonists (cimetidine, famotidine, nizatidine, ranitidine)	Increased acid production in the gut, resulting in decreased or negated effect of the H_2-receptor antagonists
Insulin	Decreased subcutaneous insulin absorption, possibly requiring an increase in insulin dosage
Psychotropics (barbiturates, benzodiazepines, phenothiazines, and tricyclic antidepressants)	Decreased efficacy, delayed effects, or increased dose required
Theophylline	Increased metabolism of theophylline, requiring increased doses because of the decreased half-life of theophylline and its derivatives; when the smoker successfully stops smoking, the dose of theophylline should be decreased
Vitamins	Decreased levels of vitamin C

aware of the influence of smoking on many physiologic, therapeutic, and disease state processes. Studies have identified many interactions between smoking and medications. One interaction, the effect of smoking on drug metabolism, is well documented. The primary mechanism for interactions appears to be the induction of hepatic microsomal enzymes by compounds present in tobacco smoke. Table 42–2 lists the medications affected by smoking and the subsequent effects.[34–37]

Alternate therapy may be available for some patients who cannot stop smoking. For example, the ulcer patient could instead take sucralfate. It does not influence acid production, but rather coats the site of ulceration with a spongy film, thus allowing the ulcerated lesion to heal. The patient's continuing to smoke, however, will delay healing. Patients who have other conditions and who stop smoking may need to decrease their medication dosages (e.g., diabetes patients who take insulin, or patients who take theophylline).

The precise mechanisms of these interactions remain unclear. It is not known whether the effect is caused by tobacco substrates (nicotine or others) or perhaps by other byproducts of smoking (polycyclic aromatic hydrocarbons). Nevertheless, it is important for patients to be aware of what is occurring and why. They may try to stop smoking if they can be convinced that it is futile to try to influence other disease states and attendant drug therapies while continuing to smoke. Despite a medication's demonstrated efficacy in nonsmokers or appropriate compliance by the smoking patient, the negative health effects of smoking and the associated lack of response to the medication can eventually overcome and negate any drug therapy.

Treatment of Nicotine Addiction

To become a nonsmoker, the individual must overcome the powerful addiction to nicotine. Nicotine addiction is difficult to overcome even after a period of successful abstinence. Research has shown that relapse can occur years after cessation of use because of the complex character of nicotine addiction.[38] Maintaining cessation remains a difficult task for many individuals regardless of the smoking cessation method they used.[39] Few individuals are successful in their first attempt. In fact, smoking cessation may be regarded as a cycle in which the individual smoker has to attempt to stop smoking several times before achieving the goal permanently.[40] Similar to heroin, morphine, cocaine, or alcohol, nicotine is an addictive drug of abuse, and, as such, treatment of nicotine addiction should address nicotine-related withdrawal symptoms.[41]

Treatment Outcomes

The goals of any treatment for smoking cessation are to (1) have the individual quit smoking and (2) maintain the cessation. Nicotine addition is very powerful, so the person attempting to quit can greatly benefit from the knowledge and expertise of the pharmacist.

General Treatment Approach

In 1996, the Agency for Health Care Policy Research (AHCPR) published a clinical practice guideline titled *Smoking Cessation. Clinical Practice Guideline No. 18.*[42] The guidelines contain the following six major recommendations:

- Every person who smokes should be offered smoking cessation treatment at every office visit.
- Clinicians should ask and record the tobacco-use status of every patient.
- Cessation treatment even as brief as 3 minutes is effective.
- The more intense the treatment, the more effective it is in producing long-term abstinence from tobacco.
- Nicotine replacement therapy (NRT) using nicotine patches or gum, clinician-delivered social support, and skills training are effective components of smoking cessation treatment.
- Health care systems should be modified to routinely identify and intervene with all tobacco users at every visit.[42]

The treatment algorithm in Figure 42–1 is based on the AHCPR guidelines and available product information.

Nicotine is similar to other addictive substances because of its psychoactive effect, compulsive use, and requirement to take more of the substance over time to obtain the same level of "high."[44] Researchers have noted that in such addictions the chemical factor is in control of behavior, and treatment is helped by dealing with the drug-related factors. In the case of nicotine, the withdrawal symptoms that occur upon abstinence must be dealt with if smoking cessation is to be successful.[44]

The response to withdrawal symptoms is highly variable among patients and depends on the length of exposure (i.e., how long the patient has been a smoker), dose (i.e., how much the patient smoked per day), and other unquantifiable effects. As with many other drugs, the individual's physiologic response to nicotine varies from person to person. Thus, the addiction and response to nicotine are also patient specific. Some smokers can stop and suffer virtually no withdrawal symptoms; others are dramatically influenced by withdrawal symptoms. Recognizing this interindividual variation plus the subsequent occurrence of withdrawal symptoms in some patients is key to pharmacists and others who help patients to successfully stop smoking. Successful programs address both the physical (pharmacologic) and psychologic (nonpharmacologic) aspects of nicotine addiction. None of the interventions will work optimally unless the smoker wants to stop smoking and maintain cessation.

Currently, there is controversy about the use of NRT during pregnancy. Cigarette smoking is a preventable cause of fetal morbidity and mortality; however, the pharmacologic adjuncts to smoking cessation that are now available are contraindicated during pregnancy. Benowitz[45] has recommended examining in clinical settings the use of NRT in pregnant women who smoke, particularly in those who smoke 20 or more cigarettes per day and who have been unsuccessful with behavioral smoking cessation therapies.

Other exclusions to self-treatment for nicotine gums and patches include breast-feeding, presence of cardiovascular disease, use of antidepressants, or use of nicotine in patients younger than 18 years. Contraindications specific to nicotine gum include esophagitis, peptic ulcer disease, and use of insulin or asthma medications. Contraindications specific to nicotine patches include skin problems or allergies to adhesive tape.

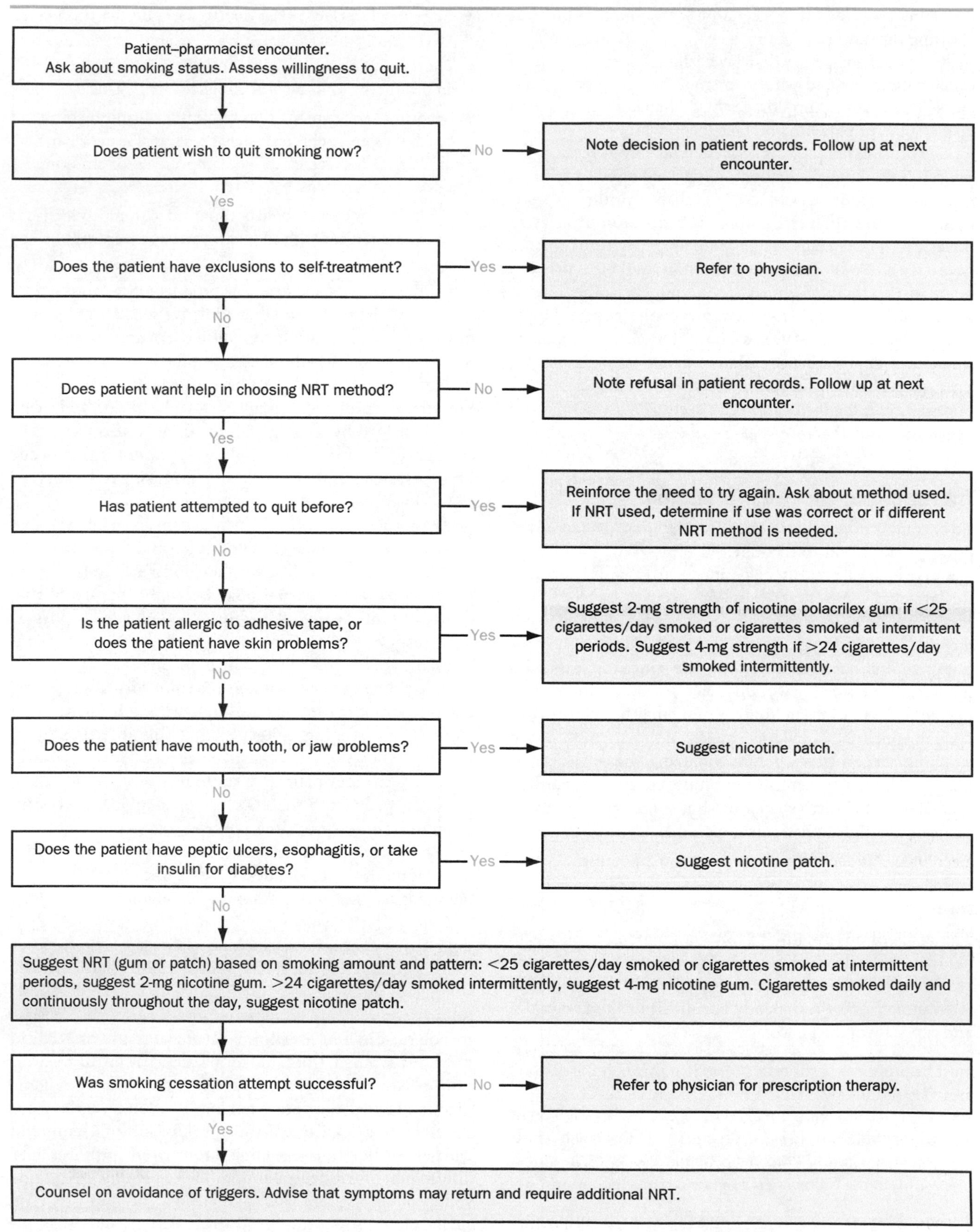

Figure 42–1 Self-care of nicotine addiction.

Nonpharmacologic Therapy

Behavioral interventions used in smoking cessation therapies have included aversion therapy, educational programs, group therapy, hypnosis, and self-help literature. The success rate for each of these modalities varies; as would be expected, each is patient dependent. Some smokers can stop smoking through behavioral modification alone. Programs have been developed to help smokers learn to avoid certain stimuli to smoking. Patients are counseled to deal with the urge to smoke after a meal by taking a walk or doing exercise and by practicing stress management as a method to control their responses to stimuli, such as anxiety, that would normally result in their smoking. Patients are also advised to avoid places or environments in which they usually smoked and to substitute alternate behaviors when the urge to smoke does occur. However, the more highly addicted smoker usually needs pharmacologic assistance.

Pharmacologic Therapy

When a patient presents for help in quitting smoking, NRT is a recommended first option to try. Currently, four dosage forms of nicotine replacement are approved by the Food and Drug Administration (FDA): (1) nicotine transdermal systems (nonprescription and prescription), (2) nicotine nasal spray (prescription only), (3) nicotine polacrilex gum (nonprescription), and (4) nicotine inhaler (prescription only). The initial intent of NRT is to substitute pharmacologically dosed nicotine for "smoked" nicotine. Through a tapering of nicotine doses from cigarettes to NRT, the patient is gradually weaned from higher to lower doses. Because the nicotine addiction is decreased, smokers should have successfully modified their behavior to the point that environmental and behavioral stimuli to smoke are no longer effective. Pharmacologic treatment with NRT should optimally be accompanied by behavioral counseling and patient counseling.

Although replacing nicotine from smoking with a pharmacologic source and dose reduces the craving and withdrawal symptoms, the pharmacologic dose usually does not relieve these symptoms to the same degree as smoked nicotine. Thus, any smoker who expects the same "smoking effect" from NRT products may be disappointed.[52] NRT is designed to be used short term (6 months or less) to reduce the magnitude of the nicotine withdrawal syndrome experienced by smokers who stop smoking "cold turkey."

After a patient completes a course of NRT, the pharmacist must be prepared to support the patient through the discontinuance of therapy. The true measure of success lies in examining the cessation rate after the patient is weaned from the product. The cessation rate can be improved through appropriate behavioral counseling of the former smoker.

Nicotine Polacrilex Gum

In 1996, the FDA approved nonprescription use of nicotine polacrilex resin.[53] This agent was first approved for prescription use in the United States in 1984. When used correctly, nicotine polacrilex gum (Nicorette) has been shown to reduce withdrawal symptoms and to increase cessation rates when compared with the use of a placebo. Patients must understand how to use the resin dosage form (gum), how much to use per day, how long to use it, and how to stop use gradually. Strict patient adherence and cessation of product use are required if patients are to become free of nicotine use. Ensuring a patient's adherence with any therapy is difficult, let alone a therapy that requires an initial dosing of 12 units to 24 units per day.

Dosage/Administration Guidelines Nicotine polacrilex gum is available in two package sizes: a starter kit containing 108 units and a supplemental package containing 48 units. Each package size is available in either the 2-mg or the 4-mg dose. The 4-mg dosage packages are targeted to those individuals who smoke more than 24 cigarettes per day.

The Nicorette package contains a cassette tape that provides instructions for use as well as a printed user's guide. The FDA considers these items to be part of the product labeling. Table 42–3 provides specific guidelines for using nicotine gums.[54]

The bite-and-park method described in the table permits nicotine in the saliva to be absorbed into the bloodstream through the buccal mucosa. If the patient swallows the nicotine with saliva or washes it down when drinking a hot or cold liquid, it will not be effective and may cause side effects such as heartburn, upset stomach, or hiccups. A basic pH is required for the nicotine to be properly released from the dosing piece into the saliva and then through the buccal mucosa. Thus, the patient must avoid consuming acidic liquids while the dosing piece is in the mouth. Nicotine polacrilex gum is sugar free and, although somewhat sticky, is suitable for use by many denture wearers.

Adverse Effects If the nicotine gum causes hiccups, nausea, an upset stomach, or a sore throat, the patient is probably not using the product properly. The pharmacist should counsel the patient not to chew the dosing piece like regular chewing gum, but to park and retrieve the dose of nicotine polacrilex gum sporadically. After a few days, the patient will automatically adjust the rate of dosing through the park and retrieval process.

Contraindications/Precautions/Warnings Several of the same warnings appear on the product labeling for nicotine polacrilex gum and for nicotine transdermal system. Such products are contraindicated for pregnant or breast-feeding patients, as well as for patients with cardiovascular disease. Nicotine can increase heart rate in patients who have heart disease or an irregular heartbeat, or who have had a recent heart attack. It can also increase blood pressure in patients with hypertension that is not controlled with medication. Such products are also contraindicated in patients who take medications for depression. Dosages of these medications may have to be adjusted during NRT. Patients younger than 18 years of age and those who continue to use other forms of nicotine are also warned not to use NRT products.[54]

Table 42-3

Administration Guidelines for Nicotine Polacrilex Gum

- Before using this product, carefully read the user's guide.
- Do not start using nicotine polacrilex gum until you have stopped smoking.
- Do not smoke cigarettes or use other forms of nicotine (e.g., nicotine patches, snuff, chewing tobacco, pipes, cigars, etc.) while using nicotine polacrilex gum.
- Be aware that nicotine polacrilex gum is purposely made not to taste like ordinary chewing gum. It is a dose delivery device, not a chewing gum.
- Be aware that it may take several days to adjust to the product's taste and the special manner in which it should be used.
- Use the product on a scheduled rather than an as-needed basis.
- Follow the dosage regimen carefully and reduce the dosage at the recommended intervals.
- Use this product according to the following 12-week schedule:
  —*Weeks 1–6*: Use one piece every 1–2 hours.
  —*Weeks 7–9*: Use one piece every 2–4 hours.
  —*Weeks 10–12*: Use one piece every 4–8 hours.
- Do not use more than 24 pieces per day.
- Do not eat or drink for 15 minutes before using this product or while using it.
- If acidic drinks (e.g., fruit juices, cola drinks, coffee) or foods (e.g., catsup, soy sauce, salsa, or hot sauce) have been consumed, rinse the mouth with water before placing the gum in the mouth.
- To take advantage of the product's slow release formula, use the bite-park-bite rotation method:
  —Bite each piece slowly (10–15 times) until a peppery taste or tingling sensation occurs.
  —When this sensation begins, place the gum between the upper or lower cheek and gums for approximately 1 minute.
  —After the peppery taste fades, retrieve the dosing piece and repeat the process. (Keep the dosing piece in the mouth for approximately 30 minutes.)
  —If biting the gum becomes tedious, push the gum from the outside of the cheek with a finger to expose a new surface of the gum to the saliva.
- Be aware that chewing the gum too quickly will result in an unpleasant taste caused by too much nicotine in the saliva and, if the nicotine is swallowed, may cause effects similar to those produced by excess smoking (e.g., nausea [especially if the stomach is empty], irritation of the throat, hiccups, light-headedness).
- Carry at least one full sleeve of nicotine polacrilex gum (12 doses per sleeve) at all times. Keep it in the same place where cigarettes were normally kept (e.g., shirt pocket or purse).
- Do not expose the product to extreme temperatures (i.e., place in a glove box, next to a source of heat, etc.).
- Remember to keep an extra sleeve of the product in the car, at work, or by the telephone.
- Keep this product out of the reach of children or pets.
- Stop using the product at the end of week 10. If you still feel the need for its use, talk with your physician.
- If a problem or severe symptoms develop, report them to a pharmacist or physician.

Source: Reference 43.

Contraindications specific to nicotine polacrilex gum include patients with esophagitis or peptic ulcer disease and patients taking insulin for diabetes or asthma medications.[13] Use of nicotine polacrilex gum should stop if (1) mouth, teeth, or jaw problems develop; (2) irregular heartbeat or palpitations occur; and (3) symptoms of nicotine overdose (e.g., nausea, vomiting, dizziness, weakness, and rapid heartbeat) occur.

Nicotine Transdermal Systems

On April 19, 1996, an FDA advisory panel voted that two nicotine transdermal systems (NTS) products, Nicotrol and Nicoderm CQ, should be available for nonprescription use. Subsequently, both products have been made available as nonprescription products. In addition, ProStep is now available as a nonprescription therapy. Habitrol is a nonprescription product in Canada.

Nicotrol, ProStep, and generic formulations have a recommended treatment period of 6 weeks, and Nicoderm CQ has a recommended treatment period of 10 weeks. Nicoderm CQ is a tapered (step) therapy. Nicotrol, ProStep, and generic formulations (22-mg and 11-mg patches) are a one-step dosage therapy. It is recommended that the 22-mg patch be used daily for 6 weeks if the patient smokes equal to or more than 16 cigarettes per day, and that the 11-mg patch be used daily for 6 weeks if 15 or fewer cigarettes are smoked daily.

If an NTS is used, the patient must understand the purpose of the patches, their proper application, and the appropriate time to stop using them. Table 42–4 lists specific instructions for using this dosage form of NRT.

Contraindications/Precautions/Warnings As with the nicotine gum, contraindications for the use of NTS include patients who are pregnant or breast-feeding, have cardiovascular disease, use antidepressants, or are younger than 18 years of age. Contraindications specific to NTS include patients who are allergic to adhesive tape or have dermatologic problems.

The use of NTS should stop and a physician should be consulted if (1) skin redness caused by the patch does not go away after 4 days, (2) the skin swells or a rash develops, (3) irregular heart beat or palpitations occur, or (4) signs of nicotine overdose (e.g., nausea, vomiting, dizziness, weakness, or rapid heart beat) develop.

Nicotine Nasal Spray

In March 1996, the FDA approved nicotine nasal spray for use as a prescription smoking cessation therapy. The patient using this therapy must understand the purpose of the spray, its proper use, and the appropriate method of stopping its use (i.e., stopping use gradually at the appropriate time).

Table 42–4

Administration Guidelines for Nicotine Transdermal Systems

- Each day apply a new patch to a different place on skin that is dry, clean, and hairless.
- If the application site is washed with soap, rinse and dry the skin. Soap will increase penetration of nicotine into the skin.
- Wash your hands after applying or removing the nicotine transdermal systems. Do not touch the eyes or mouth with your fingers before washing them.
- Apply the patch to the chest, upper arms, shoulders, or hips.
- Be aware that a 24-hour patch may be worn for 16 or 24 hours, whereas a 16-hour patch should be only worn for 16 hours.
- If you crave cigarettes upon awakening, wear the 24-hour patch for 24 hours.
- If you have vivid dreams or other sleep disruptions, use either the 16-hour hour patch or remove the 24-hour patch after 16 hours (during waking hours).
- Do not leave the 24-hour patch on for more than 24 hours, or leave the 16-hour patch on for more than 16 hours.
- Remove and replace the patch at the same time each day.
- Discard the removed patch in the pouch the new patches come in. Keep the discarded patches away from children and pets.

Nicotine Inhaler

In September 1998, the FDA approved a nicotine inhaler for use as a prescription smoking cessation therapy. The Nicotrol inhaler (nicotine inhalation system) is the first FDA-approved smoking cessation that provides smokers with the comfort of the hand-to-mouth smoking ritual, although the clinical importance of such behavior in quitting smoking is, as yet, unknown.

Other Prescription Therapies

In May 1997, an oral anti-depressant drug (bupropion, Zyban), was approved for use as a smoking cessation therapy. This drug is available only by prescription. Nicotine replacement therapies in combination with prescription-only therapies (bupropion or a nicotine nasal spray) have also been used with success. Also, both forms of nonprescription nicotine replacement (nicotine polacrilex gum and nicotine transdermal systems) have been used concurrently in recalcitrant smokers. Patients who have been unsuccessful in quitting while attempting nonprescription NRTs may be candidates for referral to their primary care physician so they can consider using combination therapies.

Effectiveness of Nicotine Replacement Therapies

It is estimated that smoking cessation interventions are extremely cost-effective when one considers other preventive health interventions. Further, the more extensive the intervention, the more cost-effective the interventions become.[55] Researchers have examined NRT, and have suggested that—in comparison with prescription availability of NRT—nonprescription availability would result in more successful quitters, fewer smoking-attributable deaths, and increased life expectance for current smokers.[56] Elsewhere, researchers have found that potential quitters who are willing to use NRT as a nonprescription therapy may have fewer or less-severe factors for relapse.[56]

A comparison of the success rates achieved with the various NRTs can be found in Table 42–5.

Product Selection Guidelines

Based on contraindications, nicotine polacrilex gum is the best choice for patients with allergies to adhesive tape or skin problems, whereas nicotine transdermal systems are the best choice for patients who have esophagitis or peptic ulcer disease or who take insulin for diabetes or asthma medications. Some patients, however, may object to the taste of the nicotine gum or the frequency of doses. Others may derive oral gratification from the tactile nature of the gum.

Barring the presence of contraindications, the faster onset of nicotine delivery through the gum also makes it the best choice for patients who smoke intermittently throughout the day or smoke intensely for short periods followed by periods of no smoking. Similarly, patients who smoke continuously throughout the day would benefit most from the sustained and steady release of nicotine from a transdermal system. Finally, the level of dependence should influence the choice of

Case Study 42–2

Patient Complaint/History

Imogene, a 35-year-old woman, presents to the pharmacist holding a carton of cigarettes and a 108-unit 4-mg package of Nicorette. Numerous earlier attempts to help the patient stop smoking have been unsuccessful. When questioned about the Nicorette, the patient indicates she wishes to try to stop smoking "a little at a time" using this product. She says she smokes a pack per day, usually on work breaks and in the evening. On separate occasions, she previously tried a 24-hour and a 16-hour NTS without success. The patient admits she just could not stop smoking, even when using the NTS.

A review of the patient profile reveals the following current prescriptions: propranolol 40 mg, one tablet bid for hypertension (#60 filled monthly); and Nordette, one tablet daily (#28 filled monthly). While filling the oral contraceptive prescription, the pharmacist notes the presence of tobacco flakes behind the tape covering the label on the container.

Clinical Considerations/Strategies

Readers can use the following considerations/strategies to determine whether treatment of the patient's condition with nonprescription drugs is warranted:

- Counsel the patient on potential interactions between smoking and her current medications.
- Assess the willingness of the patient to stop smoking.
- Determine why the NTS therapies might have failed.

Patient Education/Counseling

Readers can use the following strategies to develop a patient education/counseling plan that will help ensure optimal therapeutic outcomes:

- Develop a pharmaceutical care plan for the patient's smoking cessation efforts.
- Continue to educate and counsel the patient on smoking cessation options.
- Contact the patient's physicians and explain the pharmaceutical care plan.

Table 42–5

Success Rates Achieved with Nicotine Replacement Therapies

Type of NRT	Rate of Success (%)	Period of Assessment
Nicotine polacrilex gum, 4 mg	39	12 months[a]
Nicotine polacrilex gum, 2 mg	16	12 months[a]
Nicotine transdermal patch	22–42	6 months[b]
Nicotine transdermal patch	27	6 months[c]
(Estimates for transdermal patch based on meta-analysis of studies including 5098 patients.)		
Nicotine nasal spray	27	12 months[d]
Nicotine inhaler	15	12 months[e]
All forms of nicotine replacement	19	12 months[f]
(Estimates for sprays and inhalers based on meta-analysis of studies including 18,000 patients.)		

[a] Source: Reference 46.
[b] Source: Reference 47.
[c] Source: Reference 48.
[d] Source: Reference 49.
[e] Source: Reference 50.
[f] Source: Reference 51.

strength of the therapy chosen. For example, a person on NTS therapy who craves cigarettes upon awakening should wear the 24-hour patch for the entire period. Patients with a heavy dependence on nicotine who choose the gum may need the 4-mg strength to cope with cravings for cigarettes.

Table 42–6 lists examples of commercially available products for both types of nonprescription NRT.

Patient Assessment of Nicotine Addiction

To help the smoker succeed at smoking cessation, the pharmacist must help patients evaluate how they smoke, what they have or have not tried in the past, and what their willingness is to try differing smoking cessation therapies. Analyzing smoking patterns and the reasons for smoking helps in assessing the degree of nicotine dependence. A valuable tool to help pharmacists determine the degree of patient nicotine dependence is the validated Fagerström Test for Nicotine Dependence. (See Table 42–7.) The pharmacist can use this short assessment (six questions) tool to help patients choose the appropriate NRT. For example, less-dependent smokers may be best aided by lower dosage forms of NRT. Conversely, heavily addicted smokers may need the highest strength of NRT, or perhaps prescription strength therapies.[57]

Concerning assessment, the American Psychiatric Association (APA)[58] recommends the diagnostic criteria in Table 42–8 be coupled with the Fagerström test to determine the degree of nicotine dependence. Again, such assessments are potential aids to help patients understand the addictive nature of nicotine and the various smoking cessation methods.

Table 42–6

Selected Products for Nicotine Replacement Therapy

Trade Name	Primary Ingredients
NicoDerm CQ Transdermal Patch	Nicotine 7 mg; 14 mg; 21 mg
Nicorette Gum	Nicotine polacrilex 2 mg
Nicorette DS Gum	Nicotine polacrilex 4 mg
Nicotrol Transdermal Patch	Nicotine 15 mg

Table 42–7

Fagerström Test for Nicotine Dependence

Questions/Responses	Points
1. How soon after you wake up do you smoke your first cigarette?	
Within 5 minutes	3
6–30 minutes	2
31–60 minutes	1
After 60 minutes	0
2. Do you find it difficult to refrain from smoking in places where it is forbidden (e.g., in church, at the library, in a movie theater, etc.)?	
Yes	1
No	0
3. Which cigarette would you hate most to give up?	
The first one in the morning	1
All others	0
4. How many cigarettes per day do you smoke?	
10 or less	0
11–20	1
21–30	2
>31	3
5. Do you smoke more frequently during the first hours after waking than during the rest of the day?	
Yes	1
No	0
6. Do you smoke if you are so ill that you are in bed most of the day?	
Yes	1
No	0

Source: Reference 57; used with permission from Carfax Publishing Ltd., PO Box 25, Abingdon, Oxfordshire OX14 3UE UK.

Asking patients the following additional questions will help elicit further information needed to accurately assess the level of nicotine dependence and to recommend the appropriate smoking cessation method for the patient's health status and lifestyle.

Table 42–8

Diagnostic Criteria for Nicotine Dependence

Nicotine dependence is a maladaptive pattern of substance use that leads to clinically significant impairment or distress, as manifested by three or more of the following criteria, which can occur at any time in the same 12-month period.

1. Tolerance is defined by either of the following:
   —A need for markedly increased amounts of the substance to achieve intoxication or desired effect, or
   —Markedly diminished effect with continued use of the same amount of the substance.
2. Withdrawal is manifested by either of the following:
   —The characteristic withdrawal syndrome for the substance, or
   —The same (or a closely related) substance taken to relieve or to avoid withdrawal symptoms.
3. The substance is often taken in a larger amount or over a longer period than was intended.
4. There is a persistent desire or unsuccessful efforts to cut down or control substance use.
5. A great deal of time is spent in activities necessary to obtain the substance, use the substance (e.g., chain-smoking), or recover from its effects.
6. Important social, occupational, or recreational activities are given up or reduced because of substance abuse.
7. The substance use is continued despite knowledge of having a persistent or recurrent physical or psychologic problem that is likely to have been caused or exacerbated by the substance (e.g., nicotine use despite physician's orders to cease smoking because of emphysema, chronic obstructive pulmonary disease, peptic ulcer, or heart disease).

Source: Adapted from Reference 58; used with permission.

Q~ Do you currently smoke?

A~ Tailor recommendations for smoking cessation to the patient's smoking status. For example, advise patients who have stopped smoking but are experiencing withdrawal symptoms how to cope with the symptoms. For patients who are still smoking, inform them of the initial steps in smoking cessation.

Q~ How many cigarettes do you smoke per day? How long have you smoked?

A~ Use the patient's answers to these questions, along with the results of the Fagerström Test, as a guide to estimating level of dependence. (See Table 42–7.) Remember, however, the level of dependence is patient specific.

Q~ Have you tried to stop smoking before? If yes, which smoking cessation methods did you use?

A~ If a particular method was used, evaluate whether the patient implemented it properly. If the use was improper, advise the patient of the proper method of implementation. In cases in which implementation was correct, either rule out the method or consider it as an adjunctive measure in the new smoking cessation plan.

Q~ If you have not tried to stop smoking before, are you ready to do so now?

A~ Advise the patient that quitting smoking requires a high level of commitment. If the patient is not ready to make the commitment, suggest postponing the attempt to quit until a later time.

Q~ Have you sought help from a physician or other health professional?

A~ If so, find out what methods were recommended and whether the patient implemented them correctly.

Q~ What other prescription or nonprescription medications are you currently taking?

A~ *Identify potential nicotine–drug interactions. (See Table 42–2.)* Advise patients taking such medications to see a physician for possible adjustments to the drug therapy.

The following questions are appropriate for patients who choose NRT as a smoking cessation method.

Q~ Are you interested in trying nicotine replacement therapies (nicotine polacrilex gum or nicotine transdermal systems)? If so, do you understand how to use these products?

A~ Make sure the patient knows that this therapy precludes the use of nicotine in any form: smoking cigarettes, cigars, or pipes; dipping snuff ; chewing tobacco; or using nicotine prescription products (nicotine inhaler or nicotine nasal spray).

Q~ If the patient is a woman, are you pregnant or breast-feeding?

A~ Advise a pregnant patient that the use of nicotine replacement therapy during pregnancy is a much safer option than continuing to smoke. But advise her to get her physician's approval for using this therapy.

Q~ Do you have heart disease or an irregular heartbeat, or have you had a recent heart attack? Do you have high blood pressure not controlled with medication?

A~ Advise a patient with cardiovascular disease that the disorder does not preclude use of nicotine replacement therapy. Stress that the patient's physician should, however, approve use of this therapy.

Q~ Do you have, or have you had, esophagitis or peptic ulcer disease? Do you have tooth, mouth, or jaw problems such as active temporomandibular joint disease?

A~ Advise a patient with any of these disorders that nicotine polacrilex gum may aggravate esophagitis or peptic ulcer disease and that oral problems will make chewing the gum difficult. Recommend transdermal nicotine systems instead.

Q~ Are you allergic to adhesive materials that are present in first aid bandages or tape?

A~ Advise a patient who has such hypersensitivity to use nicotine polacrilex gum instead.

Patient Counseling for Nicotine Addiction

The success of any NRT depends on a behavioral change in the patient. The patient must truly desire to stop smoking and must alter habits and behaviors to accommodate a nicotine-free existence. Support and encouragement (from family, friends, and health care providers) and proper patient counseling are also important so the patient can achieve success with any of the smoking cessation therapies.

Various associations and societies (e.g., American Cancer Society, American Heart Association, American Lung Association) offer self-help literature to help smokers grapple with the periods before, during, and after smoking cessation. Available information helps smokers understand the reasons to stop smoking and how to do it. Again, success varies and depends on individual motivations. Phone numbers for each of these organizations are listed in telephone directories in most communities.

Table 42–9 lists other information sources for smoking cessation or for people with nicotine dependence. As is noted, many sources are now available through the internet to allow the smoker, family member, or health professional to obtain further information about how to help smokers quit.

It is professionally important for pharmacists to encourage and counsel patients who smoke or use other forms of nicotine to become nicotine free. Pharmacists may be reluctant to counsel patients to stop smoking because they fear alienating them. However, as health professionals, pharmacists should not fear letting their patients understand that they care enough about each patient to encourage this important health promotion and disease prevention activity. Pharmacists can set a good example by not using nicotine and by discouraging colleagues from doing so as well. The sale of tobacco products in pharmacies has been much debated and remains an ethical and individual decision for pharmacists. Making the pharmacy area a "smoke-free" area establishes a good example. Signs and reminders indicating that the area is smoke free can communicate the message without offending anyone. For patients who indicate that they do not want to stop smoking, pressing the issue can only lead to potential frustration. However, for the current smoker, even one who professes not to want to stop smoking, counseling on the benefits of smoking cessation should

Table 42–9

Information Sources on Smoking Cessation

Disease-Based Organizations
American Cancer Society 1599 Clifton Road, NE Atlanta, GA 30329-4251 (800) ACS-2345 ([800] 227-2345) www.cancer.org www.cancer.org/gasp
American Heart Association 7320 Greenville Avenue Dallas, TX 75231 (214) 750-5300 www.americanheart.org
American Lung Association 1740 Broadway New York, NY 10019-4374 (212) 315-8700 (800) LUNG-USA ([800] 586-4872) www.lungusa.org
U.S. Federal Government Agencies
Office on Smoking and Health Centers for Disease Control and Prevention Mail Stop K-50, 1600 Clifton Road, NE Atlanta, GA 30333 (404) 488-5705 www.cdc.gov/tobacco
National Cancer Institute 9000 Rockville Pike Building 31, 4A-18 Bethesda, MD 20892 (800) 4-CANCER ([800] 422-6237) www.cancernet.nci.nih.gov
Other Information Sources
The Foundation for Innovations in Nicotine Dependence (FIND) www.findhelp.com
Action on Smoking and Health (ASH) 2013 H Street NW Washington, DC 20006 (202) 659-4310 www.ash.org
The QuitNet www.quitnet.org
Community Intervention, Inc. www.youthtobacco.com

be performed tactfully at every pharmacist–patient encounter.

Because of pharmacists' accessibility, trustworthiness, and knowledge base, patients view them as valued sources of information on any number of health concerns. Patients who smoke will not be surprised when a pharmacist asks questions about their nicotine use and counsels them to stop its use. The pharmacist should note on patient profiles any information about nicotine use.

If patients express a desire to stop nicotine use, pharmacists should advise them of available options (such as pharmacotherapy or support groups in the community), as well as explaining effective nondrug measures for smoking cessation. Such measures include (1) behaviors to avoid that traditionally reinforced the urge to smoke, (2) places or activities to avoid in which the individual previously would smoke, and (3) social and psychologic stimulators to avoid that previously influenced smoking.

The box "Patient Counseling for Nicotine Addiction" lists specific information about nonprescription NRT therapies to provide patients.

Evaluation of Patient Outcomes for Nicotine Addiction

The pharmacist should contact the patient regularly by phone to encourage compliance with the NRT if the patient does not present in person at the pharmacy during the first weeks of therapy. Such follow-up will strongly indicate concern about the attempt to quit smoking and will help the patient sustain his or her level of commitment to continue as a nonsmoker. Throughout the NRT, the patient will need praise for any progress made and encouragement to stay with the therapy.

CONCLUSIONS

Smoking continues to extract a tremendous toll on everyone in the United States. The economics alone are staggering. This is not just a U.S. problem: An estimated 3 million tobacco-related deaths occurred in the world during the 1990s alone.[59]

There has never been a better time for pharmacists to become involved as smoking cessation and patient advocates. Pharmacists must first identify which patients are smokers and then counsel those who wish to stop about the various options available and the success potential of each option.

Pharmacists should feel comfortable in recommending NRTs as smoking cessation nonprescription pharmacotherapy. After a treatment plan (whatever the makeup) is started, the pharmacist should be prepared to deliver pharmaceutical care by helping the patient follow through on the therapeutic plan. Helping the smoking patient stop smoking is one of the most needed and rewarding activities for pharmacists. Encouraging smoking cessation, monitoring patients who are using pharmacologic treatment for smoking cessation, and supporting the patients throughout the withdrawal symptom stage can provide therapeutic benefits for patients, savings on health care costs, economic benefits for pharmacists, and long-term enhancement of the patients' quality of life.

Patient Counseling for Nicotine Addiction

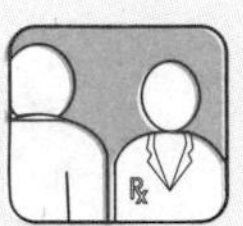

The objectives of self-treatment are to quit smoking and not start again. For most patients, carefully following product instructions for the selected nicotine replacement therapy, as well as the self-care measures listed below, will help ensure optimal therapeutic outcomes.

Nicotine Polacrilex Gum

- See Table 42–3 for guidelines on using this product.
- Do not use this product if you continue to smoke, chew tobacco, use snuff, or use a nicotine patch or other nicotine-containing product.
- Consult a physician before using this product if you
  —Are pregnant.
  —Are under 18 years of age.
  —Have heart disease or an irregular heartbeat or have had a recent heart attack. Nicotine can increase your heart rate.
  —Have high blood pressure not controlled with medication. Nicotine can increase blood pressure.
  —Have a history of, or currently have, esophagitis or peptic ulcer disease.
  —Take insulin for diabetes.
  —Take prescription medications for depression or asthma. The prescription dose may need to be adjusted.

Stop using this product and see your physician if you have

—Mouth, teeth, or jaw problems.

—Irregular heartbeat or palpitations.

—Symptoms of nicotine overdose such as nausea, vomiting, dizziness, weakness, and rapid heartbeat.

Nicotine Transdermal Patch

- See Table 42–4 for guidelines on using this product.
- Do not use this product if you continue to smoke, chew tobacco, use snuff, or use a nicotine patch or other nicotine-containing product.
- Consult a physician before using this product if you
  —Are pregnant.
  —Are under 18 years of age.
  —Have heart disease or an irregular heartbeat or have had a recent heart attack. Nicotine can increase your heart rate.
  —Have high blood pressure not controlled with medication. Nicotine can increase blood pressure.
  —Take insulin for diabetes.
  —Take prescription medications for depression. The prescription dose may need to be adjusted.

Stop use of the patch and see a physician if

—Skin redness caused by the patch does not go away after 4 days, or if skins swells or a rash develops.

—You develop irregular heartbeat or palpitations.

—You have symptoms of nicotine overdose such as nausea, vomiting, dizziness, weakness, and rapid heartbeat.

References

1. Lee EW, D'Alonzo GE. Cigarette smoking, nicotine addiction, and its pharmacologic treatment. *Arch Intern Med.* 1993;153:34–48.
2. Tobacco use – United States, 1900–1999. *MMWR Morb Mortal Wkly Rep.* 1999;48:986–93.
3. Giovino GA, Schooley MW, Zhu BP, et al. Surveillance of selected tobacco-use behaviors—United States, 1900–1994. *MMWR Morb Mortal Wkly Rep CDC Surveill Summ.* 1994;43:1-43.
4. Adams EK, Young TL. Costs of smoking: a focus on maternal, childhood, and other short-run costs. *Med Care Res Rev.* 1999;56:3–29.
5. Miller VP, Ernst C, Collin F. Smoking-attributable medical care costs in the USA. *Soc Sci Med.* 1999;48:375–91.
6. Goodwin PJ, Shepherd FA. Economic issues in lung cancer: a review. *J Clin Oncol.* 1998;16:3900–12.
7. Centers for Disease Control. State tobacco prevention and control activities: Results of the 1989–1990 Association of State and Territorial Health Officials (ASTHO) survey final report. *MMWR Morb Moral Wkly Rep.* 1991;40(RR–11):1–41.
8. Distefan JM, Gilpin EA, Sargent JD, et al. Do movie stars encourage adolescents to start smoking? Evidence from California. *Prev Med.* 1999;28:1–11.
9. Gottlieb A, Pope SK, Rickert VI, et al. Patterns of smokeless tobacco use by young adolescents. *Pediatrics.* 1993;91:75–8.
10. Coultas DB. The physician's role in smoking cessation. *Clin Chest Med.* 1991;12:755–68.
11. Haire-Joshu D, Morgan G, Fisher EB Jr. Determinants of cigarette smoking. *Clin Chest Med.* 1991;12:711–25.
12. Marwick C. Advocates say smoke free society eventually may result from more curbs, taxes on tobacco use. *JAMA.* 1993;269:724.
13. Cohen C, Pickworth WB, Henningfield JE. Cigarette smoking and addiction. *Clin Chest Med.* 1991;12:701–10.
14. Volle RL. Nicotine and ganglion blocking drugs. In: Smith CM, Reynard AM, eds. *Textbook of Pharmacology.* Philadelphia: WB Saunders; 1991:119–126.
15. Brunton SA, Henningfield JE. *Nicotine Addiction and Smoking Cessation.* New York: Medical Information Services; 1991.
16. Public Health Service, Office on Smoking and Health. *The Health Consequences of Smoking: Cardiovascular Disease.* DHHS (PHS) Pub No 84–50204. Washington, DC: US Department of Health and Human Services; 1983.
17. Glantz SA, Parmley WW. Passive smoking and heart disease. Epidemiology, physiology, and biochemistry. *Circulation.* 1991;83:1–12.
18. Lesmes GR, Donofrio KH. Passive smoking: the medical and economic issues. *Am J Med.* 1992;93:38S–42S.
19. Stimmel B. *Cardiovascular Effects of Mood-Altering Drugs.* New York: Raven Press; 1979:200.
20. Doll R. Uncovering the effects of smoking: historical perspective. *Stat Methods Med Res.* 1998;7:87–117.
21. Hecht SS. Tobacco and cancer: approaches using carcinogen biomarkers and chemoprevention. *Ann NY Acad Sci.* 1997;833:91–111.
22. Clark KD, Wardrobe-Wong N, Elliott JJ, et al. Cigarette smoke inhala-

tion and lung damage in smoking volunteers. *Eur Respir J.* 1998;12:395–9.

23. Golding J. Sudden infant death syndrome and parental smoking—a literature review. *Paediatr Perinat Epidemiol.* 1997;11:67–77.
24. Haglund B, Cnattingius S. Cigarette smoking as a risk factor for sudden infant death syndrome: a population-based study. *Am J Public Health.* 1990;80:29–32.
25. McGill HC Jr. The cardiovascular pathology of smoking. *Am Heart J.* 1988;115(1 Pt z):250–7.
26. Alderson MR, Lee PN, Wang R. Risks of lung cancer, chronic bronchitis, Ischaemic heart disease, and stroke in relation to type of cigarette smoked. *J Epidemiol Community Health.* 1985;39:286–93.
27. Amler RW, Eddins DL. Cross-sectional analysis: precursors of premature death in the United States. In: Amler RW, Dull HB, eds. *Closing the Gap: The Burden of Unnecessary Illness.* New York: Oxford University Press; 1987:181–7.
28. Lane MR, Lee SP. Recurrence of duodenal ulcer after medical treatment. *Lancet.* 1988;1:1147–9.
29. Hankinson SE, Willett WC, Colditz GA, et al. A prospective study of cigarette smoking and risk of cataract surgery in women. *JAMA.* 1992;268:994–8.
30. Breslau N, Kilbey MM, Andreski P. Nicotine dependence and major depression: new evidence from a prospective investigation. *Arch Gen Psychiatry.* 1993;50:31–5.
31. Locker D, Leake JL. Risk indicators and risk markers for periodontal disease experience in older adults living independently in Ontario, Canada. *J Dent Res.* 1993;72:9–17.
32. Prummel MF, Wiersinga WM. Smoking and the risk of Graves' disease. *JAMA.* 1993;269:479–82.
33. Bateson MC. Cigarette smoking and Helicobacter pylori infection. *Postgrad Med J.* 1993;69:41–4.
34. Lipman A. How smoking interferes with drug therapy. *Modern Med.* 1985;53:141–2.
35. Pelkonen O, Maenpaa J, Taavitsainen P, et al. Inhibition and induction of human cytochrome P450 (CYP) enzymes. *Xenobiotica.* 1998;28:1203–53.
36. Schein JR. Cigarette smoking and clinically significant drug interactions. *Ann Pharmacother.* 1995;29:1139–48.
37. Shoaf SE, Linnoila M. Interaction of ethanol and smoking on the pharmacokinetics and pharmacodynamics of psychotropic medications. *Psychopharmacol Bull.* 1991;27:577–94.
38. Stapleton J. Cigarette smoking, prevalence, cessation, and relapse. *Stat Methods Med Res.* 1998;7:187–203.
39. McIlvain HE, McKinney ME, Thompson AV, et al. Application of the MRFIT smoking cessation program to a healthy, mixed-sex sample. *Am J Prev Med.* 1992;8:165–70.
40. Jorenby DE. New developments in approaches to smoking cessation. *Cur Opin Pulm Med.* 1998;4:103–6.
41. Thompson GH, Hunter DA. Nicotine replacement therapy. *Ann Pharmacother.* 1998;32:1067–75.
42. Fiore MC, Bailey WC, Cohen SJ, et al. Smoking Cessation. Clinical Practice Guideline No. 18. Rockville, Md; U.S. Department of Health and Human Services, Public Health Service, Agency for Health Care Policy Research. AHCPR Publication No. 96–0692. April 1996:1.
43. Fincham JE, Smith MC. The role of the pharmacist in smoking cessation counseling. *Drug Topics.* 1989;133(suppl):1S–24S.
44. Fattinger K, Verotta D, Benowitz NL. Pharmacodynamics of acute tolerance to multiple nicotinic effects in humans. *J Pharmacol Exp Ther.* 1997;281:1238–46.
45. Benowitz NL. Nicotine replacement therapy during pregnancy. *JAMA.* 1991;262:3174–7.
46. Herrera N, Franco R, Herrera L, et al. Nicotine gum, 2 and 4 mg, for nicotine dependence. A double-blind placebo-controlled trial within a behavior modification support program. *Chest.* 1995;August 108:447–51.
47. Fiore MC, Jorenby DE, Baker TB, et al. Tobacco dependence and the nicotine patch. Clinical guidelines for effective use. *JAMA.* 1992;268:2687–94.
48. Fiore MC, Smith SS, Jorenby DE, et al. The effectiveness of the nicotine patch for smoking cessation. A meta-analysis. *JAMA.* 1994;June 22/29:1940–7.
49. Hjalmarson A, Franzon M, Westin A, et al. Effect of nicotine nasal spray on smoking cessation: randomized placebo-controlled, double-blind study. *Arch Intern Med.* 1994;154:2567–72.
50. Tonnesen P, Norregaard J, Mikkelsen K, et al. Double-blind trial of nicotine inhaler for smoking cessation. *JAMA.* 1993;269:1268–71.
51. Silagy C, Mant D, Fowler G, Lodge M. Meta-analysis of nicotine replacement therapies in smoking cessation. *Lancet.* 1994;343:139–42.
52. Gourlay SG, Benowitz NL. The benefits of stopping smoking and the role of nicotine replacement therapy in older patients. *Drugs and Aging.* 1996;9:8–23.
53. OTC Nicorette will be available in retail stores by late spring following Feb 9 approval. *F-D-C Reports—The Tan Sheet.*1996;4:4–5.
54. SmithKline Beecham Consumer Healthcare. Nicorette® product and packaging information. Pittsburgh: SmithKline Beecham Consumer Healthcare, LP. 1996.
55. Cromwell J, Bartosch WJ, Fiore MC, et al. Cost-effectiveness of the clinical practice recommendations in the AHCPR guideline for smoking cessation. Agency for Health Care Policy and Research. *JAMA.* 1997;278:1759–66.
56. Lawrence WF, Smith SS, Baker TB, et al. Does over-the-counter nicotine replacement therapy improve smokers' life expectancy? *Tob Control.* 1998;7:364–8.
57. Heatherton TF, Kozlowski LT, Frecker RC, et al. The Fagerström test for nicotine dependence: a revision of the Fagerström Tolerance Questionnaire. *Br J Addict.* 1991;86:1119–27.
58. American Psychiatric Association. *Diagnostic and Statistical Manual of Mental Disorder.* 4th ed. Washington, DC: American Psychiatric Association; 1994:242–7.
59. World Health Organization, Consultative Group on Statistical Aspects of Tobacco-Related Mortality. The future worldwide health effects of current smoking patterns. Paper presented at Perth, Western Australia: Seventh World Conference on Tobacco and Health; April 3, 1990.

Section X

Home Medical Equipment

CHAPTER 43

Home Testing and Monitoring Devices

Wendy Munroe Rosenthal and Geneva Clark Briggs

Chapter 43 at a Glance

Home testing and monitoring kits are designed to detect the presence or absence of a condition and to monitor disease therapy. The Food and Drug Administration requires home tests to be 95% to 99% accurate.[1] The products must be used properly to achieve these accuracy rates.

Editor's Note: This chapter is based, in part, on the 11th edition chapter titled "In-Home Testing and Monitoring Products," which was written by Wendy P. Munroe and Marcus D. Wilson.

In 1977, the home diagnostics market made a quantum leap when Warner-Lambert introduced the first home pregnancy test kit. The market continues to grow, with an expanded array of products and more user-friendly versions of established ones. Annual sales of home tests range from $2.2 billion to $2.4 billion.[2] Several forces are driving the growth in home diagnostics. First is the increased public interest in health, fitness, and preventive medicine: Testing and monitoring kits now allow patients to test themselves conveniently at home, which encourages active participation in their own health care. Second is reduced health care costs: Home tests help patients avoid unnecessary physician visits or allow them to seek earlier treatment of a condition. Third is the increased number of different tests available. Important advances in technology, such as monoclonal antibodies, have led to simplified tests that can be accurately and easily performed at home.

This chapter discusses home test kits that aid in detecting the following conditions: colorectal cancer (fecal blood tests), pregnancy, high cholesterol levels, urinary tract infections (UTIs), and human immunodeficiency virus (HIV), as well as illicit drug use. Other diagnostic products include ovulation prediction tests and devices to aid patients who are defined as clinically infertile to conceive a child. It also covers the proper selection and use of blood pressure monitors for patients with diagnosed hypertension. (See Chapter 10, "Asthma," and Chapter 39, "Diabetes Mellitus," for products used in self-monitoring these disorders.)

Selection and Use of Home Tests

Selection Criteria

With the variety of diagnostic products available, deciding which test to recommend to patients is quite challenging. The major variables to consider include the test's complexity, its ease of reading results, the presence of a control, and the cost.

Because human error plays such an important part in the ultimate value of these products, simplicity of use deserves major consideration. Each step required is a potential source of error. Some tests are more user friendly than others; simple tests are generally more desirable.

In most home test kits, the result is indicated by a change in color. With some products, the color change is easily discernible (e.g., the appearance of a plus sign or a check mark) whereas other products require that the user recognize subtle variations in shade. The latter results are more likely to be misinterpreted.

When possible, patients should select a test that includes a control to ensure the test is functioning correctly.

Many products provide more than one test per kit. Thus, when considering cost, patients should determine the cost per test unit. Generic or store brand kits may be available and can cost significantly less.

Usage Considerations

Testing procedures and kit contents vary among manufacturers, but the mechanism of action for each category of tests is basically the same. Patients should follow these general guidelines for using home test kits.

Because the products use monoclonal antibodies and various chemicals, reagent stability is a concern. Patients should always check the test kit's expiration date and should follow the manufacturer's instructions for storage.

Patients should read all instructions before attempting to perform a test. They should note the time of day the test is to be conducted, the length of time that is required, and any necessary equipment. This approach will allow the patient to schedule the best time and place to conduct the test.

Many kits require that the user wait a specified length of time between steps. Because the timing must be precise, patients should use an accurate timing device that measures seconds. Many kits also require the user to observe a color change to read the test results; therefore, someone must be present who does not have color-defective vision or other visual impairment.

The instructions must be followed exactly and in sequence. Patients who have questions about the testing procedure or interpretation of the results should consult a pharmacist or other health professional. Most kits offer a toll-free number to call for assistance.

Colorectal Cancer

Colorectal cancer, accounting for 15% of all cancers, is the second most common form of cancer in the United States.[3] This disorder is also hard to detect. One early and common symptom of colorectal cancer is rectal bleeding. Checking for hidden (occult) blood in the stool is an easy way to screen for a potential colon problem. Fecal blood testing products can be used as an adjunct to more invasive tests to detect colorectal cancer and other causes of gastrointestinal bleeding.

Epidemiology of Colorectal Cancer

Colorectal cancer occurs most commonly in patients with a family history of colorectal cancer, intestinal polyps, or ulcerative colitis. The incidence of colorectal cancer increases with advancing age. Consumption of high amounts of animal fat and low amounts of dietary fiber is related to colorectal cancer.[4]

Self-Detection of Colorectal Cancer with Fecal Blood Tests

Two nonprescription fecal blood tests are available: ColoCARE and EZ-Detect Stool Blood Test are noninvasive and easy to use in the privacy of the home.

Mechanism of Action

The in-home tests detect blood in feces with a colorimetric assay for hemoglobin. The heme portion of hemoglobin acts as an oxidizing agent, catalyzing the oxidation of the test reagent, tetramethylbenzidine, which produces a blue-green color. The appearance of this color indicates that the test is positive.[5,6]

Blood may be present on the surface or contained within the stool matrix. In general, matrix blood originates in the upper gastrointestinal tract while surface blood comes from the lower tract. The kits are more likely to detect blood from lower gastrointestinal abnormalities. With the available kits (ColoCARE and EZ-Detect), the reagent is sandwiched between two layers of biodegradable paper that is placed in the toilet bowl following a bowel movement. The kits are based on the premise that a significant amount of fecal blood will remain on the surface of the toilet bowl water after a bowel movement.

Interferences

Blood in the stool can signify a number of conditions in addition to cancer of the colon and rectum, including ulcers, Crohn's disease, colitis, anal fissures, diverticulitis, and hemorrhoids. Any of these conditions can give a positive result for a fecal blood test. If present in the toilet bowl water, menstrual blood can also produce a false positive result.

Aspirin, nonsteroidal anti-inflammatory drugs, steroids, and reserpine may cause sufficient gastric bleeding to produce false positive results. These medications should be avoided for at least 2 to 3 days before testing as well as during the test period. Rectally administered medications should also be avoided. However, patients should consult their physician before discontinuing any prescribed medications.

Vitamin C ingestion in excess of 250 mg per day may interfere with the peroxidase action of hemoglobin, causing false negative results in the ColoCARE test.[5] This test is not specific for human blood and may produce positive results if red meat is consumed. Toilet bowl cleaners may also produce false positive results.[5,6] The box "Patient Education for Fecal Blood Tests" lists measures for avoiding false test results.

Usage Guidelines

See the box "Patient Education for Fecal Blood Tests."

Product Selection Guidelines

Patients who wish to avoid restricting their diet or stopping vitamin C may prefer the EZ-Detect product. Both EZ-Detect and ColoCARE are similar in cost.

Patient Assessment of Fecal Blood Tests

Assessing the degree of risk a patient has for colorectal cancer is a major consideration in determining whether to recommend a fecal blood test. Patients with a personal or family history of colorectal cancer have a higher risk of developing the disease and would most likely benefit from testing. Patients with a family history should start testing annually at age 40; everyone should test yearly starting at age 50. Determining the potential for false test results is another important consideration. False negative tests could delay necessary treatment whereas false positive tests could cause unwarranted anxiety. Finally, to further ensure accurate test results, the patient should be assessed for any physical limitations that could interfere with performing the test. Asking the patient the following questions will help elicit the information needed to determine whether testing is appropriate and which product best meets the patient's needs or preferences.

Q~ Have you ever suffered from any bowel disorder? Have you or anyone in your family had colorectal cancer?

A~ *Identify the risk factors for colorectal cancer. (See the section "Epidemiology of Colorectal Cancer.")* If the patient is at risk for colorectal cancer, recommend testing for fecal blood.

Q~ Are you currently experiencing known bleeding such as bleeding hemorrhoids or menstruation?

A~ If yes to either condition, advise the patient that the condition could be the source of blood on the stool and that testing should be delayed to avoid false test results. *Identify other disorders that can cause blood in the stool. (See the section "Interferences.")*

Q~ What nonprescription or prescription medications are you currently taking?

A~ *Identify which medications can interfere with the test. (See the section "Interferences.")*

Q~ Do you have any visual limitations?

A~ If yes, advise patient to obtain assistance in performing the test and interpreting the results.

Patient Counseling for Fecal Blood Tests

When counseling a patient on fecal blood tests, the pharmacist should do the following: (1) emphasize to the patient the importance of strictly following test instructions to avoid false results; (2) explain any steps that are unclear; and (3) reiterate the medical and environmental factors that can affect test results. The box "Patient Education for Fecal Blood Tests" lists specific information to provide patients.

Evaluation of Patient Outcomes with Fecal Blood Tests

Patients evaluating the results of fecal blood tests must remember that the test is a screening method and is not specific

Patient Education for Fecal Blood Tests

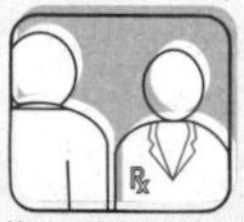

The objective of self-testing is to screen for blood in the stool. For most patients, carefully following product instructions and the self-care measures listed below will help ensure accurate test results.

Avoidance of Incorrect Results

EZ-Detect and ColoCARE Tests

- Do not perform test during times of known bleeding, such as hemorrhoidal or menstrual bleeding.
- Increase dietary fiber intake for several days before testing. Roughage increases the accuracy of the test by stimulating bleeding from lesions that might not otherwise bleed.
- Because bleeding from cancerous lesions may be intermittent, perform the test on three consecutive bowel movements to increase the chance of detecting a possible lesion.
- Complete all three stool tests even if the first two produce negative results. Flush testing pads when testing is completed.
- Do not take nonprescription medications such as aspirin and nonsteroidal anti-inflammatory drugs for 2 to 3 days before testing and during testing.
- Some prescription medications can cause bleeding and may need to be stopped before testing. Consult a physician about which medications to stop before performing the test.
- Chemicals in the toilet can interfere with the test. Following the instructions carefully can prevent this problem.

ColoCARE Test

- Do not eat red meat 2 to 3 days before testing and during the test period.
- Do not take more than 250 mg of vitamin C for 2 to 3 days before and during the test period.

Usage Guidelines

EZ-Detect Test

- Remove toilet tank cleansers or deodorizers; then flush toilet twice before testing.
- Before testing, use one test pad to perform a water quality check. If any trace of blue appears in the cross-shaped area when the pad is placed in the toilet water, use another toilet to complete the testing.
- Immediately after a bowel movement, place a pad in the toilet bowl, printed side up. After 2 minutes, check for the appearance of a blue cross on the test pad (positive result).
- Repeat the test on the next two bowel movements.
- If results are negative for all three tests, use remaining pad to perform a quality check of the test pads: Flush the toilet and empty the contents of the positive control chemical package into the bowl as it refills. Float the remaining test pad in the water, printed side up. After 2 minutes, check for a blue cross, which indicates that the test pads were working properly. If the blue cross does not appear, call the assistance line provided with the product.

ColoCARE Test

- Remove toilet tank cleansers or deodorizers and flush toilet twice before testing.
- Immediately after a bowel movement, place a pad in the toilet bowl, printed side up. Observe pad for 30 seconds for the appearance of a blue or green tint in the test area. This color change should be considered a positive sign of the presence of hemoglobin.
- Two control areas on the bottom of each pad indicate whether the test is functioning properly. Check that the left area has turned blue or green and that the right area did not change color. If color changes differ from these, discard the pad and repeat the test after the next bowel movement.
- Be sure to test three consecutive bowel movements.

⚠ Notify a physician if any of the three tests is positive.

Source: References 5 and 6

to a particular disease. A positive test result may indicate any medical condition that causes a loss of blood through the gastrointestinal system. The primary value of fecal blood tests is to alert patients and physicians that a thorough work-up may be needed. The kits are not intended to replace other diagnostic procedures. Patients should be advised to contact their physician if a positive test result is obtained.

Infertility

Women who have difficulty becoming pregnant use various methods of predicting ovulation. Such methods are useful because they allow women to detect ovulation so they can time sexual intercourse to coincide with optimal fertility. In

1998, about 1.5 million ovulation test kits were sold in the United States.[7] This section will discuss the use of basal thermometers, ovulation prediction test kits, and fertility microscopes. These tests and devices are also useful for women who are not infertile but wish to be better aware of their time of ovulation.

Epidemiology of Infertility

Infertility, the medical inability to conceive after 1 year of unsuccessful attempts, is estimated to occur in 5.3 million American men and women.[8] In addition, it takes many fertile women several months to become pregnant.

Physiology of the Female Reproductive Cycle

The female reproductive cycle, which is approximately 28 days long, is hormonally controlled. At the beginning of the cycle (day 1 through approximately day 13), low levels of circulating estrogen and progesterone cause the hypothalamus to secrete gonadotropin-releasing hormone (GnRH). GnRH stimulates the release of follicle-stimulating hormone (FSH) and low levels of luteinizing hormone (LH) from the anterior pituitary gland. This combination of hormones promotes the development of several follicles within an ovary during each cycle. At one point in the development, one follicle is singled out and continues to mature while the others regress. At midcycle (approximately day 14 or 15), circulating LH levels significantly increase and cause final maturation of the follicle. Ovulation (rupturing of the follicle and release of the ovum) occurs approximately 20 to 48 hours after the LH surge. Cells in the ruptured follicle then luteinize and form the corpus luteum, which begins to secrete progesterone and estrogen. For approximately 7 to 8 days after ovulation, the corpus luteum continues to develop and to secrete estrogen and progesterone, which inhibits further secretion of FSH and LH.[9]

Once ovulation occurs, the ovum remains viable for fertilization for only 12 to 24 hours.[8] Because sperm may live up to 72 hours, the optimal days for fertilization are the 2 days before ovulation, the day of ovulation, and the day after ovulation. For the greatest chance of achieving pregnancy, intercourse should take place within the 24 hours after the LH surge.

If fertilization occurs, trophoblastic cells produce human chorionic gonadotropin (hCG) hormone. This hormone causes the corpus luteum to continue to produce progesterone and estrogen, which forestalls the onset of menses while the placenta develops and becomes functional. As early as day 7 after conception, the placenta produces hCG, the concentration of which continues to increase during early pregnancy. Some hCG is excreted in the urine, while maximum levels of hCG are reached 6 weeks after conception. The hCG levels decline over the following 4 to 6 weeks and then stabilize for the remainder of the pregnancy.[9]

If fertilization does not occur during a cycle, the corpus luteum degenerates, circulating levels of progesterone and estrogen diminish, and menstruation occurs (days 1 to 5). Resulting low levels of progesterone and estrogen cause the release of GnRH from the hypothalamus, and the hormonal cycle begins again.[9]

Methods for Self-Detection of Ovulation

Available nonprescription products for ovulation prediction include basal thermometers, ovulation prediction tests, and fertility microscopes. (See Table 43–1 for examples of commercially available ovulation prediction tests.) Each detection method has a different mechanism of action and method of use. Women may pick a method that best suits their lifestyle or philosophy of self-care.

Table 43–1

Selected Ovulation Prediction Tests

Trade Name	Reaction Time (minutes)	Product Features
Answer 1-Step Ovulation	5	5-day kit: uses test sticks; predicts ovulation within 24–36 hours
Clearplan Easy	3	5-day kit: uses test sticks; predicts ovulation within 24–36 hours
Conceive Ovulation Test	3	5-day kit: provides test cassette, dropper, plastic cup; predicts ovulation within 24–40 hours
First Response 1-Step Ovulation Predictor Test	5	5-day kit: uses test sticks; predicts ovulation within 24–36 hours
HealthCheck Ovulation Detection Test	5	6-day kit: uses test sticks; predicts ovulation within 20–44 hours; provides two pregnancy tests
OvuKIT Self-Test	60	6-day or 9-day kit: uses test sticks; predicts ovulation within 24–40 hours
OvuQUICK One Step	4	6-day or 9-day kit: uses test pads; predicts ovulation within 24–40 hours
Q Test for Ovulation Prediction	35	5-day kit: uses test pads; predicts ovulation within 20–44 hours

Basal Thermometry

For many years, women have measured basal body temperature to predict the time of ovulation. Resting basal body temperature is usually below normal during the first part of the female reproductive cycle. After ovulation, it rises to a level closer to normal (i.e., 98.6°F [37°C]).

Mechanism of Action

When using basal thermometry, women take their temperature (orally, rectally, or vaginally) with a basal thermometer each morning before arising. These temperature measurements are then plotted graphically. A rise in temperature signals that ovulation has occurred. When the increase occurs, women who want to become pregnant should have intercourse as soon as possible to maximize their chances of conception.

The only equipment necessary for monitoring basal body temperature is a basal thermometer. Although basal thermometry is a relatively simple method of ovulation prediction, recording and interpreting temperature data can be confusing. In addition, some women may have difficulty reading mercury thermometers accurately. Because the temperature increase that follows ovulation is small (0.4°F to 1.0°F [0.2°C to 0.6°C]), women who have trouble reading a thermometer may miss the rise altogether.[10]

The Bioself Fertility Indicator uses computer technology to provide a digital temperature reading in just 2 minutes. This device can store temperature readings in its memory for 120 consecutive days. The user must input the date of the first day of menses each month. The device then processes temperature measurements and cycle information to calculate the user's average cycle length and to predict the user's most fertile days. Each morning when the temperature is taken, the indicator lights activate and display the predictions. A green light means that a woman is in the most infertile period of her cycle, a red light indicates that fertility is low but conception is possible, and a flashing red light signals that a woman is in her most fertile period and the likelihood of conception is highest.[10]

The Bioself Fertility Indicator has a unique feature: a modem that allows transmission of stored temperature data to the manufacturer by telephone. The company then mails a printout to the user that indicates the number of days the device was used, the lengths of the past six menstrual cycles, a graphic plot of daily temperature measurements for the past 120 days, and fertility-level estimates for the same period. The woman may then provide this information to her fertility specialist as a starting point for consultation.

Two clinical studies have demonstrated that the Bioself Fertility Indicator is 90% effective in indicating a time window that signals a woman's highly fertile period.[11,12] However, knowing this time window does not guarantee that a woman will conceive, even when the device is used properly.

Interferences

Several factors, such as emotions, movements, and infections, can influence the basal metabolic temperature. Eating, drinking, talking, and smoking should be postponed until after each measurement is obtained.

Usage Guidelines

See the box "Patient Education for Ovulation Prediction Tests and Devices" for instructions on using basal thermometers.

Product Selection Guidelines

Although it is significantly more expensive, the Bioself Fertility Indicator may be of benefit for women who cannot accurately read a thermometer but wish to use basal thermometry. It would be a good choice for a woman who does not want to keep track of her temperature readings.

Ovulation Prediction Tests

Ovulation prediction tests, which estimate the time of ovulation, are marketed to women who are having difficulty conceiving and need to pinpoint ovulation.

Mechanism of Action

Ovulation prediction tests use monoclonal antibodies specific to LH to detect the surge of this hormone . An enzyme-linked immunosorbent assay (ELISA) elicits a color change indicating the amount of LH in the urine.[8] The LH surge is revealed by a difference in color or color intensity from that noted on the previous day of testing. The intensity of color on the test stick is directly proportional to the amount of LH in the urine sample. Generally, early morning collection of urine is recommended because the LH surge usually begins early in the day and the urine concentration is relatively consistent at this time. Some products do not specify a time of day, requiring only that a consistent time be used.

Testing should begin 2 to 4 days before ovulation. The kit contains directions to determine when to begin testing according to the average length of the past three menstrual cycles. If the cycle varies by more than 3 to 4 days each month, the woman should use the shortest cycle to determine the starting date.

The ClearPlan Easy Fertility Monitor increases the specificity of ovulation prediction by measuring both LH and E3G, a component of estrogen. E3G levels rise and fall in a similar pattern to LH. This product uses test sticks that the woman exposes to her urine stream and then inserts into a small, palm-sized monitor with a light-emitting diode screen. She must establish baseline data about her hormone-level fluctuations. For the first month, she tests for 20 consecutive days, starting on approximately the sixth day after the beginning of menstruation. Using these data, the monitor calculates the time window during which the woman is most likely to conceive. After establishing her baseline, she tests for 10 to 20 days each month, depending on her cycle length. The results each day are displayed as low, high, or peak fertility.[13] A low result indicates a small chance of conception; a high result indicates increased chance of conception. This reading is typically given for 1 to 5 days leading up to peak fertility for each cycle. A "peak" reading indicates the highest chance of conception and is usually given 2 days before ovulation.

Interferences

Because LH levels are artificially elevated, medications used to promote ovulation (e.g., menotropins) may cause false positive results in ovulation prediction tests that measure only LH. The true LH surge can be detected in patients receiving clomiphene as long as testing does not begin until the second day after drug therapy ends. Medical conditions associated with high levels of LH, such as menopause and polycystic ovary syndrome, may also cause false positive results. Pregnancy can give a false positive result.[14] If the patient has recently discontinued using oral contraceptives, the start of ovulation may be delayed for one to two cycles. Thus, it would not be appropriate for this individual to use a home ovulation prediction test until fertilization has been attempted unsuccessfully for 1 to 2 months following discontinuation of the oral contraceptives.

Polycystic ovary syndrome; medications that affect the cycle (hormonal contraception, certain fertility treatments, and hormone replacement therapy); impaired liver or kidney function (which alter levels of E3G); breast-feeding; tetracycline (not oxytetracycline or monocycline); and perimenopause may produce false positive results when using the ClearPlan Easy Fertility Monitor.[13] Recently pregnant women who have stopped breast-feeding or stopped using hormonal contraception may wish to wait until they have at least two natural menstrual cycles in a row (lasting 21 to 42 days) before using the ClearPlan Easy Fertility Monitor.[13]

Usage Guidelines

See the box "Patient Education for Ovulation Prediction Tests and Devices" for instructions on using ovulation prediction tests.

Product Selection Guidelines

The available ovulation prediction tests vary in the length of time needed to complete the test, the method of applying urine to the test stick, and the number of individual tests provided. Patients with longer cycles may benefit from purchasing the kits that contain more testing sticks.

Traditional ovulation prediction kits identify the 24- to 48-hour window around ovulation, whereas the ClearPlan Easy Fertility Monitor identifies a larger window of several days. This monitor has no patient interpretation of color changes. The Clearplan Easy Fertility Monitor is effective for women with monthly cycle length of 21 to 42 days[15] because the monitor calculates the fertility period on the basis of each individual's hormone levels.

The initial cost of the Clearplan Easy Fertility Monitor is higher than that of the ovulation prediction kits that detect only LH, but it is reusable for an indefinite period with only the additional expense of more test sticks.

Fertility Microscopes

Fertility microscopes (OVU-Tec Fertility Detector and CycleView) are reusable devices that analyze the woman's saliva to predict ovulation.

Mechanism of Action

OVU-Tec Fertility Detector and CycleView allow women to examine saliva ferning patterns. These lipstick-sized illuminated microscopes allow the woman to examine her dried saliva on a slide. The hormonal changes that occur before, during, and after ovulation directly affect dried saliva patterns.[15] During fertile periods, sample patterns resemble fern leaves (straight lines with railroad track-like crosshatches). Dotted or bubble-like structures appear during nonfertile periods. The characteristic fern pattern appears in samples approximately 3 to 4 days before ovulation and persists until 2 to 3 days after ovulation.

A woman should track her cycle daily to get a clear picture of the changes that occur in saliva samples. Randomly using the microscope can give a misleading interpretation.[16] Some women may notice an occasional day of light ferning before the start of menstruation.

Interferences

Smoking, alcohol consumption, anticholinergic medications, or food consumption can affect the quality of saliva specimens.[17] The woman should not collect saliva samples within 2 hours of smoking, eating, or drinking. Conditions such as polycystic ovary syndrome and perimenopause, which cause increased LH levels, may result in consistent ferning throughout the cycle.[16]

Usage Guidelines

See the box "Patient Education for Ovulation Prediction Tests and Devices" for instructions on using fertility microscopes.

Product Selection Guidelines

Examining ferning patterns can identify a larger fertility window than traditional ovulation prediction kits, but the identification of saliva ferning is subjective. Additionally, testing must be done daily. CycleView provides an instructional videotape and a chart for daily recording of saliva sample interpretations to assist the woman in identifying changes.

The initial cost for fertility microscopes is higher than for ovulation prediction kits that detect LH in the urine, but the microscopes are reusable indefinitely, if the slide surface is taken care of appropriately.

Patient Assessment of Ovulation Prediction Tests and Devices

The pharmacist should privately ask a patient the reasons for using an ovulation prediction test. If the reason is difficulty in conceiving, the pharmacist should find out whether a physician has diagnosed infertility and whether the patient has previously used ovulation prediction tests or devices such as basal thermometers or fertility microscopes. Questions about other possible pathology and medication use are appropriate for determining possible interference with test results or temperature measurements. Asking the patient the following questions will help elicit the information needed to determine whether testing is appropriate and which product best meets the patient's needs or preferences.

Q~ Do you have any chronic medical conditions? Are you taking any medications?

A~ *Identify which disorders or medications can affect test results. (See the sections that discuss interferences with ovulation prediction methods.)*

Q~ Are you consulting or have you consulted a doctor who specializes in fertility problems?

A~ Find out whether the patient is taking fertility medications. Such medications can interfere with the results of ovulation prediction tests.

Q~ How "regular" are your periods?

A~ Drawing on the patient's response, determine the appropriate timing for her using an ovulation prediction test.

Q~ Have you ever used a product like this? If so, which one? Did you have difficulty using the product?

A~ Tailor instructions to the patient's level of experience and success with these tests. If use was successful, recommend the same type of product. If unsuccessful, clarify any instructions that the patient had difficulty following. Advise the patient to read all instructions carefully each time the product is bought because the instructions might have changed.

Q~ Do you have any visual limitations?

A~ If yes, advise the patient to obtain assistance when reading a basal thermometer or interpreting results of the ovulation prediction and saliva ferning tests. Subtle temperature changes may be difficult to see on a basal thermometer.

Patient Education for Ovulation Prediction Tests and Devices

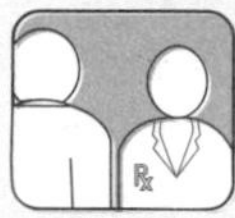

The objective of self-testing is to more accurately determine the time of ovulation and to increase the chances of conception. For most patients, carefully following product instructions and the self-care measures listed below will help increase the chances of achieving this goal.

Basal Thermometers

Avoidance of Incorrect Results

- Do not move while taking temperature measurements.
- Note that emotions can affect temperature measurements.
- If an infection is suspected, discontinue the measurements until the disorder is resolved. Begin taking temperatures again on the first day of menstruation of the cycle following resolution of the disorder.
- Do not eat, drink, talk, or smoke while taking temperature measurements.

Usage Guidelines

- Read the instructions thoroughly before using the thermometer, and follow instructions carefully.
- Choose one method of taking temperatures (orally, vaginally, or rectally), and use that method consistently.
- Take temperature readings at approximately the same time each morning. Take temperatures just before rising each morning after at least 5 hours of sleep. If using a regular basal thermometer, plot the temperatures on a graph. A rise in temperature indicates that ovulation has occurred.
- If using the Bioself Fertility Indicator, input the first day of menses each month. Check the Bioself's indicator lights each morning for an indication—flashing red light—that ovulation has occurred.
- If conception does not occur after using the Bioself thermometer for three consecutive cycles, consider using the modem feature to transmit data stored in the device to the manufacturer by telephone. The manufacturer will supply a printout of the stored information, which will be useful in consultations with fertility specialists.

Ovulation Prediction Tests Excluding ClearPlan Easy Fertility Monitor

Avoidance of Incorrect Results

- Note that fertility medications, polycystic ovary syndrome, menopause, and pregnancy can cause false positive results.
- Recent pregnancy or discontinuation of oral contraceptives or breast-feeding will delay ovulation for one or two cycles. Start testing after two natural menstrual cycles have occurred.

Usage Guidelines

- Start using the test 2 to 3 days before ovulation is expected.
- Follow the manufacturer's specific directions regarding the timing of urine collection. If not collecting morning urine, avoid urinating until ready to test the urine. Restrict fluid intake for at least 4 hours before testing so that the urine will not be diluted.
- Test the urine sample immediately after collection.

- If immediate testing is not feasible, refrigerate urine for the length of time specified in the directions for each product. Allow refrigerated sample to stand at room temperature for 20 to 30 minutes before beginning the test.
- Do not redisperse any sediment that may be present in the sample.
- If using a kit designed to be passed through the urine stream, either hold a test stick in the urine stream for the specified period of time, or collect urine in a collection cup and dip the stick in the urine.
- If using a kit not designed to be passed through the urine stream, collect urine in a collection cup; then place the urine in the testing well using the dropper provided.
- After the urine is placed on the testing device, read the results in 3 to 5 minutes depending on the manufacturer's instructions.
- Watch for the test's first significant increase in color intensity, which indicates that the LH surge has occurred and that ovulation will occur within a day or two.
- Once the LH surge is detected, discontinue testing. Remaining tests can be used at a later date, if necessary.
- If the LH surge is not detected, carefully review the testing instructions to ensure they were performed properly. If the testing procedure was accurate, ovulation may not have occurred or testing may have occurred too late in the cycle. Consider testing for a longer period in the next cycle to increase the chances of detecting the LH surge.

ClearPlan Easy Fertility Monitor Test

Avoidance of Incorrect Results

- Note that fertility medications, polycystic ovary syndrome, menopause, and pregnancy can cause false positive results.
- Oral contraceptives, hormone replacement therapy, impaired liver or kidney function, breast feeding, tetracycline (but not oxytetracycline or monocycline), and perimenopause can cause false positive results with the ClearPlan Easy Fertility Monitor.
- Recent pregnancy or discontinuation of oral contraceptives or breast-feeding will delay ovulation for one or two cycles. Start testing after two natural menstrual cycles have occurred.

Usage Guidelines

- For the first month, begin testing on the sixth day after beginning menstruation and test for 20 days.
- For subsequent months, test the number of days indicated by the monitor.
- Remove test stick or cassette from packaging just before use.
- Hold the test stick in the urine stream; insert stick in monitor.
- Discard test stick after use.

Fertility Microscopes

Avoidance of Incorrect Results

- Do not smoke, drink, or eat within 2 hours of testing the saliva.
- Note that polycystic ovary syndrome and perimenopause may interfere with the test results.

Usage Guidelines

- Wash and dry hands. Place saliva on the slide area of the microscope eyepiece. Allow saliva to dry for 5 to 7 minutes.
- Compare the observed saliva pattern with drawing A (fertile period) and B (nonfertile period).
- Clean the round slide surface after each use with a cotton swab soaked with water or alcohol. Be careful not to scratch the glass.
- Do not wash or soak the eyepiece as water may be trapped between the lens of the microscope and the slide.
- To improve accuracy in identifying the fertile period, combine saliva examination with basal thermometry.

A

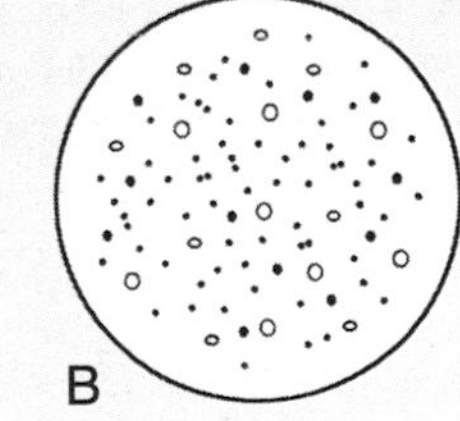

If pregnancy does not occur after 3 months of using these products, see a physician.

Source: References 8, 13, 16, and 17.

Patient Counseling for Ovulation Prediction Tests and Devices

To use ELISA-based ovulation prediction products effectively, a woman must know approximately when ovulation occurs or must be willing to track three menstrual cycles to determine when it occurs. The pharmacist should explain the hormonal fluctuations during the cycle and how they relate to the use of ovulation prediction tests, basal thermometers, and fertility microscopes. The pharmacist should also explain the reason for the number of tests or measurements that must be performed with each type of product. The pharmacist should emphasize that the woman must consistently use the products for at least 3 months. The box Patient Education for "Ovulation Prediction Tests and Devices" lists specific information to provide patients.

Evaluation of Patient Outcomes with Ovulation Prediction Tests and Devices

Ovulation prediction products should not be used for more than 3 months. If conception does not occur within this period, the woman should see a physician.

Pregnancy Detection

One-third of women who think they may be pregnant have reportedly used a home pregnancy test.[18] Early detection of pregnancy is desirable for many reasons, including allowing the woman to make decisions regarding prenatal care and lifestyle changes to avoid potential harm to the fetus.

Epidemiology of Pregnancy

In 1996, the crude birth rate in the United States was 14.7 live births per 1,000 population.[19] The largest numbers of births are for women between 18 and 34 years old.

Self-Detection of Pregnancy with Pregnancy Tests

Human chorionic gonadotropin (hCG) is a hormone produced by the trophoblast of the fertilized ovum and is detectable in the urine within 1 to 2 weeks after conception. It is considered a diagnostic indicator of pregnancy. More than a dozen pregnancy tests with a variable number of steps and reaction times are available for home use. (See Table 43–2 for examples of commercially available products.)

Mechanism of Action

Home pregnancy tests are designed to detect the presence of hCG in the urine.[8] The tests use monoclonal or polyclonal antibodies in an enzyme immunoassay. The antibodies are bound to a solid surface such as a stick, bead, or filter. If urinary hCG is present, it will form a complex with the antibodies. Another antibody, one linked to an enzyme that will react with a chromogen to produce a distinctive color, is added. The hCG is "sandwiched" between the antibody linked to the enzyme and the antibodies bound to the solid surface. Washing or filtering the testing device removes unbound substances; a chromogen that will react with the enzyme is then added. These antibody-based tests are very sensitive and specific. If correctly used, they have a reported accuracy of 98% to 100%.[8] However, in studies of consumer use of home pregnancy tests, the accuracy rate was found to be 50% to 75% because the directions were not followed carefully.[20]

Interferences

False negative results may occur with home pregnancy tests if they are performed before the first day of a missed period or if refrigerated urine is not allowed to warm to room temperature before testing. Waxed cups or soap residue in household containers can also cause erroneous results. A false positive may occur if the woman has had a miscarriage or given birth within the previous 8 weeks because hCG will still be present in the body. Medications such as Pergonal (menotropins for injection) and Profasi (chorionic gonadotropin for injection) can produce false positive results. Unreliable results may occur in patients with ovarian cysts or an ectopic pregnancy.[8]

Usage Guidelines

See the box "Patient Education for Pregnancy Tests."

Product Selection Guidelines

Some pregnancy tests are one-step procedures. Some tests have clear test sticks that allow the woman to see the reaction occurring as a check that sufficient urine was absorbed by the

Table 43–2

Selected One-Step Pregnancy Tests

Trade Name	Reaction Time (minutes)	Product Features
Answer	3	1 test; uses test sticks
Answer Quick & Simple	2	1 or 2 tests; uses test sticks
Clearblue Easy	2	1 or 2 tests; uses test sticks
Confirm	1	1 or 2 tests; uses test stick
e.p.t.	3	1 or 2 tests; uses test sticks
early Pregnancy test	1	1 test; uses test cassette; provides dropper and urine cup
Fact Plus One Step	1	1 or 2 tests; uses test sticks; can verify negative results in 3 minutes
First Response 1-Step	2	1 or 2 tests; uses test sticks
Nimbus Quick Strip	1–5	25 tests; uses test strips
RapidVue	1	1 test; uses test cassette
Qtest	1	1 test; uses test sticks

stick. Other tests include two devices, which can be helpful if a negative test is obtained first. The time to obtain test results varies from 1 minute to 5 minutes. The woman may use most tests on the market as early as the first day of a missed menstrual period. Generic (store-brand) kits are available, are usually less expensive than the brand-name kits, and are just as reliable.

Patient Assessment of Pregnancy Tests

The pharmacist should first determine whether the timing for using the pregnancy test is appropriate. If product use is appropriate, the pharmacist should ask about previous use of pregnancy tests and any difficulties the patient had with those tests. The pharmacist must ask questions about medical disorders and medication use to determine whether special measures are required to protect the unborn child. Asking the patient the following questions will help elicit the information needed to determine whether testing is appropriate and which product best meets the patient's needs or preferences.

Q~ How late is your period?

A~ *Identify the time frame in which pregnancy tests should be used. (See the section "Interferences.")* If testing is appropriate, recommend a product preferred by the patient. If not, advise the patient when testing would be appropriate.

Q~ What nonprescription or prescription medications are you currently taking?

A~ If the patient is taking teratogenic medications, advise her to discuss with her physician and the pharmacist any possible effects of the drugs if she is pregnant. If the patient is on chronic medications, advise her to see her physician as early as possible after obtaining a positive test result.

Q~ Have you ever used a pregnancy test before? If so, which one?

A~ Tailor instructions to the patient's level of experience and success with such tests. If use was successful, recommend the same type of product. If unsuccessful, clarify any instructions the patient had difficulty following. Advise the patient to read all instructions carefully each time the product is bought because the instructions might have changed.

Q~ Do you have any visual limitations?

A~ If yes, advise patient to obtain assistance in interpreting results of the pregnancy tests.

Patient Education for Pregnancy Tests

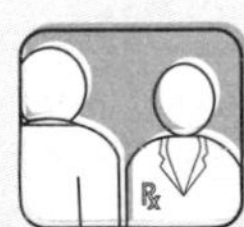

The obvious objective of self-testing is to determine whether a patient is pregnant. For most patients, carefully following package instructions and the self-care measures listed below will help ensure accurate test results.

Avoidance of Incorrect Results

- Wait the specified number of days after a missed period before performing the test. Performing the test too early may produce false negative results.
- Be sure to use the urine collection device provided in the kit. Wax particles in waxed cups can clog the test matrix, causing false results. Soap residue in household containers can also interfere with test results.
- Try to test the urine sample immediately after collection.
- If the sample must be tested later, store it in the refrigerator, but allow the sample to warm to room temperature before testing. Chilled urine may produce false negative results. Be careful not to redisperse any sediment present in the sample.

Usage Guidelines

- Unless package instructions specify otherwise, use the first morning urine because the levels of hCG, if present, will be concentrated at that time.
- If testing occurs at other times of the day, restrict fluid intake for 4 to 6 hours before urine collection.
- Remove test stick or cassette from packaging just before use. For test sticks, remove cap, if present, from absorbent tip.
- Apply urine to testing device using whichever of the following methods is specified in package instructions: (1) hold test stick in the urine stream for designated time, (2) urinate into testing well of test cassette, (3) collect urine in a collection cup and dip the strip or use a dropper to apply the urine.
- After the urine is applied, lay the testing device on a flat surface. Wait the recommended time before reading results (1 to 5 minutes).
- After reading the results, discard the testing device. If the test is negative, test again in 1 week if menstruation has not started.

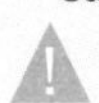

If the second test is negative, see a physician.

Patient Counseling for Pregnancy Tests

Counseling on pregnancy tests requires the same privacy as that for ovulation prediction tests. The pharmacist should emphasize the importance of following package instructions carefully, especially the instruction for when to begin testing. Pregnancy tests are very sensitive; therefore, the patient should be advised of medical and environmental factors that can cause inaccurate test results. The box "Patient Education for Pregnancy Tests" lists specific information to provide patients.

Evaluation of Patient Outcomes with Pregnancy Tests

If the pregnancy test result is positive, the woman should assume she is pregnant and contact her family physician or an obstetrician as soon as possible. If the test result is negative, the woman should review the procedure and make sure she performed the test correctly. She should test again in 1 week if menstrual flow has not begun. If the results of the second test are negative and menses still has not begun, the woman should seek the advice of a physician.

Hypercholesterolemia

A 1988 FDA survey found that only 30% of people with high cholesterol were aware of their condition. The U.S. Department of Health and Human Services recommends efforts to increase to 60% the proportion of adults with high blood cholesterol who not only are aware of their condition but also are taking action to alleviate the problem.[21] Consistent with this goal, the National Cholesterol Education Program recommends that all adults ages 20 and older have their total cholesterol measured at least every 5 years.[22] A home cholesterol test is one means of achieving this first critical step to minimize the risk for cardiovascular heart disease.

Because elevated cholesterol is a chronic condition that requires lifestyle modification and, frequently, medication for treatment, adhering to a treatment plan can be difficult for patients. Home cholesterol tests can monitor the efficacy of and adherence with diet, exercise, and medication plans.

Epidemiology of Hypercholesterolemia

More than 15% of Americans have elevated serum cholesterol values of greater than 240 mg/dL.[19] Forty percent of women ages 55 to 64 years have high cholesterol. Twenty-eight percent of men in this same age group have high cholesterol.

Etiology/Complications of Hypercholesterolemia

Elevated cholesterol levels result from excessive production of cholesterol by the liver, deficient removal of the cholesterol from the bloodstream, and excessive intake of cholesterol-rich foods such as eggs and red meat. Elevation of cholesterol and other lipids is a major predisposing factor for developing atherosclerotic heart disease, which can contribute to developing heart attack and stroke.[23]

Self-Detection of Hypercholesterolemia with Cholesterol Tests

One nonprescription test kit, CholesTrak Home Cholesterol Test, allows patients to measure their total blood cholesterol levels at home. The test kit includes all the items necessary to run the test on a finger stick, whole-blood specimen: test cassette, lancet, and chart for interpreting test results. Each chart is specific for that test cassette and should be used only for interpreting results with that test cassette.

Mechanism of Action

Cholesterol present in a blood sample of one to two drops is converted into hydrogen peroxide through two chemical reactions involving cholesterol esterase and cholesterol oxidase. The peroxide then reacts with horseradish peroxidase and a dye to produce the color that rises along the cholesterol test's measurement scale. The test cassette has two separate indicator spots that change color to show that the test is functioning properly. One of the indicator spots also indicates completion of the test, which signals it is time to read the scale.

Interferences

Good finger-sticking technique is necessary to avoid erroneous results with cholesterol tests. Two or three hanging drops of blood are needed, but excessive squeezing and milking of the finger will negatively affect the quality of the blood sample. If sufficient blood cannot be obtained from the first finger stick, the patient should use a different finger. A low cholesterol value may result if the blood sample is too small or if it takes longer than 5 minutes to collect the necessary amount of blood. Excessive bleeding from a finger stick can occur in patients who have coagulation disorders or use anticoagulants. These patients should not self-test for cholesterol levels.

The patient should avoid doses of 500 mg or more of vitamin C or standard doses (e.g., 325 to 1000 mg) of acetaminophen for 4 hours before the test because they may cause an artificially low result.

Usage Guidelines

See the box "Patient Education for Cholesterol Tests."

Product Selection Guidelines for Cholesterol Tests

Only one product for testing cholesterol levels is available. According to the product literature, CholesTrak is 97% accurate when performed according to package directions.[24]

Patient Assessment of Cholesterol Tests

Before recommending a cholesterol test, the pharmacist should first determine whether the patient has been diagnosed with heart disease or has some reason to be concerned about hypercholesterolemia. Conscientious monitoring of cholesterol is imperative for patients with heart disease because elevated cholesterol levels have a significant impact on the disorder. The pharmacist should also ask about lifestyle and other factors that can affect test results. Asking the patient the following questions will help elicit the information needed to determine whether testing is appropriate and which product best meets the patient's needs and preferences.

Q~ Do you have any medical conditions? Are you pregnant?

A~ *Identify medical conditions that can affect cholesterol levels. (See the section "Etiology/Complications of Hypercholesterolemia.")* If the patient has heart disease, encourage the patient (1) to follow the physician's guidelines for controlling hypercholesterolemia and (2) to use the cholesterol test to monitor effectiveness in meeting the guidelines. If other conditions are present that can affect cholesterol levels, advise the patient to test more than once to obtain accurate results.

Q~ Have you recently lost or gained weight? Do you exercise? Are you under stress?

A~ Advise the patient that such factors can affect test results and that more than one test is required to obtain accurate readings of cholesterol levels.

Q~ Do you have any conditions that cause excessive bleeding from a finger prick?

A~ *Identify conditions that can cause excessive bleeding. (See the section "Interferences.")* Advise patients with these conditions that finger sticks may cause excessive bleeding. Refer them to their physician for testing of cholesterol levels.

Q~ Have you ever used this product before?

A~ Tailor instructions to the patient's level of experience and success with these tests. If use was successful, recommend the same type of product. If unsuccessful, clarify any misunderstanding of directions. Advise the patient to read all instructions carefully each time the product is bought because the instructions might have changed.

Q~ Do you have any visual limitations?

A~ If yes, advise patients to obtain assistance in performing the test and accurately interpreting the results.

Q~ Do you have difficulty collecting your own blood samples?

A~ If yes, advise the patient to obtain assistance in performing the finger stick and blood collection.

Patient Education for Cholesterol Tests

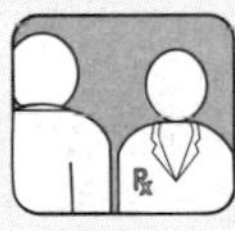

One objective of self-testing is to screen for high total cholesterol levels, allowing patients with elevated levels to start making lifestyle changes that can prevent heart attack and stroke. Another objective is to monitor the effects of diet, exercise, or medication in patients with diagnosed hypercholesterolemia. For most patients, carefully following package instructions and the self-care measures listed below will help ensure achievement of accurate test results, which, in turn, can help patients achieve their medical goals.

Avoidance of Incorrect Results

- Do not use cholesterol tests if you have hemophilia or take anticoagulants because of the risk of excessive bleeding from the finger stick. Have a physician perform the test.
- If two or three hanging drops of blood cannot be obtained or if it takes longer than 5 minutes to collect this amount of blood, do not perform the test. Such problems could cause low readings. If taking vitamin C in doses of 500 mg or more, do not take the dose within 4 hours of testing.
- Do not take standard doses (325 to 1000 mg) of acetaminophen within 4 hours of testing.

Usage Guidelines

- Before starting the test, wash your hands thoroughly with soap and warm water and dry them.
- To stabilize the cholesterol level, sit and relax for 5 minutes before performing the test.
- After washing and drying your hands, select the outside of one fingertip for the test.
- Lance your fingertip, wipe away the first sign of blood with the gauze pad, and fill the well of the test cassette as indicated as quickly as possible.
- Wait at least 2 but no more than 4 minutes before pulling the clear plastic tab on the right side of the cassette until it clicks into place and a red line appears. Use a timepiece with a second hand for accurate timing.
- After another 10 to 12 minutes, when the "END" indicator turns green, measure the height of the purple column against the scale printed on the cassette. Use the paper result chart included in the kit to interpret the reading.
- Dispose of used cassettes and finger-sticking devices appropriately; they are considered potentially biohazardous.

⚠ If the reading is 200 mg/dL or greater, see a physician for evaluation and further testing.

Patient Counseling for Cholesterol Tests

When counseling a patient on cholesterol tests, the pharmacist should emphasize the importance of properly collecting blood samples and should advise the patient to seek assistance with the finger stick, if needed. The pharmacist should also explain the purpose of the well and indicator spots on the test cassette. To further ensure accurate test results, the pharmacist should advise the patient of medical and lifestyle factors that can cause inaccurate test results. The box "Patient Education for Cholesterol Tests" lists specific information to provide patients.

Evaluation of Patient Outcomes with Cholesterol Tests

Home cholesterol tests measure only total cholesterol. Any consumer who obtains a result of 200 mg/dL or greater should see a physician for a repeat measurement, lipid profile, and appropriate medical work-up. Patients should not adjust their cholesterol-lowering medications on the basis of the results of this test.

Urinary Tract Infections

Urinary tract infections (UTIs) are the cause for 7 million visits to physicians every year.[25] Two primary uses for UTI tests are (1) early detection of such infections in patients with a history of recurrent UTIs or risk factors associated with UTI and (2) confirmation that an infection has been cured by antibiotic therapy.

Epidemiology of Urinary Tract Infections

Women have a shorter urethra than do men and are therefore more likely to contract UTIs than men. After the age of 50, men have a greater likelihood of contracting UTIs than women because of prostate problems. Conditions that increase the risk of UTI include pregnancy, diabetes, urinary stones, urinary obstructions such as those caused by an enlarged prostate, presence of urinary catheters, and a history of UTIs.[25]

Etiology/Signs and Symptoms of Urinary Tract Infections

UTIs result from bacteria entering the bladder and other structures of the urinary tract and multiplying. The gram-negative bacteria *Escherichia coli* causes 80% of urinary tract infections.[25] Both gram-positive and gram-negative bacteria account for the other 20% of the causative organisms.

The symptoms of a urinary tract infection include pain on urination, feeling an urgent need to urinate, frequent urination, and lower abdominal pain or discomfort.

Self-Detection of Urinary Tract Infections with Urinary Tract Infection Tests

Two types of UTI tests are available. The mechanism of action is the primary difference between the two.

Mechanism of Action

The first type of UTI test detects nitrites in the urine by using the principle that nitrate in the urine is reduced to nitrite by gram-negative bacteria.[25–27] Uri-Test and UTI Home Screening Test are two products that detect nitrites. The other type of test detects both nitrite and leukocyte esterase (LE), an enzyme unique to leukocytes (white blood cells).[28] White blood cells may also be found in the urine when a urinary tract infection is present. One product, AZO Test Strips, detects UTIs by this method.

The nitrite strips detect only infections caused by gram-negative bacteria. In the strip, aursanilic acid reacts with urinary nitrite to form a diazonium compound, which in turn reacts with another chemical on the strip to form a pink color. A positive test requires a bacterial concentration of 10^5 per milliliter of urine. Based on the presence of white blood cells in the urine, the nitrite and LE strips can detect infections caused by non–nitrate-reducing organisms.

Interferences

A strict vegetarian diet that provides insufficient urinary nitrates can cause false negative nitrite results with a UTI test. False negative results can also be caused by doses of ascorbic acid (vitamin C) in excess of 250 mg, because ascorbic acid blocks the nitrite test reaction. The patient should allow 10 hours between the last dose of ascorbic acid and the test procedure. Doses of ascorbic acid in excess of 500 mg within 24 hours of testing may result in a false negative result for the LE test.[28] Tetracycline may produce a false negative reading for nitrites. Dyes or drugs, such as phenazopyridine, may cause a false positive result by changing the sensor pad to pink.

Usage Guidelines

See the box "Patient Education for Urinary Tract Infection Tests."

Product Selection Guidelines

The combination of nitrite and LE tests in AZO Test Strips enhances the specificity and sensitivity of this UTI test. The Uri-Test and UTI Home Screening Test include urine collection cups whereas the AZO Test Strips does not. The UTI Home Screening Test includes twice as many test strips as the other kits. All are similar in cost. Patient preference will determine the selection.

Patient Assessment of Urinary Tract Infection Tests

Before recommending a UTI test, the pharmacist should first determine the patient's reason for using the test. If the patient is testing for a suspected UTI, the pharmacist should evaluate the patient's symptoms and risk factors for UTIs. If the patient is testing to find out if a treated UTI has been cured, the pharmacist should assess patient compliance with the therapy. The patient's diet and medication use are important factors to evaluate for possible interference with test results. Asking the patient the following questions will help elicit the information needed to determine whether testing is appropriate and which product best meets the patient's needs or preferences.

Q~ Have you been treating a urinary tract infection? When did you stop taking the antibiotic? Did you take the antibiotic as instructed? What symptoms, if any, are you having now?

A~ If the patient's responses indicate adherence with the prescribed therapy, recommend a UTI test on the basis of the patient's responses to the following questions.

Q~ For patients who are not treating a diagnosed UTI, ask the following questions: Why do you want to use this test? Do you have a history of urinary tract infections?

A~ *Identify the symptoms that indicate a possible UTI. (See the section "Etiology/Signs and Symptoms of Urinary Tract Infections.")* If the patient's responses warrant it, recommend a product on the basis of the patient's answers to the following questions.

Q~ What types of food do you eat daily?

A~ If the patient's diet is primarily vegetarian, explain the effect of diet on the UTI test. (See the section "Interferences.") If the patient is not receptive to changing the diet, refer the patient to a physician for evaluation.

Q~ What prescription and nonprescription medications, including vitamins, are you taking?

A~ *Identify medications that can interfere with the test. (See the section "Interferences.")* If the patient's medication history indicates possible interference, emphasize measures that will ensure accurate test results. (See the box "Patient Education for Urinary Tract Infection Tests.")

Q~ Do you have any visual difficulties?

A~ If the patient is colorblind, advise the patient to obtain assistance in interpreting the test results.

Patient Counseling for Urinary Tract Infection Tests

Counseling on the use of UTI tests should emphasize the importance of collecting a clean sample of midstream urine if

Patient Education for Urinary Tract Infection Tests

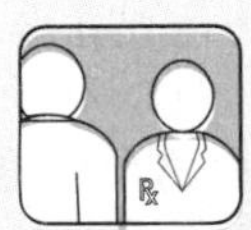

The objective of self-testing is to detect urinary tract infections in the early stages or to confirm that an infection was successfully treated. For most patients, carefully following the package instructions and the self-care measures listed below will help ensure achievement of accurate test results and allow prompt treatment of a detected urinary tract infection.

Avoidance of Incorrect Results

- Note that persons on a strict vegetarian diet may not get accurate results.
- Note that dyes or drugs, such as phenazopyridine, may cause a false positive result by changing the sensor pad to a pink color.
- If using UriTest and UTI Home Screening Test, do not take 250 mg or more of ascorbic acid (vitamin C) within 10 hours of testing.
- If using AZO Test Strips, do not take 500 mg or more of vitamin C within 24 hours of testing. Note also that tetracycline may produce a false negative result for this test.

Usage Guidelines for Urinary Tract Infection Tests

- Clean the genital area thoroughly before collecting a urine sample.
- Test the first urine of the morning or, if tested later, urine held in the bladder for at least 4 hours.
- To improve sensitivity, test urine samples on 3 consecutive days.
- Depending on the test purchased, pass the test strip through the urine stream, or collect a clean midstream sample of urine in the collection cup provided with the test.
- Do not touch the sensor pad on the strip because skin oils can interfere with the test reaction. If urine is collected in a cup, immerse the sensor pad on the test strip into the cup for 1 second.
- Make sure urine completely covers the pad.
- Wait the indicated time (30 to 60 seconds); then compare the color on the sensor pad to the color chart provided. For Uri-Test and UTI Home Screening Test, a pink color on the pad indicates a positive result. For AZO-Test, a dark tan to purple color on the leukocyte pad indicates a positive result.
- Wait no longer than 3 minutes to read the test strip; ignore any color changes that occur after that time.

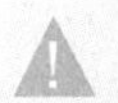
If the test is positive, see a physician immediately for evaluation and treatment.

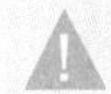
If the test is negative but symptoms persist, see a physician immediately for evaluation and treatment.

the sensor pad is to be immersed in a cup of urine. The pharmacist should advise a colorblind patient to seek assistance in interpreting test results. To further ensure accurate test results, the patient should be advised of medical and dietary factors that can cause inaccurate test results. The box "Patient Education for Urinary Tract Infection Tests" lists specific information to provide patients.

Evaluation of Patient Outcomes with Urinary Tract Infection Tests

The patient should contact a physician if a negative test is obtained but UTI symptoms persist because the test will detect only about 90% of infections. If a positive test is obtained, the patient should contact a physician immediately for evaluation and treatment.

Acquired Immunodeficiency Syndrome (AIDS)

More than 1 million Americans are infected with type 1 human immunodeficiency virus (HIV-1) and the number of cases is rising each year.[15] Home HIV-1 tests allow a patient to test for this virus in privacy.

Epidemiology of AIDS

Women, especially minority women, are experiencing a significant increase in the number of cases of AIDS.[29]

Etiology of AIDS

AIDS is an incurable disease caused by HIV-1.[15] The disease destroys the body's immune system. AIDS can be contracted by contact with infected body fluids such as blood or semen. People at risk for contracting the virus include those who (1) share needles or syringes for the purpose of injecting drugs, including steroids; (2) have sex with a person infected with HIV-1; (3) have sex with someone who injects drugs; (4) had a blood transfusion anytime between 1978 and May 1985; and (5) have sex with multiple partners.

Self-Detection of AIDS with HIV-1 Tests

Two test kits for HIV-1 detection are currently available: Home Access HIV-1 Test System and Home Access Express HIV-1 Test System.

Mechanism of Action

The HIV-1 tests detect antibodies to the virus. Because 3 weeks to 6 months can be required for developing sufficient antibodies for detection, the time since possible exposure to the virus must be considered in determining when to perform the test.

After collection, the home HIV-1 test samples are mailed to a certified laboratory for processing using an enzyme-linked immunoassay (ELISA). Positive samples are rescreened twice. Repeatedly positive samples are confirmed using an immunofluorescent assay.[30]

Interferences

No factors are known to interfere with home HIV-1 tests.

Usage Guidelines

See the box "Patient Education for HIV-1 Tests."

Product Selection Guidelines

The two available HIV-1 tests differ in price and turnaround time to obtain results. The first test, Home Access, takes approximately 7 business days to obtain the results. The second, Home Access Express, takes approximately 3 business days. The Home Access sample is sent to the testing laboratory by regular mail, whereas the Home Access Express sample is shipped by Federal Express. Consequently, the Home Access Express version costs more.

Patient Assessment of HIV-1 Tests

Before recommending an HIV-1 test, the pharmacist should first determine how much time has elapsed since the patient was possibly exposed to the HIV-1 virus. The patient may not know all the risk factors for AIDS; therefore, the pharmacist should tactfully find out whether the patient has engaged in any activities that can cause the disease. The patient should be asked about medical disorders that might rule out use of the test or physical limitations that might interfere with performing the test. Asking the patient the following questions will help elicit the information needed to determine whether testing is appropriate and which test best meets the patient's needs or preferences.

Q~ Do you have hemophilia or a bleeding disorder?

A~ If yes, discourage the patient from using the test because of the risk of excessive bleeding. Advise that a physician perform the test.

Q~ Do you have any risk factors for AIDS?

A~ *Identify the risk factors for this disorder. (See the section "Etiology of AIDS.")* Using the patient's response, determine whether the patient is at risk for HIV-1 infection.

Q~ (If applicable) When do you think you were exposed to AIDS?

A~ *Identify the appropriate time frame after exposure to test for HIV-1. (See the section "Mechanism of Action.")* If sufficient time has not elapsed, advise the patient to wait at least until the minimum time for antibody formation has passed.

Q~ Do you have difficulty collecting your own blood samples?

A~ If yes, advise the patient to obtain the assistance of a trusted person in performing the finger stick and blood collection. Explain that the person assisting should wear gloves and avoid sticking himself or herself with the lancing device.

Patient Counseling for HIV-1 Tests

Counseling on the use of HIV-1 tests should emphasize the importance of applying enough blood on the specimen card to ensure an accurate reading. The pharmacist should also advise the patient of the fragility of blood samples and to not delay in sending the specimen card. The box "Patient Education for HIV-1 Tests" lists specific information to provide patients.

Evaluation of Patient Outcomes with HIV-1 Tests

A patient with a positive result should see a physician to be retested for confirmation of HIV-1 infection. Patients with negative results should confirm that sufficient time had passed since potential exposure before they tested themselves.

Illicit Drug Use

An estimated 13 million Americans use illicit drugs. Drug abuse, in turn, leads to higher accident and absentee rates at work.[31] Drug abuse by adolescents is often never diagnosed, only partially diagnosed, or diagnosed too late for proper intervention.[32] Drug abuse tests allow parents and caregivers to detect such use early enough to affect the course of addiction.

Epidemiology of Illicit Drug Use

Illicit drug use is a problem in the United States regardless of socioeconomic status. In 1996, 5% of people ages 12 and over admitted they had used marijuana during the past month and 0.8% had used cocaine.[19]

Signs and Symptoms of Illicit Drug Use

The symptoms of illicit drug use are varied but may include withdrawal from activities, fatigue, red eyes, drowsiness, slurred speech, and chronic cough.[33–35]

Self-Detection of Illicit Drug Use with Drug Abuse Tests

Three products are available for detecting the use of illicit drugs: PDT-90 Personal Drug Testing Service uses hair as the sample material and both Parent's Alert Home Drug Testing Service and Dr. Brown's Home Drug Testing Service use urine to test for drug abuse. Table 43–3 lists the substances each test identifies.

Home drug tests are marketed primarily to parents as an aid for determining illicit drug use in their children. Home drug testing, however, is not a substitute for open communication between parents and children regarding drug use.

Patient Education for HIV-1 Tests

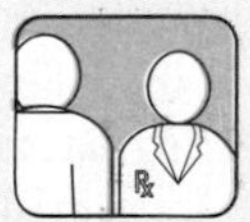

The objective of self-testing is to determine whether an HIV-1 infection is present. For most patients, carefully following package instructions and the self-care measures listed below will help ensure the achievement of accurate test results. Self-testing will allow prompt treatment of a detected infection.

Precautions

- Do not share the test lancet with other individuals. Do not allow the blood being tested to contact other individuals.
- The lancet is considered a biohazard; dispose of it appropriately.

Usage Guidelines

- Call the product manufacturer's toll-free number to register and to receive pretest counseling. The manufacturer's customer representative will ask for the confidential code included in the kit.
- With alcohol, clean the fingertip chosen for puncture.
- Prick the cleaned fingertip using the lancet provided, and place a few drops of blood on the blood specimen card. Fill the circle on the card completely to ensure a readable test. Examine the back of the card to ensure the blood soaked through. If it did not, place more blood on the front of the card. If a second blood stick is needed, use the second lancet provided in the kit.
- Allow the card to air-dry for 30 minutes, place sample in specimen return pouch, and seal in the prepaid and addressed shipping package. Be sure that the processing laboratory receives the specimen within 10 days of sampling.
- Call the manufacturer's toll-free number in 3 to 5 business days to obtain the results.

⚠ If the test is positive, see a physician right away for evaluation and treatment. Avoid activities that can result in transfer of blood or other body fluids to other individuals.

Table 43–3

Substances Detected by Home Drug Abuse Tests

Product	Substances Detected
PDT-90 Personal Drug Testing Service	Marijuana, cocaine, opiates, methamphetamine, phencyclidine (PCP)
Parent's Alert Home Drug Testing Service	Marijuana, cocaine, opiates, methamphetamine, ecstasy, barbiturates, benzodiazepines, lysergic acid diethylamide (LSD)
Dr. Brown's Home Drug Testing System	Marijuana, cocaine, amphetamine, PCP, codeine, morphine, heroin

These tests are a way to obtain results anonymously when drug use by a child is suspected.

Samples of urine or hair are collected at home and mailed to a clinical laboratory. Results are obtained by telephone. Some of the test kits include telephone counseling to (1) help parents recognize the signs of drug use, (2) assist in creating a family drug policy, and (3) emphasize to parents that they should use the test as a way to develop trust and open communication within their families rather than to threaten random testing.[31] Some telephone counseling programs provide referrals to rehabilitation and counseling services in the community.

Mechanism of Action

Clinical laboratories test the urine samples collected with a home drug abuse test for evidence of adulteration before processing the sample for the presence of illicit drugs. (Substances such as water or household chemicals can be added to urine samples in an attempt to mask drug use.) The laboratories use an enzyme-multiplied immunoassay technique to detect illicit drugs in the urine samples. Gas chromatography–mass spectrometry (GC–MS) is then used to identify the specific drug. Home urine tests detect drug use that occurred from several hours before testing to within 2 to 3 days before testing. The amount of drug found in the urine is affected by the time since consumption, the amount taken, and the amount of water consumed before sampling.[33–35] Test results are reported only as positive or negative for a drug. Quantity or route of ingestion is not determined.

Hair testing detects trace amounts of ingested drugs that become trapped in the core of the hair shaft as it grows at an average rate of ½ inch per month. Drug use over a 90-day period can be determined from a 1½ inch hair sample. The presence of drugs is determined by radioimmunoassay techniques, and then GC–MS analysis identifies the specific substance. Hair tests report positive or negative results for a drug. Positive results are reported as a number indicating low, medium, or high levels of use for all drugs except marijuana.

Usage Guidelines

See the box "Patient Education for Drug Abuse Tests."

Interferences

Ingestion of codeine-containing cough medicines, decongestants, antidiarrheals, and poppy seeds can cause false positive results for home drug abuse tests. These items contain substances structurally related to certain drugs of abuse.

Product Selection Guidelines

The criteria for selecting one drug abuse test over another include the drugs that are suspected of being used, the type of suspected use (casual versus chronic), the length of time since last use, and the possibility of the suspected drug user tampering with the sample. The list of drugs that may be identified with each kit varies. (See Table 43–3.) In general, urine tests are better for detecting low-level, casual drug use. Urine testing detects drugs from several hours before testing to the previous 2 to 3 days. Hair testing detects drugs from 5 to 90 days of use. It takes at least 5 to 7 days for hair to grow long enough away from the scalp for testing purposes.

Urine samples are subject to tampering by adding chemicals, by diluting with water, or by substituting someone else's sample. Hair samples, if taken directly from the person being tested, are not subject to tampering. Parents should weigh the possibility of tampering when deciding which type of test to choose.

Patient Assessment of Drug Abuse Tests

To determine which type of drug abuse test to recommend, the pharmacist should ask about the length of suspected drug use and the types of drugs that are suspected. The pharmacist should also ask whether the suspected user is likely to tamper with urine samples. The pharmacist should determine if the suspected user takes legal medications that are prescription and nonprescription. Asking the parent or caregiver the following questions will help elicit the information needed to determine whether testing is appropriate and which test is appropriate.

Q~ Who are you planning to test and why?

A~ Advise the parent or caregiver to use the tests to improve lines of communication rather than to punish the suspected drug user.

Q~ Have you already sought professional advice? If test results confirm suspected drug use, are you prepared to seek counseling?

A~ If the parent or caregiver has not sought professional advice, provide information about community rehabilitation resources.

Q~ Do you suspect casual or chronic drug use?

A~ *Identify which test is appropriate for each type of drug use. (See the section "Product Selection Guidelines.")* Recommend an appropriate test that is based on the degree of suspected drug use.

Q~ How long ago did the suspected drug use occur?

A~ Recommend an appropriate test that is based on the time frame of the suspected drug use. (See the section "Product Selection Guidelines.")

Q~ What are the suspected substances?

A~ Recommend a test that is based on the suspected substance of abuse. (See Table 43–3.)

Q~ What medications does the person being tested take?

A~ *Identify medications that can interfere with the test. (See the section "Interferences.")* Advise the parent or caregiver that these medications could cause false positive results.

Patient Counseling for Drug Abuse Tests

When parents or caregivers ask for assistance in selecting a drug abuse test, the pharmacist should be prepared to offer information about family counseling agencies as well as clinical advice. The pharmacist should emphasize the limitations of the tests when confirming illicit drug use and, in the case of urine tests, when identifying anything more than the type of drug that is being abused. The box "Patient Education for Drug Abuse Tests" lists specific information to provide patients.

Evaluation of Patient Outcomes with Drug Abuse Tests

If a positive result is obtained with a drug abuse test, parents or caregivers need to consider potential problems with the test itself before concluding that drug use is confirmed. They must not assume that a negative result is accurate. Parents should also consider the testing window when evaluating results.

Miscellaneous Home Tests

Hepatitis C Home Test

In April 1999, FDA approved a home test for detection of the hepatitis C virus. Home Access Hepatitis C Check is a single-use test kit containing two lancets, a gauze, a blood sample

Patient Education for Drug Abuse Tests

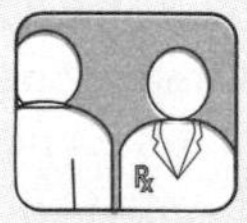

The objective of self-testing is to detect and to identify abuse of illicit drugs. For most patients, carefully following package instructions and the self-care measures listed below will help ensure achievement of accurate test results. Self-testing will allow prompt intervention to rehabilitate a confirmed drug user.

Avoidance of Incorrect Results

- Note that urine samples can be tampered with by adding water or household chemicals, possibly giving false results.
- Note that drug tests on urine samples report only a positive or negative outcome. The quantity of drug taken and the method in which it was taken are not determined.
- Note that drug tests on hair samples can report low, medium, or high level of use, but the use could have occurred as long as 90 days before testing.
- Note that poppy seeds, codeine-containing cough medicines, decongestants, and antidiarrheals can cause false positive test results.

Usage Guidelines

Urine Drug Abuse Tests

- Collect urine using the collection device included with the test. Do not take urine from the toilet.
- Check the temperature of the urine sample immediately after collection using the temperature strip included in the package. If the sample is not between 90°F to 100°F, adulteration may have occurred.
- Make sure the collection device is tightly closed. Put device in the collection package as directed and mail package.
- Results are available 2 to 3 business days after the laboratory receives the sample. To obtain the results, call the toll-free number provided in the kit and relay the code number accompanying the kit.

Hair Drug Abuse Tests

- Collect a hair sample that is ½-inch wide and one strand deep from the crown of the head as close to the scalp as possible.
- Align the cut ends of the hair sample, and place the sample in the collection package as directed. Do not collect hair from a hairbrush because there is no guarantee the hair is actually from the person to be tested.
- Results are available approximately 5 days after receipt by the laboratory. To access results, call the toll-free number and relay the code number accompanying the kit.

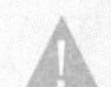

If the test is positive, seek the services of a drug rehabilitation organization.

card, gauze pad, an adhesive bandage, and a postage-paid envelope. Each kit also includes a unique personal identification number (PIN). The purchaser uses the PIN to register the kit and access test results.[36]

A recent study[37] reports that an estimated 4 million Americans are infected with hepatitis C. The hepatitis C virus is also responsible for 8000 to 10,000 deaths per year[38] (CDC unpublished data). This infection accounts for approximately one-third of all deaths due to chronic liver disease each year. Of people infected with hepatitis C, 85% are likely to progress to the chronic disease state. Clinically, hepatitis C may go undetected for many years; liver disease may be advanced by the time symptoms arise. Hepatitis C induces liver damage by causing hepatic cell necrosis and inflammation, which over time may progress to fibrosis, cirrhosis, and hepatocellular carcinoma.[39]

Current risk factors for transmission of the hepatitis C virus include high-risk sexual activity (e.g., unprotected intercourse),[40–42] and illicit drug use,[37,43] especially parenteral drug abuse and intranasal cocaine use, possibly via "straw-sharing."[44] Patients who received blood transfusions before 1992 are also at increased risk for developing hepatitis C.[38,43]

The kit tests for the presence of antibodies to the hepatitis C virus, not the virus itself. The Hepatitis C Check uses an enzyme linked immunosorbent assay (ELISA) to test for antibodies, then confirms the results with a recombinant immunoblot assay (RIBA). A patient who has recently been infected may receive a false negative result because antibodies have not had sufficient time to form against the virus. Clinical studies on file with the manufacturer report no false positive results. Patients who test positive should be referred to a physician, because treatment options are available only by prescription. These patients should also be vaccinated against other forms of hepatitis, such as the hepatitis A virus and hepatitis B virus.[36]

The pharmacist should counsel infected patients on precautions to avoid infection of others. These patients should also be advised to avoid alcohol and other drugs that may advance the progression of liver disease. Reviewing the illustrated product instructions with the patient will help ensure adherence with the following product usage guidelines:[36]

- Read all instructions carefully before using the test.
- Register the PIN with the manufacturer by calling the enclosed toll-free telephone number and following the automated directions.
- Remain seated during the testing process to prevent falling if dizziness occurs.
- Wash hands with warm, soapy water.
- Lance the side of one of the middle fingers.
- Apply a sufficient number of blood drops until both the front and back of the circular area on the testing card are saturated.
- Allow the sample to dry at least 30 minutes before sealing in the pouch and mailing.
- After 4 to 10 business days, call the 800 number provided and use the PIN number to access the test results. Test results are available for up to 1 year.
- Note that counseling is available 24 hours per day, for both negative and positive results, and is included in the cost of the testing unit.

Other Home Tests

The HealthCheck Skin Growth Monitoring System is available for patients to monitor skin growths while using a measuring device, color chart, body map, and journal. The HealthCheck Vision Screening test allows patients to test vision while using a vision screener or an Amsler grid. The Sensability Breast Self-Examination Aid is a 10-inch diameter, two-layer polyurethane breast shield containing a small amount of silicone lubricant that is meant to make breast self-examination easier and more comfortable.

Hypertension

Hypertension, which is defined as a blood pressure greater than 140/90,[45] is an asymptomatic disease. Its treatment often involves significant lifestyle changes (diet and exercise) and the institution of drug therapies. These measures inevitably produce side effects, so the patient who was without symptoms of disease is suddenly symptomatic. Patient education and empowerment play a large role in improving patient adherence with antihypertensive efforts. Adherence, in turn, helps reduce morbidity and mortality, maintains or improves the patient's quality of life, and improves the patient's use of health care resources.[46]

Teaching patients to take their own blood pressure at home is an excellent means of achieving these goals because home blood pressure monitoring (HBPM) gives patients a sense of control over their health. Patients can measure their progress toward a goal blood pressure level. In addition, HBPM provides valuable data on blood pressure values that occur away from the physician's office. Although the office measurement of blood pressure is still the mainstay of monitoring, hypertension experts strongly encourage the use of HBPM in the routine care of most patients with hypertension or suspected hypertension.[45,47] The sixth report of the Joint National Committee on the Detection, Evaluation, and Treatment of High Blood Pressure (JNC–VI) noted four general advantages of measuring blood pressure outside of the clinician's office: (1) distinguishing sustained hypertension from "white-coat hypertension," (2) assessing response to antihypertensive medication, (3) improving patient adherence to treatment, and (4) potentially reducing health care costs.

The market for HBPM devices has grown steadily over the past decade. Sales of home blood pressure monitors were $175 million in 1996.[48] Sales are expected to grow to $282 million by the year 2001.

Epidemiology of Hypertension

Between 1988 and 1994, hypertension affected nearly one in four U.S. adults over the age of 20.[19] A significant number of adults with hypertension have uncontrolled hypertension (20% of men and 17% of women with hypertension).[19] The reasons for this are multiple, but a significant factor is lack of patient motivation, which leads to nonadherence.

Complications of Hypertension

The consequences of untreated hypertension are well documented. Long-standing elevations in blood pressure can lead to damage of the heart, kidney, lungs, eyes, and vessels, and to an increase in morbidity and mortality.[45,49,50]

Self-Monitoring of Hypertension with Blood Pressure Monitors

Of the three categories of blood pressure monitors—mercury column, aneroid, and digital—aneroid and digital monitors are the most popular choices for home use. Table 43–4 lists examples of these two types of blood pressure monitors.

Mechanism of Action

Blood pressure readings include two types of pressures: systolic, which indicates contraction of the heart cavities, and diastolic, which indicates dilation of the heart cavities. Blood pressure is measured indirectly by two methods: auscultatory

Table 43–4

Selected Blood Pressure Monitors

Trade Name	Product Features
Aneroid Monitors	
Health Team Manual Monitor	Manual inflation; includes stethoscope and blood pressure log
Marshall One Person Monitor	Includes stethoscope and blood pressure log
Tycos Home Blood Pressure Monitor	Trigger-release inflation; includes stethoscope and tape of heart sounds
A&D UA-702 Manual Inflation Monitor	Manual inflation/deflation; low-battery indicator
A&D UA-777 One-Step Auto-Inflation Monitor	Automatic inflation/deflation; fuzzy logic operation; single-button operation
Digital Monitors	
A&D UB 211 Finger Digital Monitor	Automatic inflation; adjustable finger cuff
A&B UB-325 Wrist Digital Monitor	Automatic inflation/deflation; jumbo display; memory recall of 14 readings for 2 persons
Lumiscope 1060 Digital Monitor	Manual inflation/preset automatic deflation valve; D-bar cuff; memory recall of last reading
Lumiscope 1083N Finger Monitor	Automatic inflation/preset automatic deflation valve; adjustable finger cuff; memory recall of last reading
Lumiscope 1085M Auto Inflation Monitor	Automatic inflation/preset automatic deflation rate; D-bar cuff; jumbo LCD display; memory recall of last reading
Lumiscope 1090 Wrist Monitor	Automatic inflation/deflation; fuzzy logic operation; large LCD display of blood pressure, pulse, time, and date; memory recall of fourteen readings for two persons
Omron HEM-412C Manual Inflation Monitor	Manual inflation/automatic deflation; contoured D-ring cuff; digital display
Omron HEM-602 Wrist Monitor	Automatic inflation/deflation; jumbo digital display; memory recall of seven readings in digital and bar-graph form; built-in cuff storage feature
Omron HEM-705CP Monitor	Automatic inflation/deflation; curved contour D-ring cuff; large digital display; memory recall of 14 readings
Omron HEM-711 Smart-Inflate	Automatic inflation to ideal cuff level/automatic deflation; curved contour D-ring cuff; large display
Omron HEM-815F Finger Monitor	Automatic inflation/deflation; adjustable finger cuff
Sunbeam 7624 Manual Monitor	Manual inflation/deflation; one-touch operation; jumbo display; memory recall of last reading
Sunbeam 7654 Digital Monitor	Automatic inflation/deflation; jumbo display; fuzzy logic operation; memory recall of last reading
Sunbeam 7655-10 Digital Finger Monitor	Automatic inflation/deflation; adjustable finger cuff; over- or under-inflation indicator
Sunbeam 7684 Digital Wrist Monitor	Automatic inflation/deflation; jumbo display; fuzzy logic operation; memory recall of 14 readings for 2 persons

(measurement of sound) and oscillometric (measurement of vibration). Mercury and aneroid meters involve auscultation with the use of a stethoscope to detect Korotkoff's sounds, which are produced by the motion of the arterial wall in response to changes in arterial pressure. Oscillometric sensors, which are often used with digital meters, measure blood pressure by detecting blood surges underneath the cuff as it is deflated. The detection device, which is usually indicated on the cuff with a tab or other marking, is placed directly over the brachial artery. The brachial artery can be found by palpating 1 to 2 inches above and just to the inside of the antecubital space. As cuff pressure increases during the measurement procedure, the brachial artery is compressed and blood flow is obstructed. As cuff pressure is gradually released, blood flow is reestablished and Korotkoff's sounds can be heard in different phases. Phase I, which corresponds to systolic pressure, can be identified when at least two consecutive "beats" are heard as cuff pressure is decreased. The nature of the sounds changes over the next three phases. Diastolic pressure is identified as phase V, the disappearance of sound.

Interferences

Stress, smoking of tobacco and ingestion of caffeine-containing beverages can increase blood pressure. Conversely, eating or taking a hot bath can lower blood pressure.

Usage Guidelines

The actual measurement of blood pressure is a relatively simple procedure; however, many people consistently do it incorrectly. Blood pressure is naturally variable and can change in seconds. Thus, proper technique is essential to reduce measurement variability and to improve the quality of results. The normal range for blood pressures is established with patients sitting in the resting state; thus, any variation from this setting can produce inaccurate results.

Using the appropriate size cuff is essential for accurately measuring a patient's blood pressure. (See Table 43–5.) If the cuff is too small, blood pressure readings can be significantly overestimated by as much as 20 mm to 30 mm Hg. Several monitors are supplied with a large cuff; many others allow for the purchase of a large cuff separately. A thigh cuff for home monitoring is currently not available. For those patients requiring a thigh cuff, a wrist monitor may be a useful alternative. To obtain accurate readings with wrist cuffs, the patient must hold the wrist at heart level during the reading. Because these devices are also highly sensitive to changes in wrist level, it is best to support the arm on a table with a pillow that will raise the wrist to the appropriate level. For the person who is doing the actual monitoring, following the steps outlined in the box "Patient Education for Self-Monitoring of Blood Pressure" will help improve the accuracy of blood pressure readings whether they are taken in the physician's office, in the pharmacy, or in the home by the patient.

Table 43–5

Arm Circumferences for Determining Appropriate Cuff Size

Arm circumference (adult)[a]	Cuff size
<31 cm	Regular adult cuff
31–40 cm	Large adult cuff
>40 cm	Thigh cuff[b]

[a] Determine arm circumference by measuring around the midpoint of the upper arm. Remeasure the patient's arm periodically, especially if he or she has recently gained or lost significant weight.

[b] Consider a wrist monitor for patients whose arm circumference is >40 cm.

Source: References 46 and 51.

Product Selection Guidelines

Of the three types of blood pressure–measuring devices, no single device is best for every patient. The choice of device is individualized according to characteristics such as the patient's ability and willingness to learn, physical handicaps, patient preference, and the cost of the device. Mercury column devices are expensive and, as discussed below, have other disadvantages for home use. In general, aneroid devices are the least expensive. Depending on the features, a digital device can cost as much as a mercury column device. (See Table 43–4 for examples of commercially available aneroid and digital devices.) A discussion of the pros and cons of all three types of devices follows.

Mercury Column Devices

The mercury column blood pressure monitor is still the reference standard in blood pressure measurement. (See Figure 43–1.) This monitor typically comes with a cuff and an inflation bulb. The tubing from the cuff is attached to a column of mercury encased in a glass gauge.

Although mercury monitors are the most accurate and reliable of the devices, their routine use for home measurement is discouraged because they are cumbersome and pose the risk of mercury toxicity should the glass tubing break. They also require good eyesight and hearing for effective use. If the mercury does not rest at zero when the cuff is lying flat and completely deflated, the device needs recalibration.

Aneroid Devices

Next to the mercury column monitors, the aneroid devices are the most accurate and reliable. They are light, portable, and very affordable, and they pose no risk from mercury toxicity. They include several features that make patient teaching much easier. First, many devices now come with a stethoscope attached to the cuff. (See Figure 43–2.) This feature keeps the patient from having to hold the bell of the stethoscope in place. Second, a D-ring on the cuff allows a single user to place the cuff on the arm easily. Third, a few manufacturers offer a gauge that is attached to the inflation

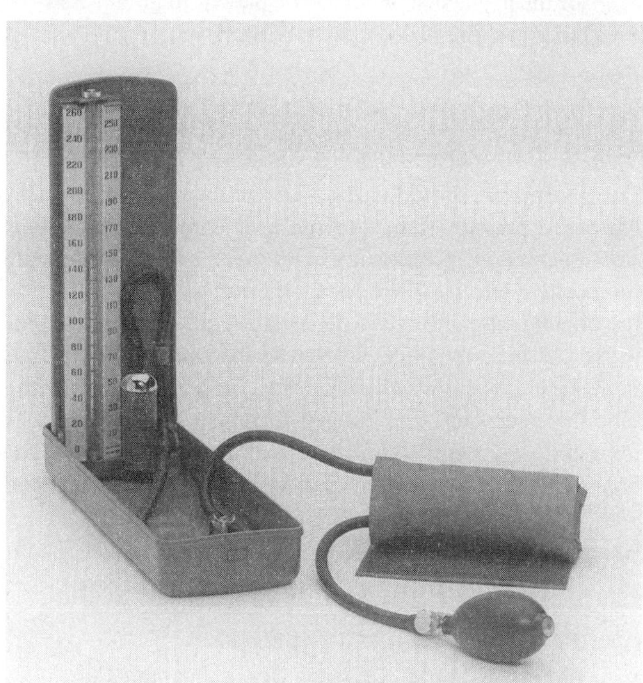

Figure 43–1 Mercury blood pressure monitor. Reprinted with permission from *Am Pharm.* 1989;NS29:578.

bulb; again, this gauge makes it easier to manipulate the equipment because there are fewer pieces to control. Such monitors are considered the option of choice for home use, but they do require careful patient instruction and follow-up. Good eyesight and hearing are necessary for accurate readings when using standard models. For patients with reduced visual capacity, however, devices with large-type print on the face of the gauge are available.

At the bottom of the face of each aneroid device is a small box. When the cuff is completely deflated and lying on the table, the needle of the gauge should rest in the box. If the needle is outside the box, the gauge needs recalibration. Many manufacturers sell recalibration tools to allow health care professionals to adjust the devices themselves.

Digital Devices

With advancing technology, digital devices are more accurate, reliable, and easy to use, and as a result have skyrocketed in popularity. (See Figure 43–3.) Such devices include semiautomatic (manually inflating), fully automatic (auto-inflating), wrist, and finger blood pressure monitors. Features such as printouts, a pulse monitor, a digital clock, automated inflation and deflation, memory, a large display, and a D-ring for the cuff differentiate many of the devices. These features add significantly to the price.

A major drawback to the digital monitors is the user's inability to determine whether the device is out of calibration. Many devices on the market lack extensive accuracy and reliability data, and they are often found to be inade-

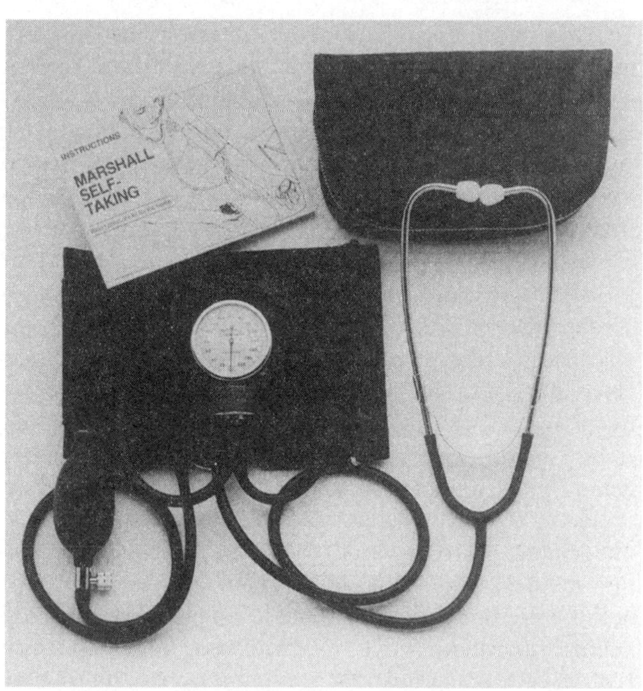

Figure 43–2 Aneroid blood pressure monitor. Photograph provided by Omron Healthcare, Inc., Vernon Hills, Ill. Reprinted with permission.

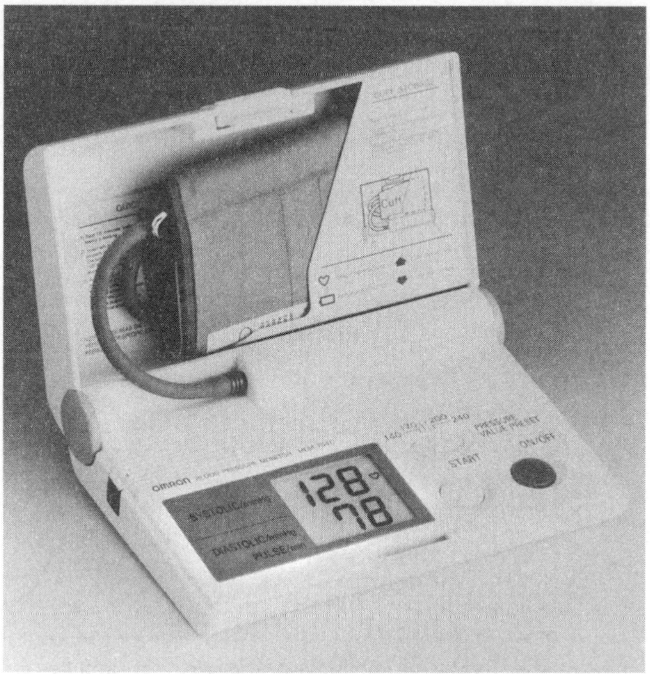

Figure 43–3 Digital blood pressure monitor. Photograph provided by Omron Healthcare, Inc., Vernon Hills, Ill. Reprinted with permission.

quate for routine use.[51,52] As a result, many clinicians recommend the use of the aneroid devices over the easier-to-use digital products. The JNC–VI report approves the use of both aneroid and digital monitors for home use. A recent study comparing blood pressure devices found that with a digital monitor only 34% of systolic and 48% of diastolic pressures measured were within ± 5 mm Hg of a mercury monitor.[53] Fifty-four percent of systolic and 58% of diastolic readings with an aneroid device were within ±5 mm Hg of a mercury monitor. The JNC–VI report notes that finger monitors are inaccurate and should not be used for home monitoring.[45]

Patient Assessment of Self-Monitoring of Blood Pressure

The pharmacist should first determine why a patient wishes to use a blood pressure monitor. If the use is warranted, the pharmacist should determine whether the patient has physical impairments that can interfere with proper use of the monitor. The pharmacist should also evaluate the patient's ability to comprehend and follow instructions. Asking the patient the following questions will help elicit the information needed to determine whether self-monitoring is appropriate and which monitor best meets the patient's needs or preferences.

Q~ Why do you want to take your blood pressure?

A~ If the patient thinks his or her blood pressure is elevated, ask whether a physician has diagnosed hypertension. If not, refer the patient to a physician. If the patient is diagnosed as hypertensive, ask the following questions to aid in selecting the appropriate device.

Q~ Have you been instructed on the use of a blood pressure monitor?

A~ Tailor the level of instruction to the patient's level of experience in using such devices.

Q~ Have you monitored your own blood pressure in the past? If so, what type of device did you use?

A~ If past use of a particular device was successful, recommend that the patient use that type of device again unless the patient prefers to use another device. If so, instruct the patient on the proper use of the new device.

Q~ Do you have difficulty with your hearing or vision? Do you have difficulty using your hands?

A~ *Identify which type of monitor or which monitor features are appropriate for patients with these physical impairments. (See the section "Product Selection Guidelines" and Table 43–4.)* If a patient has one or more such impairments, recommend a monitor that compensates for the problems, or advise the patient to obtain assistance in using a blood pressure monitor.

Patient Counseling for Self-Monitoring of Blood Pressure

The pharmacist should emphasize the importance of tracking blood pressure values to monitor control of hypertension. Regular self-monitoring of blood pressure will illustrate the positive effects of proper diet, exercise, and medication use on controlling the disorder. Such reinforcement can improve patient adherence with prescribed therapies. The patient should be shown the proper technique for monitoring blood pressure and encouraged to return to the pharmacy for a follow-up evaluation of the patient's technique. The box "Patient Education for Self-Monitoring of Blood Pressure" lists specific information to provide patients.

Evaluation of Patient Outcomes for Self-Monitoring of Blood Pressure

Patients measuring blood pressure for diagnostic purposes should be instructed how to track values and to discuss the values with a physician. Patients using home blood pressure measurement for monitoring of therapy should also track values. However, they should be cautioned not to adjust their medications unless instructed otherwise.

CONCLUSIONS

To advise patients properly on selecting and using home testing or monitoring products, pharmacists must be familiar with the procedures for each available product. Manufacturers are continually introducing new products and modifying current ones to provide more user-friendly versions. To keep up-to-date, pharmacists should request product information from manufacturers by calling their toll-free numbers or contacting their sales representatives.

Patients who are using diagnostic tests should be encouraged to follow instructions carefully and to contact either the pharmacist or the manufacturer's toll-free number for assistance if needed. The pharmacist should stress that the patients are self-testing, not self-diagnosing. Positive test results should be reported to a physician immediately for definitive diagnosis and management. Negative test results should be questioned when the patient is experiencing definite symptoms of a suspected condition. If there is any question about the results, the patient should seek the advice of a health professional. The pharmacist can play a major role in aiding hypertensive patients by motivating them to perform HBPM; by guiding them in product selection; by training them to use the device appropriately; and by facilitating communication between the patient, the patient's family, and the patient's primary care provider regarding any antihypertensive therapy.

Patient Education for Self-Monitoring of Blood Pressure

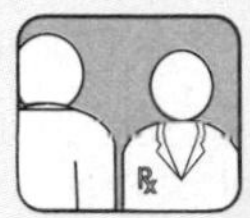

The objective of self-testing is to identify elevated blood pressure or to monitor the efficacy of diet, exercise, or medication in managing hypertension. For most patients, carefully following product instructions and the self-care measures listed below will help ensure accurate blood pressure readings.

Precautions/Avoidance of Incorrect Results

- Keep a log of blood pressure readings and of any circumstances that might have affected the reading (e.g., nervous, late for work).[54]
- If home readings are being done for diagnostic purposes, take readings at different times throughout the day and under different circumstances.[47]
- If readings are being done to determine adequacy of antihypertensive therapy, take the reading at the same time of day, preferably in the early morning soon after arising from bed.[47] Allow plenty of time to relax before taking a blood pressure reading. Feelings of stress or pressure can elevate the blood pressure.
- Do not smoke tobacco or drink caffeine-containing beverages for at least 30 minutes before taking a measurement. These activities can increase blood pressure.
- Wait 10 to 15 minutes after a bath and 30 minutes after eating to take a measurement. These activities can lower blood pressure.

Usage Guidelines

- Make sure the room is at a comfortable temperature.
- Sit in a comfortable chair, with the back supported and with the feet straight ahead and flat on the floor.
- If using an arm cuff, place the arm to be measured on a table, making sure the upper arm is at heart level as shown in the drawing.
- Remove restrictive clothing from the arm.
- If using a wrist cuff, place a pillow (or two pillows) under the arm to be measured so you bring the wrist up to heart level.
- Place the cuff on the arm to be measured. The cuff should be snug but not tight enough to restrict blood flow. Use the guidelines in Table 43–5 for selecting cuff size.
- Rest for at least 5 minutes in this position.
- Measure the blood pressure as directed by the product instructions. If using a stethoscope, listen for the Korotkoff's sounds as defined below:

  —Phase 1: Sound begins as a soft tapping. Record the systolic pressure at the point when two taps are heard in sequence.

  —Phase 2: Tapping sound gets louder and is accompanied by a swishing sound or murmur.

  —Phase 3: Tapping sounds persist but the swishing or murmur sound stops.

  —Phase 4: Muffling or softening of tapping sounds marks the start of phase 4.

  —Phase 5: Sound stops. Record the diastolic pressure at the point when sound stops.
- Take two to three measurements separated by at least 2 minutes using the same arm.
- Record the results, arm used, and the time and date of the measurement, as well as any medications, including antihypertensive medications, currently being taken plus the time of the last dose of each.

⚠ Do not adjust blood pressure medications on the basis of home measurements unless specifically instructed to do so by a physician.

References

1. Miller SW. Update on self-monitoring products. *NARD J.* 1992;114:51–4.
2. When it comes to choosing home tests, pharmacists can help. *Drug Topics.* 1998;142:54.
3. Centers for Disease Control and Prevention. Screening for colorectal cancer—United States, 1997. *MMWR Morb Mortal Wkly Rep.* 1999;48:116–21.
4. Williamson J, Wyandt C. Making a difference in cancer prevention. *Drug Topics.* 1999;143:71–80.
5. ColoCARE product information. Beaumont, TX: Helena Laboratories; 1991.
6. EZ-Detect product information. Newport Beach, CA: NMS Pharmaceuticals, Inc; 1994.
7. Frandzel S. Unipath Diagnostics. *Retail Pharmacy News.* 1999;March:34.
8. Quattrocchi E, Hove I. Ovulation and pregnancy home testing products. *US Pharm.* 1998;23(9):54–63.
9. Inglis JK. *A Textbook of Human Biology.* 3rd ed. New York: Pergamon Press; 1986:252–3.
10. Bioself product information. Thonex-Geneva, Switzerland: Bioself SA.
11. Labrecque M, Drevin J, Rioux JE. Validity of the Bioself 110 fertility indicator. *Fertil Steril.* 1989;63:604–8.
12. Ismail M, Arshat H, Pulcrano J, et al. An evaluation of the Bioself 110 fertility indicator. *Contraception.* 1989;30:53.

13. ClearPlan Easy Fertility Monitor product information. New York: Unipath Diagnostics; 1999.
14. Engle JP. Ovulation predictors. *Am Druggist.* 1993;207:55–6.
15. Newton GD, Pray S, Popovich NG. OTC 1997 review. *J Am Pharm Assoc.* 1998;38:199–209.
16. OVU-Tec Fertility Detector product information. Ocala, FL: Gennex Healthcare Technologies.
17. CycleView product information. Midvale, OH: Stilson Natural Products.
18. Gannon K. Who is most apt to turn to a home pregnancy test? *Drug Topics.* 1992;136:46.
19. *Health, United States, 1998 with Socioeconomic Status and Health Chartbook.* Hyattsville, MD: National Center for Health Statistics; 1998.
20. Bastian L, Nanda K, Hasselblad V, et al. Diagnostic efficiency of home pregnancy test kits: a meta-analysis. *Arch Fam Med.* 1998;7:465–9.
21. *Healthy People 2000.* Washington, DC: US Department of Health and Human Services; 1990:402.
22. Summary of the second report of the National Cholesterol Education Program (NCEP) Expert panel on detection, evaluation, and treatment of high blood cholesterol in adults: Adult Treatment Panel II. *JAMA.* 1993;269:3015–23.
23. McKenney JM, Hawkins DW, eds. *Handbook on the Management of Lipid Disorders.* Springfield, NJ: Scientific Therapeutics Information, Inc; 1995.
24. Cholestrak product information. Sunnyvale, CA: Chemtrak; 1995.
25. Bacheller CD, Bernstein J. Urinary tract infections. *Med Clin North Am.* 1997;81:719–30.
26. Uri-Test Nitrite in Urine product information. Miami, FL: Crosswell International Corporation; 1997.
27. UTI Home Screening Test product information. Bellevue, WA: Consumers Choice Systems; 1997.
28. AZO test strips product information. Woburn, MA: PolyMedica Corporation; 1997.
29. Segal M. Women and AIDS. *FDA Consumer.* 1993;27:9.
30. Home Access Express HIV-1 test system product information. Hoffman Estates, IL: Home Access Health Corporation; 1996.
31. Floren AE. Urine drug testing and the family physician. *Am Fam Physician.* 1994;49:1441.
32. Macdonald DI. Diagnosis and treatment of adolescent substance abuse. *Curr Prob Pediatr.* 1989;19:395.
33. Dr. Brown's Home Drug Testing System product information. Baltimore: Personal Health & Hygiene, Inc.
34. Parent's Alert Home Drug Test Service product information. Sunnyvale, CA: ChemTrak; 1997.
35. PDT-90 Personal Drug Testing Service product information. Cambridge, MA: Psychemedics Corporation; 1997.
36. Newton GD, McCullough JA, Pray WS, et al. New OTC drugs and devices 1999: A selective review. *J Am Pharm Assoc.* 2000:40(2):231–2.
37. Alter M, Kruszon-Moran D, Nainan O, et al. The prevalence of hepatitis C virus infection in the Unites States, 1988 through 1994. *N Eng J Med.* 1999;341:556–62.
38. FDA Licenses Improved Supplemental Test for Hepatitis C. *FDA Talk Paper.* Rockville, MD: Food and Drug Administration; February 12, 1999.
39. FDA Approves First Home Test for Hepatitis C Virus. *FDA Talk Paper.* Rockville, MD: Food and Drug Administration; April 29, 1999.
40. Recommendations for Prevention and Control of Hepatitis C Virus (HCV) and HCV-Related Chronic Disease. *MMWR Morbid Mortal Wkly Rep.* 1998;47(RR9):1–39.
41. Bresters D, Mauser-Bunschoten E, Reesink H, et al. Sexual transmission of the hepatitis C. *Lancet.* 1993;342:210–1.
42. Piazza M, Sagliocca L, Tosone G, et al. Sexual transmission of hepatitis C and efficacy of prophylaxis with intramuscular immune serum globulin: A randomized controlled trial. *Arch Intern Med.* 1997;157: 1537–44.
43. Conry-Cantilena C, VanRaden M, Gibble J, et al. Routes of infection, viremia, and liver disease in blood donors found to have hepatitis C virus infection. *N Eng J Med.* 1996;334:1691–6.
44. *Pharmacist's Letter.* Detail #151115; November 1999.
45. Joint National Committee on Detection, Evaluation, and Treatment of High Blood Pressure. The sixth report of the Joint National Committee on the Detection, Evaluation, and Treatment of High Blood Pressure (JNC–VI). *Arch Intern Med.* 1997;157:2413–46.
46. Soghikian K, Casper SM, Fireman BH, et al. Home blood pressure monitoring: effect on use of medical services and medical care costs. *Med Care.* 1992;30:855–65.
47. Kaplan NM. Measurement of blood pressure. In: Kaplan NM, ed. *Clinical Hypertension.* Baltimore: Williams and Wilkins; 1998:19–39.
48. Stickel AL. Opportunities abound in home blood pressure monitoring market. *Am Druggist.* 1998;215:33–6.
49. Stamler J, Neaton JD. Blood pressure, systolic and diastolic, and cardiovascular risk: US population data. *Arch Intern Med.* 1993;153:598–615.
50. Pyorala K, De Backer G, Graham I, et al. Prevention of coronary heart disease in clinical practice. Recommendations of the task force of the European Society of Cardiology, European Atherosclerosis Society and European Society of Hypertension. *Atherosclerosis.* 1994;110:121–61.
51. von Egmond J, Lenders JW, Weernink E, et al. Accuracy and reproducibility of 30 devices for self-measurement of arterial blood pressure. *Am J Hypertens.* 1993;6:873–9.
52. O'Brien E, Mee F, Atkins N, et al. Inaccuracy of seven popular sphygmomanometers for home measurement of blood pressure. *J Hypertens.* 1990;8:621–34.
53. Johnson KA, Partsch DJ, Gleason P, et al. Comparison of two home blood pressure monitors with a mercury sphygmomanometer in an ambulatory population. *Pharmacotherapy.* 1999;19:333–9.
54. King DS, Evans YQ, Noble SL. Educating patients on hypertension and blood pressure monitoring. *Drug Topics.* 1998;142(Nov suppl):1–15.

CHAPTER 44

Adult Urinary Incontinence Supplies

Martin D. Higbee

Chapter 44 at a Glance

Urinary incontinence is defined as the involuntary loss of urine in an amount or with a frequency that is sufficient to be a social or health problem.[1] The consequences of this problem are considerable. First, many elderly people are embarrassed by such a condition and refrain from discussing their urinary problems with their primary health care providers. Second, elderly people often accept the myth that urinary incontinence is a normal consequence of aging, rather than a symptom of underlying disease or anatomic change. This acceptance leads to depression and low self-esteem. Social isolation occurs because the incontinent elderly patient refuses social interaction to avoid the embarrassment and rejection that often accompany urinary incontinence. Intimate contact and sexual activity with the patient's partner can also decrease. Thus, the patient's social and psychologic well-being are compromised. Third, attempts to limit episodes of involuntary urine loss by restricting fluid intake can cause dehydration and hypotension, while skin irritation and ulceration caused by long exposure to urine results in "diaper rash" and, perhaps worst of all, pressure ulcers.[1]

The caregivers of incontinent elderly patients are under stress because of the tedious and time-consuming care needed to deal with the problem at home. Often the loss of urine control leads to premature institutionalization or to elder abuse.[1,2] It is, therefore, important that health care professionals, patients, and caregivers recognize that urinary incontinence is a symptom and not a single disease process. Urinary incontinence must always be medically evaluated because it can often be treated and resolved.[1,2] For some patients, protective undergarments and pads allow independence and mobility. These products can also be used in the care of bedridden, incontinent patients.

Epidemiology of Urinary Incontinence

As illustrated by the discussion of predisposing factors in the following section, the incidence of urinary incontinence is high among the elderly population, afflicting 30% of the elderly in the community, 35% of those in hospitals, and approximately 60% of those in nursing homes.[1] The annual costs associated with this problem are staggering: $7 billion for care in the community and $3.3 billion for nursing home residents, according to 1987 costs.[3]

Physiologic Changes in the Urinary Tract

Age-related changes in the bladder and urinary tract may contribute to an elderly person's vulnerability to urinary incontinence. This vulnerability is especially true for women. With age, the kidney's ability to concentrate urine dimin-

Editor's Note: This chapter is based, in part, on the 11th edition chapter titled "Diaper Rash, Prickly Heat, and Adult Incontinence Products," which was written by Gary H. Smith, Victor A. Elsberry, and Martin D. Higbee.

ishes, resulting in larger urine volumes. In addition, age-related hypotrophic changes in bladder tissue lead to frequent urination and nocturia (urinating at night), while decreases in the muscle tone of the bladder, as well as of the bladder sphincters and pelvic muscles, contribute to the potential for decreased urine control. This loss of control, combined with diminished mobility and reaction time, sets the stage for many elderly people to develop urinary incontinence.[2,4]

Certain chronic and acute illnesses encountered in the elderly may enhance the potential for urinary incontinence. Parkinson's disease, stroke, and conditions of cerebrovascular degeneration can disrupt parasympathetic control of the bladder, leading to bladder instability and a decline in bladder capacity.[4] Conditions that cause peripheral neuropathy (e.g., vascular disease, diabetes mellitus, and nutritional deficiencies) may also decrease bladder capacity, leading to an increased need to urinate.[4]

In women, the loss of estrogen with age causes a decrease in bladder outlet and urethral resistance, as well as a decline in pelvic musculature—all of which increase the likelihood of urinary incontinence. Additionally, estrogen loss results in atrophic changes in the vaginal and urethral mucosa, disrupting the vaginal flora and leading to atrophic vaginitis and chronic urethritis. These conditions, in turn, may cause urinary frequency and urgency, dysuria (difficult or painful urination), urinary tract infections, and urinary incontinence.[2,4] The woman's short urethra exerts less resistance to intravesicular pressure than does the longer male urethra. Childbirth, gynecologic procedures, and obesity also weaken the woman's pelvic floor muscles, thereby decreasing support for the bladder. As a consequence, the anatomy of the bladder becomes distorted, resulting in cystocele, rectocele, or uterine prolapse. These conditions result in chronic obstruction to the bladder, again leading to incontinence.[4] For their part, men often have prostatic enlargement, which results in urethral obstruction leading to decreased urinary flow rates, increased residual volumes, detrusor instability, and overflow incontinence.[2] Urologic surgical procedures, such as prostatectomy, may also contribute to urine leakage in men.

Types of Urinary Incontinence

Part of the difficulty in understanding and communicating about urinary incontinence is the number of synonyms used to describe the same condition. The basic types of incontinence and their associated synonyms are as follows:[1]

- Detrusor instability: detrusor hyperactivity, detrusor overactivity, detrusor hyperreflexia, unstable bladder, spastic bladder, uninhibited bladder, urge incontinence.
- Stress incontinence: sphincter insufficiency, outlet impotence.
- Overflow incontinence: detrusor areflexia, atonic bladder, impaired contractility, urge incontinence.
- Functional incontinence: reflex incontinence.
- Iatrogenic incontinence.
- Mixed incontinence.

Transient and *established* are other terms occasionally used to describe the type of urinary incontinence manifested.[5,6] Transient incontinence usually occurs suddenly and is secondary to acute illness,(e.g., urinary tract infections) or to any disease that causes acute confusion (e.g., respiratory disease, myocardial infarction, septicemia) or immobility so that the person cannot reach a toilet independently or in time.[5,6] Established incontinence is persistent and related to neurologic or other chronic conditions, such as prostatic hypertrophy, cystocele, or uterine prolapse.[4–6] *Urge incontinence* is another term often used by the public. The condition is a sudden desire to void, resulting often in uncontrolled urine loss. This term is medically imprecise because both detrusor instability and overflow incontinence have associated urgency as a symptom.[1]

Pathophysiology/Etiology of Adult Urinary Incontinence

Detrusor Incontinence

Detrusor instability is a common form of incontinence caused by uninhibited contractions of the detrusor muscle, which are bundles of smooth muscle fibers that form the body of the bladder and cause urine expulsion when they contract.[1] The primary symptoms of detrusor instability are an urgent sensation to void urine and an inability to delay voiding when the sensation occurs. The etiology of this incontinence is most often related to local irritants or central nervous system diseases, such as dementias, stroke, Parkinson's disease, and demyelinating diseases (e.g., multiple sclerosis).[5,7]

Stress Incontinence

Stress incontinence is the most frequently encountered type of urinary incontinence in women. It is characterized by involuntary leakage of small amounts of urine during sudden increases in intra-abdominal pressure which occurs with sneezing, laughing, coughing, exercising, and lifting.[1,5,7] This involuntary leakage is thought to be caused by hypermobility of the bladder neck or weakness of the bladder sphincter and pelvic floor muscles.[1] Hypermobility refers to displacement of the bladder neck and urethra during exertion, and it occurs when the supporting pelvic muscles have been weakened as a result of childbearing and aging. The weakening of the sphincter can be secondary to surgery or trauma, or it may be neurogenic in etiology.[1]

Overflow Incontinence

Overflow incontinence results in dribbling, urgency, and sometimes stress incontinence. It occurs when the bladder cannot be emptied properly because of an obstruction (prostate hypertrophy, cystocele, fecal impaction) or a contractile state (diabetes mellitus, drugs) and when the bladder is thus overdistended.[1,5]

Functional Incontinence

Functional incontinence is associated with the inability to reach toileting facilities in time or to perform toileting tasks. Causes of this type of incontinence are many and include stroke, diminished mobility, impaired cognitive function or perception, environmental barriers, and psychologic unwillingness to release urine in the proper place.[1,5,7]

Iatrogenic Incontinence

Iatrogenic causes of incontinence should be considered because many medications are capable of causing transient incontinence. Incontinence may result from the medical use of physical restraints that make using the toilet without assistance impossible. Drugs with anticholinergic action (phenothiazines, antihistamines, and antidepressants) may inhibit bladder function (emptying). Decongestants may cause retention of urine by stimulating α- and β-receptors, which enhance bladder filling and increase the bladder's sphincter tone. The α-receptor agonists used for hypertension treatment may also enhance the action of adrenergic receptors in the bladder. Diuretics, particularly if given late in the evening, may overwhelm the elderly person's ability to visit the toilet. Sedating medications (hypnotics) may decrease the older patient's awareness of bladder filling.[1,7]

Mixed Incontinence

It is important for health care professionals to understand that urinary incontinence is rarely one isolated type of incontinence, but rather it is often a mixture of types. Elderly women frequently have stress incontinence with an element of detrusor instability (urge incontinence). Among men with outlet obstruction (prostate enlargement), 50% have detrusor instability.[1,5,7]

Treatment of Adult Urinary Incontinence

Treatment Outcomes

The goals of self-treatment in urinary incontinence are to (1) control or treat skin breakdown (diaper rash), (2) control the odor of leaked urine, and (3) control leakage of urine from undergarments.

General Treatment Approach

After medical evaluation has occurred and a diagnosis has been established, treatment with appropriate agents and nonpharmacologic measures can be implemented for each type of urinary incontinence. Most medications used to treat these disorders are prescription products, but in some cases nonprescription medications may be appropriate.

Nonprescription medications such as skin protectants are used to control or treat skin breakdown caused by the irritating effects of urine. Adult diaper rash was not addressed by the Food and Drug Administration (FDA) during its 1990 review of products for infant diaper rash. Therefore, since FDA has no guidelines for such products, the pharmacist may interpolate from the FDA's proposed skin protectant monograph for use of ingredients in infant products.[8] (See Chapter 30, "Diaper Dermatitis and Prickly Heat," for a discussion of these agents.)

Chlorophyll-containing products control urine odor, and absorbent undergarments or briefs prevent the leakage of urine.

Although not many nonprescription products are available for this medical problem, pharmacists should be familiar with this disease process to advise patients and caregivers appropriately. Oral nonprescription medications may be useful in some cases of detrusor instability and stress incontinence. Diphenhydramine and pseudoephedrine can be used, for example, to help control urine loss. However, these medications should be used only after a thorough evaluation has determined the cause and/or type of incontinence. Inappropriate use of systemic nonprescription products and incorrect use of absorbent undergarments and pads before a proper evaluation has been made may result in unnecessary expense, inappropriate treatment, and possibly unnecessary changes in the patient's lifestyle and psychologic well-being.

Type-Specific Treatment Approaches

The type of incontinence will influence the choice of treatments. For that reason, an overview of the nonpharmacologic and pharmacologic measures for specific types of urinary incontinence is presented here.

Detrusor Incontinence

Detrusor instability may be treated with anticholinergic medications, which facilitate urine storage by decreasing uninhibited detrusor contractions. Most often a prescription medication such as oxybutynin chloride, flavoxate hydrochloride, or hyoscyamine will be initiated for this type of incontinence.[1,5] However, diphenhydramine is occasionally used as initial drug therapy. (See Chapter 9, "Disorders Related to Cold and Allergy.") Pharmacists should counsel patients about the potential side effects that occur more frequently with diphenhydramine than with the other prescription products. Sedation, dry mouth (a problem for denture use), constipation, and confusion can be significant problems in elderly patients. In addition, the patient should be instructed to do pelvic floor muscle exercises and encouraged to adhere to a "timed voiding" schedule to increase the efficacy of treatment.[1] Contraindications to the use of diphenhydramine (and other anticholinergic medications) include many conditions (e.g., narrow-angle glaucoma, peptic ulcer, urinary tract obstruction, and hyperthyroidism) that occur more often in elderly individuals than in other patients.

Stress Incontinence

Stress incontinence is often treated with agents that increase outflow resistance through α-receptor stimulation that enhances contraction of the bladder neck muscles. Commonly recommended drugs are often nonprescription agents such as ephedrine, pseudoephedrine, phenylephrine, and phenylpropanolamine. (See Chapter 9, "Disorders Related to Cold and Allergy.") Caution should be used, however, when initiating such therapy in patients with hypertension and/or cardiac arrhythmias. The pharmacist should advise patients to monitor their blood pressure and pulse, and to report any new occurrences of heart palpitations or fainting. As in detrusor instability, the use of pelvic floor muscle exercises and a timed voiding schedule will assist in controlling stress incontinence.[1]

In women, estrogen therapy may be used; benefits are usually seen in 4 to 6 weeks. Estrogen can be used in combination with α-adrenergic agonists. Pharmacists should counsel female patients about the common side effects of estrogen therapy, such as weight gain, fluid retention, increased blood pressure, and vaginal spotting. Should medical treatment fail, surgical correction may be possible.[1]

Overflow Incontinence

The treatment of overflow incontinence is directed by the underlying cause. Surgery is often necessary. Prescription agents such as bethanechol chloride with or without metoclopramide may be initiated if the bladder has insufficient contractile strength.[1] Catheterization, a last resort, is used when medical and surgical corrections have failed.[1]

Functional/Iatrogenic Incontinence

Treatment of functional and iatrogenic incontinence requires evaluating the patient's entire medical status and medication history. Side effects from medications can often be eliminated by initiating alternative treatments. Underlying dysfunctions such as rheumatoid arthritis and decreased mobility can be remedied by medical as well as environmental changes that make using the toilet easier and possible within the limitations of the patient's functional status. Often an assessment by physical or occupational therapists can remedy many problems caused by physical limitations of the patient.

Use of Urinary Incontinence Supplies

Protective undergarments and pads are used to protect clothing, bedding, and furniture, while allowing the patient to have independence and mobility. Although absorbent products are very beneficial, they should be used only after a thorough and complete examination.[5] If patients or caregivers prematurely initiate the use of absorbent protective products, they treat the symptom and obscure the cause. Because correction may be possible, the premature acceptance of urinary incontinence may have significant financial, social, and psychologic consequences.

Product Selection Factors

The type of absorbent product used depends on several factors:[7]

- Type and severity of incontinence.
- Functional status.
- Sex.
- Availability of caregivers.
- Patient preference.
- Convenience.

The pharmacist needs to discuss these factors with patients and their caregivers while helping to select absorbent products. Absorbent garments and pads are available as reusable or disposable products. (See Table 44–1 for examples of commercially available products.) The disposable product market has become a multimillion dollar industry during the past decade.[9] These products work in the same manner as children's disposable diapers. They are designed to absorb urine; to provide a moisture barrier to protect clothes, bedding, and furniture; and to minimize skin contact with urine. Urine is jelled in the matrix, which minimizes urine contact with skin.

The capacity of each disposable product corresponds to the needs of the patient:

- Guards/shields: 2 to 12 ounces (60 to 360 mL), light to heavy capacity.
- Briefs: 28 to 36 ounces (840 to 1100 mL), moderate to heavy capacity.
- Undergarments: 12 to 18 ounces (360 to 540 mL), moderate to heavy capacity.

Patients with small amounts of leakage, as occurs in stress or overflow incontinence and following urologic surgical procedures (e.g., dribbling), may require only a shield. If larger amounts of urine are lost with incontinence, as often occurs with detrusor instability, products with a larger capacity would be more appropriate. Many products are designed for overnight (heavy) use and tend to have the largest capacities.[9,10]

Another important issue is the functional capacity of the patient. If the patient needs assistance with the absorbent garments, the caregiver may find that briefs or diapers with "roll-on" bed application and adhesive closures are useful. Securing the product may be an important issue. Some garments or shields have adhesive strips or belts to hold them in place. Belts may require assistance from a caregiver. Of course, comfort and leg security from urine leakage are important. Many product lines offer elastic legs or contoured shapes. The anatomic differences between men and women are another consideration. Caregivers and patients should consider products designed with these differences in mind when using large-capacity products.[9,10]

Protective underpads are often used in conjunction with briefs and undergarments for extended duration activities,

Table 44–1

Selected Adult Incontinence Products

Trade Name	Product Features[a]
Attends Briefs	For heavy leakage; sizes S, M, L; refastenable tapes
Attends Guards Super Absorbency	For light/moderate leakage; curved fit
Attends Pads	For light leakage
Attends Undergarments Regular Absorbency	For moderate leakage; reusable elastic belts
Attends Undergarments Super Absorbency	For heavy leakage; reusable elastic belts
Depend Fitted Briefs Regular Absorbency	For heavy leakage; sizes S, M, L; six refastenable tapes plus elastic leg and waist
Depend Fitted Briefs Super Absorbency	For heavy leakage (absorbs 30% more urine than regular absorbency); sizes M, L; six refastenable tapes plus elastic leg and waist
Depend Guards for Men	For light/moderate leakage; one size; anatomic design with elasticized pouch and cup-like fit
Depend Undergarments Easy Fit Elastic Leg Regular Absorbency	For moderate leakage; soft, cloth-like outer cover; one size; reusable hook and hoop strap tabs
Depend Undergarments Easy Fit Elastic Leg Extra Absorbency	For moderate leakage; soft, cloth-like outer cover; one size; reusable hook and hoop strap tabs
Depend Undergarments Elastic Leg Regular Absorbency	For moderate leakage; soft, cloth-like outer cover; one size; reusable button strap tabs
Depend Undergarments Elastic Leg Extra Absorbency	For moderate leakage; soft, cloth-like outer cover; one size; reusable button strap tabs
Poise Thin Pads Light Absorbency	For light leakage; maxipad size; elasticized sides
Poise Pads Regular Absorbency	For light leakage; maxipad size; elasticized sides
Poise Pads Extra Absorbency	For light leakage; maxipad size; elasticized sides
Poise Pads Extra Plus Absorbency	For light leakage; maxipad size; elasticized sides
Poise Pads with Side Shields Ultra Absorbency	For heavy leakage; padlike comfort with guard-like absorbency
Stayfree Serenity Curved Pads Extra Absorbency	For light/moderate leakage; curved fit
Stayfree Serenity Curved Pads Extra Plus Absorbency	For light/moderate leakage; curved fit
Stayfree Serenity Guards Regular Absorbency	For moderate leakage
Stayfree Serenity Guards Super Absorbency	For moderate/heavy leakage
Stayfree Serenity Guards Super Plus Absorbency	For heavy leakage
Stayfree Serenity Thin Pads	For light leakage
Stayfree Serenity Pads	For light/moderate leakage

[a] S = small, M = medium, and L = large.

such as sleeping and sitting. Both bed and chair pads are available, and the pharmacist should inquire about the need for additional protection. The underpad should have a known capacity, a waterproof duration of several hours, and an ability to remain intact when wet. Bed pads are available in sizes from 16 × 24 inches to 24 × 24 inches. For chairs, a pad that is 16 × 18 inches should be used.[10]

Complications from Absorbent Products

Because the use of absorbent products increases the risk of skin irritation and maceration, such products should be checked every 2 hours. With continual urine loss, it is recommended that the absorbent material be changed every 2 to 4 hours. The use of skin protectants (barrier creams and ointments) as in diaper rash is appropriate. Should a rash occur, the same treatment is indicated as that described for infants in Chapter 30, "Diaper Dermatitis and Prickly Heat."

Odor is an embarrassing problem. Nonprescription products containing chlorophyll (e.g., Derifil, Pals, and Nullo) can be recommended to help decrease urine odor. However, frequent checks and changes are better than efforts to disguise the odor.

Pressure ulcers may occur if the patient is immobile. Any skin breakdown with the development of lesions needs to be reported to the primary care provider. This serious compli-

Case Study 44–1

Patient Complaint/History

MR, a 72-year-old woman, presents to the pharmacy with a complaint of "urine release"; she reveals that the first incident occurred 2 weeks earlier during lunch with friends. The patient goes on to explain that the "leakage" occurs when she laughs, coughs, or sneezes. As a result, she has become depressed and declines social invitations.

MR recalls that a friend who also experienced urine leakage was treated by a physician with a "cold medicine." The patient pleads for help, exclaiming, "I can't go on like this! I'm missing so much because of this problem, and I'm so depressed and embarrassed."

The patient's known medical problems include hypertension and congestive heart failure for which she has taken hydrochlorothiazide 25 mg once daily for 6 years, digoxin 0.25 mg once daily for 3 years, potassium chloride 20 mEq once daily for 6 years, and ofloxacin 200 mg twice daily for 7 days. Other medications include an unidentified cough medicine as needed, aspirin taken occasionally for headache, and chlorpheniramine sustained-release capsules 8 mg as needed for allergies.

Clinical Considerations/Strategies

Readers can use the following considerations/strategies to determine whether treating the patient's condition with nonprescription medications is warranted:

- Determine what additional information is needed and formulate the appropriate questions.
- On the basis of information provided, assess the most likely explanation for this patient's symptoms/condition.

Patient Education/Counseling

Readers can use the following strategies to develop a patient education/counseling plan that will help ensure optimal therapeutic outcomes:

- Provide the patient with information to help her understand the condition.
- Define a care plan for the patient.
- Identify the type of absorbent garment that could be used if applicable.
- Define nonpharmacologic treatments that could resolve the problem.
- Counsel the patient on the appropriate use of medications prescribed by the physician.
- Advise the patient of adverse effects that may occur with pharmacologic therapy.

cation should not be treated with nonprescription products without medical supervision.

Because most pharmacies do not carry a full line of products for the urine incontinent patient, the pharmacist can direct patients to the National Association for Continence, PO Box 8310, Spartanburg SC 29305-8310; 864-579-7900, 800-BLADDER, or fax 864-579-7902.

Patient Assessment of Adult Urinary Incontinence

Pharmacists must obtain enough patient history to ensure that requests for nonprescription products are made under the proper medical supervision. Because of the public's general lack of sufficient medical knowledge about the different types of urinary incontinence, some patients (or their caregivers) may attempt self-diagnosis and treatment without consulting their primary care providers. This self-diagnosis could obviously lead to inappropriate assessment and treatment. Thus, it is imperative that pharmacists inquire about a proper medical evaluation before recommending nonprescription products, including absorbent products.

Armed with the patient's history and proper diagnosis, the pharmacist can answer questions appropriately and can help in the selection and proper use of devices and medications for treating this disorder. Before recommending nonprescription products, even absorbent undergarments, for incontinent patients, the pharmacist should ask the following questions.

Q~ Has a physician evaluated your incontinence?

A~ If no, encourage the patient or caregiver to consult a physician to ensure that the disorder is being treated properly. An early evaluation may lead to resolution of the urinary incontinence.

Q~ What type of urinary incontinence does the patient have?

A~ Base recommendations for nonprescription products, especially absorbency of garments, on the degree of bladder control associated with each type of incontinence. This approach allows the pharmacist to estimate volume of urine loss in order to determine the type of incontinence product needed (e.g. guards/shields versus undergarments).

Q~ What time of day is the protection needed most?

A~ If nighttime protection is the greatest need, recommend undergarments with large absorption capacities.

Q~ Does the patient use the toilet and change undergarments independently?

A~ If no, recommend briefs or diapers with roll-on bed application and adhesive closures.

Q~ What products have been used to treat or prevent rash? Odor?

A~ On the basis of the patient's response, determine whether the appropriate products are being used for these problems and whether they are being used properly. Advise the patient accordingly.

Patient Counseling for Adult Urinary Incontinence

The pharmacist's role in self-treatment of urinary incontinence is limited primarily to assisting patients and caregivers in selecting products to manage the overflow of urine. The box "Patient Education for Urinary Incontinence" lists specific information to provide patients.

Evaluation of Patient Outcomes for Adult Urinary Incontinence

At follow-up, the pharmacist should find out whether the recommended incontinence product is comfortable and easy to use, and whether leakage from the undergarment or odor is a problem. If leakage is occurring, the absorbency and/or type of product may need to be changed. Patients who have problems with odor may need to use deodorizers. The patient or caregiver should also be asked whether the skin, especially in the perivaginal and perianal areas, is being checked for breakdown. Redness or skin fissures call for the use of skin protectants. Questioning about occurrence of urinary tract or vaginal infections is also appropriate. Such infections may indicate a need to change garments more often or to use another type of garment. These measures will prevent prolonged skin contact with urine.

The pharmacist should also evaluate whether the use of incontinence products has allowed the patient to resume his or her normal life style and social interactions. If these objectives are not being met, the cause of the incontinence should be reevaluated. Other undergarment options should also be considered.

CONCLUSIONS

Urinary incontinence is common in the elderly community. Because various processes can cause this complex urinary disorder, the patient should receive a full medical evaluation before treating the problem. At that point, a variety of treatments—both pharmacologic and nonpharmacologic—can be prescribed, depending on the etiology and type of the disorder. The pharmacist can assist the patient or caregiver by

Patient Education for Urinary Incontinence

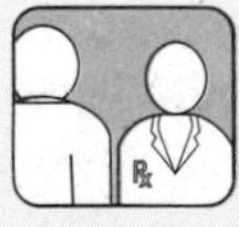

The objectives of self-treatment are to (1) control or treat skin irritation caused by contact with urine, (2) control the odor of urine leaked from the bladder, and (3) control leakage of urine from undergarments. For most patients, carefully following product instructions and the self-care measures below will help ensure optimal therapeutic outcomes.

- Consult a physician for a thorough examination before using absorbent undergarments or shields. Many cases of urinary incontinence are reversible with treatment.
- Be aware that these products are designed to absorb urine; to provide a moisture barrier to protect clothes, bedding, and furniture; and to minimize skin contact with urine.
- Base selection of absorbent products on the amount of leaked urine:
  —Guards/shields: 2 to 12 ounces (60 to 360 mL), light to heavy capacity.
  —Briefs: 28 to 36 ounces (840 to 1000 mL), moderate to heavy capacity.
  —Undergarments: 12 to 18 ounces (360 to 540 mL), moderate to heavy capacity.
- Choose briefs or diapers with roll-on bed application and adhesive closures for patients who are unable to change themselves.
- If additional protection is needed during sleeping and sitting, select absorbent bed or chair pads to use with absorbent undergarments.
- Check skin for irritation or maceration every 2 hours, even when absorbent garments are used.
- If urine loss is continual, change absorbent undergarments every 2 to 4 hours.
- If desired, use skin protectants labeled for diaper rash to protect the patient's skin.
- If desired, use products containing chlorophyll, such as Derifil, Pals, and Nullo to help decrease odor. However, continue frequent skin checks and frequent changes of absorbent undergarments.

⚠ If pressure ulcers (open sores) occur in an immobile patient, consult a physician. Do not attempt to treat the ulcers with nonprescription products.

providing medication counseling, advice on the complications, and assistance in selecting appropriate absorbent devices for patients with urinary incontinence.

References

1. Rosenthal AJ, McMurtry CT. Urinary incontinence in the elderly: often simple to treat when properly evaluated. *Postgrad Med.* 1995;97:109–21.
2. Pickell GC, Ham RJ, Smith MR, et al. Genitourinary and sexual problems of the elderly. In: Ham RJ, Holtzman JM, Marcy ML, et al., eds. *Primary Care Geriatrics: A Case-Based Learning Program.* Littleton, MA: PSG Inc; 1983:203–13.
3. Hu TW. Impact of urinary incontinence on health-care costs. *J Am Geriatr Soc.* 1990;38:292–5.
4. Houston KA. Incontinence and the older woman. *Clin Geriatr Med.* 1993;9:157–71.
5. Brocklehurst JC. The bladder. In: Brocklehurst JC, Tallis RC, Fillit HM, eds. *Textbook of Geriatric Medicine and Gerontology*, 4th ed. New York: Churchill Livingstone; 1992:629–46.
6. Plymat KR, Turner SL. In-home management of urinary incontinence. *Home Healthc Nurse.* 1988;6:30–4.
7. US Department of Health and Human Services. *Urinary Incontinence in Adults: Clinical Practice Guideline.* AHCPR Pub No. 96-0682. Washington, DC: Public Health Service, Agency for Health Care Policy Research; US Dept of Health and Human Services; March 1996.
8. *Federal Register.* 1990;55:25204.
9. Smith DA. Devices for continence. *Nurse Pract Forum.* 1994;5:186–9.
10. Brink CA, Wells TJ. Environmental support for geriatric incontinence. Toilets, toilet supplements, and external equipment. *Clin Geriatr Med.* 1986;2:829–41.

SECTION XI

ALTERNATIVE THERAPIES

CHAPTER 45

Herbal Remedies

George Nemecz and Wendell L. Combest

Chapter 45 at a Glance

After an absence of nearly half a century, herbs and phytomedicinals have returned to the shelves of pharmacies. The herb market in the United States has grown exponentially since 1992 when the annual sales in pharmacies amounted to only $53.1 million, a small portion of the retail market.[1] In 1997 sales of herbs in retail stores (pharmacies, grocery stores, mass merchandiser retail stores) amounted to $441.5 million. A survey conducted in 1997 revealed that the use of at least 1 of 16 alternative therapies increased from 33% in 1990 to 42% in 1997.[2] Therapies that showed the greatest increases were herbal medicine, massage, homeopathy, folk remedies, and megavitamins.[2] Alter-

Editor's Note: This chapter is based, in part, on the 11th edition chapter titled "Herbs and Phytomedicinal Products," which was written by Varro E. Tyler and Steven Foster.

native therapies were used most frequently for chronic conditions, including back problems, anxiety, depression, and headache. The popularity of herbal products continues to increase with certain products being in high demand. Among the best sellers are ginkgo, echinacea, goldenseal, St. John's wort, garlic, and ginseng products.[3] The list of available herbal remedies from different companies is extensive and has expanded greatly in the past 2 years.

The number of annual visits to practitioners of alternative therapies increased by 32% from 1990 to 1997, while the number of visits to primary care physicians remained unchanged. Studies have shown that more than 40% of the U.S. population now uses some form of unconventional medicine, if unconventional is defined in such broad terms as to include nutrition and other subjects not normally found in medical school curricula.[4] It is difficult to characterize the use of botanicals and phytomedicinals as unconventional when they are used so extensively by about three-quarters of the world's population—in many cases, as the only medicines for those people. No single factor accounts for the increasing popularity of herbal medicine. The reasons are probably an extension of the antiestablishment mentality of the 1960s: increased appreciation of things "organic" and "natural" by members of the green movement; disenchantment with modern medicine (i.e., its inability to cure everything); reduced side effects caused by many gentle herbal remedies; and the low cost of herbal products, at least in comparison with patented single-chemical entities.

Herbs are defined in several ways, but for medical purposes they are simply botanicals used to treat health-related problems, often of a chronic nature, or to attain or maintain a condition of improved health. Phytomedicinals are galenicals: preparations made by extracting herbs with various solvents (usually a hydroalcoholic menstruum) to produce tinctures, fluidextracts, extracts, and the like to be used as prepared or manufactured as other dosage forms.

Obviously, pharmacists must master the essentials of this complicated field in order to advise patients on the safe and effective use of these popular remedies. The demand for pharmacist assistance is needed to avoid the consequences of self-medication and to avoid drug–herb interactions following concomitant use of herbs and conventional drug therapy. This task is not easy because of (1) the abundance of misinformation currently circulating and (2) the lack of courses about herbal products in past curriculums of pharmacy schools. A recent survey of pharmacy colleges in the United States showed that 74% of the schools now offer at least one course addressing herbs.[5]

In the sections that follow, some of the more significant herbs are classified according to the disease syndromes or conditions they are intended to treat. This chapter briefly discusses the identity, chemical constituents, physiologic activity and therapeutic use, appropriate cautions concerning use, and dosage of each.

Specific Considerations for Herbal Remedies

Safety and Effectiveness of Herbal Remedies

Despite their intended use, most herbs and phytomedicinals are sold in the United States not as drugs but as dietary supplements because insufficient data have been submitted to the Food and Drug Administration (FDA) to permit that agency to classify them as safe and effective therapeutic agents. This lack of classification does not necessarily mean that the herbs and phytomedicinals are unsafe and/or ineffective. It simply means that FDA lacks data to place these products in Category I. An understanding of this technicality is important; otherwise, one might think that peppermint is an unsafe and ineffective carminative and that prune concentrate (juice) is an unsafe and ineffective laxative. What these categorizations mean is that FDA has simply not evaluated these and many other herbal products, primarily for economic reasons.

Having been used for hundreds—even thousands—of years, most classic herbs and their long-known constituents are not patentable. Therefore, no prospective marketer is willing to invest the hundreds of millions of dollars required to obtain sufficient clinical evidence to convince FDA of their safety and utility. To do so would place that marketer at a distinct disadvantage compared with competitors who make no such investment.[6]

Although FDA has been requested to adopt more reasonable standards of proof of efficacy for the long-used botanicals, it has been unwilling to do so and, in 1993, even threatened to remove many products from the market. Lobbied intensively by an irate public, Congress passed the Dietary Supplement Health and Education Act of 1994, allowing herbs and phytomedicinals to be sold as "dietary supplements" but without any labeled therapeutic or health claims. Under the act, a statement may appear on the label that describes the product's role in affecting structure or function in humans. However, this statement must be followed by a disclaimer noting that the statement has not been evaluated by FDA and that the product is not intended to diagnose, treat, cure, or prevent any disease. In addition to the label, accurate scientific information of a generic nature may be passed along to the consumer with the product.[7]

The situation is quite different in advanced European nations. Following World Health Organization guidelines, relevant literature and research studies, and the experience of individual health care practitioners and patients, these nations have considered additional parameters along with clinical evidence to evaluate the efficacy of herbs and phytomedicinals. The best system has been developed in Germany, where a special, broadly based Commission E (appointed by the Federal Health Agency) has been actively studying the safety and utility of botanicals since 1978. Using information derived from clinical trials, field studies, case collections, scientific literature, and the opinions of medical associations, Commission E has published about 300 monographs on herbs in the *Bundesanzeiger*, the German equivalent of our *Federal Register*. These monographs normally include nomenclature, part(s) used, constituents, range of application, contraindications, side effects, incompatibilities, dosage, use, and action of the herb.

Approximately two-thirds of the monographs provide positive assessments of herbs found to be safe and effective. The remaining monographs are negative, usually because the drug—and these products are considered to be drugs in Germany—presents an unsatisfactory risk:benefit ratio. Although not perfect, the Commission E monographs represent the most accurate summaries of information available anywhere about the safety and efficacy of herbs and phytomedicinals. Their conclusions will be cited extensively in the monographs that make up the bulk of this chapter.[8]

Precautions for Herbal Remedies

Certain precautions must be observed when using herbal dietary supplements. Because these products are not approved drugs in the United States, neither information about proper use nor essential cautionary warnings appear on all labels. Consequently, prospective users should make every effort to obtain accurate information about the specific product before purchasing it. This task is complicated by the prevalence of hyperbolic literature, which in many cases is written to promote the sale of the product rather than to accurately inform the consumer.

FDA neither establishes nor regularly enforces any standards of quality for herbal products, forcing the consumer to rely on the reputation of the marketer for quality assurance. Products are often misbranded, and often the quantities of the ingredients are not listed. Mixtures containing a large number of herbal constituents often lack quantities sufficient to render a therapeutic effect. The consumer is best advised to purchase a preparation containing a specified amount of a standardized extract marketed by a reputable firm. For example, Food and Drug Canada has recommended that feverfew products contain not less than 0.2% parthenolide. A 1993 study showed that some feverfew products purchased in Louisiana contained no parthenolide at all.[9] Reputable companies are now beginning to market in the United States feverfew preparations that contain 125 mg of an extract that is standardized to have 0.2% parthenolide. Standardization of products offers a distinct improvement.

Other concerns about herbal consumption must include a general prohibition related to use by pregnant or nursing mothers and by young children, especially infants. This precaution applies particularly to stimulant laxatives and similar products that may lack adequate warning labels. Many botanicals lack the necessary long-term toxicity testing to ensure safety in cases of prolonged administration. Despite the deceptive legal classification as "dietary supplements," herbs used for therapeutic purposes are drugs, and patients must carefully observe the proper dosage recommendations.

Dosage Forms of Herbal Remedies

Among the various dosage forms available, the most common is the coarsely comminuted botanical that is used to prepare an infusion (tea) or a decoction. This dosage form is also used to prepare poultices for external application. Finely powdered herbs are either encapsulated or used to prepare compressed tablets. Some of these latter dosage forms may be enteric coated if their active constituents are inactivated by stomach acid. Herbs are extracted with various solvents to produce liquid or solid phytomedicinals. Such extracts (galenicals) permit both concentration and standardization of the active principles, which are often highly desirable features. Because some herbal consumers are highly concerned about the nature of the products they ingest, special preparations, such as nongelatin capsules that are not prepared from animal byproducts, along with glycerites that do not use ethanol in their production, are occasionally encountered. Herbs derived from sources said to be "organic" (grown without synthetic chemical fertilizers or pesticides) are often advertised. Table 45–1 lists examples of the primary ingredients and available dosage forms of the major herbal remedies.

Digestive System Disorders

Ginger

Ginger (*Zingiber officinale*) is a perennial that reaches a height of 2 to 3 feet and is thought to have originated in the tropical jungles of Asia. It has been grown in India and China for thousands of years and today is widely cultivated around the world. The underground rhizomes are the part of the plant used medicinally.

Chemical Constituents

Ginger rhizomes contain a volatile oil (1% to 3%) dominated by sesquiterpene hydrocarbons, including mainly zingiberene and a-curcumene with lesser amounts of farnesene, β-sesquiphellandrene, and β-bisabolene. Also present is an oleoresin (4% to 7.5%) with nonvolatile pungent components including gingerol, shogaols, and zingerone.[6,10]

Physiologic Activity and Therapeutic Use

The most-established therapeutic use of ginger is as an antiemetic to relieve nausea and vomiting associated with motion sickness, following surgery, or during pregnancy. Results from at least four clinical studies (three positive and one negative) support its use in preventing nausea associated with motion sickness. In one study,[11] powdered ginger (940 mg) was found to be as effective as 100 mg of the nonpre-

Table 45–1

Selected Herbal Products

Trade Name	Primary Ingredients
Bilberry (*Vaccinium myrtillus*)	
Bilberry 2020 Capsules	Anthocyanosides 25% (60 mg 100 : 1 extract)
Bilberry-Power 475-mg Capsules[a,b]	Anthocyanosides 25% (40 mg standardized extract)
Capsicum (*Capsicum* species)	
Cayenne Extract Tincture[a,b]	Alcoholic extract of dried mature fruit
Cayenne Power-Herb 450-mg Capsules[a,b]	Cayenne 100000 STU (450 mg standardized)
Chaste Tree Berry (*Vitex agnus-castus*)	
Chasteberry-Power 566-mg Capsules[a,b]	Glycosides 0.9%–1.1% (100 mg standardized); dong quai root; Siberian ginseng
Vitex Extract 560-mg Capsules[a,b]	Agnusides 0.5 mg (100 mg standardized extract); dong quai root; Siberian ginseng powder
Cranberry (*Vaccinium macrocarpon*)	
Cran Support Capsules	Cranberry 400 mg; uva ursi 115 mg; fructooligosaccharides 100 mg; vitamin C 100 mg; cat's claw root 50 mg; corn silk 30 mg; kava kava 8.5 mg
Cranberry-Power 505-mg Capsules	Organic acids 40 mg (200 mg standardized extract); vitamin C; freeze-dried cranberries
Echinacea (*Echinacea* species)	
Celestial Seasonings Herbal Comfort Lozenges	Total phenols 4% (standardized powdered root extract); ginsenosides 7% (standardized powdered root extract)
EchinaCare Tincture	Fresh juice of echinacea purpurea stems, leaves, and flowers in 22% alcohol
Echinacea-Power 505-mg Capsules[a,b]	Echinacoside 3.2%–4.8% (125 mg standardized *Echinacea angustifolia* extract); parthenium root; unstandardized *Echinacea angustifolia; Echinacea purpurea* root
Echinex Caplets	Total phenolic compounds 4% (250 mg *Echinacea purpurea* root and herb); eleutherosides 0.8% (100 mg Siberian ginseng root); gingerols 5% (100 mg ginger root)
Sundown Standardized Echinacea 400-mg Capsules	Phenolic compounds 4% (25 mg standardized whole herb)
Eleuthero (*Eleutherococcus senticosus*)	
Siberian Ginseng Extract Tincture[a,b]	Extract of dried root (2 : 1)
Siberian Ginseng Power-Herb 404-mg Capsules[a,b]	Eleutheroside D 400 mcg; eleutheroside B 300 mcg (100 mg standardized extract); Siberian ginseng root
Evening Primrose Oil (*Oenothera biennis*)	
Natrol Evening Primrose Oil Softgels	*cis*-Linoleic acid 350 mg; oleic acid 50 mg; *cis*-ω-lineolenic acid 45 mg
Primrose-Power 1300-mg Softgels[a,b]	*cis*-Linoleic acid 962 mg; ω-linolenic acid 1300 mg
Feverfew (*Tanacetum parthenium*)	
Herb Pharmaceuticals Feverfew Tincture[a,b]	Alcohol extract of dried leaf and flower
Feverfew-Power Softgels[a,b]	Sesquiterpene lactones 100 mg (standardized extract)
Garlic (*Allium sativum*)	
Garlic-Power Tablets[a,b]	Allicin total potential 3 mg (400 mg standardized extract)
Kwai 100-mg Tablets	Allicin yield 600 mcg
One-A-Day Garlic 600-mg Softgels	Garlic oil macerate 600 mcg
Ginger (*Zingiber officinale*)	
Herb Pharmaceuticals Ginger Extract Tincture[a,b]	Alcoholic extract of dried rhizome
Ginger-Power 480-mg Capsules[a,b]	Gingerols 5% (100 mg standardized extract); ginger root
Ginkgo (*Ginkgo biloba*)	
Natrol Ginkgo Biloba Liquid	Ginkgo flavone glycosides 24% (60 mg/mL 50 : 1 extract); terpene lactones 6%

Table 45–1

Selected Herbal Products (continued)

Trade Name	Primary Ingredients
Herb Pharmaceuticals Ginkgo Extract Tincture[a,b]	Alcoholic extract of fresh leaf
Ginkgo-Power 389-mg Capsules[a,b]	Ginkgo flavone glycosides 24% (40 mg standardized extract); ginkgolic acid-free ginkgo biloba leaf
Ginkoba Tablets	Ginkgo flavone glycosides 24% (40 mg standardized leaf extract; 50 : 1 concentration)
Ginseng (*Panax ginseng*)	
NaturPharma Daily Ginseng 495-mg Capsules[a,b]	Ginsenosides 7% (standardized extract); eleutheroside B1 (standardized); eleutheroside D (standardized); Siberian ginseng root
Korean Ginseng Power-Herb 535-mg Capsules[a,b]	Ginsenosides 7% (100 mg standardized); Korean panax ginseng powder
Panaxin 100-mg Capsules[b]	Saponins 7% (calculated as ginsenoside Rg1; standardized extract)
Sundown Standardized Korean Ginseng 560-mg Capsules	Ginsenosides 77% (100 mg standardized root extract)
Lemon Balm (*Melissa officinalis*)	
Herpalieve Cream	Melissa (70 : 1 extract); allantoin 1%
Herb Pharmaceuticals Lemon Balm Extract Tincture[a,b]	Alcoholic extract of fresh flowering plant
Milk Thistle (*Silybum marianum*)	
DTX 300-mg Caplets	Silymarin 80% (240 mg standardized extract)
Herb Pharmaceuticals Milk Thistle Extract Tincture[a,b]	Alcoholic extract of dried mature seed
Oligomeric Proanthocyanidins	
Grape Seed-Power 100 227-mg Capsules[a,b]	Oligomeric proanthocyanidins 95% (100 mg standardized extract); polyphenols 14% (standardized grape skin extract)
PCO Phytosome 50-mg Tablets[b]	Procyanidolic oligomers (from *Vitis vinifera* seed coat bound to phosphatidylcholine)
St. John's Wort (*Hypericum perforatum*)	
Harmonex Caplets	Hypericin 0.3% (450 mg standardized extract); eleutherosides 0.8% (90 mg Siberian ginseng root)
Mood Support Capsules	Hypericin 0.3%; ginseng 100 mg; 1-tyrosine 50 mg; vitamin E 30 IU; DMAE 25 mg; lemon balm 25 mg; folic acid 400 mcg; vitamin B12 50 mcg; selenium 25 mcg
Herb Pharmaceuticals St. John's Wort Extract Tincture[a,b]	Alcoholic extract of fresh flowering and budding top
Saw Palmetto (*Serenoa repens*)	
Propalmex Softgels	Fatty acids and sterols 85%–95% (160 mg berry); free fatty acids 85%–95% (40 mg pumpkin seed oil extract); zinc 7.5 mg
Herb Pharmaceuticals Saw Palmetto Extract Tincture[a,b]	Alcoholic extract of dried mature berry
Saw Palmetto-Power 160 Softgels[a,b]	Fatty acids and sterols 85%–95% (320 mg standardized extract); pumpkin seed oil
Valerian (*Valeriana officinalis*)	
Celestial Herbal Extracts Sleepytime Extra Capsules	Valerenic acid 0.8% (320 mg standardized extract); hypericin 0.3% (150 mg standardized extract); kava kava extract 100 mg; passion flower extract 100 mg; chamomile extract 100 mg; hawthorne berry extract 50 mg
Rest Easy Tincture	Alcoholic root extract 10%
Valerian Plus Tablets[a]	Valerenic acid 0.8% (37.5 mg standardized valerian root extract); passion flower; German chamomile

[a] Dye-free product.

[b] Gelatin-free product.

scription antiemetic, dimenhydrinate. For postoperative nausea, ginger was found to be as effective as metoclopramide.[12] In a study[13] of nausea during pregnancy, 1 g of ginger reduced the frequency of vomiting in 19 of 27 women. However, its use during pregnancy should not be recommended because of a lack of long-term toxicity studies.

In the United States, ginger is commonly used as a digestive aid to treat indigestion and ulcers. Although no clinical trials support this use, several animal studies document its ability to enhance gastrointestinal (GI) motility and protect against gastric lesions. Some clinical and animal studies have shown that ginger can potentially reduce the pain and swelling in inflamed tissue associated with arthritis.[14] The results from a few in vitro and animal studies indicate that certain compounds in ginger have potential antitumor, antimicrobial, antiparasitic, antioxidant, and cardiotonic activity.[15]

Precautions

No reports exist that show significant side effects or toxic reactions following the consumption of ginger in usual therapeutic doses. The German Commission E has approved ginger for dyspeptic complaints and as a prophylactic for motion sickness. Ginger has also been shown to inhibit platelet aggregation, through inhibition of thromboxane synthetase, in some studies but not in others.[16] Therefore, ginger should be avoided before and after operative procedures because of possible prolongation of bleeding times, and should be used with caution in the presence of drugs that inhibit platelet aggregation.

Dosage

For nausea associated with motion sickness, a typical dose is two 500 mg capsules taken 30 minutes before travel departure, followed by one or two more 500 mg capsule(s) taken as needed every 4 hours. Fresh grated ginger (0.5 to 1 g) can be added to a cup of hot water and consumed as a tea.

Plantago Seed and Husk

Plantago, also known as plantain or psyllium seed, consists of the cleaned, dried, ripened seed of psyllium (Spanish, French, or Indian psyllium). Several different plants are used medicinally, some for their leaves and others for their seeds. Other commonly used psylliums are *Plantago arenaria* (golden psyllium), *Plantago psyllium* (brown psyllium), *Plantago indica* (black psyllium), and *Plantago ovata* (blonde psyllium), all of which are members of the plantain family (Plantaginaceae). These psylliums are primarily used for their seed husks.[16,17]

Chemical Constituents

Plantago seeds contain up to 80% insoluble fiber, and 10% to 30% of a hydrocolloid soluble fiber is concentrated in the epidermis. The hydrocolloid consists of acidic and neutral polysaccharide fractions that, upon hydrolysis, yield L-arabinose, D-galactose, D-galacturonic acid, L-rhamnose, and D-xylose.[17]

Physiologic Activity and Therapeutic Use

Plantago or psyllium seeds are bulk-forming laxatives. Swelling of the mucilaginous seed coats (husks) as they bind with fluid in the intestine increases intestinal content volume, causing a physical stimulation of the gut wall. At the same time, the bowels are lubricated by the seeds' mucilage, and accelerated transit through the colon is achieved.[16,18] Uses include treatment of chronic constipation and conditions necessitating soft stools, such as hemorrhoids, anal fissures, or rectal–anal surgery.[19] (See Chapter 12, "Constipation," for discussions of laxative products containing psyllium.)

Plantago produces a modest but significant lowering of total cholesterol and low-density lipoprotein levels, whereas high-density lipoproteins are increased.[19,20] A blood glucose lowering effect has been shown in Type II diabetes.[21] Plantago is also used topically for skin irritations.

Precautions

Rare allergic reactions are reported in patients and in individuals involved with industrial handling of the drug. Its use is contraindicated in the presence of GI tract obstructions and requires special caution in patients with diabetes mellitus.[19]

Dosage

The dose is 7.5 g (average 4 to 20 g per day), taken with at least 150 mL of water for each 5 g of drug, 30 to 60 minutes after a meal or after the administration of other drugs.[17,19]

Senna

Alexandria senna (*Cassia acutifolia*) and Tinnevelly senna (*Cassia angustifolia*), both of which are also referred to in recent botanical literature as *Senna alexandrina,* are shrubs or herbaceous perennials and members of the family Caesalpiniaceae. They are either indigenous or have been introduced to North, Central, and South America and are grown commercially in the Middle East, India, and elsewhere.[16] The leaves as well as the pods contain the medicinally active constituents.

Chemical Constituents

Dianthrone glycosides, particularly sennosides A, A_1, B, C, D, and G, are present along with various other anthraquinone derivatives. Sennosides, a complex of total glycosides, are also official in the *United States Pharmacopeia.*[6,17]

Physiologic Activity and Therapeutic Use

Senna is a laxative because of its content of sennosides and is useful in treating constipation.[6,17] Sennosides influence the motility of the colon and accelerate intestinal transit. Chloride secretion is also stimulated, which increases the water and electrolyte content in the colon. (See Chapter 12, "Constipation," for discussion of laxative products that contain senna.)

Precautions

Patients may experience cramping discomfort in the GI tract. Use of stimulating laxatives should not continue beyond 1 to 2 weeks except under medical supervision. Chronic abuse or overdose can result in potassium loss, along with electrolyte and fluid imbalances that could increase the toxicity of digoxin and certain diuretics. Senna should not be used in the presence of acute inflammatory intestinal disease, intestinal obturation, appendicitis, or in children younger than 12 years. Because of the lack of toxicologic studies, the use of senna is not recommended during pregnancy or lactation.[22]

Dosage

Fluid extracts and a syrup are commonly made from the leaflets. Capsules containing dried leaf powder or a mixture of purified sennosides are available. Senna can be consumed as a tea by steeping 1 to 2 teaspoons of dried leaves in a cup of hot water.

Peppermint

Peppermint (*Mentha piperita*), a member of the mint family Lamiaceae, originated as a natural hybrid of spearmint. Peppermint is cultivated in Europe, Egypt, and the United States, especially in Indiana, Michigan, Idaho, Oregon, and Washington.[23] Peppermint has been intensively cultivated for its fragrant volatile oil extracted primarily from its leaves.[23]

Chemical Constituents

The biologic activity of peppermint is attributed to its essential oil (0.5% to 4%, average 1.5%), which contains not less than 50% (50% to 78%) (–)-menthol and 5% to 20% menthol combined in esters, including the acetate or isovalerate. Menthol stereoisomers are also present, which include (+)-neomenthol (3%) as well as other monoterpenes such as menthone, menthofuran, eucalyptol, and limonene. The sesquiterpene viridoflorol provides a marker for oil identification.[6,17] Among other leaf constituents are flavonoids, rosmarinic acid, and tannin.[15]

Physiologic Activity and Therapeutic Use

Peppermint leaf and oil are currently in pharmaceutical use in the United States as flavoring agents. As a result of a decision by the FDA's Advisory Review Panel on Over-the-Counter (OTC) Miscellaneous Internal Drug Products, the oil was dropped from nonprescription drug status in 1990. Again, this decision does not necessarily reflect the oil's lack of safety or efficacy; it indicates only that no information on safety and efficacy was presented to the agency.[6]

Recent European interest has focused on using peppermint oil to treat irritable bowel syndrome (IBS). The oil (enteric-coated capsules) has been reported to reduce symptoms of IBS characterized by recurrent colicky abdominal pain, a feeling of distention, and variations in bowel habits with minimal attendant side effects.[23] The German health authorities allow peppermint oil for the treatment of IBS, spastic discomfort of the upper GI tract, and other related conditions.[15]

Peppermint leaf is recognized as a carminative and choleretic, with a direct spasmolytic effect on smooth muscles of the digestive tract. The leaf is the subject of a positive German monograph indicating its use for spastic GI tract complaints.[24] Traditionally, peppermint leaf tea is used to treat dyspepsia, flatulence, and intestinal colic.[10]

Precautions

Peppermint tea is considered safe for normal individuals. Excessive use of the essential oil (0.3 g, not enteric coated) may produce toxic reactions such as heartburn and relaxation of the lower esophageal sphincter.[23] Peppermint leaf tea should be used with caution in infants and small children because of possible laryngeal and bronchial spasms from volatilized menthol.[6] The oil may also irritate mucous membranes.

Dosage

The cut herb is used in hot infusions at an average daily dose of 1.5 to 3 g of the dried leaf.[24] For relief of stomach upset, an infusion is made by pouring 160 mL of boiling water on 1 to 1.5 g of the herb, steeping for up to 10 minutes, and ingesting it up to three or four times daily.[6] Each dose of enteric-coated peppermint oil is 0.2 to 0.4 mL, up to 0.6 to 1.2 mL per day.[25]

Chamomile

Two herbs are commonly called chamomile: Roman or Common Chamomile (*Chamaemelum nobile, Anthemis nobilis*) and or German or Hungarian (*Matricaria recutita, Chamomilla recutita*). *Matricaria recutita* is one of the most extensively distributed medicinal herbs and is present in all parts of the world except tropical and arctic regions. It is originally native to southeastern and southern Europe.[26] Both chamomiles are used in traditional herbalism and medicine; however, German chamomile is preferred for internal medicinal uses. Use of Roman chamomile is largely restricted to the United Kingdom, where most of the supply is grown. In addition, chamomile extract and essential oils are frequent components in several cosmetic and hygienic products.

Chemical Constituents

Different classes of active constituents have been isolated and used individually in medical practice and cosmetics. The plant contains 0.3% to 2% volatile oil, composed of several different individual oils. This oil, extracted from flower heads by steam distillation, can range in color from brilliant blue to deep green when fresh but fades over time to dark yellow. Despite fading, the oil does not lose its potency. The oil contains α-bisabolol, chamazulene cyclic sesquiterpenes, which directly reduce inflammation and are mild antibacterials. The essential oil contains bisabolol oxides, farnesene, and spiro-ether, which have anti-inflammatory and antispasmodic actions.[26] The characteristic blue color of the volatile oil results from the presence of chamazulene, which forms during steam distillation. Important flavonoids have been identified in German chamomile, including apigenin, luteolin, and quercetin. Recent research indicates inhibitory effects on certain malignant cell proliferation in vitro. These flavonoids may also contribute to the herb's antispasmodic activity.[10,27]

Physiologic Activity and Therapeutic Use

The dried flower heads and volatile oil have anti-inflammatory, antiphlogistic (inflammation reduction), spasmolytic, and antimicrobial activity. The flower preparations are used for GI spasms, GI tract inflammatory diseases, and peptic ulcers. An infusion (as a mouthwash) is used to treat inflammatory conditions of the oral cavity and gums.[28,29] Chamomile tea is also known for its sedative and hypnotic effects. Combined administration of diazepam and chamomile oil vapor decreased the stress-related elevation of adrenocorticotropic hormone in animal studies.[30,31] The authors suggested that, similar to the benzodiazepines, chamomile oil might affect the γ-aminobutyric acid (GABA) system in the rat brain.

Chamomile preparations are widely used in skin care products to reduce cutaneous and mucous membrane inflammation as well as other dermatologic diseases.[6,10,32] Wound-healing effects include promotion of granulation and tissue regeneration.

Precautions

Numerous professional and popular references during the past decade have warned of possible anaphylactic shock from drinking chamomile tea. However, only five cases of allergy attributed to German chamomile were identified between 1887 and 1982.[6] These figures would imply the drug's relative safety, although large doses of tea can be a potential emetic.

Dosage

Chamomile may be used medicinally in many forms. An infusion can be prepared from fresh or dried flower heads, usually 2 to 3 teaspoons put in a cup of boiling water, infused for 10 minutes, and taken orally three times a day. From an alcoholic tincture, 1 to 4 mL can be diluted in a cup of water and taken orally three times a day. The same preparation can be used externally as a poultice. An infusion of 1 teaspoon of flower heads (as described above) can be given to children for pain of dentition, stomachache, earache, or neuralgic pain. In aromatherapy, the essential oil of chamomile is a valued part of blended preparations and is also used as a component of massage oils.

Milk Thistle

Milk thistle (*Silybum marianum*) is a member of the aster family (Asteraceae, formerly Compositae), which grows abundantly throughout Europe and North America. The seeds and fruit contain the highest levels of medicinally active constituents. Milk thistle extract has long been popular as a hepatoprotective agent throughout Europe, especially in Germany.

Chemical Constituents

The seeds and, to a lesser extent, the leaves and stems contain several isomeric flavonolignans collectively referred to as silymarin (4% to 6% in seeds). Silymarin is composed primarily of silybin, along with isosilybin, dehydrosilybin, silydianin, and silychristin.[33] These compounds are believed to be the biologically active constituents responsible for milk thistle's antioxidant and hepatoprotective effects. Products available in the United States generally consist of capsules containing varying amounts of a concentrated seed extract, standardized to 70% to 80% flavonolignans calculated as silybin.[6,33]

Physiologic Activity and Therapeutic Use

Accumulating evidence supports the use of milk thistle seed extracts as hepatoprotective. One of the most well-documented uses in Europe is to treat poisoning by the mushroom *Amanita phalloides* (death cap). Silybin has been shown to protect patients against liver damage when administered within 48 hours of ingestion of the mushroom.[34] The mechanism of this protective effect appears to involve an alteration in the outer cell membrane of the hepatocyte, which prevents toxin penetration. Milk thistle has been shown to have liver protective effects against exposure to various toxic chemicals and drugs such as carbon tetrachloride (CCl_4), toluene, ethanol, and acetaminophen.[35] Investigators have attributed these protective effects to free-radical scavenging properties of silymarin. Several studies have shown that silymarin has potent antioxidant activity. In addition, silymarin has a stimulating effect on liver protein synthesis through its activation of DNA-dependent–RNA polymerase I and the subsequent increase in ribosomal RNA.[36] In addition to silymarin's well-described hepatoprotective effects, several animal and human studies show similar protective effects in the GI tract and in the kidney, as well as the ability to inhibit the promotion and growth of certain cancerous cells.[37]

Precautions

Toxicity studies in rats and mice have shown that silymarin, even at daily doses as high as 2500 to 5000 mg/kg, produced no adverse toxic effects.[38] Most clinical trials have reported few noticeable side effects other than minor GI disturbances and allergic reactions. Mild transient diarrhea has occasionally been reported.

Dosage

Capsules, tablets, or ethanol extracts are available containing dried or extracted seeds standardized to 70% silymarin. An intravenous formulation is available in Europe and has been used in many of the clinical trials. The average daily recommended dose is 12 to 15 g (equivalent to 200 to 400 mg of silymarin). Milk thistle is marketed in the United States most often in a capsule that contains 140 mg of silymarin. Silybin is often combined with phosphatidylcholine to increase its normally poor absorption (20% to 50%) from the intestine.

Licorice

Licorice (*Glycyrrhiza glabra*) belongs to the family Leguminoaea and is a tall shrub (4 to 5 feet) indigenous to Turkey, Iraq, Spain, Greece, and northern China. Most of the licorice imported into the United States comes from the eastern Mediterranean region. The roots contain the medicinally active constituents. Licorice has been used as a medicine for thousands of years and has been found in the tombs of ancient Egyptian pharaohs.

Chemical Constituents

Licorice contains a triterpene glycoside, glycyrrhizin (GL), at 2% to 14% of the dried root. This compound, 50 times sweeter than sugar, gives licorice its sweet taste and contributes to many of the herb's observed pharmacologic effects. GL is partially hydrolyzed by a glucuronidase in the liver to its aglycone glycyrrhetinic acid (GA). Several antioxidant compounds have been isolated from dried roots: the isoflavans hispaglabin A and B, glabridin, 4′-*O*–methylglabridin; the chalones isoprenylchalone, licochalone A, isoliquirtigenin; and the isoflavone formanonetin.[39] In addition, several compounds with antimicrobial activity have been isolated and identified in alcoholic extracts of the dried roots.

Physiologic Activity and Therapeutic Use

For hundreds of years, licorice has been used to treat peptic ulcers. GL and GA have recently been found to inhibit two enzymes, 5-hydroxy-prostaglandin dehydrogenase and δ-13-prostaglandin reductase, in the stomach, which control the degradation of prostaglandins E and F_{2a}.[40] The resulting increase in prostaglandins produces a protective effect on the gastric mucosa through promoting mucus secretion and enhancing mucosal blood flow, thereby promoting the healing of gastric ulcers.

Since 1980, accumulated evidence has supported the efficacy of several constituents in licorice in treating many types of viral infections. The results from animal studies indicate that the antiviral effect may be indirect and partly a result of the stimulation of interferon production by T cells. When splenic T cells from GL-treated mice were transplanted to mice exposed to influenza virus, 100% of the recipients survived compared with 0% of controls.[41] Clinical studies carried out mainly in Japan since 1992 have demonstrated the efficacy of GL in treating viral hepatitis types A, B, and C.[42]

Many animal and cell culture studies indicate that GL and GA have antimicrobial, antiparasitic, and antitumor activity. In addition, several compounds isolated from licorice roots were shown to prevent oxidation of low-density lipoprotein (LDL).[39] Licorice has long been used to treat numerous inflammatory conditions such as asthma, psoriasis, and rheumatoid arthritis. Experimental evidence for these effects is generally lacking, but a few animal studies support the therapeutic rationale for many of these treatments. Some of the proposed mechanisms for the anti-inflammatory effects include stabilization of lysosomal membranes, prevention of the release of proteolytic enzymes, inhibition of mononuclear leukocyte migration, and inhibition of cortisol degradation.

In addition, licorice has long been used as an ingredient in antitussive and expectorant formulations although no clinical studies support this widespread use. Many candy products labeled as licorice are flavored with the herb anise and contain no GL.

Precautions

High doses or long-term use of licorice may result in mineralocorticoid-like effects, including sodium and water retention and the resultant elevation in blood pressure, as well as potassium loss leading to hypokalemia. This effect is likely caused by the inhibition of cortisol breakdown resulting in higher peripheral and intrarenal concentrations of cortisol, which also has a high affinity for the aldosterone receptor in the kidney. The high cortisol levels in the kidney are believed to stimulate sodium and water retention, as well as excessive excretion of potassium. The German health authorities stipulate that use of licorice be limited to no longer than 4 to 6 weeks. Patients with cardiovascular or renal disease should use licorice cautiously and only under the advice of a physician. Also, patients who are prone to potassium deficiency should avoid using licorice.

Dosage

The German Commission E has approved the use of licorice to treat peptic ulcers and recommends a dosage of 200 to 600 mg of GL daily for a maximum of 4 to 6 weeks. A tea can be made by adding 2 to 4 g of dried or freshly grated licorice roots to a cup of hot water.

Kidney, Urinary Tract, and Prostate Disorders

Uva-ursi

Uva-ursi (*Aractostaphylos uva-ursi*), also known as bearberry, is a low-growing evergreen shrub with dark green leathery leaves, and it grows in cold temperate regions throughout the Northern Hemisphere.

Chemical Constituents

The dried leaf contains 5% to 15% hydroquinone derivatives, mainly arbutin and methylarbutin, which have an antiseptic action. Other constituents include flavonoids, a high level of tannins, and various organic acids such as gallic and ellagic acid. Arbutin is hydrolyzed in the intestinal tract, producing hydroquinone, which is mildly astringent and antiseptic in an alkaline urine.

Physiologic Activity and Therapeutic Use

Although bearberry is listed in most monographs as a diuretic, such activity is minimal; its primary activity is as an antibacterial agent for urinary tract infections (UTIs). Activation requires the urine pH to be alkaline, thereby releasing free hydroquinone from the conjugates. Administration should be in conjunction with a diet rich in milk, vegetables (such as tomatoes and potatoes), fruits and fruit juices, and other foods capable of inducing alkalinuria. Ingestion of 6 to 8 g of sodium bicarbonate a day will produce alkalinity during treatment. The arbutin content of uva-ursi may increase the inhibitory action of prednisolone and dexamethasone in inflammatory diseases, allergic reactions, and arthritis.[43] Other effects include expelling bile and lowering the incidence of kidney stone formation.[44]

Precautions

Large doses of hydroquinone are toxic. Ingestion of 1 g of hydroquinone could cause nausea, vomiting, ringing in the ears, cyanosis, and convulsion.

Dosage

The dried cut or powdered herb is administered in a mean daily dose of 10 g (corresponding to 400 to 700 mg arbutin) macerated overnight in 150 mL of cold water (to reduce the tannin content extracted with hot water). Use should be limited to 1 week or less.[45]

Cranberry

Cranberry (*Vaccinium macrocarpon*) of the family Ericaceae is an evergreen bush native to North America from Alaska to the Carolinas. The plant produces pink flowers that are followed by small red-black berries normally from June to July. The English are credited with the creation of cranberry sauce. Since the 1940s, dehydrated cranberries and juice cocktails (sweetened diluted juice of the fruits) have been available. Early Americans prepared wound dressings from the whole fruit. They also used cranberries for blood disorders, stomach ailments, liver function, scurvy, and cancer. In Alaska, combinations of boiled cranberries and seal oil have been used to reduce severity of gall-bladder attacks. Today the extracts of the American cranberry are used to treat UTIs.

Chemical Constituents

Organic constituents include β-hydroxybutyric acid, flavonoids, catechin, malic acid, ellagic acid, gionic acid, hippuric acid, and high levels of condensed tannins and proanthocyanidins. The constituents responsible for efficacy in the treatment of UTIs include the organic acids and the condensed tannins. They prevent the leading bacteria, *Escherichia coli*, which causes UTI, from adhering to the walls of the bladder, kidneys, and urethra. Recently, cranberry extract was discovered to inhibit oxidation of LDL.

Physiologic Activity and Therapeutic Use

Cranberry juice has long been used to self-treat UTIs. Clinical studies using 300 to 1500 mL a day of cranberry juice showed beneficial effect in UTI. One clinical study followed 153 elderly women (mean age 78.5) with bacteriuria and pyuria in which subjects were randomly assigned to consume 300 mL of cranberry juice per day. This study concluded that cranberry beverage reduced the frequency of bacteriuria in older women.[46]

It has been suggested that cranberry juice can reduce the urinary odor of incontinent patients. The cranberry juice lowers the pH enough to retard the degradation of urine by *E. coli*, which produces the offensive ammoniac odors.[47]

Precautions

No precautions are noted.

Dosage

As a UTI preventive, 90 mL of cranberry juice can be consumed daily; for UTI treatment, consumption should increase to 360 to 960 mL daily. Capsules containing dried cranberry and a dried, concentrated extract are available. Six capsules are reported to be equivalent to 90 mL of cranberry juice cocktail, about one-third of which is cranberry juice.[6]

Saw Palmetto

Saw palmetto (*Serenoa repens*) is a dwarf palm tree in the family Arecaceae, which is native to the southeast region of the U.S. Atlantic coast. The berries of this dwarf palm are gathered from September until January; the dried fruits are used for medicinal purposes.[48]

Chemical Constituents

Analysis of the 95% ethanol extract of the berries for their lipid content showed fatty acids, fatty acid esters, and phytosterols. The following sterols have been identified in the alcoholic extract: campesterol, stigmasterol, β-sitosterol, and cycloartenol. The berries also contain 1% to 2% essential oil. Other chemical constituents identified in the berries include aliphatic alcohols (C26-30), polyprenic compounds, flavonoids, glucose, galactose, arabinose, uronic acid, and other polysaccharides. The antiandrogenic constituent(s) have not been specifically identified but are found in acidic lipophilic fractions of the fruits.[6,15]

Case Study 45–1

Patient Complaint/History

Clayton, an apparently healthy and obviously vigorous 64-year-old male, enters the consulting area and asks to speak privately with a pharmacist. The patient, who has patronized the pharmacy for several years, was diagnosed 2 years ago as having BPH for which his urologist prescribed Proscar 5 mg one tablet daily. His response to the medication has been excellent, but he now admits that the drug has greatly reduced his sexual potency. He also reveals that he plans to marry a 32-year-old woman; his first wife died 10 years ago.

Clayton has read the *Physician's Desk Reference*'s monograph on finasteride and is aware that the medication is probably the cause of his impotency. A friend who has no medical or pharmaceutical training advised him to quit taking finasteride and to start taking saw palmetto standardized extract instead. The patient asks whether this change is a good idea. In addition to finasteride, he currently takes ascorbic acid (vitamin C) 250 mg one tablet daily and the standard nonprescription products for aches/pains and coughs/colds.

Clinical Considerations/Strategies

Readers can use the following considerations/strategies to determine whether treatment of the patient's condition with nonprescription medications is warranted:

- Assess the therapeutic use of saw palmetto as an alternative to finasteride.
- Assess the appropriateness of recommending a dietary supplement as a substitute for a prescription medication.
- Determine the best method for encouraging the patient's urologist to become involved, remembering that the therapeutic use of botanicals is not usually taught in U.S. medical schools.

Patient Education/Counseling

Readers can use the following strategies to develop a patient education/counseling plan that will help ensure optimal therapeutic outcomes:

- Inform the patient of the need to consult his urologist before making any therapeutic decision.
- Explain the effectiveness and limitations of saw palmetto standardized extract in treating BPH.
- Aid the patient in selecting a specific botanical product, and provide a suitable dosage regimen for the product (if the patient and his urologist collaborate and mutually approve a switch from Proscar to saw palmetto).
- Explain the efficacy, side-effect profile, and guidelines for proper use of Proscar (if the patient and his urologist decide the switch is not appropriate).

Physiologic Activity and Therapeutic Use

Saw palmetto has been used as a mild diuretic and urinary antiseptic. Recent interest in saw palmetto has been linked with the finding that sitosterols may act on steroid receptors. Remedies made from the berries gained a reputation for treating symptoms related to benign prostatic hypertrophy (BPH). Various studies have shown that liposterolic fruit extracts reduce testosterone and dihydrotestosterone in tissue samples by more than 40%.

A large-scale, 6-month, placebo-controlled double-blind study of 1098 patients was conducted to compare phytotherapy (Permixon 320 mg) with finasteride 5 mg. Patients with moderate BPH were selected, and the International Prostate Symptoms Scores (IPSS) were used as the primary endpoints. The IPSS is a seven-item questionnaire that rates urinary symptoms such as urgency, hesitancy, and frequency on a scale of 0 to 5. Both Permixon and finasteride decreased IPSS (–37% and –39%, respectively) and showed similar improved urinary flow rates and overall quality of life.[49]

According to the German Commission E, saw palmetto extracts are used to relieve symptoms associated with enlarged prostate without reducing the enlargement. However, a recent study reports results of a 505-patient trial in which prostate size was reduced.[50]

Precautions

Stomach upset from using saw palmetto has been reported in rare instances.

Dosage

Average daily dose is 1 to 2 g of the ground, dried fruits or 160 mg of a lipophilic fruit extract taken twice daily with the morning and evening meal to minimize GI disturbances.

Respiratory Tract Disorders

Ephedra

Ephedra, commonly known by its Chinese name, ma huang, is a shrub-like plant similar in appearance to horsetail. Ephedra consists of about 40 species that are native to warm, dry regions of the Americas, Asia, and Europe. Three species are found in the Mediterranean region, nine species and two hybrids are found in North American deserts, and the rest are found in South America and Asia. *Ephedra sinica* (the most often cited medicinal species), *E. intermedia*, and *E. equisetina* are the three species found in Asia. The medicinally useful parts of the plants are the young branches that are harvested in the fall. The rhizomes and roots are rarely if ever used.

The American species, *E. nevadensis*, known as Mormon or Brigham tea, is found in the southwestern deserts of the United States. Pharmacologically active alkaloids are absent in all *Ephedra* species in North and Central America. Therefore, the inherent medicinal value of these species, if any, is caused by other, unidentified compounds.[15]

Chemical Constituents

The stem of ephedra contains a number of active compounds, including small amounts of an essential oil and, most importantly, 1% to 2% of an alkaloid mixture composed mainly of ephedrine and pseudoephedrine. The contained ephedrine ranges from 30% to 90% of the total, depending on the source. *E. sinica* contains about 1.3% alkaloids with more than 60% ephedrine, *E. intermedia* contains about 1.1% alkaloids with 30% to 40% ephedrine, and *E. equisetina* contains about 1.7% alkaloids with 85% to 90% ephedrine. More than 50% of the alkaloids are concentrated in the stem internodes, with none in the root.[15]

Physiologic Activity and Therapeutic Use

Use of ephedra to treat bronchial asthma and related conditions has been known for at least 5000 years. Alkaloid-containing Asian *Ephedra* species have historically been used to promote bronchodilation, vasoconstriction, and reductions in bronchial edema, as well as acting as potent cardiovascular and central nervous system (CNS) stimulants. Ephedrine acts indirectly to stimulate the release of norepinephrine from sympathetic and CNS adrenergic neurons, as well as acting as a potent direct agonist at α- and β-adrenergic receptors in the brain and in the peripheral CNS.

Precautions

Ephedra should be avoided by patients suffering from heart conditions, hypertension, diabetes, or thyroid disease. Ephedrine and related alkaloids are CNS stimulants; overdose can result in nervousness, insomnia, palpitations, and death. Products containing ephedra, often spiked with ephedrine and/or pseudoephedrine, are commonly used in weight-loss formulations although there is no evidence to suggest that ephedra or its alkaloids are safe and effective in reducing weight or appetite. Because of reports of toxicity, FDA's regulatory action on such products is anticipated. Several states have restricted sales of ephedra because ephedrine is used as a precursor in the manufacture of the illicit drugs methamphetamine and methcathinone.[6]

Dosage

Two grams of the herb is steeped in 240 mL of boiling water for 10 minutes (equivalent to 15 to 30 mg of ephedrine) and consumed as a tea. Alcoholic stem extracts are also popular.

Slippery Elm

Slippery elm (*Ulmus rubra*) is a deciduous tree growing in the woods of North America from southern Canada to Florida. The medicinally useful part of the tree is the reddish-brown inner bark.

Chemical Constituents

The inner bark of slippery elm is high in mucilage (primarily consisting of a water-soluble polysaccharide), bioflavonoids, vitamin E, starch, and small amounts of tannins.

Physiologic Activity and Therapeutic Use

Slippery elm bark is a mucilaginous demulcent, emollient, nutrient, astringent, and anti-inflammatory. It is used traditionally to soothe irritated mucous membranes of the intestines, colon, and urinary tract, as well as ulcerations of the digestive tract. It is also effective in treating GI irritations resulting from diarrhea.[10] The ointment is used externally to soothe wounds, burns, and chapped lips. The primary use in the United States is as a soothing demulcent for sore throat; it has received FDA's approval for this purpose. A recent study suggests possible antioxidant effects of the compounds isolated from root bark. These compounds include the newly discovered davidianons A, B, and C, as well as mansonones E, F, H, and I.[51]

Precautions

No precautions are noted for slippery elm. Although once used by midwives to abort fetuses, the powdered inner bark available on the market has no abortifacient effect.

Dosage

Between 0.5 and 2 g of powdered bark steeped in 10 parts hot water (5 to 20 mL) is consumed as required. Commercially produced tablets and troches are also available.[10]

Cardiovascular System Disorders

Hawthorn

More than 100 species of hawthorn trees exist in North America, all members of the rose family (Rosaceae). The species used for medicinal purposes include *Crataegus laevigata*, *C. monogyna*, and, less often, *C. pentagyna*.[52] The dried leaves with flower and/or fruits are harvested from wild populations or cultivated trees. While studies suggest that the flower contains more cardioactive components than do the berries, total extracts of both have been recommended to treat cardiac failure, arteriosclerosis, hyperlipidemia, hypertension, angina pectoris, and a variety of geriatric conditions. Chinese medicine uses the berries of *C. pinnatifida* as a digestive and circulatory stimulant.

Chemical Constituents

Flowers and leaves contain mixtures of chlorogenic acid and flavonoids such as quercin, hyperoside (quercetin 3-galactoside), vitexin, and vitexin 4′-rhamnoside.[53] The other major constituents are triterpenoids (e.g., oleanolic acid, ursolic acid, and crataegus acid). All have anti-inflammatory and antihyperlipidemic properties.

Physiologic Activity and Therapeutic Use

In Europe, hawthorn extract gained recognition in the treatment of age-related degenerative heart diseases. The herb enhances coronary and myocardial circulation by dilating coronary vessels, relieving cardiac hypoxemia. Additional benefits are its hypotensive and hypolipidemic effects. Clinical studies compared the positively inotropic hawthorn extract with other known positive inotropic drugs, such as the β-adrenergic agonist isoprenaline or the cardiac glycoside ouabain. The effects of the hawthorn extract were significantly more economical with respect to the energy of the myocytes. The anti-inflammatory effect has been tested on a hydroalcoholic extract from the flower heads of *C. oxyacantha* and inhibited thromboxane A2 biosynthesis in vitro.

The alcoholic extract of *C. oxyacantha* has shown direct influence on the CNS, having sedative, hypothermic, and hypotensive actions.[54]

Precautions

Therapeutic doses of hawthorn did not have adverse effects. However, drug interactions are likely with other cardiovascular agents that generate undesired synergetic effects. Hawthorn can potentiate cardiac glycoside action of digitalis (or other related drugs like digitoxin, digoxin, or gitalin). Patients who take these drugs should consult a medical professional before taking hawthorn.

Dosage

The recommended daily dosage is (1) dried fruit or powdered capsule 0.3 to 1 g by infusion 2 teaspoonfuls three times daily, (2) liquid extract 0.5 to 1.0 mL three times daily (1 : 1 in 25% alcohol), or (3) tincture 1 to 2 mL three times daily (1 : 5 in 45% alcohol).[55] Tincture combinations are available such as hawthorn–cactus–motherwort–ginger; 15 to 40 drops three times daily will provide the effective dosage. Hawthorn and its extracts are slow acting and can take up to 2 weeks to produce effects. Maximum benefit comes from at least 4 to 8 weeks of use, and elderly people can be treated for several months.

Bilberry

Bilberry (*Vaccinium myrtillus*), in the family Ericaceae, is a small deciduous shrub common to central and northern Europe, Asia, and North America. Among its many common names are huckleberry, hurtleberry, and wineberry. The medicinally useful parts of the plant are the leaves and the ripe fruit (berries).

Chemical Constituents

The berries contain flavonoid compounds known as anthocyanosides (0.1% to 0.25%), which are believed to be the pharmacologically active constituents. Anthocyanosides are composed of a backbone anthocyanidin attached to one of three sugars: arabinose, glucose, or galactose. Other flavonoids such as avicuarin, hyperoside, and astragaline are present, in addition to tannins. Typical extracts of bilberry are concentrated to yield a content of 25% anthocyanidin.

Physiologic Activity and Therapeutic Use

The most popular current use of bilberry extracts is to treat various eye disorders such as cataracts, macular degeneration, and glaucoma. Many of these conditions are associated with aging. Bilberry extracts, with their high content of anthocyanosides, are believed to offer benefits by improving the delivery of oxygen and nutrients to the eye and by protecting the eye tissues from the damaging effects of free radicals through potent antioxidant activity. Interest in bilberry and vision started with reports that during World War II the Royal Air Force pilots who took bilberry claimed to have improved nighttime vision and a quicker recovery from exposure to glare. Clinical studies support at least some of these early observations, especially in terms of improving visual performances at low illumination.[56] Results were most striking in individuals who had retinitis pigmentosa or who demonstrated poor night vision. In one study, bilberry extract was found to give measurable improvement in 31 patients who had various forms of retinopathy.[57] Bilberry extract has also shown promise in treating numerous vascular disorders that are particularly related to capillary fragility and varicose veins.[58]

Anthocyanosides have been shown to have a high affinity for the pigmented epithelium or visual purple area of the retina. This part of the retina controls the adaptation to light and dark. Benefits in treating varicose veins and other vascular disorders may be caused by anthocyanidin's effects on stabilizing membrane phospholipids in endothelial cells and on increasing the biosynthesis and cross-linking of collagen, thus restoring the connective tissue sheath around the vein.

In addition, bilberry is often administered as a tea to treat diarrhea and is commonly used topically for mild inflammation of the mucous membranes of the mouth and throat.

Precautions

No significant side effects have been reported other than occasional mild GI disturbances and skin rashes in clinical studies using bilberry extracts.

Dosage

Most clinical studies were done with bilberry extracts concentrated to yield 25% anthocyanidins.

Garlic

The medicinally useful part of the plant consists of the dried or fresh bulbs of *Allium sativum* L. of the lily family (Liliaceae). Garlic has been consumed both as a food and medicine since the time of the Egyptian pharaohs.

Chemical Constituents

The bulbs contain an odorless sulfur-containing amino acid derivative alliin (S-allyl-L-cystein sulfoxide). When the bulb is crushed, the enzyme alliinase is released and converts alliin localized in adjacent cells to the pungent odoriferous allicin, which is the main component of garlic volatile oil. The characteristic derivatives of allicin are all sulfur compounds (more than 30 additional sulfur compounds). Allicin, considered the major active component, gives the characteristic odor and carries many of the characteristic pharmacologic actions of garlic such as being an antibiotic, lowering cholesterol, inhibiting platelet aggregation, and so forth. Ajoene (formed by the self-condensation of allicin) has been shown to have antiplatelet aggregation and antibacterial activity. Commercial garlic products vary greatly in chemical composition.[59]

Physiologic Activity and Therapeutic Use

Garlic is considered antibacterial, antifungal, antithrombotic, and hypotensive; it activates fibrinolysis and is anti-inflammatory. Recent interest has focused on the potential use of garlic and its preparations for several purposes, including the treatment of high blood pressure, atherosclerosis, hypoglycemia, digestive ailments, colds, flu, and bronchitis, as well as for its blood cholesterol– and triglyceride-lowering activity.[59] Of all these activities, the best substantiated are those involving garlic's antihyperlipidemic properties.

Precautions

Garlic may cause GI discomfort; rare allergic reactions have also been reported. Potential interaction between garlic and anticoagulant drugs, such as warfarin, has been reported.[60]

Dosage

The daily dosage is equivalent to 4 to 12 mg of alliin (2 to 5 mg of allicin) in appropriate formulations, 400 to 1200 mg of dried powder, or 2 to 5 g of the fresh bulb.[10,61]

Ginkgo

Ginkgo biloba is often referred to by its common names maidenhair tree or simply ginkgo. It is the only living member of the ginkgo family (Ginkgoaceae) and is recognized by its sturdiness, resistance, and longevity. In the West, the extract or tincture from the leaves is used primarily for medicinal purposes. In oriental herbalism, the seed kernel is also used.

Chemical Constituents

The typical standardized *Ginkgo biloba* concentrated (50:1) leaf extract (GBE) contains diterpene lactones such as ginkgolides (A, B, C, and M) and the sesquiterpene bilobalide. These constituents are thought to be responsible for the neuroprotective properties of the leaf extract. Ginkgolide B is also a potent platelet-activating factor (PAF) antagonist. In addition to terpenoids, the extract is rich in bioflavonoids and flavone glycosides such as quercetin, 3-methyl quercetin, and kaempferol. The flavonoid fractions of the extract have been shown to possess potent antioxidant and free radical scavenger effects.[62]

Physiologic Activity and Therapeutic Use

The extract from the leaves is traditionally known as an antimicrobial, anti-inflammatory, vasodilator, and uterine stimulant. Today, the primary therapeutic use is enhancement of various CNS functions such as short-term memory, concentration, and alertness, particularly in the elderly. Many of the recent pharmacologic and clinical studies of GBE have demonstrated a positive effect in increasing vasodilatation and the peripheral blood flow rate in capillary vessels and in various circulatory disorders. Among these are varicose conditions, postthrombotic syndrome, chronic cerebral vascular insufficiency, short-term memory loss, and cognitive disorders secondary to depression, dementia, tinnitus, vertigo, and obliterative arterial disease of the lower limbs. Ginkgo leaf extract exerts a protective effect against hypoxia, and it protects biomembranes from oxidative injury and minimizes cell loss by acting as an oxygen free radical scavenger.[62]

The increased blood flow to the brain is likely caused by GBE promotion of arterial vasodilatation through stimulation of prostaglandin biosynthesis or indirectly by stimulation of norepinephrine release. In summary, ginkgo extract has three main effects on the body:

- It improves circulation through all the vital tissues and organs, such as the heart and brain.
- It has protective effects against damaging free radicals.
- It blocks the effect of PAFs, which may contribute to the development of asthma, heart disease, skin disorders, and hearing loss.[63]

Precautions

Few, if any, significant side effects have been documented. Rarely, gastric disturbance, headache, and allergic skin reactions have been reported following prolonged administration.[64] Ginkgo extract's ability to inhibit platelet aggregation could prolong bleeding time and should be considered, especially when other anticoagulant and antiplatelet drugs are given.

Dosage

Ginkgo biloba is commonly available as capsules or tablets containing 40, 60, or 120 mg of a concentrated (50:1) leaf extract. The typical daily dose is 120 to 160 mg.

Grape Seed and/or Pine Bark

Grape seed extract is derived from the seeds of *Vitis vinifera*, a member of the family Vitaceae. Pine bark extract is known by the trade as pycnogenol, a chemical designation (as well as the trademark of a French company) for a mixture of water-soluble flavonoids derived from the bark of the European coastal pine *Pinus nigra* Arnold var. *maritima* (also known as *Pinus maritima* Lam.).[65,66]

Chemical Constituents

Both pine bark and grape seed extracts contain various proanthocyanidins (condensed tannins) that are polyphenol oligomers derived from the condensation of flavan–3–ols and flavan–3,4–diols.

Physiologic Activity and Therapeutic Use

Most of the clinical research has been conducted in France by a company that produces pycnogenol (Horphag). In vitro studies show that proanthocyanidins are potent antioxidants. Grape seed and pine bark extracts are popular in Europe and are used to treat circulatory disorders such as atherosclerosis, varicose veins, diabetic retinopathy, and cardiac or cerebral infarction.[65,66] Pycnogenol is widely used for its anti-inflammatory activity. One animal study demonstrated that pycnogenol, when injected intradermally, bound tightly to tissue elastin and decreased its degradation by elastases.[67] Thus the enhanced breakdown of elastin by elastases seen in many inflammatory processes could be potentially prevented by pycnogenol if injected or absorbed into the blood. Much additional research is required to determine with certainty the effectiveness of oligomeric proanthocyanidins in preventing or treating these various conditions.

Precautions

No precautions are noted for using grape seed or pine bark.

Dosage

Tablets or capsules (75 to 300 mg) of grape seed or pine bark are ingested daily for up to 3 weeks, followed by a maintenance dose of 40 to 80 mg daily.

Nervous System Disorders

Valerian

Valerian (*Valeriana officinalis*), belonging to the family Valerianaceae, is a tall perennial herb (3 to 5 feet) with grooved hollow stems bearing large-toothed, dark green leaves. Approximately 200 species of valerian grow in mild climate areas of North America, western Asia, and Europe. The rhizome and the attached roots, which are harvested in the fall of the second year, are the medicinally used parts of the plant.

Chemical Constituents

The two major active principles are (1) a series of lipophilic iridoid compounds known collectively as the valepotriates and (2) several compounds from the essential oil fraction. Because of their lipophilicity and instability in aqueous solutions, the valepotriates are present in only small amounts in commercially available root extracts. The essential oil fraction from valerian roots contains the compound bornyl acetate and the sesquiterpene derivatives valerenic acid, valeranone, and valerenal. Aqueous extracts containing no valepotriates and little essential oil have still proven to be effective as sedative/hypnotics, indicating there are other, as yet unidentified, active components.

Physiologic Activity and Therapeutic Use

Several clinical trials carried out since the early 1980s have demonstrated valerian's effectiveness in treating insomnia.[68] The results of these studies indicated that 400 to 450 mg of an aqueous extract of valerian decreased sleep latency (time to fall asleep) as well as improved sleep quality when compared with placebo. The German Commission E approved its use in sedative and sleep-inducing preparations to mediate states of excitation and difficulty in falling asleep as a result of nervousness. The morning hangover characteristic of some sleep-inducing sedatives is absent with valerian. Animal studies show anticonvulsive, antidepressant, and spasmolytic activity of valerian extracts although no clinical studies have been done to indicate that these effects occur in humans. Little is known about the biochemical mechanisms underlying these observed effects. However, several studies indicate that certain compounds in valerian extracts have potential effects on the inhibitory neurotransmitter GABA, thereby inhibiting its reuptake and stimulating its synthesis.[69]

Precautions

Valeriana officinalis preparations are considered safe despite the known in vitro cytotoxic activity of valepotriates.[70] However, levels of valepotriates in typical extracts are too low to cause such effects in vivo. Several clinical trials have reported isolated incidents of headaches, excitability, and cardiac disturbances. Also because of its potential effects on uterine contraction, using valerian during pregnancy could be problematic. Valerian extracts have not proven to act synergistically with alcohol as have the benzodiazepines. The interaction of valerian with other CNS depressants such as opiates, barbiturates, and benzodiazepines, although unknown, could conceivably result in potentiation.

Dosage

For the treatment of insomnia, 400 to 450 mg doses of the aqueous extract of dried valerian roots in a capsule have been given from 30 to 60 minutes before bedtime. Standardized root extracts containing 0.8% valerenic acid are commonly available. Teas can be prepared from 2 to 3 g (1 teaspoon) of dried roots per cup of boiling water. Note that as the root dries it develops a characteristic disagreeable odor, which arises from certain of its constituent volatile oils.

St. John's Wort

St. John's wort (*Hypericum perforatum*), in the family Hypericaceae, is a shrubby herbaceous perennial comprising more than 400 species. The herb is native to Europe, West Asia, and North Africa, but has been naturalized in many parts of the world including North America, South America, and Australia. The plant often invades pastures, disturbed sites along roadways, and meadows where it prefers dry and sunny locations. The numerous five-petal, star-shaped yellow flowers and the leaves contain the highest levels of medicinally useful compounds.

Chemical Constituents

The most distinctive and unique compounds are the naphthodianthrones (0.05% to 0.3%) including hypericin, pseudohypericin, protohypericin, and cyclopseudohypericin.[15] Many of the pharmacologic effects of this herb have been attributed to these compounds. The phloroglucinol derivative hyperforin is one of the most abundant compounds found in *Hypericum* flowers and leaves (2.8%). The flavonoids catechin, quercetin, rutin, kaempferol, biapigenin, and hyperin are present as a total of 11.7% in flowers and 7.4% in leaves. Tannins are present in both leaves and flowers (8% to 16%). An essential oil is present composed of methyl octane, α- and β-pinene, β-myrcene, limonene, geraniol, and humulene.

Physiologic Activity and Therapeutic Use

More than 30 German studies since the mid-1980s have confirmed *Hypericum*'s effectiveness in treating mild-to-moderate depression. These studies demonstrate that *Hypericum* is significantly more effective than placebo and as effective as tricyclic antidepressants with fewer side effects. Criticism of many of these studies includes the use of variable product and dosage formulations, inadequate blinding protocols, and unreliable inclusion/exclusion criteria. No studies have yet been published comparing *Hypericum* with the selective serotonin reuptake inhibitor agents. St. John's wort has also been shown to be effective in treating seasonal affective disorder in a limited number of studies. The Commission E of the German Federal Health Agency cites the following indications for *Hypericum:* "for psychoautonomic disturbances, depressive mood disorders, anxiety and nervous unrest." *Hypericum* does not produce acute effects so it is not suitable for use as a daily sedative or sleep aid. Certain compounds in *Hypericum*, including hypericin, are capable of inhibiting monoamine oxidase in vitro but at concentrations that could not be reached in vivo. Several in vitro studies have shown that *Hypericum* inhibits the synaptosomal uptake of serotonin, dopamine, and norepinephrine. Such an in vivo inhibition in humans would lead to an increase in these neurotransmitters in the brain.

Many studies have demonstrated that St. John's wort extracts have antibacterial, antiviral, and wound-healing activity.[6] The high tannin concentration in *Hypericum* extracts likely contributes to its wound-healing efficacy. In addition, hyperforin appears to have a mild antibiotic activity.

Precautions

Minimal side effects have been reported following the use of *Hypericum*. A small percentage of patients (less than 1%) experience GI irritation, mild allergic reactions, restlessness, and fatigue. Severe photosensitivity has been reported in grazing animals and leads to inflammation of the skin and mucous membranes. Photosensitivity has been recently reported in humans following single high doses of 3600 mg but not at normal therapeutic doses. Therefore, a caution should be extended to fair-skinned individuals, particularly if they are taking other photosensitizing drugs.

Dosage

For the treatment of mild-to-moderate depression, doses of 300 mg of a standardized extract containing 0.3% hypericin are typically taken three times a day. Significant therapeutic effects are not seen for several weeks, similar to other antidepressant drugs. Most of the German clinical trials were conducted using the German product Jarsin 300, which is a methanol extract of flowers and leaves dried to a powder and put into a capsule. Liquid ethanolic tinctures of flowers and leaves (4:1 to 7:1 in 50% to 70% ethanol) are popular among herbalists. Topical preparations of olive or sunflower oil extracted from flowers or leaves are often used to treat skin abrasions or burns.

Kava-Kava

Piper methysticum, a large shrub indigenous to the Polynesian area of Oceania, belongs to the black pepper family and was first described by botanist George Foster, who accompanied Captain James Cook during his Polynesian voyage. When the root of the plant is chewed and mixed with saliva, a hot intoxicating mixture results, hence its folk name "intoxicating pepper."

Chemical Constituents

Kava contains several pharmacologically active constituents having primarily anxiolytic and sedative CNS effects. Extracts of kava root are rich in different substituted delta lactones (also called alpha pyrones), such as yangonin, desmethoxyyangonin, methysticin, dihydromethysticin, kavain, and dihydrokavain. A number of additional pharmacologic effects have been described for these pyrones, such as local anesthetic and antiarrhythmic properties, as well as potentiation of barbiturates.[71]

Physiologic Activity and Therapeutic Use

Kava has long been used in ceremonial rites in Hawaii and Polynesia for protection and luck. Today many uses of kava have been rediscovered, especially for anxiety disorders. With moderate usage, kava has few side effects that are physiologically adverse, which accounts for kava's recent increased popularity in the United States. Studies in the rat and guinea pig indicate that kava pyrones may block different forms of epileptic activity, as well as reduce the infarct area in the brain if administered before inducing ischemia.[72] In a clinical trial in Germany, patients with anxiety disorder were treated with kava extract (90 to 110 mg dry extract). The data proved both the short- and long-term efficacy of the kava extract was superior to the placebo. These authors suggest the use of kava extract as an alternative to tricyclic antidepressants and benzodiazepines in treating anxiety disorders, because even long-term use had none of the tolerance problems associated with the tricyclics or benzodiazepines.

Precautions

Among heavy users, a scaly rash is often observed, which resolves upon discontinuation.[73] Alcohol has been reported to markedly increase the toxicity of kava. Therefore, concomitant use is discouraged, especially when driving vehicles. One case report notes a possible interaction between kava and benzodiazepines that led to lethargy and disorientation in a 54-year-old male. Caution is also advised for concomitant use of kava and anticoagulant medications until the clinical significance of kava's antithrombotic action is determined.

Dosage

The recommended daily dosage of kava preparations is equivalent to 60 to 120 mg of kava pyrones. From a standardized kava extract (70% kavalactons), the patient takes 100 mg two to three times a day.

Feverfew

Feverfew, *Tanacetum parthenium* (L.) Schulz Bip. (*Chrysanthemum parthenium* [L.] Bernh.), is a member of the aster family (Asteraceae, formerly Compositae). Native to Europe, it is commonly grown as an ornamental flower in the United States.[74] The leaves are the medicinally useful part of the plant.

Chemical Constituents

The primary chemical constituents of feverfew leaves are the sesquiterpenes, especially parthenolide (0.1% to 1.27%). While parthenolide is the dominant sesquiterpene lactone present, several chemotypes have been found in which parthenolide is absent. Selection of parthenolide-containing germ plasm is necessary for product development. Canadian regulatory authorities have proposed correctly identified whole dried leaf or leaf extract with at least 0.2% parthenolide as a minimum standard for reasonable certainty of efficacy in feverfew products.

Physiologic Activity and Therapeutic Use

Throughout history, feverfew has been used to treat many conditions including fever, headache, menstrual difficulties, stomachache, toothache, and insect bites. It is often used to treat arthritis and inflammatory diseases such as psoriasis. Current primary use is as a prophylactic to reduce the frequency, severity, and duration of migraine headaches and to relieve associated symptoms such as nausea. The pharmacologic effects of feverfew extracts on platelet aggregation and secretion, leukocyte and macrophage function, and vascular smooth muscle contraction are consistent with its reported efficacy in migraine treatment. Evidence supports an association between migraines and vascular system instability. Migraines are characterized by excessive intracranial arterial constriction, followed by rebound dilation of the extracranial blood vessels. Alternatively, the direct inhibition of vascular smooth muscle contraction by parthenolide could decrease the initial excessive intracranial arterial constriction that triggers the rebound vasodilatation. Platelet aggregation and release of serotonin may also play a role in the pathogenesis of migraine. Feverfew's inhibition of these functions would, therefore, be expected to prevent some of the vascular responses triggered by serotonin.[75]

Precautions

Some individuals may experience gastric discomfort following ingestion of feverfew. Administration of fresh leaves has produced occasional mouth ulceration.

Dosage

The average daily dose of the dried leaves with a minimum content of 0.2% parthenolide is 125 mg. Feverfew is usually consumed in tablet or capsule form.[6]

Caffeine-Containing Plants

Caffeine-containing plants include coffee (dried ripe seed of *Coffea arabica* L., a member of the family Rubiaceae); tea (leaves and leaf buds of *Camellia sinensis* [L.] O. Kuntze, a member of the tea family [Theaceae]); kola (the dried cotyledon of *Cola nitida* [Vent.] Schott & Endl. and other *Cola* species, members of the cola family [Sterculiaceae]); cocoa, also known as cacao (the roasted seed of *Theobroma cacao* L., also a member of the cola family); guarana (crushed seeds of *Paullinia cupana* H.B.K., a member of the soapberry family [Sapindaceae]); and maté, also known as yerba maté (the dried leaves of *Ilex paraguariensis* St.-Hil., a member of the holly family [Aquifoliaceae]).[6]

Chemical Constituents

These plants all contain purine alkaloids that are mainly caffeine (1,3,7-trimethylxanthine), along with varying amounts of theobromine and theophylline.[17]

Physiologic Activity and Therapeutic Use

All of these herbs are CNS stimulants. They are used alone to overcome drowsiness and in combination with nonprescription analgesics, whose effects they potentiate by as much as 40%. Combined with ergot alkaloids, caffeine has been used in preparations for treating migraine headaches. Caffeine-containing beverages also have a weak diuretic activity of relatively short duration.[6]

Precautions

At usual therapeutic doses, few significant side effects have been reported. As CNS stimulants, caffeine-containing plants should be used with caution by patients with hypertension, kidney disease, hyperthyroidism, and certain psychic disorders such as panic disorder. At quantities of caffeine greater than 500 mg/day, stomach hyperacidity and irritation, diarrhea, and reduced appetite are often seen. Other symptoms such as restlessness, irritability, sleeplessness, and palpitations are common at high daily doses of caffeine. Psychic as well as physical dependency can develop from the long-term intake of high levels of caffeine (greater than 1.5 g/day). Withdrawal symptoms include headache and sleep disturbances.

Dosage

An average daily dose is equivalent to 100 to 200 mg of caffeine (1 to 2 cups of coffee). The lethal dosage (LD50) for an adult is approximately 200 mg caffeine per kilogram of body weight.

Metabolic and Endocrine Disorders

Black Cohosh

The dried rhizome and roots of *Cimicifuga racemosa* (L.) Nutt., used by the early native Americans, is reputed to soothe sore throat, nourish the respiratory system, and ease muscular pain. The plant is indigenous to the rich woods of the eastern deciduous forest of North America. It derives its name from characteristics of the rhizome, which is black and rough.

Chemical Constituents

The primary biologically active components of black cohosh rhizomes are triterpene glycosides, including acetein and cimicifugoside (cimigoside). Isoflavones are also present, especially formononetin. Other constituents of minor importance include isoferulic and salicylic acids, tannins, resin, starch, and sugars.

Physiologic Activity and Therapeutic Use

The most recent popular use of this herb is to treat premenstrual syndrome (PMS) and menopause.

Recent small-scale clinical studies have concluded that black cohosh is a safe and effective alternative to estrogen replacement therapy for those patients in whom such therapy is contraindicated. In support of these clinical findings, several studies have shown that black cohosh reduces serum concentration of the pituitary luteinizing hormone (LH), and it inhibits the binding of LH to receptors in the hypothalamus. In Europe, particularly in Germany, black cohosh is used as an emmenagogue and for endocrine activity in treating neurovisceral and psychic problems associated with menopause, premenstrual complaints, and dysmenorrhea. It is also used as a uterine antispasmodic.

In a study involving 100 menopausal women, none of whom had received steroid replacement therapy for at least 6 months immediately preceding admission into the trial, an ethanolic extract of the rhizome was found to cause a selective reduction of serum concentrations of pituitary LH.[76] Black cohosh extracts have also been shown to bind to estrogen receptors in rat uterine tissue. The German Commission E monograph approves black cohosh for treating premenstrual discomfort and dysmenorrhea.[77]

Precautions

GI disturbances have been reported from the use of black cohosh in some patients. Use is contraindicated during pregnancy and lactation.

Dosage

The dried rhizome is used in appropriate formulations, such as decoctions or tinctures (1:10, 60% ethanol), in amounts corresponding to a daily dosage of 40 to 200 mg. The German health authorities specify that duration of use should not exceed 6 months (presumably because information on long-term effects is lacking).[10]

Chaste Tree Berry

Chaste Tree (*Vitex agnus-castus*), commonly referred to as Vitex, is in the family Verbenaceae. This shrub or small tree is native to the Mediterranean area, West Asia, and southwestern Europe but has become naturalized in much of the southeastern United States. The dried ripe fruits or berries and the leaves are the medicinally useful parts of the plant.

Chemical Constituents

The fruits contain flavonoids, which are considered to be the primary active components. These fruits include the major flavonoids casticin, orientin, and quercetagetin.[78] The dried fruits also contain an essential oil (up to 1.22%) composed of limonene, cineole, and sabinene, as well as the iridoid glycosides, aucubin, eurostoside, and agnuside.[79]

Physiologic Activity and Therapeutic Use

The results of at least eight clinical studies indicate that Vitex is effective in treating symptoms of irregular menstruation and PMS. These symptoms are often associated with hyperprolactemia, with low levels of progesterone, and with corpus luteum insufficiency. A recent double-blind, placebo-controlled study in 175 women suffering from PMS revealed that Vitex was more effective in alleviating PMS symptoms than was pyridoxine (vitamin B_6).[80] Additional observational studies support the above finding, the largest involving 1542 German women with PMS.[81] Vitex treatment for 166 days improved symptoms in more than 90% of patients in this study. Vitex appears to work at the level of the hypothalamus–pituitary axis, causing an increase in LH, which increases progesterone blood levels.[82] Vitex has been shown to decrease the secretion of prolactin from anterior pituitary cells in vitro by acting as a dopamine agonist.[83]

Precautions

Several human studies indicate that Vitex is safe for most women of menstruation age. Side effects have been rare but include itching, headache, GI complaints, and skin rashes. Some women have reported an increased menstrual flow during Vitex treatment. There has been one report of a 32-year-old woman who was taking Vitex and who developed mild ovarian hyperstimulation in the luteal phase of her cycle.[84] Vitex should not be used during pregnancy.

Dosage

Most of the clinical trials were carried out in Europe using a proprietary alcohol-based tincture (Agnolyt or Strotan). A typical dose of Vitex extract for treating PMS or menstrual abnormalities is 40 drops (20 mg) daily usually taken in the morning with some beverage. Solid formulations of the alcohol extracts are also available. The glycoside agnuside is often used as a reference compound for standardization in the manufacture of Vitex extracts.

Evening Primrose (Black Currant, Borage Seed) Oil

Evening primrose (*Oenothera biennis* L.), native to eastern North America and widely naturalized elsewhere, is a member of the primrose family (Onagraceae). Although evening primrose is used mainly for its high content of essential fatty acids, this plant contains additional medicinally active ingredients used by herbalists. The seed oils of black currant (*Ribes nigrum* L.) and borage (*Borago officinalis* L.) are also used for similar purposes.

Native Americans consumed the leaves, roots, and seed pods as food and prepared extracts for use as a painkiller and asthma treatment.[85] Modern uses include treatment for rheumatoid arthritis, eczema, multiple sclerosis, PMS, cardiovascular disorders, chronic fatigue syndrome, Raynaud's syndrome, weight loss, and diabetes.

Chemical Constituents

The freshly pressed oil from evening primrose seeds is light yellow and has at least 85% to 92% unsaturated fatty acids. Most of the polyunsaturated fatty acids are composed of the essential *cis*-linoleic acid (LA) and the rare *cis*-gamma-linolenic acid (GLA) forms. Depending on the brand, the oil contains a minimum of 8% to 12% GLA. The seed oil contains smaller amounts of palmitic, oleic, and stearic acids, as well as steroids, including campesterol and β-sitosterol.[15]

Physiologic Activity and Therapeutic Use

Studies suggest that the GLA found in dietary supplement sources, especially evening primrose oil (EPO), can be directly converted to the prostaglandin precursor dihomo-GLA and could be of benefit to individuals who are unable to metabolize *cis*-linoleic acid in addition to patients whose diets are low in that acid.[86]

GLA is present only in small amounts in normal dietary sources although it is a major component of human milk. Conversion of LA into GLA can be reduced by a number of factors such as aging, high cholesterol levels, high intake of saturated fats and *trans*-fatty acids, viral infections, stress, high alcohol intake, diabetes, eczema, and PMS.[87]

Recent theories about the causes of PMS include hormonal imbalances involving estrogen–progesterone, pyridoxine deficiency, elevated serum aldosterone, hypoglycemia, abnormal magnesium metabolism, and varying prostaglandin levels in the female reproductive tract. A study conducted in a London hospital using Efamol (primrose oil as a source of GLA) involved 68 women who had failed to respond to other therapeutic regimens. Of those women, 61% experienced total remission and 23% experienced partial remission.

Atopic eczema might be related to abnormal essential fatty acid (EFA) metabolism; an imbalance in the two EFAs in the plasma phospholipids has been shown. LA level is somewhat higher than normal, and GLA and its derivatives are reduced. A meta-analysis of nine controlled trials of EPO therapy that assessed the severity for eczema by scoring measures of inflammation, dryness, scaliness, and overall skin improvement showed a highly significant improvement ($P < .0001$) in patient and doctor scores over baseline as a result of primrose oil treatment.[88]

Other plant oils, including those from the seeds of black currant and borage, also contain large amounts of GLA. However, the results of EPO research are difficult to apply to these species because the patterns of fatty acids present in these oils are different. Unlike the oils of the other plants, EPO contains no ω-3 EFAs and almost no saturated fatty acids. Fatty acids are known to interfere with the biologic activity and metabolism of ω-6 EFAs and may diminish the biologic activity of the GLAs present in the oil. The triglyceride structures of the oils are also different and could produce different effects.[87]

Precautions

The only side effects reported for EPO were possible worsening of temporal lobe epilepsy or schizophrenia if administered with conventional drug therapy such as phenothiazines.

Dosage

The recommended daily dosage of EPO for adults should not exceed 4 g (containing approximately 300 to 360 mg GLA). In some cases, such as in atopic eczema, the dosage could temporarily be higher (i.e., 4 to 8 g/day). For children, the advisable dose is 2 to 4 g/day. Both LA and GLA are present in breast milk. A breast-fed baby consumes 23 to 65 mg GLA/kg/day; therefore, to provide sufficient amounts of EFA for both the mother and the baby, EPO may be taken during pregnancy and while breast-feeding. No toxic effects have been observed, even at high dosages (5 mL/kg/day).

Arthritic and Musculoskeletal Disorders

All of the effective plant derivatives, mustard oil, methyl salicylate, and so forth, are covered in Chapter 5, "Musculoskeletal Injuries and Disorders."

Disorders of the Skin, Mucous Membranes, and Gingiva

Witch Hazel

Witch hazel (*Hamamelis virginiana*), a member of the family Hamamelidaceae, is a tree-like deciduous shrub (10 to 12 feet) found in the eastern deciduous forest of North America. It is commercially cultivated in Europe. Vernal witch hazel (*Hamamelis vernalis*) may be involved in the commercial supply of witch hazel products. The preparation most commonly available in the United States is distilled witch hazel extract (also referred to as hamamelis water), which is prepared by steam distillation of the recently harvested, dormant twigs macerated in water, with 14% alcohol subsequently added. Conversely, hydroalcoholic extracts are commonly used in Europe.[6]

Chemical Constituents

Witch hazel leaves contain 8% to 10% tannin (the bark has 1% to 3%) composed of hamamelitannin or digallyhamamelose, gallotannins, and proanthocyanidins. Tannins are considered responsible for the astringent activity of the herb; however, they are absent from the commonly available steam distillate, which relies on the added alcohol for its astringent effect.[6,15]

Physiologic Activity and Therapeutic Use

Witch hazel preparations are used to treat local inflammation of the skin and mucous membranes.[6] In Europe, hydroalcoholic extracts are used for their astringent and anti-inflammatory activity as well as local hemostyptics for minor skin injuries, hemorrhoids, and varicose veins.[89]

Precautions

No precautions are noted for using witch hazel.

Dosage

Witch hazel preparations are applied topically as needed for the described therapeutic disorders.

Aloe Vera Gel

Aloe vera gel consists of a mucilaginous gel obtained from the parenchymatous tissue in the center of the leaf of *Aloe vera* (L.) N. L. Burm., a member of the lily family (Liliaceae). It is also referred to in the literature as *Aloe barbadensis* Mill. The gel should not be confused with the yellow latex or juice occurring in specialized cells just below the leaf epidermis, which is the source of the cathartic drug aloe that contains the anthraquinone aloin.

Chemical Constituents

The gel primarily consists of several types of polysaccharides, including an acidic galactan, a mannan, a glucomannan, an arabinan, and/or a glucogalactomannan. Polysaccharides constitute 0.2% to 0.3% of the fresh gel and are thought to be responsible for the antiviral and immunoprotective properties. The reported ratios of hexoses in each polysaccharide, as well as the molecular weights of the polysaccharides themselves, differ widely in various studies. The alcoholic extract contains saponins, triterpenoids, naphthoquinones, anthraquinones, and sterols. Several of these compounds have anti-inflammatory activity. A serine carboxypeptidase has been suggested as an antithermic agent in aloe gel.[15]

Physiologic Activity and Therapeutic Use

Fresh aloe gel, perhaps the most widely used folk medicine in the United States, is applied to first-degree burns and minor skin irritations. It has anti-inflammatory and emollient properties, and it also enhances wound healing. A recent review of the pharmacologic and clinical studies of aloe gel concluded a possible therapeutic value in burns and a wide variety of soft tissue injuries. The authors found that it prevented progressive dermal ischemia following thermal injury, frostbite, and electrical trauma. Aloe gel penetrates injured tissue, relieves pain, and is anti-inflammatory. It acts to dilate capillaries, thus increasing the blood supply to the injury.[90] The juice made from freshly cut leaves can be used internally as a laxative or to eliminate intestinal parasites.

Precautions

No precautions are noted when aloe is used externally.

Dosage

Fresh aloe gel is applied topically as necessary. When taken orally, it is usually combined with tamarind or fennel.

Essential Oils, Including Tea Tree Oil

Essential oils are more or less fluid, odorous, and volatile. They occur in roots, leaves, flowers, barks, resins, and the rind of some fruits. Their composition differs from fatty oils in that essential oils contain terpenoids, phenyl propane–derived compounds, aldehydes, ethers, ketones, and esters other than glycerates. These components barely dissolve in water, but they dissolve well in alcohol and fatty oils. The original function of secreted/excreted essential oils, to protect the plant from disease and parasites, more or less determines their therapeutic function. In general, essential oils are antibacterial and antiparasitic; some are antiviral and antifungal. The oils are obtained primarily by steam distillation but other methods of extraction are also used.

The essential oils are highly concentrated and very potent medicines used both internally and externally. For a patient to avoid irritation and harmful effects resulting from direct contact on mucous membrane or skin, the proper dilution and administration of essential oils are very important.

Table 45–2 presents a few of the most frequently used essential oils and their therapeutic effects. Featured are the oils of eucalyptus, lavender, peppermint, rosemary, and tea tree. These oils have been used for treating a wide variety of external and internal conditions.

As an example of the essential oils, tea tree oil is a volatile oil that is steam distilled from the leaves of *Melaleuca alternifolia* (Maiden & Betche) Cheel (family Myrtaceae), which is a shrub or small tree growing up to 18 feet in height. The plant is found in swampy or wet ground on the northern coast of New South Wales (north of Port Macquarie), as well as in adjacent areas of southern Queensland in Australia. Production of the oil is generally limited to this region.

Chemical Constituents

Tea tree leaves contain about 2% of volatile oil, with terpene hydrocarbons including pinene, terpinene, cymene (about 30%), and 65% or more of oxygenated terpenes, particularly terpinen-4-ol (30% to 60%).[4] High-quality volatile oil (Australian Standard. "Oil of Melaleuca, Terpinen-4-ol type," AS 2782) contains 30% to 47% terpinen-4-ol and less than 15% cineole as major components. Cineole-rich oils are considered to be of inferior quality.[15]

Physiologic Activity and Therapeutic Use

Oil high in terpinen-4-ol is considered bacteriostatic and germicidal. The oil has been used for treating boils, abscesses,

Table 45–2

Traditional Therapeutic Effects of Selected Essential Oils

Effect	Eucalyptus	Lavender	Peppermint	Rosemary	Tea Tree
Antibacterial	√				√
Anti-inflammatory		√	√	√	√
Antirheumatic	√	√		√	
Antispasmodic	√	√	√	√	
Antiviral	√		√		√
Asthma	√	√			
Bronchitis	√	√	√	√	√
Calming		√			
Colds	√		√	√	
Depression		√		√	
Fevers	√			√	√
Headache	√	√	√	√	
Insomnia		√			
Menstrual cramps		√	√	√	
Mental activity			√	√	
Nervousness		√			
Premenstrual syndrome			√		
Pain relief	√	√	√	√	
Stress		√			
Wounds/burns	√	√			√

sores, cuts, and abrasions, as well as for wounds with pus discharge. During World War II, the oil was mixed with machine-cutting oils in Australian ammunition factories to reduce infections from metal filing injuries.[6]

Other conditions for which use of the oil has been promoted include acne, arthritis, bruises, burns, cystitis, dermatitis, fungal infections, herpes, insect bites, muscular aches and pains, respiratory tract infections, sunburn, vaginal infections, varicose veins, and warts.[6] However, the oil's utility in many of these conditions requires verification.

A 1990 clinical trial involving 124 patients provided evidence that *Melaleuca alternifolia* oil is effective in treating acne vulgaris. A 5% tea tree oil in a water-based gel was less effective (because of slower onset of action) than a 5% benzoyl peroxide in water-based lotion. However, clinical assessment and self-reporting of side effects suggested that tea tree oil was better tolerated on facial skin with less skin scaling, dryness, pruritus, and irritation. The results of this study were less than conclusive.[91] Tea tree oil products are widely marketed, often with hyperbolic claims.

Precautions

Tea tree oil may cause skin irritation or allergies in sensitive individuals. Generally, the oil has not been associated with toxicity.[6]

Dosage

The oil is applied topically in concentrations from 0.4% to 100%, depending on the condition and area of treatment.[6]

Goldenseal

Goldenseal (*Hydrastis canadensis*), is a member of the buttercup family, Ranunculaceae, and is found in the rich, deciduous forests of the eastern United States. Settlers learned from the American Indians about its use as a bitter, a stomach aid, and an eye wash. Modern use includes the treatment of congestion and various inflammatory conditions of the mucous membranes that line the respiratory, gastrointestinal, and digestive tracts. The medicinally useful parts of the plant are the roots and the rhizomes. An infusion of the roots is typically used as a wash for sore eyes and skin diseases.

Chemical Constituents

The rhizome and roots contain a number of isoquinoline alkaloids, including hydrastine (1.5% to 4%), berberine (1.7% to 4.5%), and canadine (0.5%) and related alkaloids.[10]

Physiologic Activity and Therapeutic Use

Root preparations have traditionally been used for their antimicrobial, astringent, and antihemorrhagic activities when treating mucosal inflammation. The activity of goldenseal is largely caused by the presence of hydrastine and, to a lesser extent, berberine. Hydrastine is considered to be vasoconstrictive, and hydrastine and berberine are thought to have choleretic, spasmolytic, and antibacterial properties.

A modern folk use for goldenseal has been to mask illicit drugs in urinalysis tests. The herb's activity in this regard is a myth that has grown out of the fictional plot of the novel *Stringtown on the Pike*, published in 1900 by pharmacist John Uri Lloyd (1849–1936). No scientific evidence supports this use; in fact, goldenseal may instead promote false positive readings. Some laboratories are now testing for the presence of hydrastine during urinalysis.[92]

Precautions

The use of goldenseal is contraindicated during pregnancy.

Dosage

The dosage for goldenseal is 0.5 to 1 g of the dried root or 2 to 4 mL of tincture (1:10, 60% ethanol) three times per day.[10]

Melissa

Melissa or lemon balm (*Melissa officinalis*) is a member of the mint family Lamiaceae. The medicinally useful parts of the plant are the leaves.

Chemical Constituents

Melissa contains about 0.1% to 0.2% volatile oil composed mainly of oxygenated compounds such as citral (a and b), citronellal, geraniol, caryophyllene oxide, and polyphenols (caffeic acid, protocatechuic acid, etc.); a tannin composed of chlorogenic, caffeic, and rosmarinic acids; flavonoids; and other compounds.[15]

Physiologic Activity and Therapeutic Use

Historically, the leaves (primarily in tea form) have been used for their calmative, spasmolytic, and carminative activity. The German Commission E approves the use of lemon balm preparations to (1) alleviate difficulty in falling asleep because of nervous conditions and (2) treat functional GI symptoms.[15]

More recently, antibacterial and antiviral activities have been confirmed. Oxidative products of caffeic acid and derivatives were found to have antiviral activity against herpes simplex virus type 1 (cold sores) and type 2 (genital herpes).[6] A European ointment corresponding to 0.7 g of leaf per gram has recently become available on the American market.

Two dermatologic centers carried out a randomized, placebo-controlled, double-blind study on the effect of a cream containing 1% dried extract of lemon balm leaves (drug extract 70 : 1) on herpes lesions. The study evaluates case reports of 116 patients using lemon balm cream. The physicians and patients judged the lemon balm cream to be superior to the placebo. At the critical initial stage of treatment as well as during the second day, when the swelling began to decline, the treatment group showed significant improvement compared with the placebo group. To achieve efficacy, treatment must be started at very early stages of the infection. Accelerated healing was most pronounced in the first 2 days of treatment.[93]

Precautions

No precautions are noted for lemon balm.

Dosage

Appropriate formulations of lemon balm preparations are applied topically as needed.

Performance and Endurance Enhancers

Ginseng

One of the most popular herbal remedies is the dried root of Asian ginseng (*Panax ginseng* C.A. Meyer) and American ginseng (*Panax quinquefolius* L.), both members of the ginseng family (Araliaceae). Wild Asian ginseng is rare in its indigenous northeast Asian habitats, which include northeastern China, the Korean peninsula, and adjacent Russia. It is, however, extensively cultivated in China and Korea.[94] The American species is scarce in the wild in the eastern United States but is cultivated successfully in Wisconsin and Pennsylvania.

Chemical Constituents

Asian ginseng contains as its primary active components at least 18 triterpenoid saponins, including ginsenosides R_0, R_{b-1}, R_{b-2}, R_{b-3}, R_c, R_d, R_e, R_f, $R_{20\text{-gluco-}f}$, R_{g-1}, and R_{g-2}. Traditionally, the root is harvested in the sixth year of growth. A recent 5-year study showed that the highest levels of ginsenosides were obtained at the end of the summer of the fifth year of growth. The root weight doubles between the fourth and fifth years of growth. The steamed ginseng root, which is also called red ginseng, contains saponins that are degradation products as a result of heat and processing. Other constituents include a trace of volatile oil, sesquiterpenes, starch, polysaccharides (panaxans A–U in a concentration of 7% to 9%), pectin, mono- and disaccharides, and polyacetylenes.[15]

Physiologic Activity and Therapeutic Use

Traditionally characterized as an aphrodisiac and a tonic, ginseng has a documented use dating back more than 2000 years. Ginseng is surrounded by controversy as a result of the different source and quality of the products and because of attached claims. Numerous pharmacologic and clinical benefits have been attributed to the root and its preparations, including its antitumoral and antiviral activity. Ginseng root is also used to enhance liver metabolic functions; to improve functions of the CNS, reproductive, and cardiovascular systems; to protect against ischemia; and to enhance the immune and endocrine systems.[95,96]

Ginseng is now designated as an adaptogen (i.e., an agent facilitating resistance to various kinds of stress). Extracts that have been standardized to contain between 4% and 7% ginsenosides have been subjected to several clinical studies in Europe. Reported positive results include shortened reaction time to visual and auditory stimuli, elevated respiratory quotient, increased alertness, improved power of concentration, enhanced grasp of abstract concepts, and better visual and motor coordination.[97] Conflicting results of various studies have been attributed to differences in the type of preparation, route of administration, dosage, and presence or absence of biologically active compounds, among other factors.[95,96] The German Commission E monograph allows ginseng's use as a tonic to treat fatigue, diminished work capacity, and loss of concentration, in addition to its use as a general aid during convalescence.[97]

Precautions

Ginseng is generally considered safe. However, acute illness, hypertension, use of large amounts of stimulant (including caffeine-containing beverages), and concurrent use of antipsychotic drugs would contraindicate the use of ginseng.[55] Ginseng should be used with caution in circumstances such as cardiac disorders, diabetes, hypertensive and hypotensive disorders, and steroid therapy. Safety of ginseng during pregnancy has not been firmly established.

Dosage

The daily dosage is 1 to 2 g of root or equivalent preparations. For short-term use in young and healthy individuals 0.5 to 1 g daily in two divided dosages is common.

Eleuthero

Eleuthero (*Eleutherococcus senticosus*), a member of the family Araliaceae, grows up to 9 feet tall and is found in eastern Siberia, northeastern China, adjacent Korea, and Hokkaido Island in Japan. In traditional Chinese medicine, the bark of the root was the plant part used; today, all parts of the root as well as the stems are used. Eleuthero is widely marketed in the United States under the name "Siberian ginseng," although it is not related to true ginseng, *Panax ginseng*.

Chemical Constituents

The main active compounds in root and stem extracts are designated eleutherosides A–G. Their concentrations range from 0.6% to 0.9% in the roots and from 0.6% to 1.5% in the stems.[9] Eleutherosides B and E account for about 80% of the total eleutherosides and are thought to be responsible for most of the plant's pharmacologic activity. Although the common name *eleutheroside* would seem to imply similarity in chemical structure, such is not the case. This group of compounds is chemically heterogeneous. Eleutheroside A is the sterol daucosterol; eleutheroside B is syringin, a phenylpropanoid; and eleutheroside B_1 is isofraxidin-7-*O*-α-L-glucoside (β-calycanthoside). Lignans include eleutheroside B_4 [(−)-sesamin], eleutheroside D [(−)-syringaresinol-di-*O*-β-

D-glucoside], and eleutheroside E (acanthoside D). Triterpenes include eleutherosides I–M. Senticosides A–F represent incompletely characterized oleanolic acid glycosides (possibly identical to other triterpenoid components).[15,98]

Physiologic Activity and Therapeutic Use

The most prominent therapeutic effect reported for eleuthero is its action as an adaptogen. The German Commission E has approved eleuthero for use as a tonic for invigoration during fatigue, debility, and declining work capacity, as well as during convalescence.

Essentially all the studies relating to eleuthero's potential therapeutic effects have been carried out in Russia since the early 1960s and involve more than 2000 normal and stressed human subjects. Many of these studies have a deficient experimental design, often lacking in adequate controls. Many of the clinical studies[99] published in Russian journals in the 1960s by Drs. Brekhman and Petkov reported improved recoveries of patients under stress from various diseases such as diabetes and cancer. Normal healthy subjects treated for 4 weeks with eleuthero showed an increase in immunocompetent cells, principally T lymphocytes.[99] In addition, eleuthero polysaccharides, similar in quality and quantity to those found in echinacea, have been shown to stimulate phagocytic activity in human granulocytes.[100] Well-designed, randomized clinical trials with standardized preparations are required to determine which of the numerous claims of utility for eleuthero can be verified.

Precautions

The Russian studies reported no significant adverse side effects except for an occasional transient rise in blood pressure. The German Commission E thus has indicated high blood pressure as a contraindication for using eleuthero. Eleuthero is often adulterated with other plants (particularly the silk vine, *Periploca sepium*) or with caffeine to enhance its stimulant effects. A recent report of eleuthero elevating plasma digoxin levels in a single patient may have been a case of adulterated product.[101]

Case Study 45–2

Patient Complaint/History

Jessie, a 16-year-old male student who participates actively in football, wrestling, and track and field events, asks the pharmacist about the availability of preparations that will enhance his physique and increase his performance and endurance in sports. He explains that body-building magazines regularly advertise dioscorea, sarsaparilla, and yohimbe as "natural testosterone sources." He then displays an advertisement that calls these products "steroid alternatives" and requests recommendations for suitable products containing the advertised or other related botanicals.

The patient is obviously a healthy teenager; his patient profile shows that he uses no prescription medications on a regular basis. His infrequent use of nonprescription products is limited to Advil 200 mg tablets as needed for athletic aches or pains and Robitussin as needed for symptoms related to occasional colds.

Clinical Considerations/Strategies

Readers can use the following considerations/strategies to determine whether treatment of the patient's condition with nonprescription medications is warranted:

- Assess this patient's actual versus perceived need for effective physique-enhancing drugs.
- Inform the patient of inaccuracies in herbal advertisements in a manner that will not cause the patient to "turn off" from seeking professional advice or that will cause the patient to order useless products by mail.
- Advise the patient that certain steroidal compounds may be converted to active substances in the laboratory but not in the human body.
- Advise the patient that, in most instances, the safety and effectiveness of many products touted as wondrous cures or enhancers of mental and physical prowess—which are commonly sold by mail order, telephone order, or health food stores, or by nutrition centers—have not been clinically tested or proven in objective, controlled studies.

Patient Education/Counseling

Readers can use the following strategies to develop a patient education/counseling plan that will help ensure optimal therapeutic outcomes:

- Explain appropriate non–drug-assisted techniques for body building.
- Help the patient understand that there are no shortcuts to improving the mind and/or body and that all such "quick fixes" (promises) are irrational and without a basis in fact.
- Further enlighten the patient as to the serious physical consequences that accompany the improper use of androgenic steroids to improve athletic performance.
- Encourage the patient to seek professional advice on the safety and effectiveness of plant-derived products. Also, ask the patient to encourage friends to seek professional advice if they have questions or concerns about these products.

Dosage

The average daily dose of eleuthero is 2 to 3 g of the powdered root. In Russian studies using a 33% ethanol extract of the root, dosages of 2 to 16 mL were taken one to three times a day for up to 60 consecutive days (with a 2- to 3-week resting interval between courses of administration). Up to five courses of the herb were administered within a period of 1 year.[102]

Echinacea

Echinacea, or purple coneflower, is an indigenous North American perennial that grows from Canada to as far south as northern Texas. Three species are of medicinal value: *Echinacea angustifolia*, *Echinacea purpurea*, and *Echinacea pallida*, all in the family Asteraceae. The roots, leaves, and flowers of echinacea are the medicinally useful parts of the plant.

Chemical Constituents

Echinacea purpurea, the best-studied species, contains cichoric acid, 1.2% to 3.1% in the flowering tops and 0.6% to 2.1% in the roots. It also contains other caffeic acid derivatives such as chlorogenic acid and cynarin, which may play roles in stimulating phagocytosis. An essential oil containing humulene, echinlone, vanillin, germacrene, and borneol is also present. Alkylamides, such as echinacein and several isobutylamides, are believed to be responsible for the local anesthetic effect and for some of the anti-inflammatory activity. The presence of several high molecular weight polysaccharides such as heteroxylan, arabinogalactan, and fucogalactoxyloglucan has been shown to stimulate macrophages and to possess anti-inflammatory activity. *Echinacea angustifolia* and *Echinacea pallida* have similar constituent profiles.

Physiologic Activity and Therapeutic Use

Echinacea products (oral dosage forms) are used as nonspecific immunostimulants, especially as prophylactics at the first sign of cold and flu symptoms, as well as in other upper respiratory infections such as tonsillitis, otitis media, sore throat, and whooping cough. A recent double-blind, placebo-controlled study indicates that a daily dose of 450 mg of *Echinacea purpurea* root extract (1:5 in 55% ethanol) significantly relieved the severity and duration of flu symptoms.[103] A double-blind, placebo-controlled clinical trial examined the immune-stimulating influence of an expressed fresh juice preparation of *Echinacea purpurea* on the course and severity of colds and flu-like symptoms in patients deemed to have greater than normal susceptibility to infections. At a dose of 2 to 4 mL per day, patients with diminished immune response (expressed by a low T4/T8 cell ratio) were found to benefit significantly from preventive treatment with the echinacea preparation.[104] Echinacea extracts have also been shown to reduce the growth of *Trichomonas vaginalis* and lower the recurrence rates of *Candida albicans* infections.[105]

The pharmacologic mechanisms underlying these antimicrobial effects appear to be related to Echinacea's ability to stimulate the body's immune defense system rather than to any significant direct antimicrobial action. A major part of this stimulation involves the enhancement of macrophage phagocytosis as well as the increased production and secretion of immune-potentiating substances such as interferon, interleukins, and tumor-necrosis factor (TNF).[106] Echinacea extracts also promote nonspecific T-lymphocyte activation with resultant increased cell replication and enhanced production of interferon and an increase in antibody binding sites.

Topical preparations (ointment) of the fresh aboveground parts of *Echinacea purpurea* are used for the external treatment of hard-to-heal wounds, eczema, burns, psoriasis, and herpes simplex.[107] (These preparations are available in Germany but are not usually available in the United States.) The direct wound-healing effect of echinacea is most likely caused by inhibition of the enzyme hyaluronidase, thus preventing the spread of invading microorganisms.

Precautions

Echinacea, as well as nonspecific immunostimulants in general, are contraindicated in tuberculosis, leukosis, collagenosis, multiple sclerosis, human immunodeficiency virus (HIV) infections, and other autoimmune diseases.[71] Also, prolonged administration of echinacea may lead to overstimulation and eventual suppression of the immune system. Individuals with known allergies to plants in the daisy family should be cautious when using echinacea. Historical confusion about plant identity in scientific studies and persistence of adulterated supplies of *Echinacea purpurea* with *Parthenium integrifolium* have resulted in the publication of negative (not recommended) German therapeutic monographs on *Echinacea purpurea* root, as well as on *Echinacea angustifolia* root and *Echinacea angustifolia/Echinacea pallida* aerial parts. Positive monographs have been published for preparations containing aerial parts of *Echinacea purpurea* and the roots of *Echinacea pallida*.[107]

Dosage

Of the expressed fresh juice of *Echinacea purpurea*, the dose is 6 to 9 mL per day for not longer than 8 weeks; after that period, the immunostimulatory effects decline.[108] For *Echinacea pallida* root preparations, the average daily dose corresponds to 900 mg per day, often administered in the form of a tincture (1 : 5) prepared with 50% ethanol. The dosage of *Echinacea angustifolia* root in the form of capsules, tablets, or a tincture is 1 gram, three times daily for up to 10 days. Most of the German clinical trials over the past 10 years have used an injectable preparation of fresh stabilized extract of *E. purpurea* known as Echinacin. Because injectable preparations are not available in the United States, caution should be used when comparing German clinical results with treatment results using orally active preparations.

Astragalus

Astragalus (*Astragalus membranaceous*), commonly called milk vetch or yellow vetch, is in the family Leguminosae. This perennial legume has yellow flowers and grows to a height of 2 to 4 feet. The genus *Astragalus* is composed of more than 2000 species. Astragalus is native to China and is referred to as huang qi (yellow leader). The plant's black roots with pale yellow center have been used for 2000 years in Chinese traditional medicine as a general tonic and to strengthen the immune system. Astragalus root has recently become popular in the West mainly for its immune-stimulating and cardiovascular benefits.

Chemical Constituents

Astragalus roots contain bioflavonoids such as astraisoflavin, choline, and several polysaccharides with Astragalan B being the most noted.[108] The polysaccharides are believed to be responsible for the plant's immune-stimulating properties.

Physiologic Activity and Therapeutic Use

Many animal and human studies carried out both in vivo and in vitro give strong experimental evidence for the immune-stimulating potential of *Astragalus membranaceous* (AM) root extracts. Several in vitro investigations since 1988 have demonstrated that AM extracts potentiate the stimulating effect of recombinant interleukin–2 (rIL-2) on lymphokine activated killer (LAK) cell antitumor activity.[109] This potentiation would allow a lower level of excessively toxic rIL-2 to be used for immunotherapy. Polysaccharide-rich extracts of AM have also been shown to stimulate the secretion of TNF from peripheral blood mononuclear cells and to promote a blastogenic response of lymphocytes in vitro.[110] Studies in rats and mice have demonstrated an immune-stimulating effect of AM in animals immunodepressed by cyclophosphamide or radiation treatment.[111] Astragalus root extracts given orally increased the abnormally low blood levels of T lymphocytes in patients with viral myocarditis.[112] In addition, natural killer activity of isolated peripheral blood mononuclear cells from 28 patients with systemic lupus erythematosus was enhanced following incubation with AM.[113]

Several animal studies in China from 1990 to 1994 have documented the protective effect of Astragalus on Coxsackie B3 viral myocarditis. Mice infected with Coxsackie B3 virus and treated with AM showed significantly fewer histologic signs of myocardial tissue damage, as well as a lower copy number of Coxsackie virus–RNA.[114] Another mouse study showed significant electrophysiologic improvements in the right ventricular myocardium of mice infected with Coxsackie B3 virus after treatment with AM.[115] These studies support earlier findings, one in cultured rat heart cells and another in mice, that showed an improvement in myocyte function as well as a reduction in the virus titer following infection with Coxsackie B3 virus.[116,117]

Several Chinese clinical studies have shown an improvement in cardiac function in patients with congestive heart failure or angina pectoris, as well as in patients suffering an acute myocardial infarct following AM treatment.[118,119] Certain constituents in Astragalus roots appear to exert a positive inotropic effect on the myocardium, possibly by activating the Na^+, K^+-ATPase. Other constituents have potent antioxidant activity that is beneficial in a number of cardiovascular diseases.

In addition to AM having immune-stimulating and cardiovascular effects, some experimental evidence supports its effectiveness as a hepatoprotectant. Isolated polysaccharides from Astragalus were shown to protect against *E. coli* endotoxin-induced liver damage in mice.[120] This protective effect was reflected in enhanced glutathione levels in the liver and was thought to be a result of antioxidant activity. Another study in mice showed a hepatoprotective effect of an ethanol extract of AM against the damaging effects of stilbenemidine on the liver.[121]

Precautions

Astragalus membranaceous has no reported dangerous side effects. Occasional abdominal bloating and loose stools were the most commonly reported adverse reactions in clinical trials. However, many flowering species in the *Astragalus* genus are toxic. One American species is referred to as locoweed by cattle ranchers because of its behavioral effects.

Dosage and Formulations

Astragalus root preparations are commonly available as capsules, teas, and tinctures. Chinese practitioners often combine astragalus with ginseng and other herbs. Popular formulations in China are pan roasting the roots in honey or including the roots in a soup. Most Chinese clinical trials used AM extracts taken orally, whereas most animal studies used injected doses of AM.

Green Tea

Green tea (*Camellia sinensis*), an evergreen shrub native to eastern Asia, is cultivated extensively in India, China, Japan, Indonesia, Sri Lanka, Turkey, and Pakistan, as well as in other parts of the world such as Africa and South America. The Chinese have used the leaves to prepare beverages for more than 4000 years. Green tea is prepared from steamed and dried leaves, and the method of curing determines the final product. Black tea is withered, rolled, fermented, and then dried. The so-called oolong tea is semi-fermented and considered an intermediate product between green and black tea.[122,123]

Tea was introduced to Europe in the 17th century and became a favorite beverage, especially in the form of black tea. The Chinese have regarded the tea infusion as a cure for many diseases and as a way to prevent heart problems and cancer. Tea has been used to flavor food, and the essential oil is applied in perfumes and cosmetics.

Chemical Constituents

Several chemical constituents of green tea have been identified. The variation in chemical composition is further complicated with fermentation and other treatments. The most characteristic components are polyphenols such as gallic acid and catechin, and their derivatives theogallin, gallocatechin, epiatechin, and epigallo catechin. The fresh leaves contain caffeine (3% to 4% depending on the development process), theobromine (0.15% to 0.2%) and theophylline (0.02% to 0.04%), and other methylxanthines.[124] During fermentation, catechins partially change into either oligomeric quinones (e.g., theaflavine, theaflavine acid, and thearubigene) or non–water-soluble flavonoids (e.g., quercetin, kaempferol, and myrecetin).[124] Green tea contains B vitamins and ascorbic acid, which are destroyed in the process of making black tea. The essential oil contains more than 300 components including aldehydes, phenylethyl alcohols, phenols, hexenal, hexenol, linalool, dihydroactinidiolide, and p-vinylphenol.[125]

Physiologic Activity and Therapeutic Use

Tea drinking in Asian countries has evolved into a cultural habit and a part of everyday life. Freshly brewed green tea has an aromatic smell with a slight bitter taste that stimulates the nervous system and works as a diuretic. Current knowledge of the pharmacology of tea includes its antimicrobial, antioxidant, antimutagenic, and numerous anticancer actions, as well as its effect on lipid metabolism.

In vitro and animal studies evoked high hope that regular consumption of tea, especially green tea, would have a direct lowering effect on plasma LDL level and LDL oxidation in vivo in humans. However, research has not supported such claims.

Extensive examinations of the antimutagenic and anticarcinogenic activities of green tea show that the polyphenol components of tea may possess chemopreventive properties.[126] The antimutagenic activity was demonstrated against various mutagens. The mechanisms of antimutagenesis and anticarcinogenesis by which tea polyphenols act include the modulation of extracellular and intracellular metabolic and proliferative processes.[126,127] The antibacterial effects against oral bacteria and several pathogenic strains common in the GI tract have also been well documented. An in vitro test showed that green tea was effective against some pathogenic fungi.[127]

Studies of the antioxidant activity of catechins in various experimental and human conditions show that catechins possess antioxidant activity in different in vitro and in vivo conditions. A Japanese longevity study suggests that regular green tea consumption contributes to an extended life span.[127]

Other components of green tea such as caffeine and tannin can be effective in treating different pathologic conditions. Caffeine is an effective stimulant of the central nervous system and can be used to treat headache, to enhance stomach acid production, and to enhance renal excretion of water. Caffeine is frequently included in weight-loss pills and used as a cardiotonic agent.

Green tea is also used to treat hepatitis, protect the liver against chemical toxins, and treat various skin disorders topically.

Precautions

Moderate consumption of green tea does not pose any hazard. However, pregnant women should avoid caffeine-containing products. Also, evidence suggests that highly condensed tannins and catechin could induce esophageal cancer. Tea combined with milk can possibly prevent the undesired effects of tannins. People with high blood pressure, insomnia, asthma, heart problems, and elevated cholesterol should consult with their physician before becoming a regular tea drinker.

Dosage

The beneficial effects of tea infusion are typically seen at the dosages normally consumed by humans. Overdose (quantities more than 300 mg caffeine, more than 5 cups/day) can lead to negative effects on the CNS and to irritation of the stomach.

Patient Assessment/Counseling for Herbal Remedies

The assessment process for patients seeking advice on herbal remedies differs little from that for patients using nonprescription medications. Because FDA has not approved herbal products for any indications, the pharmacist's major challenge is determining which remedies are safe to use for a particular indication. Books such as this one and the various available herbal references are for now the pharmacist's best resources for such information.

The pharmacist should ask patients the following general questions about their previous or intended use of herbal remedies as well as whether they have seen a physician about their symptoms. Because herbs and phytomedicinals have a broad range of therapeutic use, many of the questions presented in other chapters are also applicable to these products. Once the complaint is delineated, the assessment questions listed in the chapter covering that disorder should also be asked.

Q~ Have you used this product before? If so, for how long and in what dosage form?

A~ Determine whether the patient exceeded the recommended length of therapy and, as a result, is no longer achieving symptomatic relief. Determine whether the most effective dosage form or proper dosages were taken.

Q~ Are you allergic to any plant materials? If so, which specific materials or products?

A~ If plant allergies exist, steer the patient away from products in plant families to which a known allergy exists.

Q~ Is this product for personal use or for someone else (e.g., a child)?

A~ Determine whether the product is appropriate for use by children or, if applicable, elderly patients.

Q~ Are you pregnant or breast-feeding?

A~ If yes, determine whether the product is recommended for use in these situations.

Q~ Have you seen a health care professional, or are you self-medicating?

A~ Determine whether the patient has a diagnosed condition. If so, encourage the patient to involve the physician in the use of herbal remedies, if such use is appropriate.

Q~ Are you taking prescription or nonprescription medications intended for the same purpose as this herb? What other remedies have you tried for this problem?

A~ If a medication is being taken, find out whether it is providing symptomatic relief. If so, determine why the patient wishes to use herbal remedies. Find out whether other remedies were effective in treating the complaint.

As with any request for advice on self-treating a disorder, the pharmacist should tailor the counseling to the patient's knowledge and understanding of the condition. Maintaining a nonjudgmental attitude will prevent the patient from "going it alone" with herbal remedies. Just as with nonprescription medications, the pharmacist should explain why a particular herbal remedy is appropriate for the present situation, how to use the product, and what precautions to take. Potential interactions, adverse effects, contraindications, and the maximum duration of treatment should also be explained. Finally, the pharmacist should explain the signs and symptoms that indicate medical attention is needed.

References

1. The right stuff: *Drug Store News* picks the categories taking off in '94. *Drug Store News.* 1994;16:15.
2. Eisenberg D, Kessler R, Foster C, et al. Unconventional medicine in the United States. *N Engl J Med.* 1993;328:246–52.
3. Bartels M. *Nutr. Clin Pract.* 1998;13:5–19.
4. Eisenberg D, Davis R, Ettner S, et al. Trends in alternative medicine use in the United States, 1990–1997: results of a follow-up national survey. *JAMA.* 1998;280:1569–75.
5. Miller LG, Murray WJ. Herbal instruction in the United States pharmacy schools. *Pharm Education.* 1998;61:160–2.
6. Tyler VE. *Herbs of Choice: The Therapeutic Use of Phytomedicinals.* Binghamton, NY: Pharmaceutical Products Press; 1994.
7. Schepers A. Reading between the lines of the new "pill bill." *Environ Nutr.* 1994;17:2.
8. Schilcher H. The significance of phytotherapy in Europe. *Z Phytother.* 1993;14:132–9.
9. Castañeda-Acosta J, Fischer NH, Vargas D. Biomimetic transformations of parthenolide. *J Nat Prod.* 1993;56:90–8.
10. Govindarajan V. Ginger-chemistry, technology and quality evaluation: Part I. CRC. *Crit Reviews in Food Science and Nutrition.* 19;17:1–96.
11. Mowrey D, Clayson D. Motion sickness, ginger, and psychophysics. *Lancet.* 1982;22:655–7.
12. Bone M, Wilinson D, Young J, et al. The effect of ginger root on postoperative nausea and vomiting after gynecological surgery. *Anesthesia.* 1990;45:669–71.
13. Fisher-Rasmussen W, Kjaer S, et al. Ginger treatment of hyperemesis gravidarum. *Eur J Ob & Gyn & Rep Biol.* 1990;38:19–24.
14. Srivastava K, Mustafa T, et al. Ginger (*Zingiber officinale*) in rheumatic disorders. *Med Hypotheses.* 1989;29:25–8.
15. Leung AY, Foster S. *Encyclopedia of Common Natural Ingredients Used in Foods, Drugs, and Cosmetics.* 2nd ed. New York: John Wiley & Sons; 1995.
16. Bordia A, Verma S, Srivasteve K, et al. Effects of ginger (*Zingiber officinale* Rosc) and fenugreek (*Trigonella foenumgraecum* L.) on blood lipids, blood sugar, and platelet aggregation in patients with coronary artery disease. *Prost Leuko Essen Fatty Acids.* 1997;56:379–84.
17. Tyler VE, Brady LR, Robbers JE. *Pharmacognosy.* 9th ed. Philadelphia: Lea and Febiger; 1988.
18. European Scientific Cooperative on Phytotherapy (ESCOP). *Proposal for European Monographs.* Vol. 2. Beurijdingslaan, The Netherlands: ESCOP Secretariat; 1992.
19. Monographie: Plantaginis ovatae testa (Indische Flohsamenschalen); Plantaginis ovatae semen (Indische Flohsamen). *Bundesanzeiger.* 1990 Feb 1.
20. Sprecher DL, Harris BV, Goldberg AC, et al. Efficacy of psyllium in reducing serum cholesterol levels in hypercholesterolemic patients on high- or low-fat diets. *Ann Intern Med.* 1993;119:545–54.
21. Rodriguez-Moran M, Guerrero-Romero F, Lazcano-Burciegie G., et al. Lipid and glucose-lowering efficacy of *Plantago psyllium* in Type II diabetes. *J Diabetes Complications.* 1998;12:273–8.
22. Monographie: Sennae folium (Sennesblatter). *Bundesanzeiger.*1993 Jul 21.
23. Foster S. *Peppermint: Mentha x piperita.* Botanical Series 306. Austin, TX: American Botanical Council; 1991:1–7.
24. Monographie: Menthae piperitae folium (Pfefferminzblatter). *Bundesanzeiger.* 1985 Nov 30;rev 1990 Mar 13.
25. Monographie: Menthae piperitae aetheroleum (Pfefferminzol). *Bundesanzeiger.* 1990 Mar 13.
26. Isaac VO, Schimpke H. Wissenverte fur die pharmazeutische. *Praxis Mitt Dtsch Pharmaz Ges.* 1965;35:133–47.
27. Agullo G, Gamet-Payraste L, Manenti S., et al. Relationship between flavonoid structure and inhibition of phosphatidylinositol 3-kinase: a comparison with tyrosine kinase and protein kinase C inhibition. *Biochem Pharmacol.* 1997;11:1649–57.
28. ESCOP. *Proposal for European Monographs.* Vol 1. *Beurijdingslaan.* The Netherlands: ESCOP Secretariat; 1990.
29. Foster S. *Chamomile: Matricaria recutita and Chamaemelum nobile.* Botanical Series 307. Austin, TX: American Botanical Council; 1991: 1–7.
30. Roberts A, Williams JMC. The effect of olfactory stimulation on fluency, vividness of imagery and associated mood: a preliminary study. *Br J Med Physiol.* 1992;65:197–9.
31. Yamada K, Miura T, Mimaki Y, et al. Effect of inhalation of chamomile oil vapor on plasma ACTH level in the ovariectomized rat under restriction stress. *Biol Pharm Bull.* 1996;9:1244–6.
32. Monographie: Matricarie flus (Klamillenbluten). *Bundesanzeiger.* 1984 Dec 5;rev 1990 Mar 13.
33. Foster S. *Milk Thistle: Silbum marianum.* Botanical Series 305. Austin, TX: American Botanical Council; 1991:1–7.

34. Floersheim G. Treatment of human Amatoxin mushroom poisoning: myths and advances in therapy. *Medical Tox.* 1987;2:1–9.
35. Muriel P, Garciapina T, Perez-Alvarez V, et al. Silymarin protects against paracetamol-induced lipid peroxidation and liver damage. *J Applied Tox.* 1992;12:439–42.
36. Sonnenbichler J, Zetl I. *Hoppe Seyler's Z Physiol Chem.* 1984;365:555.
37. Combest W. Milk thistle. *US Pharmacist.* September 1998; 86–90.
38. Katiyar S, Korman N, Mukhtar H, et al. Protective effects of silymarin against photocarcinogenesis in a mouse skin model. *J National Cancer Institute.* 1997;89:556–66.
39. Vaya J, Belinky P, Aviram M. Antioxidant constituents from licorice roots: isolation, structure elucidation, and antioxidant capacity toward LDL oxidation. *Free Radic Biol Med.* 1997; 23:302–13.
40. Baker M. Licorice and enzymes other than 11 beta-hydroxysteroid dehydrogenase: an evolutionary prospective. *Steroids.* 1994;59:136–41.
41. Utsunomiya T, Kobayashi M, Hemdon D, et al. Glycyrrhizin, an active component of licorice roots, reduces morbidity and mortality of mice infected with lethal doses of influenza virus. *Antimicrob Agents Chemother.* 1997;41:551–6.
42. Combest W. Licorice. *US Pharmacist.* April 1998:125–31.
43. Matsuda H, Nakate H, Tanake T, et al. Pharmacological study on *Arctostaphylos uva-ursi* (L.) Spreng. II. Combined effects ofarbutin and prednisolone or dexamethazone on immuno-inflammation. *Yakugaku Zasshi.* 1990;110:68–76.
44. Grases F, Melero G, Costo-Bauzo A, et al. Urolithiasis and phytotherapy. *Int Urol Nephrol.* 1994;26:507–11.
45. Monographie: Uvae ursi folium (Barentraubenblatter). *Bundesanzeigar.* 1984 Dec 5.
46. Avorn J, Monane M, Gurwitz JH, et al. Reduction of bacteriuria and pyuria after ingestion of cranberry juice. *JAMA.* 1994;271:751–4.
47. Cranberry [monograph]. In: Marderosian A, ed. *The Review of Natural Products.* St. Louis: Wolters Kluwer Co; July 1994.
48. Bricell C, ed. *The American Horticultural Society Encyclopedia of Garden Plants.* New York: Macmillan; 1996:568.
49. Carraro JC, Raymond J, Chisholm G, et al. Comparison of phytotherapy (Permixon) with finasteride in the treatment of benign prostate hyperplasia: a randomized international study of 1,098 patients. *Prostate.* 1996;29:231–40.
50. Braeckman J. The extract of *Serenoa repens* in the treatment of benign hyperplasia: a multicenter open study. *Curr Ther Res.* 1994;55:776–85.
51. Kim JP, Kim W, Koshino H, et al. Sesquiterpene O-naphthoquinones from the root bark of *Ulmus davidiana. Phytochemistry.* 1996;43: 425–30.
52. Wichtl M. Herbal drugs and phytopharmaceuticals. In: Bisset NG, ed. *A Handbook for Practice on a Scientific Basis.* Boca Raton, FL: Medpharm Scientific Publications CRC; 1996:161–6.
53. Ficarro P, Ficarra R, Tsmmasini A, et al. High-performance liquid chromatography of flavonoids in *Crataegus oxycantha* L. I. Reversed-phase high-pressure liquid chromatography. *Farmacon.* 1984;39:148–57.
54. Rewerski W, Piechocki T, Rylski M, et al. Einige Pharmakologische Eigenschaften der aus Weisdorn (*Crataegus oxycantha*) isolierten oligomeren procyanidine. *Arzneim-Forsch Drug Res.* 1971;21:886–8.
55. Newall CA et al. *Herbal Medicines: A Guide for Health-Care Professionals.* London: Pharmaceutical Press; 1996.
56. Sala D, Rolando M, et al. Effects of anthocyanosides on visual performances at low illumination. *Minervaa Oftalmol.* 1979;21:283–5.
57. Scharrer A, Ober M. Anthocyanosides in the treatment of retinopathies. *Klin Monatsbl Augenheikd.* 1981;178:386–9.
58. Mian E, Curri S, Lietti A, et al. Anthocyanosides and the walls of microvessels: further aspects of the mechanism of action of their protective effect in syndromes due to abnormal capillary fragility. *Minerva Med.* 1977;68:3565–81.
59. Foster S. *Garlic: Allium sativum.* Botanical Series 311. Austin, TX: American Botanical Council; 1991:1–7.
60. Koch HP, Lawson LD, eds. *Garlic: The Science and Therapeutic Application of* Allium sativum *and Related Species.* 2nd ed. Baltimore: Williams & Wilkins; 1996.
61. Monographie: Allii sativi bulbus (Knoblauchswiebel). *Bundesanzeiger.* 1988 Jul 6.
62. Foster S. *Ginkgo: Ginkgo biloba.* Botanical Series 304. Austin, TX: American Botanical Council; 1991:1–7.
63. Nemecz G, Combest W. Ginkgo biloba. *US Pharmacist.* September 1997:144–51.
64. Warburton DM. Clinical psychopharmacology of *Ginkgo biloba* extract. In: Funfgeld EW, ed. *Rokan (Ginkgo biloba): Recent Results in Pharmacology and Clinic.* Berlin: Springer-Verlag; 1988:327–45.
65. Liviero L, et al. Antimutagenic activity of procyanidins from *Vitis vinifera. Fitoterapia.* 1994;65:203–9.
66. Grape Seed [monograph]. In: DerMarderosian A, ed. *The Review of Natural Products.* St. Louis: Wolters Kluwer Co; September 1995.
67. Tixier J, Godeal G, et al. Evidence by in vivo and in vitro studies that binding of pycnogenols to elastin affects its rate of degradation by elastases. *Biochemical Pharmacology.* 1984;33:3933–9.
68. Combest W. Valerian. *US Pharmacist.* December 1997: 62–8.
69. Santos M, Ferreira F, Ceurha A, et al. An aqueous extract of valerian influences the transport of GABA in synaptosomes. *Planta Med.* 1994;60: 278–9.
70. Bountanh C, Bergman C. Valepotriates: a new class of cytotoxic and antitumor agents. *Planta Med.* 1981;41:21–8.
71. Meyer HJ, Kretzschmar R. Kawa pyrone—a new kind of substance group of central muscle relaxants of the mephenesin type. *Klin Wochenschr.* 1966;44:902–3.
72. Schmitz D, Zhang C, Chatterjee S, et al. Effects of methysticin on three different models of seizure like events studied in rat hippocampal and entorhinal cortex slices. *Naunyn Schmiedebergs Arch Pharmacol.* 1995;351:348–55.
73. Mathews JD, Riley M, Fejo L, et al. Effects of the heavy usage of kava on physical health: summary of a pilot survey in an aboriginal community. *Med J Aust.* 1988;148:548–55.
74. Foster S. *Feverfew: Tanacetum parthenium.* Botanical Series 310. Austin, TX: American Botanical Council; 1991:1–8.
75. Olesen J. The ischemic hypothesis of migraine. *Arch Neurol.* 1987;44: 321–2.
76. Duker E, Kopanski L, Tarry H, et al. Effects of extracts from *Cimicfuga racemosa* on Gonadotropin release in menopausal women and ovariectomized rats. *Planta Med.* 1991;57:420–4.
77. Monographie: Cimicifugae racemosae rhizoma (Cimicifugawurzelstock). *Bundesanzeiger.*1989 Mar 2.
78. Wollenweber E, Mann K. Flavonols from fruits of *Vitex agnus-castus. Planta Med.* 1983;48:126–7.
79. Gorler K, Oehlke D, et al. Iridoidfuhrung von *Vitex agnus-castus. Planta Med.* 1985;51:530–1.
80. Lavritzen C, Reuter H, et al. Treatment of premenstrual tension syndrome with *Vitex agnus-castus:* controlled, double-blind study versus pyridoxine. *Phytomedicine.* 1997;4:183–9.
81. Dittman F, Bohnert K, et al. Premenstrual syndrome: treatment with a phytopharmaceutical. *TW Gynakol.*1992;5:60–8.
82. Milewiez A, Gejdel E, et al. Vitex agnes-castus extract in the treatment of luteal phase defects due to hyperprolactinemia: results of a randomized placebo-controlled double-blind study. *Arzneim-Forsch Drug Res.* 1993;43:752–6.
83. Sliutz G, Speiser P. *Agnus-castus* extracts inhibit prolactin secretion of rat pituitary cells. *Horm Metab Res.* 1993;25:253–5.
84. Cahill D, Fox R. Multiple follicular development associated with herbal medicine. *Human Reproduction.* 1994;9:1469–70.
85. Briggs CJ. Evening primrose: la belle de nuit, the king's cureall. *Canadian Pharm Journal.* May 1986;249–54.
86. Nemecz G. Evening primrose. *US Pharmacist.* November 1998:85–94.
87. Horrobin DF. Gamma linolenic acid, an intermediate in essential fatty acid metabolism with potential as an ethical pharmaceutical and as a food. *Rev Contemp Pharmacother.* 1990;1:1–41.
88. Morse PF, Horrobin DF, Mankee M, et al. Meta analysis of placebo-controlled studies of efficacy of Epogam in the treatment of atopic eczema: relationship between plasma essential fatty acid changes and clinical response. *Br J Dermatol.* 1989;121:75–90.
89. Monographie: Hamamelidis folium et cortex (Hamamelisblatter undrinde). *Bundesanzeiger.* 1985 Aug 21;rev 1990 Mar 13.
90. Heggers JP, Pelley RP, et al. Beneficial effects of Aloe in wound healing. *Phytother Res.* 1993;7:548–52.
91. Bassett IB, Pannowitz DL, Barnetson P, et al. A comparative study of tea-tree oil versus benzoyl peroxide in the treatment of acne. *Med J Aust.* 1990;153:455–8.

92. Foster S. *Goldenseal: Hydrastis canadensis.* Botanical Series 309. Austin, TX: American Botanical Council; 1991:1–8.
93. Wobling RH, Leonhardt K. Local therapy of herpes simplex with dried extract from *Melissa officinalis. Phytomedicine.* 1994;1:25–31.
94. Foster S. *Asian ginseng: Panax ginseng.* Botanical Series 303. Austin, TX: American Botanical Council. 1991:1–7.
95. Ng TB, Yeung HW. Scientific basis of the therapeutic effects of ginseng. In: Steiner RP, ed. *Folk Medicine: The Art and the Science.* Washington, DC: American Chemical Society; 1986:139–52.
96. Shibata S, et al. Chemistry and pharmacology of Panax. In: Wagnor H, Hikino H, Farnsworth NR, eds. *Economic and Medicinal Plant Research.* Vol 1. Orlando, FL: Academic Press; 1985:217–84.
97. Monographie: Ginseng radix (Ginsengwurzel). *Bundesanzeiger.* 1991 Jan. 17.
98. Farnsworth NR, et al. Siberian ginseng (*Eleutherococcus senticosus*): current status as an adaptogen. In: Wagnor H, Hikino H, Farnsworth NR, eds. *Economic and Medicinal Plant Research.* Vol. 1. Orlando, FL: Academic Press; 1985:155–215.
99. Wagner W, Proksch A, et al. Immunostimulierend Wirkende polysaccharide heteroglykane aus ho hern pflanzen. *Arzneim-Forsch Drug Res.* 1984;34:659–61.
100. Brekhman I, Dardymov I. Pharmacological investigation of glycosides from Ginseng and Eleutherococcus. *Lloydia.* 1969;32(1):46–50.
101. McRae S. Elevated serum digoxin levels in a patient taking digoxin and Siberian ginseng. *Can Med Assoc J.* 1996;155:293–5.
102. Monographie: Eleutherococci radix (Eleutherococus-senticosus-wurzel). *Bundesanzeiger.* 1991 Jan 17.
103. Braunig B, Dorn M, et al. *Echinaceae purpurea radix:* zur Starkung der Korpereigenen Abwehr bei grippalen Infekten. *Z Phytother.* 1992;13: 7–13.
104. Schoneberger D. Einfluss der immunostimulierenden Wirkung von Prebsaft aus Herba Echinaceae purpureae auf Verlauf und Schweregrad von Erkaltungskrankheiten. *Forum Immunologie.* 1992;8:2–11.
105. Samuchowhec E, et al. Evaluation of the effect of *Calendula officinalis* and *Echinacea angustifolia* extracts on *Trichomonas vaginalis* in vitro. *Wiad Parazytol.* 1979;25:77–81.
106. Bauer R, et al. Immunological in vivo and in vitro examinations of Echinacea extracts. *Arzneim-Forsch Drug Res.* 1988;38:76–81.
107. Monographie: Echinaceae purpureae herba (Purpursonnenhutkraut). *Bundesanzeiger.* 1989 Mar 2.
108. He Z, Wang B. Isolation and identification of chemical constituents of *Astragalus* root. *Yao Hsueh Hsueh Pao.* 1990;25:694–8.
109. Chu D, Lepe-Zuniga J, Wong W, et al. Fractionated extract of *Astragalus membranaceous,* a Chinese medicinal herb, potentiates LAK cell cytotoxicity generated by a low dose of recombinant interleukin-2. *J Clin Lab Immunol.* 1988;26:183–7.
110. Zhoa K, Kong H. Effect of *Astragalus* on secretion of tumor necrosis factors in human peripheral blood mononuclear cells. *Chung Kuo Chung His I Chieh Ho Tsa Chih.* 1993;13:263–5.
111. Chu D, Wong W, Mavligit G, et al. Immunotherapy with Chinese herbs II: reversal of cyclophosphamide-induced immune suppression by administration of fractionated *Astragalus membranaceous* in vivo. *J Clin Lab Immunol.* 1988;25:125–9.
112. Huang Z, Qin N, Ye W, et al. Effect of *Astragalus membranaceous* on T-lymphocyte subsets in patients with viral myocarditis. *Chung Kuo Chung His I Chieh Ho Tsa Chih.* 1995;15:328–30.
113. Zhao X. Effects of *Astragalus membranaceous* and *Tripterygium hypoglancum* on natural killer cell activity of peripheral blood mononuclear cells in systemic lupus erythematosus. *Chung Kuo Chung His Chieh Ho Tsa Chih.* 1992;12:669–71.
114. Peng T, Yang Y, Randolf R, et al. Effect and mechanism of *Astragalus membranaceous* on Coxsackie B3 virus RNA in mice. *Chung Kuo Chung His I Chieh Ho Tsa Chih.* 1994;14:664–6.
115. Rui T, Yang Y, Zhou T, et al. Effect of *Astragalus membranaceous* on electrophysiological activities of acute experimental Coxsackie B3 viral myocarditis in mice. *Chung Kuo Chung His I Chieh Ho Tsa Chih.* 1994;14:292–4.
116. Yuan W, Chen H, Yang Y, et al. Effect of *Astragalus membranaceous* on electrical activities of cultured rat beating heart cells infected with Coxsackie B-2 virus. *Chin Med J.* 1990;103:177–82.
117. Yang Y, Jin P, Guo Q, et al. Treatment of experimental Coxsackie B3 viral myocarditis with *Astragalus membranaceous* in mice. *Chin Med J.* 1990;103:14–8.
118. Lei Z, Qin H, Liao J. Action of *Astragalus membranaceous* on left ventricular function of angina pectoris. *Chung Kuo Chung His Chieh Ho Tsa Chih.* 1994;14:199–202.
119. Chen L, Liao J, Guo Q, et al. Effects of *Astragalus membranaceous* on left ventricular function and oxygen free radical in acute myocardial infarction patients and mechanism of its cardiotonic action. *Chung Kuo Chung His I Chieh Ho Tsa Chih.* 1995;15:141–3.
120. Wang L, Han Z. The effect of *Astragalus* polysaccharide on endotoxin-induced toxicity in mice. *Yao Hsueh Hsueh Pao.* 1992;27:5–9.
121. Zhang Z, Wen Q, Liu C. Hepatoprotective effects of *Astragalus* root. *J Ethnopharmacol.* 1990;30:145–9.
122. Graham H. Green tea composition, consumption, and polyphenol chemistry. *Prev Med.* 1992;21:334–50.
123. Bokuchava M, Skobeleva N. The biochemistry and technology of tea manufacture. *Crit Rev Food Sci Nutr.* 1980;12:303–70.
124. Gruenwald S, Brenoller T, Jaenicke L, eds. *PDR for Herbal Medicine.* Montvale, NJ: Medical Economics Co; 1999:710.
125. Duke J. *Handbook of Medicinal Herbs.* Boca Raton, FL: CRC Press; 1985.
126. Antimutagenic and anticarcinogenic activity of tea polyphenols. *Mutat Res.* 1999;436:69–97.
127. Tea, green tea [monograph]. In: DerMarderosian A, ed. *The Review of Natural Products.* St. Louis: Wolters Kluwer Co; February 1999.

CHAPTER 46

Homeopathic Remedies

Kathryn L. Grant and Richard N. Herrier

Chapter 46 at a Glance

Homeopathic remedies are specially prepared, highly diluted substances derived from botanical, zoological, or chemical sources that are thought to trigger healing processes in the body. Both single and combination remedies are available as nonprescription products. A nonprescription homeopathic remedy is by definition a nontoxic homeopathic drug used to treat a self-limiting condition that does not require medical diagnosis or monitoring.[1] The Food and Drug Administration (FDA) has regulated that homeopathic remedies included in the Homeopathic Pharmacopoeia of the United States (HPUS) are official, and that unlisted remedies are nonofficial. About 1350 remedies currently exist in HPUS. Of those, 440 are considered prescription in some potencies, while 20 are prescription regardless of potencies. Sales of homeopathic remedies totaled $165 million in 1994, with sales rising more than 20% annually.[2] One survey reported that homeopathy use in the United States increased from 0.7% in 1990 to 3.4% in 1997 ($P < .001$).[3]

Some practitioners want a ban on homeopathy while others are admonishing pharmacists not to sell homeopathic products, but the public's use of and interest in homeopathy continues to grow.[4,5] Pharmacists, therefore, need to be knowledgeable about the pros and cons of this alternative medicine, even though it is not taught in most pharmacy schools. Pharmacists have had little exposure to homeopathy, but an increasing number carry homeopathic preparations in their inventory.

The purpose of this chapter is to provide a basic introduction to the very complicated subject of homeopathy. The reader will not be able to practice homeopathy or—simply on the basis of the information provided here—to comfortably make recommendations for homeopathic product selection in a retail or clinical setting. It would take much more than the space allotted here to accomplish such goals. The aim of this chapter is to objectively provide information on homeopathy, not to serve as an advocate for homeopathic practice.

Homeopathy has developed more as a complex art than a science, and practitioners of homeopathy vary greatly in their practice styles. Clinical studies do not support any one particular practice type. For more information on the practice of homeopathy, the pharmacist or pharmacy student is encouraged to explore other references or to seek out certification programs.

Patient Preferences for Homeopathic Remedies

Patient preference for homeopathy over conventional medicine or nonprescription products has not been well documented in the professional literature. However, the rapidly increasing interest in all complementary therapy, including homeopathy, is well documented.[3] The reasons for this increased interest are complex and include changes in generational and cultural values, as well as dissatisfaction with the increasingly impersonal and brief encounters that occur with many conventional medicine practitioners. Expanded-role practitioners such as nurse practitioners get high marks from patients because they tend to spend more time with the patient and have a more holistic approach. Because the tenets of homeopathy require a more detailed and personal history, the homeopathic practitioner gives more time and attention to the patient's recitation.[6] This increased time and attention also tend to be true for many practitioners of nonhomeopathic alternative therapy and may represent one of the factors that contributes to increased interest in alternative remedies.

Leaders in conventional medicine have noted the deterioration of patient–provider relationships, a decline caused by inadequate communication skills. Also there has been a rebirth in training physicians to listen more effectively to the patient.[7,8] Some patients appear to be turning to alternative medicine not because of dissatisfaction with conventional medicine, but because the alternative medicine is more consistent with their philosophical values and beliefs.[9]

A survey of new patients being seen by homeopathic physicians showed that most patients were seeking homeopathic care for their chronic conditions for which 80% of the respondents had unsuccessfully used conventional medicine.[10] Those surveyed had limited knowledge about homeopathy but believed that most of their problems could be resolved by homeopathy. On follow-up 3 months after the initial visit and treatment, 59% (52/88) reported feeling better or much better. Regarding their primary problem, 18% reported they were completely healed, 24% reported partial healing, and 29% were somewhat healed. As other surveys on the general use of alternative medicine show, women (68%) and college graduates (69%) are more likely to use homeopathy.[3,10] Patients who have diseases for which conventional medicine does not offer a cure (e.g., serious illnesses or common illnesses such as the common cold) are most likely to use alternative medicine. In Switzerland, 56 out of 100 patients infected with human immunodeficiency virus (HIV) used alternative medicine.[11] The most frequent alternative used was homeopathy ($n = 22$). Homeopathy is more accepted as a primary health care practice in Switzerland than in the United States. Of 65 cancer patients queried about their use of alternative medicine, 16 (25%) used homeopathy.[12]

History and Basic Laws of Homeopathy

Samuel Hahnemann (1755–1843) was a German physician who developed homeopathy in response to his concerns about the unsafe and unproven drugs (e.g., mercury) and therapies (e.g., blood-letting) being used at the time.[13] Having left conventional clinical practice, Hahnemann used his extensive language skills and chemistry background to translate medical and chemical texts into German. While translating William Cullen's *Treatise of the Materia Medica,* he disagreed with Cullen's explanation of the reason for quinine's effectiveness in treating malaria. Cullen contended that quinine was effective because it was bitter and astringent. Because many other drugs are bitter and astringent but have no efficacy against malaria, Hahnemann sought another explanation. He took 4 drams of Peruvian bark twice daily for several days and developed the symptoms of malaria. In consulting Hippocrates, Hahnemann found that Hippocrates had written that what cures a condition will also cause it. From this, Hahnemann developed a medical philosophy of *homeo* (similar) *pathos* (suffering).[14] He then began to systematically test hundreds of substances on himself, colleagues, and medical students. In an era of empiricism, Hahnemann emphasized quantitative and systematic procedures involving clinical trials with controls.[15]

Hahnemann developed the theory that the symptoms experienced by the patient are a manifestation of an underlying disease that is affecting the individual.[13] He stated that the symptoms (i.e., fever) are the body's attempt to heal itself from the illness-producing agent. Thus, the symptoms should not be suppressed, but aided. Once the symptoms have been "worked through," the disease is considered cured. This opinion is in contrast to conventional medicine, which first identifies the cause of disease (a diagnosis) before a treatment can be selected. From this initial theory, Hahnemann developed the Law of Similars: A substance that causes a set of symptoms in a healthy individual will also alleviate the same set of symptoms in an ill individual. This theory is sometimes referred to as "like cures like." In homeopathy, the totality of the symptoms is important to determine the appropriate remedy to use. At first, Hahnemann used the normal doses prescribed by conventional physicians, but soon decided that this dosage overstimulated the desired healing response.

Next Hahnemann developed the idea that the body needs only a slightly extra therapeutic stimulus to achieve the desired effect. From this theory came the Law of Infinitesimals: The correct dose to use is the smallest one necessary to achieve the desired effect while minimizing the potential adverse effects.

Growth in the popularity of homeopathy was stimulated by such successes as the lower mortality rates witnessed in the homeopathic hospitals compared with regular hospitals during the cholera epidemics of 1831–1832 in the United States and the 1854 epidemic in England.[14] However, because a common feature of treatment in the conventional medicine hospitals was blood-letting and emetics, these data may support the ineffectiveness and counterproductive effects of the treatments used by the conventional medicine hospitals rather than effectiveness on the part of the primary homeopathic remedies, namely camphora or *Veratrum album.*[13,14]

Scope of Homeopathic Practice

While Hahnemann and his colleagues looked at homeopathy as appropriate treatment for all medical disorders, current practitioners focus primarily on its use in treating common, non–life-threatening disorders. Responsible homeopathic practice screens patients for serious or life-threatening disorders that require referral to a conventional medical practitioner.

Classical versus Clinical Homeopathy

Two main types of homeopathy are practiced: classical and clinical. First, in classical homeopathy, the practitioner seeks to find a single remedy to treat the patient.[15] The single remedy may be a similimum or the patient's constitutional remedy. (See Table 46–1 for definitions of basic homeopathic

Table 46–1

Glossary of Homeopathic Terms

Term	Definition
Aggravation	A temporary increase in symptoms experienced by the patient after taking a homeopathic remedy. This increase is usually followed by amelioration of the symptoms.
Allersodes	A homeopathic remedy prepared from antigens including toxins, precipitinogens, agglutinogens, opsonogens, lysogens, venins, agglutinins, complements, opsonins, amboceptors, precipitins, and most native proteins.
Antidote	A substance that neutralizes or counteracts the action of a homeopathic remedy.
Attenuation	Potency or dilution of the homeopathic remedy. (For scales of dilution, see Centesimal scale, Decimal scale, and Fifty millesimal scale.)
Avogadro's number	The number of molecules in one mole or 6×10^{23}. A homeopathic dilution greater than 24X or 12C would be unlikely to contain even one molecule of the original substance.
Centesimal scale	The scale used when preparing succussed serial dilutions (attenuations) where the dilution ratio is 1:100. Such dilutions are designated 1C (1×10^{-2} mg starting material/mg dose), 6C (1×10^{-12} mg starting material/mg dose), 30C (1×10^{-60} mg starting material/mg dose), etc. Letter designations are C or M.
Constitutional remedy	A homeopathic remedy that fits the totality of the patient and the state of his or her health over the course of life (i.e., emotionally, mentally, and physically). Distinguish from similimum and simile, although in any given patient the constitutional remedy and similimum may be the same.
Decimal scale	The scale used when preparing succussed serial dilutions (attenuations) where the dilution ratio is 1:10. Such dilutions are designated 1X (1×10^{-1} mg of starting material/mg dose), 6X (1×10^{-6} mg of starting material/mg dose), 30X (1×10^{-30} mg starting material/mg dose), etc. Letter designations are either X or D.
Engraftment	The appearance of symptoms caused by use of the remedy by the patient; similar to the appearance of symptoms in a healthy individual during a homeopathic proving. Primarily a problem with mid- to high-potencies taken over a long period of time.
Fifty millesimal scale	The scale used to prepare succussed serial dilutions (attenuations) in which a three-step process results in a calculated dilution ratio of 1:50,000. Dilutions are designated 1LM, 6LM, 30LM, etc. Letter designation can be LM or Q. Preparation process is complex and differs from that used for the centesimal and decimal methods.
Hering's Laws of Cures	Healing takes place from the interior to the exterior, from the center to the periphery, from above downward, from more-important to less-important organs and in reverse order of appearance.
Homeopathy	A system of medicine developed and practiced by Dr. Samuel Hahnemann and based on the central principle of the Law of Similars.
HPUS	The Homeopathic Pharmacopoeia of the United States.
Individualization	The prescribing of a homeopathic remedy on the basis of the patient's unique symptoms.
Isodes	A homeopathic remedy of botanical, zoological, or chemical substances including drugs, excipients, or binders that have produced a disease or disorder that interferes with homeostasis.
Isopathy	Literally means equal cures equal. Generally used to mean potentizing a specific allergen for the patient on the basis of history and/or allergy tests. Other isopathic uses are potentizing the pathogenic substance that caused the illness. (See isodes.)
Keynote	Specific symptom(s) associated with a homeopathic remedy that make the remedy unique and identifiable from other homeopathic remedies. For example, for bryonia the keynote symptoms are stitching or bursting pains that are worse with motion.
Law of Infinitesimals	A dilution that is regarded in homeopathy to be beyond Avogadro's number.
Law of Similars	A substance that can cause a characteristic set of symptoms in a healthy individual will cure that set of symptoms when experienced by an ill individual.
Materia medica	A reference that describes the various homeopathic remedies and the symptoms they produce. May also contain suggested doses and antidotes. Distinguish from repertory.
Nosodes	A homeopathic remedy prepared from diseased organs or tissues; causative agents such as bacteria, fungi, ova, parasites, virus particles, or yeast; products of disease; excretions; or secretions. Almost all nosodes are prescription only.
Palliation	A homeopathic remedy that will alleviate symptoms but totally restore the patient to health, thus the symptoms may return or the weaknesses may be experienced by the patient with development of new symptoms.

(continued)

Table 46–1

Glossary of Homeopathic Terms (continued)

Term	Definition
Polycrest	A homeopathic remedy that has many uses covering a wide variety of symptoms and is commonly used in clinical practice (e.g., sepia). (See Table 46–2.)
Potentization	Dilution or trituration of a substance followed by succussion for preparing a homeopathic remedy. (See succussion.)
Proving	A test in which a homeopathic remedy is administered to healthy volunteers. Symptoms that develop are rigorously recorded, compiled, and included into a materia medica.
Remedy	A homeopathic preparation used to treat a patient. Typically prepared from botanical, zoological, or chemical sources.
Repertory	A book of symptoms that is organized by body system and that lists the homeopathic remedies associated with each symptom. Distinguish from materia medica.
Sarcode	A homeopathic remedy prepared from healthy tissue or secretions.
Simile	The remedy that is similar to, but not the most similar to, the totality of the case. Distinguish from similimum and constitutional remedy.
Similimum	The remedy that is most similar to the totality of the case. Distinguish from constitutional remedy and simile, although in any given patient, the similimum and constitutional remedy may be the same.
Succussion	To vigorously shake with impact during each dilutional step during the manufacturing process.
Totality	The comprehensive picture of the whole patient encompassing the emotional, environmental, mental, physical, and spiritual aspects.
Trituration	Solid attenuations. (See attenuations.)

Source: References 16, 17, and 18.

terms.) Even though about 3000 homeopathic single remedies exist, it is possible that no single remedy will match the patient's symptoms exactly. However, the closer the remedy fits the patient's symptom picture, the greater the chance it will be effective in treating the problem(s). A great deal of time and patience are needed to determine single constitutional remedies.

Second, in clinical homeopathy, the practitioner may be a physician who is using a combination of homeopathy and other approaches. For treating acute illnesses, or because they are using homeopathy in addition to other modalities, those physicians may not have the time to make a classically based determination. Thus, practitioners will use single or combination homeopathic remedies on the basis of the literature, their training, and their clinical experience. Such a remedy would be one that fits the most obvious of the patient's symptoms (e.g., allergies, trauma) but would not necessarily treat all symptoms.

Theories of Homeopathic Mechanism of Action

Despite publication of clinical trials that appear to document the efficacy of some homeopathic remedies, conventional practitioners are still very skeptical about the potential overall efficacy or utility of homeopathy because of a lack of a "plausible" mechanism of action. Several potential mechanisms have been proposed. One proposed mechanism is based on the theory of systemic memory.[19] This theory, using general systems theory, contends that recurrent feedback interactions will result in information storage and will create systemic memories in dynamic systems such as water.

Another theory, using the paradigm of signifiers, contends that living beings communicate with the world nonverbally on a somatic and a psychological level.[20] The specially prepared, highly diluted solutions manufactured with a molecular representation of the disease carries this information to the body even though no actual molecules of the remedy are present.

A third theory involves a molecular mechanism. Matsumoto[21] hypothesizes that cell-surface proteins of the human body can be activated by hydration-shell structures that exist in solution even though the molecules that formed the crystal structures, called clathrates, are no longer present. Clathrates may be formed in high dilutions subjected to succussion that would induce continued crystal formation in subsequent dilutions. A group of researchers found that human polymorphonuclear basophils would release histamine in response to high dilution of anti-immunoglobulin E antibodies, despite the absence of these antibodies in most of the dilutions.[22] Others were not able to replicate this research and were criticized by the original researchers as not having followed the original methodology.[23,24] It is important to emphasize that none of the hypotheses attempting to explain a mechanism for homeopathy has been scientifically validated.

Treatment with Homeopathic Remedies

Use of homeopathic remedies or combination products may be warranted in several situations including when serious illness that can be adequately and safely treated by conventional medicine has been ruled out.[17] Homeopathic remedies might be tried when conventional medicine has not been able to adequately address the patient's problems. For example, homeopathic remedies may be tried for physical symptoms such as allergies, chilblains, impotence, influenza, injuries, premenstrual syndrome, teething, and tinnitus[17,25,26] or for mental symptoms such as anger, fears or phobias, grief, and nightmares.

Also, homeopathic remedies may be tried in non–life-threatening situations where conventional medicine may provide effective medications, but where the side-effect profile is unacceptable to the patient. Examples include anxiety, depression, morning sickness in pregnancy, night cramps, and osteoarthritis. Homeopathic remedies might be used to reduce conventional medications if the remedy would help reduce the symptoms. For example, it would be desirable to reduce medication use in asthma, dysmenorrhea, eczema, migraine, neuralgias, and psoriasis. Table 46–2 lists some potential remedies for given conditions. Case Study 46–1 illustrates the approach to selecting a combination homeopathic remedy for a patient with multiple symptoms. This table does not list all remedies for all conditions that are amenable to treatment with homeopathic products. The pharmacist who wants more information should consult one of several repertories.[27]

Even though homeopathic remedies are relatively safe and economical, patients will benefit most when a pharmacist can help them determine the best option(s) for the condition presented, including conventional or homeopathic nonprescription products, or can refer them to a medical or homeopathic practitioner. Other chapters in this text handle the first two scenarios in detail by disorder, but pharmacists need to know what conditions warrant referral to a homeopathic practitioner and how to select the practitioner. If the pharmacist has ruled out using a conventional nonprescription product and a referral to a conventional practitioner, the situations that could warrant referral to a homeopathic practitioner would include the following considerations:

- The patient has expressed a desire to see a homeopathic practitioner.
- The patient has tried several homeopathic remedies as self-treatment either with no results or with problems that have developed and that sound like aggravation (or possibly engraftment).
- The patient is chronically taking one or more homeopathic remedies without being under the care of a homeopathic practitioner.
- The patient has tried several conventional nonprescription or prescription drug products without success or with unwanted side effects.

Homeopathic practitioners must be licensed in Washington, D.C., and in the states of Alaska, Arizona, Connecticut, Florida, Hawaii, Maine, Montana, Nevada, New Hampshire, Oregon, Utah, and Washington.[28] The Board of Homeopaths in these states will connect callers to licensed practitioners. In other states, it would be useful to develop a knowledge of, or professional relationship with, licensed physicians, doctors of osteopathy, or naturopaths who use homeopathic preparations. Designation of homeopaths varies by state or national certification. For example, the American Board of Homeotherapeutics uses the designation of Dht, while the Arizona Board of Homeopathic Medical

Case Study 46–1

Alonzo, a 45-year-old man, comes into the pharmacy on a Sunday morning in April and is sneezing. He has bloodshot eyes with bilateral tearing and red, swollen eyelids. He is constantly blowing his nose. You ask if you can help him. He says he does not know if he has a cold or what, but could you please find something to relieve his symptoms that will not make him drowsy. You determine that he is not feverish and has no chest congestion, but he has a dry cough that occurs only during the day and does not keep him awake at night. You ask if his family or associates have had colds, and he replies no. His symptoms are more consistent with allergies than the common cold.

Taking a homeopathic viewpoint, you ask if he works outdoors. Alonzo explains he is a long-distance truck driver and is just passing through, which is why he cannot take Chlortrimeton because he gets too drowsy to drive. You ask if his tears or nasal discharge burns, and he says the tears feel like they are filled with acid, but the nasal discharge is bland. His nose itches. He sneezes again and again, shivering as if he is chilly. Because all nonprescription antihistamines will cause drowsiness, perhaps even those combined with a decongestant, you decide to ask if he would like to try a homeopathic remedy. He appears interested.

Going over his symptoms (see Table 46–2), you realize he is giving you a very mixed picture from a homeopathic point of view, so you offer a combination product that contains *Euphrasia, Sabadilla, Allium cepa,* and *Urtica urens*. You counsel him on how to take the product following label instructions, but caution him to discontinue use if there is no symptomatic relief after a few doses. You also counsel him on what substances to avoid. (See the box "Patient Education for Homeopathic Remedies" presented later in this chapter.)

Table 46–2

Examples of Homeopathic Remedies for Common Non–Life-Threatening Clinical Conditions

Clinical Condition	Potentially Useful Remedy	Keynote or Grade 4 Symptoms[a]	Grade 3 Symptoms[b]
Allergies	Isopathy[c]		
	Urtica urens (stinging nettles)	Urticarial eruptions worse with bathing, warmth, violent exercise.	Worse with snow-air, yearly, cool moist air; cold bathing.
	Allium cepa (red onion)	Excoriating nasal discharge with bland lacrimation.	Sneezing worse with returning to a warm room. Catarrhal hoarseness. Cough compels patient to grasp larynx.
	Euphrasia (eyebright)	Profuse and acrid lacrimation with profuse bland coryza.	Photophobia. Daytime cough.
	Sabadilla (Cevadilla seed; *Asagroa officialis*)	Paroxysmal sneezing. Itching in nose.	Chilly. Conjunctivitis. Desires hot drink.
Anger	*Nux vomica* (poison nut)	Anger and digestive disturbances.	Fastidious. Angry and impatient. Hard-working, hard-living individual. Craves stimulants.
	Staphysagria (stavesacre)	Ailments from suppressed anger with indignation.	Sweet individuals who believe they have been unfairly treated and suppress their anger.
	Hepar sulphuris calcareum (Hahnemann's calcium sulphide)		Violent rage leading to violent deeds. Oversensitive to all impressions. Hurried. Dissatisfied. Disposition to contradict
Anxiety	Arsenicum album (arsenic trioxide)		Anxiety about health. Worrier. Fastidious.
	Calcarea carbonica (calcium carbonate)		Fears particularly of insanity and poverty. Slow.
	Natrum muriaticum (sodium chloride)	Ailments from grief.	Anxiety worse in cold places and in crowds. Wringing of hands. Worse with consolation.
Asthma	Arsenicum album (arsenic trioxide)		Anxious. Restless. Asthma worse from midnight to 2 am. Chilly. Thirst for small quantities frequently.
	Kali carbonicum (potassium carbonate)		Sharp, cutting stabbing pains. Better with sitting forward. Startles at noise.
	Natrum sulphuricum (sodium sulfate)		Worse every time weather changes from dry to damp. Asthma in children. Asthma worse from 4 to 5 am. Must hold chest while coughing.
Chilblains	*Agaricus muscarius* (Amanita muscaria; fly agaric)		Very sensitive to cold. Stitching, splinter-like pain.
	Petroleum	Cracking eczema in cold weather.	Rough, hard, thickened and fissured skin.
	Zincum metallicum (zinc)		Worse with rubbing and touch. Restless, fidgety feet.
Depression	Calcarea carbonica (calcium carbonate)		Slow. Sluggish. Low energy.

(continued)

Table 46–2

Examples of Homeopathic Remedies for Common Non–Life-Threatening Clinical Conditions (continued)

Clinical Condition	Potentially Useful Remedy	Keynote or Grade 4 Symptoms[a]	Grade 3 Symptoms[b]
Depression (*continued*)	Sepia (cuttlefish ink)	Feelings of sadness during menstruation, bearing down sensation.	Irritable. Weary. Cannot be bothered. Averse to loved ones.
	Aurum metallicum (gold)	Suicidal depression.	Black despondency. Hopelessness. Suicidal
Dysmenorrhea	Magnesia phosphorica (magnesium phosphate)	Dysmenorrhea better with local heat.	Severe cutting pain. Must bend over. Better with pressure.
	Colocynthis (bitter cucumber)	Colic	Severe pain. Better with pressure. Angry or suppressed anger. Colicky in nature.
	Sepia (cuttlefish ink)	Feelings of sadness during menstruation, bearing down sensation.	Cramping low abdominal discomfort. Bearing down feeling. Must cross legs. Wants to be left alone.
Eczema	Sulphur		Itchy. Hot. Sticks hot feet out of bed at night. Red orifices. Excoriations. Untidy.
	Petroleum	Cracking eczema in cold weather.	Painful cracks especially in fingertips. Worse in cold and winter.
	Arsenicum album (arsenic trioxide)		Restless. Chilly. Fastidious. Anxious. Burning pain better with hot applications.
Fears/phobias	Argentum nitricum (silver nitrate)	Anticipation anxiety with diarrhea and flatulence.	Impulsive, hurried. Worse with anxiety, sugar.
	Gelsemium (yellow jasmine)	Stage fright.	Anticipatory anxiety. Paralysis of mind, voice, and body.
	Phosphoricum acidum (phosphoric acid)	Mental, then physical weakness.	Fears that something will happen, imaginary things, dark, thunderstorms.
Grief	*Ignatia* (St. Ignatius bean)	Ailments from disappointed love and silent grief.	Sighing. Incredible changeability of mood, laughter to tears.
	Natrum muriaticum (sodium chloride)	Ailments from grief.	Worse with consolation. Cannot cry. Irritable.
	Causticum (potassium bisulfate)		Ailments from long-lasting grief. Intensely sympathetic individuals who weep easily.
Impotence	*Lycopodium* (club moss)		Apprehensive about new things. Lack of confidence. Desire to be in control.
	Conium (poison hemlock)		Stopping or starting of urinary flow. Hard, sore glands.
	Phosphoricum acidum (phosphoric acid)		Ailments from disappointed love. Silent grief.
Influenza	*Gelsemium* (yellow jasmine)		Slow onset. Thirstless. Aching, heavy weakness and soreness of limbs.
	Mercurius (mercury)	Cannot tolerate extremes of heat or cold.	Profuse sweating/salivation. Metallic taste in mouth.

(*continued*)

Table 46–2

Examples of Homeopathic Remedies for Common Non–Life-Threatening Clinical Conditions (continued)

Clinical Condition	Potentially Useful Remedy	Keynote or Grade 4 Symptoms[a]	Grade 3 Symptoms[b]
Influenza (*continued*)	Influenzinum	Single dose after influenza when patient complains of being "never well since" a bout of influenza.	
Injuries	*Arnica montana* (leopard's bane)	Bruises.	Very painful, bruised soreness. Never well since injury. Fears being struck, touched, or approached.
	Hypericum (St. John's wort)	Injuries to nerves or nerve-rich areas.	Crush injuries to fingers. Punctured or penetrating wounds. Lacerations. Complaints from fright.
	Ruta graveolens (rue-bitterwort)	Tendon and ligament injuries and sprains.	Bruised, sore, aching, and restless. Worse with cold and damp. Violent thirst for ice-cold water.
	Ledum (marsh tea)	Puncture wounds better with cold.	Pain in small joints. Worse with motion of joints. Migraines.
	Natrum muriaticum (sodium chloride)		Recurrent hammering headache with visual disturbances. Worse with sunlight. Must wear hat in the sun. Irritable. Averse to consolation.
	Glonione (nitroglycerin)	Bursting, pounding headache.	Confusion. Disorientation. Time passes too slowly.
	Sanguinaria (blood root)	Migraine.	Right-sided, sick headache. Settles over right eye. Begins in morning and settles by evening. Better with lying down. Better with sleep.
Morning sickness of pregnancy	Ipecac	Continuous nausea unrelieved by vomiting.	Violent spasmodic cough causing vomiting. No better after vomiting or lying down.
	Sepia (cuttlefish ink)		Nausea worse with smell of food. Worse with hands in water. Desires vinegar, pickles, and acids.
	Nux vomica (poison-nut)		Fastidious. Angry and impatient. Nausea better after vomiting. Sensation of stone in abdomen.
Night cramps	Cuprum metallicum (copper)	Cramps.	Spasmodic violent cramps and convulsions. Cold feet.
	Arnica montana (leopard's bane)		Cramps at night after overuse of muscles.
	Veratrum album (white hellebore)		Night cramps occurring during a diarrheal illness.
Nightmares	*Atropabelladonna* (deadly nightshade)		Delirium. Throbbing head. Jerks and spasms.
	Carcinosin	Family history of cancer.	Waking screaming or shrieking during sleep. Familiar things seem strange.

(*continued*)

Table 46–2

Examples of Homeopathic Remedies for Common Non–Life-Threatening Clinical Conditions (continued)

Clinical Condition	Potentially Useful Remedy	Keynote or Grade 4 Symptoms[a]	Grade 3 Symptoms[b]
Nightmares (*continued*)	Sulphur		Waking at night with nightmares. Hot, sticks feet out of bed at night.
Osteoarthritis	*Rhus toxicodendron* (poison ivy)	Joint pain worse after rest; better with motion.	Worse with cold, damp weather.
	Bryonia (wild hops)	Stitching or bursting pains worse with motion.	Pain better with rest.
	Causticum (potassium bisulfate)		Tearing pains around the joint. Contractions. Better with damp, wet weather.
Premenstrual syndrome	Lachesis (bushmaster snake venom)	Jealousy.	Cannot bear tight clothing, especially around the neck. Heat flushes. Loquacity.
	Sepia (cuttlefish ink)	Feelings of sadness during menstruation, bearing down sensation.	Depressed and irritable. Aversion to loved ones. "Cannot be bothered." Worse with consolation.
	Pulsatilla (wind flower)	Changeability of symptoms.	Timid. Weepy. Better with company; consolation.
Psoriasis	Sulphur		Itchy. Hot. Sticks hot feet out of bed at night. Red orifices. Excoriations. Untidy. Offensive discharges.
	Graphites	Thickened scaly or crusty patches on skin.	Chilly. Obese. Timid. Weepy. Sensitive to music. Cracks and excoriations, especially around the ears. Honey-like oozing and/or scales.
	Psorinum (scabies vesicle)	Itchy skin condition.	
Teething	*Chamomilla* (German chamomile)	Teething infant.	Child wants to be carried and then is more quiet. Twitching and convulsions during teething. Angry.
	Calcarea phosphorica (calcium phosphate)	Headache of schoolchildren with diarrhea.	Craves salt. Coldness or soreness in spots. Thin, brittle bones and swollen glands.
	Mercurius (mercury)	Cannot tolerate extremes of heat or cold.	Profuse sweating/salivation. Metallic taste in mouth.
Tinnitus	*China officinalis*		Ringing in ears, weak/debilitated, associated with fluid loss.
	Graphites		Ringing in ears. Weeping to music. Timidity. Worse with cold weather and around menses.
	Spigelia (pinkroot)		Noises in ear. Left-sided headache. Worse with tobacco smoke.

[a] Keynote symptom(s) may not always be that closely related to listed condition in column one, thus the remedy would be selected for the condition in column one on the basis of the Grade 3 symptom(s) and/or clinical experience. When that is the case, the keynote symptom(s) for the remedy were omitted.

[b] Some of the symptoms listed may be Grade 2 or 1, and the choice is based more on clinical experience than strict interpretation of a repertory. A remedy may appear in this table more than once with different symptoms showing the diversity for which the remedy may be used (i.e., polycrest).

[c] See Table 46–1 for definition.

Source: References 17, 25, and 26.

Examiners uses MD(H). The National Center for Homeopathy annually publishes a list of more than 500 medical doctors and other practitioners who recommend homeopathic remedies. Table 46–3 lists the contact information for homeopathic organizations.

Qualifications, experience, and competence of homeopathic practitioners vary widely; therefore, to make sound referrals, pharmacists are encouraged to meet with potential practitioners and to make a personal assessment of their qualifications and abilities. Making a referral on the basis of a patient's testimony would not necessarily represent the best method of practitioner selection.

Homeopathic training varies widely. Many certificate programs and schools are available. Two examples of more than 15 schools teaching homeopathy in the United States include the Hahnemann College of Homeopathy located in Port Richmond, California, and John Bastyr College of Naturopathic Medicine in Seattle, Washington.[29]

Methods of Selecting a Homeopathic Remedy

Homeopathic practitioners can rely on two types of references when selecting remedies for a patient's symptoms: a repertory and a materia medica. Some of the information in a materia medica is gathered through a process called proving.

Repertory

A homeopathic repertory indexes symptoms organized by body system (e.g., circulatory, respiratory). Remedies associated with that symptom are listed. Typically, the remedy is cataloged by its abbreviation (e.g., Ars. for arsenic) and is graded for the strength of association with that symptom.[25,27]

Table 46–3

Homeopathic Organizations

The National Center for Homeopathy
801 North Fairfax St., Ste. 306
Alexandria, VA 22314-1757
703-548-7790
703-548-7792 (fax)
nchinfo@igc.apc.org (e-mail)
www.homeopathic.org

American Institute of Homeopathy
1585 Glencoe St.
Denver, CO 80220
303-898-5477

Homeopathic Academy of Naturopathic Physicians
PO Box 69565
Portland, OR 97201
803-795-0579

American Homeopathic Pharmaceutical Association
PO Box 174
Norwood, PA 19074

Homeopathic Pharmacopoeia Convention of the United States
www.hpus.com

Figure 46–1 shows a repertory listing for acrid tears. If the symptom is a keynote, or the most important, symptom for that remedy, the remedy is either designated as Grade 4 or is transcribed in boldface type and capital letters. A Grade 3 remedy is associated with important symptoms but not with keynote symptoms; this remedy will be transcribed using boldface type. A Grade 2 remedy is transcribed in italic typeface, whereas a Grade 1 remedy, which is associatd with the least important symptoms, is noted in plain typeface. Some repertories designate a remedy's keynote symptom as Level 1; a Level 4 remedy would be associated with the least important symptom.

When analyzing the information obtained in taking a patient's case, the practitioner must also grade the symptoms in respect to their importance to the overall case. Therefore, the practitioner uses the symptoms or characteristics believed to be most unusual or most important for the patient, finds each of the symptoms in the repertory, and notes the remedies that match the symptoms. The more the patient's symptoms or characteristics match a remedy, the better the remedy will benefit the patient. However, some practitioners select the most appropriate remedy concentrating on the keynote, mental, and unusual symptoms. Because of the complexity and time that selecting a remedy can take, several computer programs are now available to aid the practitioner.

For acute illnesses, the practitioner will use primarily the most notable symptoms of the patient's condition. Using the training, literature, or clinical experience, the practitioner will choose a remedy from several remedies (e.g., *Allium cepa, Euphrasia, Sabadilla,* or *Urtica urens* for allergies) or a combination of remedies that have often been successfully used in that acute condition. Examples of classic remedies for acute problems include (1) *Arnica* for muscle trauma with bruising (even for residual pain when the trauma occurred months or years in the past), (2) *Hypericum* for painful nerve injury of the extremities, and (3) *Symphytum* for bone healing.[28]

Materia Medica and Provings

A materia medica describes the various homeopathic remedies and the symptoms they induce. This information comes from three different sources: (1) toxicological data, (2) provings, and (3) clinical experience.[30] The provings conducted

TEARS, acrid: All-s., **Ars.,** bell., bry., *calc., caust.,* cedr., clem., *colch., coloc.,* dig., eug., euph., **Euphr.**, fl-ac., gamb., graph., *ham., ign.,* iod., kali-ar., *kreos., led., lyc.,* merc., **Merc-c.**, *nat-m., nit-ac.,* ph-ac., pic-ac., plb., puls., rhus-t., sabin., spig., staph., **Sulph.**, syph., teucr.

Figure 46–1 Sample repertory listing for acrid tears. Reprinted with permission from reference 27.

by Hahnemann were very systematic, considering the lack of scientific rigor in the medical professions in the 1700s. The concept that a remedy will produce, in a healthy individual, the symptoms to be treated in a sick individual is the basis of the provings process. The basic rules for provings—as Hahnemann eventually developed them—were to use specially prepared, highly diluted substances in healthy individuals. The substance was stopped as soon as symptoms appeared, and all symptoms were written down verbatim, using precise descriptions.[31]

The methodology for modern day provings varies widely, but is based on Hahnemann's original method of observation and detailed recording.[31–33] The methodology promoted by David Riley in the United States incorporates blinding and placebo controls.[18,32] A modern proving uses a 12C dilution (see definition of Centesimal scale in Table 46–1) in 17 to 22 healthy male and female subjects.[32] (See the section "Dosages of Homeopathic Remedies" for an explanation of dilutional or potency nomenclature.) Subjects are enrolled on the basis of strict inclusion and exclusion criteria and are required to take extremely detailed daily records of all physical symptoms, emotions, phobias, personality changes, and more.

The first 14 days are used to gather baseline data on each subject to determine their "normal" constellation of emotions, physical symptoms, and so forth. The main trial begins with randomization of the subjects to the remedy or matching placebo given three times daily in a double-blind design until symptoms occur or the remedy has been taken for 3 days. In some trials, only two subjects will receive placebo; the rest will receive the substance to be proved. The main trial lasts for 28 days, although women may be asked to collect data over several months to determine the influence of their menstrual cycle. The trial ends with 14 days of follow-up. Only the symptoms or the mental/emotional changes that appeared in the active remedy group in more than one subject over the 28-day period are used to develop a materia medica monograph. The symptom selection criteria are listed in Table 46–4.

Table 46–4

Symptom Selection Criteria in a Proving

The following criteria are used to select symptoms in a proving:

- The symptom occurs shortly after taking the remedy.
- The symptom occurs in more than one subject.
- The symptom has specific modalities associated with its occurrence.
- The symptom is strange, rare, or peculiar—either in general or for that person.
- The symptom is described with clarity.
- The symptom occurs for several days or at intervals.
- The symptom is intense.
- Concomitant symptoms are described.
- The symptom is a new symptom or a recurrent symptom.

Source: Reference 32.

Preparation of Homeopathic Remedies

Since 1938 when the Federal Food Drug and Cosmetic Act was passed, FDA has been required to regulate homeopathic manufacturers.[28] The official monographs for homeopathic remedies are published by the Homeopathic Pharmacopoeia Convention of the United States (HPCUS) in HPUS. HPCUS publishes more than 1300 official monographs. Each official monograph includes the official name, official abbreviation, name in contemporary use, chemical formula, atomic or molecular weight, description, range and habitat, preparation, classification, and prescription/nonprescription status of the remedy. HPUS also contains general pharmacy guidelines that specify the weights, measures, units of medicinal strength, solvents, diluents, and general methods of preparation.

HPCUS has designated the dry crude substance as the unit on which to calculate strength for ensuring uniformity.[18] Botanical homeopathic remedies are prepared from freshly gathered whole plants, flowers, or roots and are made into the starting tincture as soon as possible. The plants must be free from insects, animal material, animal excreta, mold, discoloration, abnormal odor, or deterioration. The starting tincture is most often made by maceration. Briefly, the specified plant material is chopped or mashed together and covered with the correct solvent. The amount of alcohol in the tincture depends on the starting moisture content of the plant, as well as on the types of constituents to be extracted. Alcohol content ranges from 35% volume per volume (v/v) to 90% v/v. The maceration jar is tightly sealed and placed in a dark room at normal room temperature. The jar is shaken at specified intervals. Maceration time varies with the specific botanical ingredients but in general lasts 2 to 4 weeks. The clear liquid is decanted and the residue is pressed out. Zoological substances are prepared similarly with a 65% v/v hydroalcoholic solution that is stored for not less than 3 weeks and is then decanted. Insoluble substances such as minerals are most often triturated with lactose up to 6X. They can be converted to liquid attenuations.

Subsequent attenuations (liquid) or triturations (solid) are made from the tincture or the starting material. The scales (ratios) of attenuations are decimal, centesimal, and fifty millesimal. The tincture contains 1 part of plant material (dry weight) in 10 parts of liquid, which corresponds to the 1X attenuation (1×10^{-1} mg starting material/1 mg dose). One part of this tincture (or 1X) is added to 9 parts of solvent (water, alcohol) or lactose (for solids). This dilution is a 2X attenuation, representing 1×10^{-2} mg starting material per 1 mg dose. For the practitioner to make a 3X attenuation, 1 part of 2X is added to 9 parts of solvent or lactose, resulting in 1×10^{-3} mg starting material per 1 mg dose. This process is repeated as needed. After each dilution, the flask is succussed either manually or by machine.

The centesimal attenuations are prepared in a manner similar to the decimal attenuations, except 1 part of the preceding attenuation is added to 99 parts of the diluting medium. The fifty millesimal attenuations are more complicated to manufacture in each step and are usually not used for homeopathic therapy except under the direct care of a qualified practitioner.

Once the final attenuation has been made, the dosage form is then prepared.[18] The most common dosage forms are medicated tablets, tablet triturates, compressed tablets, globules, or pellets. Globules are made from 85% sucrose and 15% lactose. Tablet triturates are 100% lactose. Either the final solution may be atomized over the solid dosage form and then bottled (0.2%), or one drop of the attenuation per 2 g may be added to a bottle of the solid dosage forms in 3 aliquots and shaken to distribute. Globules come in several standardized sizes. Some tablets are manufactured with the remedy mixed throughout the carrier. Nonprescription homeopathic remedies are also available as oral liquids, tinctures, ophthalmic preparations, or topical creams or ointments.

Dosages of Homeopathic Remedies

The dosing regimen is based primarily on the potency and not on the specific remedy.[17] The definition of low versus high potency has been variously defined. Some practitioners use the following definitions: Low-potency remedies are less than 12X, mid-potency remedies are from 12X to 30X, and high-potency remedies are anything greater than 30X.[34] Others have defined low-potency remedies as dilutions less than 30C, mid-potency remedies as 30C, and high-potency remedies as greater than 30C.[17] Potency selection is based on several factors. For acute illness, for illnesses that are more physical than mental, for patients who are more debilitated, and for patients where aggravation is of concern, the lower potencies are used. Higher potencies are more likely to produce aggravations and should not be used if the practitioner is unsure of the remedy, if a non-expert is recommending the remedy, or if the patient is using the remedy as self-treatment without the aid of a homeopathic practitioner.[35]

The number of tablets, globules, pellets, or drops to take for a single dose is not considered to be as important compared with conventional dosing of medications.[35] The general recommendation is for 1 large tablet, 6 to 7 globules, or 5 to 15 tiny pellets or drops for a single dose.

Dosing frequency is determined by the length of time required for the remedy to wear off.[17] For acute illnesses, this effect may result in frequent dosing (e.g., every 15 to 30 minutes or so initially). Rarely does the patient need to take a remedy for longer than 3 days. For chronic disorders, the dose might be repeated as infrequently as every few months. Classical homeopaths prescribe a single dose and wait for follow-up to determine if more doses are required. Others may give a "split single dose," meaning that three separate doses are given over 24 hours or over 3 days. Nonclassical practitioners may dose twice daily until the symptoms disappear. Nonprescription homeopathic remedies are labeled for the dose to be taken from three times daily to every 4 hours. Some labels state that for acute conditions the dose should be repeated every hour until symptoms are relieved.

Interactions with and Antidotes to Homeopathic Remedies

Pharmacists are often asked if a homeopathic preparation can be taken with other medications. From a conventional medicine point of view, it is difficult to imagine a drug–drug interaction because the dilution is so extreme. If we use the concept of Avogadro's number (the number of molecules in a mole is 6×10^{23}), potencies that are 24X or 12C (i.e., 1×10^{-24}) or higher are unlikely to contain even one molecule of the starting substance. However, for potentially highly toxic substances that are dosed in micrograms (e.g., 1–3X), the theoretical possibility does exist. Reports of such interactions, however, are not found in the medical literature.

From the homeopathic practitioner's perspective, however, "antidotes" can negate the effects of homeopathic remedies. For example, the antidote for *Arnica* is camphor, and the antidotes for camphor are opium and phosphorus.[25] (See the section "Patient Counseling for Homeopathic Remedies" for substances to avoid while taking homeopathic remedies.)

Precautions for Homeopathic Remedies

Occasionally, a patient will initially experience a brief intensifying of symptoms called an aggravation, which is often taken as a good sign that the correct remedy has been chosen. However, if homeopathic remedies are taken for too long an interval, the result can be like a "proving" and may induce symptoms in a process called engraftment. Usually such symptoms will abate once the homeopathic remedy is discontinued. Obviously, homeopathic remedies are meant to be taken only until the symptoms improve. Usually the symptoms improve after a single dose (high-potency remedy) or after only 3 days (low- to mid-potency) of therapy as discussed above.

Because homeopathic remedies are administered in such dilute solutions (from the conventional medicine viewpoint), adverse effects should not be possible. However, problems have been reported. For example, a chiropractor dispensed to a 34-year-old patient 100 BHI Regeneration Tablets (Biological Homeopathic Industries, Albuquerque, NM) to treat neck pain.[36] The package insert promoted the product as a treatment for cancer. The patient was instructed to take 2 tablets every 15 minutes until he felt better, then 2 tablets four times daily. After 16 tablets, the patient experienced signs and symptoms of pancreatitis. Other causes were ruled out. This report may represent a case of aggravation rather than a case of drug-induced adverse effects in the conventional sense. Either way, the company stated that nearly 50% of the people taking this remedy reported abdominal pain as part of the "healing crisis," which is another term for aggravation.

Two patients with stable multiple sclerosis ingested nonofficial homeopathic remedies containing cerebral, nerve, and tissue extracts. One patient took the preparation to treat insomnia and anxiety.[37] The second patient began to chronically take a similar homeopathic treatment to help prevent recurrences of his multiple sclerosis. Between a few days to 2 weeks later, both patients developed exacerbations of their multiple sclerosis. In either patient, a spontaneous relapse cannot be ruled out, but the temporal relationship bears consideration of the fact that the homeopathic remedies may have contributed to or induced the relapse.

Efficacy of Homeopathic Remedies

Nearly 200 clinical trials have been published on the use of homeopathic remedies, but their efficacy is still hotly debated. In 1991, a group of researchers collected and scored the methodology of 107 controlled trials.[38] Among these trials, 14 evaluated a form of classical homeopathy, and 58 trials used the same single homeopathic remedy to treat a specific conventional diagnosis. Because of the heterogeneity of the data a meta-analysis could not be performed. The authors rated each article on a 100-point scale to determine research methodology quality. They found that most trials scored greater than 55 points out of 100. Of the trials that received higher scores, 15 showed positive results and 7 showed negative results.

Two meta-analyses on homeopathic treatments have been published.[39,40] The first examined 186 placebo-controlled trials and incorporated another rating system for determining the quality of the clinical trials.[39] Of these trials, 26 showed better methodological quality. Of the 26 trials, the homeopathic remedy was greater than 1.5 times more likely to be effective compared with placebo.

The second meta-analysis specifically looked at the trials of homeopathy to treat postoperative ileus.[40] Using the methodology developed by Kleijnen, the authors included six studies. For four of the six studies of higher methodological quality, the authors found that the homeopathic remedy shortened the duration of postoperative ileus ($P < .05$). Table 46–5 summarizes the methodology and results of a selected group of trials reported in English.[41–59]

Overall, homeopathic trials have been criticized by conventional practitioners when the results are positive and by homeopathic practitioners when the results are negative. Trials that did not allow individualized treatments were not following the tenets of classical homeopathy and, thus, may not have been a fair evaluation of homeopathy. Even in those that were individualized to a specific remedy, the dose and duration were often standardized, which is also not how classical homeopathy is practiced.[60] Any trial that used a crossover design and did not thoroughly evaluate a carryover effect is also problematic. From the homeopathic viewpoint, if the appropriate remedy is found, the effects are very long lasting and a set washout period of even several weeks may not be sufficient to truly "wash out" the effects if the remedy was given first.[31]

In summary, some homeopathic remedies appear to have better effect than a placebo. Although many trials with positive results have been published, the overall quality of the trials is low. Many studies are not available in English and are, thus, not available for personal evaluation by the individual practitioner.

Product Selection Guidelines for Homeopathic Remedies

Remedies are often sold with the product's display describing a clinical condition and/or the remedy's keynote symptom. Table 46–6 lists examples of such displays. Effective use of homeopathic remedies requires accurate assessment of the patient's keynote symptoms. Moreover, single remedies that do not fit a patient's clinical picture should not induce any effects, positive or negative.

Combination products are not typically used by the classical homeopath.[16] They are most often used by nonclassical homeopaths or are sold in stores directly to the public.[15,16] Combinations are generally developed drawing on a practitioner's experience. Some combination products are developed using groups of individual agents that are most likely to be the correct remedy. The others that do not match the patient's symptoms have no action. Especially in France, some combination products are used that combine remedies with different symptomatic indications relevant to the patient's condition.[16] Other formulas are thought to target the corresponding illness with either a cumulative and/or synergistic action.[15] When combination products are used, fewer patient details are needed and thus a remedy can be chosen in less time or can be self-selected by a consumer. Table 46–7 provides some examples of combination products used for the treatment of premenstrual syndrome.

Homeopathic Method of Patient Assessment

Historically, both conventional medicine and homeopathy relied on interviews with the patient as the primary method of assessment. Both use the same methods to obtain specific details about the patient's symptoms such as location, quality (sharp versus dull pain), severity, onset, frequency, timing, and aggravating and ameliorating factors. However, for certain disorders, the homeopathic practitioner seeks even more detailed information. For example, the homeopathic practitioner assessing a patient with allergies would ask about the quality of the tears or nasal discharge, particularly whether the tears or nasal discharge felt acrid or bland, whether the patient was photophobic (intolerant of light), whether the sneezing was worse when the patient entered a cold room, and whether the patient desired hot drinks or felt worse drinking cold water. In the homeopathic practitioner's terms, practitioners are using individualization of the patient's symptoms to decide on the most appropriate specific remedy.

Table 46–5

Selected Controlled Trials on Homeopathic Remedies

Disease State/Reference	Intervention	Design	Population	Numbers	Primary Endpoints	Results	Comments/Critique
Upper respiratory tract infections/De Lange de Klerk, 1994[41]	Individualized, constitutional remedies and remedies to treat acute upper respiratory illnesses.	Randomized, placebo-controlled, double-blind trial.	Children ages 1.5 to 10 years.	Remedy (R) = 86 Placebo (P) = 84	Mean daily symptom scores from diaries kept by the parents, lifetime prevalence rates of otitis media, mean number of antibiotic courses, adenoidectomies, and tonsillectomies.	For all endpoints R = P	Trends favored the homeopathic remedy but were not statistically significant. Specific remedies were not published. Did not achieve sample size to avoid a type II error.
Otitis media/ Friese, 1997[42]	Individualized remedy versus conventional treatment.	Open, nonrandomized, observational.	Children with a median age of 5 and 6 years.	R = 103 Conventional (C) = 28	Duration of pain, duration of therapy, and number of recurrences over 1 year.	R = C (trend toward fewer recurrences and earlier improvement in symptoms in R group)	The conventionally treated patients were slightly older and more likely to have both ears involved. The homeopathically treated patients included more males.
Asthma/Reilly, 1994[43]	Individualized allersodes based on the patient's largest skin-test weal.	Randomized, placebo-controlled, double-blind trial with a single-blind placebo run-in.	Adults with asthma with positive skin tests for allergies.	R = 13 P = 15	Pulmonary function tests' (PFT) visual analog scale (VAS) for symptoms; digital scales for nighttime asthma, daytime asthma (0–4); peak flow rates.	PFT R = P VAS R > P (P = .003) Digital daily scores & peak flow rates R = P	Did not achieve sample size.
Hayfever/Reilly, 1986[44]	Mixed grass pollens 30C.	Randomized, placebo-controlled, double-blind trial with a single-blind placebo run-in for 1 week; 5 weeks.	Children older than 5 years and adults with symptoms of hayfever.	R = 79 P = 79 Complete 5-week data R = 70 P = 68	100 mm VAS of overall symptom intensity, physician's global assessment week 0 and week 5.	R > P (P = .02 on VAS) R = P (P = .05 on physician's global assessment)	Similar groups at baseline. Did not calculate sample size. Confirmed pollen allergy objectively in 106 (46 not tested). Did not do intent-to-treat analysis. More patients on remedy showed initial aggravation (21 vs. 11; P <.05).
Hayfever/ Wiesenauer, 1985[45]	Galphimia 6X versus Galphimia conventional dilution 10^{-6} (i.e., obtained by simple dilution without potentization).	Randomized, placebo-controlled, double-blind trial; 4 weeks.	Children older than 14 years and adults with symptoms of hayfever.	R = 50 Dilution (D) = 55 P = 57	4-item rating scale (symptom-free, obvious relief, slight improvement, no improvement)	Ocular and nasal symptoms R > D = P (P >.05)	Similar groups at baseline. Did not calculate a sample size.

Disease State/Reference	Intervention	Design	Population	Numbers	Primary Endpoints	Results	Comments/Critique
Influenza/Ferley, 1989[46]	Ana Barbariae Hepatis and Cordis Extractum 200C (Oscillococcinum).	Randomized, placebo-controlled, double-blind trial; 1 week.	Children older than 11 years and adults with symptoms of influenza.	R = 237 P = 241	Morning and evening temperature and presence/absence of 5 cardinal symptoms; overall global rating by the patient.	R > P (P = .03)	Similar groups at baseline. Recovery better in younger patients (ages 12 to 29 years) with mild to moderate symptoms.
Warts/Labrecque, 1992[47]	Thuya 30C, Antimony 7C, and Nitric acid 7C.	Randomized, placebo-controlled, double-blind trial; 6 weeks; patients were followed to 18 weeks.	Children older than 5 years and adults ages 59 years and younger.	R = 86 P = 88	Healing of wart. Physician and self-assessment.	R = P	Sample size calculated and achieved. The group receiving the homeopathic treatment was older, had the warts for a longer duration, and had not used as many other alternative treatments.
Warts/Smolle, 1998[48]	Individualized remedy.	Randomized, placebo-controlled, double-blind trial; 8 weeks.	Children—ages not provided.	R = 34 P = 33	Size of the wart pre- and post-treatment.	R = P	Sample size not calculated.
Pain and infection after total abdominal hysterectomy/Hart, 1997[49]	*Arnica* 30C.	Randomized, placebo-controlled, double-blind trial; acutely and followed for 2 weeks.	Women ages 25 to 76 years.	R = 38 P = 35	Pain and discomfort (10-cm VAS) every 12 hours starting 12 hours post-surgery; antibiotic and analgesic use.	R = P	Sample size not calculated.
Postpartum/Hofmeyr, 1990[50]	*Arnica* 6X, *Arnica* 30X.	Randomized (1:1:2), placebo-controlled, double-blind trial.	Women.	*Arnica* 6X = 37 *Arnica* 30X = 39 P = 85	Pain, analgesic use, mood, perineal appearance.	R = P	Groups were comparable at baseline except that the arnica 6X group had more assisted deliveries.
Mosquito bites/Hill, 1995[51]	*Echinacea angustifolia*, *Ledum paulster*, *Urtica urens* in a topical gel.	Randomized, placebo-controlled, double-blind trial.	Adults age 18 years or older.	R = 68 P = 68 C = 68	Area of erythema, VAS of pruritus at 0, 1, and 3 hours, then again at 6, 26, and 31 hours.	R = P = C	The mosquitos were laboratory raised and placed on the volunteers in three spots. Spots 1 and 3 were treated by a research technician with either R or P. Spot 2 remained untreated as a control.

(*continued*)

Table 46–5

Selected Controlled Trials on Homeopathic Remedies (continued)

Disease State/Reference	Intervention	Design	Population	Numbers	Primary Endpoints	Results	Comments/Critique
Primary fibromyalgia/ Fisher, 1989[52]	*Rhus toxicodendron* 6C determined as appropriate for the patient before enrollment.	Randomized, placebo-controlled, double-blind, cross-over trial.	Not provided.	N = 30	Number of tender spots, VASs for pain, sleep, and overall assessment.	Number of tender spots R > P ($P < .005$) Pain/sleep R > P ($P = .0052$)	Sample size not calculated. No washout period. Authors maintain carry-over effects were not noted.[52]
Bilateral oral surgery/Lokken, 1995[53]	Individualized remedy (all remedies dosed at 30X).	Randomized, placebo-controlled, double-blind, cross-over trial (27 days between surgery and about 20 days between treatments).	Adults ages 19 to 28 years.	N = 24	VAS for pain, facial swelling, postoperative bleeding, wound healing, and bruising.	R = P	Sample size not calculated.
Acute or chronic vertigo/Weiser, 1998[54]	Ambra grisea 6X, Anamirta cocculus 4X, Conium maculatum 3X, and Petroleum rectificatum 8X (Vertigoheel).	Randomized, double-blind; compared with betahistine (B) using a double dummy technique to blind the taste and smell of the active control; per protocol analysis.	Adults ages 18 to 83 years.	R = 59 B = 60 Per protocol R = 53 B = 52	Five-point rating scales for frequency, duration, and intensity; secondary outcomes were quality of life and impairment of daily life measures; patient and investigators 5-point global assessment.	R = B	Sample size calculated and achieved.
Osteoarthritis/ Shipley, 1983[55]	*R. toxicodendron* 6X (patients were assessed that they were likely to respond to the remedy).	Randomized, placebo-controlled, double-blind, cross-over, double-dummy trial; compared with fenoprofen (F); each treatment given to each subject for 2 weeks; per protocol analysis.	Adults ages 18 to 85 years. Fifteen were enrolled from a homeopathic hospital, and 21 were enrolled from a conventional hospital.	N = 36 Per protocol Group I – 13 Group II – 20	VASs for pain at rest, pain on movement, and night pain; 4-point pain scale; patient preference.	F > R = P	Sample size not calculated. Two dropouts while on R because of apparent aggravation. Third dropout for reasons unrelated to the study.

Disease State/Reference	Intervention	Design	Population	Numbers	Primary Endpoints	Results	Comments/Critique
Rheumatoid arthritis/Andrade, 1991[56]	Individualized remedy, dose, and duration.	Randomized, placebo-controlled, double-blind study; per protocol; 6 months.	Adults (range not provided).	R = 23 P = 21 Per protocol R = 17 P = 16	Ritchie's articular index, duration of morning stiffness, grip strength, functional class, and 15-meter walking time; global assessment of improvement; daily use of steroids and NSAIDs.	R > baseline on ⅗ clinical variables and steroid use; P > baseline on ⅕ clinical variables, steroid use and NSAID use	Sample size not calculated. The patients in the R group tended to be older and with slightly more severe disease.
Rheumatoid arthritis/Gibson, 1980[57]	Individualized remedy, dose, and duration.	Randomized, placebo-controlled, double-blind; 3 months.	Adults ages 24 to 76 years.	R = 23 P = 23	VAS for pain, articular index of joint tenderness, grip strength, digital joint circumference, duration of morning stiffness, and functional index. Patient global assessment.	Global assessment R = 19/23 slightly better to much better; P = 5/23 slightly better (none much better); R > P on all clinical measurements	Sample size not calculated. Subjects were classified into two groups: Group I had subjects with good homeopathic prescribing symptoms, and group II had poor prescribing symptoms. At baseline, patients receiving placebo had higher mean rheumatoid factor titers.
Postoperative ileus/Mayaux, 1988[58]	Opium (O) 30X, Raphanus (Ra) 10X.	Randomized, placebo-controlled, double-blind; double dummy; a fourth group was no treatment (control).	Adults? (ages not reported)	N = 150 divided into four groups	Time to passage of the first stool.	O = Ra = P = control	Sample size not calculated. Baseline comparisons similar except more laxative use in the placebo group.
Childhood diarrhea/Jacobs, 1994[59]	Individualized remedy, all 30C.	Randomized, placebo-controlled, double-blind; 5 days.	Children ages 6 months to 5 years.	R = 43 P = 44	Duration of diarrhea, number of days until <½ the amount of stools at baseline, number of days until first formed stool, diarrhea-index score, and average number of stools per day.	R > P on ¾ assessments (P <.05)	All children received oral rehydration therapy. Sample size not calculated. Groups comparable at baseline.

Key:

B = betahistine; C = conventional; D = dilution; F = fenoprofen; N = number; NSAID = nonsteroidal anti-inflammatory drug; O = opium; P = placebo; PFT = pulmonary function test; R = remedy; Ra = Raphanus; VAS = visual analog scale.

Table 46–6

Examples of Selection Guidelines as Part of the Display for Single Homeopathic Remedies

Clinical Condition (Keynote Symptoms)	Homeopathic Remedy
Muscle and joint pain improved by rest and firm local pressure	*Bryonia* (wild hops)
Pain in small joints associated with arthritis in the hands	*Caulophyllum thalictroides* (blue cohosh)
Pain and feeling of weakness in the lower back	Kali carbonicum (potassium carbonate)
Joint pain improved by motion, worsened by rest and humidity	*Rhus toxicodendron* (poison ivy)

Table 46–7

Examples of Combination Homeopathic Remedies for Premenstrual Syndrome (PMS)

Clinical Condition (Common Name)	Ingredients with Potency
PMS by Hyland (tablets)	*Viburnum opulus* 2X (high cranberry)
	Caulophyllum thalictroides 3X (blue cohosh)
	Cocculus indicus 3X (Indian cockle)
	Gelsemium 3X (yellow jasmine)
PMS by Nova (20% USP alcohol by volume, a.a.)	*Apis mellifica* 4X (honeybee)
	Atropium sulphuricum 6X (atropine sulfate)
	Calcarea carbonica 12X (calcium carbonate)
	Caulophyllum thalictroides 4X (blue cohosh)
	Colocynthis 4X (bitter cucumber)
	Cuprum aceticum 4X (copper acetate)
	Gelsemium 4X (yellow jasmine)
	Hamamelis virginiana 3X (witch hazel)
	Helonia diodica 4X (false unicorn)
	Ignatia 12X (St. Ignatius bean)
	Nux vomica 12X (poison nut)
	Pulsatilla 12X (wind flower)
	Stannum metallicum 8X (tin)
	Viburnum opulus 3X (high cranberry)
PMS by Bioforce, A. Vogel (alcohol content 30% or tablet)	*Aristolochia clematis* 12X (birthwort)
	Cimicifuga racemosa 6X (black snake root or black cohosh)
	Cyclamen europa 6X (sow-bread)
	Hydrastis canadensis 6X (goldenseal)
	Lachesis mutus 10X (bushmaster snake venom)
	Potentilla anserina 1X (cinquefoil)
	Pulsatilla 6X (wind flower)
PMS by Dolisos (granules)	*Caulophyllum thalictroides* 4C (blue cohosh)
	Ignatia 4C (St. Ignatius bean)
	Phytolacca 4C (poke root)
	Platina 4C (platinum)
	Viburnum opulus 4C (high cranberry)

After World War II, training in conventional medicine increasingly focused on the organic causes of illness. The interview process correspondingly became more diagnosis-focused, provider-oriented, and provider-controlled. Biopsychosocial aspects of interviewing decreased in importance as scientific advances made a priority of identifying the physical causes of a patient's illness. Homeopathic practitioners have continued to use a holistic approach that includes the discovery of an individual patient's psychosocial characteristics that are key elements in determining which treatment should be used.

In the assessment, the homeopathic practitioner includes additional factors such as whether the patient was late or early for the appointment, was untidy or extremely neat, was passive or dominant during conversation, or was eager or reluctant to volunteer information. The practitioner listens carefully to the patient to make sure the patient means what he or she says and that the practitioner understands what the patient means. How the patient describes something or relates an event is as important as the symptom or the event. In addition, details on the patient's appetite, thirst, sleep patterns, and dreams are elicited, as well as the patient's food, temperature, and weather preferences. How a patient feels during different times of the day, during different seasons, or during different times of the month is also discussed. The patient's emotional or mental state is often more important in determining the specific remedy to use than are the physical symptoms. Figure 46–2 illustrates the type of information gathered during a holistic patient interview. Case Study 46–2 illustrates the procedure for obtaining such information.

After the symptoms are determined and organized, they are graded. Grading assists in selecting the symptoms that will provide the key indicators for choosing the most appropriate remedy.[16]

The homeopathic practitioner will not make a diagnosis, but will determine the specific remedy to use to eliminate the symptoms by triggering the healing process to cure the illness. A conventional medical practitioner prescribes a medication that has the opposite effect of the symptom to be treated (e.g., antihistamines for a runny nose). A homeopathic practitioner treats the same condition by giving a patient a remedy that would cause the symptoms in a healthy

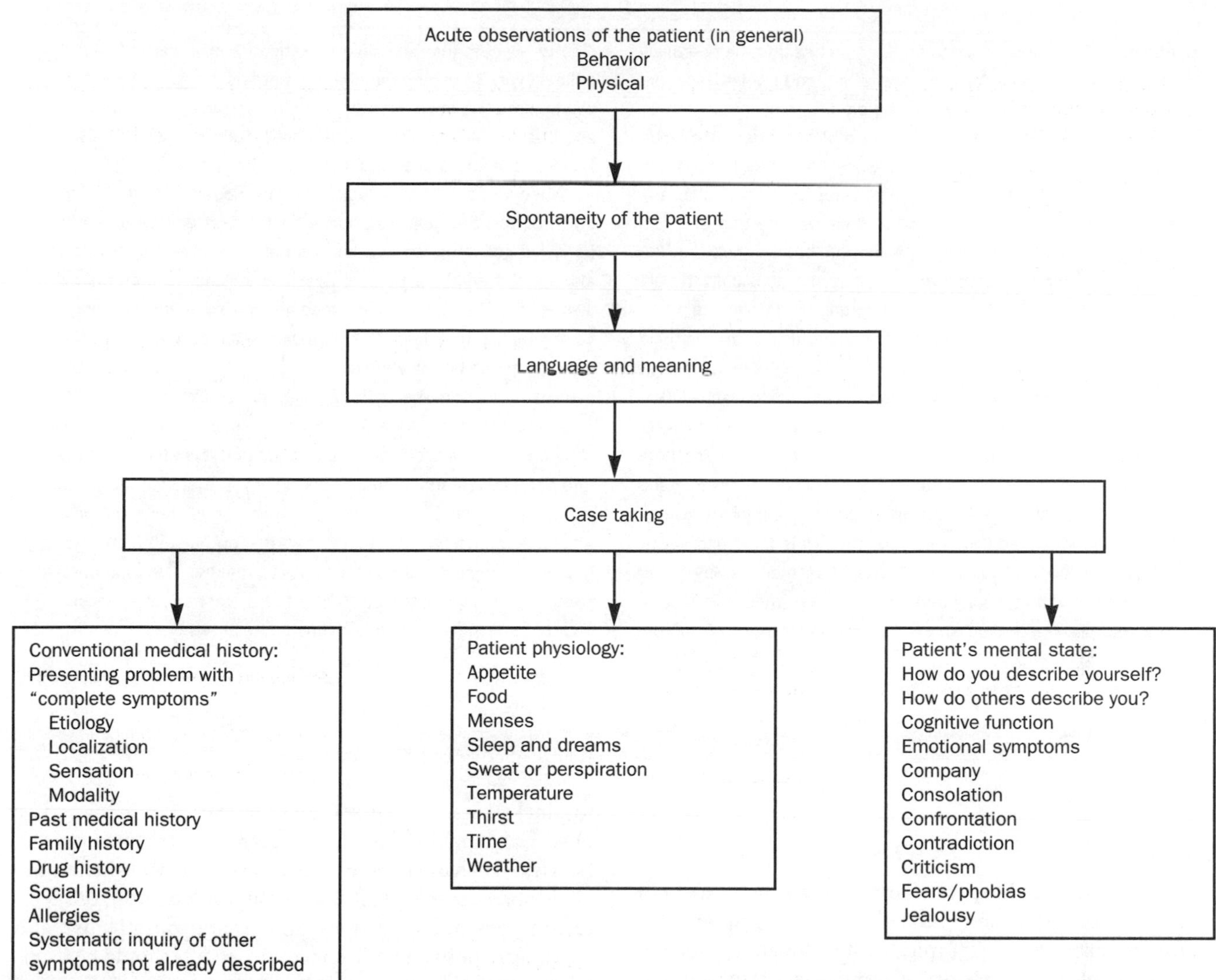

Figure 46–2 Homeopathic patient interview process. Adapted from references 16 and 17.

individual if given in a higher dose or for a longer period. (See Table 46–1 for an explanation of the Law of Similars.)

The classical homeopathic practitioner is often interested in determining a patient's constitution.[16] A patient's constitution is his or her overall mental, emotional, and physical makeup, including temperament, appearance, and behavior. Knowing a patient's constitution not only helps to select a very specific remedy based on these characteristics but also helps predict vulnerability to diseases. Popular books on homeopathy imply that everyone fits into 1 of 10 or so constitutional types, but such is not the case. Finding a constitutional remedy is not always possible. There may not be a remedy that fits a particular individual's constitution, or the clinical picture may distort the individual's constitution. For example, a person who is placid and easy-going when healthy, may be apathetic or assertive and quarrelsome when ill. A long-term relationship with the patient is necessary for the practitioner to know the patient's "true self." In these situations, the best remedy is based on the clinical picture (i.e., a simile or similimum). Evaluating symptoms can be further complicated by patients experiencing side effects from conventional medications. For example, a patient who takes propranolol may have nightmares and decreased libido.

In summary, homeopathic practitioners use a holistic approach to patient assessment because selection of appropriate treatment is based on finding distinctly individual symptoms. In contrast, conventional practitioners look for symptom complexes that fit a known diagnostic pattern in order to identify the cause of the patient illness, so appropriate treatment can be prescribed.

Case Study 46–2

Andrea, a 20-year-old college student, comes into the pharmacy stating that she is having problems with mood swings, bloating, and weight gain for 1 to 2 weeks before every menstrual period. She also tells you that her menses are always late and painful. When asked to describe the pain, she says it feels like a downward pressure with pain in her abdomen and back. You ask about previous treatments, and Andrea reveals that she has tried large amounts of aspirin or ibuprofen, but they help only the feelings of pain and pressure, not what she considers the primary problems of mood changes, bloating, and weight gain.

From a homeopathic viewpoint, you note that Andrea is timid and soft-spoken. Periodically during the conversation she becomes weepy. You ask about her eating habits and discover that she normally does not like to eat fatty foods but craves chocolate milkshakes during this time. You offer sympathy and note that she immediately seems to feel better. Andrea says that she does find that she feels better when she has company. You refer to Table 46–6 and you note that Andrea is timid and weepy (rather than loquacious and irritable), has mood swings, and feels better with company and consolation (rather than worse). Because she has asked about a homeopathic remedy, you decide to suggest that she take pulsatilla 6X in a dose of 3 to 5 pellets every 30 minutes until the symptoms are gone. If the first two to three doses do not substantially decrease the symptoms, she should call you. You explain how to take the remedy. (See the box "Patient Education for Homeopathic Remedies.")

When you call her the next day, she appears to be feeling much better. She tells you that after the first dose, the symptoms did get worse as you had warned. Because she felt very sleepy, she slept for 60 minutes, but still had symptoms on awakening. She took the next dose and felt some improvement, so she took a third dose 30 minutes after the second dose. She then felt much better and went out for the evening. During the evening, she felt herself getting teary and feeling bloated again, so she took a fourth dose. The rest of the evening was fine, and she has been fine today despite the fact that it is still 5 days before her menses should begin. She tells you that even after the first dose, she felt better and happier even though her symptoms were still bothering her. You tell her to keep pulsatilla on hand to use if the symptoms occur again. You make a note in her profile that pulsatilla appeared to help her premenstrual syndrome and that pulsatilla may be her constitutional remedy.

Patient Counseling for Homeopathic Remedies

The pharmacist should encourage the self-treating patient to set clear outcomes to determine if the target symptoms are improving or worsening. Typically, homeopathic remedies are sold in potencies of 6X or 30C for single remedies and in lower dilutions for combinations (e.g., 1X to 12X). The patient should be counseled to take the remedies according to the dosing guidelines presented on the label. Labeling guidelines on many nonprescription remedies are potentially confusing. The dose is often given as 3 to 5 tablets three times daily with no guidance on how many doses or for how long it should be taken. If the dosing guidelines are not clear, patients should be advised to seek the recommendation of a pharmacist, homeopathic practitioner, or a physician for symptoms that do not improve after 3 to 4 days. This advice appears on the labels of some products.

In addition, self-treating patients need to be warned about the potential for initial aggravation of symptoms. They should be counseled to call the pharmacist or their homeopathic practitioner for advice if aggravation occurs. Patients can be assured that this phenomenon is usually transient and a signal that the correct remedy has been selected, but the pharmacist should be alert to the possibility that it may represent a true worsening of the condition that requires referral to a conventional medical practitioner. The pharmacist should advise the patient that certain substances are known to block the action of some homeopathic remedies. The pharmacist should have a homeopathic materia medica (e.g., Boericke) on hand to help determine potential antidotes. Because homeopathic practitioners vary in their opinions concerning general guidelines on the appropriate use and handling of homeopathic remedies, patients should be counseled, where appropriate, to consult their homeopathic practitioner for that practitioner's preferences.

The box "Patient Education for Homeopathic Remedies" lists other potential guidelines to provide patients.

Evaluation of Patient Outcomes with Homeopathic Remedies

After prescribing a remedy, the practitioner closely follows the patient to determine the response to treatment as well as what adjustments to make based on the response. The practitioner may repeat the dose if symptoms appear again after the response has worn off. On the basis of less than optimal responses, the potency may be adjusted or a new remedy selected.

The expected outcome is amelioration of symptoms for either a constitutional or a clinical remedy. However, an initial, transient aggravation of symptoms may occur.[16] If aggravation occurs, it represents an intensification of the original symptoms (as opposed to development of new symptoms), and practitioners take this aggravation as a sign

Patient Education for Homeopathic Remedies

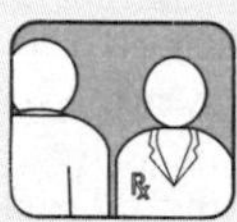

As with conventional medications, improvement of symptoms is the objective of self-treatment with homeopathic remedies. To obtain maximum benefit from these products, patients should carefully follow label instructions and the general self-care guidelines listed below.[7,61]

- Do not eat or drink anything, brush your teeth, or smoke for 15 minutes before and after the remedy is taken.
- If the remedy to be used is a single remedy or small globule or small tablet, do not touch the remedy. Instead, pour the dose into the cap, and place the tablets into your mouth without letting your lips or tongue touch the cap. If the product comes in a dispenser vial, dispense the tablet directly into your mouth without touching your lips or tongue to the vial.
- Store the remedy out of direct sunlight, and avoid extremes of hot or cold. Also, store the remedy away from aromatic medications, cleaners or other household products, perfumes, or essential oils. Any of these can "antidote" the remedy and render it ineffective.
- Avoid other homeopathic remedies unless needed for an emergency (e.g., *Arnica*). Note that homeopathic remedies can antidote the actions of other homeopathic remedies.
- Avoid both caffeinated and decaffeinated coffee products. The aromatic principles, not the caffeine, can function as an antidote.
- Avoid medications, cosmetics, or hair care products that are strongly aromatic, including aromatherapies. Avoid menthol and peppermint when given Natrum muriaticum (sodium chloride). In general, nonaromatic herbal teas, many teas containing mint, and cooking herbs do not present a problem.
- Avoid recreational drugs, but, if desired, you can use alcohol in moderation.
- Avoid major dental work unless it is an emergency. Manual cleaning without electrical equipment is acceptable.
- Although acupuncture and other "energetic" therapies can be beneficial, avoid them during homeopathic treatment.
- Do not stop taking prescription or over-the-counter medications. Discuss discontinuing or decreasing dosages of prescription medications with a physician. Discuss such actions for nonprescription medications with a pharmacist.
- Avoid taking any new medications unless they are for an emergency condition. New medications can change your clinical picture and subsequently your response to the homeopathic remedy that was chosen on the basis of your presenting clinical picture.

Consult a pharmacist, homeopathic practitioner, or physician if symptoms do not improve in 3 to 4 days.

that the correct remedy was chosen. Another sign that a correct remedy was chosen before actual evidence of healing occurs is that the patient feels sleepy. This feeling is not fatigue, but a healthy need for rest because the body has started to heal. When the correct remedy is chosen, healing is thought to occur along the lines outlined by the American homeopath, Constantin Hering.[16,28] Hering's laws are outlined briefly in Table 46–1.

What may occur—indeed, can occur even though the patient is experiencing symptom aggravation—is an increase in the sense of well-being, especially for a constitutional remedy.[16] That is, the patient senses an overall feeling of benefit that ameliorates distress or anxiety. Once again, this feeling usually indicates that the correct remedy was chosen. Conversely, if patients experience a decrease in their sense of well-being, it is usually a signal that the wrong remedy was chosen. Another sign that a constitutional remedy is working is that changes in the constitution show the patient is moving toward normalcy. For example, a chronically chilly patient feels warm or cravings for salt diminish.

If the patient and practitioner discern no change, several things can be happening.[17] First, the lack of change could signal that the wrong remedy was used. Second, the wrong potency could have been chosen. Third, the response could have been blocked by some other factor. For example, as Hahnemann outlined, chemical substances in the environment or used by the patient could be obstacles to a cure as could medications that may block the response (e.g., immunosuppressants or anti-inflammatory agents). Other obstacles to cures are lifestyle excesses such as diet, stress, hygiene, or sexual behavior. When there is no change or incomplete symptomatic control, the practitioner will screen for potential obstacles to cure, will consider a different potency, and, after reviewing the case notes, may try another remedy.

The patient may become worse[16] and may progress in severity of the original symptoms or the appearance of new symptoms. Even though, in general, it is believed that giving the wrong homeopathic remedy will not be harmful, in certain situations it can be (such as the inappropriate use of a conventional nonprescription product), especially if it delays the recognition and treatment of a serious or life-threatening disorder. Patients may need to be referred to their conventional medical practitioner for evaluation. Administering high potencies in debilitated or sensitive individuals may weaken the patient. The patient initially feels better, then becomes more debilitated. When the patient worsens, the practitioner reviews the case and determines whether a new remedy needs to be chosen or makes an adjustment in potency.

CONCLUSIONS

Patients are attracted to homeopathy and, like conventional nonprescription interventions, homeopathy is safe as long as serious and life-threatening disorders that require conventional medical interventions are ruled out. Homeopathy uses specially prepared highly diluted solutions that are thought to trigger the healing process. While the efficacy of homeopathy remains controversial, it represents an alternative for patients who are without serious or life-threatening diseases, who have not experienced symptomatic relief from other treatment modalities including conventional medical care, or who wish to minimize the potential for adverse effects from conventional medical therapies. In addition, patients who desire a holistic approach to their primary health care may find homeopathy in keeping with their lifestyle choices. The pharmacist's role is to ensure that patients appropriately select and take homeopathic remedies to maximize the potential for beneficial effects.

References

1. Homeopathic Pharmacopoeia Convention of the United States. Homeopathic Pharmacopoeia of the United States. Available at: http://www.hpus.com.1998.
2. Ernst E, Kaptchuk TJ. Homeopathy revisited. *Arch Intern Med.* 1996;156:2162–4.
3. Eisenberg DM, Davis RB, Ettner SL, et al. Trends in alternative medicine use in the United States, 1990–1997: results of a follow-up national survey. *JAMA.* 1998; 280:1569–75.
4. Anonymous. FDA petitioned to "stop homeopathy scam." *JAMA.* 1994;272:1154–5.
5. Barrett S, Tyler VE. Why pharmacists should not sell homeopathic remedies. *Am Health Sys Pharm.* 1995;52:1004–5.
6. Lepine P. Homeopathy's potential for enriching the medical interview: looking beyond the tiny white pill. *Can Fam Physician.* 1995;41: 1649–51.
7. Roter DL, Hall JA. *Doctors Talking with Patients/Patients Talking with Doctors.* Westport, CT: Auburn House; 1992.
8. Smith, RC. *The Patient's Story; Integrated Patient–Doctor Interviewing.* New York: Little Brown and Company; 1996.
9. Astin JA. Why patients use alternative medicine: results of a national survey. *JAMA.* 1998; 279:1548–53.
10. Goldstein MS, Glik D. Use of and satisfaction with homeopathy in a patient population. *Altern Ther Health Med.* 1998;4:60–5.
11. Langewitz W, Ruttimann S, Laifer G, et al. The integration of alternative treatment modalities in HIV infection: the patient's perspective. *Psychosom Res.* 1994;38:687–93.
12. Downer SM, Cody MM, McCluskey P, et al. Pursuit and practice of complementary therapies by cancer patients receiving conventional treatment. *Br Med J.* 1994;309:86–9.
13. Wittern R. The origins of homeopathy in Germany. *Clio Medica.* 1991;22:51–63.
14. Rothouse H. History of homeopathy reveals discipline's excellence. *Alternative and Complementary Ther.* June 1997:223–7.
15. Driehsen HW, Foxman EL, Hebisch C, et al. *Homeotherapy: Definitions and Therapeutic Schools.* Baden-Baden, Germany: European American Coalition on Homeopathy; 1997.
16. Swayne J. *Homeopathic Method: Implications for Clinical Practice and Medical Science.* New York: Churchill Livingstone; 1998.
17. Leckridge B. *Homeopathy in Primary Care.* New York: Churchill Livingstone: 1997.
18. Homeopathic Pharmacopoeia Convention of the United States. *The Homeopathic Pharmacopoeia of the United States.* Boston: O. Clapp; 1998.
19. Schwartz GER, Russek LGS. The plausibility of homeopathy: the systemic memory mechanism. *Integrative Medicine.* 1998;1:53–9.
20. Bastide M, Lagache A. A communication process: a new paradigm applied to high-dilution effects on the living body. *Altern Ther Health Med.* 1997;3:35–9.
21. Matsumoto J. Molecular mechanism of biological responses to homeopathic medicines. *Med Hypotheses.* 1995;45:292–6.
22. Davenas E, Beauvais F, Amara J, et al. Human basophil degranulation triggered by very dilute antiserum against IgE. *Nature.* 1988;333:816–8.
23. Hirst SJ, Hayes NA, Burridge J, et al. Human basophil degranulation is not triggered by very dilute antiserum against human IgE. *Nature.* 1993;366:525–7.
24. Benveniste J, Ducot B, Spira A. Memory of water revisited. *Nature.* 1994;370:322.
25. Boericke W. *Pocket Manual of Homeopathic Materia Medica and Repertory and a Chapter on Rare and Uncommon Remedies.* New Delhi, India: B. Jain Publishers, Ltd; 1995 [reprint].
26. *The Smart Guide to Homeopathy: The Gentle Medicine for the Generation of Harmony and Well Being.* Newtown Square, PA: Boiron; undated brochure.
27. Kent JT. *Repertory of the Homeopathic Materia Medica and a Word Index.* New Delhi, India: B. Jain Publishers Ltd; 1997 [reprint].
28. Frye J. Homeopathy in office practice. *Complementary and Alternative Therapies in Primary Care.* 1997;24:845–65.
29. Homeopathy Home Directory. Available at: http://www.homeopathy-home.com/directory/usa/training_colleges. 1999.
30. Belon P. Provings: concepts and methodology. *Br Homoeopathic J.* 1995;84:213–7.
31. Walach H. Provings: the method and its future. *Br Homoeopathic J.* 1994;83:129–31.
32. Riley D. Contemporary drug provings. *J Am Inst Homeopathy.* 1994;87: 161–5.
33. Sankaran R. A protocol for provings. *Homeopathic Links.* 1995;8:15–6.
34. Jounnay J. *Essentials of Homeopathic Therapeutics.* Newtown Square, PA: Boiron; 1994.
35. Ullman D. *The Consumer's Guide to Homeopathy: The Definitive Resource for Understanding Homeopathic Medicine and Making It Work for You.* New York: G.P. Putnam's Sons; 1995.
36. Kerr HD, Yarborough GW. Pancreatitis following ingestion of a homeopathic preparation. *N Eng J Med.* 1986;314:1642–3.
37. Moore N, Coquerel A, Hannequin D, et al. Exacerbation of multiple sclerosis during therapy that included brain extracts. *Med J Aust.* 1988;149:343–4.
38. Kleijnen J, Knipschild P, ter Riet G. Clinical trials of homeopathy. *Br Med J.* 1991;302:316–23.
39. Linde K, Clausius N, Ramirez G, et al. Are the clinical effects of homeopathy placebo effects? A meta-analysis of placebo-controlled trials. *Br Med J.* 1997;350:834–43.
40. Barnes J, Resch KL, Ernst E. Homeopathy for postoperative ileus? A meta-analysis. *J Clin Gastroenterol.* 1997;25:628–33.
41. De Lange de Klerk ESM, Blommers J, Kuik DJ, et al. Effect of homeopathic medicines on daily burden of symptoms in children with recurrent upper respiratory tract infections. *Br Med J.* 1994;309:1329–32.
42. Friese K-H, Kruse S, Ludtke R, et al. The homoeopathic treatment of otitis media in children: comparisons of conventional therapy. *Int J Clin Pharmacol Ther.* 35:296–301.
43. Reilly DT, Taylor MA, Beattie NGM, et al. Is evidence for homeopathy reproducible? *Lancet.* 1994;344;1601–6.
44. Reilly DT, Taylor MA, McSharry C, et al. Is homeopathy a placebo re-

sponse? Controlled trial of homeopathic potency, with pollen in hayfever as a model. *Lancet.* 1986;2:881–6.
45. Wiesenauer M, Gaus W. Double-blind trial comparing the effectiveness of the homeopathic preparation Galphimia potentisation D6, Galphimia dilution 10^{-6}, and placebo on pollinosis. *Arzneimittelforschung.* 1985;35:1745–7.
46. Ferley JP, Zmirou D, D'adhemar D, et al. A controlled evaluation of a homoeopathic preparation in the treatment of influenza-like syndromes. *Br J Clin Pharmacol.* 1989;27:329–35.
47. Labrecque M, Audet D, Latulippe LG, et al. Homeopathic treatment of plantar warts. *Can Med Assoc J.* 1992;146;1749–53.
48. Smolle J, Prause G, Kerl H. A double-blind, controlled clinical trial of homeopathy and an analysis of lunar phases and postoperative outcome. *Arch Dermatol.*1998;134:1368–70.
49. Hart O, Mullee MA, Lewith G, et al. Double-blind, placebo-controlled, randomized clinical trial of homeopathic arnica C30 for pain and infection after total abdominal hysterectomy. *J Royal Society Med.* 1997;90:73–8.
50. Hofmeyr GJ, Piccioni V, Blauhof P. Postpartum homoeopathic *Arnica montana*: a potency finding pilot study. *Br J Clin Practice.* 1990;44:619–21.
51. Hill N, Stam C, Tuinder S, et al. A placebo-controlled clinical trial investigating the efficacy of a homeopathic after-bite gel in reducing mosquito bite–induced erythema. *Eur J Clin Pharmacol.* 1995;49:103–8.
52. Fisher P, Greenwood A, Huskisson EC, et al. Effect of homoeopathic treatment of fibrositis (primary fibromyalgia). *Br Med J.* 1989;299:365–6.
53. Lokken P, Straumsheim PA, Tveiten D, et al. Effect of homoeopathy on pain and other events after acute trauma: placebo-controlled trial with bilateral oral surgery. *Br Med J.* 1995;310:1439–45.
54. Weiser M, Strosser W, Klein P. Homeopathic versus conventional treatment of vertigo: a randomized double-blind controlled clinical study. *Arch Otolaryngol Head Neck Surg.* 1998;124:879–85.
55. Shipley M, Berry H, Broster G, et al. Controlled trial of homoeopathic treatment of osteoarthritis. *Lancet.* 1983;1:97–8.
56. Andrade LE, Ferraz MB, Atra E, et al. A randomized controlled trial to evaluate the effectiveness of homeopathy in rheumatoid arthritis. *Scand J Rheumatol.* 1991;20:204–8.
57. Gibson RG, Gibson SLM, MacNeill AD, et al. Homoeopathic therapy in rheumatoid arthritis: evaluation by double-blind clinical therapeutic trial. *Br J Clin Pharmacol.* 1980;9:453–9.
58. Mayaux MJ, Guihard-Moscato ML, Schwartz D, et al. Controlled clinical trial of homoeopathy in postoperative ileus. *Lancet.* 1988;1:528–9.
59. Jacobs J, Jimenez LM, Gloyd SS, et al. Treatment of acute childhood diarrhea with homoeopathic medicine: a randomized clinical trial in Nicaragua. *Pediatrics.* 1994;93:719–25.
60. Ernst E. Effects of homoeopathy: trial did not evaluate "true" homoeopathy. *Br Med J.* 1995;311:510–1.
61. Spector IM. Personal communication of patient counseling information. Tucson, AZ: Osteopathic and Homeopathic Physician; 1998.

APPENDIX I

FDA Pregnancy Risk Categories for Selected Nonprescription Medications

Drug therapy during pregnancy may sometimes be necessary. However, because most drugs cross the placenta to some extent, a mother who takes a drug might expose her fetus to it. Medications should be used during pregnancy only under the supervision of a physician and only when the potential benefits outweigh the potential risks.

The table on the following pages lists FDA categories for evaluating the safety of drugs during pregnancy for many of the nonprescription medications discussed in this book. The listed categories pertain to the particular strengths or formulations in which the nonprescription medications are available. Prescription strengths or formulations of a medication may have different pregnancy risk categories. Categories that bear a subscript M (e.g., C_M) were assigned by the manufacturer. The majority of the remaining categories were assigned by drug information sources based on available clinical information. *Drugs in Pregnancy and Lactation: A Reference Guide to Fetal and Neonatal Risk* is the primary information source.

The pregnancy risk categories are defined as follows:

A Adequate studies in pregnant women have not demonstrated a risk to the fetus in the first trimester of pregnancy, and there is no evidence of risk in later trimesters.

B Animal studies have not demonstrated a risk to the fetus, but there are no adequate studies in pregnant women . . . or . . . Animal studies have shown an adverse effect, but adequate studies in pregnant women have not demonstrated a risk to the fetus during the first trimester of pregnancy, and there is no evidence of risk in later trimesters.

C Animal studies have shown an adverse effect on the fetus, but there are no adequate studies in humans; the benefits from the use of the drug in pregnant women may be acceptable despite its potential risks . . . or . . . There are no animal reproduction studies and no adequate studies in humans.

D There is evidence of human fetal risk, but the potential benefits from the use of the drug in pregnant women may be acceptable despite its potential risks.

X Studies in animals or humans demonstrate fetal abnormalities, or adverse reaction reports indicate evidence of fetal risk. The risk of use in a pregnant woman clearly outweighs any possible benefit. Use of drugs with this rating is contraindicated in women who are or may become pregnant.

FDA Pregnancy Risk Categories for Selected Nonprescription Medications

Agent	FDA Category
Acetaminophen	B
Aluminum hydroxide	C[a]
Aminobenzoic acid (PABA)	C
Ammonium chloride	C
Aspartame	B (C in women with phenylketonuria)[a]
Aspirin	C (D if full-doses taken in 3rd trimester)
Bacitracin	C
Benzocaine	C
Benzoyl peroxide	C
β-Carotene	C
Bisacodyl	B
Bismuth	C (D in 3rd trimester)
Brompheniramine	C_M
Butoconazole	C_M (for use only in 2nd or 3rd trimester)
Caffeine	B
Calcium carbonate	C[a]
Calcium gluconate	C
Camphor	C
Capsaicin	No rating[b]
Carbamide peroxide	No rating[b]
Casanthranol	C
Cascara sagrada	C
Castor oil	X
Charcoal, activated	No rating[b]
Chlorhexidine gluconate	B
Chlorpheniramine	B
Chlortetracycline	D
Choline salicylate	C
Chondroitin sulfate–glucosamine	No rating[b]
Cimetidine	B_M
Clemastine	B_M
Clotrimazole	B
Coal tar	C
Codeine	C (D if used for prolonged periods or in high doses at term)
Cromolyn	B_M
Cyclizine	B
Dexbrompheniramine	C
Dexpanthenol	C
Dextromethorphan	C
Dimenhydrinate	B_M
Diphenhydramine	B_M
Docusate calcium	C
Docusate potassium	C
Docusate sodium	C
Doxylamine	B
Dyclonine	C
Ephedrine	C
Epinephrine	C
Ethanol	D (X if used in large amounts or for prolonged periods)[a]
Famotidine	B_M
Ferrous fumarate	C
Ferrous gluconate	C
Ferrous sulfate	C
Folic acid	A (C if doses exceed RDA)[a]
Glycerin	C
Guaifenesin	C
Hydrocortisone	C
Hydroquinone	C
Ibuprofen	B (D if used in 3rd trimester or near delivery)
Insulin	B
Iodine	See potassium iodide
Ipecac syrup	C
Iron	See ferrous fumarate, ferrous gluconate, ferrous sulfate
Kaolin	C
Ketoconazole	C_M
Ketoprofen	B_M (D if used in 3rd trimester or near delivery)
Lidocaine	B
Loperamide	B_M
Lysine	C
Magnesium citrate	No rating[b]
Magnesium hydroxide	No rating[b]
Magnesium oxide	No rating[b]
Manganese	No rating[b]
Meclizine	B_M
Methylcellulose	No rating[b]
Miconazole	C_M
Mineral oil	C
Minoxidil	C_M
Naphazoline	C
Naproxen sodium	B (D if used in 3rd trimester or near delivery)[a]

FDA Pregnancy Risk Categories for Selected Nonprescription Medications (continued)

Agent	FDA Category	Agent	FDA Category
Neomycin	C	Simethicone	C
Niacinamide (Nicotinamide)	A (C if doses exceed RDA)[a]	Sodium bicarbonate	C
Nicotine transdermal system	D_M	Sodium chloride	C
Nicotine polacrilex gum	C_M	Sodium citrate	C
Nizatidine	B_M (C according to some drug references)	Sodium fluoride	C
		Sodium phosphate	C
Nonoxynol-9	C	Sodium salicylate	C
Octoxynol-9	C	Terbinafine	B
Oxymetazoline	C	Terpin hydrate	D
Pantothenic acid	A (C if doses exceed RDA)[a]	Tetracaine	C
Permethrin	B	Tioconazole	C
Phenazopyridine	B	Tolnaftate	No rating[b]
Pheniramine	C	Triethanolamine	C
Phenylephrine hydrochloride	C	Triprolidine	C_M
Phenylpropanolamine	C	Urea	C
Phenyltoloxamine	C	Vitamin A	A (X if doses exceed RDA)[a]
Polyethylene glycol	C	Vitamin B_1 (thiamine)	A (C if doses exceed RDA)[a]
Polymyxin B	B	Vitamin B_2 (riboflavin)	A (C if doses exceed RDA)[a]
Povidone–iodine	D	Vitamin B_3 (niacin)	A (C if doses exceed RDA)[a]
Pseudoephedrine	C	Vitamin B_6 (pyridoxine)	A (C if doses exceed RDA)[a]
Psyllium hydrocolloid	B	Vitamin B_{12} (cyanocobalamin)	A (C if doses exceed RDA)[a]
Pyrantel pamoate	C	Vitamin C (ascorbic acid)	A (C if doses exceed RDA)[a]
Pyrethrins	C	Vitamin D (calciferol)	A (D if doses exceed RDA)[a]
Pyrilamine	C	Vitamin D_2 (ergocalciferol)	A (C if doses exceed RDA)[a]
Ranitidine	B_M	Vitamin D_3 (cholecalciferol)	A (D if doses exceed RDA)[a]
Saccharin	C	Vitamin E (tocopherol)	A (C if doses exceed RDA)[a]
Salicylic acid	C	Vitamins, multiple	A (risk factor varies for amounts exceeding RDAs)[a]
Selenium sulfide	C		
Senna	C	Xylometazoline	C

[a] Source references did not provide pregnancy risk category. Category is instead based on available clinical information.

[b] Source references did not provide pregnancy risk category. Insufficient clinical information is available to support a rating.

Source:

Briggs GG, Freeman RK, Yaffe SJ. *Drugs in Pregnancy and Lactation: A Reference Guide to Fetal and Neonatal Risk*. 5th ed. Philadelphia: Lippincott Williams & Wilkins; 1998.

Hebel SK, ed. *Drug Facts & Comparisons*. St. Louis: Wolters Kluwer Co; 2000.

Lacy CF, Armstrong LL, Goldman MP, Lance LL. *Drug Information Handbook*. 7th ed. Hudson, OH: Lexi-Comp; 1999.

Micromedex Healthcare Series, [database online]. Volume 104. Englewood, CO: Micromedex, Inc; 2000.

Pagliaro LA, Pagliaro AM. Drugs as human teratogens and fetotoxins. In: *Problems in Pediatric Drug Therapy*. 4th ed. Washington DC: American Pharmaceutical Association; 2000. In press.

Schrefer J, ed. *Mosby's GenRx 2000*. St. Louis: Mosby, Inc; 2000.

USP-DI Volume I: Drug Information for the Health Professional. 20th ed. Englewood, CO: Micromedex, Inc; 2000.

APPENDIX II

Suggested Treatment Approaches for Case Studies

Note: The following chapters do not feature case studies: 1, 25, 37, 38, and 43. The case studies in Chapter 2 support discussion in the text, whereas those in Chapter 46 illustrate the homeopathic approach to assessment of disorders.

For the remaining case studies, readers should refer to the patient assessment sections, patient education boxes, and pertinent tables in the appropriate chapters for additional information on assessment of the disorders, administration guidelines for suggested treatments, and counseling/education information for patients.

Case Study 3–1

The patient complains of pain in his right leg that is related to a muscle strain. Instruct the patient to begin nonpharmacologic therapy, such as RICE (resting the leg, applying ice and compression bandages, and elevating the leg), immediately for the muscle strain to help minimize the trauma to the affected tissues. Advise the patient to rest his leg for 48 to 72 hours and to begin ice/cold therapy right away. Explain that heat therapy may also relieve the swelling, but that this therapy should not start until 2 to 3 days after the injury. Caution the patient to avoid nonsalicylate nonsteroidal anti-inflammatory drugs (NSAIDs) and salicylates since he is on lithium therapy.

Determine whether the patient's alcohol use is of a chronic nature. If alcohol is used only occasionally, recommend acetaminophen 650 mg to 1 g every 6 hours for 3 days. Caution against the use of alcohol while taking acetaminophen. Advise the patient to seek appropriate medical attention if the pain persists after 10 days, or if it intensifies at any time.

Case Study 4–1

The 4-year-old patient with fever has a history of seizures. Using nonprescription antipyretics to treat her fever is inappropriate. Advise the mother that fever can induce seizures and to notify her child's physician immediately about the fever. Explain also that the recent bacterial infection could have caused the fever. Advise her to remind the physician of the recent illness and the amoxicillin prescription. Further, advise her that the physician will probably order antipyretic therapy every 4 hours for 24 hours and may alter the regimen for the anticonvulsant medication.

Case Study 5–1

The 18-year-old athlete complains of pain and swelling in his left ankle. Nondrug measures such as RICE (rest, ice, compression, and elevation) can reduce the swelling, and external or internal analgesics can help alleviate the pain. Because the patient has seasonal allergies, determine whether he has asthma, nasal polyps, or salicylate allergy before recommending a product. Methyl salicylate, aspirin, or other salicylates would not be appropriate choices if any of these situations apply.

Counsel the patient on proper use of the recommended analgesic, as well as the proper implementation of RICE therapy. Advise the patient not to apply an occlusive bandage to the injury because it will enhance the absorption of the external analgesic.

Case Study 5–2

The 75-year-old patient with a history of congestive heart failure received emergency treatment for vaginal bleeding, irregular heartbeat, and orthostatic hypotension. An interaction between warfarin and methyl salicylate is the most probable cause of the patient's vaginal bleeding. This patient should not use methyl salicylate or trolamine salicylate to treat her joint pain. Capsaicin-containing products are appropriate alternative external analgesics.

Explain to the patient that concomitant use of nonprescription salicylates and warfarin predisposes her to bleeding. Explain also that the bleeding is an overt sign of complications related to the drug interaction. Caution that the bleeding could lead to hypotension and tachycardia. Advise the patient that external analgesics that do not contain salicylate are appropriate for her joint pain. Explain the proper use of the recommended agent.

Case Study 6–1

The patient's vaginal symptoms of a clumpy white discharge that is not malodorous and intense vulvar pruritis are consistent with vulvovaginal candidiasis (VVC). A previous episode of VVC two years earlier was clinician diagnosed. Other than the localized vaginal symptoms, which are mild to moderate and have been present for 1 to 2 days, this woman is a healthy, nonpregnant (inferred from the use of oral contraceptives) patient.

The oral contraceptives and the amoxicillin are predisposing medications for VVC; however, the patient is not taking any corticosteroids, immunosuppressant agents, or medications for diabetes mellitus. In the absence of chronic VVC and with the patient in apparent good health, the pharmacist can infer that the patient is not HIV positive (pharmacist inquiry possible, but somewhat unwarranted).

The patient is a suitable candidate for self-treatment based on the present vaginal symptoms, the previously diagnosed case of VVC, and the patient's medical and medication histories. Recommend a topical antifungal based on either the patient's preference or the best product for the significant vulvar itching. A cream product or a combination suppository/cream product, which is applied topically to the labia and the vagina, is the best choice. An alternative for the vulvar symptoms is a sodium bicarbonate sitz bath.

Counsel the patient on the proper use of the product. Advise the patient that she may wait until after her menses to begin treatment but that the significant vulvar itching may prove too uncomfortable for such delay. Explain that symptom resolution should be rapid, generally within hours and should take no longer than 24 to 48 hours. Advise the patient to seek medical attention if the symptoms do not improve within 3 days or if the symptoms worsen.

Case Study 7–1

The patient's symptoms of severe cramping, backache, and diarrhea are clinician diagnosed as primary dysmenorrhea. The duration of her symptoms (since late adolescence or about 10 years) and their timing (begin at onset of menses and last for 2 days) are consistent with primary dysmenorrhea. Symptom improvement while using an oral contraceptive is also consistent with primary dysmenorrhea. The symptoms are moderately severe, causing her to miss work.

The patient is healthy, not pregnant, and has no contraindications to use of nonsalicylate NSAIDs. These factors make her a suitable candidate for self-treatment. No medications or other medical conditions prohibit self-treatment; therefore, recommend that she begin taking a nonsalicylate NSAID if her menses begin. Consider the patient's previous use and experience with these agents in making product recommendations. Base product selection on patient preference, or choose a product on the basis of cost and dosing frequency.

Advise the patient on proper usage and common side effects of the selected product. Because the patient is trying to become pregnant, advise her to wait until her menses begin to take the NSAID and to take it on a scheduled basis for 2 days, the usual length of time she has symptoms.

Explain that symptom resolution should be rapid—generally within hours of taking the medication—and that taking several scheduled doses may show even greater improvement. If symptoms do not improve during the first cycle, advise her to take a higher dose next cycle or to switch to a different NSAID. Emphasize that she should not exceed nonprescription dosing limits without consulting a physician. If the nonprescription NSAIDs do not provide adequate resolution of symptoms, suggest medical evaluation.

Case Study 7–2

The patient's symptoms of abdominal bloating, irritability, breast tenderness, food cravings, and fatigue include physical, emotional, and behavioral symptoms. The duration of symptoms (about 6 months) and timing of symptoms (begin the week before menses and do not occur at other times of cycle) are consistent with premenstrual syndrome (PMS). Because the symptoms are relatively mild, medical referral is not indicated initially.

Although this woman appears healthy, confirm that she is not pregnant. Pregnancy is a general consideration when treating a woman in her reproductive years. If pregnancy is not an issue, the patient is a suitable candidate for self-treatment.

The patient is already taking vitamin E in the quantity recommended for management of breast tenderness. Suggest that she also take 1200 mg daily of calcium. The multiple vitamin that she is taking supplies 60 mg. Find out whether her diet is supplying additional calcium. If needed, suggest a calcium supplement to bring her daily intake to 1200 mg. Advise her to limit calcium doses to 500 mg at a time for best absorption. A recent trial of calcium supplements showed calcium to be beneficial in treating PMS and in preventing osteoporosis; it is also a nontoxic substance. If calcium is not effective, recommend that she try magnesium or vitamin B_6 or a combination of these three agents.

Before recommending a diuretic for the bloating, suggest that the patient weigh herself during the premenstrual phase (several times to get an average weight) and again at another time in her cycle to see whether her bloating is the result of fluid retention or just hormone-induced fluid shifting. If fluid is being retained, recommend limiting salt intake as a nondrug alternative. If the patient wishes to use a nonprescription diuretic, advise her to avoid combination products that contain an antihistamine.

Explain that side effects of calcium (gastrointestinal upset, constipation) are uncommon. Emphasize that calcium is taken daily, not just at the time of symptoms. Educate the patient about PMS in general, and suggest some nonpharmacologic measures to reduce symptoms (e.g., stress reduction techniques, ingestion of carbohydrate-rich foods during the luteal phase). Explain that symptom resolution from calcium may take several cycles. If the nonpharmacologic measures and vitamin/mineral supplements do not provide adequate symptom resolution, suggest medical evaluation.

Case Study 8–1

The patient is interested in nonprescription contraceptives, but her sexual partner will not use male condoms. The pharmacist must consider several points when discussing contraceptive products with her. The patient seems interested in contraception to prevent consequences of unprotected sexual activity. The initial discussion revealed that her partner does not want to use a male condom. With this fact in mind, ask the patient if she has had any experience with other modes of contraception. In the area of nonprescription products, the female condom, contraceptive foams, and other products (all depend on the woman to use) might be viable alternatives. In the discussion, it can also be useful to ask the patient what she knows of other contraceptive options. Her answers may help to tailor the discussion according to her potential readiness to consider other products.

In addition to suggesting nonprescription contraception, the pharmacist might refer the patient to her obstetrician/gynecologist or family practitioner for further discussion of prescription products such as oral contraceptives and injectable products. The severity of the patient's hypertension must be considered though. Ask about her history of further cardiovascular disease to determine her relative risk of exacerbation of disease secondary to prescription hormonal contraceptives.

Once the patient selects a contraceptive product, provide appropriate counseling guidelines. Consider referring to the text *Contraceptive Technology*, an excellent book that is listed in the references for Chapter 8.

Case Study 8–2

Although the patient complains of vaginal itching, two components of her medical history suggest that the itching is not related to a yeast infection: (1) She has no discharge consistent with a yeast infection. (2) The symptoms clear up regardless of whether she uses an antifungal product.

Other possible causes of the vaginal itching include latex allergy or spermicide allergy/irritation. Differentiation between the two possible causes requires additional information from the patient. Does the irritation occur only when she uses latex condoms, or does it also occur when she uses vaginal spermicides? Occurrence with only the latex condoms suggests a latex allergy, even if it does not occur with every incidence of condom use—allergenicity differs between various condom brands. Does she develop itching or a rash if she wears rubber gloves or blows up a balloon? If yes, this information would further indicate a possible allergy to latex. If the itching occurs with or without latex condom use, is there a difference when she uses spermicide-treated condoms versus plain condoms? This question would help identify a spermicide-related problem. This patient has dual contraceptive needs: (1) the prevention of pregnancy and (2) the prevention of transmission of sexually transmitted diseases (STDs), specifically genital herpes. To make an appropriate recommendation, the pharmacist must determine the patient's risk for other STDs by finding out if she is in a mutually monogamous relationship. If yes, then a reasonable alternative for this couple is the use of polyurethane male or female condoms. Natural membrane male condoms could be recommended for pregnancy prevention if she does not have an outbreak of herpes; however, a polyurethane condom should be used during herpes outbreaks. The female condom may provide greater protection against transmission of herpes because of greater coverage of the perineum during intercourse. Provided that the patient is not allergic to spermicide, adding a vaginal spermicide should provide increased contraceptive benefit. If the patient is not in a mutually monogamous relationship, polyurethane condoms, male or female, should be used during all acts of intercourse.

This patient seems to be aware of the issues of contraception and STD transmission. Counsel on the issues of latex allergy and the use of alternate methods of contraception to protect herself. Stress the need for protection with each act of intercourse.

Case Study 9–1

The patient's history and symptoms of fever, muscle aches, and a dry, hacking cough suggest an acute nonproductive cough secondary to a viral infection. She has no exclusions to self-care with nonprescription medications. She has no history or symptoms that suggest a chronic underlying condition associated with cough, nor is she taking medications that can induce cough. Further, she is not taking any prescription or nonprescription medications known to interact with nonprescription cough medications.

Appropriate nondrug therapy includes adequate hydration and rest. The patient may also benefit from a cough suppressant, especially at bedtime. Available nonprescription cough suppressants include dextromethorphan, diphenhydramine, and codeine. (The patient lives in a state in which codeine-containing cough suppressants are available without a prescription.) Although all three agents may provide effective cough suppression, diphenhydramine and codeine cause significant drowsiness and impaired performance. However, the patient says codeine has been the most effective antitussive for her in the past.

Recommend a codeine-containing nonprescription antitussive but warn the patient about the side effects of codeine, such as drowsiness, dizziness, impaired performance, constipation, and stomach upset including nausea and vomiting. The initial dose is 10 mg every 4 hours as needed for cough. Advise the patient to drink eight to ten glasses of fluids (water, juices, milk) per day and to get adequate rest for the duration of the viral illness. She may wish to add fiber to her diet and/or take a stool softener while taking codeine. Advise the patient to avoid alcohol and any medications that cause drowsiness while taking codeine.

The patient's selection of Contac Night Cold and Flu caplets, which contain pseudoephedrine 60 mg, diphenhydramine 50 mg, and acetaminophen 650 mg, is not appropriate because the patient is not congested and may not always require the analgesic and/or antipyretic relief of acetaminophen. Recommend instead that the patient treat the fever and aches with acetaminophen 325 to 650 mg every 4 to 6 hours as needed.

Advise the patient to see her physician if (1) the cough persists for more than 7 to 10 days, (2) the cough becomes productive with thick yellow or green phlegm, (3) she develops a fever higher than 101.5°F, (4) she loses weight without trying, (5) she has drenching night sweats, (6) she coughs up blood, or (7) she develops a rash or any other new symptom.

Case Study 9–2

The patient's history and symptoms of nasal congestion; rhinorrhea; sneezing; itchy nose and throat; and red, itchy, swollen eyes suggest seasonal allergic rhinitis. He has no exclusions to self-care with nonprescription medications. He has no history or symptoms that suggest a chronic underlying condition that would be potentially exacerbated by the nonprescription medications commonly recommended to treat seasonal allergic rhinitis symptoms, and he is taking no medications that could be causing his symptoms.

Management of seasonal allergic rhinitis consists of avoiding exposure to allergens, pharmacotherapy, and immunotherapy. The patient has not received maximal pharmacotherapy. Whether he will comply with or can tolerate the recommend drug therapy is not known; therefore, immunotherapy is not an appropriate option at this time.

Counsel the patient about the role of pollen in causing his symptoms; tell him how to access and interpret local reports about daily pollen counts. Advise him that pollen counts are lowest in the evening and after rainstorms. Advise him to avoid outdoor activities as much as possible until after the first fall frost. Tell the patient to keep the windows in his house and car closed and to stay in an air-conditioned environment as much as possible during the allergy season.

Pharmacotherapy is targeted at specific symptoms. Advise the patient that an antihistamine–decongestant combination will provide convenient symptomatic relief for most of his symptoms but emphasize that drug treatment is symptomatic, not curative, and that no single drug or combination of drugs will alleviate all symptoms. The antihistamine will prevent the itching, sneezing, and rhinorrhea; the decongestant will treat the congestion. Advise him to take the medication regularly for the duration of his allergy season. Recommend a sustained-release product for convenience.

Counsel the patient about the sedation and impaired performance associated with all sedating antihistamines; advise him to avoid alcohol and all medications that may cause drowsiness while taking the sedating antihistamine. Inform the patient that less-sedating antihistamine–decongestant combination products are available by prescription. Caution him that nasal decongestant sprays are not useful in long-term conditions such as seasonal allergy because they cause rebound congestion when used for more than 3 to 5 days. Nasal and ocular allergy medications may help nasal and ocular symptoms, respectively, but will have little effect on this patient's other allergy symptoms. Advise the patient to start his allergy medications about a week before his symptoms usually start.

Caution the patient to see a physician if symptoms do not improve or if they worsen while taking the combination antihistamine–decongestant, or if he develops signs or symptoms of a secondary bacterial infection (purulent upper or lower airway secretions, fever higher than 101.5°F, chest congestion, shortness of breath, wheezing, significant ear pain, or rash).

Case Study 10–1

The 35-year-old patient, who was diagnosed with asthma at age 10 years, complains that his prescription asthma medication is not effective. Ask the patient about the frequency and severity of his asthma symptoms. Also, find out how long the effects of the inhaled bronchodilator last. Patients who require frequent doses of β-agonists have poorly controlled asthma and other interventions are recommended.

This patient's pattern of medication use is consistent with that of many patients with asthma. Patients rely on "rescue" therapies that provide immediate but temporary relief of symptoms. In this case, the patient is using a combination of rescue inhalers, albuterol and epinephrine. Nonprescription products for asthma contain nonselective, shorter-acting medications. Prescription medications are generally preferred for all patients with asthma. This patient's nonadherence to the inhaled corticosteroid is also common and may be related to a lack of understanding of the role of or concerns about the safety of inhaled steroids. The patient already has a prescription for a selective β-agonist, but may be trying to limit use by combining it with the nonprescription inhaler. This strategy is inappropriate. Monitoring the frequency of refills of short-acting β-agonist or the purchase of nonprescription inhalers is a good strategy for evaluating asthma control.

This patient has signs of poorly controlled asthma. Poor adherence with his inhaled corticosteroid therapy, poor inhalation technique, or failure to employ environmental control measures may be responsible for the poor control.

Caution the patient that overuse of albuterol, while not optimal, is not dangerous but that overuse of epinephrine, which is more likely because of its short half-life, may be associated with greater risk of cardiovascular adverse effects since it is a nonselective β-agonist.

One of the cornerstones of asthma management includes minimization or avoidance of triggers of asthma. Question the patient about his exposure to known triggers, and his adherence with avoidance techniques. Environmental control strategies can reduce the frequency and severity of asthma symptoms.

At this point, it is unknown whether the patient exhibits good inhalation technique. Such evaluation is appropriate since his technique will effect the benefit that he gets from each of his inhalation therapies. Poor inhalation technique with metered-dose inhalers is a common problem.

Review with the patient the role, purpose, and proper use of each medication to ensure that he understands the various beneficial effects of each. Counsel him about long-term control therapies and quick relief agents, and provide a written self-management plan and action plan to follow. These strategies help the patient be an active participant in his own care, improve asthma control, and reduce utilization of resources. Pharmacists are in an excellent position to collaborate with other clinicians and the patient in developing these plans.

Pharmacists should focus on other services that can be offered to the patient with asthma. Educational materials and programs can be provided, strategies and products to reduce exposure to asthma triggers, and self-monitoring devices (e.g., peak flow meters) are all examples of how pharmacists can help patients. In special situations, pharmacists could also provide other equipment, such as nebulizers for home use.

The patient's symptoms warrant evaluation by a physician. A short course of prednisone may be needed to regain control of his asthma. The pharmacist should contact the physician and discuss the findings about the patient's adherence with therapy and his inhalation technique.

Case Study 10–2

A history of frequent, recurrent colds, as in this 7-year-old patient, can be an indication of undiagnosed asthma. Viral upper respiratory tract infections are the most common trigger of an acute asthma exacerbation, especially in children. A brief review of the patient's history can also provide additional information about triggers that will be valuable in developing a management strategy. Information about allergies to drugs, foods, and other substances, which should be recorded in the patient profile, will be useful in advising about management strategies.

Consider other potential causes of the symptoms. The presence of upper airway allergies can also be investigated since they frequently coexist with asthma. Inquire about emergency department visits to obtain some indication about the severity of past symptoms.

Determine whether any previous therapies, including nonprescription medications, have been helpful. The mother has previously suggested some cold symptoms, however, the only apparent symptoms have been wheezing, chest congestion, cough, and shortness of breath. The decongestant and antihistamine that she has selected will not provide direct benefit for these symptoms.

At this point, the patient is not diagnosed. The most appropriate intervention may be referring the patient to a physician for assessment and diagnosis and implementing therapy with a short-acting selective β-agonist. It is appropriate to encourage the mother to see a physician and to contact the physician to discuss the information gathered during the intervention.

Counsel the mother and the patient on common asthma symptoms. The onset, intensity, and duration of asthma symptoms vary from patient to patient. Collecting information about a specific patient's pattern is helpful in educating and counseling about asthma and in developing an action plan. The action plan should indicate when the patient and mother should seek medical attention based on the severity and duration of symptoms.

Cigarette smoke is one of the most common irritants identified as an asthma trigger. Children of parents who smoke have a higher incidence of allergies and asthma. The father should be encouraged to stop smoking in the interest of his child's health.

Nonprescription medications for asthma would not be appropriate in this case. Allergy medication may be needed intermittently if allergies are also present. Antihistamines can be taken safely by the asthma patient. A peak flow meter may also be useful in the self-monitoring of asthma.

Educating the patient about asthma, allergen avoidance, and self-monitoring using the peak flow meter are cornerstone activities in asthma management. These activities can be performed by a pharmacist who is providing pharmaceutical care for patients with asthma. In this case, the patient should be advised not to use nonprescription asthma inhalers, particularly if he participates in organized sports activities. Ingredients in nonprescription inhalers are usually not approved for use by various sport authority bodies.

Nonprescription products for asthma contain nonselective, shorter-acting medications. Prescription medications are generally preferred for all patients with asthma.

Case Study 11–1

The patient's substernal chest pain should cause concern about abdominal versus cardiac causes. The occurrence of pain after meals and when the patient lies down strongly suggests reflux. Further questioning could help elucidate factors that contribute to or eliminate the pain.

Advise the patient to lose weight, avoid fatty foods (e.g., "fast foods"), and decrease or eliminate caffeine intake, alcohol, smoking, and foods known to exacerbate reflux. Also, recommend that dinner be eaten sooner than 3 hours before sleeping and that the head of the bed be elevated.

If pharmacologic therapy is necessary or desired, any of the available histamine$_2$-receptor antagonists (H_2RAs)—famotidine, cimetidine, ranitidine, or nizatidine—could be tried in addition to the nondrug measures. Warn the patient to take no more than the recommended dose of the selected product and not to take it during pregnancy, should that be or become an issue.

The nondrug measures and nonprescription H_2RAs constitute a basic plan of action. Antacids could also be used as needed. Base antacid selection on the patient's preference for taste; recommend a dose that would provide between 40 to 80 mEq ANC. Advise the patient to consult a physician if her symptoms worsen or persist.

Ensure that the patient understands the importance of the dietary and lifestyle modifications. Explain the proper use of the recommended nonprescription medications, and ensure that the patient knows the signs and symptoms that require medical attention.

Case Study 11– 2

The patient's fatigue and abdominal pain are alarming symptoms. She has a history consistent with the possibility of peptic ulcer disease (PUD). Contributing factors include family history and use of NSAIDs, among others. Blood loss from a bleeding ulcer or gastritis could be contributing to her fatigue. Typical signs of bleeding include dark-colored stools; however, she is also taking an iron preparation, which can produce the same effect. Her weight gain could be a sign of overeating as a way to ameliorate the abdominal pain. Gastric acid output is greatest at night. The absence of food or antacids in the stomach to act as buffers appears to be causing the abdominal pain. Further questioning could help elucidate factors that contribute to or eliminate the pain.

Aluminum hydroxide has a low acid-neutralizing capacity and can cause constipation, one of the patient's complaints. The patient's iron supplement can also contribute to developing constipation. An antacid containing a mixture of magnesium and aluminum salts would be a better choice in this case.

Cigarette smoking and the use of ethanol and caffeine can contribute to enhanced gastric acid production. Advise the patient to stop these activities.

Refer the patient to a physician for further evaluation of the likelihood of PUD and possible upper gastrointestinal bleeding. PUD will require prescription drug management. If a gastric ulcer has resulted from NSAID use, prostaglandin therapy may be necessary. In the interim, recommend an antacid product with a mixture of magnesium and aluminum salts to control pain.

Stress the importance of discontinuing cigarette smoking and of dietary modifications. Ensure that the patient knows the signs and symptoms that require medical attention.

Case Study 12–1

Because the patient has recently retired from a physically demanding job, his initial complaints of constipation may have developed as a result of reduced physical activity. The patient associated poor sleep with the constipation, so he initiated a course of therapy of Benadryl to help him sleep better. Unfortunately, the Benadryl's anticholinergic activity has likely contributed to his problem with constipation, rather than cured it. The patient is also taking prescription medications that have constipating side effects: Capoten and Pravachol.

Neither of the patient-selected laxatives—Fleet Mineral Oil Enema and Kondremul—would be the best choice for this patient. The mineral oil enema, although of some usefulness, may lead to soiling and rectal irritation beyond the time of the bowel movement that the patient desires. Kondremul also contains mineral oil. Even though it is emulsified, mineral oil can lead to problems in elderly patients, especially aspiration of the droplets into the lungs when reclining. Any patient with a history of, or characteristics that might suggest the occurrence of, nighttime reflux would be at risk. A lipoid pneumonia may result.

Administering the Kondremul would be easier for the patient than would the Fleet's enema. If an enema had been the best choice, the pharmacist would have to instruct the patient on the appropriate use of the enema.

The patient's retirement 2 years earlier indicates his physical activity may have declined. As a result, he has become more susceptible to constipation. Encourage the patient to increase his physical activity as a countermeasure to developing constipation. Also, evaluate his dietary fiber and fluid intake; then counsel him on how to increase fiber and fluid intake. Advise the patient to increase physical activity if only by walking 30 minutes every day. If your assessment suggests his dietary fiber is not likely to increase, recommend a bulk-forming laxative. Advise the patient to take the bulk-forming laxative with a full glass of liquid, such as fruit juice or water, and to follow it with another full glass. Instruct him not to take any other medication within 2 hours of taking the laxative. Because the client is elderly, advise him not to take mineral oil, saline cathartics, or stimulant laxatives.

Case Study 12–2

Several factors are possibly contributing to this patient's constipation: late pregnancy, use of Vitron–C, and irritable bowel syndrome. Ask the patient to describe her usual bowel movement in terms of frequency, consistency, and quantity. Within the scope of the patient's physical tolerance, exercise is allowed during pregnancy. Ask about the obstetrician's instructions regarding exercise. Ensure that the patient is not exceeding the limits of what has been prescribed for her stage of pregnancy.

Advise the patient to avoid using the milk of magnesia and cascara. Milk of magnesia could lead to excessive fluid loss and resultant electrolyte abnormalities, while cascara could lead to discomforting abdominal cramping. This patient is a candidate for a stool softener.

Encourage the patient to eat foods that promote healthy gastrointestinal function and to add fiber to the diet, either by increasing the daily amount of dietary fiber or by adding a bulk-forming laxative to her drug regimen. These laxatives now have dual labeling as a laxative and a nutritional supplement, so adding a bulk-former as a nutritional supplement is now possible. Encourage the patient to drink eight or more glasses of water daily. Recommend docusate as an alternative to soften the stool.

Case Study 13–1

The patient's complaints of sudden onset of watery stool, nausea, vomiting, and fever of 99°F (37°C) indicate infectious diarrhea, either viral or bacterial. Fever is the key indicator of infectious diarrhea. The patient's history rules out food intolerance and drug side effects. The patient describes the diarrhea as sudden onset that suggests an "acute" type of diarrhea, excluding chronic diarrhea causes. Because the patient does not report travel outside the United States or to mountainous or lake areas, traveler's diarrhea and *Giardia* are less likely causes.

Etiology of the complaint and degree of dehydration are the primary criteria for determining whether self-treatment is appropriate. Mild and moderate dehydration can usually be managed with oral rehydration therapy, but severe diarrhea needs intravenous therapy. The passing of four to five watery stools, plus low-grade fever, indicates moderate dehydration. The pharmacist should recommend household fluids (e.g., sport drinks) and salty crackers or oral rehydration products (e.g., Rehydralyte or Pedialyte) to manage the diarrhea.

For the next 24 hours, the patient should follow the rehydration therapy plan as described above. The patient can eat easily digestible foods such as soups, broths, bananas, cereal, potatoes, and rice but should avoid spicy, fatty, and dairy foods.

Loperamide, 4 mg initially, then 2 mg after each loose stool up to 16 mg/day, would provide symptomatic relief. Used as indicated, loperamide has minimal side effects except for dizziness and constipation. If the diarrhea persists beyond 48 hours, the patient should seek medical care. If the patient has an invasive (e.g., *Shigella*) or inflammatory (e.g., *Clostridium difficile*) bacterial infection, the diarrhea may worsen. In this case, the patient should seek medical care.

Instruct the patient to follow label directions for loperamide and the oral rehydration solution and to adhere to the dietary plan. Advise the patient to seek medical care if the condition worsens or persists beyond 48 hours. Explain that an antipyretic drug (e.g., aspirin or acetaminophen) may be taken for the fever.

Case Study 13–2

The onset of the patient's symptoms (loose, watery stools and abdominal cramps) after 3 days of taking amoxicillin indicates antibiotic-associated diarrhea. If the diarrhea continues, the patient may have pseudomembranous colitis secondary to *Clostridium difficile* overgrowth, a condition that requires medical treatment.

According to physical findings, the patient is mildly dehydrated. As in Case Study 13–1, consumption of household fluids or commercial rehydration solutions are appropriate treatment.

The patient can manage her diet with household remedies such as soups, sport drinks, and a low-residue diet but should avoid fatty, spicy, and dairy foods. After the diarrhea subsides, she can return to her normal diet, as tolerated.

An adsorbent such as attapulgite 30 mL taken after each loose stool is appropriate. If bacterial gastrointestinal infectious diarrhea is suspected, the pharmacist should not recommend loperamide. Antiperistaltic drugs may prolong certain invasive or inflammatory gastrointestinal infections.

Advise the patient to contact her physician to discuss the continued use of amoxicillin or an alternative antibiotic. Also advise her to seek medical care if her condition worsens or persists after 48 hours of treatment. Explain that she may continue the ibuprofen as needed for muscle aches, but that she should consult a physician if she develops a fever.

Case Study 14–1

The patient's signs and symptoms include red blood in the stool and rectal irritation, burning, and itching. Hemorrhoids and anal fissures can cause bleeding during defecation. Also, bleeding without pain during defecation is one of the most common symptoms of hemorrhoids. External hemorrhoids can be painful; however, internal hemorrhoids rarely cause pain. Bleeding from anal fissures is usually accompanied by pain. Patients with an anal fissure will probably see blood on the bathroom tissue.

Peptic ulcers and colorectal cancer are less likely causes of the bleeding. Black tarry stools are more common with bleeding peptic ulcers; however, red blood may appear in the stool if the condition is severe enough.

Rectal irritation, burning, and itching are commonly associated with hemorrhoids. Allergic reactions and pinworm infection are less likely causes of these symptoms. The allergic reactions are usually to dyes in clothing, laundry detergent, or perfumed bathroom tissue. Although rectal itching is common with pinworms, pinworm infection is much more common in young children.

Further questioning might help to identify the cause of the signs and symptoms; however, patients presenting with blood in the stool should be referred to a physician immediately.

Case Study 14–2

The patient's signs and symptoms include rectal itching and constipation, so she may have hemorrhoids. First, the mechanical and physiologic body changes that occur during pregnancy frequently cause constipation. Second, a common side effect of iron supplementation is constipation. A third likely cause is hemorrhoids, which may lead to constipation or vice versa.

To better determine the cause of the constipation, ask the patient to describe her normal bowel habits and her diet. Ask whether she had constipation with previous pregnancies. Then, ask how long she has been taking the iron supplement and docusate and whether they were recommended by her physician. Next, ask about her use of other medications, especially those that may cause constipation. Finally, to rule out hemorrhoids, ask whether she has seen blood in the stool or on the bathroom tissue and whether she has had lower gastrointestinal problems before.

If the stool softener is not relieving the constipation, recommend a bulk-forming laxative (e.g., psyllium) taken with adequate fluid, as well as an increased consumption of dietary fiber. If the constipation persists, refer the patient to a physician.

Hemorrhoids are a likely cause of the rectal itching, a disorder that often occurs during pregnancy. In fact, pregnancy is the most common cause of hemorrhoids in young women.

Less likely causes of the rectal itching are pinworm infection or allergies to dyes in clothing, laundry detergent, or perfumed bathroom tissue. Pinworm infection, however, is much more common in young children.

To better determine the cause of itching, ask the patient whether other symptoms are present and, if so, to describe them. Determine whether the patient has a history of allergies. If so, remind the patient of the causes of allergic reactions in the anal area. (See Case Study 14–1.)

Whether rectal itching was caused by an allergic reaction or hemorrhoids, recommend a topical external analgesic or hemorrhoidal preparation to relieve it. Explain the proper use of the recommended product, as well as good hygiene habits for the anal area. Advise the patient to use the anorectal product for no more than 7 days and to consult a physician if the itching is not alleviated. (Protectants are the only intrarectal products that should be used by pregnant women.)

Case Study 15–1

Intense perianal itching, especially at night, is the primary complaint of the 5-year-old patient. If the presence of pinworms has not been confirmed, ask the mother to visually inspect the child's anal area after the child has gone to bed. Treatment begins with an accurate assessment. If pinworms are suspected as the cause of symptoms, pyrantel pamoate is the only nonprescription product approved for pinworm infection. Pinworm infections can be easily spread to others; therefore, treatment of the patient requires treating all household contacts.

Provide information about treating family members and methods of preventing reinfection. Explain that the dose of pyrantel pamoate is based on body weight (5 mg/pound or 11/mg/kg, not to exceed 1 g). Refer children under 2 years of age to a physician for treatment.

Explain the proper administration and possible adverse effects of the recommended product. Educate the patient about drug and nondrug measures.

Case Study 15–2

The patient's passing of a large (6 inch) worm could be related to the use of human fertilizer ("night soil") and poor handwashing. These activities increase the risk of ascariasis. If other household members have similar symptoms, the infection was probably transmitted through poor hygiene practices. Fever, weight loss, and failure to grow are common symptoms of worm infections. Refer this patient to a health care provider.

Case Study 16–1

The treatment of nausea and vomiting in a child or adult should focus on identifying and correcting the underlying cause. Most cases of acute vomiting require no specific treatment since they are mild, self-limiting, resolve spontaneously, and require only symptomatic treatment. One of the more common causes of vomiting in children is acute viral gastroenteritis. Treatment of gastroenteritis is directed primarily at preventing and correcting dehydration and electrolyte disturbances. Lost fluids should generally be replaced within 24 hours. Oral rehydration solutions may be used in mild cases. If severe diarrhea or vomiting persists for more than 24–48 hours, the child should be referred to a health care provider for evaluation.

The use of antiemetics in children is controversial. Some clinicians question the wisdom and value of treating children with antiemetics in an acute, self-limiting disorder. It is suggested that vomiting in gastroenteritis is a host defense process that sheds the pathogen and should therefore not be suppressed. Therefore, recommending the use of an oral rehydration solution would be an appropriate step in the self-treatment of nausea and vomiting in this child.

Signs and symptoms or medical conditions associated with nausea and vomiting that necessitate referral to a health care provider for evaluation and treatment include:

- Blood in the vomitus. (No blood reported by parent.)
- Abdominal pain or distention. (No pain or distention reported by parent.)
- Prolonged nausea and vomiting (longer than 24–48 hours), especially for children under 1 year of age, or projectile vomiting. (Child's vomiting began less than 24 hours earlier.)
- Dehydration. (Question parent regarding signs of dehydration, such as dry mouth, excessive thirst, little or no urination, dizziness, and lightheadedness.)
- Weight loss of more than 5% of body weight. (Assess for signs and symptoms of dehydration or possible underlying medical condition such as diabetes.)
- Fever. (Parent reports that child is afebrile.)
- Severe headache. (No headache reported by parent; however, headache is difficult to determine in a 2-year old child due to communication issues.)
- Change in behavior or alertness. (No change in behavior or alertness reported by parent.)
- Pregnancy. (Not applicable in this case.)
- Presence of diabetes or other medical conditions that may be affected by lack of nutritional intake or missed doses of oral medications. (Parent reports no medical conditions or medication use.)
- Recent trauma, particularly a significant head injury. (No recent trauma reported by parent.)
- Suspected poisoning. (No poisoning reported by parent. However, this is important to assess. Question parent about the potential for poison ingestion.)

Since vomiting has lasted less than 24 hours and the child has no medical conditions and takes no medications, she may be a candidate for self-treatment. Consider self-treatment if there are no signs or symptoms of dehydration or underlying medical condition and poison ingestion is not suspected.

In a child with vomiting, the oral rehydration solution should be given very slowly, starting with 5 to 10 mL every 10 minutes. The quantity of fluid may be increased as tolerated. If vomiting and diarrhea stop after 12 to 24 hours of clear liquids, the child should be gradually returned to a regular diet over the next 2 or 3 days.

Advise the child's parent that

- Nausea and vomiting is a common, usually self-limiting condition.
- Most cases of acute vomiting require only symptomatic treatment since they are self-limiting and resolve spontaneously.
- Prolonged nausea and vomiting (more than 24 to 48 hours) or a change or worsening of symptoms requires immediate referral to a health care provider.
- Loss of fluids and inability to eat or drink associated with nausea and vomiting can result in dehydration and electrolyte disturbances.
- Oral rehydration solution can be used to prevent dehydration secondary to vomiting and diarrhea.

Assist the parent with the selection of an appropriate oral rehydration solution product. Provide both written and verbal instruction for proper administration of oral rehydration solution. Offer further assistance if necessary. Provide parent with a method to reach someone if she has additional questions or concerns. Review signs and symptoms that require medical evaluation. Perform a telephone follow-up assessment of patient within 24 hours to determine whether symptoms have improved, changed, or worsened.

When a child experiences nausea and vomiting, the child's health care provider should be contacted if

- The child is less than 1 year of age.
- The child refuses to drink.
- Urination has not occurred in the past 8 to 12 hours.
- The child appears lethargic or is crying.
- Weight loss or dehydration occurs.
- Vomiting occurs with each feeding.
- Vomiting is repeatedly projectile.
- Vomitus contains red, black, or green fluid.
- Vomiting is associated with diarrhea, distended abdomen, fever, or severe headache.
- Vomiting occurs following a head injury.
- Poisoning is suspected.
- Vomiting occurs with recurrent, severe, acute abdominal pain.

Case Study 17–1

Robitussin DM, which was consumed by the 18-month-old patient, contains guaifenesin (100 mg/5 mL) and dextromethorphan HBr (15 mg/5 mL). Although guaifenesin is essentially nontoxic, dextromethorphan can product significant toxicity, including depression of the central nervous and respiratory systems. Gastrointestinal decontamination is normally considered for ingestions of 10 mg/kg or more.

The first step in assessing this situation is to obtain more information from the parents, particularly the child's weight and amount of medication ingested. Assuming the patient weighs 11 kg, gastrointestinal decontamination should be considered if 100 mg/kg (a little more than 7 teaspoons) of the medication was ingested. Assuming that 2 ounces of medication are missing from the bottle (the mother is sure she has given 3 teaspoons of the medication and some has spilled), the amount ingested is less than 10 mg/kg. Therefore, observation at home is the appropriate recommendation. If more than that was ingested, treatment at an emergency treatment facility would have been appropriate given that the child is drowsy and is not a good candidate for use of an at-home emetic. Provide information about poison prevention to the parent and advise that a bottle of ipecac syrup be kept in the home.

Case Study 18–1

Skin problems such as the patient's itching around the stoma are usually caused by pouches that fit improperly, leakage of stool on the skin, hair follicle irritation, perspiration, misuse of skin barriers, or fungal overgrowth caused by antibiotic therapy.

The primary cause of the irritation should be corrected first, which may require consultation with a physician or WOCN. The following techniques may provide symptomatic relief: (1) using a heat lamp or hair dryer to dry the skin before applying the appliance; (2) sprinkling a small amount of powder (e.g., karaya, Stomahesive) on the skin, wiping off the excess, and then blotting with a skin sealant to seal the powder to the skin (powder the skin on which the pouch lies, not under the face plate); and (3) discontinuing the Benadryl because it is a cream and the area should be kept dry.

Concerning the patient's other complaints, the most likely cause of the diarrhea is the antibiotic therapy. Treatment of the diarrhea with Pepto-Bismol is the most likely cause of the black stools.

Refer the patient to a physician or WOCN to assess itching, diarrhea, swollen stoma, and appliance fit and application. Encourage the patient to increase fluid and electrolyte consumption. Recommend care in removing the appliance so that the patient does not irritate the stoma.

Case Study 18–2

The Lasix therapy is the probable cause of the patient's increased urine output. Vitamin B complex is a possible cause of her other complaint: the odor in her pouch.

Contact the patient's physician to discuss the use of Lasix in a patient with a urinary diversion. Suggest an alternative antihypertensive. Ask the patient whether Tums is being taken at a physician's suggestion. If not, suggest that the patient discontinue taking Tums because of the risk of urinary calculi or calcium-stone formation. If yes, contact the patient's physician to discuss the use of Tums. Suggest the use of a non–calcium-containing antacid (e.g., Amphojel, Riopan).

Determine whether the onset of stomach distress coincided with any change in therapy such as the initiation of Vitamin B complex. If Vitamin B complex is to be continued, suggest adding a deodorant to the pouch or using a pouch with a charcoal filter.

Make sure that the patient understands the importance of using the non–calcium-containing antacid as well as the effects that her medication(s) are having on her condition. Advise her to contact her physician or WOCN if the increased output continues.

Case Study 18–3

The patient's complaint of irritation of the skin around the stoma may be related to the use of Dial soap. Cleansing the area with warm water only should be adequate. Make sure that the patient understands the importance of a rigorous regimen to clean the ostomy as well as the recommended cleaning procedures.

Advise the patient that removing all of the cement or skin barrier left on the skin is not necessary. Aggressive cleaning may abrade the skin. Suggest that the patient visit his WOCN to review his pouching procedure.

The two-piece appliance system is a good choice for this patient because it allows for quick pouch changes, flexibility in positioning the pouch, and extended wearing time. The latter reduces the number of times the skin around the stoma is cleaned.

The patient's medication history indicates a possible drug-absorption problem. Long-acting medications such as Chlor-Trimeton 12 mg are often not completely absorbed in patients with an ostomy. More dependable absorption may be obtained with the use of a short-acting product such as Chlor-Trimeton 4 mg.

Case Study 19–1

The patient's complaint of facial flushing is likely related to the use of niacin. Although niacin is used to lower cholesterol levels, the patient should use immediate-acting niacin tablets, rather than the long-acting niacin tablets that were purchased. Further, buying niacin and other vitamins from a health food store provides no assurance of the release pattern of the drug. In other words, depending on the release-mechanism and the quality control procedures of the company, the purchased niacin may disintegrate rapidly and dissolve, causing rapid absorption, high blood levels, and the resultant flushing experienced by the patient. Advise the patient to work with the physician in developing a dosing schedule for immediate-release niacin tablets.

Case Study 19–2

The patient's primary complaint is fatigue. The hemoglobin level of 9.5 g/dL confirms that the patient's diet is insufficient in iron and supports the prescribing of the iron supplement. The long-acting iron preparations are generally more expensive, however, and may not have been a wise choice for the patient's financial circumstances.

Advise the patient that the switch to the nonprescription iron supplement and the subsequent use of an antacid for stomach distress has decreased the bioavailability of the iron. Recommend that the patient take the nonprescription iron product with meals to lessen the stomach distress. Although less iron will be absorbed when taken with food, this action is preferable to stopping the iron or taking it concurrently with an antacid.

Case Study 20–1

The infant's symptoms of the past 2 days—frequent spitting up; irritability; frequent loose, watery stools; and mild fever—are consistent with those of self-limited viral gastroenteritis. They may also be signs of a non-self-limiting condition.

While the infant's pediatrician should be contacted about these symptoms, the pharmacist can perform a more thorough assessment. The following questions may provide important additional assessment information: Which formula was your baby eating prior to his spitting up and loose stools? How long has he been taking this formula? Have you been preparing it according to the label instructions or other specific instructions from your baby's physician? The pharmacist can take note of the type of formula being used (e.g. standard milk-based, soy, therapeutic, hypercaloric) and the formula preparation procedure, since this gastrointestinal symptomatology may be related to formula intolerance, use of a hypercaloric formula, or an inappropriate formula concentration resulting from improper preparation.

Regardless of the cause of the clinical symptoms, the infant is at risk for dehydration. The pharmacist can assess the presence of symptoms of dehydration by asking about or observing whether mucous membranes are dry, the fontanelle is sunken, urine output (or number of wet diapers) is significantly decreased, or weight loss has occurred in conjunction with the 2-day symptomatology. If one or more of these symptoms are present, the infant's physician should be contacted for further follow-up and treatment.

If the symptoms are determined to be related to a self-limiting viral gastroenteritis, the usual formula should be discontinued and the infant should receive an oral electrolyte solution for 24 hours. The gastrointestinal symptoms will likely subside; then the usual formula can be resumed at half-strength or full-strength depending on the severity of the symptoms. If the diarrhea continues, it may be due to a secondary lactase deficiency associated with viral gastroenteritis. In this case, a lactose-free formula (soy-based or lactose-free variety of standard) may be beneficial for an additional 1 to 3 weeks. Once the diarrhea is resolved, the usual formula can be resumed. If the diarrhea still persists after these measures are taken, the infant's pediatrician may desire to change formulas or consider further evaluation.

Case Study 21–1

The patient obviously has high weight-loss expectations from the chromium product. Anytime a reference is made using terminology such as "miracle," "breakthrough" or other similar language, it suggests that a patient is looking for the "quick fix." Since this patient often comes into the pharmacy asking about the latest diet plan or product, she has probably tried other weight-loss measures without success. She probably does not have good insight into the concept of an integrated approach to losing weight. Like many individuals, she wants something that will safely and rapidly "melt away" extra pounds, but require little effort on her part. The reality is, any weight-loss program requires tremendous discipline by the dieter to be effective.

At 5 foot 2 inches tall and 182 pounds, this patient's body mass index (BMI) is 33.3. She is obese by current standards. If she has a waist circumference of greater than 88 cm, she is at very high risk for Type 2 diabetes, hypertension, and cardiovascular disease. If her waist circumference is less than or equal to 88 cm, she is still at high risk for these disorders. Her desire to lose weight should be applauded and she should be encouraged to find the right weight-loss program. If she already has any risk factors (e.g., established coronary heart disease, other atherosclerotic diseases, Type 2 diabetes, and sleep apnea), she should be apprised of her special risk for future health problems.

The patient probably has had difficulty adhering to a restricted-calorie diet and a suitable exercise program. Referral to a nutritionist or dietitian would be a good recommendation if she is open to this advice. Participation with a support group might provide the help that she needs to stay with a weight-loss regimen.

The medical evidence for chromium's effectiveness is meager. Explain that this is no "miracle" drug and that more proven medications would be a better idea, if pharmacologic management is desired.

If the pharmacist feels that an appetite suppressant would help the patient stick to her diet and exercise program, a product containing phenylpropanolamine (PPA) 75 mg in sustained-release dosage form is appropriate. If the patient has high blood pressure, heart disease, thyroid disease or diabetes, she is not a good candidate for PPA. Emphasize in clear and certain terms that this medication is only an adjunct to the caloric restriction and exercise program. She must understand that there are no weight-loss medications that will work without restricting dietary caloric intake.

Case Study 21–2

This patient, who is 5 foot 6 inches tall and weighs 128 pounds, does not need to lose weight. Her BMI is 20.7 and, if anything, she is underweight. She should be instructed to cease taking the diet caplets.

With young women, there is always the chance of an underlying eating disorder. The patient's body image (note her reference to the "ugly fat") may be distorted. The pharmacist should explore in more detail why the teenager thinks she needs to lose weight. In the final analysis, it would be inappropriate to even imply that she should be dieting to lose weight.

Even if she were overweight, the patient suffers from seasonal allergies for which she takes a medicine containing PPA. Recommending a nonprescription weight-loss product that also contains PPA would be imprudent. Because most patients are unaware that PPA is both an oral nasal decongestant and an appetite suppressant, it is predictable that some patients will be "doubling up" on this ingredient. By taking a thorough medication history, including all nonprescription drugs used, therapeutic duplications can be avoided.

Encourage the teenager and her mother to see the family physician if the teenager insists on dieting. Malnutrition, electrolyte disturbances, and bone loss can accompany certain eating disorders. Make sure the patient is not engaging in dangerous weight-loss methods such as taking strong laxatives or self-inducing vomiting. Counsel the teenager and her mother about taking medications, either prescription or nonprescription, without fully understanding their potential risks and benefits.

Case Study 22–1

The patient presents with a chronic eye condition that, according to her medical history, is amenable to self-treatment. The patient's age, postmenopausal status, and symptoms of burning and watering eyes make dry eye a likely diagnosis. Assess whether the patient has used eye drops or ointment to manage previous occurrences of similar symptoms. If so, ask the patient whether the medications were effective.

The patient chose a nonpreserved ophthalmic ointment, a preserved ophthalmic ointment, and a decongestant solution to treat her symptoms. However, first-line therapy of dry eye is typically an artificial tear solution. Ointments are added if drop therapy is inadequate. Accordingly, assess her need to use an artificial tear solution during waking hours, as well as her need for a preserved versus nonpreserved solution. Other factors to assess include whether she needs to apply a lubricating ointment at bedtime, what the cost-versus-benefit ratio is of the selected product(s), and whether a single product will relieve the symptoms.

If an ointment is indicated, select only one product and instruct the patient when (at bedtime) and how to apply the ointment. During patient counseling/education, explain the limited effectiveness of ophthalmic decongestants for the symptoms (i.e., discourage their use); explain the chronic nature of the condition; suggest environmental modifications if fans, air conditioners, etc., exacerbate symptoms; and advise the patient to see an eye practitioner if the symptoms persist.

Case Study 22-2

The patient presents with a known diagnosis of pediculosis. He has chosen three nonprescription products as an adjunct to the prescription product. Both ophthalmic products are good choices for the condition. The lid scrub product will mechanically remove lice and nits, and the ophthalmic lubricant will suffocate any remaining organisms.

Explain the methods of applying the products, as well as the fact that the ophthalmic lubricant may blur vision and that the nonophthalmic product (Nix) should not contact the eye surface. In addition, emphasize strategies to prevent spread of the infestation, such as washing bed linens or contaminated clothing.

Case Study 23–1

The patient, who began wearing contact lenses 2 months earlier, complains of eye discomfort. Although the patient is complying with most steps of her prescribed lens care regimen, she needs to add an enzymatic cleaner to the regimen. Because she uses Ultra-Care to disinfect her lenses, the enzymatic cleaner of choice is Ultrazyme. Advise the patient that this product can be used concurrently with Ultra-Care, thus eliminating adding an extra step to the care regimen. Instruct her to add one Ultrazyme tablet to the lens case containing the Ultra-Care solution at least once a week.

Advise her to contact her lens care prescriber if the lens discomfort continues.

Case Study 23–2

The patient, who has been wearing soft contact lenses for only 3 weeks, asks about the proper care of his lenses. The patient is presently not cleaning his soft contact lenses properly. He should clean his lenses with Opti-Clean II immediately after removing them from the eyes. He should also add an enzyme cleaner to his regimen and disinfect his lenses daily.

After consulting with the lens prescriber, recommend a chemical preservative or hydrogen peroxide disinfection regimen. A suitable chemical preservative disinfection regimen for this patient includes the concurrent use of Opti-Free disinfecting solution and Opti-Free Supra-Clens, an enzymatic cleaner. Advise the patient to (1) add one drop of Supra-Clens to the disinfecting solution in each well of the storage case and (2) disinfect the lenses for at least 4 hours to ensure elimination of all microorganisms.

Advise the patient not to store his lenses in the aerosolized saline although the saline can be used to rinse his lenses just before insertion. Stress that he should also follow the care regimen for the lens case as described in Chapter 23.

If the patient continues to experience blurred vision or other lens-related problems develop, refer him to his lens prescriber for further follow-up.

Case Study 24–1

The patient's lack of other symptoms besides mild, partial hearing loss coupled with her previous history of excessive earwax does not indicate cerumen impaction, nor does her medical history suggest other reasons for her slight hearing loss. Thus the FDA-approved nonprescription cerumen-softening agent, carbamide peroxide 6.5% in anhydrous glycerin, can be tried. The patient should be congratulated for not making matters worse by trying to dislodge the earwax using a foreign object.

Explain to the patient the purpose of earwax and the potential dangers of improper removal attempts, such as earwax impaction or infection subsequent to skin damage. Advise that using a washcloth-draped finger is the only recommended method for cleaning the ear canal and preventing this damage. Explain that cerumen-softening agents do not dissolve cerumen but do soften it so that it can readily be removed with gentle flushing, using body temperature water and a rubber bulb ear syringe. Give proper directions for use of the agents and ear syringes. Monitor for adverse reactions and follow up in 4 days to assess effectiveness. If symptoms persist after 4 days of proper treatment, refer the patient to a physician.

Case Study 24–2

The patient's symptoms, pain, inflammation, itching, and discharge occurring together, indicate a high likelihood of external otitis. The FDA has approved no nonprescription products to treat external otitis (swimmer's ear). Referral to a physician is warranted for proper diagnosis and treatment.

Repeated exposure of the ear canal to water can cause tissue maceration and/or swelling of cerumen, thereby trapping water in the canal. Bacteria and fungus grow well under these conditions. While hydrogen peroxide may be useful as an anti-infective, it is not effective at removing water from the ear. Furthermore, repeated use of undiluted or aqueous solutions of hydrogen peroxide can cause tissue maceration, which, in turn, provides access for pathogens. Using a foreign object to scratch the inner ear canal can also further abrade the skin.

For the patient's future use, explain proper ear hygiene and appropriate treatment for water-clogged ear. While not appropriate in this case, appropriate agents for treating water-clogged ears are 95% isopropyl alcohol in 5% anhydrous glycerin or a 50:50 mixture of 95% isopropyl alcohol and 5% acetic acid.

Case Study 26–1

The patient reports tooth pain that is in two quadrants and that occurs when drinking hot liquids and brushing teeth. Tooth pain triggered or worsened by hot, cold, or contact (chewing, brushing) may indicate pulpal response to decay, damaged dentition, or hypersensitivity. In this case, the patient's dentist diagnosed hypersensitivity. Although the patient used the sample desensitization toothpaste provided by the dentist, she does not think the problem is resolved.

Explain to the patient that exposed dentin allows stimuli (e.g., heat, cold, sweetness, contact) to reach nerve fibers within the pulp. Explain also that recession of gum tissue, braces, or trauma (e.g., excessive brushing with abrasive dentifrices or hard brushes) can erode the enamel layer of the teeth, thereby exposing areas of the dentin.

Tooth desensitization ingredients act on the dentin to block hyperperception of stimuli. The effect is cumulative and takes several days or up to 2 weeks to occur. The patient has not used the desensitization toothpaste long enough to see results. Recommend a nonabrasive formula that contains potassium nitrate 5% as the desensitization agent in combination with fluoride for prevention of caries. Because the exposed areas of dentin are susceptible to root caries, a nonprescription fluoride rinse can be recommended for an anticaries effect.

Explain to the patient that she must use the dentifrice for as long as the sensitivity is present or as directed by her dentist. About one-fourth of adults develop chronic tooth sensitivity.

Stress that the dentifrice is a therapeutic, not a cosmetic, agent. Suggest that she experiment with flavors or brands to find a more pleasant flavor, but advise her that she may have to get used to the medicinal flavor. Counsel her to apply a 1-inch strip of dentifrice to a soft toothbrush and to brush for at least 1 minute twice a day. Explain that a soft toothbrush prevents further gum recession or enamel damage.

Advise the patient not to use a cosmetic toothpaste with whitening or stain-removing properties at the same time that she is using a desensitization toothpaste. Explain the abrasive properties of these cosmetic toothpastes. Although not applicable in this case, do not recommend desensitization toothpastes for children younger than 12 years.

Case Study 26–2

The adult patient presents with a crusted, erythematous lesion visible on the skin bordering his upper lip. The lesion's location and appearance are consistent with that of herpes simplex labialis. The tingling sensation in the area of the lesion before its appearance is a prodrome typical of a herpes virus lesion. As the patient's three outbreaks this year attest, herpes simplex labials is a recurrent problem that may be triggered by certain factors. The correlation of the patient's outbreaks with sun exposure indicates such exposure is a predisposing factor for him. Question the patient about the duration of previous episodes. A duration of 2 to 3 weeks is consistent with herpes virus labialis. Also, ask what products were used in the past to treat the lesions and whether he has allergies other than to aspirin. An allergy to a caine-type anesthetic would preclude recommending topical products containing local anesthetics.

Explain to the patient that cold sores are usually caused by the herpes simplex virus 1 (HSV-1) and that they usually occur on the lip or areas bordering the lip. Explain that herpesvirus lesions are contagious and that fluid from the herpes blisters contains live virus. The fluid may serve to transmit the virus to other people. Advise the patient that about 50% of patients who have had an initial herpesvirus lesion will have recurrent lesions after some unpredictable period of dormancy. Explain that primary infection usually occurs in childhood and may have gone unnoticed.

Advise the patient that herpes simplex lesions are self-limiting and usually resolve in 2 weeks with or without treatment. Explain that nonprescription products (1) control discomfort, (2) protect or lubricate the lesion to allow healing, and (3) prevent secondary bacterial infection. Recommend a skin protectant (e.g., allantoin, petrolatum, cocoa butter) to keep the lesion moist. Depending on the patient's level of discomfort, recommend topical local anesthetics in a bland emollient base. These agents will relieve pain and itching and will keep the lesion moist. Explain that drying and fissuring of the lesion can make it more susceptible to secondary infection, can delay its healing, and can contribute to discomfort. Advise the patient not to use either astringents (they cause drying) or hydrocortisone (herpesvirus lesions do not respond to steroids).

If the patient can identify predisposing factors for the outbreaks, advise eliminating or providing protection from these factors. In this case, sun exposure seems to be a predisposing factor. Recommend use of lip balm with sunscreen and a brimmed hat during sun exposure. Advise the patient to seek medical attention if the condition worsens (increased redness, sign of infection, or increased level of discomfort) or does not improve in 10 days.

Case Study 27–1

The patient's symptoms of pruritus and erythema are related to irritant contact hand dermatitis without infection. Thus, the FDA-approved nonprescription 1% hydrocortisone ointment is recommended for application to the irritated skin areas. Since the patient's skin is dry, an ointment, rather than a cream, is suggested to achieve the concomitant emollient effect on the dry skin component of hand dermatitis.

Advise the patient to apply the hydrocortisone by rubbing a thin layer into the skin gently, but thoroughly, at least 3 times per day until acute symptoms are relieved. Rubbing the agent into the skin is important in ensuring a vasoconstrictive response in the dermis.

Recommend alternate applications of an emollient to allow for tapering of and discontinuing the corticosteroid once the itching and redness have subsided. Encourage the patient to wear cotton-lined gloves while working with the mortar and to particularly avoid direct skin contact with mortar.

Explain to the patient the pathogenesis of his reaction and the importance of fully restoring a functional skin barrier. Once the barrier (the stratum corneum or outer layer of skin) has been disrupted by the irritant reaction, moisture retention by the dermatitic skin is greatly reduced and symptoms such as erythema, pruritus, and fissuring are common. Treating the acute symptoms with a topical corticosteroid assists in restoring barrier function. Institution of an emollient regimen will provide barrier function until the normal barrier is restored.

Follow up after 2 to 4 days of treatment. If the symptoms have not improved or have worsened after 4 days of compliant treatment, refer the patient to a physician.

Case Study 28–1

The initial assessment of the patient's signs and symptoms—excessive dandruff, with itchy, flaky scalp, and yellow, oily scales around the nose and mouth—suggests dandruff with possible seborrheic dermatitis. Inform the patient of the proper types of shampoos to use: Those that contain zinc pyrithione, coal tar, or salicylic acid. Explain that the scalp should be shampooed with regular shampoo first to cleanse the hair and scalp of any oils or dirt; then the medicated shampoo is applied and allowed to remain in contact with the scalp for 5 to 10 minutes. Advise that alternating products and using them two to four times per week as opposed to using them daily would probably result in a faster response.

Concerning the scales around the nose and mouth, ask the patient if he has similar lesions on other parts of his body. Find out if he has recently been exposed to extreme temperature changes or possibly has vitamin deficiencies. Recommend a soap or cleanser containing zinc pyrithione or selenium sulfide.

Case Study 28–2

The patient complains about the appearance of new scales on her legs and around her knees. Ask the patient where else on her body the scales are located. Also, ask her to describe their appearance. The presence of dry, silvery scales on the scalp, elbows, knees, fingernails, and lower back and in the genitoanal region suggests psoriasis. The bleeding marks that occur after the patient picks at the lesions are characteristic of psoriasis. The β-blocker could be unmasking psoriasis vulgaris, or it could be inducing psoriasiform lesions. Ask the patient when the scales first appeared.

Advise the patient that the β-blocker could be related to the skin disorder and that she should see her physician for evaluation of the skin lesions and the hypertension therapy. In the meantime, recommend the use of emollients and lubricating bath products for relief of dryness and itching. Explain that gentle rubbing with a soft cloth after bathing helps to remove scales but that vigorous rubbing will only aggravate the condition.

If the physician approves treatment of the skin disorder with nonprescription products, several products can be used. Scaly plaques can be treated with topical hydrocortisone, coal tar products, and keratolytic agents such as salicylic acid, depending on the anatomic site. Topical 1% hydrocortisone ointment is applied sparingly to body lesions and massaged thoroughly but gently into the skin. Coal tar products are applied to the body, arms, and legs at bedtime, followed by a bath in the morning to remove the remaining coal tar and loosen the scales. Salicylic acid products are usually more cosmetically acceptable than coal tar products and are most useful if thick scales are present. Soaking the affected area in warm (not hot) water for 10 to 20 minutes before applying salicylic acid enhances its keratolytic activity. Of these products, only hydrocortisone, applied sparingly two or three times a day and less often as the lesions improve, may be used on intertriginous areas if needed. Emollients and hydrocortisone are recommended when lesions are erythematous. Coal tars, salicylic acid, and ultraviolet radiation therapy must be used cautiously because they could exacerbate this type of lesion.

The guidelines presented in Case 28–1 for use of medicated shampoos also apply to treating scalp psoriasis. If the nails are involved, advise the patient that nonprescription treatments are not usually effective for nail psoriasis. Also, stress that flares can be prevented by minimizing or avoiding known precipitating factors such as emotional stress, skin irritation, and physical trauma.

Advise the patient to consult the physician if the lesions become more widespread or if the condition does not improve or worsens after 1 week of using nonprescription products.

Case Study 29–1

The pharmacist should ask the patient whether *Toxicodendron* plants grow at the site where the brush was cleared and burned. The patient should also be asked about possible exposure to other noxious chemicals. The key facts in this case are (1) it is the growing season for poison ivy, (2) the pruritis is localized to exposed and protected areas, and (3) the pruritis affects the genitalia. Strongly encourage the patient to see a physician as soon as possible. If exposure to noxious chemicals is excluded, deposition of urushiol on the patient's skin from the smoke of the burning bush may well be causing the symptoms.

Although self-care may not be appropriate, recommend several therapeutic options for temporary relief of the itching and erythema until the patient visits a physician. Such options include taking tepid or cold showers, soaking in either sodium bicarbonate or colloidal oatmeal baths, and, if the itching is localized and patchy, applying topical hydrocortisone cream. Advise the patient that oral sedating antihistamines can be used to relieve nighttime itching if there is a delay in seeing a physician.

Discourage the practice of burning brush. Advise the patient to instead bury the plants at a remote site on his property or contact the state extension service to determine whether a safe herbicide can be used to control *Toxicondendron* plants.

Case Study 30–1

The pharmacist should refer this infant to a pediatrician because of the extent and spread of the diaper rash: The rash is on its way to developing out of the diaper region, and the skin is starting to peel. Diaper rash accompanied by diarrhea and diarrhea in a child who is significantly underweight are other compelling reasons for referring this infant. An urgency exists for physician referral because diarrhea is a potentially life-threatening problem in newborns and infants.

The fact that the child has not been back to the pediatrician in the past 3 months would indicate that well-baby visits are not occurring. For normal birth-weight infants, well-baby visits generally occur monthly, but such visits might be required more frequently for a low-birth-weight infant. This situation presents another reason for a physician's attention.

Questions to determine whether the weight loss was recent and related to the diarrhea revealed no connection; therefore, the pharmacist pursued the search for another possible cause. The duration of the diarrhea and whether it was coincident with the diaper rash could establish that they were connected, because diarrhea can lead to diaper rash. The matter of prescription medications is obvious.

The issue of breast-feeding is threefold. Diaper rash is more common in bottle-fed babies than in those who are breast-fed. The diarrhea may have been caused by something that the mother consumed and was subsequently secreted in the breast milk, or by something that is absent from the breast milk. Only one previous episode of diaper rash was noted, and it occurred in a time frame that does not support a suspicion of chronic diarrhea.

Questioning about allergies is a search for atopy or hypersensitivity of the immune system that could account for the diaper rash as a contact dermatitis or the diarrhea as an intolerance to a food. Questioning about fever was intended to determine whether an infectious process was present. The mother's answer was not consistent with acute infection but could be consistent with a chronic low-grade infection or a more generalized inflammatory process. No other children are in the home who may be sharing some disease process. The number of diaper changes is reasonable. The questions are not necessarily in the most logical order, but enough information was elicited to make a case for referral.

Note that this case is based on a report in which the diaper dermatitis was an early manifestation that progressed to a seborrheic distribution and an exfoliative erythroderma. (See reference 2 in Chapter 30.) Diarrhea and failure to thrive are common symptoms. The dermatitis eventually covered the whole body and was complicated by a gram-negative urinary tract infection. The child was later determined to have the Leiner's disease phenotype with severe combined immunodeficiencies, hypogammaglobulinemia, and hyperimmunoglobulinemia. The treatment was administration of fresh-frozen plasma.

Case Study 30–2

The infant's mother reports a recalcitrant case of diaper dermatitis. The child also has occasional mild fever, and the mother has a history of candidal infection. The recurrence of diaper rash after prophylactic use of corn starch and good diaper hygiene suggests that the physician's diagnosis of diaper dermatitis is wrong. Suspected causes include (1) candidal infection being passed back and forth between the mother and child or (2) a dermatitis such as impetigo or erysipelas.

Encourage the mother to take the child back to the physician for reevaluation. Advise her to continue the zinc oxide therapy and good diaper hygiene while waiting for the appointed visit. Recommend that she ask the physician to look for possible infection and do a work-up for possible metabolic or GI diseases. If the results are negative, it may be time to recommend that the mother consider getting the opinion of another physician. Do not recommend any new therapies in this situation.

Case Study 30–3

The appearance and patient's description of the rash—small, red, itchy "bumps" on the upper chest, upper back, and inner surface of the upper arm—are typical of prickly heat. The probable precipitating factors are sweating associated with dancing combined with 6 hours of wearing a shirt made of fabric or material that does not easily dissipate moisture.

Given that the rash was better after the shower and that the symptoms had subsided enough for the patient to almost forget that he had the problem, this patient may not need any medication. Explain to the patient the likely cause of the problem and how to prevent recurrences. Reassure the patient that this disease is not life-threatening and that if he wears loose clothing over the area and keeps the skin dry for a few days, the rash should resolve itself. Advise the patient to consult a pharmacist or physician if the rash worsens. Explain the signs/symptoms that indicate medical attention is needed: The lesions enlarge, the itching returns, the area of involvement enlarges, pustules form, and so forth.

If the patient had still been symptomatic (itching or burning) or had desired a medicine, the pharmacist could have recommended a product for itching. Cooling or soothing water-washable lotions might also have been useful if used sparingly. The primary need in this case is to explain the disease state to the patient, make sure that no further occlusion occurs during the healing process, and educate the patient about signs that warrant other medical intervention.

Case Study 31–1

The patient's reaction to the wasp sting—difficulty in breathing, nausea, and dizziness—was not limited to the site of the sting. Reactions to previous bee stings were milder, but they indicate that the patient is sensitized to Hymenoptera venom. The patient's hay fever and his mother's asthma indicate that the reaction to insect stings is allergic in nature. Self-treatment of a sting is not appropriate when sensitization has occurred.

The patient's failure to tell his physician or pharmacist of previous milder allergic reactions to insect stings indicates that he does not understand his progressively severe hypersensitivity reaction to insect stings. Explain the pathogenesis of anaphylactic reactions to the patient. Advise him to avoid Hymenoptera insects and to consult with an allergist.

Explain also the limitations of nonprescription drugs in treating anaphylactic reactions and the importance of having immediate access to epinephrine injection.

Advise the patient to let family members, friends, and co-workers know of his hypersensitivity, and stress the importance of immediate medical intervention if he is stung again. Advise the patient to wear a bracelet or carry a card showing the nature of the allergy.

Case Study 31–2

The intense itching of the child's scalp occurring 2 weeks after a sleepover could indicate a lice infestation. The salivary secretions of a louse contain allergenic substances that trigger itching. In addition, the louse's mouthparts pierce the skin, which can cause itching.

Explain to the mother how to identify a louse. Stress that the presence of live lice must be confirmed before self-treatment is recommended. Once the lice infestation is confirmed, recommend a pediculicide according to the child's allergy history, if one exists.

Stress the contagious nature of lice infestations. Advise the mother to instruct her child to avoid direct physical contact with an infested individual and not to share clothing, towels, caps, or bed sheets.

Case Study 32–1

Because the patient is outside the 12- to 24-year-old range of the typical acne patient, the pharmacist should consider other conditions and causes of the reddened, rough skin of the cheeks accompanied by lesions resembling closed comedones. The androgenic balance of the oral contraceptive might be causing the symptoms. The coincidence of worsening of the condition before menstrual periods, plus the presence of eye irritation and telangiectasis, strongly suggest rosacea. Although often called "adult acne," rosacea is not a true acne. The initial treatment of rosacea is similar to that of acne vulgaris; however, the patient should be encouraged to obtain a definite diagnosis from a dermatologist.

Case Study 32–2

The patient's use of tetracycline for his acne could be problematic on a trip during spring break to a southern climate. Tetracycline may cause sensitivity to sunlight. Because this effect may last from weeks to months after discontinuing the tetracycline, switching to a nonsensitizing antibiotic is not appropriate in the given time frame of 2 weeks. Instead counsel the patient on protecting himself from sun exposure.

Prescription drug therapy is appropriate for acne consisting of both noninflammatory and inflammatory lesions. The supplemental treatment with a nonprescription, topical product is appropriate if suggested by the dermatologist. A benzoyl peroxide product is an appropriate recommendation. Counsel the patient on appropriate use of this agent.

Case Study 33–1

The 23-year-old patient has systemic lupus erythematosus (SLE), an autoimmune disease primarily of young women. Although it has many clinical presentations, arthritis and arthralgias are most common. Ultraviolet radiation (UVR)—primarily UVB but also UVA—can exacerbate the condition. In addition, a high degree of photosensitivity is common in many patients with SLE. If the patient is taking any photosensitizing drugs, the chances of having such a reaction are even greater. This patient is currently taking an NSAID. NSAIDs can cause photosensitivity reactions even in patients without lupus. Use of an NSAID by a patient with lupus most likely increases the risk of photosensitivity.

The fact that the patient has brown hair and eyes and that she tans fairly well does not change the clinical management of her situation. Advise her that the best approach is to avoid UVR exposure as much as possible. However, it may be difficult to convince a young person in the heat of summer to avoid the beach. If the patient is going to be out of doors for any length of time, advise her to wear protective clothing: A shirt with long sleeves, pants, and a hat are important. Recommend the use of a broad-spectrum sunscreen product. Even though UVB is the primary precipitating factor, UVA can aggravate the condition. A sunscreen that protects throughout the entire UVB spectrum and as much of the UVA spectrum as possible is recommended. Assuming the patient has never had a reaction to a sunscreen product before, menthyl anthranilate, any of the benzophenones, or any of the cinnamates would give adequate UVB protection. The addition of avobenzone and/or titanium dioxide would provide complete UVA coverage. Ideally, the SPF of the selected product should be 30+, which signifies that maximal UVB protection is provided. Because of the potential for sweating, a "very water-resistant" product is best. Explain to the patient that sun exposure could exacerbate her disease and could precipitate a photosensitivity reaction; thus, she might be more motivated to adhere to this regimen.

Counsel the patient on the following general guidelines for avoiding UVR exposure:

- Avoid UVR as much as possible. This avoidance includes tanning beds and booths.
- If you must be out in the sun, wear long sleeves, pants, and a hat.
- Note that you are exposed to UVR even on a cloudy day and that you must follow the same precautions as those for a sunny day.
- Cover all exposed areas of the body with a broad-spectrum, high-SPF product.
- Reapply the sunscreen (approximately 1ounce) every 80 minutes or more frequently if you rub a towel against your skin.

Stress the following points during patient counseling:

- When riding in a car, remember that, although UVB is screened out by window glass, UVA is not. Therefore, cover exposed areas of the body with the sunscreen product even with the window closed.
- Many drugs, especially antibiotics, can increase the risk of a photosensitivity reaction. The NSAID that you are taking can cause such reactions. Therefore, you are at greater risk and extra care is warranted.

In the case of SLE, evaluation of outcomes is based on two considerations. First, if the condition gets worse, it may be because of exposure to UVR. If the patient experiences a flaring of her condition but has avoided UVR, the symptoms are probably related to the SLE alone and not much else can be done. If, however, she spends time in the sun and her condition gets worse or she has a photosensitivity reaction (usually a rash), she must reduce her UVR exposure and perhaps change to a different formula of sunscreen product.

Case 33–2

The patient, who requests help in selecting a sunscreen product, apparently spends much time out of doors, especially on the golf course. Although he says that he wears a hat, the sunburn on his head and neck indicates that he may not be very compliant in covering his head. The removal of several growths (probably premalignant actinic keratoses) indicates that he has been subjecting his body to significant amounts of UVR for a long time without adequate protection. This indication is supported by the fading sunburn on his arms. The development of skin growths and presence of numerous nevi put the patient at greater risk for skin cancer.

The patient's current and past history indicate that avoiding UVR as much as possible is the best clinical management approach. Because he is an avid golfer, this approach is probably not an option. Therefore, the patient must use protective clothing such as a shirt with long sleeves, pants, and a hat. The use of a high-SPF product to protect against sunburn is best. However, a broad-spectrum sunscreen product is recommended because, even though UVB is primarily responsible for skin cancer, UVA can contribute to its occurrence. The pharmacist should recommend a sunscreen that protects throughout the entire UVB spectrum and protects as much as possible of the UVA spectrum. Assuming the patient has never had a reaction to a sunscreen product before, menthyl anthranilate, any of the benzophenones, or any of the cinnamates would give adequate UVB protection. The addition of avobenzone and/or titanium dioxide would provide complete UVA coverage as well. Ideally, the SPF of the selected product should be 30+, which signifies maximal UVB protection. Because of the potential for sweating, a "very water-resistant" product is best. Explain to the patient his continuing risk of skin cancer so that his adhering to a prevention program will be enhanced. Also, explain the general guidelines for avoidance of UVR given in Case Study 33–1.

Stress the following points during patient counseling:

- Keep sunscreen products out of high heat (such as in a golf bag) for extended periods of time because they can lose their potency just like any other drug.
- Note that the prior history of skin growths increases the risk of others developing in the future.
- Have your physician immediately check any new growths; a change in the size, shape, or color of an existing growth; or a growth that bleeds.

The patient should be aware that skin redness, even if it is not a painful sunburn, indicates inadequate protection. He must adhere to the prevention program. If he still experiences redness, he should reevaluate the sunscreen product he is using.

Case Study 34–1

The use of benzoyl peroxide and tetracycline could be related to erythema on the patient's face, neck, arms, and legs. Both medications are photosensitizing agents. However, because benzoyl peroxide is used to treat acne, it is unlikely that the patient applied it to all the erythematous areas. Tanning beds emit primarily UVA radiation, and UVA is most often associated with phototoxic reactions. This patient probably experienced an exaggerated or phototoxic response to tanning bed exposure resulting from tetracycline administration.

Advise the patient to consult her prescriber about discontinuing tetracycline and avoiding tetracycline products in the future. Should tetracycline products be required, advise her to avoid sun exposure and apply sunscreen agents during such use. Advise her to also avoid further use of keratolytic agents such as benzoyl peroxide until the sunburn is healed. Explain that use of keratolytic agents may make her skin more susceptible to sunburn and that she should consider sunscreen agents.

Explain that obtaining a tan may be an unrealistic goal because of her fair complexion. Because she is more susceptible to photoaging, advise her to use sunscreen products.

Case Study 34–2

The presence of erythema, blisters, and edema in the burned areas indicate superficial and superficial partial-thickness burn injuries. In this case, the burn covers about 2% of the patient's body surface area. Because her hand is injured, specialized care is required to ensure full functional recovery. The pharmacist should refer this patient to a surgeon for evaluation of the burn injury because self-care is inappropriate.

Explain to the patient that the depth and severity of the burn injury and the potential for scarring could cause reduced functionality of her hand. Advise her to avoid rupture of the blisters and to use a skin protectant such as white petrolatum. An internal analgesic such as ibuprofen may be administered to help reduce pain and swelling.

Explain that burn care centers and hospitals care for many indigent patients. Lack of insurance should not dissuade this patient from seeking medical attention.

Case Study 35–1

Irrigating this child's abrasion with normal saline may be a better alternative than harsh scrubbing of the wound bed with Dial soap and water. Further, antisepsis with hydrogen peroxide may not be necessary in this case because signs of infection are not present.

The presence of warmth and pinkness in the skin surrounding the wound is part of the normal inflammatory process in wound healing. Explain to the mother that use of triple-antibiotic ointment is optional when infection is not present. Caution that sensitization with neomycin may be a concern for this 5-year-old. If the mother elects to use an antibiotic ointment, recommend a preparation without neomycin such as Polysporin to minimize the risk of sensitization. Advise the mother to use the agent when the wound becomes slightly exudative. She should apply the ointment after cleansing three times daily and should cover the wound with an appropriate adhesive bandage. Stress that proper cleansing and closure are the most important components in wound healing in this case. Caution the mother to watch for signs of systemic infection (green or foul-smelling discharge, fever, or flulike symptoms) and to consult a physician if they occur.

Case Study 35–2

Delayed healing of the patient's puncture wound may be related to use of the corticosteroid fludrocortisone. Also the patient's thin stature may suggest an underlying nutritional deficiency or medical problem that can impair proper wound healing.

The yellow and odorous exudate may indicate an infection in the wound bed. *Staphylococcus aureus* and *Staphylococcus epidermidis* are the most common organisms infecting this type of wound. *Candida albicans* may be possible if the patient is immunocompromised.

Explain the appropriate procedure for cleaning and dressing the wound. Advise the patient to consult a physician promptly if local infection continues along with the presence of systemic signs and symptoms (fever, flulike symptoms).

Explain that—even when treated superficially with topical antibiotics—some wounds become infected by nonsusceptible bacteria. The most common bacteria implicated in community-acquired wound infections include *S. aureus* and *Streptococcus pyogenes*, which, depending on the strain, may be resistant to the topical triple-antibiotic preparation. In some cases, *C. albicans* may be the causative organism if the host is immunocompromised, thus rendering antibiotics completely ineffective.

Case Study 36–1

The patient's symptoms of painful, red, raised bumps on the dorsal surfaces of her fourth toes are typical of corns. Repeated irritation from wearing high-heeled shoes that tend to crowd the toes into a small toe space probably caused the lesions. Treatment options include referring the patient to a physician, recommending a nonprescription corn-removal product, suggesting that the patient avoid wearing high-heeled shoes, or taking no action.

Clearly, the severity of the symptoms rule out taking no action. The patient's medical and medication histories show no contraindications to self-treatment with corn-removal products. Because the patient is sensitive to adhesive tape, suggest a salicylic acid product in a collodion base or a pad form. To prevent recurrent corns, advise the patient to use Dr. Scholl's Corn Pads with Cushlin to protect the toes from further irritation once the corn is removed and to avoid wearing high-heeled shoes.

Case Study 36–2

The patient's symptoms (itching between the toes, redness, irritation) are characteristic of athlete's foot. Additional questioning about the nature of the skin in the affected area (e.g., flaky, wet) might help confirm the first impression. Retention of moisture around and between the toes has probably provided an entry for topical fungi. Further, showering in public facilities (residence hall and gymnasium) bolster a strong suspicion that the patient has contracted athlete's foot.

Although the patient describes the symptoms as bothersome, particularly at bedtime, they have not yet made walking difficult. The patient's description of his toenails (no apparent discoloration or brittleness) indicates that the infection has not spread to the toes. Given that the patient has no known diseases or allergies, he seems to be a good candidate for topical antifungal treatment.

Advise the patient that the failure of the agent he selected previously—Lotrimin-AF—to resolve the infection is related to the intermittent application of the agent. Advise the patient to apply the medication twice daily for 2 to 4 weeks. Stress that resolution of the disorder may take this long. Stress also the importance of good foot hygiene during and after the treatment. Explain the cause of the infection and the role that foot moisture plays in the infection's development. Be sure to ask the patient if he has any questions about the therapy and ask him to repeat the instructions for product use. Encourage him to return in 4 weeks for follow-up of the therapy.

Case Study 39–1

The patient is demonstrating an interest in getting more involved in self-management of her diabetes. Her log of blood glucose readings indicates that she is taking steps to achieve good diabetes control and that she may be a good candidate for an insulin pump. Additional information is needed, however, before making this recommendation. The patient must have an interest in and understanding of the effects of insulin, physical activity, and nutrition on blood glucose control. While the pump provides an opportunity for excellent control, significant problems can occur if the pump is not used properly.

At this visit, consider reviewing with the patient the use of insulin pens and determine whether she is interested in this type of insulin injection device. However, the patient's insulin requirements must match the insulin in the pen. If they do not, she would need to continue using insulin in a vial and administer it with a syringe.

The patient's high blood glucose levels at 10 pm and the slight swings at noon indicate the possible need to add regular insulin with the two injections of NPH in the morning and afternoon. It is usually prudent to add or change only one dose of insulin per visit. At this visit, advise the patient to add a small amount of regular insulin to the afternoon dose of NPH and monitor the response. The amount added should be less than 10% of the total daily dose. For example, add 4 U if the daily dose is 50 U.

Case Study 39–2

The patient does not understand the need to calibrate his blood glucose monitor when using new test strips. Demonstrate how to enter the batch number for the box of new strips. Stress that the patient should check the batch number for each box of strips he uses, and, if appropriate, recalibrate the monitor.

Base recommendations for nonprescription cold medications on a review of the impact each ingredient could have on glucose control and diabetes-related complications.

Encourage the patient to call with any questions about the diabetes care plan. Finally, instruct the patient to bring in his monitor in 1 month to review his use of the instrument. If the patient is using his monitor properly, this quality control visit should take about 10 minutes.

Case Study 40–1

Probable causes of the patient's difficulty in falling asleep are environmental stress (i.e., anxiety about his upcoming presentation at work) and increased caffeine consumption. Advise the patient as follows: (1) Consume no caffeine after 2:00 pm. (2) Participate in light, early evening exercise (e.g., walking). (3) Take a warm bath and/or relax by reading before bedtime. (4) Establish a regular bedtime schedule. (5) Assess the bedroom and make sure that the environment is restful (e.g., no light, no noise, comfortable bed, no distractions, etc.). It is important to emphasize that, whenever possible, nondrug measures should be used to treat sleep disturbances. Review with the patient the points outlined in Table 40–3 in Chapter 40. If possible, also give the patient a handout regarding sleep hygiene for future reference. However, it is important that the patient receive verbal reinforcement of these principles.

Although the patient has not used a sleep aid (nonprescription or prescription), he does drink an occasional beer at bedtime when he has difficulty falling asleep. Advise the patient that sleep aids offer advantages over the use of alcohol: (1) Sleep aids give symptomatic relief. (2) With his age and no concomitant medications, his relative risk of medication adverse effects is low. (3) Sedating antihistamines are effective in treating transient insomnia, particularly if the primary complaint is difficulty falling asleep. The disadvantages of using sleep aids in this patient are minimal. His insomnia is likely to resolve after the presentation, so sleep hygiene measures alone may be an adequate and appropriate intervention.

Counsel the patient as follows on the proper use of sleep aids:

- Take 25 to 50 mg of diphenhydramine 1 to 2 hours before your anticipated bedtime. Do not exceed 50 mg per night. Doses above 50 mg are no more effective, but side effects increase with higher doses.
- Take the medication for 2 to 3 nights; then skip a night and see how you sleep. However, with the work presentation occurring in four days, take the medication the night before the presentation as well.
- Do not take the medication longer than 7 to 10 nights. If insomnia persists after taking these measures, please consult your primary care physician.
- Note that common potential side effects include dry mouth and potential "hang over" effects in the morning upon awakening. Do not take the medication before driving or using any other machinery or performing activities that require high levels of attention or concentration.

- Do not take diphenhydramine with alcoholic beverages, other sleep aids, or other medications that can cause sedation (without consulting a physician or pharmacist).

Advise the patient that nonprescription sleep aides work only for cases of difficulty falling asleep that are of short duration. Also emphasize that tolerance to medications occurs rapidly and that, if the sleep disturbance lasts longer than 7 to 10 days, he should see a physician. Emphasize that when insomnia lasts more than a few weeks it is critical to identify and resolve the underlying cause.

Case Study 41–1

In general, caffeine consumption is not a substitute for adequate sleep in resolving the patient's complaint of not being able to stay awake at night. Question the patient about her sleep habits. (See Chapter 40.) For example: Please describe your sleep habits for me. What time do you usually go to bed? Get up in the morning? Do you feel groggy or refreshed when you get up in the morning?

Encourage the patient to sleep more if she is not functioning well. Additionally, advise her that staying up late to study may actually decrease her test performance if she is drowsy and fatigued during the examination. Stress that her performance is more likely to be positive if she goes to bed at an established bedtime (e.g., 10:00 to 11:00 pm) and gets up early to study if additional study is required.

The patient already ingests moderate daily amounts of caffeine through coffee, sodas, and chocolate; additional caffeine ingestion could increase nervousness, anxiety, and jitteriness. Recommend that she not consume more than the current amount of caffeine and that she consider decreasing consumption to a total of two cups of coffee or two caffeinated sodas daily. Similarly, women who are pregnant or seeking to become pregnant should limit caffeine consumption to the equivalent of one or two cups of coffee daily.

Although estrogen has been reported to possibly inhibit caffeine metabolism through CYP 1A2, thus potentially increasing the effects of caffeine ingestion, the clinical significance of this interaction is unclear. Since both caffeine and hydrochlorthiazide (ingredient in Dyazide) are diuretics, the patient may experience increased polyuria as a result of the combination. Advise the patient that caffeine can impair the metabolism of some medications, and that a pharmacist or physician should be consulted about potential drug interactions before caffeine (either dietary or from nonprescription products) is taken. Explain that caffeine may interfere with iron absorption and that it is best not to take caffeinated beverages with iron tablets or with vitamin supplements that contain iron.

Ask the patient about nonprescription stimulant use. If used, ask about the frequency of use and her effects from taking it. Excess caffeine consumption may result in a variety of undesirable effects including anxiety, nervousness, jitteriness, difficulty concentrating, headache, palpitations or pounding of the chest and stomachache among other symptoms. Advise that if these effects occur, the patient should immediately stop taking caffeine or caffeinated beverages. Caution the patient not to take alcohol or other CNS depressants to counteract the symptoms. Stress that medical attention is needed if chest pains or severe panicky symptoms (uncommon) occur.

Case Study 42–1

The patient's symptom of a racing heart beat should be evaluated by a physician before nicotine replacement therapy (NRT) is continued. Chances are good that the racing heart is related to ingestion of excess nicotine; however, elevated levels of theophylline that might occur after asthmatic patients stop smoking may also be the cause.

When any additional serious abnormalities are ruled out, the patient can then attempt smoking cessation again.

The good news is that the patient has stopped smoking. He now needs to choose an NRT that is best for him and his smoking behavior. Because of the quantity of cigarettes the patient smoked before his attempt to quit, a sustained and steady release of nicotine will most likely be successful. This type of nicotine delivery is best achieved through nicotine transdermal systems. Either the 16-hour or 24-hour patch would be appropriate. If sleep disturbances occur, the 16-hour patch (or a 24-hour patch worn for 16 hours) is the better choice. If the patient craves cigarettes upon awakening in the morning, the 24-hour patch might be a better choice.

Because of the decline in the rate of metabolism of theophylline after a successful attempt to quit, the dose of theophylline may need to be decreased by as much as 25%. Also, the symptoms and severity of asthma may diminish with the successful attempt to quit. The patient's sore throat may be related to ingesting nicotine orally while consuming large quantities of acidic coffee. Although the nicotine polacrilex gum is buffered with sodium carbonate to enhance buccal absorption, coffee is acidic; thus, the combination of coffee and nicotine polacrilex gum increases the amount of swallowed nicotine. This combination, in turn, can irritate the throat.

Contact the patient regularly to determine his success or perhaps the need for further coaching. Advise the patient to focus on the behaviors necessary to avoid a relapse to smoking. Using NRT to diminish withdrawal symptoms will help the patient avoid temporal or situational triggers. Praise and encourage the patient's attempt to stop smoking and for the success achieved. These follow-ups will strongly indicate your concern about the patient's smoking cessation attempt and will help him sustain his level of commitment to continue as a nonsmoker. Encourage the patient to follow the suggested pattern of weaning off the patches. Ultimate success in quitting smoking is not achieved until all nicotine is eliminated from the body.

Case Study 42–2

Before using nicotine replacement therapy (NRT), the patient must decide to quit smoking abruptly. Trying to quit "a little at a time" simply is not an effective approach. The chances of success are minimal, and the risk for relapse is great.

The combination of smoking while consuming oral contraceptives is a deadly one. The patient is at a real risk for deep vein thrombosis or cardiovascular problems. Reinforcement of these potential dangers could help the patient decide to try to quit smoking with renewed vigor.

Actually, the patient's choice of nicotine gum is the best choice for her smoking behavior. Patients who smoke intermittently or smoke intensely for periods of time (during breaks, after work, in the car, or other places) and then do not smoke for a while may benefit most from the faster onset of nicotine delivery found with nicotine polacrilex gum. Also, the tactile nature of the gum might soothe the oral gratification necessary for some smokers when they quit smoking.

Counsel the patient on the proper use of the gum, and discourage her from smoking during the NRT. Also counsel her on how to reduce use and taper off the gum. Ultimate success in quitting smoking is not achieved until all nicotine is eliminated from the body.

Explain to the patient that she should focus on the behaviors necessary to avoid relapse. Using NRT to diminish the withdrawal symptoms will help her avoid temporal or situational triggers to smoking.

Praise and encourage the patient for trying to quit smoking and for her ultimate success in the endeavor. Notify the patient's physician about the smoking cessation attempt and the method chosen. Contact the patient by phone regularly to encourage adherence if she does not present in person at the pharmacy during the first few weeks of therapy. Such follow-up will strongly indicate your concern about her attempt to quit smoking and will help her to sustain her level of commitment to continue as a nonsmoker.

Case Study 44–1

To help determine the cause of the patient's problem with urine release, ask her whether she has had children and whether she has consulted her physician or gynecologist about the problem. The patient's age (72 years) and the likelihood of multiple births indicate that stress incontinence may be the cause of her complaint; however, she should be referred to her physician for evaluation. If stress incontinence is the final diagnosis, appropriate nonpharmacologic and pharmacologic therapy can be initiated. Use of absorbent products may be appropriate during the treatment period.

Case Study 45–1

The patient was diagnosed 2 years earlier by his urologist with benign prostatic hypertrophy (BPH) and has been taking finasteride (Proscar) 5 mg daily with success. The patient also takes 250 mg of vitamin C daily. Other than the BPH, the patient seems to be in good health; however the patient reports problems with sexual potency, a likely side effect of the Proscar. Because of this side effect, he is considering discontinuing his current medication and substituting the popular herbal product, saw palmetto. Saw palmetto is widely used to treat common symptoms of BPH and reportedly has few, if any, side effects.

First, advise the patient to inform his urologist of his desire to try saw palmetto primarily because of the undesirable side effects of Proscar. The physician may be able to lower the dose to lessen or eliminate the side effects. Although many European clinical studies show that saw palmetto is effective in treating BPH, the physician may not be familiar with the herbal product. Many of these trials have directly compared saw palmetto and Proscar with reported similar results. Ideally, the pharmacist, physician, and patient should all discuss these results before deciding to switch the patient's therapy.

Case Study 45–2

The patient, a 16-year-old healthy teenager who is active in sports, expresses a strong desire to increase his body strength and appearance and to improve his athletic performance. His interest in "natural testosterone sources" and "steroid alternatives" is likely a result of misleading advertisements that promise quick results. These claims are rarely backed by clinical evidence and, for the most part, can be considered unsubstantiated. The majority of popular claims that certain plants and dietary supplements contain precursors of testosterone that can be converted to testosterone by the body are unfounded. Many plants do, however, contain certain steroid precursors that can be converted to testosterone in the laboratory. An exception would be dehydroepiandrosterone (DHEA) or androstenedione (not found in plants), which are intermediates in testosterone biosynthesis and can be converted to testosterone by the body.

Advise the patient to use caution in taking these agents since they can lead to possibly harmful alterations in hormone levels. Evidence for their benefit in improving athletic performance is controversial. This case presents a good opportunity for the pharmacist to counsel the individual on effective nonpharmacologic methods for enhancing body strength that emphasize weight training techniques possibly combined with certain nutritional supplements.

Index

Note: Page numbers followed by an italic "f" or "t" denote figures or tables, respectively.

D

F

H

I

O

Q

W

X

Y

Z